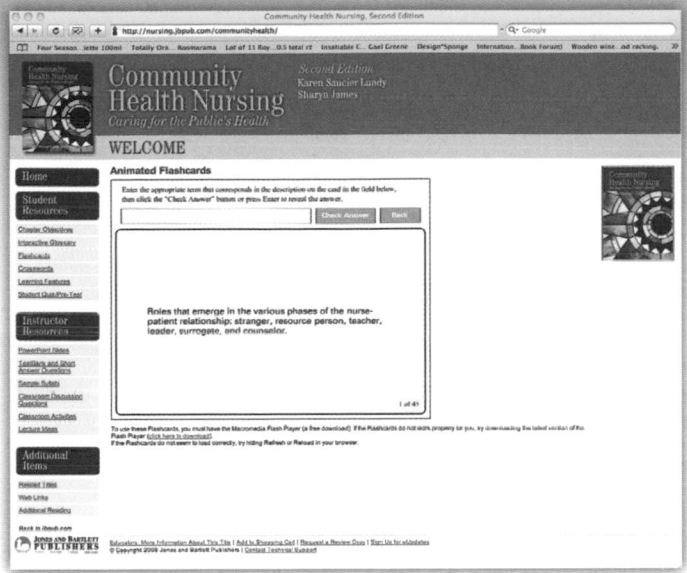

## For Instructors and Students

### Web Links
Applicable evidence-based nursing Web resources for easy clicking and linking!

### Related Titles
Additional Jones and Bartlett titles in related areas that might be of interest to the student and the instructor.

### Additional Reading
A compilation of chapters from Jones and Bartlett titles in related areas—great for further studying or for research projects. Instructors can also package these related chapters with this textbook for required reading on a particular topic.

# Community Health Nursing
## *Caring for the Public's Health*

# Welcome to

## Along with useful tables and figures, each chapter includes:

**Reflections** A combination of quotes, statements, and questions that are presented at the beginning of each chapter to prompt the reader to reflect upon the topic(s) to be addressed in the chapter.

CHAPTER FOCUS

**A Closer Look at Health**
- Historical Insights

**Nursing in the Twenty-First Century**
- Educating Nurses for Community Health Nursing Practice

**Community-Based, Population-Focused, Community Health Nursing: What's in a Name?**
- Communities and Populations
- Acute Care Versus Community Health Nursing

**Reform and Reinvention of Systems of Care**
- *Nursing's Agenda for Health Care Reform*
- Managed Care and the Future of Nursing

**Back to the Future: From Hospital to Community, from Cure to Prevention**
- Home Health Care
- Care and Prevention: Can We Really Do It All?
- Benefits Versus Costs
- *Healthy People 2010:* Goals for the Nation
- Influences on a Community's Health: Culture, Environment, and Ethics

**Epidemiol...**

**Measuri...**
**When W...**

**Chapter Focus** Highlights important content noted throughout the chapter and provides instructors and students with a quick look at key information they will encounter in each chapter. Students and instructors can use the chapter focus to help guide and focus the learning process.

**Questions to Consider** Offers a list of questions for the student to consider while reading the chapter and to be answered after completion of the chapter. This feature allows students to focus their study on key information discussed within each chapter.

**Key Terms** These terms introduce essential vocabulary in community health nursing, and are bolded throughout the chapter. Visit http://nursing.jbpub.com/communityhealth to see these key terms in an interactive glossary, and use flashcards and word puzzles to nail the definition!

**Cultural Connection** Explores cultural influences on the public's health and illness and the effects of cultural beliefs on healthcare delivery and the interactions between healthcare provider and patient. Also engages readers in self-reflection on their own cultural beliefs and how those beliefs will color their interactions with patients in the clinical setting.

# Community Health Nursing: Caring for the Public's Health, Second Edition!

## ETHICAL CONNECTION

Every community is an association of some kind and e
community is established with a view to some good; for ev
one always acts in order to obtain that which they think g
But, if all communities aim at some good, the state or poli
community, which is the highest of all, and which embraces
all the rest, aims at good in a greater degree than any other
and at the highest good

**Ethical Connection** Boxed features
which delve into specific ethical and
legal issues and interactions between
nurses and their patients, and their
effects on the community's health and
illness.

## ENVIRONMENTAL CONNECTION

The work we are speaking of has nothing to do with nu
disease, but with maintaining health by removing the th
which disturb it . . . dirt, drink, diet, damp, draughts,
drains.

—*Florence Nightingale, 1860*

**Environmental Connection** This feature
reviews specific environmental issues
and concerns and their effects on the
community's health and illness. Also examined are varying healthcare systems
within different environments such as
rural communities versus metropolitan
areas.

**Global Connection** Looks at the impact
of a global society and how issues
within one's own community are affected by global events. It also allows
insight into various healthcare systems
internationally as well as locally.

## GLOBAL CONNECTION

**The Three Ps of Global Health**
Pollution
Population
Poverty

*Source:* Turnock, 1997.

*❝I enjoy situations where I have to adjust to the environment,
learn the culture, and develop interpersonal relationships
quickly. Being able to experience a particular area of nursing
through the eyes of someone from another region is one of the
best benefits of traveling.❞*

—*Mary Jo Alessio, RN*
*Travel Nurse*
*Supplemental Health Care*

**Quotes** Quotes from prominent people
in the community related to health care.

## EPIDEMIOLOGY in Practice

**Epidemiology in Practice** This feature
examines the epidemiological process
of researching factors affecting the
health and illness of a community and
preventative medicine in relation to
nursing practice.

...ditional epidemiological triad has focused on infectious
...as agent, human host, and physical environment.
...developed countries, in the past century there has
...epidemiological transition from infectious to chronic
..., such as cardiovascular disease, cancer, diabetes,
...and depression, and the environment has broadened
to include the social and psychological environment, such as
prejudice, racism, and stress.

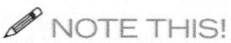
## NOTE THIS!
Common Definitions in Community Health Nursing

**Community Health Nursing** is a systematic process of delivering
nursing care to improve the health of an entire community (Nehls et
al., 2001, p. 305).

**Community-Based Nursing** refers to both the setting and the practice of the nursing role. The focus of community-based nursing care
is primarily at the individual and family levels, which contribute to
the health of the community. Community-based nursing often refers
to nursing care provided outside of acute care settings.

**Population-Focused Care** refers to interventions aimed at health
promotion and disease prevention that shape a community
health status.

**Note This!** Quick tidbits and facts called
out to highlight important aspects of the
chapter topic.

Just remember, Mr. Potter, that this rabble you're talking about, they do most of the working and paying and living and dying in this community.

—*It's a Wonderful Life*, 1947

**Waking Ned Divine, (1998)**
When a lottery winner dies of shock, his fellow townsfolk attempt to claim the money.

**Where the Heart Is, (2000)**
A pregnant 17-year-old rebuilds her life after being abandoned by her boyfriend at a Wal-Mart in Sequoyah, Oklahoma.

**The Straight Story, (1999)**
An old man makes a long journey by lawnmower to mend his relationship with an ill brother.

**Local Hero, (1983)**
An American oil company sends a man to Scotland to buy up an entire village where the company wants to build a refinery, but things don't go as expected.

**Erin Brockovich, (2000)**
An unemployed single mother becomes a ░░░ almost single-handedly brings down a ░░░ company accused of polluting a city's wa░

**Media Moment** This feature uses various forms of media to discuss broader health-related issues within the community such as mental health, substance abuse, and disease.

 *Got an Alternative?*

Research indicates that at least 62% of the U.S. public uses some form of nontraditional or alternative medicine—yet few patients mention such measures when visiting their healthcare providers. Why do you think people are reluctant to share their use and interest in alternative health practices with nurses and physicians?

*Source*: Barnes, P. M., Powell-Griner, E., McFann, K., & Nahin, R. L. (2004). Complementary and alternative medicine use among adults: United States, 2002. *Advance Data, 343*, 1–19.

**Got an Alternative?** Examines alternative methods for dealing with preventing and healing illness and disease.

 Research Alert

Research has shown that children wearing Heelys sustain the same types of injuries as those wearing inline skates or riding skateboards or scooters. According to ░ Iannelli, MD, two recent medical studies report ░ children wearing Heelys had injuries ranging from radius fractures and elbow injuries to a head inj░ required surgery."

**Research Alert** Each research alert contains an abstract of a research article for further reading in a wide array of topics related to health and illness in the population.

Although the manufacturer recommends w░░░ safety gear such as a helmet, wrist guards, and knee pads, very few children wear safety gear with Heelys. To prevent injuries, children should wear safety gear, remove the wheels when using Heelys in shoe mode, and avoid using the Heelys in skate mode in traffic, on stairs, or on uneven surfaces. Children should also avoid crowded areas and rolling faster than they can walk.

Many public places, including schools, ban the use of Heelys in skate mode and require children to take the wheels out of the Heelys before entering. Heelys should not be used in skate mode indoors. Falling into such indoor hazards as a table or display case can cause serious injury.

Parents should also know that W.A.T.C.H (World Against Toys Causing Harm) included Heelys on their "10 worst toys" list.

*Sources*: Iannelli, V., MD. (2007). *Heelys—Staying safe and preventing injuries*. Retrieved October 16, 2008, from http://pediatrics.about.com/od/safety/a/0407_heelys_inj.htm; Lenehan, B., Callendar, A., McIntyre, A., Boran, S., Moore, D., Fogarty, E., & Dowling, F. (2007). Heely injuries: A new epidemic warranting a government health warning! *Injury, 38*(8), 923–925; Oh, D. (2006). Heelys injuries in children. *Singapore Medical Journal, 47*(5), 373–375; Korioth, T. (2007). Heely shoe users: Take heed of risks. *AAP News, 28*(4), 29.

**❝❝** *a conversation with . . .* **❞❞**

**Professor Martha Rogers**
Nursing's story is a magnificent epic of service to mankind. It is about people: how they are born, and live and die; in health and in sickness; in joy and in sorrow. Its mission is the translation of knowledge into human service.

Nursing is compassionate concern for human beings. It is the heart that understands and the hand that soothes. It is the intellect that synthesizes many learnings into meaningful administrations.

For students of nursing, the future is a rich repository of far-flung opportunities around this planet and toward the further reaches of man's explorations of new worlds and new ideas. Theirs is the promise of deep satisfaction in a field long dedicated to serving the health needs of people.

—Martha Rogers, PhD
The Education Violet, June 1966,
New York University

**A Conversation With...** Interviews with influential people within nursing, health care, and the general community discussing topics related to health care.

### Application to Practice

**Community-Based Care: An Example from Practice**

A 3-year-old child is brought to a public health department for her first set of immunizations. As the nurse assesses the child, she finds that the child has a generalized red rash all over her body. The mother complains that the child scratches and cries about the rash. She has been using a cortisone skin cream for three days, but the rash has worsened.

The nurse attends to the immediate concerns of the mother about home care comfort measures and possible causes. The nurse then delivers direct care to the child and to her family, while considering the following community implications:

- Does anyone else in the family exhibit those symptoms?
- Does the child go to d...
- Have there been any c... cently with similar sy... case compare with ca...
- What is the likely p... rash?
- Are there any pregnant women in the clinic or in the home setting?
  1. What are possible conclusions that the nurse can make that have individual implications?

**Application to Practice** Case studies designed to enhance the reader's learning experience by giving them a hands-on feel for situations they may encounter in clinical practice.

 **I THINK ABOUT THIS**

In the case of heart transplantation, people typically focus on the dramatic stitching in of a transplanted heart as the "breakthrough." Few notice that the intensive medical and nursing follow-up—solving the day-to-day problems of living with a transplanted organ, treating sores in the mouth due to immunosuppression, coping with a new hormonal milieu, promptly recognizing and responding to infection and rejection—were all caring "breakthroughs" that led to the eventual success of heart transplantation. These essential day-to-day nursing care issues had to be solved in order to make heart transplantation a viable therapy. Yet they are all but overlooked in the scientific and popular media coverage of the transplant story.
— Benner and Wrub...

**Think About This** Research briefs and situational narratives that prompt the reader to think critically and objectively.

 **Evidence-Based Practice Content** Includes all features within the book. Those with evidence-based practice content will have an icon indicating this content.

---

 A Good Read

**Working as a Nurse and Family Nurse Practitioner in Alaska: Just Another Day in a Frozen Paradise**
*Amanda Traver, FNP, MSN*

The first word that comes to my mind after taking a job as a nurse in Alaska as a new BSN graduate is diversity—diversity in opportunities, diversity in the people I worked with, diversity in the type of injuries and illnesses, and diversity in my patients. I first came to Alaska as an Army nurse and functioned primarily in medical-surgical roles in military health care facilities. I saw more than my share of frostbite victims and all types of injuries related to living in this frigid environment. Once I completed my Army obligation, I realized just how even more diverse nursing could be. My options were numerous and diverse: working at the Army hospital as a civilian nurse, working in the local hospital, doing Medevac flights from rural villages in Alaska to regional medical centers such as Fairbanks or Anchorage, or working in the regional medical centers with Medevac flights from Fairbanks to Anchorage. What amazing choices! I eventually chose to work in the emergency room (ER) in the Fairbanks hospital.

As an ER nurse in Fairbanks, I was challenged with many diverse and complex patients. I will mention here only a few of my unique cases. There was the man who ran out to his outhouse "real quick" without his shoes at 30 degrees below zero and locked himself out of his house; he suffered severe frostbite on his feet. There was the man who was working for the forest service chopping down trees, when he turned around and looked straight into the eyes of a grizzly bear. He endured massive claw marks on his back and four deep teeth marks in his thigh before he could get his gun out of his pocket to shoot the bear. One of the highlights of my ER time...

was getting to know all the local alcoholics by name and their "drinks of choice." There were the usual gunshot wounds, car accidents, and domestic violence cases, but even with these typical ER cases, many were unique to Alaska's culture and environment, such as moose-versus-car accidents and harpoons impaled in patients' chests and limbs.

I returned to nursing school and successfully completed a family nurse practitioner (FNP) program. As I write this, I am in King Cove, Alaska, a small fishing village on the Aleutian chain, working as an FNP. Last night we had a tsunami warning (it was only a 6-inch tsunami, thank goodness!). Recent patients included a man who had fallen, had a neck and head injury, and needed to be transported to a regional hospital. The wind was blowing at 35 miles per hour, with gusts up to 65 miles per hour, and snow squalls that made driving even more treacherous than usual. Only small, six-se...

fly w... the Coast Guard helicopter arrived with a medic onboard.

My next assignment will be in Nome, where I will work in the clinic and ER at the hospital for five months. My next assignment will be in Fairbanks for six months. Such is the life of a traveling FNP in Alaska—never a dull moment!

Even my time off in Alaska is diverse. I have learned to mountain bike and mountain climb; I have had a close encounter on a peripheral vision, feel her breath on my leg as I was pedaling, and feel the ground shaking as the bear ran. Fortunately, the bear left me alone.

I have learned to ice climb and mountain climb; I have backpacked in amazing, treacherous landscapes; and cross-country skiing is as close as my front yard. There are more pilots in Alaska per capita than anywhere else, and many places in Alaska are accessible only by plane. So I am now a licensed pilot and look forward to even more adventures in the remote, frozen wilderness. Who knows, perhaps one day...

**A Good Read** Additional reading designed to further stimulate the interest of the reader in order to garner additional insight into the relationship between health care and the community.

---

### ■ CRITICAL THINKING ACTIVITIES

1. After reading "Think About This" on page 23 respond to the following questions:
   - What are three risks described in the essay that were unknown a century ago?
   - What is the responsibility of the individual in creating a safe environment?
   - What are three public safety measures mentioned in the essay that do not exist in underdeveloped countries?
2. Ho...
   lem...

3. For several decades now, nurses have worked primarily in hospitals using a medical model approach to health and illness. Does nursing have a vision of the profession with community at the center, or has nursing become so institutionalized into hospital-based practice over the past decades that we will resist the tremendous opportunities to care for people in a myriad of settings and situations?
4. How has the ethic of caring for a patient's environment changed from Florence Nightingale's era?

**Critical Thinking Activities** Questions presented at the end of each chapter that test the ability of the reader to think critically about topics discussed in the chapter.

---

### ▥ HEALTHY PEOPLE 2010

**Promote Healthy Behaviors**
1. Physical activity and fitness
2. Nutrition
3. Tobacco use

**Promote Healthy and Saf...**
4. Educational and commu...
5. Environmental health
6. Food safety
7. Injury/violence prevention
8. Occupational safety and health
9. Oral health

**Improve Systems for Personal and Public Health**
10. Access to quality health care services
    1. Preventive care
    2. Primary care
    3. Emergency services
    4. Long-term care and rehabilitative services

**Healthy People 2010 boxes** Highlights information from the Healthy People 2010 initiative that is pertinent to each chapter.

# *Dedication*

I AM HONORED TO DEDICATE THIS BOOK TO MY FAMILY and friends who make up my life community and who provided me with the love and commitment needed to see this book come to life. To bring a text of this size and breadth to print consumes time, energy, and focus from many. Special recognition to my husband, Dr. Joel Christopher Lundy, who acted as gentle critic and editor and gave me the time and space when I needed it. Thank you for staying the distance with me and making my dream, your dream. For my son, Parker Lundy, who still believes that anything is possible; You are the joy of my existence and my connection to the faculty of wonder. Thank you for sharing your childhood with this text and now, serving as my assistant and connection to the academic life of today's student. For my late father, Marshall Saucier, from whom I learned the value of intellectual curiosity and the importance of the circle of community that gives life meaning. You continue to be my inspiration and I am eternally grateful for your love and intellectual presence in my life. And I am most grateful to Marcelle Saucier Stinson, Wayne Saucier, and John Lundy for the encouragement needed to complete this second edition. To my friend and coauthor, Dr. Sharyn Janes, without your commitment and unwavering belief in the power of lifelong discovery, this book would not have happened. Thank you for helping me to believe that anything was possible, even when the rest of the world seemed to suggest otherwise. For your friendship and shared vision of this second edition, I remain eternally grateful.

—*Karen Saucier Lundy*

THIS BOOK IS DEDICATED TO ALL OF MY FAMILY, friends, and students who have encouraged and supported me along the way and who gave me the strength to continue on the many personal and professional pathways that make up the journey of my life. Special recognition goes to my mother, Joan Janes, for always believing in me and helping me to believe in myself; to my daughter, Heather Rakauskas Sherry, for always making me proud of her in every way and being the continuous light in my life; to my son-in-law Cliff Sherry for being the son I would have chosen, and to my beautiful granddaughter, Sydney Ellen Sherry, who is a gift sent to us to make us believe in miracles. Nothing can match the joy of being her "Grammy." I want to recognize my dancing teacher, Darian Chancellor, for helping me to discover a piece of my spirit I didn't know was there. And to my friend and coauthor, Dr. Kay Lundy, who has given me both professional and personal opportunities that I could only have imagined in my dreams. We have shared laughter, tears, and most of all the belief in a common dream. She is much more than a friend. She is part of my family.

—*Sharyn Janes*

# Community Health Nursing
## *Caring for the Public's Health*

### Second Edition

**Karen Saucier Lundy, PhD, RN, FAAN**
Professor
School of Nursing
The University of Southern Mississippi
Hattiesburg, Mississippi

**Sharyn Janes, PhD, RN, ACRN**
Professor
School of Nursing
Florida Agricultural and Mechanical University
Tallahassee, Florida

**JONES AND BARTLETT PUBLISHERS**
*Sudbury, Massachusetts*
BOSTON    TORONTO    LONDON    SINGAPORE

World Headquarters
Jones and Bartlett Publishers
40 Tall Pine Drive
Sudbury, MA 01776
978-443-5000
info@jbpub.com
www.jbpub.com

Jones and Bartlett Publishers Canada
6339 Ormindale Way
Mississauga, Ontario L5V 1J2
Canada

Jones and Bartlett Publishers International
Barb House, Barb Mews
London W6 7PA
United Kingdom

Jones and Bartlett's books and products are available through most bookstores and online booksellers. To contact Jones and Bartlett Publishers directly, call 800-832-0034, fax 978-443-8000, or visit our website www.jbpub.com.

Substantial discounts on bulk quantities of Jones and Bartlett's publications are available to corporations, professional associations, and other qualified organizations. For details and specific discount information, contact the special sales department at Jones and Bartlett via the above contact information or send an email to specialsales@jbpub.com.

The authors, editor, and publisher have made every effort to provide accurate information. However, they are not responsible for errors, omissions, or for any outcomes related to the use of the contents of this book and take no responsibility for the use of the products and procedures described. Treatments and side effects described in this book may not be applicable to all people; likewise, some people may require a dose or experience a side effect that is not described herein. Drugs and medical devices are discussed that may have limited availability controlled by the Food and Drug Administration (FDA) for use only in a research study or clinical trial. Research, clinical practice, and government regulations often change the accepted standard in this field. When consideration is being given to use of any drug in the clinical setting, the health care provider or reader is responsible for determining FDA status of the drug, reading the package insert, and reviewing prescribing information for the most up-to-date recommendations on dose, precautions, and contraindications, and determining the appropriate usage for the product. This is especially important in the case of drugs that are new or seldom used.

Production Credits
Publisher: Kevin Sullivan
Acquisitions Editor: Emily Ekle
Acquisitions Editor: Amy Sibley
Associate Editor: Patricia Donnelly
Editorial Assistant: Rachel Shuster
Production Editor: Wendy Swanson
Marketing Manager: Rebecca Wasley
V.P., Manufacturing and Inventory Control: Therese Connell
Composition: Shepherd, Inc.
Text and Cover Design: Anne Spencer
Assistant Photo Researcher: Jessica Elias
Cover Image: © Annelene Oberholzer/age fotostock
Printing and Binding: Courier Kendallville
Cover Printing: Courier Kendallville
Additional photo credits appear on page 1130 which constitutes a continuation of the copyright page.

Library of Congress Cataloging-in-Publication Data
Lundy, Karen Saucier.
  Community health nursing : caring for the public's health / Karen Saucier Lundy, Sharyn Janes. — 2nd ed.
      p. ; cm.
  Includes bibliographical references and index.
  ISBN-13: 978-0-7637-1786-5 (hardcover : alk. paper)
  ISBN-10: 0-7637-1786-X (hardcover : alk. paper)
  1.  Community health nursing.  I. Janes, Sharyn. II. Title.
  [DNLM: 1.  Community Health Nursing.  WY 106 L962c 2010]
  RT98.L86 2010
  610.73'43—dc22
                        2008054190
6048
Printed in the United States of America
13  12  11  10  09    10  9  8  7  6  5  4  3  2  1

# Contents

**PART 1 Community-Focused Nursing . . . . . 2**

**UNIT 1 The Context . . . . . . . . . . . . . . . . . . . 3**

**CHAPTER 1 Opening the Door to Health Care in the Community . . . . . . . . . . . . . . . . . . . . . . . 4**
*Karen Saucier Lundy, Sharyn Janes, and Sherry Hartman*

A Closer Look at Health . . . . . . . . . . . . . 9
Historical Insights . . . . . . . . . . . . . . . . . 10
**Nursing in the Twenty-First Century . . . . . . . . 11**
Educating Nurses for Community Health Nursing Practice . . . . . . . . . . . 12
**Community-Based, Population-Focused, Community Health Nursing: What's in a Name? . . . . . . . . . . . . . . . . . . . . . . . . . . . . 12**
Communities and Populations . . . . . . . 14
Acute Care Versus Community Health Nursing . . . . . . . . . . . . . . . . . . . . . . . . 15
**Reform and the Reinvention of Systems of Care . . . . . . . . . . . . . . . . . . . . . . . . . . . . 16**
Nursing's Agenda for Health Care Reform . . . . . . . . . . . . . . . . . . . . . . . 16
Managed Care and the Future of Nursing . . . . . . . . . . . . . . . . . . . . . . . 16
**Back to the Future: From Hospital to Community, from Cure to Prevention . . . . . . 17**
Home Health Care . . . . . . . . . . . . . . . . . 18
Cure and Prevention: Can We Really Do It All? . . . . . . . . . . . . . . . . . . . . . . . . . 18
Benefits Versus Costs . . . . . . . . . . . . . . . 19
HEALTHY PEOPLE 2010: Goals for the Nation . 20
Influences on a Community's Health: Culture, Environment, and Ethics . . . 20
**Epidemiology: The Science of Public Health . . 24**
**Measuring a Community's Health: How Do We Know When We Get There? . . . . . . . . . . . . . 25**
**Conclusion . . . . . . . . . . . . . . . . . . . . . . . . . . . 27**
**Appendix: Standards of Care . . . . . . . . . . . . . 29**
Standard I. Assessment . . . . . . . . . . . . . . 29
Standard II. Diagnosis . . . . . . . . . . . . . . 29
Standard III. Outcomes Identification . 29
Standard IV. Planning . . . . . . . . . . . . . . . 29
Standard V. Assurance: Action Component of the Nursing Process for Public Health Nursing . . . . . . . . . 29
Standard VI. Evaluation . . . . . . . . . . . . . 29

**CHAPTER 2 Community and Population Health: Assessment and Intervention . . . . . . . 30**
*Karen Saucier Lundy and Judith A. Barton*

Communities and Populations . . . . . . . . . . . . 33
The Health of Communities and Populations . . . . . . . . . . . . . . . . . . . . . 34
Differences and Similarities Among Communities and Populations . . . . . . 36
**Community Assessment Frameworks . . . . . . . 37**
Community Empowerment . . . . . . . . . 37
Community Assessment Frameworks/ Models . . . . . . . . . . . . . . . . . . . . . . . . . 38
**Using the Nursing Process for the Community . 41**
Conducting a Community Assessment 41
Community Diagnosis . . . . . . . . . . . . . . 46
Planning and Prioritization Phase . . . . 47
Implementation Phase . . . . . . . . . . . . . . 47
Evaluation Phase . . . . . . . . . . . . . . . . . . . 52
**Conclusion . . . . . . . . . . . . . . . . . . . . . . . . . . . 52**
**Appendix: The Lundy–Barton General Systems Model for Community and Population Assessment and Intervention . . . . . . . . . . . . 56**
Database (Assessment Phase: Nursing Process) . . . . . . . . . . . . . . . . . . . . . . . . 56
Community Profile . . . . . . . . . . . . . . . . . 56
Comparison of the Profile . . . . . . . . . . . 57
Review of Systems . . . . . . . . . . . . . . . . . 58
Problem List (Nursing Diagnosis: Nursing Process) . . . . . . . . . . . . . . . . 59
Problem Assessment and Plan Formulation (Planning: Nursing Process) . . . . . . . . . . . . . . . . . . . . . . . . 59
Progress Notes (Evaluation: Nursing Diagnosis) . . . . . . . . . . . . . . . . . . . . . . 59

**CHAPTER 3 History of Community Health and Public Health Nursing . . . . . . . . . . . . . 62**
*Karen Saucier Lundy and Kaye W. Bender*

**Classical Era . . . . . . . . . . . . . . . . . . . . . . . . . . . 64**
**The Greeks and Health . . . . . . . . . . . . . . . . . . 65**
**Roman Era . . . . . . . . . . . . . . . . . . . . . . . . . . . . 66**
**Middle Ages . . . . . . . . . . . . . . . . . . . . . . . . . . . 66**
Black Death . . . . . . . . . . . . . . . . . . . . . . . 67
The "Witch Craze" of the Early Middle Ages . . . . . . . . . . . . . . . . . . . . . . . . . . . 68
**The Renaissance . . . . . . . . . . . . . . . . . . . . . . . 68**
**The Advancement of Science and Health of the Public . . . . . . . . . . . . . . . . . . . . . . . . . . . . . . 69**
**The Emergence of Home Visiting . . . . . . . . . . 69**
**The Reformation . . . . . . . . . . . . . . . . . . . . . . . 69**
**The Dark Period of Nursing . . . . . . . . . . . . . . 70**
**Early Organized Health Care in the Americas: A Brave New World . . . . . . . . . . . . . . . . . . . . . 71**
The Chadwick Report and the Shattuck Report . . . . . . . . . . . . . . . . . . . . . . . . . 71

The Industrial Revolution ................ 71
John Snow and the Science of Epidemiology . . 72
And Then There Was Nightingale .......... 72
    The Crimean Experience: "I Can Stand
      Out the War with Any Man" ....... 74
    Florence Nightingale and Sanitation. . . 75
Returning Home a Heroine: The Political
    Reformer ........................... 77
    Nightingale and Military Reforms .... 77
    The Nightingale School of Nursing at
      St. Thomas: The Birth of Professional
      Nursing ....................... 77
    Taking Health Care to the Community:
      Nightingale and Wellness ......... 78
    Nightingale's Legacy ............... 79
Early Nursing Education and Organization in the
    United States ....................... 80
The Evolution of Nursing in the United States: The
    First Century of Professional Nursing ...... 81
The Emergence of Community and Public Health
    Nursing............................ 83
    Lillian Wald, Public Health Nursing, and
      Community Activism ............. 83
    Dorothea Linde Dix ............... 85
    Clara Barton .................... 86
    Birth of the Midwife in the United
      States ........................ 87
    The Nursing Profession Responds to the
      Great Depression and World War II . . 88
    Early Education and Standardization of
      Practice of Public Health Nursing ... 88
    Challenges of the 1930s ............. 89
    Progressive Initiatives After the War
      Years.......................... 89
    Social and Political Influence of the 1960s
      and 1970s ...................... 91
    Public Health Nursing Services in the
      1980s and 1990s ................. 93
Science and Health Care, 1945–1960: Decades of
    Change............................ 95
Years of Revolution, Protest, and the New Order,
    1961–2000 ......................... 96
The New Century: An Era of Managed Care ... 96

**CHAPTER 4**    **Epidemiology of Health
    and Illness** ..................... **100**
    *Gail A. Harkness and Demetrius J. Porche*
Epidemiology Defined .................. 102
Scope of Epidemiology ................. 103
The Epidemiological, Research, and Nursing
    Processes ......................... 104
Natural History of Disease.............. 104

Descriptive Epidemiology ............... 105
    Use of Rates..................... 106
    Sources of Data.................. 110
Person, Place, and Time ............... 111
    Person ........................ 111
    Place.......................... 111
    Time.......................... 112
Analytic Epidemiology ................. 114
Conclusion .......................... 118

**CHAPTER 5**    **Health Care Systems in Transition. . 120**
    *Bonita R. Reinert*
The Evolving U.S. Healthcare Delivery System 122
    Private Health Care Delivery ........ 123
    Public Health Care ................ 124
    Military Health Care............... 125
    Health Care Reform ............... 125
The Current U.S. Health Care Delivery System 126
    Levels of Care ................... 126
    Health Care Providers ............. 127
    Health Care Settings............... 128
Issues Affecting the Delivery of Health Care
    Services........................... 130
    Deregulation .................... 130
    Emphasis on Secondary and Tertiary
      Health Care Services ............. 130
    Increasing Consumerism........... 130
    Technological Advances ........... 130
    Increasing Longevity of Americans. . . 131
    Defensive Health Care and Government
      Regulation..................... 131
Managed Care......................... 131
    The Concept of Managed Care ...... 132
    Managed Care Organizations ....... 132
    Patient Care Outcomes............. 133
Health Politics and Policy ............... 136
    Government Policy................. 136
    Public Opinion and Special-Interest
      Groups........................ 136
    Nursing and Health Care Policy ..... 137
New Nursing Opportunities .............. 137
    Advanced Practice Nurses .......... 137
    Entrepreneurs ................... 137
    Data Management ................ 138
    Research........................ 138
Conclusion .......................... 138

**CHAPTER 6**    **Managed Care .................... 140**
    *Ann H. Cary*
What Is Managed Care?................. 142
Principles of Managed Care ............. 142
Managed Care Models.................. 143

Indemnity Plans . . . . . . . . . . . . . . . . . . 143
Point-of-Service Plans . . . . . . . . . . . . . 143
Health Maintenance Organizations . . 144
Preferred Provider Organizations . . . . 145
**Community Nursing Organizations . . . . . . . . 145**
**Management Mechanisms . . . . . . . . . . . . . . 146**
**Credentialing: Regulation and Accreditation . 146**
**Ethical Issues . . . . . . . . . . . . . . . . . . . . . . 148**
**Nurses' Roles in Managed Care . . . . . . . . . . 149**
**Managed Care and Healthy Communities:**
  **Nursing's Approach. . . . . . . . . . . . . . . . 151**
**Managed Care Nursing as a Specialty with**
  **Membership and Certification Benefits . . . . 152**
**Conclusion . . . . . . . . . . . . . . . . . . . . . . . . 152**

## UNIT 2     Influences on a Community's Health 155

**CHAPTER 7     Economics of Health Care . . . . . . . . . 156**
*Sherry Hartman*
**An Economic Approach to Health Care . . . . . 159**
Competition in the Market . . . . . . . . . 159
Competition Versus Regulation . . . . . . 159
Market Failure in Health Care . . . . . . . 160
**Rising Costs and Today's Healthcare System . 162**
From Private Pay to Government
  Involvement . . . . . . . . . . . . . . . . . . . 162
Increased Costs: The Economic
  Indicators . . . . . . . . . . . . . . . . . . . . . 163
Decreased Access: The Economic
  Barriers . . . . . . . . . . . . . . . . . . . . . . . 164
Influences on Costs and Access . . . . . . 167
**Paying for Health Care . . . . . . . . . . . . . . . 168**
Out-of-Pocket Payments and Charity. 168
Health Insurance. . . . . . . . . . . . . . . . . 169
Publicly Funded Insurance and Direct
  Care Programs . . . . . . . . . . . . . . . . . 170
**Cost Containment, Cost Analysis, and Quality  174**
**Public Health, Managed Care, and the**
  **Economics of Prevention . . . . . . . . . . . . 176**
Opportunities for Collaboration. . . . . 177
Counterforces to Collaboration . . . . . 178
Economics of Alternative Therapies . . 179
**Significance of Economics for Community**
  **Health Nursing Practice . . . . . . . . . . . . . 180**
**Economics and Nightingale's Legacy. . . . . . 181**

**CHAPTER 8     Politics and the Law . . . . . . . . . . . . . . 186**
*Sharyn Janes, Heather Rakauskas Sherry, and*
*Karen Saucier Lundy*
**Government Authority . . . . . . . . . . . . . . . . 188**
Protection of the Public's Health. . . . . 188
Power, Authority, and the Health

of the Public . . . . . . . . . . . . . . . . . . . 188
Evolution of the Government's
  Role in Health Care . . . . . . . . . . . . . . 190
**Government . . . . . . . . . . . . . . . . . . . . . . . . 191**
Federal Government. . . . . . . . . . . . . . . 191
State Government. . . . . . . . . . . . . . . . . 196
Local Government . . . . . . . . . . . . . . . . 197
Different Types of Law . . . . . . . . . . . . . 197
How an Idea Becomes a Law . . . . . . . . 198
**Regulation and Licensing of Nursing**
  **Practice . . . . . . . . . . . . . . . . . . . . . . . . . 203**
The Regulatory Process . . . . . . . . . . . . 203
Licensure . . . . . . . . . . . . . . . . . . . . . . . 204
**Nursing Practice and the Law . . . . . . . . . . . 204**
Nursing Practice in Correctional
  Settings . . . . . . . . . . . . . . . . . . . . . . . 205
Forensic Nursing: An Emerging Nursing
  Role . . . . . . . . . . . . . . . . . . . . . . . . . . 205
**Conclusion . . . . . . . . . . . . . . . . . . . . . . . . 205**

**CHAPTER 9     Health Policy . . . . . . . . . . . . . . . . . . . . 208**
*Nancy Milio and Sharyn Janes*
**Health Policy and Public Policy . . . . . . . . . . 210**
Goals and Policies. . . . . . . . . . . . . . . . . 210
Purpose of Public Policy . . . . . . . . . . . 211
Choosing Policies . . . . . . . . . . . . . . . . . 211
History of Health Policy in the
  United States. . . . . . . . . . . . . . . . . . . 212
Present Need for Public Health Policy 213
**Public Health and Public Policy . . . . . . . . . . 214**
**Policy Development. . . . . . . . . . . . . . . . . . . 215**
Policy Environment . . . . . . . . . . . . . . . 215
Public Health Advocacy and Action . . 217
Policy Shape and Setting . . . . . . . . . . . 217
Policy Goals, Tools, and Resources . . . 217
The Players as Stakeholders . . . . . . . . . 218
Player Connections. . . . . . . . . . . . . . . . 219
**Information for Action. . . . . . . . . . . . . . . . . 219**
**Policy Development Strategies . . . . . . . . . . . 219**
Bargaining . . . . . . . . . . . . . . . . . . . . . . 219
Information Through the Mass
  Media. . . . . . . . . . . . . . . . . . . . . . . . . 220
Health Information . . . . . . . . . . . . . . . 220
Mass Media and the Case of Health Care
  Reform: A Cautionary Tale . . . . . . . . 221
**Implementation. . . . . . . . . . . . . . . . . . . . . . 222**
Evaluation . . . . . . . . . . . . . . . . . . . . . . 222
**Nurses in Communities, Public Health**
  **Policy, and Primary Prevention. . . . . . . . . 223**
Advocacy Tools of the Future . . . . . . . 224
**Conclusion . . . . . . . . . . . . . . . . . . . . . . . . 224**

**CHAPTER 10**    Transcultural Nursing Care in the Community ........................ 228
*Madeleine Leininger*

Community-Based Transcultural Nursing .... 230
Scope of Transcultural Nursing Cultures .... 234
Transcultural Nursing Principles ......... 234
Transcultural Concepts ................ 235
Leininger's Theory of Culture Care Diversity and Universality ............. 238
    Development of the Theory ......... 238
    Goal of the Theory ............... 239
    Assumptions of Theory ............ 239
    The Sunrise Model: A Visual Guide for the Theory ................... 240
    Application of the Theory and Model ........................ 241
Conclusion ......................... 245

**CHAPTER 11**    Ethics and Health ................ 248
*Pat Kurtz and Ronald L. Burr*

Virtue or Character Ethics .............. 251
Principle-Based Ethics: Developing Moral Rules ............................ 252
    Utilitarian Theories: Doing the Most Good for the Most People ......... 252
    Deontological Theories: Balancing Rights and Obligations ........... 253
Communitarian Ethic ................. 256
    Justice in Health Care ............. 258
    Values and Health Policy .......... 259
Ethics of Care ....................... 261
Ethical Problems Faced by Community Health Nurses: The Research .......... 262
Ethical Decision Making ............... 263
Service Learning: Discovering the Self and Developing Community Values ......... 264
Conclusion ......................... 265

**CHAPTER 12**    Environmental Health ........... 270
*Carol J. Nyman, Patricia Butterfield, and Jean Shreffler-Grant*

Trends in Exposure and Disease ......... 272
A World View ....................... 272
The Environment and Health ........... 273
    Environmental Health Policy: Historical Perspectives ........... 274
    Recent Environmental Health Issues . 275
    Historical Perspectives on Environment and Health .......... 276
    Origins of Environmental Health Policy ........................ 276
    Environmental Policy: Governmental and Public Roles ................. 278
Nursing and the Environment ........... 279
Roles of the Community Health Nurse ...... 281
    Identifying Risks ................. 281
    Assessing Exposures .............. 282
    Communicating Risks ............. 282
    Assessing and Referring Patients ..... 285
Upstream Thinking: Making Connections Between Environmental and Human Health . 286
Ethical Principles Addressing Environmental Health Nursing ..................... 286
Conclusion ......................... 288
Appendix: Environmental Agents and Their Adverse Health Effects ............... 293

**UNIT 3**    Care of Communities and Populations ................ 301

**CHAPTER 13**    Health Promotion and Wellness .... 302
*Joan H. Baldwin and Cynthia O'Neill Morgan*

Basic Concepts of Health and Health Promotion ......................... 304
    Selected Definitions of Health Promotion and Wellness .......... 305
    Community Health Promotion and Wellness ...................... 306
Factors Influencing Health Promotion and Wellness ........................... 307
    Changes in Societal Expectations .... 307
    Shifting Sands of the Healthcare Delivery System ...................... 308
    U.S. Government Initiatives ......... 309
    Public–Private Partnerships ......... 309
    Growing Consumerism and Emphasis on Self-Care ............ 310
Models of Health Promotion and Wellness ... 311
    Holistic Wellness: Self-Inventory of Personal Wellness Using the Medicine Wheel ........................ 312
    The 4+ Model of Wellness .......... 314
    How to Use the 4+ Model of Wellness with Individuals, Families, Populations, and Communities .... 317
Conclusion ......................... 321

**CHAPTER 14**    Nursing Informatics in Community Health Nursing Practice ........... 324
*Russell C. McGuire and Sandra L. Walker*

The Science of Nursing Informatics ....... 326
Community Health Nursing and Nursing Informatics ........................ 328
Benefits of Nursing Informatics for

Community Health Nursing . . . . . . . . . . . . 328
   Nursing Classification Systems . . . . . . 328
Patient Information Management . . . . . . . . 330
   Efficiency and Time Benefits . . . . . . . . 330
Computer Applications in Community Health
   Nursing. . . . . . . . . . . . . . . . . . . . . . . . . . 330
   Electronic Mail . . . . . . . . . . . . . . . . 330
   Databases. . . . . . . . . . . . . . . . . . . . . . 330
   Electronic Spreadsheets . . . . . . . . . . . 331
Internet Applications in Community-Based
   Nursing Practice . . . . . . . . . . . . . . . . . 332
Healthcare Delivery System Management
   Software. . . . . . . . . . . . . . . . . . . . . . . . . 332
   Networked Patient Care . . . . . . . . . . . . 333
Communication Technology and Community
   Health Nursing . . . . . . . . . . . . . . . . . . . 335
   Telehealth Care Benefits. . . . . . . . . . . . 335
   Community Health Nursing Benefits
     of Telehealth Care. . . . . . . . . . . . . . 336
The Future of Informatics and Telehealth . . . 336
Conclusion . . . . . . . . . . . . . . . . . . . . . . . . 338

**CHAPTER 15**    Health Education in the
           Community . . . . . . . . . . . . . . . . . . . . . . 340
           *Lucy Bradley-Springer*
Theoretical Bases . . . . . . . . . . . . . . . . . . . 342
   Concepts . . . . . . . . . . . . . . . . . . . . . . 342
   Learning Theory . . . . . . . . . . . . . . . . . 343
   Behavior Change Theory . . . . . . . . . . . 344
The Health Education Process. . . . . . . . . . . 346
   Assessment . . . . . . . . . . . . . . . . . . . . 348
   Planning. . . . . . . . . . . . . . . . . . . . . . . 350
   Implementation . . . . . . . . . . . . . . . . . 352
   Evaluation . . . . . . . . . . . . . . . . . . . . . 352
Health Education in Communities . . . . . . . . 353
   Individuals, Families, and Groups. . . . 353
   Community. . . . . . . . . . . . . . . . . . . . . 355
   Beyond Community. . . . . . . . . . . . . . . 358
Ethical Issues in Health Education. . . . . . . . 359
Conclusion . . . . . . . . . . . . . . . . . . . . . . . . 360

**CHAPTER 16**    Complementary and Holistic
           Health . . . . . . . . . . . . . . . . . . . . . . . . . 364
           *Margaret A. Burkhardt*
Holistic Framework. . . . . . . . . . . . . . . . . . 367
Historical Influences. . . . . . . . . . . . . . . . . 367
Complementary Modalities: What Are They? . 369
   Alternative Medical Systems . . . . . . . . 370
   Mind–Body Interventions . . . . . . . . . . 370
   Biologically Based Therapies . . . . . . . . 370
   Manipulative and Body-Based
     Methods . . . . . . . . . . . . . . . . . . . . . 371

Energy Therapies . . . . . . . . . . . . . . . . . 371
Complementary Health and Community
   Nursing Practice . . . . . . . . . . . . . . . . . 372
   The Right to Choose. . . . . . . . . . . . . . 372
   Nursing Assessment . . . . . . . . . . . . . . 372
Potential Barriers to Use of Complementary
   Therapies . . . . . . . . . . . . . . . . . . . . . . 373
Integrating Complementary Therapies into
   Community Nursing Care . . . . . . . . . . . 374
   Spirituality. . . . . . . . . . . . . . . . . . . . . 375
   Music Therapy . . . . . . . . . . . . . . . . . 375
   Imagery . . . . . . . . . . . . . . . . . . . . . . 376
   Herbal Therapies . . . . . . . . . . . . . . . . 377
   Touch Therapy . . . . . . . . . . . . . . . . . 378
Conclusion . . . . . . . . . . . . . . . . . . . . . . . . 379

**CHAPTER 17**    Global Health . . . . . . . . . . . . . . . . . . . . 382
           *Sharyn Janes*
Globalization and International Health . . . . . 384
Role of International Agencies . . . . . . . . . . . 384
   United Nations . . . . . . . . . . . . . . . . . 384
   United Nations Children's Fund . . . . . 386
   World Health Organization . . . . . . . . 387
   World Bank . . . . . . . . . . . . . . . . . . . . 388
   Carter Center. . . . . . . . . . . . . . . . . . . 390
   Bill and Melinda Gates Foundation . . 390
Global Health Issues . . . . . . . . . . . . . . . . . 391
   Disease Burden . . . . . . . . . . . . . . . . . 391
   Violence and War . . . . . . . . . . . . . . . 393
   Poverty. . . . . . . . . . . . . . . . . . . . . . . 394
   Women's Rights. . . . . . . . . . . . . . . . . 394
Global Initiatives. . . . . . . . . . . . . . . . . . . . 395
   Declaration of Alma Ata. . . . . . . . . . . 395
   Millennium Developmental Goals . . . 396
Global Nursing. . . . . . . . . . . . . . . . . . . . . 396
   Nursing Shortages. . . . . . . . . . . . . . . 396
   International Council of Nurses . . . . . 396
   Nursing and Human Rights. . . . . . . . 396
Appendix. . . . . . . . . . . . . . . . . . . . . . . . . . 399
Canada . . . . . . . . . . . . . . . . . . . . . . . . . . . 399
Cuba. . . . . . . . . . . . . . . . . . . . . . . . . . . . . 400
Jordan . . . . . . . . . . . . . . . . . . . . . . . . . . . 401

**CHAPTER 18**    Groups in the Community. . . . . . . . . . 402
           *Margaret J. Hickman, Marilyn Givens King,*
           *and Karen Saucier Lundy*
Characteristics of Effective Groups. . . . . . . . 406
   Collective Identity. . . . . . . . . . . . . . . . 406
   Shared Purpose. . . . . . . . . . . . . . . . . 406
   Communication . . . . . . . . . . . . . . . . 406
   Group Norms . . . . . . . . . . . . . . . . . . 406
   Participation . . . . . . . . . . . . . . . . . . . 406

Shared Leadership. . . . . . . . . . . . . . . 407
Cohesion . . . . . . . . . . . . . . . . . . . . . 407
Shared Decision Making . . . . . . . . . . 407
Conflict Management. . . . . . . . . . . . . 408
Problem Solving . . . . . . . . . . . . . . . . 408
Stages of Group Development . . . . . . . . . . . 408
Group Formation . . . . . . . . . . . . . . . 408
Group Maintenance: Cohesion, Norms,
and Conflict Resolution. . . . . . . . . . 409
Group Dissolution . . . . . . . . . . . . . . 410
Group Stages and Formation. . . . . . . 410
Group Functions . . . . . . . . . . . . . . . . . . . 410
Group Tasks. . . . . . . . . . . . . . . . . . . . 410
Roles of Group Members . . . . . . . . . . 410
Groups as Change Agents . . . . . . . . . 411
Concepts Related to Change . . . . . . . 412
Types of Groups. . . . . . . . . . . . . . . . . . . . 413
Working with Groups . . . . . . . . . . . . . . . . 415
Group Leadership . . . . . . . . . . . . . . . 415
Ethical Considerations . . . . . . . . . . . 416
Evaluating Groups . . . . . . . . . . . . . . 416
Conclusion . . . . . . . . . . . . . . . . . . . . . . . 417

UNIT 4    Common Community Health
Problems . . . . . . . . . . . . . . . . . . 421

CHAPTER 19    Communicable Disease . . . . . . . . . . 422
Sharyn Janes and Gale A. Spencer
The Problem of Communicable Disease. . . . . 424
Transmission of Infectious Agents. . . . . . . . 426
Chain of Infection . . . . . . . . . . . . . . 426
Routes of Infection . . . . . . . . . . . . . . 427
Susceptibility Versus Immunity. . . . . . 428
Communicable Disease Prevention . . . . . . . 429
Primary Prevention . . . . . . . . . . . . . 429
Secondary Prevention. . . . . . . . . . . . 430
Tertiary Prevention. . . . . . . . . . . . . . 431
Control of Diseases. . . . . . . . . . . . . . . . . . 431
Vaccine-Preventable Diseases . . . . . . 431
Routine Vaccines Indicated for Adults 435
Emerging and Reemerging Infectious
Diseases. . . . . . . . . . . . . . . . . . . . . . . 436
Health Care–Associated Infections . . . 437
Food-Borne Diseases . . . . . . . . . . . . 438
Vector-Borne Diseases . . . . . . . . . . . 440
Zoonoses . . . . . . . . . . . . . . . . . . . . . 442
Parasitic Diseases . . . . . . . . . . . . . . . 444
Bioterrorism . . . . . . . . . . . . . . . . . . 445
HIV/AIDS . . . . . . . . . . . . . . . . . . . . 445
Tuberculosis . . . . . . . . . . . . . . . . . . 446
The HIV/TB Connection . . . . . . . . . . 447

Global Disease Eradication Efforts . . . . . . . . 447
Conclusion . . . . . . . . . . . . . . . . . . . . . . . 447

CHAPTER 20    Sexually Transmitted Diseases and
HIV/AIDS . . . . . . . . . . . . . . . . . . . . . . 452
Sharyn Janes, Janet St. Lawrence, and
Julia B. St. Lawrence
Scope of the Problem . . . . . . . . . . . . . . . . 454
Common STDs . . . . . . . . . . . . . . . . . . . . . 454
Syphilis. . . . . . . . . . . . . . . . . . . . . . . 454
Chlamydia . . . . . . . . . . . . . . . . . . . . 455
Gonorrhea. . . . . . . . . . . . . . . . . . . . . 455
Herpes Simplex Virus. . . . . . . . . . . . 456
Human Papillomavirus . . . . . . . . . . . 456
Health Consequences of STDs . . . . . . . . . . 457
Cancers . . . . . . . . . . . . . . . . . . . . . . 457
Reproductive Health Problems . . . . . . 457
Health Consequences for Pregnant
Women and Infants . . . . . . . . . . . . . 458
Health Consequences for Men. . . . . . 458
HIV/AIDS . . . . . . . . . . . . . . . . . . . . . . . . 458
Scope of the Problem . . . . . . . . . . . . 459
Populations at Risk for HIV/AIDS . . . 463
Nursing Care of Families with HIV . . 469
STDs and the U.S. Healthcare System . . . . . 470
Problems of Access . . . . . . . . . . . . . . 470
Health Services . . . . . . . . . . . . . . . . 470
Screening and Prevention . . . . . . . . . 472
The Role of Community Health Nurses . . . . . 472
Conclusion . . . . . . . . . . . . . . . . . . . . . . . 475

CHAPTER 21    Substance Abuse as a Community
Health Problem . . . . . . . . . . . . . . . . . 478
Jean Haspeslagh and Judith A. Barton
The Nature of Substance Abuse as a
Community Health Problem . . . . . . . . . . 480
Definitions of Substance Abuse. . . . . . 480
Scope of Substance Abuse . . . . . . . . . 481
Impact of Substance Abuse on
Society . . . . . . . . . . . . . . . . . . . . . . 483
Impact of Substance Abuse on the
Individual . . . . . . . . . . . . . . . . . . . . 483
Risk Factors for Substance Abuse . . . . . . . . 484
Society's Influence . . . . . . . . . . . . . . 484
The Family's Influence . . . . . . . . . . . 486
The Workplace's Influence. . . . . . . . . 486
Personal Factors . . . . . . . . . . . . . . . . 487
Nursing Assessment . . . . . . . . . . . . . . . . . 488
Nurses' Attitude Self-Assessment . . . . 488
Drug History. . . . . . . . . . . . . . . . . . . 488
Recognizing the Signs of Substance
Abuse. . . . . . . . . . . . . . . . . . . . . . . 488

Interventions . . . . . . . . . . . . . . . . . . . . . . . . 489

   Society's Response . . . . . . . . . . . . . . . 489

   Interventions with Special

   Populations. . . . . . . . . . . . . . . . . . . . 493

Conclusion . . . . . . . . . . . . . . . . . . . . . . . . . 502

**CHAPTER 22**    **Violence and Nursing's Response. . .506**

*Sherry Hartman, Sharyn James, and Anne*
*Troy*

From Criminal Justice to Public Health . . . . . 508

Defining and Explaining Violence . . . . . . . . . 509

Types of Violence in U.S. Society . . . . . . . . . 513

   Violence in the Family . . . . . . . . . . . . . 513

   Youth Violence . . . . . . . . . . . . . . . . . . 521

   Workplace Violence . . . . . . . . . . . . . . . 529

   Mass Violence and War . . . . . . . . . . . . 530

Interventions to Prevent Violence . . . . . . . . . 532

   Microlevel Interventions with

   Individuals and Families . . . . . . . . . . 533

   Mesolevel Interventions: Community

   Structures . . . . . . . . . . . . . . . . . . . . . 535

   Macrolevel Interventions: Society and

   Culture . . . . . . . . . . . . . . . . . . . . . . . 536

Conclusion . . . . . . . . . . . . . . . . . . . . . . . . . 537

**CHAPTER 23**    **Chronic Illness . . . . . . . . . . . . . . . . . . .542**

*Edith Hilton, Kristin Ramsey, and Linda L.*
*Morris*

Chronic Illness in the United States. . . . . . . . 545

Caregivers for Individuals with Chronic

   Conditions . . . . . . . . . . . . . . . . . . . . . . . 548

   Prevention Measures . . . . . . . . . . . . . . 549

Vulnerable Populations . . . . . . . . . . . . . . . . 549

   Disability . . . . . . . . . . . . . . . . . . . . . . 550

   Disability Versus Chronic Illness . . . . . 552

   Experiences of Chronic Illness . . . . . . 552

Caring for Persons with Long-Term Health

   Problems . . . . . . . . . . . . . . . . . . . . . . . . 555

Quality of Life in Disability and Chronic

   Illness . . . . . . . . . . . . . . . . . . . . . . . . . . 556

The Chronic Care Model . . . . . . . . . . . . . . . 558

Roles for Community Health Nurses . . . . . . . 559

   Change Agent . . . . . . . . . . . . . . . . . . . 559

   Advocate . . . . . . . . . . . . . . . . . . . . . . 559

   Professional Caregiver . . . . . . . . . . . . . 560

Role Models . . . . . . . . . . . . . . . . . . . . . . . 560

   Interdisciplinary Roles and

   Responsibilities. . . . . . . . . . . . . . . . . . 560

Financing Costs of Chronic Illness . . . . . . . . 560

Self-Determination: The Patient as Partner . . 561

Sensitivity in Community-Based Caring . . . . . 561

   Gender-Specific Considerations . . . . . 561

Issues Community Health Nurses Encounter . 562

   Supporting Community-Based

   Caregivers . . . . . . . . . . . . . . . . . . . . . 562

   The Advanced Practice Nurse with a

   Community Health Focus . . . . . . . . . 563

   Palliative and Hospice Care . . . . . . . . . 564

   Institutionalization. . . . . . . . . . . . . . . . 564

   Health Promotion in Chronic Illness and

   Disability. . . . . . . . . . . . . . . . . . . . . . 565

The Future Role of Community Health in

   Chronic Illness and Disability . . . . . . . . . 566

Conclusion . . . . . . . . . . . . . . . . . . . . . . . . . 566

**CHAPTER 24**    **Disasters in the Community . . . . . . .570**

*Karen Saucier Lundy and Janie B. Butts*

The Nature of Disasters. . . . . . . . . . . . . . . . . 576

   Definitions and Types of Disasters . . . 576

   NA-TECH . . . . . . . . . . . . . . . . . . . . . 577

   Disaster Characteristics . . . . . . . . . . . . 577

   Global Disaster Issues. . . . . . . . . . . . . . 580

   Natural Disaster Reduction . . . . . . . . . 581

   Disaster as a Global Public Health

   Problem. . . . . . . . . . . . . . . . . . . . . . . 581

   Populations at Risk in Disasters . . . . . 582

Stages of Disaster. . . . . . . . . . . . . . . . . . . . . 583

Disaster Planning . . . . . . . . . . . . . . . . . . . . 586

   Steps in the Disaster Process . . . . . . . . 586

   The Disaster Plan . . . . . . . . . . . . . . . . 587

   Disaster Management. . . . . . . . . . . . . . 589

Disaster Response . . . . . . . . . . . . . . . . . . . . 590

   Response and Recovery . . . . . . . . . . . . 590

   Levels of Disaster Response . . . . . . . . . 590

   National Disaster Medical System. . . . 590

   Federal Emergency Management Agency

   and Disaster Responsiveness and

   Recovery . . . . . . . . . . . . . . . . . . . . . . 591

   Other Disaster Agencies . . . . . . . . . . . 592

   Evacuation. . . . . . . . . . . . . . . . . . . . . . 593

   Rescue . . . . . . . . . . . . . . . . . . . . . . . . 595

   Triage. . . . . . . . . . . . . . . . . . . . . . . . . 595

   Disaster Shelters . . . . . . . . . . . . . . . . . 595

Role of the Community Health Nurse in

   Disasters . . . . . . . . . . . . . . . . . . . . . . . . 596

   General Functions of the Community

   Health Nurse. . . . . . . . . . . . . . . . . . . 597

   Specific Nursing Approaches. . . . . . . . 597

   Shelter Management and Care . . . . . . 598

Disaster Recovery. . . . . . . . . . . . . . . . . . . . . 599

   Effects on Survivors . . . . . . . . . . . . . . 601

   Special Survivor Populations: Elders and

   Children . . . . . . . . . . . . . . . . . . . . . . 604

Collective Trauma: The Loss of
  Community . . . . . . . . . . . . . . . . . . . 604
  Nurses' Reactions to Disasters . . . . . . . 605
  Prevention Strategies for Nurses . . . . . 608
**Conclusion** . . . . . . . . . . . . . . . . . . . . . . . . 609

**UNIT 5    Vulnerable Populations . . . . . . . . 613**

**CHAPTER 25    Vulnerability: An Overview . . . . . . . 614**
*Angeline Bushy*
**Basic Concepts Related to Risk and
  Vulnerability** . . . . . . . . . . . . . . . . . . . . . 616
  Risk . . . . . . . . . . . . . . . . . . . . . . . . . . . . 616
  Vulnerability . . . . . . . . . . . . . . . . . . . . 616
  Persons with Special Needs . . . . . . . . 616
  Vulnerable Populations . . . . . . . . . . . 616
**Web of Causation: The Interrelationship of
  Risk and Vulnerability** . . . . . . . . . . . . . . 617
**Poverty: Impact on Risk and Vulnerability** . . . 618
  Historical Perspectives . . . . . . . . . . . . 619
  Cultural Perspectives . . . . . . . . . . . . . 619
  Policy Perspectives . . . . . . . . . . . . . . . 620
  Health-Related Perspectives . . . . . . . . 620
  Community Perspectives . . . . . . . . . . 621
**Vulnerable Populations with Special Needs** . . 621
  Children and Adolescents . . . . . . . . . 622
  Elders . . . . . . . . . . . . . . . . . . . . . . . . . 623
  Underrepresented Ethnic Groups . . . . 623
  Women . . . . . . . . . . . . . . . . . . . . . . . . 624
  Disenfranchised Populations . . . . . . . 625
  Uninsured and Underinsured
    Populations . . . . . . . . . . . . . . . . . . . 625
**Nursing Considerations** . . . . . . . . . . . . . . 626
  Limited Access to Care . . . . . . . . . . . 626
  Ethical and Legal Considerations . . . . 626
  Patients' Strengths and Resources . . . . 627
**Nursing Roles** . . . . . . . . . . . . . . . . . . . . . 627
  Advocate and Activist . . . . . . . . . . . . . 628
  Case Manager . . . . . . . . . . . . . . . . . . . 628
  Educator and Counselor . . . . . . . . . . 628
  Collaborator and Partner . . . . . . . . . . 629
  Researcher . . . . . . . . . . . . . . . . . . . . . 630
**Conclusion** . . . . . . . . . . . . . . . . . . . . . . . . 630

**CHAPTER 26    Urban and Homeless Populations . . 632**
*Janie B. Butts and Karen Saucier Lundy*
**Urban Populations** . . . . . . . . . . . . . . . . . . 634
  Health and Social Problems . . . . . . . . 634
  Programs for Healthier Urban
    People . . . . . . . . . . . . . . . . . . . . . . . 635
  Urban Sprawl and Health . . . . . . . . . . 636
**The Homeless Population** . . . . . . . . . . . . . 636

Scope of the Problem . . . . . . . . . . . . . 637
  Definitions of Homeless People . . . . . 638
  Historical Perspective . . . . . . . . . . . . . 639
  The Health Problems of Homeless
    People . . . . . . . . . . . . . . . . . . . . . . . 643
**Nursing Care of Urban and Homeless People** . 647
  Be Committed . . . . . . . . . . . . . . . . . . 648
  Use Leadership Skills . . . . . . . . . . . . . 648
  Use Available Resources . . . . . . . . . . . 649
  Be an Advocate . . . . . . . . . . . . . . . . . . 649
  Foster Communication and Trust . . . . 650
  Assess the Problem . . . . . . . . . . . . . . . 650
  Plan and Give Care . . . . . . . . . . . . . . . 652
**Conclusion** . . . . . . . . . . . . . . . . . . . . . . . . 652

**CHAPTER 27    Rural Populations . . . . . . . . . . . . . . 656**
*Gale A. Spencer and Lindsay Lake Morgan*
**Definitions of Rural** . . . . . . . . . . . . . . . . . 658
**Rural Population Characteristics** . . . . . . . . 659
**Perspectives and Stereotypes** . . . . . . . . . . . 661
**Issues, Concepts, and Populations** . . . . . . . 661
  Lifestyle: Adolescents . . . . . . . . . . . . . 662
  Isolation: Rural Elders . . . . . . . . . . . . 666
  Culture: Migrant Farm Workers . . . . . 667
  Housing: Homeless People . . . . . . . . . 667
  Confidentiality: Persons with HIV/
    AIDS . . . . . . . . . . . . . . . . . . . . . . . . 669
  Access to Health Care: Agricultural
    Workers . . . . . . . . . . . . . . . . . . . . . . 671
**Conclusion** . . . . . . . . . . . . . . . . . . . . . . . . 673

**CHAPTER 28    Adolescent Pregnancy . . . . . . . . . . . . 676**
*Loretta Sweet Jemmott, Michelle Cousins
  Mott, Susan Oliver Dodds, Karen Saucier
  Lundy, and Lynn Reynolds Stabler*
**Sexual Behavior and Pregnancy Rates** . . . . . 678
  Teen Birth Rates: How Does the United
    States Compare? . . . . . . . . . . . . . . . . 678
  Teen Sexual Activity in the United
    States . . . . . . . . . . . . . . . . . . . . . . . . 679
**Factors Contributing to Adolescent
  Pregnancy** . . . . . . . . . . . . . . . . . . . . . . . 679
  Developmental Stage . . . . . . . . . . . . . 679
  Social and Environmental Factors . . . . 680
**Impact of Adolescent Pregnancy** . . . . . . . . 684
  Psychosocial and Health Outcomes
    of the Mother . . . . . . . . . . . . . . . . . . 684
  Impact on the Family . . . . . . . . . . . . . 686
  Impact on the Adolescent Father . . . . . 686
  Psychosocial and Health Outcomes
    of the Newborn . . . . . . . . . . . . . . . . . 687
**Role of the Nurse** . . . . . . . . . . . . . . . . . . . 687

Primary Prevention . . . . . . . . . . . . . . . 688
Adolescent Pregnancy Prevention
    Community-Based Programs . . . . . . 690
Program Evaluation . . . . . . . . . . . . . . 692
Secondary and Tertiary Prevention. . . 692
Conclusion . . . . . . . . . . . . . . . . . . . . . . . 698

**CHAPTER 29  Disabilities and Health . . . . . . . . . . . . 702**
*Valerie M. Rachal and Linda G. McDowell*
Definitions. . . . . . . . . . . . . . . . . . . . . . . . . 704
Incidence of Disabilities . . . . . . . . . . . . . . 704
Historical Context of Disability Services and
    Disability Legislation. . . . . . . . . . . . . . . 706
Current Situation for People with
    Disabilities . . . . . . . . . . . . . . . . . . . . . . 707
    Situation for Adults . . . . . . . . . . . . . . 707
    Situation for Children . . . . . . . . . . . . . 708
Legislation Protecting the Rights of People
    with Disabilities . . . . . . . . . . . . . . . . . . 708
Appropriate Language for Communicating
    About Persons with Disabilities. . . . . . . . . 711
    Community Living Needs of People Who
        Have Disabilities. . . . . . . . . . . . . . . . 713
    Homes of Their Own . . . . . . . . . . . . . . 715
    An Accessible Community. . . . . . . . . . . 716
    Meaningful Work . . . . . . . . . . . . . . . . 716
    Relationships. . . . . . . . . . . . . . . . . . . . 717
    Recreation . . . . . . . . . . . . . . . . . . . . . . 717
Services for Individuals with Disabilities . . . . 718
    Case Management. . . . . . . . . . . . . . . . . 718
    Educational Programming. . . . . . . . . . 719
    Transition from Education to Work and
        Living in the Community . . . . . . . . . 720
    Rehabilitation . . . . . . . . . . . . . . . . . . . 720
    Medical Technology . . . . . . . . . . . . . . 720
    Nonmedical Assistive Technology. . . . 721
    Assistance Animals . . . . . . . . . . . . . . . 722
Ethical Issues Related to Disabilities. . . . . . . 723
    HEALTHY PEOPLE 2010: Objectives Related to
        Disabilities . . . . . . . . . . . . . . . . . . . . 724
Roles of the Community Health Nurse . . . . . 724
Conclusion . . . . . . . . . . . . . . . . . . . . . . . 727

**PART 2  Community-Based Nursing Care  732**

**UNIT 6  Care of Families. . . . . . . . . . . . . . 733**

**CHAPTER 30  Foundations of Family Care . . . . . . . 734**
*Ruth A. O'Brien and Karen Saucier Lundy*
Definition of Family . . . . . . . . . . . . . . . . . . 736
Health Responsibilities of the Family. . . . . . 737

Development of Members' Sense of
    Personal Identity and Self-Worth . . . 737
Emotional Support and Guidance
    During Life-Cycle Transitions. . . . . . 738
Socialization of Family Members
    to Value and Maintain Health . . . . . . 739
Education About When and How to
    Use the Healthcare System . . . . . . . . 739
Care Provision and Management for
    Chronically Ill, Disabled, and Aging
    Family Members. . . . . . . . . . . . . . . . . 740
Theoretical Approaches to the Family . . . . . . 740
    Human Ecology Theory. . . . . . . . . . . . 740
    Family Systems Theory. . . . . . . . . . . . . 741
    Family Development Theory. . . . . . . . . 742
Family-Oriented Versus Family-Focused
    Nursing Role. . . . . . . . . . . . . . . . . . . . . 742
A Conceptual Framework for Family
    Assessment . . . . . . . . . . . . . . . . . . . . . . 743
    Energy . . . . . . . . . . . . . . . . . . . . . . . . 744
    Consciousness. . . . . . . . . . . . . . . . . . . 745
    Role Structure . . . . . . . . . . . . . . . . . . . 745
    Decision-Making Processes . . . . . . . . . 746
    Communication Patterns. . . . . . . . . . . 747
    Values. . . . . . . . . . . . . . . . . . . . . . . . . 749
    Family Boundaries . . . . . . . . . . . . . . . 750
A Self-Efficacy Model for Nurse–Family
    Intervention . . . . . . . . . . . . . . . . . . . . . 752
    Identification of Family Health
        Concerns and Needs . . . . . . . . . . . . 752
    Mutual Setting of Goals . . . . . . . . . . . . 752
    Delineation of Alternatives . . . . . . . . . 752
    Implementation of the Plan. . . . . . . . . 753
    Evaluation . . . . . . . . . . . . . . . . . . . . . . 753
Conclusion . . . . . . . . . . . . . . . . . . . . . . . 755

**CHAPTER 31  Caring for the Family in Health and
    Illness . . . . . . . . . . . . . . . . . . . . . . . . . . 758**
*Linda Beth Tiedje and Karen Saucier Lundy*
Thinking Differently About Family Health . . . . 760
    Thinking Upstream . . . . . . . . . . . . . . . 760
    Thinking of a Bottom-Down Health
        System . . . . . . . . . . . . . . . . . . . . . . . 761
    The Human Ecology Model: Thinking
        in Layers . . . . . . . . . . . . . . . . . . . . . . 762
Community-Based Services for Promoting
    Family Health . . . . . . . . . . . . . . . . . . . . 763
    Preventive Support Services for All
        Families. . . . . . . . . . . . . . . . . . . . . . . 763
    Targeted Programs for More
        Vulnerable Families . . . . . . . . . . . . . 764

Families in Crisis. . . . . . . . . . . . . . . . . 766
**Characteristics of Successful Interventions: Creating Healthy Families and Communities** . . . . . . . . . . . . . . . . . . . . . 766
Relationship-Focused Care . . . . . . . . 766
Intensity and Timing of Interventions . . . . . . . . . . . . . . . . . . 766
Nursing Skills and Strategies . . . . . . . 767
**Issues in Family Nursing Today** . . . . . . . . . . 769
**Values: A Challenge for the Future** . . . . . . . . 770
**Conclusion** . . . . . . . . . . . . . . . . . . . . . . . . . 774

## UNIT 7 Care of Individuals. . . . . . . . . . . 777

**CHAPTER 32 Women's Health** . . . . . . . . . . . . . . . . . . .778
*Karen Saucier Lundy, Norma G. Cuellar, and Venus Callahan*
**Profile of Women's Health** . . . . . . . . . . . . . . 780
Education . . . . . . . . . . . . . . . . . . . . . . . 781
Employment . . . . . . . . . . . . . . . . . . . . . 781
Poverty. . . . . . . . . . . . . . . . . . . . . . . . . 782
Marital Status/Family Configuration . 783
Reproductive Health and Risks . . . . . . 785
Patterns of Health and Illness . . . . . . . 786
**Health Issues, Health Promotion, and Health Prevention Across the Life Span** . . . . . . . . . 789
Adolescence (12 to 18 Years Old) . . . . 789
Young Adulthood (19 to 35 Years Old) 792
Perimenopausal/Menopausal (36 to 55 Years Old) . . . . . . . . . . . . . . . . . . . . 793
Mature (55 and Older). . . . . . . . . . . . . 796
**Specific Disease Conditions of Women Throughout the Life Span** . . . . . . . . . . . . . . 797
Cancer . . . . . . . . . . . . . . . . . . . . . . . . . 797
Osteoporosis . . . . . . . . . . . . . . . . . . . . 797
**Diversity and Women's Health** . . . . . . . . . . . 799
Cultural Influences . . . . . . . . . . . . . . . . 799
Sexual Orientation . . . . . . . . . . . . . . . . 800
Women and Aging . . . . . . . . . . . . . . . . 800
Global Issues and Women's Health . . . 802
**Special Issues Affecting Women's Health** . . . 803
Violence. . . . . . . . . . . . . . . . . . . . . . . . 803
Homelessness . . . . . . . . . . . . . . . . . . . 806
Incarceration. . . . . . . . . . . . . . . . . . . . 806
Poverty. . . . . . . . . . . . . . . . . . . . . . . . . 807
Workplace Health . . . . . . . . . . . . . . . . 807
**Toward the Future.** . . . . . . . . . . . . . . . . . . . 808
Women's Ways of Knowing . . . . . . . . 808
Feminism. . . . . . . . . . . . . . . . . . . . . . . 809
Empowerment. . . . . . . . . . . . . . . . . . . 809
Health Care Policy . . . . . . . . . . . . . . . 810
**Conclusion** . . . . . . . . . . . . . . . . . . . . . . . . . 812

**CHAPTER 33 Men's Health** . . . . . . . . . . . . . . . . . . . . .814
*Sharyn Janes, A. Serdar Atav, Joseph E. Farmer, and Karen Saucier Lundy*
**Men's Health** . . . . . . . . . . . . . . . . . . . . . . . . 816
Genetic Factors . . . . . . . . . . . . . . . . . . 816
Sociocultural and Ethnic Factors . . . . 816
Environmental Factors. . . . . . . . . . . . . 818
Behavioral Factors . . . . . . . . . . . . . . . . 818
Healthy People 2010. . . . . . . . . . . . . . . 820
**Healthcare System Utilization** . . . . . . . . . . . 821
Ambulatory Care . . . . . . . . . . . . . . . . . 822
Hospital Care . . . . . . . . . . . . . . . . . . . . 822
Preventive Care . . . . . . . . . . . . . . . . . . 823
**Specific Male Health Issues.** . . . . . . . . . . . . 823
Prostate Cancer . . . . . . . . . . . . . . . . . . 823
Testicular Cancer. . . . . . . . . . . . . . . . . 824
Erectile Dysfunction (Impotence). . . . 825
Cardiovascular Disease. . . . . . . . . . . . . 828
**Selected At-Risk Populations** . . . . . . . . . . . . 829
Men with HIV/AIDS . . . . . . . . . . . . . . 829
Homosexual Men and Families. . . . . . 830
**Community Health Nursing Roles.** . . . . . . . . . 832
Patient Advocate . . . . . . . . . . . . . . . . . 832
Educator . . . . . . . . . . . . . . . . . . . . . . . 832
Facilitator. . . . . . . . . . . . . . . . . . . . . . . 833
**Men's Health Research Issues.** . . . . . . . . . . . 833
**Conclusion** . . . . . . . . . . . . . . . . . . . . . . . . . 833

**CHAPTER 34 Children's Health** . . . . . . . . . . . . . . . . .836
*Carole Hanks, Harriet J. Kitzman, and H. Lorrie Yoos*
**Improving Childrens' Health: Working with Families** . . . . . . . . . . . . . . . . . . . . . . . . . . 838
Preventing Mother and Infant Deaths . . . . . . . . . . . . . . . . . . . . . . . 839
Immunizing Children. . . . . . . . . . . . . . 840
Preventing Childhood Injuries . . . . . . 840
Promoting Children's Mental Health . 840
**Selected Nursing Interventions** . . . . . . . . . . 841
Transition from Hospital to Home . . . 841
Weaving Spirituality into Nursing Interventions . . . . . . . . . . . . . . . . . . 841
School-Based Programs . . . . . . . . . . . . 842
Home-Based Programs . . . . . . . . . . . . 843
**Improving Children's Health: Systems of Care** . . . . . . . . . . . . . . . . . . . . . . . . . . . 844
**Ecology of Children's Health: Contexts for Growth and Development.** . . . . . . . . . . . 848
Poverty. . . . . . . . . . . . . . . . . . . . . . . . . 848
Neighborhood Contexts. . . . . . . . . . . . 851
Parents' Work Context . . . . . . . . . . . . . 852

Childcare Context . . . . . . . . . . . . . . . . 852
Public Policy Context . . . . . . . . . . . . . 852
**Conclusion** . . . . . . . . . . . . . . . . . . . . . . 852

**CHAPTER 35**     **Elder Health . . . . . . . . . . . . . . . . . . . . 856**
*Virginia Lee Cora*

**Aging . . . . . . . . . . . . . . . . . . . . . . . . . . . 858**
Aging Terminology . . . . . . . . . . . . . . . 858
Gerontological Nursing . . . . . . . . . . . 859
Aging and Health . . . . . . . . . . . . . . . . 859
**Nursing of Elders . . . . . . . . . . . . . . . . . 860**
Elders in the Community . . . . . . . . . . 860
Elders in the Family . . . . . . . . . . . . . 862
Elders as Individuals . . . . . . . . . . . . . 865
**Preventive Health Care . . . . . . . . . . . . 869**
Sensory Integrity . . . . . . . . . . . . . . . . 869
Nutrition and Sleep . . . . . . . . . . . . . . 871
Elimination . . . . . . . . . . . . . . . . . . . . 874
Mobility and Communication . . . . . . 876
Cognition and Affect . . . . . . . . . . . . . 878
Employment and Retirement . . . . . . . 881
Thermal Regulation and Skin
Integrity . . . . . . . . . . . . . . . . . . . . . 883
Comfort and Spirituality . . . . . . . . . . 885
**Special Elder Health Issues . . . . . . . . . . 886**
Immunizations . . . . . . . . . . . . . . . . . 886
Medications . . . . . . . . . . . . . . . . . . . . 886
Chemical Addictions . . . . . . . . . . . . . 887
Ethical Dilemmas . . . . . . . . . . . . . . . 887
**Conclusion** . . . . . . . . . . . . . . . . . . . . . . 890
**Appendix A: Selected Theories of Aging . . . . 892**
Biological Theories . . . . . . . . . . . . . . 892
Sociological Theories . . . . . . . . . . . . 892
Psychological Theories . . . . . . . . . . . 892
**Appendix B: Activities of Daily Living . . . . . 892**
**Appendix C: Tinetti Fall Assessment Scale . . . 893**
**Appendix D: Mini-Mental State Exam . . . . . . 894**
**Appendix E: Geriatric Depression Scale . . . . . 895**
**Appendix F: Home Safety Checklist . . . . . . . 896**
Home Interior . . . . . . . . . . . . . . . . . . 896
Communication . . . . . . . . . . . . . . . . . 896
Kitchen . . . . . . . . . . . . . . . . . . . . . . . 896
Bathroom . . . . . . . . . . . . . . . . . . . . . . 896
Medications . . . . . . . . . . . . . . . . . . . . 896
Outside . . . . . . . . . . . . . . . . . . . . . . . 896

**CHAPTER 36**     **Psychiatric Care and Mental Health in
the Community . . . . . . . . . . . . . . . . . . 898**
*Sarah Steen Lauterbach and Janna Lesser*

**The Unique Role and Perspective of
Psychiatric–Mental Health Nursing in
Caring for the Public's Health . . . . . . . . . 901**

Definitions of Mental Health . . . . . . . . . . . . 902
History of Mental Health in the Community . . 903
Early Humanitarian Reform in Mental
Health . . . . . . . . . . . . . . . . . . . . . . . . 904
Community Mental Health Reform in the
1960s . . . . . . . . . . . . . . . . . . . . . . . . 904
**Historical Context for Professional Nursing . . 907**
**History and Spirit of Psychiatric–Mental
Health Nursing in the Community . . . . . . . 907**
State of the Science of Psychiatric–
Mental Health Nursing . . . . . . . . . . 909
Levels of Psychiatric–Mental Health
Nursing Practice . . . . . . . . . . . . . . . 911
**Individuals and Population Groups Needing
Psychiatric–Mental Health Services . . . . . 913**
**Current Assessment of the Public's Mental
Health Status . . . . . . . . . . . . . . . . . . . . 915**
Ethics of Psychiatric–Mental Health
Services . . . . . . . . . . . . . . . . . . . . . 919
**Psychiatric–Mental Health Nursing's Roles and
Phenomena of Concern . . . . . . . . . . . . . 919**
Guiding Philosophical and Theoretical
Frameworks for Mental Health
Nursing . . . . . . . . . . . . . . . . . . . . . 920
**Models for Psychiatric–Mental Health Nursing
Practice . . . . . . . . . . . . . . . . . . . . . . . . 921**
Public Health Model . . . . . . . . . . . . . 922
Primary Care Model . . . . . . . . . . . . . 923
Primary Mental Health Care Model . . 923
Using Reflection in Nursing Education
and Practice . . . . . . . . . . . . . . . . . . 924
Using a Phenomenological Perspective:
Understanding the Public's Mental
Health Lived Experience, One
Person at a Time . . . . . . . . . . . . . . . 926
**The Future of Psychiatric–Mental Health
Nursing Practice . . . . . . . . . . . . . . . . . . 927**
**Conclusion** . . . . . . . . . . . . . . . . . . . . . . . . 928

---

**PART 3**     **Diversity in Community Health
Nursing Roles . . . . . . . . . . . . . 932**

---

**UNIT 8**     **Community Health Nurse Roles . . . 933**

**CHAPTER 37**     **Public Health Nursing: Pioneers of
Healthcare Reform . . . . . . . . . . . . . . . . 934**
*Kaye W. Bender and Marla E. Salmon*

**History of Public Health Nursing . . . . . . . . . 936**
Early Healthcare Reform . . . . . . . . . . 936
The Later Years . . . . . . . . . . . . . . . . . 938

Public Health Nursing Philosophy . . . . . . . . 939
    Institute of Medicine Study . . . . . . . . 939
    Conceptual Basis for Public Health
      Nursing Practice . . . . . . . . . . . . . . . . 940
    Definition and Development of
      Public Health Nursing . . . . . . . . . . . 944
    Essential Public Health Services . . . . . 944
    Activities for Essential Services . . . . . . 944
**Challenges and Issues for Public Health**
**Nursing in the New Millennium** . . . . . . . . . 944
    Impact of the Nursing Shortage on
      Public Health Nursing . . . . . . . . . . . 944
    Further Development of Public Health
      Nursing Models and Competencies . 945
    National Public Health Performance
      Standards . . . . . . . . . . . . . . . . . . . . . 946
    Other Challenges for Public Health
      Nursing . . . . . . . . . . . . . . . . . . . . . . . 946
**Conclusion** . . . . . . . . . . . . . . . . . . . . . . . . . . 948

CHAPTER 38    **The Home Visit** . . . . . . . . . . . . . . . . . . . . **952**
    *Karen Saucier Lundy*
**The Home Visiting Process** . . . . . . . . . . . . . . 954
**Advantages of Home Visits** . . . . . . . . . . . . . . 955
**Effectiveness of Home Visits** . . . . . . . . . . . . . 959
**Challenges of Home Visits** . . . . . . . . . . . . . . . 961
**Distractions in the Home Environment** . . . . . . 965
**Conclusion** . . . . . . . . . . . . . . . . . . . . . . . . . . 966

CHAPTER 39    **Home Health and Hospice Nursing** . **968**
    *Karen Saucier Lundy, Karen B. Utterback,*
    *Debra K. Lance, and Ilene Purvis Bloxsom*
**Home Health Nursing** . . . . . . . . . . . . . . . . . . 970
    Standards of Home Health Nursing . . 973
**The Medicare Era** . . . . . . . . . . . . . . . . . . . . . 974
**Types of Home Health Agencies** . . . . . . . . . . . 976
    Home Health Care Documentation . . 977
**Financing and Payment Systems for Home**
**Health Services** . . . . . . . . . . . . . . . . . . . . . 979
    Medicare . . . . . . . . . . . . . . . . . . . . . . 979
    Medicaid . . . . . . . . . . . . . . . . . . . . . . 980
    Private Insurance . . . . . . . . . . . . . . . . 980
    Payment by Individual . . . . . . . . . . . . 981
**Quality Assurance and Public Accountability** . 981
    Regulation and Licensure . . . . . . . . . . 981
    Quality Assurance in Home Health . . 981
    Accreditation . . . . . . . . . . . . . . . . . . . 983
    Managed Care and Home Health . . . . 984
**Interdisciplinary Team Approach in Home**
**Health** . . . . . . . . . . . . . . . . . . . . . . . . . . . 985
**Role of Family Caregivers in Home Health** . . . 986
**Legal and Ethical Issues in Home Health** . . . . 987

    Home Care Bill of Rights . . . . . . . . . . . 988
    Advance Medical Directives . . . . . . . . . 988
**Information and Technology in Home Health** . 990
    Communication and Data
      Management . . . . . . . . . . . . . . . . . . . 990
    Delivery of Care . . . . . . . . . . . . . . . . . 990
**Hospice Care in the Home** . . . . . . . . . . . . . . 991
    Quality Assurance and Hospice . . . . . . 991
    Hospice Care for Children . . . . . . . . . . 993
    Holistic Care . . . . . . . . . . . . . . . . . . . 993
**The Future of Health Care in the Home** . . . . . 994
**Conclusion** . . . . . . . . . . . . . . . . . . . . . . . . . . 995

CHAPTER 40    **School Health Nursing** . . . . . . . . . . . **1000**
    *Frances Martin*
**History of School Health Nursing** . . . . . . . . . 1005
    Origins . . . . . . . . . . . . . . . . . . . . . . . . 1005
    Evolution of School Nursing . . . . . . . 1007
    Federal Mandates in School Health . 1007
**The Education System and the School**
**Nurse** . . . . . . . . . . . . . . . . . . . . . . . . . . . 1008
**Education and Credentials of the**
**School Nurse** . . . . . . . . . . . . . . . . . . . . . 1010
    Continuing Professional Education of the
      School Nurse . . . . . . . . . . . . . . . . . . 1010
**Role Definition of the School Nurse** . . . . . . . 1010
    Provider of Health Care . . . . . . . . . . . 1010
    Communicator . . . . . . . . . . . . . . . . . 1011
    Planner and Coordinator of Student
      Health Care . . . . . . . . . . . . . . . . . . . 1012
    Teacher . . . . . . . . . . . . . . . . . . . . . . . 1012
    Investigator . . . . . . . . . . . . . . . . . . . . 1012
    Role within the Profession . . . . . . . . . 1013
**Healthy People 2010** . . . . . . . . . . . . . . . . . . 1013
    At-Risk Populations . . . . . . . . . . . . . . 1015
    Nurse as Team Member . . . . . . . . . . . 1015
**School Health Nursing Practice** . . . . . . . . . . 1015
    Health-Related Services . . . . . . . . . . . 1016
    Case Finding . . . . . . . . . . . . . . . . . . . 1016
    Practice Issues in School Health . . . . 1017
**Legal Issues in School Nursing** . . . . . . . . . . 1019
    Documentation . . . . . . . . . . . . . . . . . 1020
    Delegation . . . . . . . . . . . . . . . . . . . . 1021
    Supervision and Accountability . . . . 1021
    Funding Issues in School Health . . . . 1021
    Violence and Terrorism in U.S.
      Schools . . . . . . . . . . . . . . . . . . . . . . 1022
**Community Issues in School Health** . . . . . . . 1023
    School–Health Linkages . . . . . . . . . . . 1023
    Collaboration . . . . . . . . . . . . . . . . . . 1023
    Resources . . . . . . . . . . . . . . . . . . . . . 1025
**Innovations** . . . . . . . . . . . . . . . . . . . . . . . . 1025

School-Based Clinics and Primary
Health Care . . . . . . . . . . . . . . . . . . . . 1025
Increased Role of the Media in School
Health . . . . . . . . . . . . . . . . . . . . . . . 1025
Technology . . . . . . . . . . . . . . . . . . . . 1026
**Conclusion** . . . . . . . . . . . . . . . . . . . . . . . . 1026

**CHAPTER 41   Occupational Health Nursing . . . . . 1030**
*Bonnie Rogers*
**History of Occupational Health Nursing** . . . . 1032
Definition . . . . . . . . . . . . . . . . . . . . . . 1034
**Work and Workplace Hazards** . . . . . . . . . . 1034
Allergic and Irritant Dermatitis . . . . . 1036
Asthma and Chronic Obstructive
Pulmonary Disease . . . . . . . . . . . . . 1036
Fertility and Pregnancy
Abnormalities . . . . . . . . . . . . . . . . . 1037
Hearing Loss . . . . . . . . . . . . . . . . . . . 1038
Infectious Diseases . . . . . . . . . . . . . . 1038
Low Back Disorders . . . . . . . . . . . . . 1039
Musculoskeletal Disorders of the
Upper Extremities . . . . . . . . . . . . . 1040
Traumatic Injuries . . . . . . . . . . . . . . 1041
**Work/Workplace Change** . . . . . . . . . . . . . 1041
**Occupational Health Nursing Practice** . . . . . 1042
Scope of Practice . . . . . . . . . . . . . . . . 1044
Occupational Health Nursing Roles . 1050
**Governmental Influence** . . . . . . . . . . . . . . . 1052
**Professionalism in Occupational Health
Nursing** . . . . . . . . . . . . . . . . . . . . . . . . . 1054
Education and Certification . . . . . . . 1054
Nurse-Managed Models in
Occupational Health . . . . . . . . . . . 1054
**Future Expansions** . . . . . . . . . . . . . . . . . . . 1056
Environmental Health . . . . . . . . . . . . 1056
Migrant Health . . . . . . . . . . . . . . . . . 1056
Health Promotion in the Workplace . 1057
**Conclusion** . . . . . . . . . . . . . . . . . . . . . . . . 1058

**CHAPTER 42   Advanced Nursing Practice in the
Community** . . . . . . . . . . . . . . . . . . . . . 1060
*Karen Saucier Lundy and Mary H. Huch*
**Advanced Practice Defined** . . . . . . . . . . . . . 1062
**Historical Development of Advanced
Practice Roles** . . . . . . . . . . . . . . . . . . . . 1064
Certified Registered Nurse
Anesthetists . . . . . . . . . . . . . . . . . . 1064
Certified Nurse Midwives . . . . . . . . . 1064
Clinical Nurse Specialists . . . . . . . . . 1064
Nurse Practitioners . . . . . . . . . . . . . . 1065
**Education Issues and Scope of Practice** . . . 1066
Certified Registered Nurse

Anesthetists . . . . . . . . . . . . . . . . . . 1066
Certified Nurse Midwives . . . . . . . . . 1066
Clinical Nurse Specialists . . . . . . . . . . 1066
Nurse Practitioners . . . . . . . . . . . . . . . 1067
**Healthy People 2010** . . . . . . . . . . . . . . . . . . 1068
**Credentials** . . . . . . . . . . . . . . . . . . . . . . . . 1068
**Reimbursement** . . . . . . . . . . . . . . . . . . . . . 1069
Medicare . . . . . . . . . . . . . . . . . . . . . . 1069
Medicaid . . . . . . . . . . . . . . . . . . . . . . 1069
Private Insurance . . . . . . . . . . . . . . . . 1069
**Role Differentiation** . . . . . . . . . . . . . . . . . . 1070
**Practice Arenas** . . . . . . . . . . . . . . . . . . . . . 1070
Acute Care Settings . . . . . . . . . . . . . . 1070
Clinics . . . . . . . . . . . . . . . . . . . . . . . . 1071
Long-Term Care Facilities . . . . . . . . . 1071
Educational Institutions . . . . . . . . . . . 1072
**Innovations in Healthcare Delivery in the
Community** . . . . . . . . . . . . . . . . . . . . . . . 1073
Nursing Centers . . . . . . . . . . . . . . . . 1073
Case Management . . . . . . . . . . . . . . . . 1073
Holistic Practice . . . . . . . . . . . . . . . . 1074
**Conclusion** . . . . . . . . . . . . . . . . . . . . . . . . 1074

**CHAPTER 43   Health Ministries: Health and Faith
Communities** . . . . . . . . . . . . . . . . . . . 1078
*Emily Chandler, Ruth D. Berry, and Karen
Saucier Lundy*
**Development of Health Ministries** . . . . . . . . 1080
History of Ministering. Hospitals,
Hospitality, and Religious
Communities . . . . . . . . . . . . . . . . . 1080
Nightingale's Legacy: Relationship of
Nursing to Early Models . . . . . . . . . 1082
Philosophical Underpinnings . . . . . . 1083
**Health Ministry in Action** . . . . . . . . . . . . . . 1084
The Faith Community . . . . . . . . . . . . 1084
Models of Health Ministry . . . . . . . . . 1085
Structure of Health Ministries . . . . . . 1085
**Relationship Between Community Health
Nursing and Faith Communities** . . . . . . . 1088
Parish Nursing . . . . . . . . . . . . . . . . . . 1088
Activities of Parish Nurses . . . . . . . . . 1090
Missionary Nursing . . . . . . . . . . . . . . 1093
Roles and Practice of Missionary
Nurses . . . . . . . . . . . . . . . . . . . . . . 1093
Conclusion . . . . . . . . . . . . . . . . . . . . 1098
**Appendix: Parish Nurse Services** . . . . . . . . 1100
Health Questionnaire . . . . . . . . . . . . 1100
**Index** . . . . . . . . . . . . . . . . . . . . . . . . . . . . 1103
**Photo Credits** . . . . . . . . . . . . . . . . . . . . . 1130

**Karen Saucier Lundy, PhD, RN, FAAN** is currently a Professor at the University of Southern Mississippi School of Nursing in Hattiesburg, Mississippi. She has practiced in community and public health in diverse settings, such as state health departments, migrant health programs, the U.S. Public Health Service, school health, and high-risk maternity and child health. She has also functioned in neonatal intensive care as a staff nurse, clinical instructor, and transport nurse in regional referral medical centers. Dr. Lundy has taught community health at the baccalaureate and master's levels. She has been responsible for undergraduate and graduate courses in community health nursing and doctoral courses in philosophy of science and qualitative research. Dr. Lundy served as Dean at Delta State University School of Nursing in Cleveland, Mississippi, and was on faculty at the University of Mississippi, Loretta Heights College in Denver, Colorado, and the University of Colorado School of Nursing in Denver. Dr. Lundy has also taught sociology at the University of Colorado in Boulder, including courses in family, gender roles, deviance, and social theory. Her scholarly presentations and publications have been in the areas of community health, historical inquiry, philosophy of science, European medieval historical research, gender role and the family, media, and international health and education in Great Britain, Germany, Jamaica, France, and Cuba. Dr. Lundy also holds a teaching appointment in sociology at the University of Southern Mississippi where she most recently taught at the USM Abbey in Pontlevoy, France. Her current research involves the transformation of women healers to social deviants in the systematic torture and killing of "labeled" witches in 11th- and 12th-century Europe. She holds a BS in nursing from the University of Southern Mississippi School of Nursing, an MS in community health nursing from the University of Colorado School of Nursing in Denver, and an MA and PhD in sociology from the University of Colorado in Boulder. Dr. Lundy is the author of *Perspectives in Family and Community Health*, which was named an *American Journal of Nursing* Book of the Year in 1990.

**Sharyn Janes, PhD, RN, ACRN** is currently a professor in the School of Nursing at Florida Agricultural and Mechanical University in Tallahassee, Florida, where she teaches community/public health nursing at the baccalaureate level and research and theory at the master's level. Prior to her position at Florida A & M University, she was a case manager in the Division of Organizational Planning and Improvement at Tallahassee Memorial Hospital. She has held the rank of professor of nursing at Thomas University, Thomasville, GA, Louisiana State University Health Sciences Center, New Orleans, LA, and the University of Southern Mississippi, Hattiesburg. While at LSUHSC, she held the positions of Associate Dean for Professional Practice and Community Relations and Director of the MSN Programs. While at USM, she was the Director of the School of Nursing. She taught community health/public health nursing at the baccalaureate and master's levels, health care policy and philosophy of science at the doctoral level, international health courses in Cuba and Jamaica, and graduate and undergraduate courses in transcultural nursing. Dr. Janes was the Director of the Cuba Studies Program in the University of Southern Mississippi College of International and Continuing Education. She earned her BSN at Marywood College, Scranton, Pennsylvania; her MS in community health nursing at the State University of New York at Binghamton; and her PhD in Higher Education at Florida State University, Tallahassee. Dr. Janes has practiced nursing in a variety of community settings, including home health, hospice, and school health and in several acute care settings, including medical-surgical units and emergency departments. Her scholarly presentations and publications are predominantly in the areas of HIV/AIDS education and prevention; cultural issues in nursing education, practice, and research; and international health and education.

# Contributors

## Chapter Contributors

**Barbara Aranda-Naranjo, PhD, RN, ACRN, FAAN**
Branch Chief
SPNS/HIV/AIDS Branch
Health Resources and Services
Administration
U.S. Department of Health and Human
Services
Rockville, Maryland

**A. Serdar Atav, PhD**
Associate Professor
Decker School of Nursing
Binghamton University
Binghamton, New York

**Joan H. Baldwin, DNSc, RN**
Professor Emeritus
College of Nursing
Brigham Young University
Provo, Utah

**Judith A. Barton, PhD, RN**
Associate Professor
School of Nursing
University of Colorado Health Sciences
Center
Denver, Colorado

**Kaye W. Bender, PhD, RN, FAAN**
Dean and Professor
Associate Vice Chancellor for Nursing
School of Nursing
University of Mississippi Medical Center
Jackson, Mississippi

**Ruth D. Berry, RN, MSN**
Professor Emeritus
College of Nursing
University of Kentucky
Parish Nurse, Second Presbyterian Church
Lexington, Kentucky

**Ilene Purvis Bloxsom, RN, BSN, MSHA**
Chief Nursing Officer
Dale Medical Center
Ozark, Alabama

**Lucy Bradley-Springer, PhD, RN, ACRN, FAAN**
Associate Professor and Director
Mountain Plains AIDS Education and
Training Center
Associate Professor of Medicine
Adjunct Associate Professor of Nursing
Editor, *Journal of the Association of Nurses
in AIDS Care*
University of Colorado Health Sciences
Center
Denver, Colorado

**Margaret A. Burkhardt, PhD, RN, CS, HNC**
Director
Healing Matters
Beckley, West Virginia

**Angeline Bushy, PhD, RN, CS**
Bert Fish Endowed Chair
Professor
School of Nursing
University of Central Florida–Daytona
Beach
Daytona Beach, Florida

**Ronald L. Burr, PhD**
Professor Emeritus
Department of Philosophy
University of Southern Mississippi
Hattiesburg, Mississippi

**Patricia Butterfield, PhD, RN, FAAN**
Professor and Dean
Washington State University
Intercollegiate College of Nursing
Spokane, Washington

**Janie B. Butts, DSN, RN**
Associate Professor
School of Nursing
University of Southern Mississippi
Hattiesburg, Mississippi

**Venus Callahan, RNC, MSN, FNP, WHNP**
Family Nurse Practitioner
Mississippi State Department of Health
Mississippi Family Health Care Center
Instructor, School of Nursing
University of Southern
Mississippi
Hattiesburg, Mississippi

**Ann H. Cary, PhD, MPH, RN, A-CCC**
Director
School of Nursing
Loyola University
New Orleans, Louisiana

**Emily Chandler, MS, MDIV, PhD, RN**
Professor Emeritus
MGH Institute of Health Professions
Boston, Massachusetts

**Virginia Lee Cora, DSN, RN, CS**
Adult/Geriatric Nurse Practitioner
Assistant Professor
Division of Geriatrics
School of Medicine
University of Mississippi Medical Center
Jackson, Mississippi

**Norma G. Cuellar, DSN, RN**
Assistant Professor
University of Pennsylvania
School of Nursing
Philadelphia, Pennsylvania

**Susan Oliver Dodds, MSN, RN, CRNP**
Family Nurse Practitioner
Private Practice
Marlton, New Jersey

**Joseph E. Farmer, RN, MSN, ACRN, PhD(c)**
Clinical Assistant Professor
Community and Mental Health Nursing
College of Nursing
The University of South Alabama
Mobile, Alabama

**Carole Hanks, DrPH, RN**
Research Associate
University of Rochester
School of Nursing
Rochester, New York

**Gail A. Harkness, DrPH, RN, FAAN**
Professor Emeritus
University of Connecticut
Storrs, CT
Adjunct Professor, Boston College
Boston, Massachusetts

**Sherry Hartman, DrPH, RN**
Professor Emeritus
School of Nursing
University of Southern Mississippi
Hattiesburg, Mississippi

**Jean Haspeslagh, DNS, RN**
Professor Emeritus
School of Nursing
University of Southern Mississippi
Hattiesburg, Mississippi

**Margaret J. Hickman, EdD, RN, CCD**
Associate Professor
College of Nursing
University of Kentucky
Lexington, Kentucky

**Edith Hilton, PhD, DSN, MS, APRN, BC**
Advanced Practice, Neurosciences
Northwestern Memorial Hospital
Chicago, Illinois

**Mary H. Huch, PhD, RN, ANP**
Professor Emeritus
School of Nursing
University of Southern Mississippi
Family Nurse Practitioner
Hattiesburg Clinic, P.A.
Hattiesburg, Mississippi

**Loretta Sweet Jemmott, PhD, RN, FAAN**
van Ameringen Professor
Psychiatric Mental Health Nursing
Director, Center for Health Disparities
  Research
School of Nursing
University of Pennsylvania
Philadelphia, Pennsylvania

**Marilyn Givens King, DNSc, RN**
Associate Professor
College of Nursing
Medical University of South Carolina
Charleston, South Carolina

**Harriet J. Kitzman, PhD, RN, FAAN**
Professor of Nursing
School of Nursing
University of Rochester
Rochester, New York

**Pat Kurtz, PhD, RN**
Professor Emeritus
School of Nursing
University of Southern Mississippi
Hattiesburg, Mississippi

**Debra K. Lance, RN, MSN**
Agency Director
St. Luke Home Health Services
McComb, Mississippi

**Sarah Steen Lauterbach, MSPH, EdD, RN**
Professor
College of Nursing
Valdosta State University
Valdosta, Georgia

**Madeleine Leininger, PhD, RN, LHD, DS, CTN, FAAN, FRCNA, LL**
Founder of Transcultural Nursing
Leader of Human Care Research
Adjunct Professor, University of Nebraska
  Medical Center (Omaha) College of
  Nursing
Professor Emerita, Wayne State University–
  Detroit
Omaha, Nebraska

**Janna Lesser, PhD, RN**
Assistant Professor
Department of Family Nursing Care
University of Texas Health Science Center
San Antonio, Texas

**Frances Martin, PhD, FNP**
School of Nursing
Medical College of Georgia
Athens, Georgia

**Linda G. McDowell, PhD**
Associate Professor
College of Education and Psychology
Department of Curriculum, Instruction and
  Special Education
University of Southern Mississippi
Long Beach, Mississippi

**Russell C. McGuire, PhD, RN**
Director, Clinical Services
Appalachian Regional Healthcare, Inc.
Hazard, Kentucky

**Nancy Milio, PhD, MA, RN, FAPHA, FAAN**
Professor Emeritus
Nursing and Health Policy and
  Administration
School of Public Health, Nursing
University of North Carolina at Chapel Hill
Chapel Hill, North Carolina

**Cynthia O'Neill Morgan, PhD, RN**
Pandemic Influenza Program Coordinator
Texas Department of State Health Services
Austin, Texas

**Lindsay Lake Morgan, PhD, RN, GNP**
Assistant Professor and Director
O'Connor Office of Rural Health Studies
Decker School of Nursing
Binghamton University
Binghamton, New York

**Linda L. Morris, PhD, APN, CCNS**
Clinical Nurse Specialist, Respiratory Care
Northwestern Memorial Hospital
Chicago, Illinois

**Michelle Cousins Mott, RN, MSN, CRNP**
Family Nurse Practitioner
Penn Nursing Network Practices
School of Nursing Center for Urban Health
  Research
University of Pennsylvania
Philadelphia, Pennsylvania

**Carol J. Nyman, CRN, FNP, MPH**
Family Nurse Practitioner
U.S. Public Health Service
White Earth Indian Reservation
White Earth, Minnesota

**Ruth A. O'Brien, PhD, RN, FAAN**
Professor
School of Nursing
University of Colorado Health Sciences
  Center
Denver, Colorado

**Demetrius J. Porche, PhD, RN**
Dean and Professor
Louisiana State University
School of Nursing
New Orleans, Louisiana

**Valerie M. Rachal, PhD, RN**
Grant Specialist
University of Southern Mississippi
Hattiesburg, Mississippi

**Kristin Ramsey, CRNP, MSN, MPPM, CNA, BC**
Director, Nursing Operations and Neuro/
  Ortho Nursing
Northwestern Memorial Hospital
Chicago, Illinois

**Bonita R. Reinert, PhD, RN, FAAN**
Professor Emeritus
School of Nursing
University of Southern Mississippi
Hattiesburg, Mississippi

**Bonnie Rogers, DrPH, COHN-S, FAAN**
Associate Professor of Nursing and Public
  Health
Director, Occupational Health Nursing
  Program
Director, NC Education and Research
  Center
University of North Carolina at Chapel Hill
School of Public Health, Curriculum in
  Public Health Nursing
Chapel Hill, North Carolina

**Marla E. Salmon, ScD, RN, FAAN**
Robert G. and Jean A. Reid Endowed Dean
  and Professor
University of Washington
School of Nursing
Seattle, Washington

**Jean Shreffler-Grant, PhD, RN**
Associate Professor & Campus Director
Montana State University, College of
  Nursing
Missoula/Flathead Valley Campus
Missoula, Montana

**Heather Rakauskas Sherry, PhD**
Director, Office of Articulation
Florida Department of Education
Former Legislative Analyst
Florida House of Representatives
Tallahassee, Florida

**Gale A. Spencer, PhD, RN**
Distinguished Teaching Professor
Decker Chair in Community Health
  Nursing
Decker School of Nursing
Binghamton University
Binghamton, New York

**Lynn Reynolds Stabler, MSN, RN**
Assistant Administrator Physician Relations/
  Joint Commission Compliance
Memorial Hospital & Manor
Bainbridge, Georgia

**Julia B. St. Lawrence, MSN, RN, CNM**
Certified Nurse Midwife
Maternal Health Center
Bettendorf, Iowa

**Janet St. Lawrence, PhD**
Chief of Behavioral Interventions and
  Research Branch
Division of STD Prevention
National Center for HIV, STD, TB
  Prevention
Centers for Disease Control and Prevention
Atlanta, Georgia

**Linda Beth Tiedje, PhD, RN, MA, FAAN**
Adjunct Associate Professor
College of Human Medicine
Department of Epidemiology
Michigan State University
East Lansing, Michigan

**Anne Troy, RN, MN, FNP-C, SANE, LNC**
Assistant Professor of Nursing
School of Nursing
Louisiana State University
New Orleans, Louisiana

**Karen B. Utterback, RN, MSN**
Vice President, Clinical Strategy
McKesson-Extended Care Solutions Group
Springfield, Missouri

**Sandra L. Walker, PhD, RN, APRN**
Family Nurse Practitioner
Tallahassee, Florida

**H. Lorrie Yoos, PhD, CPNP**
Professor, University of Rochester School of
  Nursing
Professor of Pediatrics, University of
  Rochester School of Medicine and
  Dentistry
Rochester, New York

# Contributors to Chapter Special Features

**Margaret M. Aiken, PhD, RN**
Sexual Assault Nurse Examiner (SANE)
Memphis Sexual Assault Resource
  Center
Memphis, Tennessee

**Jason Beasley, DSN, RN**
Forrest General Hospital
Hattiesburg, Mississippi

**Miriam Cabana, MSN, RN**
Coordinator of Learning Center
School of Nursing
University of Southern Mississippi
Hattiesburg, Mississippi
Former Nursing Supervisor
Mississippi State Penitentiary
Parchman, Mississippi

**Lynne Cameron, ANP**
Skagway Medical Center
Skagway, Alaska

**David Cartwright, LLB, DipEd, MSW**
Social Worker and Grief Counselor
Southern Care Hospice
Hattiesburg, Mississippi

**Alvara Leonard Castillo**
Assistant Professor of Nursing
Instituto Superior de Ciencias Medicas
President of Havana Chapter of Cuban
  Nurses Society
Havana, Cuba

**Pamela N. Clarke, PhD, MPH, RN, FAAN**
Past President, Association of Community
  Health Nursing Educators (ACHNE)
Professor, University of Wyoming
Fay W. Whitney School of Nursing
Laramie, Wyoming

**Waddah Demeh, PhD, RN**
Faculty of Nursing
University of Jordan
Amman, Jordan

**Betty Dickson**
Lobbyist
Mississippi Nurses Association
Jackson, Mississippi

**Donna Beard Doherty, RN, BSN, MSN**
Forrest General Hospital
Adjunct Faculty
William Carey University
Hattiesburg, Mississippi

**Mary Fisher**
Author and AIDS Activist
Washington, DC

**Betty Ford**
Former First Lady
Founder of the Betty Ford Center
Rancho Mirage, California

**Loretta C. Ford, EdD, RN, FAAN**
Cofounder, First Nurse Practitioner
  Program
Dean and Professor Emerita
University of Colorado School of Nursing
Wildwood, Florida

**Barbara Foster, RN, MSN**
Division of Associate Degree Nursing
Copiah-Lincoln Community College
Wesson, Mississippi

**Toni D. Frioux, MS, CNS, ARNP**
Chief, Nursing Service
Oklahoma State Department of Health
Oklahoma City, Oklahoma

**Sherry Hartman, DrPH, RN**
Professor Emeritus
School of Nursing
University of Southern Mississippi
Hattiesburg, Mississippi

**Jim Jones, BEd, RN**
Case Manager
Pine Grove Recovery Center
Forrest General Hospital
Hattiesburg, Mississippi

**Noah Seth Jordan, RN, BSN**
Baptist Memorial Hospital
Memphis, Tennessee

**Carolyn Keil, PhD, RN**
Associate Professor
School of Nursing
University of Alaska
Anchorage, Alaska

**Felton Keyes, BSN, RN**
Forrest General Hospital
Hattiesburg, Mississippi

**Debbie Konkle-Parker, PhD, RN, FNP**
Assistant Professor of Nursing
The University of Mississippi Medical
    Center
Jackson, Mississippi

**Ann Thedford Lanier, PhD**
Adjunct Professor
Department of Sociology
Texas Tech University
Lubbock, Texas
National Science Foundation (Ret.)
Washington, DC

**Jerri Laube, PhD, RN, CS, FAAN**
Director, Personal Growth Center
Professor Emerita and Former Dean
College of Nursing
University of Southern Mississippi
Hattiesburg, Mississippi

**Judith K. Leavitt, MEd, RN, FAAN**
Consultant
Health Policy and Strategic Development
Asheville, North Carolina

**Mollie Little, BSN, MSN, RN**
University of Virginia Medical Center
Charlottesville, Virginia

**David Lyon, RN, BSN**
Gulfport, Mississippi

**Susan Mayfield-Johnson, PhD, MPH, CHES**
Center for Sustainable Health Outreach
University of Southern Mississippi
Hattiesburg, Mississippi

**James A. Lopresti, PhD**
Poet
Denver, Colorado

**Cynthia H. Luther, DSN, FNP, GNP**
Assistant Professor
Director of Geriatric and Psychiatric
    Mental/Health Nurse Practitioner Tracks
The University of Mississippi Medical
    Center
Jackson, Mississippi

**Lic. Juana Daisy Berdayes Martinez**
Associate Dean for Graduate Studies and
    Research
Julio Trigo School of Nursing
Instituto Superior de Ciencias Medicas
Havana, Cuba

**Arlene McFarland, DNS, RN**
Family Therapist and Author
Fort Payne, Alabama

**Anayda Fernandez Naranjo, MD**
Dean
Julio Trigo School of Medical Sciences
Instituto Superior de Ciencias Medicas
Havana, Cuba

**Regina Hood Posey, MSN, RN**
Community Health Private Practice
Hattiesburg, Mississippi

**Johnny R. Purvis, EdD**
Professor and Director of Education Service
    Center
College of Education and Psychology
The University of Southern Mississippi
Hattiesburg, Mississippi

**Karen Rich, PhD, RN**
Assistant Professor
School of Nursing
University of Southern Mississippi–Gulf
    Park
Long Beach, Mississippi

**James Ryan, MSN, RN, ANP**
Memorial Hospital at Gulfport
Gulfport, Mississippi

**Julie Tanner Sanford, DNS, RN**
Associate Professor
College of Nursing
University of South Alabama
Mobile, Alabama

**Imani Shareef**
New Medinah
Sumrall, Mississippi

**Amanda Traver, BSN, ARNP-BC**
Family Nurse Practitioner
Fairbanks, Alaska

**Connie Thompson, BSN, RN, ACRN**
Consulting Nurse Advocate–Wellness
International Health Ministries
Patient Advantage, LLC
Tonawanda, New York

**Jean Watson, PhD, RN, FAAN, HNC**
Distinguished Professor of Nursing
Endowed Chair in Caring Science
University of Colorado Health Sciences
    Center
Denver, Colorado

**Marge Whaley, MEd, RN**
Pasco County Board of Education
Land O'Lakes, Florida

**Serena Williamson, RN, BSN**
Portneuf Medical Center
Pocatello, Idaho

**Anna Frances Z. Wenger, PhD, RN, FAAN**
Affiliate Faculty, Neil Hodgson Woodruff
    School of Nursing
Faith and Health Consortium Coordinator
Interfaith Health Program
Rollins School of Public Health
Emory University
Atlanta, Georgia

## Ancillary Contributors

**Lisa D. Wagnes, MSN, RN**
School of Nursing
University of North Carolina at Charlotte
Charlotte, North Carolina

**Kim Clevenger, MSN, RN, BC**
Assistant Professor of Nursing
Morehead State University
Morehead, Kentucky

**Nathania Bush, MSN, APRN, BC**
Assistant Professor of Nursing
Morehead State University
Morehead, Kentucky

**Valerie Clift**
Cambridge, Massachusetts

# Reviewers

# Foreword

The health of people is a reflection of the communities in which they live, play, work, and learn. Communities shape the lifestyles that people adopt and their likelihood of living safe, fulfilling, and productive lives. For those who seek to understand human health, the community is an important force to understand. For those who wish to improve the health of others, the community is an essential factor in the equation of people's health and well-being.

The relationship between the health of people and their communities lies at the core of nursing's work. As a profession whose hallmark is concern for human health, nursing has had a long history of engagement in the community. Nurses have practiced in this context, have exercised social activism and advocacy for community causes, and are themselves active members of their communities. Many of nursing's greatest leaders have come from the ranks of nurses working in community and public health.

Despite the close relationship between nurses and the community, the advancement of medical technology, the rise of institutions in which people receive care, and the financial systems supporting services have overshadowed the roles that nurses play in the community context. The public perception of nurses is frequently one in which the nurse is seen as a provider of services to people in hospitals. This view, coupled with the fact that the majority of nurses do work in institutional settings, has had a negative impact on the development of specialties within the community—and the education that prepares them for these roles. One indication of this is the relatively small number of outstanding texts available for teaching community health nursing.

Fortunately, community health nursing is now moving into its renaissance. The fastest growing context for nursing services is now the community. And, there is widespread recognition that the challenges facing health care today can only be addressed if early interventions to populations at risk are delivered in the community context. In short, the day of community health nursing has arrived.

This text heralds the arrival of this new era for community health nursing. It does so in a manner that sets it apart from previous works of this type. It is an exciting and innovative collection of important information, ideas, and perspectives that promise to meet the challenge of educating nurses for effective, population-based, community health nursing practice. It is also a text that makes significant connections between theory, practice, and learning, in ways that are grounded in the emerging reality of community health nursing.

There are many important and useful features to this text. First, it has value as a text specifically designed for undergraduate BSN nursing programs. Second, the text is designed to support education that integrates community health nursing across content and specialty practice areas. It can also support individual specialty course work in community health nursing. This is a text that has widespread applicability across types of education and curricular designs.

The contributors to this book are also noteworthy in that they represent some of the very best thinkers in the field. They are practitioners, researchers, educators, policy makers, and innovators in the field. They bring important viewpoints, challenging readers to think beyond conventional views of community health.

Perhaps most important is that this book is a significant and timely contribution to the advancement of the public's health. The theme that ties this work together is one that focuses on the real goal of nursing education and practice: meeting the health needs of people everywhere. This theme is one that recurs throughout the text with great clarity.

The editors of this book are really its architects—they have conceptualized and brought to fruition a wonderfully designed project that serves its mission very well. They had the foresight to see the movement of community health nursing into new importance in the health of people and to help move the field forward through enhancing the education of those practicing in its specialties.

**Marla E. Salmon, ScD, RN, FAAN**
Robert G. and Jean A. Reid Endowed Dean
 and Professor
University of Washington
School of Nursing
Seattle, Washington

Former Director, Division of Nursing
U.S. Department of Health and
 Human Services

# Preface

Community health nursing has historically responded to changes in healthcare needs of the population and met those needs in a variety of diverse roles and settings. As the first decade of the twenty-first century reaches its end, healthcare needs of the public can seem overwhelming to the beginning nurse. Since the publication of our First Edition, the events of 9/11 and Hurricane Katrina have changed the way we look at the public's health, security, and well-being. For those of us in community health, political, social, economic, cultural, and environmental issues have always been connected to population health outcomes. With recent national and global events, the public has become increasingly aware of the fragility of these interwoven influences on our existence within a global community. The healthcare system in the United States has produced technological advancements never thought possible at the beginning of the last century. Public health, along with scientific and technological progress, has resulted in an ever-increasing average life span for Americans, while other parts of the world struggle to meet basic healthcare needs. Greater life expectancy of individuals with chronic and acute conditions has continued to challenge the healthcare system's ability to provide efficient and quality care for its population. As the population of the United States has become increasingly more diverse, the need for change in community health nursing is imperative; practice must now reflect an awareness of these diverse values and beliefs of populations from homeless female veterans to children with HIV/AIDS. Morbidity and mortality statistics reveal significant disparities among population groups, while socioeconomic and cultural factors contribute to persistent public health problems stemming from violence and substance abuse. Health care must be provided within a population's cultural context, whether influenced by age, gender, race, or ethnicity. In the Second Edition of this text, we have attempted to represent diversity among our authors, in the selection of chapter content, and in the general visual presentation of the text.

In spite of the overwhelming availability of health information to most of the U.S. population, we continue to be plagued with preventable illnesses that are largely a result of unhealthy lifestyles. In essence, despite advanced technology and unprecedented access to knowledge about health, our society remains unhealthy. We are faced with escalating obesity and diabetes rates, family violence, alcohol and drug abuse, high teen pregnancy rates, the reemergence of infectious diseases from last century, and chronic illnesses unknown in previous generations. Although the United States is the most advanced country in the world, it is far from being the healthiest. What can we do as nurses to promote healthy lifestyles, when all of our advanced diagnostics, therapies, surgeries, pharmacological agents, and an educated public present such great challenges? Public health has historically addressed these questions, with a focus on population health and the social and cultural environment. As student nurses in community health, sensitivity to one's own thoughts, feelings, and experiences are necessary for successful nurse interventions. Through our unique pedagogical approach to learning, this text will offer the student a variety of ways to learn through self-reflection. Features such as poetry, art, music, films, literature, and narratives can help students move to greater understanding of self through the shared experiences of others. This text will challenge the student to be fully engaged in the health of populations. Students will be confronted with their own values and prejudices about poverty, racism, sexism, distribution of health resources, and personal and cultural beliefs. Personal beliefs affect one's ability to connect with and promote positive health changes in groups, families, and populations. Although text chapters can stand alone, students should become aware of the connections of all systems among the social, economic, historical, and political contexts that influence our effectiveness in connecting with patient populations in the promotion of our society's health. By doing so, we hope to continue the tradition of a textbook that is more representative of what communities are in the United States—a unified society made up of many different populations and unique health perspectives.

This book is intended to serve as a primary text for undergraduate BSN nursing students throughout the curriculum with an emphasis on population-based nursing, directed toward health promotion and primary prevention in the community. It is both community based and community focused, reflecting the current dynamics of the healthcare system. The Association of Community Health Nursing Educators' Essentials of Baccalaureate Nursing Education for Entry Level Practice in Community/Public Health Nursing (2000) guided the conceptual development of chapter selection, structure, and content of the book.

Rising costs and an aging population have both contributed to the shift toward a population-based healthcare system. As the large cohort of baby boomers move into their aging years, their rising expectations for a healthy lifespan have resulted in a shift from episodic, acute care management to a more chronic focus on health and well-being. Such a change has contributed to population-based outcomes and evidence-based practice. The community has largely become the setting for chronic illness management and prevention. BSN nurses, to provide care for defined populations in all settings, must have the additional skills and knowledge in such areas as epidemiology and environmental sciences. Nurses will need to demonstrate skills in managed care at both the individual and group level, keeping an ever-vigilant eye on population-influenced variables, such as age, gender, and cultural factors.

The cost and quality of health care in the United States continues to be the primary concern of its citizens. No longer just the interests of economists and policy makers, everyone has joined the debate about how to pay for the public's increasing expectations of quality health care at every life stage. More than 40 million U.S. citizens lack adequate health insurance while certain health indicators lag behind those of other comparable advanced countries who are spending far less for health care. The growing economic and health disparity between competing segments of the population has taken on national political significance, as all political parties struggle to find acceptable solutions. Health policy is no longer confined to nurses in leadership or government positions. Although nurses have historically remained uninvolved in the policy arena, this too is changing. The impact of federal and state policy on the delivery of community health services cannot be ignored if nurses in the community expect to influence the delivery of appropriate services to the population. This text provides chapters on economics, managed care, and health policy by prominent nurse scholars who help beginning nurses understand how the knowledge of these often abstract forces can be used in everyday clinical practice.

With the technological explosion of the twentieth century, advances in digital technology have increased applications in telehealth, bringing together health providers and patients, without regard to geographical proximity. The community health nurse of the twenty-first century must use computer technology as the public health nurse of the eighteenth century used quill and ink. With faster and more current data access in community and acute care settings, new dimensions are emerging in patient assessment and intervention. As a result, we continue in our tradition of including a chapter on nursing informatics in the community.

With advances in information technology and global travel, global health issues create challenges for all nurses, not just those working in international settings. With the global community becoming smaller with every passing day, the spread of disease as well as health information occurs in hours rather than the years of the past. These dramatic risks have created the need for different approaches for the community health nurse. Travel nursing, both domestic and abroad, is one of the fastest growing areas in the nursing profession and challenges nurses to adapt quickly to changing physical and cultural environments. Vast opportunities now exist for nurses in global health, as formerly inaccessible populations throughout the world may now be reached through the advent of telehealth and telecommunications.

The passive health consumer of yesterday has given way to the well-informed, fully participating patient of today. With digital and media access to health information, which until recently had been available only to health professionals and scientists, individuals can participate as full partners in their care decisions and in the management of their health. This has raised expectations of care outcomes for patients and nurses. Through the phenomenal proliferation of the World Wide Web, most individuals can access unlimited information about health and health choices. This has greatly increased the power of consumer groups in health and has resulted in greater demands for services and access. The nurse in the community setting will have even greater responsibilities in the educator role as community populations demand the most current information and become more assertive about securing services.

The increased interest in the use of complementary and alternative, non-Western health practices among Americans to enhance health, healing, and a more holistic sense of well-being continues to influence the healthcare system. Nurses in the community are now confronted much more frequently with unfamiliar health practices that may or may not have a research basis for use. Attempts to legitimize many unconventional approaches to health are occurring at research medical centers and through the federal government. A greater interest in the spiritual aspects of health is part of the movement among healthcare consumers for more emphasis on the subjective experience of health. With greater awareness of health information and greater participation in alternative health practices, community health nurses must be more prepared to understand these revolutionary changes. Nurses in the community are in an ideal position to help families and populations navigate through these uncharted and unfamiliar areas, making ethically sound and informed decisions. This text include chapters on holistic health and health ministries to prepare the nurse for these challenges, breaking new ground for community health nursing textbooks.

With the extension of life through technology and improved living conditions, end-of-life issues have changed dramatically as well. The traditional approaches to caring for the dying are no longer as acceptable to patients accustomed to having more control in healthcare decisions. More patients and families are electing to die at home with hospice services and nurses as part of this team approach to a more dignified and humane end of life. In recognition of these needs, this text includes an extended section on hospice in the chapter on home health nursing. Recognizing the increased need for detailed information about home visiting, the Second Edition offers a separate chapter on home visiting.

Nursing education is moving to integrate a more collaborative and interdisciplinary practice in the curriculum; therefore, this text features a unique collaborative model of chapter authorship. The BSN nurse will take the leadership role in such coordinated care in an increasingly complex healthcare system. Although most of our authors are community health nurse specialists, we also use other specialists in chapters that benefit from diverse perspectives. We believe that by securing well-known authors from nursing and other community health–related fields, we present a strong text and support our ideology of a more integrated approach to community health nursing. Further, student nurses are included as authors of special features, providing the reader with narrative accounts of the authenticity of student experiences in the community. The inclusion of clinical practitioners as authors further provides a clinical authenticity that is often missing from nursing textbooks.

A further strength of this text was in our review process. In addition to the traditional review process by community health nurse authors and faculty, we included nurses in other specialties; student nurses at all levels, including RN-to-BSN students; and beginning practicing nurses and experienced nurses in community health practice. These reviews were extremely enlightening, and we believe that through such an extensive and diverse group of reviewers, the text is more accessible for a broader section of nursing students and this second edition of our text is more grounded in current practice.

Change has always been a certainty in the U.S. healthcare system. These changes present community health nurses with unlimited opportunities to influence the public's health. It is up to the student nurses of today to fully realize such possibilities. Nurses of the future must be in partnership with the healthcare system, which requires a broad understanding of community structure and process. The need for a commitment to lifelong learning and critical thinking skills emerge as vital for the nurse who will be successful in the challenging nursing roles of the future. We challenge faculty and students to use this text as the basis for their future professional practice, whatever the setting or role.

## Organization

The book is organized into 3 parts with 8 units and 43 chapters and is designed to be used throughout the undergraduate nursing curricula, as well as in the traditional community/public health nursing theory and clinical courses. The central focus of the 5 units and 29 chapters in Part 1 is community-/population-focused health care. Unit 1 provides an overview of community and public health, which includes the history of public and community health nursing, the Lundy-Barton Model for community and population health assessment and intervention, the science of epidemiology, and an examination of the current U.S. healthcare system.

Unit 2 addresses the major influences on the health of a community. Health care and nursing are viewed through the lenses of economics, ethics, and culture. Environmental influences on community health are explored and discussed. The influence of politics and the law on healthcare delivery is described and examined, along with the role of the community/public health nurse in the formation of health policy.

Unit 3 presents the nursing care of communities and populations. The increasing use of complementary therapies as well as innovative health-promotion and health-education concepts and models are discussed within the context of public health nursing. Nursing informatics, along with the use of technology in the practice of community and public health nursing, is introduced and examined. A definition of groups and an explanation of group process assist the new community health nurse in working with groups in the local community. World health issues are examined, and the global initiative of primary care as delineated by the Declaration of Alma Ata is explored. A unique and interesting feature of the global health chapter includes essays on the healthcare systems of selected developing nations.

Common community health problems provide the focus for Unit 4. Communicable diseases, including sexually transmitted diseases and HIV/AIDS, are examined from a global public health perspective. Violence—the number one public health problem in the United States—and substance abuse are addressed within both family and community nursing frameworks. Chronic health problems in the community are examined, and examples of population-focused nursing interventions are provided. Disaster preparedness and population-focused interventions are addressed in a post-9/11 world, as essential components of public health nursing practice.

Unit 5 presents an overview of vulnerability, including social, economic, cultural, and political factors. Specific needs of homeless and migrant populations, pregnant teens, and people living with disabilities are addressed in both rural and urban settings.

Part 2 contains two units and eight chapters with a focus on community-based nursing care. This part of the book can be used to supplement learning throughout nursing curricula. The emphasis is on the health care of families and individuals as they move between acute care and community settings. Unit 6 is focused on the foundations of family care and nursing interventions for both healthy and unhealthy families, whereas the chapters in Unit 7 address the health issues specific to women, men, children, and elders, as well as mental health issues in the community.

Part 3 provides a view of the diversity in community health nursing roles and functions. The seven chapters in this unit describe the rapidly changing and constantly evolving functions of nurses in many community settings, including public health departments, homes, schools, and workplaces. Advanced practice roles for nurses working with populations are explored. Health ministries have appeared in recent years as a method of delivering health care to faith communities using a spiritual framework; therefore the successful role of nurses within this framework is examined.

## Pedagogy

The First Edition of *Community Health Nursing: Caring for the Public's Health* broke new ground in our efforts to produce a readable, relevant, and interesting text that reflected our passion for the fascinating and challenging field of public health. The Second Edition continues this tradition in our attempt to produce a book that both students and faculty should actually enjoy reading. Faculty are faced with a new generation of media-savvy students who often eschew reading long, dry passages in traditional texts. We are committed to creating a text that is visually appealing while presenting current information that transcends the traditional knowledge-based text in a variety of ways that students learn and experience the world of public and community health. Traditional texts that have virtually unchanged in format for decades no longer meet the needs of learners in the twenty-first century. Students are confronted with a myriad of information sources, from the Internet and social networking websites, to media technology that appeals to all their senses. In order to meet the needs of students so that they will actually read texts, nursing educators must evolve with these ever-changing forms of communication, technology, and options for knowledge acquisition. This requires that we promote partnerships with students in their learning, rather than continue to perpetuate the authority hierarchy of teacher to student that has existed for centuries. Both the National League for Nursing and the American Association of Colleges of Nursing have called for new paradigm development and nursing education innovation to meet the demands of our future professional nurses. The shift to reflecting, learning, connecting, and thinking together with students drives the pedagogical changes in the Second Edition of our text. (See AACN, 1998; Brown, Kirkpatrick, Mangum, & Avery, 2008; Diekelmann, 2003; NLN, 2002).

As a result of our commitment to create a text that addresses these critical changes in pedagogical approach, we have structured the text around reflective and connected learning through the inclusion of art, poetry, narratives, stories, media, and literature. We believe this approach can be a successful integration with traditional course content, either online or in the classroom, recognizing that students learn best using a variety of learning options. Chinn and Watson (1994) advance that "art allows us to locate ourselves in another space and place, to change our perception, our points of view" (pp. xv–xvi). Although our text encourages community health nursing to include diversity in knowing, learning, and caring, we are not breaking new ground. More than 140 years ago, Florence Nightingale wrote that "nursing is an art and if it is to be made an art, it requires as exclusive devotion, as hard a preparation, as any painter's or sculptor's work." In this text, we define art broadly, from photographs, film, and music to cartoons, poetry and literature, and personal narratives. We have included various personal narratives from nursing students and others in the text to capture interest and allow the student to place themselves in these personal stories. Further, through reading poetry or narratives, students can develop ethical knowledge and sensitivity, as well as promoting caring in a cultural context. Reading the chapter content for information and assuming a more active role through reflective reading and engagement of ideas will provide the student with opportunities to observe, experience, and analyze their own reactions to the broad field of public and community health. The depictions of illness, health, and healing through art, literature, and narratives can be powerful enhancements to student understanding of such human experiences as chronic illness, aging, and poverty. In short, they will have the opportunity to explore art, literature, music, and narrative, connect these with their own lives, and interpret the material according to their personal and professional life experiences.

Public and community nurses, perhaps more than other nursing specialties, require that we enter the "other's world," armed not only with theoretical knowledge, but with a greater awareness of the human experiences of suffering, vulnerability, and life-sustaining health practices. This greater awareness that human experiences are more than diagnoses or risk factors will further develop students' collaborative behaviors between nurses and the populations we serve. This qualitative expression of the human experience in aesthetic knowing is "transformative and creative and promotes caring intention which can transform the learning experience of student nurses" (Purnell & Lynn, 2006, p. 9). Community health nursing is perhaps the oldest of all specialties; its historical roots lie in caring for people where they live, work, and play, long before the development of hospital-based, "professional" care. As Jean Watson illuminates:

*Because we are humans, our Truths are cocreated through a process of values and meaning-making through language. When those values become human values of caring for self, others, and all living things, including planet Earth, and when the meaning-making of Truth involves humans and cocreation of meaning via language, then another scenario, different than the one we are used to, reveals the possibility of poeticizing as Truth . . . by inverting the paradigm and understanding human experiences from the inside out, we come full circle—from modern, detached, sterile language to postmodern connections, interpretations, and aesthetics. We see the beginning of a new dynamic of understanding human experience. Nursing's subject matter becomes, for nursing authentically and poetically expressed. (Watson, 1994, p. 4, 15)*

We hope that through the inclusion of these aesthetic expressions of human experiences and health, our text can contribute to nurses' different ways of knowing and learning and thus, sensitize them to the development of holistic nursing practice in their selected fields, wherever they practice in the community.

## ■ References

American Association of College of Nursing (AACN). (1998). *Essentials of baccalaureate education for professional nursing practice.* Washington, DC: Author.

Brown, S. T., Kirkpatrick, M. K., Mangum, D., & Avery, J. (2008). A review of narrative pedagogy strategies to transform traditional nursing education. *Journal of Nursing Education, 47*(6), 283–286.

Chinn, P. L., & Watson, J. (1994). *Art and aesthetics in nursing.* New York: National League for Nursing Press.

Diekelmann, N. (2003). *Teaching the practitioners of care: New pedagogies for the health professions.* Madison, WI: University of Wisconsin Press.

National League for Nursing (NLN). (2002). *Position statement: Innovation in nursing education: A Call to reform.* New York: Author.

Purnell, J. J., & Lunn, C. E. (2006). Development of a model of nursing education grounded in caring and application to online nursing education. *International Journal for Nursing Caring, 10*(3), 8–16.

Watson, J. (1988). *Nursing: Human science, human care.* New York: National League for Nursing.

# Acknowledgments

Many people have contributed to the development and completion of both editions of this text. The chapter authors have honored us with their contributions to this text and have enriched our lives through our interactions with them. We thank them for helping this book come to life. The ideas and eventual structure of this text have evolved over countless conversations and interactions with faculty, colleagues, patients, and students over many years. We thank those who have inspired us and given us the hope and confidence that the unique format and presentation of this text meets the challenges of students and faculty in the twenty-first century. Our students continue to be the main inspiration for writing a text in community health nursing; as our future, they represent our best hope for a nurse-centered healthcare system for all. They have shared their stories, personal accounts, and daily reminders of what a textbook should be. We are honored to share many of their written narratives, poems, songs, and essays in the Second Edition. We remain in debt to the following people for their encouragement and belief in seeing us through the Second Edition with their professional support: Dr. Marie Farrell, Dr. Katherine Nugent, Dr. Kathleen Masters, Ms. Betty Anderson, Dr. Karen Rich, Ms. Cathy Hughes, Ms. Lois Williamson, and the University of Southern Mississippi School of Nursing faculty and students. And for Jones and Bartlett Publishers who believed in the continued importance of this project, especially Wendy Swanson, for her insights and infinite patience, which go far beyond the critical eye of a manuscript editor—you saved us in so many ways, our debt is immeasurable; Anne Spencer, who endured endless challenges of working with over-involved authors in the resulting graphic design of this Second Edition; and Dr. Penny Glynn, for her insights and valuable critical evaluation of the First Edition. For those who participated in the critical review of this text, we thank them for their interest, enthusiasm, and courage to produce candid, detailed evaluations of this Second Edition throughout the many stages—and years—of development: Dr. Sherry Hartman; Dr. Kaye Bender; University of Southern Mississippi undergraduate and graduate students; Dr. Judith A. Barton; Dr. Ann Thedford Lanier; Dr. Heather R. Sherry; Dr. Joel Christopher Lundy; Marshall Parker Lundy; and Michael Peerboom and Wayne Saucier for technical, graphic, and production support. We would also like to acknowledge our colleagues in the Association of Community Health Nursing Educators (ACHNE) who provided valuable contributions through insightful and visionary input throughout the development of the Second Edition. Our best hope is that our Second Edition of the text in some small measure reflects the effort of so many who contributed to the final printed version. Our names appear on the cover but the truest sense of authorship is shared with those named above and many unidentified friends, patients, family, and colleagues who are part of our life journey.

And lastly, we honor and acknowledge the work of our colleague and friend, Dr. Sherry Hartman, who contributed her energy and passion during both editions of this text. Her global insights, belief in humanity and justice for all, philosophical wisdom and humor are woven throughout the text. We remain eternally grateful for her intellectual and personal presence in our lives.

## Special Acknowledgment

The Publisher would like to thank Kim Clevenger, MSN, RN, BC, of Morehead State University for her assistance in reviewing this text in its entirety. Her work on the project was invaluable to the quality of this Second Edition and greatly appreciated.

# PART 1

# Community-Focused Nursing

WHAT DOES IT MEAN to take care of a community? Community-focused nursing care is often difficult to define and even more difficult to practice. Baccalaureate nurses are educated to practice nursing in all healthcare settings. Community health nurses care for populations. Since the late 1800s, professional public health nurses have cared for communities. Those communities have changed over time, and the practice of community health nursing has changed as well. Community health nursing has evolved into a complex, multifaceted nursing specialty that is constantly challenged by rapidly changing delivery systems. While reading about the history of community and public health nursing, both similarities and differences in today's community health nursing practice will emerge. Community health nursing, which evolved from public health nursing and is accountable to the public for meeting the population's healthcare needs, has responded to changes in society to include the care of such diverse populations as school children, women with HIV/AIDS (human immunodeficiency virus/acquired immunodeficiency syndrome), and the homeless. Part One introduces the student to the world of the community health nurse: the focus, the settings, and the historical issues relevant to today's community health practice. As a broadly based specialty, community health nursing practice is more affected by structural changes in society than are other nursing specialties. The community health nurse must be aware of the healthcare system, social trends, economics, and culture to deliver effective care to the public. Part One assists the student in understanding the uniqueness of community health nursing and the structural influences that must be considered when delivering effective care for an entire community.

# UNIT 1

# The Context

CHAPTER 1
Opening the Door to Health Care
in the Community
*Karen Saucier Lundy*
*Sharyn Janes*
*Sherry Hartman*

CHAPTER 2
Community and Population Health:
Assessment and Intervention
*Karen Saucier Lundy*
*Judith A. Barton*

CHAPTER 3
History of Community Health
and Pulic Health Nursing
*Karen Saucier Lundy*
*Kaye W. Bender*

CHAPTER 4
Epidemiology of Health and Illness
*Gail A. Harkness*
*Demetrius J. Porche*

CHAPTER 5
Health Care Systems in Transition
*Bonita R. Reinert*

CHAPTER 6
Managed Care
*Ann H. Cary*

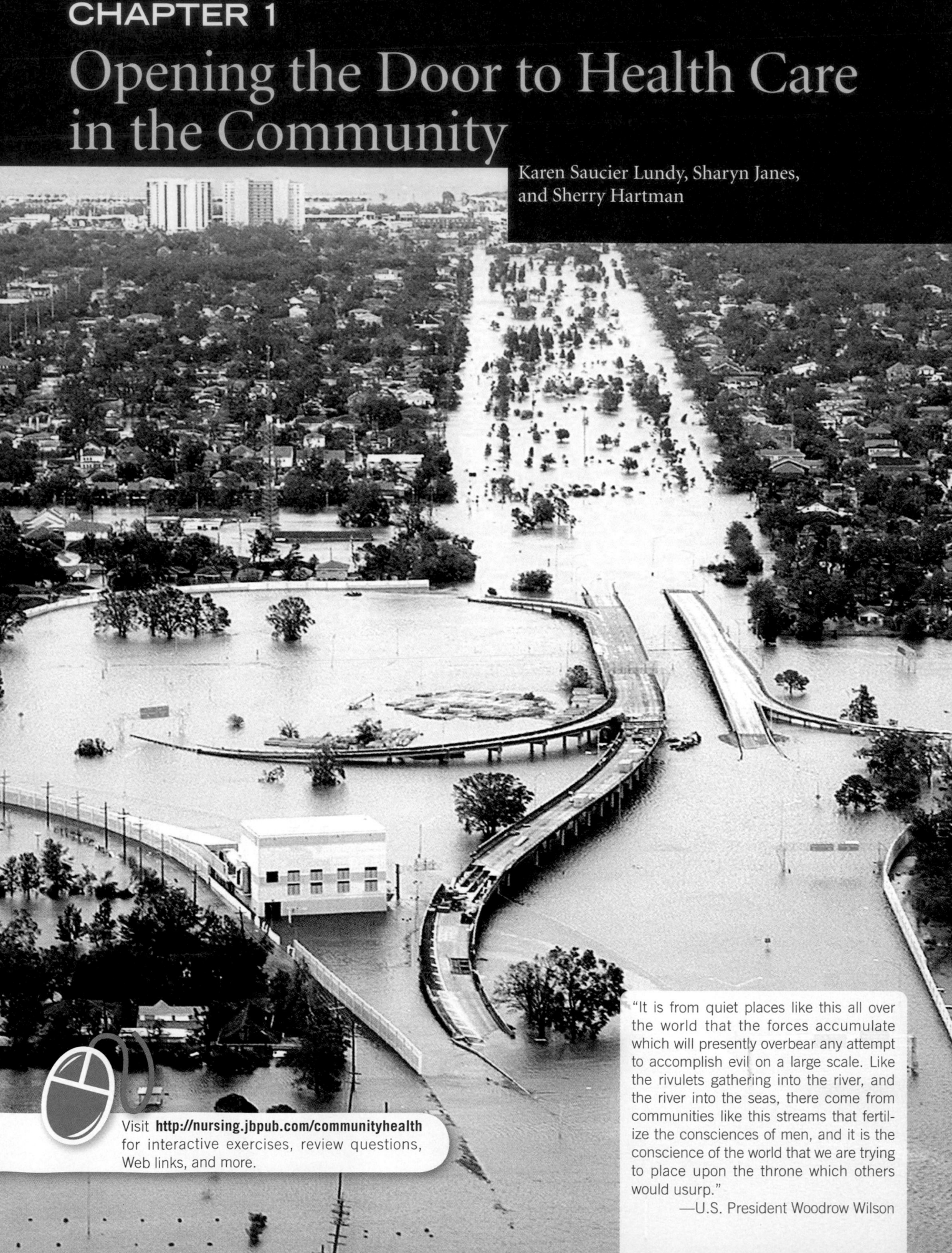

## CHAPTER 1

# Opening the Door to Health Care in the Community

Karen Saucier Lundy, Sharyn Janes, and Sherry Hartman

Visit **http://nursing.jbpub.com/communityhealth** for interactive exercises, review questions, Web links, and more.

"It is from quiet places like this all over the world that the forces accumulate which will presently overbear any attempt to accomplish evil on a large scale. Like the rivulets gathering into the river, and the river into the seas, there come from communities like this streams that fertilize the consciences of men, and it is the conscience of the world that we are trying to place upon the throne which others would usurp."

—U.S. President Woodrow Wilson

- Firefighters who responded to the terrorist attacks on September 11, 2001, have a higher risk for suicide two years after the experience.
- The Hurricane Katrina disaster has contributed to skyrocketing homicide rates in New Orleans.
- Children who were in the Hurricane Katrina disaster area are experiencing higher rates of stress-related illnesses, such as ulcers, night terrors, and school absences.
- Coffee Linked to Lower Cancer Risks
- Marburg Bacteria Outbreak Still Rages, with Nearly 300 Dead
- Allergens Found High in Daycare Centers
- Moderate Alcohol Consumption Appears to Slow Cognitive Decline in Older Women
- States Wrestle with How to Accommodate Children Born in the U.S. to Illegal Immigrants
- Dull, Low-Level Jobs Linked to Heart Problems
- Teens Say Oral Sex Not Really Sex
- Cosmetic Surgeons Focus More on Teen Set
- Proximity to Power Lines at Birth May Increase Leukemia Risk
- Middle-Age Obesity Predicts Old-Age Dementia
- WHO Just Says No to Tanning Beds for Teens
- Days Off in Fine Weather Linked to Melanoma-Courting Behavior

- CDC Finds Unsafe Drinking Water on Most U.S. Airlines
- VA Report Links Gulf War Illnesses to Neurotoxins
- TB Has Small Presence in America, but Remains Huge Worldwide
- Is Your Desk Making You Sick? Computer Keyboards and Office Equipment Swarm with Germs
- Cruise Ships May Be Hazardous to Your Health
- Few Americans Following "Big Four" Healthy Lifestyle
- Obesity in U.S. at Pandemic Level, May Decrease Life Expectancy for Younger Generations
- Autism Linked to Allergic Disease During Pregnancy
- Mental Disorders Strike Nearly Half of All Americans
- Experts: AIDS Vaccine Years Away
- Most Prescription Bottles Difficult for Elders to Read
- Majority of Elders Do Not Take Drugs as Prescribed
- Methamphetamine Now "Drug of Choice" in Rural U.S.
- FDA Bans Dietary Supplements Containing Ephedra
- Drug Safety Fears Prompt Some Patients to Seek Alternative Pain Remedies
- Antibiotics, Sex Hormones and Tranquilizers Found in Major U.S. Cities' Drinking Water

These headlines are all actual headlines from the last few years. Sometimes it may seem that as nurses, the larger social issues are unrelated to our practice. As you will see in this text, however, community health nurses define health very broadly so that the connections between these headlines and our work in the community will become clearer. Almost every problem in the news can be linked to larger issues in public health.

After reading these headlines, think about the following questions:

- Why are illness and disease the focus of most health care in the U.S. healthcare system?
- Are you more interested in the "drama of trauma" in health care than community health nursing, such as educating people about prevention of disease and injury? If you are, you are not alone! Most student nurses and the public are more impressed with high-tech health care than with prevention.
- Think about why nurses might find self-care and prevention to be less interesting. Why do you?

## CHAPTER FOCUS

**A Closer Look at Health**
- Historical Insights

**Nursing in the Twenty-First Century**
- Educating Nurses for Community Health Nursing Practice

**Community-Based, Population-Focused, Community Health Nursing: What's in a Name?**
- Communities and Populations
- Acute Care Versus Community Health Nursing

**Reform and Reinvention of Systems of Care**
- *Nursing's Agenda for Health Care Reform*
- Managed Care and the Future of Nursing

**Back to the Future: From Hospital to Community, from Cure to Prevention**
- Home Health Care
- Cure and Prevention: Can We Really Do It All?
- Benefits Versus Costs
- *Healthy People 2010:* Goals for the Nation
- Influences on a Community's Health: Culture, Environment, and Ethics

**Epidemiology: The Science of Public Health**

**Measuring a Community's Health: How Do We Know When We Get There?**

## QUESTIONS TO CONSIDER

After reading this chapter, you will know the answers to the following questions:

1. How does the definition of health affect the way we care for populations?
2. How have settings for health care changed in recent decades?
3. What implications does managed care have for nurses?
4. What is health care reform and prevention, and how has it influenced the U.S. health care system?
5. What is the significance of *Nursing's Agenda for Health Care Reform?*
6. What is *Healthy People 2010,* and how does it influence the health care system related to a policy of prevention?
7. What are the distinctions between the concepts of community health, population-focused care, and acute care?
8. What is a community and a population?
9. What are the three major influences on community health?
10. What is epidemiology?
11. What is the relationship between the natural history of disease and the three levels of prevention?
12. How is a population's health measured?

## KEY TERMS

Care management
Community
Community-based nursing
Community health nursing
Culture
Environment

Epidemiology
Ethics
Florence Nightingale
Health
Health care reform
*Healthy People 2010*

Home health care
Managed care
*Nursing's Agenda for Health Care Reform*
Population
Population-focused care

Populations of interest
Primary prevention
Public health nursing
Secondary prevention
Tertiary prevention
World Health Organization (WHO)

> **"***We hear much of 'contagion and infection' in disease. May we not also come to make health contagious and infectious?***"**
> —*Florence Nightingale, 1890*

THE WORLD OF NURSING and the nurse's role are always changing, but it is probably safe to say that those who choose nursing in the twenty-first century are caught in unprecedented currents of change: changes in health care, changes in nursing, and changes in settings of care. The post–September 11 world has forever changed our feelings about security in our communities. The health care system has been challenged like never before to respond to bioterrorist threats unknown to nurses just a few years earlier. The unprecedented "disaster of disasters" Hurricane Katrina forced us as a society to question our ability to respond to natural threats as well. Many of us watched in shock, and some of us experienced firsthand, the disintegration of an entire region along the Mississippi Gulf Coast and New Orleans. How could this happen in the United States? Even more importantly, how can we respond more efficiently and effectively with future disasters?

These and other health crises have left us as a nation questioning our ability to respond to the public health needs of the new millennium. In this climate of disillusionment, Americans feel even more vulnerable than ever in terms of their safety, despite living in the most advanced nation in the world.

These forces for change have been developing for some time now, engulfing all health care professionals in the shifting sands of practice. In response to new demands, new opportunities, new possibilities, and a more complex health care environment, current nursing students pursue a curriculum

### ✎ NOTE THIS! •

**Common Definitions in Community Health Nursing**

**Community Health Nursing** is a systematic process of delivering nursing care to improve the health of an entire community (Nehls et al., 2001, p. 305).

**Community-Based Nursing** refers to both the setting and the practice of the nursing role. The focus of community-based nursing care is primarily at the individual and family levels, which contribute to the health of the community. Community-based nursing often refers to nursing care provided outside of acute care settings.

**Population-Focused Care** refers to interventions aimed at health promotion and disease prevention that shape a community's overall health status.

**Public Health Nursing** is the practice of promoting and protecting the health of populations using knowledge from nursing, social, and public health sciences. The practice is population-focused, with the goals of promoting health and preventing disease and disability for all people through the creation of conditions in which people can be healthy (American Public Health Association, Public Health Nursing, Section, 1996; American Nurses Association, 2007).

that their predecessors might not recognize. The nurse's place in the health care system is at the patient's side, not just in the hospital, but in any setting where people work, play, learn, worship, shop, surf on the World Wide Web, or call a hotline; the nurse has an opportunity to educate and promote health for people in broad and diverse communities. Further, travel nursing has emerged as a new trend that provides nurses with opportunities to work in different cultures, settings, and locales—a new role in the health care system.

Chapter author Dr. Karen Saucier Lundy assists nursing students learning individual assessment skills. Community health nursing skills often involve additional data collection, such as morbidity and mortality statistics.

---

**BOX 1-1**

**Cornerstones of Public Health Nursing**

Public health nursing practice:

- Focuses on entire populations.
- Reflects the community's priorities and needs.
- Establishes caring relationships with the community, families, individuals, and systems that comprise the populations public health nurses (PHNs) serve.
- Is grounded in social justice, compassion, sensitivity to diversity, and respect for the worth of all people, especially the vulnerable.
- Encompasses mental, physical, emotional, social, spiritual, and environmental aspects of health.
- Promotes health through strategies driven by epidemiological evidence.
- Collaborates with community resources to achieve those strategies, but can and will work alone if necessary.
- Derives its authority for independent action from the Nurse Practice Act.

*Source*: Minnesota Department of Health Center for Public Health Nursing. (2004). *Cornerstones of public health nursing*. Retrieved October 15, 2008, from http://192.70.175.126/oll/intro/PDF/CornerstonesDefinitionRevised2004.pdf

---

❝*The answer to health will not be found in more drugs, more technology, or more hospitals.*❞

—Martha E. Rogers

As health care moves towazrd a more community-driven system, a change in focus becomes vital as we embrace a growing mindfulness to form partnerships with those served by community health nurses. New directions in health care are occurring internationally as well with community-based partnerships between health care providers and communities (Nehls & Vandermause, 2004). Even if the world around us appears to remain chaotic and complex, as some suggest, nursing ideals and commitments will fulfill the promise of the dreams that bring most nurses to the profession.

With the headlines often heralding hospital closures, mergers, and downsizing, where does that leave nurses? What is the story behind where we are today? What kind of job will there be for you after graduation? When you graduate from nursing school, you will join more than 2.4 million registered nurses (RNs) in the United States. The good news is that the federal government predicts that registered nurse will be one of the top 10 careers with the most job openings *of any job* in the coming decade (Bureau of Labor Statistics, 2008). Rapid growth in this job market will be driven by technological advances in patient care, which permit a greater number of health problems to be treated, coupled with an increasing emphasis on preventive care as we learn more about what keeps people healthy.

A critical nursing shortage exists today in all areas of nursing and is projected to extend into the coming decades, especially for positions requiring a BSN. Travel nursing positions are in great demand in the United States and throughout the world. Nurses who can respond to different cultures and practice settings and adjust quickly to diverse care situations requiring community-health and population-based skills will be in the greatest demand. In addition, the number of older people, who are much more likely than younger people to need nursing care, is projected to grow rapidly.

Although nearly 60% of RNs still work in hospitals, that percentage has dropped more than six percentage points since 1992, according to the Bureau of Labor Statistics (2008). The greatest changes have been an increase in the percentage of nurses who work in community-ambulatory care, home health, public health, and other community-based settings (DHHS, 2000). Dramatic changes in the way health care is delivered have led to the discharge of sicker patients to their homes. As managed care continues to result in

❝*I enjoy situations where I have to adjust to the environment, learn the culture, and develop interpersonal relationships quickly. Being able to experience a particular area of nursing through the eyes of someone from another region is one of the best benefits of traveling.*❞

—Mary Jo Alessio, RN
Travel Nurse
Supplemental Health Care

## A Good Read

# Working as a Nurse and Family Nurse Practitioner in Alaska: Just Another Day in a Frozen Paradise

*Amanda Traver, FNP, MSN*

The first word that comes to my mind after taking a job as a nurse in Alaska as a new BSN graduate is diversity—diversity in opportunities, diversity in the people I worked with, diversity in the type of injuries and illnesses, and diversity in my patients. I first came to Alaska as an Army nurse and functioned primarily in medical-surgical roles in military health care facilities. I saw more than my share of frostbite victims and all types of injuries related to living in this frigid environment. Once I completed my Army obligation, I realized just how even more diverse nursing could be. My options were numerous and diverse: working at the Army hospital as a civilian nurse, working in the local hospital, doing Medevac flights from rural villages in Alaska to regional medical centers such as Fairbanks or Anchorage, or working in the regional medical centers with Medevac flights from Fairbanks to Anchorage. What amazing choices! I eventually chose to work in the emergency room (ER) in the Fairbanks hospital.

As an ER nurse in Fairbanks, I was challenged with many diverse and complex patients. I will mention here only a few of my unique cases. There was the man who ran out to his outhouse "real quick" without his shoes at 30 degrees below zero and locked himself out of his house; he suffered severe frostbite on his feet. There was the man who was working for the forest service chopping down trees, when he turned around and looked straight into the eyes of a grizzly bear. He endured massive claw marks on his back and four deep teeth marks in his thigh before he could get his gun out of his pocket to shoot the bear. One of the highlights of my ER time

was getting to know all the local alcoholics by name and their "drinks of choice." There were the usual gunshot wounds, car accidents, and domestic violence cases, but even with these typical ER cases, many were unique to Alaska's culture and environment, such as moose-versus-car accidents and harpoons impaled in patients' chests and limbs.

I returned to nursing school and successfully completed a family nurse practitioner (FNP) program. As I write this, I am in King Cove, Alaska, a small fishing village on the Aleutian chain, working as an FNP. Last night we had a tsunami warning (it was only a 6-inch tsunami, thank goodness!). Recent patients included a man who had fallen, had a neck and head injury, and needed to be transported to a regional hospital. The wind was blowing at 35 miles per hour, with gusts up to 65 miles per hour, and snow squalls that made driving even more treacherous than usual. Only small, six-seater planes can land on the runway in King Cove, and that is in good weather. No planes can land on the runways at night. We had to request a Coast Guard helicopter to fly the patient across the bay to a town with a larger, lighted runway. A fishing boat was standing by to take the patient across the bay in case the helicopter could not get in. Fortunately, the Coast Guard helicopter was able to land. As we loaded the patient into the helicopter, the snow was blowing hard in our faces and the wind was howling. He was flown by helicopter to Fairbanks, where a plane picked him up and flew him to the larger medical center in Anchorage. I initially planned to fly with him on the Coast Guard transport, but fortunately the Coast Guard helicopter arrived with a medic onboard.

My next assignment will be in Nome, where I will work in the clinic and ER at the hospital for five months. My next assignment will be in Fairbanks for six months. Such is the life of a traveling FNP in Alaska—never a dull moment!

Even my time off in Alaska is diverse. I have learned to mountain bike and have been chased by a bear on a mountain biking trip. It was so close I could see the bear in my peripheral vision, feel her breath on my leg as I was pedaling, and feel the ground shaking as the bear ran. Fortunately, the bear left me alone.

I have learned to ice climb and mountain climb; I have backpacked in amazing, treacherous landscapes; and cross-country skiing is as close as my front yard. There are more pilots in Alaska per capita than anywhere else, and many places in Alaska are accessible only by plane. So I am now a licensed pilot and look forward to even more adventures in the remote, frozen wilderness. Who knows, perhaps one day I will be working as a nurse and a pilot transporting patients in the wild and beautiful state I now call home!

## ◉ MEDIA MOMENT

View an episode of a current medical show on television such as *Scrubs*, *ER*, or *House*. Can you identify a situation on the show where preventive interventions such as patient or family education by a community health nurse could have reduced or prevented the occurrence of an injury or disease? Why are these shows so popular with audiences when the worst-case scenario tends to occur?

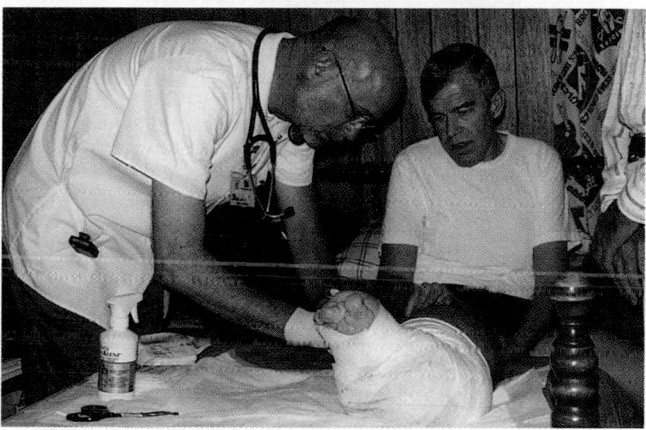

Home health nursing practice is the fastest growing community health nursing role.

fewer hospitalizations, nurses in acute care settings are facing assignments on a daily basis to different units and in diverse settings, including outpatient, home health, and other community-based agencies housed in or associated with their own facility. As the patient census (the number of occupied beds in a hospital on a daily basis) fluctuates, nurses must be flexible, willing, and competent in multiple settings. So, no matter where you ultimately choose to work as a nurse, community health will be an influence on your choice of position, your role, and on your patients' lives. According to Gebbie (1996), the U.S. vision of public health is that of healthy people in healthy communities because individual health can be fully realized only if the community itself is in good shape as well. For a closer look at how much our health is influenced by public health measures, see "Think About This" on page 23.

In this chapter, the history, context, and setting for nursing practice are discussed, as well as some of the current controversies and confusions specific to the new move to the patient's side in the community. So many things influence health: In this century we continue to find out through research how much in the environment, in our own behavior, and in the kind of health care we deliver affects whether we are healthy or ill. Why some people get sick and some people don't has intrigued health care providers for centuries. This chapter introduces health as a concept, presents the historical insights we have learned, and reveals what we can expect nursing and health care to look like in this new millennium.

Sometimes the ways in which we use terms can confuse and obscure the focus of community and public health nurs-

### ❝ *a conversation with . . .* ❞

**Professor Martha Rogers**

Nursing's story is a magnificent epic of service to mankind. It is about people: how they are born, and live and die; in health and in sickness; in joy and in sorrow. Its mission is the translation of knowledge into human service.

Nursing is compassionate concern for human beings. It is the heart that understands and the hand that soothes. It is the intellect that synthesizes many learnings into meaningful administrations.

For students of nursing, the future is a rich repository of far-flung opportunities around this planet and toward the further reaches of man's explorations of new worlds and new ideas. Theirs is the promise of deep satisfaction in a field long dedicated to serving the health needs of people.

—Martha Rogers, PhD
The Education Violet, June 1966,
New York University

ing. In this chapter the terms related to community, population, and nursing roles are discussed in the context of health care delivery. The ways in which a population's health is determined are introduced as well as concepts related to disease and illness prevention and health promotion.

The term *community health nursing* will be used throughout this text to represent care directed toward improving the health of communities and population groups.

❝*It is cheaper to promote health than to maintain people in sickness.*❞

—*Florence Nightingale, 1894*

## A Closer Look at Health

Before we can talk in more detail about the U.S. health care system and nursing roles in today's health care arena, we need an understanding of what health is. That seems simple; after all, everyone knows what health is. However, there are many definitions and descriptions of health depending on one's perspective and purpose.

The most well-known and widely cited description of health is the **World Health Organization's (WHO)** definition of **health** as a state of complete physical, mental, and social well-being, and not merely the absence of disease or infirmity (WHO, 1958). When this definition was drafted in 1948, it began a trend that has persisted for more than 50 years to define health more broadly, including social terms in addition to medical terms.

In 1986, the WHO definition of health was expanded to include a community concept of health. WHO now defines health as the extent to which an individual or group is able, on the one hand, to realize aspirations and satisfy needs; and on the other hand, to change or cope with the environment. Health is, therefore, seen as a resource for everyday life, not the objective of living; it is a positive concept emphasizing social and personal resources, as well as physical capacities (WHO, 1986). An individual or community then must be able to attain and use resources effectively and exhibit a resilience when facing change.

Although WHO's definition of health is the most widely accepted, many other definitions also imply a social or community focus. Health has been defined as a purposeful and integrated method of functioning within an environment (Hall & Weaver, 1977, p. 7), and as the common attainment of the highest level of physical, mental, and social well-being consistent with available knowledge and resources at a given time and place (Hanlon & Pickett, 1984). Even Florence Nightingale's definition of health as not only to be well, but also to use well every power that we have, can be used to describe health for both individuals and communities (Nightingale, 1860).

Many social issues surround the concept of health, making it difficult to limit it to only one definition and perspective. Health is defined by the society and culture in which we live. How individuals, families, and communities perceive what health means is often determined by social, cultural, and economic conditions that limit health choices (Kuss, Proulx-Girouard, Lovitt, Katz, & Kennelly, 1997). Put another way, health is highly dependent on where and how we live. A 20-year-old man may consider himself healthy only if he can run up the stairs at work. For an 80-year-old woman, retrieving her own mail at the mailbox may be her idea of health.

> **❝** *[Health is] a way of life, an attitude, an outlook, a history, a context with socio-cultural norms, a belief, and a tradition. Being healthy is managing, negotiating, achieving, growing, becoming, and helping others grow and become. Being and becoming healthy may be parts of a whole perception of health. Becoming healthy is hopefulness, transcending worries, realizing options, advocating, and accessing resources.* **❞**
> —A. L. Meleis, 1996

> **❝** *[Health is] a modus vivendi enabling imperfect men to achieve a rewarding and not too painful existence while they cope with an imperfect world.* **❞**
> —Rene Dubos, 1968

Young Florence Nightingale

Nurses differ in their perception of health and are influenced by their own background, age, and experiences. In a study that explored the perceptions of community health nurses about health, the nurses interviewed described health as an "interactive vision" between nurses and patients (Leipert, 1996). This vision of health varies with each nurse–patient relationship, depending on the values and characteristics of the nurse, the patient, and the setting where the interaction occurs. Some of the characteristics that can greatly affect the vision of health are age, culture, social environment, and economic status. Patients in this context include individuals, families, groups, and communities.

## ■ Historical Insights

Sickness and suffering have always been a part of human existence. As a result, from the beginning there have been men and women who served as caregivers to the sick and injured. Early on, most care was provided by family members. As human society evolved, moral consciousness became formalized into religious codes, and religious groups assumed more responsibility for the ill. Although their efforts were commendable, they were limited because so little was known about disease causation or prevention. In Chapter 3, we explore the history of community and public health more fully.

**Florence Nightingale** is recognized as the founder of modern professional nursing, as well as for developing the first school of nursing at London's St. Thomas Hospital in 1860. Although her initial efforts focused on preparing nurses to care for the sick in hospitals and infirmaries, she continued throughout her life to promote well nursing in the community. Nightingale's directive was to manipulate the patient's environment to allow nature to take its course in the healing process.

Through scientific inquiry during the nineteenth century, causes of the devastating communicable diseases of these earlier centuries began to emerge and professional intervention became possible. During the mid- to late 1800s, public health measures were established as the process of contagion between human hosts and the environment became better understood.

Throughout the twentieth century, medical science grew in leaps and bounds, and the manipulation of nature became the drive that resulted in significant medical discoveries and inventions. The United States experienced unprecedented growth in technology and medical science in this century. We learned more about the causes of diseases and generated a broad knowledge base about disease and injury detection, treatment, and prevention. The resulting health care system, which early on was divided into public and private sectors, focused on the diagnosis and treatment of disease in the highly specialized and centralized setting of the hospital. For most individuals, health care was synonymous with the local hospital.

During the twentieth century, most nurses were employed in hospital settings as skilled caregivers for the acutely ill; nursing education was mostly focused on care of the sick. Nursing students gained experience almost exclusively in hospitals.

Nevertheless, even as the United States was credited worldwide with having the most advanced health technology for treating disease, and while health care spending vastly increased during the 1960s and 1970s, health professionals and the public increasingly expressed a growing concern that the health care needs of all citizens were not being met. As the twentieth century came to a close, we came to realize that as a society our obligation is to provide an environment in which achievement of good health for all is not only possible but expected. Yet there are population groups—such as the homeless, the elderly, and the poor—whose illness and death rates exceed those of the general population and may require additional resources to achieve good health.

Health care costs in the United States already amount to more than 14% of the gross domestic product (GDP), more than twice that of other countries that can boast better health statistics. Americans would probably be willing to live with the high price tag of health care if it made us all healthier than people in other countries. However, that is not the case. In the United States, where the health care system is heralded as the most sophisticated in the world, when compared with similar countries such as the United Kingdom, Germany, or France, we are lagging behind:

- The United States has high infant mortality rates relative to other highly developed industrialized nations.
- The United States ranks twenty-fifth in the world in life expectancy, behind Japan, Italy, France, and the Scandinavian countries.
- At least one third of the U.S. population has limited access to basic health services and one third of the uninsured are children.
- The United States is the only industrialized nation in the world without guaranteed access to basic health care services.

> **"**It is from quiet places like this all over the world that the forces accumulate which presently will overbear any attempt to accomplish evil on a large scale. Like the rivulets gathering into the river, and the river into the seas, there come from communities like this streams that fertilize the consciences of men, and it is the conscience of the world that we are trying to place upon the throne which others would usurp.**"**
>
> —U.S. President Woodrow Wilson, address in Carlisle, England, December 29, 1918

> **"**The awareness that health is dependent upon habits that we control makes us the first generation in history that to a large extent determines its own destiny.**"**
>
> —U.S. President Jimmy Carter

Much must be done in this country for many to achieve levels of health that are acceptable and equitable. Many deaths and disabilities could be reduced by environmental improvements and lifestyle changes. One hundred years ago, most deaths were caused by infectious diseases; today, the leading causes of death are related to societal influences, lifestyle, and behavioral choices. Progress in technology, while making our everyday lives easier and safer, has created environmental threats to our air, water, products, and food. Health problems such as addiction and violence have emerged as serious threats to our well-being and even survival. As Keck contends, "Good health cannot be achieved without a social concern for ethical, humane decision-making . . . a just and caring society does not withhold health care from its citizens; sickness, after all, is never something people deserve" (1994, p. 4).

Beyond looking at our own country's struggle with internal decisions about health care delivery and connecting it with the broader determinants of health, there has been a concurrent recognition of the global connectedness and importance of concerns for health. The achievement of world health has increasingly become a global expectation. Although nurses are still needed as skilled caregivers who improve the health of individual patients, a broader perspective has evolved as population health interventions are realized to be at least equally, if not more significant, in the attainment of health for all. Solutions to the health problems of populations worldwide now exceed the resources and control of any one individual (McKenzie & Pinger, 1997; Gostin, 2004).

## Nursing in the Twenty-First Century

Hospitals in the early part of the new millennium are relinquishing their role as the recognized hub of care delivery, while delivery of health care services at home, at work, at play, in schools and churches, online with the World Wide Web through the Internet, and on the telephone continues to increase. Who delivers health care, what is provided, and when and where patients are seen have changed. Trends related to cost containment, managed care systems, technology, societal expectations, and politics have all influenced these changes. Patients stay less often in the hospital, and when they do, they stay for fewer days. Patients are generally sicker both when they are admitted and when they are discharged than they have been in the past. There has not been a significant decrease in patient numbers, but rather the settings for care have changed; with this shift, population health issues have become more of a focus.

There are greater demands on the health care system now than ever before, including evidence-based practice, as health care becomes more focused on efficiency and quality in patient care (Ferguson & Day, 2007). Nurses, as the translators and caregivers for patients with more complex needs, are needed more than ever. Nurses, as always, continue to meet the needs of patients; we move to care for populations in whatever setting they are found.

### Got an Alternative?

Research indicates that at least 62% of the U.S. public uses some form of nontraditional or alternative medicine—yet few patients mention such measures when visiting their healthcare providers. Why do you think people are reluctant to share their use and interest in alternative health practices with nurses and physicians?

*Source*: Barnes, P. M., Powell-Griner, E., McFann, K., & Nahin, R. L. (2004). Complementary and alternative medicine use among adults: United States, 2002. *Advance Data, 343*, 1–19.

In a study conducted by the American Nurses Association's (ANA) Department of Labor Relations and Workplace Advocacy, nurse executives from acute, home health, extended, and managed care settings reported on the skills seen as most important for the next generation of nurses. According to this study, nurses should possess skills of self-reliance, independence, flexibility, and decision making, as well as a systems-thinking approach to health care, patient education, critical thinking skills, and computer skills. The conclusion of the study was that nurses need to be prepared to provide the four rights of nursing practice: give the *right* care, in the *right* setting, at the *right* time, and at the *right* cost (Canavan, 1996).

Trossman, in *American Nurse*, stated that "Hospitals will still be a major place of employment for nurses. The type of work will slowly change, though, as these hospitals become the care zones for the nation's oldest and sickest individuals. At the same time, other settings, such as home health and community based care, will provide increased opportunities for R.N.s" (1998, p. 1).

❝ *What life have you if you have not life together? . . .*

*There is no life that is not in community.* ❞

—T. S. Eliot

### ■ Educating Nurses for Community Health Nursing Practice

The *Essentials of Baccalaureate Nursing Education for Entry Level Community/Public Health Nursing Practice*, a document endorsed by the Association of Community Health Nursing Educators (ACHNE) in 2000, provides recommendations regarding the baccalaureate educational content essential for entry level in community health nursing practice. ACHNE is the only organization that represents community health nurse educators throughout the United States and many other parts of the world. For nursing to survive as a profession, ACHNE recognizes that nursing must evolve along with the changing health care system. Nursing of the future will practice in a more complex health care system that involves both care of individuals outside of acute care and traditional hospital settings (community-based care) and care of populations (community-focused care). Details of the *Essentials* can be found in the appendix at the end of this chapter. This text uses the ACHNE document as the basis for its content and organization (ACHNE, 2000).

One of the most intriguing and challenging aspects of the health problems that we face in the twenty-first century is that we already know about effective interventions for many diseases and conditions in our society. According to Salmon and Vanderbush (1990), never before have we known as much about health as we do now; what we don't know is how to put this knowledge into action (p. 192).

## Community-Based, Population-Focused, Community Health Nursing: What's in a Name?

What does it mean that health care is moving to the community? Why are there so many terms to describe nurses who work with a community focus? Much of the confusion over the title of a nurse who focuses on prevention in non-acute populations reflects the diversity that has created new roles for nurses in the community. Both the terms *public health nursing* and *community health nursing* are used to describe a nurse who works with populations and toward goals associated with improving the health of communities, families, and individuals. The primary difference may mean little to you as a student nurse at this point. Community health nursing has been the accepted title for the past few decades. In recent years, public health nursing has reemerged as an accepted title for nurses who work with the entire public, not just in an official public health agency, to improve the health of populations. Various groups representing all community and public health nurses in the United States through the Quad Council of Public Health Nursing Organizations continue to debate the appropriate title for the nurse who works with a community focus (American Nurses Association (ANA), 2007; American Public Health Association, 1996; Association of Community Health Nurse Educators, 2000). The term *community health nursing* will be used throughout this text.

### ⌨ Research Alert

Aspirin does not protect women against heart attacks in the same way it does men, but the venerable painkiller does cut women's chances of suffering a stroke, researchers reported yesterday.

A long-awaited, 10-year study of nearly 40,000 women, the biggest and best such study to date, provides healthy women with the first authoritative assessment of the benefits of taking regular aspirin, a practice many have already begun based largely on studies of men.

The study found that aspirin does not reduce the risk of a first heart attack for middle-aged women, as it does for men, but does cut the risk of strokes, which is not the case for women. For women 65 and older, aspirin does lower the chances of having a heart attack, and its stroke-preventing benefits appear to be the greatest.

The findings suggest the benefits of aspirin may not outweigh the risks for healthy women in their forties and fifties, but once they hit their sixties the balance shifts enough to make it worthwhile. Aspirin's major risk is of bleeding, which can cause serious problems including rare but deadly bleeding strokes. Women with high blood pressure and problems with stomach bleeding may be at particular risk.

"The bottom line is that for younger women it's not clear that there would be an overall benefit," said Julie Buring of the Brigham and Women's Hospital in Boston, who led the study. "But for those age 65 and older, that's where we may see it being useful."

The results also add powerful new evidence to the growing body of data showing that men and women differ in fundamental ways on various aspects of health, and that research on men does not necessarily translate directly to women.

"This truly underscores the importance of studying medical therapies among women as well as men," said Buring, whose findings were released early by the *New England Journal of Medicine* to coincide with a presentation at an American College of Cardiology meeting in Orlando. "We can't assume studies involving men apply to women."

It remains unclear why women respond differently, although some researchers have speculated that it may be due to hormonal differences or the fact that women tend to develop heart disease later in life.

"Age 50 in men is biologically about age 60 in women in terms of their risk of cardiovascular disease," Buring said.

Aspirin, an ancient medicine known for a century mainly as a way to alleviate headaches and fevers, became a key player in the fight against cardiovascular disease—the nation's leading killer—after doctors discovered its powers to prevent and help dissolve blood clots and reduce inflammation.

Previous research has clearly demonstrated that aspirin can help stop heart attacks as they are happening in both men and women by dissolving blood clots blocking blood flow to the heart muscle. Also, men and women who have already had a heart attack can sharply cut their chances of having another by taking low doses of aspirin regularly.

But the value of having healthy people take low doses of aspirin on a regular basis to prevent a first heart attack has been less clear. Five studies have indicated it may have that effect, prompting aspirin makers to begin promoting that use and many men and women to start taking it. Very few women were involved in those studies, however, raising concerns that many women could be needlessly exposing themselves to the drug's risks.

"We know millions of people take aspirin thinking it will prevent them from having a heart attack," said Scott M. Grundy of the University of Texas Southwestern Medical Center in Dallas. "But there are risks, and there might be a huge number of women who might be taking aspirin who shouldn't be, because the risks may outweigh the benefit. We just hadn't had the data."

In the new, federally funded Women's Health Study, about half of a group of 39,876 women age 45 and older took 100 milligrams of aspirin every other day, while the other half took a placebo. After 10 years, the researchers found that aspirin did not reduce the overall risk of heart attacks. But aspirin did reduce by 17% the overall risk of strokes, which tend to strike women more than men, and cut the risk for the most common type of strokes by 24%.

When the researchers did a separate analysis of women 65 and older, however, they found that those taking aspirin were 34% less likely to suffer heart attacks, and that the protection against strokes increased as well.

Other researchers said the findings represent a watershed.

"This is the definitive trial that we've been waiting for," said Lori Mosca, a women's heart expert at Columbia University. "This answers a big question about whether healthy women have benefits from taking low-dose aspirin."

Mosca and other experts emphasized that the potential risks of aspirin can be significant, particularly for women, making it especially crucial that they consult their doctors. In the study, women taking aspirin did suffer from more bleeding strokes.

"This is exactly the type of study that doctors need when they are sitting across the desk from a patient trying to decide about the best course of action," said Larry Goldstein of Duke University, speaking for the American Heart Association.

The same study also found that vitamin E does not protect women against heart disease. That finding is the latest in a series of major blows to the theory that the vitamin, an antioxidant, might provide that benefit. ◓

*Source*: Ridker, P. M., Cook, N. R., Lee, I. M., Gordon, D., Gaziano, J. M., Manson, J. E., et al. (2005). A randomized trial of low-dose aspirin in the primary prevention of cardiovascular disease in women. *New England Journal of Medicine, 552*(13), 1293–1304.

### ■ Communities and Populations

When we think of the word "community," we may have many pictures in our mind, because the word has a variety of meanings. Andy Griffith lived in the community of Mayberry, and Mr. Rogers' neighborhood is also a community. Most television situation comedies revolve around a community, such as the television shows *Seinfeld*, *Friends*, *Sesame Street*, or even *The Simpsons* and *South Park*. In this text, the word **community** is defined as a group of people who share something in common and interact with one another, who may exhibit a commitment with one another and may share a geographic boundary. A **population** is defined as a group of people who have at least one thing in common and who may or may not interact with one another. See Box 1-2.

Examples of communities include the following:

- Lesbians in a communal living setting
- The town of Golden, Colorado
- The faculty at Florida State University School of Nursing
- The Devil's Own neighborhood urban gang
- Sunshine Heights Retirement Village
- Elders with disabilities living in urban high-rise apartments

Examples of populations include the following:

- Teens who remain sexually abstinent
- Sexually active teenagers
- Nurses who work the night shift
- Female long-distance runners
- Teenagers with Down syndrome
- First-time mothers older than age 35
- People who use cell phones while driving

According to Schultz (1994), *interaction* is essential in a community, whereas members of a population may or may not interact with one another. To put it another way, communities are usually aware of their "communityness," which binds them into a collective entity and to which they give a name (Cottrell, 1976, pp. 114–115). Some populations evolve into communities over time. Elderly persons who participate in a water aerobics class, for example, may develop into a cohesive community of older women who share other common activities and interests.

❝*Small communities grow great through harmony, great ones fall to pieces through discord.*❞

—*Gaius Sallustius Crispus (c. 86–35/34 B.C.), Roman historian*

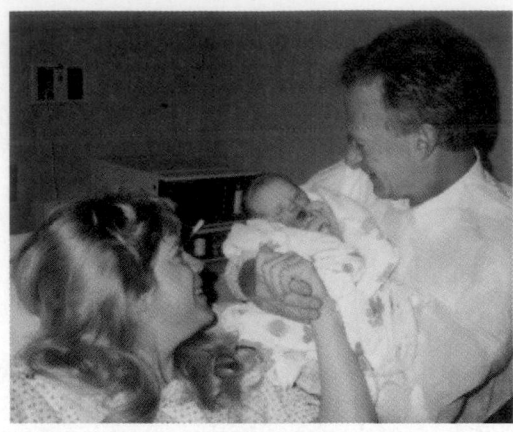

"The true sense of community lies in understanding our interconnectedness and acting from a sense of relatedness. It is a challenge. Let's begin at the beginning. That is where we can start to reweave the sacred web of life so that it once again becomes whole."—Suzanne Arms

The average life span of Americans increased from 45 years to 75 years during the twentieth century, but it is interesting to note that only five of those years are attributable to individual preventive or curative interventions such as cardiac surgery. Twenty-five of the additional years of life expectancy have resulted from public health efforts to provide for safe water, effective waste disposal, adequate housing, and other improvements in the overall health of communities (Bunker, Frazier, & Mosteller, 1994; CDC, 2002).

There are many ways in which nurses are moving into new settings and expanding their application of community health nursing skills. Although these nurses are bringing expertise of acute care and technology to community settings, they are often lacking in their knowledge of community dynamics and public health concepts (Gebbie, 1996). If nurses are to continue to be a dynamic part of health care in the future, we must be able to understand the complex and community-focused nature of health promotion, illness prevention, recovery from illness and injury, and health restoration (Kurtzman et al., 1980). We need to expand our knowledge and expertise in the care of individuals and our skills in hospital-based clinical management of illness and injury to include care of individuals in community settings (Hall & Stevens, 1995; Keller et al., 2004). By using our expert knowledge and experience in medical–surgical, maternal–child, and psychiatric nursing, we can assist individuals, families, and groups to make choices that promote health and wellness (Smith, 1995).

❝*Measures to improve public health, relating as they do to such obvious and mundane matters as housing, smoking, and food, may lack the glamour of high-technology medicine, but what they lack in excitement they gain in their potential impact on health, precisely because they deal with the major causes of common disease and disabilities.*❞

—*Geoffrey Rose, 1992*

---

**BOX 1-2**

**Terms to Know**

A **community** is a group of people who share something in common and interact with one another, who may exhibit a commitment with one another, and who may share a geographic boundary.

A **population** is a group of people who have at least one thing in common and who may or may not interact with one another.

## ■ Acute Care Versus Community Health Nursing

Let's compare acute care and community health nursing to more fully understand how these nursing roles differ both in setting and practice focus. In the acute care setting, there is the issue of provider control. Patients are well aware of who is in control in the hospital setting—the health care professional. The patient is in a subordinate position to the nurse, who remains the ultimate authority regarding when to go to sleep, what to wear, when and how much to urinate, what kind of diet to eat and when, and whether visitors are allowed. Treatments and interventions are done to the patient and scheduled at staff and hospital convenience. Patients, who are often identified by their condition (e.g., "the gallbladder in room 214"), are isolated from friends, family, and pets, who are excluded from the health care setting. Little individualized care that takes into consideration the patient's lifestyle and preferences is given. When a person changes into a hospital gown, the role of patient is assumed. Personal items such as medications, glasses, and false teeth are often relinquished, and self-care is limited, with permission often required from nurses for activities taken for granted at home. Many questions are asked, sometimes over and over by different health professionals, and most often these questions are of a very personal and intimate nature. Rarely does the patient receive any explanation for why information is needed, for to question is to risk being labeled a "difficult" patient—and we know what that means (Armentrout, 1998)! Refer to Table 1-1 for differences in nursing interventions by setting.

The controlled environment of the acute care setting, however, has many benefits for the nurse:

- Predictable routine
- Maintenance of hospital policy
- Predictability of nursing and medical goals
- Resource availability, both human and material
- Collegial collaboration and consultation
- Controlled patient compliance with the plan of care: the patient takes correct medicine and treatment on time
- Standardization of care

The community setting is very different from acute care, especially in regard to the nurse–patient relationship. Nurses tend to be dependent on patients' willingness to share health information and to adhere to the plan of care, and patients on their own turf act very differently than they do in the acute care setting. A significant advantage is that the nurse is able to assess environmental conditions, food and other

Community nurses work with patients in their homes to improve health. For many elders, pets are considered family.

critical resources, lifestyle influences, and the social support system, such as friends, family, and pets. Transportation issues, which may affect the ability to adhere to medical and nursing goals, often become overriding concerns that are not even considered in the hospital setting.

In a community-based setting such as a school clinic, the nurse is dependent on the child's willingness to share information about his or her health concerns and the teacher regarding any relevant learning issues that may affect the child's health. Educational goals are the primary concerns of the school, and the nurse must consider health in this total context.

The lack of colleagues to consult about problems and challenges encountered in community settings is often a cause of stress among new graduates and nurses who have

| Table 1-1 | Differences in Nursing Interventions by Setting | |
| --- | --- | --- |
| **Health Problem** | **Acute Care Setting: Hospital** | **Community-Based Setting: Home Health** |
| ■ Osteoporosis resulting in degenerative hip disease | ■ Treatment<br>■ Surgery and recovery (total hip replacement) | ■ Teach patient how to walk after surgery.<br>■ Involve family with encouraging activity and flexibility exercises. |

never worked outside the controlled environment of the hospital and acute care settings (Armentrout, 1998).

Benefits for the community-based patient include the following:

- Familiar and comfortable environment
- Routine that is less determined by the nurse or health professional
- Diverse resources, including friends, family, and pets, available for support and comfort
- Autonomy and choice in health decisions

## Reform and the Reinvention of Systems of Care

Our health care system is but one of the many overlapping and interacting systems created by society. Societies create systems that reflect the commonly held values of that society. This is the realm of policy, politics, and power. For example, since September 11, 2001, and the terrorists' attacks on the United States, U.S. priorities have changed dramatically regarding safety and well-being. Bioterrorism and threats such as anthrax require public officials to use resources previously earmarked for other health priorities. Nurses have functioned in situations with increased stress, coping with the effects of national diseases themselves while still helping others deal with the ongoing trauma of a post–September 11 world (Davidhizar, Eshleman, & Wolff, 2003).

Health care reform initiatives have arisen in this realm of competing and conflicting values. Groups that advocate values related to protection, well-being, sustenance, quality of life, equity, fairness, and justice must often compete with other values related to economic self-interest. Even when values do not seem to be in conflict, the methods recommended to act on those values often cannot be agreed upon.

The capitalistic values of the health care delivery system in the United States have also been questioned by health care leaders and policy makers in other countries (Moon, 1993; Morse, 2003). They often do not understand how the United States can consider itself a highly industrialized and civilized country and not provide basic, essential health care for all. A caring society would not allow individuals (especially children) to be deprived of health care. Many find our nonsystems approach to health care confusing. In a post–September 11 world, these chaotic times require even more thoughtful and prioritized planning to meet critical population health needs of the most vulnerable groups in our society (Gustin, Boufford, & Martinez, 2004; Morse, 2003).

Indeed, few Americans would not argue that, although the health–illness system has changed, it still needs improvement. Many of the authors throughout this text make reference to **health care reform**. Enacted reforms, proposed reforms, and preferred reforms all have actual and possible effects on the populations for which nurses provide care and the conditions under which they provide it. Reform is not new, nor is it controlled; rather, it is episodic, responding to multiple forces for change. Reform implies some major change in the process of the delivery of health care. We often refer to reform as change that originates at the national level but is implemented by the states, by payers, or by provider systems. When change is not a "broad" and "sweeping" reform, it is considered an "incremental change," meaning smaller adjustments occur over time. This is the type of health care reform that occurred during the 1990s.

Historically, there have been numerous reform proposals. Major health care reform was attempted following World War II—in 1948, President Harry Truman proposed national health insurance. What many thought were the beginnings of broad health coverage were introduced in the 1960s as Medicaid and Medicare. In the 1970s, Senator Edward Kennedy (D-Massachusetts) was one of the major supporters of nationwide reform. Most recently, the presidential campaign of 2008 was marked by health reform issues.

Despite various proposals from both political parties, no reform initiatives have been passed. Even though there was initial support from diverse stakeholders, many of these stakeholders—such as businesses, physicians, and insurance companies—eventually opposed the reform approaches. In addition, the public was confused and did not recognize the cost and choice consequences to individuals (Starr, 1993; IOM, 2003).

### ■ Nursing's Agenda for Health Care Reform

The failed effort of the 1990s to redesign the U.S. health care system had at least one positive consequence for nursing. In an unprecedented collaboration, more than 75 nursing associations endorsed the document jointly developed by the ANA and the NLN, *Nursing's Agenda for Health Care Reform.* This document was significant in terms of its expression of nursing's values and in furthering an understanding of the profession itself. Values such as health services for all, illness prevention, and wellness were identified as prominent concerns. Many nurses played influential and visible roles during the health care reform attempts. Nursing supported the need for cost containment but wanted assurance of quality of care, reduced barriers to advanced practice nursing, and promotion of nursing care as the link between consumers and the health care system. According to the document, "the cornerstone of nursing's plan for reform is the delivery of primary health care services to households and individuals in convenient, familiar places" (ANA, 1991, p. 9).

### ■ Managed Care and the Future of Nursing

Although major health care reform proposals are still debated, significant change at the national level is unlikely in the near future. The controversial issues most debated are expanding federal coverage (access), controlling costs, and the move to evidence-based practice. Evidence-based practice directs care through verifiable research (Ferguson & Day, 2007). Many policy and regulation changes, however, have had a significant impact on health care delivery systems and providers. **"Managed care"** and a market approach based on "managed competition" have emerged as major strategies to control costs in the United States. These connected strategies have together transformed the organization and methods of care delivery.

**Care management** is a growing practice arena for nurses. Within the managed care environment, care management attempts to provide more timely and coordinated care for individuals. Individuals move among the following possible states: being well and promoting that state, having acute care needs, needing outpatient surgery, needing follow-up home care, and so on (ANA, 1994).

Health care organizations now see the economic and quality outcome benefits of caring for patients and managing patient care over a continuum of possible settings and needs. Traditional health care was episodic, with individuals moving with little connection from one episode of need to the next (often waiting until the need for care was acute) and one facility to another. When care is managed, the term "discharge planning" is now more accurately referred to as "transition planning" (Ferguson & Day, 2007). The patient does not leave the system, but merely requires another type of care, including wellness care or health promotion. Patients are followed much more closely both during illness care and with follow-up when well. Care managers can practice from a base in many settings, including the offices of a payer. To more clearly conceptualize this change in thinking, instead of a patient being discharged from the hospital, he or she is described as being admitted *back* to the community.

When the health care providers in a system have the responsibility for all types of care for the plan's enrolled population, they have a financial incentive to coordinate or manage that care efficiently. The goal is to provide the best value in the most efficient way to be competitive in the health care market. A market economy for health care delivery dramatically changes health care services and incentives. For nurses who are historically committed to doing whatever it takes for their patients, cost-consciousness is an unfamiliar and often resisted viewpoint.

---

👆 THINK ABOUT THIS ·····················

In the case of heart transplantation, people typically focus on the dramatic stitching in of a transplanted heart as the "breakthrough." Few notice that the intensive medical and nursing follow-up—solving the day-to-day problems of living with a transplanted organ, treating sores in the mouth due to immunosuppression, coping with a new hormonal milieu, promptly recognizing and responding to infection and rejection—were all caring "breakthroughs" that led to the eventual success of heart transplantation. These essential day-to-day nursing care issues had to be solved in order to make heart transplantation a viable therapy. Yet they are all but overlooked in the scientific and popular media coverage of the transplant story.

—Benner and Wrubel, *The Primacy of Caring*, 1989

---

Nurses in today's health care system must remain informed about the complexities of managed care if they are to sustain their professional identity and to assist patients in navigating this market system. The continued growth of managed care as a system for health financing and delivery provides unique challenges and opportunities for nurses, especially those prepared in community health. Nurses remain the only health care professionals who are specifically educated to assess health status and risks, unhealthy lifestyles, and health education needs for patients and families; who provide support and reassurance while caring for present and potential health problems; and who act as advocates for primary and preventive care services. Managed care organizations, as well as all agencies that provide health care services in a managed care environment, have come to value quality and recognize the importance of prevention, wellness, and early intervention. The community health nurse is especially well prepared to provide managed care with the direction needed to focus on providing a full range of quality, cost-effective services in the promotion of a population's health (ANA, 1994).

❝ *Money would be better spent in maintaining health in infancy and childhood than in building hospitals to cure diseases.* ❞

—Florence Nightingale, 1894

······················································

## Back to the Future: From Hospital to Community, from Cure to Prevention

As we have learned from the history of health care, early attempts to improve health, treat disease, and prevent disability occurred primarily in the home. The primary characteristic of the emerging system has been the move back to the community practice setting. Perhaps the major force behind much of the change has been economic, with efforts to contain what many see as the exploding costs of the U.S. health care system. One cost-related factor encouraging a community focus has been the movement of patients out of expensive acute care facilities and into community settings, where many of their illness needs can be adequately met at a much lower cost. This movement has encouraged the growth of home care, hospice care, outpatient treatment clinics, and outpatient surgeries. Another among the many results of cost-containment efforts has been the recognition of the connection between prevention and keeping populations healthy. Healthy populations have lower morbidity (disease rates) and mortality (death rates) statistics.

❝ *My view, you know, is that the ultimate destination of all nursing is the nursing of the sick in their own homes. . . . I look to the abolition of all hospitals and workhouse infirmaries. But no use to talk about the year 2000.* ❞

—Florence Nightingale, 1867

Opening Doors. While the majority of RNs still work in hospitals, the number of them working in community-based settings continues to grow.

## ■ Home Health Care

**Home health care** is the fastest-growing community-based nursing role outside of the acute care setting. It is just one of many roles available in community health and is covered in depth in various chapters of this book. Home health nursing is an example of an emerging role that has resulted from changes in the way health care is delivered and paid for.

One attempt at major health care cost containment in the early 1980s was the shift from cost reimbursement to prospective payment for hospital care, which means that payment is based on standard disease categories. Because of this change, hospitals could make money if they were efficient in taking care of patients' problems and could discharge them more quickly. Home health boomed as patients were discharged while still needing nursing care in their homes. Even with recent government attempts to regulate the growth of home health by changing reimbursement patterns, home health continues to grow and present new and challenging opportunities for nursing (Trossman, 1998).

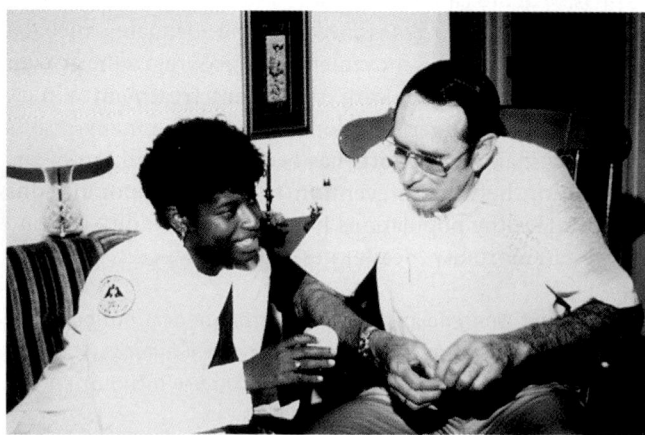

Home health nurses deliver care in the patient's home. A goal of home care is to teach patients and their families self-care.

## ❝ *a conversation with . . .* ❞

### Melanie C. Dreher

I am more convinced than ever that the major health problems in this and future decades—chronicity, aging, the personal and public health problems generated by social and economic dislocations, the prevention of illness, and the promotion of healthy communities—are all within the nursing genius to address and ameliorate. These are the very things that we are known for. They are the things we do best and we are the best to do them. . . . I truly believe that we are at a place in nursing that we will never see again. This is our big chance. . . . We cannot wait for anybody to let us do anything. . . . We have more capacity to play in the health care game, we have the obligation to take charge, to endorse professional values and improve health outcomes.

—Melanie C. Dreher, PhD, RN, FAAN, Past President of Sigma Theta Tau International, December 6, 1997, Indianapolis, Indiana; cited in *Reflections* (1998), first quarter, pp. 36–37

## ■ Cure and Prevention: Can We Really Do It All?

Most people—even nurses—spend little time thinking about or planning for their own good health or the community's health. Research tells us that our health is influenced more by our social and biological environment, lifestyle choices, and self-care initiatives than by our inherited traits, yet we continue to pour money into newer and better treatments rather than into learning about what we can do to promote health and prevent illness from the beginning. We are discovering that we have overemphasized cure with a disease-based medical model for health care.

As early as 1977, the Centers for Disease Control and Prevention (CDC) reported an analysis of the proportional contributions to mortality in the United States of four health field elements: lifestyle, human biology, environment, and health care. Its conclusions were that approximately 50% of premature mortality in the United States is due to lifestyle, 20% to human biology, 20% to environment, and only 10% to inadequacies in health care. Seventy percent of the potential for reducing premature mortality lies in the areas of health promotion and disease prevention, but only about 3.5% of the health care dollar is spent in those areas. Therefore, although the health status of a population is related more to the determinants of health than it is to the causes of disease, we have developed a system that pays for illness care rather than a system designed to create the healthiest population possible.

❝*What we have to do . . . is to find a way to celebrate our diversity and debate our differences without fracturing our communities.*❞

—*Hillary Rodham Clinton*

Certainly, access to competent and skilled health practitioners and technologies related to the diagnosis and treatment of disease is important, but no more so than having clean water to drink, safe food to eat, meaningful and safe employment with an adequate wage, adequate housing and child care, a good education, a life free of discrimination, and a safe environment. Such insights are leading to a "reinvention" of health services organizations at all levels—from single facilities organized to serve sick patients to complex networks organized to serve populations of mostly well people (Shortell & Gilles, 1995).

Prevention activities and population-focused care are often contrasted with the more immediately gratifying and exciting acute care. Community-focused care is long term, often behind the scenes, taken for granted, and largely unseen unless something goes amiss. Nurses have always promoted the welfare and health of those in their care. Wolf (1989) contends that nursing has difficulty being visible because much of the work of nursing goes unnoticed. Health care reform and the move to health promotion and illness prevention may provide the opportunity for nursing to shine as a profession.

Despite the excitement of acute care, many economic, social, and political factors suggest that the future focus of health care should be on health promotion and disease prevention in a health-based model with a community orientation (Procnca, 1998). These areas and such networking have traditionally been the domain of the less visible and less financially supported practice of public health. Mechanic (1998) has pointed out that an alignment of public health with the growing managed care health plans would be a logical and potential benefit to the mission of the U.S. public health system. The vision of public health for more than a century has been one of health promotion and disease prevention that depends on a community perspective to activate identification of risks and protective and restorative interventions.

Healthcare providers in managed care plans are increasingly subject to competition and are evaluated on their successes in improving outcomes for their plan's enrollees. They have become more interested in the population activities and methods long carried out by public health. Acknowledging the economic value of population health promotion and disease prevention activities within the health care marketplace encourages the adoption of these approaches. Thus, for many nurses caring for individuals, the focus on community health nursing roles represents a transition to the community in practice setting.

Nurses have been optimistic about the trends in health care practice and reform. With the increasing impetus for health promotion, nurses seem well poised as a result of their longstanding commitment to and expertise in keeping people healthy. In the past, when nurses have made claims about the benefits of health promotion and disease prevention strategies, the thoughts have been on benefits to the individual, not on any financial benefit or loss. Now we as nurses are beginning to embrace the possibilities of teaming up with a market-driven business world to also realize financial benefits and improved health for populations.

## ■ Benefits Versus Costs

Anderson (1997) cautions against a naive understanding of what we take for granted. Indeed, she describes the case of smoking cessation programs, which have been proven to have economic benefits. However, a potential financial loss scenario is possible for preventing cardiopulmonary disease in middle-aged individuals. Prevention may actually increase managed care costs by prolonging a person's life and thus incurring greater costs for the complex medical problems of old age. Similarly, early detection of HIV in at-risk populations should permit early drug treatment to prevent costly AIDS-related illnesses. For a managed care organization, early detection would imply antiviral treatment costing thousands of dollars annually. Nondetection and an early death would actually save money for a private health care provider and increase its profits. Nurses are socialized to value life; health care companies are in business to make a profit first.

### 💻 Research Alert

Research has shown that children wearing Heelys sustain the same types of injuries as those wearing inline skates or riding skateboards or scooters. According to Vincent Iannelli, MD, two recent medical studies reported that children wearing Heelys had injuries ranging from "distal radius fractures and elbow injuries to a head injury that required surgery."

Although the manufacturer recommends wearing safety gear such as a helmet, wrist guards, and knee pads, very few children wear safety gear with Heelys. To prevent injuries, children should wear safety gear, remove the wheels when using Heelys in shoe mode, and avoid using the Heelys in skate mode in traffic, on stairs, or on uneven surfaces. Children should also avoid crowded areas and rolling faster than they can walk.

Many public places, including schools, ban the use of Heelys in skate mode and require children to take the wheels out of the Heelys before entering. Heelys should not be used in skate mode indoors. Falling into such indoor hazards as a table or display case can cause serious injury.

Parents should also know that W.A.T.C.H (World Against Toys Causing Harm) included Heelys on their "10 worst toys" list.

*Sources:* Iannelli, V., MD. (2007). *Heelys—Staying safe and preventing injuries.* Retrieved October 16, 2008, from http://pediatrics.about.com/od/safety/a/0407_heelys_inj.htm; Lenehan, B., Callendar, A., McIntyre, A., Boran, S., Moore, D., Fogarty, E., & Dowling, F. (2007). Heely injuries: A new epidemic warranting a government health warning! *Injury, 38*(8), 923–925; Oh, D. (2006). Heelys injuries in children. *Singapore Medical Journal, 47*(5), 373–375; Korioth, T. (2007). Heely shoe users: Take heed of risks. *AAP News, 28*(4), 29.

With such dire warnings, nurses must realize the competing values often at work in the health care arena. Community-focused health promotion strategies also can face ideological, political, and religious differences that cause conflict. Much-needed sex education to prevent teenage pregnancy has long met with resistance from some groups. Strategies must be developed at the individual and societal levels to bring about change that aligns with all interested parties' goals and needs.

In the case of smoking cessation, for example, other community groups could be approached to encourage health promotion interventions and policies. Employers could be motivated to realize the financial gain of less employee illness and fewer work days lost. They would then negotiate for managed care plans that cover health promotion activities.

### ■ *Healthy People 2010:* Goals for the Nation

Even before the more recent reform efforts and regulations encouraged increased use of prevention practices, it became obvious in the 1970s, based on the CDC's study of premature deaths, that health promotion and disease prevention could save lives and perhaps reduce health care costs. In 1980, the federal government issued a set of national health objectives that were evaluated to measure progress in U.S. health goals and health care services. The process proved valuable and was repeated with the issuing of a new set of objectives to guide the 1990s. That plan was titled *Healthy People 2000: National Health Promotion and Disease Prevention Objectives.*

The process was again repeated, culminating in the release of a ***Healthy People 2010*** document in October 2000. Two overarching goals—increase years of healthy life and eliminate health disparities—are proposed. Four enabling goals provide support; they are concerned with promoting healthful behaviors, protecting health, achieving access to quality health care, and strengthening community prevention. These objectives provide a tool that the creators envision for public health policy makers and all policy makers at both state and local levels as well. Meeting these objectives requires that all health care providers move toward a community-based practice or focus. That is, providers must move from a focus on illness and cure to a focus on health promotion and illness prevention not only for populations at risk, but also for **populations of interest**—those people who are essentially healthy but whose health status could be improved or protected (Keller et al., 2004).

❝ *Of all the forms of inequality, injustice in health care is the most shocking and inhumane.* ❞

—*Martin Luther King, Jr.*

❝ *Preventable disease should be looked on as a social crime.* ❞

—*Florence Nightingale, 1894*

## HEALTHY PEOPLE 2010

**Promote Healthy Behaviors**
1. Physical activity and fitness
2. Nutrition
3. Tobacco use

**Promote Healthy and Safe Communities**
4. Educational and community-based programs
5. Environmental health
6. Food safety
7. Injury/violence prevention
8. Occupational safety and health
9. Oral health

**Improve Systems for Personal and Public Health**
10. Access to quality health care services
    1. Preventive care
    2. Primary care
    3. Emergency services
    4. Long-term care and rehabilitative services
11. Family planning
12. Maternal, infant, and child health
13. Medical product safety
14. Public health infrastructure
15. Health communication

**Prevent and Reduce Diseases and Disorders**
16. Arthritis, osteoporosis, and chronic back conditions
17. Cancer
18. Diabetes
19. Disability and secondary conditions
20. Heart disease and stroke
21. HIV
22. Immunization and infectious diseases
23. Mental health and mental disorders
24. Respiratory diseases
25. Sexually transmitted diseases
26. Substance abuse

*Source*: DHHS 2000.

### ■ Influences on a Community's Health: Culture, Environment, and Ethics

So many different factors influence health care that it is difficult to decide which are the most important. For the nurse to isolate any one factor for assessment and intervention with both individuals and communities is like the captain of a ship seeing only the tip of the iceberg and not looking for the real threat to the ship's safety that lies underneath. However, three major components of health care are addressed in this first chapter because they have a profound effect on all aspects of patient care: culture, environment, and ethics. The factors are discussed in greater detail in later chapters.

## Culture

The numerous global, social, demographic, economic, and political changes in recent years have alerted health care professionals to the need to provide attention to the increasing diversity in our society and the effect of that diversity on people's health (Meleis, 1996). International travel and advances in communication through the Internet and satellite television make it essential for today's nurses to develop the skills needed to provide care that recognizes complexities and differences among patients (Janes & Hobson, 1998).

The United States is the most culturally diverse nation in the world. In fact, in 1994, *Time* magazine designated the United States the first universal nation (Grossman, 1994). In 2000, almost 30% of Americans were members of ethnic minority groups, including 12.1% African American, 12.5% Hispanic/Latino, and 3.7% Asian/Pacific Islander. In that same year, however, less than 13% of the RN population were members of ethnic minority groups, including 4.9% African American, 2% Hispanic/Latino, and 3.7% Asian/Pacific Islander (Vilschick, 2003). Nursing has traditionally been a female-dominated profession, with male nurses making up only 5.4% of the total number of RNs in the United States. Although this percentage has increased by 226% since 1980 (DHHS, 2000), greater gender diversity should clearly be sought in the nursing profession.

It is clear that nurses must be sensitive to cultural differences to be able to provide the best possible care to individuals, families, and communities. But what, exactly, do we mean by the term "culture"? According to Leininger (1995), **culture** refers to the learned and shared beliefs, values, and lifeways of a designated or particular group that are generally transmitted intergenerationally and influence one's thinking and action modes. Giger and Davidhizar (1995) say that culture is a patterned behavioral response that develops over time as a result of imprinting the mind through social and religious structures and intellectual and artistic manifestations.

Purnell and Paulanka (2003) define culture as the totality of socially transmitted behavioral patterns, art, beliefs, values, customs, lifeways, and all other products of human work and thought characteristics of a population of people that guide their worldview and decision making. Obviously, culture is more than just ethnicity. Culture is language, religion, food, traditions, customs, clothing, and everything that make one group of people unique and distinguish it from other groups. Cultural values, beliefs, and behaviors can also be related to age, gender, sexual orientation, socioeconomic status, and profession. There is a culture of nursing that all nurses belong to, with its own language, values, and traditions, that often clashes with patients whose cultural beliefs about health care differ from those of their nurses.

When considering cultural issues, we need to look beyond the borders of our own country. Those who hold privileged and recognized positions in societies by virtue of specialized expertise, such as nursing, have an obligation to give back to those societies. To make such contributions, nurses should become "global citizens" holding a broad vision of international health. In today's connected world, no profession can be truly effective without interactions and viewpoints that include international perspectives. Community health nurses especially, who by definition practice within a broad systems perspective, must incorporate understandings from international health efforts in their own interventions. Comparing and drawing insights from methods and successes of nurses in delivering care in other countries holds the promise of improving the care to U.S. patients. In addition, there is a need to understand and support collaborating agencies at the international level. Principles of pluralism, consultation, coherence, consensus, compassion, partnership, and cooperation are the hallmarks of nurses who practice and embrace global citizenship (Neufield, 1992). For example, control measures for effectively reducing AIDS have involved the active cooperation of most countries worldwide.

 CULTURAL CONNECTION

After reviewing the section on culture in Chapter 1, why do you think nursing has had difficulty recruiting minorities and males into the profession?

## Environment

The environment has been a concern for nursing since the days of Florence Nightingale. In *Notes on Nursing* (1860), Nightingale emphasizes the fact that recovery from illness can occur only in a bright, clean, well-ventilated environment. She states:

> The very first canon of nursing, the first and the last thing upon which a nurse's attention must be fixed, the first essential to a patient, without which all the rest you can do for him is nothing, with which I had almost said you may leave all the rest alone, is this: TO KEEP THE AIR HE BREATHES AS PURE AS THE EXTERNAL AIR, WITHOUT CHILLING HIM.

When Nightingale spoke of the patient's environment, she meant the room in the hospital or home in which the patient stayed during the course of illness. In more recent years, the public health definition of **environment** has come

 ENVIRONMENTAL CONNECTION

The work we are speaking of has nothing to do with nursing disease, but with maintaining health by removing the things which disturb it . . . dirt, drink, diet, damp, draughts, and drains.

*—Florence Nightingale, 1860*

**How Safe Is Airline Drinking Water?**

The Environmental Protection Agency (EPA) is the federal agency responsible for safe drinking water in communities, in public places, and on airplanes. In the summer and fall of 2004, the EPA tested drinking water aboard hundreds of randomly selected domestic and international passenger aircraft. The summer data showed that 13% of tested aircraft water failed to meet EPA standards; the fall 2004 testing showed that 17% failed the standards. Coliform bacteria, usually harmless, indicate that harmful organisms could be present and were found in unacceptable levels.

In response to these findings, the EPA embarked on a process to tailor the existing regulations for aircraft public water systems. In 2008, the EPA proposed the Aircraft Drinking Water Rule for public review and comment. The EPA will now have domestic airlines test themselves and submit results to the agency to see if the trend continues. Some self-sampling has begun, and airlines are adapting their routine disinfections to meet EPA guidance. Airlines now must disinfect water systems every three months and water carts and hoses leading to aircraft monthly.

Passengers with compromised immune systems should request canned or bottled beverages and avoid drinking coffee, tea, and other drinks prepared with tap water while on board airplanes. In the interim, to further protect the traveling public, the EPA placed 45 air carriers under Administrative Orders on Consent (AOC), which will remain in effect until tailored aircraft drinking water regulations are final. These protocols will protect the public while existing regulations are being reviewed and data are being collected and analyzed from the aircraft drinking water. The air carrier AOCs combine sampling, best management practices, corrective action, public notification, and reporting and recordkeeping.

*Source*: Environmental Protection Agency (EPA). (2008). *Airline water supplies*. Retrieved August 28, 2008, from http://www.epa.gov/safewater/airlinewater

to mean all the surroundings and conditions that affect the health of individuals, families, and communities. The environment has many different components, including social, cultural, political, economic, and ecological factors.

Environmental issues have been in the forefront of many political campaigns during the last few years and seem to be gaining momentum, with many governmental and private community groups supporting legislation to protect the environment. Most of this activity has been focused on the ecological component of environmental health—primarily clean air and water and a safe food supply.

Nurses are beginning to take a more active role in promoting environmental health, reducing environmental health risks, and protecting the earth's resources. In fact,

several nursing organizations, such as the American Holistic Nurses Association and the International Council of Nurses, have developed position statements to delineate the nurse's role in promoting environmental health. A specialty organization called Nurses for Environmental and Social Responsibility has been formed specifically to educate nurses and the public about environmental health hazards.

### Ethics

Since the time of Florence Nightingale, the nursing profession has been addressing **ethics** concerns related to patient care issues. The ANA's (2001) *Code of Ethics for Nurses with Interpretive Statements* provides guidance for ethical decisions made by nurses in the clinical setting.

Ethical dilemmas have traditionally included such issues as informed consent and individual freedom of choice, autonomy, truth telling, protection of privacy and confidentiality, and discrimination. In addition, public health nurses have had to make ethical decisions related to the dual obligation to protect the public's welfare while respecting the rights of individual patients (Folmar, Coughlin, Bessinger, & Sacknoff, 1997).

 ETHICAL CONNECTION

Every community is an association of some kind and every community is established with a view to some good; for everyone always acts in order to obtain that which they think good. But, if all communities aim at some good, the state or political community, which is the highest of all, and which embraces all the rest, aims at good in a greater degree than any other, and at the highest good.

—*Aristotle (384–323 B.C.)*

Public health is concerned with ensuring the safety of the public's "good"—for example, through protection from hazards such as known infectious diseases where the administration of vaccinations ensure population and public protection. Such public interventions often inspire highly politicized legal debates, where the delicate balance between individual rights and freedom of choice is sacrificed for the sake of the community's right to good health. One such debate is over smoking bans in public places versus the right of individual tobacco users to exercise their rights to smoke in restaurants and bars. How do you think Aristotle would respond to such a debate?

**❝***Throughout the 1980s, we did hear too much about individual gain and the ethos of selfishness and greed. We did not hear enough about how to be a good member of a community, to define the common good, and to repair the social contract. And we also found that while prosperity does not trickle down from the most powerful to the rest of us, all too often indifference and even intolerance do.* **❞**

—*Hillary Rodham Clinton, Senator and former First Lady, 1993*

## ☞ THINK ABOUT THIS

The first rays of sunlight peek through your bedroom curtains, accompanied by the fresh air of a new day. You breathe deeply and enjoy the clean air that public health protects by monitoring radiation levels and developing strategies to keep them low.

Rousing the children, you usher them into the bathroom for their showers. You brush your teeth, knowing the water won't make you sick because safe drinking water is the responsibility of public health.

You check your smile in the mirror. You can't remember your last cavity, thanks in part to the fluoride public health helps add to the water. Through similar programs, public health has always sought to promote good health by preventing disease altogether.

The family clambers to the table just as you finish pouring the milk, which is safe to drink because the State Department of Health checks and monitors it from the dairy to the grocery store.

After breakfast, you call your sister, who is pregnant with her first child, and find out her routine doctor's visit went perfectly. Even in the small town where she lives, your sister can visit a local doctor. Public health recognized the need for doctors in rural areas and helped place one there.

Your sister tells you her doctor suggested she visit the county health department and enroll in the Women, Infants, and Children Program, another public health service that ensures children get the proper nutrition to prevent sickness later in life.

You walk outside and guide the children into the car. You buckle their seatbelts without realizing it. Seatbelts have become a habit now, because public health has explained how proper seatbelt use has greatly reduced automobile-related deaths nationwide.

Playmates greet your children at the child care center with yelps of youthful joy. As you watch the children run inside to play, you know they'll stay safe while you're away at work. Public health has licensed the center and made certain the staff knows the proper ways to avoid infectious disease outbreaks that can occur among young children.

And thanks to the immunizations your children have gotten, you know they'll be safe from life-threatening diseases like polio and whooping cough. In fact, public health has eliminated the deadly smallpox virus worldwide, so your children will never catch it. Maybe your children's children won't have to worry about polio or whooping cough.

You arrive at work and find a flyer for a new exercise program tacked to the bulletin board. You decide to sign up, remembering the public health studies that show you can reduce the risks of chronic disease by staying physically active.

The morning goes well, and you feel good because your company became a smoke-free workplace this month. Science shows that tobacco can cause cancer and other ailments in those who use tobacco and among those who breathe second-hand smoke. Public health encourages people and organizations to quit smoking so that all people can live more healthful lives.

Walking to a nearby fast-food restaurant for lunch, you pass a bike rider with a sleek, colorful helmet—another example of a public health message that can influence healthy behaviors. Inside, you order a hamburger and fries.

You notice the food service license signed by the State Health Officer on the wall, and you know the food is sanitary and free of disease-causing organisms. Still, a State Department of Health public service announcement from TV rings in your head, and you make a mental note to order something with a little less cholesterol next time.

You finish your day at work, pick up the kids, and head to the community park to let the children play. You watch the neighborhood children launch a toy sailboat into the park pond, knowing public health protects lakes and streams from dangerous sewage runoff.

At home, your spouse greets you at the door. You sort the mail and discover a letter from your uncle. He's doing fine after his surgery in the hospital and will head back to the nursing home in 2 days. You know he's getting quality care at both facilities because public health monitors and licenses them to ensure a commitment to quality standards. Even the ambulance that transported him to the hospital met public health standards for emergency medical services.

After dinner, you put the children to bed and sit to watch the evening news. The anchor details a new coalition dedicated to preventing breast and cervical cancer. A representative of the State Department of Health issues an open invitation for members from all walks of life. You jot down the telephone number and promise yourself you'll call first thing tomorrow.

As you settle into bed, you decide that public health is more than a point-in-time recognition. Without even realizing it, you'll rely on public health every day for an entire lifetime. ◉

*Source: Mississippi State Department of Health Annual Report (1997), pp. 2–3.*

---

Today's changing health care delivery system brings with it additional ethical dilemmas for nurses. We are now concerned with problems related to equity in health care delivery, environmental safety, politicization of health care interventions, euthanasia, elder abuse in nursing homes, provider–patient relationships, and community partnerships (Graham, 1997). Recent advancements in science and technology are presenting ethical dilemmas that Florence Nightingale could not have envisioned in even her wildest fantasies—for example, physician-assisted suicide, living wills, stem cell research, gene therapy, in vitro fertilization, and human cloning. All nurses would do well to follow Spicer's advice to nursing students in an editorial in *Imprint* (1998): "As you prepare for your careers, remember your professional commitment to place your patient first in all decisions. Take time to establish your ethical boundaries. . . . Base your decisions from your head and your heart."

## Epidemiology: The Science of Public Health

Whether a person is healthy or ill results from numerous constantly changing interacting forces. The actual occurrence of disease results from a triad of factors, referred to as the epidemiological model or triangle. This triad is composed of the host, the agent, and the environment. The *host* is the human body influenced by such variables as gender, age, race, and behavior. The *agent* is a physical, chemical, or biological element that can cause illness or injury. Examples might include tuberculosis bacilli or nicotine. The *environment* is perhaps the most complex component. As we learn more about health and its determinants, the environment holds more and more keys to explaining health risks to our human hosts. The environment not only includes the physical environment, such as climate and terrain, but also the sociocultural–political environment, such as poverty, racism, and other stressors that influence health.

Prevention strategies are made up of measures that protect people from disease and take the form of efforts that we use to protect ourselves and others from specific diseases and conditions and their resulting consequences. There are three levels of prevention: primary, secondary, and tertiary. Nurses in all settings use all three levels of prevention as a basis for practice. The nurse caring for patients in an acute care setting may primarily use secondary and tertiary interventions, whereas the occupational health nurse may use primary and secondary interventions in his or her role. These levels of prevention were originally conceptualized by Leavell and Clark in 1953 and were tied to what these authors described as the natural history of disease. Their assumption was that disease in humans is a process: The conditions that promote either health or disease are present in the human's biological, physical, emotional, and social environments as well as in the human host itself.

The relationship between levels of prevention and the natural history of any given disease condition or health state is the basis for community health interventions. Disease occurs in two stages: pre-pathogenesis and pathogenesis. The intervention strategies or levels of prevention must coincide with predictable events within the stages of pre-pathogenesis (predisease) and pathogenesis (disease, condition, or injury). One can readily see that applying the levels of prevention

 EPIDEMIOLOGY in Practice ——————

The traditional epidemiological triad has focused on infectious disease as agent, human host, and physical environment. In most developed countries, in the past century there has been an epidemiological transition from infectious to chronic disease, such as cardiovascular disease, cancer, diabetes, asthma, and depression, and the environment has broadened to include the social and psychological environment, such as prejudice, racism, and stress. ◯

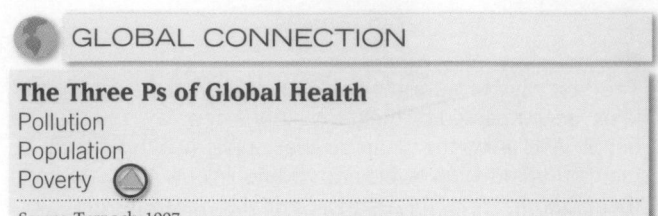

GLOBAL CONNECTION

**The Three Ps of Global Health**
Pollution
Population
Poverty ◯

*Source*: Turnock, 1997.

requires that the nurse know the natural history of a given disease or condition. The less known about the disease or condition, the greater the likelihood of interventions occurring in secondary or tertiary prevention levels. In other words, the more we learn about disease, disability, and injury, the earlier we can intervene to prevent the illness from occurring. The goal of preventive health, then, is to intervene at the earliest possible stage in the natural history of disease to prevent complications, limit disability, and halt irreversible changes in health status (Leavell & Clark, 1979).

**Primary prevention** refers to those measures that focus on prevention of health problems before they occur. Primary prevention is not therapeutic, which means that it does not consist of symptom identification and use of the typical therapeutic skills of the nurse (Shamansky & Clausen, 1980). This level includes both generalized health promotion and specific protection against certain identified diseases or conditions. The purpose is to reduce the person's vulnerability to the illness by strengthening the human host's capacity to withstand physical, emotional, and environmental stressors. An example would be teaching a person about adequate nutrition, exercise, and hygiene. Specific protection includes numerous interventions associated with public health nursing: immunizations, bicycle helmets, auto seatbelts, safety caps on electrical outlets, handrails on bathtubs, and drug education for children.

**Secondary prevention** begins when pathology is involved and is aimed at early detection through diagnosis and prompt treatment. This level of prevention is aimed at halting the pathological process, thereby shortening its duration and severity and getting the person back to a normal state of functioning. All screening tests, such as breast self-examinations, hypertensive assessments, and Pap smears, are included in this level of prevention. The goal of this level is to identify groups of individuals who have early symptoms of disease so that they may be treated as soon as possible in the natural history of the disease, condition, or injury. If the disease, condition, or injury cannot be cured, further complications and disability move the level of prevention to that of tertiary prevention.

**Tertiary prevention** consists of activities designed around rehabilitation of a person with a permanent, irreversible condition. The goal of tertiary prevention goes beyond halting the disease process to restoring the person to an optimal level of functioning within the constraints of the disability. Nursing strategies at this level might include teaching a stroke patient how to ambulate with assistance or assisting a child with cystic fibrosis how to reduce risks of respiratory infection while maintaining an active lifestyle.

The boundaries between secondary and tertiary prevention are often fuzzy and more difficult to identify as either one or the other. One feature that helps in this identification is that tertiary intervention takes place only if the condition results in a permanent disability (Shamansky & Clausen, 1980). This outcome may be influenced by the age or development of the patient rather than by the condition itself. For example, if a 15-year-old high school athlete suffers a simple broken femur during a soccer game, intervention would occur at the secondary prevention level. Although the athlete may require extensive physical rehabilitation after the cast is removed, unless there are serious complications, she should eventually be able to return to her normal state of health. Compare this situation with a 75-year-old man who falls from a roof and suffers the identical injury. Most likely, this patient would need both secondary and tertiary intervention strategies because of the aging process, recovery, and the likelihood of permanent disability resulting from this fall.

Shamansky and Clausen (1980) use the following example to illustrate how all levels of prevention are often used with the same patient and family:

A nurse is conducting a group session with young parents and uses values clarification as a method to discuss issues of parental responsibility for providing a safe yet stimulating environment for the young, curious child. This is primary prevention: Health promotion occurs, because the discussion is general and directed toward nonspecific efforts to ensure the well-being of the young child.

Later, on a home visit, the nurse encourages a mother to use screens on a second-story window, because she perceives the window is dangerously accessible to the active three-year-old. This, too, is primary prevention, an example of specific protection, because the nurse is attempting to remove a risk factor from the environment of a vulnerable child.

If the screen is not used and the child falls out of the window onto a cement driveway below, the mother's and emergency personnel's use of appropriate emergency first aid would be secondary prevention through the use of prompt treatment. If the child sustained a severe head injury, was hospitalized (and secondary measures were used in the hospital), and later released to home care, teaching the mother to turn, feed, and give range-of-motion exercises would represent the disability limitation aspect of secondary prevention.

Several months later, if the child is found to have some permanent brain damage, tertiary prevention would take the form of referrals to special education classes, or physical or speech therapy to increase the child's maximum potential level of functioning, although the damage itself is irreversible. (pp. 106–107)

### NOTE THIS!

Why are American children getting heavier every year? Each day, most 8- to 18-year-olds spend an average of 4 hours watching television, videos, and DVDs; more than 1 hour on the computer; and about 50 minutes playing video games.

## Measuring a Community's Health: How Do We Know When We Get There?

Outcomes and measurements of community health interventions take the form of health statistics such as birth rates, infant mortality rates, and incidence and prevalence rates for various diseases and age groups. Most threats to health do not occur at random (i.e., by chance). Natural forces influence health threats, but by no means do they dictate the outcome. In this century we have learned through epidemiological research that most threats or risks to our health and well-being are associated with patterns of human activity and behavior. It is those patterns that we use to evaluate health interventions and the multitude of influences on people's health (Cohen, 1989).

For example, breast cancer rates in the United States are high compared with other countries such as Japan and China. In other words, breast cancer is not universal among all females, nor is it randomly distributed in the female population (Cohen, 1989).

> **"** We allow our ignorance to prevail upon us and make us think we can survive alone, alone in patches, alone in groups, alone in races, even alone in genders. **"**
>
> —Maya Angelou

We can see from epidemiological research that individual behavior has a significant effect on a person's chance of developing breast cancer. Breast cancer may be associated with a high-fat, high-protein, high-calorie diet, and with high levels of estrogen (either produced by the woman's own body or ingested in diet and medication). Women who do not have or nurse children or have them later in life also have higher rates of breast cancer. These lifestyle factors clearly influence the chances of a woman's contracting breast cancer in her lifetime. The availability of cutting-edge technology and diagnostic interventions cannot prevent women from contracting breast cancer; these measures can improve chances of survival only after cancer is detected (Kolata, 1987; Marx, 1986; Winick, 1980).

In another example, maternal death risk in childbirth plummeted during the twentieth century in developed countries as a result of application of prenatal care, use of antibiotics, and infectious disease control. In the United States, a woman has a 1 in 3,700 chance of dying in childbirth. By contrast, in Latin America, a woman's mortality risk is 1 in 130, and women in parts of Africa have an alarming 1 in 16 chance of dying as a result of childbearing (Whaley & Hashim, 1995).

Table 1-2 provides an illustration of the links among all levels of care. You will learn in this text how these group rates of disease, health, injury, and disability reflect more accurately the values of a society and how health professionals measure not only their interventions but the influences of many variables on health.

| Table 1-2 | A Comparison of Individual, Family, Community, and Global Population-Focused Care | | |
|---|---|---|---|
| **Individual Care** | **Family** | **Community** | **Global** |
| ■ Injuries suffered by women in violent spousal domestic relationship | ■ Family dysfunctions, such as inability to provide appropriate behavioral roles for conflict resolution<br>■ Children exhibiting early and inappropriate use of firearms | ■ Children unable to function in school setting because of disruptive behavior in classroom<br>■ Gang violence resulting in neighborhood isolation, decreased population, diminished economic base because of business closure and decreased funds available for education and family assistance | ■ Women and children refugees in war-torn Pakistan and Afghanistan suffering from injuries as a result of acts of war violence |

## " a conversation with . . . "

### Dr. Richard Carmona

I am Richard Carmona. I am the U.S. Surgeon General and I am a registered nurse. I recalled that President Bush introduced me once as a former nurse and I quietly reminded him that there is no such thing as a former nurse. I am a nurse, and the past, present, and future of nursing are my passion.

As Surgeon General, I have three priorities: health problem prevention, improved health literacy, and elimination of health disparities. The country needs to convert from embracing treatment to embracing prevention. When we prevent health problems, we will have more money for the underserved. Another top priority is to decrease health illiteracy: Health issues are complex. People don't understand what to do, where to go, how to manage their health. The United States has great science, but lacks the translational element to be accessible.

Now is the best time to be a nurse. ◯

—Richard Carmona, RN, MD, MPH, FACS,
U.S. Surgeon General, National Student Nurses
Association Annual Meeting, April 7, 2005

### Application to Practice

### Community-Based Care: An Example from Practice

A 3-year-old child is brought to a public health department for her first set of immunizations. As the nurse assesses the child, she finds that the child has a generalized red rash all over her body. The mother complains that the child scratches and cries about the rash. She has been using a cortisone skin cream for three days, but the rash has worsened.

The nurse attends to the immediate concerns of the mother about home care comfort measures and possible causes. The nurse then delivers direct care to the child and to her family, while considering the following community implications:

- Does anyone else in the family exhibit those symptoms?
- Does the child go to day care?
- Have there been any other children in the clinic recently with similar symptoms? If so, how does this case compare with cases in recent months?
- What is the likely pathogen that is causing the rash?
- Are there any pregnant women in the clinic or in the home setting?
  1. What are possible conclusions that the nurse can make that have individual implications?
  2. Are there community and public health issues that may be present that the nurse must address? ◯

## Conclusion

In community-based care, community patients are the focus wherever they live, work, or reside. The focus of nurses' practice may be on the individual, but various influences on a community's health and the way in which the health care system has organized services around societal needs and expectations must also be considered. Nurses will play a critical role in the future of managed care, which is organized around prevention and a healthy population. **Epidemiology** is the science that provides community and public health with a framework for addressing the primary, secondary, and tertiary health needs for a population and directs community health nursing practice. The personal well-being of individuals is more than an individual matter. Humankind does not live in isolation, unaffected by others. Community health is a dynamic of the community and is influenced by the context of where and how the population lives, works, and addresses health care needs.

## ■ CRITICAL THINKING ACTIVITIES

1. After reading "Think About This" on page 23 respond to the following questions:
   • What are three risks described in the essay that were unknown a century ago?
   • What is the responsibility of the individual in creating a safe environment?
   • What are three public safety measures mentioned in the essay that do not exist in underdeveloped countries?
2. How can heart disease be both a personal health problem and a community health problem?

3. For several decades now, nurses have worked primarily in hospitals using a medical model approach to health and illness. Does nursing have a vision of the profession with community at the center, or has nursing become so institutionalized into hospital-based practice over the past decades that we will resist the tremendous opportunities to care for people in a myriad of settings and situations?
4. How has the ethic of caring for a patient's environment changed from Florence Nightingale's era?

## ■ REFERENCES

American Nurses Association (ANA). (1991). *Nursing's agenda for health care reform: Executive summary.* Washington, DC: Author.

American Nurses Association (ANA). (1994). *Managed care: Challenges and opportunities for nursing.* Washington, DC: Author.

American Nurses Association (ANA). (2001). *Code of ethics for nurses with interpretive statements.* Washington, DC: Author.

American Nurses Association (2007). *Public health nursing: Scope and standards of practice.* Washington, DC: Author.

American Public Health Association. Public Health Nursing Section. (1996). *The definition and role of public health nursing: A statement of the APHA Public Health Nursing Section.* Washington, DC: Author.

Anderson, C. (1997). The economics of health promotion. *Nursing Outlook, 45*(3), 105–106.

Armentrout, G. (1998). *Community-based nursing: Foundation for practice.* Stamford, CT: Appleton & Lange.

Bunker, J. P., Frazier, H. S., & Mosteller, F. (1994). Improving health: Measuring effects of medical care. *Milbank Quarterly, 72,* 225–258.

Bureau of Labor Statistics. (2008). *Occupational outlook handbook, 2008–2009 edition.* U.S. Department of Labor. Retrieved Septemeber 20, 2008, from http://www.bls.gov/oco/ocos083.htm

Canavan, K. (1996). Nursing education on cusp of shift in focus: Faculty grapple with preparing students for changing health care delivery. *American Nurse, 28*(6), 1, 11.

Centers for Disease Control and Prevention (CDC). (2002). *Public health infrastructure: A status report.* Atlanta: Author.

Cohen, M. (1989). *Health and the rise of civilization.* New Haven, CT: Yale University Press.

Cottrell, K. (1976). The competent community. In B. H. Kaplan, R. N. Wilson, & A. H. Leighton (Eds.), *Further explorations in social psychology.* New York: Basic Books.

Davidhizar, R., Eshleman, J., & Wolff, L. (2003). Living with stress since 9/11. *Caring, 22*(4), 26–28, 30.

Department of Health and Human Services (DHHS), Division of Nursing, Bureau of Health Professions, Health Resources and Services Administration. (2000). *National sample survey of registered nurses.* Washington, DC: U.S. Government Printing Office.

Ferguson, L. M., & Day, R. A. (2007). Challenges for new nurses in evidence-based practice. *Journal of Nursing Management, 15*(1), 107–113.

Folmar, J., Coughlin, S. S., Bessinger, R., & Sacknoff, D. (1997). Ethics in public health practice: A survey of public health nurses in southern Louisiana. *Public Health Nursing, 14*(3), 156–160.

Gebbie, K. M. (1996, November 18). *Preparing currently employed public health nurses for changes in the health care system: Meeting report and suggested action steps.* New York: Columbia University School of Nursing Center for Health Policy and Health Sciences Research. (Report based on meeting in Atlanta, GA, July 11, 1996.)

Giger, J. N., & Davidhizar, R. E. (1995). *Transcultural nursing: Assessment and intervention* (2nd ed.). St. Louis: Mosby.

Gostin, L. O. (2004). Health of the people: The highest law? *Journal of Law, Medicine and Ethics, 32*(3), 509–515.

Gostin, L. O., Bufford, J. I., & Martinez, R. M. (2004). The future of the public's health: Vision, values and strategies. *Health Affairs, 23,* 96–107.

Graham, K. Y. (1997). Ethics: Do we really care? *Public Health Nursing, 14*(1), 1–2.

Grossman, D. (1994). Enhancing your cultural competence. *American Journal of Nursing, 94*(7), 58–62.

Hall, J. E., & Weaver, B. R. (1977). *Distributive nursing practice: A systems approach to community health.* Philadelphia: Lippincott.

Hall, J. M., & Stevens, P. E. (1995). The future of graduate education in nursing: Scholarship, the health communities, and health care reform. *Journal of Professional Nursing, 11*(6), 332–338.

Hanlon, J. J., & Pickett, G. E. (1984). *Public health: Administration and practice* (8th ed.). St. Louis: Mosby.

Institute of Medicine (IOM). (2003). *The future of the public's health in the twenty-first century.* Washington, DC: National Academy Press.

Janes, S., & Hobson, K. (1998). An innovative approach for affirming cultural diversity among baccalaureate nursing students and faculty. *Journal of Cultural Diversity, 5*(4), 132–137.

Keck, E. W. (1994). Community health: Our common challenge. *Family and Community Health, 17*(2), 1–9.

Keller, L. O., Strohstein, S., Lia-Hoagberg, B., & Shaeffer, M. A. (2004). Population-based public health interventions: Practice-based and evidence-supported. Part I. *Public Health Nursing, 21*(5), 453–468.

Kurtzman, C., Ibgui, D., Pogrund, R., & Monin, S. (1980). Nursing process at the aggregate level. *Nursing Outlook, 28*(12), 737–739.

Kuss, T., Proulx-Girouard, L., Lovitt, S., Katz, C. B., & Kennelly, P. (1997). A public health nursing model. *Public Health Nursing, 14*(2), 81–91.

Leavell, H. R., & Clark, E. G. (1953). *Preventive medicine for the doctor in his community.* New York: McGraw-Hill.

Leavell, H. R., & Clark, E. G. (1979). *Preventive medicine for the doctor in his community: An epidemiological approach* (3rd ed.). Huntington, NY: RE Dreges.

Leininger, M. (1995). *Transcultural nursing: Concepts, theories, research, and practices* (2nd ed.). New York: McGraw-Hill.

Leipert, B. D. (1996). The value of community health nursing: A phenomenological study of the perceptions of community health nurses. *Public Health Nursing, 13*(1), 50–57.

McKenzie, J. F., & Pinger, R. R. (1997). *An introduction to community health.* Boston: Jones and Bartlett.

Mechanic, D. (1998). Topics of our times: Managed care and public health. *American Journal of Public Health, 88*(6), 84–85.

Meleis, A. L. (1996). Culturally competent scholarship: Substance and rigor. *Advances in Nursing Science, 19*(2), 1–16.

Moon, M. (1993). Health care reform. *Future of Children, 3*(2), 21–36.

Morse, S. S. (2003). Building academic-practice partnerships: The Center for Public Health Preparedness at the Columbia University Mailman School of Public Health, before and after 9/11. *Journal of Public Health Management & Practice, 9*(5), 427–432.

Nehls, N., Owen, B., Tipple, S., & Vandermause, R. (2001). Lessons learned from developing, implementing and evaluating a model of community-driven nursing. *Nursing and Health Care Perspectives, 22,* 304–307.

Nehls, N., & Vandermause, R. (2004). Community driven nursing: Transforming nursing curricula and instruction. *Nursing Education Perspectives, 25*(2), 81–85.

Neufield, V. (1992). Training: A Canadian perspective. In Pan American Health Organization (Ed.), *International health: North–south debate.* (Human Resource Development Series, pp. 95, 193–203). Washington, DC: Pan American Health Organization.

Nightingale, F. (1860). *Notes on nursing: What it is and what it is not.* London: Harrison.

Proenca, E. J. (1998). Community orientation in health services organizations: The concept and its implementation. *Health Care Management Review, 23*(2), 28–38.

Purnell, L. D., & Paulanka, B. J. (2003). *Transcultural health care: A culturally competent approach* (2nd ed.). Philadelphia: F. A. Davis.

Salmon, M., & Vanderbush, P. (1990). Leadership and change in public and community health nursing today: The essential intervention. In J. C. McCloskey & H. K. Grace (Eds.), *Current issues in nursing* (3rd ed., pp. 187–193). St. Louis: Mosby.

Schultz, P. R. (1994). On the matter of populations, aggregates, and communities. Unpublished manuscript, University of Washington, Seattle.

Shamansky, S. L., & Clausen, C. L. (1980). Levels of prevention: Examination of the concept. *Nursing Outlook, 28*(2), 104–108.

Shortell, S. M., & Gilles, R. R. (1995). Reinventing the American hospital. *Milbank Quarterly, 73*(2), 131.

Smith, C. M. (1995). Responsibilities for care in community health nursing. In C. M. Smith & F. A. Maurer (Eds.), *Community health nursing: Principles and practice* (pp. 3–29). Philadelphia: Saunders.

Spicer, G. (1998). Learning right from wrong. *Imprint, 45*(3), 4.

Starr, P. (1993). The framework of health care reform. *New England Journal of Medicine, 329,* 1666–1672.

Trossman, S. (1998, March/April). Self-determination: The name of the game in the next century. *American Nurse,* 1.

Turnock, B. (1997). *Public health: What it is and how it works.* Baltimore: Aspen.

Vilschick, J. (2003, January/February). Lack of minority role models affects nursing shortage. Closing the gap, First Summit Packs the House, pp. 16–17.

Wolf, Z. R. (1989). Uncovering the hidden work of nursing. *Nursing and Health Care, 10*(8), 462–467.

World Health Organization (WHO). (1958). *The first ten years of the World Health Organization.* New York: Author.

World Health Organization (WHO). (1986). Health promotion: A discussion document on the concept and principles. *Public Health Reviews, 14*(3–4), 245–254.

## APPENDIX
# Standards of Care

Scope and Standards of Public Health Nursing Practice
Author: Quad Council of Public Health Nursing
    Organizations
American Nurses Association
Washington, DC
1999

## Standards of Care

### Standard I. Assessment

The public health nurse assesses the health status of populations using data, community resources identification, input from the population, and professional judgment.

### Standard II. Diagnosis

The public health nurse analyzes collected assessment data and partners with the people to attach meaning to those data and determine opportunities and needs.

### Standard III. Outcomes Identification

The public health nurse participates with other community partners to identify expected outcomes in the populations and their health status.

### Standard IV. Planning

The public health nurse promotes and supports the development of programs, policies, and services that provide interventions that improve the health status of populations.

### Standard V. Assurance: Action component of the nursing process for public health nursing

The public health nurse assures access and availability of programs, policies, resources, and services to the population.

### Standard VI. Evaluation

The public health nurse evaluates the health status of the population.

# CHAPTER 2
# Community and Population Health: Assessment and Intervention

Karen Saucier Lundy and Judith A. Barton

Visit **http://nursing.jbpub.com/communityhealth** for interactive exercises, review questions, Web links, and more.

Organized sports such as soccer provide children and teens with beneficial exercise and social interaction with peers.

"We are all longing to go home to some place we have never been—a place, half-remembered, and half-envisioned we can only catch glimpses of from time to time. Community: Somewhere, there are people to whom we can speak with passion without having the words catch in our throats. Somewhere a circle of hands will open to receive us, eyes will light up as we enter, voices will celebrate with us whenever we come into our own power. Community means strength that joins our strength to do the work that needs to be done. Arms to hold us when we falter. A circle of healing. A circle of friends: Someplace where we can be free."

—Starhawk from *Dreaming in the Dark*

After reading the quote, think about what living in a community means to you. How has it shaped your beliefs about health and what you do when you are sick? Did you spend your childhood and teen years in a small town, an urban area, or a suburb, or did you move around and spend time in many different types of communities? As a nursing student, think about the different communities where you feel most "at home" now. Describe these communities and indicate how they differ from those you grew up in terms of health values.

## CHAPTER FOCUS

**Communities and Populations**
- The Health of Communities and Populations
- Differences and Similarities Among Communities and Populations

**Community Assessment Frameworks**
- Community Empowerment
- Four Community Assessment Frameworks/Models

**Using the Nursing Process for the Community**
- Conducting a Community Assessment
- Community Diagnosis
- Planning and Prioritization Phase
- Implementation Phase
- Evaluation Phase

## QUESTIONS TO CONSIDER

After reading this chapter, you will know the answers to the following questions:

1. What is a population-focused approach to health care?
2. How does the baccalaureate-prepared nurse use population assessment in health care settings?
3. What is the "community as patient"?
4. What is the difference between a community and a population?
5. What do the terms *status, structure,* and *process* refer to?
6. What is the Healthy Cities initiative?
7. How are community assessment frameworks or models used in the assessment process?
8. What are examples of community assessment frameworks or models?

9. How does a community health nurse gain entry into the community?
10. What are the five methods of collecting community data?
11. What is a community diagnosis, and what is an example of one?
12. What occurs in the planning and prioritization phase of the community assessment process?
13. What occurs in the implementation phase of the community assessment process?
14. What are examples of strategies that the community health nurse can use to assist communities in healthy change?
15. What is media advocacy?

## KEY TERMS

Collaborative arrangement
Community
Community- and population-focused care
Community as patient
Community assessment
Community assessment frameworks and models

Community competency
Community empowerment
Community-focused intervention
Community forums
Community health diagnoses
Constructed surveys
Focus groups
Healthy change

Healthy communities
Informant interviews
Key informant
Media advocacy
Observation
Planning phase
Population
Population assessment

Population-level interventions
Primary informant
Process
Secondary analysis of existing data
Secondary data
Status
Structure
Windshield surveys

COMMUNITY NURSES HAVE TRADITIONALLY conducted nursing assessments of entire geopolitical communities and of vulnerable populations within communities. The focus of the nursing assessment is on the community or population's health status rather than the individual's health status, and consequently the assessment takes on a different form and process. Perhaps the best and most dramatic example was the post–Hurricane Katrina public health disaster that occurred in New Orleans as a result of a lack of attention to planning for this vulnerable population's health needs. Public health nurses, along with other disciplines, are challenged to balance these short-term crises with progress toward longer-term goals, as we seek newer and better ways of solving health problems in our communities (Carney, 2006).

Today more than ever, the community health nurse has the unique responsibility of defining problems and proposing solutions at the community/population level (Baldwin, Conger, Abegglen, & Hill, 1998; Gebbie, 1996; Keck, 1994; Williams & Highriter, 1978). Furthermore, baccalaureate-prepared nurses will be expected to practice population-based nursing in all settings as managed care of populations becomes the basis of organizational survival.

The U.S. health care system's trend toward community- and population-focused care was well documented in the previous chapter. The shift from location-based care (e.g., hospital, outpatient clinic care) to community-based care will demand a greater emphasis on nursing assessments of both geopolitical communities and high-risk populations. In other words, to plan care, carry out interventions, and evaluate care outcomes when the patient is either a geopolitical community or population at risk, there is a need for all nurses to have skills in community and population assessment. Although community and population assessment, planning, intervention, and evaluation are receiving greater attention in today's health care system, these skills have always been associated with community health nursing role expectations (Hegyvary, 1990).

Historically, community/population assessment, the initial step in community-/population-focused care, was first seen as a nursing practice role by Florence Nightingale. Nightingale was concerned with assessing the physical and social environment as a possible cause of illness. Nightingale's own community assessments included an analysis of the 1861 census data of England, which served as the foundation of England's sanitary reform acts (Kopf, 1986). She also included community assessment as a nursing role for district nurses. These nurses were to assess both the physical and social environments of the community to determine which health teaching and social reform programs were needed by the community (Montero, 1985). From its earliest history, the nursing profession has viewed community and population assessment as an important role directed toward improving the health of entire communities.

Today, recommitment toward community and population assessment is a vital nursing practice role, as identified by all organizations that set standards for community health nursing (AACN, 1986; ACHNE, 2000; ANA, 1986; APHA, 1981). This recommitment to seeing the community as patient has emerged as a critical function of the community health nurse as more and more research connects the important role that physical and social environments play in health and disease (Cassel, 1976; Gordon, 1990, 1993; Lalonde, 1974; Rodgers, 1984). Such findings also influence health policy formation, the establishment of priorities when financing health care, and the potential of the nursing community to establish itself as a leader in health care reform. Knowledge of community and population assessment is now considered essential for the baccalaureate nurse (Ruth, Eliason, & Schultz, 1992; Eide et al., 2006). The diagnoses and interventions that result from the community and population assessment process are population-based, community-focused interventions. Such interventions are directed at groups of persons within a community; activities are geared toward changes in community norms, greater consciousness about health issues and solutions, and healthy practices and behaviors, to name a few (Keller, Strohschein, Lia-Hoagberg, & Schaffer, 1998).

This chapter introduces the **community as patient**, explains how to get to know the community patient, and describes how to practice skills of community and population assessment in actual community assessment examples. The future of nursing depends to a large degree on our understanding of the "big picture" of health care delivery (Aiken & Salmon, 1994). As we become more and more dependent on outcome and evidence-based measures, such as evaluation of morbidity and mortality statistics, this chapter will help the beginning nurse use the community/population assessment process in all practice settings (Reinhart, 1984) (Box 2-1).

---

## BOX 2-1

**Ways in Which the Community Assessment/Population Assessment Can Be Used in the "Everyday Life" of a Practicing Nurse**

- Applying for grants to provide health care for specific populations, such as pregnant adolescents
- Conducting a "mini" assessment during orientation to a new position in any setting to be better prepared for serving the agency's target population
- Avoiding burnout by going beyond personal care of patients, identifying better ways of delivering care, and using staff and material resources
- Justifying new projects by establishing the needs of a selected population
- Joining a community group such as the Parent Teacher Organization or American Cancer Society, volunteering to do an assessment and follow-through program planning
- Conducting an assessment of unfamiliar locales, both national and international, to determine possible relocation possibilities

This chapter also discusses how to interpret community- and population-level data and plan interventions more appropriately and efficiently as we work within the limited resources of the present health care environment. Our health care system can no longer rely on quick fixes. For example, in developed countries the nature of fatal diseases has changed. In the course of recent human history, when people were fighting diseases such as smallpox, diphtheria, or polio, immunizations were an easy, quick, and sure prevention. As we learned more about infectious disease and the contribution of human factors, such as lifestyle, heredity, and behavior, solutions became more complex. Chronic disease and disabling conditions are continuing to grow as we extend the life span through technology and advancement of diagnosis and treatment. Today many diseases and conditions require that we are much more attentive to the totality of variables that influence health and illness (Gebbie, 1996). Achieving prevention and control requires much more effort on the part of communities and changes in thinking about the impact of the structure of society (e.g., economics, culture, and politics) on the health of community (Community Health Advisor Network, 1999).

## Communities and Populations

The significance of the community/population nursing process becomes evident only when community health nurses define the community as patient. A nurse would not even consider omitting individual patient assessment and basing interventions only on intuition or a standard formula, but this is what happens when community health nurses fail to do a focused community/population assessment when planning and implementing health care for patients. For example, we would not even consider examining just the arm of a patient and totally ignoring the other systems of the body when we plan our nursing care. And yet by looking at only a few aspects of a selected community or population, such as the number and availability of hospitals, we are examining just the "arm" and ignoring the rest of the "body" of the community or population.

The first step in delivering **community- and population-focused care** is to define the boundaries of the group to be assessed. We often use the term **community** in various ways, as was discussed in Chapter 1, so defining the boundaries of a community or population becomes critical in the early stages of **community-focused intervention**. Community is defined in this text as a group of people who share something in common, who interact with one another, and who may exhibit a commitment to one another. A population is defined as a group of people who have at least one thing in common and who may or may not interact with each other. From these definitions one can see that *interaction* is essential in a *community*, whereas members of a *population* may or may not interact with one another. To put it another way, community members are usually aware that they are part

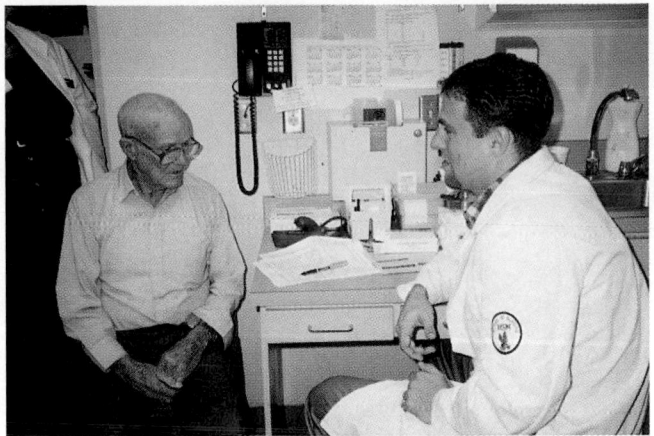
Nurse providing individual care.

### BOX 2-2

**Examples of Communities**
- Retirement apartment community
- Corvette Club of San Francisco
- Town of Blackhawk, Colorado

**Examples of Populations**
- Cross-country truck drivers
- Elders with chronic asthma
- College soccer players
- Street musicians
- Ice skaters

of a community and most often have an identified name. **Populations** may or may not have such self-awareness (Box 2-2). Some populations do evolve into communities. For example, adults who have disabilities and attend a day program in a certain community may develop into a cohesive, interactive group over time. Whether the population being assessed has self awareness, the environment (e.g., the social, cultural, ecological environment of a particular community or the greater society) of the target population must be considered for effective health interventions to occur (Baldwin et al., 1998).

❝ *The 'sayings' of a community, its proverbs, are its characteristic comment upon life; they imply its history, suggest its attitude toward the world and its way of accepting life. Such an idiom makes the finest language any writer can have; and he can never get it with a notebook. He himself must be able to think and feel in that speech—it is a gift from heart to heart.* ❞

—*Willa Cather*

This college tennis team has formed a community after one year of common and meaningful interactions.

## The Health of Communities and Populations

Public health professionals often describe **healthy communities** and populations in three different ways: status, structure, and process. See Box 2-3 for a summary of these components.

**Status** is what we most commonly use to describe communities and populations and is the component you are most familiar with. When we talk about life expectancy rates and the morbidity (or illness) rates of a community or population, these are the "outcome" measures of *physical* or *biological* determinants of health. The *emotional aspects* of a community's or population's health status are often measured by such indices as specific mental health rates (e.g., suicide or drug addiction). The *social* determinants are reflected by such indices as crime rates and juvenile delin-

An example of a noninteracting population of young concertgoers.

> ### BOX 2-3
>
> **Basic Components of Community and Population Health with Example Indicators**
>
> **Dimensions**
>
> ***Status***
> - Vital statistics
> - Leading causes of death
> - Mental health statistics
> - Crime rates
>
> ***Structure***
> - Hospitals, community health clinics
> - Health professionals, government structures, and so on
> - Statistics related to use of health resources
> - Population characteristics (e.g., gender, age, socioeconomic status)
>
> ***Process***
> - Commitment of members
> - Self and other awareness
> - Articulateness
> - Effective communication
> - Conflict resolution
> - Active participation by members
> - Management of social interactions with larger society/environment
> - Machinery for effective resource procurement and utilization
>
> *Source*: Schuster, G. F., & Goeppinger, J. (1996). Community as patient: Using the nursing process to promote health. In M. Stanhope & J. Lancaster (Eds.), *Community health nursing: Promoting health of aggregates, families, and individuals* (pp. 289–314). St. Louis: Mosby.

quency. As we have learned more about the health and the "ills" of modern society, we have discovered that most status outcome measures reflect the influences of all three status components. For example, teen drug use is associated with risky behavior such as unprotected sex, which may result in high rates of teen pregnancy, sexually transmitted diseases, and associated higher infant mortality rates.

**Structure** refers to aspects of a community's or population's health such as health organizations, health professionals, utilization rates of health services and facilities, and characteristics of the community structure itself. How the community or population is structured is reflected in such measures as socioeconomic and educational levels; demographics of race, age, and gender; and the ways in which the members of a community access and use resources related to health. Research has linked education, socioeconomic status, and health outcomes, so these components are aspects that reflect the health status of a group to that end (Schuster & Goeppinger, 1996).

**Process** is a measure of community or population health that reflects how well a community/population functions to keep healthy. Just as the care of the individual patient commonly includes an assessment of personal competence to maintain health, so a community or population can be described in relation to **community competency**. This notion of community competency has been around for some time. George Herbert Mead (1934), the noted sociologist, linked our individual behaviors to what eventually emerges as collective behavior. These collective behaviors ultimately take the form of social institutions, such as a church, the Microsoft Corporation, or the American Red Cross. Mead contends that it is only this "organized self" and the resulting group response that makes communities possible and survival likely. For example, people exhibit varying degrees of competency at meeting social needs. Each individual who is intrinsically tied to the group through social interaction is changed by the interaction—each participant then not only becomes a part of the "other," but also learns his or her part as well as the part of the other (Mead, 1934). Cottrell (1976) defines community competence as a process in which the components of a community—families, organizations, and populations—"are able to collaborate effectively in identifying the problems and needs of the community; can achieve a working consensus on goals and priorities, can agree on ways and means to implement the agreed-on goals; and can collaborate effectively in the required action" (p. 197).

An important distinction must be made between individual competence and community competence: Although we often assume that a community made up of competent citizens and health professionals results in a competent community, these are not sufficient conditions. The complexity of community requires that we look not only beyond the individual parts of a community but also to the "whole" and the interactions between and among community constituents (Goeppinger, Lassiter, & Wilcox, 1982). Goeppinger, Lassiter, and Wilcox (1982) developed a nursing process–related model for community assessment designed to address the importance of community processes and community competence. To assess community competencies, the nurse examines the health capabilities and potential health actions of the community. The basic assumption of the community competency model is that health assessments need to include the community's strengths and abilities to improve their own health status. The model is based on research conducted by Goeppinger and Baglioni (1986) that was designed to discover indices of community competence. These competencies are not considered mutually exclusive, but are interrelated. Table 2-1 summarizes essentials for community competency and includes examples from Goeppinger and Baglioni's research on indices of community competency (1986).

**❝**What is a slum? . . . it is something that mostly exists in the imaginations of middle-class do-gooders and bureaucrats: people who do not have to live in them in the first place and do not have to live in what they put up afterwards once they have pulled them all down. One person's slum is another person's community.**❞**

—May Hobbs

## Healthy Cities

The World Health Organization (WHO) developed the Healthy Cities initiative as a global approach to community-focused health promotion and preventive health. The Healthy Cities movement began in 1984 in Canada; in 1986, WHO initiated the project in Europe. The largest Healthy City in Europe in the WHO project is St. Petersburg, Russia, while Indiana and California have the longest history with Healthy Cities in the United States. Approximately half the world's population lives in urban areas, where health problems are the most complex. As an international movement, Healthy Cities (Box 2-4) now involves more than 1,000 cities throughout the world where public, private, and not-for-profit partnerships work together to address the complex

| **Table 2-1** | **Essential Conditions for Community Competence** |
|---|---|
| ■ Commitment | ■ Evidence that community members are attached to their community—people within the community demonstrate loyalty and pride. |
| ■ Self–other awareness | ■ Evidence that community members are aware of how they fit into their community—as outsiders or insiders, as having power or not having power. |
| ■ Articulateness | ■ Evidence that the community is able to clearly express its own issues, needs, and strengths as compared with other similar communities so as to effectively secure resources to meet needs. |
| ■ Effective communication | ■ Evidence of good communication within a community—the people say that they feel they are always well informed about issues ahead of time so that good decisions can be made. |
| ■ Conflict containment and accommodation | ■ Evidence that the community has been able to deal effectively with conflicts within the community such as growth policies or taxes for local school districts. |
| ■ Participation | ■ Evidence that all populations (e.g., different age groups, ethnic groups) participate in community organizations and governmental decisions. |
| ■ Management of relations with larger society | ■ Evidence that the community is able to secure resources from county, state, or federal governments as needed. |
| ■ Machinery for facilitating participant interaction and decision making | ■ Evidence that a community's governmental structure has built-in processes that encourage participation by the members of the community for good decision making. |

*Source*: Adapted from Goeppinger, J., Lassiter, P. G., & Wilcox, B. (1982). Community health is community competence. *Nursing Outlook, 30*(8), 464–467.

"If our American way of life fails the child, it fails us all."
—Pearl S. Buck

health and environmental problems in urban areas (Flynn, Ray, & Rider, 1994). Based on the belief that the health of a community is largely influenced by the social and physical environments in which people live and work, Healthy Cities projects promote change in the complex web of city life (Flynn & Dennis, 1996). Community assessment is a critical and early step in the process of identifying the health needs of cities and working with residents to develop realistic and community-identified solutions (Hancock, 1993). The underlying philosophy of such an approach is based on the belief that when residents work out their own locally defined health issues, they will find sustainable solutions to those problems (Flynn, 1994; Lia-Hoagberg et al., 1999).

### Differences and Similarities Among Communities and Populations

Chapter 1 introduced the idea that baccalaureate nurses are prepared to deliver population-focused care. The Association of Community Health Nursing Educators (ACHNE) has identified in its *Essentials of Baccalaureate Nursing Education for Entry Level Practice in Community/Public Health Nursing* (2000) community assessment, diagnosis, and community planning as essential skills for the BSN nurse.

For advanced-degree nurses specializing in community-based public health nursing, population-focused care becomes the primary focus of the role. For baccalaureate-prepared nurses not specializing in public health nursing, such care may be a secondary focus. However, baccalaureate-prepared nurses practicing in all settings (hospital settings as well as community settings) will need to have skills in population-focused care. Baccalaureate-prepared nurses will be expected to move beyond being able to just provide care for individual patients. They will be expected to move

beyond incorporating only pathophysiological, psychological, pharmacological, and family factor knowledge into their nursing assessments of individual patients. They will need to incorporate population knowledge—population knowledge that includes an understanding of the common needs of all patients who share one or more characteristics (Salmon, 1993).

These characteristics may include, for example, a common disease, gender, occupation, or age range. For example, an emergency room nurse noted that most of the patients she was caring for had some condition related to substance abuse. Perhaps they had been involved in an automobile accident caused by drunk driving, or perhaps they suffered a gunshot wound that occurred during a drug deal. Conducting a **population assessment** to better understand the demographic, political, economic, and health system factors affecting this population will eventually lead to **population-level interventions** such as an initiative to coordinate care of substance abusing patients with mental health professionals. Such efforts may improve not only the health of the individuals within this population, but also the efficiency of the health care system (Keller, Strohschein, Lia-Hoagberg, & Schaffer, 2004; Keller, Strohschein, Schaffer, & Lia-Hoagberg, 2004).

Nurses also participate as team members in communitywide health assessments. **Community assessments** differ from population assessments only in that they are not focused on a specific group of individuals who share one or more common characteristics. City municipalities are an example of a community. The individuals in a city municipality interact to achieve goals of employment, the exchange of goods and services, law and order, and so on. A hospital is an example of a community. The individuals within the hospital environment interact to achieve the goals of the organization. You could think of community assessment as more expansive, more complex than a population assessment. In addition, the process of community assessment usually requires a team of researchers to complete a comprehensive analysis of the health of a community.

In the following section, four models for community assessment are presented. Please note that although these models use the language of community assessment and were developed for community assessment, they can be and are adapted for use in population assessments.

**❝***It is by knowing where you stand that you grow able to judge where you are. Place absorbs our earliest notice and attention. It bestows on us our original awareness; and our critical powers spring up from the study of it and the growth of experience inside it. One place comprehended can make us understand other places better.***❞**

—Eudora Welty

## Community Assessment Frameworks

Just as there are models, theories, and organizing frameworks that guide nursing practice for individual and family care, there are theoretical perspectives for understanding community dynamics and assessing the needs and strengths or assets of communities. In addition to providing guidance on the criteria or systems to be assessed when the patient is a community, these theoretical perspectives provide guidance for the development of community diagnoses, program planning, and the process for data collection, analysis, and dissemination of the findings. All **community assessment frameworks and models** presented in this chapter are based on the underlying assumption that successful health programs are those that emerge from empowered communities that participate in all phases of program planning, implementation, and evaluation, with community assessment being the first phase of the empowerment process (Eisen, 1994).

### ■ Community Empowerment

The WHO has provided leadership in the use of **community empowerment** as a means toward health for all. WHO's International Conference on Primary Health Care,

## EPIDEMIOLOGY in Practice

During the community assessment process, data can be organized by the epidemiological triad of host, agent, and environment. The interaction of these factors determines the health status of the community and can be used with any of the models described in this chapter. For example, the host is made up of the members of the community or population; the agent takes many forms, including influences as stress, diet, racism, physical fitness, and access to health services; and the environment includes pollution, water quality, and weather conditions. ⬤

held in 1978 at Alma-Ata, U.S.S.R., concluded that people throughout the world have little control over their own health care and that more positive health outcomes would occur if people had a greater sense of power over programs that address their needs (Glick, Hale, Kulbok, & Shettig, 1996). The term *community empowerment* means "a social-action process in which individuals and groups act to gain mastery over their lives in the context of changing their social and political environment" (Wallerstein & Bernstein, 1994). Based on the work of Brazilian educator Paulo Freire, community empowerment involves a participatory educational process in which people are not just the recipients of political, educational, or health care projects, but become active participants in naming their problems and proposing solutions. For example, empowerment projects should not begin with a nurse-conducted assessment of an at-risk population. Instead, participants from the identified population at risk are recruited by nurses to co-conduct the assessment. Of course, this recruitment process involves a level of trust that has developed between the nurses and the identified population at risk. For more information on building trust when the patient is a community, see "Gaining Entry into the Community" later in this chapter.

Community empowerment is also considered the prerequisite to health promotion. Indeed, the World Health Assembly observes that "the effective participation of the community is indispensable to guarantee the development of health activities and the prevention and control of disease" (WHO, 1984, p. 75). Just as individual patients cannot participate in health promotion until their basic needs are met and they feel some control over their lives, populations and communities must also feel empowered to participate in prevention and health promoting projects.

Community assessment, viewed within the context of community empowerment, is just one part of the methodology that hopefully will lead to health for all. It is an essential component leading to effective, acceptable, affordable health care for our society and all other societies. It is one of the core competencies for nursing practice directed toward communities.

Keck (1994) believes that for community health to become a reality, all health care professionals will need to learn how to empower citizens to take responsibility for decision making related to the community's health, as well as their own. Empowering our patients requires that health professionals give up some of their power and rely on true partnership and collaboration for the community good. Such thinking brings resistance because to promote "power sharing" means to rely on community involvement, not just "lip service," for the advancement in a community's health status. An example of giving up power to the community is when the nurse facilitates the establishment of a board of directors for a community health center made up entirely of community members as the voting members with health care professionals as ad hoc members. Keck (1994, p. 8) contends that "our common challenge [in community health] is the facilitation of that [empowering] process."

## ■ Community Assessment Frameworks/Models

Many community assessment frameworks and models have been designed to guide the process of community assessment. Two theoretical perspectives described here have either been developed by public health nurses or are often used by public health nurses when conducting a community assessment. Other important approaches to community assessment not included in this chapter are *Community Competence: A Positive Approach to Needs Assessment* by Goeppinger and Baglioni (1986) and *The Sunrise Model* by Leininger, which will be addressed in Chapter 10.

Use of a framework or model to help guide a community assessment project is an essential step in the process. A framework/model provides a frame of reference for data collection. Concepts or elements within a theoretical framework or model can be transposed into categories for data collection, diagnosis, and planning. Example concepts or elements that can be transposed into categories for data collection include safety, community boundaries, lines of resistance, and government systems. The following sections of this chapter give examples of how theoretical concepts can be used as criteria for assessment, community diagnoses, and planning.

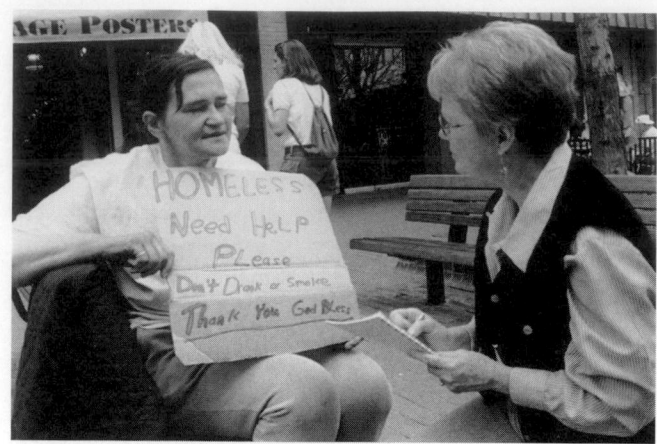

Chapter author Dr. Judith Barton conducting an interview, using the Lundy–Barton Systems Model as a theoretical guide to conduct a community health assessment with a community member who is homeless.

> ### ■■ CULTURAL CONNECTION
>
> We know very little about many communities in the United States because of their "marginal" relationship to the larger society. Sometimes these communities experience self-imposed isolation through their religion, such as the Amish, or by their lifestyle, such as the homeless. Using Kauffman's (p. 43) five phases of "getting in" to a community, how would a community health nurse go about conducting an assessment with these challenging groups?

### Community-as-Partner Model

The *community-as-partner model* includes community assessment as the first phase of the nursing process to be used when the patient is a community. The model is based on nursing theorist Betty Neuman's (1989) total-person model for viewing individual patient problems. Nurse-authors Anderson and McFarlane (2003) developed the model to help guide public health nurses in their practice with communities. The authors explain that the title of the model is purposeful in that the underlying philosophy of the model is primary health care with an emphasis on community empowerment. The model is also intended to be a synthesis of public health and nursing.

The community-as-partner model is a systems perspective that gives direction to types of community systems (e.g., educational system and transportation system) that need to be assessed when conducting a community assessment. It also provides direction for the analysis of the data collected to illuminate community dynamics related to health. Concepts in the model include the *community core*, eight interacting community *subsystems*, community *stressors*, and boundaries titled *normal level of defense*, *flexible line of defense*, and *lines of resistance*.

The *core* of any community is its people. Included in the core are the demographics of the population and their values, beliefs, and history. The core, in turn, affects and is affected by eight interacting subsystems. Those subsystems are physical environment, education, safety and transportation, politics and government, health and social services, communication, economics, and recreation. In addition to assessing the core people within a community and the eight interacting subsystems, the community-as-partner model directs the nurse to assess current stressors that are producing tension within the community, the normal level of defense or current level of health within the community, the flexible line of defense representing current temporary responses to stressors or threats to health within the community, and lines of resistance or established community strengths that weave through all the interacting subsystems. Table 2-2 is a summary of all concepts or elements included in the community-as-partner model and their definitions.

After assessing *all* elements in the model, the researchers are directed to develop community diagnoses that include

> ### ◗ ENVIRONMENTAL CONNECTION
>
> Research has demonstrated a relationship between urban sprawl and greater risk of being overweight and obese. Urban sprawl is defined as a pattern of development across a metropolitan area where large percentages of the population live in lower-density residential areas. Houses are on larger lots; cultural values reflect urban living and emphasize auto use. Consequences include a greater reliance on automobiles and decreased ability to walk to destinations, decreased neighborhood cohesion, and environmental degradation (e.g., greenhouse gas emissions and destruction of open spaces, decreased parks). The CDC has also released findings connecting urban sprawl with obesity, especially in the southern United States.
>
> *Source:* Lopez, R. (2004). Urban sprawl and risk for being overweight or obese. *American Journal of Public Health, 94*(9), 1574–1579.

| Table 2-2 | Community-as-Partner Model: Concepts for Assessment |
|---|---|
| ■ **Community core**  | ■ The people who reside in a geopolitical community or the population of a community. Criteria to evaluate when assessing the core include the community's history, current demographics, and the values and beliefs of community residents. |
| ■ **Interrelated subsystems:** | |
| Physical environment | ■ Observations of the climate, terrain, natural boundaries, commercial systems, neighborhoods, religious symbols, planning studies, and so on. |
| Health and social services | ■ Hospitals and clinics, home health care, extended care facilities, public health services, counseling and support services, clothing, food, shelter, and special needs services. |
| Economics | ■ Household median income, percentage of persons living in poverty, employment status, occupational categories, and union activity. |
| Safety and transportation | ■ Information about protection services (fire, police, water treatment, solid waste) and air quality. Information on public transportation. |
| Politics and government | ■ Type of city government, political action groups, and political party affiliation. |
| Communication | ■ Formal communication sources (e.g., newspapers) and informal communication sources (e.g., bulletin boards, posters). |
| Education | ■ Educational status of community members and educational sources. |
| Recreation | ■ Recreational facilities. |
| ■ **Stressors** | ■ Tension-producing situations within the community, such as an increase in substance abuse among teens within the community. |
| ■ **Normal level of defense** | ■ Health statistics for the community (e.g., mortality and morbidity). |
| ■ **Flexible line of defense** | ■ Community responses to current stressors. |
| ■ **Lines of resistance** | ■ Established strengths within the community (e.g., shelters, food banks). |

*Source:* Anderson, E. T., & McFarlane, J. (2003). *Community as partner: Theory and practice in nursing.* Philadelphia: Lippincott.

| Table 2-3 | Community Diagnosis for Health Planning Using the Community-as-Partner Model | |
|---|---|---|
| **Response (Problem)** | **Related to (Causes)** | **As Manifested by (Data)** |
| ■ Community disorganization and health/social services economic crisis | ■ Increase in illegal immigrant workers from Mexico not eligible for government benefits<br>■ Noncoordinated efforts between agencies within one community and among neighboring communities | ■ Increase in nonreimbursed emergency room care at community hospital<br>■ Increase in free school lunches at local schools<br>■ Increase in delayed prenatal care and lower-birth-weight infants |
| **Goal** | **Objective(s)** | **Evaluative Indicators** |
| ■ Regional coordination of efforts to meet the needs of medical and social underserved populations | ■ Establish a task force made up of service providers and community leaders representing the medically and socially underserved populations to design appropriate and feasible solutions/programs to deal with current community disorganization and health/social services economic crisis | ■ Reduced nonreimbursed emergency room costs, free school lunches, and low birth weight rates<br>■ Increase in first-trimester prenatal care |

community responses to stressors (i.e., problem identification), causative factors leading to each problem, and a list of supporting data to validate each community diagnoses. In other words, the outcome of the community assessment using the community-as-partner model is a set of community diagnoses developed in the same format as nursing diagnoses. In turn, these community diagnoses lay the groundwork for health planning. For an example community diagnosis and plan see Table 2-3.

Although the community-as-partner model does not specifically direct the nurses to develop an interview guide

based on the model's elements, an interview guide using an ethnographic open-ended approach has been developed and can be found in Box 2-5.

### General Systems Model for Community Assessment

Lundy and Barton's (1995) *General Systems Model for Community and Population Assessment and Intervention* is based on general systems theory as originally conceived by Von Bertalanffy (1968). A general systems approach is the basis for many nursing theories and has widespread usage in

**Example Key Informant Ethnographic Interview Guide Based on Community-as-Partner Model**

**Introduction by Interviewer**

*Explain the purpose of the interview (i.e., to better understand the culture and the customs of your community). In addition, confirm that you will be taping the interview so that you do not have to take notes the whole time. Tell the informant that he or she may ask you to stop the taping at any time. Finally, assure the informant that his or her identity will remain confidential in all reports.*

*Grand Tour Question: What is it like to live in your community?*

*Mini-Tour Questions* (some of the following questions, which target community subsystems, may have been thoroughly covered in response to grand tour question):

- What do you do for fun?
- What would you tell someone new to your community about the natural resources (environment) in your community?
- What are the schools like? Where do people go if they want to further their education?
- How safe do you feel in your community? How do you get around (transportation) in your community?
- Who has the political power in the community (i.e., who is the most powerful figure[s] in your community)? Discuss your rationale (reasons).
- Describe your perceptions of the health of your community. Where do you personally go for your health care needs? How adequate are the services available to you?
- Please describe the formal and informal types of communication in your community.
- How would you describe the economic trends/future for your community? If I moved here, how easy would it be to make a living, buy groceries and clothes, and have a place to live?
- Can you tell me something about the cultural and spiritual/religious aspects of your community (e.g., family life, philosophy of community)?
- Is there anything else you would like to tell me about your community?

*Source*: Copyright 1996 The Regents of the University of Colorado. Used by permission.

most all scientific disciplines. This approach to community assessment directs the research team to focus on the whole community, not on the parts of a community. Two broad concepts for assessment using this model include community structure and process.

The structure of any system can be defined as an arrangement of *interacting subsystems* or parts at a given point in time. The system as a whole has specified boundaries that determine what is inside the system and what is outside the system. In turn, each subsystem has boundaries that specify what is inside the subsystem and what is outside. Similar to the community-as-partner assessment model, subsystems within the community system include schools, churches, self-help groups, health systems, and so on. Systems also have a *suprasystem*, the larger construct of which the system is a part. For example, if the community system is identified as a municipality or a city, the county and state where the municipality is situated become suprasystems to the community system and have great relevance to the community system and the community assessment process.

Community health nurses using the general systems assessment approach to community assessment begin by identifying the target system and its boundaries. For example, if the assessment is to be carried out on a geopolitical community named Jonestown, the researchers must ask the following questions:

1. Do the boundaries for Jonestown stop at the city's geopolitical limits or does the community consider a neighboring smaller crossroads community as within its boundaries?
2. What are the critical subsystems within the target community system?
3. What are the critical suprasystems impacting the community?
4. What types of relationships exist among the subsystems and between the target community and its suprasystems?
5. Are the boundaries between subsystems, the system, and its suprasystems open and cooperative, or is there a lack of cooperation and support between these systems?
6. Does the target community system and its subsystems have a sense of integrity or are the boundaries too open?

In assessing *community process*, nurses need to determine how the community system works to meet its needs or goals. Questions to be asked include the following: How is the community system responding (termed *throughput*) to internal and external stimuli or *inputs*? What are the results or *outputs* of the community system's response? (An example of a result or output to a stressor such as air pollution might be stricter auto emission policies.) Is the output successful (negative feedback) or does the Environmental Protection Agency fine the community for having too many poor air quality days per year (positive feedback). In other words, does the community return to a *steady state* or does it continue to experience *disequilibrium*? and How can the community continue to grow from the ongoing processes of *input*, *response*, *output*, and *feedback*?

The Lundy–Barton Model also includes a process for the nurse to use as a follow-through to the community assessment. This process is a familiar one to both nursing and medicine. One assesses the patient (i.e., the community), arrives at several diagnoses, develops a plan of action, evaluates the outcomes, and revises the plan as needed. Table 2-4 is a

| Table 2-4 | Lundy–Barton Model: Concepts for Assessment with Example Questions |
|---|---|

**Community Structure**

| | |
|---|---|
| ■ Target system | ■ *Observations*: Are the boundaries for the target community geopolitical or geographic? How would you describe the natural environment? Describe cultural symbols noted.<br>■ *Measurements*: Demographics, health and social service statistics.<br>■ *Interactions*: History of community, values and beliefs. |
| ■ Subsystems | ■ *Observations*: Windshield survey of public institutions such as schools, churches, businesses, recreational facilities, and so on.<br>■ *Measurements*: Literature on various subsystems within community.<br>■ *Interactions*: Interview key community leaders to find out how the community subsystems interact. |
| ■ Suprasystems | ■ *Observations*: Compare and contrast target community environment with suprasystems (e.g., in comparison to other cities within county).<br>■ *Measurements*: Demographic and health statistic data for most relevant suprasystem (e.g., state statistics) to compare target system with suprasystem.<br>■ *Interactions*: Interview key community leaders to find out how the target community interacts with state or county agencies. |

**Community Process**

| | |
|---|---|
| ■ Goals | ■ *Observations*: Windshield survey may reveal new construction sites indicating growth direction.<br>■ *Measurements*: Seek community planning documents, interview key community leaders concerning goals of community.<br>■ *Interactions*: Does there seem to be agreement among key community leaders about community goals?<br>■ *Observations*: Attendance at community meetings to gain information about particular community stressors (inputs). Windshield survey to observe for environmental hazards. |
| ■ Inputs<br>■ Responses/<br>  throughputs<br>■ Results/outputs<br>■ Feedback | ■ *Measurements*: Review of literature obtained from various community agencies to determine ongoing community initiatives (responses or throughputs). Interviews with key community members to learn more about final outcomes of initiatives and if the initiatives met their objectives (results or outputs and feedback).<br>■ *Interactions*: Is the community experiencing a steady state or is it experiencing disequilibrium? |

*Source*: Lundy, K. S., & Barton, J. A. (1995). Assessment: Data collection of the community patient. In P. J. Christensen & J. W. Kenney (Eds.), *Nursing process: Application of conceptual models* (4th ed., pp. 102–119). St. Louis: Mosby.

---

**ETHICAL CONNECTION**

What about a population that chooses to ignore a critical health problem, as identified by the assessment? Considering the principle of autonomy, how would the community health nurse approach this challenge?

---

summary of all concepts found in the Lundy–Barton Model, their definitions, and examples of types of data to collect. A community assessment guide based on the Lundy–Barton Model can be found in Appendix A.

## Using the Nursing Process for the Community

### ■ Conducting a Community Assessment

More often than not, a community assessment project will be guided by a blend of two or more theoretical perspectives. In addition, a community assessment model or blended

model can be used to conduct a population assessment *in any practice setting*. For example, a nurse in a postpartum unit of a regional medical center noted that there had been an influx of Mexican immigrants. These immigrants were Spanish-speaking only, and no staff spoke Spanish, nor was patient education literature available in Spanish. The nurse in this case realized that she needed to provide the leadership role in conducting a population assessment. Her population assessment included an examination of population demographics in both the hospital and the general community. She then examined the hospital's human resources for language translation and available Spanish-language educational materials. She also interviewed personnel (key informants familiar with the population) on the unit and some of the inpatients as well (**primary informants**). The nurse, with the support of the nurse manager of the unit, raised the consciousness of the hospital administration that patient educational materials and translators should be available for Spanish-speaking patients. The nurse then developed a culturally sensitive child education program including written materials in Spanish. The program was implemented by nurses on the postpartum unit and was well accepted by the immigrant patients and nurses on the unit. Recommendations were made to administration for the program's continuation with support from the Hispanic community. The nurse conducted key and primary informant interviews, gathered secondary data (e.g., community resources for the population and some census data on the population), and analyzed both sources of data to define the strengths and limitations of the population and recommendations for interventions at the population level. Clearly this nurse used her understanding of the connection between population health and individual care regardless of setting (Baldwin et al., 1998).

Once a theoretical perspective or a combination of theoretical perspectives has been chosen to guide the community assessment process, general tenets from the nursing process (i.e., assessment techniques, planning based on the assessment, interventions implemented at the community or population level, and evaluation) will apply. Box 2-6 summarizes steps in the process of a community health assessment.

### Gaining Entry into the Community

The collection of meaningful data about a community depends on the nurse's successfully gaining entry into the community. According to Goeppinger and Schuster, "gaining entry or acceptance into the community is perhaps the biggest challenge in assessment" (1988, p. 202).

Just as you would never just enter a patient's room in a hospital or knock on the door of a home health patient and say, "Turn over in bed, I am here to give you a 'shot,'" the population-focused nurse should not expect to just walk into a community and plan to conduct a community-focused intervention without going through some stages of getting to know the community as patient. As Kauffman (1994) explains in her study of the experience of white nurse researchers who conducted an ethnography of a senior citizen center in a poor, inner-city black ghetto, "getting in" a community is "a process of gaining, building, and maintaining trust with the group under study" (p. 179). Differences in characteristics such as social status, ethnicity, age, and class between the researchers, who are the *outsiders*, and the community being studied, the *insiders*, may create an environment of prejudicial and discriminatory responses that impede *getting in*. In other words, would the community be willing to share their issues with a community assessment team that just barged in and said they were here to study their health and health care needs? Would the results of an assessment set up in this manner produce valid results? Is it not possible that the outsiders could commit flagrant errors in their interpretations that might even promote prejudice and discrimination toward the very community that they intended to assist?

Another strategy found to be helpful is to use a variety of communication channels to "reach" the target population. Using existing personal networks (e.g., clubs, social groups)

---

## BOX 2-6

### Steps in Community-Focused Intervention
*Community defined; partnership established*
*Identification of the community*
*Promotion of the partnership of the community*

**Assessment**
What are the characteristics of the population (age, gender, race)?
Which changes are occurring in the characteristics of the people in the community (births, deaths, migrations)?
Which health problems exist in the community (morbidity rates)?
Which health problems are causing deaths in the population (mortality rates)?
How do these health problems compare with other populations? Are they increasing or decreasing?

**Nursing Diagnoses**
Name the:
Risk of (a specific problem or health risk in the community)
Among (the specific group or population affected by the problem/risk)
Related to (strengths and weaknesses in the community that influence the specific health risk in the community)

**Planning**
Which factors that are changeable (environmental, behavioral) increase the risk of the health problem?
What can most effectively reduce risk among the population?
What can be done in the community to reduce risk?
How much change in the health problem is desired over what period of time in the population (goals and objectives)?
Who can most effectively affect the outcome of the plan?

**Implementation**
What is the role of the community health nurse in the action phase?
Which strategies can facilitate healthy change in the community?

**Evaluation**
Was the plan carried out?
Was it acceptable to the community or population?
Was the health problem changed as planned?
Was the program effective?
What would be done differently?
What are recommendations for future community health promotion?

*Source*: Watson, N. M. (1984). Community as client. In J. A. Sullivan (Ed.), *Community health nursing*. Boston: Blackwell.

---

and social institutions (e.g., voluntary health organizations, churches, schools) that the target population depends on for support and information can both yield positive access results. If the target group has an established health network (e.g., a group of diabetic elders), contacting those medical/health

**"**_It was the world of Southern, rural, black growing up, of folks sitting on porches day and night, of folks calling your mama, 'cause you walked by and didn't speak, and of the switch waiting when you got home so that you could be taught some manners. It was a world of single black older women schoolteachers, dedicated, tough; they had taught your mama, her sisters, and her friends. They knew your people in ways that you never would and shared their insight, keeping us in touch with generations. It was a world where we had a history._**"**

—bell hooks, on growing up in a small
African American Southern community

societies to seek support and approval can provide valuable entry. The nurse must be aware, however, that all members of a subgroup may not be reached through any one organization, thus necessitating the use of diverse means in attempts to initially establish contact with the target population (Keller, Strohschein, Lia-Hoagberg, & Schaffer, 2004). With the Internet, many new opportunities for developing contact and securing information about target groups are possible and hold great promise in this stage of community assessment. Another way to demonstrate the community team's commitment to reach the community is to participate in community activities. Community team members may stay in local motels, rather than chains, and patronize local eateries.

If the community assessment team is very different in social characteristics from the community under study, it would be easy for the outsiders to err by underestimating the effects of ethnicity, age, and class on insiders' responses (Richards et al., 2002). They may use inappropriate data collection tools, or they may assume the insiders are just not knowledgeable enough or educated enough to be able to articulate their health beliefs and health issues. If the assessment team believes the community is not knowledgeable, they may patronize the group (i.e., treat the community with unseemly deference rather than as equals). Locals and important leaders in communities and target populations can function as valuable "cultural brokers," controlling entry into the group, especially to underserved populations. These brokers are often laypersons who might be called "natural helpers," people to whom the community turns for help in times of health concerns and other crises. Identifying these significant persons takes time because they may not be the formal leaders of a group. These brokers can impede "outside" projects or provide invaluable assistance in accessing the group. By serving as local "interpreters," these brokers can translate culture for both the health team and residents and promote collaboration for assessment activities.

Note that it is not detrimental to be an outsider when studying a community. The sociological concept of the "professional stranger" has taught us that being an outsider studying the group allows the researcher to not be caught up in the commitments of the group and therefore to be able to raise questions unlikely to be raised by insiders.

Kauffman (1994) proposes five phases of "getting in" to a community to build trust that will lead to a valid study of the community. These five phases are impressing, behaving, swapping, belonging, and "chillin' out." Kauffman points out that several phases may sometimes occur simultaneously. However, at all times the processes are mutual, interactive, and context specific.

_Impressing_ is the initial and sometimes lengthy process of outsiders and insiders evaluating one another. Social myths are explored; stereotypes and traits of the other (e.g., skin color, clothes, social courtesies) are observed. Rejection is possible by either side. Strategies for the community assessment team to maintain include (1) maintaining political, institutional, and personal neutrality; (2) avoiding obligations to any sponsor or patron of the assessment project; (3) following the rules or customs of all the insiders, not just the leaders; (4) continuing to return to the community and clarifying the assessment process; (5) keeping abreast of local events; and (6) identifying key informants who represent all different groups within the community. An important aspect of a cultural system is its members' valued ideas—those notions about how things should be done. As is so often the case, community members and the community assessment team have different "valued ideas," and cultural clashes occur.

_Behaving_ occurs when actions and interactions between outsiders and insiders begin to erode myths about each other, and each sees the other as fellow human beings, although each side may still guard against rejection. Strategies for continuing the trust-building process in this phase include (1) demonstrating nonjudgmental and unconditional regard, (2) being genuine and avoiding trying too hard to be accepted, (3) learning the language of the group (e.g., the meaning of cultural slang words, perhaps phrases of a foreign language), and (4) placing the insider as the esteemed teacher of community life and health. The gender and age of team members and community members can also play an important part in this phase. For example, using a very young community interviewer in an elderly population may be less effective than using a middle-aged person. Wax (1986) found that middle-aged or older women are more able than any other age or gender to collect data across ages and gender categories. Of course, generalizations must be avoided in any context; however, ignoring age and gender influences can often impede or distort data collection.

_Swapping_ involves reciprocal giving and sharing between the outsiders and insiders. Giving and sharing helps break down the remaining barriers to mutual acceptance and trust between the outsiders and insiders. Strategies used in the swapping process include telling insiders more about the roles of the outsiders (e.g., health programs involved in, outcomes of previous community assessments). Going to community events is an important swapping activity that often allows for informal interviews.

*Belonging* is the culmination of the process. During this phase, outsiders and insiders are able to talk about issues that heretofore provoked discomfort. Issues such as racism, prejudice, and discrimination are open to discussion. Insider language no longer seems foreign to the outsider, who understands the meaning of the language. Greetings and good-byes include physical displays of affection such as hugging. Socially deviant acts such as drug use may no longer be hidden from the outsider.

*Chillin' out* begins as the outsiders near the end of their community assessment phase and begin (hopefully) a long-term partnership with the community for the improvement and maintenance of community health. Outsiders should give insiders an idea of what to expect in the future, such as the amount of help that will always be available from health care experts.

 GLOBAL CONNECTION

International travel nursing is rapidly becoming a growing field. How would knowing the community assessment process benefit a nurse who is traveling to a new city or country for the first time?

### Collecting Data

What kinds of data do nurses look for when conducting a community assessment, and where do they find it? The primary goal of data collection is to acquire meaningful and useful information about the community and its health. A systematic and informed nursing assessment in partnership with the community involves a variety of techniques and resources. The scope of a community or population assessment is determined by the purpose of the assessment and the complexity and nature of the identified community or population. For community assessments of large geopolitical communities, the process may take several months to a year or more and may require an interdisciplinary team.

Confidentiality regarding sensitive or controversial data is a critical issue for nurses conducting a community assessment (Goeppinger & Schuster, 1988). Just as a nurse must safeguard information obtained from the individual patient as an ethical and legal responsibility, the information derived from the community may involve a more concerted effort. Because there are often many team members collecting information from a variety of sources, it may be necessary to assign anonymous names to community members and even to other organizations within the community.

There are seven methods of collecting community data: **informant interviews**, **observation**, **secondary analysis of existing data**, **constructed surveys**, **focus groups**, **community forums**, and **windshield surveys**. The community health nurse should attempt to collect data using several different methods because no method is without bias. The process of using multiple complementary methods is termed *triangulation*.

> **"** *If you don't ask, you don't get.* **"**
> —Stevie Wonder

Informant interviews involve directly questioning community residents. **Key informants** should be identified and interviewed early in the assessment process. These key informants are formal and informal leaders in the community who represent a cross section of age groups and ethnic groups. They include town officials, elected members, student and group leaders, and informal "spokespersons" such as barbers or postal carriers. The nurse uses appropriate communication techniques in directed conversations with selected members of a community. These interviews can be structured, with planned questions, or unstructured, in which the informants guide the interviews. Data gathered through informant interviews are considered subjective and can yield valuable information about the residents' perspectives on health values and health care; for example, how do the residents perceive their community health care services? Such data are recorded in the resident's own words and noted as direct quotations in the interaction column of the assessment tool. Both formal and informal leaders of groups and communities will yield important information about the community.

The nurse uses observation by purposefully looking and listening for significant events that are taking place in the community. Examples include city council meetings, high school basketball games, county fairs, barber shop conversations, and other similar social events. The nurse systematically records these observations. Relevant conversations of community residents are recorded in the interaction column of the assessment tool.

Secondary analysis is analysis of records, documents, and other previously collected data. The nurse may not have to collect new data when conducting the community assessment. Such data may already exist in the form of census data, historical accounts, diaries, previous studies of the community or aggregate, court records, minutes from community meetings, and research studies on population risks. The following research alert describes risks for cross-country truck drivers. The results of this research can be incorporated in a population assessment of cross-country truck drivers and is an example of the use of **secondary data** in a population health assessment. These are invaluable sources of information that can reveal the characteristics of the community as well as the attitudes of people in the community and how they cope with their lives on a daily basis.

Voluntary agencies, such as the American Heart Association, can provide aggregated data on specific health issues. These data are often organized in a more useful and focused format than official agencies. *Healthy People 2010* can be an excellent resource for specific health issues, including baselines and progress in preventive health. State health departments, the U.S. Public Health Service, the National Center for Health Statistics, and the U.S. Census provide a wide array of mortality and morbidity statistics and demographic

## ⊙ MEDIA MOMENT

Just remember, Mr. Potter, that this rabble you're talking about, they do most of the working and paying and living and dying in this community.

— *It's a Wonderful Life*, 1947

**Waking Ned Divine, (1998)**
When a lottery winner dies of shock, his fellow townsfolk attempt to claim the money.

**Where the Heart Is, (2000)**
A pregnant 17-year-old rebuilds her life after being abandoned by her boyfriend at a Wal-Mart in Sequoyah, Oklahoma.

**The Straight Story, (1999)**
An old man makes a long journey by lawnmower to mend his relationship with an ill brother.

**Local Hero, (1983)**
An American oil company sends a man to Scotland to buy up an entire village where the company wants to build a refinery, but things don't go as expected.

**Erin Brockovich, (2000)**
An unemployed single mother becomes a legal assistant and almost single-handedly brings down a California power company accused of polluting a city's water supply.

---

profiles of populations. The CDC is an excellent source for information about national illness and health patterns as well as aggregated state health information.

 ### Research Alert

Long-haul truck drivers spend long hours on the road separated from family and other support systems, drive in hazardous conditions, and are often sleep deprived. Due to the demands of truck driving as an occupation, long-distance truck drivers are considered a population at risk for increased rates of drug use. Researchers and policy makers are especially interested in truck drivers' rates of drug use, the influence of drugs on truck accidents, and the link between drug use and fatigue. Studies have focused on identifying truck drivers at risk for abusing alcohol and drugs and investigating the drug use patterns of long-distance truck drivers.

Researchers interviewed 35 long-haul truck drivers at truck stops and loading facilities in cities and towns across Queensland, Australia. The majority of truck drivers interviewed reported high rates of over-the-counter, prescription, and illicit drug use. Reported use of amphetamines was particularly high.

In contrast to earlier studies that focused on fatigue as the motivating factor in drug use, the researchers found overlapping and changing motivations for drug use among the individual drivers. Using Becker's model of a drug use "career," they found that some of the drivers began using illicit drugs before they joined the truck driving occupation. They were motivated to use drugs by peer pressure, socialization, relaxation, wanting to fit their image of a truck driver, and addiction.

The results of this study indicate that social factors as well as fatigue should be considered when developing drug prevention and treatment programs and policies for truck drivers.

*Source*: Davey, J. J., Richards, N., & Freeman, J. (2007). Fatigue and beyond: Patterns of and motivations for illicit drug use among long-haul truck drivers. *Traffic Injury and Prevention*, 8(3), 7–18; Gay Anderson, D., & Riley, P. (2008). Determining standards of care for substance abuse and alcohol use in long-haul truck drivers. *Nursing Clinics of North America*, 43(3), 357–365.

In constructed surveys, community or aggregate members in a random sample of the population provide answers to written or oral questions. This technique is costly and time-consuming and is used only when other resources have been exhausted. Survey tools are available at the CDC website (www.cdc.gov) for a variety of attitude and opinion surveys with established reliability and validity for community data collection. For example, if a nurse is interested in abortion attitudes and if very little information is available through other techniques, a survey of community members may provide useful information about this issue.

A focus group can be used very effectively to derive information about health needs of specific groups in the community or population. The focus group is a qualitative approach to learning about subgroups within the population regarding sociocultural and other specific characteristics (Clark et al., 2003). Members of a focus group differ from other small groups in that the members are usually chosen to be fairly homogenous in regard to specific characteristics, such as gender, age, or other social variables. By being highly selective about the membership of a focus group, the nurse can learn a great deal about that particular subpopulation's needs and perceptions about viable, acceptable solutions to health problems. The average group meeting lasts 2 to 3 hours and can be a very efficient way to determine group perceptions (Basch, 1987).

A community forum, which involves having an open meeting for all members of a community or population, can also be used to obtain information concerning the needs and perceptions of community members. In contrast to the focus group, a community forum is open to all; no attempt is made to structure a homogenous group. A town hall meeting is a variation of the community forum and was used by President Bill Clinton to bring his health care reform package to the grass-roots level. Even though community forums are not necessarily representative of the entire target population, they can be used effectively in a short period of time, with little cost, as one strategy for community members to voice their views.

The nurse can conduct a windshield survey of the geopolitical community as a technique for data collection.

These observations through the window of an automobile are a way of collecting information about a community's environment. As an initial data collection technique, a windshield survey often reveals common characteristics about how people live (e.g., transportation primarily by automobile, little pedestrian traffic), where they live, and the type of housing they live in.

### ■ Community Diagnosis

Conclusions about data collected on the community patient are a natural outcome of the assessment process. Eventually, these stated analyzed conclusions identify "labels" or names for the health problems in the community; these are called **community health diagnoses** (Higgs & Gustafson, 1985). The gathered data and generated data form a composite database. At this phase of the nursing process, as raw data are analyzed, themes begin to emerge and needs are noted, as are problems, strengths, and community resources. Community members continue to be involved in this process as both subjective and objective data are compiled (Keller, Strohschein, Lia-Hoagberg, & Schaffer, 2004; Keller, Strohschein, Schaffer, & Lia-Hoagberg, 2004).

Written community health diagnoses differ significantly from those written for the individual patient. Most systems of classification developed for nursing diagnoses have focused on the individual. Hamilton (1983) analyzed various theories and diagnostic classification schemata and concluded that research is needed in both the application of individual models of diagnoses and the clarification of the *target* of care, whether that be the community, individuals in the community, or individuals influenced by the community. Viewing the community as a patient who has varying degrees of ability to meet its own needs extends the focus to include response to illness and change, social problems, or any areas in which the community patient needs assistance in order to function optimally (Higgs & Gustafson, 1985). Data from the target community or population are compared with similar populations in other settings. Comparing data such as infant mortality rates or accident rates can reveal significant differences and point to specific disparate health risks in the target population. During this phase, the community health nurse compares conclusions about the community's health status with accepted standards of health and judgments are made as to strengths and concerns of a community's functioning (Lundy & Barton, 1995).

Identified problems are now stated in the form of a community health diagnosis. Each diagnosis is documented, the recipient of care is identified (the community as opposed to the individual), and factors contributing to the problem are explicated.

A common nursing diagnosis format that has been modified for community use has been developed by Schuster and Goeppinger (1996) and Muecke (1984). Here the diagnosis takes the following form:

1. Risk of (a specific problem or health risk in the community)

2. Among (the specific group or population that is affected by the problem/risk)

3. Related to (strengths and weaknesses in the community that influence the specific problem or health risk in the community)

The following are some sample community/population diagnoses using the aforementioned format:

- Risk of lung infections among disaster workers related to debris from Hurricane Katrina recovery
- Risk of hearing loss among studio musicians related to constancy of loud music in occupational settings and nonuse of hearing protection
- Risk for increased incidence of pregnancy among teens at Rydell High School related to increased sexual activity and nonuse of contraceptive services or methods
- Risk for lung damage among migrant farm workers in the Louisiana delta related to presence of pesticide pulmonary irritants in the occupational environment
- Risk of eating disorders among professional ballet dancers related to occupational pressure to stay underweight for professional advancement
- Risk of sleep deprivation among nurses who are permanent night shift workers at Bayview Medical Center related to erratic and interrupted day sleep
- Build on community strength of coordination among community agencies to address all risks or identified community health issues
- Support beginning efforts by faith communities within community to address family solidarity through church-sponsored day-care facilities

### A Good Read

## The Healing Heart: Communities Storytelling to Encourage Caring and Healthy Families (2003)

*By A. Cox and D. Alperts, British Columbia, Canada: New Society Publishers*

This book is a "basket of memories" that is meant to trigger memories for storytelling for use in personal and professional communities. The stories are for sharing among people of all ages, and many of the contributors preface their stories with work-related discussions about programs, projects, agencies, the use of storytelling with their patients, and its impact upon them. Communities include battered women, substance abuse and recovery patients, sex offenders, refugees, immigrants, and an adult prison group. The editors of the book maintain that the book is for people who work with communities so that they may learn to use storytelling in their work.

## ■ Planning and Prioritization Phase

During the **planning phase**, priorities are established, goals and objectives are identified based on those priorities, and community-focused interventions are developed. Unlike a clinical individual diagnosis, a community diagnosis requires more than simple establishment of the presence of a health problem. More than one health problem is always present in a community or population; consequently, diagnoses require prioritizing problems for community action. Criteria must be established to determine how resources and energies will be allocated toward addressing the identified needs (Watson, 1984).

The WHO has published criteria that may be used to prioritize health problems identified in communities. These criteria are listed in Box 2-7.

Goeppinger (1984) has also developed a set of criteria to guide the prioritization of community health problems. Those criteria are as follows:

- Community awareness of the problem
- Community motivation
- Nurse's or team's ability to influence problem solution
- Availability of expertise
- Severity of consequences to society if problems left unresolved
- Quickness with which the problem can be resolved

Reviewing the identified health problems using a set of criteria is a critical step in the process to address complex community health problems. In addition, community members representing multiple subpopulations within the community (e.g., different age groups, ethnic groups), community leaders, and assessment team members should be involved at this stage.

Once the prioritized problem list emerges, goals, objectives, strategies, and plans are developed. *Goals* are broad and general statements of concern that are usually considered long range. *Objectives* are specific, measurable statements of desired outcomes and are often viewed as short term.

All planning group members, community representatives, and other experts within the appropriate areas are involved in this process, especially those who will be most affected and who are in a position to influence the implementation of solutions. The importance of this involvement cannot be overemphasized. Many community interventions have failed and undermined future professional assistance because community teams excluded community members from participating in this process (Goodman et al., 1998). We know from research that when communities and populations develop a vested interest in the identification of health needs and proposed solutions, there is a greater likelihood of sustaining these intervention strategies over time. In other words, the community must be willing to "pay the price" of whatever objectives and goals are proposed (Watson, 1984).

Community health nurses are often members of teams who are conducting community or population level assessments, and as such the identified health problems and concerns are rarely limited to the use of nursing interventions (Robinson, 2005). The complexity of group-identified health concerns requires an interdisciplinary approach, and planning and intervention strategies usually reflect the involvement of other professionals (e.g., social workers, audiologists, physicians, and psychologists) and community resources' utilization (Smith and Barton, 1992).

### 🖥 Research Alert

Catholic Healthcare West (CHW) of San Francisco has developed a national Community Need Index (CNI) to identify and address barriers to health care access in communities. The CNI aggregates five socioeconomic indicators known to contribute to health disparity—income, culture/language, education, housing status, and insurance coverage—and applies them to every ZIP code in the United States. Each ZIP code is then given a score ranging from 1.0 (low need) to 5.0 (high need). Residents of communities with the highest CNI scores have been shown to be twice as likely to experience preventable hospitalization for manageable conditions—such as ear infections, pneumonia, or congestive heart failure—as residents of communities with the lowest CNI scores.

The CNI provides evidence for addressing socioeconomic barriers when considering health policy and local health planning. This tool links health care disparities between geographic regions and illustrates the acute needs of inner-city and rural areas. It may enable health care providers, policy makers, and others to allocate resources where they are most needed, using a standardized, quantitative tool. ◯

*Source*: Roth, R. (2005). The "Community Need Index": A new tool pinpoints health care disparities in communities throughout the nation. *Health Progress*, 86(4), 32–38

## ■ Implementation Phase

The implementation phase is the action phase. It translates the objectives and strategies into reality. Strategies should be selected based on not only currently available resources in the community but also the likelihood that the means will have some long-term availability. During imple-

---

### BOX 2-7

**Criteria for Selecting a Health Problem for Community Intervention**

- Significance of the problem (in terms of numbers affected or consequences)
- Level of community awareness and priority
- Ability to reduce risk
- Cost of reducing risk (economic, social, ethical)
- Ability to identify the target population
- Availability of resources to intervene in the reduction of risk

*Source*: Adapted from World Health Organization (WHO). (1976, October 11–15). Criteria to be considered in selecting a preventive health action. In *Report of the first interdisciplinary workshop on psychosocial factors and health*. Stockholm: Author.

**❝** *When the best leader's work is done, the people say, 'We did it ourselves.'* **❞**

—Lao-Tzu

mentation, lay leaders in the communities, professionals, and organizations must be included and their support acquired. In the long run, it is always better to educate others on how to implement these strategies than for the nurse and other team members to control the implementation (Barton, Smith, Brown, & Supples, 1993). The tendency toward paternalism is strong among health professionals and for many has been reinforced through acute care organizational structures and roles; one must safeguard against the problems of paternalism. In the implementation phase, those community leaders who have greatest probability of achieving success—those whom the community respects and looks to for guidance—are identified. In general, a pilot test should be planned if possible as a trial run of the implementation. In this way, using a few individuals from target groups for feedback, delivery and design issues may be discovered that can be ironed out before the major investments of time, energy, and resources (Clark, 1996). Pilot studies often reveal that more training is needed, along with more or different types of resources and more time. Minor flaws can be corrected; feedback can be collected from the pilot participants with ideas about how the implementation might be changed or improved; and fine-tuning can increase likelihood for success in the implementation (Schuster & Goeppinger, 1996). The following three boxes are all examples of community-focused interventions implemented through a **collaborative arrangement** between health professionals and community leaders.

### Role of the Community Health Nurse

The roles of the community health nurse (CHN) and other professionals depend on the nature of the health problem, the community's ability to make decisions, and professional and personal values and preferences. Also important is the history of the community's ability to solve its own problems. The nurse will play a different role in an established population where there is a history of successful health

Alaskan child with husky puppy.

problem management, as opposed to one that is poorly organized and loosely connected to each other or that has vague community identity. In one case the nurse may serve only as advisor, whereas in another, the nurse must work with the community first to teach the community how to solve problems (Richards et al., 2002).

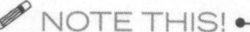

### 🖉 NOTE THIS! ●

**Alaskans Race to Vaccinate: Children as a Population at Risk— A Community-Focused Intervention Implemented Through Collaboration Between Health Professionals and Target Population**

A population assessment revealed that only 52.7% of the young children in Alaska were fully immunized. Through collaboration with several groups, including the University of Alaska Anchorage School of Nursing, the Iditarod Trail Committee, and the Indian Health Service, the Alaska Nurses Association established the "I Did It By TWO Race to Vaccinate" as a health project analogous to the Iditarod Sled Dog Race. The original Iditarod, in 1925, was an appropriate focus event because that relay, in which mushers and dogs carried antitoxin across 700 miles of Alaskan wilderness, halted a diphtheria epidemic. Alaska's "checkpoints" are two, four, and six months of age. The best possible "finishing time" is 12 to 15 months. Any child who reaches the long-distance goal by age two wins an Iditarod certificate autographed by a musher. The Iditarod is the most famous sled dog race in the world, and the mushers who drive the sleds are influential spokespersons. The geographic outreach to connect with the target population was extensive, since the Iditarod Race runs from Anchorage to Nome, covering more than 1,049 miles. The immunization project has become the largest in the nation in conjunction with a sporting event. Outcome evaluation revealed first and second year immunization rates improved to more than 80% in targeted areas.

The Vaccinate Alaska Coalition (VAC), which cosponsors the Race to Vaccinate campaign, along with the Alaska State Health Department, received national recognition for their efforts to promote and provide immunization to people of all ages. Vaccinate Alaska Coalition (VAC) was a recipient of a 2003 Excellence in Immunization Award from the National Partnership for Immunization (NPI) in recognition of its sponsorship of the I Did It By Two! Campaign and the Race to Vaccinate Campaign with the Iditarod Trail Sled Dog Race, which heightens public awareness of the critical need for timely immunization of children from birth through 2 years of age. For the campaign, children pass immunization "checkpoints" in order to cross the finish line and are declared "Winners in the Race to Vaccinate," just as mushers must pass checkpoints in the actual race. Since its inception, the Race to Vaccinate and the I Did It By Two campaign participate in the Iditarod race by providing sled dogs and their mushers with race bibs, which display the Race to Vaccinate slogan. Four-time Iditarod champion Martin Buser and mushers Jon Little and Paul Gebhardt speak throughout Alaska about the crucial role of immunizations in lifelong good health. ◯

Carolyn Keil, PhD, RN
Associate Professor, University of Alaska Anchorage
Project Director, Race to Vaccinate, 1992–1996

*Sources*: Adapted from: Alaskans Race to Vaccinate. (1996). *Reflections* (4th Quarter). Roberts K. (2003). Going the Distance: An itinerant nurse takes health care to the corners of Alaska, *American Journal of Nursing, 103*(12), 102–103; Alaska Department of Health and Social Services. (2005). *Strategic plan 2005–2007*. Juneau, AK: Division of Public Health.

**❝** *The 21st century should be the 'century of the community' and the emphasis of efforts to improve theory and practice ought to reflect this paradigm.* **❞**

*—Robinson, R. G. (2004, April). Response to S. Leonard Syme's essay [Letter to the editor]. Preventing Chronic Disease. Retrieved from http://www.cdc.gov/pcd/issues/2004/apr/04_0005.htm*

 NOTE THIS!

### Carter Center's Interfaith Health Program: Faith Population as Target Community, a Community-Focused Intervention Implemented Through a Collaborative Arrangement Between Health Professionals and Community Leaders

President Jimmy Carter and the Carter Center in Atlanta, Georgia, along with leaders from the Atlanta Interfaith Health Program, have developed a highly successful collaborative project to help faith communities nationwide to prevent disease and promote wellness in their congregations. Through this program, Starting Point, religious groups and health professionals work together to identify risk factors, such as economics or age, and link resources to the church congregations. Dr. Fran Wenger of the Emory School of Nursing in Atlanta is one of the original organizers of this program and is responsible for training lay church leaders in identification of risk and the development of interventions. Religious groups across the country are building an impressive network of leaders, scholars, and community activists who share a common goal: to help people through their churches and religious groups lead more healthful lives. This effort uses a step-by-step training program in which lay volunteers in the church are prepared to be "health promoters." These volunteers then help identify group needs and then work to find appropriate resources, such as the American Cancer Society or the local Red Cross, to meet them. Jimmy Carter sums up the program in this way: "The key to empowering any community, be it religious or otherwise, is team work and a strong spirit of collaboration." ◯

*Source: Starting Point: Empowering Communities to Improve Health. A Manual for Training Health Promoters in Congregational Coalitions. Interfaith Health Program. (1997). Atlanta: The Carter Center.*

## Social Change and Community Action

The age-old question of how to "teach an old dog new tricks" leads us inevitably to the process of change. There are two types of change: unplanned or spontaneous change and planned change. There is considerable debate about the ultimate benefits of unplanned change, but the CHN is most interested in planned and directed change. Such community changes imply that the activities of the CHN are directed toward some goal or goals set in the planning stage of the nursing process (Richards et al., 2002). Intervention activities based on the concepts of planned change center on conscious, deliberate, and intentional actions directed toward **healthy change** in the community (Chin & Benne, 1989). Several forces influence the process of creating meaningful change.

A community assessment report should be shared with target community. Dr. Judith Barton shares County Health Assessment with residents in rural Colorado

The CHN intervenes in changing attitudes, values, knowledge, and skills of the community or population. Kurt Lewin (1951), in his force field theory, postulated that there are always two types of forces that affect the likelihood of change in any situation: driving forces and restraining forces. These two types of forces work in opposition to each other, and Lewin theorized that it is the relative strength of each force that determines whether change will occur. Force field theory postulates that when driving forces are stronger than restraining forces, change occurs.

Driving forces are those influences that favor change. Restraining forces, by contrast, impede change. For example, a group of restless teens, frustrated with the lack of unorganized recreational settings, may be a driving force that motivates a community to establish safe socialization sites for teens to gather. However, the same teen population might feel threatened by adults making the decisions about how these safe socialization sites operate and would, therefore, serve as a restraining force operating against change.

The role of the CHN in promoting healthy change involves manipulating the driving and restraining forces in ways that increase the likelihood of positive changes in the population. This occurs by increasing the driving forces while minimizing the restraining forces. The nurse in the change agent role can promote these changes through an understanding of the process. An underlying assumption of this process is that the community or population must participate in the planning of change (Tembreall & Schaffer, 2005). Some resistance to change can be assumed in most situations. To counter this resistance, the nurse engages the population members in planning the change. Such participation can result in decreased resistance to that change (Lippitt, Langseth, & Mossop, 1985). You will learn more about change theory in Chapter 18.

### Lay Advisors

Community members who hold more status and prestige in the community and are looked to by community members as the "movers and shakers" are the lay advisors who can make or break community intervention. By promoting new ideas and representing positive change, lay advisors provide the connection to the community while often displaying natural leadership abilities that can be encouraged and reinforced by the community health nurse (McKinley, 1973).

 THINK ABOUT THIS ·······································

The virtual community assessment . . . try a community assessment board game!

Dr. Kathleen Masters has developed a board game based on the Lundy–Barton General Systems Tool for Community Assessment; it enables students to apply knowledge and practice skills necessary for performing a community assessment. Students are divided into teams who answer questions about their community by moving along spaces in "cars" through drawing "data" cards. Data include observations related to environment, demographic data, interviews with community residents, and observations of resident behavior. To advance, team members must answer correctly, move to interventions, and eventually reach the evaluation spaces on the board. Teams vote on correct diagnoses based on subjective and objective data presented.

This game helps students learn how to use the community assessment process in a fun way for a trial run before getting out in the real world! ◢

*Source*: Masters, K. (2005). Development and use of an educator-developed community assessment board game. *Nurse Educator, 30*(5), 189–190.

### Focus Groups

Small groups in the community are often the selected mechanism by which change is introduced and sustained. Existing community groups or new groups formed specifically around the community objectives are often successful in implementing healthy change. These groups link the individual to the community. Through formal groups such as church-related organizations or special interest groups, such as the Parent–Teacher Organization, nurses can provide the leadership both in initiating healthy change and promoting the group's efforts toward autonomy and self-care.

### Policy and Legislation

To effect change at the governmental level, collective needs must be translated into a grass-roots power base of influence. Nurses are often unfamiliar with this level of intervention and often need to build coalitions with other influential professional and organizational constituents to effect change. *Policy* refers to the principles and values that govern actions directed toward given ends; policy statements set forth a plan, direction, or goal for action. Because politics is always about scarce resources, the CHN involved in policy changes whether at the local, state, national, or global level effects healthy change in communities by influencing the distribution of resources, the amount of resources allocated, and the recipients of the allocated resources, that is, the target community (Chitty, 1997). Although different from politics, policy is shaped by politics (Mason, Talbott, & Leavitt, 1993).

Through the assessment process, the CHN identifies, along with the community or population, health needs or problems. Depending on the nature of the problem, the CHN can use his or her knowledge of the political process to influence the policy process, such as drafting legislation, providing formal testimony as an advocate for the community, and lobbying governmental officials to make certain that those health issues are a priority for action. All activities are done with the community, by serving as both advocate and educator for the population in efforts to meet those identified goals (Chitty, 1997).

### Mass Media

The most common use of the mass media to promote healthy change in communities has been to communicate specific health information to larger audiences. Using a combination of media forms (television, radio, Internet, newspapers, newsletters, and magazines) provides a greater possibility for exposure and contact with the population. Some community members are more oral, whereas others read more, watch or view television, read newsletters, or notice posters in selected community sites. Some population members might be more likely reached through the Internet. Websites are the latest in media resources that can be successful communication tools for health issues.

Media coverage of health issues and events can be a successful strategy for informing and motivating large numbers of the population (Box 2-8). A well-constructed, focused media campaign can be an excellent means for disseminating and modifying values about health. Such activities can be as simple as a well-timed letter to the editor, which can provide an excellent forum for airing of health concerns and eliciting feedback from the community. Securing the local newspaper's editorial support can be a major factor in soliciting legislators' and other policy makers' attention, particularly with controversial community issues. Press releases should also be considered standard fare for most community projects that serve a targeted population (Box 2-9). In addition, feature writers for local and state newspapers are always looking for stories of interest. Novel approaches to community programs, even the community or population

---

**BOX 2-8**

**Steps in Using the Media for a Health Policy Intervention**

1. Designate one member of the community team who has experience with media relations as spokesperson.
2. Identify health issues from goals that would be appropriately advanced in the media.
3. Work in conjunction with professional organizations and specialty groups to develop a media strategy.
4. Build coalitions with consumer groups and lay leaders in the community.
5. Go public through newspapers, television, radio spots, and websites.
6. Evaluate effectiveness through community response: letters to the editor, phone calls, chat groups on the Internet, and so on.

---

**BOX 2-9**

**Sample Press Release**

*For immediate release. October is Breast Cancer Awareness month. The focus on breast cancer targets all age groups of women and their partners in an effort to educate the public about the importance of early detection and treatment of breast cancer. The American Cancer Society sponsors the national campaign, and local health organizations, schools of nursing, and voluntary health groups working with the American Cancer Society provide speakers, materials, promotional media messages, and community-focused events. The Breast Cancer Awareness Committee of the greater Hattiesburg, Mississippi, area is a group of representatives from health care agencies, voluntary agencies, schools of nursing, and health care consumers who develop various projects in the community to enhance the public's awareness about breast cancer survival in the Pine Belt. Students in the University of Southern Mississippi College of Nursing BSN and RN students are involved in this collaborative effort as part of their community health educational experiences in their senior course, community health nursing. They have developed activities and projects that raise awareness on the college campus about the importance of breast self-examination (BSE). The students learn about the use of the media in community health education. Activities include sorority and fraternity presentations, newspaper press releases, television interviews, a website development focusing on men and breast cancer, and information booths at the student center and post office throughout the month of October.*

*Contact Persons:*
*Breast Cancer Awareness Team, Chairperson, Karen S. Lundy, 601-266-4452*
*American Cancer Society Regional Director, Robert Nerraro*

---

assessment itself, should be of interest to readers, particularly when the newspaper has a large readership. Other media tools include television talk programs, beginning with local television stations and expanding to the networks. The coverage of community health issues not only helps inform the population about health issues but also is an excellent way of promoting positive, accurate public images of nursing in a health promotion role. Publicizing these nursing roles, goals, concerns, and accomplishments in the policy arena will serve to increase the likelihood of public support of nurse-initiated policy recommendations (Hanley, 1984).

### Media Advocacy

**Media advocacy** is the strategic use of the mass media to advance healthy public policy by applying pressure to legislators and other policy makers (Wallack, Dorfman, & Woodruff, 1997). By focusing the attention of those who have the power to change policy, the media become a powerful tool for drawing attention to the actions of a specific group (e.g., the town council, a governing body, or a planning commission). This can also occur when the news story alerts people in the target population to an issue or an action and mobilizes community and population support. The goal in media advocacy is to have the news story told from a public health perspective. This means emphasizing the public policy dimensions of prevention and shifting the focus away from the individual health behavior to the cultural, social, economic, and political context of health issues. When the health issue is visible to large numbers of people, the issue becomes part of the public agenda. Thus, once a health issue is on the public agenda, media advocacy helps advance the goals of community policy by directing public attention to the actions of those responsible for enacting or opposing the policy. For example, one of the problems in lack of initiative concerning the AIDS epidemic was the lack of media attention. The issue did not make it to the national policy agenda as a result of complicated influences, primarily because

the population at perceived risk was the male homosexual community, which had little success accessing the media. Without public attention on an issue or an event, the broader community remains in the dark, along with those who have the power to make the desired change (Wallack, Dorfman, & Woodruff, 1997). According to Daniel Schorr, National Public Radio commentator, "If you don't exist in the media, for all practical purposes, you don't exist" (Communications Consortium Media Center, 1991, p. 7). By using the media to promote healthy change, Flynn (1998) advocates that nurses continue to think "upstream" and focus on fairness and equity in targeting those populations at risk.

### Education

Educational strategies are perhaps the most common strategies used by CHNs in promoting health and preventing illness in both individuals and communities. Educating the target population about available knowledge and community resources is common (Syme, 2004). The purpose of educating the target population about health issues and possible solutions is ultimately to create greater self-sufficiency and a community that is better prepared to make appropriate health-related decisions in the future (Magee, 2005). These include decisions about personal health behaviors, decisions about the use of available health resources, and decisions about societal health issues (Clark, 1996). Education strategies take many forms, including formal presentations, printed materials, community billboards, media, and the Internet. When current information and research are provided about health issues, people can become more involved in their own self-care and make informed decisions regarding personal behaviors that promote health; for example, should ear protection be used by persons in a rifle club, or should teens be held to a higher standard regarding alcohol use and driving automobiles? Health education can be viewed as a means of freeing people in populations from influences that lead them to unhealthy behaviors. Education is much more than merely imparting knowledge and skills; it includes helping people change their attitudes to those more conducive to healthful behavior. People learning to use resources—learning not only what is available in the community but how to apply that knowledge in promoting healthy change—is an even more empowering strategy (Greenberg, 1989).

On a more global level, populations can be educated about decisions related to social health issues, such as AIDS or teen suicide risks. For example, educating the target population can assist people in determining whether they support legislation that requires motorcyclists to wear helmets or that bans smoking in public buildings. An informed population is better able to make decisions about major health issues that affect their lives (Clark, 1996).

## ■ Evaluation Phase

To evaluate the effectiveness of implementations, the nurse evaluates the responses of the community to the interventions, the progress that has been made in affecting outcome measures, such as statistical changes, and how well the efforts have fared in comparison to the goals and objectives. Evaluation data are collected in various formats and should come from diverse viewpoints, both from the target population and from the team members (Anderson & McFarlane, 2003). Because the nursing process is cyclical instead of linear, evaluation as the final step in the process ultimately affects the next assessment. In community health interventions, there rarely is a true end point, but rather there is a dynamic interplay of the steps in a process. The effectiveness of community nursing interventions depends on continuous reassessment of the community's health and on appropriate revisions in the planning interventions. Essentially, evaluation boils down to this: What has been the intervention's impact on the health of the target population or community? Because the community is so complex and so many variables affect the outcome of health measures, it is often difficult to measure all the variables, including the interventions, that

shaped the outcomes. The nurse must be cautious about attributing changes to the interventions, or denying influence because of lack of concrete evidence that changes occurred. Was it worth the time and effort and resources? What would or could be done differently in the future? Equally important, the community must have an opportunity to shape the evaluation conclusions. Before a final analysis and evaluation report is finished, the team should seek input from the community and population members. Does the community deem the process a success? After all, the perceived results are most important in the final analysis and should be reported in the formal conclusions.

The evaluation process entails both formative evaluation and summative evaluation. *Formative evaluation* measures focus on the process *during* the community interventions (Clark, 1996). For example, perhaps a strategy had been devised in which parents of young children would be offered a safety class on accident prevention at home. This class was initially offered on Saturday mornings. In the first two classes, only a few parents attended. It was discovered that Saturday mornings were often taken up with Little League sports and dancing lessons. The class was rescheduled for a weekday after work and attendance doubled within a week. In contrast, *summative evaluation* refers to the outcomes of the interventions, those measures that include end of intervention evaluations. Such measurements as satisfaction surveys, self-reports from parents of changes in their use of safety information in the home, or changes in the number of home accidents reported by the local hospital are all summative evaluation strategies (Benner & Meleis, 1978).

Putting the evaluation into lay terms in the final report to the community is expected of all community assessment team projects. The media (e.g., newsletters, local newspapers, television stations, and the Internet) and churches are appropriate resources for distributing the final report to the community. Whatever the outcome, because of the community assessment process, both the team members and the target population are changed (Magee, 2005). Closure in the form of a final report can have a critical impact on the future of the populations or community's response to health challenges and interventions.

## Conclusion

Assessment of communities or populations is a critical nursing skill in the rapidly evolving U.S. health care system. The need for nurses to be able to assess communities and populations as the focus of nursing care has always been an integral skill for public health nurses working in official public health agencies. With an increasing focus on keeping participants of health care plans healthy, an emphasis on health promotion and prevention brings evidence-based, community-focused interventions to the forefront for professional nursing. In addition, health care agencies receiving federal funding to offset expenses incurred for treating the underinsured or noninsured are now required to assess the communities and populations they serve. In other words, there is a new emphasis on prevention rather than illness care pervading the U.S. health care system as outcome measures form the basis of reimbursement and service continuations. Preparation in community/population assessment is essential for nurses at the BSN level in all settings to promote the health of their patients.

Explore Community Health Nursing on the Web! To learn more about the topics in this chapter, use the passcode provided to access your exclusive website: **http://nursing.jbpub.com/ communityhealth.** If you do not have a passcode, you can obtain one at this site.

## ■ CRITICAL THINKING ACTIVITIES

Population Assessment Guide for Community Health Nursing Students: An Introductory Field Experience for a Local Geopolitical Community

1. Before beginning your community assessment, identify the conceptual framework you would like to use in organizing your community assessment. Remember, a conceptual framework for community assessment will help you in knowing what data to collect, how you should collect the data, and how to interpret the analysis of data for community planning.

2. Go to the local library or to the Internet and access census data for your community before going out to the community so that you have a feel for the social status of your community. Necessary demographic data to collect include the following:
   - Total population for catchment area
   - Racial composition (%) for catchment area
   - Ethnic composition (%) for catchment area
   - Age distribution (% by category) for catchment area
   - Educational attainment (% by category) in catchment area
   - Percentage of all persons living below poverty level
   - Percentage of children younger than age of 5 living below poverty level
   - Percentage of persons 65 years and older living below poverty level
   - Percentage of females 16 years and older who have children younger than 6 years of age and who work outside the home

   Use census data to compare to your catchment area.

3. Meet with a key informant at the designated time. Ask the key informant to tell you what he or she knows about the immediate community in which the health center is located. What kind of people live in the community? What are some of the health issues (views of health are broad, including economic, political, cultural, education issues)? What does the key informant see as a primary strength of the community?

   Ask your key informant about specific gathering places within the community where you might talk to community members, such as fire stations, housing offices, recreation centers, and so on.

   Ask your key informant if it would be okay if you talked to a few of the patients waiting in the clinic area. Explain that you will introduce yourself as a student nurse who is conducting a community health needs assessment and you will then ask the waiting patients to just describe what it is like to live in this community.

4. Spend a little time in the clinic setting meeting some of the patients in the waiting rooms. Many of the clerks working in these clinics live in the neighborhood, and they may also be willing to talk to you. Be brave! Find out all you can about what it is like to live in the community. What is a strength of the community? What is a need? How has the community changed across time (history)? What is currently happening in the community? These are general "round the world" questions that can open up a full discussion. Write down the questions mentioned in this guide on an index card. When in doubt as to what to say next, just ask the person to more fully describe what they are talking about. For example, if the person is talking about gang crimes in the neighborhood, you can ask, "Can you tell me some more about this problem with gangs?"

5. Gather outside the clinic and take a windshield survey of your community (census tract boundaries). Pay attention to environmental characteristics such as range of housing, industry, recreation facilities, and so on.

6. Spend some time talking to members of the community who are located outside the clinic area. For

example, you may venture into the recreation center and talk to a few people. Venture into a daycare center and ask to talk to the workers, children, and parents. Ask again about what it is like to live in the neighborhood.

7. Review any secondary data (e.g., health status reports) you were able to obtain from your key informant or others in the community.

8. Meet for lunch or an afternoon snack to analyze the findings from the secondary and primary sources. As a group, brainstorm about strengths and needs of the community assembled from observations, interviews, census data, and any previous reports you have been able to obtain. Develop two to three community diagnoses. Decide on an outline for a written report on your community assessment, and write a report on your community assessment as a group or divide up the outline for section writing.

9. Do an oral presentation of your community assessment. Share your findings with the "target" community and with your classmates.

*Source*: Adapted from Barton, J. (1997). "Undergraduate Mini Community Health Assessment." University of Colorado School of Nursing Health Sciences Center.

## ■ REFERENCES

Aiken, L. H., & Salmon M. E. (1994). Health care workforce priorities: What nursing should do now. *Inquiry, 31*, 318.

American Association of Colleges of Nursing (AACN). (1986). *Essentials of college and university education for professional nursing: Final report*. Washington, DC: Author.

American Nurses Association (ANA). (1986). *Standards of community health nursing practice*. Kansas City, MO: Author.

American Public Health Association (APHA), Public Health Nursing Section. (1981). *The definition and role of public health nursing in the delivery of health care. A position paper*. Washington, DC: Author.

Anderson, E. T., & McFarlane, J. (2003). *Community as partner: Theory and practice in nursing* (4th ed.). Philadelphia: Lippincott.

Association of Community Health Nursing Educators (ACHNE). (2000). *Essentials of baccalaureate nursing education for entry level practice in community health nursing*. Louisville, KY: Author.

Baldwin, J. H., Conger, C. O., Abegglen, J. C., & Hill, E. M. (1998). Population-focused and community-based nursing—moving toward clarification of concepts. *Public Health Nursing, 15*(1), 12–18.

Barton, J. A., Smith, M., Brown, N. J., & Supples, J. M. (1993). Methodological issues in a team approach to community health needs assessment. *Nursing Outlook, 41*(6), 252–261.

Basch, C. (1987). Focus group interview: An underutilized research technique for improving theory and practice in health education. *Health Education Quarterly, 14*(Winter), 411–448.

Benner, P., & Meleis, A. (1978). Process or product evaluation? *Nursing Outlook, 23*, 302–307.

Bernal, H., Shellman, J., & Reid, K. (2004). Essential concepts in developing community-university partnerships carelink: The partners in caring model. *Public Health Nursing, 1*, 21, 32–40.

Carney, J. K. (2006). *Public health in action: Practicing in the real world*. Sudbury, MA: Jones and Bartlett.

Cassel, J. (1976). The contribution of the social environment to host resistance. *American Journal of Epidemiology, 104*(2), 107.

Chin, R., & Benne, K. D. (1989). General strategies for effecting changes in human systems. In W. L. French, C. H. Bell, & R. A. Zawacki (Eds.), *Organization development: Theory, practice and Research* (pp. 89–95). Homewood, IL: BPI Irwin.

Chitty, K. (1997). *Professional nursing: Concepts and challenges* (2nd ed.). Philadelphia: W. B. Saunders.

Clark, M. J. (1996). *Nursing in the community* (2nd ed.). Stamford, CT: Appleton and Lange.

Clark, M. J., Cary, S., Diemart, G., et al. Involving communities in community assessment. *Public Health Nursing, 20*(6), 456–463.

Communication Consortium Media Center. (1991). *Strategic communication for non-profits: Strategic media—Designing a public interest campaign* (p. 7). Washington, DC: Benton Foundation and the Center for Strategic Communications.

Community Health Advisor Network. (1999). *Community facilitator implementation manual*. Jackson, MS: Freedom from Hunger.

Cottrell, L. S. (1976). The competent community. In B. H. Kaplan, R. N. Wilson, & A. H. Leighton (Eds.), *Further explorations in social psychology*. New York: Basic Books.

Eide, P. J., Hahn, L., Bayne, T., Allen, C. B., & Swain, D. (2006). The population-focused analysis project for teaching community health. *Nursing Education Perspectives, 27*(1), 22–27.

Eisen, A. (1994). Survey of neighborhood-based, comprehensive community empowerment initiatives. *Health Education Quarterly, 21*(2), 235–252.

Flynn, B. C. (1994). Partners for healthy cities. *Healthcare Forum Journal, 37*(3), 55–56.

Flynn, B. C. (1998). Communicating with the public: Community-based nursing research and practice. *Public Health Nursing, 15*(3), 165–170.

Flynn, B. C., & Dennis, L. I. (1996). Health promotion through healthy cities. In M. Stanhope & J. Lancaster (Eds.), *Community health nursing: Promoting health of aggregates, families and individuals*. St. Louis: Mosby.

Flynn, B. C, Ray, D., & Rider, M. (1994). Empowering communities: Action research through healthy cities. *Health Education Quarterly, 21*(3), 395–405.

Gebbie, K. M. (1996, November 18). *Preparing currently employed public health nurses for changes in the health care system: Meeting report and suggested action steps*. New York: Columbia University School of Nursing Center for Health Policy and Health Sciences Research. (Report based on meeting in Atlanta, July 11, 1996.)

Glick, D. F., Hale, P. J., Kulbok, P. A., & Shettig, J. (1996). Community development theory: Planning a community nursing center. *Journal of Nursing Administration, 26*(7/8), 44–50.

Goeppinger, J. (1984). Primary health care: An answer to the dilemmas of community health nursing? *Public Health Nursing, 3*, 129–140.

Goeppinger, J., & Baglioni, A. J. (1986). Community competence: A positive approach to needs assessment. *American Journal of Community Psychology, 13*, 507.

Goeppinger, J., Lassiter, P. G., & Wilcox, B. (1982). Community health is community competence. *Nursing Outlook, 30*(8), 464.

Goeppinger, J., & Schuster, G. (1988). Community as patient: Using the nursing process to promote health. In M. Stanhope & J. Lancaster (Eds.), *Community health nursing: Process and practice for promoting health*. St. Louis: Mosby.

Goodman, R. M., Speers, M. A., McLeroy, K., et al. (1998). Identifying and defining the dimensions of community capacity to provide a basis for measurement. *Health Education Behavior, 2*(33), 258–278.

Gordon, L. J. (1990). Who will manage the environment? *American Journal of Public Health, 80*, 904–905.

Gordon, L. J. (1993). The future of environmental health and the need for public health leadership. *Journal of Environmental Health, 56*(5), 38–40.

Greenberg, J. S. (1989). *Health education: Learner-centered instructional strategies.* Dubuque, IA: W. C. Brown.

Hamilton, P. (1983). Community health diagnosis. *Advances in Nursing Science, 5*(3), 21–36.

Hancock, T. (1993). The evolution, impact and significance of the Healthy Cities/Healthy Communities movement. *Journal of Public Health Policy, 14*(1), 5–18.

Hanley, B. (1984). Legislation and policy. In J. A. Sullivan, *Directions in community health nursing.* Boston: Blackwell.

Hegyvary, S. T. (1990). Education: Redefining community. *Journal of Professional Nursing, 6*(1).

Higgs, Z. R., & Gustafson, D. D. (1985). *Community as patient: Assessment and diagnosis.* Philadelphia: F. A. Davis.

Kauffman, K. S. (1994). The insider/outsider dilemma: Field experience of a white researcher "getting in" a poor black community. *Nursing Research, 43*(3), 179–183.

Keck, C. W. (1994). Community health: Our common challenge. *Family and Community Health, 17*(2), 1–9.

Keller, L. O., Strohschein, S., Lia-Hoagberg, B., & Schaffer, M. (1998). Population-based public health nursing interventions: A model from practice. *Public Health Nursing, 15*(3), 207–215.

Keller, L. O., Strohschein, S., Lia-Hoagberg B., & Schaffer, M. A. (2004). Population-based public health interventions: Practice-based and evidence-supported. (Part I). *Public Health Nursing, 21*(5), 453–468.

Keller, L. O., Strohschein, S., Schaffer, M. A., & Lia-Hoagberg, B. (2004). Population based public health interventions: Innovations in practice, teaching, and management. (Part II). *Public Health Nursing, 21*(5), 469–487.

Kopf, E. W. (1986). Florence Nightingale as statistician. In B. W. Spradley (Ed.), *Readings in community health nursing.* Boston: Little, Brown.

Lalonde, M. (1974). *A new perspective on the health of Canadians—a working document.* Ottawa: Government of Canada.

Leininger, M. M. (1988). Leininger's theory of nursing: Cultural care diversity and universality. *Nursing Science Quarterly, 1*(4), 152–160.

Lewin, K. (1951). *Field theory in social science.* New York: Harper.

Lia-Hoagberg, B., Schaffer, M., & Strohschein, S. (1999). Public health nursing practice guidelines: An evaluation of dissemination and use. *Public Health Nursing, 16*(6), 397–404.

Lippitt, G. L., Langseth, P., & Mossop, J. (1985). *Implementing organizational change.* San Francisco: Jossey-Bass.

Lundy, K. S., & Barton, J. A. (1995). Assessment: Data collection of the community patient. In P. J. Christiansen & J. W. Kenney (Eds.), *Nursing process: Application of conceptual models* (4th ed.). St. Louis: Mosby.

Magee, C. G. (2005). Public health consequences of imprisonment: Preventive care for women in prison: A qualitative community health assessment of the Papanicolaou test and follow-up treatment at a California state women's prison. *American Journal of Public Health, 95*, 10.

Mason, D., Talbott, S., & Leavitt, J. (Eds.). (1993). *Policy and politics for nurses: Action and change in the workplace, government, organization and community* (2nd ed.). Philadelphia: W. B. Saunders.

McKinley, J. B. (1973). Social networks, lay consultation, and help-seeking behavior. *Social Forces, 53*(1), 275.

Mead, G. H. (1934). *Mind, self, and society.* Chicago: University of Chicago Press.

Montero, L. A. (1985). Florence Nightingale on public health nursing. *American Journal of Public Health, 75*(2), 181.

Muecke, M. A. (1984). Community health diagnosis in nursing. *Public Health Nursing, 1*(1), 23–35.

Neuman, B. (1989). *The Neuman systems model: Application to nursing theory and practice.* Norwalk, CT: Appleton-Century-Crofts.

Reinhart, U. W. (1984). Rationing the health-care surplus: An American tragedy. *Nursing Economics, 1*(4), 210.

Richards, L., Kennedy, P. H., Krulewitch, C. J., et al. (2002). Achieving success in poor urban minority community-based research: Strategies for implementing community-based research within an urban minority population. *Health Promotion Practice, 3*(3), 410–420.

Robinson, R. G. (2005). Community development model for public health applications: Overview of a model to eliminate population disparities. *Health Promotion Practice, 6*(3), 338–346.

Rodgers, S. (1984). Community as patient—a multivariate model for analysis of community and aggregate health risk. *Public Health Nursing, 1*(4), 210.

Ruth, J., Eliason, K., & Schultz, P. R. (1992). Community assessment: A process of learning. *Journal of Nursing Education, 31*(4), 181.

Salmon, M. E. (1993). Public health nursing—the opportunity of a century. *American Journal of Public Health, 83*, 1674–1675.

Schuster, G., & Goeppinger, J. (1996). Community as client: Using the nursing process to promote health. In M. Stanhope & J. Lancaster, *Community health nursing: Promoting health of aggregates, families and communities* (pp. 289–314). St. Louis: Mosby.

Smith, M. C., & Barton, J. A. (1992). Technologic enrichment of a community needs assessment. *Nursing Outlook, 40*(1), 32–37.

Sweeney, N., & de Peyster, A. (2005). Assessing environmental health risk in the home. *Nurse Educator, 30*(3), 104–108.

Syme, S. L. (2004, January). Social determinants of health: The community as an empowered partner. *Preventing Chronic Disease.* Retrieved from http://www.cdc.gov/pcd/issues/2004/jan/syme.htm.

Tembreull, C. L., & Schaffer, M. A. (2005). The intervention of outreach: Best practices. *Public Health Nursing, 22*(4), 347–353.

Von Bertalanffy, L. (1968). *General systems theory.* New York: George Braziller.

Wallack, L., Dorfman, L., & Woodruff, K. (1997). Communications and public health. In F. D. Scutchfield & C. W. Keck (Eds.), *Principles of public health practice.* Albany, NY: Delmar.

Wallerstein, N., & Bernstein, E. (1994). Introduction to community empowerment, participatory education, and health. *Health Education Quarterly, 21*(2), 141–148.

Watson, N. M. (1984). Community as patient. In J. A. Sullivan (Ed.), *Directions in community health nursing.* Boston: Blackwell.

Wax, R. H. (1986). Gender and age in fieldwork and field work education: "Not any good thing is done by one man alone." In T. L. Whitehead & M. E. Conaway (Eds.), *Self, sex and gender in cross-cultural fieldwork.* Urbana: University of Illinois Press.

Williams, C. A., & Highriter, M. E. (1978). Community health nursing: Population focus and evaluation. *Public Health Reviews, 7*(2–4), 197.

World Health Organization (WHO). (1985). *Handbook of resolutions and decisions by the World Health Assembly and the Executive Board, 1972–1984* [Vol. 2(31), 42]. Geneva: World Health Assembly.

## The Lundy–Barton General Systems Model for Community and Population Assessment and Intervention

The unique responsibility of community health nursing practice is defining problems and proposing solutions at the population level. The process of making this connection from the individual to the community has proven to be an especially difficult task for the nurse conducting a community or population assessment. The community health assessment process is based on the understanding of the community as patient. Although nurses wouldn't consider the omission of individual patient assessment and base intervention on intuition, this is almost precisely what happens when we fail to do a thorough assessment when planning and delivering health care services to community populations. For example, we would not ever consider just examining the arm of a patient and totally ignoring the rest of the body when we plan nursing interventions. And yet by looking at only one aspect of the community, such as the physical parameters, we are just examining the "arm" and ignoring the "body" and "mind" of the community. One of the major difficulties in conducting a community assessment is that students and practicing nurses alike have often been limited to individualistic patient care. This focus on personal care sometimes presents difficulty in the transference of those skills to assessment and problem solving at the community and population levels.

The Lundy–Barton Model uses familiar systems theory and the nursing process to guide the collection and interpretation of data, development of problems and areas of need, and evaluation of nursing strategies to promote community health. The model includes a database, a needs list, assessment, and a plan to address each need with progress notes delineated for selected problems. Each of these components will be discussed in relation to community assessment with concurrent identification of the nursing process components.

## Database (Assessment Phase: Nursing Process)

The collection of data corresponds to the assessment phase of the nursing process. The collection of data has one primary goal–to learn about the patient. The exploration of available data about the community can be general or quite specific, depending on the definition of the community or population as well as the purpose of the project. An example of how the definition of community can affect the assessment of a community can be illustrated by the distinction of the community as a *place* or *nonplace*. A *place* community, according to Anderson and Carter (1974), refers to a specific geographic locality, one that can be defined by physical boundaries. This definition is the one most often used in health planning projects for specific urban or rural locales. A *nonplace* community is defined as one based on cooperation and commitment by its members to common goals and ideologies. A nonplace community is in a sense a "mind" community, such as the academic community or the nursing community. The distinction can also be made on the degree of attachment to a specific locale and the scope of activities, interest, and needs. Place communities have the greatest attachment to a specific locality, whereas nonplace communities usually have limited geographic ties. Nonplace communities generally are narrow in their scope of activities, interests, or needs, whereas place communities have a wider scope of activities, interests, and needs. Defining the community as a place or nonplace will thus affect the direction and method of assessment (Anderson & Carter, 1974).

There are eight categories of data, which are presented in the following section and are considered necessary for the database of a community or population assessment.

## Community Profile

What makes the identified community different from any other community? The "community patient" is somewhat harder to get to know than the individual patient. Instead of using temperature, pulse, respiration, blood pressure, and so on, the indices of a community will take the form of *demographics* and *vital statistics*, such as morbidity/mortality rates, sex, age, ethnic and racial distributions, educational levels, occupation/employment patterns, and socioeconomic patterns. *Mortality rates* are important indices because they provide a picture of the health and living conditions of a community. The *infant mortality rate* is considered perhaps the most sensitive indicator of a community's health status. According to Taylor, "such indices require a basic readjustment in thinking. A woman is either pregnant or not pregnant; a community is about 3% pregnant. A patient has or does not have heart disease; the community always has heart disease though the rate may go up or down" (Mattison, 1968).

Demographic data can be found in local and state health departments and on the Internet. United States census data are an excellent source for demographic data concerned with population density, population age distribution, occupational distribution, socioeconomic characteristics (income, education, employment), and marital status. Information concerning the kinds of family forms that are prevalent—young families with small children, percentage of women working, and so on—is also available through the U.S. Census and can provide useful information for the identification of family needs.

Information about how the population is distributed spatially is extremely important in considering the location, distribution, and delivery of health services. Whether a population is densely or sparsely populated has been shown to affect other aspects of people's lives such as norms, values, and types of health problems. Population density can also affect behavior and the emotional health of residents.

Information about the percentage of persons in each age category contributes to the assessment of health needs. Many times, when the age distribution is examined in a historical context, it becomes evident that there has been a population shift over time.

Morbidity and mortality statistics can help provide a statistical picture of the community or population in terms of the incidence and prevalence of specific diseases and deaths within a community. These statistics can be obtained through local and state health departments and the CDC (for specific population groups such as teenagers) as well as from special-interest groups, such as the American Cancer Society or the American Heart Association, or the various population interest groups such as women with HIV/AIDS. Most can be obtained from the Internet.

## Comparison of the Profile

Demographics and other statistics *should be compared* with adjoining communities or similar populations, the state, and/or the nation to ascertain the relative significance of the statistics. Not only can these comparisons provide clues as to what kinds of health problems and needs exist in a particular community, but they can also provide an evaluation of the effectiveness of existing health services and programs.

### ■ Psychological Climate

Just as an evaluation of an individual patient includes an examination of his or her psychological status, an assessment of the community is incomplete without evaluating the psychological aspects. There are three areas: (1) self-concept, (2) attitude toward health, and (3) history and changes over time. How the community views itself is usually based on history and traditions from the past. How does one find out what kind of *self-concept* the community or population has? Ask the members! Each community often thinks of itself in terms of descriptors such as "we are a friendly place," or "we just leave each other well-enough alone," which can reflect

whether the inhabitants see themselves as being connected to adjoining communities or separate from them. Listen to the people talking with one another–are the inhabitants proud of their community or are they somewhat distanced and seemingly apathetic? Does the population express powerlessness or worthlessness, such as women who have been abused by parents? Focus groups are an excellent means of listening to the voices of the often "hidden" community members; elderly, mothers of small children, people with disabilities, and so on (Clark et al., 2003).

In addition to evaluating the community's self-image as an indicator of the psychological climate, it is useful to determine the *community's attitude toward health in general*. Is health care a priority in the community? Indicators such as safety and public service media messages (e.g., radio, television, billboards) are evidence of the degree of voluntary efforts for the development of health programs and should aid in the assessment of where health fits into the community priority structure. What is the website of the community or group like? Is it current? Do members of community interact with each other—either online on "blogs" or in person? Populations have a wide variety of attitudes and values about health. Teens may have very little interest in health because of their developmental level of self-awareness.

A third area to assess in terms of the psychological database is information concerning the *historical changes that a community has experienced* and its response to those changes. Understanding the history of the community or population—how and when it came to be, how it has responded to change (e.g., industrial growth, highway construction, rapid population growth or decline), and how it has dealt with health problems in the past—would all be helpful in planning realistically for health services. A community's experiences, its ability to mobilize resources, and dominant patterns of solutions to health problems all significantly affect how that community will respond to intervention. For example, the population of homosexual men has a long history of discrimination in the United States and may exhibit a distrust of the traditional health care system as a result. Knowledge about the community's past can give perspectives on the present and future. A community recovering from a catastrophic natural disaster, such as a major flood, may take years to recover.

### ■ Nutritional Evaluation

A history and evaluation of the community's nutritional status, as a part of the community assessment process, includes identification of sources of food (e.g., homegrown, imported into community, processed foods, fast foods), ethnic or regional food prevalence, and food preparation customs (e.g., vegetarian, seafood availability, wild game). Morbidity/mortality statistics related to nutritional status and resources (e.g., goiter, cardiac disease, cancer) are also vital information to include in the nutritional assessment. A population of truck drivers, for example, may have nutritional patterns of consumption related to their erratic pattern of eating on the run.

### Physical Fitness

In examining the community's "fitness," the presence or absence of exercise/fitness facilities available and/or used by the public, such as jogging and bicycling trails, are most certainly a reflection of its inhabitants' interest in physical fitness. Although most communities do not fall into a clear-cut category of either sedentary or active, one pattern usually tends to dominate and can provide important health status information. As a population, elders tend to be more sedentary than their younger counterparts.

### Physical Examination

A physical examination of the community patient involves a hands-on type of approach. This obviously applies only to a geographic community. Shumway and Wisehart (1969) suggest using a walking tour to know a community at the resident level. They advise that getting "a feel for a community" involves a *systematic approach of observations* that can ultimately increase one's sensitivity to the surrounding ecological elements. If the community can be defined as a place community, the *geographic boundaries should be defined* and described as clearly as possible. Parameters can be defined in several ways: census tracts, natural boundaries (e.g., mountains, rivers), or roads and streets, specifically noting terrain, proximity to needed resources, and *isolation/proximity* to other communities. The *climate* has been demonstrated to have a significant effect on the health risks of a population. Whether the climate is desert or mountainous can affect the lives of the inhabitants in dramatic ways. Such factors as road conditions, animal vectors, housing conditions, and general appearances of the community should be noted in the physical assessment of the community.

## Review of Systems

Once the "physical examination" has been done, it is important to conduct a review of systems within the community or population. This review should include an assessment of the services and facilities, human power, government (federal, state, county), and leadership (formal and informal) of both health and nonhealth systems that affect the population or community.

The *health system* should include all organizations and services that provide health care. The private health services and public health services should be examined not only for availability and quality, but also for the degree of coordination between the services. The availability of homes for the elderly, services for the disabled (including accommodation in the community, such as access ramps), mental health services, and disaster preparedness for the community are examples of such services to be assessed. As community workers know all too well, it is often not a case of availability of needed services, but rather a lack of coordination within agencies, a lack of awareness of the services by the community members, an unwillingness by the members to use the facilities, or unacceptability of resources or services as a result of cultural differences. The source of health care is another important aspect of this assessment of health care systems specific to the community. Particularly in rural communities, the local pharmacist may be the primary source for health information and should be included in the assessment. Most members of population seek health care and advisement on health issues from nonprofessionals daily. These sources should be identified in the assessment.

*Nonhealth systems*, such as the political system, the economic system, the educational system, and the religious system, should be assessed as critical influences on the health of a community. Health care does not exist in a vacuum apart from the other social structures within a community; it is influenced by and influences other systems within the community.

The *political system/atmosphere* of a community can be assessed through various sources: the local newspaper, community action groups, and/or previous history and political activities. The community should be assessed as liberal or conservative.

Klein (1965) identifies three important components of the political system that reflect interaction patterns of a community. This can also be applied to a population. *Authority* within a community can be often identified by the political leaders of a community—both elected, official leaders and nonofficial leaders (e.g., religious leaders). *Power* is often associated with authority but is not by any means limited to it. Power patterns in a community can often be identified by examining how formal decisions are made and who makes or vetoes them. *Prestige* is often based on social status, family class designation, and wealth. These three concepts—authority, power, and prestige—are closely linked.

The *social system* includes the prevalent norms and values as well as the dominant ethnic makeup of the community or population. Values influence norms and are often difficult to determine. Norms and values are intangible, so the community worker has to get a real feel for the group through direct involvement before they become apparent. Customs, specific town laws, and cultural patterns are reflective of that community's value system.

*Communication patterns*, both formal and informal, are an integral component of the social system. Communication as a necessary process by which people exchange information and interact with each other is basic to community living. *Informal* communication tends to occur wherever people collect—post offices, local cafes, recreation centers, barbershops, and so on. How information is disseminated can be reflected in community bulletin boards, supermarket notice boards, and the like. Often, asking community residents where information is obtained will yield the most accurate information. The beauty shop or local bar might serve as the center for information dissemination. Without an understanding of who the key people and places are in terms of informal communication, meaningful, realistic programs can seldom be created.

Formal communication channels include all forms of media, including newspapers, television, radio, telephone, the Internet, and postal systems. These channels of communication can be used very effectively in the dissemination of health information, as well as in the identification of community ideas, attitudes, and health knowledge.

Information about *educational systems* includes public and private educational facilities, libraries, special educational services (pregnant teens, handicapped, adult education), and available resources. The *economic system* includes major businesses and industries as well as the census information previously mentioned—median family income, unemployment rates, major occupations, and percentage of families living below the poverty level.

The *religious system* is an important part of the community and can have a major influence on the political ideology and social norms and values of a community. Major denominations should be identified along with the major religious leaders of a community.

Services and community health programs sponsored by religious groups are an integral part of the community's health care delivery system.

## Problem List (Nursing Diagnosis: Nursing Process)

The problem list corresponds to the nursing diagnosis component of the nursing process. As with individual nursing diagnoses, community diagnoses should specifically indicate that (1) *no* problems exist that demand intervention by the nursing discipline or by any other members of the health team or (2) needs exist as stated in terms of community problems that have evolved when basic human needs are either not being met or are being met inadequately.

Nursing diagnoses on the community level (as with the individual) use a humanitarian approach when specifying basic human needs. Examples of nursing diagnoses at the community level are as follows:

- Increased number of respiratory diseases related to air pollution
- Increased infant mortality rate related to increased teenage pregnancies
- Lack of neighborhood participation related to apathy

## Problem Assessment and Plan Formulation (Planning: Nursing Process)

The integration of the two problem-solving methods of Problem-Oriented Medical Recording (POMR) and the nursing process requires that the nurse reassess each community diagnosis using the SOAP format. During this phase, each problem is individually described and evaluated with an intervention plan formulated for each problem. The specific components of the SOAP format follow:

**Subjective data:** encompasses the community's point of view; how do persons in the community express the problem?

**Objective data:** a summarization of vital statistics, health statistics, review of systems, environmental realities, and so on related to identified problem

**Assessment:** includes an analysis of the identified needs or problem in terms of origination of the problem, overall impact, possible intervention points, and community parties that may have an interest in the problem and its solutions

**Plan:** further diagnostic plans or an initial intervention plan developed for the identified problem in terms of short- and long-term goals/objectives with specific actions to be taken to accomplish each objective; health team members, community members, or organizations are designated to carry out specific actions

After each problem has been reassessed using the SOAP format, the problems are then prioritized. A committee of community members, experts, and community leaders should be involved in problem prioritization.

## Progress Notes (Evaluation: Nursing Diagnosis)

The evaluation of the community assessment process should be documented in the form of progress notes. Progress notes are simply an appraisal of the effects of some predetermined plan to accomplish some measurable objective. During this phase of the POMR, new objectives and plans for each problem may be determined.

## The Lundy–Barton General Systems Model for Community and Population Assessment and Intervention

I. Database (Assessment Phase)
A. Definition of community or population
B. Profile
1. Demographics (census data)
2. Morbidity (illness patterns)
3. Birth rate
4. Death rates by age
5. Mortality rate (death rate)
6. Socioeconomic characteristics
   a. Occupation/employment patterns
   b. Median income
   c. Percentage of families below poverty level income
C. Psychological climate
1. Self-concept
2. Attitude toward health
3. Historical changes of community over time
D. Nutritional evaluations
1. Sources of food
2. Statistics related to nutritional status
E. Physical fitness
1. Facilities
2. Attitudes of residents
F. Physical examination (for geographic communities)
1. Systematic observation of community
2. Defined parameters/boundaries
3. Climate
4. Location, topography, rural/urban
5. Area in miles
6. Environmental conditions
   a. General description
   b. Housing, quality and condition
   c. Sanitation, water supply, sewage, and trash disposal
   d. Degree of pollution (air, water)
   e. Presence of vectors
   f. Safety/protection
      (1) Police
      (2) Fire
      (3) Other
   g. Transportation

G. Review of systems
1. Health system
   a. Private, public services
      (1) Hospitals
      (2) Long-term care
      (3) Ambulatory service
         (a) Primary care
         (b) Mental health/substance abuse
         (c) Home health
         (d) Public health
   b. Resources for specific health needs (e.g., elderly, teen parents)
   c. Human power—need versus availability, type (health workers)
   d. Other health care or related resources
      (1) Occupational health service
      (2) School health
      (3) Voluntary agencies
      (4) Welfare agencies
      (5) Disaster preparedness services
      (6) Other
2. Nonhealth systems
   a. Political system/atmosphere
      (1) Dominant values
      (2) Authority formal, nonformal leadership
      (3) Current political issues in community
   b. Social system
      (1) Prevalent norms
      (2) Cultural patterns/variables
      (3) Dominate values
      (4) Customs
      (5) Recreational/social facilities/activities
   c. Communication patterns
      (1) Informal and formal communication sources (e.g., newspapers, bulletin boards, Internet)
   d. Educational system
      (1) Public, private schools (number, type, student population, availability)
      (2) Values
      (3) Special educational services (e.g., pregnant teens, disabled, adult learners)
      (4) Libraries

e. Economic system
   (1) Major businesses/industries
   (2) Marketing and shopping facilities
   (3) Leading occupations
   (4) Employment patterns
f. Religious systems
   (1) Major denominations
   (2) Religious leadership

II. Problem List (Nursing Diagnosis)
  A. Identification of needs and assets from the assessment

III. Problem Assessment and Plan Formulation (Plan)
  A. Subjective data: community's point of view
  B. Objective data: nurse's point of view

C. Assessment: interpretation of data
D. Plan
  1. Short-term goals/objectives
  2. Long-term goals/objectives
  3. Specific actions for each objective/goal
E. Prioritization of nursing diagnoses

IV. Progress Notes (Evaluation)
  A. Specification of any intervention implemented and evaluation of effectiveness
  B. Formulation of new objectives and plan

## ■ REFERENCES

Anderson, R. E., & Carter, I. E. (1974). *Human behavior in the social environment: A social systems approach.* Chicago: Aldine.

Clark, M. J., Cary, S., Dicmart, G., et al. (2003). Involving communities in community assessment. *Public Health Nursing, 20*(6), 456–463.

Klein, D. C. (1965). Community and mental health: An attempt at a conceptual framework. *Community Health Journal, 1,* 301–308.

Mattison, B. (1968, June). Community health planning and the health professions. *Journal of Public Health, 58,* 1015–1021.

Shumway, S. M., & Wisehart, D. (1969). How to know a community. *Nursing Outlook, 17,* 63–64.

# CHAPTER 3
# History of Community Health and Public Health Nursing

Karen Saucier Lundy and Kaye W. Bender

Visit **http://nursing.jbpub.com/communityhealth** for interactive exercises, review questions, Web links, and more.

For as long as humanity has existed, so has the nursing of the sick. Health practices of early humans most likely evolved as a way for groups to survive. Many of these early causal links between humans and environment were attributed to superstition and religion. Early evidence from these primitive societies suggests that techniques such as mind–body connectins (e.g., voodoo or spells), isolation or banishment from the group, and fumigation (e.g., smoke) were used to manage disease and protect the health of the community (Hanlon & Pickett, 1984).

"Women have always been healers. Cultural myths from around the world described a time when only women knew the secrets of life and death and therefore they alone could practice the magical art of healing. In crises and calamity, or so some of the stories go, women's revered position as keepers of the sacred wisdom was deliberately and forcibly wrested away from them."

*—Achtenberg, 1990, p. 1*

What is your image of public health nursing as you begin this course? How do you define healing and its association with history? How do you think Florence Nightingale would react if she were alive today regarding nursing, healing, and health care?

## CHAPTER FOCUS

**Classical Era**

**The Greeks and Health**

**Roman Era**

**Middle Ages**
- Black Death
- The "Witch Craze" of the Early Middle Ages

**The Renaissance**

**The Advancement of Science and Health of the Public**

**The Emergence of Home Visiting**

**The Reformation**

**The Dark Period of Nursing**

**Early Organized Health Care in the Americas: A Brave New World**
- The Chadwick Report and the Shattuck Report

**The Industrial Revolution**

**John Snow and the Science of Epidemiology**

**And Then There Was Nightingale . . .**
- The Crimean Experience: "I Can Stand Out the War with Any Man"
- Florence Nightingale and Sanitation

**Returning Home a Heroine: The Political Reformer**
- Nightingale and Military Reforms
- The Nightingale School at St. Thomas: The Birth of Professional Nursing

- Taking Health Care to the Community: Nightingale and Wellness
- Nightingale's Legacy

**Early Nursing Education and Organization in the United States**

**The Evolution of Nursing in the United States: The First Century of Professional Nursing**

**The Emergence of Community and Public Health Nursing**
- Lillian Wald, Public Health Nursing, and Community Activism
- Dorothea Linde Dix
- Clara Barton
- Birth of the Midwife in the United States
- The Nursing Profession Responds to the Great Depression and World War II
- Early Education and Standardization of Practice of Public Health Nursing
- Challenges of the 1930s
- Progressive Initiatives After the War Years
- Social and Political Influence of the 1960s and 1970s
- Public Health Nursing Services in the 1980s and 1990s

**Science and Health Care, 1945–1960: Decades of Change**

**Years of Revolution, Protest, and the New Order, 1961–2000**

**The New Century: An Era of Managed Care**

## QUESTIONS TO CONSIDER

After reading this chapter, you will know the answers to the following questions:

1. When did humans first begin thinking about the causes of illness?
2. What were the contributions of the Greeks and Egyptians to our health practices today?
3. What are the origins of public health?
4. Who did the first home visits?
5. What were major health concerns of the Middle Ages?
6. What were Florence Nightingale's contributions to nursing as a profession?
7. What was the Chadwick Report, and why is it significant to community health nursing?
8. What role did William Rathbone play in the evolution of community health nursing?
9. Who is Lillian Wald, and why is she considered a prominent figure in the development of community health nursing in the United States?
10. What led to early standardization of public health nursing practice in the United States?
11. What are the major legislative events that occurred in the 1960s?

## KEY TERMS

American Journal of Nursing (AJN)
American Nurses Association (ANA)
Clara Barton
Black Death (bubonic plague)
Frances Payne Bolton
Mary Breckenridge
Mary Brewster
Cadet Nurse Corps
Case management
Deaconesses

Jane A. Delano
Dorothea Linde Dix
Lavinia Lloyd Dock
Frontier Nursing Service
Goldmark Report
Annie Goodrich
Greek era
Health visiting
Henry Street Settlement
Edward Jenner

Kaiserwerth Institute
Edwin Klebs
Robert Koch
Joseph Lister
Managed care
Nightingale School of Nursing at
   St. Thomas
Nursing's Agenda for Health
   Care Reform
Louis Pasteur

William Rathbone
Reformation
Isabel Hampton Robb
Roman era
Margaret Sanger
Jessie Sleet Scales
Saint Vincent de Paul
Elizabeth Tyler
Lillian Wald

## Classical Era

More than 4,000 years ago, Egyptian physicians and nurses used an abundant pharmacological repertoire to cure the ill and injured. The Ebers Papyrus lists more than 700 remedies for ailments from snake bites to puerperal fever. The Kahun Papyrus (circa 1850 B.C.) identified suppositories (e.g., crocodile feces) that could be used for contraception (Kalisch & Kalisch, 1986).

Healing appeared in the Egyptian culture as the successful result of a contest between invisible beings of good and evil (Shryock, 1959). The physician was not a shaman; instead there was specialization and separation of function, with physicians, priests, and sorcerers all practicing separately and independently. Some patients would consult the physician, some visited the shaman, and others sought healing from magical formulas. Many tried all three approaches. The Egyptians, quite notably, did not accept illness and death as inevitable but rather believed that life could be indefinitely prolonged.

Because Egyptians blended medicine and magic, the concoctions believed to be the most effective were often bizarre and repulsive by today's standards. For example, lizard's blood, swine's ears and teeth, putrid meat and fat, tortoise brains, the milk of a lactating woman, the urine of a chaste woman, and excreta of donkeys and lions were frequently used ingredients. At least some explanation for these odd ingredients can be found in the following:

> These pharmacological mixtures were intended to sicken and drive out the intruding demon which was thought to cause the disease. Drugs containing fecal matter were in fact used until the end of the eighteenth century in Europe as common practice. (Kalisch & Kalisch, 1986)

As early as 3000 to 1400 B.C., the Minoans created ways to flush water and construct drainage systems. Circa 1000 B.C., the Egyptians constructed elaborate drainage systems, developed pharmaceutical herbs and preparations, and embalmed the dead. The Hebrews formulated an elaborate hygiene code that dealt with laws governing both personal and community hygiene, such as contagion, disinfection, and sanitation through the preparation of food and water. Hebrews, although few in number, exercised great influence

> **"**For as long as humanity has existed, so has the nursing of the sick. Health practices of early humans most likely evolved as a way for groups to survive. Many of these early causal links between humans and environment were attributed to superstition and religion. Early evidence from these primitive societies suggests that techniques such as mind-body connections (e.g., voodoo or spells), isolation or banishment from the group, and fumigation (e.g., smoke) were used to manage disease and protect the health of the community.**"**
>
> —Hanlon & Pickett, 1984

in the development of religious and health doctrine. According to Bullough and Bullough (1978), most of their genius was religious, giving birth to both Christianity and Islam. The Jewish contribution to public health is greater in sanitation than in their concept of disease. Garbage and excreta were disposed of outside the city or camp, infectious diseases were quarantined, spitting was outlawed as unhygienic, and bodily cleanliness became a prerequisite for moral purity. Although many of the Hebrew ideas about hygiene were Egyptian in origin, Moses and the Hebrews were the first to codify them and link them with spiritual godliness. Their notion of disease was rooted in the "disease as God's punishment for sin" idea.

The civilization that grew up between the Tigris and Euphrates Rivers is known geographically as Mesopotamia (modern Iraq) and includes the Sumerians. Disease and disability in the Mesopotamian area, at least in the earlier period, was considered a great curse, a divine punishment for grievous acts against the gods. Having such a curse of illness resulting from sin did not exactly put the sick person in a valued status in the society. Experiencing illness as punishment for a sin linked the sick person to anything even remotely deviant: Such things as murder, perjury, adultery, or drunkenness could be the identified sins. Not only was the person suffering from the illness, but he or she was also branded by society as having deserved it. The illness made the sin apparent to all; the sick person was isolated and disgraced. Those who obeyed God's law lived in health and happiness. Those who transgressed the law were punished, with illness and suffering thought to be consequences. The sick person then had to make atonement for the sins, enlist a priest or other spiritual healer to lift the spell or curse, or live with the illness to its ultimate outcome. In simple terms, the person had to get right with the gods or live with the consequences (Bullough & Bullough, 1978). Nursing care by a family member or relative would be needed in any case, regardless of the outcome of the sin/curse/disease–atonement/recovery or death cycle. This logic became the basis for explanation of why some people get sick and some don't for many centuries, and it still persists to some degree in most cultures today (Achterberg, 1990).

**❝**I have an almost complete disregard of precedent and a faith in the possibility of something better. It irritates me to be told how things always have been done . . . I defy the tyranny of precedent. I cannot afford the luxury of a closed mind. I go for anything new that might improve the past.

You must never so much as think whether you like it or not, whether it is bearable or not; you must never think of anything except the need, and how to meet it. **❞**
—Clara Barton, Civil War nurse and founder of the American Red Cross

## The Greeks and Health

In Greek mythology, the god of medicine, Asclepias, cured disease. One of his daughters, Hygeia, from whose name we derive the word "hygiene," was the goddess of preventive health and protected humans from disease. Panacea, Asclepias's other daughter, was known as the all-healing "universal remedy"; today her name is used to describe any ultimate "cure-all" in medicine. Panacea was known as the "light" of the day, and her name was invoked and shrines built to her during times of epidemics (Brooke, 1997).

During the **Greek era**, Hippocrates emphasized the rational treatment of sickness as a natural, rather than god-inflicted, phenomenon. Hippocrates of Cos (460–370 B.C.) is considered the father of medicine because of his arrangements of the oral and written remedies and diseases, which had long been secrets held by priests and religious healers, into a textbook of medicine that was used for centuries (Bullough & Bullough, 1978). Hippocrates's contribution to the science of public health was his recognition that making accurate observations of and drawing general conclusions from actual phenomena formed the basis of sound medical reasoning (Shryock, 1959).

In Greek society, health was considered to result from a balance between mind and body. Hippocrates wrote a most important book, *Air, Water and Places*, which detailed the relationship between humans and the environment. It is considered a milestone in the eventual development of the science of epidemiology as the first such treatise on the connectedness of the web of life. This topic of the relationship between humans and their environment did not reoccur until the development of bacteriology in the late nineteenth century (Rosen, 1958).

Perhaps the idea that most damaged the practice and scientific theory of medicine and health for centuries was the doctrine of the four humors, first spoken of by Empedodes of Acragas (493–433 B.C.). Empedodes was a philosopher and a physician, and as a result, he synthesized his cosmological ideas into his medical theory. He believed that the same four elements (or "roots of things") that made up the universe were found in humans and in all animate beings (Bullough & Bullough, 1978). Empedodes believed that each human was a microcosm, a small world within the macrocosm, or external environment. The four humors of the body (blood, bile, phlegm, and black bile) corresponded to the four elements of the larger world (fire, air, water, and earth) (Kalisch & Kalisch, 1986). Depending on the prevailing humor, a person was sanguine, choleric, phlegmatic, or melancholic.

Because of this strongly held and persistent belief in the connection between the balance of the four humors and health status, treatment was aimed at restoring the appropriate balance of the four humors through the control of their corresponding elements. By manipulating the two sets of opposite qualities—hot and cold, wet and dry—balance was the goal of the intervention. Fire was hot and dry, air was hot and wet, water was cold and wet, and earth was cold and dry. For example, if a person had a fever, cold compresses would be prescribed for a chill and the person would be warmed. Such doctrine gave rise to faulty and ineffective treatment of disease that influenced medical education for many years (Taylor, 1922).

Plato, in *The Republic*, detailed the importance of recreation, a balanced mind and body, nutrition, and exercise. A distinction was made among gender, class, and health as early as the Greek era; that is, only males of the aristocracy could afford the luxury of maintaining a healthful lifestyle (Rosen, 1958).

In *The Iliad*, Homer's poem about the attempts to capture Troy and rescue Helen from her lover Paris, 140 different wounds are described. The mortality rate averaged 77.6%, with the highest mortality resulting from sword and spear thrusts and the lowest mortality resulting from superficial arrow wounds. There was considerable need for nursing care, and Achilles, Patroclus, and other princes often acted as nurses to the injured. The early stages of Greek medicine reflected the influences of Egyptian, Babylonian, and Hebrew medicine. Therefore, good medical and nursing techniques were used to treat these war wounds: The arrow was drawn or cut out, the wound washed, soothing herbs applied, and the wound bandaged.

### ■■ CULTURAL CONNECTION

During the Early Middle Ages, Europeans seldom washed or changed their clothes more than once or twice a year. This lack of personal sanitation set up ideal conditions for the bubonic plague where one out of three faces disappeared from these human communities. ◯

*Source:* Kelly, J. (2005). *The great mortality: An intimate history of the Black Death, the most devestating plague of all time.* New York: HarperCollins.

However, in sickness in which no wound occurred, an evil spirit was considered the cause. For example, the cause of the plague was unknown, so the question became how and why affected soldiers had angered the gods. According to *The Iliad*, the true healer of the plague was the prophet who prayed for Apollo to stop shooting the "plague arrows." The Greeks applied rational causes and cures to external injuries, while internal ailments continued to be linked to spiritual maladies (Bullough & Bullough, 1978).

## Roman Era

During the rise and the fall of the **Roman era** (31 B.C.–A.D. 476), Greek culture continued to be a strong influence. The Romans easily adopted Greek culture and expanded the Greeks' accomplishments, especially in the fields of engineering, law, and government. The development of policy, law, and protection of the public's health was an important precursor to our modern public health systems. For Romans, the government had an obligation to protect its citizens, not only from outside aggression such as warring neighbors, but also from inside the civilization in the form of health laws. According to Bullough and Bullough, Rome was essentially a "Greek cultural colony" (1978, p. 20).

During the third century B.C., Rome began to dominate the Mediterranean, Egypt, the Tigris–Euphrates Valley, the Hebrews, and the Greeks (Boorstin, 1985). Greek science and Roman engineering then spread throughout the ancient world, providing a synthesized Greco-Roman foundation for eventual public health policies (Bullough & Bullough, 1978).

Galen of Pergamum (A.D. 129–199), often known as the greatest Greek physician after Hippocrates, left for Rome after studying medicine in Greece and Egypt and gained great fame as a medical practitioner, lecturer, and experimenter. In his lifetime, medicine evolved into a science; he submitted traditional healing practices to experimentation and was possibly the greatest medical researcher before the seventeenth century (Bullough & Bullough, 1978). Galen was considered the last of the great physicians of antiquity (Kalisch & Kalisch, 1978).

The Greek physicians and healers certainly made the most contributions to medicine, but the Romans surpassed the Greeks in promoting the evolution of nursing. Roman armies developed the notion of a mobile war nursing unit as their battles took them too far from home to be cared for by their wives and family. This portable hospital was a series of tents arranged in corridors; as battles wore on, these tents gave way to buildings that became permanent convalescent camps along the battle sites (Rosen, 1958). Many of these early military hospitals have been excavated by archaeolo-

gists along the banks of the Rhine and Danube Rivers. They had wards, recreation areas, baths, pharmacies, and even rooms for officers who needed a "rest cure" (Bullough & Bullough, 1978). Coexisting were the Greek dispensary forms of temples (*iatreia*), which started out as a type of physician waiting room. These eventually developed into a primitive type of hospital—that is, places for surgical patients to stay until they could be taken home by their families. Although nurses during the Roman era were usually family members, servants, or slaves, nursing had strengthened its position in medical care and emerged during the Roman era as a separate and distinct specialty (Minkowski, 1992).

During this era, the Romans developed massive aqueducts, bath houses, and sewer systems. Even though these engineering feats were remarkable at the time, poorer and less fortunate residents often did not benefit from the same level of public health amenities, such as sewer systems and latrines (Bullough & Bullough, 1978). However, the Romans did provide many of their citizens with what we would consider public health services.

## Middle Ages

Many of the advancements of the Greco-Roman era were reversed during the Middle Ages, after the decline of the Roman Empire (A.D. 476–1453). The Middle Ages, or the

As one of the oldest hospitals in existence, Hotel Dieu, in Paris, France, was founded in A.D. 650. The hospital is located adjacent to Notre Dame Cathedral on the Seine River and continues to provide state-of-the-art health care services. The motto of Hotel Dieu translates "Liberty, Equality, Brotherhood."

> 🖉 NOTE THIS! •——
>
> Did you know that engineers during the Roman era developed an aqueduct system capable of providing 40 gallons of water person per day to Rome's 1 million residents, comparable to our consumption rates today? (Rosen, 1958)

medieval era, served as a transition between ancient and modern civilizations. Once again, myth, magic, and religion were explanations and cures for illness and health problems. The medieval world was the result of fusion among three streams of thought, actions, and ways of life—Greco-Roman, Germanic, and Christian—into one (Donahue, 1985).

Nursing was most influenced by Christianity with the beginning of **deaconesses**, or female servants, doing the work of God by ministering to the needs of others. Deacons in the early Christian churches were apparently available only to care for men, deaconesses cared only for the needs of the women. This role of the deaconess in the church was considered a forward step in the development of nursing and in the nineteenth century would strongly influence the young Florence Nightingale.

During this era, Roman military hospitals were replaced by civilian ones. In early Christianity, the *diakonia*, a kind of combination outpatient and welfare office, was managed by deacons and deaconesses and served as the equivalent of a hospital. Jesus served as the example of charity and compassion for the poor and marginal of society.

Communicable diseases were rampant during the Middle Ages, primarily because of the walled cities that emerged in response to the paranoia and isolation of the populations. Infection was next to impossible to control. Physicians had little to offer, deferring to the church for management of disease. Nursing roles were carried out primarily by religious orders. The oldest hospital (other than military hospitals in the Roman era) in Europe was most likely the Hotel Dieu in Lyons, France, founded about 542 by Childbert I, king of France. The Hotel Dieu in Paris was founded about 652 by St. Landry, bishop of Paris.

During the Middle Ages, charitable institutions, hospitals, and medical schools increased in number, with the religious leaders as caregivers. The word "hospital" which derives from the Latin *hospitalis*, meaning "service of guests," was most likely used for a shelter for travelers and other pilgrims as well as the occasional person who needed extra care (Kalisch & Kalisch, 1986). Early European hospitals were more like hospices or homes for the aged, sick pilgrims, or orphans. Nurses in these early hospitals were religious deaconesses who chose to care for others in a life of servitude and spiritual sacrifice (Minkowski, 1992).

## ■ Black Death

During the Middle Ages, a series of horrible epidemics, including the **Black Death (bubonic plague)**, ravaged the civilized world (Diamond, 1997). In the fourteenth century, Europe, Asia, and Africa saw nearly half their populations lost to the bubonic plague. According to Bullough and Bullough (1978), an interesting account of the arrival of the bubonic plague in 1347 claims that the disease had started in the Genoese colony of Kaffa in the Crimea. The story passed down through the ages was that the city was being besieged by a Mongol khan. When the disease broke out among the

 THINK ABOUT THIS

The Pima Indians of the American Southwest referred to the plague as *oimmeddam* or "wandering sickness." Below is an ancient Indian legend that describes the horror of their ancestors suffering from *oimmeddam*.

"Where do you come from?" an Indian asks a tall, black-haired stranger.

"I come from far way," the stranger replies, "from . . . across the Eastern Ocean."

"What do you bring?" the Indian asks.

"I bring death," the stranger answers. "My breath causes children to wither and die like young plants in the spring snow. I bring destruction. No matter how beautiful a woman, once she has looked at me, she becomes as ugly as death. And to men, I bring not death alone, but the destruction of their children and the blighting of their wives. . . . No people who look upon me are ever the same."

khan's men, he catapulted the bodies of its victims into Kaffa to infect and weaken his enemies. The soldiers and colonists of Kaffa then carried the disease back to Genoa.

Worldwide, more than 60 million deaths were eventually attributed to this horrible plague. In some parts of Europe, only one fourth of the population survived, with some places having too few people to bury the dead. Families abandoned sick children, and the sick were often left to die alone (Cartwright, 1972).

Nurses and physicians were powerless to avert the disease. Black spots and tumors on the skin appeared, and petechia and hemorrhages gave the skin a darkened appearance. There was also acute inflammation of the lungs, burning sensations, unquenchable thirst, and inflammation of the entire body. Hardly anyone afflicted survived the third day of the attack. So great was the fear of contagion that ships were set to sail with bodies of infected persons without a crew, drifting through the North, Black, and Mediterranean seas from port to port with their dead passengers (Cohen, 1989). Bubonic plague is caused by the bacillus *Pasteurella pestis*, which is usually transmitted by the bite of a flea carried by an animal vector, typically a rat. After the initial flea bite, the infection spreads through the lymph nodes, and the nodes swell to enormous size; the inflamed nodes are called bubos, from which the bubonic plague derives its name. Medieval

 ETHICAL CONNECTION

The Gallup Poll organization named nurses as the most "ethical" profession in the United States in 2005, according to a recent survey of 1,002 American adults. Eighty-two percent of respondents categorized nurses as having very high or high ethics. Nurses have been ranked the most ethical profession six of the last seven years, passed only in 2001 by fire fighters in the wake of the 9/11 terrorist attacks.

people knew that this disease was in some way communicable, but they were unsure of the mode of transmission (Diamond, 1997)—hence the avoidance of victims and a reliance on isolation techniques. The practice of quarantine in city ports was developed as a preventive measure and is still used today (Bullough & Bullough, 1978; Kalisch & Kalisch, 1986).

### ■ The "Witch Craze" of the Early Middle Ages

As respected "wise women" through the centuries, during the Middle Ages midwives and women healers gradually transformed into members of a "demonized" avocation. As formal training in medicine gradually developed in Europe, leaders of the church and officials at the time restricted such education to men only, consequently creating a legal male monopoly of the practice of medicine and healing (Briggs, 1996; Achterberg, 1990; Barstow, 1994). As women found themselves "ineligible" to practice in their roles as healers, they faced an even greater threat as they were labeled as witches.

A revival of the Holy Inquisition, a body formed in France in 1022 and codified by the Catholic Church in the 1486 *Malleus maleficarium* (Hammer of Witches) by Pope Innocent VIII, allowed the persecutions to take form. By formalizing the legal punishment of witches and midwives, the Pope codified this "step-by-step, how-to manual" for dealing with the witch problem. Achterberg describes this significant endorsement in this way: "We are dealing here with an evil that surpasses rational understanding. Here was, indeed, the worst aberration of humanity and it trickled down the hierarchy of authority" (1990, p. 86). The legal system throughout Europe became increasingly harsh with each new conviction and as the distinction between sorcery and heresy was further blurred: Those accused of witchcraft and heresy were guilty of devil worship. With the support of both the church and civil authorities, as many as 250,000 women were accused, "tried," and tortured into making confessions and eventually burned at the stake simply for being women healers (Briggs, 1996). The accusers linked women's special healing "powers" to an alliance with Satan, and over three centuries they punished and eliminated women as perceived threats to their medical supremacy in society.

Our stereotype of a witch today reflects these ancient and deadly associations of women healers and evil magic: the elderly, unattractive woman dressed in black on a broomstick with a black cat at her side. Women in Europe who practiced as healers often used empirically sound herbal and alternative health practices (hence the caldron association), provided gynecological and obstetric care of women at all hours (hence the broom, because proper women did not go out at night and were presumed to "fly"), and relied on other women for advice and shared practices of healing (hence the "coven" association) (Achterberg, 1990; Barstow, 1994). As described by Briggs, "To this end they have allegedly flown by night to meetings where orgiastic, blasphemous or cannibalistic rituals symbolized their defection from social and personal virtue" (1996, p. 4).

Briggs estimates that 100,000 trials of witches occurred in Europe between the years 1450 and 1750, with at least 50% of the accused being executed in brutal hangings and burnings. This "witch craze" reached its height during the twelfth through fourteenth centuries in France, Germany, and other European countries (Achterberg, 1990; Barstow, 1994; Briggs, 1996). Religion, magic, healing, and witchcraft were inextricably linked throughout human history, but during this era dramatic changes in cultural values, and paranoia about women's perceived powers resulted in a mass cultural movement to eliminate women as healers (Briggs, 1996; Minkowski, 1992).

❝*Witches have haunted the human imagination with remarkable persistence. Destructive and malicious figures, they have always represented the opposite of all positive value . . . it is therefore hard for us to understand the ways village and small town societies used to work, when their members were far less mobile and interacted in a much closer fashion at many levels. For good or ill, people could not easily escape one another, something which played a vital role in breeding charges of witchcraft. This was the case because the core of the belief lay in the notion that witches had peculiar powers to harm their neighbors and the community at large.*❞

—Briggs, 1996, p. 3

❝*The position held by the Church and enforced by civic bodies— that women who practiced without appropriate study must die—had a catch of course. Women were not allowed access to education. All women healers therefore were suspect. Any woman with exceptional talent was suspect; any woman who had acquired her knowledge through the oral tradition of woman's domestic healing was suspect; any woman who had studied independently with a master healer (even a man) was suspect. Any woman who had the bad luck to be associated by proximity or reputation with a physician's failure to cure his patient was suspect.*❞

—Achterberg, 1990, p. 83

## The Renaissance

During the rebirth of Europe, great political, social, and economic advances occurred along with a tremendous revival of learning. Donahue contends that the Renaissance has been "viewed as both a blessing and a curse" (1985, p. 188). There was a renewed interest in the arts and sciences, which helped advance medical science (Boorstin, 1985; Bullough & Bullough, 1978). Columbus and other explorers discovered new worlds, and belief in a sun-centered rather than earth-centered universe was promoted by Copernicus (1473–1543); Sir Isaac Newton's (1642–1727) theory of gravity changed the world forever. Gunpowder was introduced, and social and religious upheavals resulted in the American and French revolutions at the end of the 18th century.

In the arts and sciences, Leonardo da Vinci, known as one of the greatest geniuses of all time, made a number of anatomical drawings based on dissection experiences. These drawings have become classics in the progression of knowledge about the human anatomy. Many artists of this time left an indelible mark and continue to exert influence today, including Michelangelo, Raphael, and Titian (Donahue, 1985; Minkowski, 1992).

 *Got an Alternative?*

Ehrenreich and English (1973), in their seminal work, *Witches, Midwives, and Nurses: A History of Women Healers*, note that in the Middle Ages it was the women who were testing new herbs and innovative ways of healing, leading to the adoption of humane, empirical paradigms of healing. All the while, they contend, their male counterparts clung to their ritualistic and outdated procedures, such as leeching, use of mercury, and purgation.

These authors contend that the witch craze, where thousands of women were tried and put to death, was a ruling-class campaign of terror against the female peasant healers who dared to introduce what is now considered holistic or complementary healing modalities. Given that God considered illness and suffering as payment for sin, anyone who offered healing interventions, such as boiling up herbs and potions in big pots, must be anti-God and, therefore, must be working for the "other side" or the Devil. It is hardly surprising, according to Ehrenreich and English, that nursing fell into disrepute by the eighteenth century, and that the only women who had any status for being involved in healing were those in holy orders. Yet for many poor people, their only remedies were these traditional healing "potions." As medicine grew with scientific models of illness management, these tired and tested remedies were held up as "old wives' tales."

*Source:* Ehrenreich, B., & English, D. (1973). *Witches, midwives, and nurses: A history of women healers.* Old Westbury, NY: Feminist Press.

## The Advancement of Science and Health of the Public

It took the first 50 years of the eighteenth century for the new knowledge from the Enlightenment to be organized and digested, according to Donahue (1985). In Great Britain, **Edward Jenner** discovered an effective method of vaccination against the dreaded smallpox virus in 1798. Psychiatry developed as a separate branch of medicine, and instruments such as the pulse watch and the stethoscope were invented that measured and allowed for assessment of the body.

One of the greatest scientists of this period was **Louis Pasteur** (1822–1895). A French chemist, Pasteur first became interested in pathogenic organisms through his studies of the diseases of wine. His discovery, that if wine was heated to a temperature of 55° to 60°C, the process killed the microorganisms that spoiled wine, was critical to the wine industry's success in France. This process of pasteurization led Pasteur

to investigate many fields and save many lives from contaminated milk and food.

**Joseph Lister** (1827–1912) was a physician who set out to decrease the mortality resulting from infection after surgery. He used Pasteur's research to eventually arrive at a chemical antiseptic solution of carbolic acid for use in surgery. Widely regarded as the father of modern surgery, he practiced his antiseptic surgery with great results, and the Listerian principles of asepsis changed the way physicians and nurses practice to this day (Dietz & Lehozky, 1963).

**Robert Koch** (1843–1910), a physician known for his research in anthrax, is regarded as the father of microbiology. By identifying the organism that caused cholera, *Vibrio cholerae*, he also demonstrated its transmission by water, food, and clothing.

**Edwin Klebs** (1834–1913) proved the germ theory—that is, that germs are the causes of infectious diseases. This discovery of the bacterial origin of diseases may be considered the greatest achievement of the nineteenth century. Although the microscope had been around for two centuries, it remained for Lister, Pasteur, and Koch—and ultimately Klebs—to provide the missing link (Dietz & Lehozky, 1963; Rosen, 1958).

## The Emergence of Home Visiting

In 1633, **Saint Vincent de Paul** founded the Sisters of Charity in France, an order of nuns who traveled from home to home visiting the sick. As the services of the sisters grew, St. Vincent appointed Mademoiselle Le Gras as supervisor of these visitors. These nurses functioned as the first organized visiting nurse service, making home visits and caring for the sick in their homes. De Paul believed that for family members to go to the hospital was disruptive to family life and that taking nursing services to the home enabled health to be restored more effectively and more efficiently.

## The Reformation

Religious changes during the Renaissance were to influence nursing perhaps more than any other aspect of society. Particularly important was the rise of Protestantism as a result of the reform movements of Martin Luther (1483–1546) in Germany and John Calvin (1509–1564) in France and Geneva. Although the various sects were numerous in the Protestant movement, the agreement among the leaders was almost unanimous on the abolition of the monastic or cloistered career. The effects on nursing were drastic: Monastic-affiliated institutions, including hospitals and schools, were closed, and orders of nuns, including nurses, were dissolved. Even in countries where Catholicism flourished, seizures of monasteries by royal leaders occurred frequently.

Religious leaders, such as Martin Luther in Germany, who led the **Reformation** in 1517, were well aware of the lack of adequate nursing care as a result of these sweeping changes. Luther advocated that each town establish something akin to a "community chest" to raise funds for hospitals and nurse visitors for the poor (Dietz & Lehozky, 1963). For example, in

MEDIA MOMENT

**Troy, (2004)**

This movie starring Brad Pitt as Achilles, is based on the epic poem *The Iliad* by Homer. The movie recounts the legend of the Trojan War, as the fortress city is attacked by a Greek army led by Menelaus of Sparta and Agamemnon of Mycenae.

Achilles, the mighty Greek warrior, had been dipped as an infant by his mother in the River Styx so that he would be invincible to iron weapons. Because his mother had held him by his heel, this was the only vulnerable part of his body. In the adaptation of Homer's *Iliad*, the Trojan warrior Paris (played by Orlando Bloom) shoots Achilles in the heel with a poison arrow and brings about his death. A simple superficial wound to the heel would not have been deadly; consequently, history provides us with an early account of biochemical warfare.

 NOTE THIS!

The Reformation had a devastating effect upon nursing . . . imagine our situation in the United States if a decree went out that hospitals would be closed in two years. There would be no places available to care for the ill. Such were the conditions in England from 1538–1540 during the reign of Henry VIII. No provision was made for the sick and poor, there was no lay organization to replace those who had fled, and no one to develop or teach others to carry on.

*Source:* Dietz and Lehozky, 1963.

England, where there had been at least 450 charitable foundations before the Reformation, only a few survived the reign of Henry VIII, who closed most of the monastic hospitals (Donahue, 1985). Eventually, Henry VIII's son, Edward VI, who reigned from 1547 to 1553, was convinced and did endow some hospitals—namely St. Bartholomew's Hospital and St. Thomas's Hospital, which would eventually house the Nightingale School of Nursing in the nineteenth century (Bullough & Bullough, 1978).

## The Dark Period of Nursing

The last half of the period between 1500 and 1860 is widely regarded as the "dark period of nursing" because nursing conditions were at their worst (Donahue, 1985). Education for girls, which had been provided by the nuns in religious schools, was lost. Because of the elimination of hospitals and schools, there was no one to pass on knowledge about caring for the sick. As a result, the hospitals were managed and staffed by municipal authorities; women entering nursing service often came from illiterate classes, and even then there were too few to serve (Dietz & Lehozky, 1963). The lay attendants who filled the nursing role were illiterate, rough, inconsiderate, and often immoral and alcoholic. Intelligent women and men could not be persuaded to accept such a degraded and low-status position in the offensive municipal hospitals of London. Nursing slipped back into a role of servitude as menial, low-status work. According to Donahue (1985), when a woman could no longer make it as a gambler, prostitute, or thief, she might become a nurse. Eventually, women serving jail sentences for crimes such as prostitution and stealing were ordered to care for the sick in the hospitals instead of serving their sentences in the city jail (Dietz & Lehozky, 1963). The nurses of this era took bribes from patients, became inappropriately involved with them, and survived the best way they could, often at the expense of their assigned patients.

During this era, nursing had virtually no social standing or organization. Even Catholic sisters of the religious orders throughout Europe "came to a complete standstill" professionally because of the intolerance of society (Donahue, 1985, p. 231). Charles Dickens, in *Martin Chuzzlewit* (1910), created the immortal characters of Sairey Gamp and Betsy Prig. Sairey Gamp was a visiting nurse based on an actual hired attendant who Dickens had met in a friend's home.

 A Good Read

## Martin Chuzzlewit (1843)

*By Charles Dickens, New York: Penguin Books.*

She was a fat old woman, this Mrs. Gamp, with a husky voice and a moist eye, which she had a remarkable power of turning up and showing the white of it. Having very little neck, it cost her some trouble to look over herself, if one may say so, to those to whom she talked. She wore a very rusty black gown, rather the worse for snuff, and a shawl and bonnet to correspond. . . . The face of Mrs. Gamp—the nose in particular—was somewhat red and swollen, and it was difficult to enjoy her society without becoming conscious of the smell of spirits. Like most persons who have attained to great eminence in their profession, she took to hers very kindly; insomuch, that setting aside her natural predilections as a woman, she went to a lying-in [birth] or a laying-out [death] with equal zest and relish.

Sairey Gamp was hired to care for sick family members but was instead cruel to her patients, stole from them, and ate their rations; she was an alcoholic and has been immortalized forever as a reminder of the world in which Florence Nightingale came of age (Donahue, 1985; Minkowski, 1992).

## Early Organized Health Care in the Americas: A Brave New World

In the New World, the first hospital in the Americas—the Hospital de la Purisima Concepcion—was founded some time before 1524 by Hernando Cones, the conqueror of Mexico. The first hospital in the continental United States was erected in Manhattan in 1658 for the care of sick soldiers and slaves. In 1717, a hospital for infectious diseases was built in Boston; the first hospital established by a private gift was the Charity Hospital in New Orleans. A sailor, Jean Louis, donated the endowment for the hospital's founding (Bullough & Bullough, 1978).

During the seventeenth and eighteenth centuries, colonial hospitals were often used to house the poor and downtrodden, though they bore little resemblance to modern hospitals. Hospitals called pesthouses were created to care for people with contagious diseases; their primary purpose was to protect the public at large, rather than to treat and care for the patients. Contagious diseases were rampant during the early years of the American colonies, often being spread by the large number of immigrants who brought these diseases with them on their long journeys to America. Medicine was not as developed as in Europe, and nursing remained in the hands of the uneducated. Average life expectancy at birth was only around 35 years by 1720. Plagues were a constant nightmare, with outbreaks of smallpox and yellow fever. In 1751, the first true hospital in the new colonies, Pennsylvania Hospital, was erected in Philadelphia on the recommendation of Benjamin Franklin (Kalisch & Kalisch, 1986).

By today's standards, hospitals in the nineteenth century were disgraceful, dirty, unventilated, and contaminated by infections; to be a patient in a hospital actually increased one's risk of dying. As in England, nursing was considered an inferior occupation. After the sweeping changes as a result of the Reformation, educated religious health workers were replaced with lay people who were "down and outers," in prison, or had no option left except to work with the sick (Kalisch & Kalisch, 1986).

### ■ The Chadwick Report and the Shattuck Report

Edwin Chadwick became a major figure in the development of the field of public health in Great Britain by drawing attention to the cost of the unsanitary conditions that shortened the life span of the laboring class and posed threats to the wealth of Britain. Although the first sanitation legislation, which established a National Vaccination Board, was passed in 1837, Chadwick found in his classic study, *Report on an Inquiry into the Sanitary Conditions of the Laboring Population of Great Britain*, that death rates were high in large industrial cities such as Liverpool. A more startling finding, from what is often referred to simply as the Chadwick Report, was that more than half the children of labor-class workers died by age 5, indicating poor living conditions that affected the health of the most vulnerable. Laborers lived only half as long as members of the upper classes.

One consequence of the report was the establishment of the first board of health, the General Board of Health for England, in 1848 (Richardson, 1887). More legislation followed that initiated social reform in the areas of child welfare, elder care, the sick, the mentally ill, factory health, and education. Soon sewers and fire plugs, based on an available water supply, appeared as indicators that the public health linkages from the Chadwick Report had an impact.

In the United States during the nineteenth century, waves of epidemics of yellow fever, smallpox, cholera, typhoid fever, and typhus continued to plague the population as in England and the rest of the world. As cities continued to grow in the industrialized young nation, poor workers crowded into larger cities and suffered from illnesses caused by the unsanitary living conditions (Hanlon & Pickett, 1984). Similar to what occurred with Chadwick's classic study in England, Lemuel Shattuck, a Boston bookseller and publisher who had an interest in public health, organized the American Statistical Society in 1839 and issued a census of Boston in 1845. Shattuck's census revealed high infant mortality rates and high overall population mortality rates. In his *Report of the Massachusetts Sanitary Commission* in 1850, Shattuck not only outlined his findings on the unsanitary conditions, but also made recommendations for public health reform that included the keeping of population statistics and development of a monitoring system that would provide information to the public about environmental, food, and drug safety as well as infectious disease control (Rosen, 1958). He also called for services such as well-child care, school-age children's health, immunizations, mental health, health education for all, and health planning. The Shattuck Report was revolutionary in its scope and vision for public health, but it was virtually ignored during Shattuck's lifetime. It would not be until 19 years later, in 1869, that the first state board of health was formed (Minkowski, 1992; Kalisch & Kalisch, 1986).

## The Industrial Revolution

During the mid-eighteenth century in England, capitalism emerged as an economic system based on profit. This emerging system resulted in mass production, as contrasted with the previous system of individual workers and craftsmen. In the simplest terms, the Industrial Revolution was the application of machine power to processes formerly done by hand. Machinery was invented during this era and ultimately standardized quality; individual craftsmen were forced to give up their crafts and lands and become factory laborers for the capitalist owners. All types of industries were affected; this newfound efficiency produced profits for owners of the means of production. As a result, the era of invention flourished, factories grew, and people moved in record numbers to work in the cities. Urban areas grew, tenement housing projects emerged, and overcrowded cities became serious threats to well-being (Donahue, 1985).

Workers were forced to go to the machines, rather than the other way around. Such relocations meant giving up not only farming, but also a way of life that had existed for centuries. The emphasis on profit over people led to child labor, frequent layoffs, and long workdays filled with stressful, tedious, unfamiliar work. Labor unions did not exist, nor was there any legal protection against exploitation of workers, including children (Donahue, 1985). All of these rapid changes and often threatening conditions were described in the work of Charles Dickens; in his book *Oliver Twist*, for example, children worked as adults without question.

According to Donahue (1985), urban life, trade, and industrialization contributed to these overwhelming health hazards, and the situation was confounded by the lack of an adequate means of social control. Reforms were desperately needed, and the social reform movement emerged in response to the unhealthy by-products of the Industrial Revolution. It was in this world of the nineteenth century that reformers such as John Stuart Mill (1806–1873) emerged. Although the Industrial Revolution began in England, it quickly spread to the rest of Europe and to the United States (Bullough & Bullough, 1978). The reform movement is critical to understanding the emerging health concerns that were later addressed by Florence Nightingale. Mill championed popular education, the emancipation of women, trade unions, and religious toleration. Other reform issues of the era included the abolition of slavery and, most important for nursing, more humane care of the sick, the poor, and the wounded (Bullough & Bullough, 1978). There was a renewed energy in the religious community with the reemergence of new religious orders in the Catholic church that provided service to the sick and disenfranchised.

Epidemics had ravaged Europe for centuries, but they became even more serious with urbanization. Industrialization had brought people to cities, where they worked in close quarters (as compared with the isolation of the farm) and contributed to the social decay of the second half of the nineteenth century. Sanitation was poor or nonexistent, sewage disposal from the growing population was lacking, cities were filthy, public laws were weak or nonexistent, and congestion of the cities inevitably brought pests in the form of rats, lice, and bedbugs, which transmitted many pathogens. Communicable diseases continued to plague the population, especially those who lived in these unsanitary environments. For example, during the mid-eighteenth century typhus and typhoid fever claimed twice as many lives each year as did the Battle of Waterloo (Hanlon & Pickett, 1984). Through foreign trade and immigration, infectious diseases spread to all of Europe and eventually to the growing United States.

## John Snow and the Science of Epidemiology

John Snow, a prominent physician, is credited with being the first epidemiologist. In 1854, he demonstrated that cholera rates were linked with water pump use in London (Cartwright, 1972). Snow investigated the area around Golden Square in London and arrived at the conclusion that cholera was not carried by bad air, nor necessarily by direct contact. He formed the opinion that diarrhea, unwashed hands, and shared food somehow played a large part in spreading the disease.

People around Golden Square in London were not supplied with water by pipes, but rather drew their water from surface wells by means of hand-operated pumps. A severe outbreak of cholera occurred at the end of August 1853, resulting in at least 500 deaths in just 10 days in Golden Square. By identifying rates of cholera, Snow for the first time linked the sources of the drinking water at the Broad Street pump to the outbreaks of cholera, thereby proving that cholera was a waterborne disease. Snow's epidemiological investigation started a train of events that eventually would end the great epidemics of cholera, dysentery, and typhoid (Minkowski, 1992).

When Snow attended the now-famous community meeting of Golden Square and gave his evidence, government officials asked him what measures were necessary. His reply was, "Take the handle off the Broad Street pump." The handle was removed the next day, and no more cholera cases occurred (Snow, 1855). Although he did not discover the true cause of the cholera—the identification of the organism—he came very close to the truth (Rosen, 1958).

## And Then There Was Nightingale . . .

Florence Nightingale was named one of the 100 most influential persons of the last millennium by *Life* magazine (1997), one of only eight women so identified. Of those eight women, who included such luminaries as Joan of Arc, Helen Keller, and Elizabeth I, Nightingale was identified as a true "angel of mercy," having reformed military health care in the Crimean War and used her political savvy to forever change the way society views the health of the vulnerable, the poor, and the forgotten. She is probably one of the most written-about women in history (Bullough & Bullough. 1978). Florence Nightingale has become synonymous with modern nursing.

Florence Nightingale was the second child born to the wealthy English family of William and Frances Nightingale on May 12, 1820, in her namesake city, Florence, Italy. As a young child, Florence displayed incredible curiosity and intellectual abilities not common to female children of the Victorian age. She mastered the fundamentals of Greek and Latin, and she studied history, art, mathematics, and philosophy. To her family's dismay, she believed that God had called her to be a nurse. Nightingale was keenly aware of the suffering that industrialization created; she became obsessed with the plight of the miserable and suffering. Conditions of

✎ NOTE THIS! •————————————————
Florence Nightingale never made a public appearance, never issued a public statement, and did not have the right to vote.

## ⦿ MEDIA MOMENT

### The Lady with the Lamp: Florence Nightingale

*Country Joe McDonald*

In 1981 while attending a conference on post–Vietnam War problems of Vietnam veterans, Lynda Van Devanter, Vietnam War nurse and author of *Home Before Morning: The Story of an Army Nurse in Vietnam*, accused the audience of "ignoring women in the military." I felt I was certainly guilty of that in spite of the fact that I was ex-military myself. I began to research nursing and started with the life of the English woman credited with inventing "professional nursing" as we know it today, back in the Crimean War, 1854–1856: Florence Nightingale.

I wanted to write a Florence Nightingale song but it was years to come. As a break from reading about the Crimean War, Florence Nightingale, and the Vietnam War, I took to reading a book about the famous American woman who was a Civil War nurse and the person credited with starting the American Red Cross. This turned into the song "Clara Barton." Then one day, lo and behold, out of the blue came my Florence Nightingale song, "The Lady with the Lamp."

I now had three "war nurse songs." I realized that I was in a rut. I felt bad that my brother was a nurse practitioner and my wife a labor and delivery nurse but I had no non-military nurse song. I was struck with the fact that nurses are seldom given thanks for the work that they do. Nursing is often just taken for granted. So after much thought and effort out came "Thank the Nurse."

I have always wanted to advocate for people who seemed to be "taken for granted" and seemed to have no voice of their own in the public. So it has been a very interesting and rewarding experience these last 20 years studying about nursing and working on my Florence Nightingale website.

—Joe McDonald

First they use us
And then they throw us away.
Only Miss Nightingale
Knows the price that we pay,
The lady with the lamp.

*Source:* From the albums *Carry On* (Shanachie) and *Thank the Nurse*; lyrics by Joe McDonald; sung by Joe McDonald and Jerry Garcia.

To order the recording of the song and find out more about Joe McDonald's Web tribute to Florence Nightingale, go to http://www.countryjoe.com/nightingale/fnstore.htm.

---

general starvation had accompanied the Industrial Revolution, along with overflowing prisons and workhouses, and displaced persons in all sections of British life. Nightingale wrote in the spring of 1842, "My mind is absorbed with the sufferings of man; it besets me behind and before. . . . All that the poets sing of the glories of this world seem to me untrue. All the people that I see are eaten up with care or poverty or disease" (Woodham-Smith, 1951, p. 31).

 Research Alert

As part of her work, Florence Nightingale collaborated with William Farr, the eminent medical statistician. Nightingale's epidemiological investigations, supported by Farr, illustrated that attention to environmental cleanliness was an important factor in preventing spread of disease. Nightingale channeled her investigations to support hospital reforms and the need for educated nurses who could provide better management of the hospital environment. Statistical support and solicited criticism allowed Nightingale to argue more forcefully for her reforms. ◐

*Source:* Keeling, A.W. (2006). "Carrying ointments and even pills!" Medicines in the work of Henry Street Settlement visiting nurses, 1893–1944. *Nursing History Review, 14.*

For Nightingale, her entire life would be haunted by this conflict between the opulent life of gaiety that she enjoyed and the plight and misery of the world, which she was unable to alleviate. She was, in essence, an "alien spirit in the rich and aristocratic social sphere of Victorian England" (Palmer, 1977, p. 14). Nightingale remained unmarried, and at the age of 25, she expressed a desire to be trained as a nurse in an English hospital. Her parents emphatically denied her request, and for the next 7 years, she made repeated attempts to change their minds and allow her to enter nurse training. She wrote, "I crave for some regular occupation, for something worth doing instead of frittering my time away on useless trifles" (Woodham-Smith, 1951, p. 162).

During this time, Nightingale continued her education through the study of math and science, and she spent 5 years collecting data about public health and hospitals (Dietz & Lehozky, 1963). During a tour of Egypt in 1849 with family and friends, Nightingale spent her thirtieth year in Alexandria with the Sisters of Charity of St. Vincent de Paul, where her conviction to study nursing was only reinforced (Tooley, 1910). While in Egypt, Nightingale studied Egyptian, Platonic, and Hermetic philosophy; Christian scripture; and the works of poets, mystics, and missionaries in her efforts to understand the nature of God and her "calling" as it fit into the divine plan (Calabria, 1996; Dossey, 1985).

The next spring, Nightingale traveled unaccompanied to the **Kaiserwerth Institute** in Germany and stayed there for 2 weeks, vowing to return to train as a nurse. In June 1851, Nightingale took her future into her own hands and announced to her family that she planned to return to Kaiserwerth and study nursing. According to Dietz and Lehozky (1963, p. 42), her mother had "hysterics" and "scene followed scene." Her father "retreated into the shadows," and her sister, Parthe, expressed that the family name was forever disgraced (Cook, 1913).

In 1851, at the age of 31, Nightingale was finally permitted to go to Kaiserwerth. She studied there for 3 months with Pastor Fliedner. Her family insisted that she tell no one outside the family of her whereabouts, and her mother forbade her to write any letters from Kaiserwerth. While there, Nightingale learned about the care of the sick and the importance of discipline and commitment of oneself to God (Donahue, 1985). She returned to England and cared for her then-ailing father, from whom she finally gained some support for her intent to become a nurse—her lifelong dream.

In 1852, Nightingale wrote the essay "Cassandra," which stands today as a classic feminist treatise against the idleness of Victorian women. Through her voluminous journal writings, Nightingale reveals her inner struggle throughout her adulthood with what was expected of a woman and what she could accomplish with her life. The life expected of an aristocratic woman in her day was one she grew to loathe; throughout her writings, she poured out her detestation of the life of an idle woman (Nightingale, 1979, p. 5). In "Cassandra," Nightingale put her thoughts to paper, and many scholars believe that her eventual intent was to extend the essay to a novel. She wrote in "Cassandra," "Why have women passion, intellect, moral activity—these three—in a place in society where no one of the three can be exercised?" (Nightingale, 1979, p. 37). Although uncertain about the meaning of the name "Cassandra," many scholars believe that it came from the Greek goddess Cassandra, who was cursed by Apollo and doomed to see and speak the truth but never to be believed. Nightingale saw the conventional life of women as a waste of time and abilities. After receiving a generous yearly endowment from her father, Nightingale moved to London and worked briefly as the superintendent of the hospital Establishment for Gentlewomen During Illness, finally realizing her dream of working as a nurse (Cook, 1913).

### ■ The Crimean Experience: "I Can Stand Out the War with Any Man"

Nightingale's opportunity for greatness came when she was offered the position of female nursing establishment of the English General Hospitals in Turkey by the British Secretary of War, Sir Sidney Herbert. Soon after the outbreak of the Crimean War, stories of the inadequate care and lack of medical resources for the soldiers became widely known throughout England (Woodham-Smith, 1951). The country was appalled at the conditions so vividly portrayed in the *London Times*. Pressure increased on Sir Herbert to rectify the situation. He knew of one woman who was capable of bringing order out of the chaos and wrote the following now-famous letter to Nightingale on October 15, 1854, as a plea for her service:

There is but one person in England that I know of who would be capable of organising and superintending such a scheme. . . . The difficulty of finding women equal to a task after all, full of horrors, and requiring besides knowledge and good will, great energy and great courage, will be great. Your own personal qualities, your knowledge and your power of administration and among greater things your rank and position in Society give you advantages in such a work which no other person possesses. (Woodham-Smith, 1951, pp. 87–89)

Nightingale took the challenge from Sir Herbert and set sail with 38 self-proclaimed nurses with varied training and experiences, of whom 24 were Catholic and Anglican nuns. Their journey to the Crimea took a month. On November 4, 1854, the brave nurses arrived at Istanbul and were taken to Scutari the same day. Faced with 3,000 to 4,000 wounded men in a hospital designed to accommodate 1,700 patients, the nurses went to work (Kalisch & Kalisch, 1986). This is the scene that the nurses faced: There were 4 miles of beds 18 inches apart. Most soldiers were lying naked with no bed or blanket. There were no kitchen or laundry facilities. The little light present took the form of candles in beer bottles. The hospital was literally floating on an open sewage lagoon filled with rats and other vermin (Donahue, 1985).

The barrack "hospital" was more of a death trap than a place for healing before Nightingale's arrival. In a letter to Sir Herbert, Nightingale, demonstrating her sense of humor, wrote, with tongue in cheek, that "the vermin might, if they had but unity of purpose, carry off the four miles of beds on their backs and march them into the War Office" (Stanmore, 1906, pp. 393–394).

By taking the newly arrived medical equipment and setting up kitchens, laundries, recreation rooms, reading rooms, and a canteen, Nightingale and her team of nurses proceeded to clean the barracks of lice and filth. Nightingale was in her element: She set out not only to provide humane health care for the soldiers, but also to essentially overhaul the administrative structure of the military health services (Williams, 1961). Nightingale and her nurses faced overwhelming odds and deplorable conditions. No accommodations had been made for their quarters, so they ended up in one of the hospital towers, 39 women crowded into six small rooms. In addition to having no furniture, one of the rooms even contained a long-neglected, forgotten corpse swarming with vermin! Ever the disciplinarian, Nightingale insisted on strict adherence to a standard nurse uniform: gray tweed dresses, gray worsted jackets, plain white caps, short woolen cloaks, and brown scarves embroidered in red with the words "Scutari Hospital" (Bullough & Bullough, 1978).

## Florence Nightingale and Sanitation

Although Nightingale never accepted the germ theory, she demanded clean dressings; clean bedding; well-cooked, edible, and appealing food; proper sanitation; and fresh air. After the other nurses were asleep, Nightingale made her famous solitary rounds with a lamp or lantern to check on the soldiers. Nightingale had a lifelong pattern of sleeping few hours, spending many nights writing, developing elaborate plans, and evaluating implemented changes. She seldom believed in the "hopeless" soldier; instead, she saw only one that needed extra attention. Nightingale was convinced that most of the maladies that the soldiers suffered and died from were preventable (Williams, 1961).

Before Nightingale's arrival and her radical and well-documented interventions based on sound public health

> **❝** *Bad sanitary, bad architectural, and bad administrative arraignments often make it impossible to nurse.* **❞**
>
> —*Florence Nightingale*

principles, mortality rates for the Crimea War were estimated to range from 42% to 73%. Nightingale is credited with reducing that rate to 2% within 6 months of her arrival at Scutari. She did so by conducting careful, scientific epidemiological research (Dietz & Lehozky, 1963). Upon arriving at Scutari, Nightingale's first act was to order 200 scrubbing brushes. The death rate fell dramatically once Nightingale discovered that the hospital was built literally over an open sewage lagoon. A dead horse was even retrieved from the sewer system under Scutari (Andrews, 2003).

According to Palmer (1982), Nightingale possessed the qualities of a good researcher: insatiable curiosity, command of her subject, familiarity with methods of inquiry, a good background of statistics, and the ability to discriminate and abstract. She used these skills to maintain detailed and copious notes and to codify observations. Nightingale relied on statistics and attention to detail to back up her conclusions about sanitation, management of care, and disease causation. Her now-famous "cox combs" are a hallmark of military health services management, through which she

---

 **GLOBAL CONNECTION**

*I made up my mind that if the army wanted nurses, they would be glad of me, and with all the ardor of my nature, which ever carried me where inclination prompted, I decided that I would go to the Crimea; and go I did, as all the world knows.*

—*Mary Seacole*

Mary Seacole, contemporary of Florence Nightingale, was named in 2004 the greatest black Briton of all time. Although few have heard of Seacole, she was an important figure in the establishment of nursing as a profession. The Royal College of Nursing President Sylvia Denton said of this honor: "Mary Seacole stood up against the discrimination and prejudices she encountered. Against all odds, Mary had an unshakeable belief in the power of nursing to make a difference."

Seacole was born in the early 1880s as Mary Grant, in Kingston, Jamaica, to a Scottish father and a free black Jamaican mother. Her mother taught her about Creole medicine and she grew up well educated. In 1838, she married Edward Seacole, who died shortly afterward. During their short marriage, they traveled around the Caribbean and Central America. After her husband's death, she returned to Kingston to help run the family boardinghouse. During two epidemics of cholera and one epidemic of yellow fever, she sharpened her skills as a nurse, even performing a postmortem autopsy of a baby who had died of cholera.

Seacole eventually traveled with her brother to other South American countries, establishing hotels and providing care for the sick. When she learned of the Crimean War, she traveled to England, at her own expense, and offered her services to the British Army. She was refused because of the color of her skin. The put-down did not deter Seacole, who funded her own 3,000-mile trip to Crimea, where she offered her services to Florence Nightingale. Nightingale refused her offer as a nurse, so Seacole set up a "hotel for invalids"—called the British Hotel—in nearby Baklava.

At her hotel, Seacole banned drunkenness and gambling, dispensed medicines, fed soldiers meals, and tended to the wounded on the battlefield under fire, making home visits to campsites in the area. Seacole's hotel was a financial disaster, because she did not require payment for services and did not have the support of the British government. She used all of her savings to secure medicine and other needed supplies for the sick. When the Crimean War ended in 1856, Seacole was in severe debt and struggled in her lifetime residence in England. Her writings provided some financial support.

Through the years, historians have come to recognize Seacole's heroic and strong commitment to the development of war nursing. It is possible that Nightingale and Seacole never met. Historical evidence is unconclusive regarding the exact nature of their personal contact at Scutari. Nightingale's refusal to accept Seacole's offer to join her nurses at Sebastopol reflected the discrimination and prejudice of the day. Seacole received the Crimean Medal, the French Legion of Honor, and a Turkish Medal. She died in 1881 and is buried in London.

**Selected References on the Life of Mary Seacole**

Crawford, P. (1992). The other lady with the lamp: Nursing legacy of Mary Seacole. *Nursing Times, 88*(11), 56–58.

Gustafson, M. (1996). Mary Seacole, the Florence Nightingale of Jamaica. *Christian Nurse International, 12*(4), 9.

King, A. (1974). Mary Seacole, part I: A matter of life. *Essence, 4*(11), 32.

King, A. (1974). Mary Seacole, part II: The Crimea. *Essence, 4*(12), 68, 94.

Messmer, P. R., & Parchment, Y. (1998). Mary Grant Seacole: The first nurse practitioner. *Clinical Excellence for Nurse Practitioners, 2*(1), 47–51.

Payne, D. (1999). Face to face: Florence Nightingale and Mary Seacole battle it out face to face. *Nursing Times, 95*(19), 26–27.

## BOX 3-1

### Singing to Promote a Healthy Body and Soul: "The Nightingale's Song to the Sick Soldier"

Florence Nightingale set an example to all with her commitment and compassion to the weary and the sick. She had a special fondness for animals and birds and regularly showed compassion for them in correspondence. In one such letter to her cousin, she said, "There is nothing that makes my heart thrill like the voice of birds, much more than the human voice. It is the angels calling us with their songs." After her extraordinary acclaim resulting from her heroic actions during the Crimean War, numerous articles, songs, and poems of praise were written that linked Nightingale's compassion to the beautiful song of a nightingale. One such broadside that circulated after the war was published anonymously by *Punch* magazine entitled "The Nightingale's Song to the Sick Soldier." A broadside was a song or poem that was written to reflect the feelings and sentiment of the community.

> Singing succour to the brave and a rescue from the grave,
> Hear the nightingale that's come to the Crimea,
> 'Tis nightingale as strong in her heart as in her song,
> To carry out so gallant an idea.

The title of this poem is used as a metaphor for Nightingale's contribution to the war as a beautiful song. Last summer while preparing to enter nursing school, I volunteered at a hospital where my job was to help conduct recreational activities for the patients on the hospice ward. My favorite part of the day was when I got the chance to sing hymns to the patients. They would reach their hands out to me and smile. The nurses often remarked that many of these patients had not smiled in weeks. I was able to use singing as a way to touch the souls of the sick and bring comfort to those who were sad. After realizing how the singing touched my patients, I thought about how I could integrate singing, my other profession, into my nursing practice as a way to focus on the needs of the soul and the body. I believe that a nurse can communicate the joy that is inside us to the patient through the use of music as an act of compassion.

In this poem, Nightingale's legacy as a model, compassionate caregiver is conveyed through singing and the song of a nightingale. A song that was to keep a weary soldier alive and hopeful. It is this song that should be kept in the hearts of each nurse. It should radiate outwardly to "infect" all those around and emit a joyful spirit that is highly contagious.
Shandi Shiver, Senior BSN Nursing Student
Professional singer
The University of Southern Mississippi
School of Nursing

---

diagrammed deaths in the Army from wounds and from other diseases and compared them with deaths that occurred in similar populations in England (Palmer, 1977).

Nightingale was first and foremost an administrator: She believed in a hierarchical administrative structure with ultimate control lodged in one person to whom all subordinates and offices reported. Within a matter of weeks of her arrival in the Crimea, Nightingale was the acknowledged administrator and organizer of a mammoth humanitarian effort. From her Crimean experience on, Nightingale involved herself primarily in organizational activities and health planning administration. Palmer contends that Nightingale "perceived the Crimean venture, which was set up as an experiment, as a golden opportunity to demonstrate the efficacy of female nursing" (1982, p. 4). Although Nightingale faced initial resistance from the unconvinced and oppositional medical officers and surgeons, she boldly defied convention and remained steadfastly focused on her mission to create a sanitary and highly structured environment for her "children"—the British soldiers who dedicated their lives to the defense of Great Britain. Proving her resilience and insistence on absolute authority regarding nursing and the hospital environment, Nightingale was known to send nurses home to England from the Crimea for suspicious alcohol use and character weakness.

It was her success at Scutari that enabled Nightingale to begin a long career of influence on the public's health through social activism and reform, health policy, and the reformation of career nursing. Using her well-publicized successful "experiment" and supportive evidence from the Crimean War, Nightingale effectively argued the case for the reform and creation of military health that would serve as the model for people in uniform to the present (D'Antonio, 2002). Nightingale's ideas about proper hospital architecture and administration influenced a generation of medical doctors and the entire world, in both military and civilian service. Her work in *Notes on Hospitals*, published in 1859, provided the template for the organization of military health care in the Union Army when the U.S. Civil War erupted in 1861. Her vision for health care of soldiers and the responsibility of the governments who send them to war continues today; her influence can be seen throughout the last century and into the twenty-first century, as health care for the women and men who serve their countries is a vital part of the well-being of not only the soldiers but also society in general (D'Antonio, 2002). See Box 3-1.

**❝***Many soldiers wrote about their experiences of the Angel of Mercy, Florence Nightingale. One soldier wrote perhaps one of the most revealing tributes to this "Lady with the Lamp":*

*What a comfort it was to see her pass even. She would speak to one and nod and smile to as many more, but she could not do it all, you know. We lay there by hundreds, but we could kiss her shadow as it fell, and lay our heads on the pillow again content.* ❞

—Tyrell, 1856, p. 310

An African nurse from Jamaica, Mary Grant Seacole, offered her services to Nightingale after hearing of the need for nurses in Scutari. Although Nightingale rejected Seacole as a part of her nursing staff, Seacole persisted in her passion to provide care to the British military (Payne, 1999). Using her own money, she set up a type of inn that provided food and lodging for soldiers and their families near Scutari (Hine, 1989). Although Seacole is less well known than Nightingale, her contributions to nursing in wartime were significant in the history of minority nursing. Seacole is often referred to as "the other lady with the lamp" and "the Florence Nightingale of Jamaica." The School of Nursing in Kingston, Jamaica, is today named in her honor (Crawford, 1992).

Scores of books and articles have been written about Nightingale—she is an almost mythic figure in history. She truly was a beloved legend throughout Great Britain by the time she left the Crimea in July 1856, 4 months after the war ended. Longfellow immortalized this "Lady with the Lamp" in his poem of "Santa Filomena" (Longfellow, 1857).

> ❝ *Miss Nightingale had stamped the profession of nurse with her own image . . . in the midst of the muddle and the filth, the agony and the defeats; she had brought about a revolution.* ❞
> —Woodham-Smith, 1951, p. 179

## Returning Home a Heroine: The Political Reformer

When Nightingale returned to London, she found that her efforts to provide comfort and health to the British soldier succeeded in making heroes of both Nightingale and the soldiers (Woodham-Smith, 1951). Both had suffered from negative stereotypes: The soldier was often portrayed as a drunken oaf with little ambition or honor; the nurse was perceived as a tipsy, self-serving, illiterate, promiscuous loser. After the Crimean War and the efforts of Nightingale and her nurses, both returned with honor and dignity, never more to be downtrodden and disrespected.

After her return from the Crimea, Florence Nightingale never made a public appearance, never attended a public function, and never issued a public statement (Bullough & Bullough, 1978). Even so, she single-handedly raised nursing from, as she put it, "the sink it was" into a respected and noble profession (Palmer, 1977). As an avid scholar and student of the Greek writer Plato, Nightingale believed that she had a moral obligation to work primarily for the good of the community. Because she believed that education formed character, she insisted that nursing must go beyond care for the sick; the mission of the trained nurse must include social reform to promote the good. This dual mission of nursing—caregiver and political reformer—has shaped the profession as we know it today, especially in the field of community health nursing. LeVasseur (1998) contends that Nightingale's insistence on nursing's involvement of a larger political ideal in the historical foundation of the field distinguishes us from other scientific disciplines, such as medicine.

How did Nightingale accomplish this transformation? You will learn throughout this text how nurses effect change through others. Florence Nightingale is the standard by which we measure our effectiveness. She effected change through her wide command of acquaintances: Queen Victoria was a significant admirer of her intellect and ability to effect change, and she used her position as national heroine to get the attention of elected officials in Parliament. She was tireless and had an amazing capacity for work. She used people. Everyone who could be of service to her was enlisted to help her meet her goals. Her brother-in-law, Sidney Herbert, was a member of Parliament and often delivered her "messages" in the form of legislation. When Nightingale wanted the public incited, she turned to the press, writing letters to the *London Times* and having others of influence write articles. She was not above threats to "go public" by certain dates if an elected official refused to establish a commission or appoint a committee. And when those commissions were formed, Nightingale was ready with her list of selected people for appointment (Palmer, 1982).

### ■ Nightingale and Military Reforms

The first real test of Nightingale's military reforms came in the United States during the "War Between the States"—the Civil War. Nightingale was asked by the Union to advise on the organization of hospitals and care of the sick and wounded. She sent recommendations back to the United States based on her experiences and analysis in the Crimean War, and her advisement and influence gained wide publicity. Following her recommendations, the Union Army set up a sanitary commission and provided for regular inspection of camps. Nightingale also expressed a desire to help with the Confederate military but, unfortunately, had no channel of communication with them (Bullough & Bullough, 1978).

### ■ The Nightingale School of Nursing at St. Thomas: The Birth of Professional Nursing

The British public honored Nightingale by endowing 50,000 pounds in her name upon her return to England from the Crimea. The money had been raised from the soldiers under her care and donations from the public. This Nightingale Fund eventually was used to create the **Nightingale School of Nursing at St. Thomas**, which was to be the beginning of professional nursing (Donahue, 1985).

Nightingale, at the age of 40, decided that St. Thomas's Hospital was the place for her training school for nurses. While the negotiations for the school went forward, she spent her time writing *Notes on Nursing: What It Is and What It Is Not*, which was published in 1859. The small book of 77 pages, written for the British mother, was an instant success. An expanded library edition was written for nurses and used as the textbook for the students at St. Thomas. The book has since been translated into multiple languages, although it is believed that Nightingale refused all royalties earned from the publication of the book (Tooley, 1910; Cook, 1913).

The nursing students chosen for the new training school were handpicked; they had to be of good moral character, sober, and honest. Nightingale believed that the strong emphasis on morals was critical to gaining respect for the new "Nightingale nurse," with no possible ties to the disgraceful association of past nurses. Nursing students were monitored throughout their 1-year program both on and off the hospital grounds; their activities were carefully watched for character weaknesses, and discipline was severe and swift for violators. Accounts from Nightingale's journals and notes revealed instant dismissal of nursing students for such behaviors as "flirtation, using the eyes unpleasantly and being in the company of unsavory persons." Nightingale contended that "the future of nursing depends on how these young women behave themselves" (Smith, 1934, p. 234). She knew that experiment at St. Thomas to educate nurses and raise nursing to a moral and professional calling represented a drastic departure from the past images of nurses and would take extraordinary women of high moral character and intelligence. Nightingale knew every nursing student (called a probationer), personally, often having the students at her house for weekend visits. She devised a system of daily journal keeping for the probationers; Nightingale herself read the journals monthly to evaluate their character and work habits. Every nursing student admitted to St. Thomas had to submit an acceptable "letter of good character," and Nightingale herself placed graduate nurses in approved nursing positions.

One of the most important features of the Nightingale School was its relative autonomy. Both the school and the hospital nursing service were organized under the head matron. This was especially significant because it meant that nursing service began independently of the medical staff in selecting, retaining, and disciplining students and nurses (Bullough & Bullough, 1978).

Nightingale was opposed to the use of a standardized government examination and the movement for licensure of trained nurses. She believed that schools of nursing would lose control of educational standards with the advent of national licensure, most notably those standards related to moral character. Nightingale led a staunch opposition to the movement by the British Nurses Association (BNA) for licensure of trained nurses, which the BNA believed critical to protecting the public's safety by ensuring the qualification of nurses by licensure exam. Nightingale was convinced that qualifying a nurse by examination tested only the acquisition of technical skills, not the equally important evaluation of character. She believed nursing involved "divergencies too great for a single standard to be applied" (Woodham-Smith, 1951; Nutting & Dock, 1907).

## ■ Taking Health Care to the Community: Nightingale and Wellness

Early efforts to distinguish hospital from community health nursing include Nightingale's views on "health nursing," which she distinguished from "sick nursing." She wrote two influential papers: "Sick-Nursing and Health-Nursing," was

**❝** *I look to the day when there are no nurses to the sick but only nurses to the well.* **❞**

—Florence Nightingale, 1893

read in the United States at the Chicago Exposition in 1893, and "Health Teaching in Towns and Villages" in 1894 (Monteiro, 1985). Both papers praised the success of prevention-based nursing practice. Winslow (1946) acknowledged Nightingale's influence in the United States by being one of the first in the field of public health to recognize the importance of taking responsibility for one's own health. As she wrote in 1891, "there are more people to pick us up and help us stand on our own two feet" (Attewell, 1996). According to Palmer (1982), Nightingale was a leader in the wellness movement long before the concept was identified. Nightingale saw the nurse as the key figure in establishing a healthy society, and she envisioned a logical extension of nursing in acute hospital settings to the broadest sense of community used in nursing today. Writing in *Notes on Nursing*, she visualized the nurse as "the nation's first bulwark in health maintenance, the promotion of wellness, and the prevention of disease" (Palmer, 1982, p. 6).

**William Rathbone**, a wealthy ship owner and philanthropist, is credited with the establishment of the first visiting nurse service, which eventually evolved into district nursing in the community. He was so impressed with the private-duty nursing care that his sick wife had received at home that he set out to develop a "district nursing service" in Liverpool, England. At his own expense, in 1859, he developed a corps of nurses who were trained to care for the sick poor in their homes (Bullough & Bullough, 1978; Minkowski, 1992; Howse, 2007). He divided the community into 16 districts; each was assigned a nurse and a social worker who provided nursing and health education. Rathbone's experiment in district nursing was so successful that he was unable to find enough nurses to work in the districts. Rathbone then contacted Nightingale for assistance. Her recommendation was to train more nurses, and she advised Rathbone to approach the Royal Liverpool Infirmary with a proposal for opening another training school for nurses (Rathbone, 1890; Tooley, 1913). The infirmary agreed to Rathbone's proposal, and district nursing soon spread throughout England as successful "health nursing" in the community for the sick poor through voluntary agencies (Rosen, 1958).

Ever the visionary, Nightingale (1893) contended that "Hospitals are but an intermediate stage of civilization. The ultimate aim is to nurse the sick poor in their own homes" (Attewell, 1996). She also wrote in regard to visiting families at home (1894), "We must not talk to them or at them but with them" (Attewell, 1996). A service similar to that begun by Rathbone, **health visiting**, began in Manchester, England, in 1862 by the Manchester and Salford Sanitary Association. The purpose of placing "health visitors" in the home was to provide health information and instruction to families. Eventually, health visitors evolved to provide preventive

❝ *Florence Nightingale believed in Work with a capital W and her legacy of nurses as workers is with us to this day. I sometimes think that it [work] has on occasions stood in the way of healing. Maybe there have been times when we've been too busy looking as we were working to spend time healing.* ❞

—*Mary Chiarella*

........................................................

health education and district nurses to care for the sick at home (Bullough & Bullough, 1978; Howse, 2007).

Although Nightingale is best known for her reform of hospitals and military health care, she was a great believer in the future of health care, which she anticipated should be preventive in nature and would more than likely take place in the home and community. Her accomplishments in the field of "sanitary nursing" extended beyond the walls of the hospital to include workhouse reform and community sanitation reform. In 1864, Nightingale and Rathbone once again worked together to lead the reform of the Liverpool Workhouse Infirmary, where more than 1,200 sick paupers were crowded into unsanitary and unsafe conditions. Under the British Poor Laws, the most desperately poor of the large cities were gathered into large workhouses. When they became sick, they were also sent to the workhouse. Trained nursing care in these venues was all but nonexistent. Through legislative pressure and a well-designed public campaign describing the horrors of the workhouse infirmary, reform of the workhouse system was accomplished by 1867. Although it was not as complete as Nightingale had wanted, nevertheless nurses were in place and being paid a salary (Seymer, 1954).

## ■ Nightingale's Legacy

When Nightingale returned to London after the Crimean War, she remained haunted by her experiences related to the soldiers dying of preventable diseases. She was troubled by nightmares and had difficulty sleeping in the years that followed. She wrote in her journal: "Oh my poor men; I am a bad mother to come home and leave you in your Crimean graves. . . . I can never forget. . . . I stand at the altar of the murdered men and while I live, I fight their cause" (Woodham-Smith, 1983, pp. 178, 193). Nightingale became a prolific writer and a staunch defender of the causes of the British soldier, sanitation in England and India, and trained nursing.

As a woman, Nightingale was not able to hold an official government post or to vote. Historians have had varied opinions about the exact nature of the disability that kept her homebound for the remainder of her life. Recent scholars have speculated that she experienced post-traumatic stress disorder from her experiences in the Crimea; there is also considerable evidence that she suffered from the painful disease brucellosis (Barker, 1989; Young, 1995). Nevertheless, Nightingale exerted incredible influence through friends and acquaintances, directing from her sickroom sanitation and poor law reform. Her mission to "cleanse" spread from the military to the British Empire; her fight for improved sanitation both at home and in India consumed her energies for the remainder of her life (Vicinus & Nergaard, 1990).

According to Monteiro (1985), two recurrent themes are found throughout Nightingale's writings about disease prevention and wellness outside the hospital. *The most persistent theme is that nurses must be trained differently and instructed specifically in district and instructive nursing.* Nightingale consistently wrote that the "health nurse" must be trained in the nature of poverty and its influence on health, something she referred to as the "pauperization" of the poor. She also believed that above all, health nurses must be good teachers about hygiene and helping families learn to better care for themselves (Nightingale, 1893). She insisted that untrained, "good intended women" could not substitute for nursing care in the home. Instead, Nightingale pushed for an extensive orientation and additional training, including prior hospital experience, before someone was hired as a district nurse. She outlined the qualifications in her paper "On Trained Nursing for the Sick Poor," in which she called for 1 month's "trial" in district nursing, 1 year's training in hospital nursing, and 3 to 6 months training in district nursing (Monteiro, 1985). According to Nightingale, "There is no such thing as amateur nursing."

The second theme that emerged from her writings was the focus on the role of the nurse. *Nightingale clearly distinguished the role of the health nurse in promoting what we today call self-care.* In the past, philanthropic visitors under the aegis of Christian charity, would visit the homes of the poor and offer them relief (Monteiro, 1985). Nightingale believed that such activities did little to teach the poor to care for themselves and further "pauperized" them—keeping them dependent and vulnerable, unhealthy, prone to disease, and reliant on others to keep them healthy. The nurse had to help the families at home manage a healthy environment for themselves, and Nightingale saw a trained nurse as being the only person who could pull off such a feat. She stated, "Never think that you have done anything effectual in nursing in London, till you nurse not only the sick poor in workhouses, but those at home."

---

### ✎ ETHICAL CONNECTION

There are five essential points in securing the health of houses:
- Pure air
- Pure water
- Efficient drainage
- Cleanliness
- Light

........................................................

*Sources:* Nightingale, F. (1860). *Notes on nursing: What it is and what it is not.* London: Harrison; Cook, 1913, p. 133.

---

❝ *To set these poor sick people going again, with a sound and clean house, as well as with a sound body and mind, is about as great a benefit as can be given them—worth acres of gifts and relief. This is depauperizing them.* ❞

—*Florence Nightingale*

❝*My view you know is that the ultimate destination of all nursing is the nursing of the sick in their own homes. . . . I look to the abolition of all hospitals and workhouse infirmaries. But no use to talk about the year 2000.*❞

—*Florence Nightingale, letter to Henry Bonham Carter, 1867*

By 1901, Nightingale lived in a world without sight or sound leaving her unable to write. Over the next 5 years, she lost her ability to communicate and most days existed in a state of unconsciousness. In November 1907, Nightingale was honored with the Order of Merit by King Edward VII, the first time the award was ever given to a woman. In May 1910, the Nightingale Training School of Nursing at St. Thomas celebrated its Jubilee. By that time, there were now more than 1,000 training schools for nurses in the United States alone (Tooley, 1910; Cook, 1913).

Nightingale died in her sleep around noon on August 13, 1910, and was buried quietly and without pomp near the family's home at Embley, her coffin carried by six sergeants of the British Army. Only a small cross marks her grave at her request: "FN. Born 1820. Died 1910." (Brown, 1988). The family refused a national funeral and burial at Westminster Abbey out of respect for Nightingale's last wishes. She had lived for 90 years and 3 months.

❝*Money would be better spent in maintaining health in infancy and childhood than in building hospitals to cure disease.*❞

—*Florence Nightingale, 1894*

❝*It is cheaper to promote health than to maintain people in sickness.*❞

—*Florence Nightingale, 1894*

👆 THINK ABOUT THIS ·······························

Some nurses believe that the legacy of Florence Nightingale is holding nursing back and represents the negative and backward elements of nursing. This view cites as evidence Nightingale's support for the subordination of nurses to physician, opposition to registration of nurses, and failure to see mental health nurses as part of the profession. Wheeler has gone so far as to say, "The nursing profession needs to exorcise the myth of Nightingale, not necessarily because she was a bad person, but because the impact of her legacy has held the profession back too long." After reading this chapter, what do you think? Is Nightingale relevant in the twenty-first century to the nursing profession? Why or why not?

*Source:* Wheeler, W. (1999). Is Florence Nightingale holding us back? *Nursing 99, 29*(10), 82–23.

❝*Preventable disease should be looked upon as a social crime.*❞

—*Florence Nightingale, 1894*

❝ *a conversation with . . .* ❞

**Barbara Dossey**

Barbara Dossey is a noted Nightingale scholar and the author of the book *Florence Nightingale: Mystic, Visionary, Healer* (Philadelphia: Lippincott, Williams & Wilkins, 2000).

Was Nightingale a mystic? Mysticism is often defined as an individual's direct, unmediated experience of God. A mystic is a person who has such an experience, to a greater or lesser degree. Nightingale received her fire call from God at age 16, and received three more direct calls from God in her life. She believed the messages of Christianity, but was tolerant and ecumenical in her attitude toward world religions. She wrote, "To know God we must study Him in the Pagan and Jewish dispensations as in the Christian."

*Source*: Manthey, M. (1999). A Nightingale legacy: The art of nursing: Interview with Barbara Dossey. *Creative Nursing, 5*(3), 7–15.

 THINK ABOUT THIS ·······························

What would Florence Nightingale's resume or vita look like? Find out what Nightingale herself wrote in her vita online at http://www.countryjoe.com/nightingale/cv.htm.

## Early Nursing Education and Organization in the United States

In the United States, the first training schools for nursing were modeled after the Nightingale School of Nursing at St. Thomas in London. Bellevue Training School for Nurses in New York City; Connecticut Training School for Nurses in New Haven, Connecticut; and the Boston Training School for Nurses at Massachusetts General Hospital in Boston were the earliest programs for trained nurses in the United States (Dock & Nutting, 1907; Christy, 1975). Based on the Victorian belief in the natural affinity for women to be sensitive, possess high morals, and be caregivers, early nursing training required that applicants be female. Sensitivity, high moral character, purity of character, subservience, and "ladylike" behavior became the associated traits of a "good nurse," thus setting the "feminization of nursing" as the ideal standard for a good nurse. These historical roots of gender-and-race based caregiving excluded males and minorities from the nursing profession, a trend that continued for many years and still influences career choices for men and women today. These early training schools provided a stable, subservient, white female workforce, as student nurses served as the primary nursing staff for these early hospitals.

A significant report, known simply as the **Goldmark Report** (more formally, *Nursing and Nursing Education in the United States*), was released in 1922; it advocated the

☞ THINK ABOUT THIS ⋯⋯⋯⋯⋯⋯⋯

There have been many theories about the cause of Nightingale's chronic illness, which led her to being an invalid for most of her adult life. Many people have interpreted her condition as hypochondriacal, something of a melodrama of the Victorian times. Nightingale was rich and could take to her bed. Rumors have floated around among nursing students for years that she suffered from tertiary syphilis. She became ill during the Crimean War in May 1855 and was diagnosed with a severe case of Crimean fever. Today Crimean fever is recognized as Mediterranean fever and is categorized as brucellosis. Nightingale also developed alter spondylistis, or inflammation of the spine.

For the next 34 years, Nightingale managed to continue her writing and advocacy, often predicting her imminent death. Some have claimed that she suffered from a bipolar disorder, causing her to experience long periods of depression and remarkable bursts of productivity. Read about the various theories of her chronic disabling condition and reflect on your own conclusions about her mysterious illness.

*Sources:* Dossey, B. (2000). *Florence Nightingale: Mystic, visionary, healer* (Philadelphia: Lippincott, Williams & Wilkins); Nightingale suffered bipolar disorder. (2004). *Australian Nursing Journal, 12,* 2.

establishment of university schools of nursing to train nursing leaders. The report, initiated by Nutting in 1918, was an exhaustive (500-page) and comprehensive investigation into the state of nursing education and training. Author Josephine Goldmark, a social worker and pioneer in research into nursing preparation in the United States, stated, "From our field study of the nurse in public health nursing, in private duty, and as instructor and supervisor in hospitals, it is clear that there is need of a basic undergraduate training for all nurses alike, which should lead to a nursing diploma" (Goldmark, 1923, p. 35).

The first university school of nursing was established at the University of Minnesota in 1909. Although the new nurse training school was under the college of medicine and offered only a 3-year diploma, the Minnesota program nevertheless represented a significant leap forward in nursing education.

*Nursing for the Future* (the so-called Brown Report), authored by Esther Lucille Brown in 1948 and sponsored by the Russell Sage Foundation, was critical of the quality and structure of nursing schools in the United States. The Brown Report ultimately became the catalyst for the implementation of educational nursing program accreditation through the National League for Nursing (NLN) (Brown, 1936, 1948).

Positive changes also occurred for minority and male nurses. As a result of the post–World War II nursing shortage, the Associate Degree in Nursing (A.D.N.) was established by Mildred Montag in 1952 as a 2-year program for registered nurses (Montag, 1959). In 1950, nursing became the first profession for which the same licensure exam, the State Board Test Pool, was used throughout the nation to license registered nurses. This increased mobility for the registered nurse resulted in a significant advantage for the relatively new profession of nursing (State Board Test Pool Examination, 1952).

## The Evolution of Nursing in the United States: The First Century of Professional Nursing

Early nurse leaders of the century included **Isabel Hampton Robb**, who in 1896 founded the Nurses' Associated Alumnae. In 1911, this organization officially became known as the **American Nurses Association (ANA). Lavinia Lloyd Dock** was a militant suffragist who linked women's roles as nurses to the emerging women's movement in the United States. By contrast, Isabel Hampton Robb—like Nightingale herself—opposed the women's suffragist movement, instead focusing on the need for women to own property in Great Britain. Her well-reasoned position was that property ownership was the link to women's voting power.

Mary Adelaide Nutting, Lavinia Lloyd Dock, Sophia Palmer, and Mary E. Davis were instrumental in developing the first nursing journal, **American Journal of Nursing (AJN),** in October 1900. Through the ANA and the *AJN*, nurses then had a professional organization and a national journal with which to communicate with one another (Kalisch & Kalisch, 1986).

State licensure of trained nurses began in 1903 with the enactment of North Carolina's licensure law for nursing. Shortly thereafter, New Jersey, New York, and Virginia passed similar licensure law for nursing. Professional nursing was well on its way to public recognition of practice and educational standards, as state after state passed similar legislation over the next several years.

**Margaret Sanger** worked as a nurse on the Lower East Side of New York City in 1912 with immigrant families. She was astonished to find widespread ignorance among these families about conception, pregnancy, and childbirth. After a horrifying experience with the death of a woman from a failed self-induced abortion, Sanger devoted her life to teaching women about birth control. A staunch activist in the early family planning movement, Sanger is credited with founding Planned Parenthood of America (Sanger, 1928).

By 1917, the emerging nursing profession was driven by two significant events that dramatically increased the need for additional trained nurses in the United States: World War I and the influenza epidemic. Nightingale's work and the devastation of the Civil War had firmly established the need

> ❝ *As the modern nursing movement is emphatically an outcome of the original and general woman's movement . . . it would be a great pity for them [nurses] to allow one of the most remarkable movements of the day to go on under their eyes without comprehending it. . . . Unless we possess the ballot we shall not know when we may get up in the morning to find all that we had gained has been taken from us.* ❞
>
> —*Lavinia Lloyd Dock, 1907*

**A Good Read**

## African American Nurses in History

Read more about the contributions of African American nurses . . .

Alexander, Z., & Dewjee, A. (1981). Mary Seacole. *History Today, 31*, 45.

Bell, P. L. (1993). "Making do" with the midwife: Arkansas's Mamie O. Hale in the 1940s. *Nursing History Review, 1*, 155–169.

Brewman, M. P. (1952). The Negro nurse. *Nation, 175*(8), 160.

Buhler-Wilkerson, K. (1992). Caring in its "proper place": Race and benevolence in Charleston, SC, 1813–1930. *Nursing Research, 41*(1), 14–20.

Campinha-Bacote, J. (1988). The Black nurses' struggle toward equality: An historical account of the National Association of Colored Graduate Nurses. *Journal of National Black Nurses Association, 2*(2), 15–25.

Carnegie, M. E. (1992). Black nurses in the United States: 1879–1992. *Journal of National Black Nurses Association, 6*(1), 13–18.

Chayer, M. E. (1954). Mary Eliza Mahoney. *American Journal of Nursing, 54*(4), 429–431.

Davis A. T. (1999). *Early black American leaders in nursing: Architects for integration and equality*. (National League for Nursing Series.) Sudbury, MA: Jones and Bartlett.

Doona, M. E. (1986). Glimpses of Mary Eliza Mahoney (7 May 1845–4 January 1929). *Journal of Nursing History, 1*(2), 20–34.

Elmore, J. A. (1976). Black nurses: Their service and their struggle. *American Journal of Nursing, 76*(3), 435–437.

George, V. D., Bradford, D. M., & Battle, A. (2000). Yesterday, today, and tomorrow: Transitioning through time with the Cleveland Council of Black Nurses. *Nursing & Health Care Perspectives, 21*(5), 219–227.

Goldstein, R. L. (1960). Negro nurses in hospitals. *American Journal of Nursing, 60*(2), 215–217.

Mabel Staupers, who led battle to end prejudice, dies at 99. (1990). *American Journal of Nursing, 9*(2), 121.

Mosley, M. O. P. (1995). Beginning at the beginning: A history of the professionalization of black nurses in America, 1908–1951. *Journal of Cultural Diversity, 2*(4), 101–109.

Mosley, M. O. P. (1995). Despite all odds: A three-part history of the professionalization of black nurses through two professional nursing organizations, 1908–1955. *Journal of National Black Nurses Association, 7*(2), 10–20.

Mosley, M. O. P. (1995). Mabel K. Staupers: A pioneer in professional nursing. *N & HC Perspectives on Community, 16*(1), 12–17.

Mosley, M. O. P. (1996). A new beginning: The story of the National Association of Colored Graduate Nurses, 1908–1951. *Journal of National Black Nurses Association, 8*(1), 20–32.

Smith, S. L. (1994). White nurses, black midwives, and public health in Mississippi, 1920–1950. *Nursing History Review, 2*, 29–49.

Staupers, M. K. (1937). The Negro nurse in America. *Opportunity, 15*(11), 339–341.

Staupers, M. K. (1961). *No time for prejudice: A story of the integration of Negroes in nursing in the United States.* New York: MacMillan.

Tucker-Allen, S. (1997). The founding of the Association of Black Nursing Faculty: My memories of the first five years. *ABNF Journal, 8*(4), 73–80.

Washington, B. T. (1910). Looking through the years: 1910. Training colored nurses at Tuskegee. *American Journal of Nursing, 11*, 167–171. Reprinted by permission. *Creative Nursing: A Journal of Values, Issues, Experience & Collaboration, 3*(1), 16, 1997.

Wilkins, R. (1943). Black women in white. *Negro Digest, 1*(6), 61–63.

---

for nursing care in war. Mary Adelaide Nutting, now Professor of Nursing and Health at Columbia University, chaired the newly established Committee on Nursing in response to the call for more nurses as the United States entered the war in Europe. U.S. nurses realized early on that World War I was unlike previous wars: It was a global conflict that involved coalitions of nations against nations, involving vast amounts of supplies and demanding the organization of all the nation's resources for military purposes (Kalisch & Kalisch, 1986). Along with **Lillian Wald** and **Jane A. Delano**, Director of Nursing in the American Red Cross, Nutting initiated a national publicity campaign to recruit young women to enter

nurse training. The Army School of Nursing, headed by **Annie Goodrich** as dean, and the Vassar Training Camp for Nurses prepared nurses for the war as well as home nursing and hygiene nursing through the Red Cross (Dock & Stewart, 1931). The Committee on Nursing estimated that there were at most 200,000 active "nurses" in the United States at the beginning of World War I, both trained and untrained, which was inadequate to support the military effort abroad (Kalisch & Kalisch, 1986). At home, the influenza epidemic of 1917–1919 led to increased public awareness of the need for public health nursing and public education about hygiene and disease prevention.

The successful campaign to attract nursing students focused heavily on patriotism, which ushered in the new era for nursing as a profession. By 1918, nursing school enrollments were up by 25%. In 1920, Congress passed a bill that provided nurses with military rank (Dock & Stewart, 1920). Following close behind, the passage of the Nineteenth Amendment to the U.S. Constitution granted women the right to vote. According to Stewart,

> Probably the greatest contribution of the war experience to nursing lies in the fact that the whole system of nursing education was shaken for a little while out of its well-worn ruts and brought out of its comparative seclusion into the light of public discussion and criticism. When so many lives hung on the supply of nurses, people were aroused to a new sense of their dependence on the products of nursing schools, and many of them learned for the first time of the hopelessly limited resources which nursing educators have had to work with in the training of these indispensable public servants. Whatever the future may bring, it is unlikely that nursing schools will willingly sink back again into their old isolation or that they will accept unquestionably the financial status which the older system imposed on them. (Stewart, 1921, p. 6)

While nursing as a profession was emerging in the United States, it remained a "white, female only" career choice during these early years. Men and minorities were excluded from the field, and those who wanted to enter nursing school found themselves essentially "locked out." Eventually, quotas were established in select nursing programs to permit African Americans' and other minorities' admission. Even when these nurses graduated, they had very few employment opportunities owing to segregationist policies of hospitals and other health agencies. Males faced the same challenges, and eventually schools of nursing were developed specifically for male nurse training. Early roles for male nurses were limited to psychiatric facilities, where their strength and larger stature were considered advantages in dealing with these populations.

These early discriminatory policies both reflected the era and were patterned after Nightingale's belief that nursing was best suited for women and their nurturing instinct. Nightingale did not write specifically about the inclusion of minorities in the nursing profession. However, as indicated by her attitude toward Mary Seacole (as discussed earlier in chapter), she seemed to have a preference for white female nurses as the face of the emerging profession of nursing.

## The Emergence of Community and Public Health Nursing

The pattern for health visiting and district nursing practice outside the hospital was similar in the United States to that in England (Roberts, 1954). U.S. cities were besieged by overcrowding and epidemics after the Civil War. The need for trained nurses evolved as in England, and schools throughout the United States developed along the Nightingale model. Visiting nurses were first sent to philanthropic organizations in New York City (1877), Boston (1886), Buffalo (1885), and Philadelphia (1886) to care for the sick at home. By the end of the century, most large cities had some form of visiting nursing program, and some headway was being made even in smaller towns (Heinrich, 1983). Industrial or occupational health nursing was first started in Vermont in 1895 by a marble company interested in the health and welfare of its workers and their families. Tuberculosis (TB) was a leading cause of death in the nineteenth century; nurses visited patients bedridden from TB and instructed persons in all settings about prevention of the disease (Abel, 1997).

### ■ Lillian Wald, Public Health Nursing, and Community Activism

Lillian Wald, a wealthy young woman with a great social conscience, graduated from the New York Hospital School of Nursing in 1891 and is credited with creating the title "public health nurse." After a year working in a mental institution, Wald entered medical school at Woman's Medical College in New York. While in medical school, she was asked to visit immigrant mothers on New York's Lower East Side and instruct them on health matters (see Box 3-2). Wald was appalled by the conditions there. During one now famous home visit, a small child asked Wald to visit her sick mother.

A nurse makes her "rounds" on the street of New York City for the Henry Street Visiting Nurse Services.

## BOX 3-2

### Lillian Wald Takes a Walk

From the schoolroom where I had been giving a lesson in bed-making, a little girl led me one drizzling March morning. She had told me of her sick mother, and gathering from her incoherent account that a child had been born, I caught up the paraphernalia of the bed-making lesson and carried it with me.

The child led me over broken roadways . . . between tall, reeking houses whose laden fire-escapes, useless for their appointed purpose, bulged with household goods of every description. The rain added to the dismal appearance of the streets and to the discomfort of the crowds which thronged them, intensifying the odors which assailed me from every side. Through Hester and Division Streets we went to the end of Ludlow; past odorous fish-stands, for the streets were a market-place, unregulated, unsupervised, unclean, past evil-smelling, uncovered garbage cans . . .

All the maladjustments of our social and economic relations seemed epitomized in this brief journey and what was found at the end of it. The family to which the child led me was neither criminal nor vicious. Although the husband was a cripple, one of those who stand on street corners exhibiting deformities to enlist compassion, and masking the begging of alms by a pretense of selling, although the family of seven shared their two rooms with boarders—who were literally boarders, since a piece of timber was placed over the floor for them to sleep on—and although the sick woman lay on a wretched, unclean bed, soiled with a hemorrhage two days old, they were not degraded human beings, judged by any measure of moral values.

In fact, it was very plain that they were sensitive to their condition, and when, at the end of my ministrations, they kissed my hands (those who have undergone similar experiences will, I am sure, understand), it would have been some solace if by any conviction of the moral unworthiness of the family I could have defended myself as a part of a society which permitted such conditions to exist. Indeed, my subsequent acquaintance with them revealed the fact that miserable as their state was, they were not without ideals for the family life, and for society, of which they were so unloved and unlovely a part.

That morning's experience was a baptism of the fire. Deserted were the laboratory and the academic work of the college. I never returned to them. On my way from the sick-room to my comfortable student quarters my mind was intent on my own responsibility. To my inexperience it seemed certain that conditions such as these were allowed because people did not know, and for me there was a challenge to know and to tell. When early morning found me still awake, my naive conviction remained that, if people knew things—and "things" meant everything implied in the condition of this family—such horrors would cease to exist, and I rejoiced that I had a training in the care of the sick that in itself would give me an organic relationship to the neighborhood in which this awakening had come.

*Source*: *The House on Henry Street*. (1915). New York: Henry Holt and Company.

And the rest, as they say, is history. According to Wald: "Nursing is love in action and there is no finer manifestation of it than the care of the poor and disabled in their own homes" (Wald, 1915, p. 14).

What Wald found changed her life forever and secured a place for her in American nursing history. Wald said, "all the maladjustments of our social and economic relations seemed epitomized in this brief journey" (1915, p. 6). Wald was profoundly affected by her observations; she and her colleague, **Mary Brewster**, quickly established the **Henry Street Settlement** in this same neighborhood in 1893. She quit medical school and devoted the remainder of her life to "visions of a better world" for the public's health.

This effort later evolved into the Visiting Nurse Service of New York City, which laid the foundation for the establishment of public health nursing in the United States. The health needs of the population were met through addressing social, economic, and environmental determinants of health, in a pattern after Nightingale. The nurses helped educate families about disease transmission and stressed the importance of good hygiene. They provided preventive, acute, and long-term care. As such, the Henry Street Settlement went far beyond the care of the sick and the prevention of illness: It aimed at rectifying those causes that led to the poverty and misery.

Wald was a tireless social activist for legislative reforms that would provide a more just distribution for the marginal and disadvantaged in the United States (Donahue, 1985). She began her work with 10 nurses in 1893, which grew to 250 nurses serving 1,300 patients each day by 1916. During this same period, the budget for the service grew from nothing to more than $600,000 per year, all from private donations.

Wald hired African American nurse **Elizabeth Tyler** in 1906 as evidence of her commitment to cultural diversity. Although unable to visit white patients, Tyler made her own way by "finding" African American families who needed her service. In 3 months, Tyler had so many African American families in her caseload that Wald hired a second African American nurse, Edith Carter. Carter remained at Henry Street for 28 years until her retirement (Carnegie, 1991).

During her tenure at Henry Street, Wald demonstrated her commitment to racial and cultural diversity by employing 25 African American nurses over the years, and she paid them salaries equal to white nurses, and provided identical benefits and recognition to minority nurses (Carnegie, 1991). This practice was exceptional during the early part of the twentieth century, a time when African American nurses were often denied admission to white schools of nursing and membership in professional organizations and were denied opportunities for employment in most settings. Because hospitals of this era often set quotas for African American patients, those nurses who managed to graduate from nursing schools found themselves with few patients who needed or could afford their services. African American nurses struggled for the right to take the registration examination available to white nurses.

Wald submitted a proposal to the city of New York after learning of a child's dismissal from a New York City school for a skin condition. Her proposal was for one of the Henry Street Settlement nurses to serve for free for 1 month in a New York school. The results of her experiment were so convincing that salaries were approved for 12 school nurses. From this beginning, school nursing was born in the United States and became one of many community specialties credited to Wald (Dietz & Lehozky, 1963).

In 1909, Wald proposed a program to the Metropolitan Life Insurance Company to provide nursing visits to its industrial policyholders. Statistics kept by the company documented the lowered mortality rates of policyholders attributed to the nurses' public health practice and clinical expertise. The program demonstrated savings for the company and was so successful that it lasted until 1953 (Hamilton, 1988).

---

### 🖥 Research Alert

Three exceptional African American nurses—Jessie Sleet, Elizabeth Tyler, and Edith Carter—are considered pioneers in community health nursing. This research article details how these three African American community health nurses made significant contributions to the development of New York City's community health nursing by providing much needed health care to unserved members of the African American community (1900–1937). They provided strong leadership in diverse roles such as supervisors, administrators, and educators in patient's homes, babies' health stations, settlement houses, and clinics. Their work occurred during a period of rapid industrialization, immigration, and great population growth in the midst of teeming slums, diseases, and death. In community health nursing history, it was a period of establishment, activism, expansion, and development. For these African American nurse pioneers, it was a time of significant challenges and growth. They faced educational, professional, and racial barriers and increased mortality among people of their own race. This research chronicles their brave and skilled efforts to transcend these barriers and improve the health of African American citizens during the early part of the twentieth century.

*Source*: Mosley, M. O. (1996). Satisfied to carry the bag: Three black community health nurses' contributions to health care reform, 1900–1937. *Nursing History Review, 4*, 65–82.

---

Wald's other significant accomplishments include the establishment of the Children's Bureau, set up in 1912 as part of the U.S. Department of Labor. She was also an enthusiastic supporter of and participant in women's suffrage, lobbied for inspections of the workplace, and supported her employee, Margaret Sanger, in her efforts to give women the right to birth control. She was active in the American and International Red Cross and helped form the Women's Trade Union League to protect women from sweatshop conditions.

Wald first coined the phrase "public health nursing" and transformed the field of community health nursing from the narrow role of home visiting to the population focus of today's community health nurse (Robinson, 1946). According to Dock and Stewart (1931), the title of "public health nurse" was purposeful: The role designation was designed to link the public's health to governmental responsibility, not private funding. As state departments of health and local governments began to employ more and more public health nurses, their role increasingly focused on prevention of illness in the entire community. A distinction was made between the visiting nurse, who was employed by the voluntary agencies primarily to provide home care to the sick, and the public health nurse, who concentrated on preventive measures (Brainard, 1922). Early public health nurses came closer than hospital-based nurses to the autonomy and professionalism that Nightingale advocated. Their work was conducted in the unconfined setting of the home and community, they were independent, and they enjoyed recognition as specialists in preventive health (Buhler-Wilkerson, 1985). Public health nurses from the beginning were much more holistic in their practice than their hospital counterparts. They were involved with the health of industrial workers, immigrants, and their families, and were concerned about exploitation of women and children. These nurses also played a part in prison reform and care of the mentally ill (Heinrich, 1983).

Considered the first African American public health nurse, **Jessie Sleet Scales** was hired in 1902 by the Charity Organization Society, a philanthropic organization, to visit African American families infected by TB. Scales provided district nursing care to New York City's African American families and is credited with paving the way for African American nurses in the practice of community health (Mosley, 1996).

### ■ Dorothea Linde Dix

**Dorothea Linde Dix**, a Boston schoolteacher, became aware of the horrendous conditions in prisons and mental institutions when asked to do a Sunday school class in the House of Correction at Cambridge, Massachusetts. She was appalled at what she saw and went about studying if the conditions were isolated or widespread; she took 2 years off to visit every jail and almshouse from Cape Cod to the Berkshire Mountains (Tiffany, 1890, p. 76). Her report was devastating. Boston was scandalized by the reality that the most progressive state in the union was now associated with such horrible conditions. The shocked legislature voted to allocate funds to build hospitals. For the rest of her life, Dorothea Dix stood out as a tireless zealot for the humane treatment of the insane and imprisoned. She had exceptional savvy in dealing with legislators: She acquainted herself with the legislators and their records and displayed the "spirit of a crusader." For her contributions, she is considered one of the pioneers of the reform movement in the United States, and her efforts are felt worldwide to the present day (Dietz & Lehozky, 1963).

Dix was also known for her work in the Civil War, having been appointed superintendent of the female nurses of the Army by the secretary of war in 1861. Her tireless efforts

Nurse midwives in rural areas contributed to the decline in maternal and infant mortality during the 1950s.

led to the recruitment of more than 2,000 women to serve in the army during the Civil War. Officials had consulted Florence Nightingale concerning conditions in military hospitals and were determined not to make the same mistakes. Dix enjoyed far more sweeping powers than Nightingale, in that she had the authority to organize hospitals, to appoint nurses, and to manage supplies for the wounded (Brockett & Vaughan, 1867). Among her most well-known nurses during the Civil War were the poet Walt Whitman and the author Louisa May Alcott (Donahue, 1985).

### ■ Clara Barton

The idea for the International Red Cross was the brainchild of a Swiss banker, J. Henri Dunant, who proposed the formation of a neutral international relief society that could be activated in time of war. The International Red Cross was ratified by the Geneva Convention on August 22, 1864.

**Clara Barton**, through her work in the Civil War, had come to believe that such an organization was desperately needed in the United States. However, it was not until 1882 that Barton was able to convince Congress to ratify the Treaty of Geneva, thus becoming the founder of the American Red Cross (Kalisch & Kalisch, 1986). Barton also played a leadership role in the Spanish–American War in Cuba, where she led a group of nurses to provide care for both U.S. and Cuban soldiers and Cuban civilians. At the age of 76, Barton went to President McKinley and offered the help of the Red Cross in Cuba. McKinley agreed to allow Barton to go with Red Cross nurses, but only to care for the Cuban citizens. Once in Cuba,

the U.S. military saw what Barton and her nurses were able to accomplish with the Cuban military, and American soldiers pressured military officials to allow Barton's help. Along with battling yellow fever, Barton was able to provide care to both Cuban and U.S. military personnel and eventually expanded that care to Cuban citizens in Santiago. One of Barton's most famous patients was young Colonel Teddy Roosevelt, who later became the president of the United States.

Barton became an instant heroine both in Cuba and in the United States for her bravery, tenaciousness, and organized services for the military and civilians torn apart by war. On August 13, 1898, the Spanish–American War came to an end. The grateful people of Santiago, Cuba, built a statue to honor Clara Barton in the town square, where it stands to this day. Tales of the work of Barton and her Red Cross nurses were spread through the newspapers of the United States and in the schools of nursing. A congressional committee investigating the work of Barton's Red Cross staff applauded the work of these nurses and recommended that the U.S. Medical Department create a permanent reserve corps of trained nurses. These reserve nurses became the Army Nurse Corps in 1901.

Barton also led the disaster recovery of the deadliest natural disaster in U.S. history, which surpassed even the recent Hurricane Katrina in its devastating death toll. On September 8, 1900, before hurricanes were even named, a vast storm with wind speeds exceeding 140 miles per hour blew into Galveston Bay. In 24 hours time, wind and water had killed an estimated 6,000 people and destroyed an estimated 6,000 buildings. There was no federal help or resources, and the grieving survivors were faced with a federal government that "didn't do" relief for disasters. The only resources came from outside private donors, churches, and philanthropic organizations—and Clara Barton and her Red Cross nurses. One sixth of the city's population was dead, and the sandbar of Galveston had no place to bury them. Clara Barton arrived on the scene quickly, and she organized efforts to comfort the survivors and provide health care services and community based relief (Baker, 2006).

Clara Barton will always be remembered both as the founder of the American Red Cross and the driving force behind the creation of the Army Nurse Corps.

## Birth of the Midwife in the United States

Women have always assisted other women in the birth of babies. These "lay midwives" were considered by communities to possess special skills and somewhat of a "calling." With the advent of professional nursing in England, registered nurses became associated with safer and more predictable childbirth practices. In England and in other countries where Nightingale-system nurses were prevalent, most registered nurses were also trained as midwives with a 6-month specialized training period. In the United States, the training of registered nurses in the practice of midwifery was prevented primarily by physicians. U.S. physicians saw midwives as a threat and an intrusion into medical practice. Such resistance indirectly led to the proliferation of "granny wives" who were ignorant of modern practices, were untrained, and were associated with high maternal morbidity (Donahue, 1985).

The first organized midwifery service in the United States was the **Frontier Nursing Service** founded in 1925 by **Mary Breckenridge**. Breckenridge graduated from the St. Luke's Hospital Training School in New York in 1910 and received her midwifery certificate from the British Hospital for Mothers and Babies in London in 1925. She had extensive experience in the delivery of babies and midwifery systems in New Zealand and Australia. In rural Appalachia, babies had been delivered for decades by granny midwives, who relied mainly on tradition, myths, and superstition as the bases of their practice. For example, they might use ashes for medication and place a sharp axe, blade up, under the bed of a laboring woman to "cut" the pain. The people of Appalachia were isolated because of the terrain of the hollows and mountains, and roads were limited to most families. They also had one of the highest birth rates in the United States. Breckenridge believed that if a midwifery service could work under these conditions, it could work anywhere (Donahue, 1985).

Breckenridge had to use English midwives for many years and only began training her own midwives in 1939, when she started the Frontier Graduate School of Nurse Midwifery in Hyden, Kentucky, with the advent of World War II. The nurse midwives accessed many of their families on horseback. In 1935, a small 12-bed hospital was built at Hyden and provided delivery services. The nurse midwives under the direction of Breckenridge were successful in

Mary Breckenridge, founder of the Frontier Nursing Service.

lowering the highest maternal mortality rate in the United States (in Leslie County, Kentucky) to substantially below the national average. These nurses, as at Henry Street Settlement, provided health care for everyone in the district for a small annual fee. A delivery was assessed an additional small fee. Nurse midwives provided primary care, prenatal care, and postnatal care, with an emphasis on prevention (Wertz & Wertz, 1977).

Once they were armed with the right to vote, the "Roaring Twenties" ushered American women into the new freedom of the "flapper era"—shrinking dress hemlines, shortened hairstyles, and the increased use of cosmetics. Hospitals were used by greater numbers of people and the scientific basis of medicine became well established as most surgical procedures were done in hospitals. Penicillin was discovered in 1928, creating a revolution in the prevention of infectious disease deaths (Kalisch & Kalisch, 1986; Donahue, 1985). The previously mentioned Goldmark Report recommended the establishment of college and university based nursing programs.

Mary D. Osborne, who functioned as supervisor of public health nursing for the state of Mississippi from 1921 to 1946, had a vision for a collaboration with community nurses and granny midwives, who delivered 80% of the African American babies in Mississippi. The infant and maternal mortality rates were both exceptionally high among African American families, and these granny midwives, who were also African American, were untrained and had little education.

Osborne took a creative approach to improving maternal and infant health among African American women. She developed a collaborative network of public health nurses and granny midwives in which the nurses implemented training programs for the midwives, and the midwives in turn assisted the nurses in providing a higher standard of safe maternal and infant health care. The public health nurses used Osborne's book, *Manual for Midwives*, which contained guidelines for care and was used in the state until the 1970s. They taught good hygiene, infection prevention, and compliance with state regulations. Osborne's innovative program is credited with reducing the maternal and infant mortality rates in Mississippi and in other states where her program structure was adopted (Sabin, 1998).

## The Nursing Profession Responds to the Great Depression and World War II

With the stock market crash of 1929 came the Great Depression, which resulted in widespread unemployment of private-duty nurses and the closing of nursing schools, while simultaneously creating an increasing need for charity health services for the population. Nursing students, who had previously been the primary source of staff for hospitals, become scarcer. Unemployed graduate nurses were hired to replace them for minimal wages, a trend that was to influence the profession for years to come (MacEachern, 1932).

Other nurses found themselves accompanying troops to Europe as the United States entered World War II. Military nurses were a critical presence at the invasion of Normandy in 1938, as well as in North Africa, Italy, France, and the Philippines, where Navy nurses provided care aboard hospital ships. More than 100,000 nurses volunteered and were certified for military service in the Army and Navy Nurse Corps.

The resulting severe shortage of nurses on the home front resulted in the development of the **Cadet Nurse Corps**. **Frances Payne Bolton**, congresswoman from Ohio, is credited with the founding of the Cadet Nurse Corps through the Bolton Act of 1945. By the end of the war, more than 180,000 nursing students had been trained through this Act, while advanced practice graduate nurses in psychiatry and public health nursing had received graduate education to increase the numbers of nurse educators (Kalisch & Kalisch, 1986; Donahue, 1985).

Ernie Pyle, a famous correspondent in World War II, offered Americans a "front-seat view" of the war through his detailed journalistic accounts of daily life on the front. Pyle was the first journalist who put his own life in danger by reporting from the battlefront; he spent a great deal of time with soldiers during active combat and was killed during a sniper attack in Ie Shima, Japan, in 1942. Chaplin Nathan Baxter Saucier was assigned to retrieve his body, conduct his service, and assist the soldiers with building his coffin. The funeral service lasted only about 10 minutes. Pyle was buried with his helmet on, at Saucier's request. The Navy, Marine Corps, and Army were all represented at the service. Pyle was a highly regarded and humanistic voice for those serving America during World War II. Here is an example of his accounts of life for nurses in a field hospital in Europe:

The officers and nurses live two in a tent on two sides of a company street—nurses on one side, officers on the other. . . . The nurses wear khaki overalls because of the mud and dust. Pink female panties fly from a line among the brown warlike tents. On the flagpole is a Red Cross flag made from a bed sheet and a French soldier's red sash. The American nurses—and there were lots of them—turned out just as you would expect: wonderfully. Army doctors and patients too were unanimous in their praise of them. . . . Doctors told me that in the first rush of causalities they were calmer than the men. For the first ten days they had to live like animals, even using open ditches for toilets but they never complained. One nurse was always on duty in each tentful of 20 men. She had medical orderlies to help her. The touch of femininity, the knowledge that a woman was around, gave the wounded man courage and confidence and a feeling of security. (Pyle, 1944)

During the midst of the Depression, many nurses found that the expansion and advances in aviation opened up a new field for nurses. In an effort to increase the public's confidence in the safety of transcontinental air travel, nurses were hired in the promising new role of "nurse-stewardess" (Kalisch & Kalisch, 1986). Congress created an additional relief program, the Civil Works Administration (CWA), in 1933 that provided jobs to the unemployed, including placing nurses in schools, public hospitals and clinics, public health departments, and public health education community surveys and campaigns.

The Social Security Act of 1935 was also passed by Congress to provide old age benefits, rehabilitation services, unemployment compensation administration, aid to dependent and/or disabled children and adults, and monies to state and local health services. The Social Security Act included Title VI, which authorized the use of federal funds for the training of public health personnel. This led to the placement of public health nurses in state health departments and the expansion of public health nursing as a viable career path.

While nurses were forging new paths for themselves in various fields, Hollywood began featuring nurses in films during the 1930s. The only feature-length films to ever focus entirely on the nursing profession were released during this decade. *War Nurse* (1930), *Night Nurse* (1931), *Once to Every Woman* (1934), *The White Parade* (1934 Academy Award nominee for Best Picture), *Four Girls in White* (1939), *The White Angel* (1936), *and Doctor and Nurse* (1937) all used nurses as major characters. During the bleak years of the economic depression, young women found these nurse heroines who promoted idealism, self-sacrifice, and the profession of nursing over personal desires particularly appealing. No longer were nurses depicted as subservient handmaidens who worked as nurses only as a temporary pastime before marriage (Kalisch & Kalisch, 1986).

## Early Education and Standardization of Practice of Public Health Nursing

After the turn of the century in the United States, infectious diseases such as smallpox, TB, malaria, cholera, and typhoid were practice priorities for public health nurses. The public health nurse often initially detected an infectious disease, then referred those patients to physicians for treatment, provided follow-up care to patients when indicated, and tried through education and demonstrations to family and caregivers to prevent the spread of disease. Progress for early education efforts was largely gained through experience. A 3-month orientation and observation process was established in the early 1920s for nurses new to the concepts and policies of public health nursing. The philosophy was simple: Public health nursing was about prevention of disease, the promotion of health, care of the sick, and rehabilitation to productive life (Erickson, 1996).

By 1927, the Rockefeller Foundation provided private funding for a training station for health workers in conjunction with several local county health departments. Nurses, physicians, and sanitarians from many states and foreign countries received public health orientation and training through this initiative before it was discontinued in 1932. In 1929, the Rockefeller Foundation provided grants through the Rosenwald Fund designated for programs to improve the health and lower the death rates of the African American population in the South. These funds, used to establish permanent public health nursing positions for African American nurses, targeted children in areas where nursing and sanitation would make a profound impact on health and health practices (Forbes, 1946).

## Challenges of the 1930s

In 1933, President Roosevelt initiated the New Deal to relieve the economic hardship of the country. The Social Security Act in 1935 (Public Law No. 99-271) provided funding to increase public health programs, particularly to extend services and improve health care for mothers and children in rural areas suffering from economic stress. State boards of health secured funds in 1934 through the Children's Bureau of the U.S. Department of Labor for state supervisory nurses, regional supervisory nurses, and local county nurses. The goal of this special project was to place at least one public health nurse in each county in every state. The efforts to reach this goal were remarkable, but qualified public health nurses continued to be few in number (ASTDN, 1993).

The U.S. Public Health Service (USPHS), under the nursing consultation of Pearl Melver, provided leadership in the development of public health nursing services to the states. This effort was encouraged by the National Organization of Public Health Nursing and the Nursing Section of the American Public Health Association. Joint efforts became the federal public health nurses and those who were becoming organized in the states became the impetus for the growth of the specialty of public health nursing (ASTDN, 1993).

Another provision of the Social Security Act of 1935 was the establishment of Crippled Children's Services. Through this initiative, public health nurses were trained in rehabilitation nursing, primarily in orthopedics. These nurses visited crippled children in their homes, held conferences with parents, and assisted in the field clinics (Roberts, 1985a).

Syphilis had also been recognized as a major source of morbidity and mortality for many years. In 1938, the USPHS and state boards of health cooperated in a major project to attempt to conquer the disease through case finding, treatment, follow-up contact, and education. Public health nursing was in the vanguard of this effort. Educational con-

---

### BOX 3-3

**Public Health Milestones of the 1920s and 1930s**

| | |
|---|---|
| 1920s | Frost established epidemiology as science basic to community health |
| 1920s | National Organization for Public Health Nursing formed |
| 1920s | Public Health Nursing Section of American Public Health Association formed |
| 1921 | First federal monies allocated for health and social welfare |
| 1923 | Health Organization of League of Nations founded |
| 1925 | Frontier Nursing founded |
| 1930s | Association of State and Territorial Directors of Nursing formed |
| 1930 | Crippled Children's Programs established |
| 1930 | National Institutes of Health established |
| 1935 | Social Security Act passed |
| 1938 | American Public Health Association set standards for school health |

*Source*: From Public Health Milestones in the 1920s and 1930s. APHA, 2006. Reprinted with permission from the American Public Health Association.

---

ferences were planned so that all public health nurses would have an opportunity to attend. Prenatal screening of patients for syphilis was being introduced as a standard nursing intervention at this time. These efforts were particularly successful in the South (Erickson, 1940) (Box 3-3).

The country was gradually recovering from the Depression, and economic progress was accelerating. Farm production had broadened through diversification. New industries expanded the economy. The southern states, along with some of the eastern states, began to recognize the importance of nursing service in industrial hygiene programs. The U.S. Division of Industrial Hygiene asked for a public health nurse to plan and help institute nursing services. The prevention of disease, improvement of hazardous work conditions, promotion of health practices including nutrition, and first aid were the interventions to be provided through industrial nursing. As these nurses were employed, short-term educational and direct experience opportunities in areas with industrial nurses were planned so that the nurses could receive the best preparation possible to the role (Morton, Roberts, & Bender, 1993; Roberts, 1985a, 1985b; Smith, 1934).

## Progressive Initiatives After the War Years

By 1942, state boards of health and education began to enter on operative agreements to strengthen public health nursing service to the school-age population. The role of the public health nurse in the school was generalized, but much emphasis was placed on health promotion, immunizations, nutrition, and correction of physical defects. Landmark legislation was passed by the U.S. Congress in March 1943, establishing the Emergency Maternity and Infant Care (EMIC) program for the care of the dependents of enlisted men of the U.S. armed services. The program was designed to provide for maternity care and acute illness care of the infants and was administered through the United States Children's Bureau. In less than a month, the program was initiated in almost all states. Training for public health nurses was once again funded by the federal government, and the role of the public health nurse expanded to include mothers and babies in a more formal way (ASTDN, 1935–1993).

The USPHS Division of Public Health Nursing conducted research during the mid-1940s to study public health nursing. The most significant recommendations included the designation of public health nursing in states a major division of nursing, the recognition of public health nursing as a service delivery system to all public health divisions and programs, and the importance of educational and practice issues related to professional nursing. The studies cited a low educational level for public health nurses and strongly recommended upgrading educational qualifications. The studies critiqued the established expenditure of nursing time and activities, determining that many duties carried out by public health nurses could be delegated to clerical staff and health aides. Health aides were introduced to the public health team with high school graduates employed to support public health nursing. These individuals quickly became a valuable resource and support to public health nursing, performing both clerical and clinical support activities (ASTDN, 1935–1993).

In December 1947, senior cadet nurses had a 6-month general training in public health and polio care through the training center of the state boards of health. The purpose of the Cadet Nurse Corps Program, funded through the USPHS, was to encourage young women to study nursing and to augment the supply of nurses in all health services.

Nurses were returning to work following the close of World War II, although the overall demand for nurses continued to exceed the supply. Newly constructed hospitals, industry, and public health agencies were all clamoring and vying for the short supply of nurses. While more active professional nurses and more students in schools existed by the early 1950s than at any previous time, the increase in numbers and caliber of nurses had not kept pace with the need for service (ASTDN, 1935–1993).

Throughout the 1950s, the nursing home industry began to emerge, with licensure requirements for standards of operation developed to ensure quality of services and care. Communities were accommodating an increase in the number of elderly persons living with chronic and degenerative diseases. Public health nurses provided training courses for nurses' aides employed in nursing homes. Country public health nurses regularly visited the nursing homes within their communities, providing TB skin testing, administering flu vaccines, and providing technical assistance in nursing care. Nutritionists and physical therapists provided additional expertise to improve care processes and support public health nurses in the areas of rehabilitation and nutrition (Hanlon & Pickett, 1974a, 1974b; Morton, Roberts, & Bender, 1993).

A national trend began in the 1960s to release psychiatric patients from institutional care as improved psychotropic drugs and treatment modalities were available. Inadequate staffing at the state mental health institutions as a result of the nursing shortage was a complicating factor. The National Institute of Mental Health funded projects to study the impact that public health nurses might have on mental health care. A mental health nurse consultant was employed by many states to spearhead the research efforts of these projects. The projects public health nursing activity was defined as "aftercare" and was designed to determine the effectiveness of integrating follow-up services to mental health patients and their families into general public health nursing service. Public health nursing services included case finding and referral, hospital discharge planning, home and family assessments before and after discharge to the home, and medication monitoring (Amendt & White, 1965; Cottrell, 1948). Mental health services remained an integral part of public health service delivery throughout this decade, with new activities enhancing the communities focus (Box 3-4).

Great emphasis was placed on child health, growth, and development in the early 1960s. Communicable disease, intestinal parasites, and physical defects that had been so prevalent in the school-age population were greatly diminished. Evaluations of this population found the new concerns to be dental and oral defects, vision and hearing defects, mental and emotional disturbances, accidents, and serious nutritional deficiencies. Continuing education was provided to enhance public health nurses' skills in observation, assessment, and nursing interventions in the care of children. Public health nurses began to be trained to assess developmental progress of children. Child health services provided by public health nurses included screening for physical defects, administration of immunizations, follow-up to correct physical defects, referral for mental health evaluations, consultation

---

### BOX 3-4

**Public Health Milestones of the 1940s and 1950s**

| | |
|---|---|
| 1940s | Public health programs focused on health needs of the war period |
| 1946 | Centers for Disease Control and Prevention established by Congress |
| 1946 | Mahoney introduced use of penicillin for treatment of syphilis |
| 1948 | National Heart, Lung, and Blood Institute established |
| 1948 | World Health Organization established |
| 1950s | Policy emphases on health and federal funds for states, environmental health issues, housing, behavior, medical care, and children's health |
| 1950 | Tuberculosis outpatient treatment becomes acceptable |
| 1950 | Introduction of the Salk vaccine |
| 1950 | White House Conference on Children and Youth |

*Source*: From Public Health Milestones in the 1940s and 1950s. APHA, 2006. Reprinted with permission from the American Public Health Association.

Public health nurses implemented the Salk vaccine beginning in 1955 in efforts to eradicate polio.

with teachers, and health promotion in nutrition, accident prevention, and mental health (Roberts, 1985a).

An evaluation of the school health programs in the mid-1960s identified the need for additional nursing personnel to provide more direct preventive health services. Specialized federal funding through Title V grants was provided through the state departments of education to promote public health initiatives. Many schools recruited their nursing staff from the public health nursing workforce. Those public health nurses who went to schools took a broad view of child health and served as emissaries to school administrators and local boards' members. County public health nurses continued to serve as consultants to the schools in the areas of immunizations and communicable disease and as a referral source for Crippled Children's Services (Roberts, 1985a).

Immunizations administered by public health nurses were proving effective, yet surveys showed that many preschool and school-age children were not completely immunized. Boards of health, continuing their vigilance regarding children's health status, received federal grants under the Vaccination Assistance Act. In 1965, public health nurses administered an increased number of immunizations. The oral polio vaccine, known as the Sabin vaccine, became available in a sugar cube administration form. A measles vaccine became available in 1966 and rubella in 1969. Following mass initial immunization campaigns for both measles and rubella, the new vaccines were incorporated into routine immunization schedules for children (ASTDN, 1935–1993).

By the mid-1960s, federal funding for maternal/child health services required the incorporation of contraceptive information and general reproductive health into public health services. The objective was to reduce maternal and infant mortality and to generally improve the health and well-being of mothers and children. Some states had already identified the health problems associated with multiple

unplanned and unwanted pregnancies and had been early leaders in efforts to repeal federal and state laws restricting birth control services. By 1944, these efforts had resulted in integrated family planning counseling and issuing of select supplies with maternity and postpartum services into many of the county health departments. Contraceptive supplies at that time included condoms and diaphragms. However, because of the wide divergence of public opinion the development of the program was slow and unpublicized (ASTDN, 1935–1993: Morton, Roberts, & Bender, 1993).

## ■ Social and Political Influence of the 1960s and 1970s

By 1965, county health departments routinely provided contraceptive counseling and supplies. Oral contraceptives were also available by this time and gave women more convenient and accepted choices. Public health nurses promoted family planning and were key in identifying women at highest risk and need for such services. Family planning nursing visits increased across the country. Eventually, the federal government appropriated monies for additional education of public health nurses to function as family planning nurse practitioners.

Landmark legislation in 1965 amended the Social Security Act of 1935 by establishing Medicare, a health insurance plan for people 65 years of age and older and for those with long-term disabilities. The insurance plan included reimbursement for intermittent skilled nursing services provided to homebound persons. The purpose of home health services was twofold. Health care costs were beginning to skyrocket; home care would reduce costly hospitalization stays with the added benefit of patients' being in familiar home settings, enhancing quality of life. The goal of the program was to rehabilitate patients to their maximum potential and to teach families to care for the physical and emotional needs of patients.

Public health nurses had been providing home nursing services on a limited basis since the inception of public health nursing, but this would be the first reimbursement established for direct nursing services. In addition, the reimbursable home health nursing services to be provided would require public health nurses to learn new assessment and rehabilitative technical skills. Federal regulations established for certification were monumental, however. Continuing education for the nurses and nurses' aides who were directly providing care was just one of the regulations that in itself would be an immense task once service delivery was fully implemented (Buhler-Wilkerson, 1993; Ericson, 1996; IOM, 1988).

Federal grants through the USPHS were made available to support the implementation of home health. Nurse consultants, supervising nurses, and staff nurses attended university-supported educational offerings in rehabilitation care and techniques. Educational workshops were designed to upgrade nursing skills and techniques in rehabilitative care and on the conditions of participation of home health services. Additional workshop topics included documentation of skilled care and nursing care plans, medication administration and side effects, and the disease processes of many chronic health conditions.

After federal costs studies were implemented by the public health nurses in home health care, it was demonstrated that additional auxiliary staff, including health aides and clerks, would allow public health nurses more time for nursing activities. Action was taken to create additional clerical and aide positions to support the nursing staff.

More liberal social values emerged, and the 1960s became known for having spawned a sexual revolution. These effects were recognized by the early 1970s. Communities were faced with tremendous increases in sexually transmitted diseases and teen pregnancy rates. Social programs in response to these increases were initiated in the 1960s and were formalized in public and community health efforts in all states. The establishment of Medicaid through the amendment to the Social Security Act, Title XIX, enhanced the delivery of health care services to a wider range of recipients. The quantity and variance of activities in public health nursing continued to increase.

All the while, the traditional programs of health protection and disease control moved forward, many with an accelerated pace. Collaboration with other agencies, institutions, and groups continued at a high level in an effort to coordinate resources to achieve the best possible public health service delivery. Medicaid programs enhanced the expansion of Crippled Children's Services as a payment mechanism for many previously uncovered services. Additional screening and specialty treatment clinics for neurology, heart, and orthopedics were established throughout the United States. Other initiatives also centered the delivery of child health services. Particularly in states with high infant mortality rates, state boards of health entered cooperative agreements in the 1970s to establish public health nursing positions in newborn intensive care units. The goal was to improve the communication, referral, and follow-up mechanisms for these high-risk infants after discharge from the hospital.

Title XIX of the Social Security Act (Medicaid) established Early Periodic Screening Diagnosis and Treatment (EPSDT) in 1969 to improve the access to preventive and primary health care for low-income children. State boards of health used this opportunity to strengthen the delivery of well-child services. These physical screenings were made available primarily by public health nurses and were reimbursable nursing services, another recognition of the value of public health nursing service. The Denver Developmental Screening Test (DDST) was incorporated into the physical assessment, giving public health nurses a new tool to help find potential developmental delays and provide early intervention in the newborn to 6-year age groups. Workshops and in-service programs were conducted to teach the DDST standardized procedures.

---

**BOX 3-5**

**Public Health Milestones of the 1960s and 1970s**

| | |
|---|---|
| 1960s | Public health policy issues focused on inequality, integration, poverty, "the pill," housing environmental health, consumer protection, human rights, and peace |
| 1960 | Tuberculosis sanatoriums phased out and mainstream treatment begun |
| 1961 | First White House Conference on Aging |
| 1961–1962 | Sabin vaccine introduced |
| 1962 | National Institute of Child Health established |
| 1964 | *Surgeon General's Report on Smoking and Health* published |
| 1965 | Medicaid and Medicare programs enacted |
| 1970 | *Roe v. Wade* |
| 1970 | Occupational Safety and Health Administration established |
| 1973 | HMO Act passed |
| 1976 | National immunization program for "swine flu" |
| 1978 | Association of Community Health Nursing Educators formed |
| 1979 | Last outbreak of poliomyelitis in the United States |
| 1979 | First *Healthy People* report |

*Source*: From Public Health Milestones in the 1960s and 1970s. APHA, 2006. Reprinted with permission from the American Public Health Association.

---

Medical technology continued to advance rapidly, including advances in genetic diagnostics and treatment. Routine screening for sickle cell anemia was introduced and was integrated with EPSDT services. Other genetic technological advances determined that a contributing factor to the high incidence of mental retardation resulted from genetic disorders such as hypothyroidism and phenylketonuria. Medication and dietary treatments were developed for these genetic disorders that would improve the quality of life and life expectancy. Nursing interventions included a home assessment, treatment modalities ordered by the attending physician, provision of dietary supplements, and teaching basic child health care and special health care based on the genetic diagnosis derived from the screening (ASTDN, 1935–1993; Hanlon & Pickett, 1974b). Please refer to Box 3-5 for milestones of the 1960s and 1970s.

A dramatic increase in home health nursing visits began at the close of the 1970s as a result of Medicare's implementation of diagnosis-related groups (DRGs), which were designed to lower costs through reduced institutionalization. Medicaid also reimbursed for home health services to eligible individuals not on Medicare and for some children with special health care needs. Private medical insurance plans and the Veteran's Administration were beginning to reimburse for home health services as well. Additional nursing positions were essential to meet the demand and to balance the quantity relationship with quality nursing care. As more acutely ill patients were cared for in the home and more advanced technological care was introduced into home health care, this specialty increased (ASTDN, 1935–1993).

## Public Health Nursing Services in the 1980s and 1990s

As the 1980s began, the United States was experiencing an economic recession with skyrocketing interest rates and rising unemployment rates. National leadership was reducing funding for many of the social programs begun in the 1960s; the philosophy was that less governmental spending would enhance the national economy. The increased number of homeless persons became a national concern. Continuing concerns included illicit drug use, rising teen pregnancy rates, and alterations in family unit structures. Inadequate health care resources were also a continuing concern requiring cost containment, management of resources, and careful evaluation and incorporation of advancing technology. During this era, public health nursing services became varied throughout the country. In some states, basic services included both traditional preventive health services and family health services directed at high-risk mothers and babies and a reduction of unplanned pregnancies (ASTDN, 1935–1993).

Fortunately, public health nursing continued to grow and was a strong workforce in the country by the 1980s. Infant death rates declined significantly. Public health nurses participated in many research studies on public health problems such as congenital syphilis and TB preventive studies. Federal funding requirements changed from categorical grants to block grants. Categorical funding of the 1960s and 1970s had required that resources be restricted to the program that funded the resource; a nursing position funded by family planning, for example, was limited to family planning activities. Block funding allowed agencies more discretion on the use of these funds; therefore, services could be offered more efficiently to the public. Integrated public health nursing delivery systems were born. The integration of services allowed public health nurses to return to the more patient-oriented or family-oriented care that had been the traditional philosophy of public health nursing (ASTDN, 1993; Buhler-Wilkerson, 1993).

Genetics screening programs expanded as a result of advanced technology in the early 1980s. The first initiative was newborn screening for sickle cell anemia. The goal was early detection of disease because early intervention could prevent common infections or premature deaths. State legislatures mandated hospitals to collect newborn screening specimens before infant discharge from the hospital. Screening included at least three genetic disorders: sickle cell anemia, phenylketonuria (PKU), and hypothyroidism. Public health nurses were given the responsibility for following up with the newborns with a questionable or positive screen. Question-able screens for PKU and hypothyroidism require prompt attention because early treatment with diet and/or medication will prevent irreversible mental retardation and growth delay. The availability of public health nurses provided an effective means for timely follow-up of screenings and for the implementation of medical and nursing care plans when indicated (ASTDN, 1993).

A crucial indicator of any state's quality of life is infant mortality. Public health nursing became a viable resource during the 1980s for delivering services (either personal or preventive) aimed at reducing infant mortality. The major cause of infant mortality was prematurity. Contributing factors included poor nutrition, smoking, teen pregnancy, and inadequate prenatal care. Socioeconomic factors such as inadequate housing, drug abuse, and lack of education were also contributing factors. Maternal risk scoring and documentation to ensure referrals to appropriate levels of care were standards of care. Tracking systems were intensified to ensure adequate levels of care.

Family planning services during the 1980s were also identified as a priority to reduce infant mortality. Risk factors included age and/or inadequate income to purchase contraceptive supplies. Public health nurses continued to promote family planning services, provide health promotion and education in their communities, and intensify tracking systems of teens and others at risk. The Special Supplemental Food Program for Women, Infants, and Children (WIC) continued to address infant mortality. WIC certification and nutrition education were integrated into maternal and child health nursing services' standards of care.

Congressional authorization gave states the option to expand their Medicaid programs in 1987. The services' expansion included case management of high-risk mothers and infants to ensure comprehensive care as a reimbursable service. Nutritionists, social workers, and public health nurses formed teams to establish care plans and assume case manager roles based on the patient's risk factors. Public health nursing activities included nursing assessments, home visits, health education, and communication with medical providers in an effort to improve the overall status of this high-risk population. Documentation of the care process was essential for continuity of care from the initial assessment and plan of care through implementation of services and ongoing evaluation.

*Case management* emerged during this decade as a new term, but the concept and the related activities of case management were the principles and foundations upon which public health nursing practice had been built. **Case management** is a program for intensive individual supervision, follow-up, and referrals to appropriate levels of care. Public health nurses had been providing a form of case management through the years to many patients, such as those receiving TB treatment, those receiving home health services, and children with special health care needs.

School health nurses also became stronger in this era. School nurses strengthened the educational process of students by assisting them in improving or adapting to their health status. School nurses were available during school hours to serve as counselors and to provide case finding and referral to physicians, health departments, and other agencies as appropriate to meet the needs of school-age children. Activities included general health screening and referral, hearing and vision screening, identification of suspected abuse and neglect, substance abuse counseling, and appropriate decision making and support. In addition, school nurses provided classroom presentations on health issues and provided emergency care for injuries and illnesses at school.

Communicable disease had renewed public health interest in the nation throughout the 1980s. Tuberculosis case rates were increasing. Measles cases were being reported among college-age students. New communicable disease concerns emerged in the 1980s, including increased incidence of hepatitis B, human immunodeficiency virus (HIV) infection, and acquired immune deficiency syndrome (AIDS). Case conferences with private medical consultants were established on a district level for initiation and ongoing review of treatment plans carried out by public health nurses. Drug resistance and failure to take medication were identified as major hindrances to individual cure and subsequent eradication of TB. In 1986, public health nurses initiated directly observed therapy (DOT) for TB cases. Rather than self-administration, patients would present to the health department or the public health nurse would visit the home for administration of medications. Later in the decade, public health officials recognized that the increase in TB cases was, in part, associated with the emerging HIV and AIDS cases. HIV screening became a standard of nursing care for all active TB cases.

Many states took an early stance to address measles among the college-age population in the mid-1980s as a result of the increased incidence of disease reported throughout the nation. The college-age population was at greatest risk for disease because they had been immunized with less-than-effective immunizations in the late 1960s or had not received the immunization. Collaboration with state college boards resulted in requirement of measles and rubella immunity for college admission. Public health nurses reviewed immunization records, provided screening tests when indicated, and administered immunizations to assist in the control of measles.

The first cases of AIDS were diagnosed in the early 1980s. Research soon unraveled part of the mystery of the disease. Risk factors for transmission of disease were identified, and a screening test for HIV, the virus that leads to AIDS, became available. Screening provided a means to detect HIV infection earlier and to provide appropriate counseling and education to alter risk behaviors and reduce transmission. Education of the public and high-risk

individuals was the only effective weapon that public health had to address this disease. Public health nurses attended educational workshops to gain knowledge and skills for testing and counseling patients who requested testing. Health education materials were developed to support counseling and educational strategies. In addition, public health nurses implemented standards of care by integrating assessment of risk factors for patients receiving other public health services and by disseminating information through public presentations in schools and community organizations.

Progress continued for public health nurses during this era, yet dilemmas remain. A national nursing shortage was recognized, with all states feeling the effects. Public health felt the effects of the nursing shortage greatly, with the vacancy rates reaching 20% at times. A commission on nursing was organized by the Secretary of the U.S. Department of Health and Human Services to examine and make recommendations regarding the nursing shortage. The commission's report, completed in 1989, cited the reality of the shortage and the impact on health care delivery. The shortage was determined to result from the increasing demand for nurses, and the report urged agencies to be attentive to using measures aimed at reducing the barriers to effective recruitment and retention (DHHS, 1988).

One of the commission's recommendations was that nursing should have greater representation in the policy and decision-making activities of health care institutions. Acting on this recommendation, both public health nurses and their administrations developed mechanisms whereby public health nurses moved into broader policy-making roles. At the close of the decade, public health nursing continued as a strong force in the delivery of health care in many states and in health promotion and disease prevention in others. Public health nurses were instrumental in establishing and integrating new initiatives in public health to combat old public health problems as well as to address new public health concerns. The value of public health nursing activities continued to be recognized as reimbursement for selected activities and for nurse practitioner services were expanded.

The federal government's staggering budget deficits were the major national focus as the 1990s began. Health care costs were escalating, and governmental measures attempting to control increasing costs were not proving effective. The gloomy financial picture was exacerbated by Desert Storm, the U.S. military troops' assignment by President George H. W. Bush to protect Saudi Arabia and to retaliate for Iraq's invasion of Kuwait.

Current and emerging health care issues of the 1990s lay close to the heart of public health. The percentage of the population older than 65 continued to rise. Life expectancy in the United States had risen from 47 years in 1900 to 75 years in 1990. Infant mortality, although significantly declining through the years, required continued vigilance. The increased incidence of syphilis and other sexually transmitted diseases was of chief concern to public health. The number of persons infected with HIV and/or diagnosed with AIDS was increasing at alarming rates. Substance abuse continued to be a major problem, with studies identifying it as a contributing factor in 50% of all traffic accidents, in the transmission of HIV infection, and in infant morbidity and mortality.

Yet federal funding reductions were inevitable for public health as a result of the sluggish national economy as the United States entered the 1990s. Without significant infusions of money for additional staff, medications, vaccines, and health promotion/disease prevention activities, states faced increases in preventable diseases and deaths and a reversal of the recent favorable trends in lowering infant mortality and teen pregnancy. Difficult economic times resulted in the careful reviews of resources and the utilization of those resources. Focus was again directed toward enhancing nursing education and staff development, strengthening relationships with schools of nursing, and developing a quality assurance process for the integration of public health nursing services. Because of the large number of nurses employed, public health nurses were afforded greater access to approved continuing education opportunities specific to their area of practice. Select continuing education offerings, including TB updates, HIV testing and counseling courses, and community assessment, became required orientation for newly employed public health nurses (Gebbie, 1996).

The nation experienced a significant increase in the incidence of syphilis. Case rates were climbing and were higher than they had been since the late 1940s. Much of the increased incidence was associated with drug abuse—the exchange of sex for drugs. Congenital syphilis was again an issue of public health concern for infant morbidity and mortality. Public health nursing protocols included standards of care for infected maternity patients and follow-up for their newborn infants. Public health nurses increased their assessment for signs and symptoms of disease and for risk status of patients in their care, assisted disease intervention specialists with follow-up of patients with positive laboratory results, and assisted with accessing medical treatment.

The incidence of another communicable disease, hepatitis B, was also increasing. With the advent of hepatitis B vaccination, public health nurses implemented new protocols to screen maternity patients for hepatitis B and to provide follow-up and immunization administration to the infants of infected mothers. Standing orders were written to effectively carry out the immunization and follow-up of these infants. This was a major new public health initiative. See Box 3-6 for a summary of activities during the years.

Federal monies increased for public health to address preventive intervention strategies for persons infected with HIV during 1990s. States initiated programs to make select drugs available to patients. These programs required private physicians to submit medication orders for the patient. Public health nurses assisted patients with completing applica-

---

### BOX 3-6

**Public Health Milestones of the 1980s and 1990s**

| | |
|---|---|
| 1980s | Public policy centered around AIDS, Medicare, Medicaid, tobacco control, international health, minority health, national health care reform, and national health objectives |
| 1982 | Warning labels on aspirin for Reye's syndrome prevention |
| 1986 | First antitobacco initiative by public health community |
| 1988 | *The Future of Public Health* published by the Institute of Medicine |
| 1989 | *Year 2000 Health Objectives* published |
| 1990 | *Healthy People 2000* report published |
| 1991 | *Healthy Communities 2000: Model Standards* published |
| 1993 | AZT sanctioned as able to reduce perinatal HIV |
| 1996 | *War and Public Health* published |
| 1997 | Plans under way for modern microbiological/biomedical laboratory capabilities |
| 2000 | *Healthy People 2010* published |

*Source:* From Public Health Milestones in the 1980s and 1990s. APHA, 2000. Reprinted with permission from the American Public Health Association.

---

tion forms, consulting private physicians regarding program guidelines, and adding medication.

Immunization administration had been a priority health effort for public health nurses since the early part of the century. A national emphasis reemerged in the early 1990s to meet a national objective to complete the immunization of 90% of all children by 2 years of age. The Centers for Disease Control and Prevention (CDC) identified barriers to children receiving their basic immunization series. The national discussion provided public health nurses with current knowledge on their assessment of simultaneous administration of several vaccines when indicated and on contraindications for immunization administration (DHHS, 1992).

## Science and Health Care, 1945–1960: Decades of Change

Dramatic technological and scientific changes characterized the decades following World War II, including the discovery of sulfa drugs, new cardiac drugs, surgeries, and treatment for ventricular fibrillation (Howell, 1996). The Hill–Burton Act, passed in 1946, provided funds to increase the construction of new hospitals. A significant change in the health care system was the expansion of private health insurance coverage and the dramatic increase in the birth rate, coined the "baby boom" generation. Clinical research, both in medicine and in nursing, became an expectation of health providers and more nurses sought advanced degrees. The *Journal of Nursing Research* was first published, heralding the arrival of nursing scholarship in the United States.

Owing to increased numbers of hospital beds, additional financial resources for health care, and the post–World War II economic resurgence, an acute shortage of nurses occurred, and the existing staff faced increasingly stressful working conditions. Nurses began showing signs of the strain, engaging in debates about strikes and collective bargaining demands.

The composition of the nursing profession also changed. The American Nurses Association (ANA) accepted African American nurses for membership, consequently ending racial discrimination in the dominant nursing organizations. The National Association of Colored Graduate Nurses was disbanded in 1951. Males entered nursing schools in record number, often as a result of previous military experience as medics. Prior to the 1950s and 1960s, male nurses had suffered minority status and were discouraged from nursing as a career. Seemingly forgotten by modern society, including Florence Nightingale and early U.S. nursing leaders, males made up more than one half of the nursing care during medieval times. The Knights Hospitalers, Teutonic Knights, Franciscans, and many other male nursing orders had provided excellent nursing care for their societies. In fact, St. Vincent de Paul had first conceived of the idea of social service. Pastor Theodor Fliedner, teacher and mentor of Florence Nightingale at Kaiserwerth in Germany; Ben Franklin; and Walt Whitman (during the Civil War) all either served as nurses or were strong advocates for male nurses (Kalisch & Kalisch, 1986).

## Years of Revolution, Protest, and the New Order, 1961–2000

During the social upheaval of the 1960s, nursing was influenced by many changes in society, such as the woman's movement, the organized protest against the Vietnam War, the civil rights movement, President Lyndon Johnson's "Great Society" social reforms, and increased consumer involvement in health care. Specialization in nursing, such as cardiac intensive care unit (ICU), nurse anesthetist training, and the clinical specialist role for nursing emerged as a trend that affected both education and practice in the health care system. Medicare and Medicaid, enacted in 1965 under Title XVIII of the Social Security Act, provided access to health care for the elderly, the poor, and disabled. The ANA took a courageous and controversial stand in that same year (1965) by approving its first position paper on nursing education, advocating for all nursing education for professional practice to take place in colleges and universities (ANA, 1965). Nurses returning from Vietnam faced emotional challenges through the recognition of post-traumatic stress disorder (PSTD), which affected some nurses' postwar lives.

With the increased specialization in medicine, the demand for primary care health care providers exceeded the supply (Christman, 1971). As a response to this need for general practitioners, Dr. Henry Silver (MD) and Dr. Loretta Ford (RN) collaborated to develop the first nurse practitioner program in the United States at the University of Colorado (Ford & Silver, 1967). Nurse practitioners (NP) were initially prepared in pediatrics with advanced role preparation in common childhood illness management and well-child care. Ford & Silver (1967) found that NPs could manage as much as 75% of the pediatric patients in community clinics, leading to the widespread use of NPs and growth of educational programs for NPs. The first state in 1971 to recognize diagnosis and treatment as part of the legal scope of practice for NPs was Idaho. Alaska and North Carolina were among the first states to expand the NP role to include prescriptive authority (Ford, 1979). By the new century, NP programs were offered at the MSN level in family nursing, gerontology, adult, neonatal, mental health, and maternal–child care; they have since expanded to include the acute care practitioner as well (Huch, 2001). Certification of NPs now occurs at the national level through the ANA and many specialty organizations, and NPs are licensed throughout the United States by state boards of nursing.

Escalating health care costs resulting from the explosion of advanced technology and the increased life span of Americans led to the demand for health care reform in the late 1980s. The nursing profession heralded the way in health care reform when an unprecedented collaboration of more than 75 nursing associations, led by the ANA and NLN, published *Nursing's Agenda for Health Care Reform.* This document addressed the challenge of managed care in the context of cost containment and quality assurance of health care service for the nursing profession (ANA, 1991). **Managed care** is a market approach based on managed competition as a major strategy to contain health care costs; it remains the dominant approach today (Lundy, Janes, & Hartman, 1991).

## The New Century: An Era of Managed Care

The Institute of Medicine's (IOM) report *Assuring the Health of the Public in the 21st Century* (2008a) builds upon its 1988 report and is anticipated to have major implications for public health policy development. The report contains several specific recommendations for strengthening the relationship between the vital sectors charged with protecting the public's health. The report proposes an ecological model upon which to base health professional education (including nursing education), clinical activities, and research with a population focus. Multiple determinants of health form the basis for an ecological model, which operates on the assumption that health is affected on several levels by these factors. Given that nurses make up the largest single workforce within the health system, the report's recommendations and the potential use of an ecological model as part of a population-focused practice have significant potential for creating new paths in nursing practice, education, and research.

A companion study by the IOM, *Who Will Keep the Public Healthy?* (2008b), builds on the ecological model and considers factors likely to affect public health in the twenty-first century, such as globalization, technological and scientific advances, and demographic shifts in the U.S. population. It defines a public health professional as a person educated in public health or a related discipline who is employed to improve health through a population focus. Eight new content areas for public health professionals to master are identified in this study: informatics, genomics, communication, cultural competence, community-based participatory research, policy and law, global health, and ethics.

Even as these studies were being conducted, public health history was being changed. Seasoned public health professionals, experiencing the erosion of the basic public health infrastructure created by state and local budget cuts, had predicted that the United States would be challenged significantly should any of the dilemmas of the past return. None of those predictions, however, accurately portrayed the impact that the events of September 11, 2001, and the subsequent anthrax threats would have on public health. Almost overnight, public health agencies and their partners became immersed in emergency preparedness activities that have now become routine. Public health professionals were challenged to place a high priority on such activities as syndromic surveillance, mass-casualty planning, handling of biological and chemical agents that would also be considered evidentiary material, and other similar work. New partners such as postal workers, law enforcement, and communication experts emerged. Public health nurses were also called upon to administer smallpox vaccine, something that had not been done in almost two decades. The beginning of the twenty-first century had dawned with improved health status and a new public health threat: terrorism.

Although health care reform continues to be debated, it is unlikely that there will be significant changes at the national level in the immediate future. The U.S. health care system today continues to focus on federal coverage, including improving access to care and controlling health care costs. Health care organizations in a managed care environment, such as preferred provider organizations (PPOs) and health maintenance organizations (HMOs), now see the economic and quality outcome benefits of caring for patients and managing their care over a continuum of possible settings and needs. Patients are followed more closely within the system, during both illness and wellness. Hospital stays are shorter, and more health care services are being provided in outpatient facilities and through community-based settings such as home health, occupational health, and school health (Lundy, Janes, & Hartman, 1991). Since September 11, 2001, terrorism is a constant threat to the United States and to the global community. War, bioterrorism, and emerging epidemics are just some of the challenges for today's nurses. Consensus regarding basic education and the entry level of registered nurses has not occurred. Relating to the global community as well as our own diverse population demands that nurses remain committed to cultural sensitivity in care delivery. The history of health care and nursing provides us with ample examples of the wisdom of our forebears in the advocacy of nursing in these challenging settings and the unknown future. Nurses today, by considering the lessons of the past, become part of a profession that is well prepared to provide the full range of quality, cost-effective services needed in the promotion of health throughout the new century. See Box 3-7.

### The Nurse

Starch white,
 lipstick, capped nurse.
She thanks the old man.
Six hen-brown eggs, half slab home-cured bacon, jar of last
 years peach.
Carefully placed on the front seat of the old black ford beside her.
Pay as he can, for the old woman's dying.

—*Ann Thedford Lanier*

---

**BOX 3-7**

**Public Health Milestones in the 21st Century**

| | |
|---|---|
| 2001 | 9/11 terrorist attacks (New York City and Washington, DC) and bioterrorist attacks lead to new initiatives in state and federal public health policies, organizational responses, and initiatives. |
| | CDC investigates first anthrax case; the victim was a 63-year-old Florida man. Patient first in a series of domestic terrorism victims of infection by anthrax sent through the mail. |
| 2003 | Severe acute respiratory syndrome (SARS) coronavirus identified. |
| 2004 | First state laws restricting access to over-the-counter medications used in methamphetamine production in Georgia. |
| 2005 | Hurricane Katrina hits New Orleans and Mississippi Gulf Coast resulting in unprecedented public heath disaster and response at state and federal level. |
| | Rubella eliminated in the United States. |
| 2006 | CDC recommends 15th and 16th routine immunizations for children and adolescents (rotavirus and human papillomavirus, respectively). |

## ■ CRITICAL THINKING ACTIVITIES

1. Take a walk through your neighborhood and college campus. Identify public health measures that exist that can be traced to the Greek and Romans eras.

2. How do you think Lillian Wald would react to present-day public health departments?

3. How does the current interest in alternative and complementary health care relate to the Greeks' ideas about health?

## ■ REFERENCES

Abel, E. K. (1997, November). Take the cure to the poor: Patients' responses to New York City's tuberculosis program, 1894–1918. *American Journal of Public Health, 87*, 11.

Achterberg, J. (1990). *Woman as healer: A panoramic survey of the healing activities of women from prehistoric times to the present.* Boston: Shambhala.

Amendt, J. A., & White, R. P. (1965, July). Continued care services for mental patients. *Nursing Outlook*, pp. 57–60.

American Public Health Association (APHA). (2006, November). *Public health milestones.* Washington, D.C. Unpublished paper.

Andrews, G. (2003). Nightingale's geography. *Nursing Inquiry, 10*(4), 270–274.

Association of State and Territorial Directors of Nursing (ASTDN). (1993). *Historical summary of the Association of State and Territorial Directors of Nursing (1935–1993).* Unpublished manuscript.

Association of State and Territorial Directors of Nursing (ASTDN). *Selected reports from annual meeting and correspondence, 1935–1993.*

Attewell, A. (1996). Florence Nightingale's health-at-home visitors. *Health Visitor, 69*(10), 406.

Baker, K. (2006, April/May). The future of New Orleans: Can the disasters that befell other cities help save this one? *American Heritage.*

Barker, E. R. (1989). Care givers as casualties. *Western Journal of Nursing Research, 11*(5), 628–631.

Barstow, A. L. (1994). *Witchcraze: A new history of the European witch hunt.* New York: Harper Collins.

Boorstin, D. J. (1985). *The discoverers: A history of man's search to know his world and himself.* New York: Vintage.

Brainard, A. M. (1922). *The evolution of public health nursing.* Philadelphia: W. B. Saunders.

Briggs, R. (1996). *Witches and neighbors: The social and cultural context of European witchcraft.* New York: Penguin Books.

Brooke, E. (1997). *Medicine women: A pictorial history of women healers.* Wheaton, IL: Quest Books.

Brown, E. L. (1936). *Nursing as a profession.* New York: Russell Sage Foundation.

Brown, E. L. (1948). *Nursing for the future.* New York: Russell Sage Foundation.

Brown, P. (1988). *Florence Nightingale.* Herts, UK: Exley Publications.

Buhler-Wilkerson, K. (1985). Public health nursing: In sickness or in health? *American Journal of Public Health, 75*, 1155–1156.

Buhler-Wilkerson, K. (1993). Bringing care to the people: Lillian Wald's legacy of public health nursing. *American Journal of Public Health, 83*(12), 1778–1786.

Bullough, V. L., & Bullough, B. (1978). *The care of the sick: The emergence of modern nursing.* New York: Prodist.

Calabria, M. D. (1996). *Florence Nightingale in Egypt and Greece: Her diary and "visions."* Albany: State University of New York Press.

Carnegie, M. E. (1991). *The path we tread: Blacks in nursing 1854–1990* (2nd ed.). New York: National League for Nursing Press.

Cartwright, F. F. (1972). *Disease and history.* New York: Dorset Press.

Chiarella, M. (1995). The magic of nursing. *Australia Nursing Journal, 3*(3), 22–23.

Cohen, M. N. (1989). *Health and the rise of civilization.* New Haven, CT: Yale University Press.

Cook, E. (1913). *The life of Florence Nightingale* (Vols. 1 and 2). London: Macmillan.

Cottrell, H. (1948). *Mental health principles in the state and local health programs: A Commonwealth Fund demonstration* (Record Group 51, Vol. 36). Mississippi Department of Archives, Division of Public Health Nursing, Historical Files.

Crawford, P. (1992). "The other lady with the lamp": Nursing legacy of Mary Seacole. *Nursing Times, 88*(11), 56–58.

D'Antonio, P. (2002). Nurses in war. *Lancet, 360*(9350), 7–12.

Department of Health and Human Services (DHHS). (1988, December). *Final report of the Secretary's Commission on Nursing.* Washington, DC: Author.

Department of Health and Human Services, Public Health Services, Centers for Disease Control and Prevention. (1992, May). *Standards for pediatric immunization practice.* Atlanta: Author.

Diamond, J. (1997). *Guns, germs, and steel: The fates of human societies.* New York: W. W. Norton.

Dickens, C. (1844). *Martin Chuzzlewit.* New York: Macmillan.

Dietz, D. D., & Lehozky, A. R. (1963). *History and modern nursing.* Philadelphia: F. A. Davis.

Dock, L. N., & Stewart, I. M. (1931). *A short history of nursing* (3rd ed.). New York: G. P. Putnam.

Donahue, M. P. (1985). *Nursing: The finest art.* St. Louis: Mosby.

Erickson, G. P. (1996, June). To pauperize or empower: Public health nursing at the turn of the 20th and 21st century. *Public Health Nursing, 13*(3), 163–169.

Erickson, P. (1940). *The role of the public health nurse in the syphilis research project in Washington County.* Presented at the 1940 annual meeting of the Mississippi Nurses Association, Jackson, MS.

Forbes, M. D. (1946). *Report of a review of public health nursing in the Mississippi Board of Health* (Record Group 51, Vol. 36). Mississippi Department of Archives, Division of Public Health Nursing, Historical Files.

Gebbie, K. M. (1996, November 18). *Preparing currently employed public health nurses for change in the health care system: Meeting report and suggested action steps.* New York: Columbia University School of Nursing Center for Health Policy and Health Sciences Research. (Report based on meeting in Atlanta, GA, July 11, 1996.)

Goldmark, J. C. (1923). *Nursing and nursing education in the United States.* New York: Macmillan.

Hamilton, D. (1988). Clinical excellence, but too high a cost: The Metropolitan Life Insurance Company Visiting Nurse Service (1909–1953). *Public Health Nursing, 5*, 235–240.

Hanlon, J. J., & Pickett, G. E. (1974a). Community nursing services. In *Public health administration and practice* (pp. 533–547). St. Louis: Mosby.

Hanlon, J. J., & Pickett, G. E. (1974b). Historical perspectives. In *Public health administration and practice* (pp. 22–44). St. Louis: Mosby.

Hanlon, J. J., & Pickett. G. E. (1984). *Public health administration and practice* (8th ed.). St. Louis: Mosby.

Heinrich, J. (1983). Historical perspectives on public health nursing. *Nursing Outlook, 32*(6), 317–320.

Hine, D. C. (1989). *Black women in white: Racial conflict and co-operation in the nursing profession 1890–1950.* Bloomington: Indiana University Press.

Howse, C. (2007). "The ultimate destination of all nursing": The development of district nursing in England, 1880–1925. *Nursing History Review, 15,* 65–94.

Institute of Medicine (IOM). (1988). *The future of public health.* Washington, DC: National Academy Press.

Institute of Medicine (IOM). (2008a, November). *Assuring the health of the public in the 21st century.* Retrieved September 20, 2008, from http://www.iom.edu/8/cms/3793/4720.aspx

Institute of Medicine (IOM). (2008b, November). *Who will keep the public healthy?: Educating public health professionals for the 21st century.* Retrieved September 20, 2008, from http://www.iom.edu/CMS/3793/4723/4307.aspx

Kalisch, P. A., & Kalisch, B. J. (1986). *The advance of American nursing* (2nd ed.). Boston: Little, Brown.

Le Vasseur, J. (1998). Plato, Nightingale, and contemporary nursing. *Image: Journal of Nursing Scholarship, 30*(3), 281–285.

Longfellow, H. W. (1857, November). Santa Filomena. *Atlantic Monthly, 1,* 22–23.

MacEachern, M. T. (1932). Which shall we choose: Graduate or student service? *Modern Hospital, 38,* 97–98, 102–104.

Minkowski, W. I. (1992). Women healers of the Middle Ages: Selected aspects of their history. *American Journal of Public Health, 82*(2), 288–295.

Montag, M. L. (1959). *Community college education for nursing: An experiment in technical education for nursing.* New York: McGraw-Hill.

Monteiro, L. A. (1985). Florence Nightingale on public health nursing. *American Journal of Public Health, 75*(2), 181–185.

Morton, M., Roberts, E., & Bender, K. (1993). *Celebrating public health nursing: Caring for Mississippi's communities with courage and compassion, 1920–1993.* Jackson: Mississippi State Department of Health.

Mosley, M. O. P (1996). Satisfied to carry the bag: Three black community health nurses' contribution to health care reform, 1900–1937. *Nursing History Review, 4,* 65–82.

Nightingale, F. (1893). Sick-nursing and health-nursing. In *Women's mission* (pp. 184–205). Arranged and ed. by Baroness Burdett-Coutts. London: Sampson, Law, Marston and Co.

Nightingale, F. (1979). Cassandra. In M. Stark (Ed.), *Florence Nightingale's Cassandra* (original work published in 1928). Old Westbury, NY: Feminist Press.

Nutting, M. A., & Dock, L. L. (1937). *A history of nursing* (Vol 1). New York: G. P. Putnam.

The 100 people who made the millennium. (1997). *Life Magazine, 20*(10a).

Palmer, I. S. (1977, March/April). Florence Nightingale: Reformer, reactionary, researcher. *Nursing Research,* pp. 13–18.

Palmer, I. S. (1982). *Through a glass darkly: From Nightingale to now.* Washington, DC: American Association of College of Nursing.

Payne, D. (1999). Face to face: Florence Nightingale and Mary Seacole battle it out face to face. *Nursing Times, 95*(19), 26–27.

Pyle, E. (1944). *Here is your war: The story of G. I. Joe.* Cleveland, OH: World Publishing.

Rathbone, W. (1890). *A history of nursing in the homes of the poor.* Introduction by Florence Nightingale. London: Macmillan.

Richardson, B. W. (1887). *The health of nations: A review of the works of Edwin Chadwick* (Vol. 2). London: Longmans, Green and Company.

Roberts, E. (1985a). *Highlights: Maternal and child health and crippled children's service, 1935–1985.* Jackson: Mississippi Department of Health.

Roberts, E. (1985b, March). *The role of the southern nurse in public health.* Symposium on Southern Science and Medicine at the Education and Research Center, Jackson, MS. Education and Research Center.

Roberts, M. (1954). *American nursing: History and interpretation.* New York: Macmillan.

Robinson, V. (1946). *White caps: The story of nursing.* Philadelphia: J. B. Lippincott.

Rosen, G. (1958). *A history of public health.* New York: M. D. Publications.

Sabin, L. (1998). *Struggles and triumphs: The story of Mississippi nurses 1800–1950.* Jackson: Mississippi Hospital Association Health, Research and Educational Foundation.

Sanger, M. (1928). *Motherhood in bondage.* New York: Brentano's.

Seymer, L. (1954). *Selected writings of Florence Nightingale.* New York: Macmillan.

Shryock, R. H. (1959). *The history of nursing: An interpretation of the social and medical factors involved.* Philadelphia: W. B. Saunders

Smith, E. (1934). *Mississippi special public health nursing project made possible by federal funds.* Paper presented at the 1934 annual Mississippi Nurses Association meeting, Jackson, MS.

Stanmore, A. H. G. (1906). *Sidney Herbert of Lea: A memoir.* New York: E. P. Dutton.

The state board test pool examination. (1952). *American Journal of Nursing, 52,* 613.

Stewart, I. M. (1921). Developments in nursing education since 1918. *U. S. Bureau of Education Bulletin, 20*(6), 3–8.

Taylor, H. O. (1922). *Greek biology and medicine.* Boston: Marshall Jones.

Tiffany, F. (1890). *The life of Dorothea Linda Dix.* Boston: Houghton Mifflin.

Tyrell, H. (1856). *Pictorial history of the war with Russia 1854–1856.* London: W. and R. Chambers.

Vicinus, M., & Nergaard, B. (1990). *Ever yours, Florence Nightingale: Selected letters.* Boston: Harvard University Press.

Wald, L. D. (1915). *The house on Henry Street.* New York: Henry Holt.

Wertz, R. W., & Wertz, D. C. (1977). *Lying-In: A history of childbirth in America.* New Haven, CT: Yale University Press.

Williams, C. B. (1961, May). Stories from Scutari. *American Journal of Nursing, 61,* 88.

Winslow, C. E. A. (1946). Florence Nightingale and public health nursing. *Public Health Nursing, 38,* 330–332.

Woodham-Smith, C. (1951). *Florence Nightingale.* New York: McGraw-Hill.

Woodham-Smith, C. (1983). *Florence Nightingale.* New York: Atheneum.

Young, D. A. (1995). Florence Nightingale's fever. *British Medical Journal, 311,* 1697–1700.

# CHAPTER 4
# Epidemiology of Health and Illness

Gail A. Harkness and Demetrius J. Porche

Visit **http://nursing.jbpub.com/communityhealth** for interactive exercises, review questions, Web links, and more.

To understand the changes that can occur in the health of individuals or in various populations, it is necessary to identify the relationships between the various biological and psychosocial phenomena that underlie health and illness. Epidemiology, the basic science of preventive medicine, has provided a process for understanding these relationships by studying different populations of people in various situations. Through study of health problems as they occur in groups or populations, many characteristics of specific illness or disabilities can be identified that may not be evident in the study of individuals alone.

"The work we are speaking of has nothing to do with nursing disease, but with maintaining health by removing the things which disturb it . . . dirt, drink, diet, damp, draughts, and drains."

*—Florence Nightingale, 1860*

"When we try pick out anything by itself, we find it is tied to everything else in the universe."

*—John Muir*

After reading the quotes, think about this question: How are the "connections" in your life related to your health? Think about your environment, your personal identity (such as gender), and the changing variables that can make you sick (e.g., stress) or keep you well (e.g., exercise).

## CHAPTER FOCUS

**Epidemiology Defined**

**Scope of Epidemiology**

**The Epidemiological, Research, and Nursing Processes**

**Natural History of Disease**

**Descriptive Epidemiology**
- Use of Rates
- Sources of Data

**Person, Place, and Time**
- Person
- Place
- Time

**Analytic Epidemiology**

## QUESTIONS TO CONSIDER

After reading this chapter, you will know the answers to the following questions:

1. What is the contribution of epidemiology to public health?
2. How do nurses use the principles of epidemiology?
3. How is the epidemiological process related to nursing and research?
4. What is the usefulness of rates in community health nursing?
5. What is the natural history of disease and levels of prevention?
6. What are the *incidence* and *prevalence* rates?
7. What are the characteristics of a population by person, place, and time?
8. What are the characteristics of the four types of epidemiological research studies?
9. How can epidemiological research be used in community health nursing?

## KEY TERMS

| | | | |
|---|---|---|---|
| Adjusted rates | Epidemiological triad | Period prevalence | Retrospective |
| Case-control | Incidence | Point prevalence | Risk factors |
| Cross-sectional | Intervention | Primary prevention | Secondary prevention |
| Crude rates | Morbidity | Prospective | Specific rates |
| Epidemic | Mortality | Rate | Tertiary prevention |
| Epidemic curve | | | |

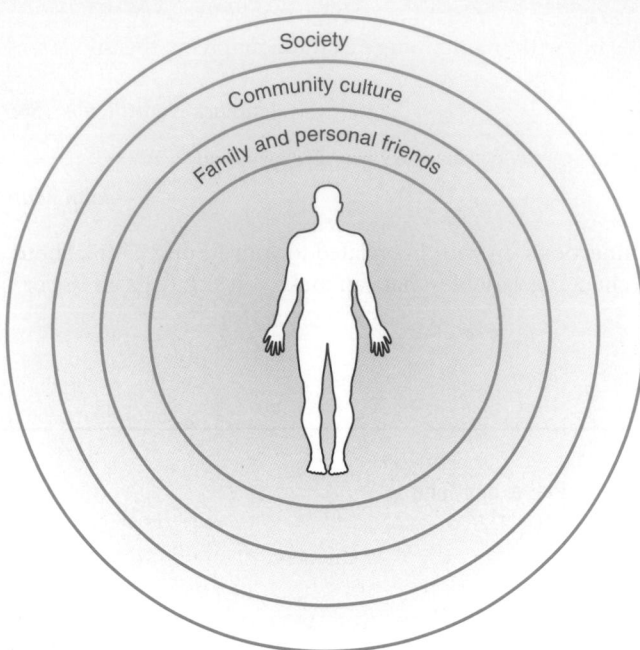

Individual within the framework of life

HEALTH CARE FOR ALL individuals should be planned within the framework of family and personal friends, the immediate community culture where they live, and the larger world society. Any individual's health care needs cannot be completely or correctly defined unless these broader factors are analyzed and appropriately incorporated into a plan of care. Just as information must be collected about individuals in assessing health problems, so data must be collected about groups, communities, and populations to assess the broader health needs of society.

For instance, the association between lung cancer and smoking might not have been ascertained by studying individual cases of lung cancer. Many smokers never develop lung cancer, and some nonsmokers do develop lung cancer. However, in 1950, Doll and Hill contrasted a group of lung cancer patients with a group of people who did not develop lung cancer. They clearly demonstrated that more people with lung cancer had smoked cigarettes than those people without the disease. This was substantiated by further research, and cigarette smoking is now considered a primary risk factor for lung cancer. This information has been the basis for national campaigns to decrease smoking among Americans. This example demonstrates the value of identifying certain characteristics or behaviors that increase risk of health problems even if the pathophysiology is not precisely known. Health care personnel can implement preventive health measures for both individuals and groups of people who are at high risk even if the causative factors are not known.

## Epidemiology Defined

*Epidemiology* is the study of the distribution and the determinants of states of health and illness in human populations (Gordis, 2004; Valanis, 1999). *Distribution* refers to the frequency of occurrence of states of health and illness; *determinants* refers to agents or factors that contribute to the cause of various states of health and illness. The word *epidemiology* is derived from the Greek word meaning **epidemic: epi,** upon; *demos,* people; and *logos,* treatise. The ultimate goal of epidemiology is to use the information obtained from the study of the distribution and determinants of states of health and illness to prevent or limit the consequences of illness and disability in humans and maximize their state of health. Although the influence of the environment on the occurrence of disease and the contagious nature of many diseases can be traced to Hippocrates, the techniques of modern epidemiological investigation were first developed in the mid-nineteenth century.

William Farr, a physician from London, established the field of medical statistics. In 1839, he was appointed to the Office of the Registrar General for England and Wales. He set up a system for compilation of the numbers and causes of deaths and compared the deaths of workers in different occupations, the difference in mortality between men and women, and the effect of imprisonment on the frequency of death. He realized that studying the data from populations of people would provide much more information about human disease than studying individual cases (Humphreys, 1885).

During the mid-nineteenth century, infectious diseases such as cholera and plague were still killing much of the population of Europe. The primary goal then was to limit the spread of these devastating diseases and prevent their recurrence. John Snow, another British physician, investigated the epidemic of cholera that took place from 1848 to 1854. His classic investigation of the outbreak clearly established the rate as a fundamental tool of epidemiology. Snow investigated cholera outbreaks associated with water supplied from two different water companies. He demonstrated statistically that cholera was associated with the water company that obtained its water from an area of the Thames River that was heavily polluted with sewage, and not with the company that obtained its water farther upstream (Snow, 1855).

Florence Nightingale was a contemporary of Farr and Snow and was significantly influenced by their statistical methods. Nightingale is probably best known for her work at the British military hospital in Scutari. British and French troops had invaded the Crimea on the north coast of the Black Sea, supporting Turkey in its dispute with Russia. Nightingale and her 38 nurses found the conditions appalling. Buildings were infested with rats and fleas, streams of sewage flowed under the buildings, linens were filthy, and

■■
■■ CULTURAL CONNECTION

African Americans as a group have a higher mean blood pressures than white Americans. Various hypotheses have been proposed to explain the differences between the races, such as genetic, social, economic, diet, and behavioral factors. To date, epidemiological studies have been inconclusive as to the exact causes for the differences. ◕

Nightingale's polar-area diagram

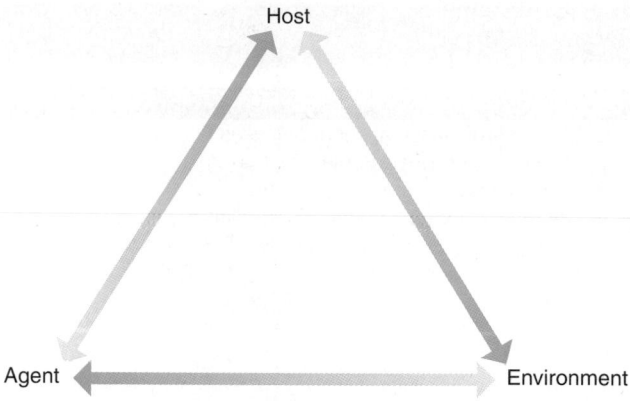

The epidemiological triad

supplies were scarce. They initiated sanitary reforms, keeping records of illness and deaths. The following figure shows a polar-area diagram designed by Nightingale to dramatize the needless deaths that occurred during the war and the effect of her reforms (Aiken, 1988; Cohen, 1984).

As a result of these early investigations, epidemiology traditionally has been associated with infectious diseases, with a focus on the **epidemiological triad:** agent, host, and environment. This model is based on the belief that health status is multifactorial, determined by the interaction of many agent, host, and environment characteristics, and not by any single factor. For example, factors influencing the development of a heart attack include heredity, high cholesterol levels, dietary excess, cigarette smoking, emotional stress, physical exercise, and many other factors. No one factor is considered a causative factor for the illness. Therefore, the epidemiological triad remains a fundamental conceptual framework for the contemporary study of health problems.

 EPIDEMIOLOGY in Practice

Florence Nightingale has been called one of the first epidemiologists as a result of her use of statistics to document health care needs.

Epidemiology can be considered both as a *methodology* used to study health-related conditions and as a *body of knowledge* that results from research into a specific health-related condition (Gordis, 2004; Volanis, 1999). Using epidemiological research methodology to investigate health

problems leads to the accumulation of a body of knowledge about that particular problem. (Epidemiological research methods are discussed later in the chapter.) Practitioners then can use this body of knowledge in their clinical decision making and in developing health services. For example, epidemiological research has associated hypertension, obesity, and smoking with increased incidence of heart disease. These are all potentially modifiable risk factors that often are associated with lifestyle and behavior choices. Nurses and other health professionals can use this information when assessing individual patients and helping them make choices about intervention techniques that may reduce their risk of heart disease. Also, community health nurses may initiate community-level programs to identify hypertension at an early stage, to stop smoking, or to decrease weight in an attempt to decrease the risk of heart disease for the population as a whole.

## Scope of Epidemiology

The scope of epidemiology has been expanded and therefore changed in recent years. Not only are the distribution and determinants of illness and disease investigated, but variables that contribute to the maintenance of health are also studied. The evolving changes in demographic characteristics, the patterns of disease, methods of control and prevention of health problems, and the need for maintaining wellness have contributed to this shift in the scope of epidemiology. *Healthy People 2010* uses determinants of health to derive the objectives for the nation. The depth of topics covered by the objectives reflect the diversity of critical influences that determine the health of persons who live in communities.

 ENVIRONMENTAL CONNECTION

Nature has no mercy at all. Nature says, "I'm going to snow. If you have on a bikini and no snowshoes, that's tough. I am going to snow anyway."

—*Maya Angelou*

| Table 4-1 | Comparison of the Leading Causes of Death in the United States Between 1900 and 2000 |
|---|---|

| 1900 | 2000 |
|---|---|
| 1. Major cardiovascular-renal diseases | 1. Heart disease |
| 2. Influenza and pneumonia | 2. Cancer—maligant neoplasms |
| 3. Tuberculosis | 3. Cardiovascular disease (strokes) |
| 4. Gastritis, duodenitis, enteritis, cholitis | 4. Chronic lower respiratory disease |
| 5. Accidents | 5. Unintentional injuries (accidents) |
| 6. Malignant neoplasms | 6. Diabetes mellitus |
| 7. Diphtheria | 7. Alzheimer's disease |
| 8. Typhoid and paratyphoid fever | 8. Influenza and pneumonia |
| 9. Measles | 9. Kidney disease |
| 10. Cirrhosis of the liver | 10. Septicemia |

*Source:* Kung, H. C., Hoyert, D. L., Xu, J., & Murphy, S. L. (2008). Deaths: Final data for 2005. *National Vital Statistics Report, 56*(10), 1–120.

Improved public health services, increased life expectancy, increased frequency of noninfectious disease and chronic degenerative conditions, and advances in technology are continually changing the health needs of society. (See Table 4-1 for a comparison of the leading causes of death in the United States over time.) Provision of present and future health care depends on (1) identifying health problems and needs, (2) collecting and analyzing data to identify factors that influence those health problems or needs, and (3) planning, implementing, and evaluating methods for prevention and control. These steps form the basis of the epidemiological process.

## The Epidemiological, Research, and Nursing Processes

The epidemiological process, the research process, and the nursing process have all evolved from steps in the problem-solving process. All three processes have similar basic components: defining the problem, gathering data, analyzing the data, and evaluating the results. The research process focuses on obtaining new knowledge about a health condition. The epidemiological process and the nursing process are more focused on planning for control, for prevention, or for intervention activities that will mediate a health condition (Table 4-2). The cyclical nature of the epidemiological process is illustrated in the following figure.

## Natural History of Disease

In 1958, Leavell and Clark, two public health physicians, championed the cause of preventive medicine by emphasizing that prevention is required at every phase of the disease process. They called the course of any disease process as it develops in humans the "natural history of the disease." HIV disease progression or natural history of HIV disease encompasses HIV infection, asymptomatic HIV infection, period with symptoms, and finally AIDS diagnosis (see the figure on p. 106). During the prepathogenesis period, there are factors within individuals and their environments that may predispose or precipitate the disease. The initial interactions among agent, host, and environment occur during this

| Table 4-2 | Similarities Between the Epidemiological Process, the Research Process, and the Nursing Process |
|---|---|

| Epidemiological Process | Research Process | Nursing Process |
|---|---|---|
| ■ Define problem | ■ Define problem | ■ Assessment: |
| ■ Gather information from reliable sources | ■ Review literature | Establish patient database |
| ■ Describe problem by person, place, time | ■ Conceptualize problem | |
| ■ Formulate tentative hypothesis | ■ Define variables | ■ Diagnosis: |
| | ■ Identify methodology | Interpret data |
| ■ Analyze descriptive data to test hypothesis | | Identify health care needs |
| | | Select goals of care |
| ■ Plan for control of the problem | | ■ Planning: |
| | | Select process for achieving goals |
| ■ Implement control plan | ■ Collect data | ■ Implementation: |
| | | Initiate and complete actions to achieve goals |
| ■ Evaluate control plan | ■ Analyze data | ■ Evaluation: |
| ■ Prepare appropriate report | ■ Publish report | Determine extent of goal achievement |
| ■ Conduct further research | ■ Conduct further research | |

Model of the epidemiological process

**ETHICAL CONNECTION**

Epidemiological studies consistently show that Americans are getting fatter. The percentage of Americans who were obese in 1971 was 14.5%; in 2005, that percentage had climbed to a staggering 30.9%. The number of deaths per year associated with being overweight is estimated at 400,000. Adult women are now eating 335 more calories per day than they did in 1971, while adult men have upped their daily intake by 168 calories.

What ethical responsibilities do community health nurses have in the prevention of obesity versus the treatment of obesity-related diseases? Where are most of the resources spent in the health care system related to this serious, yet preventable health problem?

period. For example, an individual may have an inherited predisposition to high cholesterol levels and may be obese, a smoker, and under excessive pressure at work in the prepathogenesis period. The period of pathogenesis begins when the host begins to respond with biological, psychological, or other changes. It is manifested by signs and symptoms that continue until the condition is resolved by recovery, disability, or death. If this individual is not able to modify the factors that predispose to disease, he or she is at high risk for a heart attack.

Leavell and Clark identified levels of prevention for the prepathogenesis and pathogenesis periods as primary prevention, secondary prevention, and tertiary prevention.

**Primary prevention** includes activities that prevent a disease from becoming established and occurs during the prepathogenesis period. These activities include both health promotion activities and specific protection activities such as immunizations and protection from hazards and hygiene. Because no symptoms of illness exist, primary prevention programs are directed toward either the general healthy population or toward a group of healthy people who are known to be at high risk for a particular disease, illness, or injury. For example, public health organizations and voluntary agencies have emphasized the importance of regular exercise, a low-fat diet, and smoking cessation programs in an attempt to prevent coronary artery disease.

**Secondary prevention** includes activities designed to detect disease and provide early treatment. These activities involve early diagnosis, prompt treatment, and measures to limit disability. Screening programs for high cholesterol are an example of secondary prevention of coronary artery disease. If high levels are found, early treatment can be effective in lowering cholesterol levels. For example, screenings such as monograms and prostate-specific antigen (PSA) tests are secondary prevention activities.

**Tertiary prevention** includes the treatment, care, and rehabilitation of people with acute and chronic illness to achieve their maximum potential. If coronary artery disease is not prevented, a myocardial infarction may occur. A coronary artery bypass graft may be required, followed by a cardiac rehabilitation program.

Both secondary and tertiary prevention occur during the pathogenesis period. However, tertiary prevention is initiated after irreversible changes have resulted from the disease process. A detailed outline of the natural history can be created for any illness, and it becomes a helpful guideline for health professionals at all three levels of prevention (Leavell & Clark, 1965).

## Descriptive Epidemiology

Descriptive epidemiology focuses on the frequency and distribution of states of health within a population. By describing characteristics of groups of people who have or do not have certain illnesses, factors that are associated primarily

| The natural history of any disease affecting humans | | | |
|---|---|---|---|
| Interrelations of agent, host, and environmental factors<br><br>Production of *stimulus* ⟶ | Reaction of the *host* to the *stimulus* ⟶<br><br>Early pathogenesis ⟶ Discernible early lesions ⟶ Advanced disease ⟶ Convalescence ⟶ | | |
| Prepathogenesis period | Period of pathogenesis | | |

**Health promotion**
- Health education
- Good standard of nutrition adjusted to developmental phases of life
- Attention to personality development
- Provision of adequate housing, recreation, and agreeable working conditions
- Marriage counseling and sex education
- Genetics
- Periodic selective examinations

**Specific protection**
- Use of specific immunizations
- Attention to personal hygiene
- Use of environmental sanitation
- Protection against occupational hazards
- Protection from accidents
- Use of specific nutrients
- Protection from carcinogens
- Avoidance of allergens

**Early diagnosis and prompt treatment**
- Case-finding measures, individual and mass
- Screening surveys
- Selective examinations

*Objectives:*
- To cure and prevent disease processes
- To prevent the spread of communicable diseases
- To prevent complications and sequelae
- To shorten period of disability

**Disability limitation**
- Adequate treatment to arrest the disease process and to prevent further complications and sequelae
- Provision of facilities to limit disability and to prevent death

**Rehabilitation**
- Provision of hospital and community facilities for retraining and education for maximum use of remaining capacities
- Education of the public and industry to utilize the rehabilitated
- As full employment as possible
- Selective placement
- Work therapy in hospitals
- Use of sheltered colony

| Primary prevention | Secondary prevention | Tertiary prevention |
|---|---|---|

**Levels of application of preventive measures**

Levels of application of preventive measures in the natural history of disease

*Source:* Leavell & Clark, 1965.

with the people who have the illness can be identified. These are called **risk factors.** Knowledge regarding risk factors provides supporting data to plan primary and secondary prevention activities. Generally, descriptive data can tell us what kind of people are at risk of developing certain health problems; what diseases, disabilities, or needs they have; how these problems are distributed in the population, who goes where for different kinds of health service; and who provides the health services they need in the community. Health professionals then use this information to set priorities for health programs, to find ways of using health resources more effectively, to plan strategies to meet emerging health care needs, and to evaluate the effectiveness of measures used to control or prevent specific disorders. However, it is important to emphasize here that descriptive epidemiology can be used to study states of wellness. For example, identifying factors such as diet and exercise that are associated with healthy, community-dwelling elderly people older than 85 years of age can provide the information necessary to enhance wellness in other elderly populations.

## ■ Use of Rates

All epidemiological investigations depend on the ability to quantify the occurrence of a health problem. The most basic measure of frequency is to count the number of affected individuals. However, this may be misleading. The number of people in the population who could have been affected, but were not, should be taken into consideration. For example, five people in a community may have developed human immunodeficiency virus/acquired immune deficiency syndrome (HIV/AIDS). The implications of this event would be interpreted very differently if those people came from a community of 500 people versus a community of 100,000 people. Also, the time frame in which the problem has occurred is important. The use of ratios, proportions, and rates provide a more valid description of health problems.

A *ratio* is a fraction that is obtained by dividing one quantity by another quantity; it represents the relationship between the two numbers. The numerator is not included in the denominator. For example, the number of boys on a pediatric unit could be contrasted with the number of girls on the same unit using a ratio: 10 boys and 5 girls would result in a 2:1 ratio of boys to girls. A *proportion* is a type of ratio that includes the quantity in the numerator also as a part of the denominator. Therefore, it is the relationship of a part to the whole. Dividing the number of boys on the pediatric unit by the total number of boys and girls on the unit results in a proportion: 10 boys out of 15 boys and girls would result in a proportion of boys equal to 67%.

 ## Research Alert

The purpose of this research study was to determine whether county syphilis rates were increased along I-95 in North Carolina during an epidemic. Data on syphilis cases, demographics, drug activity, and highways were used to conduct a longitudinal study of North Carolina counties from 1985 to 1994. Crude and adjusted incidence rates were calculated and adjusted for sociodemographic factors and drug use. A cross-section design was used. Ten-year syphilis rates in the I-95 counties greatly exceeded rates in non-I-95 counties: 38 versus 16 cases per 100,000 persons, and remained high even after adjustment for race, age, sex, poverty, urban area designation, and drug activity. Syphilis rates were stable until 1989, but increased sharply in I-95 counties after 1989. Increased drug activity in I-95 counties preceded the rise in syphilis rates. The authors offer possible explanations for these results: spread of syphilis through contact between truck drivers and local sex workers at truck stops and rest stops; cocaine distribution; and the use of crack cocaine, which increases risky behaviors such as higher numbers of sexual partners and less frequent condom use owing in part to the exchange of sex for drugs. Although the authors do not state specifically which factors were responsible for the increase in syphilis rates along I-95, cocaine distribution along the highway seems the most likely explanation. Further study is recommended to determine the specific associations along I-95. A better understanding of the cause of the association has public health applications where more resources and interventions can be focused.

*Source:* Cook, R. L., Royce, R. A., Thomas, J. C., & Hanusa, B. H. (1999). What's driving in epidemia. The spread of syphilis along an interstate highway in rural North Carolina. *American Journal of Public Health, 89*(3), 369–373.

 ### ENVIRONMENTAL CONNECTION

Many nursing students note that the environment gets little attention, compared to the person and agent parts of the epidemiological triangle in the nursing curriculum. What do you think?

A **rate** is a proportion that includes the factor of time. It is a measure of the quantity of a health problem in a specific population within a given period. Rates are the best indicators of the probability that a disease, condition, or event will occur; therefore, rates are the primary measurements used to describe occurrence. Rates take into consideration the population statistics and are frequently a more precise measure than is frequency. By using rates, it is possible to compare events that happen at different times and places and with different people. For example, rates make it possible to compare the occurrence of HIV/AIDS in two or more locations.

A rate consists of two parts: a *numerator* and a *denominator*. The numerator is composed of the number of cases of the health problem being investigated within a given period. The denominator is the population at risk during the same period. If the period is long, the population at risk is often estimated at a midperiod, such as midyear. There are four basic principles that apply to the calculation of rates:

1. The numerator should include all events being measured; therefore, adequate information must be available.
2. Everyone in the denominator must be at risk for the event in the numerator.
3. A specific period must be indicated during which observations are made.
4. To make the rate a reasonable size to interpret and remove decimal points, the rate is multiplied by a base, usually a multiple of 10. Any base multiple of 10 may be chosen that results in a rate above the value of 1.

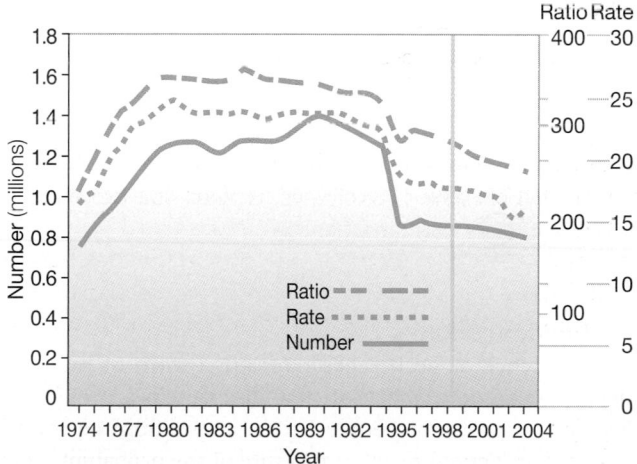

Number, ratio,* and rate† of legal abortions performed, by year— United States, 1974–2004
*Number of abortions per 1000 live births
†Number of abortions per 1000 women aged 15–44 years

*Source:* Centers for Disease Control and Prevention. (2007). Abortion surveillance— 2004. *Morbidity and Mortality Weekly Report, 56*(SS9), 1–36.

**Table 4-3**    Calculating and Comparing Rates Between Two Cities

| City A | City B |
|---|---|
| ■ Number of hepatitis cases (conditions) = 45 | ■ Number of hepatitis cases (conditions) = 341 |
| ■ Population of City A = 153,000 | ■ Population of City B = 1,326,000 |
| ■ Hepatitis rate = 45 ÷ 153,000 = 0.000294 | ■ Hepatitis rate = 341 ÷ 1,326,000 = 0.000257 |
| ■ 0.000294 × 100,000 (base multiple of 10) = 29.4 | ■ 0.00257 × 100,000 (base multiple of 10) = 25.7 |
| ■ Hepatitis rate = 29.4 cases/100,000 people | ■ Hepatitis rate = 25.7 cases/100,000 people |

Counting only cases, City B has a higher frequency of hepatitis. However, when the population at risk is included in the rate calculation, City A has more cases per population than City B.

The formula for rate calculation follows. Table 4-3 illustrates the calculation of rates that can be compared between cities.

$$Rate = \frac{\text{Number of conditions or events occurring in a period of time}}{\text{Population at risk during the same period of time}} \times \text{Base multiple of 10}$$

An example of the difference between rates and ratios is shown in the figure on p. 107. Legal abortion rates are defined as the number of legal abortions per 1,000 women age 15 to 44 years. Women experiencing legal abortions are in the numerator, and all women of childbearing age are in the denominator. The abortion ratio is the number of legal induced abortions per 1,000 live births. The numerator, the number of legal induced abortions, is not a part of the denominator, live births. Therefore, it is a ratio and not a rate. However, the number of legal induced abortions per 1,000 women of childbearing age is a rate, the abortion rate. The graph on p. 107 shows the changes in the rates and ratio over a 27-year period (CDC, 2003a).

 GLOBAL CONNECTION

People living in Japan have from one half to one third the risk of dying from heart disease in comparison to people living in the United States, even when their mean cholesterol levels remain the same. When Japanese immigrants settle in the United States, within 5 years their risk for heart disease equals that of native U.S. citizens. How do you explain this difference?

### Incidence Rates

**Incidence** or occurrence rates are a form of rate that measures the occurrence of new illnesses in a previously disease-free group of people within a specific time frame, often a year. Therefore, it is a measure of the probability that people without a certain condition will develop the condition over a period of time. The numerator of incidence rates includes only the number of *new* conditions or events occurring within a period of time; therefore, the date of onset

must be known. The general rules that apply to rates apply to incidence rates. Incidence rates and incidence ratios, especially **mortality** (death) rates, are often indices of the health of communities.

Incidence rates can be used to determine trends over time. For example, the following figure shows the rates of group B streptococcal (GBS) infection among infants in the United States (CDC, 2007b). This infection is the leading cause of bacterial disease and death among newborns in the United States and can cause illness and death in peripartum women and in adults with chronic medical conditions. Therefore, the incidence of this disease has been tracked in selected cities and their surrounding regions in different geographic locations. This incidence rate has been calculated as the number of infants infected per 1,000 live births. The figure shows that while the incidence of GBS disease decreased among white infants after guidelines for preventing perinatal GBS disease were issued, it increased significantly among black infants. Continued surveillance is necessary to deter-

Rate* of early-onset[†] group B streptococcal (GBS) disease by race and year—Active Bacterial Core Surveillance System, United States, 2000–2005[§]

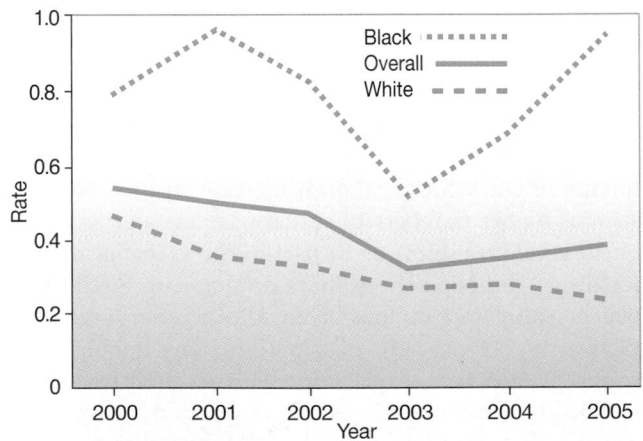

* Per 1,000 live births.
[†] Occurring in infants aged 0-6 days.
[§] Rates for 2000-2005 correspond to surveillance areas participating since 2000, with the addition of Colorado in 2001. New Mexico, where surveillance began in 2004, is not included in comparison of incidence over time.

**NOTE THIS!** •————————————————

The mortality rate of lung cancer has surpassed the mortality rate of breast cancer among women.

———————————————————————————————

mine if this trend continues and to identify possible barriers to universal screening among black women (CDC, 2007b).

### Prevalence Rates

Prevalence rates measure the number of people in a given population who have an existing health problem within a specified time frame. There are two types of prevalence rates. **Period prevalence** indicates the existence of a condition during an interval of time. **Point prevalence** refers to the existence of a condition at a specific point in time. Prevalence measures the amount of illness or **morbidity** that exists in a community as a result of the health problem under investigation. Many health care workers believe that prevalence rates are more important than incidence rates in determining the total burden of the illness on the community. Community health nurses use prevalence data to plan for the allocation of resources in a community based on the amount of disease burden present. Knowledge of the prevalence of a condition such as diabetes mellitus within a population can lead to the prioritizing of facilities, services, and personnel to meet the special needs of diabetics in the community.

Prevalence is influenced by two factors: the number of people who have developed the condition in the past and the duration of their illness. A formula for prevalence is

Prevalence = Incidence × Duration of Illness

The longer the duration of a condition, the higher the prevalence rate in the community. This is best illustrated with chronic diseases. For example, there are many more cases of diabetes in a community than would be indicated by calculation of the incidence rate, which reflects new cases only. Although the incidence rate for diabetes is low, people live for many years with the illness, and the duration is high. Therefore, in calculating prevalence rates, the numerator consists of the number of *existing* cases of the condition or event that occur within a specified period. For example, the existing cases of diabetes mellitus include new cases that were recently diagnosed plus those cases diagnosed in the past who are currently living with the illness.

 *Got an Alternative?*

Life doesn't cease to be funny when people die any more than it ceases to be serious when people laugh.

—George Bernard Shaw

•  •  •  •  •  •  •  •  •  •  •  •  •  •  •  •  •  •  •  •  •  •  •  •  •  •  •

### Crude, Specific, and Adjusted Rates

Other common rates include crude, specific, and adjusted rates. **Crude rates** measure the experience of health problems in populations of designated geographic areas. These broad descriptive statistics may obscure significant differences in the risk of developing various conditions. Factors such as age, gender, ethnicity, and other demographic factors are not taken into consideration. Therefore, **specific rates** for subgroups of the population may be calculated. These more detailed rates are commonly calculated to describe the distribution of health problems by age, gender, ethnicity, and other demographic characteristics. **Adjusted rates** have been standardized, removing the differences in composition of populations, such as age. The following figure (part a) illustrates the prevalence of diabetes in four

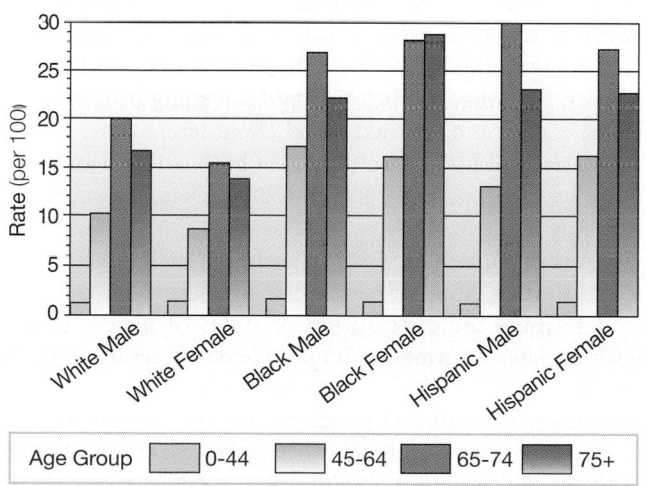

Age-specific prevalence of diagnosed diabetes, by race/ethnicity and sex, United States, 2005

*Source:* Centers for Disease Control and Prevention. (2007). *Data and trends: Diabetes surveillance system.* Retrieved October 21, 2008, from http://www.cdc.gov/diabetes/statistics/prev/national/fig2004.htm

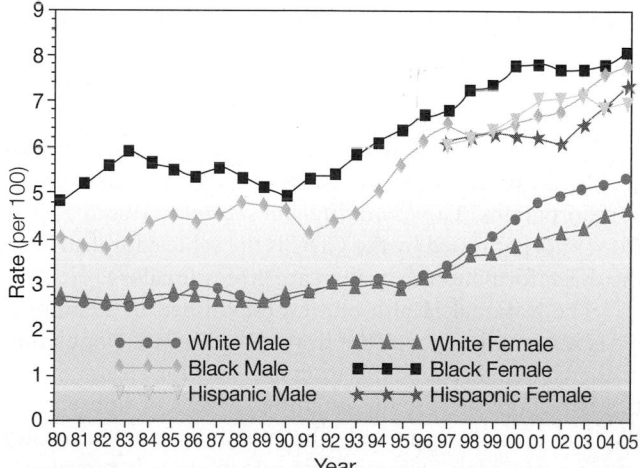

Age-adjusted prevalence of diagnosed diabetes, by race/ethnicity and sex, United States, 1980–2005

*Source:* Centers for Disease Control and Prevention. (2007). *Data and trends: Diabetes surveillance system.* Retrieved October 21, 2008, from http://www.cdc.gov/diabetes/statistics/prev/national/figraceethsex.htm

specific age groups. The rates are highest in the 65 to 74 and 75 plus categories. Part b of the figure illustrates age-adjusted rates of self-reported diabetes by race (CDC, 2007a). In this example, age adjustment removes age as a factor in the calculation of the rates. Therefore, the differences shown reflect a rather dramatic increase in diabetes mellitus in African American females. Knowledge of these factors can be helpful in assessing individual patients for their health care needs, as well as group needs for prevention and control programs.

## ■ Sources of Data

To describe a specific condition or event appropriately, it is necessary to collect data from reliable sources. Traditionally, epidemiologists have used the census of the population as a reliable source for the denominators in the calculation of rates. The census is required once every 10 years by the U.S. Constitution and is the basis for apportionment of seats in the House of Representatives. It has been performed every 10 years since 1790. The twenty-second census was completed in 2000. Through the years, the census has expanded, including characteristics of housing, nativity, migration, education, employment, income, and other information that is gathered from random samples of the population. Census information is analyzed and reported for the nation as a whole and in progressively small regions down to municipalities, census tracts, and blocks. Results are also reported in regions known as standard metropolitan statistical areas (SMSA). These regions are densely populated and are not necessarily bound by traditional state or county lines. The majority of the population of the United States lives within these areas.

Vital statistics are data collected from the continuous recording of events such as births, deaths, marriages, divorces, and adoptions, usually by state agencies. This information can be used to provide valid numerators and denominators for calculation of rates. The Centers for Disease Control and Prevention (CDC) in Atlanta collects all information regarding reportable diseases from state health departments. A sample of common reportable communicable diseases is found in Box 4-1. However, reportable diseases may vary somewhat from state to state. The CDC also collects information about other infectious and non-infectious health problems through a series of more than 100 national surveillance programs. The *Morbidity and Mortality Weekly Report (MMWR)* published by the CDC is the vehicle for distributing this information to health care professionals.

The National Health Survey, established in 1956, provides information about the health needs of the population of the United States. The National Center for Health Statistics is responsible for the ongoing surveys of households, physical examinations and laboratory reports, and health services providers. Most of this information is prevalence

> ❝*It is more important to know what sort of patient has a disease than what sort of a disease a patient has.*❞
> —*Sir William Osler*

---

| BOX 4-1 | |
|---|---|
| **Common Reportable Communicable Diseases** | |
| AIDS | Malaria |
| Amebiasis | Measles |
| Anthrax | Meningitis |
| Botulism | Meningococcal |
| Brucellosis | infection |
| Campylobacteriosis | Mumps |
| Chancroid | Pertussis |
| Chickenpox—zoster | Plague |
| Chlamydia | Poliomyelitis |
| Cholera | Psittacosis |
| Diphtheria | Rabies |
| Encephalitis | Reye's syndrome |
| Food-associated | Rocky Mountain |
| illnesses | spotted fever |
| Giardiasis | Rubella |
| Gonorrhea | Salmonellosis |
| Granuloma inguinale | Shigellosis |
| Hemophilus | Syphilis |
| influenzae | Tetanus |
| Hepatitis A, B, non-A, | Toxic shock syndrome |
| non-B, unspecified | Trichinosis |
| Legionellosis | Tuberculosis |
| Leprosy | Tularemia |
| Leptospirosis | Typhoid fever |
| Lyme disease | Typhus |
| Lymphogranuloma | Yellow fever |
| venereum | |

data and is the only nationwide source of data on chronic illness, minor conditions, and functional problems.

The Behavioral Risk Factor Surveillance System (BRFSS) was established in 1984 to collect, analyze, and interpret behavioral risk factor data from all states. Information is gathered about health behaviors such as obesity, lack of physical activity, smoking, seat belt use, and screening programs for breast cancer and elevated blood cholesterol. These BRFSS data were used in the formulation of both national and state objectives for the year 2000 and 2010. Data are published regularly in the *MMWR*.

Any health-related information that has been collected about a group of people can be a source of data used to determine the distribution of states of health. Often, health-related information is found in databases from health care institutions, disease registries, insurance companies, industries, accident and police records, private doctors offices, local surveys, and any other place where information is gathered. Community health nurses are likely to use these data when planning programs for groups of people with specific health needs and information about the population is needed. These records reflect only those conditions or events that are characteristic of the people that sought the services of that agency or participated in the survey. These data are helpful in establishing health services to meet their needs and in evaluating outcomes, but data must be interpreted carefully when applying the information to the community as a whole.

### Got an Alternative?

Both green tea and black tea contain antioxidant chemicals that help block oxidation of LDL in the blood; herb teas do *not* contain antioxidants. Consuming green tea daily can protect the coronary arteries in a manner similar to that of the C and E antioxidant vitamins. Asian people drink green tea daily, which may account for their reduced risk of cardiovascular disease.

## Person, Place, and Time

One of the first steps in investigating the distribution and determinants of a health care problem is to describe the problem *(what occurs)* in terms of person, place, and time. Descriptive epidemiology deals primarily with the study of the distribution of health problems. However, research studies that attempt to identify the determinants of a problem *(why it occurs)* depend on the accurate collection of descriptive data. Examining the information about person, place, and time can help identify the characteristics of people who develop a disease or illness and those who do not.

### ■ Person

Describing the person characterizes *who* develops the health problem. There are many variations among people based on genetic factors, biological characteristics, behavioral choices, lifestyle, and socioeconomic conditions. Because so many variations exist, incidence and prevalence rates should be calculated according to these factors. This can be done by examining individual case data and examining specific and adjusted rates. Age is the most important characteristic affecting health status, followed by sex. Therefore, age-specific rates and sex-specific rates are usually calculated when describing a problem. Age-specific rates are calculated using the number of people in a given age group who have the problem being investigated in the numerator, and the population at risk in the given age group in the denominator.

An example of age-specific rates follows. The study describes heat-related deaths in Missouri, New Mexico, Oklahoma, and Texas when temperatures elevated for several consecutive days during July and August of 2001. The figure above is a bar graph that demonstrates that the average rate of heat-related deaths each year is greatest in the newborn to 1, 75 to 84, and 85 age groups (CDC, 2002).

Using this knowledge, community health nurses could initiate multiple actions, either for individuals in their care or for groups. When a heat wave is forecast, primary prevention messages about how to avoid heat-related illness should be disseminated to the public. The elderly should be encour-

Average annual rate* of heat-related deaths attributed to weather conditions[†] and exposure to excessive natural heat[§], by age group, United States, 1979–1999.

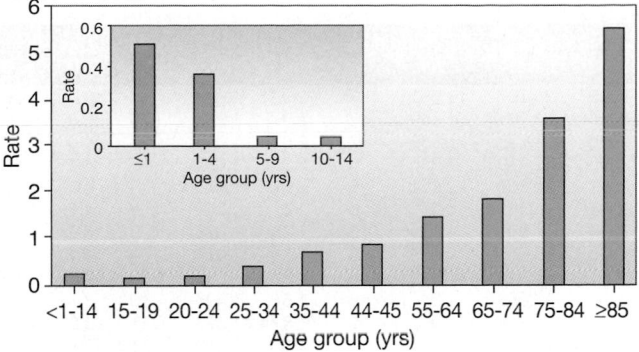

* Per million population.
[†] *International Classification of Diseases, Ninth Revision* (ICD-9), code E900.0.
[§]ICD-10, code X30.

*Source:* Centers for Disease Control and Prevention. (2002). Heat-related deaths—four states, July–August 2001, and United States, 1979–1999. *Morbidity and Mortality Weekly Report, 51*(26), 567–570.

aged to maintain their fluid intake and assisted to increase their time in air-conditioned environments, making use of shopping malls and public libraries, even for part of the day. Alcohol consumption should be discouraged because it may cause dehydration and increase the risk for heat-related illnesses. Parents of young children should be educated about the increased heat sensitivity of young children and their need for adequate fluids. Daycare centers could be primary sites for dissemination of information.

Often, specific rates are presented in table form, combining characteristics of persons and changes over time. Table 4-4 indicates the number of reported tuberculosis cases and the age characteristics of the cases by year, as well as the percentage change from 1993 to 2006 (CDC, 2003b). This information shows that people older than 65 are the most vulnerable to tuberculosis. Nurses use this knowledge in establishing primary prevention programs and in assessing their elderly patients for signs and symptoms that may be indicative of the infection.

### ■ Place

*Where* the rates of the health problem are the highest or the lowest can be determined by examining the characteristics of place. Understanding where illness occurs is a primary factor to be considered in planning prevention and control measures and making decisions about distribution of health care

THINK ABOUT THIS

**The Paradox of Life**

A bit beyond perception's reach
I sometimes believe I see
that Life is two locked boxes, each
containing the other's key.

—*Piet Hein, Danish mathematician and physicist*

**Table 4-4**    Tuberculosis Cases, Percentages, and Case Rates per 100,000 Population by Age Group, United States, 1992–2006

| Year | Total Cases | 0–14 No. | % | Rate | 15–24 No. | % | Rate | 25–44 No. | % | Rate | 45–64 No. | % | Rate | ≥65 No. | % | Rate | Unknown[1] No. | % |
|---|---|---|---|---|---|---|---|---|---|---|---|---|---|---|---|---|---|---|
| 1993 | 25,107 | 1,661 | 7 | 2.9 | 1,823 | 7 | 5.0 | 9,587 | 38 | 11.5 | 6,197 | 25 | 12.4 | 5,820 | 23 | 17.7 | 19 | 0 |
| 1994 | 24,205 | 1,659 | 7 | 2.9 | 1,833 | 8 | 5.0 | 9,043 | 37 | 10.7 | 6,125 | 25 | 11.9 | 5,539 | 23 | 16.6 | 6 | 0 |
| 1995 | 22,728 | 1,536 | 7 | 2.6 | 1,698 | 7 | 4.6 | 8,201 | 36 | 9.7 | 5,960 | 26 | 11.3 | 5,328 | 23 | 15.8 | 5 | 0 |
| 1996 | 21,210 | 1,356 | 6 | 2.3 | 1,637 | 8 | 4.4 | 7,564 | 36 | 8.9 | 5,572 | 26 | 10.2 | 5,076 | 24 | 14.9 | 5 | 0 |
| 1997 | 19,751 | 1,251 | 6 | 2.1 | 1,675 | 8 | 4.5 | 6,884 | 35 | 8.0 | 5,277 | 27 | 9.4 | 4,663 | 24 | 13.6 | 1 | 0 |
| 1998 | 18,287 | 1,077 | 6 | 1.8 | 1,542 | 8 | 4.1 | 6,335 | 35 | 7.4 | 4,956 | 27 | 8.5 | 4,377 | 24 | 12.6 | 0 | 0 |
| 1999 | 17,501 | 1,039 | 6 | 1.7 | 1,518 | 9 | 3.9 | 6,063 | 35 | 7.1 | 4,858 | 28 | 8.0 | 4,020 | 23 | 11.6 | 3 | 0 |
| 2000 | 16,310 | 964 | 6 | 1.6 | 1,617 | 10 | 4.1 | 5,575 | 34 | 6.6 | 4,637 | 28 | 7.4 | 3,516 | 22 | 10.0 | 1 | 0 |
| 2001 | 15,945 | 929 | 6 | 1.5 | 1,597 | 10 | 4.0 | 5,609 | 35 | 6.6 | 4,515 | 28 | 7.0 | 3,293 | 21 | 9.3 | 2 | 0 |
| 2002 | 15,056 | 944 | 6 | 1.6 | 1,497 | 10 | 3.7 | 5,288 | 35 | 6.3 | 4,182 | 28 | 6.3 | 3,141 | 21 | 8.8 | 4 | 0 |
| 2003 | 14,838 | 912 | 6 | 1.5 | 1,573 | 11 | 3.8 | 5,073 | 34 | 6.0 | 4,283 | 29 | 6.2 | 2,994 | 20 | 8.3 | 3 | 0 |
| 2004 | 14,502 | 954 | 7 | 1.6 | 1,602 | 11 | 3.8 | 4,940 | 34 | 5.9 | 4,194 | 29 | 5.9 | 2,811 | 19 | 7.7 | 1 | 0 |
| 2005 | 14,080 | 857 | 6 | 1.4 | 1,544 | 11 | 3.7 | 4,739 | 34 | 5.6 | 4,125 | 29 | 5.7 | 2,815 | 20 | 7.7 | 0 | 0 |
| 2006 | 13,779 | 807 | 6 | 1.3 | 1,540 | 11 | 3.6 | 4,702 | 34 | 5.6 | 4,053 | 29 | 5.4 | 2,676 | 19 | 7.2 | 1 | 0 |

[1]Includes unknown and missing.

Note: Previously published rates for 1993–1999 have been updated using Bridged-Race 1990–1999 Intercensal Population Estimates (http://www.cdc.gov/nchs/about/major/dvs/popbridge/popridge.htm) (accessed May 18, 2007). Denominators for computing 2000–2006 cases rates were obtained from the Annual Estimates of the Population by Sex and Five-Year Age Groups for the United States: April 1, 2000, to July 2, 2006 (http://www.census.gov/popest/national/asrh/NC-EST2006/NC-EST2006-01.xls) (accessed May 18, 2007). Data for all years updated through April 6, 2007.
See Technical Notes (page 9).
Zero % (0) denotes <0.5%.
See Surveilliance Slides #5 and #6.

*Source*: Centers for Disease Control and Prevention. (CDC). (2007). Retrieved November 19, 2008, from http://www.cdc.gov/tb/surv/surv2006/pdf/table4.pdf

resources. Place can be a neighborhood, a health care facility, a town, a region, a nation, or any other natural or political boundary. The identification of health differences between urban and rural sectors or between similar localities are often helpful in investigating specific health needs of a community.

Place often is illustrated through the use of maps. For example, in an attempt to monitor progress to reduce the risk of severe adverse effects in children of mothers who consume alcohol, the CDC published the prevalence by state of reported frequent alcohol consumption among women of childbearing age. Table 4-5 illustrates the prevalence of this risk factor (CDC, 1997). State health departments have used these data to determine priorities for their health objectives for 2010. For example, Michigan, Iowa, and Pennsylvania have the highest prevalence rates and should have targeted primary prevention programs toward this risk factor. Community health nurses would participate in the various efforts to reduce alcohol consumption in this age group.

## ■ Time

*When* health problems occur can be described by identifying short-term fluctuations measured in hours, days, weeks, or months; by periodic changes that are seasonal or

**Table 4-5**

Prevalence of reported frequent alcohol consumption among childbearing-age women (18–44 years)—United States, Behavioral Risk Factor Surveillance System, 1995

| Reported consumption level | Pregnant women 1991 (n = 1,053) | (95% CI[1]) | 1995 (n = 1,313) | (95% CI) | p value | All women 1991 (n = 26,105) | (95% CI) | 1995 (n = 30,415) | (95% CI) | p value |
|---|---|---|---|---|---|---|---|---|---|---|
| ■ Any drinking[§] | 12.4 | (9.5–15.2) | 16.3 | (13.1–19.4) | 0.07 | 49.4 | (48.4–50.3) | 50.6 | (49.7–51.6) | 0.02 |
| ■ <7 Drinks per week | 12.2 | (9.4–15.0) | 14.6 | (11.5–17.6) | 0.27 | 43.9 | (43.0–44.9) | 45.7 | (44.8–46.5) | 0.01 |
| ■ 7–14 Drinks per week | —[¶] | | 0.9 | (0.0–1.8) | — | 3.4 | (3.1–3.8) | 3.0 | (2.6–3.3) | 0.04 |
| ■ >14 Drinks per week | 0.1 | (0.0–0.3) | 0.3 | (0.0–0.7) | 0.28 | 1.4 | (1.2–1.6) | 1.1 | (0.9–1.3) | 0.04 |
| ■ ≥5 Drinks on occasion** | 0.7 | (0.2–1.2) | 2.9 | (1.5–4.3) | 0.003 | 10.5 | (10.0–11.1) | 10.5 | (9.9–11.1) | 0.96 |
| ■ Frequent drinking[††] | 0.8 | (0.3–1.4) | 3.5 | (1.9–5.1) | 0.002 | 12.4 | (11.8–13.1) | 12.6 | (12.0–13.3) | 0.67 |

*Because weighted data are used in this analysis, results for 1991 may be slightly different from those reported previously. For consistency, national analyses were restricted to the 47 states that participated in the BRFSS in both 1991 and 1995.
[†]Confidence interval.
[§]Levels of any drinking may not add to the total prevalence of any drinking because some women did not respond to questions about consumption frequency and amount. One additional state was eliminated from the breakdown of any drinking because questions regarding consumption frequency and amount were not asked in that state in 1995.
[¶]Too few observations to calculate a reliable estimate.
**Five or more drinks on at least one occasion during the preceding month.
[††]Consumption of an average of seven or more drinks per week or five or more drinks on at least one occasion during the preceding month.

## MEDIA MOMENT

Your health is bound to be affected if, day after day, you say the opposite of what you feel.

—Boris Pasternak, *Doctor Zhivago*

### Epidemic (1987)

The movie *Epidemic* is director Lars von Trier's unconventional treatment of a plague epidemic. The film comes close to being a horror movie, telling the story of a director who receives a government grant to create a script about a mysterious plague that engulfs Europe, only to find the horrific scenario coming true in real life.

---

cyclical; or by long-term changes over decades that reflect gradual changes. Describing the time of short-term outbreaks of infectious diseases is often performed by developing an **epidemic curve.** These graphs provide indications as to the mode of transmission and spread of the organism. The following figure is an example of an epidemic curve. It depicts an outbreak of *Escherichia coli* O157:H7 associated with eating spinach in Utah and New Mexico in 2006 (Grant et al., 2008). Nationally, this outbreak involved 205 people. A multistate investigation was initiated, and the US Food and Drug Administration (FDA) and the CDC advised the public not to eat bagged spinach. A case-control study and laboratory investigation conducted by the Utah and New Mexico Departments of Health confirmed 18 cases in Utah and 5 in New Mexico. Illness onset dates ranged from August 22 to September 11. *E. coli* O157:H7, which matched the national strain, was detected in three bags of spinach provided by case patients.

*Periodic* and *cyclical* changes also occur. For example, respiratory diseases are more common in the winter and spring (periodic), and hepatitis often increases in incidence every 7 to 9 years (cyclical). The following figure reflects both periodic and cyclical changes in pneumonia and influenza mortality. A seasonal baseline is developed, and variations from this baseline determine whether an epidemic is occurring.

These types of data are the evidence base for many of the control, prevention, and surveillance activities that are initiated by public health departments and community agencies initiated to keep the public healthy.

*Long-term changes* or trends over time are shown in the figure on p. 114. Significant changes in life expectancy at birth occurred between the years 1970 and 2003. The figure includes gender, a characteristic of persons to make the graph more meaningful.

**❝**There is never time to do it right, but there is always time to do it over. **❞**

—Carl N. Buechner

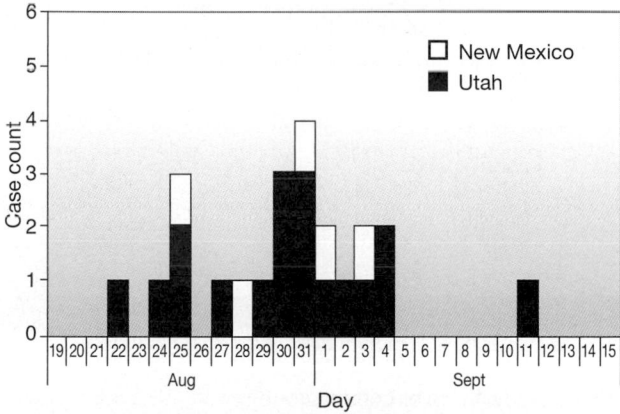

Epidemic curve by date of onset of confirmed cases, *Escherichia coli* O157:H7 spinach-associated outbreak, Utah and New Mexico, 2006.

*Source:* Grant, J., Wendelboe, A.M., Wendel, A., Jepson, B., Torres, P., & Smelser, C. (2008). Spinach-associated *Escherichia coli* O157:H7 outbreak, Utah and New Mexico, 2006. *Emerging Infectious Diseases, 14*(10). Retrieved October 22, 2008, from http://www.cdc.gov/EID/content/14/10/1633.htm

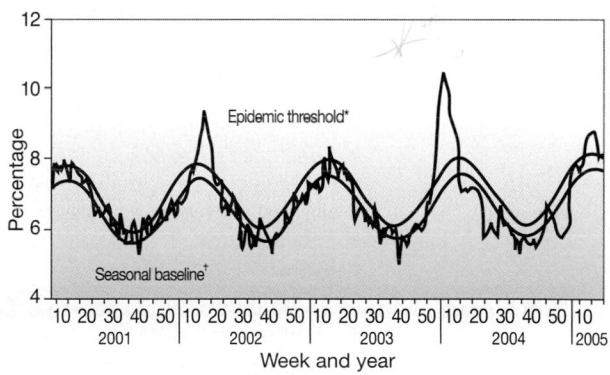

\* The epidemic threshold is 1.645 standard deviations above the seasonal baseline percentage.

† The seasonal baseline is projected by using a robust regression procedure that applies a period regression model to the observed percentage of deaths from P&I during the preceding 5 years.

*Source:* Centers for Disease Control and Prevention (CDC). (2005). Update: Influenza activity—United States, 2004–2005 season. *Morbidity and Mortality Weekly Report, 54*(13), 328–331.

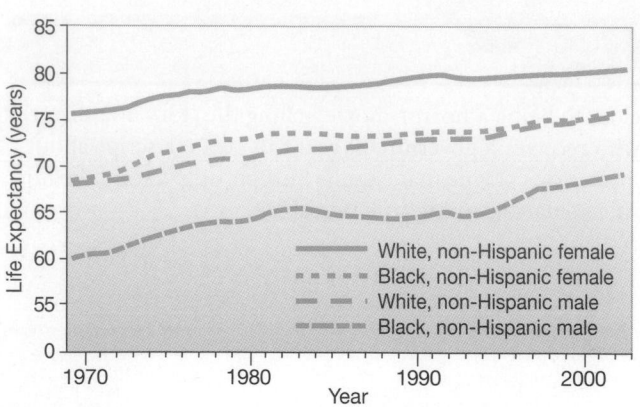

Life expectancy at birth by year, United States, 1970–2003

*Source*: Centers for Disease Control and Prevention (CDC). (2005). QuickStats: Life expectancy at birth, by year—United States, 1970–2003. *Morbidity and Mortality Weekly Report, 54*(14), 363.

## Analytic Epidemiology

Analytic epidemiology focuses on the determinants of health problems, or the *why*. When descriptive data are analyzed, the variations in person, place, and time often suggest tentative explanations or hypotheses. These hypotheses can then be tested through application of research methods in an attempt to find the reasons, or determinants, for these variations. This is a cyclical process because new knowledge may require further descriptive or analytic analysis. Four types of studies are used in epidemiological analytic investigations: **cross-sectional, retrospective (case-control), prospective,** and **intervention** (experimental) studies. The basic characteristics of these studies are outlined in Table 4-6.

| Table 4-6 | Characteristics of Epidemiological Analytic Studies |
|---|---|

**Cross-Sectional Studies**

| | |
|---|---|
| ■ Purpose | ■ Describe health states and provide a measure of the burden of a disease (prevalence) in a population |
| ■ Design | ■ All data are collected at the same time |
| ■ Data collection | ■ Interviews, observation, questionnaires |
| ■ Advantages | ■ Flexible, broad, economical, uncomplicated; rapid results, large samples possible |
| ■ Disadvantages | ■ Superficial, cannot infer cause and effect |

**Case-Control (Retrospective)**

| | |
|---|---|
| ■ Purpose | ■ Identify possible causes or risk factors of a disease by comparing the difference in two groups: one with the disease (cases) and one without the disease (controls) |
| ■ Design | ■ Select case and control samples according to specific criteria. The dependent variable (case or not) has already occurred |
| ■ Data collection | ■ Trace past experience to determine relevant exposure factors (independent variables) |
| ■ Advantages | ■ First step in hypothesis testing, inexpensive, relatively small samples can be used, results obtained quickly |
| ■ Disadvantages | ■ Information about past exposure may not be available |
| | ■ Selection of appropriate control groups may be difficult |
| | ■ Temporal association between exposure and outcome may be difficult to determine |
| | ■ Potential selection, recall, and observation bias |

**Prospective, Cohort, or Longitudinal Studies**

| | |
|---|---|
| ■ Purpose | ■ Determine the incidence of the health problem in a population at baseline, then follow the population over time to document the incidence of an outcome among exposed and non-exposed persons |
| ■ Design | ■ Samples chosen and observed forward in time |
| ■ Data collection | ■ Information on outcome variables obtained at specific intervals |
| ■ Advantages | ■ Incidence rates can be calculated directly |
| | ■ Time sequence easier to obtain |
| | ■ Effects of rare exposure can be investigated |
| | ■ Multiple outcomes may be studied |
| ■ Disadvantages | ■ May extend over a long period |
| | ■ Expensive |
| | ■ Cases lost to follow-up |

**Clinical, Experimental, or Intervention Studies**

| | |
|---|---|
| ■ Purpose | ■ Determine whether a group with particular characteristics will benefit from interventions when compared with a group or groups who do not receive the intervention |
| ■ Design | ■ Randomly choose and assign groups to either a study group or control group |
| | ■ Introduce an intervention (independent variable) to the study group and compare with controls |
| ■ Data collection | ■ Collect data prospectively on a number of dependent variables |
| ■ Advantages | ■ Cause and effect can be examined |
| | ■ Control over confounding variables |
| ■ Disadvantages | ■ Possible reactivity (Hawthorne effect) |
| | ■ Possible noncompliance with study protocols |
| | ■ Observation bias, placebo effect |

## NOTE THIS!

The Framingham Heart Study is a prospective study that has continued to follow the health characteristics of a community for more than 30 years. Much of the information about risk factors for coronary heart disease that underlies preventive programs was obtained from the results of this study.

Ideally, the epidemiologist is seeking to establish a cause-and-effect relationship between the health problem or outcome that is being studied (dependent variable) and exposure factors (independent variables) that preceded it in time. Often, associations can be made between a condition and a specific factor, but a direct cause-and-effect relationship is weak or does not exist. More than one factor must be present for any illness to occur (multifactorial causation). Even in an infectious process, such as tuberculosis, presence of the organism alone is not sufficient to cause the disease. Characteristics of the agent, the host, and the environment all interact to determine the onset of the infection. The more factors that can be identified as contributors to a disease process, the weaker the cause-and-effect relationship will be.

*There are in fact two things, science and opinion; the former begets knowledge, the latter ignorance.*
—Hippocrates (circa 460–377 B.C.)

*Facts do not cease to exist because they are ignored.*
—Carl N. Buechner

**Application to Practice**
Using the Ethical Connection on page 105, identify primary and secondary interventions that would be feasible and appropriate for a group of elementary school children related to the risk of obesity. What additional information would you need regarding risk factors and interventions prior to designing health promotion programs for addressing them? How would you evaluate these interventions in terms of outcome effectiveness?

## Research Alert

Many factors, including viewing smoking in movies, employment status, and gender, have been studied to ascertain whether they influence adolescents to begin smoking cigarettes. Cross-sectional studies linked viewing smoking in movies to initiation of smoking among adolescents. Researchers assessed 3547 adolescents who were 10 to 14 years old and who reported that they had never tried smoking. Based on the number of smoking occurrences viewed in 50 selected movies, researchers estimated the adolescents' exposure to smoking in movies. The researchers interviewed 2603 students (73%) 13–26 months later to determine if they had begun smoking. Among those in the highest quartile of movie exposure to smoking, 17% had begun smoking, while only 3% of those in lowest quartile of exposure had begun smoking. After controlling for baseline characteristics, it was determined that there is a strong link between viewing smoking in movies and smoking initiation among adolescents.

Another research study investigated the link between working for pay and tobacco usage among adolescents. Researchers performed retrospective and prospective analyses using data obtained from 799 predominately African-American students in Baltimore who had been followed since the first grade. When the adolescents were 14 to 18 years old, the data showed a positive relationship between the time spent working for pay and tobacco use. Students who worked for pay for more than 10 hours per week tended to start smoking cigarettes earlier than their peers did. Students who started to work one year after assessment and those who worked over two consecutive assessments were more likely to start smoking than those adolescents who did not work. A strong link was found between working for pay and adolescent tobacco use.

A secondary analysis of the National Longitudinal Study of Adolescent Health investigated the relationship between variables such as mother-daughter connectedness, self-concept, and residential mother's smoking behavior as well as known risk factors such as friends' smoking behavior and race/ethnicity on smoking initiation in female adolescents. This secondary analysis found that the influential and protective factors related to smoking vary with race and ethnicity.

*Sources*: Dalton, M. A., Sargent, J. D., Beach, M. L., Titus-Ernstoff, L., Gibson, J. J., Ahrens, M. B., Tickle, J. J., & Heatherton, T. F. (2003). Effect of viewing smoking in movies on adolescent smoking initiation: A cohort study. *Lancet, 362*(9380), 281–285; Ialongo, N. S., & Chilcoat, H. D. (2007). The effect of working for pay on adolescent tobacco use. *American Journal of Public Health, 97*(11), 2056–2062; Faucher, M. A. (2003). Factors that influence smoking in adolescent girls. *Journal of Midwifery & Women's Health, 48*(3), 199–205.

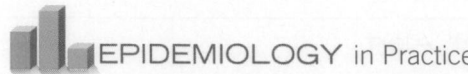

EPIDEMIOLOGY in Practice

### "If I Have to Explain, You Would Not Understand": Real Bikers Are an Endangered Species
*Charlene Pippin, MSN, RN*

Bikers are a vulnerable population. In 2006, 4,810 motorcyclists were killed in the United States. This figure represents 11% of all traffic fatalities, even though motorcycles account for less than 2.2% of all U.S. vehicles (NHTSA, 2007). During severe accidents, 85% of motorcyclists are killed compared to 45% of occupants of passenger cars, 32% of occupants of SUVs, 25% of occupants of vans, and 36% of occupants of pickup trucks (Shankar, 2004; NHTSA, 2007).

### Never Ride Faster Than Your Guardian Angel Can Fly
Motorcycles do not kill people. In this particular epidemiological triad (host, agent, environment), the agent is unintentional, accidental injuries. The host is the motorcyclist—biker and rider. The environment includes the actual roadways and physical environment, including other vehicles with human drivers. Motorcycle fatalities are caused by interactions of the characteristics of unintentional injuries (agent), motorcyclists/bikers (host), and the physical surroundings including the roadways and other vehicles (environment) (Harkness, 1995).

### Remember When Sex Was Safe and Motorcycles Were Dangerous
Death rates from motorcycle accidents are increasing despite the inclusion of additional safety features on new motorcycles. Motorcyclist deaths from unintentional injuries decreased steadily each year from 1993 to 1997 (National Center for Statistics and Analysis, 2001). In 1998 and 1999, however, this trend reversed. Motorcyclist fatalities overall increased for the ninth year in a row compared to 1997. Contributing to the increase in fatality rates for this at-risk population of motorcyclists is an increase in the number of people who ride motorcycles, particularly baby boomers who are older and buying larger bikes, and the weakening of helmet laws in many states. Several states in recent years have repealed mandatory helmet requirements for motorcyclists.

### Fifteen Grand and Fifteen Miles Do Not Make You a Biker
In 2006, there were 5,381,338 registered motorcycles in the United States (NHTSA, 2007). In 2002, the overall mean age of all motorcycle riders was 40 years. The average purchaser of a new Harley Davidson motorcycle was 46 years old. This group includes many retired persons who are purchasing large motorcycles after an absence from riding after a number of years or who are starting riding for the first time. Seventy percent of fatal accidents occur in rural areas on undivided roads—that is, during recreational motorcycling rather than commuting motorcycling. These motorcyclists are referred to as "weekend warriors" because of limited riding experience, especially related to adverse road and weather conditions.

Bikers are a subgroup of motorcyclists distinguished based on culture. In an interview with a recognized Harley expert, the following criteria usually must be present to be considered a true "biker":

Charlene Pippin, MSN, RN, on her Harley after graduating with her Master of Science in community health nursing. The article by Pippin raises many issues about the epidemiology of motorcycle accidents. How do you feel about the mandatory use of protective gear such as helmets for riders?

- A person must own and ride a motorcycle, a Harley Davidson.
- A person must have an appreciation for, and skill with, the mechanical aspects of motorcycles.
- A person must have a lifestyle of the biker subculture and treat fellow motorcyclists with respect as brothers and sisters.

The biker lifestyle depends more often on actual riding experience and skills than the amount of money spent on the motorcycle. Therefore, anyone who rides a motorcycle is a *motorcyclist,* but only dedicated riders become *bikers* (DeGroat, 2003).

### You Can't Ride If You Are Fried
Of motorcycle riders killed in single-vehicle crashes in 2006, 33% were intoxicated (NHTSA, 2007). Simply put, alcohol affects motorcyclists more profoundly than drivers of other types of vehicles. This difference is believed to be related to the increased skill level required to operate a motorcycle and the effects the environment (weather) has on the motorcyclist (Motorcycle Safety Foundation, 2007). Motorcyclists' own beliefs, attitudes regarding drinking, and riding also increase their risks. Motorcyclists have a culturally reinforced respect for rider freedom even if intoxicated (Syner & Vegega, 2001). Another commonly held belief is that the impaired rider's concern for the safety and security of the motorcycle nearly always overshadows the rider's concern for his or her own personal safety. Bikers prefer to ride drunk rather than leave their motorcycle behind (Becker, McKnight, Nelkin, & Piper, 2003). This same principle of freedom to choose also applies to mandatory helmet use laws.

### Helmet Laws: Let Those Who Ride Decide
In the United States, 20 states currently have full helmet-use laws; another 26 states have helmet-use laws that apply only to minors or passengers. In recent years, many states have

repealed or eliminated helmet requirements (Richardson & Houston, 2007). Some states also require motorcyclists to be covered by additional insurance policies of at least $10,000 in medical benefits specifically set aside for motorcycle injuries (Stolzenberg & Stewart, 2003).

Most bikers do not support mandatory helmet laws. Bikers believe prevention should be directed toward preventing motorcycle accidents instead of simply preventing head injuries by wearing helmets (American Motorcyclist, 2008). Current public health opinion considers the use of helmets to be a means of primary prevention (American Medical Association, 2004).

### In Case of Accident, Do Not Remove This Helmet

Preventing motorcycle accidents and their consequential injuries and death should be guided by the levels of prevention, including primary, secondary, and tertiary prevention.

Primary prevention includes stricter alcohol-related traffic laws for both bikers and the public, mandatory education and licensure, all-vehicle driver education, vehicle conspicuity measures, mandatory inspections, and improved roadway design and maintenance. Primary prevention is referred to as "pre-crash" measures.

Secondary prevention deals with preventing injury once an accident occurs. During-the-"crash" measures include the use of protective gear, such as leather jackets, gloves, pants, vest, boots, eye goggles, and helmets. CPR at the accident scene, including leaving helmets on to splint skull fractures, is also part of secondary prevention (NHTSA, 2007).

"Post-crash" (tertiary) care includes rehabilitation for disabling, permanent motorcycle injuries; allowing motorcycle clubs to visit these patients without unnecessary resistance from health care professionals; and modifying motorcycles for the disabled bikers (Disabled Bikers Association, 2004).

The number of motorcyclists and bikers is unlikely to decrease in the future; indeed, current projections predict an increase in both the age and the number of bikers who can afford bigger and faster motorcycles. The title of this article comes from a common bumpersticker found on bikers' motorcycles: "If I have to explain, you won't understand." As community health nurses, by educating ourselves about the risks for this population—including the host, agent, and environment of motorcycle accidents—as well as implementing interventions at all levels of prevention, perhaps we can better understand this at-risk population and promote safer roads and highways for everyone.

### References

American Medical Association. (2004). *Options for improving motorcycle safety.* Retrieved from www.ama-assn.org

American Motorcyclist. (2008). *AMA position in support of voluntary helmet use.* Retrieved September 20, 2008, from http://www.amadirectlink.com/legis/tn/positions/helmet.asp

Becker, L., McKnight, A., Nelkin, V., & Piper, D. (2003). *Drinking, riding, and prevention: A focus group study.* Washington, DC: U.S. Department of Transportation.

DeGroat, R. (2003). *What is a biker?* Unpublished manuscript. Personal interview, December 26, 2003, Gulfport, MS.

Disabled Bikers Association. (2004). Bikes. Retrieved March 7, 2004, from http://www.nabd.org

Harkness, G. (1995). *Epidemiology in nursing practice.* St. Louis: Mosby-Year Book.

Motorcycle Safety Foundation. (2007). *The effects of alcohol and other drugs.* Retrieved September 20, 2008, from http://www.msf-usa.org

National Highway Traffic Safety Administration (NHTSA). (2001). *Traffic safety facts 2001* (DOT HS 808953) [Brochure]. Washington, DC: U.S. Department of Transportation.

National Highway Traffic Safety Administration (NHTSA). (2008). *Traffic Safety Facts, 2001: Motorcyclists.* Retrieved September 20, 2008, from http://www.nrd.nhtsa.dot.gov/Pubs/809473.pdf

Richardson, L. & Houston, D. J. (2007). Motorcycle safety and the repeal of universal helmet laws. *American Journal of Public Health, 97*(11), 2063–2069.

Shankar, U. (2004). Alcohol involvement in fatal motorcycle crashes. Traffic Review Board Seminar, January 13, 2004, Washington, DC.

Stolzenberg, L., & Stewart, J. (2003). "Born to be wild": The effect of the repeal of Florida's mandatory motorcycle helmet use law on serious injury and fatality rates. *Evaluation Review, 27*(2), 131–150.

Syner, J., & Vegega, M. (2001). *Impaired motorcycle riding: What motorcyclists think about alcohol and motorcycling.* Washington, DC: U.S. Department of Transportation.

## Conclusion

Promoting and preserving the health of populations are fundamental characteristics of community health nursing. Although nursing is a profession that focuses primarily on the individual, the person's health care needs cannot be completely or correctly defined unless family, personal friends, and the characteristics of the community and the society are considered. *Epidemiology,* the science of preventive medicine, provides a framework for studying and understanding these interactions. *Epidemiology* is the study of the distribution and the determinants of states of health and illness in human populations. The basic conceptual framework of epidemiology is the interaction among the agent, host, and environment—the epidemiological triad. Epidemiology is considered both as a methodology used to study health-related conditions and as an accumulated body of knowledge about a state of health. Nurses use the body of knowledge about health problems in their clinical decision making and may become involved in epidemiological research methods to gather new health-related information.

Descriptive epidemiology examines the distribution of states of health in the population. The primary tool that is used in epidemiology is the rate, a proportion that includes the factor of time. Incidence rates measure the probability that people without a certain condition develop the condition during a specific time frame. The number of new conditions or events is measured in an incidence rate. Prevalence rates measure the extent of an existing health problem within a specific period including new and existing cases in a specific time period. These rates are often calculated according to characteristics of person (who), place (where), and time (when). Analytical epidemiology attempts to define the determinants of health problems (why) through rigorous research techniques. Types of analytical studies include cross-sectional, retrospective, prospective, and intervention studies.

Explore Community Health Nursing on the Web! To learn more about the topics in this chapter, use the passcode provided to access your exclusive website: **http://nursing.jbpub.com/ communityhealth.** If you do not have a passcode, you can obtain one at this site.

## ■ CRITICAL THINKING ACTIVITIES

1. Using an example from your practice, identify two examples that illustrate how the epidemiological body of knowledge is used in clinical decision making.
2. Between January 1 and December 1, 2000, 25 new cases of tuberculosis were diagnosed in Boon Town, population 450,000. A prevalence survey taken the first week in January 2000 indicated that there were 250 cases on the list of active tuberculosis cases. There were 20 deaths due to tuberculosis recorded during this 1-year period. Using this information, calculate the following rates.

- What was the incidence rate per 100,000 population for tuberculosis during 2000?
- What was the prevalence rate per 100,000 population for tuberculosis during 2000?
- What was the cause-specific death rate per 100,000 for tuberculosis in 2000?

3. Discuss how nurses could use the case-control research methodology to answer questions in their practice.

## ■ REFERENCES

Aiken, L. (1988). Assuring the delivery of quality patient care. State of the Science Invitational Conference: Nursing resources and the delivery of patient care (NIH Publication No. 89-3008, pp. 3–10). Washington, DC: U.S. Department of Health and Human Services, Public Health Service.

Alanis, B. (1999). *Epidemiology in health care* (3rd ed.). Stamford, CT: Appleton and Lange.

Centers for Disease Control and Prevention (CDC). (1997). Alcohol consumption among pregnant and childbearing-aged women—United States, 1991 and 1995. *Morbidity and Mortality Weekly Report, 46*(16), 346–350.

Centers for Disease Control and Prevention (CDC). (2002). Heat-related deaths—four states, July–August 2001, and United States, 1979–1999. *Morbidity and Mortality Weekly Report, 51*(26), 567–570.

Centers for Disease Control and Prevention (CDC). (2003a). Abortion surveillance—United States, 2000. *Morbidity and Mortality Weekly Report, 52*(5512), 1–32.

Centers for Disease Control and Prevention (CDC). (2003b). Reported tuberculosis in the United States, 2002. *Surveillance Reports.*

Centers for Disease Control and Prevention (CDC). (2007a). Data and trends: National diabetes surveillance system. Retrieved September 20, 2008, from http://www.cdc.gov/diabetes/statistics/prev/national/tableraceethsex.htm

Centers for Disease Control and Prevention (CDC). (2007b). Perinatal group B streptococcal disease after universal screening recommendations—United States, 2003–2005. *Morbidity and Mortality Weekly Report, 56*(28), 701–705.

Cohen, B. (1984). Florence Nightingale. *Scientific American, 250*(3), 129.

Doll, R., & Hill, A. B. (1950). Smoking and carcinoma of the lung: Preliminary report. *British Medical Journal,* 2739.

Gordis, L. (2004). *Epidemiology* (3rd ed.). Philadelphia: Elsevier/Saunders.

Humphreys, N. A. (1885). *Vital statistics: A memorial volume of selections from the reports and writings of William Farr.* London: Sanitary Institute of Great Britain.

Kung, H. C., Hoyert, D. L., Xu, J., & Murphy, S. L. (2008). Deaths: Final data for 2005. *National Vital Statistics Report, 56*(10), 1–120.

Leavell, H. R., & Clark, H. G. (1958). *Preventive medicine for the doctor in his community* (3rd ed.). New York: McGraw-Hill.

Leavell, H. E., & Clark, H. G. (1965). *Preventive medicine for the doctor in his community: An epidemiologic approach.* New York: McGraw-Hill.

Snow, J. (1855). *On the mode of communication of cholera.* London: Churchill. (Reproduced in *Snow on cholera.* [1965]. New York: Hafner.)

# CHAPTER 5
# Health Care Systems in Transition

Bonita R. Reinert

Visit **http://nursing.jbpub.com/communityhealth** for interactive exercises, review questions, Web links, and more.

Health care is one of the largest industries in the United States, employing an estimated 10 million workers. The healthcare system in the United States includes the most technology-rich facilities and the most advanced practices in the world. The most well-educated physicians, nurses, and other healthcare workers use sophisticated treatments on a daily basis to prolong life and restore function.

Like the Roman god Janus, America has two faces. Despite being the richest nation on the planet, we suffer from higher rates of poverty, infant mortality, homicide, and HIV infection, and from greater economic inequality, than other advanced democracies. We have far more uninsured citizens, and a lower life expectancy. On a per capita basis, we spend a much larger percentage of our GNP on health care than other like countries and yet have poorer health statistics on those that matter most.

—*Ted Halstead. (2003, January-February). The American paradox.* Atlantic Monthly, *p. 123.*

What has been your experience with health care in the United States both as a nursing student and as a patient? Have you seen evidence of any of the problems mentioned by Halstead? What has it been like as an "insider" compared to your experience before you became a nursing student?

## CHAPTER FOCUS

### The Evolving U.S. Health Care Delivery System
- Private Health Care Delivery
- Public Health Care
- Military Health Care
- Health Care Reform

### The Current U.S. Health Care Delivery System
- Levels of Care
- Health Care Providers
- Health Care Settings

### Issues Affecting the Delivery of Health Care Services
- Deregulation
- Emphasis on Secondary and Tertiary Health Care Services
- Increasing Consumerism
- Technological Advances
- Increasing Longevity of Americans
- Defensive Health Care and Government Regulation

### Managed Care
- The Concept of Managed Care
- Managed Care Organizations
- Patient Care Outcomes

### Health Politics and Policy
- Government Policy
- Public Opinion and Special-Interest Groups
- Nursing and Health Care Policy

### New Nursing Opportunities
- Advanced Practice Nurses
- Entrepreneurs
- Data Management
- Research

## QUESTIONS TO CONSIDER

After reading this chapter, you will know the answers to the following questions:

1. How did the current U.S. health care system evolve to its present form?
2. What is the difference between private and public health care?
3. What are some of the current issues affecting health care delivery in the United States?
4. How do politics and policy influence the health care delivery system?
5. What are some of the current and evolving health care settings?
6. What impact is managed care having on health care delivery?
7. What are some potential roles for some nurses within the changing health care system?

## KEY TERMS

Capitation
Diagnosis-related groups (DRGs)
Fee-for-service
Healthcare delivery system
Health maintenance organization (HMO)

Integrated health care system
Managed care
Managed care organization (MCO)
Managed competition

Point-of-service (POS) plan
Preventive care
Primary care
Preferred provider organization (PPO)

Prospective payment system (PPS)
Shelter nurse
Third-party payer

HEALTH CARE IS ONE of the largest industries in the United States, employing an estimated 14 million workers (National Center for Health Statistics, 2007). The U.S. health care system includes the most technology-rich facilities and the most advanced practices in the world. The best-educated physicians, nurses, and other health care workers use sophisticated treatments on a daily basis to prolong life and restore function. As a result of the cutting-edge nature of this health care, the U.S. system is the most costly, in terms of resources, in the world (Organization for Economic Cooperation and Development, 2000).

The current patterns of health care delivery have resulted in an annual cost that exceeds $2 trillion, a figure that is significantly higher than the expenditures of any other industrialized nation. This figure represents more than 15% of this country's gross domestic product (GDP). Expenditures for hospital care accounted for 31% of all national expenditures in 2005. Physician and clinical services accounted for 21%, prescription drugs for 10%, and nursing home care for 6% (National Center for Health Statistics, 2007).

Despite the advances in health care technology and high health care costs, clinical outcomes are not always significantly better in the United States when compared to other industrialized nations. In the National Scorecard on U. S. Health System Performance, 2008, which measures and monitors health care outcomes, quality, access, efficiency, and equity in the United States, the U. S. ranked 65 out of a possible 100. This score is a decrease from the 67 received in 2006. For one indicator, preventable mortality, the U. S. fell to last place among 19 industrialized nations (The Commonwealth Fund Commission on a High Performance Health System, 2008). Access to health care is believed to be one of the determinants of the less than auspicious health indicators in the United States.

Lack of access to quality health care services can take several forms. For example, needed services may simply not be available in an accessible location or during hours when individuals are able to use them. The health care site may not be organized in a user-friendly manner so that individuals can obtain timely and acceptable services. For example, providers may not be as culturally sensitive or as multilingual as is needed in certain locations in the United States.

Routine health care may also not be accessible because of a lack of personal funds and/or insurance coverage. Medications and special treatments may be beyond the financial resources of the individual despite a provider's carefully developed plan of care. Based on recent data, 19% of Americans were without health care insurance during a typical month in 2005 (National Center for Health Statistics, 2007).

Finally, individuals may not have a regular provider and may have to receive care from a variety of providers in a number of unconnected facilities. Thus care may not be comprehensive or timely.

Although leaders in government, health care, and consumer groups continue to express concern over access issues, inequities in the current system are readily apparent. By most accounts, more than 47 million Americans are uninsured (U.S. Census Bureau, 2008b). In addition, many more U.S. citizens are underinsured, and this figure is growing. Individuals working at part-time and minimum-wage jobs make up a large part of the uninsured and underinsured in this country.

A lack of insurance frequently results in a lack of prevention services and early interventions. Lack of adequate prenatal care and infant immunizations, especially for the poor and minority populations, has sometimes led to illness and disability and, ultimately, increased financial demands on the public health care system. Statistically, African Americans fare worse in virtually every condition that affects health (Donatiello, Droese, & Kim, 2004). The rates of infectious disease such as tuberculosis, sexually transmitted diseases, and HIV continue to rise, especially within at-risk populations. A lack of accessible community mental health services has also resulted in a number of tragedies and untold stress for families.

Attempts to contain spiraling costs, deal with the dissatisfaction of consumers and providers, and address issues of uneven access and poor clinical outcomes have resulted in cost-containment legislation, new configurations of providers, and new ways of providing care. Because nursing care holds the answer to many of the current dilemmas, the nursing profession appears to be poised on the edge of an exciting and challenging future.

## The Evolving U.S. Healthcare Delivery System

The term **healthcare delivery system** refers to a multilevel industry that transforms a variety of resources into essential services designed to meet the health care needs of a population. This transformation occurs through a complex set of interactions among consumers, providers, payers, employers, and the government. Resources include physical structures, personnel, technology, supplies, and financing, among other things. The system is both guided and, in some instances, undermined by competition, demands for profit, technological innovation, standards, and government regulations.

Many critics suggest that the U.S. health care system is not actually a system at all—that is, it is not a coordinated whole with interrelated parts. Instead, health care in this country often occurs as a series of fragmented episodes that may be isolated, unrelated, confusing, or even competing. Furthermore, in the United States there is no single source of oversight, policies, or goals, nor is there a set of shared values and concerns among the various entities in the delivery system.

Services in the United States may be provided in traditional settings, such as hospitals or physicians' offices, and in less traditional settings, such as shelters, specially equipped vans, or shopping malls. Patient care information may or may not be shared among the providers in the subsystems or even between providers at separate sites in a single subsystem. Furthermore, follow-up contact between providers and patients is rare.

Reimbursement may come from one or more of the following sources: private insurance companies, managed care organizations, government agencies, foundations, and the patient. The patient is often the one who has to decide who to bill, what to do when reimbursement is denied, or who to talk to when the bill is only partially reimbursed.

Finally, services may need to be accessed in one or more of the following health care systems: private, public, and/or the military. Each system has a unique set of rules and requirements. Coverage may be overlapping, costs of care are different, and reimbursement occurs in different ways.

## ■ Private Health Care Delivery

Our complicated private health care system has changed dramatically in the last 100 years. In the nineteenth century, family, servants, or close friends cared for patients in the home, with physicians making visits as needed. Treatment involved medicinal herbs and comfort measures. Medical knowledge was limited, and most medical practitioners in the United States lacked a standardized education. Medical treatments were based on common sense, and physicians often lacked acceptance as professionals. Care was purchased out of private funds or provided on a charity basis. The few hospitals that existed basically served indigent patients (i.e., without family or support) who found themselves at death's door. The medical treatments delivered in these early hospitals were often crude and seldom very effective.

After the middle of the nineteenth century, large leaps in medical knowledge occurred. These advances paved the way for significant gains in surgical interventions and the treatment of disease. The new, more sophisticated procedures required centralized facilities to house the new technology and train the personnel needed to provide patient care. This resulted in an era of extensive hospital construction, the institutionalization of health care, and the establishment of the hospital as the center of health care delivery (see Box 5-1).

After World War I, the medical profession in this country grew in prestige and power. This transformation was based on several trends: movement to cities away from family and friends, advances in medical science and technology, organization of medicine and adoption of state licensing requirements, establishment of worker's compensation and growth of health insurance, and educational requirements for providers.

---

### ENVIRONMENTAL CONNECTION

While clean drinking water is taken for granted in the United States due to a long-standing commitment to public health and the availability of resources, nearly 22% of the world's people lack clean drinking water and close to one third lack sanitation services. The United Nations reported in 2006 that the number of people lacking potable water was more than 1 billion worldwide.

---

### BOX 5-1

**Phases of Health Care System Development**

Development of the private health care delivery system occurred in four phases:

- Prior to the 1850s: Illness and disability were handled at home. Few hospitals and clinics existed, and they provided mostly indigent care.
- 1850–1930: Significant gains in medical knowledge occurred. Technology advances necessitated an increase in the number of hospitals and nurses.
- 1930–1980: Health care became more organized. Insurance became available so people were more likely to go to hospitals for care.
- 1980 to present: Soaring costs resulted in reorganization, restructuring, reallocation of scarce resources, and difficult ethical decisions.

---

To ensure that hospital bills would be paid, insurance companies such as Blue Cross were formed. With the establishment of broader health insurance coverage, providers were at less financial risk and insurance policies provided for the reimbursement of increasing numbers of patients. Patients selected the provider. Providers simply decided on the appropriate course of care for the patient, implemented that care, and then submitted bills at the end of the illness episode. This form of payment was known as fee-for-service.

**Fee-for-service** is a form of retrospective payment for health care in which a facility or provider submits a bill for services rendered at the completion of the health care episode. An advantage of this type of billing is that care is reimbursed according to the acuity of the patient's condition based on the services required. However, some health care experts now believe that paying a fee for each service performed encourages unnecessary services and frequent return visits, which in turn increases health care costs.

The Hill–Burton Act was passed in 1946 to help communities build hospitals. In the 1950s, National Institutes of Health became a major funding source for health care research. The Medicare Act was passed in 1965 to provide hospital insurance for the elderly. Each of these efforts increased the organizational strength of the U.S. health care system.

Two acts passed by Congress have significantly affected the methods by which hospitals are reimbursed for care. The Tax Equity and Fiscal Responsibility Act of 1982 (TEFRA) established a cost-per-case basis for Medicare-reimbursed inpatient services. The 1983 amendments to the Social Security Act established a prospective payment method of paying for inpatient services for Medicare patients based on a system of admitting diagnoses known as **diagnosis-related groups (DRGs)**.

Under the **prospective payment system (PPS)**, an annual fixed (prospective) rate was established for reimbursing providers for care based on 467 diagnoses or procedures. The prototype for the prospective payment system was developed at Yale University. Under the Yale program, reimbursement amounts bore "little or no relationship to length of stay, services rendered, or costs of care" (Williams & Torrens, 2008, p. 112). Rules stated that costs above the established amount for a given DRG would be absorbed by the hospital. If the care was delivered for less than the established amount, however, the hospital could keep the difference and make a profit.

**Third-party payers** are agencies or organizations such as insurance companies or HMOs that are responsible for all or part of an insured individual's health care costs. Third-party payers also adopted the DRG system as apart of their cost-saving measures. It has been suggested that prospective payment legislation introduced a new era of fiscal constraints, demands for accountability, and pressure to provide services in innovative ways. This new era involved the constant evaluation of practices, policies, and procedures to limit costs whenever possible and has resulted in concerns about access, equitable treatment decisions, and quality of care.

As a result of the need to control costs, provide quality care, and meet the needs of increasing numbers of individuals, a variety of creative and innovative health care organizations have developed. Often called alphabet health care, acronyms such as HMOs (health management organizations), PPOs (preferred provider organizations), POS (point-of-service plans), and MCOs (managed care organizations) have become part of the new health care vocabulary (Feldstein, 2007). With these new health care models have come some difficult ethical questions. Is health care a right? If a treatment or procedure is available and you want it, should your insurance be required to pay for it? Who should decide on the appropriateness of medical treatment plans, the physician or the insurance company? These questions are probably going to be with us for a long time, as there are no easy answers.

## ■ Public Health Care

Public health can be defined as the health outcomes of a group of individuals, including the distribution of such outcomes within the group; the field of population health, which includes health outcomes, patterns of health determinants, and policies; and the interventions that link these two (Kindig & Stoddart, 2003). The U.S. public health system is an interwoven local, state, and national governmental agency designed to look at broad community-based health issues and protect the general public from the hazards that result from living in populated urban areas.

Massachusetts was the first state to establish a state department of health modeled, in part, after the British General Board of Health. Lemuel Shattuck, from Massachusetts, produced a visionary report in 1850 entitled *Report of the Sanitary Commission of Massachusetts*. In that report, Shattuck outlined the health needs of the state and offered recommendations related to the need for sanitary engineers, accurate vital statistics, inspectors, food and drug regulations, public health education, and routine preventative

---

### ■■ CULTURAL CONNECTION

Immigration issues have always affected health care. Following Hurricane Katrina in 2005, many Hispanic immigrants, documented and undocumented, flowed into the United States seeking work opportunities in the Gulf Coast region. Prior to Katrina, New Orleans' Hispanic population was estimated to be 5% of the city's total population; after Katrina, it was as high as 30%. What are the challenges for community health nurses in caring for this population?

---

health care for all citizens. Despite its carefully written and documented recommendations, however, this report was virtually ignored for almost 20 years.

In 1872, the Public Health Association was formed. Its membership focused on interdisciplinary efforts to improve health and developed a number of health promotion and illness prevention materials for the public. In the 1880s, based on work by Pasteur and Koch, public health moved from having a narrow emphasis on environmental sanitation to taking a broader view that included bacteriology and immunology.

During the first decades of the twentieth century, public health services began to expand in the United States. The Social Security Act of 1935 provided federal funding for support of local health departments and marked the first step toward the development of a nationwide network of public health agencies. Public health agencies were responsible for providing health care services to special populations such as urban poor, mothers, babies, and Native Americans, among others (Fairbanks & Wiese, 1998).

Today, public health agencies range in size and scope from local health departments to the Centers for Disease Control and Prevention (CDC) in Atlanta and focus on ensuring that the public health of the community is protected, promoted, and restored (see Chapter 3). To meet that overall goal, public health departments currently have a wide range of population-based goals (see Box 5-2). To meet the goal of healthy communities, public health agencies have expanded their core functions to include community assessment, policy

---

### BOX 5-2

**Public Health Goals**
The public health system is responsible for the following activities:
- Prevent epidemics and the spread of disease
- Reduce environmental hazards
- Prevent injuries
- Promote healthy behaviors
- Provide disaster services
- Ensure the quality and accessibility of health services

*Source*: Fairbanks & Wiese, 1998.

## Research Alert

Many Native American nations, tribes, and bands are at an elevated risk for premature death from unintentional injury. The purpose of this study was to identify and characterize any association between prior injury and/or alcohol use contacts with the Indian Health Service (IHS) and subsequent alcohol-related injury death. Death certificates of Native Americans who died from injury in a rural IHS area over six consecutive years were linked to IHS acute care facility records and toxicology reports. Of the 526 injury deaths involving Native Americans in the IHS area studied, 411 (78%) were successfully linked to IHS records. Of these cases, 152 met the inclusion criteria, with an additional 98 cases identified as a comparison group.

No differences in alcohol use at time of death between groups with and without prior health care contact (for injury or alcohol) could be determined (81% versus 73%). A significant relationship was found between previous visits for acute or chronic alcohol use and subsequent alcohol-related fatalities ($P = .01$).

Based on these findings, injury-prevention activities in the population studied should be initiated at the time of any health-system contact in which alcohol use is identified. Community health nursing interventions should be developed to educate patients and families about the risk of alcohol use and injury risk with any contact at point of service for this at-risk population.

*Source:* Sanddal, T. L., Upchurch, J., Sanddal, N.D., & Esposito, T. J. (2005). Analysis of prior health system contacts as a harbinger of subsequent fatal injury in American Indians. *Journal of Rural Health, 21*(1), 65–69.

development, limited medical services (i.e., immunizations, well-baby check-ups, sexually transmitted disease treatment and surveillance), and program evaluation (Keck & Scutchfield, 1997).

## Military Health Care

One of the most important fringe benefits of military life is a system of well-organized comprehensive health care services provided at little or no extra cost (Williams & Torrens, 2008). Military personnel are also covered for service-connected problems for life. Health care is always available when needed, although personnel may have little choice of provider. Finally, the military health care system emphasizes prevention in addition to illness care. The National Defense Authorization Act for fiscal year 2005 was designed to improve the comprehensiveness of the overall health benefits available to members of the National Guard, reservists, and their families.

Ambulatory care is provided in military base and regional clinics. Simple hospital services, including short-term stays, are available through base dispensaries or sick bays on board ships. More advanced care is available in regional hospitals. Well-trained medics, nurses, and physicians, working in facilities owned by the U.S. government, provide most of the care. This system of care is well organized, integrated, and sophisticated.

Dependents and families of active-duty personnel are covered by an extensive health insurance plan known as Tri-Care. This program allows dependents and families to obtain health care from private clinics and practitioners, local hospitals, and health maintenance organizations when similar services are not available from a nearby military base.

A second program, the Veterans Administration (VA) health care system, is a hospital and long-term care system that exists to care for retired and disabled military personnel. Whereas a hospital clinic system is available for complicated ambulatory services, most simple ambulatory services are obtained through other systems of care. The VA health care system is probably the largest long-term care provider in the United States and is funded through an annual appropriation from Congress.

## Health Care Reform

The current U.S. health care delivery system is undergoing dramatic changes. Advances in research and technology have resulted in the most sophisticated care in the world, and the most costly. At the same time, millions of Americans have limited or no access to health care services. When the uninsured do receive care, it is often in costly emergency rooms and after the condition has become unnecessarily complex. Uncompensated care is on the rise, and many providers are limiting their numbers or refusing to care for uninsured or underinsured patients. Patients without a regular provider are often forced to seek care in emergency rooms after their conditions have become serious and where care is often fragmented. Consequently, it was not surprising that health care reform has drawn the attention of many supporters.

Health care reform is not a new issue. The administrations of Franklin Roosevelt, Truman, Kennedy, Nixon, Ford, Carter, George H. W. Bush, Clinton, and George W. Bush all attempted to design some type of health care reform. Only the Social Security Act, supported by President Kennedy before his death, was passed without undergoing major changes.

Each time, the need for health care reform was based on the need to control health care costs while providing access to quality health care services to increasing numbers of people. Prior to 1993, the prototypes for Clinton's health care reform bill had been debated through three elections and defeated by two legislatures because of concerns about increased costs and governmental control.

A massive reorganization attempt was started during the first year of President Clinton's administration under the direction of First Lady Hillary Rodham Clinton. This plan would have guaranteed all individuals access to a basic benefit package of selected primary and preventive services while ensuring cost containment and quality care.

---

### ETHICAL CONNECTION

According to the Institute of Medicine:

- Uninsured Americans get about half the medical care of those with health insurance. As a result, they tend to be sicker and to die sooner.
- Approximately 18,000 unnecessary deaths occur each year because of lack of health insurance.
- Only half of uninsured children visited a physician during 2001, compared with three-fourths of insured children. Lack of regular care can result in more expensive care for preventable or treatable conditions, and disruptions in learning and development.
- When even one family member is uninsured, the entire family is at risk for the financial consequences of a catastrophic illness or injury.
- Tax dollars paid for an estimated 85% of the roughly $35 billion in unreimbursed medical care for the uninsured in 2001.
- The burden of uncompensated care has been a factor in the closure of some hospitals and the unavailability of services in others. Disruptions in service can affect all who are served by a facility, including those who have health insurance.
- The United States loses the equivalent of $65 billion to $130 billion annually as a result of the poor health and early deaths of uninsured adults.

"In light of the adverse consequences that uninsurance has for individuals, families, communities, and society as a whole, it should be painfully clear that our nation can no longer afford to ignore this problem," said committee co-chair Arthur Kellermann, professor and chair of emergency medicine at Emory University School of Medicine, Atlanta. "We must find a way to cover the uninsured."

The committee's five guiding principles to judge proposed solutions are as follows:

1. Health care coverage should be universal.
2. Health care coverage should be continuous.
3. Health care coverage should be affordable to individuals and families.
4. The health insurance strategy should be affordable and sustainable to society.
5. Health care coverage should enhance health and well-being by promoting access to high-quality care that is effective, efficient, safe, timely, patient centered, and equitable.

Based on the above, what are our ethical responsibilities to providing basic health care to our citizens? Who is responsible? Who is most vulnerable?

*Source*: Committee on the Consequences of Uninsurance. (2004). *Insuring America's health: Principles and recommendations*. Washington, DC: National Academies Press.

---

The failure of the Clinton plan is generally attributed to a number of structural, strategic, and tactical mistakes. The opposition was well organized, the president had critics within his own party, the plan was too complex, the drafters of the plans were politically naive, and the president's political base of support was narrow. The arguments that were most often heard were that the plan was too expensive, it was too confusing, and taxpayers did not want to pay for health care for poor people. The failure of the plan left the United States and South Africa as the only major industrialized countries in the world without some form of universal insurance coverage. Although the reform package was never passed, health care changes did eventually occur. President Clinton's incremental initiatives such as the Health Insurance Portability and Accountability Act of 1996 have succeeded.

In his health policy agenda, President George W. Bush focused less on broad, sweeping reform, and more on market-based, individualistic, incremental policies. Bush promoted health savings accounts, which allow people to create tax-free accounts to pay for out-of-pocket medical expenses, efforts to increase transparency in health care pricing and quality, and health information technology (Shi & Singh, 2008).

## The Current U.S. Health Care Delivery System

In response to a need for change, a number of new and innovative organizations are emerging, and many traditional components of the system are in transition. A single hospital operating independently or a physician in an individual practice is becoming unusual. Hospitals, physicians, clinics, and other providers have been forced into a variety of interrelated systems. Growth and consolidation of smaller providers into larger organizations, horizontal and vertical integration of services within organizations, changes from government-owned facilities to private nonprofit and for-profit facilities, and diversification of traditional health care services are occurring at an amazingly rapid pace (Lee & Estes, 2003). Large purchasers of medical services are demanding wholesale prices for services and even dictating terms to providers. Insurance coverage is constantly changing, and patient choices have been reduced.

### ■ Levels of Care

The U.S. health care delivery system provides six basic levels of care: preventive, primary, secondary, tertiary, restorative, and continuing or long-term health care.

**Preventive care** includes education and screening programs. **Primary care** includes services directed at reducing the potential for a disease through continuous, coordinated, and comprehensive care. Preventive and primary care generally take place in the primary care provider's office.

Secondary care is concerned with early detection and treatment of acute illness and injury to prevent disability and mortality. This type of care usually occurs in the primary care provider's office or in a community hospital.

Tertiary care is concerned with slowing the progression of established disease, preventing further disability, and improving the individual's degree of functioning. It sometimes occurs in community hospitals and sometimes in large medical referral centers.

Restorative care includes hospice and chronic care and occurs in hospitals or special rehabilitation facilities. Long-term care occurs in long-term care facilities such as nursing homes and hospice facilities.

Historically, the United States has focused most of its resources on tertiary care provided in large medical care institutions.

## ■ Health Care Providers

Registered nurses and physicians are the two largest groups of health care professionals. As health care has become more complex, however, the number and variety of providers has increased proportionately. The Commission on Accreditation of Allied Health Education Programs (CAAHEP) is the largest programmatic/specialized provider of accreditation in the health sciences field. In collaboration with its Committees on Accreditation, CAAHEP accredits more than 2,000 educational programs in 19 health sciences occupations across the United States and Canada (CAAHEP, 2008).

### Physicians

Physicians are the second-largest group of health care professionals. A total of 921,904 physicians are currently practicing in the United States and its possessions (AMA, 2008). They diagnose and treat patients in an attempt to cure or improve the health of their patients. Physicians may be allopathic (MDs) or osteopathic (DOs).

In the past, most physicians were in solo practice. Today, many physicians are joining group practices or contracting with health care corporations. By joining groups, physicians are able to spread out both their workloads and their risks.

### Nurses

Nurses are the largest group of health care providers. Approximately 2.9 million individuals hold nursing licenses in the United States (ANA, 2007). A nursing degree prepares an individual to work in many areas. For example, in 2004, approximately 56% of all nurses worked in hospitals, 5%

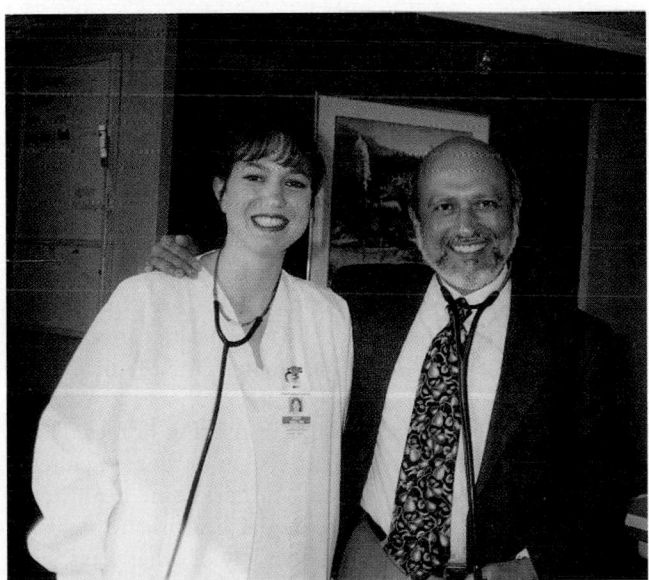

Physicians and nurses work in acute care settings in collaboration to improve health of patients.

worked in home health, 14.9% in community/public health settings, 11.5% in ambulatory settings, 6.3% in nursing homes, and 2.6% in nursing education (ANA, 2007). Nurses both deliver and coordinate health care for patients within settings and across sites, collaborate with physicians, and carry out day-to-day treatments and care.

More than 200,000 registered nurses have the education and credentials to call themselves advanced practice nurses (ANA, 2007). The category of advanced practice nurse contains several different specialty areas, including clinical nurse specialists, nurse practitioners, nurse midwives, and nurse anesthetists. These advanced-level roles have grown over the years, usually in response to a physician shortage or a physician misdistribution. Each role has its own certification, rules and regulations, and state recognition process.

Nurses are currently at an important juncture in the development of the profession. They currently have the opportunity to show their value in providing quality care at a reasonable cost while obtaining positive patient outcomes.

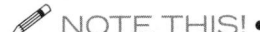 NOTE THIS! ●————————————

The American health care bill in 2004, according to government sources, was around $1.79 trillion. That amounts to approximately $6,167 per person.

### Physician Assistants

Approximately 61,910 physician assistants (PAs) are currently practicing in the United States (American Academy of Physician Assistants, 2004). The first training program for PAs was started at Duke University in 1965. In 2004, the American Academy of Physician Assistants' website reported that it had accredited 133 PA programs in 43 states. The PA training program is typically the last two years of an undergraduate degree program, and focuses on medical science and clinical skills. PAs work directly under the supervision and license of physicians, who are responsible for their performance. PAs can provide a variety of medical services as part of their role, such as history and physical examinations, minor medical diagnoses and care, follow-up care for acute and chronically ill patients, hospital rounds, and surgical assistance, among other things.

### Specialized Care Providers

Within the health care delivery system, certain groups of professionals provide focused care services. Examples are clinical psychologists, dentists, podiatrists, and optometrists. These professionals are licensed, although standards vary from state to state. They are usually addressed as "doctor," and in some areas they may have prescriptive authority and hospital privileges (i.e., they can admit and treat patients in a hospital setting). Their education is in depth in their specialty areas at a master's level or higher.

### Technicians/Therapists

Many people who provide ancillary health care services are called technicians or technologists; examples include the medical laboratory technician or medical technologist, the medical record technician, the x-ray technician, and the dietary technician. Other ancillary health care professionals are called therapists; examples are respiratory, occupational, physical, mental health, and speech therapists. Each is educated and licensed to provide a specific service and is educated at a bachelor's level or higher.

### Other Providers

Other health care providers include professionals such as pharmacists and social workers. Pharmacists are specialists in the science of drugs and can make recommendations about drug therapy. Most programs preparing pharmacists are five years long and include an internship. Pharmacists are the third largest group of health care providers.

Social workers are assuming increasingly important roles in today's health care delivery system. These professionals counsel patients and families, often directing them to various health care resources. They may also be involved in discharge planning. Chaplains address the spiritual and emotional needs of patients and families from a nondenominational perspective.

## ■ Health Care Settings

Services may be provided in traditional settings, such as hospitals, nursing homes, physicians' offices, ambulatory clinics, and homes. In addition, services may be provided in less traditional settings such as shelters, shopping malls, homeless shelters, pharmacies, schools, and job sites.

### Acute Care Facilities

Hospitals, or acute care facilities, make up the largest component of the U.S. health care delivery system and accounted for 31% of total U.S. health expenditures in 2002 (National Centers for Medicare and Medicaid, 2004). Hospitals include federal, state, and local government facilities as well as those owned by private organizations. Privately owned hospitals include voluntary (not-for-profit) or proprietary (for-profit) hospitals. Religious and charitable groups operate voluntary hospitals and may be independent or represent health maintenance organizations or cooperatives. Individuals, partnerships, or corporations own proprietary hospitals. The last decade has seen an increase in investor-owned hospital corporations; the stock of these large corporations is traded on stock exchanges.

In the current health care market, many hospitals have established home health agencies to help patients as they transition from the hospital to the home environment. Community health nurses can provide a critical link between hospital care and home care.

### Short-Term Specialized Care Facilities

Some facilities, such as mental health centers, substance abuse facilities, and rehabilitation centers, offer very specialized services. Patients are admitted to these facilities for a short-term stay to learn how to function with their disability. Another example of a short-term facility is a respite care facility that provides temporary inpatient services for individuals who usually are cared for at home. The purpose of respite care is to offer relief to the informal caregiver, usually a family member.

A short-term facility may be part of a network of coordinated services or a single independent entity. Centers may be staffed with a variety of health care providers, including physicians, nurses, and social workers. Short-term specialized care facilities discharge patients into the community after short stays. Community health nurses could provide family and home assessments to determine the patient's needs upon discharge and serve as a resource to patients once they are at home.

### Long-Term Care Facilities

Long-term care may be defined as a wide range of social, personal, and health care services in addition to medical care. These services may include arranging social functions, exercise classes, and shopping trips to improve mental and physical function. Services might also include assistance with eating and bathing, arranging for therapy sessions, dental treatments, and visits by health care providers. Such services may be needed by older individuals or individuals who have lost their ability to care for themselves through disease or injury. Long-term care focuses on maintaining as much function as possible and emphasizes activities of daily living (basic needs such as eating, dressing, bathing, and ambulating). Nursing home and home health care expenditures make up approximately 9% of the total health care expenses in the United States (National Centers for Medicare and Medicaid Services, 2004).

Most long-term care occurs in nursing homes. However, as the prospective payment system has forced patients to be discharged from hospitals earlier, home health care has become an essential part of the health care delivery system. Care may take place in a variety of other ways, such as through assisted living facilities and home health care agencies. Care is provided by registered nurses skilled in assessment and practical nurses and aides trained to provide safe patient care. Agencies receiving Medicare reimbursement must be certified and must meet specified conditions and federal standards.

Technology previously found only in hospitals is now provided by home care agencies. These treatments may include intravenous feedings and medications, ventilators, portable dialysis machines, and cardiac monitoring, for example. Although home health care has changed dramatically, it is still the traditional practice area for community health nurses. In addition to skilled nursing care, home health care may include physical, occupational, or speech therapy; homemaker services; and home-delivered meals (see Chapter 3). Community health nurses must have excellent skills related to assessing community resources and individualized patient needs in each of these long-term care modalities.

### Ambulatory Care Sites

Patients can receive care for conditions not requiring hospitalization at ambulatory care sites. Physician and clinical services account for 22% of the total health care expenses in the United States (National Centers for Medicare and Medicaid Services, 2004). Many ambulatory care sites are affiliated with hospitals, whereas others operate independently. Traditional "walk-in" clinics have existed for many years and are often supported by government funding or charitable organizations. People often use these clinics in lieu of having a personal physician. Centers may operate on an appointment or drop-in basis. Some clinics are specialized, such as family-planning clinics or those offering only women's health care services, and nurse practitioners or physician assistants frequently provide the care. Community health nurses can provide essential services in assisting patients while they try to meet their health care needs and stay at home.

Rural health centers were developed as a result of federal funding and to meet the need for care in rural, impoverished areas with few or no local physicians. Teams of residents and physicians from medical centers, along with nurse practitioners and physician assistants, frequently provide much of the care in these centers. These providers may cover several clinics on a rotating basis. Community health nurses play an important role in providing continuity in the care of patients who are often seen by many different providers. See "Ambulatory Care Center Nursing" section on page 135 for further discussion on ambulatory care in the community.

### Daycare Centers

Daycare centers target specific patient populations. For instance, many daycare centers serve elderly persons who cannot be left alone for long periods of time but who can carry out activities of daily living. Other daycare centers serve patients who are physically or mentally challenged, such as those with cerebral palsy or Down syndrome, or chemical dependencies. They care for individuals when family members are working and offer services such as meals, rehabilitation, and occupational therapy. Because the primary

needs of these patients are in the area of personal care needs, nurses play an important role in these facilities.

### Hospices

A hospice, whether run by a public or private agency, is designed to care for terminally ill patients and their families by providing noncurative, supportive, and palliative services. Many patients receiving these services are suffering from cancer, although conditions such as AIDS, multiple sclerosis, or end-stage renal disease may also require hospice care. Although nurses play the major role in hospice care, a team approach including physicians, therapists, volunteers, and clergy is often used. Nursing activities focus on managing pain, treating symptoms, and preparing the patient and family for death and bereavement.

Hospice care has been the fastest-growing segment of Medicare-reimbursed care in recent years. The percentage of hospice enrollees without cancer nearly doubled between 1992 and 2000 (National Centers for Medicare and Medicaid Services, 2002). The percentage of hospice enrollees in nursing homes increased from 11% to 36% (AMA, 2004).

### Retirement Communities

In the last 20 years, the number of retirement communities in the United States has increased significantly. These communities take many forms, such as entire small towns, retirement subdivisions, apartments or condominiums, and continuing-care communities. Although the services vary, retirement communities usually provide a number of levels of care.

In an arrangement known as assisted living, older people live independently with care nearby if needed. A convalescent center may be associated with the facility, and services such as physical and occupational therapy may be provided. Other health care services such as dental care may also be available. Residents are guaranteed access to various health care services, and the financial responsibilities are spread over the entire community. Some of the fees, such as entry fees, must be prepaid and may be very expensive. Entry fees and monthly maintenance fees are often high, thus limiting access to some of these facilities to the more affluent retirees.

### Complementary/Alternative Health Care

Complementary and alternative health care involves nontraditional treatments such as acupressure, acupuncture, therapeutic touch, herbal treatments, hypnosis and imagery, and homeopathy. Complementary and alternative health care treatments are now being studied to see how they can be used to support more traditional medical plans of care.

Congress established the Office of Alternative Medicine in 1992 to sponsor research in this field to attempt to determine the value of nontraditional treatments on patient outcomes. Nurses have often been supportive of and practiced alternative health care. Current research has recently focused more attention on some of these modalities and made them more acceptable in mainstream health care.

 *Got an Alternative?*

The National Center for Complementary and Alternative Medicine (NCCAM) was established by Congress in 1992 to sponsor research into complementary and nontraditional treatments and their effects on patient health outcomes. The NCCAM is one of the 27 institutes and centers that make up the National Institutes of Health (NIH). The NIH is one of eight agencies under the Public Health Service (PHS) in the Department of Health and Human Services (DHHS).

NCCAM is dedicated to exploring complementary and alternative healing practices in the context of rigorous science, training complementary and alternative medicine (CAM) researchers, and disseminating authoritative information to the public and professionals.

## Issues Affecting the Delivery of Health Care Services

Many issues have contributed to the growth, complexity, and expense of the U.S. health care delivery system, such as deregulation, consumerism, technology, the graying of America, and our litigious society. (See Box 5-3.) Local, state, and federal governments have attempted to address these issues at one time or another. However, short-term fixes for any one factor have had little impact on the overall problem.

### ■ Deregulation

In the last few years, the United States has experienced deregulation of health care. The result has been a proliferation of facilities and technology (i.e., CAT scans and MRIs) in some urban areas, which has resulted in excess capacity and, in turn, increased competition. This expense is inevitably passed along to the patients. Also, the trend leads to misdistribution of essential services in underserved areas. Competition as a price control strategy has not helped to control health care costs. Americans still want the specialist, the newest technology, the cutting-edge treatment, and the hospital that looks like a four-star hotel: They simply hope their insurance will pay for it.

### ■ Emphasis on Secondary and Tertiary Health Care Services

Historically, the U.S. health care system has allocated the majority of its resources to the care that occurs after the patient has become critically ill. Vast amounts of money have been spent on critical care units, technical procedures, and sophisticated surgical techniques, but little money has been devoted to preventing the illness in the first place. Education and screening services are often not reimbursed by third-party payers and are undervalued by busy providers. Although managed care organizations frequently say they value what these preventive services can accomplish, the cost is often more than they wish to pay. As a result, managed care often makes decisions about which preventive services are the most valuable and ignores the rest.

### ■ Increasing Consumerism

Health care consumerism encompasses the public's involvement in determining the type, quality, and cost of their health care. Today, consumers are reading, looking up information, subscribing to newsletters specializing in their health care problem, and attending support groups. They are better informed and asserting their right to have an active role in decisions related to their care.

In the past, the poor often either went without health care or had to be satisfied with a lesser quality of care. Values are now changing, and equal access to health care is now viewed by many as a right.

### ■ Technological Advances

Advances made in technology have drastically changed health care and altered how physicians treat hospitalized patients. For example, the life expectancy of a person with diabetes has increased considerably in recent decades. New chemotherapy treatments have extended cancer patients' lives and, in some cases, greatly increased the quality of their lives. Heart, lung, and liver transplants—all of which were unheard of three decades ago—have become commonplace. The latest antibiotic therapies ward off deadly diseases. Taken collectively, advances have reduced hospital stays and allowed people to live longer.

The new technology is expensive, and some advances have raised formidable ethical questions. If you can extend the life of an 80-year-old man for a short time by putting him on a ventilator, should you do it? If you can keep a premature baby alive on life support, but you know that the child has multiple irreparable problems that will result in incredible future costs, should you do it? For the cost of the care of one elderly man on a ventilator for several weeks, you could provide prenatal care to a large group of pregnant women.

**❝** *It is no measure of health to be well adjusted to a profoundly sick society.* **❞**

—*Krishnamurti*

Research Alert

### Public Not Doing Things to Protect Their Health

Reeves and Rafferty found in their study of 153,000 Americans that only 3% of Americans follow the four basic healthy lifestyle habits that public health experts consider the cornerstones to a longer and better life: engaging in regular exercise, refraining from smoking, eating five or more fruits and vegetables daily, and maintaining a healthy weight. Many public health authorities believe that a person who follows the big four will have gone a long way toward reducing the risks of life-threatening chronic illnesses.

"These data illustrate that a healthy lifestyle—defined as a combination of four healthy lifestyle characteristics—was undertaken by very few adults in the United States, and that no subgroup followed this combination to a level remotely consistent with clinical or public health recommendations," said Mathew J. Reeves, PhD, of Michigan State University, and colleagues.

The findings, they added, "support the need for comprehensive primary prevention activities to increase healthy lifestyles and to reduce the prevalence of chronic risk factors at the population level."

The researchers analyzed data from the 2000 Behavioral Risk Factor Surveillance System, which included 164,940 respondents aged 18 to 74 years. Participants were randomly telephoned and questioned about lifestyle habits, such as how often they drank fruit juice, ate green leafy vegetables, and the frequency and duration of physical activity.

Survey results showed the prevalence (95% confidence interval) of participants' four healthy lifestyle characteristics were as follows: nonsmoking, 76% (75.6%–76.4%); healthy weight, 40.1% (39.7%–40.5%); five fruits and vegetables a day, 23.3% (22.9%–23.7%); and regular exercise 22.2% (21.8%–22.6%). The overall prevalence of people engaging in all four healthy habits was a mere 3% (95% CI, 2.8%–3.2%) with little variation among subgroups (range, 0.8%–5.7%).

Researchers noted that one of the drawbacks to this study was its reliance on self-reported data. Still, it suggests health care providers have their work cut out for them.

"We believe that these findings serve to illustrate the health promotion crisis in the United States, characterized by excessive caloric intake, inadequate leisure time physical activity, increasing obesity, and high rates of cigarette use," the researchers wrote.

Currently, two thirds of the entire U.S. population is overweight or obese. According to the Centers for Disease Control and Prevention, 22.5% of all U.S. adults (or 46 million people) smoke cigarettes. More men smoke than women, 25.2% compared to 20%, respectively. ◉

*Source:* Reeves, M. J., & Rafferty, A. P. (2000). Healthy lifestyle characteristics among adults in the United States. *Archives of Internal Medicine, 5*(165), 854–857.

---

**BOX 5-3**

**Key Concepts: Factors Affecting Health Care Delivery**
- Failure of competition as a strategy following deregulation of health care
- Emphasis on secondary and tertiary health care instead of prevention
- Increasing consumerism
- Escalating cost of technology
- Aging of the population
- Cost of defensive medicine
- Government regulation and administrative costs

### ■ Increasing Longevity of Americans

In the 2000 census, approximately 35 million individuals reported that they were 65 years of age or older. This represents 12.4% of the total U.S. population (U.S. Census Bureau, 2008a). The fastest-growing age group in the United States is people 85 and older. Because the heaviest users of health services are the elderly, more emphasis is being placed on their needs, the need for services has increased, and gerontology has become a significant branch of medicine and nursing. Topics such as living wills and powers of attorney are becoming more widely discussed, as people become concerned about their ability to maintain life and the quality of that life.

### ■ Defensive Health Care and Government Regulation

The cost of defensive health care and government regulations has been a major factor affecting the delivery of health care in the United State. Physicians are often forced to pay extremely high costs for malpractice insurance and attorney's fees when they are sued. As a result, some physicians have simply stopped offering high risk services such as obstetrics or have stopped providing care to indigent patients as a way to increase their profits.

Physicians also tend to practice defensive health care by ordering more tests or more expensive treatments. In addition, increased government regulation has caused many physicians to increase their office staff, reduce their patient load, or join health care systems where billing services are provided. The result of the increased costs is the physician must become much more cost-conscious and health care has become a business rather than a service.

## Managed Care

Total integration of services is expected to be the future economic structure of the health care delivery system. Networks are expected to compete for patients by becoming more efficient, charging lower prices, offering a wider range of services, and insuring quality care for a fixed cost for the individual. They will maintain a central database to ensure that comprehensive care is delivered as the patient moves from provider to provider within the system. These networks are called managed care.

**❝** *The health plan [was] constructed to be deconstructed. [Instead,] it was described as an ultimatum by our opponents and therefore used to undermine the process of reaching agreement.* **❞**

—Hillary Rodham Clinton, 1994

### ■ The Concept of Managed Care

The concept of managed care encompasses a wide variety of organizational structures and is quickly becoming the dominant management strategy in the U.S. health care delivery system. By definition, **managed care** refers to a system that, for a set fee, assumes responsibility and accountability for the health of a population through the use of effective, responsible, and cost-efficient care. "Managed care integrates the financing and delivery of health care services to covered individuals, most often by arrangements with providers. These systems offer packages of health care benefits, explicit standards for the selection of health care providers, formal programs for ongoing quality assurance and utilization review, significant financial incentives for its members to use providers, and procedures associated with the plan" (ANA, 1998).

**Managed care organizations (MCOs)** first made their appearance in the 1970s and 1980s, when the insurance industry was faced with employers starting to self-insure and health care costs were soaring. The huge reserves of money that insurance companies had previously invested were being depleted. Strategically thinking insurance companies redefined their market and began developing managed care organizations.

The goals of managed care are achieved by keeping patients healthy and treating them in the lowest-cost setting using providers that have also agreed to provide services at a reduced rate. Under this system, primary care replaces the hospital as the center of care. The goal is to keep people out of the hospital—not to keep the hospital beds full. More treatments and care are provided in clinics and physicians' offices. Ambulatory patients go home to recover from surgery rather than upstairs in the hospital for a leisurely recovery in a private room.

Managed care has transformed health care from a service industry into a competitive, market-driven business. The question now is whether health care decisions are made based on the patient's needs or on the need to show a profit for the organization and its stakeholders. Who is making the decisions about treatment options, and who is caring for the patient with complex, multisystem problems? Is the cheapest treatment always the best treatment? All of these questions are currently without answers.

**❝** *The care of human life and happiness, and not their destruction, is the first and only object of good government.* **❞**

—Thomas Jefferson

If managed care is considered the long-term answer to patient care questions, the answer lies in the premise that a healthy patient is cheaper to care for than an unhealthy one. Therefore, preventive care is the only answer. If managed care looks at the short-term answer, then cheaper is better.

### ■ Managed Care Organizations

The majority of managed care organizations can be categorized into three basic types: health maintenance organizations (HMOs), preferred provider organizations (PPOs), and point-of-service plans (POSs). **Capitation** refers to the amount of money that is paid to a health maintenance organization to cover the cost of health care for a group of patients. An agency or organization representing a group of individuals seeking health care contracts with a group of providers and pays a predetermined fee periodically, usually quarterly.

**❝** *Health is my expected heaven.* **❞**

—John Keats

### Health Maintenance Organizations

Federally recognized **health maintenance organizations (HMOs)** are prepaid health management plans that offer an organized system for providing a predetermined set of health care services in a geographic area to a voluntarily enrolled group of people for an established fee. This system combines traditional insurance and health care delivery in one organization and provides a wide range of services, including inpatient and outpatient hospital care, infertility and mental health services, therapeutic x-ray treatments, alcohol and drug addiction treatment, and physical therapy.

HMOs were first established in 1973 under a federal program. The number of HMOs in existence grew dramatically over the next 30 years. Enrollment is voluntary; members have the option to select another plan. Because the fee paid by members is fixed annually, the organization tries to minimize costs. To do so, HMOs must place greater emphasis on health promotion and disease prevention. Some HMOs hire providers as employees, whereas others contract with providers for services.

### Preferred Provider Organizations

A **preferred provider organization (PPO)** is a type of managed care plan composed of a group of physicians, and possibly one or more hospitals, which join forces to offer a prepaid health care plan to employers. In preferred provider arrangements, patients select their health care providers from the list of preferred providers and receive services at a discounted cost. If a consumer chooses to seek services from a provider who has not contracted with the plan, either a substantial deductible fee is assessed or the service is not covered. In the future, PPOs are likely to grow larger and include a wider range of providers.

### Point-of-Service Plans

**Point-of-service plans (POSs)** are also known as open-ended HMOs. POSs provide a set of services that are covered under the established fee, but members are also given the choice of going out of the network for services. Members share in costs with the HMO if they decide to go out of the network for care.

### Multilevel Integrated Systems

The **integrated health care systems** of the future will consist of a mix of many types of health care facilities and providers connected through different types of contractual arrangements. These complex systems will be able to supply a broad range of services, from in-house care to outpatient care, from traditional to nontraditional care, within their own system (vertically integrated) or arrange for the services to be provided by other systems (horizontally integrated). Primary care providers, hospitals, retirement communities, wellness centers, pharmacies, health food outlets, rehabilitation centers, counseling centers, and many other types of providers from a large geographical area will be connected and accessible to members of these systems.

The process of changing traditional systems into new, multilevel integrated systems is often complicated and emotionally difficult. The literature is full of words designed to make the transformation process sound less cold and calculating. The first term to appear was "downsizing," which was immediately changed to "rightsizing." This term simply refers to cutting the number of funded positions to decrease costs. "Redesigning" was the next term to make an appearance; it referred to the process of examining all job descriptions to ensure equitable distribution of activities and reduce role overlap, excess specialization, and waste. The next term to appear was "restructuring," which refers to an assessment of the overall organizational structure in an attempt to improve productivity. Finally, "reengineering" refers to a comprehensive and often-radical process to look at jobs and organizational structure as a way to form new relationships, new visions, and improved functioning and productivity. As the evolution of these terms suggests, future integrated health care systems will be larger and more comprehensive.

## ■ Patient Care Outcomes

The term "patient care outcomes" refers to the consequences of care that the patient receives or does not receive. Outcomes studies are becoming very popular in managed care organizations as a way to predict and provide effective patient care. These studies look for trends over time in patient status and adverse events. Adverse patient care outcomes are occurrences that are not expected as a result of the patient's disease process or treatment. Data obtained from patient care studies are then used as a basis for decisions, the development of policies and procedures, and changes in health care practice.

Efforts to improve patient care outcomes involve assessing individual patients' care and recovery as well as analyzing large data sets from across the country and world. Large national databases will be used in the future to provide predictive information on which to base treatments, types of care, lengths of care, and level of provider needed to achieve positive outcomes.

 Research Alert

Health care amounts to 14% of our GNP—a lot of money. It is the size of the Italian economy. And the president turned it over to his wife.

—*Jack Kemp, U.S. Republican congressman from New York, Secretary of Housing and Urban Development, at the National Press Club, November 21, 1994*

### Community-Based Health Care Settings

#### Shelters in the Community

Another focus of community-based health nursing is that of the **shelter nurse**. Shelters are facilities established to assist people, who for one reason or another have found themselves to be homeless. While some shelters simply provide a place to get out of the weather, other shelters offer a wide range of services, often specializing in the concerns of specific populations such as the homeless, victims of abuse, or runaway youth.

Shelters are usually run by a combination of paid professionals and volunteer staff, including psychologists, nurses, attorneys, and others. Shelters may be sponsored by churches, community governments, and a variety of social agencies and are designed to provide a variety of services to people who often suffer from a variety of problems (Townsend, 2000). There is really no such thing as a typical shelter. Shelters are housed in warehouses, churches, government buildings, and single-family homes that have been converted to supervised residences (Carson, 2000). The location of many shelters is kept secret to protect the safety of the residents (Lundy et al., 2003).

#### Abuse Shelters

Most cities in the United States now have shelters, or "safe houses," where women can go to obtain protection for themselves and their children. Most battered women who reside in shelters have experienced multiple traumatic events, with some even suffering from post-traumatic stress disorder (Humphreys, Lee, Neylan, & Marmar, 2001). Shelters not only provide a haven of safety to the abused and battered woman, they provide health care, counseling, a milieu to express the intense emotions she may be experiencing, and a wealth of support including financial, social, and spiritual (Humphreys et al., 2001; Townsend, 2000).

#### Homeless Shelters

In the United States, the homeless population is "among the poorest of the poor" (Zuvekas & Hill, 2000, p. 153) and consists not just of adult men and women but also countless numbers of children (Huang & Menke, 2001). A large segment of this population faces potential barriers to work, as many have serious mental and physical disabilities and others have single or multiple drug addictions (Hatton, 2001). In addition to meeting the medical and mental health needs of the homeless, shelters provide a safe, supportive environment for individuals who simply have no other place to go. While a small percentage of the homeless use the resources available to improve their lives, others become dependent on the provisions that the shelter offers (Townsend, 2000; Lundy et al., 2003).

### Disaster Shelters

When major flooding, tornadoes, landslides, and earthquakes strike, thousands of families are often displaced from their homes. For some families, displacement may be on a short-term basis. For others, their homes and all their belongings are gone. The greatest immediate need usually reported by most disaster victims is shelter (Daley, Karpati, & Sheik, 2001). This need is closely followed by food and hygiene requirements. Disaster victims include the young and the very old as well as those who are ill and those who are pregnant. Because of this, there is also a great demand in shelters for medications along with medical and nursing care (Daley et al., 2001).

The community health nurse, as a provider of care and manager of care in shelters, is in a unique position to help meet the needs of those people for whom shelters are their lifeline—the difference between life and death. It is essential that the shelter nurse exhibit the following competencies when working with all persons who enter a shelter in search of help and hope.

Professional behaviors essential to the shelter nurse would include crisis intervention and counseling; health promotion and maintenance; screening and evaluation; provision of a therapeutic environment; assisting patients with self-care activities; administering and monitoring treatment regimens; health teaching; and outreach activities including home visits and community action (Townsend, 2000).

Shelter nurses must be able to accurately assess the needs of the population for whom they provide care. Depending on the type of shelter, nurses may care for patients with a multitude of physical needs, ranging from bruises and broken bones to pneumonia, STDs, AIDS, substance abuse, tuberculosis, and dysentery.

Too often, however, it is the patient's spiritual and mental needs that are harder to assess. Shelter patients often suffer from mental illness, depression, anger, guilt, poor coping mechanisms, a multitude of stressors, and low self-esteem. Shelter nurses must be able to use therapeutic communication skills to develop a trusting relationship with their patients. It is the shelter nurse who is in the best position to let the shelter patient know that his or her feelings of anger and despair are normal and that others have

experienced these same emotions in similar situations (Townsend, 2000). Through collaboration with the health care team, the nurse works with the patient in individual and group settings in an effort to develop coping skills that will serve as a stable base upon which the patient can begin to build a future.

One of the most important tasks of the shelter nurse is simply to care for the shelter patient. This starts with being nonjudgmental. It probably goes without saying that none of the shelter patients desire to be at the station in life in which they find themselves when they come to the shelter. Among the caring behaviors the shelter nurse must exhibit are listening, providing feedback, helping the patient to recognize available choices, and accepting and supporting the patient in whatever he or she chooses to do. One of the most important roles for nurses who work in shelters is that of educator, with emphasis on providing information about the availability of resources in the community (Townsend, 2000).

In addition to not having a place to live, shelter patients often lack the knowledge and skills that will help them to leave the shelter and function on their own. Patients may need assistance with completing paperwork to get federal or local assistance that will enable them to find a permanent home. They may need training or education to get a job, and many of the mentally ill lack the knowledge as to how to get the medications that will treat their mental illness. The shelter nurse may need to teach parenting skills, methods of building self-esteem, and alternative coping mechanisms to many of the shelter's patients. The mentally ill often need information about their medications to promote compliance. This includes when and how to take their medications as well as ways to reduce troublesome side effects. Some patients need assistance with hygiene as well as teaching about how to socially interact with others.

Nurses often serve as case managers for a selected group of patients who have been seen in shelters (Townsend, 2000). As case manager, the nurse coordinates services that are required to meet the needs of the patient. This is done in an effort to prevent avoidable episodes of illness—physical and mental—among these at-risk patients. Responsibilities include negotiating with many health care providers to obtain whatever services are needed by the patient. This coordination of services by the shelter nurse is done in an effort to optimize patient functioning and problem solving, improve work and socialization skills, promote leisure-time activities, and enhance the overall independence of the individual (Townsend, 2000).

The shelter nurse can participate in the research process at multiple levels. Areas of research involvement include identifying problem areas; collecting, analyzing, and interpreting data; applying findings; helping to evaluate, design, and conduct research; and using research available on the needs of shelter patients to formulate clinical pathways that will help to maximize outcomes for shelter patients (Hitchcock, Schubert, & Thomas, 1999). The shelter nurse can also keep abreast of current literature, share findings with other members of the health care team, and, when appropriate, apply findings to the care of shelter patients (Lundy et al., 2003).

For specific information about shelter nursing, see additional text chapters on specific populations, such as the homeless, patients of abuse, and services for disasters.

## Ambulatory Care Center Nursing

Perhaps one of the most innovative and dramatic changes in community-based health care is in the diversity in care delivered in ambulatory care centers, from ambulatory surgical centers to ambulatory oncology care settings. These free-standing centers provide acute care to walk-in (ambulatory) patients without the custodial feel of traditional hospital care. These alternative sites for acute care have been very successful because of their efficiency, cost-effectiveness, and high degree of patient satisfaction. They can provide faster service with less paperwork and administrative time involvement. These ambulatory care centers are smaller in size than hospitals, employ fewer personnel, and have less technical equipment, which keeps costs down (Lundy et al., 2003).

### Ambulatory Emergency/Trauma and Primary Care Centers

These centers, often referred to as "urgent care," "urgicare," "minute clinics," or "walk-ins" do not perform major surgeries. Most are located in urban areas, shopping centers, and, most recently, retail stores. These community-based health care services have seen significant growth in the first part of the twenty-first century due to consumer demands for quick and inexpensive services. For example, when patients are unable to make an appointment with their primary caregiver, they can visit these "minute clinics" in Wal-Mart, get a five-minute strep test, and fill any prescriptions at the same location. Referrals can be made, based on diagnosis, to local full-service hospitals when patients need additional care.

As a relatively new resource for immediate and primary care, ambulatory centers are often staffed by family nurse practitioners, family practice physicians, registered nurses, licensed practical nurses, lab technicians, diagnostic technicians, and clerks. Ambulatory care centers try to enhance consumer satisfaction by being convenient, cost-effective, and caring. They do so by providing the four "A's": They are affable, available, accessible, and affordable. These centers are often open seven days a week, for 12 to 16 hours per day.

Minor illnesses, such as upper respiratory tract illnesses, impetigo, diarrhea, dehydration, urinary tract infections, asthma, and cellulites can be easily diagnosed and treated at these clinics. Many also see more serious symptoms and illnesses such as chest pain, back pain, seizures, and anaphylaxis. Pregnancy tests are offered, along with suturing of lacerations, casting and splinting of fractures, and treatment of wounds, burns, and eye injuries. These centers offer limited diagnostic services, such as routine radiologic services, complete blood cell counts, bacteriology, electrolytes, and toxicology tests.

The majority of patients are adults, although most centers see children as well. Return visits can be arranged but most customers are referred back to their family physician, nurse practitioner, or a specialist (Seidel, Henderson, & Lewis, 1991).

These relatively new health care services have been subjected to considerable criticism, especially from the medical community. Many critics view these "one-stop" services as inappropriate for children and others who need the comprehensive and continuous care delivered by a family health care provider (Lundy et al., 2003).

### Ambulatory Surgery Centers

Ambulatory surgery refers to a surgical process in which patients have surgery, recover, and are discharged home on the same day. Because of advances in anesthesia, surgical techniques, and a desire for convenience, these centers have grown significantly in the past 10 years. Cost containment is a major factor in the proliferation in same-day surgical centers. Approximately 65% of all surgical procedures are now performed safely on an ambulatory basis without compromising the quality of care (Atkinson & Fortunato, 1995). Surgical procedures generally do not exceed 90 minutes in length and do not require more than four hours of recovery time. Each center has emergency equipment and trained personnel, including registered nurses. Pharmacy services are also available. Laboratory and radiological services may be performed on site or by referral to nearby facilities.

The American Academy of Ambulatory Care Nursing provides standards and guidelines for ambulatory centers in the community. Because of the brevity of patient contact in these centers, nurses must be focused and well educated as professionals in caring for persons who are frightened, stressed, and quickly discharged. The amount of time during which the ambulatory care center nurse stays with patients in these centers is short, so good communication skills are of special significance, both to patients and their families and other health professionals. Remaining focused and precise, nurses in these settings should communicate with deliberate and yet compassionate purpose due to the short length of time with the patients.

The ambulatory health center nurse conducts assessments, serves as an assistant to physicians as either a scrub or circulating nurse for surgical procedures, and takes histories during admission. Assessments after procedures are especially important at surgical centers because the collected data assist the physician in making the decision to discharge the patient.

The ambulatory center nurse makes quick decisions based on well-thought-through clinical assessments and uses multiple interventions depending on the setting and diagnosis. Such a nurse analyzes data and integrates knowledge about the specific risks associated with the illness or procedure and takes appropriate action.

The nurse in the ambulatory care center must possess good interpersonal skills in which complex health and safety information can be conveyed in an understandable and concise manner to patients and their families, and in a respectful way to other workers and administration. Compassion for the patient and family is critical, as they are aware that they will be under medical supervision and care for only a short time. Nurses must promote self-care and confidence in the patient's ability to follow through with post-discharge instructions.

Much of the nurse role in an ambulatory care setting involves teaching of appropriate discharge measures. The nurse often follows up the following day to evaluate the health status of the patient after services have been delivered.

The nurse in the ambulatory care setting collaborates with other health professionals to share and manage critical information about the patient before, during, and after procedures. This team approach provides the patient with comprehensive care so that upon discharge, successful healing is more likely.

The ambulatory care center nurse manages a quick turnaround for patients with acute illnesses, which requires excellent organizational skills and a knowledge of critical information related to the specific illness or injury. Evaluation using outcome measurement can provide vital information about how to make the system work more efficiently while maintaining quality levels (Williams, 1993; Lundy et al., 2003).

*Source*: Lundy, K. S., Sutton, V., & Foster, B. (2003). The nurse's role in ambulatory health settings. In K. S. Lundy & S. Janes (Eds.), *Essentials of community-based nursing* (pp. 258–295). Sudbury, MA: Jones and Bartlett.

## Health Politics and Policy

How did the U.S. health care delivery system become so expensive? Who should pay for the ever-increasing costs of health care and hospitalization? These questions have become the basis for untold numbers of legislative reports, articles, studies, and documentaries. The astronomical costs of some forms of treatment have made it impossible for the average patient to pay personally for needed medical, surgical, and nursing services. Single illness-episode bills well above $10,000 are no longer the exception. Many people rely on government interventions to help them deal with soaring costs and inaccessible services.

### ■ Government Policy

Health insurance provides protection against the high cost of medical care and hospitalization arising from illness or injury. Most Americans look to their jobs for health insurance, but increasingly insurance benefits are not available at work sites. The number of Americans who are uninsured or underinsured is increasing at an alarming rate. In response, Americans have appealed to their legislators for help.

Government policy focuses on health care on several levels. For example, federal legislation establishes boards to govern the practice of health care professionals and health care agencies, establishes commissions to examine health care delivery and make recommendations, and sets guidelines for the payment of Medicare benefits. State guidelines influence Medicaid benefits. Medicare and Medicaid guidelines affect the entire health care industry because the government is the third-party payer for more than 40% of all U.S. expenditures for health care (National Centers for Medicare and Medicaid Services, 2002).

The publication of *Healthy People 2010*, based on the progress made under *Healthy People 2000* goals, again moved forward the U.S. agenda of disease prevention and health promotion for all citizens. The majority of the goals for the year 2010 still fall into three categories: increasing the healthy life span, reducing health disparities, and increasing access to service (American Public Health Association, 2004). Prior to the publication of *Healthy People 2000*, these goals were not central in health legislation. However, in a time of increasing fiscal austerity, these goals make increasing economic sense: Keeping people well is much less costly than trying to cure or rehabilitate them.

Finally, there have been many debates about whether the United States should adopt a national health insurance plan or support market competition. Under a national plan, taxpayers would pay the government for the coverage, much as insurance companies currently collect funds from subscribers, and everyone would be covered at a predetermined basic level of services. The disadvantage is that government plans rarely operate very efficiently and many people feel that it is inappropriate for government to meddle in individuals' health care decisions.

**Managed competition** has been promoted as another way to keep health care costs at a reasonable level while insuring quality care. Under this system, the government would allow a rivalry between health care providers for the purpose of attracting patients. However, an unequal distribution of the most ill patients might keep corporations from wanting to insure the very patients who need care the most.

### ■ Public Opinion and Special-Interest Groups

Public opinion expressed through special-interest groups is very influential in the development of public policy. Many special-interest groups, such as the American Hospital Association, the American Medical Association, and the American Insurance Association, spend huge amounts of time and money providing legislators with information on which to base health care decisions. Many legislators lack an in-depth understanding of health care issues. As a result, the information provided by special-interest groups often serves as a basis for health care decisions. When that happens, decisions may fail to reflect the best interests of the majority.

### Nursing and Health Care Policy

As the largest health care provider group, it is important for nurses to be both visible and vocal advocates for quality health care. To meet that important goal, the American Nurses Association (ANA) has worked tirelessly over the years to develop an effective special-interest group infrastructure. In response to the health care reform issue, the ANA (2007) formulated a position paper stating that the U.S. health care system needs restructuring, wellness promotion must become our emphasis, and universal access to health care services must be developed.

The ANA has been politically active in several other areas, including the area of health care rationing. When resources are limited, the question of health care rationing must be addressed. Of course, the well-insured individuals will worry about restrictions under such a system, and the uninsured or underinsured will worry that they will be excluded. Rationing can mean limiting access to care or limiting contact to the more expensive providers.

Through the years, ANA and state nurses organizations have continued to support legislation that aims to ensure basic health care services for everyone. To influence policy, nurses need to vote, be politically active in their states, and know which bills are being considered. To be politically active, you can work on someone's campaign, run for political office, support candidates financially, or simply stay in contact with elected state and federal officials and provide them with information when needed.

## New Nursing Opportunities

As health care changes, the practice of nursing must also change. Nurses must stay knowledgeable about health care trends to make decisions about future careers. Those trends include things such as the growth in the health care workforce, the role of economics as a driving force, the changing U.S. demographics, the transformation of individual providers into multilevel corporations, the trend of physicians becoming employees, the philosophic move from "everything for a few" to "an adequate amount for many," and the increased importance of ambulatory care and home health care (Huston & Fox, 1998). Some of the nursing roles related to these trends are discussed here. However, many future roles are yet to be created.

### Advanced Practice Nurses

Advanced practice nursing is not a new category for nurses, but many of the traditional roles for nurses are changing. Nurse practitioners are moving into specialized

### Application to Practice

A pregnant woman with severe epilepsy has presented to the health department from a local obstetrical practice. She had been working part-time at a local grocer until her seizures became unmanageable, and she is no longer employed. The patient has been referred to the health department so that she can qualify for state funds for high-risk maternity care. The patient's husband works for a local manufacturing company and has HMO coverage for both himself and his wife through a company-sponsored managed care plan. The deductible and co-payment are more than the couple can afford to pay, and they would like to find other resources to pay for the additional services needed to manage the epilepsy. The public health nurse checks with the state high-risk maternity care program and finds that the couple exceeds the income criteria and most likely will not qualify.

1. What are possible health and economic consequences if the patient's health is not managed appropriately during pregnancy?
2. Which system problems can you identify from the situation that result in ethical issues of treatment and care?
3. Who is responsible for seeing that this patient receives appropriate care at an affordable cost?

areas such as geriatrics, acute care, and correction facilities health care. Clinical nurse specialists are becoming experts in case management, genetics, and comprehensive cancer care. Nurse anesthetists and nurse midwives are managing patients with specialized needs. Advanced practice nurses are prepared to work with physicians, not for them. As specialties develop, nurses are finding ways to become experts in those area. As more emphasis is placed on controlling health care costs, more providers will look to advanced practice nurses as providers of effective, quality, lower-cost care. The Doctorate of Nursing Practice (DNP) has emerged as the entry level for all advanced practice nurses. How this will impact the healthcare delivery system remains to be seen.

### Entrepreneurs

In the future, more nurses than ever before will own nursing businesses. In areas such as home health, health care management, insurance evaluation, nursing clinics, environmental evaluation, workplace health care, caregiver support,

## A Good Read

### Balanced Choice: A Common Sense Cure for the U.S. Health Care System (2006)

*By Ivan J. Miller, Bloomingdale, IN: Healthcare Authorhouse.*

Miller turns a very critical eye toward the current U.S. health care system. He critically examines the broken system of industrialized HMOs and other versions of managed care.

He calls for a reformation of health care, with a vision that places people ahead of corporate profits. Miller discusses the assets and liabilities of the variety of available health care models. He proposes a new national model that uses both market forces and a national regulatory board (not unlike the Federal Reserve) to save on massive administrative costs, promote improved services for patients, allow professionals the freedom to practice, and reduce costs to a stable, predictable level for employers.

program evaluation, and respite care, the opportunities are endless. Nurses will be in a position to contract with larger systems for consulting services and the application of specialized knowledge and skills.

### Data Management

Public and private agencies are looking for nurses who are skilled at creating and managing large databases containing patient information, a field known as informatics. Every health care organization is struggling with the need to maintain information in a safe, yet easily accessible manner. Data must be available for evaluation and decision making. Nurses with an understanding of patient care data coupled with a working knowledge of computers, the workings of databases, and the use of evaluative statistics will be in the perfect position to fill these critical slots.

### Research

We can no longer make decisions on the basis of what we have done before or what we think will work. Decisions must be based on data that can be seen, measured, and reproduced as needed, integrated with sound clinical practice experience. We are moving into an age of evidence-based patient care. Consequently, patient care research is more important today than at any time in the past. Nurse researchers try to develop an understanding of essential patient care issues on which to base practice. They may be employees of an organization or working on a research project funded by the government or other organizations that fund research. Their work provides the structure for future practice that will identify efficient and effective health care practices that improve the lives of patients.

> **❝** *Our ancestors tithed in the hope of life after death; we hope for more and better life before death.* **❞**
>
> —Robert G. Evans

> **❝** *I don't know the key to success, but the key to failure is trying to please everybody.* **❞**
>
> —Bill Cosby

### Conclusion

Some critics suggest that the U.S. health care system, which is supposed to guarantee access, innovation, and quality care, has instead become a system in crisis. A crisis exists in several areas: cost, availability, equity, efficiency, and responsiveness to public needs. This chapter discussed the history of the U.S. health care delivery system and described the changing components of that system. New roles for nursing are emerging as this health care system moves from one that was measured by the cost of its components to a system measured by the effectiveness of the care provided by its components.

Explore Community Health Nursing on the Web! To learn more about the topics in this chapter, use the passcode provided to access your exclusive website: **http://nursing.jbpub.com/communityhealth.** If you do not have a passcode, you can obtain one at this site.

### ■ CRITICAL THINKING ACTIVITIES

1. You are a 28-year-old single mother with three children. You are having pain in your stomach and trouble sleeping. You have no money and no insurance. How will you get someone to help you? What will you do if you need medication?

2. You are a 22-year-old single parent with two children ages 1 and 3. Your mother is unemployed and watches the children while you work. Your job does not provide you with insurance. Your pay is too high to allow you

to be eligible for Medicaid and too low to allow you to afford insurance. Which types of services do you need from the Health Department?

3. In a world of limited resources, developing equitable health policies involves many difficult decisions. How would you answer the following questions?

- Should an 85-year-old man with debilitating emphysema be placed on a respirator?

- Should a 78-year-old woman with breast cancer be put on chemotherapy?
- Should major health insurance plans reimburse for experimental treatments?
- Should an insurance plan be required to pay for a liver transplant for an alcoholic?
- Should a baby with multiple incurable birth defects be placed in a neonatal intensive care unit?

## ■ REFERENCES

American Academy of Physician Assistants. (2004). *Physician assistants—statistics.* Retrieved May 23, 2008, from http://www/aapa.org/

American Medical Association (AMA). (2008). *Physician characteristics and distribution in the U.S.* Retrieved May 23, 2008, from http://www.ama-assn.org/ama/pub

American Nurses Association (ANA). (1998). *Managed care: Challenges and opportunities for nursing. Nursing Facts.* Retrieved May 23, 2008, from http://www.nursingworld.org/readroom/fsmg

American Nurses Association (ANA). (2007). *About nursing.* Retrieved April 15, 2008, from http://nursingworld.org/MainMenuCategories/CertificationandAccreditation/AboutNursing.aspx

American Public Health Association. (2004). *Healthy people 2010 objectives* Washington, DC: Author.

Atkinson, L. J., & Fortunato, N. H. (1995). Ambulatory surgery. In L. J. Atkinson & N. H. Fortunato (Eds.), *Berry and Kohn's operating room technique* (pp. 833–839). St Louis, MO: Mosby Year Book.

Commission on Accreditation of Allied Health Educational Programs (CAAHEP). (2008). *What is CAAHEP?* Retrieved September 8, 2008, from http://www.caahep.org/

The Commonwealth Fund Commission on a High Performance Health System. (2008). *Why not the best? Results from the national scorecard on U. S. health system performance, 2008.* Retrieved October 26, 2008, from www.commonwealthfund.org/publications/publications_show.htm

Daley, W. R., Karpati, A., & Sheik, M. (2001). Needs assessment of the displaced population following the August 1999 earthquake in Turkey. *Disasters, 25*(1), 67–75.

Donatiello, J. E., Droese, P. W., & Kim, S. H. (2004). A selected, annotated list of materials that support the development of policies to reduce racial and ethnic health disparities. *Journal of the Medical Library Association, 92*(2), 257–265.

Fairbanks, J., & Wiese, W. H. (1998). *The public health primer.* Thousand Oaks, CA: Sage Publications.

Feldstein, P. J. (2007). *Health policy issues: An economic perspective* (4th ed.). Chicago: Health Administration Press.

Hatton, D. C. (2001). Homeless women and children's access to health care: A paradox. *Journal of Community Health Nursing, 18,* 25–35.

Hitchcock, J. E., Schubert, P. E., & Thomas, S. A. (1999). *Community health nursing: Caring in action.* Albany, NY: Delmar.

Huang, C. Y., & Menke, E. M. (2001). School-aged homeless sheltered children's stressors and coping behaviors. *Journal of Pediatric Nursing, 16,* 102–109.

Humphreys, J., Lee, K., Neylan, T., & Marmar, C. (2001). Psychological and physical distress of sheltered battered women. *Health Care Women International, 22,* 401–414.

Huston, C., & Fox, S. (1998). The changing healthcare market: Implications for nursing education in the coming decade. *Nursing Outlook, 46,* 109–114.

Keck, C. W., & Scutchfield, E. D. (1997). *Principles of public health practice.* Albany, NY: Delmar.

Kindig, D., & Stoddart, G. (2003). What is population health? *American Journal of Public Health, 93*(3), 380–383.

Lee, P. R., & Estes, C. L. (2003). *The nation's health* (7th ed.). Sudbury, MA: Jones and Bartlett.

National Center for Health Statistics. (2007). *Health, United States, 2007 with chartbook on trends in the health of Americans.* Hyattesville, MD: U.S. Department of Health and Human Services.

National Centers for Medicare and Medicaid. (2002a). *Complementary and alternative medicine use among adults: United States 2002.* Retrieved May 23, 2008, from http://www.cms.hhs.gov/

National Centers for Medicare and Medicaid. (2002b). *National home and hospice care survey: 2000.* Office of the Actuary. Retrieved May 23, 2008, from http://www.cms.hhs.gov/

National Centers for Medicare and Medicaid. (2004, January/February). National health expenditures 2002. *Health Affairs, 23*(1).

National Institute for Occupational Safety and Health. (2001). *NIOSH safety and health topics: Health care workers.* Retrieved May 23, 2008, from http://www.cdc.gov/niosh/topics/healthcare/

Organization for Economic Cooperation and Development. (2000). *OECD data 2000: A comparative analysis of twenty-nine countries.* Paris, France: Author.

Seidel, J. S., Henderson, D. P., & Lewis, J. B. (1991). Emergency medical services and the pediatric patient: Resources of ambulatory care centers. *Pediatrics, 88*(2), 230–235.

Shi, L., & Singh, D. A. (2008). *Delivering health care in America: A systems approach* (4th ed.). Sudbury, MA: Jones and Bartlett.

Starfield, B. (2000). *America's healthcare system is the third leading cause of death.* Retrieved October 8, 2008, from http://www.health-care-reform.net/causedeath.htm

Thorpe, K. E. (2004). Protecting the uninsured. *New England Journal of Medicine, 15*(351), 1479–1481.

U.S. Census Bureau. (2008a). *The 65 years and over population: 2000, Census 2000 brief.* Retrieved October 8, 2008, from http://www.census.gov/prod/2001pubs/c2kbr01-10.pdf

U.S. Census Bureau. (2008b). *Health insurance coverage: 2006.* Retrieved April 15, 2008, from http://www.census.gov/hhes/www.hlthins/hlthin06.html

Williams, S. J. (1993). Ambulatory health care services. In S. J. Williams & P. R. Torrens (Eds.), *Introduction to health services* (4th ed., pp. 108–133). Albany, NY: Delmar.

Williams, S., & Torrens, P. (2008) *Introduction to health services* (7th ed.). Clifton Park, NY: Cengage Delmar Learning

Zuvekas, S. H., & Hill, S. C. (2000). Income and employment among homeless people: The role of mental health, health and substance abuse. *Journal of Mental Health Policy Economics, 3,* 153–163.

# CHAPTER 6
# Managed Care

Ann H. Cary

Visit **http://nursing.jbpub.com/communityhealth** for interactive exercises, review questions, Web links, and more.

Nursing is managed care. . . . Since the early 1900s, expert nurses have been shepherding the care of acute and chronic patients in homes, clinics, and hospitals. Much has changed since those early days, but much has stayed the same. It's our job as nurses to develop a strong enough understanding of the needs of the system, of our own skills and strengths and those of our communities, that we can—collectively and individually—actively help craft the emerging system.

—B. B. Gray

Managed care is rapidly dominating the health care financing and delivery system in the United States. Managed care has also become big business. . . . Increasingly, the arrangements are difficult to characterize, let alone profile statistically, in a meaningful manner.

*—P. D. Fox in Kongstvedt, 2001, pp. 3–4.*

What comes to mind when you think of "managed care"? How do you see the future of nursing being shaped by managed care?

## CHAPTER FOCUS

**What Is Managed Care?**

**Principles of Managed Care**

**Managed Care Models**
- Indemnity Plans
- Point-of-Service Plans
- Health Maintenance Organizations
- Preferred Provider Organizations
- Community Nursing Organizations

**Management Mechanisms**

**Credentialing: Regulation and Accreditation**

**Ethical Issues**

**Nurses' Roles in Managed Care**

**Managed Care and Healthy Communities: Nursing's Approach**

**Managed Care Nursing as a Specialty with Membership and Certification Benefits**

## QUESTIONS TO CONSIDER

After reading this chapter, you will know the answers to the following questions:

1. What are the forces driving the development of managed care delivery systems?
2. What are the key principles of managed care?
3. What are the differences among managed care delivery models?
4. What are the requirements for credentialing for delivery systems?
5. What are the roles/skills of nurses working in managed care?
6. How can information about managed care be accessed via websites?

## KEY TERMS

Benefits interpreter
Patient advocate and educator
Case or care manager
Community nursing organizations (CNOs)
Fee-for-service plans
Gatekeeper
Health maintenance organization (HMO)

Health plan employer data and information set (HEDIS)
Indemnity plans
Managed care
National Committee on Quality Assurance (NCQA)
Pathfinder

Patient advocate
Physician hospital organization (PHO)
Point-of-service (POS) plan
Preferred provider organization (PPO)
Primary care provider
Provider liaison

Quality Compass
Risk manager
Safety net system
Triage nurse
Utilization and resource reviewer

## What Is Managed Care?

**Managed care** is a healthcare system that incorporates both financing and delivery of services. Typically, individuals join, enroll, or subscribe to a managed care plan. These individuals are known as the *covered lives* or *population* of the managed care organization (MCO). Subscribers or enrollees have health services provided by the organization in accordance with the coverage (services) identified in their contracts.

Financing and payment for managed care are typically prepaid so that a specific dollar amount is established to cover the costs of all health care for the enrollee. Payment to the plan/provider may be on a monthly or annual basis. In return for the capitated payment (per-person payment fee) arranged between the plan/provider and the payer (employer, government funder, and/or self-payer) enrollees receive a package of health care benefits, providers, quality and medical management reviews of their care, and financial incentives for using the plan procedures (URAC, 2008).

Managed care clearly targets a population of patients who are enrolled in or subscribed to a particular system and who value population-based outcomes by providers. Examples of this view of population-practice as a defining characteristic of managed care employers may include immunization and mammogram rates, access to primary care practitioners, and arrangements with public health, educational, and social service organizations.

Healthcare delivery continues to respond to market demands and state and federal policies. It is likely that health care systems in your community may look different from systems in other states or communities. Managed care systems have not appeared overnight and have been shaped by many architects. These systems are responding to employer demand to reduce the costs of the health care benefit for employees. Federal and state funding of Medicare and Medicaid services have followed the lead of non-government employers to demand cost-effective and quality access to appropriate health services. Consumers in communities without managed care systems have seen out-of-pocket expenses for their own care needs rise. Health care system boards and corporate stockholders have argued for the financial health of the corporation as well as corporate investment in the community.

The values of stakeholders have encouraged the presence of managed care in communities; however, the degree of penetration or market presence of managed care is dissimilar, especially relative to the Medicaid population. While costs of health services are the initial drivers of managed care systems, only those that provide cost-effective, quality plans will remain viable to the community. Clearly, nurses play a role in designing, implementing, and evaluating health care services for managed care populations.

The fee-for-service system, dominant in the twentieth century, has been viewed as a major force in escalating costs and strained employer, government, and individual budgets. Managed care, initiated in the 1920s, has moved from a gradual to a frantic pace in U.S. health care and is now a corrective force for reestablishing a balance in cost, quality, and access to services for patients, payers, and providers. Most employees now receive care from managed care plans. Additionally, legislation provides incentives for Medicare and Medicaid enrollees to access managed care systems.

## Principles of Managed Care

The following are the fundamentals of managed care systems:

1. All health care choices have a price, and choices for service are made by providers, patients/consumers, and administrators of health plans. All parties who choose are held accountable for the financial burden of the resources chosen. The more one party exercises the freedom of choice in health-related services (or selects services outside those services covered by an insurance plan), the greater the cost to that party (Packard, 1997; Spitzer-Lehmann, 1996).

2. Care is population based. The health status and actuarial data of enrolled and targeted populations support the structure and process of health care delivery. For example, the construction of health care teams and use of disease management protocols will be influenced by the number of diabetics or asthmatics represented in the health plan. Population-based outcomes such as health plan employer data and information set (HEDIS) measures are inherent values of mature managed care providers and credentialing bodies (Spitzer-Lehmann, 1996).

3. An MCO uses financial, clinical, community, policy, personal, and administrative information as the basis for ensuring quality and value (Spitzer-Lehmann, 1996). Obtaining and managing information are critical.

4. Primary care is central. Patients seek referrals from a primary care provider who is responsible for coordinating care before receiving services of a medical specialist (Spitzer-Lehmann, 1996).

5. Integration and interdependence from a systems perspective are critical (e.g., provider mix, seamless information flow, coordination). Continuity and integration of clinical and financial services are important to strong managed care.

6. Financing, insurance, delivery, and payment are linked in managed care systems (Shi & Singh, 2008).

7. Consumers have rights in managed care systems. In December 1997, President Clinton's Advisory Commission on Consumer Protection and Quality in the Health Care Industry issued its *Principles and Consumer Bill of Rights*, which are now incorporated in all federally supported health care activities (see Box 6-1). Four principles guiding the *Consumer Bill of Rights and Responsibilities* in accessing and receiving health care include the following:
   • All health care consumers are created equal.
   • Quality comes first in health care.

- The parts of the health care system that work are preserved.
- Costs matter and must be identified and related to outcomes of health care.

Beck and Dempsey (1996) reveal that successful managed care models are noted for pricing practices, defined provider networks, risk sharing of costs, and care management techniques. For instance, when an MCO sets prices, it may use mathematical models to predict what costs will be influenced by the cost of living data for the region, will use and encounter patterns of enrollees, will determine the age and sex of enrollees, and will examine the nature of health care management in the system. Discounts are typically applied to providers in the system because this is a method to increase volume or reduce the chance of losing volume of payment. Managed care models use capitation pricing to pay providers a fixed amount per member per month to provide all defined services. Providers may be protected from situations where premiums do not cover costs, such as in catastrophic cases (e.g., patients with human immunodeficiency virus [HIV], transplants, multisystem failure), with the MCO agreeing to pay the provider by a fee-for-service method above a certain amount (e.g., $15,000). Conversely, providers (physicians and nurse practitioners) share in the risks of using more resources than forecasted or budgeted by having payments withheld from them; however, when the MCO has a financial surplus, providers may share in the distribution of bonuses or stock. For the MCO to provide for all needed services, it contracts with myriad providers (psychiatrists, home health agencies, pharmacies, durable medical equipment suppliers) to guarantee coverage for benefits.

Care management techniques examine the use of services, costs, and performance measures of providers. Some of these measures include controls on referrals, preauthorization for services (e.g., for diagnostics and emergency care), number and costs of prescriptions written, and frequency of office visits. As is apparent, each of these activities requires capabilities in database information development and management to provide answers to the following questions: What do we provide; to whom; what are the outcomes; how do we compare; what do patients think of services; how can we perform consistent with our targets; and what are our trends?

## Managed Care Models

The health plan and service marketplace is becoming more specialized and fragmented based on the expectations of patients, providers, employers, and other stakeholders. The ultimate challenge is to ensure the continued integrity and accountability of health care to consumers and patients.

Of course, the wide variety of health plan and insurance options makes it more difficult for consumers to fully understand the health care system. In fact, the definitional labels and constructs used—PPOs, HMOs, POS, and indemnity—in some ways may be more appropriate for a history book than describing current and future events.

That is why it is so important for consumers and patients to understand the various "functions" that make up their health plan arrangement. As a result, a more useful way to look at the current health insurance system is to look at the specific services and activities that underpin each health care offering (see Table 6-1), rather than simply at the product label. This should empower consumers to receive better health care for their specific needs.

Managed care comes in many forms, each with nuances that affect eligibility, access, patient costs, benefits, and management processes (URAC, 2008). Rules and policies of a specific managed care plan will guide the functions of your nursing practice.

### ■ Indemnity Plans

**Indemnity plans** are also known as fee-for-service (FFS) plans. In such a plan, patients access their provider of choice. The provider submits a claim to the insurance company, which then reimburses the provider for covered services. There is no network or group of providers who have agreed to accept patients by contract. This type of managed care is managed only by the patient, who must be cognizant of the degree to which services will be reimbursed (typically 80% is paid and patient pays the difference). Patients will usually contribute to the charges for health care through coinsurance (the portion the patient pays) and deductibles (the amount the patient pays annually before any reimbursement is received).

### ■ Point-of-Service Plans

Reacting to the backlash against managed care gatekeeping, **point-of-service (POS) plans** typically allow the patient to receive care within a network of (preauthorized) providers or to go "out of network" for care. By going "out of network," the patient absorbs additional costs and receives less coverage

---

**BOX 6-1**

**Consumer Bill of Rights and Responsibilities, 1997**

Consumers' rights in health care include the following:

- Accurate, literacy-appropriate information
- Choice of providers sufficient to ensure quality care
- Access to appropriate (a prudent layperson's definition of) emergency care
- Participative decision making relative to health care options
- Respectful and nondiscriminatory care
- Confidentiality and access to own health information
- Fair and efficient process for complaints/appeals
- Assumption of responsibility for health, decision making, and treatment plans

*Source:* Advisory Commission on Consumer Protection and Quality in the Health Care Industry. (1997). *Consumer bill of rights and responsibilities: Report to the President of the United States.* Washington, DC: U.S. Government Printing Office.

**Table 6-1**    The ABCs of Health Plan Coverage

| Activity | | PPO | HMO | POS | Indemnity |
|---|---|---|---|---|---|
| **Market Share** | Change in recent market share | Rapid expansion | Holding steady or slightly decreasing | Increasing | Decreasing |
| | Employer-based coverage | 49% | 31% | 14% | 6% |
| | Medicare coverage | Low to none | Moderate | Low to none | High (government assumes risk) |
| | Medicaid coverage | Low | Moderate | Low | High (government assumes risk) |
| | Federal health employee program | High | High | ? | Low to moderate |
| **Regulation** | State | Moderate: 35 states have some requirements | High: All 50 states have some requirements | Moderate | High: All 50 states have some requirements |
| | Federal | Infrequent | High | Some | Moderate |
| **Typical Features** | Network-based health care offering | Yes | Yes | Usually | No |
| | Provider credentialing for network panel | Basic verification | Yes | HMO-sponsored: Yes Other: basic verification | Not applicable |
| | Active enrollment of covered life and dependents? | Usually not | Yes | Depends on product sponsor | Usually not |
| | Primary care physician? | No | Yes | Yes, if HMO-sponsored | No |
| | Insurance function: assumes risk? | Usually not | Yes | Most states no, unless POS also has indemnity license | Yes |

for services. Some health maintenance organizations have a POS option. The POS product is growing in the United States as a managed care approach.

### ■ Health Maintenance Organizations

A **health maintenance organization (HMO)** is a prepaid networking delivery system. Typically care provided outside the network is not covered. Due to the federal HMO Act of 1973, HMOs are heavily regulated at the state level. Even within the HMO classification, several types of plans exist. Some contract with independent provider groups while employing staff to administer operations and clinical support. Other HMOs hire providers as employees. Patients are assigned to a primary care provider who coordinates referrals

to specialists. HMOs have been industry leaders in providing appropriate quality processes, including utilization management, care management, and disease management.

 THINK ABOUT THIS

Five percent of health plan members account for 50% of total plan expenditures. One percent or less of health plan members generate 20% to 23% of all costs. Highest-risk population case management in a managed care system is critical to managing quality of care, prevention, and costs.

*Source*: Glynn, K., & Patel, K. (2004). Ensuring quality of highest-risk population care management in a teleworking environment. *Case Manager, 15*(3), 61–64.

**Table 6-1**     The ABCs of Health Plan Coverage

| | Activity | PPO | HMO | POS | Indemnity |
|---|---|---|---|---|---|
| | Patient cost sharing through copayments or deductibles? | Moderate | Low | Moderate | High |
| **Benefits** | Preventive health care | Low to moderate | High | Moderate | Moderate |
| | Customized product offering for different clients? | High | Low | Some | Some |
| **Accessibility** | Typical network size | Large | Moderate | Depends on product offering | Not applicable |
| | Access to specialty care | High | Moderate | Depends on product sponsor | High |
| | Out-of-network option? | Yes | No | Yes | Yes (but no network to begin with) |
| **Medical Management** | Gatekeeper function? | Usually not | Yes | Usually yes | No |
| | Utilization or case management? | Usually yes | Yes | Usually yes | No (Managed indemnity may have some basic utilization review procedures) |
| | Case management? | Sometimes | Often | Usually yes | Usually not |
| | Disease management? | Sometimes | Sometimes | Sometimes | Usually not |
| | Accreditation (e.g., URAC, NCQA, JCAHO) | Sometimes | Often | Sometimes | Infrequent |
| | Quality reporting (e.g., J. D. Power, CAHPS, HEDIS) | Sometimes | Often | Sometimes | Infrequent |

*Source*: Adapted from the ABC's of health coverage: The four basic types of health plans. URAC. (2004). Retrieved September 15, 2004, from www.URAC.org.

## ■ Preferred Provider Organizations

In a **preferred provider organization (PPO)**, a network of health care providers agrees to provide care at a contracted reimbursement rate. In return for access to volumes of patients, discounted charges are typically offered to the employee or insurance carrier. PPOs will customize the types of benefits depending on the plan sponsor, thereby allowing the employer to control costs and benefits. There are many variations in the PPO models.

## Community Nursing Organizations

Although not widely identified in health systems and health services literature, **community nursing organizations (CNOs)** constitute a type of managed care. In 1987, Congress authorized through budget act legislation (the Omnibus Reconciliation Act [OBRA]) the funding of a CNO demonstration project composed of four national sites, which remain in existence today: Carle Clinic, Carondoler Health Services, Visiting Nurse Service of New York, and Living at Home/Block, Nurse Program. These projects examined the role of nursing in providing high-quality care with capitated payments for Medicare beneficiaries through a nurse-centered managed care model of financing and delivery at each site. The goals of these CNOs were to prevent unnecessary institutionalization, provide preventive and health promotion services, coordinate care to promote continuity, and demonstrate effective use of prospective (prepaid) and capitation payment methods. Medicare recipients had to obtain all nonemergency services through the CNO, which included home health services (nursing, therapies, aides, supplies, dressings); prosthetics and durable medical equipment; ambulance service; outpatient visits to physical therapists, clinical psychologists, or social workers; primary nursing services (in-person consultations, care plan development, coordination of services, care monitoring); consultations with family and physicians; and homemaker/personal care (May, Schraeder, & Britt, 1996).

In these CNOs, the nurse partner and nurse case manager were key. Nurse partner caseloads were linked with primary care physicians to optimize collaboration on enrollees' health care plans. This collaboration attempted to achieve efficiency and effectiveness of service type, level, intensity, and frequency. The nurse case manager authorized any CNO service for the patient. Because community-based services are important to reduce inappropriate institutionalization, the CNO nurse partner managed transitional services among sites and supported member access to little-known community resources. Nurse partners strongly emphasized health promotion activities for improved lifestyles and recommended prevention activities.

Examples of nursing actions in the CNO environment include assessment of health status and authorization for service; phone calls to monitor care; education by telephone, face to face, and electronic mail; use of advocacy skills to initiate and monitor referrals with patients; and evaluations of caseloads and individuals, based on service authorization and use to establish best-evidence practice patterns. Many of these functions are considered case management activities.

## Management Mechanisms

Managed care models embrace a large variation in organizational structure, consumer choices, financial risks, consumer rights, and grievance procedures (Kongstvedt, 2001). However, all use one or more management mechanisms to regulate incentives and behavior:

- Contracts between insurers and providers to ensure comprehensive services but only necessary treatments
- Utilization, care, and decease management
- Explicit provider selection and monitoring of standards and financial incentives for consumers to use designated providers
- Direct contracting with cost-effective and evidence-based providers
- Discounted provider reimbursement
- Cost sharing by enrollees for more expensive services
- Pharmacy benefit management
- Integrated information systems

Nurses employed in these systems must be able to assess the effectiveness and efficiency of these services and be advocates for the benefit of populations of service. Consumers and employees with regular options to change enrollment among the managed care plans are increasingly challenged to compare benefit and liability implications as well as to make judgments of quality performance among providers.

 **Research Alert**

Case management (CM) is a systems management process used in a variety of managed care settings, with a variety of populations and conditions. This research demonstrates the benefits—both resource consumption and financial savings—of using nurse case managers. A **physician hospital organization (PHO)** used registered nurse case managers to study the effect of case management processes on acute and community-based resource consumption during one year for patients who had more than one emergency room or inpatient admission or an inpatient stay of 10 days or more. Patients were assessed for physical, social, financial, and caregiver issues, and case managers ensured that appropriate levels of support were provided, including community resources offered by church groups. Patients experiencing CM rated their health as good 60.3% of the time compared with 24.7% who rated their health as good before CM services. Emergency room visits, hospital days, and admissions also decreased. The "frail elderly" were admitted less often and for shorter lengths of stay. Finally, the average saving per patient was $3,963.94, which included emergency room and hospital admissions as well as pharmacy charges.

*Sources*: Hanbury, M., Seyler, E., & Upham, S. (2002) Hartford physician hospital organization community case management program improves patient care while decreasing medical costs. *Connecticut Medicine, 9,* 549–552; Markle, A. (2004). The economic impact of case management. *Case Manager, 15*(4), 54–58.

## Credentialing: Regulation and Accreditation

Organizations and systems delivering health care services are subject to oversight activities by external bodies. Typical regulatory oversight includes licensure by the state, certification by a government agency, and/or accreditation by a voluntary accrediting organization. Each oversight mechanism requires that certain conditions must be met. The aim of the regulatory mechanism is to ensure integrity of the organization and activities as well as the safety of the public's health.

Organizational credentialing is required in addition to the credentialing of an individual provider required by the practice discipline. Credentialing of providers is an important legal obligation of the MCO. Credentialing can include verification of provider's license, certification, malpractice coverage, charting procedures, and practice privileges, to name a few. As you may recall, nurses are licensed by the state and may be certified in an area of specialty practice by voluntary professional organizations. To meet regulatory standards, organizations typically require that health professional employees (e.g., nurses) hold current licensure and certification credentials to practice in that system.

Several voluntary organizations offer accreditation processes (organizational credentialing) and designations to managed care plans and networks:

**The National Committee on Quality Assurance (NCQA)** is a nonprofit organization created to improve

(See Box 6-2 for a comprehensive list.)

## CULTURAL CONNECTION

Consider the possibility that specific cultural values of families may be in opposition to seeking assistance from outside professional resources. How can the community health nurse work within a managed care environment to provide mutual optimal care for these families?

patient care quality and health plan performance in conjunction with managed care plans, purchasers, consumers, and the public. In some states NCQA accreditation of managed care plans is mandated and used by most of the Fortune 500 employers and by federal and state governments (NCQA, 2008c). The process targets quality improvement, credentialing, members' rights and responsibilities, utilization management, preventive services, and medical records. NCQA has constructed a national database of information on the quality of managed care plans so that performance and accreditation information for each plan can be compared by the public. More than 90% of managed care plans submit data congruent with the NCQA-sponsored HEDIS, which contains performance measures (NCQA, 2008a). As an example, clinical HEDIS measures reflect important performance contributions to the health status of U.S. consumers—screening for breast cancer, screening for cervical cancer, performing childhood and adult immunizations, performing diabetic eye examinations, and helping patients control cholesterol.

Data on HEDIS measures provide a global performance picture for clinical quality in general and for specific plans for which the public may query. The *Healthy People 2010* objectives can serve as a national gold standard against which clinical HEDIS measures are designed, monitored, and evaluated (e.g., immunization rates). The NCQA **Quality Compass** is the name of the database that contains accreditation and HEDIS information from more than 250 health plans that cover more than 60 million Americans. Updated CD-ROMs for Quality Compass are available periodically to provide current information from existing and new participants. These statistics are important to employers and consumers in choosing among managed care plans. The data also assist managed care plans to set performance goals and monitor improvement and accountability. Finally, NCQA makes health care quality information accessible without charge by website and other media (NCQA, 2008d).

URAC (American Accreditation Healthcare Commission, Inc.) is the largest accreditation organization for health care (URAC, 2008). It accredits managed care organizations, other types of organizations, and even programs within organizations such as case management. URAC

publishes standards developed by experts who represent diversity within the health care community. A comparison of these standards as well as a site visit by the accreditation team constitute the accreditation process. The summary of the URAC standards can be accessed online at www.urac .org. As a nurse working in managed care, you are likely to be involved in some manner in the accreditation process.

Other accreditation bodies offering credentialing to various types of managed care plans include the Joint Commission on Accreditation of Health Care Organizations (JCAHO) for integrated delivery networks and health plans (JCAHO, 2004). (See Box 6-2 for a comprehensive list.)

As managed care penetration has increased nationally, consumer advocates, the media, and lawmakers have voiced issues of clinical integrity, access, and satisfactory performance within the mantra of public safety. Although HMOs are heavily regulated by state and federal legislation, other models are less stringently regulated. The debate concerning whether voluntary accreditation mechanisms are sufficient to ensure the health of the "enrolled" public has generated a demand for legislative regulation of the managed care industry. A Presidential Advisory Commission on Consumer Protection and Quality in the Health Care Industry issued

### BOX 6-2

**Public/Private Credentialing of Managed Care**

**AAAHC:** American Association for Ambulatory Health Care is a private organization that conducts voluntary quality reviews of ambulatory health centers including HMOs.

**CHAP:** Community Health Accreditation Program is a private voluntary accreditation program for home care agencies and community nursing organizations.

**CMS:** Centers for Medicare and Medicaid Services is a government agency that reviews federally qualified HMOs under the Federal HMO Act.

**JCAHO:** Joint Commission on Accreditation of Healthcare Organizations conducts a voluntary, private accreditation for health care networks.

**NAIC:** National Association of Insurance Commissioners is a private organization that publishes a model act to help state legislatures adapt licensure laws for HMOs.

**NCQA:** National Committee for Quality Assurance (see text).

**OPM:** Office of Personnel Management audits HMOs and health plans under Federal Employees Health Benefits Programs.

**PROs:** Peer review organizations provide mandatory quality reviews of inpatient and outpatient care for Medicare beneficiaries enrolled in Medicare risk contracting HMOs.

**State licensure of PPOs:** Many states require the PPO and PPO-like plans to go through a licensure process.

**URAC:** American Accreditation Healthcare Commission is a private organization made up of health care associations and labor groups whose goal is to improve the quality and efficiency of interactions among the utilization review industry, providers, payers, and purchasers of health care. It establishes accreditation standards for managed health care in the United States.

 ENVIRONMENTAL CONNECTION

A part of the managed care approach is assessing the environmental needs of the patient, such as physical accommodations in the home for specific health conditions.

Research Alert

After reading many articles on ethics, the author recognized a need for a common understanding of what constitutes ethical decision making. Through her exploration of the philosophical and cultural origins of ethics, the author attempts to clarify the domain of healthcare ethics and examines how these ideas apply to administrative practice. ◯

*Source*: Taft, S. H. (2001). An inclusive look at the domain of ethics and its application to administrative behavior. *The Online Journal of Issues in Nursing*. Retrieved October 27, 2008, from http://www.nursingworld.org/MainMenuCategories/ANAMarketplace/ANAPeriodicals/OJIN/TableofContents/Volume62001/No1Jan01/ArticlePreviousTopic/DomainofEthics.aspx

the *Patient's Bill of Rights* in 1997, and federal legislative efforts have since addressed issues of preexisting conditions, transportable health insurance coverage for uninsured children, and changes in Medicare to encourage more elderly patients to seek managed care. Internally, health industry leaders are attempting to ensure voluntary compliance with quality standards as an alternative to additional government regulations for the industry. Clearly, there is not consensus that voluntary standards are sufficient in the absence of a regulatory framework. Such a framework in the future may include government oversight and/or quasi-governmental bodies as regulatory structures.

## Ethical Issues

Four major stakeholders are typically affected by managed care systems. Situations abound in which the goals among stakeholders conflict, resulting in ethical issues and dilemmas not easily resolved to the satisfaction of all parties. Stakeholders include patients, providers, investors/stockholders, and the community. Silva (1998) identifies six problem areas related to MCOs:

1. Limited numbers of within-system providers
2. Financial penalties for out-of-network provider use
3. Imposition of gag rules to limit information on choice of treatments
4. Restrictive formularies for drugs
5. Lack of accountability of MCO to external assurance organizations or regulators
6. Inadequate appeals procedures for complainants

In addition, MCO saturation in a market may rob the community of resources to deliver uncompensated care. For example, physicians in a community may not be able to provide as much uncompensated care because of the decline of their own incomes when they become employers in managed care systems. The safety net system of providers in voluntary and public health systems is then stressed to provide additional services. Another concern is price competition, which requires sacrificing quality to meet price requirements that cannot be met except through denial of appropriate care. Finally, MCOs may engage in deceptive advertising and enrollment strategies, selecting and aggressively enrolling only healthy participants. These examples illustrate the ethical

### Application to Practice

*Maintaining Tom's Functional Status: Managed Costs, Managed Care, or Both?*

Tom is a disabled skier living in Vermont and working at Maple, Inc. His employer, provides two options for health plans, MAC-MCO and SHMO-MCO, both managed care entities. Tom has worn a high leg prosthesis since adolescence, when he lost his left leg in an auto accident. Lately Tom has sensed that the bearings on his prosthesis are disintegrating, causing difficulty in functioning. He contacts his primary care provider at MAC-MCO Systems and both agree to an evaluation for replacement. Tom asks the managed care plan to cover the services of Eli Prostotic, of Prostotic, Inc., because Eli crafted and fit his original and subsequent prostheses and accomplished a perfect fit each time.

1. Initially MAC-MCO denied the referral to Prostotics because it was an out-of-network provider. Tom wrote a letter of appeal. You are the nurse in charge of the appeals section at MAC-MCO.
   • What type of evidence would you require in the appeal letter to justify coverage of Tom's out-of-network referral?
2. Based on the estimate of $37,670 submitted by Prostotic, Inc., for the prosthetic device and services, you recognize this is 20% higher than your network provider. You authorize half the payment by MAC-MO and half paid by Tom. Tom appeals this decision.
   • What type of evidence would you require in the second appeal letter to justify MAC-MCO expending $37,670 on this prosthesis?
   • What other negotiations would you orchestrate to meet the financial guidelines of Tom's benefit under the MAC-MCO contract?
   • Who are the parties who will be financially impacted by these negotiations for a new prosthesis?
   • Which aspects of patient advocacy conflict with your role as systems allocator?

dilemmas for communities when cost and market share are the overriding values in market competition.

Within MCOs, nurses simultaneously fulfill the role of **patient advocate** and system/services allocator. As a nurse fulfilling these dual roles, you may confront dilemmas in practice when you implement or witness the activities within the MCO system. Cary (1998) notes the conundrums apparent when the allocator and advocate roles work discordantly with patient care and systems resources. Box 6-3 highlights the barriers to access for enrollees based on systems resource constraints.

## Nurses' Roles in Managed Care

When you explore the systems of managed care as your potential employer, the roles of the managed care nurse will have likenesses and dissimilarities to nurses seeking employment in acute care, long-term care, and other health care settings. However, the use of a systematic process of care management based on the context of biopsychosocial, environmental, informatics, and organizational theories as applied through the nursing process reflect the strength of

> **"**The gap between ideals and actualities, between dreams and achievements, the gap that can spur strong men to increased exertions, but can break the spirit of others—this gap is the most conspicuous, continuous landmark in American history. It is conspicuous and continuous not because Americans achieve little, but because they dream grandly. The gap is a standing reproach to Americans; but it marks them off as a special and singularly admirable community among the world's peoples. **"**
>
> —George F. Will

nursing to ensure managed care successes. Opportunities and specific skills for nurses working with managed care systems are listed in Box 6-4.

As an additional resource, the ANA describes eight roles and subsequent functions of nurses in managed care as explicated below (ANA, 1995):

1. **Benefits interpreter**. This role is key to the education of members in managed care organizations so that they clearly understand the benefits available to them. Likewise, the nurse explains the grievance procedures available to clarify or dispute interpretations. Because member satisfaction is a critical component of stable enrollment, the effectiveness of the nurse as a benefits interpreter is essential to the organization.

2. **Patient advocate and educator**. Of all disciplines employed in managed care, nurses with their educational background in clinical and behavioral science can ensure a variety of skillful educational and empowerment strategies in working with clientele. Advocacy helps identify needed care and education, including prevention of diseases, promotion of health, and the protection of groups of people from environmental risks. Advocacy activities may entail educating clientele on the existence and use of covered services, educating management on the collective and exceptional needs of enrollees, and educating payers and communities about the emerging gaps in essential and supportive services that can undermine a population's health status.

3. **Triage nurse**. Triaging is an activity that directs access to services so that they are efficiently and effectively used. Nurses may use telecommunications to process

---

**BOX 6-3**

**Barriers to Access/Utilization in Managed Care: Advocacy and Allocation Dilemmas**

- Few choices of plans and no point-of-service options in a benefit package
- Absence of services in a plan
- Employees limited to choice of providers selected by the insurer
- Providers excluded or rotated from panels for reasons unrelated to quality performance/efficiency measures
- Provider behaviors predicated on economic incentives and threats
- "Gag" rules for providers (withholding information)
- Administrative rules that limit visit times, services, and referrals
- Administrative controls on providers to reduce utilization
- Waste in administrative activities and duplication in clinical processes
- Culturally insensitive providers of care
- Inadequate staffing
- Less-than-competent provider substitution
- Lack of communication between and within information systems
- Providers who fail to assert the ethical guidelines and codes of the profession

*Source*: Adapted from Cary, 1998.

## BOX 6-4

### New Opportunities and the Accompanying Skills

Nurses can position themselves to accept the emerging roles in managed care systems. To assist in this process, the following seven areas of opportunity for nurses in a managed care environment and the skills needed to take on these new roles have been identified.

#### Consumer Advocacy
- Use of decision trees/tools
- Projection of statistical probabilities
- Negotiation skills
- Group interaction and facilitation
- Patient teaching using new media
- Understanding of principles of ethics

#### Change Agent
- Understand chaos theory/change theory
- Leadership skills versus management skills
- Self-managed team abilities
- Grasp of organizational behavior and development theory

#### Individual Growth
- Self-empowerment
- Professional image
- New self-accountability for lifelong learning and relevancy in a changing environment
- Computer literacy
- Networking ability
- Business-related skills: verbal and written presentation skills, communication technology familiarity, publication/media production, economics/finance forecasting skills
- Sensitivity to cost and quality, total quality management process, benchmarking, utilization management cost analysis, data integrity, tracking and manipulation, "best practices"

#### Community-Based Care
- Cultural competence
- Assessment
- Population-focused care
- Innovative approaches to enhancing health of a community
- Epidemiology and environmental health
- Understanding concepts of risk

#### Information Systems
- Computer-related skills
- Informatics
- Decision support systems
- Ability to access and process data

#### Entrepreneurs/Intrapreneurs
- Understanding of contracts
- Abilities in innovative program development
- Marketing/selling
- Program budgeting
- Business plan development
- Problem identification and costing of solutions

#### Public Health  Policy and Regulatory Bodies
- Legislative skills
- Knowledge of civics
- Understanding of administrative, legislative, and judicial roles of government
- Knowledge of key regulatory bodies related to nursing and health care
- Basic skill in legal interpretation and drafting

*Source*: ANA, 1996, p. 19.

---

 ETHICAL CONNECTION

Too many Americans feel trapped in a system which does not put their health care needs first. They believe that HMOs value a paper dollar more than they do a human life. We cannot continue to ignore the rights of patients. We have allowed the health care reform debate to be determined by special interest groups.

—John McCain, 1999

How have special-interest groups influenced how health care is delivered in the United States? Does this affect the practice of nursing? How?

inquiries as well as onsite visits for complex, sudden, or acute events. Anchored in a firm knowledge base of clinical health and disease states and established best practice guidelines, the triage nurse assists the patient to identify problems and symptoms, reviews the medical record, provides clinical decisions on appropriate op-tions, advises patients, and secures appropriate services. In many cases, the triage nurse is the first point of contact for entry to a service of the health plan.

4. **Utilization and resource reviewer.** Utilization managers help control health care costs by assessing the appropriateness of care and ensuring use of the least costly treatments known to be effective. Utilization review includes a number of data-gathering activities that measure the appropriateness, necessity, and quality of care. Mechanisms of review may include preadmission certification, concurrent review with discharge planning, retrospective review of care, length of stay, site of care, and treatment appropriateness. Nurses have been historically employed in this role for insurance companies.

5. **Risk manager.** The risk manager's goal is to decrease the occurrence of unintended adverse events and outcomes for patients and the organization. In achieving risk management outcomes, the nurse identifies potential risk factors and situations detrimental to patients' health; analyzes patterns and frequencies of events to detect system, structure, and process deficits; evaluates alternative

approaches to reducing risks; and implements corrective action. Monitoring sentinel events/patterns is essential to this role of detecting emergent disease patterns or risks to quality in the system.

6. **Provider liaison.** The administrative, clinical, and financial structures and processes in a managed care organization require collaboration, teaming, cooperation, and coordination among providers to achieve clear intended outcomes. The role of provider liaison requires the nurse to provide information and to interact with a variety of health professionals. This ensures that patients understand the functions and responsibilities of each team member as they receive coordinated care from interdisciplinary providers at different sites of care.

7. **Primary care provider.** In this role, the nurse is the first point of contact and identifies further steps to manage a patient's presentation of complaints and history as well as initiates referrals to other providers or specialists. Terms that are used for this role are **gatekeeper**, **pathfinder**, or provider of first contact. Because of the advanced clinical skills required in this role, MCOs may employ advanced practice registered nurses to fill these roles and positions.

8. **Case or care manager.** "If you have seen a case manager you have seen one case manager." The roles of case managers vary considerably among different systems. Some case managers monitor the long-term needs of enrollees, whereas while others manage the current episode of care. Case managers use critical pathways, care maps, and disease management protocols to identify key events that must occur to achieve outcomes. This ensures that the patient progresses through the restoration/maintenance goals appropriately or that needed readjustments in the plan are made.

In community-based case management, the role of case manager requires a comprehensive knowledge of complementary community resources, eligibility requirements, and expected outcomes. For catastrophic illnesses, closely managed care provides patients with appropriate monitoring, the matching of resources to the stage of illness, monitoring of financial impact, and utilization of the right service at the right time for the desired outcome. Highly developed communication skills, multi-method assessment and monitoring tools to gauge need and progress, negotiation and advocacy strategies, information management, and financial forecasting are essential. The ultimate risks to be avoided by case managers include fragmentation or duplication of service, inappropriate utilization of providers and intensity of service, and denial of appropriate care (Cary, 1998, 2008; Steinhauser, 1999).

**Research Alert**

Chronic disease prevention, early treatment, and reduced complications are all targeted in the *Healthy People 2010* report. People with diabetes are at high risk for comorbidity as well as complications. Quality health care systems can reduce complications. Continuity of care, which involves a usual site of care as well as a usual provider of care, may contribute to better diabetic control.

This study analyzed data from the Third National Health and Nutrition Examination Survey (NHANES III) using a national sample of 1,400 adult diabetics to examine the effects of continuity of care on control of diabetes and associated chronic conditions. Continuity of care was associated with better glycemic control but not better blood pressure or lipid control among diabetics. These results were the same whether there was a usual site of care or a usual provider of care.

*Source:* Mainous, A. G., Koopman, R. J., Gill, J. M., Baker R., & Pearson, W. S. (2004). Relationship between continuity of care and diabetic control: Evidence from the Third National Health and Nutrition Exam Survey. *American Journal of Public Health, 94*(1), 66–77.

## Managed Care and Healthy Communities: Nursing's Approach

In the absence of a policy of universal access to health care in the United States and the emergence of market-based health care, certain populations continue to need public support to obtain necessary health and social services. The term *health care safety net* includes the institutions, programs, and professionals who harness resources to serve the uninsured or the socially disadvantaged. Typical providers include urban public hospitals, community health centers, inner-city teaching hospitals, and local health departments. Populations in our communities using the safety-net systems include the uninsured, Medicaid recipients, persons with acquired immune deficiency syndrome (AIDS), substance abusers, frail elderly, children from low-income families, low-income pregnant women, the homeless, and the mentally ill (Baxter & Mechanic, 1997).

There are major concerns in communities where managed care reduces the revenue streams for safety-net systems and providers. These cross-subsidies that have supported the safety-net services are in danger of disappearing. This means that fewer of the most vulnerable, who are in most need of services, will be able to obtain care from a shrinking safety net of community services and providers. The impact of market-driven managed care on the safety-net options for health and social services in a community must be monitored by community health nurses, who often serve on the front line of providing care to marginalized populations.

In 1998, the ANA issued a guide for nurses endorsing principles of managed care on which policies and social action could be interpreted. Within the emerging systems of

**THINK ABOUT THIS**

- Workers with the following characteristics are most likely to be uninsured: self-employed, working in small businesses, low wage earners, part-time workers.
- The risk of being uninsured is relative to the size of the business. You are more likely to be uninsured in a business with fewer than 25 employees.
- Workers earning less than $10 per hour were at greater risk for lacking health insurance.

*Source*: Carroll, W. (2001). Statistical Brief No. 11. *The Health Insurance of US Workers, 2001.* Center for Cash and Financing Studies, AHRQ Medical Expenditures Panel Survey.

managed care in our communities and with large numbers of both acute and community-based nurses encountering the challenges of delivering appropriate health care, these principles offer an emphasis on patient advocacy and consumer protection, enhanced quality of care accountability, and increased access to an appropriate array of services (ANA, 1998).

Market-driven managed care will ultimately survive only if consumers and providers work to achieve quality outcomes substantiated by evidenced-based practices with populations. Nurses working in MCOs and with patients covered by MCO and/or safety-net providers must maintain the broad view of health to include environments for education, behavior, income, housing, community needs, and social services. Nurses must remain responsive to community needs and faithful to the application of principles that support health care access, quality, and cost efficiencies in an effort to achieve healthy communities.

### Got an Alternative?

Complementary health practices utilized by patients as part of self-care management, such as meditation, relaxation, and yoga, can be an important aspect of the overall managed care plan.

## Managed Care Nursing as a Specialty with Membership and Certification Benefits

In contrast to a direct service provider to individual patients, managed care nurses advocate for all patients in the system, administer benefits within the limits of the system, and provide customer service for all nurse encounters in the system (AAMCN, 2008). Because these nurses may be implementing demand management, quality management, disease management, and case management programs as well as wellness and prevention programs, the population perspective is critical to effective practice.

The American Association of Managed Care Nurses (AAMCN) is a membership organization of nurses as-

sociated with managed care. In 2004, AAMCN published *Managed Care Nursing Practice Standards* (AAMCN, 2004a, 2004b), which describes standards used at all levels of managed care nursing and includes the following information:

- Philosophy of managed care nursing
- Opportunities in managed care nursing
- Individuals involved in managed care nursing
- Quality and legal issues involved in managed care nursing
- Managed care acronyms
- Source key and references
- Managed care nursing model and components

Another resource developed by AAMCN is the study guide *A Comprehensive Introduction to Managed Care Nursing*, which informs nurses of the issues, roles, industry products, and quality processes used in managed care systems (AAMCN, 2004, 2008). The *Journal of Managed Care Medicine* is a part of the AAMCN membership benefit.

You can access information about this specialty organization by contacting www.aamcn.org.

Nurses can be certified in the specialty of managed care nursing by successfully passing the Certified Managed Care Nurse (CMCN) certification exam sponsored by the American Board of Managed Care Nursing (ABMCN). Nurses who pass the exam use the initials CMCN as part of their professional signatures. A current RN who seeks the designation of CMCN must meet the required score of knowledge on four components: managed care overview, health care economics, health care management, and patient issues. For additional information about certification requirements and processes, see www.abmcn.org.

## Conclusion

Managed care delivery systems have swept across the United States; there is even evidence in Europe, the Middle East, and Malaysia to suggest that managed care is being implemented alongside existing delivery systems. Patients enrolled in managed care systems are likely to experience fewer medical procedures, greater standardization of care, less opportunity to select a provider of choice without personal financial risks, shorter hospital stays, and greater numbers of outpatient and ambulatory care procedures. Nurses employed in these systems are offered greater staff development and continuing education opportunities as organizations attempt to "right-skill" their employees. New skills in technology, information systems, case management, delegation of patient care activities, performance assessment and improvement activities, advocacy, and allocation functions will be required of nurses employed by these systems.

There are many structures and types of managed care organizations operating in communities. Nurses must understand the structure, processes, goals, and outcomes expected by the MCO seeking to employ a nurse. Additional skill development may enhance a nurse's competitive chance for employment positions in these systems. Opportunities to apply clinical and program development skills in wellness and prevention are expected to rise in MCOs. However, nurses must be alert to ethical dilemmas that occur when access to care is prescribed by organizational financial goals in contrast to a patient's need for appropriate services. Nurses will hold roles as both patient advocate and service allocator in these new systems of care to communities.

Explore Community Health Nursing on the Web! To learn more about the topics in this chapter, use the passcode provided to access your exclusive website: **http://nursing.jbpub.com/ communityhealth.** If you do not have a passcode, you can obtain one at this site.

## ■ CRITICAL THINKING ACTIVITIES

1. You are a nurse employed by Start-Up Managed Care attempting to sell the Start-Up managed care plan to the local cabinet production company called CPC in your community. This employer will have 35,000 potential covered lives if you are successful in securing a contract.
   - Explain the Wellness Program and Services (WPS) feature of your benefit plan. What types of services are offered? Why would CPC be interested in the WPS feature of your plan? What data could you provide to convince the CPC health benefits administrator of the value of WPS for the company, for employees, for the community?
   - Discuss four "rights" that patients of managed care organizations can expect to receive.
   - Discuss two "rights" that stockholders and/or investors in managed care organizations can expect to be honored by MCO corporations.
   - Discuss three "rights" that providers in managed care organizations can expect to be honored by MCO corporations.
   - Name three potential conflicts in "rights" among the patients, stockholders, and providers in managed care organizations.
   - Explore one of the websites listed on the companion website or the website of a managed care company serving your community. Make a presentation to your classmates of the scope of information in the website that would be useful to patients, providers, employers, and potential consumers. What additional information should be added to make the website more informative?

## ■ REFERENCES

American Association of Managed Care Nurses (AAMCN). (2004). *Managed care nursing practice standards.* Glen Allen, VA: Author.

American Association of Managed Care Nurses (AAMCN). (2008). Retrieved October 8, 2008, from http://www.aamcn.org

American Board of Managed Care Nursing (ABMCN). (2004). *What is the American Board of Managed Care Nursing? The value of certification.* Retrieved September 9, 2004, from http://www.abmcn.org

American Nurses Association (ANA). (1995). *Nursing facts.* Washington, DC: Author.

American Nurses Association (ANA). (1996, May/June). *Task force on standards and regulation of managed care report* (pp. 11–13, 82, 86). Washington, DC: Author.

American Nurses Association (ANA). (1998). *Managed care: Nursing's blueprint for actions principles.* Washington, DC: Author.

Baxter, R. J., & Mechanic, R. E. (1997). The status of local health care safety nets. *Health Affairs, 16*(4), 7–23.

Beck, D. E., & Dempsey, J. (1996). The managed care time clock. What's making it tick? *Health Care Supervisor, 14*(3), 1–12.

Cary, A. H. (2008). Case management. In M. Stanhope & J. Lancaster (Eds.), *Public health nursing: Population-centered health care in the community* (7th ed.). Phildelphia: Elsevier.

Cary, A. H. (1998). Advocacy or allocation? *Nursing Connections, 11*(1), 1–4.

Fox, P. D. (2001). An overview of managed care. In P. R. Kongstvedt (Ed.), *Essentials of managed health care* (14th ed., pp. 3–16). Gaithersburg, MD: Aspen.

Joint Commission on Accreditation of Health Care Organizations (JCAHO). (2004). *About managed care organization accreditation.* Retrieved September 9, 2004, from http://www.jcaho.org/ generalpublic.

May, C. A., Schraeder, C., & Britt, T. (1996). *Managed care and case management: Roles for professional nursing.* Washington, DC: American Nurses Publishing.

NCQA. (2008a). *HEDIS & Quality Management.* Retrieved October 8, 2008, from http://www.ncqa.org/tabid/59/Default.aspx

NCQA. (2008b). *NCQA releases Quality Compass 2004 and updated Quality Dividend Calculator.* Retrieved October 8, 2008, from http://www.ncqa.org/tabid/315/Default.aspx

NCQA. (2008c). *New health plan report card.* Retrieved October 8, 2008, from http://www.ncqa.org/tabid/143/Default.aspx

NCQA. (2008d). *What is NCQA?* Retrieved October 8, 2008, from http://www.ncqa.org

Packard, N. J. (1997). The price of choice: Managed care in America. *Nursing Administration Quarterly, 17*(3), 8–15.

Shi, L., & Singh, D. A. (2008). *Delivering health care in America: A systems approach* (4th ed.). Sudbury, MA: Jones and Bartlett.

Silva, M. C. (1998). Ethics and managed care: A select annotated bibliography. *Ethics Forum, 8*(2), 1–4.

Spitzer-Lehmann, R. (1996, September). A new framework for managed care: Marrying finance and service delivery. Paper presented at the pre-conference meeting of the Nursing Management Congress, Chicago.

Steinhauser, E. K. (1999). Developing a strategy to win with a difficult load. *Continuing Care, 18*(5), 20–25, 32.

URAC. (2004). *The ABCs of health coverage: The four basic types of health plans.* Retrieved September 15, 2004, from http://www.urac.org

URAC. (2008). *Frequently asked questions about URAC's pharmacy benefit management accreditation.* Retrieved September 8, 2008, from http://www.urac.org/programs/faqs.aspx

# UNIT 2

# Influences on a Community's Health

CHAPTER 7
Economics of Health Care
*Sherry Hartman*

CHAPTER 8
Politics and the Law
*Sharyn Janes*
*Heather Rakauskas Sherry*
*Karen Saucier Lundy*

CHAPTER 9
Health Policy
*Nancy Milio*
*Sharyn Janes*

CHAPTER 10
Transcultural Nursing Care in the Community
*Madeleine Leininger*

CHAPTER 11
Ethics and Health
*Pat Kurtz*
*Ronald L. Barr*

CHAPTER 12
Environmental Health
*Carol J. Nyman*
*Patricia Butterfield*
*Jean Shreffler*

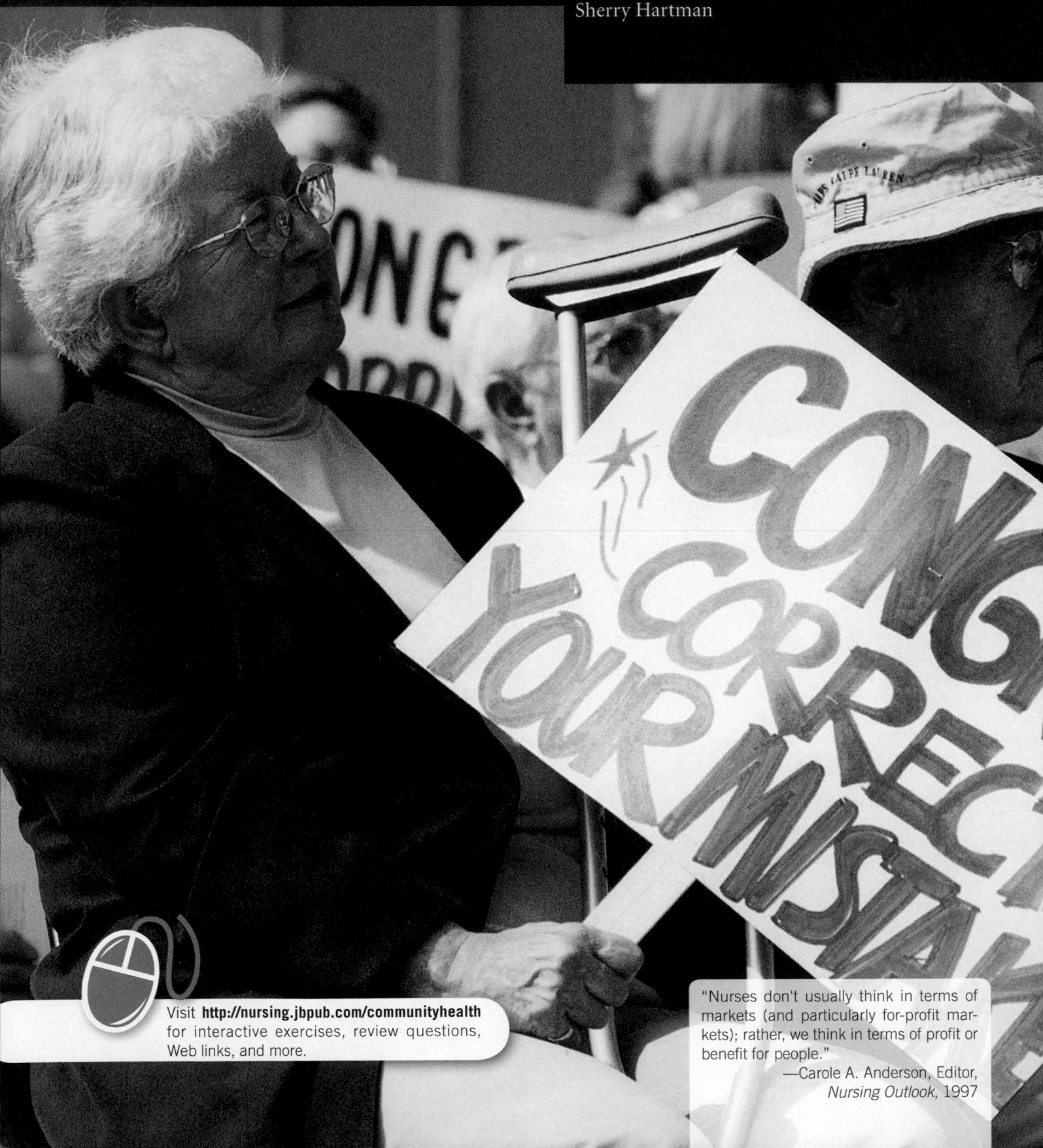

Sherry Hartman

"Nurses don't usually think in terms of markets (and particularly for-profit markets); rather, we think in terms of profit or benefit for people."

—Carole A. Anderson, Editor, *Nursing Outlook*, 1997

"Money talks" because money is a metaphor, a transfer, and a bridge. Like words and language, money is a storehouse of communally achieved work, skill, and experience. Money, however, is also a specialist technology like writing; and as writing intensifies the visual aspect of speech and order, and as the clock visually separates time from space, so money separates work from the other social functions. Even today money is a language for translating the work of the farmer into the work of the barber, doctor, engineer, or plumber. As a vast social metaphor, bridge, or translator, money—like writing—speeds up exchange and tightens the bonds of interdependence in any community. It gives great spatial expansion and control to political organizations, just as writing does, or the calendar.

*—Marshall McLuhan, 1964*

How much do you know about the real costs of health care and how nursing fits into the larger picture of economic markets? Why have nurses historically rejected the "irrelevant" knowledge about how the economic system of health care affects their practice and patient care?

Not so long ago, economic concerns were not considered an appropriate topic for basic nursing education or perhaps even for advanced nursing. In-depth knowledge was essential only for nurse administrators who needed to deal with budgets and financial resources. In today's health care environment, however, nurses need to understand health care problems from many approaches and viewpoints. The science of economics is one of those approaches that has become increasingly important. Even though "money concerns" have traditionally been resisted by practitioners whose focus has been on meeting patient needs, most now acknowledge the impact of economics on health care problems and solutions. All care providers need at least a rudimentary understanding of the economic workings of the system in which they practice at the institutional, national, and sometimes even global levels. Controlling costs while maintaining quality and access has become the major challenge of the new century. To do this, an understanding of economic descriptions and explanations of the health care market are necessary.

## CHAPTER FOCUS

### An Economic Approach to Health Care
- Competition in the Market
- Competition versus Regulation
- Market Failure in Health Care

### Rising Costs and Today's Health Care System
- From Private Pay to Government Involvement
- Increased Costs: The Economic Indicators
- Decreased Access: The Economic Barriers
- Influences on Costs and Access

### Paying for Health Care
- Out-of-Pocket Payments and Charity
- Health Insurance
- Publicly Funded Insurance and Direct Care Programs

### Cost Containment, Cost Analysis, and Quality

### Public Health, Managed Care, and the Economics of Prevention
- Opportunities for Collaboration
- Counterforces to Collaboration
- Economics of Alternative Therapies

### Significance of Economics for Community Health Nursing Practice

### Economics and Nightingale's Legacy

## QUESTIONS TO CONSIDER

After reading this chapter, you will know the answers to the following questions:

1. Why is the U.S. health care market referred to as an "imperfect" market?

2. What are the major roles of government and private enterprise in the U.S. health care market?

3. What factors are contributing to high and rising health care costs?

4. What are the strategies used for cost containment of national health expenditures?

5. What are the financing, eligibility, and covered benefits of Medicare and Medicaid?

6. What other health care financing is covered by the government?

7. Why is it that, in spite of the availability of public and private health insurance programs, some U.S. citizens are without any coverage?

8. How and why might public health and managed care organizations collaborate?

9. How are community health nurses affected by the economic environment of their practice?

## KEY TERMS

Benefit period
Categorically needy
Community rating
Competition
Cost–benefit analysis
Cost containment
Cost-effectiveness analysis
Cost-of-illness analysis
Cost sharing

Demand
Entitlement
Experience rating
Free market competition
Gross domestic product (GDP)
Health care market
Health insurance purchasing
　cooperative (HIPC)
Market

Market failure
Market justice
Medically needy
Medigap insurance
Price
Quasi-market (imperfect market)
Relative value scale
Resource utilization groups,
　version 3

Self-insurance
Social justice
Standards of participation
Supplier-influenced demand
Supply
Technology assessment
Third-party payer
Welfare

❝*The challenge for nurses and the nursing profession is to develop strategies to refuse to give in to the dominance of economic interests over the need to prevent harm.*❞
—Heggen & Wellard, 2004

NOT SO LONG AGO economic concerns were not considered a topic in basic nursing education or perhaps even in advanced nursing. Nurses grew up in an environment out of which "grew expectations and behaviors that simply ignored or neglected cost issues in their provision of services" (Malloch & Porter-O'Grady, 1999). In-depth knowledge was essential only for nurse administrators who needed to deal with budgets and financial resources.

In the current health care environment, however, nurses need to understand health care problems from many approaches and viewpoints. The science of economics is one of those approaches that has become increasingly important. Even though "money concerns" were traditionally resisted by practitioners whose focus was on meeting patient needs, there is no escape now from acknowledging the impact of economics on health care problems and solutions. All care providers need at least a rudimentary understanding of the economic workings of the system in which they practice at the institutional, national, and even sometimes global levels. Controlling costs while maintaining quality and access remains a major challenge for nurses to incorporate in their practice. To do so, an understanding of economic descriptions and explanations of the health care market is necessary.

Several chapters in this text, describing the context of and influences on health care practice, also highlight aspects of health problems from an economic point of view rather than strictly a biological or psychosocial perspective. Health care system analysts are concerned with the best structures for delivering the various needed health care services; health policy makers are concerned with deciding the best actions to take from among possible alternatives; health economists are concerned with the distribution of scarce resources among a defined population. These areas are interrelated: economic analysis influences policy decisions, which often drive the resulting health care delivery structures. The resultant structures, in turn, are analyzed in terms of how efficiently they distribute resources.

### Research Alert

According to many critics, the answer to the problems with the United States' health care system is to adopt a government-run, national health care system similar to those found in other countries. Those systems spend less on health care and seem to have better health outcomes. A closer look at international health care systems, though, shows that most countries are struggling with rising health care costs and lack of access to care.

Michael Tanner, director of health and welfare studies at the Cato Institute, identifies some trends from national health care systems that focus on access to care and costs:

- National health insurance does not guarantee universal access to care. Many countries ration care or there are long waiting periods for care.
- Health care costs are rising almost everywhere. Although other countries do spend less than the United States on health care, their costs are rising and affecting budgets, taxes, and benefits offered.
- In countries where the government has a high degree of control over the national health plan, people often deal with waiting lists for care, rationing, restrictions on physician choice, and other obstacles.
- More effective national health plans are successful to the degree that they incorporate competition, cost sharing, market prices, and consumer choice into the system and avoid centralized government control. The broad trend is to move away from centralized government control of health care.

Avoiding centralized control of health care and increasing consumer incentives and choice will help to solve the United States' health care problems.

*Source:* Tanner, M. D. (2008). The grass is not always greener: A look at national health care systems around the world. *Cato Policy Analysis, 613.* Retrieved October 29, 2008, from www.cato.org/pub_display.php?pub_id=9272

This chapter provides a basic understanding of the economic approach to health problems. After an explanation of economic theory and principles applied to health care, the current state of financing of health care in the United States is considered, along with some of the history that has brought us to today's increased and continued reliance on market economics in health care. The many sources of funding and reimbursement for heath care are explained. Approaches to cost containment and methods of economic analysis are described, followed by a look at some of the relationships between private-sector health care and public health care. Finally, some of the implications of economics for community health nursing are summarized.

# An Economic Approach to Health Care

## ■ Competition in the Market

Like most sciences, economics is complex and broad in its scope. It looks at how finite goods and services are distributed to those who want or need them. A major way of conceptualizing this process is to see it as a **market**. In a marketplace, those who have something to sell and those who have needs or wants come together to make exchanges. There are various "markets" depending on the commodity being exchanged: the automobile market, the entertainment market, the housing market, and the **health care market.** In health care, the market includes all health care–related services that need to be distributed among the total U.S. population. Within that overall market are specific markets: the health care labor market, the home care market, the hospital care market, the pharmaceuticals market, the personal health insurance market, the employer-paid health insurance market, and so on. A single hospital can also focus on its market: those potential users of its service and competing sellers in its service area. A market could also be defined geographically, such as the home health care market within a certain region.

Whatever organization a nurse works in, and particularly in a for profit system, firms are concerned with their position and success in the market. Nurses play a key role in determining their quality and financial outcomes. At the broadest levels, market mechanisms are important to understanding the total health care picture of a single state and of the whole nation.

The essence of any market is buyers and sellers. There is a particular amount of a product or service such as health care that buyers are willing and able to purchase and consume, which is referred to as the **demand** for the product. There is a certain amount that sellers or providers are willing to make available, which is referred to as the **supply** of the product. In both cases the amount demanded or supplied is related to the **price** (or cost) of the health product.

**Competition** is the key to understanding why some policy makers and health care leaders desire more free market mechanisms in health care. Competition in the market is the mechanism for setting price and quality. Suppliers compete for buyers of their products. Those who operate most efficiently (by satisfying buyers with the quality they want at the lowest possible cost) flourish; those who do not have satisfied consumers close down. Price is most commonly the basis for competition, but competition can also be based on technical quality, amenities, access, or other factors if prices become stabilized.

## ■ Competition versus Regulation

Market mechanisms are not the only way for goods to become distributed. Centralized decision making may determine the distribution of goods and services, as a central authority determines how sellers and buyers make their exchanges. The central authority may be the only producer/seller and, therefore, control all exchanges. This was the means of allocation in the Soviet Union and Eastern European nations until nearly 20 years ago. Since the collapse of the communist bloc, capitalist, free market economics as practiced in the West has come to dominate in most developed countries.

The strong values of free market competition have influenced U.S. methods of distribution of health services. In contrast to most other developed nations, the United States has never adopted a national health care system with a global budget or centralized decision making. In the United States, the private sector fulfills essential social responsibilities related to health that in most other industrialized countries are assumed by the government (Blumenthal, 2006). The United States has mainly a private system of financing as well as delivering health services. Sources of payment for U.S. health care are 55% from private sources and 45% from government sources, and the majority of hospitals, physicians, and other health care providers are private businesses.

However, even though the origins and values of the U.S health care system lie with the free market, the last century was marked by increasing government involvement in health care. From its earliest origins in a free market of direct exchange between individuals and their private physicians, the U.S. system moved slowly to more centralized decisions through government regulation. For example, federal and state governments determine public-sector expenditures, covered services, and reimbursement rates for Medicare and Medicaid services. They also regulate participants in the market by setting **standards of participation** for certification to provide services for Medicaid and Medicare patients. Such government regulations become the minimum standards of quality in other, private sectors of the health services market (Shi & Singh, 2008).

During the Reagan presidency of the 1980s, there was growing interest in establishing more market-oriented approaches in many sectors of the economy. The free market is thought to be efficient for all goods and services in dispersing scarce resources. Following this line of thought, many economic theorists claim to show the superiority of the free market competition over government regulation for allocating scarce health care resources (Rice, 1998). Responding to escalating health care costs, in 1981—among many other changes in the health care industry—came the announcement from the Reagan administration that competition in the market (not governmental regulation) would be allowed to shape health care delivery (McKenzie, 1997). Other countries with more centralized health care systems have since looked to the U.S. changes and introduced more market mechanisms as well (LeGrand, 1999; Chen & Mastilica, 1998; Tritter & McCallum, 2006).

Nevertheless, the persistent high levels and rates of growth for health care expenditures remain dominant subjects of policy decisions in health care (Fuchs, 2005). More private and public money being spent on health care means less money available to spend on other wants or needs. In the public sector, spending more on health care leaves less to spend on education, the military, the environment, and other needed public goods. As noted by Fuchs (2005), there is concern over high U.S. spending because we may not be getting the value in improved health or patient satisfaction that other alternative choices might provide. Policy-making tensions for **cost containment** and value for spending arise because of conflicts between regulation by the government—for example, the failed Clinton plan for the government to provide universal health coverage—and reliance on market competition to distribute health care services—such as the most recent high-deductible, consumer-driven health plans and health savings accounts (HSAs). There is little agreement about the two approaches, other than that both are imperfect (Pauly, 2005).

In spite of the pressure from those who favor market forces, government regulation continues to play a large role. Some states have become frustrated with federal efforts and developed their own remedies. Massachusetts recently became the first state to require residents to carry health insurance, with employer contributions to employee coverage becoming mandatory. At this time, a few other states are also considering legislation of some form of universal coverage, and at least 25 states are considering employer mandates to increase coverage (Mantone, 2006) At the same time, there is increasing reliance on the private sector and a competitive, cost-driven market.

Between these two forces, some claim that the competitive market model in health care delivery has become the industry standard with widespread acceptance (Dowd, 2005) and will continue to have more rapid, extensive, and influential effects than any initiatives at the state or federal level (Sultz & Young, 2006). Opponents, however, continue to question the appropriateness of market forces in the health care setting. The problems are considered in the next section.

## ■ Market Failure in Health Care

Those who believe in the superiority of competitive marketplaces base their preference on what would happen in an ideal pure market. In an ideal market—called **free market competition**—the following occurs. On the demand side, consumers have a variety of choices in goods and services to purchase. For individual consumers, these include choices among doctors to visit in clinics, hospitals for surgeries, home health agencies that provide nurse visits, pharmacies to buy medicines, medical equipment suppliers, and so on. Consumers maximize their satisfaction through self-motivated behavior and pick the quality they want for the price they are willing to pay. Income, tastes, preferences, and information about the product influence their choice.

Consumers' choices tell suppliers whether their products are priced right and have the right quality. Suppliers then adjust price and quality to satisfy consumers. For suppliers in a competitive industry, there are strong incentives to minimize the costs of making their products and services. Those products and services can then be priced competitively to sell in the marketplace. Suppliers must be innovative and respond to customers' perceptions of quality. These two behaviors—benefit-maximizing behaviors of consumers and profit-maximizing behaviors of suppliers—through the mechanism of the market, produce the best patterns of production and consumption.

For the market to operate ideally as outlined above, certain conditions must exist. These underlying assumptions must hold true for the market to work as described in theory. Economists recognize that often the realities of the market violate the basic assumptions and create what is referred to as **market failure.** In a failed market, the necessary competition does not occur as it should. It fails to produce the best outcomes for achieving the best use of resources. Fair allocation, quality and cost control, and setting of social priorities that enhance social welfare—all of which are the supposed gains of an effective market—are not realized.

Box 7-1 lists some of the key conditions necessary for a classic ideal free market to exist. Each of these is discussed next, along with examples, to indicate how the U.S. health

---

### ✎ ETHICAL CONNECTION

What if treatments such as organ replacement and weight-loss surgery are not reimbursed by third-party payers if the disease has been caused by a person's risky lifestyle behaviors? In November 2005, East Suffolk, a primary trust in the United Kingdom, did just that. It announced that hip and knee replacements would not be provided for obese persons. Although the U.K. government has been reluctant to become involved in difficult policy issues such as these, modifications have been made in the policy, allowing denial of care to patients who lack clear evidence-based justifications for treatment of self-imposed health conditions.

In what circumstances would it be legitimate and ethical to refuse care and treatment to an individual because that person is seen as contributing to his or her own health problems? The U.K. effort is intended to reduce health care costs and focus on populations that have the greatest chance of improving their health in the future. But what if this list of "unacceptable activities" includes other risky behavior, such as dangerous sports like skydiving and scuba diving, traveling to countries where infectious disease is endemic, being to blame for your own accident on the road, engaging in insufficient exercise, and having poor nutrition? The list would be endless.

Examine this issue from an ethical perspective. How does it relate to our values about providing essential care for the public? Is rationing already occurring?

*Source*: Diamond, B. (2006). Rights, resources and health care [Editorial]. *Nursing Ethics, 13*(4), 335–336.

## BOX 7-1

**Factors Necessary for a Free Market in Health Care with Optimal Outcomes**

- Consumers have full information about the nature of the services they require, the results of their decisions, and the benefits they can obtain.
- Consumers and buyers act independently.
- Consumers bear the financial impact of their decisions and are aware of price differences.
- There is unrestrained competition regarding price and quality among providers.
- No single provider has monopoly power.
- Providers of services seek to operate efficiently to maximize profits.

care market fails to operate under the forces of ideal free market factors.

*In a free market, consumers have full information about the nature of the services they require, the results of their decisions, and the benefits they can obtain.* In many instances, patient services are lifetime purchases with no opportunity to learn about quality differences through repeat purchases. In those cases, providers also have little reason to woo consumers by building a reputation for quality (Howell, 2006). The complexity of medical care itself and of the health care system makes informed choices difficult for patients. A consumer cannot know if a prescription or surgery is the better buy for his or her illness. There are so many choices of treatment—perhaps an acupuncturist would be a better buy. Treatment is sometimes urgently needed. Patients often do not have the time, skills, or resources to find needed information, and such information can be costly. In choice of health plan coverage, consumers do not know the differences between plan characteristics that indicate quality, convenience, flexibility, and extent of coverage. Even after a choice is made, consumers often cannot know if they made the right decision or what would have happened under other circumstances. Did the care cause the improvement or would it have happened anyway? What would have happened if another provider or treatment had been chosen?

*In a free market, consumers and providers must act independently.* Because of the "asymmetries of information" (Blumenthal, 1994, p. 252) in the health care market, patient consumers must depend on and accept the word of providers. Indeed, the words and advice of providers are as much the product being purchased as the examination or treatment. In a truly free market, the power lies with the consumer. However, physicians (suppliers) often are viewed as agents acting on behalf of patients. Thus consumer demand is subject to artificial demand, commonly called **supplier-influenced demand** (Shi & Singh, 1998, p. 16). In some cases, physicians own laboratories and invest in health care organizations, a relationship that may affect their ability to be impartial in recommending the use of these resources. At the same time,

some managed care firms have limited the choices physicians can offer patients, which puts limits on demand.

*In a free market, consumers bear the financial consequences of their purchase decisions and are aware of price differences among products.* Most Americans rely on reimbursement by third parties that bear the financial impact of decisions to receive care. This can cause patients to be price insensitive, to feel care is free, to believe they should get their money's worth for premiums paid, and to have no incentive to "shop around" for better prices. In general, most health consumers are not aware of prices for services, variations in prices between suppliers, and the relationship between price and quality. If consumers did want to compare prices for products, it is often hard to compare because of item-based pricing and negotiation for unpublished reduced fees by individual insurance companies or health plans (Deaton, 2006). Surgery, for example, includes charges for a surgeon, supplies, use of facilities, and services of an anesthesiologist and maybe a pathologist. Exact usage of each of these items sometimes cannot be anticipated and makes it difficult to determine a price prior to the service and compare it with a competitor's price. Even though health plans now negotiate fees for "packages" of services or benefits to overcome the pricing problems, these are not standardized and thus are still difficult to compare.

*In a free market, there is unrestrained competition among providers.* Unrestricted access to the market is blocked in several ways for some health care providers. An example is the case of advanced practice nurses, who often have not been free to set up primary care practices as they wish. Many states require medical oversight of nursing practice, such as permission for prescriptive privileges of nurse practitioners. Most **third-party payer** systems have not provided direct payment for nursing care. Instead, payment for most nursing care is included in hospital or clinic charges. If consumers must personally bear the cost for any nursing services they might receive directly, then services that could be offered by entrepreneurial nurses will have a limited demand in the market. Limits on entering the market for nurses as well as for some complementary or alternative health care practitioners are the same as giving physicians control over competitors. The results are lack of competition based on lower prices or on quality (Rambur & Mooney, 1998).

*No single provider in a free market has monopoly power.* Not only must providers be able to enter the market, but for competition to work, there must also be many providers vying for customers. One response to pressures from employers and health plans for cost reduction, however, was provider alliances and formation of integrated delivery systems. Consolidation among health care networks of hospitals and multispecialty group practices give very large market shares to—and thus increased negotiating leverage for—these groups. In certain geographic areas of the United States, a single large medical system has taken over as the sole provider of major health service, restricting competition (Rice, 1998; Shi & Singh, 2008). Such mergers create local market

### CULTURAL CONNECTION

One fifth of the U.S. population lives at or below the federal poverty line. Since this "line" was set in the 1960s, how does this affect the ability of poor people to manage their health costs today?

negotiating leverage that gives the provider control over local services pricing (Berenson, 2005). In some markets, newly formed local provider monopolies have increased prices by 20% to 50%. For example, after consolidation of most of the oncology groups in one local market into a single group, the cost of one-hour chemotherapy rose 51%, from $95.76 to $145 (Halvorson, 1999).

*Providers of services in the free market seek to operate efficiently to maximize profits.* Many providers of health care operate as nonprofit organizations. Their only constraint is to make their budgets balance such that expenditures equal revenues. Some may have goals beyond maximizing services, such as extending high salaries and benefits to administration, or improving organizational status with expensive equipment regardless of whether a majority of patients need such technology. Conversely workers in for-profit organizations may have adverse incentives owing to the firm's goal of profit. In the case of physicians, such conflicting goals can be seen when they focus on a specific patient and seek to exhaust every possibility for diagnosis and order many costly tests. Such conflict was a motivation for the capitated payment systems of early managed care, which encouraged less spending on care to realize higher retained profit. Concerns for quality have limited many such managed care restrictive methods, but perverse incentives still exist.

As these examples show, the current delivery and consumption of health care in the United States occur in what has been called a **quasi-market** or an **imperfect market** (Shi & Singh, 2008). Much of the controversy over introducing more market mechanisms into health care delivery is related to how poorly the U.S. health care system measures up to the assumptions for an efficient free market (Nichols et al., 2004). Chapter 6 discusses access and utilization barriers to managed care, the popular answer throughout the 1990s to market failure in health care. Compare those barriers to the problems with the free market in health care: Many problems of access in managed care were economic problems in that they limited access to the free market and thus its efficient functioning.

Although we may have success applying free market principles to the place (market) where automobiles, condos, and refrigerators are exchanged for cash, these principles seem less appropriate for health care. The place where relief of pain, care of infections, and comfort of the spirit are exchanged for cash is thought to be very different (Rambur & Mooney, 1998; Berenson, 2005; Edwards. 2005). Yet, an economic approach to health care finds that the model of perfect competition also brings benefits to buyers and sellers.

Thus, even though we continue to have intricate governmental and social structures of health care market regulation, free competition continues to be advocated and analyzed for ways in which market failure can be overcome to improve transactions between buyers and sellers.

## Rising Costs and Today's Healthcare System

### ■ From Private Pay to Government Involvement

In the past, the patient or family expected to pay for their own health care. In 1940, 81.3% of health care was paid by the individual or the family, and 18.7% was financed by some intermediary third party. Of that 18.7%, 2.6% was from private insurance and 16.1% by public funding (Gibson & Waldo, 1982). The value system of the United States has long resisted strong government intervention in health care. Values of individualism, freedom of choice, and protection of privacy underlie this resistance. Even though the idea of a national system of health services has long been present and is implemented in much of the rest of the world, such is not the case in the United States. Instead, health care originated in the private sector, and only in times of exceptional need has the government intervened with social programs. Box 9-2 in the chapter on health policy lists major legislative actions related to health that have been taken by the federal government. This kind of legislation marks the evolution of the government from a minimal provider of services and protector of public health to that of a major financier for a public enterprise whose controls have grown over the autonomy of providers and the choices of providers of care.

The Social Security Act of 1935 established Social Security but failed to include health care. The introduction of the first indemnity insurance plans, Blue Cross for hospital care and Blue Shield for physician care, diffused political moves toward compulsory health insurance (Pulcini & Mahoney, 1998). In 1959, with the Federal Employees Health Benefit Act, Blue Cross negotiated to provide health insurance coverage for federal employees and set the stage for its later involvement in Medicare and Medicaid. In the 1960s, during a period of relative prosperity and a growing concern for poor and elderly populations, Medicaid (Title XIX) and Medicare (Title XVIII) programs were passed as amendments to the Social Security Act. At the same time, the federal government became more involved in health care with legislation establishing regional medical programs, comprehensive health planning, and extensive educational aid to medical and related health professions. In 2004, payment sources

### ENVIRONMENTAL CONNECTION

How have hospitals and community agencies changed geographical landscapes as they evolve to more community-based services? Does the way in which a health care system is funded affect city and urban communities in terms of the environment? If so, how?

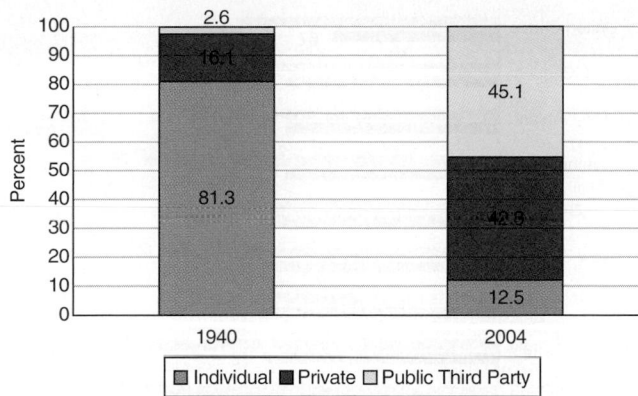

Sources of payment for health care, 1940 and 2004.

*Source*: Centers for Medicare and Medicaid Services, Office of the Actuary, National Health Statistics Group, 2006.

were completely the reverse of 1940: Individuals paid directly for 12.5% of their care and 87.4% was paid by a third party (42.3% by private insurance sources and 45.1% from public funds).

It was soon evident that the costs of health care were escalating. When the government paid for more health care expenses, the effect was as if individuals had more money to pay for care. As economic theory predicts, increased sources of funds led to increased demand, and the revenues of the industry increased as well. Government intervention had contributed to rising costs (Finkler & Kovner, 1993, p. 80). The inability of society or government to limit the rising costs continues to be one of the roots of our present fiscal challenges in health care.

## ■ Increased Costs: The Economic Indicators

One indicator of the United States' high spending for health care can be seen by comparing those expenditures to other industrialized nations' spending. The United States spends nearly one fourth more on health care than the next highest ranked country.

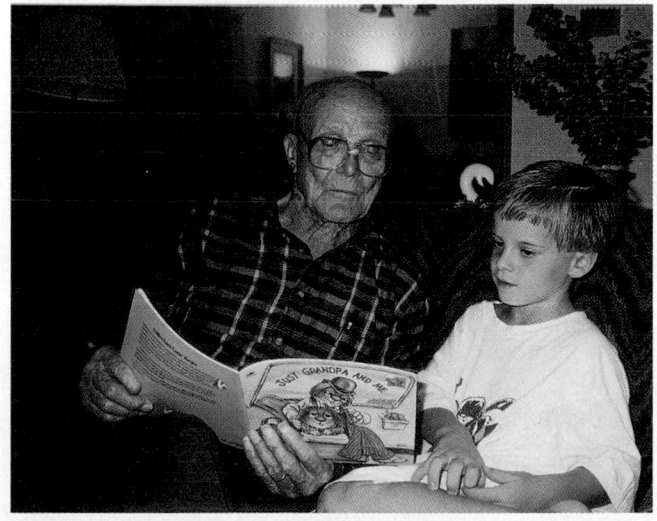

Children and elders often compete for resources in the U.S. health care system.

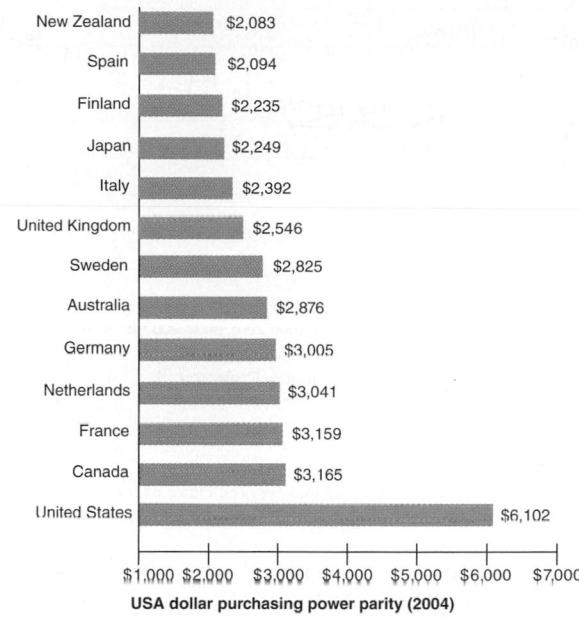

Note: Purchasing power parity is a currency conversion rate that both converts to a common currency and equalizes the purchasing power of different currencies. It eliminates the differences in price levels between countries in the process of conversion.
Data for Japan, France, Germany, and Australia are for 2003.

Total health expenditure in selected countries.

*Source*: OECD health data, 2006.

A more commonly cited indicator is related to the U.S. gross domestic product. **Gross domestic product (GDP)** is the monetary total of all finished goods and services (public and private) produced within a nation in one year. Health care expenditures (which means all funds, private and public, spent on health care) as a percentage of the GDP is a standard measure for comparing and tracking changes in expenditures (Jacobs, 1997).

In the United States health care has had a long history of escalating costs and an increasing share of the GDP. A graph of the rising amounts from all sources shows a continuing greater amount being paid by private sources but a narrowing

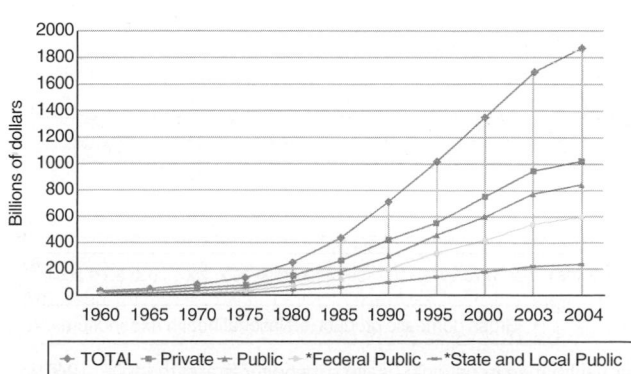

National health expenditures by source of funds, 1960 to 2004.

*Source*: Centers for Medicare and Medicaid Services, Office of the Actuary, National Health Statistics Group, 2006.

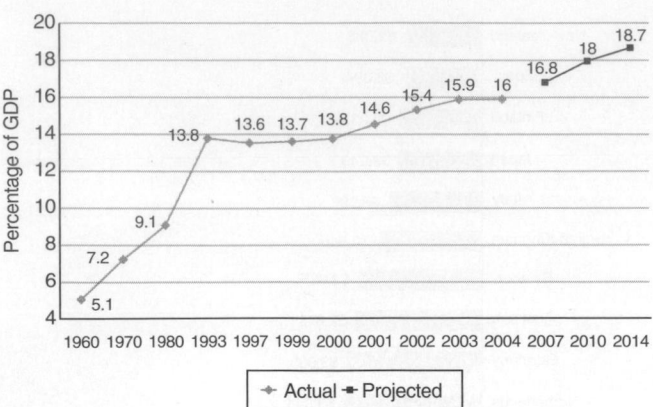

Actual and predicted national expenditures as a percentage of GDP, 1960 to 2010.

*Source*: Centers for Medicare and Medicaid Services, Office of the Actuary, National Health Statistics Group, 2006.

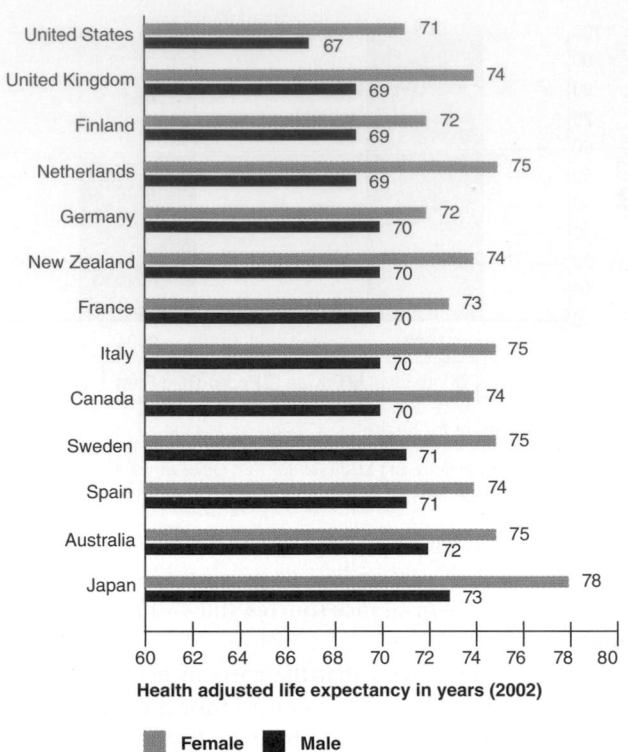

**Health adjusted life expectancy in years (2002)**

▇ Female  ■ Male

Note: Health Adjusted Life Expectancy (HALE) represents the number of expected years of life equivalent to years in full health.

Health Adjusted Life Expectancy (HALE) in selected countries.

*Source*: Statistical annex table 4, Healthy life expectancy (HALE) in all WHO member states, estimates for 2004. World Health report, 2004. Changing history. Geneva: World Health Organization, 2004.

of the gap between government and private funding. In 2004, private funding paid for 54.8% of U.S. health care ($1,030.3 billion), down from 59.5% in 1990. Currently most people are still covered by employer-based health insurance.

Health care expenditures as a percentage of the GDP grew at an alarming rate for more than 30 years. In the early 1990s, policy makers predicted that, if left to grow unchecked, health care spending would reach 19% of GDP by 2000 (White House Domestic Policy Council, 1993). This prediction proved to be high: In 2004, spending was 16% of GDP. A graph shows the continuing upward trend with some years of lower growth rates. Health care spending grew faster than the GDP for over three decades as well. In 1996, spending leveled off, with the growth rate of the overall economy exceeding, the growth rate of healthcare expenditures. In 1997, healthcare expenditures represented the smallest claim of health care on the nation's resources in 5 years (Centers for Medicare and Medicaid Services, 2008). It had been predicted that the United States would top $1 trillion in health

care spending by 1995 (Standard and Poor's Corporation, 1992), but with the slower rate of growth, it was 1996 before the $1 trillion mark was passed.

The mid-1990s progress in reducing the rate of spending growth was unexpected. Analysts disagreed over the reasons for the slowed rate, but many believed the efficiencies introduced by increased market competition and managed care were responsible. Economic analysts at the time did not view the lowered rates as a permanent trend. The limits of realizing improved efficiency without harming quality may have been reached as many factors continued to affect costs. For example, Halvorson noted that surgery fees "have been negotiated down 30–40% in many markets during the past four years. For these rock-bottom fees, there is nowhere to go but up" (1999, p. 28). Projections show future rates of growth that are in the 7% to 7.5% annual range. Currently, the pace of growth has slowed compared to the early 2000s, but spending is predicted to continue to rise (Smith et al., 2006) and to grow faster than the GDP (Heffler et al., 2005).

### ■ Decreased Access: The Economic Barriers

Services offered in the U.S. health care system are undoubtedly the best offered anywhere in the world. Yet, the United States often ranks below other developed countries in health status indicators. One author has described it this

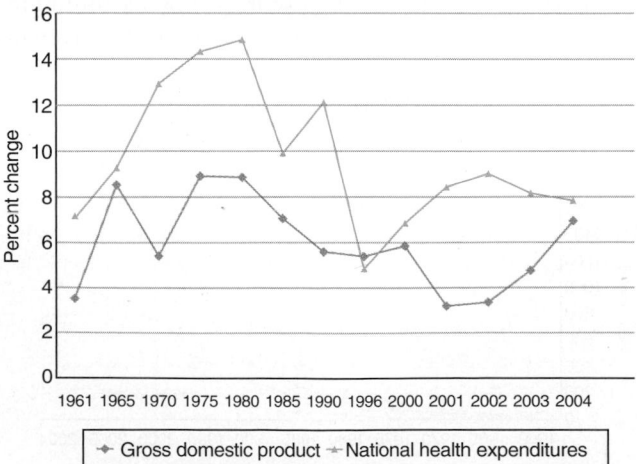

Annual change in national health expenditures and the GDP, 1961 to 2004.

*Source*: Centers for Medicare and Medicaid Services, Office of the Actuary, National Health Statistics Group, 2006.

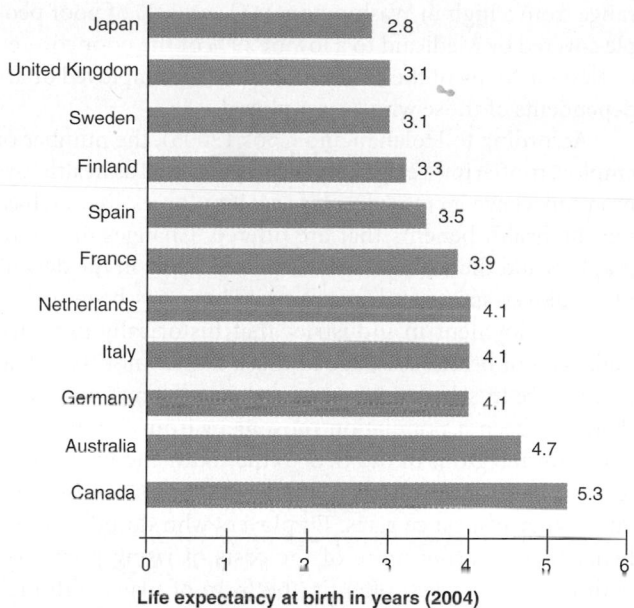

| Country | Years |
|---------|-------|
| Japan | 2.8 |
| United Kingdom | 3.1 |
| Sweden | 3.1 |
| Finland | 3.3 |
| Spain | 3.5 |
| France | 3.9 |
| Netherlands | 4.1 |
| Italy | 4.1 |
| Germany | 4.1 |
| Australia | 4.7 |
| Canada | 5.3 |

**Life expectancy at birth in years (2004)**

Note: Canada is 2003 data

Infant mortality in selected countries.

*Source*: OECD health date, 2006.

way: "The Americans who can afford health insurance, or who are well insured, can get the best care that medical technology can offer. Even so, the most expensive care is often fragmented, or insufficient, and may not restore the patient to health or adequate functioning" (Kovner & Knickman, 2005. p. 4). Even though superior services are present, the dark side of the situation is that they are not accessible to all. Access to care means that people can get health care when they need it. Inadequate access for millions of Americans is a core problem and has led to the concern for health care in the United States. The concept of access to health care has long been recognized as an issue and a responsibility for

nurses (Stevens, 1992). Gulzar (1999) examined the concept of access to health care from a nursing perspective and delineated its many dimensions. She defined access to health care as "the fit among personal, sociocultural, economic, and system related factors that enable individuals, families, and communities to have timely, needed, necessary, continuous, and satisfactory health services" (p. 17). These include, for example, age, gender, ethnic, and cultural appropriateness; understandable language, health care providers and facilities nearby where people live; available transportation; timeliness; and affordability.

### A Good Read

## The Divided Welfare State: The Battle over Public and Private Social Benefits in the United States (2004)

*By Jacob S. Hacker, New York: Oxford University Press.*

This is a book of great interest and profound scholarship from one of the country's leading thinkers on social welfare issues. Hacker makes a major contribution to the social policy literature and will most certainly provoke diverse discussions about his extensive debate on how an enabling state can transcend a commitment to promote market solutions to human ills and be worthy of the term's connotation.

Hacker's work is based on an in-depth study of comparative welfare systems and distinguishes between actual welfare tendencies and desirable utopian ambitions; it carries forward the long tradition of social decencies in the treatment of basic human needs. Politics of the welfare state, the three worlds of welfare capitalism, transformation of the welfare state, and limits to globalization are the focus of this critical and provocative book. Hacker proposes a consumer-directed, "shareholder claim" on private markets, targeting benefits in a "new social policies model approach to reducing costs and providing services for the public."

**BOX 7-2**

**Influences on Rising Health Care Costs**
- Increased government funding
- Inflation
- Imperfect market
- Third-party payment
- Rising drug costs
- Increased use of technology for care
- Increased wages for health care personnel
- Population changes
- Slow adoption of labor-saving technology
- Administrative and medical excess
- Medical practice styles
- Emphasis on treatment versus prevention
- Consumer expectations
- Indigent care

Of concern economically is the major barrier to health care access that is closely associated with the concern of rising costs—inability to pay (Bodenheimer & Grumbach, 1995). Very few people can afford to pay out of pocket for the tremendous costs of an illness episode or for the ongoing expenses of a chronic illness, and long-term institutional care is far beyond most individuals' ability to pay. In 2005, the number of people without health insurance in the United States was 46 million (17.9% of the population), an increase from 2000 of 1.3 million uninsured younger than age 65 and continuing an upward trend from the mid-1970s (Holahan & Cook, 2006). Without coverage, people either do not seek needed care or do not pay for the care they do receive. The poor and working poor without adequate access do not lack emergency or urgent care because no one needing such care is turned away if they go to a hospital. It is primary care—such as check-ups, screenings, chronic illness follow-up, and prenatal care—that they lack. Their lack of access to primary care means that many of these individuals eventually need more costly and less timely treatment.

Although the numbers of people covered by Medicare and Medicaid have grown, there has been a drop in the number covered by private health insurance. Lack of insurance is not just a problem of the poor—the numbers of uninsured are growing among the middle class (see Box 7-2). Most of the uninsured do not qualify for Medicaid. Because states set their own standards for eligibility, there are wide differences in which poor people (those with incomes below federal poverty level) are covered by Medicaid. The percentages range from a high in Washington, D.C., of 60% of poor people covered by Medicaid to a low of 29% of the poor covered in Nevada. Many of the newly uninsured are employed or are dependents of those who are employed.

According to Holahan and Cook (2006), the number of employers offering health benefits has declined as health care premiums have increased, and fewer employees are purchasing the health benefits that are offered. Changes in demographics and the workplace have played a role in the decline of employer-sponsored insurance. There has been a shift from employment in industries that historically provided high rates of health coverage to those that do not, as well as an increase in self-employment and small companies. Also, there has been a population movement from the northern and eastern regions of the U. S. to the south and west, which tend to have lower rates of employer-sponsored insurance and higher insurance rates. Employers who do offer health benefits are sharing more of the costs of rising premiums with their employees, often in the form of plans with high deductibles—$1,000 for single coverage and $2,000 for family coverage. Employee participation in high-deductible plans increased from 5% in 2007 to 8% in 2008 (Trapp, 2008).

Having private insurance does not guarantee financial access to care. Research based on data from the Commonwealth Fund Biennial Health Insurance Survey found that "the number of underinsured adults climbed to 25 million people in 2007, up from 16 million in 2003" (Collins, Kriss, Doty, & Rustgi, 2008). The study also found increases in the number of underinsured people reporting difficulty in paying their medical bills, from 34 percent of working-age adults in 2005 to 41 percent in 2007. The uninsured were twice as likely not to receive care, but three fourths of those who went without were insured, and 46% had private insurance. Those who had Medicaid were as likely to go without care as the uninsured, because many physicians do not accept the coverage offered by Medicaid. Both the insured and the uninsured cited cost as the major barrier to care (Collins et al., 2008).

Public programs are generally considered inadequate in terms of prenatal care (Hughes & Runyan, 2008) and mental health programs (Mechanic & Rochefort, 2008), and contractual arrangements for home health care can restrict needed visits in home health care services (Shaughnessy, Schlenker, & Hittle, 1997). By contrast, private coverage restricts access because of high out-of-pocket expenditures of co-payments and deductibles, fixed indemnity (maximum payment allowed), and exclusions, such as for preexisting conditions. Such an exclusion may be for a set time after enrollment or may be permanent. Changing jobs can also trigger this restriction. Most Americans are underinsured for preventive services, catastrophic illness, and long-term care (Harrington & Estes, 2008). *The Healthy People 2010* objectives that address access issues are listed on the following page.

Numerous negative outcomes for those who are uninsured or underinsured and, therefore, lack access have been documented. Chapter 24 discusses in more depth the vulnerability of the medically indigent.

**ETHICAL CONNECTION**

When a nurse has to discharge a patient from home health who is still recovering because of Medicare restrictions on reimbursement, what are the ethical dilemmas faced by the nurse and the possible solutions within a managed care system?

**OBJECTIVES RELATED TO ACCESS**

**Access to Quality Health Services**

**Clinical Preventive Care**

1.1    Increase the proportion of persons with health insurance.

1.2    Increase the proportion of insured persons with coverage for clinical preventive services.

**Primary Care**

1.3    Increase the proportion of persons who have a specific source of ongoing care.

1.4    Increase the proportion of persons with a usual primary care provider.

1.5    Reduce the proportion of families that experience difficulties or delays in obtaining health care or do not receive needed care for one or more family members.

**Educational and Community-Based Programs**

7.9    Increase the proportion of hospitals and managed care organizations that provide community disease prevention and health-promotion activities that address the priority health needs identified by their community.

**Family Planning**

9.13    Increase the proportion of health insurance policies that cover contraceptive supplies and services.

**Oral Health**

21.12    Increase the proportion of children and adults under age 19 years at or below 200% of the federal poverty level who received any preventive dental service during the past year.

**Public Health Infrastructure**

23.16    Increase the proportion of federal, tribal, state, and local public health agencies that gather accurate data on public health expenditures, categorized by essential public health service.

*Source*: U.S. Department of Health and Human Services. (2000). *Healthy People 2010*. Retrieved September 24, 2008, from http://www.healthypeople.gov/Document/tableofcontents.htm#under

◼ **Influences on Costs and Access**

No single factor explains why health spending has grown at the rate it has. Several influences collectively contribute to the situation. As discussed earlier, there was an economic effect of increased demand as a result of *increased sources of funds from government*. In addition, increases over the last few years have resulted from several sources.

*Inflation*, which is indicated by the rising consumer price index, has continued to affect all goods and services in the United States, but prices have increased at an even greater rate for health care services. Physicians and hospitals account for by far the greatest proportion. Expenditures for public health services account for only a little more than 3% of overall spending.

*Drug costs increased* nearly 14% between 2004 and 2007 (Government Accountability Office, 2007). Prices for generic drugs decreased an average of 12.8% during that time period, while prices of brand-name drugs increased an average

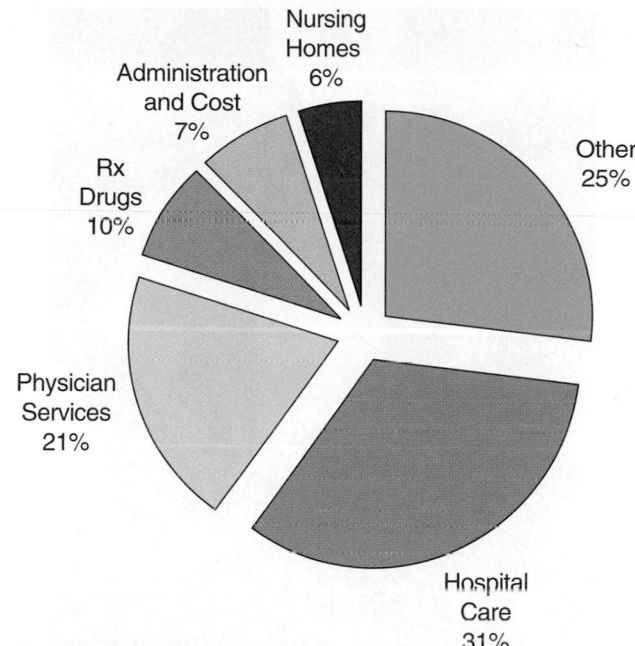

The U.S. health dollar, 2004: Where it went (Other includes dentists, other professional care, durable medical products, research, and construction).

*Source*: Centers for Medicare and Medicaid Services, Office of the Actuary, National Health Statistics Group, 2004.

of 21%. Drug companies often market new, very expensive drugs directly to consumers, who then request them from their physicians. In addition, companies raise the prices on older drugs that research shows to be most effective.

Most *advanced technology is expensive*. New and costly methods of care push prices up. One of the major contributors to health care services inflation is increased use of technology, which often consists of newer and costlier treatments and methods of care. An excellent example is the availability of new treatment for infertile, middle-aged women. A single in vitro fertilization cycle costs $12,400 in the United States, and many women require two to three cycles of treatment to conceive (American Society for Reproductive Medicine (2008). As newer technology is introduced, doctors and nurses become dependent on its use. More sophisticated technology requires more highly trained personnel to run it, and its complexity contributes to specialization among health care providers. This contributes to *higher personnel wages and benefit costs*. Consumers also become used to always having access to new technology and want the very latest in methods and equipment.

Another obvious factor in rising costs is the *change in population demographics*. The overall U.S. population is growing partly as a result of immigration. Immigrants who enter the United States are often poorer and have more health problems. Giving access to these groups increases costs. Large population numbers alone can mean greater costs, but costs per capita (per person) in the United States have grown as well. In 1960, the health care costs per capita were $143; today they are nearly $6,000. The higher costs per

Many men and women are delaying retirement in order to maintain employer-sponsored health coverage.

person can be partially explained by the changing demographics of an aging population. High-tech medicine and other factors have prolonged life. New terms, such as the "old old" and the "young old," have come into use as the population lives longer and "old" has new meaning. The over-85 group is growing at a rapid rate. Older persons require more health resources due to normal processes associated with aging as well as longstanding chronic illness. The need for more long-term care resources and personal health services are increasing proportionately with the aging population, too.

Even though some are deprived of needed health care in the United States, there is also a factor of *excess* in the system. Excess comes in a variety of forms. High-tech equipment is expensive, as is the investment in space required to house it. Such technology often becomes used more frequently than necessary to justify its high cost. In a society where providers fear litigation, even when less expensive options may be equally effective, high-tech procedures may be overused in a type of *medical excess* that is referred to as "defensive medicine." Many argue that excessive and unwanted measures are used to prolong life past what is quality life for both terminally ill persons and the elderly.

*Administrative excess* contributing to increased costs includes both inefficiencies in systems of care and high administrative costs. Inefficient systems of care can be inferred from the patterns of differentiation in treatment and costs across geographic service areas, for example. These differences, which are unexplained by other factors, are attributed to disagreement on "best practices" among direct care providers. Some practices are more expensive. For instance, the benefits of coronary artery bypass surgery over more conservative and less costly treatment are questioned. Greater numbers of hysterectomies and cesarean sections for women in some areas are explained by practice

patterns that may not be cost-effective. Even with similar population attributes and illnesses, more days are spent in the hospital in some areas than in others. All of these discrepancies point to the need to look for more cost-effective clinical practices. Administrative costs, while accounting for a small proportion of the health care dollar, still come under criticism (Bodenheimer & Grumbach, 1995).

Closely associated with clinical practice patterns has been the *emphasis on cure over prevention of illness.* Practice is often guided by reimbursement patterns, and payment from most sources in the recent past has been made only when illness is present. Many economic analyses indicate that preventing illness is more cost-effective than waiting for costly illness to be diagnosed, treated, and monitored. Managed care systems that focus on cost-effectiveness have begun to emphasize preventive care. The relationship of managed care and public health concerns for health promotion and disease prevention is addressed in detail later on.

## Paying for Health Care

Access to health care is determined by financing. Thus demand in the marketplace is directly related to the amount of financing. Services and treatments that are covered by a source of payment have greater demand than if those services were not covered. Financing of health care in the United States is complex. There are multiple sources of funds for health care. These funds, both public and private, are dispersed in a variety of programs and health plans through which resources are used to purchase services. The pie chart below indicates the major sources of funds spent on personal health care.

### ■ Out-of-Pocket Payments and Charity

Those funds that are paid directly by individuals are sometimes called out-of-pocket payments. Some individuals

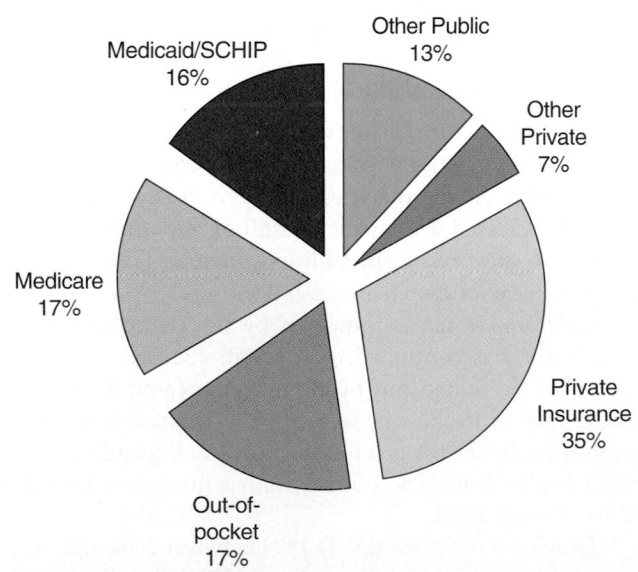

The U.S. health care dollar, 2004: Where it came from.

*Source:* Centers for Medicare and Medicaid Services, Office of the Actuary, National Health Statistics Group, 2004.

or families assume all their own costs for health care services. This is possible when costs are low. A common example is the purchase of over-the-counter drugs. However, this is the least common method of paying for services. For most individuals, who are generally covered by either private or public insurance, the more common out-of-pocket expenses are in the form of **cost sharing.** These expenses include insurance premiums, insurance deductibles, co-payment of a percentage of medical costs, costs above fixed payments, and noncovered services.

Because so many consumers are unable to meet the costs of services they need, and because providing health care to the suffering is seen by some as a moral imperative in modern societies, charity, insurance, and government sources provide funds in varying degrees (Wesson, 1999). Those who cannot afford to pay for needed care often turn to care financed by charity. Charity care has traditionally been seen as a religious duty or vocation, and various religious as well as secular organizations have offered care to the needy for little or no charge. Many physicians and other providers have also cared for the needy, either for free or based on a sliding scale. Philanthropic organizations financed by donors have established institutions to offer charitable care and special services. Another form of non-governmental funds for health care is expenditures covering health care services provided for employees in industrial settings.

## ■ Health Insurance

Risk is a notion central to the concept of insurance. Risk is the possibility of a substantial financial loss from costs of a health event that has a small probability of occurring. Health insurance is a contractual agreement for payment of such health care costs and, therefore, protection from the risk. For a prepaid premium, specific benefits or protections are covered. When the insurance company collects premiums from many subscribers, the risk is shifted from the individual to the group by pooling of resources.

Health insurance is highly regulated by both federal and state governments. For example, significant federal reform was passed in 1996 with the Health Insurance Portability and Accountability Act. Key provisions of the act were portability of health insurance (if certain conditions of prior coverage are met), mental health parity as regards lifetime limits, mandatory minimum length of stay for obstetrics, the creation of tests of new funding methods (medical savings accounts), and fraud and abuse sanctions.

### Private Insurance

Individual private health insurance is purchased by many Americans. Those who work in businesses that do not offer health insurance; the self-employed, including farmers; new college graduates; and early retirees are examples of those persons younger than age 65 who purchase their own private insurance. These types of policies do not spread risk as in group insurance, but base premiums on each individual's health risk.

### Employment-Based Insurance

The most common kind of insurance is employer provided. That is, the employer pays all or most of the insurance premium as an employment benefit. In 1994, the average share of premiums paid by employers was 72%; the remaining 28% of premiums was paid by employees. Health insurance as a fringe benefit became popular during World War II, when wages were frozen but benefits could be given. It still is favored by tax policy, which does not apply income or Social Security tax to such benefits.

Premiums paid through employment are determined by group risks. An **experience rating** is based on a group's own health insurance claims experience. One group may be at greater risk due to occupational hazards or susceptibilities. Their premiums will be higher because they can be expected to have higher utilization of health care services. In contrast, **community ratings** base premiums on the utilization experience of a whole community so that rates are the same for everyone regardless of indicators of risk such as age or occupation.

As health care costs have risen, employers' insurance costs have risen as well. After salaries and raw materials, health care is the third highest cost category in U.S. corporations (Loubeau & Maher, 1996). Employers that compete in the global market are especially concerned because competitors in other countries with government-funded health care do not have the same costs and thus can set lower prices. In response, U.S. employers have initiated more and more cost-containment strategies, such as generic-only prescriptions, second opinions, preadmission testing, and more outpatient surgery. For some employers (as well as individuals), **health insurance purchasing cooperatives (HIPCs)** help to lower costs. These organizations represent a number of employers. By consolidating purchasing power and by realizing efficiencies in enrollment and premium collection, they can help small employers get lower rates than they could alone (Chollet, 1996). However, a main strategy has been to offer managed care plans as an exclusive or an alternative health plan. Managed care plans cover nearly 75% of employees with health insurance in both small and large firms (Shi & Singh, 2008).

Some employers with large workforces have begun to rely on **self-insurance.** Instead of paying premiums to an insurance plan, they assume health care cost risks by budgeting for medical claims from their employees. Government policy stimulated this option when it passed the Employee Retirement Income Security Act of 1974, which allowed for self-funded, nonprofit health plans by corporations. Such plans were exempted from taxes and certain mandatory benefits required of regular plans (Health Insurance Association of America, 1991). For large employers, self-insurance was a better economic alternative. For employees, coverage can be less certain and they have less recourse for appealing claims that are not covered.

Some of the political debate over health care funding has centered on whether health insurance coverage should

## MEDIA MOMENT

### Fatal Care (1995)

This movie is based on the Robin Cook novel, which details the possible future of managed care. The main character has a child with cystic fibrosis and finds him in a hospital using a managed care system. Slowly, patients began to die mysteriously. Their deaths seem to follow a pattern of those who are the most costly in terms of health care and have the least chance of returning as healthy members of society. This is a mystery and fiction but does illuminate possible outcomes of a future managed health care system where costs determine patient outcomes.

### John Q. (2002)

John Quincy Archibald's (Denzel Washington) son Michael collapses while playing baseball as a result of heart failure. John rushes Michael to a hospital emergency room, where he is informed that Michael's only hope is a transplant. Unfortunately, John's insurance will not cover his son's transplant. Out of options, John Q. takes the emergency room staff and patients hostage until hospital doctors agree to do

the transplant. An excellent examination and critical assessment of the "costs" of health care and determination of who has access to our latest technology.

### Lorenzo's Oil (1992)

With this powerful 1992 drama, director–producer George Miller (*The Road Warrior*) proved that a movie about a disease does not have to be a typical disease-of-the-week movie. Based on the real-life case of the Odones family, the story concerns five-year-old Lorenzo, suffering mightily from an apparently incurable and degenerative brain illness called A.L.D. His parents, an economist (Nick Nolte) and a linguist (Susan Sarandon), refuse to accept the received wisdom that there is no hope, and set about learning biochemistry to pursue a cure on their own. The film becomes an intriguing scientific mystery mixed with a story of pain, grief, and the strain on the two adults. Miller, a doctor himself, refuses to shrink from the chaos and horrors of a child's agony, and he and his wife spend their lives trying to find alternative cures, based on their knowledge of chemistry and diseases.

---

be mandated for all firms with workers. Proponents of such a policy believe it is sound business and will attract a stable workforce. Those opposed—mostly small business leaders—believe the expense would cause small businesses to fail and jobs to be lost.

### ■ Publicly Funded Insurance and Direct Care Programs

Public financing supports **categorical programs** that are developed to benefit a certain category of people. The largest of these are Medicare for the elderly and Medicaid for the indigent. The balance of government support goes to U.S. public health service hospitals, Veterans Affairs hospitals and health services, the Department of Defense for military personnel and dependents, the Indian Health Service, state and local support for inpatient psychiatric and other long-term care facilities, worker's compensation, public health activities, and other grants and initiatives. In most cases the government provides the financing but obtains insurance and health care services through the private sector. Payments are disbursed in programs of reimbursements, direct payment, grants, matching funds, and subsidies. Some programs combine federal and state funds. The chart on this page shows the amounts of federal money spent on U.S. entitlement and welfare programs. The large impact of Medicaid, Medicare, and Social Security compared to other programs can be readily seen. Medicare and Medicaid are the primary subjects here, with other government health programs also being briefly explained to complete the picture of government financing.

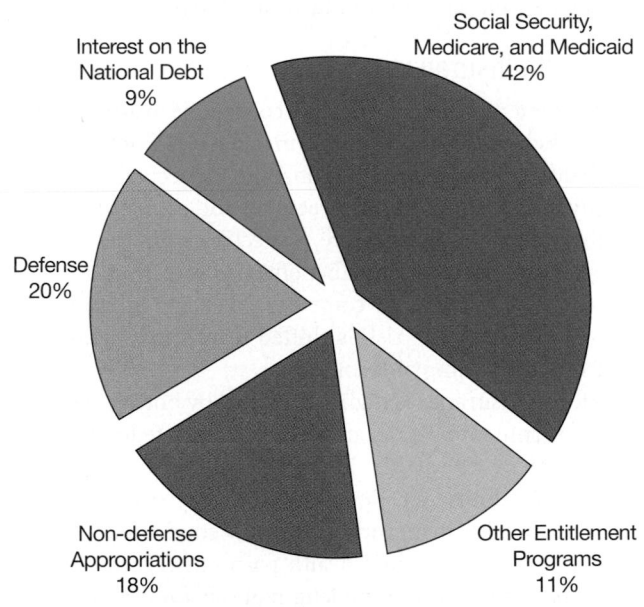

*Source*: Center on Budget and Policy Priorities.

### Medicare

Title XVIII of the Social Security Act, entitled "Health Insurance for the Aged and Disabled," is commonly known as Medicare. Its beginning in 1966 was a historical benchmark. By giving health insurance to everyone older than 65 years of age who is covered by Social Security system entitlement, it signaled a giant step for government entry into personal health care financing. In 1973, other groups became eligible for benefits: persons entitled to Social Security or Railroad Retirement disability benefits for at least 24 months, persons with end-stage renal disease (ESRD) requiring continuing dialysis or kidney transplant, and certain otherwise non-covered persons who elect to buy into Medicare. The Health Care Financing Administration (HCFA) is responsible for overseeing the total program. Medicare covers approximately 50% of the medical expenses of the elderly (Henry J. Kaiser Family Foundation, 2007a).

Medicare consists of two parts, which differ in terms of their sources of funding and benefits: Hospital Insurance (HI), known as "Part A," and Supplementary Medical Insurance (SMI), known as "Part B." A third part of Medicare, established by the Balanced Budget Act of 1997, is the Medicare+Choice program, known as "Part C," which began to provide services on January 1, 1998.

*Hospital insurance, Part A,* of Medicare is mandatory. It provides benefits for care provided in the hospital, outpatient diagnostic services, extended care facilities, and short-term care at home required by an illness for which the patient was hospitalized. HI is financed primarily by payroll taxes collected for Social Security from employees and self-employed workers. The tax is 1.45% of earnings paid by both employers and employees and 2.90% of earnings for self-employed persons. Prior to 1994, there was a ceiling on income taxed for Medicare, but in 1993 the Omnibus Budget Reconciliation Act of 1993 (OBRA-93) made all earnings subject to Medicare tax. Part A hospital insurance has limits on care and requires deductibles and co-payments based on the duration of services.

The following is an overview of the health benefits covered by Medicare's hospital insurance:

- *Inpatient hospital care* coverage covers a semi-private room, meals, regular nursing services, operating and recovery room, intensive care, inpatient prescription drugs, lab tests, x-rays, psychiatric hospital, inpatient rehabilitation, and long-term care hospitalization when medically necessary, as well as services and supplies used in the hospital. A maximum of 90 days is allowed per benefit period. Past the 90 days mark, there is a lifetime reserve of 60 inpatient days. A **benefit period** is an episode of illness starting with hospitalization and ending when the beneficiary has not been a patient in a hospital or skilled nursing facility for 60 consecutive days. There is no limit on the number of benefit periods.
- *Skilled nursing facility (SNF) care* is covered only if it follows within 30 days of a hospitalization of three or more days not including the day of discharge. Up to 100 days of care can be covered. Nursing facility care is not covered unless the required care is for skilled nursing or rehabilitation care.
- *Home health agency (HHA) care,* including care by a home health aide, can be provided intermittently in the residence of a home-bound beneficiary. Again, skilled care must be necessary. Some supplies and equipment may be provided. There are no time or visit limits. Full-time nursing, food, drugs, and blood are *not* covered as HHA services.
- *Hospice services* for terminally ill patients are covered for Medicare-certified hospices. The patient must have a life expectancy of less than six months and forgo benefits for traditional medical treatment for the terminal illness. Covered care includes pain relief, supportive medical and social services, physical therapy, nursing services, and symptom management.

*Supplemental medical insurance, Part B,* is available to almost all residents and certain aliens age 65 and older—even if not entitled to HI services; disabled who are eligible for HI are also covered by Part B. Coverage is voluntary and is financed by general tax revenues as well as a required monthly premium. Premiums are currently set at a level that covers 25% of the national expenditures for the aged beneficiaries. Although the majority of coverage goes to physician fees, SMI also covers many nonphysician services. To be covered, all services must either be medically necessary or be one of the prescribed preventive benefits (i.e., flu vaccinations). Special payment rules including deductibles, maximum amounts payable, or higher cost sharing apply to certain services and care. A yearly deductible and coinsurance of 20% of allowed charges are paid by the beneficiaries.

*Medicare+Choice* was provided by the Balanced Budget Act of 1997. This option increases the managed care plans available to Medicare beneficiaries. Beneficiaries are given the option of a variety of risk-based plans, including coordinated care plans such as health maintenance organizations (HMOs), provider-sponsored organizations (PSOs), and preferred provider organizations (PPOs), as well as other approved alternatives to traditional Medicare. From the beginning of Medicare, alternative payment methodologies have existed for HMO-type providers. In 1995, less than 8% of the total Medicare population was enrolled in such plans. The goal has been to expand the number of managed care options and increase the number of contractors (Vladeck & King, 1997). The Medicare+Choice program offers

 **GLOBAL CONNECTION**

The U.S. health care system lags behind the health care systems of virtually every comparable industrialized nation in the world. The U.S. infant mortality rate is higher and life expectancy lower than in most all countries who share similar populations and type of government. The United States is the only country in the industrialized world that does not have a national health care system, one that provides essential care to all residents with no or minimal costs to the consumer.

Why is the U.S. system different from these other countries? How does our capitalistic political system influence the economics of health?

beneficiaries a broad range of health plan options similar to those available in the private sector.

Market principles are evident in Medicare's performance as both a purchaser and a regulator of managed care. Beneficiaries are given information to allow them to compare their choices and make a selection based on individual preferences and market conditions. The Medicare Compare Database webpage, provided online by HCFA, encourages Medicare consumers to "comparison shop" and gives detailed information on Medicare's health plan options for costs and benefits effective January 1, 2000.

Electing to participate in managed care plans may serve as an alternative to purchasing **Medigap insurance**, which is often desirable if the beneficiary has traditional fee-for-service coverage. Medicare can leave beneficiaries with substantial out-of-pocket costs. Because Part B excludes coverage for prescription drugs, glasses, dentures, hearing aids, yearly physical examinations, routine foot care, and dental care, many individuals supplement their Medicare benefits. Only 12% qualify for Medicaid to pick up these extra expenses, though some retirees have employer plans that cover extra expenses. The term "Medigap" is used to mean private health insurance that pays most of the health care service charges not covered by Parts A and B of Medicare. Such policies, which are offered by Blue Cross and Blue Shield and other commercial health insurance companies, must meet federal standards.

Methods of payment to providers of services for Medicare beneficiaries continue to change as cost-containment incentives are encouraged. Currently, hospitals are paid on a prospective payment system of fixed price per case for patients in diagnosis-related groups (DRGs).

Just as DRGs were implemented to contain hospital costs, **resource utilization groups, version 3** (RUG-III) were launched in July 1998 to contain costs in skilled nursing facilities (SNFs). They are designed to differentiate patients by their levels of resource use. Payment is made on a per diem rate that varies according to the RUG-III category. The goal is to relate pay to patient care requirements and to pay SNFs with different patient caseloads equitably (Shi & Singh, 2008).

Likewise, HCFA has developed ambulatory patient groups (APGs) based on the same goals to be used in clinic settings. These have not been used in Medicare reimbursement yet, but some states have adopted the classification system for Medicaid programs (Shi & Singh, 2008).

Reimbursement for physicians prior to 1992 was for a "reasonable charge," which was the lowest of the actual charge, the customary charge, or the prevailing charge in the area. This has changed to payments based on lowest of submitted charges or a fee schedule based on a **relative value scale.** The relative values are based on time, skill, and intensity it takes to perform a service. The scale places more value on care received through primary care physicians and emphasizes prevention and health promotion. Less value is placed on surgeries and high-technology use. Outpatient and home health services are currently reimbursed

on a reasonable cost basis, but the 1997 Balanced Budget Act provided for implementing a prospective payment system for these services in the future. Claims for both HI and SMI are processed by non-government organizations that contract to serve as the fiscal agent between the federal government and providers. They function locally to apply coverage rules and are known as "intermediaries" and "carriers."

### Medicaid

Because people have contributed toward Medicare through taxes, it is considered an **entitlement** program due to them regardless of their wealth. Medicaid, however, is a **welfare** program, representing funds transferred from more economically affluent individuals to those in need.

Title XIX of the Social Security Act is a federal–state matching funds program with the intent to provide basic health care services to the economically indigent. The federal government provides matching funds based on the per capita income of each state. By law it cannot be more than 83% or less than 50% matching funds. There is no set limit on total federal outlays.

Within broad national guidelines that the federal government provides, each state (1) establishes its own Medicaid eligibility standards; (2) determines the type, amount, duration, and scope of services; (3) sets the rate of payment for services; and (4) administers its own program. Policies vary greatly from state to state; thus a person who is eligible for Medicaid in one state may not be eligible in another state. In addition, eligibility and services in a state can change during a year.

The broad federal guidelines include certain mandated coverage as part of Medicaid. These include inpatient and outpatient hospital services, skilled nursing care, physician services, home health care, family planning services, and early and periodic screening, diagnosis, and treatment services for eligible children younger than age 21.

Recipients must establish their eligibility for Medicaid based on income and assets. In 2003, 55 million individuals were provided health care assistance, with the federal government financing 57% of the costs. Children younger than 21 accounted for about half of that amount (Henry J. Kaiser Family Foundation, 2007b).

The Medicaid program provides services to two broad groups of persons: the categorically needy and the medically needy. For the **categorically needy,** federal funds are matched for mandatory eligibility groups. These would include people receiving Supplemental Security Income (SSI) in some states; those who meet the requirements for the Aid to Families with Dependent Children (AFDC) that were in effect in their state prior to July 16, 1996; children younger than age 6 and pregnant women whose family income is below 133% of the federal poverty level (FPL); and all children born after September 30, 1983, who are younger than age 19 in families with income at or below the FPL. States also have the option of providing coverage to specified other categorically related groups and receive matching federal funds. One of these is the **medically needy**—persons who incur medical expenses beyond the scope of their income.

In 1996, the Personal Responsibility and Work Opportunity Act made sweeping welfare reforms that have had consequences for the Medicaid program. Changes in eligibility for Supplemental Security Income also had an impact. For aliens who lost SSI, Medicaid can continue only if they qualify under some other eligibility status. The new legislation ended the original foundation of the welfare system, Aid to Families with Dependent Children, and replaced it with Temporary Assistance for Needy Families (TANF). TANF is a block-grant program that limits lifetime cash welfare benefits to five years (or less at a state's option). Welfare funds are no longer unconditionally guaranteed to eligible poor families, but states are allowed to impose a wide range of other restrictions as well. For example, if recipients are not involved in work-related activities by the end of their second year on welfare, they must forfeit future benefits. Single mothers have an automatic 25% reduction in benefits if they refuse to help establish paternity of their children. Of significance for Medicaid was the delinkage of its benefits from welfare cash assistance. The law does not require persons covered by TANF to receive Medicaid. Because Medicaid eligibility is not linked to welfare, it is necessary to reach needy families and children who are outside of, as well as in, the welfare system to ensure as many children and families as possible obtain health insurance coverage.

Following the initiation of TANF, some states saw a drastic reduction in the number of children enrolled in Medicaid. Many believed that families were losing Medicaid as they transitioned off of welfare (Mississippi Health Advocacy Program, 1998). Guidelines for protecting and expanding health coverage in the post–welfare reform world have been developed by the Health Care Financing Administration (U.S. Department of Health and Human Services, 2008).

Other developments in Medicaid services are related to long-term nursing home care. Increasing numbers of elderly, in addition to the excessively high expense of long-term care institutions and home-based care, led to an increasing number of people becoming newly eligible for Medicaid coverage. Many with modest resources rapidly use them up in paying for nursing homes or home care. Nursing home expenses were just under $75,000 per year for a private room in 2007 (Genworth Financial, Inc., & National Eldercare Referral Systems, Inc., 2007). Middle-class individuals paying these costs quickly become medically needy and meet state guidelines for Medicaid. With Medicare coverage limited to only three months and little use of private insurance for nursing home coverage, Medicaid currently funds approximately half of annual nursing home care expenditures. Out-of-pocket payments make up the next largest percentage of funds. Very small shares of both institutional and home-bound long-term care services are paid by private insurance. Insurance for long-term care has been difficult to market. Younger, healthier groups whose enrollment would spread the risk and costs generally do not enroll. Therefore, long-term care insurance rates stay high and policies cover only a portion of expenses. Long-term care is expected to be an increasingly utilized provision of Medicaid, with efforts being focused on more community-based long-term care alternatives (Shi & Singh, 2008; Sultz & Young, 2005; Waid, 1998).

Reimbursement under Medicaid is made directly to providers. Rate-setting formulas, procedures, and policies vary widely among states. Fee-for-service systems of payment have dominated. However, federal waivers allow states to develop innovative delivery or reimbursement systems. The last few years have seen a growth in enrollment of Medicaid beneficiaries in managed care, from 56.72% of beneficiaries in 2000 to 65.4% in 2006. As with Medicare, public policy makers have been eager to realize the cost savings reported by private buyers of managed health care services. Competitive bidding strategies allow bids to be made by provider plans. Several states have converted their entire Medicaid programs into managed care.

### Children's Health Insurance Program

One program initiated by the Balanced Budget Act of 1997 is known as the Children's Health Insurance Program (CHIP). CHIP provided federal funds for states to expand Medicaid eligibility to include more uninsured children. These mostly low-income children would not qualify for Medicaid yet their families could not afford private insurance.

Coverage could be provided by states through a Medicaid expansion, separate CHIP program, or a combination. Under a separate CHIP program, states could establish more flexible eligibility requirements. In some cases, states chose to implement coverage for low-income families—not just children—under CHIP. Also, eligibility for coverage could be expanded up to 200% of the poverty level. As with Medicare and Medicaid, managed care options were being offered.

### CHAMPUS and Other Public Direct Care Programs

Another category of persons who have publicly funded health care insurance comprises military personnel and dependents. The Military Health Services System, funded under the Department of Defense, operates to provide medical services to active and retired members of the armed forces and their dependents. Care is provided through military facilities including hospitals and clinics and is supplemented by services purchased from civilian systems and paid for by the Civilian Health and Medical Program of the Uniformed Services (CHAMPUS). Services are free at military facilities, but when care is received from civilian providers who are paid through CHAMPUS there is cost sharing (deductibles and coinsurance) by the families. CHAMPUS does not cover active-duty service members (who receive all their care from the military facilities)—only retirees and dependents.

Linked to the military health care system is the Veterans Administration (VA) health care system. Through this system, the federal government acts as a direct supplier of services to veterans for both war-related injuries and disabilities. For poor service personnel, care is also given for illness that is not related to military service.

The federal government is also involved in direct care to Native Americans living on reservations. The Indian Health Service (IHS) provides both inpatient and ambulatory clinic services through hospitals, health clinics, and ambulatory clinic facilities. These facilities operate at the local level to serve over one million Native Americans. In 1976, tribal governments were granted authority to operate IHS facilities, which are often in remote areas and have low volume. The recent trend has been to refer and contract with private providers for specialty care and diagnostic services.

### Other Public Sources of Health Care Funding

The government funds numerous health programs for specific populations and specific health problems. Many of these have come about through amendments to the Public Health Service Act of 1994. The programs in place at most local health departments come from this funding and assist vulnerable at-risk groups. These programs cover immunizations, tuberculosis, venereal diseases, and family planning along with other services. Rural health clinics, migrant health clinics, and community health centers also are publicly funded. Community health centers operate with 28% of their funds authorized from the Public Health Service Act. These clinics, which pioneered the employment of nurse practitioners, serve as the primary safety net for the poor and underserved in both rural and inner-city settings (Shi & Singh, 2008).

 *Got an Alternative?*

Alternative and complementary health care interventions, such as yoga and herbal use, are seldom reimbursed by insurance and third-party payers, in spite of growing empirical evidence that many can be as effective as traditional treatments at much lower costs and with fewer side effects. Why do you see that as being the case? How do profit motives and politics affect the way insurance providers regard nontraditional health care?

## Cost Containment, Cost Analysis, and Quality

Costs must be contained for the public to get maximum returns on prepaid private insurance, employer-sponsored insurance, and taxes paid toward health care programs. The maze of interconnecting factors related to the causes of high and rising health care costs, of course, guide the mechanisms chosen for controlling them. Mechanisms for cost containment include policy decisions at federal, state, local, and organizational levels. The forces influencing how these decisions are made are complex, as described in Chapter 9. Reform proposals described by Reinert in Chapter 5 show the policy makers' quandary in trying to rectify the cost and quality problems of the U.S. system. Proposals are for either

total or incremental system changes or for changes in the financing of health care. As has been pointed out earlier, economic trends related to costs in the last few years have so far shown results that encourage the strategy of market competition (although predictions of ability to sustain the trends vary). To quote a health services researcher, "The effects of what is now referred to as 'market driven' reform being played out through the proliferation and increasing gains by managed care in controlling costs are pervasively evident throughout virtually every component of the delivery system" (Sultz & Young, 1997, p. 196). The managed care solution is covered in detail in Chapter 6, and its relation to prevention and cost control is discussed later in the chapter.

Both regulatory and competitive strategies to control costs have been mentioned throughout the previous discussion in this chapter. Box 7-3 summarizes some of the methods of these two strategies. One economic strategy that has become increasingly important for nurses and other providers is economic evaluation, which contributes to finding the most cost-effective ways of delivering care and treatments. At the level of both practice guidelines and social policy, economic evaluation is essential. Economic evaluation can

---

### BOX 7-3

**Cost-Containment Strategies**

**Controlling quantity of supply**
- Incentives to decrease numbers of specialist physicians
- Certificate of need to limit technology duplication

**Controlling price**
- Reimbursement for lower cost providers such was nurse practitioners
- Reimbursement for example
  - DRGs: diagnosis-related groups
  - RBRVU: resource-based relative value units
  - APGs: ambulatory patient groups
  - RUGs: resource utilization groups

**Controlling quantity of demand**
- Patient cost sharing
  - increased proportion of premiums
  - Co-payments
  - Deductibles
- Managed care to provide only necessary and appropriate services

**Competition**
- Insurers to shop for best benefit plans
- Managed care plans to shop for best provider contracts

**Prioritizing through cost analysis**
- Focus on prevention
- Reduced inefficiency of interventions

### 💻 Research Alert

This study analyzed data to determine the cost-effectiveness of public nutrition education programs. Using program demographics and food-related dietary behaviors from participants in California's Expanded Food and Nutrition Education Program (EFNEP), researchers calculated benefit-cost ratios for the programs. EFNEP programs teach low-income families the basics of eating a balanced, nutritious diet, including how to shop for and prepare nutritious foods. The programs encourage increased consumption of fruits and vegetables, decreased consumption of fatty foods, and improved food safety and preparation. The long-term goal is to reduce the risk of chronic diseases and improve participants' health. To ensure continued funding, it is important to document the cost-effectiveness of EFNEP programs.

Researchers measured economic value "by comparing benefits (monetized in terms of decreased medical treatment costs) with costs (actual nutrition education expenses over a set time)." In addition to a list of program benefits and costs associated with EFNEP, the researchers assumed that there is a link between diet and chronic disease, they used a formula to quantify that relationship, and they calculated direct benefits as the money saved if treatment for a disease or condition could be prevented or delayed for five years. The initial benefit-cost ratio for California was 14.67 to 1.00, which means that for every $1.00 spent on EFNEP $14.67 was saved in future medical costs. After performing sensitivity analyses to analyze the effects of changes in key variables, researchers found benefit-cost ratios ranging from 3.67 to 1.00, to 8.34 to 1.00, which means that for every $1.00 spent on nutrition education in California, $3.67 to $8.34 is saved.

*Source:* Joy, A. B., Pradhan, V., & Goldman, G. (2006, October–December). *Cost-benefit analysis conducted for nutrition education in California*. Retrieved November 2, 2008, from http://CaliforniaAgriculture.ucop.edu

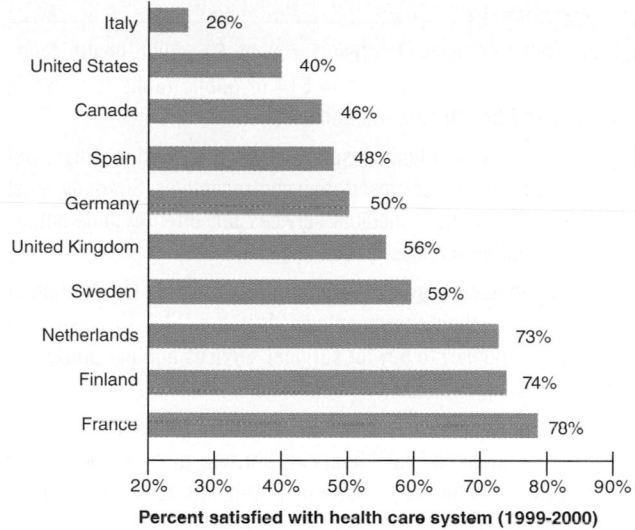

**Percent satisfied with health care system (1999-2000)**

Note: United States and Canada data from Harvard School of Public Health (2000)

Public Satisfaction with Health Care System in Selected Countries

*Source:* Blendon, R., Minah, K., & Benson, J. The public versus the World Health Organization on health system performance. *Health Affairs*, 2001, *20*(3), 10–20.

be used to help in resource allocation in delivery of nursing care and to improve the overall quality of clinical care (Stone, 1998; Spetz, 2005).

Where once the focus of health decision making was only on the effectiveness of treatments and interventions, under competition providers are now competing for contracts with consumers. Consumers look around and make choices based on information about price, quality indicators, and levels of users' satisfaction. Insurers want to know which services to cover and how much to cover. Those who pay often make the treatment decisions. Policy makers want to know how to control public expenditures. Cost-evaluation assessments can be expensive, but, for stakeholders, com-

petition provides the incentive to invest in the needed cost-effectiveness and quality outcomes data they provide. The data are used for internal decisions and now more and more often for letting potential buyers know about the "product" they are buying for "marketing" purposes.

To focus on quality and include cost in the analysis, a number of analytic techniques exist. These include cost-of-illness studies, cost–benefit analysis, and cost-effectiveness analysis.

**Cost-of-illness analysis** estimates the total monetary effects of a specific disease or condition. It takes into account all the resources used to diagnose, treat, and cope with the illness (Max, 1997).

**Cost–benefit analysis** (CBA) uses such measures to compare benefits, in terms of disease prevention, with the costs of a program. In this technique, benefits are measured in monetary terms. CBA is the principal method used to evaluate decisions involving public expenditures. Decisions are based on alternatives providing the greatest net benefit—that is, the greatest level of economic efficiency (Moore, Laufer, & Conroy, 1998).

The Research Alert is an example of a cost–benefit study. The drawback of using this method to analyze health care is the difficulty of placing a dollar value on outcomes such as pain or grief or premature loss of life. The methods for determining such costs are developed in economics, but are controversial (Thompson, 2003).

**Cost-effectiveness analysis** (CEA), sometimes considered a more acceptable health care valuation alternative,

NOTE THIS!

Contraceptives are cost-effective: For every $1 public health funds invested in family planning, $4 to $14 of public funds is saved in pregnancy and health care–related costs.

The vast majority of private insurers cover prescription drugs, but may exclude coverage for prescription contraceptives. Similarly, most policies cover outpatient medical services but often exclude outpatient contraceptive services for coverage.

Health insurance companies are more likely to cover sterilization or abortion services than contraceptives. This indicates the insurance community's tendency to pay for surgical services and not preventive care.

The Institute of Medicine Committee on Unintended Pregnancy recently recommended that "financial barriers to contraception be reduced by increasing the proportion of all health insurance policies that offer contraceptive services and supplies."

*Source*: APHA, 1998.

calculates a ratio in which health outcome is measured in health units, such as cases avoided or years of life saved. Cost of treatment or intervention is measured in dollars. Thus results are presented in terms of "cost per case prevented" or "cost per life saved." The purpose of CEA is to compare the relative value of different interventions in creating better health and/or longer life. Costs of alternative programs are compared based on a single nonmonetary outcome. CEA furnishes information that is useful in a variety of settings. In a managed care setting, an organization may wish to know the cost savings per low-birth-weight birth avoided as a consequence of a prenatal care outreach program. In addition, the organization could ask the cost of the program per year of life saved for its enrolled population. Analysis for a state health department might look at different strategies to control tuberculosis in the population. It could compare the cost-effectiveness of screening all community members versus screening only those at high risk based on history and exposure. In a larger context, the department might evaluate the costs per case of high blood lead level avoided of an educational program aimed at housing repair to reduce dust and peeling paint.

One other area in which cost–benefit and cost-effectiveness analyses are used is in the broader field of technology assessment. **Technology assessment,** a form of policy research, helps decision makers to deal with developing and using expensive health care practices and technologies. It is assessment that includes both cost–benefit analysis (CBA) and outcome effectiveness analysis (CEA). In addition, it analyzes safety and social impact of technologies (Thompson, 2003).

Cost-effectiveness analysis assists in setting priorities for the use of scarce resources. For instance, research was done on the use of cholesterol-modifying agents to compare the cost-effectiveness of primary prevention to secondary prevention of heart disease. In the study, primary prevention entailed administration of the drug to those who had never had heart disease; secondary prevention involved administration of the drug to those who had a history of angina or myocardial infarction. With primary prevention, the cost per year of life saved was more than $50,000, whereas with secondary prevention, there was actually a cost savings for some groups. Recommendations were to give priority to secondary intervention when there are scarce resources (Buerhaus, 1998).

Even though the influence of CEA on policy is not well documented, it is believed to have played a key role in some major decisions. Medicare's first preventive service—coverage of pneumococcal vaccine—was based on a CEA done by the Office of Technology Assessment. Cancer screening recommendations of the American Cancer Society are also based on CEA studies (Buerhaus, 1998; Gold, Siegel, Russell, & Weinstein, 1996).

## Public Health, Managed Care, and the Economics of Prevention

The current economic environment has had consequences for the public health sector, which, following the attacks of September 11, 2001, and the ravages of Hurricane Katrina, has found "itself again at center stage, with the spotlights focused on its performance" (Beitsch, Brooks, Menachemi, & Libby, 2006). Along with market forces playing a greater role in the total health care system, there has been a redefinition of government role. Even though government is a key instrument in community action, taxpayers appear unwilling to pay more money for publicly funded health programs (Lasker & Committee on Medicine and Public Health, 1997; Appleby, 2006). With costs rising, a tightening of public funds is the result. Although public health added new roles and responsibilities for responding to disasters, both human-made (September 11 attacks, bioterrorism) and natural (Hurricanes Katrina and Rita), and to emerging infectious diseases (avian flu and SARS), funding for public health has not increased and is very limited in contrast to financial support for the private health care system (Beitsch et al., 2006). Tightening of funds threatens support for all of the health system's public goods: research, education of health professionals, population-based programs, and safety-net care for the uninsured and underinsured. Five mechanisms for federal cost cutting have been (1) moving authority and monetary responsibility for programs to states and local governments, (2) downsizing, (3) reorganizing, (4) privatizing, and (5) linking funds to documented results. Personnel have been cut, program budgets have been cut, and total programs have been cut (Lasker & Committee on Medicine and Public Health, 1997).

### ■ Opportunities for Collaboration

In spite of the concerns about the cost-cutting effects on public health program delivery and threats of an imperfect market of privatized managed care, there are reasons for community health nurses to be encouraged by the rapid growth of managed care. One of the commonalities among all the payers of health care services has been cost-containment efforts through increased enrollment of their beneficiaries in managed care plans. The federal government has signed waivers to allow states to enroll Medicaid recipients in managed care plans; more than 60% of Medicaid beneficiaries receive healthcare services through managed care. Enrollment of Medicare beneficiaries in managed care is about 14% (Shi & Singh, 2008). Enrollment is encouraged and steadily increasing for employee-sponsored insurance as well. The positive element is the population orientation of managed care and the potential it has to strengthen public health efforts. Managed care links both the insurance and the delivery of services by paying care providers a set amount for all the services of their insured population. Thus the care providers share the financial risk of the enrolled population's health status. The incentive is to keep the population healthy.

Managed care organizations providing health care become linked in two ways to public health efforts. First, they share the interest in using population-based methods of epidemiology to study, track, and understand their enrolled populations and to keep those populations healthy. Second, to keep their enrolled populations healthy, they are aware of the benefits of collaboration in the wider public health efforts that focus on preventing illness for the total population. Their enrolled populations are a part of the total population, of course. The total population achieves better outcomes with environmental protections, greater health awareness, early detection of disease, and improved health behavior. If the total population remains or becomes healthier, their enrolled populations do the same and the managed care organizations realize the benefits of decreased use of expensive services for preventable illnesses. Plans that can improve population health will control their costs and, therefore, will have a major advantage in a competitive market.

Prior to managed care, the influence and prestige of health care professionals outside of public health disciplines did not guide public opinion or government action toward prevention and health. The emphasis on cure of diseases over which there was more biological control left social and behavioral issues of health—such as drugs, alcohol, cigarettes, AIDS, and violence—with less attention and less funding. As noted earlier, a very small percentage of the U.S. national health care expenditures goes to public health activity (slightly more than 3%). The cost-effective methods of prevention and public health have not been recognized or valued by most individuals, groups, and governments in the United States. The more cost-effective prevention strategies are less dramatic. As Sultz and Young ob-

**Application to Practice**

One of your patients at the clinic where you work comes in for a routine visit regarding her hypertension. In the midst of her visit, she tells you, "I am so confused. I have to make a decision about which Medicare plan to choose. I've only been on Medicare for two years and I've just begun to understand how it works and what they will really pay. There are gaps, but it is pretty good for me. Now they tell me I have a choice of changing plans. But I don't know what to do. How can I decide which is best for me? Surely you know more about these things than I do. What should I do?"

1. What is your role in such a situation? How would you respond?
2. What might you consider in educating this patient about care plans?
3. Are there resources you could refer her to?

serve, "Unlike the recipients of heart transplants, . . . the media cannot show pictures of the hundreds of thousands of children who have *not* been crippled and have *not* died due to poliomyelitis since the successful programs have been initiated" (1997, p. 267). Many believe that the new market incentives that led to managed care as a means of cost control will provide powerful economic incentives for a stronger alliance between managed care organizations and public health initiatives at all levels—federal, state, and local (Mechanic, 1998; Robbins & Freeman, 1999).

The shift in incentive from acute services as profitable to disease prevention as profitable is changing both who provides care and how care is provided (Shi & Singh, 2008). In contrast to most indemnity plans of insurance, managed care plans and providers are increasing preventive services such as screening, immunizations, and counseling for high-risk conditions. They encourage preventive services by increasing access to primary care providers. By making the providers accountable to the populations they care for and

### ⚑ ETHICAL CONNECTION

As the demand for alternative and complementary therapies (such as yoga, acupuncture, and Reiki) grows in our patient population, what are ethical considerations regarding patient education and the role of the community health nurse?

As a nursing student, what was your initial reaction to the term "managed care"? Did you see managed care as a way to improve patient care or as a way to save money? In your experiences as a nursing student, is the present system of cost containment working for patients, the health care providers, health care organizations, or all?

linking reimbursement for prevention to attaining certain goals, managed care methods could enhance the delivery of preventive services. If organized managed care plans, especially those enrolling public beneficiaries such as Medicaid, assume the services that have been offered by state and local health departments and publicly financed community health centers, these public services are affected. By losing Medicaid and other primary care patients to managed care plans, they must deal with shrinking budgets. Community health centers have reacted to competition by forming health plans of their own (Shi & Singh, 2004). Public health agencies are regrouping and devoting their resources to the core public health functions. If they are no longer competing for clinical patients and payments, they can focus on surveillance, community-wide interventions, and assuring and enhancing access (Robbins & Freeman, 1999).

Some see these changes as encouraging and an imperative for collaboration and cooperation through partnerships between managed care organizations and public health agencies. The Centers for Disease Control and Prevention (CDC) has brought together members of the public health and managed care sectors at national conferences that focus on prevention (CDC, 1995). In addition, the CDC has formed partnerships with the American Association of Health Plans and The HMO Group, which have encouraged the managed care community to become involved in public health and preventive measures (Schauffler & Scutchfield, 1998).

The Committee on Medicine and Public Health reported on its mission and initiatives to join medical care and public health care (Lasker & Committee on Medicine and Public Health, 1997). Through this work, which was funded by both private and public funds, the committee examined 414 examples of collaborative efforts. They described the projects and indicated how the collaborative work was done. Benefits accrued to both health sectors, as public health agencies gained from the prevention efforts of managed care organizations, and the organizations, which benefited benefit from the expertise of public health practitioners.

Managed care organizations are learning to conduct health assessments of the communities they serve and to identify areas where they can have a large influence on improving the communities' health (Shi & Singh, 1998). The

collection and analysis of population-based data are the skills of public health that make collaboration welcome. Robbins and Freeman (1999), for example, have reported on a New England joint venture between the not-for-profit managed care organizations of six states and those states' public health services. The goals these parties believe will be achieved are improved health and efficiency that reduce health care costs and, therefore, an increase in the political resolve to provide coverage for everyone.

## Counterforces to Collaboration

The opportunities are not without problems, however, and the interface of public health with the new organized systems for delivering clinical care is evolving. One pressing issue is this: Who will care for the individuals who remain uninsured? Even with policy efforts to increase coverage for all, and especially for children, there still is not access for all. If health departments are expected to be the safety net, then they must be funded to do so. With Medicaid patients moving to managed care plans, public health can no longer cross-subsidize uninsured primary and preventive care with Medicaid funds.

Another issue for health departments is the "dumping" of services covered by private managed care plans. Plans may cover immunizations in their capitated fee, yet still send their enrollees to a health department for immunizations without reimbursing the department.

Coordination of state reporting for notifiable diseases, directly observed therapy, and STD contact tracing may also be problematic, with managed care organizations seeing patients formerly seen by public health departments. Health departments must be able to obtain such patient enrollment and encounter information for surveillance and epidemiological studies. Clarification of these and other roles and responsibilities must be addressed in the midst of the new forces at work in the total system (Rosenbaum & Richards, 1996; Schauffler & Scutchfield, 1998).

Another barrier to collaboration is the nature of for-profit firms. Nonprofit providers are converting to for-profit organizations at an increasing rate. When accountability to their stockholders is their top priority, their motivation is naturally to seek short-term advantages that lead to a positive bottom line. An advantage could be realized in the short term by cutting preventive measures and increasing profits. Many know that their enrollees may change plans often and will not remain their financial responsibility if illness occurs in the future (Mechanic, 1998). Profit maximization can be socially undesirable when it leads to product quality effects. Clearly, withholding preventive services has an effect on individuals as well as the larger public. The public has loudly criticized these and other business practices: They want for-profit plans in health care to be accountable for the social responsiveness and social trust that any course in business ethics would encourage (Arrow, 1997).

## Research Alert

In the past few years, reductions in postpartum length of stay have been attempted in an effort to lower costly stays for newborns and their mothers. In spite of legislation and provider recommendations, many infants are discharged in less than 48 hours and do not have the recommended pediatrician-initiated reassessment within 48 hours of discharge.

Because practitioner compliance with recommended guidelines is inconsistent and/or impractical, the alternative of nurse home visits has been explored. Nurse visits can be more timely than office visits and can occur when jaundice or dehydration are still developing. The researchers hypothesized that home nursing visits would be cost-effective just by reducing hospital-based services for jaundice and dehydration in the first ten days after hospital discharge.

Retrospective analysis of financial records was conducted to do a cost-effectiveness analysis from the payers' perspective. This perspective was logical, as any extra costs associated with home nursing visits would be absorbed by insurers to offset any subsequent hospital-based services. Records were reviewed for all neonates born and discharged from a single center from January 2000 to December 2002 ($n = 2,967$). Outcome measures included (1) expected costs for each patient, (2) the expected number of children who did not require hospital-based care either because they did not develop symptoms or because the nurse visit led to outpatient therapy instead of the more expensive resources; and (3) the incremental cost-effectiveness ratio (ICER) of home nursing visit strategy compared to usual care.

The average cost per child *with* a home visit was $109.80 compared to $118.70 for those not visited by a nurse. Results also showed that 99.4% of children *with* a home visit did not use additional hospital services compared to 94.5% of those with no visit ($p < .0001$). Therefore, *the nurse visit strategy was concluded to be both more effective and less costly.* The ICER of the routine home nursing visit compared to no visit was –$181.82, which indicates payers will save $181.82 for each child who does not use hospital services in the first ten days of life.

*Source:* Paul, I., Phillips, T., Widome, M., & Hellenbeak, C. (2004). Cost-effectiveness of postnatal home nursing visits for prevention of hospital care for jaundice and dehydration. *Pediatrics, 114*(4), 1015–1022.

## ■ Economics of Alternative Therapies

Among the many changes driven by economics that are important to community health nursing has been the increased acceptance of alternative therapies. Insurance plans and managed care organizations, driven by consumer demand and searching for lower-cost services for their populations, have discovered alternative care methods. The economic impact of alternative care was realized with the

---

### BOX 7-4

**Cost Savings of Alternative Therapies**

In a study to test Dr. Dean Ornish's lifestyle-based treatment of heart disease, Mutual of Omaha had 200 subscribers volunteer to a structured year of exercise, meditation, group support, and a strict vegetarian diet. Almost 95% stuck to the low-technology program, which cost $5,500 versus $15,000 for angioplasty or $40,000 for bypass surgery. Mutual of Omaha estimates it has saved $6.50 for every dollar it has spent. In addition, because patients with heart problems often have several operations over the years, the company says the approach could save them up to $20 on the dollar.

*Source:* Cowley, King, Hager, & Rosenberg, 1995.

---

publication of the landmark study by Eisenberg. Although this study included only 1,539 individuals, extrapolation of its results to the larger population indicated that more visits were made to alternative providers than to conventional primary care providers; $13.7 billion was spent, mostly out of pocket; and dollars spent exceeded out-of-pocket costs for hospitalization (Weeks, 1997). These numbers indicated a potential market for insurers and managed care.

In their quest to realize economic benefits, health plans have begun to include alternative therapy providers and treatment modalities in their plans (see Box 7-4). Alternative therapies most often are focused on holistic, wellness approaches that realize the benefits of prevention. Surveys of patients of alternative providers show that there are effects on use of conventional pharmaceuticals, necessity of conventional surgeries, development of self-care abilities, and reduced visits to conventional physicians after self-care education (Weeks, 1997). Providing a popular source of care in their plans may be a strategy by which managed care organizations can achieve multiple goals: increase market share by meeting a consumer demand, realize the cost savings of less technologically advanced treatments for illnesses, and use less services due to increased wellness. There are also possibilities for linkages and collaboration with public health in including alternative approaches to health. In Washington, for example, an integrated natural medicine/conventional medicine clinic is offered as a part of county services and it may be expanded. Other states are also interested in setting up such clinics (Weeks, 1997). Washington was also the first state to mandate health plan coverage of the full range of state-licensed providers such as naturopaths, acupuncturists, and chiropractors (Hamilton, 1996).

Plans that are beginning to create benefit packages for people interested in alternative care cover such alternatives as chiropractors, naturopaths, reflexology, rolfing, herbs, acupuncture, clinical nutritionists, massage, yoga, biofeedback, and chelation, among others (Hamilton, 1996; Weeks, 1997).

For managed care organizations, these practices raise issues related to safety and efficacy documentation, which is not available in most cases.

## Significance of Economics for Community Health Nursing Practice

Throughout this chapter, we have examined the implications of economics for the individuals, families, and communities for whom nurses care. It is easy to become immersed in the immediacy of individual nursing roles and remain unaware of the outside forces affecting practice. Today, economics—even more than social and political demands—drives our practice and the results for out patients. Who gets seen? What treatment can they get? Who will treat them? What will the setting be? Who will you work with? Who will pay you? The answers to all these questions are influenced by economic considerations of financing of health and welfare services, reimbursement rates, insurance mechanisms, and means of delivery. In many ways today's environment is favorable for community nurses as care continues to move into more cost-effective sites in the community, population-focused skills are needed, and disease prevention/health promotion is needed. Following are just some of the other implications for current practice in a rapidly changing environment.

Perhaps one of the most valuable interactions with patients addresses their needs as consumers in consumer-driven health care. As indicated, earlier, informed consumers are vital for a market to work at its best. They need education, advocacy, and assistance. Beyond educating patients about their health or illness needs, nurses need to educate them for informed choices about their care. Even though Medicare covers screening mammograms, one in three women insured by Medicare did not receive a mammogram between 2004 and 2005 (Arvantes, 2008). Patients need assistance to increase their self-care knowledge, reinforce effective self-care, and partner with health providers. Nurses can reinforce the trend for consumers to be active and more informed about their health care options, including alternative therapies. As baby boomers enter the ranks of seniors, they are expected to use the Internet more than current seniors to access healthcare information (Kaiser Family Foundation, 2005).

Importantly, in a consumer-driven health system, nurses can help consumers understand price, quality issues, and more. Educating and informing health care consumers about such things as discovering treatment options, reading quality reports, navigating complicated health plans, understanding payment systems, dealing with restrictions, and finding the service amenities they want will enable them to make market comparisons and choices. In addition to educating them to meet their own needs, consumers need "trusted partners to act as their agents" (Scandlen, 2005, p. 1557) in referrals to innovative providers, advocacy in appeals processes, and good documentation to ensure reimbursement.

When considering consumers in the marketplace, there are also opportunities as a nurse provider to inform health plan purchasers about the needs of their populations and how best to meet them. Employer health plans have tended to look only at cost and not consider quality in making plan decisions (Dentzer, 1998). Nurses have knowledge about quality and can purposefully encourage quality choices.

There are dynamic changes occurring in the nursing labor market. Reimbursement patterns and cost control have been the driving forces that moved jobs into the community setting, sought to replace or substitute nurses with cheaper labor sources, and are creating new roles. Demand management through telephone triage positions staffed by nurses eliminates unnecessary visits to clinics and emergency rooms (Larson-Dahn, 1998). In market settings, positions such as case manager risk manager provider liaison, benefits coordinator, utilization review coordinator, quality assurance coordinator, and positions utilizing population assessment skills are needed. There are new opportunities in prevention counseling services, and adding alternative therapies to practice options is encouraged by reimbursement trends.

Perhaps one of the most important labor market changes for nurses was gaining third-party reimbursement for advanced practice nurses (American Nurses Association, 1997). There had been reimbursement in specific rural areas, but the Balanced Budget Act of 1997 gave Medicare coverage to nurse practitioners and clinical nurse specialists for any service that would be covered under Medicare Part B when provided by a physician, regardless of geographic area. Nurses' reimbursement is crapped at 80% of the physician rate. Direct reimbursement removed some of the barriers to entering the market, and the lower price for services made nurses more competitive. However, there are still significant labor market barriers including, for example, insurance companies that require billing under a physician's name or will credential only nurse practitioners employed by a physician and Medicare managed care organizations that will not allow nurse practitioners to be primary care providers. Free labor market competition for nurse providers still needs improvement (Ashby, 2006).

Community health nurses can optimize patient care by using economic information in coalition building, research, lobbying, negotiating with insurers, and influencing policy on health care allocation. In speaking the language of the marketplace, nurses can be more persuasive by having a broadly accepted reference point. In policy issues, nurses need to continually evaluate new or needed legislation that will affect patient care as well as themselves as consumers or providers. For example, mandatory overtime for nursing staff has become an unwelcome solution to the unmet labor market demand for nursing staff. The American Nurses Association has stated its support for legislation that limits mandatory overtime to 12 hours per 24-hour period and acknowledges that staffing concerns extend beyond acute care to community nursing as well (American Nurses Association, 2005).

Nurses can also participate in collecting, analyzing, and interpreting data for policy decisions. Spetz (2005) claims that the agenda for nursing research on cost-effectiveness is daunting. However understanding economic evaluation methods such as CEA adds to nurses' ability to explain the value-added contribution of nursing services. As a necessary adjunct to evidence-based practice, CEA techniques have the potential to refine practice and lead to nursing interventions that utilize scarce resources for the best return in terms of health (Stone, Curran, & Bakken, 2002). Measures of effectiveness alone are not sufficient for ensuring the appropriateness or feasibility of interventions for specific settings or populations (Fielding & Briss, 2006; Siegel, 1998).

❝ *Future shock is the shattering stress and disorientation that we induce in individuals by subjecting them to too much change in too short a time.* ❞

*Alvin Toffler, Future Shock, 1970*

❝ *Be enthusiastic. Remember the placebo effect—30% of medicine is show biz.* ❞

*Ronald Spark*

❝ *The art of medicine consists of amusing the patient while nature cures the disease.* ❞

—*Voltaire*

## Economics and Nightingale's Legacy

Even with the opportunities outlined previously, much in the current nursing literature reflects the uneasiness that nurses have with a health care system in which some are provided care and others, for lack of resources, go without. Historically, as well as during the failed Clinton administration attempt at comprehensive health reform, nurses have been advocates for access to quality, cost-effective health care services for all people. The gaps in access in our current system are obvious.

Nurses have also expressed misgivings about referring to those they care for as customers, buyers, or consumers. For some, the philosophy of health care as a business threatens the human interactions of nursing and creates an environment that restricts understanding of nursing's value and purpose (Heggen & Wellard, 2004; David, 1999). Nurses worry about the safety of vulnerable patients caught in cost-cutting efforts. Nurses have also questioned a system in which savings from cost cutting go into the pockets of high-salaried executives and stockholders (Gordon, 2008).

Is managed care or consumer-driven care an ethically supportable response to rising costs and giving of quality care? For community health nurses, a market system can seem at odds with the nation's public health goal to attain the highest levels of health and welfare for its citizens. Nurses appear to be struggling, as do other citizens, with the contrasting basic principles of justice underlying the production and distribution of health care resources. In broad contrast, these are market justice and social justice.

Approaching distribution by relying on capitalism and private for-profit enterprise is the **market justice** approach. Favoring the market is at the heart of the American traditions of individualism and limited government. The market solution is based on people's willingness and ability to pay. Those who cannot pay have individual accountability and do not receive services. People have the right to purchase the health goods they value. They purchase these goods with resources earned from their own efforts. The ideal results are economic efficiency. Market justice emphasizes individual rather than collective responsibility for health.

In contrast, a **social justice** approach holds health care to be a social good that should be collectively financed and available to all citizens regardless of ability to pay. Social justice favors societal responsibility for health care to be achieved through government initiative.

Elements of both market justice and social justice are present in the U.S. system, but market justice dominates (Shi & Singh, 2008). If the United States has embraced the market system in health care, does this mean that collectively we believe only those who can pay should receive care or that people can only get the amount of care they can afford? As the only developed country in the world without some measure of universal health care coverage, it would seem so. Why we have adopted such a national stance has been the subject of much debate for decades. Our policies may be accurately reflecting the ethic of the U.S. citizenry (Rice, 1998). In a reported survey, it was found that only 23% of U.S. respondents agreed with the statement, "It is the responsibility of the government to take care of the very poor people who cannot take care of themselves." The U.S. response was considerably lower than the citizens of other countries (Blendon et al., 1995). Yet, in a more recent poll, 68% of respondents said that providing coverage for everyone is more important than keeping taxes down. However, approval for coverage for all dropped considerably when it might mean loss of any treatments currently covered by insurance, limits on doctor choice, or higher premiums (Appleby, 2006). This ethics quandary could explain the present inability of our policy makers to decide who, if anyone, is to provide health care to those who do not currently have economic access to such care.

Although the two differing ethics reflect our values and beliefs about what is good or best, both beliefs seem to have flaws. Dowd (1999) has suggested that the question we really face is one of whether our problems are best solved by "imperfect government or imperfect markets" (p. 269). The United States is not alone in its struggle to deal with the economic challenges of health care. What is emerging internationally is discussion about a fundamentally different "third way" in health—a middle road between a centrally planned system and one based on market principles (LeGrand, 1999; Kritsotakis & Gamarnikow, 2004).

Nurses can better contribute to the ongoing dialogue if they understand both the opportunities and the downfalls of the two economic approaches as they operate in our present system. Nurses can look back as far as Florence Nightingale and find the origins of our public involvement in what is good for society. LeVasseur describes the Nightingale legacy as a "guardian-like stamp on nursing" (1998, p. 281). She says, "Nightingale showed a strong sense of responsibility to her society and a passion for reform. . . . It was not enough for Nightingale to have knowledge of the good, but it was important to put that knowledge into action as a guardian of the people" (p. 281). Nurses today need not and should not be passive participants in the broad marketplace of ideas about what our society values in health care.

Explore Community Health Nursing on the Web! To learn more about the topics in this chapter, use the passcode provided to access your exclusive website: **http://nursing.jbpub.com/communityhealth.** If you do not have a passcode, you can obtain one at this site.

## ■ CRITICAL THINKING ACTIVITIES

1. Explain how under imperfect market conditions, both prices and quantities of health care are higher than they would be in a highly competitive market.

2. Two emergency room nurses are debating the issue of access to health care. One is concerned about the stigma of those who are uninsured and claims that people without health insurance receive less health care and have poorer health than those with insurance. The other disagrees, claiming that hospitals, doctors, and public health clinics deliver large amounts of charity care, which allows uninsured people to have the services they need. Who has the stronger case? What does research tell us?

3. The following is a dialogue with former U.S. Health and Human Services Secretary Donna Shalala and Princeton economist Uwe Reinhardt:

**Shalala:** In fact, Medicare is the best payer in the system: It pays more quickly and better than most private systems do.

**Reinhardt:** And it operates more cheaply. Medicare passes through much more money, about 97 cents of every premium dollar, because its administrative costs are so low. No private insurer can match that record. Most providers don't know this.

**Shalala:** People just can't get the stereotype of big bureaucracy out of their heads. And the idea that Medicare's administrative expenses are 3% or 4% while the private sector spends 12% just doesn't register with many people particularly those who see health care as a business.

*Source*: Shalala & Reinhardt, 1999.

Why might the difference exist between government and private spending? How might someone in a for-profit organization respond to this conversation?

## ■ REFERENCES

American Nurses Association. (1997). *Medicare reimbursement for NPs and CNSs.* Retrieved May 23, 2008, from http://www.nursingworld.org/gova/federal/agencies/hcfa/medreimb.htm

American Nurses Association. (2005). *ANA's health care agenda 2005* [Brochure]. Washington, DC: Author.

American Public Health Association (APHA). (1998). *Fact sheet: Prescription contraceptive equity.* Retrieved May 23, 2008, from http://www.apha.org/legislative/factsheets/fs2.htm

American Society for Reproductive Medicine (ASRM). (2008). *Frequently asked questions about infertility.* Retrieved October 31, 2008, from http://www.asrm.org/Patients/faqs.html

Appleby, J. (2006, October 16). Universal care appeals to USA: But what it would cost complicates the issue. *USA Today,* p. 4B.

Arrow, K. J. (1997). Social responsibility and economic efficiency. In T. Donaldson & T. W. Dunfee (Eds.), *Ethics in business and economics.* Brookfield, VT: Ashgate.

Arvantes, J. (2008). New study finds wide disparities in Medicare's quality of care. *AAFP News Now.* Retrieved November 2, 2008, from http://www.aafp.org

Ashby, M. (2006). Barriers to nurse practitioner reimbursement. *Pennsylvania Nurse, 61*(2), 19.

Beitsch, L. M., Brooks, R. G., Menachemi, N., & Libbey, P. M. (2006). Public health at center stage: New roles, old props. *Health Affairs, 25*(4), 911–922.

Berenson, R. A. (2005). Which way for competition? None of the above. *Health Affairs, 24*(6), 1536–1542.

Blendon, R. J., Benson, J., Donelan, K., et al. (1995). Who has the best health care system? A second look. *Health Affairs, 14*(4), 220–230.

Blumenthal, D. (1994). The vital role of professionalism in health care reform. *Health Affairs, 13*(1), 252–256.

Blumenthal, D. (2006). Employer-sponsored health insurance in the United States: Origins and implications. *New England Journal of Medicine, 355*(1), 82–88.

Bodenheimer, T. S., & Grumbach, K. (1995). *Understanding health policy: A clinical approach.* Stamford, CT: Appleton and Lange.

Brown, C. (1999). Ethics, policy, and practice: Interview with Emily Friedman. *Image: Journal of Nursing Scholarship, 31,* 259–262.

Buerhaus, P. I. (1998). Milton Weinstein's insights on the development, use and methodological problems in cost-effectiveness analysis. *Image: Journal of Nursing Scholarship, 30*(3), 223–227.

Centers for Disease Control and Prevention. (1995). Prevention and managed care: Opportunities for managed care, purchasers of health care, and public health agencies. *Morbidity and Mortality Weekly Report, 44,* 1–12.

Centers for Medicare and Medicaid Services. (2008). *Table 1: National health expenditures aggregate.* Retrieved October 8, 2008, from http://www.cms.gov/NationalHealthExpendData/downloads/tables.pdf

Chen, M., & Mastilica, M. (1998). Health care reform for Croatia: For better or for worse? *American Journal of Public Health, 88*(8), 1156–1160.

Chollet, D. J. (1996). Redefining private insurance in a changing market structure. In S. H. Altman & U. E. Reinhardt (Eds.), *Strategic choices for a changing health care system.* Chicago: Health Administration Press.

Collins, S. R., Kriss, J. L., Doty, M. M., & Rustgi, S. D. (2008). *Losing ground: How the loss of adequate health insurance is burdening working families.* Findings from the Commonwealth Fund Biennial Health Insurance Surveys, 2001–2007. Retrieved October 30, 2008, from http://www.commonwealthfund.org/publications/publications_show.htm?doc_id

Cooper, P. F., & Schone, B. S. (1997). More offers, fewer takers for employment-based health insurance: 1987–1996. *Health Affairs, 16*(6), 142–149.

Cowley, G., King, P., Hager, M., & Rosenberg, D. (1995, June 26). Going mainstream. *Newsweek,* pp. 56–57.

David, B. A. (1999). Nursing's conflicting values in competitively managed health care. *Image: Journal of Nursing Scholarship, 31*(2), 188.

Deaton, A. (2006, April). Letter from America: Trying to be a good hip op consumer. *Royal Economic Society Newsletter, 133,* 3–4.

Dentzer, S. (1998, January–February). A guide to managed care, part 2. *Modern Maturity,* 35–41, 43.

Department of Health and Human Services. (1999). *Annual update of the HHS poverty guidelines.* http://aspe.hhs.gov/poverty/99fedreg.htm

Donelan, K., Blendon, R., Hill, C., et al. (1997). Whatever happened to the health insurance crisis in the United States? Voices from a national survey. In P. Lee & C. Estes (Eds.), *The nation's health.* Sudbury, MA: Jones and Bartlett.

Dowd, B. (1999). An unusual view of health economics [Review of the book *The economics of health reconsidered*]. *Health Affairs, 18*(1), 266–269.

Dowd, B. (2005). Coordinated agency versus autonomous consumers in health services markets. *Health Affairs, 24*(6), 1501–1511.

Edwards, R. (2005). Blind faith and choice. *Health Affairs, 24*(6), 1624–1628.

Fielding, J. E., & Bliss, P. A. (2006). Promoting evidence-based public health policy: Can we have better evidence and more action? *Health Affairs, 25*(4), 969–978.

Finkler, S. A., & Kovner, C. T. (1993). *Financial management for nurse managers and executives.* Philadelphia: W. B. Saunders.

Fuchs, V. R. (2005). Health care expenditures reexamined. *Annals of Internal Medicine, 143*(1), 76–78.

Genworth Financial, Inc. & National Eldercare Referral Systems, Inc. (2007). *Genworth Financial 2007 cost of care survey.* Retrieved October 31, 2008, from http://www.genworth.com

Gibson, R. M., & Waldo, D. R. (1982). National health expenditures, 1981. *Health Care Financing Review, 4*(1), 1–35.

Ginsberg, P. B. (1998). Health system change in 1997. *Health Affairs, 17*(4), 165–169.

Ginsberg, P. B., Gabel, J. R., & Hunt, K. A. (1998). Tracking small firm coverage: 1989–1996. *Health Affairs, 17*(1), 167–171.

Gold, M. R., Siegel, J. E., Russell, L. B., & Weinstein, M. C. (1996). *Cost-effectiveness in health and medicine.* New York: Oxford University Press.

Gordon, S. (2008). Advocating for nursing. In C. Harrington & C. L. Estes (Eds.), *Health policy: Crisis and reform in the U.S. health care delivery system* (5th ed.). Sudbury, MA: Jones and Bartlett.

Government Accountability Office (GAO). (2007). *Prescription drugs: Trends in usual and customary prices for drugs frequently used by Medicare and non-Medicare health insurance enrollees.*

Retrieved October 31, 2008, from http://www.gao.gov/cgi-bin/getrpt?GAO-07-1201R

Gulzar, L. (1999). Access to health care. *Image: Journal of Nursing Scholarship, 31*(1), 13–19.

Halvorson, G. C. (1999). Health plans' strategic responses to a changing market place. *Health Affairs, 18*(2), 28–29.

Hamilton, J. (1996, May). Insurance for alternative treatments. *American Health,* 44.

Harrington, C., & Estes, C. L. (Eds.). (2008). *Health policy: Crisis and reform in the U.S. healthcare delivery system* (5th ed.). Sudbury, MA: Jones and Bartlett.

Health Insurance Association of America. (1991). *Source book of insurance data.* Washington, DC: Author.

Heffler, S., Smith, S., Keehan, S., Borger, C., Clemens, M. K., & Truffer, C. (2005). U.S. spending projections for 2004–2014. *Health Affairs, 24*(1), 75–85.

Heggen, K., & Wellard, S. (2004). Increased unintended patient harm in nursing practice as a consequence of the dominance of economic discourses. *International Journal of Nursing Studies, 41,* 293–298.

Henry J. Kaiser Family Foundation. (2007a). Medicare spending and financing. *Medicare Fact Sheet.* Retrieved October 31, 2008, from http://www.amsa.org/business/Medicare%20Report.pdf

Henry J. Kaiser Family Foundation. (2007b). Medicaid and the uninsured: The Medicaid program at a glance. *Kaiser Commission on Medicaid Facts.* Retrieved October 31, 2008, from http://www.kff.org/medicaid/7235.cfm

Himmelstein, D., & Woolhandler, S. (1995). Care denied: U.S. residents who are unable to obtain needed medical services. *American Journal of Public Health, 85*(3), 341–344.

Holahan, J., & Cook, A. (2006). *Why did the number of uninsured continue to increase in 2005?* Issue Paper Report #7571. Washington, DC: Kaiser Family Foundation. Retrieved August 8, 2008, from http://www.kff.org/uninsured/upload/7571.pdf.

Howell, P. (2006). Market failure and public services. *Royal Economic Society Newsletter, 133,* 1.

Hughes, D., & Runyan, S. (2008). Prenatal care and public policy: Lessons for promoting women's health. In C. Harrington & C. L. Estes (Eds.), *Health policy and nursing: Crisis and reform in the U.S. health care delivery system* (5th ed.). Sudbury, MA: Jones and Bartlett.

Inglehart, J. K. (1996). Reform of the Veterans Affairs health care system. *New England Journal of Medicine, 335,* 1407–1411.

Jacobs, P. (1997). *The economics of health care.* Gaithersburg, MD: Aspen Publishers, Inc.

Kaiser Family Foundation. (2005). *e-health and the elderly: How seniors use the Internet for health information.* Retrieved November 3, 2008, from http://www.kff.org

Kovner, A. R., & Knickman, J. R. (2005). Overview: The state of healthcare delivery in the United States. In A. R. Kovner & J. R. Knickman (Eds.), *Jonas and Kovner's health care delivery in the United States* (8th ed., pp. 2–9). New York: Springer.

Kritsotakis, G., & Gamarnikow, E. (2004). What is social capital and how does it relate to health? *International Journal of Nursing Studies, 41*(1), 43–50.

Larson-Dahn, M. (1998). An innovative approach to appropriate resource utilization. *Nursing Economics, 16*(6), 317–319.

Lasker, R. D., & the Committee on Medicine and Public Health. (1997). *Medical and public health: The power of collaboration.* New York: The New York Academy of Medicine.

Loubeau, P. R., & Maher, V. F. (1996). Any-willing provider laws: Point and counterpoint. *Medicine and Law, 15*(2), 219–226.

LeGrand, J. (1999). Competition, cooperation, or control? Tales from the British National Health Service. *Health Affairs, 18*(1), 27–39.

LeVasseur, J. (1998). Plato, Nightingale, and contemporary nursing. *Image: Journal of Nursing Scholarship, 30*(3), 281–285.

Levit, K., Olin, G. O., & Letsch, S. W. (1992). American's health insurance coverage 1980–1991. *Health Care Financing Review, 14,* 31–57.

Malloch, K., & Porter-O'Grady, T. (1999). Partnership economics: Nursing's challenge in a quantum age. *Nursing Economics, 17*(6), 299–307.

Mantone, J. (2006). Stating the case for coverage. *Modern Healthcare, 36*(18), 6–16.

Max, W. (1997). Economic analysis in health care. In C. Harrington & C. L. Estes (Eds.), *Health policy and nursing: Crisis and reform in the U.S. health care delivery system* (2nd ed.). Sudbury, MA: Jones and Bartlett.

McKenzie, J. F. (1997). *An introduction to community health.* Sudbury, MA: Jones and Bartlett.

Mechanic, D. (1998). Topics for our times: Managed care and public health opportunities. *American Journal of Public Health, 88,* 874–875.

Mechanic, D., & Rochefort, D. (2008). A policy of inclusion for the mentally ill. In C. Harrington & C. L. Estes (Eds.), *Health policy and nursing: Crisis and reform in the U.S. health care delivery system* (5th ed.). Sudbury, MA: Jones and Bartlett.

Mississippi Health Advocacy Program. (1998). *What welfare advocates need to know about low income families' eligibility for and entitlement to Medicaid: Action alert.* Jackson, MS. www.mhap.org

Moore, S., Laufer, F. L., & Conroy, M. B. (1998). The economics of health care. In D. J. Mason & J. K. Leavitt (Eds.). *Policy and politics in nursing and health care* (3rd ed.). Philadelphia: W. B. Saunders.

National Center for Health Statistics. (1997). *Health: United States, 1996–1997.* Hyattsville, MD: Public Health Service.

Nichols, L. M., Ginsburg, P. B., Berenson, J. C., & Hurley, R. E. (2004). Are market forces strong enough to deliver efficient health care systems? Confidence is waning. *Health Affairs, 23*(2), 8–21.

Pauly, M. V. (2005). Competition and new technology. *Health Affairs, 24*(6), 1523–1535.

Pulcini, J., & Mahoney, D. (1998). Health care financing. In D. J. Mason & J. K. Leavitt (Eds.), *Policy and politics in nursing and health care* (3rd ed.). Philadelphia: W. B. Saunders.

Rambur, B., & Mooney, M. M. (1998). A point of view: Why point-of-care places are not free marketplaces. *Nursing Economics, 16*(3), 122–124, 146.

Rice, T. (1998). *The economics of health reconsidered.* Chicago: Health Administration Press.

Robbins, A., & Freeman, P. (1999). How organized medical care can advance public health. *Public Health Reports, 114,* 120–125.

Rosenbaum, S., & Richards, T. B. (1996). Medicaid managed care and public health policy. *Journal of Public Health Management Practice, 2*(3), 76–82.

Scandlen, G. (2005). Consumer-driven health care: Just a tweak or a revolution? *Health Affairs, 24*(6), 1554–1558.

Schauffler, H. H., & Scutchfield, F. D. (1998). Managed care and public health. *American Journal of Preventive Medicine, 14*(3), 240–241.

Seldon, T. M., Banthin, J. S., & Cohen, J. W. (1999). Waiting in the wings: Eligibility and enrollment in the state children's health insurance program. *Health Affairs, 18*(2), 126–133.

Shalala, D. E., & Reinhardt, U. E. (1999). Viewing the U.S. health care system from within: Candid talk from HHS. *Health Affairs, 18*(3), 47–55.

Shaughnessy, P. W., Schenkler, R. E., & Hittle, D. F. (1995). Case mix of home health patients under capitated and fee-for-service payments. *Health Services Research, 30*(1), 1–8.

Shi, L., & Singh, D. A. (2008). *Delivering health care in America: A systems approach* (4th ed.). Sudbury, MA: Jones and Bartlett.

Siegel, J. E. (1998). Cost-effectiveness analysis and nursing research: Is there a fit? *Image: Journal of Nursing Scholarship, 30*(3), 221–222.

Smith, C., Cowan, C., Heffler, S., Catlin, A., & the National Health Accounts Team. (2006). National health spending in 2004: Recent slowdown led by prescription drug spending. *Health Affairs, 25*(1), 196.

Spetz, J. (2005). The cost and cost-effectiveness of nursing services in health care. *Nursing Outlook, 53*(6), 305–309.

Standard and Poor's Corporation. (1992). *U.S. grapples with health care crisis*. Health care industry surveys, H15–H17.

Stevens, P. E. (1992). Who gets care? Access to health care as an arena for nursing. *Scholarly Inquiry for Nursing Practice, 6*(3), 185–200.

Stone, P. W. (1998). Methods for conducting and reporting cost-effectiveness analysis in nursing. *Image: Journal of Nursing Scholarship, 30*(3), 229–234.

Stone, P. W., Curran, C. R., & Bakken, S. (2002). Economic evidence for evidence based practice. *Journal of Nursing Scholarship, 34*(3), 277–282.

Sultz, H. A., & Young, K. M. (2006). *Health care USA: Understanding its organization and delivering* (5th ed.). Sudbury, MA: Jones and Bartlett.

Thompson, K. M. (2003). Economic issues in health care. In L. A. Joel (Ed.). *Kelly's dimensions of professional nursing* (pp. 220–241). New York: McGraw-Hill.

Trapp, D. (2008). Premiums for job-offered health insurance up 5% this year. *American Medical News*. Retrieved October 30, 2008, from http://www.ama-assn.org/amednews/2008/10/13/gvsb1013.htm

Tritter, J. O., & McCallum, A. (2006). The snakes and ladders of user involvement: Moving beyond Arnstein. *Health Policy, 76*, 56–168.

Vladeck, B. C., & King, K. (1997). Medicare at 30: Preparing for the future. In C. Harrington & C. Estes (Eds.), *Health policy and nursing: Crisis and reform in the U.S. health care delivery system*. Sudbury, MA: Jones and Bartlett.

Waid, M. O. (1998). *Brief summaries of Medicare and Medicaid. Title XVII and Title XIX of the Social Security Act*. Report prepared for Health Care Financing Administration, DHHS.

Waitzman, N. J., Romano, P. S., & Scheffler, R. M. (1994). Estimates of the economic costs of birth defects. *Inquiry, 31*, 188–205.

Weeks, J. (1997). The emerging role of alternative medicine in managed care. *Drug Benefit Trends, 9*(4), 14–16, 25–28.

Wesson, A. F. (1999). The comparative study of health reform. In F. D. Powell & A. F. Wesson (Eds.), *Health care systems in transition* (pp. 3–24). Thousand Oaks, CA: Sage.

White House Domestic Policy Council. (1993). *Health security: The President's report to the American people*. Washington, DC: Government Printing Office.

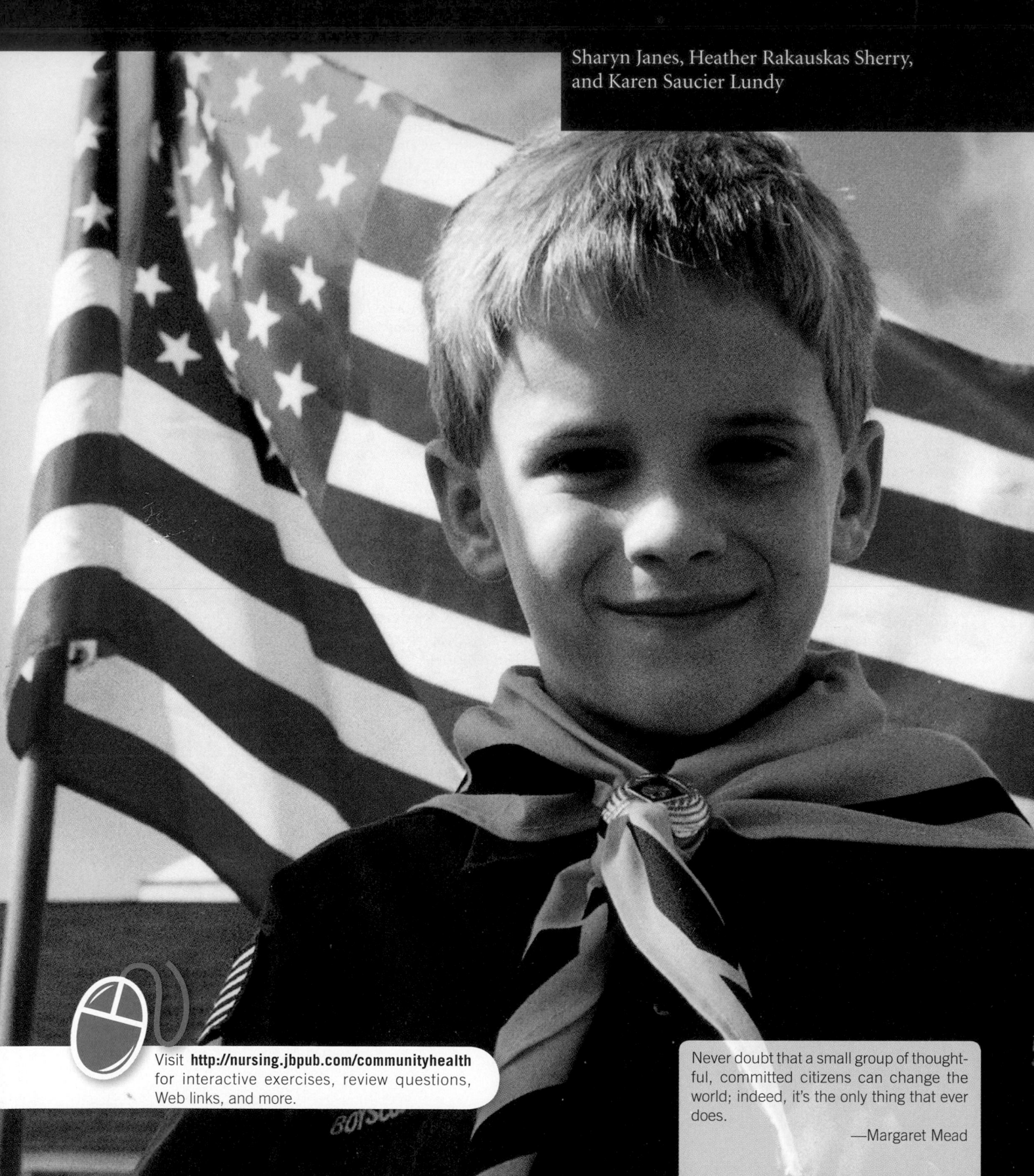

# CHAPTER 8
# Politics and the Law

Sharyn Janes, Heather Rakauskas Sherry, and Karen Saucier Lundy

Visit **http://nursing.jbpub.com/communityhealth** for interactive exercises, review questions, Web links, and more.

Never doubt that a small group of thoughtful, committed citizens can change the world; indeed, it's the only thing that ever does.

—Margaret Mead

The care of human life and happiness, and not their destruction, is the first and only object of good government.

*—Thomas Jefferson*

Abraham Lincoln did not go to Gettysburg having commissioned a poll to find out what would sell in Gettysburg. There were no people with percentages for him, cautioning him about this group or that group or what they found in exit polls a year earlier. When will we have the courage of Lincoln?

*—Robert Coles*

We often think of "politics" as something others do "for us" or "to us." Politics is always about power, who gets it, how it is used, and to what purpose. Why do you think nurses have historically avoided using their significant numbers politically? What do you think of the political system and does it relate to your work as a nurse?

## CHAPTER FOCUS

### Government Authority
- Protection of the Public's Health
- Power, Authority, and the Health of the Public
- Evolution of the Government's Role in Health Care

### Government
- Federal Government
- State Government
- Local Government
- Different Types of Law
- How an Idea Becomes a Law

### Regulation and Licensing of Nursing Practice
- The Regulatory Process
- Licensure

### Nursing Practice and the Law
- Nursing Practice in Correctional Settings
- Forensic Nursing: An Emerging Nursing Role

## QUESTIONS TO CONSIDER

After reading this chapter, you will know the answers to the following questions:

1. What is the role of the government in the health of its citizens?
2. How do the concepts of power and authority relate to public health regulation?
3. What is the history of governmental roles in health care?
4. What are the three branches of the federal government? What does each do in relation to health?
5. How is state government organized? How does it relate to health care?

6. What are the different kinds of laws?
7. What are the steps in the development of laws?
8. How can nurses be involved in the development of law and policy?
9. What are the primary issues related to regulation and licensure of nursing practice?
10. What settings are more likely to be influenced by legal issues in the practice of community health nursing and why?
11. What is the role of the nurse in correctional settings and in forensics?

## KEY TERMS

Bill of Rights
Coercive power
Connection power
Constitutional law
Correctional nursing
Democracy
Equality
Executive branch
Expert power

*Federal Register*
Forensic nursing
Freedom
Information power
Judicial branch
Judicial or common law
Legislative branch
Legitimate power
Liberty

Licensure
Lobbying
Malpractice
Negligence
Nurse Multistate Licensure Mutual
  Recognition Model
Nurse practice act
Police power
Political action committees (PACs)

Political power
Power
Preamble of the U.S. Constitution
Referent power
Regulatory process
Reward power
Statutory law
U.S. Constitution

WHILE THE POLITICAL EFFORTS of movers and shakers like Florence Nightingale, Lillian Wald, and Margaret Sanger are well documented, politics and policy have been historically seen as "outside" the scope of nursing. For most nurses, "political activism" meant voting in national and state elections. By the closing years of the twentieth century, however, nurses began to realize that they could influence public policy by using nursing knowledge and skills. In 1992, acknowledging that decisions affecting nurses and their patients were being made in the national political arena, the American Nurses Association (ANA) moved its national headquarters to Washington, D.C. (Milstead, 1999).

## Government Authority

### ■ Protection of the Public's Health

The early American colonists viewed health as controlled by divine intervention. They believed it was a result of self-care, and minimal governmental intervention was expected. Because health care was not a power granted to the federal government (such as defense or printing money), it developed into a power of the states or was left to the people themselves. Governmental health care and policies to provide funding and resources for health care were, for all practical purposes, nonexistent in the early days of the United States (Turnock, 1997).

As each new American colony was founded, the way in which it would be governed was a primary consideration. The specific problems and situations that each new colony faced varied so widely that each developed its own procedures and laws based on its own needs. From this evolved the idea of states' rights, which continues to play a critical role in the governance of health care policies, such as seatbelt laws and immunization laws. Any attempts to limit the power of the states, either by the federal government or other states, is usually strongly opposed. Most states, for instance, will have similar laws about school attendance, drinking age, and immunizations, but the regulations themselves will vary considerably.

Federal law is based on the **U.S. Constitution**, which was ratified in 1789. The creators of the Constitution were careful to limit the federal government's involvement in the daily lives of citizens. The word *health* was never mentioned in the U.S. Constitution, making health care legislation problematic, because the Constitution grants limited power in the creation of health laws. The Constitution has been amended 27 times. The first 10 amendments, known as the **Bill of Rights**, were adopted within 3 years of the Constitution's ratification. The Bill of Rights focuses on the protection of our most basic value: freedom. Freedom of speech, freedom of the press, and due process are all included. In recent years, the constitutional amendments have had relevance to health care issues. For example, the Fourteenth Amendment provides protection of personal liberty, such as a woman's right to choose to have an abortion. It is important to note, however, that neither the U.S. Constitution nor state constitutions guarantee access to health care. States retain whatever power the U.S. Constitution does not specifically define in federal law. State power concerning health care is termed **police power.** The state can use its power to protect the health, welfare, and safety of its citizens by establishing boards of nursing and medicine and passing immunization laws (Kelly & Joel, 1996).

### ■ Power, Authority, and the Health of the Public

Politics is always about **power**—who gets it, how it is obtained, how it is applied, and to what purposes it is used (Bacharach & Lawler, 1980). The German sociologist Max Weber defined power as the ability to control the behaviors of others, even in the absence of their consent (Weber, 1947). Power, then, is the capacity to participate effectively in a decision-making process. If citizens cannot or do not affect the process, they are powerless (Lenski, 1984).

Power can be classified as either legitimate or illegitimate. Power is considered legitimate if people recognize that those who apply it have the right to do so. This includes elected government officials, aristocracy, and those believed to be inspired by God. Weber referred to legitimate power as authority (Bacharach & Lawler, 1980). A simple illustration of this authority is that if the police stop you for speeding and levy a fine against you, you will recognize the law and the person carrying out the law as legitimate and you will probably obey. A political system can exist only if the people see the authority as legitimate. Most persons must see it as desirable, workable, and better than alternatives. We may complain about our legal system and its excesses or our Congress members and their self-serving interests, but most of us believe that the system works to our benefit most of the time. Once the bulk of citizens in any society no longer consider the political system legitimate, it is doomed, for its power can then rest only on coercion, which will eventually fail. Most revolutions, such as the French Revolution, the Iranian Revolution, and the American Revolution, were preceded by an erosion of the legitimacy of the existing political system (Robertson, 1981).

> **❝***Among the Indians there have been no written laws. Customs handed down from generation to generation have been the only laws to guide them. Every one might act different from what was considered right if he chose to do so, but such acts would bring upon him the censure of the Nation. . . . This fear of the Nation's censure acted as a mighty band, binding all in one social, honorable compact.***❞**
> —George Copway (Kah-ge-ga-bowh), Ojibwa Chief, 1818–1863

### ■■ CULTURAL CONNECTION

Democrats give away their old clothes; Republicans wear theirs. Republicans employ exterminators; Democrats step on the bugs. Democrats eat the fish they catch; Republicans stuff 'em and hang them on the wall.

—Sean Donlon

## Concepts of Power

**Political power** is defined by Hewison (1994) as the "ability to influence or persuade an individual holding a governmental office to exert the power of that office to [effect] a desired change" (p. 1171). What allows some people to have more influence than others? Where does such power come from? Nurses can benefit from understanding these sources of power. French and Raven (1959) identify five power bases:

1. **Coercive power**, which is the use of force to gain compliance, often born out of real or perceived fear or threat to self. Police often use coercive power.
2. **Reward power**, which involves giving something of value for compliance. Compliance then results from the perceived potential for reward or favor of someone in power. A politician may help constituents obtain money for a new hospital in exchange for their political support.
3. **Expert power,** which results from expert knowledge or skills. Bill Gates has considerable expert power because of his expertise in computers and systems.
4. **Legitimate power**, which results from a title or position, such as an elected judge or the surgeon general.
5. **Referent power**, which results from being closely associated with someone who is powerful; for example, the aide or spouse of a senator. This can also be referred to as reflected power.

Hersey, Blanchard, and Natemeyer (1979) added two additional sources of power:

6. **Information power**, which results from the desire for information held by one person from one who does not have access to the information. This is commonly seen in the diplomatic corps of the United States.
7. **Connection power**, which results from the belief that a certain person has a special connection to a person or organization believed to be powerful. Lobbyists often use this kind of power when working with legislators' staff assistants (Helvie, 1998).

One primary way of gaining power as a nurse is through knowledge. Nurses can use their knowledge of politics, power, and the change process to introduce change favoring health in the legislative process. Nurses have historically had very little interest in achieving power. Others have too long been the "voice" of nursing, and nurses and their patients have suffered through lack of appropriate nurse advocacy (Huston, 1995).

Another way that nurses can achieve power is through affiliating with others who have similar interests in health. Through networking and using the power of numbers, nurses can facilitate communication and effect change through those in power positions (Anderson, 2006). Coalitions of people and organizations are most effective in bringing about change (Helvie, 1998).

The idea of a nation-state is relatively new. The concept emerged in Europe only a few centuries ago, then spread to the Americas, and spread to most parts of Africa and Asia

> ❝When nurses fully understand the impact of policy in the health care arena, when nurses fully understand the importance of tying outcomes research to public policy and when nurses fully understand the politics of health care, and mobilize their numbers and influence behind the political process, only then will the health system thrive and with nurses as key players.❞
>
> —Betty Dickson, Executive Director and Lobbyist, Mississippi Nurses Association, 2001

only during the twentieth century. In the founding of the United States, a representative democracy was a new idea. **Democracy** comes from a Greek word meaning "rule of the people," and this is no doubt what Abraham Lincoln had in mind when he defined democracy as "government of the people, by the people, and for the people." Democracy in the United States requires that we recognize the powers of the government as being derived from the consent of the governed. We elect representatives who are responsible for making political decisions. According to Robertson, "Representative democracy is historically recent, rare and fragile" (1981, p. 488).

There are five basic conditions that must exist for a democracy to thrive:

1. Advanced economic development: This almost always involves an urbanized, literate, and sophisticated population that expects and demands participation in the political process.
2. Restraints on government power: This involves institutional checks on the power of the state (Robertson, 1981).
3. Consensus on basic values and a widely held commitment to existing political institutions.
4. Tolerance of dissent.
5. Access to information: A democracy depends on its citizens to make informed choices. There must be a free press.

> ❝Give me liberty or give me death!❞
>
> —Patrick Henry, 1775

## Liberty versus Equality

**Freedom** is defined in the United States as freedom "of"—freedom of speech, freedom of the press, and so on. In more socialist societies, freedom is defined as freedom "from"—freedom from hunger, freedom from unemployment, freedom from exploitation by people who want to make a fortune. In the United States, we equate freedom with **liberty**. Socialist societies equate freedom with **equality**. In general, the more liberty that exists in a society, the less equality. Your liberty to be richer than anyone else violates other people's right to be your equal; other people's right to be your equal violates your liberty to make a fortune. In the United States, we have chosen to emphasize liberty, which evolves from our value system. This emphasis can lead only to social inequality. Socialist societies emphasize equality, thus limiting personal liberty (Robertson, 1981).

In health care we often fail to understand why laws cannot be easily passed to impose penalties on persons who engage in risky behavior, such as requiring helmets for motorcyclists or tubal ligations for women who have injured their children through neglect or abuse. The answer lies in our emphasis on freedom in the United States and the limited power of the state. Recognizing and understanding these basic concepts about our government can help us use our skills and resources in the political process much more efficiently.

*Eternal vigilance is the price of liberty.*

—Wendell Phillips, 1852

### Evolution of the Government's Role in Health Care

The **Preamble of the U.S. Constitution** states that one of the purposes of the federal government is to "promote the general welfare" of the people. This can be found in Article 1, Section 8. The federal government derives its power to become involved in health care activities from this simple declaration. Because of this very general statement, the degree of health care services provided by the federal government

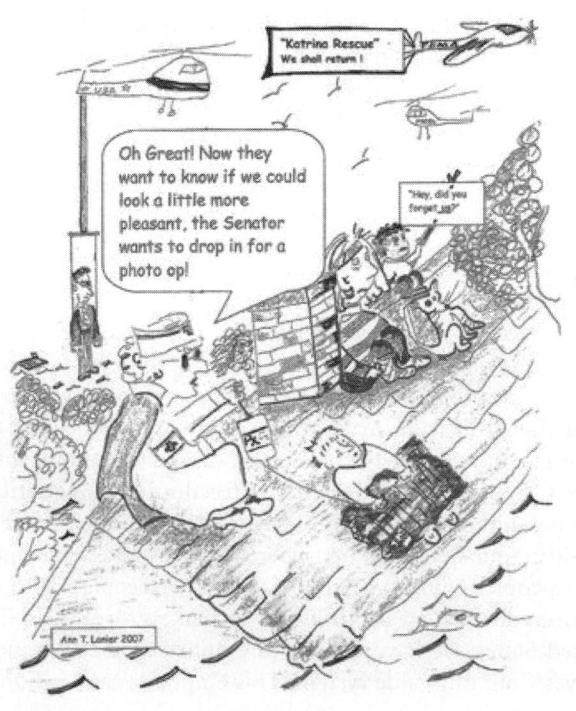

is often a source of conflict among the various constituents and political parties. As a capitalistic society, and lacking clear direction from the U.S. Constitution, the provision of health services for the general population has historically been the concern of private enterprise. Private physicians delivered services to patients, and patients in turn paid a fee for that service. This concept had been the foundation of medical care provision in the United States for nearly 200 years (Miller, 1992).

The first involvement of the federal government in health care was highly specialized for government employees. As early as 1796, the Marine Hospital Service was established to provide care for sick and disabled seamen. In 1852, St. Elizabeth Hospital in Washington, D.C., was established to provide health care for federal employees. A landmark study, the Shattuck Report, written in 1850, recommended measures such as the creation of local and state boards of health; collection of vital statistics; and supervision of housing, factories, sanitation, and communicable disease control. Soon health departments in major cities became common. The Shattuck Report is considered the basis for the development of local and state health departments (see Chapter 3). Military personnel were soon cared for through the federal government, which eventually led to the Veterans Administration (VA). The VA is currently the largest health care system in the United States.

It was not until after World War II that the federal government ventured into health care and community health programs for the general population. In 1946, the Hill–Burton Act provided funds for building hospital facilities in many communities. Government funding for specific treatments for disease did not happen until the 1960s. Be-

*If I were two-faced, would I be wearing this one?*

—Abraham Lincoln

fore the 1960s, the federal government primarily provided programs for the economically disadvantaged populations. The social welfare programs of the 1960s brought about the most dramatic changes in federal involvement in health care. The establishment of Medicare in 1965 was significant in that it became the first program to provide health services to citizens other than federal employees. The basic purpose of Medicare was to provide health care for the elderly. The Medicaid program was developed in 1965 and provided health care for low-income individuals. See Box 8-1 for a list of the most significant health legislation acts passed during the "turning point decade" of the 1960s.

The Civil Rights Act of 1964, although not directly related to health, provided fair access to health facilities for all races and genders. The Environmental Protection Agency (EPA), created through the National Environmental Policy Act, is historically one of the most significant pieces of U.S. environmental health policy. In recent years, significant legislation has been passed, including the Americans with Disabilities Act in 1990. This act increased the opportunities for Americans with disabilities to be integrated into mainstream society by removing physical barriers and improving public accommodation and services.

---

### BOX 8-1

**1965: What a Year for Health Law in the United States!**

- Drug Abuse Control Amendments of 1965 (Public Law No. 89-74)
- Federal Cigarette Labeling and Advertising Act (Public Law No. 89-92)
- Construction Act Amendments of 1965 (Public Law No. 89-105)
- Community Health Services Extension Amendments of 1965 (Public Law No. 89-109)
- Health Research Facilities Amendments of 1965 (Public Law No. 89-115)
- Water Quality Act of 1965 (Public Law No. 89-234)
- Heart Disease, Cancer, and Stroke Amendments of 1965 (Public Law No. 89-239)
- The Clean Air Act Amendments and Solid Waste Disposal Act of 1965 (Public Law No. 89-272)
- Health Professions Educational Assistance Amendments of 1965 (Public Law No. 89-290)
- Medical Library Assistance Act (Public Law No. 89-291)
- Appalachian Regional Development Act of 1965 (Public Law No. 89-4)
- Older Americans Act (Public Law No. 89-73)
- Social Security Amendments of 1965 (Public Law No. 89-97)
- Vocational Rehabilitation Act Amendments of 1965 (Public Law No. 89-333)
- Housing and Urban Development Act of 1965 (Public Law No. 89-117)

*Source:* Forgotson, 1967.

---

⚖ **ETHICAL CONNECTION**

"Health is the first of all liberties."

—Henri Amiel

"I submit to you that if a man hasn't discovered something he will die for, he isn't fit to live."

—Martin Luther King, Jr.

As a citizen of the United States, are we "free to be healthy" or to be "free from sickness"? What is the ethical responsibility of the government to safeguard such freedom?

## Government

### ■ Federal Government

The federal government consists of three separate branches—executive (Office of the President), legislative (Congress), and judicial (federal court system). All three branches have a powerful impact on the health care delivery system and nursing practice. Nurses should be aware of how the different branches of the government affect health care policy and the ways that nurses can have a voice.

#### Executive Branch

The **executive branch** consists of the president, the vice president, the Office of Management and Budget, and the administrative agencies, whose leadership is appointed by the president and approved by Congress. Presidential authority to exercise legislative leadership is clearly established

Families of the 1950s reflected a more traditional family form where mothers stayed home and fathers acted as the primary breadwinner. Children of these families make up the baby boomer generation and, as adults, now have very different values about gender roles within the family. Policies at all levels of government have been slow to respond to the dramatic changes in the diverse family forms of this century.

by the Constitution and legislation, and accepted as a practical and political necessity (Anderson, 2006). The administrative agencies that have the greatest effect on health care policy and nursing education, research, and practice are the Department of Health and Human Services, the Department of Education, and the Department of Labor.

### Department of Health and Human Services

The Department of Health and Human Services (DHHS) is the federal agency most concerned with protecting the health of all Americans and providing essential human services, especially for those who are least able to help themselves. There are more than 300 programs under DHHS supervision, with a wide spectrum of activities and services. Some of these services include the following (DHHS, 1999, 2008):

- Health and social science research
- Disease prevention, including immunization services
- Financial assistance and service for low-income families
- Child abuse and domestic violence prevention
- Medicare and Medicaid
- Food and drug safety
- Maternal and infant health improvement
- Services for older Americans
- Substance abuse treatment and prevention
- Health information technology
- Faith-based and community initiatives
- Comprehensive Native American health services
- Medical preparedness for emergencies, including potential terrorism

The DHHS employs more than 60,000 people and administers more grant dollars than all other federal agencies combined. Its Medicare program is the nation's largest health insurer, handling more than 1 billion claims per year. Medicare and Medicaid together provide health care insurance for one in four Americans.

DHHS funding for services is distributed primarily through federal, state, and local government agencies, although some services are provided through grants awarded to private-sector individuals or institutions. Programs, which are primarily located in Rockville, Maryland, are generally administered by 11 operating divisions, including eight agencies in the U.S. Public Health Service and three human services agencies. In addition, DHHS programs provide for equitable treatment of beneficiaries nationwide and enable the collection of national health and other data.

Box 8-2 lists the health offices and services under the umbrella of DHHS.

### U.S. Public Health Agencies
#### National Institutes of Health

The National Institutes of Health (NIH), located in Bethesda, Maryland, is the world's premier health research organization, supporting more than 38,000 research projects nationwide that focus on diseases such as cancer, Alzheimer's disease, diabetes, arthritis, cardiovascular diseases, and

---

### BOX 8-2

**U.S. Department of Health and Human Services Agencies**

**U.S. Public Health Service Agencies**
- National Institutes of Health
- Food and Drug Administration
- Centers for Disease Control and Prevention
- Indian Health Service
- Health Resources and Services Administration
- Substance Abuse and Mental Health Services Administration
- Agency for Health Care Research and Quality
- U.S. Public Health Service Corps

**Human Service Agencies**
- Centers for Medicare and Medicaid Services
- Administration for Children and Families
- Administration on Aging

---

HIV/AIDS. Established in 1887 as the Hygienic Laboratory located in Staten Island, New York, the NIH has grown to include 27 separate health institutes (DHHS, 2008), including the National Institute for Nursing Research (NINR). The research funded through NINR, which began as a center in 1986 and was elevated to institute status in 1993, focuses on health promotion and disease prevention, acute and chronic illness, and nursing systems (Bednash, Heylin, & Rhome, 1998).

#### Food and Drug Administration

The Food and Drug Administration (FDA) is responsible for ensuring the safety of food and cosmetics and the safety and efficacy of pharmaceuticals, biological products, and medical devices. These products account for almost 25% of U.S. consumer spending. The FDA was established in 1906 with the Pure Food and Drugs Act passed by the U.S. Congress (DHHS, 2008).

#### Centers for Disease Control and Prevention

Working with states and other partners, the Centers for Disease Control and Prevention (CDC), established in 1946 and located in Atlanta, Georgia, provides a system of health surveillance to monitor and prevent disease outbreaks (including bioterrorism), implement disease prevention strategies, and maintain national health statistics. CDC personnel, who are stationed in more than 25 countries, help guard against international disease transmission (DHHS, 2008).

The CDC director is also the administrator of the *Agency for Toxic Substances and Disease Registry* (*ATSDR*), which helps prevent exposure to hazardous substances from waste sites on the Environmental Protection Agency's National Priorities List. The ASTDR develops toxicological profiles of chemicals found at these sites (DHHS, 2008).

The CDC's focus on the community allows nurses to make significant contributions in a variety of areas. Nurses are involved in the establishment of infection control guidelines; the prevention of substance abuse, HIV/AIDS, and other sexually transmitted infections; and in the areas of violence, adolescent and school health, women's health, children's health, and immunization (Bednash, Heylin, & Rhome, 1998).

### Indian Health Service

The Indian Health Service (HIS) provides health services to 1.6 million Native Americans and Alaska Natives, who belong to more than 550 federally recognized tribes and primarily live on reservations. IHS, established in 1921, is a comprehensive health care system that includes 49 hospitals, 247 health centers, 34 health stations, satellite clinics, residential substance abuse treatment centers, Alaska Native village clinics, and 34 urban health programs (DHHS, 2008).

### Health Resources and Services Administration

The Health Resources and Services Administration (HRSA) provides access to essential health care services for people who are low income, are uninsured, or live in rural areas or urban neighborhoods where health care is scarce. HRSA-funded health centers provided medical care to almost 14 million patients at more than 3,700 sites in the United States in 2005. The agency, founded in 1982, helps prepare the U.S. health care system and providers to respond to bioterrorism and other public health emergencies, maintains the National Health Service Corps, and helps build the health care workforce through training and education programs. HRSA also administers a variety of programs to improve the health of mothers and children, serves people living with HIV/AIDS through the Ryan White Care Act pro-

grams, and oversees the U.S. organ transplantation system (DHHS, 2008).

### Substance Abuse and Mental Health Services Administration

Services to improve the quality and availability of substance abuse prevention, addiction treatment, and mental health care are provided by the Substance Abuse and Mental Health Services Administration (SAMHSA). Funding to support treatment for Americans with serious substance abuse or mental health problems is provided through block grants to states. Established in 1992, SAMHSA monitors the prevalence and incidence of substance abuse and identifies and disseminates information related to the best practices for prevention and treatment. SAMHSA replaces the Alcohol, Drug Abuse, and Mental Health Administration, which was established in 1974 (DHHS, 2008).

### Agency for Health Care Research and Quality

The mission of the Agency for Health Care Research and Quality (AHRQ), established in 1989, is to generate and distribute evidence-based information that improves health care delivery and outcomes. AHRQ supports research on health care systems, health care quality and cost issues, access to health care, and effectiveness of medical treatments (DHHS, 2008).

### U.S. Public Health Service Corps

The U.S. Public Health Service Corps (PHS) is a uniformed service of more than 6,000 health professionals who serve in many DHHS and other federal agencies. The PHS director is the Surgeon General of the United States, who is appointed by the president. PHS members, who are

---

## MEDIA MOMENT

### A Civil Action (1998)

In this true story, John Travolta stars as a personal-injury lawyer who sues a major corporation when the drinking water in Woburn, Massachusetts, is found to contain high levels of industrial solvents. Believing the contamination is responsible for the large number of leukemia deaths among the town's children, the citizens—led by a woman (Kathleen Quinlan) whose child has died—hire a lawyer to take on the corporate polluters. Beatrice and Grace are the real-life companies represented in the movie, and A Civil Action is based on Jonathan Harr's nonfiction bestseller, which won the National Book Award.

### Koyaanisqatsi (1983)

ko.yaa.nis.qatsi n. (Hopi). 1. crazy life. 2. life in turmoil. 3. life disintegrating. 4. life out of balance. 5. a state of life that calls for another way of living.

This movie, which consists of music and images, marks Godfrey Reggio's debut as a film director and producer. It is the first installment of the Qatsi trilogy. The title is a Hopi Indian word meaning "life out of balance." Created between

1975 and 1982, the film is an apocalyptic vision of the collision of two different worlds—urban life and technology versus the environment. Philip Glass composed the film's musical score. Recommended as a beginning for discussion on the political debate between government regulation of corporate interests and environmental concerns.

### Thank You for Smoking (2005)

Big Tobacco spin-doctor Nick Naylor (Aaron Eckhart) is on a mission to make the country forget the dangers of his product. Rallying for the cause, he works to promote smoking in the movies and hush former employees who bad-mouth cigarettes, all the while trying to remain a good role model for his 12-year-old son. Maria Bello, Katie Holmes, Robert Duvall, and William H. Macy co-star in Jason Reitman's movie based on Christopher Buckley's novel. Thought-provoking satire on the continued debate between tobacco companies' right to advertise and the public health concerns related to tobacco use.

commissioned officers, include many nurses. The chief nurse holds the rank of rear admiral (DHHS, 1999, 2008).

### Human Services Agencies
#### Centers for Medicare and Medicaid Services

The Centers for Medicare and Medicaid Services (CMS), originally established as the Health Care Financing Administration in 1977, administers the Medicare and Medicaid programs, which provide health care to one in every four Americans. Medicare provides health insurance for more than 43 million elderly and disabled Americans. Medicaid, a joint federal–state program, provides health coverage for 51.6 million low-income people, including 25.1 million children, and nursing home coverage for low-income elders. CMS also administers the State Children's Health Insurance Program (SCHIP), which covers more than 4.6 million children (DHHS, 2008).

#### Administration for Children and Families

The Administration for Children and Families (ACF), established in 1991 by combining several existing programs, is responsible for 60 programs that promote the economic and social well-being of children, families, and communities. Some of the programs administered by ACF are the state–federal welfare program called Temporary Assistance for Needy Families (TANF), which provides assistance to an estimated 4.4 million people, including 4 million children; the national child support enforcement system, which collected $21.2 billion in 2003 in payments from noncustodial parents; and the Head Start program, which serves more than 900,000 preschool children. ACF also funds programs to prevent child abuse and domestic violence and supports state programs to support foster care and provide adoption assistance (DHHS, 2008).

#### Administration on Aging

Administration on Aging (AoA) programs provide services to older Americans living at home in the community

### ❝ *a conversation with . . .* ❞

Practicing nursing for 30 years prepared me for service in Congress in many ways. First, legislators and nurses must both be good listeners. I believe that quality representation means taking the time to understand the views and problems of one's constituents. As a nurse, I was an advocate for my patients. Today, as a Congresswoman, I'm an advocate for my constituents. Nurses learn to withhold premature judgment, to work as a team, to set goals and priorities, and to meet them. Also, nurses are taught to put the common good before their personal ambition and ahead of political interests. I developed these important skills during my nursing career and they have served me well as a member of Congress.

—The Honorable Lois Capps,
U.S. Congresswoman from California

*Source:* Mason, D. J., Leavitt, J. K., & Chaffee, M. W. (Eds.). (2002). *Policy and politics in nursing and health care* (4th ed.). St. Louis, MO: Saunders.

Other countries have different values concerning the obligation of government to fund basic and essential health care. Why is the United States different in this respect? Why has it rejected attempts in the past to "socialize" the U.S. health care system?

through a nationwide aging services network. Services provided to elders include, but are not limited to, meals, transportation, caregiver support, personal care, information and assistance, nursing home ombudsman, elder rights protection, and health promotion. These services enable elders to remain healthy, secure, and independent (DHHS, 2008).

#### Department of Education

The U.S. Department of Education (DOE) provides billions of dollars each year for postsecondary education, including nursing education. Federal Family Education Loans (Stafford Loans), Pell Grants, and Federal Work Study programs are just a few of the sources of funding provided (Bednash, Heylin, & Rhome, 1998; White, 2002).

#### Department of Labor

The U.S. Department of Labor (DOL) is responsible for enforcing the Fair Labor Standards Act (minimum wage and overtime), the Employee Retirement Income Security Act (employee benefit and retirement plans), and the Occupational Safety and Health Act (OSHA) (job safety and health). All of these are important to nursing practice. The ANA has worked closely with the Department of Labor for over 20 years to ensure adequate funding for the health and safety of nurses in the workplace through enforcement of OSHA standards (Bednash, Heylin, & Rhome, 1998; White, 2002).

### Legislative Branch

The U.S. Congress is the **legislative branch** of the federal government. Congress has two houses with equal power: the Senate and the House of Representatives. The Senate has 100 members, two from each state. The House of Representatives membership varies according to the population. A representative is elected to represent a specific number of constituents, so states with larger populations have more representatives. The number of representatives a state has increases or decreases with corresponding changes in the state's population. The House of Representatives currently has more than 400 members. The sole legislative power of the federal government lies with the two houses of Congress (White, 2002). A partial list of the responsibilities of the U.S. Congress is outlined in Box 8-3.

### Judicial Branch

The **judicial branch** of the federal government, known as the U.S. court system, consists of 94 federal district courts, 12 circuit courts of appeals, the U.S. Supreme Court, and several specialized courts to address customs, patents, military issues, and so on. A Supreme Court justice generally keeps his or her appointment until retirement or death. At

# ❝ *a conversation with . . .* ❞

In 1991, I received a telephone call from Geraldine Ferraro asking me to come to New York City to be interviewed for a leadership position on her campaign for a United States Senate seat representing the state of New York. How did Gerry find me and why did she want a nurse to work on a major national campaign?

My connection to Gerry followed one of the most important principles of political involvement and influence—"use your connections." I had spent a sabbatical year at the ANA working in the governmental affairs department. While there, I collaborated with one of the women who had been involved in Gerry's nomination for vice president of the United States in 1984. She knew Gerry was considering a run for the U.S. Senate, so she called her to recommend my political skills to her. Gerry indicated a strong interest in working with me because of my involvement with ANA, the first group to endorse her candidacy for vice president. Gerry called me and hired me a week later.

For a year and half I worked as the upstate campaign coordinator. I was responsible for 54 of the 62 counties in the state, an area that covers over 40,000 square miles. I started with nothing except a great candidate. I had to organize an office, create a database of contacts, organize a grassroots network, raise thousands of dollars, and create fundraising and media events. Although I had been an active volunteer in numerous congressional and state legislative campaigns, I had never been a paid staff member. I did not have an appointed position in the political party, so I had to use all my communication skills, organizational skills, and nursing intuition to create a campaign presence in every one of the 54 counties under my leadership.

It helped to have a candidate with name recognition. When I called major democratic leaders and potential supporters I didn't have to introduce my candidate. I used my connections and those of Gerry to build a grass-roots structure. I focused on women's organizations, women leaders, nurses and their organizations, other health professionals, and any other men and women throughout the state who wanted to volunteer for Gerry. Gerry's candidacy energized and excited the electorate, as it had when she ran for vice president. It wasn't hard getting volunteers; it was only difficult organizing them to contribute in meaningful ways. Whether it was organizing events for fundraising, working with the media, conducting voter registration drives, or soliciting political endorsements, it took incredible planning and organizational skill and thousands of volunteer hours. I planned it all—over 200 events—supported by a grass-roots structure of over 5,000 volunteers from every profession, occupation, and interest group who held campaign events, gave money, and worked for Gerry in their home communities.

The nurses came out in droves. Nurses who had never been involved politically suddenly wanted to help Gerry

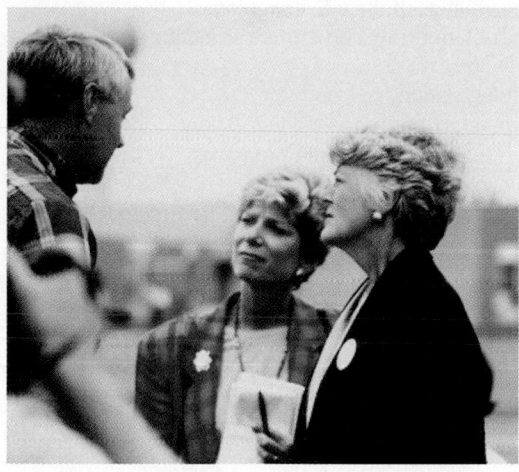

Judy Leavitt and 1984 vice presidential candidate, Geraldine Ferraro.

and listen to her message. Because I had been active in both the ANA-PAC and New York State political activities, I was able to help Gerry receive an early endorsement by the ANA-PAC and encourage the New York State Nurses Association to mobilize their members.

What was it like to work so closely for such a national and international "celebrity"? It was fun, grueling, exciting, challenging, and a once-in-a-lifetime experience. What made it easy was Gerry. She was personable, caring, and in many ways very much like her constituents. She had experienced poverty as well as success; she was a teacher and a lawyer; she was a mother, grandmother, and wife—so she knew about the issues and could relate to people throughout the country. She used me to draft her health platform and respected my expertise in teaching her about the issues. In addition, Gerry was able to bring the best political and media consultants to work with me and the campaign staff. Traveling with Gerry was the most fun of the entire year and a half. We would often spend two or three days alone traveling throughout the upstate counties, affording us an opportunity to become good friends. I was the oldest staff person, much closer in age to Gerry. That created a special bond that enabled me to have access to her and engendered mutual respect. At each event, I would sometimes look around as she was speaking and think how lucky I was to be able to have the opportunity to help elect someone whom I admired and believed could have been a fine senator. Unfortunately that never happened. Gerry lost in the primary election by less than 10,000 votes out of 4 million cast. The country lost the chance to have a great senator. I gained a friend and stories for a lifetime.

**—Judy Leavitt,**
MEd, RN, Campaign Manager for Geraldine Ferraro,
Candidate for U.S. Senate in 1992

## BOX 8-3

**Responsibilities of the U.S. Congress**
- Conduct hearings on issues that may generate federal legislation.
- Draft legislation.
- Estimate cost of proposed legislation.
- Enact legislation to create programs.
- Review legislated program operations.
- Determine the federal budget.
- Appropriate funds for federal operations.
- Decide entitlement policy (e.g., Medicare, Medicaid, Social Security).
- Confirm or reject presidential nominations for high-level federal positions (e.g., cabinet members, federal judges).

*Source:* Bednash, Heylin, & Rhome, 1998.

that time, a replacement is appointed to the position by the president and approved by Congress (White, 2002).

Although the judicial branch of the government is not involved in making policy, the way in which the courts interpret the law may have a profound effect on health care, including nursing practice. The courts are often called upon to interpret and decide the meaning of statutory provisions that are ambiguous, unclear, and open to conflicting interpretation (Anderson, 2006). Nurses can affect the outcome of court cases by serving as expert witnesses or legal consultants (Bednash, Heylin, & Rhome, 1998).

## ■ State Government

Although the role of the federal government is in the forefront of American politics, the truth is that most of the policies and laws related to nursing practice are created at the state level. The creation and enforcement of nurse practice acts and the regulation of nursing practice through licensing occurs at the state level. State governments consist of the same three branches as the federal government: executive, legislative, and judicial.

### Executive Branch

The executive branch of all state government consists of the governor and the attorney general. More than half of the states also have a lieutenant governor, who may or may not work closely with the governor, depending on the election politics of that state (Reinhard, 2002). Most governors are elected to 4-year terms and are eligible for reelection. The governor is responsible for presenting the state budget to the legislature and overseeing state spending. The governor's

### *Got an Alternative?*

Vitamins and herbal supplements are not regulated by law in the United States. Do you think the Federal Drug Administration should regulate them as other "drugs"? Why or why not?

• • • • • • • • • • • • • • • • • • • • • • • • • • • • • • •

policy initiatives are often presented as part of the state budget proposal and may contain health-related programs. The lieutenant governor presides over state affairs in the absence of the governor and can influence health and social policies within the state. The attorney general represents the public's interests in legal cases coming before the court, not including the state supreme court. The attorney general's office is often called on to interpret the nurse practice act to clarify the intent of legislation or regulations (Gaffney, 1998).

### State Agencies

The power of state agencies to influence health and social policy varies across and within states (Reinhard, 2002). Typically state agencies may be divided into five different categories:

1. Agencies led by elected officers such as secretaries of state, treasurers, and attorney generals
2. Agencies led by officers appointed by the governor or independent boards, such as secretaries of human services and commissioners of health
3. Professional licensing and regulatory boards, such as boards of nursing
4. Public authorities and corporations, such as higher education assistance authorities
5. Independent boards and commissions, such as councils of higher education and public utilities commissions

In many states, the Department of Health is a state organization whose primary purpose is to oversee and maintain the health of the community. The director of the state department of public health is appointed by the governor. In other states, the Department of Health may be a division within a larger government agency (Reinhard, 2002). There are many different functions of the department of public health, which may include data collection and surveillance, administration of Medicaid and other federally funded programs, public health programs, and hospital regulation (Gaffney, 1998).

### Legislative Branch

State legislatures are the oldest part of the American government, existing long before the drafting of the U.S. Constitution. In fact, the Declaration of Independence was signed by representatives of the legislatures of the 13 colonies that became the original 13 states. State legislatures levy taxes, appropriate funding, and create and monitor agencies to carry out state business (Gaffney, 1998). Patterned after the federal legislature, all state legislatures (excluding Nebraska) consist of two houses: a Senate and a House of Representatives. In each state, the House of Representatives is larger than the Senate because senators represent larger districts within the state than members of the House. Therefore, each senator has a greater number of constituents.

### Judicial Branch

State judicial systems are similar to that of the federal system. The state supreme courts serve to interpret the language of their state constitutions and apply it in the courtroom. In recent years, there have been many changes in state

**THINK ABOUT THIS** ·················

Something is happening to America, not something danger-ous but something all too safe. I see it in my lifelong friends. I am a child of the "baby boom," a generation not known for its sane or cautious approach to things. Yet suddenly my peers are giving up drinking, giving up smoking, cutting down on coffee, sugar, and salt. They will not eat red meat and go now to restaurants whose menus have caused me to stand on a chair yelling, "Flopsy, Mopsy, Cottontail, dinner is served!" This from the generation of LSD, Weather Under-ground, and Altamont Rock Festival! And all in the name of safety! Our nation has withstood many divisions—North and South, black and white, labor and management—but I do not know if the country can survive division into smoking and nonsmoking sections.

The forces of safety are afoot in the land. I, for one, believe it is a conspiracy—a conspiracy of Safety Nazis shouting "Sieg Health" and seeking to trammel freedom, lib-erty, and large noisy parties. The Safety Nazis advocate gun control, vigorous exercise, and health foods. The result can only be a disarmed, exhausted, and half-starved population ready to acquiesce to dictatorship of some kind.

—P. J. O'Rourke

laws related to health care. Many more malpractice suits are being brought against physicians, nurses, and hospitals by people who believe that they have been injured as a result of negligence or inappropriate action (Gaffney, 1998).

## Local Government

Local governments are the link between citizens and the state and federal governments. Local governments distribute billions of federal and state dollars to local community agen-cies to provide services. The quality of life in a community is determined by how local government officials make deci-sions about the delivery of services. Some of the services provided and monitored by local governments are public health, public education, drinking water, sewage disposal, police protection, and solid waste management (Majewski & O'Brien, 2006).

The number, size, and type of local government varies throughout the country depending on state and regional culture, economics, and geography. The U.S. Census Bureau has divided local governments into four categories: counties, municipalities, towns and townships, and special districts (Majewski & O'Brien, 2006). Local governments are divided into the same branches of government (with variations) as the federal and state governments.

*I am not an American who confuses politics with pa-triotism. I am an American who loves our country because we are all guaranteed the freedom to disagree with government decisions.*

—Natalie Maine, of the country music group Dixie Chicks, commenting on the public outcry on her negative comments about President George W. Bush and the Iraqi War

*Let the strivings of Martin Luther King, Jr., to have been correct when he said that humanity can no longer be tragically bound to the starless midnight of racism and war.*

—Nelson Mandela, Nobel Peace Prize acceptance speech, 1993

*There is no easy walk to freedom anywhere.*

—Nelson Mandela

## Different Types of Law

According to *Webster's New World College Dictionary* (Agnus, 2004), a law is a rule of conduct established and enforced by the authority, legislation, or custom of a given community, state, or other group. There are three types of laws in the United States: constitutional law, legislation and regulation, and judicial or common law.

**Constitutional law** is derived from federal and state constitutions and is the supreme law of the land. The U.S. Constitution is the highest legal authority that exists, and no other law, state or federal, may overrule it. A state consti-tution is the highest state law authority, but any provisions that conflict with the federal constitution will be invali-dated by the courts. It is not considered a conflict, however, if state constitutions provide more expansive individual rights than those guaranteed by the federal constitution (Kaplin & Lee, 2006).

Legislation and regulation, known as **statutory law,** are established through formal legislative processes. Each time the U.S. Congress or state legislatures pass legislation, the body of statutory law grows (Betts & Waddle, 2007). Statutes are enacted by both federal and state govern-ments. Local statutes, called *ordinances*, are enacted by local governing bodies, such as city and county councils (Kaplin & Lee, 2006).

**Judicial or common law**, known as case law, is derived from decisions made in the courtroom. Common law is based on the principles of justice, reason, and common sense rather than rules and regulations (Guido, 2001). Each time a judge or a jury makes a decision, the body of common law grows (Betts & Waddle, 2007). Decisions are made based on decisions from previous similar cases. Judges are bound by previous decisions (i.e., precedents) unless it can be shown that the previous rulings are no longer valid. Therefore, a de-cision made in a case with no predecessors is critical because it becomes a precedent-setting case.

Common law can be categorized as either civil or criminal. Civil law protects individuals and involves the enforcement of rights, duties, and other legal relations be-tween private citizens (Betts & Waddle, 2007). For example, an individual can sue another individual or a company for not fulfilling the terms of a legal contract. Criminal law is a crime against the state and involves public concerns against unlawful behavior that threatens society (Betts & Waddle, 2007). Murder is an example of criminal law. Although the crime was committed against an individual, it threatens the security of society as a whole.

## How an Idea Becomes a Law

In today's climate of health care reform, nurses must understand the legislative process to be able to influence the development of sound health care policy for their patients and for the profession of nursing (Abood & Mittelstadt, 2006; Santa Anna, 2006). Because the legislative process is similar at both the state and federal levels, it is described at the state level in this chapter. Although the legislative pathway may differ slightly from state to state, the basic process is the same (Abood & Mittelstadt, 2006; Santa Anna, 2006). The state of Florida is used as the example.

A bill can be introduced only by a member of the legislature. Legislators introduce bills for many reasons, which may include pleasing a constituent or a special-interest group, declaring a position on an issue, getting publicity, or simply avoiding a political attack (Abood & Mittelstadt, 2006; Santa Anna, 2006). Companion bills (or twin bills) are sometimes introduced by legislators in the Senate and House of Representatives to increase the likelihood that the bill will pass and become law.

During a legislative session, the House and Senate meet separately and attempt to pass legislation that has previously been considered by a number of legislative committees. Committees are often referred to as the "heart of the legislative process" because they allow legislators to break down into smaller groups to discuss pertinent issues (Florida Senate, 2006). This enables members to have more in-depth discussions than would be possible if all issues were discussed by the entire legislature. Committees are established by authority of rules, which are adopted separately by the House and the Senate. The Speaker of the House and the President of the Senate, both of whom are elected by each body and represent the majority party, designate a chair and a vice-chair for each committee and appoint legislators to serve as committee members. Legislators usually serve on more than one committee.

There are three basic kinds of committees: standing, select, and conference committees. Standing committees are established by both the Senate and the House of Representatives to manage their business. They can be distinguished from each other by the kind of issues that they consider. For example, the Florida House of Representatives has a standing committee on health care regulation, which is responsible for considering bills relating to that particular area. The staff of this committee is responsible for doing the fact-finding groundwork for legislation that is referred to the committee for consideration. For example, if the committee were considering a bill proposing a change in the requirements for registered nurse (RN) licensure, it would study the current licensure requirements, find out why the sponsor of the bill (one or more of the representatives) believes the change is necessary, examine what the effects of the proposed change might be, and hear testimony from nurses, as well as the broader health care community, to gain insight about how they feel about the proposed change. Once all of these things

> *"Keep, ancient lands, your storied pomp!" cries she*
> *With silent lips. "Give me your tired, your poor,*
> *Your huddled masses yearning to breathe free,*
> *The wretched refuse of your teeming shore.*
> *Send these, the homeless, tempest-tossed, to me;*
> *I lift my lamp beside the golden door.*
>
> —Emma Lazarus (1849–1887), U.S. poet, The New Colossus (1886),
> written for inscription on the Statue of Liberty

are considered, the committee passes judgment on the proposed legislation.

If the bill passes the committee, it travels either to the next committee of reference (if there is more than one) or to the floor of the House or Senate to be voted on by the respective body as a whole. If the committee does not pass the proposed legislation (reports unfavorably on the bill), the legislation will die unless two thirds of the members vote to reconsider it. This is a very high percentage, and further consideration is unlikely to occur in this situation.

Committees wield significant power in the legislative process. The chair of each committee has a great deal of influence over legislation because he or she decides which bills will be heard by the committee. If a bill is not heard, it cannot be voted on and therefore cannot be passed. Committees also have the authority to amend proposed legislation, so the original bill may look very different by the time it reaches the floor of the House or Senate.

A second type of committee is the select committee. This type of committee is appointed to perform a particular task and goes out of existence when the purpose for which it was created has been accomplished (Florida House of Representatives, 2008). Also known as an "ad hoc" committee, a select committee may last anywhere from a few minutes to several years. For example, on the opening day of each legislative session, the Senate president will appoint a select committee to inform the House of Representatives that they are ready to begin conducting business. The Speaker of the House will appoint a similar committee that completes the ritual. These select committees complete their ceremonial function in a few minutes. By contrast, when an issue arises that merits special consideration, a select committee may be established to consider that particular issue in depth. For example, the 1999 Florida Legislature had to consider a comprehensive legislative package introduced by Governor Jeb Bush regarding education. Rather than refer the large number of bills to different standing committees, the Speaker of

 THINK ABOUT THIS

Nancy Pelosi, U.S. Representative from California, became the United States' first female Speaker of the U.S. House of Representatives in January 2007.

the House of Representatives appointed a Select Committee on Transforming Florida's Schools to consider the bills as a complete educational package. This committee consisted of members of the House of Representatives (from both political parties) and was chaired by the member who sponsored the legislation. It met for 2 weeks immediately before the legislative session, heard testimony from supporters and opponents, and was responsible for amending and voting on the bills in the package.

The third type of committee is a conference committee. Before the functions of this kind of committee can be described, it is necessary to further explain the process of how a bill becomes a law. For a bill to be signed into law and become an act that is sent to the governor for consideration, it must pass both houses of the legislature in identical form. This is often more difficult than it sounds. First, the bill must have a sponsor in both the House and the Senate. These "companion" bills may be identical, similar, or very dissimilar. When a bill makes it through the committee process and is considered on the floor of the House or Senate, it goes through an amendatory process. Once amended, the bill requires a majority vote to pass.

Let's use RN licensure requirements as a hypothetical example. The House bill, after completing the committee process, increases both the level of education needed to obtain an RN license and the competencies required to pass the licensure exam. On the floor, House members amend the bill to add two more competencies. The bill, as amended, passes with a majority vote and is sent to the Senate for consideration. The Senate takes up the House bill and agrees with the increased educational requirements but decides to amend the bill because it does not agree with the competencies that the House has chosen. In the amendatory process, the Senate removes three of the competencies required in the House bill and adds two new competencies from the original Senate bill. The House bill, as amended by the Senate, then passes the Senate with a majority vote and is sent back to the House. If the House does not agree with the changes made by the Senate, they may reach an impasse. This often results in the bill's demise. However, if the proposed legislation is important to the leadership in each house, the presiding officers may appoint a conference committee in an attempt to reach a compromise agreement. If differences cannot be reconciled through the conference committee, the proposed legislation will fail. A conference committee is actually composed of two separate committees, one appointed by the president of the Senate and the other appointed by the speaker of the House. The two committees vote separately on all issues relating to the bill under consideration, and a majority of each committee must approve all changes (Florida Senate, 2008). If the conference committee can reach an agreement, the House and Senate must vote on the compromise on a "take it or leave it" basis and no amendments can be offered (Florida Senate, 2008). Usually, conference reports are submitted during the waning hours of a session, when time is short and legislators are unlikely to reject conference committee recommendations because it will most likely result in the failure of the bill (Florida House of Representatives, 2008).

It is important to realize that many bills make it through the committee process but never get heard on the floor of the House or Senate. The presiding officers of each house, through the standing committees on rules and calendar, have control over which bills will be considered by the full House or Senate. Just as in committee, if a bill is not heard on the floor, it cannot be voted on and therefore cannot pass.

If a bill makes it through the committee process and passes both houses in identical form, it is called an *act*. Each act is sent to the governor for consideration, and he or she may either sign it into law, allow it to become law without his or her signature, or veto it. If an act is vetoed, the legislature may override it with a two-thirds vote in both houses.

 NOTE THIS!

A conference committee is appointed every legislative session to consider the budget. This committee is always important because the budget is the only bill that the legislature is *required* to pass.

### A Good Read

## What We've Lost: How the Bush Administration Has Curtailed Our Freedoms, Mortgaged Our Economy, Ravaged Our Environment, and Damaged Our Standing in the World (2004)

*By Graydon Carter, New York: Farrar, Straus, and Giroux.*

Carter takes on the federal government and turns a critical eye toward recent changes in the United States since the events of September 11, 2001. He addresses the fragile state of U.S. democracy, with a critical review of the George W. Bush administration. Carter is the editor of *Vanity Fair* and has expressed his deep dissatisfaction with the current state of the nation in his monthly editor's letters in *Vanity Fair*, which have generated widespread controversy. In his book, he goes farther in a sweeping, detailed account of the ruinous effects of President Bush and his administrative policies. He looks at the war in Iraq and its costs in lives, dollars, and international standing, as well as the loss of our personal rights from the insecurity of terrorism. Hardly anything is spared in Carter's criticism of American politics and policy. This book is sure to arouse stimulating discussions from people with all political views.

However, because the governor does not consider the acts until after the legislative session has adjourned, the legislature would be forced to either call a special session or wait until the next session to take action.

### How Nurses Can Get Involved

Nurses can become involved in the political process at various levels. The first and most important thing is to be an informed voter. Nurses should watch the news, read the newspaper, surf the Internet, and be aware of what the candidates stand for on the national, state, and local levels. Nurses should also find out where candidates stand on the issues that are important to them as nurses. This can be accomplished with just a minimal amount of investigation. Nurses can contact the professional organizations to which they belong to find out which candidates they support. If a candidate is an incumbent, his or her voting record on issues of importance should be checked. Nurses must make phone calls, write letters, and ask questions!

Once legislators are in office, nurses should get to know them and make themselves and their views known to them. Box 8-4 contains some tips for effectively communicating ideas to legislators.

To have one of your ideas introduced as a bill, you must first find a sponsor in both the House and the Senate. The best scenario would be to approach a potential sponsor who is influential among legislators and who has a record of sponsoring successful legislation in your area of interest. This person will be likely to have more success in building coalitions among members than a less experienced legislator. It is also helpful if the legislator feels strongly about the issue because he or she will be more likely to fight for the proposed legislation.

---

### BOX 8-4

**Tips for Effective Communication with Legislators**

- Know who your legislators are and how to contact them.
- Make sure you understand the legislative process. Even the most basic understanding of the process will help you effectively express your ideas.
- Contact your legislator about a particular issue before the legislature takes action on it. Most matters coming before the legislature are well publicized before session.
- Use a variety of communication methods. You might choose to telephone, write e-mail, fax, or visit your legislator. You might also choose to give testimony at public hearings held by the legislature.
- Tell your legislator what effect you think a particular bill, if it becomes law, will have on you, your children, business, or community. Be concise, but specific.
- Be polite, even if you disagree strongly with the legislator you are addressing. Lawmakers cannot please everyone. Your communication will be more effective if you are reasonable in your approach.
- Suggest a course of action and offer assistance. Don't make promises or threats.

*Source:* Florida Senate, 2006.

---

Some legislative bodies place limits on the number of bills that can be filed by a particular member. It is necessary to investigate whether limitations exist and, if so, approach potential sponsors early. Timing can be crucial, especially if the issue of concern is a highly publicized one. Be aware of media coverage and strategically plan your moves.

### Lobbying

**Lobbying** is defined as "influencing or attempting to influence legislative action or non-action through oral or written communication or attempting to obtain the goodwill of a member or employee of the Legislature" (5. 11. 045 Florida, statutes). A lobbyist is a person who is employed and receives payment for the primary purpose of lobbying on behalf of another person, group, or governmental entity. Most states, if not all, require lobbyists to be registered as such. This registration allows citizens to be informed about activities that are aimed at influencing government decision making. For example, when major legislation relating to health care is being considered, it may be beneficial to know which groups have hired lobbyists to promote their interests and monitor their activities and expenditures.

For example, home health agencies may hire lobbyists whose principal responsibilities are to represent the organization's interests to the legislature and other government agencies. Nurses employed by a home health agency would not be considered lobbyists unless their most significant work responsibility dealt with governmental affairs. However, this does not mean that the nurses cannot contact their legislators and actively support or oppose legislation that affects their home health agencies. It simply means that the nurses are not be required to register because they do not receive payment for the purposes of lobbying.

Lobbyists must adhere to many rules and regulations, which may vary widely from state to state. Therefore, it is important that nurses be aware of the rules, if any, that apply in their states. Regulations may also change from year to year, which makes it necessary to keep current. For example, in Florida, rules and regulations regarding the receipt of gifts

---

### Research Alert

This study investigated the role of flight attendants and their unions in creating smoke-free air travel. Case study methodology was used to search tobacco industry documents and labor union periodicals and to interview key informants. Tobacco industry strategies against establishing smoke-free work sites failed with the airline industry, largely because of the efforts of flight attendants and their unions. This study illustrates the potential for successful partnerships between unions and tobacco control policy advocates when developing smoke-free work site policies.

*Source:* Pan, J., Barbeau, E. M., Levenstein, C., & Balbach, E. D. (2005). Smoke-free airlines and the role of organized labor: A case study. *American Journal of Public Health*, 95(3), 398–404.

## Application to Practice

### Two Mississippi Nurses Lead the Way

*Deborah Konkle-Parker, MSN, FNP*

As a nurse practitioner working in an outpatient HIV clinic in Jackson, Mississippi, Debbie Konkle-Parker and other providers depended on the federal Ryan White AIDS Drug Assistance Program (ADAP), administered by the Mississippi Department of Health (MSDH), to help many of their patients get medicines. ADAP was used primarily to help patients who had no health insurance or whose medications exceeded the Mississippi Medicaid limit of five prescriptions per month.

In early April 1997, after several years of uneventful program usage, word was received from the health department that the Ryan White program was not accepting any more referrals for ADAP assistance. The recent addition of expensive protease inhibitors to the treatment regimen for HIV had depleted the entire year of federal ADAP funding by mid-March. This news came suddenly, without warning, and with no backup plan for those with no other resources.

This sudden news sent providers and patients reeling, with no way to deal with this shortfall in services. A week later, there was a meeting of health care providers at the Mississippi Department of Health. At this meeting, the health care providers were informed that those individuals who were already receiving a protease inhibitor from ADAP would continue to receive medications, but all others would be cut off from the program. No more referrals were being accepted. This could literally mean the difference between life and death for many patients.

To deal with the problem, Debbie Konkle-Parker organized a problem-solving session to determine a way to cope with this change. She sent letters to concerned individuals, requesting their presence at a networking meeting. The meeting was attended by health care providers representing all disciplines, representatives from MSDH, representatives from the pharmaceutical industry, and persons with HIV/AIDS. The discussion at the meeting revealed that although most states provided funding from their state budgets to augment the federal ADAP dollars, Mississippi did not. It was decided that to change this policy, it was important to become an organized body to influence the legislators. The Mississippi HIV/AIDS Assembly was formed, with Debbie Konkle-Parker as its chair. The Mississippi HIV/AIDS Assembly consisted of two committees: (1) the AIDS Aware committee for mobilizing grass-roots lobbying efforts around the state and (2) the Health Provider Network of interdisciplinary health care providers who could mobilize organizational lobbying efforts. Shortly after this meeting, the Mississippi State Department of Health found a way to temporarily redirect some of the money from other parts of the Ryan White program to re-enroll some patients who had been dropped from the program. But that effort was only putting a "Band-Aid" on the problem until further funding could be obtained.

The Health Provider Network set about the task of determining the direction of the work of the assembly, and the AIDS Aware committee gathered grass-roots support for their efforts. The highest-priority goal was supporting the Health Department's request of $500,000 from the state budget for ADAP. Although this amount was much less than what was actually needed, it was determined that politically this was an amount that reasonably could be requested by the Health Department. The Mississippi AIDS Assembly requested $2 million from the legislature, which was the estimate of how much money was actually needed to meet the extent of the problem in Mississippi.

Through these two committees, several different actions were taken, including providing speakers to bring attention to the issue for the public; maintaining a "silent" presence, including media coverage at a key budget hearing meeting; attending a meeting of the legislature's public health committee where bills were decided on before being brought to the floor; and applying consistent pressure on legislators to consider this issue. Multiple mailings went out to individuals throughout the state, encouraging personal communication with their legislators and a "spreading of the word."

The result of this year-long work was the first-ever state dedication of $750,000 to the Mississippi Ryan White AIDS Drug Assistance Program, with more to follow each year. This funding allowed a return of new referrals to the program and an immediate lessening of the waiting list of individuals needing medications.

### Connie Thompson, BSN, RN

As the infection control coordinator of a medical center in Jackson, Mississippi, Connie Thompson played a big role in the efforts of the Mississippi HIV/AIDS Assembly and eagerly joined in the excitement surrounding its legislative victory. But after the excitement faded away, Thompson realized that this was only the beginning. More funding and services were needed, not only for persons living with HIV/AIDS, but for persons living with any chronic disabling disease.

In August 1998, under the leadership of Thompson, a variety of Mississippi organizations and agencies joined forces in an effort to influence legislative health care issues for disabled persons. Eventually this group formed a coalition of more than 50 organizations and agencies known as the Coalition for Uninsured Mississippians, representing thousands of Mississippians with disabilities or chronic illnesses who are denied access to health insurance each year.

*(continues)*

**Application to Practice—continued**

These individuals—persons with cancer, heart disease, HIV, diabetes, asthma, lupus, arthritis, and other diseases—earn a little more money, either from disability payments or job income, than the maximum allowed to qualify for Medicaid. However, they don't make enough money to be able to afford expensive private health insurance.

As a result, these men, women, and children are forced to make frequent visits to hospital emergency rooms for basic health care. Or worse, they do not seek care at all until a crisis occurs that requires inpatient hospitalization. Proper disease management with regular clinic visits for appropriate follow-up and networking for patient care and services would maintain optimal health standards for these individuals. Quality of life for these persons would greatly improve and health care would be more cost-effective if they had access to health insurance.

The timing for the work of the coalition was a critical factor. The Federal Balanced Budget Act of 1997 offered states the option of allowing citizens with disabilities to purchase Medicaid on a sliding fee scale according to their income. In August 1998, the U.S. Department of Health and Human Services urged state governors, state legislators, and Medicaid directors to take advantage of this important new option. The Coalition for Uninsured Mississippians sought support from Mississippi's citizens for a legislative bill that would allow disabled persons with incomes below 250% of the federal poverty level to buy in to Medicaid coverage. The purchase of this coverage would be based on a sliding scale fee. Both the Balanced Budget Act of 1997 and the encouragement from the U.S. Department of Health and Human Services were used to support the coalition's action.

Within 2 months of the coalition's initial meeting a petition supported by thousands of Mississippians had been sent to the co-chairs of the joint subcommittees of health and welfare of the state legislature. A statewide Forum for Effective Advocacy of Chronic Illnesses and Disabilities was held to discuss the issues, and a task force was formed to meet with the director of the division of Medicaid to look for solutions. Connie Thompson, as the facilitator of the Coalition for Uninsured Mississippians, was invited to serve on the attorney general's Partners for a Healthy Mississippi task force.

As a result of the coalition's efforts, a bill to expand Medicaid coverage by authorizing a buy-in opportunity to workers who are disabled and earning less than 250% of the federal poverty was drafted and signed into law by the Mississippi legislature and the governor during the 1999 legislative session.

In both of the above scenarios, nurse-led public policy strategies, starting with simple problem-solving meetings, have achieved the goal of improving health care for some of Mississippi's poor and vulnerable citizens.

Connie Thompson, BSN, RN, and Deborah Konkle-Parker, MSN, RN, FNP, work with Robert G. Clark, Mississippi State Representative.

from lobbyists are established in statute (Section 112.3148, Florida Statutes). Other states may not be so proscriptive and may outline rules only in policy manuals or employee handbooks. Some states may not even have rules for lobbyists, but most have some kind of regulation.

Best practices for lobbying as well as for concerned constituents include being aware of all applicable rules and restrictions, establishing a good rapport with legislators and legislative staff, and always backing up your position with hard data. If nurses adhere to these principles, their likelihood of successfully communicating their ideas will greatly increase.

### Political Action Committees

Through the years, the ANA and various other specialty health organizations have taken leadership roles in mobilizing nurses in grass-roots lobbying. This has required a significant effort to educate nurses about the political process and how to remain cognizant of the political issues that affect nursing and health. Because federal law requires that campaign contributions be kept as a separate fund and that no organizational membership be used for this purpose, many groups have created separate organizations for political activities. These organizations are referred to as **political action committees (PACs)**. Their work is completely separate from the rest of the organization's work. The primary purpose of a PAC is to endorse and support candidates for public office who support the legislative agenda of the organization or group making the endorsement (Curtis & Lumpkin, 1998; Malone, Chaffee, & Wachter, 2002). Nursing PACs exist at the federal and state levels, most often through the ANA (ANA-PAC) and state nurses associations.

## Regulation and Licensing of Nursing Practice

### ■ The Regulatory Process

Although it is important for nurses to be involved in the legislative process, it is equally important for nurses to understand the **regulatory process**. According to *Webster's New World College Dictionary* (Agnuo, 2004), *regulation* is the act of controlling, directing, or governing according to a rule, principle, or system. Once bills are passed into law by the legislative branch of government, they must be implemented by the administrative agencies of the executive branch (Abood & Mittelstadt, 1998; Loquist, 1999; White, 2002). Legislation is purposely expressed in broad terms to provide flexibility and adaptability of laws over time. Regulation is expressed in very specific terms describing how the administrative agency with jurisdictional authority will implement the law (Loquist, 1999; Santa Anna, 2002). The legislative process is used to create policy and laws to address a particular issue when none exist. Regulation is used to clarify and interpret existing policy and laws and decide what methods will be used to enforce them (Loquist, 1999; Santa Anna, 2002).

Regulations frame the way health policy is transposed into services and programs. Although regulations are a direct result of passed legislation, they are shaped into their final forms by the ongoing involvement of health care professionals and their professional organizations, third-party payers, consumers, and other special-interest groups. Before a federal agency can implement a law, it must publish the proposed regulation or set of regulations in the *Federal Register*. The publication of the proposed regulations affords anyone with any interest in the regulations the ability to react to them before they become finalized. Commenting on proposed regulations before they are finalized is one of the most important, but often neglected, parts of the legislative process (Abood & Mittelstadt, 1998).

The U.S. Constitution dictates that the government has a duty to protect its citizens. The Tenth Amendment to the U.S. Constitution provides the states with all the powers not specifically reserved for the federal government. Regulation of health care professions is one way that each state exercises its responsibility to protect the health, safety, and welfare of its residents.

> **❝** A small body of determined spirits fired by an unquenchable faith in their mission can alter the course of history. **❞**
>
> —Mahatma Gandi

### ▥ HEALTHY PEOPLE 2010

**OBJECTIVES RELATED TO LAW**

3.14 Increase the number of states that have a statewide population-based cancer registry that captures case information on at least 95% of the expected number of reportable cancers.

6.13 Increase the number of tribes, states, and the District of Columbia that have public health surveillance and health-promotion programs for people with disabilities and care givers.

13.9 Increase the number of state prison systems that provide comprehensive HIV/AIDS, sexually transmitted diseases, and tuberculosis (TB) education.

13.10 Increase the proportion of inmates in state prison systems who receive voluntary HIV counseling and testing during incarceration.

15.24 Increase the number of states and the District of Columbia with laws requiring bicycle helmets for bicycle riders.

18.11 Increase the proportion of local governments with community-based jail diversion programs for adults with serious mental illnesses.

23.15 Increase the proportion of federal, tribal, state, and local jurisdictions that review and evaluate the extent to which their statutes, ordinances, and bylaws assure the delivery of essential public health services.

27.14 Reduce the illegal buy rate among minors through enforcement of laws prohibiting the sale of tobacco products to minors.

*Source:* DHHS, 2000.

Nursing practice in each state is governed by a **nurse practice act,** which includes the laws and regulations that control the requirements for entry into practice, the standards for acceptable practice, the standards for continuing competence, and the disciplinary actions taken for misconduct (Loquist, 1999; Betts & Keepnews, 2002; NCSBN, 2005). The state nurse practice act is the most important piece of legislature for nurses because it governs every facet of nursing practice (Guido, 2001).

Each state legislature designates a board of nursing to administer the nurse practice act. There are boards of nursing in all 50 states, the District of Columbia, and four U.S. territories (NCSBN, 2006). The most critical role of the board of nursing is to ensure the safety of the public by monitoring the competency of practicing nurses through licensure (Loquist, 1999).

## ■ Licensure

A license is a formal permission authorized by law to do something (Agnus, 2004). Nurses must be licensed in a state in order to work as an RN, licensed practical nurse (LPN), or vocational nurse (LVN). **Licensure** provides the public with the greatest level of protection because it protects the title of RN or LPN and delineates the scope of nursing practice (Loquist, 1999; NCSBN, 2005). Requirements for licensure include proof of graduation from an approved academic program, a passing score on the licensing examination, and personal qualifications such as citizenship or visa permits, good physical and mental health, and good moral character (Barnum, 1997; Guido, 2001; Loquist, 1999).

All states administer licensing examinations using a standardized national test developed and administered by the National Council of State Boards of Nursing (NCSBN). Licensing examinations are called the National Council Licensing Examination for Registered Nurses (NCLEX-RN) and the National Council Licensing Examination for Practical Nurses (NCLEX-PN). Traditionally, nurses have been required to be licensed in the state in which they practice. If a nurse moves to a different state, he or she must obtain a license from the new state. A national examination makes seeking reciprocity (recognition of licensure from one state to another) an easy process if the nurse has a valid license in one state (Betts & Waddle, 1993; Guido, 2001).

In recent years, the use of telecommunication technology has transformed the health care delivery system and challenged the individual state licensing system. Mergers of health care systems have produced giant corporations that operate across state lines. Nurses serve as case managers for patients living in many different states and staff regional or national telephone advice and consultation hot lines (Hutcherson & Williamson, 1999; Loquist, 1999; Wakefield, 1999; Reinhard, 2002). As nurses began practicing in several states at the same time, separate licenses had to be obtained from each state. This policy is impractical and expensive.

In response to the licensing dilemma, the NCSBN adopted a new model for nursing regulation in 1997 called the **Nurse Multistate Licensure Mutual Recognition Model.** According to the ANA, multistate licensure allows a nurse to practice in several states while holding a license in only one state. States enter into interstate compact agreements to coordinate activities associated with licensure. This mutual recognition model, now called the Nurse Licensure Compact (NLC), allows nurses to practice in states that have adopted an interstate compact with each other. The nurses are held accountable for compliance with the laws and regulations of each state's nurse practice act (ANA, 1998; NCSBN, 2006). In March 1998, Utah became the first state to pass legislation to adopt the Mutual Recognition Model (ANA, 1998). By January 2007, 20 states were participating in the NLC and two more had passed legislation to join the NLC and expected implementation to begin shortly (NCSBN, 2006).

State boards of nursing are responsible not only for ensuring the competency of nurses entering into practice, but also for monitoring the competence of those nurses already in practice. Most nurse practice acts have provisions that require employers to report any violations. Procedures for reporting misconduct, conducting investigations, and issuing sanctions are outlined in the regulations of each state's or territory's nurse practice act. Licensed nurses are responsible for knowing the laws and regulations that govern nursing practice in their states (Loquist, 1999; NCSBN, 2006).

## Nursing Practice and the Law

The most common lawsuits filed against health care professionals involve the principles of **negligence** and **malpractice,** which fall under the classification of tort law. Torts are legal wrongs committed against another person or against the property of another person. The wrongdoing may be intentional or unintentional and must result in physical, emotional, or economic harm (Betts & Waddle, 1993; Guido, 2001; Pozgar, 2004).

Although the terms *negligence* and *malpractice* are often used interchangeably, there is a fine distinction between them. *Negligence* is a general term that describes the failure to act as any prudent or reasonable person would act in a specific circumstance. *Malpractice* is a more specific term that considers a professional standard of care as well as the professional status of the health care provider. To be liable for malpractice, the person committing the misconduct must be a professional acting in a professional role. Professional misconduct includes either doing something that should not be done (commission) or not doing something that should be done (omission) (Betts & Waddle, 1993; Guido, 2001; Pozgar, 2004).

For a nurse to be found guilty of malpractice in a court of law, the following must have existed:
- A duty was owed to the patient.
- There was a breach of the duty owed to the patient.

- Harm was caused to the patient.
- The harm was foreseeable.
- The action or inaction of the nurse caused the harm (Guido, 2001; Pozgar, 2004).

## ■ Nursing Practice in Correctional Settings

The role of the community health nurse in correctional settings is relatively new. Health care for this population has unique challenges for the nurse in this specialized legal setting (Box 8-5). The basis of correctional health care is providing primary care for inmates from the time of entry into the system, through transfers to other facilities, and to final release from custody back to the community (Farley, 1999). Nurses in correctional facilities provide health care to populations incarcerated in jails, prisons, juvenile detention facilities, and similar settings. Ages range from youths to aged adults. Women, although representing only 10% to 12% of the incarcerated population, make up a growing number of persons in correctional facilities (ANA, 1995; Huft, 2003; Freudenberg et al., 2005).

Although often not fully realized by the general population, the existence of health care in correctional facilities is based on the Eighth Amendment of the U.S. Constitution, which prohibits "cruel and unusual punishment" of those convicted of crimes. Furthermore, as a public health concern, correctional institutions are reservoirs of physical and mental illness, which constantly spill back into the community. Appropriate treatment must be provided, with a focus on prevention of transmission of communicable disease. The health of the general community is affected as the inmate population continues to increase.

The consequences of untreated illness in the system are not just for the inmate or even just to the correctional system. These are public health problems that require effective management and close collaboration between correctional health and the public health system (Conklin, Lincoln, & Flanigan, 1998; Freudenberg et al., 2005).

Incarcerated populations have greater health risks than the general population for communicable disease, especially HIV and tuberculosis; violence-associated risks; decreased educational levels; substance abuse; and poverty. Not only do inmates have higher risks for many of these health problems upon admission, but environmental conditions within the correctional facility and behaviors associated with incarceration lend themselves to the spread of communicable disease. The nurse in the correctional setting can provide interventions aimed at interrupting the chain of contagion and can educate the inmates about self-care and protection from these risks. Inmate education is an essential function of **correctional nursing.** The goals are for inmates to remain healthy while incarcerated and to return to the community properly educated about remaining free of communicable disease, as well as to prevent others from becoming infected. Peer education groups have been an effective strategy in the correctional system (Conklin, Lincoln, & Flanigan, 1998; Heines, 2005).

**❝** *Prisons do not exist in a vacuum: they are part of a political, social, economic, and moral order.* **❞**

—James B. Jacobs, 1977

## ■ Forensic Nursing: An Emerging Nursing Role

**Forensic nursing,** one of the fastest-growing specialties in the field of nursing, is the necessary link between health care and law enforcement. In 1992, 70 sexual assault nurses met in Minneapolis, Minnesota, and founded what would become the International Association of Forensic Nurses (IAFN). The American Nurses Association recognized forensic nursing as a nursing practice specialty in 1996. Forensic nurses can be found working in rape crisis centers, emergency departments, and nursing homes, among other places. In some parts of the United States, forensic nurses serve as coroners and death investigators to assist law enforcement officers in the investigation of homicides or other unexplained deaths.

The practice roles for forensic nurses encompass several different areas of expertise, including sexual assault nurse examiners, forensic correctional nurses, forensic pediatric nurses, and forensic psychiatric nurses. In addition to providing essential nursing services such as appropriate physical care and emotional support to victims of crime, the duties of forensic nurses include collecting and handling police evidence and providing expert testimony in court (Yost & Burke, 2006). While still a relatively new nursing specialty, forensic nurses have successfully bridged the gap between health care and law enforcement, resulting in a high demand for this valuable area of nursing expertise.

## Conclusion

Nurses in the community must remain current and informed about politics and law as related to public health nursing practice. The political system is ultimately about the distribution of power through formalized and complex

---

### BOX 8-5

**Levels of Prevention**

**Activities in Correctional Facilities**

*Primary Prevention*
Stress reduction education
Prenatal care
Immunizations
Violence prevention

*Secondary Prevention*
Treatment of infections
Trauma care for injuries

Screening for suicide risk
Disaster and emergency care

*Tertiary Prevention*
Injury rehabilitation
Diabetes foot care
Stroke rehabilitation

systems of law, policy, and regulatory control mechanisms. Settings within the community have legal implications for the nurse, and there are emerging opportunities for nurses within the political/legal community, such as correctional and forensic nursing. Furthermore, for nurses to maintain control of professional nursing practice, understanding and applying political knowledge helps secure our future in the health care delivery system.

Explore Community Health Nursing on the Web! To learn more about the topics in this chapter, use the passcode provided to access your exclusive website: **http://nursing.jbpub.com/ communityhealth.** If you do not have a passcode, you can obtain one at this site.

## ■ CRITICAL THINKING ACTIVITIES

1. Do all three types of law apply to professional nursing practice? In what ways?
2. In what ways can nurses influence legislation that affects nursing practice?
3. What types of nursing situations may lend themselves to malpractice suits?
4. What steps can you take to avoid a lawsuit?
5. Is there a particular "type" of patient who will sue? What makes you think so?

## ■ REFERENCES

Abood, S., & Mittelstadt, P. (2006). Legislative and regulatory processes. In D. J. Mason, J. K. Leavitt, & M. W. Chaffee (Eds.), *Policy and politics in nursing and health care* (5th ed.). Philadelphia: Saunders.

Agnus, M. E. (2004). *Webster's new world college dictionary* (4th ed.). New York: MacMillan.

American Nurses Association (ANA). (1998). *Multistate regulation of nurses.* Retrieved May 23, 2008, from http://www.nursingworld.org/gova/multibg.htm

Anderson, J. E. (2006). *Public policymaking* (6th ed.). Boston: Houghton Mifflin.

Bacharach, S. B., & Lawler, E. J. (1980). *Power and politics in organizations.* San Francisco: Jossey-Bass.

Barnum, B. S. (1997, August 13). Licensure, certification, and accreditation. *Online Journal of Issues in Nursing.* Retrieved May 23, 2008, from http://www.nursing world.org/ojin/tpc4/tpc4_2.htm

Bednash, G. P., Heylin, G. B., & Rhome, A. M. (1998). Federal government. In D. J. Mason & J. K. Leavitt (Eds.), *Policy and politics in nursing and health care* (3rd ed., pp. 436–457). Philadelphia: W. B. Saunders.

Betts, V. T., & Keepnews, D. (2002). Nursing and the courts. In D. J. Mason, J. K. Leavitt, & M. W. Chaffee (Eds.), *Policy and politics in nursing and health care* (4th ed., pp. 471–478). St. Louis: Saunders.

Betts, V. T., & Waddle, F. I. (2007). Legal aspects of nursing. In K. K. Chitty & B. P. Black (Eds.), *Professional nursing. Concepts and challenges* (5th ed.). Philadelphia: W. B. Saunders.

Conklin, T., Lincoln, T., & Flanigan, T. (1998). A public health model to connect correction health care with communities. *American Journal of Public Health, 88*(8), 1249–1251.

Curtis, B. T., & Lumpkin, B. (1998). Political action committees. In D. J. Mason & J. K. Leavitt (Eds.), *Policy and politics in nursing and health care* (3rd ed., pp. 546–554). Philadelphia: W. B. Saunders.

Department of Health and Human Services (DHHS). (2008). *HHS: What we do.* Retrieved October 8, 2008, from http://www.hhs.gov/about/whatwedo.html/

Earley, J. (1999, Spring/Summer). Nursing behind bars. *Minority Nurse,* pp. 22–25.

Florida House of Representatives. (2008). *The council-committee process.* Retrieved December 19, 2008, from http://www.myfloridahouse.gov/contentViewer.aspx?category=PublicGuide&file=About_The_Legislative_Process_The_Committee_Process.html

Florida Senate. (2006). Effective communication with your legislator. Retrieved May, 2006, from http://www.flsenate.gov

Florida Senate. (2008). Committees. Retrieved May, 2006, from http://www.flsenate.gov/Committees

Forgotson, E. H. (1967). 1965: The turning point in health law—1966 reflections. *American Journal of Public Health, 57*(6), 934–935.

French, J. R., & Raven, B. (1959). The basis for social power. In D. Cartwright (Ed.), *Studies in social power.* Ann Arbor: University of Michigan Press.

Freudenberg, N., Daniels, J., Crum, M., Perkins, T., & Richie, B. E. (2005). Coming home from jail: The social and health consequences of community reentry for women, male adolescents, and their families and communities. *American Journal of Public Health, 95*(10), 1725–1736.

Gaffney, T. (1998). State government. In D. J. Mason & J. K. Leavitt (Eds.), *Policy and politics in nursing and health care* (3rd ed., pp. 417–427). Philadelphia: W. B. Saunders.

Guido, G. W. (2001). *Legal issues in nursing* (3rd ed.). Upper Saddle River, NJ: Prentice Hall.

Heines, V. (2005). Speaking out to improve the health of inmates. *American Journal of Public Health, 95*(10), 1685–1688.

Helvie, C. O. (1998). *Advanced practice nursing in the community.* Thousand Oaks, CA: Sage.

Hersey, P., Blanchard, K., & Natemeyer, W. (1979). Situational leadership: Perception and impact of power. *Group Organizational Studies, 4,* 418–428.

Hewison, A. (1994). The politics of nursing: A framework for analysis. *Journal of Advanced Nursing, 20,* 1170–1175.

Huft, A. (2003, winter). Vulnerable and cultural perspectives for nursing care in correctional systems. *Journal of Multicultural Nursing & Health.* Retrieved February 2007 from http://www.findarticles.com/p/particles/mi.

Huston, C. J. (1995, Fall). Nursing and political action in the twentieth century: From separation to fusion. *Revolution: The Journal of Nurse Empowerment,* 50–53.

Hutcherson, C., & Williamson, S. H. (1999, May 31). Nursing regulation for the new millennium: The mutual recognition model. *Online Journal of Issues in Nursing*. Retrieved May 23, 2008, from http://nursingworld.org/ojin/topic9/topic9_2.htm.

Kaplin, W. A., & Lee, B. A. (2006). *The law of higher education* (4th ed.). San Francisco: Jossey-Bass.

Kelly, L. Y., & Joel, L. A. (1996). *The nursing experience* (3rd ed.). New York: McGraw Hill.

Lenski, G. E. (1984). *Power and privilege*. Chapel Hill: University of North Carolina Press.

Loquist, R. S. (1999). Regulation: Parallel and powerful. In J. A. Milstead (Ed.), *Health policy and politics: A nurse's guide* (pp. 105–146). Gaithersburg, MD: Aspen.

Majewski, J. V., & O'Brien, M. C. (2006). Local government. In D. J. Mason, J. K. Leavitt, & M. W. Chaffee (Eds.), *Policy and politics in nursing and health care* (5th ed.). Philadelphia: Saunders.

Malone, P. S., Chaffee, M. W., & Wachter, M. B. (2002). The power and influence of special interest groups in health care. In D. J. Mason, J. K. Leavitt, & M. W. Chaffee (Eds.), *Policy and politics in nursing and health care* (4th ed. pp. 627–638). St. Louis: Saunders.

Miller, D. F. (1992). *Dimensions of community health*. Dubuque, IA: Wm. C. Brown.

Milstead, J. A. (1999). Advanced practice nurses and public policy, naturally. In J. A. Milstead (Ed.), *Health policy and politics: A nurse's guide* (pp. 1–41). Gaithersburg, MD: Aspen.

National Council of State Boards of Nursing (NCSBN). (2005). *Nursing regulation and the interpretation of nursing scopes of practice*. Retrieved May 23, 2008, from http://www.ncsbn.org/NursingRegandInterpretationofSoP.pdf.

National Council of State Boards of Nursing (NCSBN). (2006). *What boards do*. Retrieved May 23, 2008, from http://www.ncsbn.org/126.htm.

Pozgar, G. D. (2004). *Legal aspects of health care administration* (9th ed.). Sudbury, MA: Jones and Bartlett.

Reinhard, S. C. (2002). State government: 50 paths to policy. In D. J. Mason, J. K. Leavitt, & M. W. Chaffee (Eds.), *Policy and politics in nursing and health care* (4th ed., pp. 491–497). St. Louis: Saunders.

Robertson, I. (1981). *Sociology* (2nd ed.). New York: Worth.

Santa Anna, Y. (2006). Legislative and regulatory processes. In D. J. Mason, J. K. Leavitt, & M. W. Chaffee (Eds.), *Policy and politics in nursing and health care* (5th ed.). Philadelphia: Saunders.

Turnock, B. J. (1997). *Public health: What it is and how it works*. Gaithersburg, MD: Aspen.

Wakefield, M. K. (1999). Have license, will travel. *Nursing Economics, 17*(2), 114–116.

Weber, M. (1947). *The theory of social and economic organization* (ed. and trans. A. M. Henderson & T. Parsons). New York: Oxford University Press.

White, K. M. (2002). The federal government. In D. J. Mason, J. K. Leavitt, & M. W. Chaffee (Eds.), *Policy and politics in nursing and health care* (4th ed., pp. 515–533). St. Louis: Saunders.

Yost, J. R., & Burke, T. L. (2006). Forensic nursing: An aid to law enforcement. *FBI Law Enforcement Bulletin*. Retrieved February 2007 from http://findarticles.com.

# CHAPTER 9
# Health Policy

Nancy Milio and Sharyn Janes

Visit **http://nursing.jbpub.com/communityhealth** for interactive exercises, review questions, Web links, and more.

"Policy is like a play in many acts, which unfolds inevitably once the curtain is raised. To declare then that the performance will not take place is an absurdity. The play will go on, either by means of the actors or by means of the spectators who mount the stage."
—Klemens von Metternich, 1880

"Manner of living, wages, the condition of industry and commerce, public administration, years of abundance and those of famine–everything that contributes to affluence and civilization—produce great variations in death rate. Affluence and wealth . . . is in truth the most important of all hygienic factors, namely that which best assures the very preservation of life."

—*Rene Villerme, mid-nineteenth century*

Nurses have been slow as a profession to view health policy as a priority in our practice. Why do you think knowledge about policy and health care is rarely considered? Do you often think of "politics" as something essential in the practice of community health nursing? In this chapter you will learn about not only the process of health care policy development but also the critical nature of such knowledge to the promotion of nursing care of populations.

## CHAPTER FOCUS

**Health Policy and Public Policy**
- Goals and Policies
- Purpose of Public Policy
- Choosing Policies
- History of Health Policy in the United States
- Present Need for Public Health Policy

**Public Health and Public Policy**

**Policy Development**
- Policy Environment
- Public Health Advocacy and Action
- Policy Shape and Setting
- Policy Goals, Tools, and Resources
- The Players as Stakeholders

- Player Connections

**Information for Action**

**Policy Development Strategies**
- Bargaining
- Information Through the Mass Media
- Health Information
- Mass Media and the Case of Health Care Reform: A Cautionary Tale

**Implementation**
- Evaluation

**Nurses in Communities, Public Health Policy, and Primary Prevention**
- Advocacy Tools of the Future

## QUESTIONS TO CONSIDER

After reading this chapter, you will know the answers to the following questions:

1. What is health policy and how is it related to the health care system?
2. What are the purposes of health policy?
3. How have health policies been developed from a historical perspective in the United States?
4. Why is health policy needed in the United States?
5. What is the policy-making process?

6. How can the tobacco control health issue be used to illustrate successful public health policy making?
7. How are policies developed and by whom?
8. How are policies evaluated in the United States?
9. Who are stakeholders and how do they influence policy development?
10. What is the role of community health nurses in the health policy-making process?

## KEY TERMS

Appropriations
Authorization
Bargaining
Collaboration
Cooperation

Fiscal policy
Health policy
Impacts
Organization policy
Outcomes

Outputs
Policy environment
Policy instruments
Public health prevention policies
Public policy

Rule making
Stakeholders
Strategic information

## Health Policy and Public Policy

To meet the social responsibility of the health professions to promote and maintain health in all segments of the population, our knowledge and skill must go beyond the biomedical and psychosocial aspects of health and illness. Today, nurses' competence requires understanding health policy—what it is and how it is made. This chapter provides an overview of health policy and its relationship to the public's health. It outlines policy-making activities and the governmental and other "players" (or stakeholders) that influence those processes. It is important for nursing as a profession and for those in practice to understand policy development in local, state, and national contexts to recognize when community health might be affected and to find ways to influence policies to promote and protect health. This awareness can guide nursing's contribution to policy action on behalf of people's health.

**Health policy** is public (governmental) policy that affects health and health care in national, state, and local arenas. It covers a broad range, including economic, housing, environmental, budgetary, and health services policy. Typically, the public, politicians, press, and professionals see health policy to include mainly those that finance and organize the delivery of personal health services; almost 13% of the U.S. gross domestic product—about $1.3 trillion per year—is devoted to supporting such services. However, much more than health services policy affects people's health (Lasker, 1997). Health is significantly related to income and other measures of socioeconomic status such as educational opportunities, affordable housing, investments in children's welfare, improvements in working conditions and benefits, and community support (Hatcher, 2003; Syme, Lefkowitz, & Krimgold, 2004; Sultz & Young, 2004).

Like all **public policy**, health policy is a guide to government action to alter what would otherwise occur, seeking more desirable or acceptable prospects. It points the way and enables effective action to coherent activity by public and private institutional systems. It is a decision about amounts and allocations (or distribution) of resources in organizations and governments.

The overall amount (i.e., the budget of governments or institutions) is a statement of commitment to a certain area of social or community or organizational relevance or concern, like health services or education. The distribution of that amount within the budget is a statement of the true priorities of the decision makers regardless of their statements about goals or mission. Together, the total amount and its allocation are called **fiscal policy**.

### ■ Goals and Policies

Goals, by themselves, are not policies. Although policies have goals, they are much more than that. For example, the goals of *Healthy People 2000* and *Healthy People 2010* were not policies because they had no instruments or resources specifically allocated to carry them out, other than having national health agencies monitor national progress toward the goals. The documents did not carry the force of law, which derives from one of the three constitutional sources of policy: Congress (legislation), the executive branch (the president's executive orders, which remain in force throughout his or her term of office and apply only to the executive branch), or independent regulatory agencies, created by Congress, having a specific jurisdiction, such as the U.S. Food and Drug Administration and the Environmental Protection Agency. None of these institutions is absolute; all are subject to constitutional checks and balances. The job of the courts is to interpret—not create—policy; however, in doing so, they inevitably influence policy, as do myriad organizations and groups in and outside government.

None of these three types of policy bodies at the national level, nor their counterparts in states and localities, is required to follow statements about national goals. Goals are useful as a framework and a source for policy ideas but are not in themselves sufficient for effective policy. They must first be fully formulated and adopted in legislation, executive order, or regulation, which are accompanied by the broad methods (or legal instruments discussed in the following) and authorized funds to carry them out. Otherwise, they remain at a voluntary level of action, dependent on the willingness of relevant groups to invest their own resources to follow them.

For example, by the late 1990s, states had adopted only some of the *Healthy People 2000* goals and were either unwilling or unable to track more than 40% of them, quite apart from authorizing funds to achieve them. In some states this monitoring capacity actually declined as a result of funding cutbacks. In addition, monies allocated to use the data often did not have high priority: Just 6 in 10 states included some environmental health objectives in their public health planning and fewer than 10 states provided air-quality data, taking more than 2 years to distribute it; fewer than half the states provided childhood poverty data and took more than 4 years to give it to local health departments; and fewer than 25 states collected data on injuries (Krieger, Chen, & Ebel, 1997; NACCHO, 1998; Public Health Foundation, 1998).

Although *Healthy People 2010* outlines 467 objectives in 28 focus areas, it has only two overarching goals: (1) to increase the number of years of healthy life and (2) to eliminate health disparities. However, *Healthy People 2010*, often called a road map for U.S. public health, is not supported by an effective or efficient public health infrastructure. The current public health system in the United States relies on a fragmented assortment of individual agencies, states, and communities to develop strategies for meeting the *Healthy People 2010* goals and to identify and provide the resources needed to accomplish them (Lurie, 2004).

The clearest and most accurate sign or indicator to determine whether actual policy change has occurred in any governmental body or other organization—health center, school, home care agency—is a change in the size and/or allocation of its resources: money, the authority and responsibilities vested in certain positions (e.g., staff nurses), and other resources. When organizations, as a result of policy changes, conduct their services differently, as staff do things differently, consumers can also behave differently: Patterns change. **Organization policy** is that of a single organization or a type of organization (e.g., public schools), either public (e.g., health department) or private (e.g., churches or child care centers or corporations), and it is closely tied to governmental policy changes.

## Purpose of Public Policy

The purpose of policy making is to shape the direction and pace of change in a preferred direction by modifying current patterns of action. It is not to change the behavior of every individual, each of whom is free to follow a policy or not, perhaps with possible personal consequences, such as refusing a vaccine or driving faster than the speed limit at the risk of injury or fine.

Rather, the aim of policy making is to change the decisions of organizations about their use of resources. This, in turn, changes the activities of managers and staff, clients, and customers from former patterns toward new patterns in governmental agencies, nonprofit organizations, and commercial organizations, whether construction firms, restaurants, regulatory agencies, schools, or clinics. A school board policy requiring the availability of healthy foods in cafeterias will change the types of foods that schools buy, the menus and methods of preparation used by kitchen staff, and the pattern of foods that students and teachers will eat, thereby promoting health.

## Choosing Policies

To address any health problem, there are always several choices (including doing nothing). We know, for example, that about 310,000 mostly low-income children aged 1–5 years in the United States have health-damaging blood levels of lead, mainly from exposure to lead-based paint in old houses and environmental contamination. The problem is three times worse in African American children, even when they are not living in old housing and are not in the lowest income bracket, indicating discrimination in the choice of neighborhoods available to some African American families (GAO, 1998; CDC, 2007). Here are the policy choices:

- Health care systems can conduct outreach, screening, and treatment.
- Community coalitions can form to conduct outreach, screening, and treatment.
- State Medicaid agencies can require Medicaid contractors to provide and report on these services for their enrollees.

These policy changes—with their goals, means, and accompanying shift in budget and program resources—would result in secondary prevention—that is, finding and treating the health problem after it exists, whether or not

| Intervention Strategy | Focus |
|---|---|
| Individual-directed, information-mediated change | • Homes and communities (e.g., computers, TV campaigns, health fairs)<br>• Organization settings (e.g., counseling; computers; small-group training of patients, clients, customers, health care practitioners, librarians, teachers, clergy) |
| Organization-directed change | • Policy bodies:<br>  – Congress, legislatures<br>  – Independent regulatory agencies<br>  – Government administration (e.g., executive orders, rule making)<br><br>• Specific organizations:<br>  – Government organizations (e.g., health departments, housing, schools)<br>  – Nongovernment organizations (e.g., managed care organizations, community health centers, companies, retailers) |

Strategies for prevention and health promotion basically aim at either (1) changing individuals' behavior or physical condition through information/education or clinical means (or changing individual practitioners) or (2) changing the decisions of organizations about their use of resources through policy efforts. This, in turn, changes the activities of managers, staff, clients, and customers in policy and service organizations in the public and private sectors.

*We all declare for liberty; but in using the same word, we do not all mean the same thing. With some the word 'liberty' may mean for each man to do as he pleases with himself, and the product of his labor; while with others the same may mean for some men to do as they please with other men, and the product of other men's labor. Here are two, not only different, but incompatible things, called by the same name—liberty.*

—*Abraham Lincoln*

 ENVIRONMENTAL CONNECTION

How has the American with Disabilities Act (ADA) changed the work environment for people with disabilities? How has it changed the work environment for people without disabilities?

overt symptoms are evident. This is basically an individual and clinical perspective.

To adopt a public health, population-oriented, primary preventive policy approach—to prevent the problem before it begins—additional choices are possible:

- Require lead paint removal and environmental code enforcement after providing information to landlords, polluting organizations, tenants, and homeowners
- Develop safe, affordable housing
- Provide for safe and effective schools and schooling, including job training and jobs development
- Work for procommunity/antidiscrimination changes

All this effort would require entry by health proponents into the complex and long-term processes that result in organizational and public policy change. Policy does not just happen. It is determined by organized groups in and outside government and, therefore, can be observed, analyzed, and understood well enough to promote health-supporting development. Policy-making processes shape policy content as groups that are affected by them (stakeholders) attempt to influence policy development to favor their own needs and priorities. See Box 9-1 for a partial list of stakeholders in health care policy decisions.

The results often have indirect or direct impact on population health. Indirect effects include access to the conditions for healthful living, such as housing, jobs, information and education, health care, protective environments, tax equity, and civil rights (Milio, 1997; Syme, Lefkowitz, & Krimgold, 2004; Hatcher, 2003). The coalition of environmental health organizations, for example, worked to influence Congress in the 1970s to pass historic laws protecting air, water, and habitats. The laws have been effective in directly improving the health of millions of Americans and indirectly affecting health by preserving the viability of agricultural land needed for sustaining food and nutrition for future generations.

*There is nothing more difficult to plan, more doubtful to success, nor more dangerous to manage than the creation of a new system.*

—*Machiavelli, The Prince, 1512*

---

### BOX 9-1

**Major Stakeholders in U.S Health Policy**

- The public (health consumers—which include patients, families, and consumer organizations such as the American Association of Retired Persons, the American Cancer Society, the American Heart Association, labor organizations, etc.)
- Employers (public and private employers and employer organizations representing small and large businesses)
- Providers (physicians, dentists, nurses, nurse practitioners, physician assistants, pharmacists, podiatrists, chiropractors, and allied health professionals)
- Hospitals (general, specialty, teaching, rural, profit or non-profit, independent, or multifacility systems)
- Alternative therapy organizations (providers of alternative health interventions such as rolfing, yoga, spiritual healing, relaxation techniques, herbal remedies, energy healing, megavitamin therapy, acupuncture, acupressure, and massage therapy)
- Insurance industry (managed care organizations, Blue Cross/Blue Shield, and other private insurance companies)
- Long-term care (nursing homes, home health agencies, rehabilitation facilities, etc.)
- Mental health (psychiatric hospitals, community mental health facilities, and many community-based ambulatory care services)
- Voluntary facilities and agencies (HIV/AIDS support groups; addiction support groups such as Alcoholics Anonymous, Narcotics Anonymous, Overeaters Anonymous; and public education and lobbying groups such as Mothers Against Drunk Driving)
- Health professions education and training institutions (schools of public health, medicine, nursing, dentistry, allied health, pharmacy, optometry, etc.)
- Professional associations (national, state, and regional organizations representing health care professionals or institutions such as the American Nurses Association, the American Medical Association, the American Public Health Association, and the American Hospital Association)
- Others health industry organizations (pharmaceutical companies, medical supply and equipment companies, and information and management system suppliers)
- Research communities (educational institutions, government agencies such as National Institutes of Health or the Agency for Healthcare Research, and not-for-profit foundations such as the Pew Charitable Trusts, The Robert Wood Johnson Foundation, and the Bill and Melinda Gates Foundation)

*Source:* Sultz & Young, 2004

---

### History of Health Policy in the United States

Historically, the United States has enacted broader health policies than those in recent years. During much of the 1990s, health policy had been viewed narrowly, focusing on health services delivery and the economics of it, while weakening environmental health, healthful living conditions, and primary public health prevention legislation (Center for the Future of Children, 1997; DHHS, 1995; Wakefield, Gardner, & Guillett, 2002).

**❝** *The master of every ship of the United States arriving from a foreign port . . . shall pay . . . twenty cents per month for every seaman employed . . . to provide for . . . the sick or disabled seamen in [government] hospitals . . . now established in the several ports.* **❞**

—*The U.S. Fifth Congress, July 16, 1798*

Some of the major steps in health policy since the start of the nation include the first national health service and national health insurance program set up before the end of the eighteenth century. This was, and in modified form continues to be, a system of government health care paid by private employer insurance for the U.S. Merchant Marine. A larger and fully tax-supported national health service is the one provided to Congress and the president, the only fully socialized medical system in the United States today. These are national governmental health care systems that are available to everyone in special groups. Most advanced countries have national systems available to their entire population, including immigrants.

Constitutional provisions in our national and state governments to protect the health, safety, and welfare of people authorize, but do not require, governments to use legal tools to realize these purposes. For example, if health were part the Bill of Rights, governments would be legally required—would be liable—early to protect health.

Other early national health policies include the Pure Food and Drug Act (1906); Social Security Act and its income support for the poor, blind, disabled, and elders and health services for mothers and children (1935); and the first environmental law, the Water Pollution Control Act of 1948. The Economic Opportunity Act was to develop poor communities and end poverty (1964); the National School Lunch and Child Nutrition Amendments included the Women, Infants, and Children's Supplemental Food Program (WIC) (1972) (Weissert & Weissert, 1996). See Box 9-2 for a partial list of health legislation that has been passed.

### 🖥 Research Alert

This study analyzed the ethical, public policy, and educational issues that arise in the United States and United Kingdom when genomic information acquired as a result of genetic testing is introduced into health care services. The research findings concluded that individual, family, and societal issues may conflict with current health care practices and policies when genetic testing is done but current health policies do not fully address these concerns. In addition, health care providers, including nurses, are not fully prepared to incorporate genetic testing into their practice.

*Source*: Williams, J., Skirton, H., & Masny, A. (2006). Ethics, policy, and educational issues in genetic testing. *Journal of Nursing Scholarship, 38*(2), 119–125.

---

### BOX 9-2

**Selected History of Important Federal Health Legislation**
- Pure Food and Drug Act, 1906
- Maternity and Infancy Act, 1921
- Social Security Act, 1935
- Nurse Training Act, 1941
- Public Health Services Act, 1944
- Hospital Survey and Construction Act (Hill–Burton Act), 1946
- Federal Employee Health Benefits Act, 1959
- Health Professions Educational Assistance Act, 1963
- Older Americans Act, 1965
- Highway Safety Act, 1966
- Child Nutrition Act, 1966
- National Environmental Policy Act, 1969
- Comprehensive Drug Abuse Prevention and Control Act, 1970
- Occupational Health and Safety Act, 1970
- Consumer Product Safety Act, 1972
- Toxic Substances Control Act, 1976
- Rural Health Clinics Act, 1977
- Comprehensive Smoking Education Act, 1984
- Emergency Medical Treatment and Active Labor Act, 1986
- Omnibus Health Act (Medicaid expansions) 1986
- Americans with Disabilities Act, 1990
- Preventive Health Amendments Act, 1992
- Health Center Consolidation Act, 1996
- Health Insurance Portability and Accountability Act, 1996
- Child Abuse and Prevention Treatment Act, 2003
- Medicare Prescription Drug Improvement and Modernization Act, 2003
- Combating Autism Act, 2006

### ■ Present Need for Public Health Policy

Although overall U.S. death rates are declining, continuing gaps in health between disadvantaged and other populations are increasing in many respects. In addition, disability from chronic illness is widespread (Cutler & Sheiner, 1999; Wakefield, Gardner, & Guillett, 2002). Health inequalities in morbidity, mortality, and disability are strongly related to poverty and income inequality. Gaps in health between low- and high-income groups are expected to increase further as wealth inequalities continue to grow (Kaplan, 1996; Montgomery, Kiely, & Pappas, 1996; Hatcher, 2003).

Widening health gaps are not accounted for by biomedical and behavioral risk factors alone. Rather, they are affected by a complex web of linked living standards as experienced in jobs and workplaces, homes, and communities. In turn, these are related to how supportive public policies are in these sectors (Hatcher, 2003; Syme, Lefkowitz, & Krimgold, 2004). Virtually all measures of health and illness are worse among poor people compared with their better-off counterparts, regardless of ethnicity, gender, or age. Because of the breadth of the determinants of health, much has been written about the need for broad social and economic policies to promote health.

Evidence shows that public health–oriented public policies make a difference. For example, Social Security retirement income has been the single most important policy to reduce poverty in the United States, especially among elders, thereby contributing to healthful living standards for millions of people. In recent years, a special tax credit for full-time working parents was supposed to be an important policy to prevent several million children from living in poverty (National Center for Children in Poverty, 1998). The federal child and dependent care tax credit reduces the amount of taxes working families with child care expenses must pay. All families at all income levels are eligible for the tax credit (NCCP, 2007).

Despite this, the tax credit was not enough to prevent an overall increase in child poverty since the 1980s because of low-wage jobs and national and state policies that cut back resources available to poor families. In addition, the credit is nonrefundable, limiting its value to low-income families. The credit cannot exceed the taxes that a family owes, and no benefit is provided for families who do not pay taxes because their income is too low. A single-parent family with two children is not required to pay taxes if their income is below $15,000 per year. To be eligible for the tax credit, a family must be responsible for paying expenses related to the care of children under the age of 13 (or older dependents who are not able to care for themselves) that occur while the parents or legal guardians are working or looking for work. In 2004, tax-paying families with two or more children could claim up to $6,000 in annual child care expenses, and families with one child could claim up to $3,000. The credit equals 20% to 35% of the amount claimed, which provided a maximum tax credit of $2,100 for families with two or more children (NCCP, 2007).

The fact remains that 28 million children in the United States are growing up in low-income families. More than 80% of these children have at least one working parent whose income is not sufficient to support the family. In most cases, it is not until a family of four reaches an income level of $40,000 per year (twice the federal poverty level) that parents are able to provide their children with the basic necessities, such as food, housing, and health care (NCCP, 2007).

## Public Health and Public Policy

Public health is a governmental (public) responsibility embodied in federal and state agencies, including the national Centers for Disease Control and Prevention, the Environmental Protection Agency, and state and local health departments. They are, in principle, accountable for the health of all the people, extending beyond the health of particular individuals, as is done in personal health services.

Public health policy involves promoting and protecting health, preventing disease, and preserving life through policies that ensure the determinants of health for all segments of the population (Rose, 1985, 1990). When it is effective, it makes healthy choices equitably available to all groups—

about where to live, work, learn, obtain needed services and information, and participate in public life in safe, supportive, and sustainable environments.

In the words of the Institute of Medicine (1988):
[The mission of public health is] . . . fulfilling society's interest in assuring conditions in which people can be healthy . . . to generate organized community efforts to address the public interest in health by applying scientific and technical knowledge to prevent disease and promote health. . . . [It] is addressed by private organizations, but the governmental public health agency has a unique function: to see to it that vital elements are in place and that the mission is adequately addressed.

This echoes the historic understanding of the public health mission:
Public health is the science and art of preventing disease, prolonging life and promoting health . . . through organizing community efforts for sanitation of the environment, the control of communicable infections, the education of the individual in personal hygiene, the organization of medical and nursing services for the early diagnosis and preventive treatment of disease, and the development of the social machinery to ensure everyone a standard of living adequate for the maintenance of health, so organizing these benefits as to enable every citizen to realize his [sic] birthright of health and longevity. (Winslow, 1920)

This public health enterprise, undertaken by government agencies and other allied groups, ranging from local health centers to national voluntary organizations like the American Health Association and public-interest groups such as Handgun Control, Inc., requires organizational and organized action directed toward all types of entities, including policy bodies and the public. This historic approach of public health during most of its first century resulted in major successes, such as regulating sewage, water supplies, and housing conditions, decades before vaccines were discovered (Institute of Medicine, 1988).

As illustrated earlier, policies change organizations (and their resource allocations and programs) so that populations can have more healthful choices about where and how to live. Examples of **public health prevention policies** include tobacco control—for example, higher cigarette taxes of 50 cents in Oregon reduced smoking by 18% in youth; communicable disease prevention, as when public and private provider subsidies produced large increases in immunization

### ENVIRONMENTAL CONNECTION

The banning of trans fats for New York City restaurants became effective in 2006. Do you support such a policy? Why or why not? How far can government policies go before the infringement of individual freedom of choice conflicts with our basic political values?

rates, especially among poor and minority children; abortion funding for poor women, which resulted in an increase in early prenatal care, fewer teen births, and lower rates of low-birth-weight babies and infant death; and containment of alcohol liberalization, handgun controls, and motorcycle safety measures, all of which achieved widespread long-term health benefits (Center for Health Economics Research, 1993; Kraus, Peek, & Williams, 1995; National Cancer Institute, 1991; Office of Disease Prevention, 1993; Pentz et al., 1989; Teh-Wei, Hai-Yen, & Keeler, 1995).

 ETHICAL CONNECTION

"There are two levers to set a man in motion, fear and self-interest."

Napoleon Bonaparte, 1769–1821,
French general and emperor

How does this quote relate to health policy? Is the fear of sickness and/or death related to national health policies on organ donation or cloning? How?

## Policy Development

What follows is first an overview of the policy-making process and then an illustration of each step in policy development.

### Policy Environment

Policy development does not occur on a clean slate. It always has precursors in earlier eras, deriving from experience with similar issues and societal assumptions about the role of government (Laumann & Knoke, 1987). Most importantly, it is formed in a context of near-term limiting and enabling circumstances. These are important to be aware of to plan effective strategies to influence policy making.

The following figure depicts the connections between policy making and health (Milio, 1976, 1986, 2000). It shows how policy works through organizational action, which shapes community environments, living patterns, and ultimately population health. This occurs in a **policy environment** or context that encompasses circumstances affecting whether and how policy making proceeds, regardless of the type of policy in question. Important factors include the demographic and epidemiological nature of the population (e.g., an aging population, high rates of smoking), the economy and technology (e.g., inflation, unemployment, extent of information technology), the socioeconomic and ethnic makeup of communities (e.g., poverty and discrimination), the distribution of resources (e.g., homelessness and extremes in wealth), political party agendas, organizational hierarchies (e.g., dominant interest groups), and even sudden disasters—national emergencies from weather or war, for example, can stop all policy development as policy mak-

U.S. Senate Building.

ers attend to (costly) emergency measures. All these things must be considered to some extent by policy participants. All this information is available and needed for effective policy work by interested nurses and is best done on an organized and thought-out basis.

Yet, however rapidly changing and uncertain the environment is, the policy-making time clock is ticking, and the electoral calendar moves on. To be effective, policy action and influence must be exerted in time and be timely, in tune with the environment.

The media are in a unique position among organizations; they are not only channels for information. They also create and shape issues (Minkler, 2004; Horton, 2006; Mason, Dodd, & Glickstein, 2006), such as portraying teen violence as a parental problem rather than a public health problem that can be effectively addressed by, among other things, elimination of handguns. For example, Japan, where handguns are banned, had two handgun killings in 1997, whereas the United States had 9,400 and Canada had 100. Media portrayals set up ideas and expectations about the kinds of solutions needed to address problems (Amundson, Lichter, & Lichter, 2005; Mason, Dodd, & Glickstein, 2006; Bomlitz & Brezis, 2008).

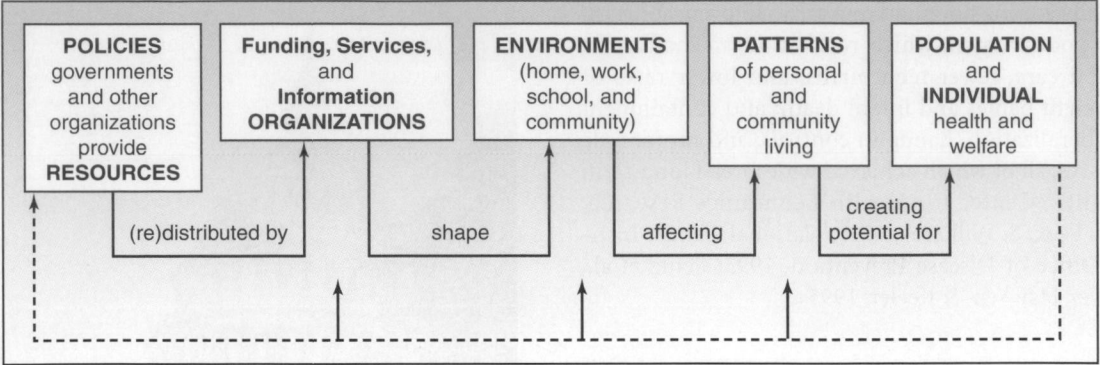

Depiction of the connections between policy making and health. Policy works through organizational action, which shapes community environments, affecting living patterns and ultimately population health. The changes that result in all these areas then feed back (*dotted lines*) and are taken into account in ongoing efforts to find acceptable and effective ways to deal with public health problems.

As global, profit-making corporations, the media seek to attract audiences and advertisers and often shape programming with this aim—news and weather have become "infotainment" rather than accurate and sometimes unpleasant depictions of complex realities (Cappela & Jamieson, 1996). Other players in the policy arena actively attempt to use the media for strategic purposes. Organized interest groups can indirectly reach policy makers and the public through the mass media (Columbia Institute, 1995; Mason, Dodd, & Glickstein, 2002).

The public in this framework consists of several populations that are affected by policy makers' decisions, such as audiences, voters, taxpayers, consumers, and donors to parties and interest groups. Policy choices set the parameters for health in the form of access to services, products, processes,

> **"** *Will Gresham's law operate in the broadcasting and political worlds, wherein the bad inevitably drives out the good? Will the politician's desire for reelection—and the broadcaster's desire for ratings—cause both to flatter every public whim and prejudice—to seek the lowest common denominator of appeal—to put public opinion at all times ahead of the public interest?* **"**
>
> —John F. Kennedy, 1960

prices, taxes, and information. Most of the public are not active members of interest groups. Through these complex processes, then, ongoing outcomes of policy making create the conditions for the health of populations, especially of disadvantaged subgroups.

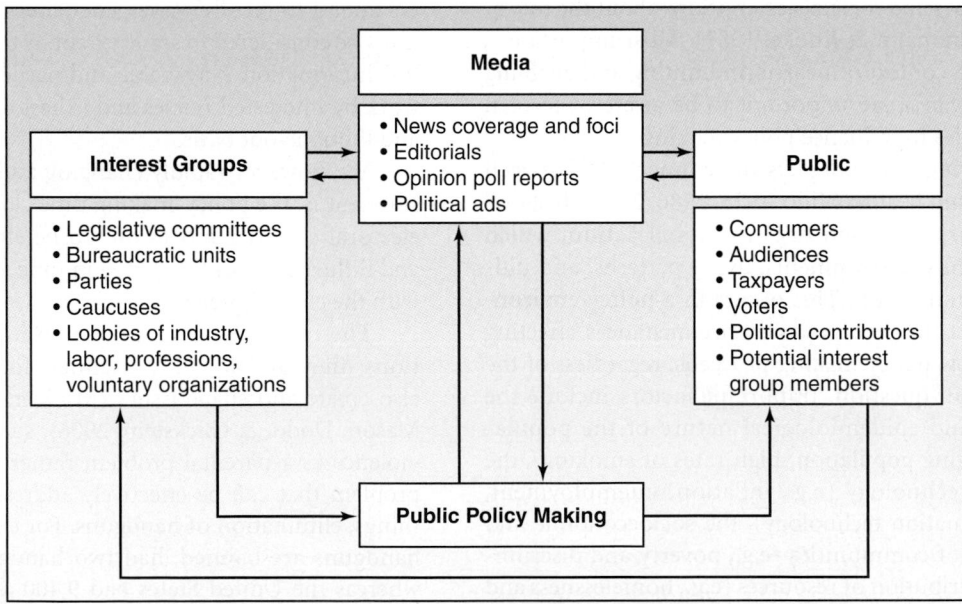

The media are not only channels for information; they also create and shape issues. Media portrayals set up ideas and expectations about the kinds of solutions needed to address problems. Other players in the policy arena actively attempt to use the media for strategic purposes. Organized interest groups within and outside government can indirectly reach policy makers and the public through the mass media. The "public" is actually several populations that are affected by policy makers' decisions, such as audiences, voters, taxpayers, consumers, and donors to parties and interest groups.

## Public Health Advocacy and Action

### The Case of Tobacco Control: A Success Story

Antismoking policy development in the United States in the 1980s and 1990s offers many lessons in public health policy making (Heiser & Begay, 1997; Jacobson, Wasserman, & Raube, 1993). Some states passed strong laws (e.g., widespread bans on smoking in public places and private work sites and large penalties), whereas others enacted weaker legislation (e.g., narrow restrictions, smokers' rights clauses, minor penalties). More effective policy making involved legislative leadership, strong coalitions, and support by top public health and government officials.

### Environmental Context

In the antitobacco case, the policy environment includes the shrinking of the U.S. tobacco market and costly legal challenges facing the tobacco industry. This impelled cigarette manufacturers to seek overseas markets, facilitated by liberal world trade policies. This offshore shift of production and marketing is weakening the once-firm alliance between cigarette manufacturers and tobacco farmers. The number of growers is shrinking, resulting in a less influential political constituency. These and other aspects of the environment make the industry increasingly vulnerable and present an opening for action by health advocates.

Successful policy-making activity must propose policies that fit the circumstances of the day. Thus, health proponents must be aware of current and changing circumstances (Rochefort & Cobb, 1993; Milio, 2002).

## Policy Shape and Setting

Health-supporting policy action also depends on how the policy issue is framed. For example, the tobacco-control issue could be framed by public health advocates in the health field and allied groups as an environmental and child health issue, or by protobacco groups as one of smokers' right to take personal risks in using a legal product. The policy outcome could be very different depending on who defines the problem (Milio, 2002).

The policy arena—that is, where the action takes place—in local, state, or national jurisdictions, is another consideration. Successful tobacco control advocates used the open arenas of legislatures or the public referendum process and sought news media coverage to amplify their position in contrast to the highly paid, behind-the-scenes activities and television advertising of the industry.

For example, for some antitobacco campaigns, local ordinances rather than state law may be more readily enacted, despite the narrower public health impact at local levels. Sufficient community-level action can be a learning laboratory and can create political conditions for stronger statewide policies. Nurses, as members of health or other groups, have been and can continue to be part of any or all such efforts.

## Policy Goals, Tools, and Resources

The design of an effective policy includes goals and the means to reach those goals. The goals should eventually be specified as measurable objectives to help focus activity and track progress. The strength (or absence) of means is important for the forward movement and implementation of a policy. Without measurable objectives, progress toward health goals becomes contentious; without sound means and resources, little program action is likely to occur.

Policy effectiveness depends on adequate financing and the choice of legislative tools used. The means to achieve policy goals involve a limited list of **policy instruments** (legal tools) that are used by most governments. These tools include economic incentives (e.g., tax breaks, subsidies) to businesses, governments, and taxpayers; mandates and regulation; and the development and provision of information, education, training, and services. Others are modeling—that

## MEDIA MOMENT

### *Sicko* (2007)

Documentary film maker Michael Moore was nominated for an Academy Award for this film in 2008. It is a raw, unflinching look at the U.S. health care system, told through the voices of everyday people faced with extraordinary and bizarre challenges in their quest for basic health coverage. Profiles of these patients whose lives have been disrupted and shattered by a health catastrophe and resulting economic and social losses are presented with sensitivity and even humor. Moore does a comprehensive job of reviewing the historical evolution of the U.S. health care system. Moore quickly moves to the health care systems of Canada, Cuba, Great Britain, and France, providing a realist and balanced examination of these systems as compared to the United States. The film ends with an emotional gathering of rescue workers from 9/11 who have been denied medical treatment and yet remain hopeful in their unusual acts of diplomacy and compassion. This is a movie that everyone who works in the health care system should see and discuss!

is, becoming exemplars (e.g., not allowing smoking in government facilities)—and market power or market management (Kessler et al., 1996).

Tools, such as market management or market power, are used when, for example, governments buy public employee health insurance plans that cover only smoking cessation programs and collaborate with public health organizations in passing clean indoor air laws (Sofaer et al., 1997). When governments buy only recycled paper or healthy foods, the market price is often lowered for everyone.

Some of these tools are clearly more powerful than others in their potential effectiveness. For example, economic and regulatory instruments are more effective than information and education to ensure healthful changes in organizations and individuals: Smoking rates drop faster with a high tobacco tax and no-public-smoking rules than with sharing of information on health effects alone, especially among teens. However, the more effective means are the most difficult to get adopted because they have a higher political cost—that is, it is riskier to offend commercial groups by using economic instruments such as a tobacco tax increase than to simply inform the public of health risks through warning labels on cigarettes. This was clear in tobacco-control cases.

### ■ The Players as Stakeholders

Policies develop through the actions of the players and their relationships as they try to shape decisions about who pays and who gets what of the determinants of health. The players are the organized groups—**stakeholders**—whose interests are affected by current and prospective policies. They include political parties, the media, bureaucracies, voluntary and commercial organizations, public-interest groups, and professional associations.

A policy issue draws the attention of public and private stakeholders who view a policy change as important to their interests. These stakeholders perceive themselves to be importantly affected by a change in policy. Their interests are the things they need to survive, including finances (from grants, contracts, dues, or sales), facilities, staff, authority, control, status, legitimacy, and image. In turn, these resources affect

## GLOBAL CONNECTION

How do U.S. health policies—for example, policies about smoking restrictions—affect global health?

a group's bargaining power. Stakeholders include elected or other officials, legislative committees, parties, and bureaus; commercial, scientific, and medical groups; and voluntary nonprofit organizations, including public interest groups (DiMaggio & Anheier, 1990; Feldstein, 1996; Jasanoff, 1993; Nathanson, 2005; Rice, 2002; Warner, 1991).

The underlying interest of political and other governmental leaders is to retain power and authority. For businesses, increased profits and market share are important. Professionals want to acquire grants, higher career status, and control over their practice. Voluntary organizations must please their boards and donors; advocacy groups must satisfy their supporters (e.g., governing board, funders, membership), both existing and potential. Each group attempts to engage in political activity in ways that will shape any particular policy to favor its own interests (Benjamin, Perfetto, & Greene, 1995; Nathanson, 2005; Rice, 2002).

In the case of tobacco policy, the involvement of major health-related organizations illustrates these self-regarding calculations and accounts for their sometimes sideline roles in the policy-making process. Neither state health departments, public health associations, medical societies, nor large voluntary organizations did more than lend their names to the antitobacco coalitions that were fighting for strong tobacco-control legislation. Each of these mainline organizations had competing priorities, such as fears of budget cuts from opposition lawmakers, lack of staff, or legal restrictions in some local health departments. The medical societies chose to use their political capital to seek better clinical payment rates, and the large nonprofit groups feared a backlash from some donors. These organizational decisions about public health advocacy were strategic choices made by each organization that took into account the tradeoffs in resources for the group and its purposes. In one state, "risk protection"

> **❝** *Each of us must choose whether to live our lives narrowly, selfishly and complacently or to act with courage and faith. We are not governed by fate or mysterious forces of history. It is the sum of our choices that will determine the kind of America and the kind of world in which we live.* **❞**
>
> —Madeleine Albright, U.S. Secretary of State, George Washington University Commencement, May 21, 2000

> **❝** *The most impressive aspect of the law of the jungle is not ruthless competition and destruction, but rather interdependence and coexistence.* **❞**
>
> —Rene Dubos, Man, Medicine, and Environment, 1968

was required before a state chapter of the American Cancer Society publicly agreed to lead a tobacco taxation campaign (Heiser & Begay, 1997).

## ■ Player Connections

Alliances are more reliable and long-lasting when they are based on written agreements, agreed rules, or intense resource exchange. **Collaboration** differs from **cooperation** by the exchange of tangible assets (e.g., part-time staff or use of printing equipment in the former, as contrasted with the verbal support and good will in cooperative ties). For example, the California Nurses Association gained much more public support than it could have otherwise in a recent referendum on state health care reform by allying with labor unions and others and sharing staff.

To influence decision makers in the face of competition by well-financed, large-scale commercial interests, as in tobacco control, requires strategic planning, continuous management, and joint efforts, despite the difficulties of coalition formation (Heiser & Begay, 1997; Kegler, 1995; Nathanson, 2005; Rice, 2002).

## Information for Action

Information is basic to policy making. It is used to monitor, analyze, evaluate, report, and critique an issue. It becomes action-oriented when used for informing, educating, persuading, mediating, activating, or mobilizing others to act (Lindblom & Cohen, 1979; Ray & Roberts, 2002).

The strategic problem for proponents of health-supporting policy is to use selected types of information to convince target groups that their policy position is economically feasible (to its supporters and users), politically acceptable (to the more powerful groups affected by it), socially approved within the milieu in which it is to operate, and administratively and technologically possible (Milio, 2000; Ray & Roberts, 2002). To do this, a wide range of **strategic information** is needed—about the policy environment and the problem, as well as the purposes, interests, and tactics of the players, and the degree of support among constituencies, as gauged by polls and endorsements. This must be sought

and developed by policy proponents, thus the need for an organized and sustained effort.

Studies can stimulate new ways to conceive policy problems and solutions and occasionally are directly incorporated into policy development, such as the knowledge that high tobacco taxes are the most effective way of reducing smoking in young people (Beyer & Trice, 1982; Brewer & De Leon, 1983; Brint, 1990; Webber, 1987). "Research that demonstrates that a course of action being contemplated by policymakers may (or may not) lead to undesirable or unexpected consequences can contribute significantly to policymaking" (Shi & Singh, 2008, pp. 554–555).

This wide array of information goes far beyond typical health status data and includes a variety of material available from all the social–political–economic disciplines and policy think tanks (institutes and centers). This information is often available on the Internet. The task, then, is to effectively use that information to influence policy making in language, formats, and amounts that are suited to each target group, including the press and the public.

 **Got an Alternative?**

Should regulation of herbal therapies be the responsibility of the U.S. Food and Drug Administration? What are advantages and possible negative consequences of regulating this type of nontraditional treatment?

> **❝** *Scientists are in general remarkably objective in reporting what they observe and measure; but the selection of their objects of study is profoundly influenced by the social environment in which they work and by the spirit of the age.* **❞**
>
> —Rene Dubos, Man, Medicine, and Environment, 1968

## Policy Development Strategies

The most effective policy-making activities, demanding the most resources, include lobbying legislative or bureaucratic policy makers directly or through their constituents; ensuring the election or appointment of supportive political leaders; and engaging in litigation. Less effective means, often used by small groups, involve developing publicity through the media and organizing demonstrations, conferences, and public education programs (Walker, 1991; Nathanson, 2005). All such activities have long been on the agendas of national, state, and, to some extent, local nursing organizations. Their voice is always stronger when allied with other groups, as occurred in the national health care reform effort of 1993–1994.

## ■ Bargaining

The central strategic activity to influence policies and move them through the phases of policy making is negotiation. This process always involves compromise. Effective

Nurses and other lobbying groups work to influence health policy through legislation.

**bargaining** requires taking account of the interests of governments and other target groups and being willing to trade away some less valued interests to gain others in the foreseeable future, such as agreeing to a 50-cent tobacco tax instead of a dollar so that political support for adoption is easier to gain.

Public distortion of facts by opponents requires prompt public rebuttal by health proponents, as when tobacco proponents maintained that there is no scientific proof of the health effects of smoking (Heiser & Begay, 1997). By contrast, to obtain political and organizational endorsement, proponents must demonstrate the political support needed by elected and bureaucratic officials—for example, by providing credible evidence of support from opinion polls and sponsorship by local groups and agencies. This involves developing information on group support for proponents' policy preferences or offering a promise by coalition members of future support for the policy maker's agenda.

### ■ Information Through the Mass Media

People's information is obtained directly from experience or through various interpersonal and technological channels. All such conduits select and shape the informa-

tion they pass on according to their own priorities (Minkler, 1997). The new media mix includes TV networks, cable, satellite, talk radio, DVDs, videos, CD-ROMs, as well as the print press, all merging on the Internet. This rapidly expanding web has implications for both policy development activities and health information/education. The interplay between information and media in policy-making arenas is another important facet that can be used to promote public policy for health (Mason, Dodd, & Glickstein, 2002).

Mass media affect policy making in many ways. They convey information and messages that influence perspectives and actions, depending on when, how, and in what social and information contexts they are received. These messages flow not only through news channels, but also through programming, videos, DVDs, talk shows, and advertising, by both expression and exclusion (Cappella & Jamieson, 1996; Mason, Dodd, & Glickstein, 2002).

The media set the agenda, telling people which issues are important to think and talk about. They also frame or focus certain aspects of issues, helping shape how people and policy makers understand them. This is especially true for the formation of short-term public opinion about public health issues, such as environmental pollution and poverty. The way in which current issues are presented on weekly television comedy and drama show can greatly influence the public's view point about even the most controversial political issues (Mason, Dodd, & Glickstein, 2002).

As commercial organizations, the media depend on advertisers. They select content and target audiences to attract viewers for their sponsors. Larger audiences mean higher prices for advertising and higher revenues. Prime-time news media focus on mainstream issues, as when they took 4 years before covering HIV/AIDS, believing that it was a minor problem of interest only to homosexuals and intravenous drug users but not to a large general audience (Edgar et al., 1992).

The media in this way reinforce mainstream views and set expectations about reality, including racial and gender stereotypes. For example, heavy viewers—those who watch more television (or videos) daily than others (more than 4 hours)—are more likely to overestimate the prevalence of divorce, illegitimacy, abortions, STDs, and crime (Edgar et al., 1992). This perception clearly has implications for the kinds of demands the public makes (or indicates in polls) for public policy action.

❝*Where is the wisdom we have lost in knowledge? Where is the knowledge we have lost in information?*❞

—T. S. Eliot, The Rock

### ■ Health Information

Education and information are part of the package of useful policy tools and are longer lasting when accompanied by other stronger tools. Public health media campaigns are usually limited to attempts to influence *individual* behavior rather than to mold public opinion about policy issues. As

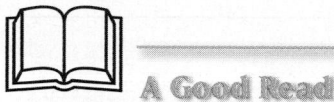

# Critical Condition: How Health Care in America Became Big Business—and Bad Medicine (2004)

*By Donald L. Barlett & James B. Steele, New York: Doubleday Publishers.*

Journalists Barlett and Steele have written a highly critical and well-documented text about the failure of the U.S. health care system today. They provide support through an examination of the U.S. health care system with other Western industrialized countries, from mortality rates to per capita income spending. Case histories of patients who reveal the gaps in insurance and government health care coverage are presented. The authors claim that health care first became driven by profits and policy at the federal level during the Reagan administration. Competing insurance plans, they contend, led not to better choices for health care consumers but to physicians who are prevented by insurers from prescribing needed treatments, a severe shortage of nurses, and unsafe hospital environments have resulted from these cost-cutting measures and policies. The authors, who strongly advocate a single-payer plan, depict a health care system in a state of near collapse.

costly as they are, however, these health education campaigns by themselves mainly affect knowledge or awareness, and only occasionally do they influence short-term behavior (Office of Technology Assessment, 1991; Rice & Atkin, 1994).

Several conditions must be in place to translate awareness of a health problem into changes in personal behavior, especially for the long term. The message must have the following characteristics:

- Targeted and attractive for specific groups
- Conveyed over multiple channels long enough for "saturation" of the target groups
- Integrated with local interpersonal communication
- Supported by environmental, organizational, and policy changes to ensure long-term behavior change, such as increases in tobacco tax and laws against smoking in public places

## ■ Mass Media and the Case of Health Care Reform: A Cautionary Tale

Policy issues raised in the mass media can have adverse public health policy effects. Issues are often defined too simply, solutions described too superficially, and legitimacy conferred on only selected groups because of what "sells" to audiences and advertisers. This in itself suggests the need for greater attention to the electronic world by the public health community as the experience of health care reform portrays.

A series of studies covering the introduction and failure of the Clinton health care plan from September 1993 to July 1994 demonstrate how mass media are woven into policy-making processes and show how important it is to take the media into account in health policy development (Braun, 1995; Cappela & Jamieson, 1994; Cappella & Jamieson, 1996; Columbia Institute, 1995). Findings show the following:

- Although the media devoted much time and space to health care reform, two thirds of all coverage was on political strategy, not content; the pros and cons of each major proposal or areas of agreement.
- Coverage was not balanced, giving more attention to the president's plan while others, like the single-payer bill, had no real public airing. Without public knowledge about options, there was little likelihood of support for a compromise bill.
- The tone of the stories was that politicians act out of self-interest rather than commitment to the public good. Randomized viewer studies showed that strategy-based (versus issue-centered) stories created perceptions of policy makers as posturing, deceptive, self-interested, and unconcerned with the welfare of citizens. Groups viewing only issue-centered stories were less cynical.
- News coverage of political advertising, by emphasizing the attack and controversial nature of the ads, dramatically enlarged the ads' audiences and collectively aired an additional 15 minutes of free nationwide television exposure. The ads' sponsors then had incentive to prepare ever more extreme ads, costing more than $50 million. These ads succeeded in reaching legislators on key committees and their media market viewers.
- The public was found to be generally poorly informed (e.g., 75% did not know the administration was the main proponent of an employer mandate requiring them to offer insurance to workers [favored by a majority of people]); fewer than half had heard of the single-payer bill; and they wanted much more information and blamed the media for not providing it.

- Reporting of opinion polls was uncritical; it magnified the impact of uninformed opinion, creating "news" out of uninformed opinion (failing to qualify the results according to people's depth of knowledge) and influencing the actions of leading members of Congress and perhaps also of undecided viewers.
- The advertising, polls, and media coverage of them ultimately had an impact on Congress's rejection of major reform. Leaders said that public opinion was as influential in the debate as the administration itself, that interest-group advertising (mainly by health insurance and business interests) was persuasive, that the public was not well informed on the issues, and that the media had done a poor job of helping people understand the issues. Despite this, leading members and staff of the House and Senate said their main sources of information about public opinion were the polls (mainly reported in the media), the trade group lobbies, and the media (Columbia Institute, 1995).

## Implementation

Congressional adoption of policies, known as **authorization**, only begins the next major phase of policy making: making a policy effective in the real world. Policies require **appropriations**, approved amounts of funds to be available over 1 year or more, to put the policy into effect. To complete the task, the monies must be allocated (i.e., distributed by an authorized agency, usually a government bureau, in the form of grants, contracts, or other payments).

Prior to this dispersal of funds, the policy must be interpreted in specific terms, known as **rule making**; opened to public comment for 30 to 60 days (always published in the weekly *Federal Register*); finalized; and then publicized to eligible recipient organizations, such as state agencies and community groups, including health centers and home health agencies. These potential users must apply for the funds by proposing what programs they will conduct with the monies. The awardees then implement programs, such as community or employee tobacco education, smoking cessation programs, or payment for the costs of setting up smoke-free workplaces.

Finally, the authorized agencies must monitor and enforce the rules that guide application of the policy and eventually feed this information back into the final phase of policy making: evaluation. At any point in implementation, groups may contest the process in court if they think it is proceeding too slowly or too quickly, fairly or unfairly.

The complexity of policy implementation processes, as federal and state funds are dispersed into programs

**❝** *In this and like communities, public sentiment is everything. With public sentiment, nothing can fail; without it, nothing can succeed.* **❞**

—*Abraham Lincoln, 1858*

 **Research Alert**

This study examined the effects of policy variables on enrollment in the Special Supplemental Nutrition Program for Women, Infants, and Children (WIC) using Aday and Anderson's framework for the study of access. Secondary analysis of data from public documents and agencies for the 50 states was done. Independent variables were the ratio of the federal WIC grant to the eligible population, state supplementation of WIC, administrative and food dollars per person, WIC population per clinic, and WIC priority categories served. The dependent variable was the eligible WIC population enrolled. State supplementation of the WIC budget, administrative and food dollars per person, cost of living, population density and distribution, and ratio of the federal WIC grant to the eligible population accounted for 85% percent of the variance in WIC enrollment. Recommendations included reorienting the federal funding formula toward enrollment incentives, state supplementation of WIC, and examination of administrative and food costs.

*Source*: Wimmer, M. (2003). The Effects of Policy on Enrollment in the Special Supplemental Nutrition Program for Women, Infants, and Children. *Policy, Politics, & Nursing Practice, 4*(3), 210–220.

across communities, means that there are infinite ways for opponents to change the pace and direction of a policy. For example, in both Massachusetts and California, where tobacco-control coalitions succeeded in passing tobacco tax referenda against strong industry lobbying, the actual use of the millions of new dollars became another source of contention. Rather than the intended use of the funds for antitobacco programs, policy makers attempted to use the monies for other, sometimes political, purposes such as financing hospital care in response to the hospital lobby (Begay & Glantz, 1997).

In one state, the antitobacco coalition sued the state in court and won, requiring authorization and allocation of the funds for the stated smoking prevention and control purposes. In the other state, the coalition negotiated a compromise on the use of the funds, but this resulted in a decline in appropriations for tobacco control over the next several years. Analysis of such experiences can help inform future public health policy efforts.

**❝** *Where there is no vision, the people perish.* **❞**

—*Proverbs, the Bible*

## ■ Evaluation

Research findings (i.e., science-based information)—in contrast to opinions and impressions—are often not available or are not used much by policy makers. Studies must be translated first into the organizational or political priorities of decision makers. The timing of findings makes a difference too in whether they are used, for instance, before interest groups have developed around a policy issue, or much later, when social acceptance improves (Brint, 1990; Brooten, Brown, Miovech, & Youngblut, 2006).

Most evaluation consists of the impressions of user groups and program reports on **outputs**, such as numbers of people served, numbers reached by public education campaigns, new smoke-free workplaces, the decline of cigarette sales, and financial reports. Policy **impacts** include the indirect effects of a policy, sometimes unintended or unwanted. For example, when strict local no-smoking laws were passed in New York, bars and restaurants did not lose business as the tobacco industry had warned (Engelen, Farrelly, & Hyland, 2006). When the WIC program was implemented, it created new local food retail jobs and improved local economies (National Farmers Association, 1996).

**Outcomes**—that is, changes in people's health—are more rare, sometimes because they can be seen only after a longer period of time than policy makers are willing to wait (such as a decline in lung cancer), and sometimes because health indicators often require additional spending for evaluation research—monies that are often not available. Evaluation is thus both a political and scientific process, and its results determine whether a policy will be revised, cut back, or repealed (Hanley, 2006; Zervigon-Hakes, 1995).

The lesson is clear: Policy making for health continues long after adoption and requires that proponents continue to monitor the processes and to take action to preserve the health effectiveness of any specific policy. This kind of "watchdog" activity is often done by public interest groups, such as the Coalition on Smoking and Health; Handgun Control, Inc.; and the Center for Public Environmental Oversight in Washington, D.C. Governments also have monitoring agencies, including the General Accounting Office of the Congress to oversee legislative results, and the Office of Management and Budget, which oversees the effectiveness of most executive branch agencies for the White House.

## Nurses in Communities, Public Health Policy, and Primary Prevention

The tobacco coalitions all succeeded to some degree in obtaining public resources to prevent the biggest single cause of death in populations. Yet the largest risk factor threatening health and life, one not often discussed or addressed by the health sector, is the gross and growing disparity in social and economic determinants of health between the nation's disadvantaged communities and others (Krieger, 1994; Link & Phelan, 1995; Wexler & Copeland, 2003). It is possible for the public health community to initiate and work with coalitions in local, state, and national strategies to improve the conditions in which people live. This includes nurses, who see the effects of poverty and discrimination based on ethnicity, age, and other factors. They have been and, to fulfill their professional duty, should continue to be involved at every level, either through their practice settings, nurse groups,

> **"** *People don't eat in the long run—they eat every day.* **"**
> —*Harry L. Hopkins, 1933*

> **"** *If you cannot convince them, confuse them.* **"**
> —*Harry S. Truman*

> **"** *Americans will always do the right thing . . . after they have exhausted all the other possibilities.* **"**
> —*Winston Churchill*

or by joining allied groups. To promote primary prevention policies, it is necessary to involve a wide range of organizations that affect living conditions and to focus on priority public, institutional, or corporate policies.

Among the many community conditions needed to support population health are housing, child welfare, and access to comprehensive primary care (Federman, 1996; Montgomery, Kiely, & Pappas, 1996; NCCP, 2007). With the kind of policy groundwork outlined previously, these issues can become priorities for health departments and other parts of the health community. Policy proposals can then be developed to ensure more healthful living conditions. A few examples follow.

Neighborhoods with high rates of unemployment, poverty, high rent, and crowded housing are associated with a high incidence of low-birth-weight babies. Adverse living situations predispose people to toxicities, infections, contagions, accidents, strains on eyesight, unhealthy food storage and use, and mental health stresses from lack of privacy, the ability to work at home, and recreation opportunities (Martin, 1977, Roberts, 1997, Sherman & Redlener, 2003).

The availability and adequacy of housing significantly affect health through the following strategies:

- The siting of housing—whether near polluting industries or near transportation routes to access job opportunities, education and health services, and stores
- Local environmental controls and maintenance, such as water supply and waste management
- Housing structure involving overcrowding, ventilation, lighting, and temperature control

Thus legitimate public health activities include improved zoning, environmental regulations, and building codes; the development of adequate low-rent housing and transportation systems; support for tenant organizations and citizen grievance processes; and open hearings on housing issues. Although not under the direct control of health departments, community health organizations and agencies can form coalitions and raise these issues by defining the type and scope of health issues and the policy changes needed to support health, as well as through work with local and state organizations in housing, economic development, land use, and the environment to advise on and advocate changes (Hardy & Satterthwaite, 1987; Rice, 2002; Slater & Carlton, 1985).

On a smaller scale, taking account of commercial establishments' interest in safe and expanding markets, local governments and community organizations, led by health departments or other health advocacy groups, can use their market power to influence the proportion of healthy foods of the local food supply as well as limit access to tobacco (CDC, 1999). For instance, they could require that cafeterias in their facilities contain low-fat, high-fiber food choices. This would encourage food suppliers to change their supplier contracts to retain their own contracts, with ripple effects on food processing corporations. The new options in these facilities would result in changes in eating habits for clients and employees while at the same time suggesting an exemplary "healthful practices" model for the public and the media. Nurses, for example, could propose healthy food options in their work site cafeterias in state and local health agencies, schools, hospitals, health maintenance organizations, prisons, military installations, vending machines, and so on.

With rising child impoverishment and lack of health care, child health and welfare are at risk (Cohen, 2002). Specific, focused policies proposed by nurses allied with child welfare proponents (Deal & Shiono, 1998) that are worthy of advocacy efforts include the following:

- An increase in cigarette excise taxes
- Strong indoor and outdoor air quality control and enforcement
- An above-poverty-level minimum wage
- Handgun control
- Repair of the welfare and prevention safety net
- Comprehensive maternal–child care and child day care

> *The new technologies hold promise for a greatly enhanced system that can meet the changing needs of an information-based society. At the same time, these technologies will generate a number of significant social problems. How these technologies evolve, as well as who will be affected positively or negatively, will depend on decisions now being made in both the public and private sectors . . . making choices about universal service is essentially making choices about equality of opportunity. Defining universal service is, in effect, making choices about the nature of society itself.*
>
> —*Office of Technology Assessment, U.S. Congress, Critical Connections, 1990*

### ■ Advocacy Tools of the Future

Electronic networks are a new set of tools to extend the sources of support and strengthen the advocacy efforts for the public's health. Community-based groups, allied with the public health community, raise and amplify issues, propose solutions, establish their legitimacy, and join larger coalitions. These advocacy networks, linked to national and local watchdog groups, supply timely and accurate information not only about problems, but also about program and policy solutions and sources of technical assistance. Perhaps most importantly, these electronic links coordinate joint advocacy efforts and alert local groups to timely actions in local, state, and national policy arenas, including coordination of e-mail, fax, phone, or letter-writing campaigns to pass, for example, a tobacco tax or handgun registration.

The case has been made in public health forums and studies for electronic networks to link public health and other community organizations to improve community health, especially in poor areas. This collaboration supports core public health functions through strengthening services delivery, education, environmental health, community mobilization, and policy advocacy (Lasker, Humphreys, & Braithwaite, 1995; Milio, 1995, 1996; Jennings, Thompson, & Roberts, 2002). Nurses are in a position to point out the importance of electronic linkages with community organizations to develop and reinforce health and community partnerships.

## Conclusion

An understanding of health policy making and the mission of public health is not merely an academic exercise. It is essential to the health professions and their institutions because practitioners in nursing and other health fields are in applied—not academic—disciplines. Our privileges are derived from our social responsibility to ensure the health of all populations. An awareness of the health effects of a wide range of public and corporate policies, the public reporting of these effects, and efforts to promote health-supporting policies fall within the scope of the health community and in our activities within other groups. Participation in any aspect of these complex and ongoing policy processes can engage us as individuals. But more often, policy work requires action through organizations to sustain the necessary long-term effort to ensure effective health-supporting policies.

The leaders in nursing of the nineteenth and twentieth centuries were great women with broad vision and understanding of the issues of their day. They engaged political, social, and health care groups in improving both the health care system and the health of all the people, especially the rural and urban poor, immigrants, and other vulnerable groups. The twenty-first century is at least as challenging and requires comparable vision, commitment, and energy.

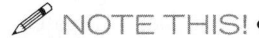 NOTE THIS!

The word *health* does not appear anywhere in the U.S. Constitution or Bill of Rights.

Explore Community Health Nursing on the Web! To learn more about the topics in this chapter, use the passcode provided to access your exclusive website: **http://nursing.jbpub.com/ communityhealth.** If you do not have a passcode, you can obtain one at this site.

## ■ CRITICAL THINKING ACTIVITIES

1. Select a community health problem, such as teen suicide or school violence. Chapter author, Dr. Milio, contends that "Media are not only channels (p. 205) for information . . . they also create and shape issues." Think of several examples from the media in which your selected health issue is presented as a problem or a solution. Who is blamed for the problem? Are there solutions identified? Who are the stakeholders in any policy making related to your identified problem?

2. If you could design a website that influences health policy for children with learning disabilities, what components would you include? How would you include the public in its development and implementation? Who would you include as experts on your website? Decide how you could link your website to other advocacy groups. Design an evaluation of this project as related to effectiveness in policy making.

## ■ REFERENCES

Amundson, D. R., Lichter, L. S., & Lichter, S. R. (2005). *What's the matter with kids today? Television coverage of adolescents in America.* Prepared for the Frameworks Institute. Retrieved November 3, 2008, from http://www.frameworksinstitute.org/assets/files/PDF/Youth_Whats_the_Matter.pdf

Begay, M., & Glantz, S. (1997). Question 1 tobacco education expenditures in Massachusetts, USA. *Tobacco Control, 6,* 213–218.

Benjamin, K., Perfetto, E., & Greene, R. (1995). Public policy and the application of outcomes assessments: Paradigms vs politics. *Medical Care, 33*(4), AS299–AS306 suppl.

Beyer, J., & Trice, H. (1982). The utilization process: A conceptual framework and synthesis of empirical findings. *Administrative Science Quarterly, 24*(4), 591–622.

Bomlitz, L. J., & Brezis, M. (2008). Misrepresentation of health risks by mass media. *Journal of Public Health, 30*(2), 202–204.

Braun, S. (1995, March/April). Media coverage of health care reform. A content analysis. *Columbia Journalism Review,* supplement, 1–8.

Brewer, G., & De Leon, P. (1983). *Foundations of policy analysis.* Homewood, IL: Dorsey.

Brint, S. (1990). Rethinking the policy influence of experts: From general characterizations to analysis of variation. *Sociological Forum, 5*(3), 361–385.

Brooten, D., Brown, L. P., Miovech, S. M., & Youngblut, J. M. (2006). Politics of nursing research. In D. J. Mason, J. K. Leavitt, & M. K. Chaffee (Eds.), *Policy and politics in nursing and health care* (5th ed.). Philadelphia: Saunders.

Brown, L. (1997). Knowledge and power: Health services research as a political resource. In E. Ginzburg (Ed.), *Health services research: Key to health policy* (pp. 20–45). Cambridge, MA: Harvard University Press.

Cappela, F., & Jamieson, K. (1996). *Media in the middle: Coverage of the health care reform debate of 1994.* Research report. Philadelphia: Annenberg School of Mass Communications.

Cappella, J., & Jamieson, K. (1994). *Public cynicism and news coverage in campaigns and policy debates: 3 field experiments.* Research report. Philadelphia: Annenberg School for Communication.

Center for the Future of Children. (1997, Spring). Welfare to work. *Future of Children, 7,* 1.

Center for Health Economics Research. (1993). *Access to health care: Indicators for policy.* Princeton, NJ: Robert Wood Johnson Foundation.

Centers for Disease Control and Prevention (CDC). (1999). *Physical activity and good nutrition.* Atlanta: Author.

Centers for Disease Control and Prevention. (CDC). (2007). *National Center for Environmental Health: General lead information.* Retrieved April 22, 2008, from http://www.cdc.gov.nceh/lead/feq/about/htm.

Cohen, S. S. (2002). Child care policy making. In D. J. Mason, J. K. Leavitt, & M. K. Chaffee (Eds.), *Policy and politics in nursing and health care* (4th ed., pp. 669–675). St. Louis, MO: Saunders.

Columbia Institute. (1995, May). *What shapes lawmakers' views? A survey of members of Congress and key staff on health care reform.* Washington, DC: Author.

Cutler, D., & Sheiner, L. (1999). *Demographics and medical care spending: Standard and non-standard effects.* Unpublished paper. Harvard School of Public Health.

Deal, L., & Shiono, P. (1998). Medicaid managed care and children: An overview. *Future of Children, 8*(2), 93–104.

Department of Health and Human Services (DHHS). (1995, April). *Personal Responsibility Act of 1995: Preliminary impacts.* Washington, DC: Author.

DiMaggio, P., & Anheier, H. (1990). The sociology of non-profit organizations and sectors. *Annual Review of Sociology, 16,* 137–159.

Edgar, T., Fitzpatrick, M. A., & Freimuth, V. S. (1992). *AIDS: A communication perspective.* Hillsdale, NJ: Lawrence Erlbaum.

Engelen, M., Farrelly, M., & Hyland, A. (2006, July). *The health and economic impact of New York's clean indoor air act.* Albany, NY: New York State Department of Health.

Federman, M., Garner, T. I., Short, K., et al. (1996, May). What does it mean to be poor in America? *Monthly Labor Review, 119*(5), 3–17.

Feldstein, P. J. (1996). *The politics of health legislation. An economic perspective.* Chico, CA: Health Administration Press.

General Accounting Office (GAO). (1998). *Blood lead levels in children.* Washington, DC: U.S. Congress.

Hanley, B. E. (2006). Policy development and analysis. In D. J. Mason, J. K. Leavitt, & M. K. Chaffee (Eds.), *Policy and politics in nursing and health care* (5th ed.). Philadelphia: Saunders.

Hardy, J., & Satterthwaite, D. (1987). Housing and health. *Cities, 4,* 221–235.

Hatcher, B. J. (2003). The Maternal and Child Health Community Leadership Institute: Putting the Health for All Framework into action. In H. M. Wallace, G. Green, & K. J. Jaros (Eds.), *Health and welfare for families in the 21st century* (2nd ed., pp. 41–51). Sudbury, MA: Jones and Bartlett.

Heiser, P., & Begay, M. (1997). Campaign to raise the tobacco tax in Massachusetts. *American Journal of Public Health, 87,* 968–973.

Horton, K. B. (2006). Lobbying: An inside view. In D. J. Mason, J. K. Leavitt, & M. K. Chaffee (Eds.), *Policy and politics in nursing and health care* (5th ed.). Philadelphia: Saunders.

Institute of Medicine. (1988). *The future of public health.* Washington, DC: National Academy Press.

Jacobson, P., Wasserman, J., & Raube, K. (1993). Politics of anti-smoking legislation. *Journal of Health Policy, Policy & Law, 18,* 787–818.

Jasanoff, S. (1993). *The fifth branch: Science advisors as policymakers.* Cambridge, MA: Harvard University Press.

Jennings, C. P., Thompson, L., & Roberts, D. (2002). Achieving health literacy. In D. J. Mason, J. K. Leavitt, & M. K. Chaffee (Eds.), *Policy and politics in nursing and health care* (4th ed., pp. 107–111). St. Louis, MO: Saunders.

Kaplan, H. (1996). Inequality in income and mortality in the US: Analysis of mortality and potential pathways. *British Medical Journal, 312,* 999–1003.

Kegler, M. (1995). *Community coalitions for tobacco control: Factors influencing implementation.* PhD dissertation. Chapel Hill: University of North Carolina School of Public Health.

Kessler, D. A., Witt, A. M., Barnett, P. S., et al. (1996). The Food and Drug Administration's regulation of tobacco products. *New England Journal of Medicine, 335*(13), 988–994.

Kraus, J., Peek, A., & Williams, S. (1995). Compliance with the 1992 California motorcycle helmet use law. *American Journal of Public Health, 85*(3), 96–99.

Krieger, N. (1994). Epidemiology and the web of causation. *Social Science & Medicine, 39,* 887–903.

Krieger, N., Chen, J. T., & Ebel, G. (1997). Can we monitor socio-economic inequalities in health? A survey of US health departments' data collection and reporting practices. *Public Health Report, 112*(6), 481–491.

Lasker, R. (1997). *Medicine and public health.* New York: New York Academy of Medicine.

Lasker, R., Humphreys, B., & Braithwaite, W. (1995, July). *Making a powerful connection: The health of the public and the national information infrastructure. Report of the Public Health Data Policy Coordinating Committee, U.S. Public Health Service.* Washington, DC: U.S. Government Printing Office.

Laumann, E., & Knoke, D. (1987). *The organizational state.* Madison: University of Wisconsin Press.

Lindblom, C., & Cohen, D. (1979). *Useable knowledge.* New Haven, CT: Yale University Press.

Link, B., & Phelan, J. (1995). Social conditions as fundamental causes of disease. *Journal of Health & Social Behavior, 2*(special issue), 80–94.

Lurie, N. (2004). The public health infrastructure: Rebuild or redesign? In C. Harrington & C. L. Estes (Eds.), *Health policy: Crisis and reform in the U.S. health care delivery system* (4th ed., pp. 184–187). Sudbury, MA: Jones and Bartlett.

Martin, A. (1977). *Health aspects of human settlements: A review.* Geneva: World Health Organization.

Mason, D. J., Dodd, C. J., & Glickstein, B. (2006). Role of the media in influencing policy: Getting the message across. In D. J. Mason, J. K. Leavitt, & M. K. Chaffee (Eds.), *Policy and politics in nursing and health care* (5th ed.). Philadelphia: Saunders.

Milio, N. (2002). Where policy hits the pavement: Contemporary issues in communities. In D. J. Mason, J. K. Leavitt, & M. K. Chaffee (Eds.), *Policy and politics in nursing and health care* (4th ed., pp. 659–668). St. Louis, MO: Saunders.

Milio, N. (1976, March). A framework for prevention: Changing health damaging to health generating life patterns. *American Journal of Public Health, 66,* 35–38.

Milio, N. (1986). *Promoting health through public policy.* Ottawa: Canadian Public Health Association.

Milio, N. (1995). Beyond informatics: Community electronic networks and public health. *Journal of Public Health Management & Practice, 2*(3), 6–11.

Milio, N. (1996). *Engines of empowerment: Using information technology to create healthy communities and challenge public policy.* Chico, CA: Health Administration Press.

Milio, N. (1997). Case studies in nutrition policymaking: How process shapes product. In B. Garza (Ed.), *Beyond nutrition information.* Ithaca, NY: Cornell University Press.

Milio, N. (2000). Evaluating health promotion policies: Tracking a moving target. In I. Rootman, M. Goodstadt, L. Potvin, & J. Springett (Eds.), *Evaluation of health promotion: Principles and perspectives.* Copenhagen: World Health Organization.

Minkler, M. (Ed.). (2004). *Community organizing and community building for health* (2nd ed.). New Brunswick, NJ: Rutgers University Press.

Montgomery, L., Kiely, J., & Pappas, G. (1996). Effects of poverty, race, and family structure of US children's health: Data from the National Health Interview Survey, 1978 through 1980 and 1989 through 1991. *American Journal of Public Health, 86*(10), 1401–1405.

Nathanson, M. D. (2005). *Health care providers' government relations handbook.* Sudbury, MA: Jones and Bartlett.

National Association of City and Council Health Officials (NACCHO). (1998). *NACCHO study of electronic communication capacity of local health departments.* Washington, DC: Author.

National Cancer Institute. (1991). *Strategies to control tobacco use in the United States: A blueprint for public health action in the 1990s.* Smoking and Tobacco Control Monographs 1. Bethesda, MD: Author.

National Center for Children in Poverty (NCCP). (1998). *Young children in poverty.* New York: Columbia University School of Public Health.

National Center for Children in Poverty (NCCP). (2007). *Federal child and dependent care tax credit.* Retrieved October 8, 2008, from http://www.nccp.org/policy

National Farmers Association Market Nutrition Programs. (1996). *Program impact report.* Washington, DC: Author.

Office of Disease Prevention and Health Promotion. (1994). *For a healthy nation: Returns on investment in public health.* Atlanta, GA: U.S. Department of Health and Human Services.

Pentz, M., Brannon, B. R., Charlin, V. R., Barrett, E. J., MacKinnon, D. P., & Flay, B. P. (1989). The power of policy: The relationship of smoking policy to adolescent smoking. *American Journal of Public Health, 79*(7), 857–862.

Public Health Foundation. (1998). *Measuring health objectives and indicators: 1997 state and local capacity survey.* Washington, DC: Author.

Public Health Service. Office of Technology Assessment. (1991). *Adolescent health* (vol. 1). Washington, DC: U.S. Congress.

Ray, M. M., & Roberts, S. (2000). Lobbying policymakers: Individual and collective strategies. In D. J. Mason, J. K. Leavitt, & M. K. Chaffee (Eds.), *Policy and politics in nursing and health care* (4th ed., pp. 551–561). St. Louis, MO: Saunders.

Rice, R. (2002). Coalitions: A powerful political strategy. In D. J. Mason, J. K. Leavitt, & M. K. Chaffee (Eds.), *Policy and politics in nursing and health care* (4th ed., pp. 121–129). St. Louis, MO: Saunders.

Rice, R., & Atkin, C. (1994). Principles of successful public communication campaigns. In J. Bryant & D. Zillman (Eds.), *Media effects: Advances in theory and research* (pp. 365–387). Hillsdale, NJ: Lawrence Erlbaum.

Roberts, E. (1997). Neighborhood social environments and the distribution of low birth weights in Chicago. *American Journal of Public Health, 87,* 597–603.

Rochefort, D., & Cobb, R. (1993). Problem definition, agenda access, and policy choice. *Policy Studies Journal, 21*(1), 56–71.

Rose, G. (1985). Sick individual and sick populations. *International Journal of Epidemiology, 14*, 32–38.

Rose, G. (1990). Future of disease prevention: British perspectives on the US Preventive Services Task for Guidelines. *Journal of General Internal Medicine, 5*, S128–S132.

Sherman, P., & Redlener, I. (2003). Homeless women and their children in the 21st century. In H. M. Wallace, G. Green, & K. J. Jaros (Eds.), *Health and welfare for families in the 21st century* (2nd ed., pp. 469–480). Sudbury, MA: Jones and Bartlett.

Slater, C., & Carlton, B. (1985). Behavior, lifestyle, and socioeconomic variables as determinants of health status: Implications for health policy development. *American Journal of Preventive Medicine, 1*, 25–33.

Sofaer, S., et al. (1997). *Models for assessing the impact of changes in health care delivery and financing on community tuberculosis prevention and control programs*. Research report. Washington, DC: George Washington University Center for Health Outcomes Improvement Research.

Sultz, H. A., & Young, K. M. (2003). *Health care USA: Understanding its organization and delivery* (4th ed). Sudbury, MA: Jones and Bartlett.

Syme, S. L., Lefkowitz, B., & Krimgold, B. K. (2004). Incorporation socioeconomic factors into U.S. health policy: Addressing the barriers. In C. Harrington & C. L. Estes (Eds.), *Health policy: Crisis and reform in the U.S. health care delivery system* (4th ed., pp. 78–82). Sudbury, MA: Jones and Bartlett.

Teh-Wei, H., Hai-Yen, S., & Keeler, T. (1995). Reducing cigarette consumption in California: Tobacco taxes vs an anti-smoking media campaign. *American Journal of Public Health, 85*, 1218–1222.

Wakefield, M.K., Gardner, D. B., & Guillett, S. E. (2002). Contemporary issues in government. In D. J. Mason, J. K. Leavitt, & M. K. Chaffee (Eds.), *Policy and politics in nursing and health care* (4th ed., pp. 421–437). St. Louis, MO: Saunders.

Walker, J. (1991). *Mobilizing interest groups in America: Patrons, professions, and social movements*. Ann Arbor: University of Michigan Press.

Warner, K. (1991). Tobacco industry scientific advisors: Serving society or selling cigarettes? *American Journal of Public Health, 81*(7), 839–842.

Webber, D. J. (1987). Factors influencing legislators' use of policy information and implications for promoting greater use. *Policy Studies Review, 6*(4), 64–80.

Weissert, C., & Weissert, W. (1996). *Governing health: The politics of health policy*. Baltimore: Johns Hopkins University Press.

Wexler, S., & Copeland, V. C. (2003). Combating family poverty: A review of the American welfare system. In H. M. Wallace, G. Green, & K. J. Jaros (Eds.), *Health and welfare for families in the 21st century* (2nd ed., pp. 119–137). Sudbury, MA: Jones and Bartlett.

Winslow, C. E. A. (1920, March). The untilled field of public health. *Modern Medicine, 183*

Zervigon-Hakes, A. (1995). Translating research into public programs and policies. *Future of Children, 5*(3), 175–191.

# Transcultural Nursing Care in the Community

Madeleine Leininger

Establishing new knowledge and practice pathways is always a major challenge, for new pathways may create fears and uncertainty; yet these pathways are essential to meet community, societal, and global human needs.

"Keep, ancient lands, your storied pomp!" cries she
With silent lips. "Give me your tired, your poor,
Your huddled masses yearning to breathe free,
The wretched refuse of your teeming shore.
Send these, the homeless, tempest-tossed, to me;
I lift my lamp beside the golden door."

*—Emma Lazarus (1849–1887), U.S. poet*
*Written for inscription on the Statue of Liberty*

Children are not born "cultured." Humans are not hard-wired genetically to their culture. Each generation transmits culture to its children through a "cultural blueprint." Our primary cultural influences come from our family and the community of our childhood. As we grow older, our blueprint also grows culturally, as we move from our family of origin to school, church, and peers. In today's media-saturated world, our cultural identity is reinforced through all forms of media. We often associate culture with the "other," those unlike ourselves. Just as a fish is unaware that he or she is "wet," so culture is largely unconscious. That which is considered "normal" exerts a powerful effect on our ideas about health and illness, even from whom and where we seek health care.

As a student nurse, how have your cultural "imprints" affected your care of "others," especially those from widely diverse cultures and population? Have you been in a situation where your own cultural beliefs have been challenged? What did this feel like, and how is it related to your role as a nurse?

## CHAPTER FOCUS

**Community-Based Transcultural Nursing**

**Scope of Transcultural Nursing**

**Transcultural Nursing Principles**

**Transcultural Concepts**

**Leininger's Theory of Cultural Care Diversity and Universality**
- Development of the Theory
- Goal of the Theory

- Assumptions of the Theory
- The Sunrise Model: A Visual Guide for the Theory
- Application of the Theory and Model

## QUESTIONS TO CONSIDER

After reading this chapter, you will know the answers to the following questions:

1. What is community-based transcultural nursing?
2. What are the principles of transcultural nursing?
3. What is culturally competent nursing care?
4. What is the theory of culture care diversity and universality?

5. How did the theory of culture care diversity and universality develop?
6. How is the sunrise model used as a guide for the theory?
7. How are the theory of culture care diversity and university and the sunrise model used to provide culturally competent nursing care?

## KEY TERMS

| | | | |
|---|---|---|---|
| Caring | Cultural ignorance | Cultural variation | Etic view |
| Cultural backlash | Cultural imposition | Culturally competent care | Generic care |
| Cultural barriers | Cultural lifeways | Culture | Immigrants |
| Cultural bias | Cultural pain | Culture bound | Professional care nursing |
| Cultural blindness | Cultural shock | Emic view | Refugees |
| Cultural clashes | Cultural values | Ethnocentrism | Stereotyping |

NURSING IS ENTERING A new century and a new millennium with many new challenges, pathways, and opportunities. In the twenty-first century, nurses are and will continue to be involved with many immigrants, refugees, travelers, and strangers coming from many different places. Many nurses will live in a variety of different geographic locations and practice nursing in largely unfamiliar cultural and physical environments.

Today's nurses are learning to use transcultural nursing concepts, principles, and practices to help them function in different community and cultural contexts. Transcultural nursing has become one of the most essential and relevant pathways to meet the holistic and special needs of people from diverse and similar cultures. As nurses learn about the essential and desired care expectations of different cultures, they become aware of different ways to provide culturally competent and sensitive care. Transcultural nursing focuses on holistic and comprehensive ways to know and serve people of diverse cultures throughout the life cycle. The primary goals of *transcultural community-based nursing* are to help people of different and similar cultures maintain their health, prevent illnesses or disabilities, and die in culturally congruent and meaningful ways. Nurses in the twenty-first century are challenged to adopt this perspective to become better professional nurses.

Transcultural community-based nursing is essential for the future of the profession. Along with transcultural definitions, concepts, principles, and practices, a brief history of transcultural nursing is provided in this chapter to describe the growth of the field over the past five decades. The theory of culture care diversity and universality is presented in the final section of this chapter as an important perspective from which transcultural nursing can be studied and assessed. The theory can be used to assist nurses in providing culturally safe, effective, and congruent nursing care. Throughout this chapter, some reflective questions and examples are posed to help nurses reflect on the cultural beliefs, values, and lifeways that exist in different cultures. Because transcultural community-based nursing is the goal for the twenty-first century, some definitions of common terms related to the field of transcultural nursing are outlined in Box 10-1 (Leininger, 1995, 2006).

**❝** *Because we have put ourselves in our own zoo, we find it difficult to break out.* **❞**

—*Edward T. Hall*

**❝** *Here the melting pot stands open—if you're willing to get bleached first.* **❞**

—*Buffy Sainte-Marie*

**❝** *Coretta Scott King seemed to be beyond the ordinary things of the world.* **❞**

—*Maya Angelou, on the death of Coretta Scott King, widow of Martin Luther King, Jr., in 2006*

---

**BOX 10-1**

**Definitions**

**Culture:** The learned, shared, and transmitted values, beliefs, norms, and lifeways of a particular group that guide their thinking, decisions, and actions in patterned ways.

**Cultural values:** The powerful directive forces that give order and meaning to people's thinking, decisions, and actions.

**Cultural variations:** The subtle or obvious variables among and between cultures that make them unique with respect to traditional or nontraditional ways of living.

**Cultural lifeways:** The patterned ways of living of a particular individual or group.

**Cultural imposition:** The tendency to impose one's beliefs, values, and lifeways on another individual or culture, due largely to ignorance about a culture.

**Ethnocentrism:** The belief that one's own ways of living or doing are the best, most preferred, or superior to others.

**Stereotyping:** The undesirable tendency to pre-judge and fix cultures into rigid and biased ways, due largely to ethnocentrism and racism.

**Cultural blindness:** The inability to recognize one's own values and lifeways or those of another culture, making culture invisible.

**Cultural clashes:** Major conflicts in valuing and understanding differences between cultures and variability among or within cultures.

**Caring:** Actions and activities directed toward assisting, supporting, or enabling another individual or group with evident or anticipated needs to improve a human condition or lifeway, or to face death.

**Nursing:** A learned humanistic and scientific profession and discipline focused on human caring.

**Emic view:** The insider's or local perspective about cultures, families, lifeways, and health care.

**Etic view:** The outsider's or external perspective about cultures, families, lifeways, and health care.

**Culturally competent care:** The deliberate and creative use of transcultural nursing knowledge and skills to assist or facilitate individuals or groups to maintain their well-being, recover from illness, or face a disability or death.

---

## Community-Based Transcultural Nursing

*Community-based transcultural nursing* refers to the creative use of transcultural nursing concepts, principles, research, knowledge, and practices that focus on large overall designated communities or geographic contexts to provide culturally competent nursing care. Most communities have many diverse cultural groups with some similar and some sharply diverse cultural lifeways.

The following fundamentals describe the nature, characteristics, and power of cultures, the concept of care, and transcultural nursing:

- Cultures tend to be stable, yet they may change over time in beliefs, values, and cultural lifeways.

- Cultural patterns, norms (rules), and practices are powerful influences on human care and transcultural community practices.
- Cultural values and beliefs vary between and within cultures and must be understood to develop culturally congruent care practices.
- Cultural rituals, symbols, taboos, and practices are important to identify and understand for transcultural nursing.
- Transcultural nursing necessitates studying the total lifeways of people, including influences on care related to religion or spirituality, politics, economics, technologies, kinship ties, environment, and specific values and practices.
- Different modes of communication; use of space, land, and property; and use of home remedies are all part of discovering the transcultural nursing care needs of people.
- Different cultures in a community have different life ways that must be considered by nurses.
- Different cultures have different caregivers to heal, cure, or assist their people.
- Cultural gatekeepers are found in communities that protect, defend, and uphold cultural values, beliefs, and desired lifeways.
- Transcultural care needs and expectations vary among communities and cannot be assumed to be alike.
- In every community there will be subcultures that are slightly different from the dominant culture and that require attention from the transcultural nurse. These subcultures include the homeless, homosexuals, gangs, drug users, individuals from poor and affluent social classes, and others.

Although nurses have traditionally worked with people in communities, providing care in homes, schools, industrial plants, clinics, and other settings, the major missing dimension has been knowledge of the cultural background of the people and how to care for them in that context. Cultural factors have been taken for granted and often viewed as less important or not even recognized. With the advent of transcultural nursing came a new and heightened awareness of the importance of culturally based knowledge. It was soon discovered that nurses prepared in transcultural community-based nursing were able to demonstrate the use of their knowledge with specific cultures in beneficial ways. Nurses working in community or public health settings found that transcultural nursing concepts were important in providing effective care. In fact, nurses who were skilled and prepared to work with different cultures realized the unique care needs of patients and became confident with individuals, groups, families, and communities (Leininger, 1981, 1988, 1995, 2006).

✎ NOTE THIS! •————————————————

The foreign born comprise 12% of the U.S. population. With their American-born children, they account for more than half of the U.S. population growth.

🏛 HEALTHY PEOPLE 2010
**OBJECTIVES RELATED TO CULTURAL DIVERSITY AND CARE**

**Access to Quality Health Services**
1.8    In the health professions, allied and associated health professions, and the nursing field, increase the proportion of all degrees awarded to members to underrepresented racial and ethnic groups.

**Educational and Community-Based Programs**
7.11    Increase the proportion of local health departments that have established culturally appropriate and linguistically competent community health-promotion and disease-prevention programs for racial and ethnic minority populations.

**Mental Health and Mental Disorders**
18.13    Increase the number of states, territories, and the District of Columbia with an operational mental health plan that addresses cultural competence.

*Source*: DHHS, 2000.

Beginning in the mid-1970s, community health nurses encountered many new cultural strangers, such as immigrants, refugees, migrant workers, and others, and felt helpless in knowing how to understand and help them. That is when many community nurses began to enroll in transcultural nursing courses. The need for transcultural community-based care was clearly evident as they told their stories about trying to help cultural strangers who seemed to suddenly come into their nursing world. Some nurses did not understand why some patients wanted their children to be cared for before any adults. Other nurses were baffled by strange terms such as *susto*, *evil eye*, and *sacred objects to heal* because they were terms specific to cultures and to cultural health care practices. Without understanding these terms and many others, nurses were disadvantaged. Many nurses said they had to almost completely relearn nursing from a

Dr. Madeleine Leininger (center), founder of transcultural nursing, with members of the Mississippi Chapter of the Transcultural Nursing Society.

**❝** *Our ambivalence with diversity has led us to bury our heads in the sand while problems escalate, causing enormous suffering. AIDS has swept away entire African communities; thousands of children are without parents. We have lost artists, musicians, designers, screenwriters, scientists, and some of our dearest friends and family members.* **❞**

—Marie Farrell

different perspective, because many of their previous nursing ideas did not fit with specific cultures. Indeed, some nursing knowledge learned earlier was counter to what some cultures needed (Leininger, 1988, 1995, 2006). Some nurses became excited and developed creative ways to use transcultural nursing knowledge and skills in community contexts. They became firm advocates of transcultural nursing and encouraged other nurses to learn how to care for diverse cultures in their community experiences.

What are some of the major reasons why transcultural nursing is important today? Which transcultural nursing concepts, principles, and research findings can help community nurses? First, any human community has people who are born, live, become ill or maintain health, and die within a community perspective (Leininger, 1981, 1988, 1995, 2006). Humans are culturally rooted, acting and making decisions daily that are based on largely unspoken values, beliefs, and cultural community lifeways (Leininger, 1970, 1978). Moreover, most cultures have beliefs about the way they prefer caregivers to care for them. They have ideas that certain decisions and actions can lead to their health and well-being or help them face illnesses, disabilities, and death. Such community beliefs and expectations are extremely important to families and individuals. Although individuals or families may not always be willing to talk openly or directly with the nurses, their expectations still exist.

As a nurse enters the home of an individual or a family, the people remain alert to see whether he or she will be responsive to their cultural beliefs, values, mannerisms, dress, language, and symbols. For example, a community nurse who was knowledgeable about Vietnamese culture allowed a young Vietnamese mother to demonstrate how she cared for her infant's upper respiratory infection. The nurse was readily accepted by the mother, the family, and the community because she understood and respected traditional Vietnamese infant care.

People do not always consciously make known their cultural values, beliefs, and lifeways to others in daily conversations. However, if important cultural practices are violated or neglected, they will often speak out. They often go back to their cultural history to support their actions and beliefs and may say things like, "Well, it has always been this way" or "This is how we have always believed and lived and my grandparents have lived that way, too." Sometimes, a nurse may not like to be told how to do things by nonprofessionals and may view the family as uncooperative, resistant, or difficult to work with when they fail to respond to the nurse's expectations. When resistance is met, the nurse should stop,

 **Research Alert**

This research investigated the nature, relationships, and implications of metaphor in the expressions of good and evil in Chinese, Vietnamese, Ethiopian, Somali, French, and English. A grounded theory research method was used in the collection of metaphoric expressions of good and evil from study participants who were fluent in both their native languages and English. The researcher, by means of dialogue and open-ended interviews with the study participants, examined both the literal and idiomatic meanings of these expressions.

From this examination, the expressions were categorized based on the underlying conceptual metaphor. The parts of the underlying metaphor were compared and contrasted with selected examples in each language group. Following this analysis, the researcher discussed the implications for moral, cognitive, and curriculum theories, which were justified based on the study results.

The results support a theory of universal moral conceptualization, with human well-being as the guiding principle for metaphoric representation of good and evil. The results also suggest a paired structure to human mental operations, which link the imagination and the reason as an interdependent dynamic of cognition. From the cognitive theory flows a curriculum theory, which makes inclusion of both the imagination and the reason imperative to moral teaching that is neither trivial nor arbitrary.

*Source:* Dunlap, R. K. (2005). *Common minds: A study of metaphors of good and evil across selected languages,* unpublished dissertation, Belmont College.

**❝** *It is utterly exhausting being Black in America—physically, mentally, and emotionally. While many minority groups and women feel similar stress, there is no respite or escape from your badge of color.* **❞**

—Marian Wright Edelman

*Source:* Edelman, M. W. (1992). *The measure of our success. A letter to my children and yours.* Boston: Beacon Press.

listen, and learn from the people who understand cultural care decisions and actions. There are many examples of why families of specific cultural backgrounds are not willing to yield to an outsider's views. Transcultural nursing gives active and serious attention to the people's views, while the professional's views are secondary.

Integrating transcultural knowledge and skills into community nursing is related to the principle that cultures have a right to have their cultural values known, respected, and appropriately used in nursing and related health care services (Leininger, 1970, 1988, 1995, 2006). Humans have a right to physical and psychological health care, and their cultural care needs should be treated with equal importance because cultural factors greatly influence how people act, feel, and perceive their environment. However, the physical and mental needs of patients are generally emphasized more in nursing education and practice than the cultural needs. A person's culture often receives limited attention or is avoided by nurses because they do not understand it. Community nurses who have been oriented to transcultural nursing are alert to cultural care factors and use specific strategies and principles to help those of different cultural backgrounds living in a community. Cultural care needs are emphasized, and physical and emotional needs are met within a cultural perspective (Leininger, 1978, 1996).

*Culturally congruent care* provides culture-specific care decisions and actions for therapeutic benefits that fit with the cultural needs and expectations of patients. Transcultural nursing knowledge can assist nurses in providing culturally congruent care for individuals and families in different communities. Nurses must remain cognizant of culture-specific care that is compatible with the values and beliefs of individual cultures. This can be accomplished by being attentive to subtle differences and similarities among cultures and recognizing care differences and similarities among patients in various living or working contexts. Maintaining a comparative perspective and not assuming all cultures are alike is important. There often is a tendency to label and lump all members of a particular culture together when considering health care needs. However, there is great variability between and within cultures and among individuals and families, and these differences must be considered when providing culture-specific and culturally congruent care. To assume that all people in a particular culture are the same is stereotyping and leads to negative outcomes. For example, to avoid stereotyping, one should not assume that all Chinese men are stoic and fit clearly into one particular behavior style. Instead, it is recommended that one observe the actual behaviors and subtle impressions that do not place the Chinese man in a rigid position at all times.

Providing culturally based community caring is directly related to the nurse's intent or desire to heal patients, prevent unnecessary illnesses, and support people in achieving their daily living goals and needs. It is impossible to achieve such important goals unless the nurse knows and practices holistic culturally based care. Holistic culturally based care includes assessing the influences of religion, politics, technology,

### Application to Practice

As a community health nurse you are making home visits twice a week to Mrs. Mendoza, who lives in a rural community. Mrs. Mendoza is an 82-year-old Mexican American woman with a below-the-knee amputation of her left leg related to her diabetes mellitus. She lives with her 50-year-old son and two teenage grandsons. It is difficult to communicate with Mrs. Mendoza or to do any diabetic teaching because you do not speak Spanish and no one in the Mendoza household speaks English. During your first five visits, the neighbor who lives down the road was willing to come to Mrs. Mendoza's house during your visits to serve as your interpreter. However, on your sixth visit, you discover that the neighbor is not at home. Because you are unable to communicate with Mrs. Mendoza, you go to each of her neighbors' houses looking for someone who can speak English but find none of them at home. Frustrated and behind schedule, you return to Mrs. Mendoza's house to learn that her son, who has been at home during all of your visits, is able to speak English fluently.

1. How do you feel when you learn that Mrs. Mendoza's son can speak English?
2. Why do you think he did not tell you he could speak English earlier?
3. What could you have done to make the situation different?

**ff***Color is what you put on your parachute when you are looking for a new path in life.***JJ**

—Richard Bolles

How does this quote relate to cultural diversity?

### NOTE THIS!

Ninety-three percent of children whose family income is $75,000 or more per year have computers in their homes. Only 32% of children have computers at home when the family income is less than $20,000 per year. A white child in a poor family is four times more likely to have Internet access than black or Latino children in poor families (Statistical Abstracts, 2002).

### THINK ABOUT THIS

While the creative implications of diversity are endless, reactions to those who are different have included fear, hatred, and war in many parts of the world. International public health workers that live and work in countries in conflict face unprecedented challenges in serving as the honest "cultural" brokers between factions unable to view diversity as a source of strength, rather than as a limitation. This is especially critical in primary health care, where health professionals attempt to stimulate governments and communities to implement primary health care strategies. Health workers must examine their own fears, prejudices, and work to strengthen especially the family, in coming to terms with the reality of an increasingly missed and diverse world.
—Marie Farrell, Ed.D., RN, MPH, past World Health Organization for European Regional Advisor for Nursing, Midwifery, and Social Work Services

*Source*: Farrell, M. (1994). Celebrating our diversity. *Community Health, 17*(2), 10–14.

education, kinship (family), and specific cultural values and beliefs within the patient's own environment. All these factors can and do influence the patient's way of living and responding to nursing care. The theory of culture care diversity and universality provides this holistic, yet specific, care perspective to heal and help people in congruent or meaningful ways. Patients have a right to have these diverse factors influencing their well-being understood and respected by health care providers. For example, if a nurse fails to explore the social and religious concerns of a Mexican American patient's family, the patient might report that he or she received no nursing care at all.

Health care in the future will become more community focused and will emphasize maintaining health and preventing as well as treating illnesses. As the largest group of health care providers, nurses will be extremely important in providing care to various cultural groups. The ways in which different cultures prevent illnesses and maintain health will be a major focus of community health nursing in the twenty-first century and beyond. The community will be recognized as the natural and familiar context for all human caring and health services, becoming the dominant mode over hospital care by the year 2010 (Leininger, 1995, 1997b, 2006). Hospital services will decrease and will largely focus on treating special diseases, chronic illnesses, and acute emergencies with costly high-tech equipment. Patients from various cultural groups will have more power in regulating health care as they gain cultural strength and visibility.

Providing transcultural community-based and community-focused care helps professional nurses gain satisfaction and rewards from their important nursing contributions to society. As community nurses incorporate transcultural nursing into their work roles, the public will more easily recognize their significant and unique contributions. Traditional community and public health principles blended with transcultural nursing principles will take on new meaning and relevance in growing multicultural communities (DeSantis, 1997; Horn, 1979; Leininger, 1988; Luna, 1998; Shapiro, Miller, & White, 2006).

> **❝** *Culturally competent care is both a message and a frame for patient care delivery. It is a concept which respects and engages people within the context of individual lifestyles, cultural heritages, and ethnic pride.* **❞**
>
> —Deborah Washington, MSN, RN, Director of Diversity, Patient Care Services, Massachusetts General Hospital, Boston

*Source:* MGH Patient Care Services. (1997). *Caring Headlines, 3*(21), 4.

## Scope of Transcultural Nursing Cultures

There are various types and sizes of community cultures. Some communities are very large (macroculture) and others are considerably smaller (microculture) (see the figure above). Nurses should make an effort to grasp the nature and scope of the communities in which they are working and be aware of the different microcultures and macrocultures that exist within a particular environment.

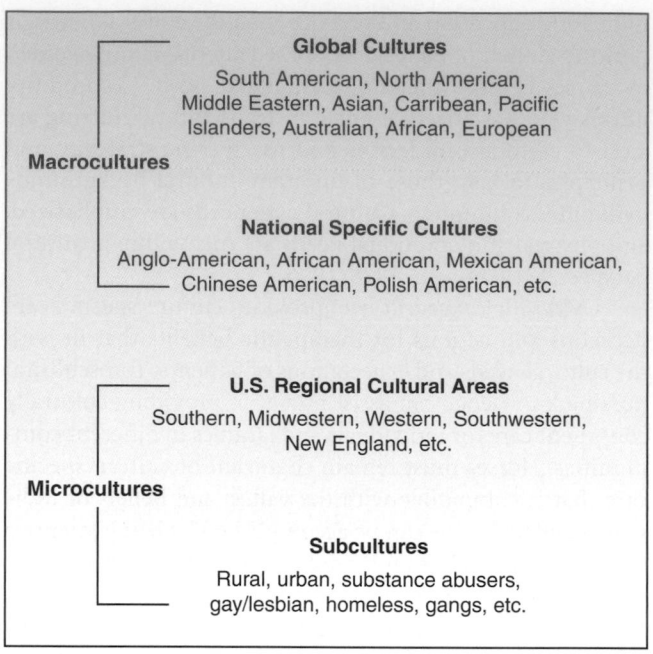

**Macrocultures**

**Global Cultures**
South American, North American, Middle Eastern, Asian, Carribean, Pacific Islanders, Australian, African, European

**National Specific Cultures**
Anglo-American, African American, Mexican American, Chinese American, Polish American, etc.

**Microcultures**

**U.S. Regional Cultural Areas**
Southern, Midwestern, Western, Southwestern, New England, etc.

**Subcultures**
Rural, urban, substance abusers, gay/lesbian, homeless, gangs, etc.

Scope of transcultural nursing cultures

## Transcultural Nursing Principles

One of the most important goals of transcultural nursing is to enter the patient's world and assist in therapeutic and beneficial ways. Providing culturally congruent care to people in a community first necessitates a careful assessment of the cultural needs of the people. After analyzing the cultural assessment data, the nurse should use transcultural principles, concepts, and research to develop and implement a culturally congruent plan of care. Working with different cultures requires that the nurse have "holding" (prelearned) knowledge about specific cultures. It is important that the nurse be able to carefully blend his or her *etic* (or professional knowledge) with the patient's *emic* (or traditional and folk knowledge). These two categories of knowledge sometimes come together, but great discrepancies can exist and need to be resolved for the safety and health of the patient. Rather than focus on medical treatments that may not fit the cultural needs of patients and may be useless or even detrimental, transcultural nursing focuses more on the information, beliefs, and practices of those being treated. Patients expect that their traditional beliefs and practices will be respected and that appropriate rituals will be used to assist them in recovery or death within their cultural environment.

 **ENVIRONMENTAL CONNECTION**

Where we live shapes our culture in ways that are seldom noticed. For example, people who live in tropical climates often express their culture through colorful clothing, art, and architecture that reflects warmth and promotes cooling.

## BOX 10-2

### Transcultural Nursing Principles

1. All human cultures have diverse living, caring, and healing modes that nurses need to study and understand to work effectively with people of different cultures.
2. Care is a basic human need, and it is the essence and dominant focus of the nursing profession.
3. Understanding one's own culture is the first essential expectation to understand other cultures or subcultures.
4. People have the right to have their cultural values known, respected, understood, and used appropriately in nursing and health care services.
5. Transcultural nursing is concerned with the comparative values, beliefs, and practices of specific cultures to provide meaningful, safe, and specific health care practices.
6. Nurses use humanistic and scientific cultural care knowledge as they provide care to different cultures. Humanistic care aspects make people remain human, and scientific research findings about cultures and care guide nurses' decisions and actions.
7. Understanding culture care differences and similarities enables the nurse to respect patients and assist them to grow, function, maintain their well-being or health, and prevent illnesses and premature death.
8. Willingness to enter the patient's world and become an active and interested participant is essential in maintaining effective nurse–patient or nurse–family relationships.
9. Listening, respecting, and being attentive to what patients of different cultures say or do are essential to understanding them and providing meaningful and beneficial nursing services.
10. A nurse's ability to speak the patient's cultural language opens the door to understanding what the patient is seeking or experiencing.
11. If the patient's cultural lifeways, values, and caring expressions do not immediately "make sense," the nurse must continue to make an effort to understand them.
12. In every culture, care, healing, and health practices are greatly influenced by patients' worldviews, environmental context, and social structure features (including the religious or spiritual beliefs, kinship ties, political–legal views, economic aspects, technologies, and specific cultural historical values).
13. Every culture usually has two major types of health care systems: generic (indigenous, traditional, folk) and professional (learned in schools). Nurses need to understand both to provide culturally congruent care.
14. Cultures have their own culturally defined ways to promote and maintain health, face death, and deal with unfavorable sociocultural conditions and crises.
15. Health care practices in Western and non-Western cultures have major differences that need to be understood when planning and providing care to patients.

*Source*: Leininger, 1995, 2006.

---

Therefore, when possible, culturally appropriate interventions should be the preferred treatment, which may create a challenge for health care professionals. Understanding general transcultural nursing principles can help nurses bridge the gap between emic and etic points of view (Box 10-2).

## Transcultural Concepts

To understand transcultural nursing as used within community nursing contexts, knowledge of several major concepts is essential. Some of these concepts come from anthropology, but others have been developed as basic transcultural nursing concepts. Although a few basic definitions were presented at the beginning of this chapter, there are some that merit further clarification with clinical examples to illustrate them.

Because an important goal of transcultural nursing is to provide culturally competent care, it needs to be considered at the outset. **Culturally competent care** refers to the use of culturally based knowledge in creative, congruent, and meaningful ways to provide beneficial and satisfying health care to diverse cultures. As nurses work with other cultures, they combine their patients' traditional knowledge with their own professional nursing knowledge to provide meaningful, safe, and responsible care. The nursing interventions must

### MEDIA MOMENT

**Selected Films About Culture**

| Film | Culture |
| --- | --- |
| *The Milagro Beanfield War* | Mexican |
| *Passion Fish* | Louisiana Cajun |
| *Belizaire the Cajun* | Louisiana Cajun |
| *Sherman's March* | Southern United States |
| *To Kill a Mockingbird* | Southern United States |
| *Crimes of the Heart* | Southern United States |
| *Do the Right Thing* | African American |
| *The Color Purple* | African American |
| *The Brothers McMullen* | Irish American |
| *Witness* | Amish |
| *Divine Secrets of the Ya Ya Sisterhood* | Southern United States |
| *Spanglish* | Mexican American |
| *A Love Song for Bobby Long* | Southern United States |
| *Barbershop* | African American |
| *Woman, Thou Art Loosed* | African American |
| *The Untold Story of Emmett Louis Till* | African American |
| *The Human Stain* | African American |

fit, or be reasonably tailored to incorporate, cultural values, beliefs, and practices to be effective and acceptable to the people. Nurses should encourage all members of the health care team to consider the cultural values of their patients when making decisions related to their health care.

The concept of cultural values is critical in health care because all cultures want their values and beliefs respected and upheld. **Cultural values** are the powerful directive forces that give order and meaning to why people think, act, and make decisions. For example, the extended family of an African American pregnant woman living in the rural South told the visiting nurse about their culture and what they valued. Several of the women said, "We value our greens, soul food, peas, pork, and special pregnancy foods." These mothers made clear the cultural values that needed to be considered by the nurse for the family's general nutrition and for the mother during pregnancy. The foods were viewed as essential for their health care, so the nurse included as many of these foods as possible in the nutritional plan for the pregnant mother, making modifications only where necessary.

Two concepts that are extremely helpful to nurses are emic and etic views. **Emic view** refers to what the local people or the "insiders" hold as important to know and believe. For example, a Philippine elderly mother and family believe that when the grandmother gets old, she should not live in a nursing home. Instead, they hold the emic view that the sons, daughters, and grandchildren should care for their elders. This emic or local Philippine view is different from Anglo-American families, who often believe that their elders will probably go to a nursing home for care and protection.

**Etic view** refers to an external or outsider's view of a culture. For example, many Anglo-American nurses believe that when Philippine elders reach about 80 years old, they should consider being placed in a nursing home so that they will not be a burden to other family members. This etic or outsider's view is very different from what the Philippine families value, wanting their elders to be cared for by family members in their homes and not in institutions such as nursing homes. The Philippine emic view and the Anglo-American nurses' etic view are very different and can often be a source of cultural conflicts and stresses.

Generic and professional care are related to emic and etic views. **Generic care** is the folk, naturalistic, or traditional health practices that cultures have known and used over time. In contrast, **professional care** is what is learned from nursing, medicine, and other health care education programs. Generic and professional care practices often have many differences that must be recognized and addressed. For example, several Mexican American families visited by a community health nurse wanted the nurse to know and integrate their generic (folk or naturalistic) care with the professional nursing care. They also wanted the community nurse to acknowledge that Mexican fathers are the ones responsible for major family decisions, such as signing treatment consents for family members. Respecting these important generic or folk family considerations was essential for the nurse to provide culturally congruent care.

Another set of closely related concepts is ethnocentrism and cultural imposition. **Ethnocentrism** refers to the belief that one's own ways are the best, most superior, or preferred ways of acting, believing, or valuing something. An example of this concept is Anglo-American nurses who contend that managed care is the best way to provide health services. Nursing students may also be ethnocentric, believing that faculty lectures are the best way to help students learn about nursing and, therefore, rejecting other methods of teaching. Ethnocentrism takes a strong position that there is only one "right" way to do things.

**Cultural imposition** refers to one group of people forcing their cultural beliefs, values, and patterns of behavior on others as a result of ethnocentrism, cultural biases, ignorance, or various other reasons. An example is an Anglo-American nurse who imposes her beliefs that women should be equal partners with their husbands in making health care decisions for the family on a Mexican American mother. This can create conflict within the family, causing difficulty for the woman and possibly leading to the family's total rejection of the nurse's care. Cultural imposition practices are one of the most common nursing care problems encountered with patients from different cultures.

**Cultural ignorance** refers to insufficient knowledge about a specific culture to provide safe and meaningful care. This chapter includes many examples of cultural ignorance as a major problem in nursing practices. Lack of knowledge often leads to destructive care practices and nontherapeutic outcomes for patients.

**Cultural bias** refers to a strong position that all decisions must be based on one's own values and beliefs. For example, nurses who firmly value nursing homes at the end of life, with no other alternative plan, can be considered culturally biased. It is a largely one-sided, rigid, and persistent stance. If nurses are not able to recognize and understand their cultural biases, these biases can greatly interfere with patients' choices, interests, and even therapeutic care practices. Both nurses and patients may have biases that should be recognized and discussed so that acceptable compromises can be reached.

**Cultural shock** refers to a state of being disoriented or unable to respond appropriately to a situation or person because of complete strangeness or unfamiliarity with what

---

### ⚒ ETHICAL CONNECTION

Gay children, especially teenage males, are committing suicide in unprecedented numbers. When you think of culture, does your idea about being a "culture" include people who have different sexual orientations, such as lesbianism, homosexuality, and bisexuality? Why or why not? What ethical implications do our ideas about what is and what is *not* a culture affect our ability to provide care for all?

was seen or experienced. This concept is often seen between nurses and patients from different cultures. For example, a community nurse entered the home of a very poor Native American family and found there were six children (ages 3 to 10 years) sleeping on the floor with dirty blankets. The nurse also discovered that the children ate only bread and beans each day and that the house was very dirty. The nurse was shocked by the conditions and did not know what to say or do, so she left the home. She reported that she found an "unbelievable home situation" and became helpless and confused. Because of her cultural shock, she was not able to assess the overall health of the children or work with the family to meet their health care needs.

**Cultural pain** refers to the considerable discomfort, suffering, or unfavorable response experienced by an individual or group belonging to a particular culture when insulting and offensive comments are made by an outsider. Cultural pain is more common than realized among health personnel (Leininger, 1997a). For example, an African American family experienced cultural pain when an Asian American community health nurse showed facial disgust when she saw the family eating "chitlins" (choice intestinal animal products). The nurse emphatically said, "That food is not good for you and you should not be eating such food." She also referred to the family as a "Negro" family, which was most offensive to them. As a consequence, the African American family experienced cultural pain from the nurse's gestures and comments.

**Cultural variation** refers to the slight or marked variability among or between cultures that makes them unique or different. This variability is often due to differences between traditional and nontraditional lifeways over time. For example, Mexicans, Puerto Ricans, and Cubans show slight or major cultural variability in beliefs and lifeways because of different historical and cultural backgrounds, yet some similarities in language, values, and beliefs have been identi-

fied that result in them being known collectively as Hispanics or Latinos. Likewise, many Native Americans show cultural variability among the nearly 540 Native American nations in the United States. Nurses need to learn about variations between and among cultures and if there are changes in these cultures over time.

**Cultural barriers** refer to obstacles that interfere with cultures accessing or achieving their desired goals or opportunities. This concept was evident when an Anglo-American community nurse always made an appointment to care for an Arab-Muslim family at noon, which was their prayer time. The nurse insisted that the family members see her at noon, when it was convenient for her to give a special medication and check the father's blood pressure. Coming at noon was a culture barrier to the Arab-Muslim family because it is their prayer time, so they refused the community nurse's services.

**Stereotyping** refers to putting a label on members of a culture or subculture that reflects fixed characteristics perceived as belonging to that particular group without considering individual or group differences or cultural variability. For example, a nurse may stereotype Native Americans as "lazy and unreliable alcoholics" or label Vietnamese as "passive, unwilling to learn English, and too difficult to understand and help." Anglo-American patients may be labeled as "pushy, selfish, and materialistic." Such rigid stereotyping statements are imprecise and crude labels that cause cultural pain and inaccurate assessments. Stereotypes are usually negative, but positive generalizations may also be harmful. For example, some nurses may assume that all Asian Americans are high achievers or that all Jewish people are wealthy. All professional nurses should be keenly aware of stereotyping to avoid its potentially negative consequences.

**Culture bound** refers to specific care, health, and illness conditions that are unique or particular to a culture and often exist within a specific geographic area. For example, Kuru is a condition observed in the Eastern Highlands of New Guinea. It is culture bound and unique to the geographic area and female gender (Leininger, 1995). Some New Guinea women who are pregnant become weak and anorexic and die within 9 to 10 months. Other examples of cultural-bound conditions, such as Arctic hysteria, running amok, *susto*, and mushroom madness, are found with specific cultures in certain geographic areas. Often, there may be no medical cure, but nursing care is essential.

**Cultural backlash** is a phenomenon that occurs when a culture has been "bought" or encouraged to use another culture's values, material goods, beliefs, and lifeways. This often proves to be unsuitable and leads to serious unfavorable outcomes. Taking on another culture's values or material goods leads to anger and disappointment because the other ideas or things do not fit the culture. For example, using self-care theory and practices in a non-Western culture may contradict cultural beliefs and lifeways. Western nursing faculty or practitioners may impose their practices on a non-Western culture, but the ideas and practices are not congruent with the cultural lifeways. As a consequence, non-Western nurses or patients may turn against the Western nurses as a cultural backlash for imposing their ideas or values on them. Cultural ignorance, cultural imposition, and culturally imperialistic behavior are often the factors contributing to cultural backlash. This is a serious and growing problem in cultural education as well as in nursing practice and exchange.

**Immigrants** and **refugees** are two different groups of people who are often confused with each other. An immigrant is a person who voluntarily chooses to come to another country for various reasons, which may include seeking new opportunities for employment. For example, Europeans immigrated to America in the early colonial days and started life anew. Today thousands of immigrants continue to come to the United States each year. In contrast, refugees are people who have been suddenly forced to leave their homeland and come to another country for survival because of political oppression, social injustices, destructive war conditions, or other threatening circumstances. For example, in the 1970s and 1980s, many Vietnamese, Cambodians, and Philippines left their homeland to escape oppressive war forces and/or because they were suddenly driven out of their country (Leininger, 1995). Nurses need to understand the historical shifts of different immigrants and refugees because their care and health needs are different. The community nurse is expected to understand and care for these strangers almost overnight as newcomers to the community.

Basic transcultural nursing ideas should be used to guide community nurses in their assessment and understanding of families and individuals from diverse cultures. All nurses should understand these fundamental concepts before beginning to work in the community so that they can avoid cultural clashes, cultural imposition, and other potentially negative outcomes with patients. It is a nurse's ethical and moral responsibility to study transcultural nursing principles before working with patients of diverse cultures and not to assume one can "luck it out" (Leininger, 1990). Self-awareness, along with the use of transcultural knowledge, can lead to successful and effective culturally congruent nursing care.

**A Good Read**

## The Culture of Fear: Why Americans Are Afraid of the Wrong Things (2000)

*By Barry Glasner, New York: Basic Books.*

Americans are afraid of many things in our culture that shouldn't frighten us, according to Barry Glasner. In this book, which is devoted to challenging conventional wisdom, Glasner critically examines such issues as violence in schools, breast cancer, environmental threats, and the influence of popular media on what we "think is true."

 NOTE THIS!

In Japan, a bow is part of a typical greeting. The depth of the bow is determined by how much respect the person bowing wishes to convey.

## Leininger's Theory of Culture Care Diversity and Universality

### ■ Development of the Theory

The development of the theory of culture care diversity and universality began in the mid-1950s in the search for a body of transcultural nursing knowledge to guide nursing decisions and actions in the care of the culturally different (Lei-ninger, 1991, 1995, 2006). As in any discipline or profession, theories are used to discover, explain, predict, and generate new knowledge or reaffirm existing knowledge. Without theories, nursing would have no scientific way to explain or interpret what happens and why. Nursing theories and clinical practices are interdependent because clinical practices need theories, and theories use clinical data to examine outcomes. These ideas led to the development of the theory of culture care diversity and universality as the scientific base for the substantive body of knowledge known as transcultural nursing (Leininger, 1970, 1991, 1995, 2006).

Interestingly, in the 1950s, there were virtually no nursing theories, and none that were focused on culture and caring phenomena. In that era nurses were preoccupied in meeting the post–World War II medical disease symptoms and treatment regimes prescribed by physicians. Very few nurses were interested in developing nursing theories to advance nursing knowledge. There were nurses interested in research, borrowing research methods from other disciplines, but few were thinking about nursing theories and nursing research methods that would focus on specific culture care phenomena. There was a need to focus on care as the essence of nursing with a transcultural nursing perspective and

*Got an Alternative?*

A Mexican American woman ties a good-luck talisman around her newborn baby's neck to protect her from "mal ojo," or bad eye. How would you assess this cultural practice?

to develop a theory that (1) focused on culture and caring, (2) was a holistic theory that would include the total human being in a cultural context, (3) would generate practical knowledge to guide nursing care decisions and practices related to specific cultures, and (4) would provide a new kind of comparative nursing care that would be meaningful to different cultures and have healing or beneficial outcomes (Leininger, 1991, 1995, 2006).

The theory of culture care diversity and universality was the first nursing theory to focus on culture and care in different cultures with multiple holistic factors influencing care (Leininger, 1991). The theory helps nurses discover and use culture care findings in community-based practices in primary, secondary, or tertiary care settings. It is useful in community nursing because it is practical and comprehensive regarding culture and care aspects. It is a theory that can be used with individual cultures or with several cultures, depending on the nurse's practice or research interests. In using the theory, nurses search for care meanings that can be used to provide culturally congruent care.

In developing the theory, it was assumed that there were cultural differences (diversities) as well as some universals (commonalities) that could be found in different cultures in which nurses were expected to provide care. It was further assumed that factors such as worldview and social structure features (e.g., religion and spirituality, kinship, philosophy of life, economics, politics, education, technology, and specific cultural values, beliefs, and lifeways) would significantly influence culture and care in different environmental contexts. In addition, transcultural nursing care would be influenced by both generic (folk or local) and professional care practices. Finally, there would be three major modes to guide cultural care decisions and actions: (1) culture care preservation or maintenance, (2) culture care accommodation or negotiation, and (3) culture care structuring or repatterning (Leininger, 1991).

*❝The issue will not be that we are diverse; it will be what we do with our diversity that is important.❞*

—Dr. Marie Farrell

## Goal of the Theory

The goal of the theory is to discover ways to provide culturally congruent and responsible transcultural nursing care (Leininger, 1991, 1995, 2006). The purpose of the theory is to discover, document, explain, and interpret culturally congruent care with individuals or groups under study (Leininger, 1991). The theory provides research findings that are tailored to meet the patients' holistic cultural needs and ex-

pectations. As a new theory, it brought together synthesized research knowledge of culture care that had not been previously discovered and had been neglected in nursing practice. Many cultures are pleased to learn that their cultural values and beliefs are used in transcultural nursing.

## Assumptions of Theory

To fully understand the theory and its relationship to transcultural community-based nursing, the following assumptions and premises that guide nurses in the use of the theory must be examined. They are specifically focused on community-based transcultural nursing care to help community nurses use the assumptions in meaningful ways (Leininger, 1991).

1. Care is the essence and the central dominant, distinct, and unifying focus of nursing.
2. Humanistic and scientific care is essential for human growth, well-being, health, survival, and the ability to face death and disabilities.
3. Care (caring) is essential to curing or healing, for there can be no curing without caring. (This assumption was held to have profound relevance worldwide.)
4. Culture care is the synthesis of two major constructs that guide the researcher to discover, explain, and account for health, well-being, care expressions, and other human conditions.
5. Culture care expressions, meanings, patterns, processes, and structural forms are diverse but some commonalities (universalities) exist among and between cultures.
6. Culture care values, beliefs, and practices are influenced by and embedded in the worldview, social structure factors (e.g., religion, philosophy of life, kinship, politics, economics, education, technology, and cultural values), and the ethnohistorical and environmental contexts.
7. Every culture has generic (lay, folk, naturalistic; mainly emic) and usually some professional (etic) care to be discovered and used for culturally congruent care practices.
8. Culturally congruent and therapeutic care occurs when culture care values, beliefs, expressions, and patterns are explicitly known and used appropriately, sensitively, and meaningfully with people of diverse or similar cultures.
9. Leininger's three theoretical modes of care offer new, creative, and different therapeutic ways to help people of diverse cultures.
10. Qualitative research paradigmatic methods offer important means to discover largely embedded, covert, epistemic, and ontological culture care knowledge and practices.
11. Transcultural nursing is a discipline with a body of knowledge and practices to attain and maintain the goal of culturally congruent care for health and well-being.

*❝In a real sense all life is interrelated. All men are caught in an inescapable network of mutuality, tied in a single garment of destiny.❞*

—Martin Luther King, Jr.

## ■ The Sunrise Model: A Visual Guide for the Theory

The sunrise model was developed to visualize the different dimensions of the theory as nurses study different cultures (see the figure on page 239) (Leininger, 1991, 1995, 2006). Nurses can use this conceptual model to see the different areas that need to be examined in assessing and planning care for patients of different cultures. Although the model is *not* the theory, it is a valuable guide to grasp the holistic aspects of humans living in a particular culture. This model can be used by community nurses to assess the cultural care factors of patients (individuals and groups, especially families) to get a holistic or complete picture of the patient's cultural world. By using this model, nurses avoid partial or incomplete assessments that fail to know the patients and their total reality in a cultural context. Patients who have had nurses who used this model often say, "At last, nurses are looking at my total life and not just my body, diseases, emotional symptoms, or other pieces of me." Patients want nurses to know what guides their daily living along with their cultural values, beliefs, and practices.

By using the sunrise model, nurses remain focused on the theory to identify differences and similarities of care dimensions as expressed and practiced in the culture. Whether working with individuals, families, or groups, nurses should be aware that the traditional physical, psychological, and social components of care are not specifically identified in the sunrise model because these factors are embedded within the social structure and worldview and are included in both

### Research Alert

the generic and professional aspects of care. Moreover, gender, class, sexual orientation, and other factors are likewise an integral part of the areas identified in the model, but they are not specifically labeled. The environmental, historical, and language contextual aspects are given attention in the model as they provide holistic ideas relative to community-based transcultural nursing and health practices.

Community nurses generally use this model to assess patients' needs. Nurses can start anywhere in the model with what patients want to talk about. It is the patients or families who take the lead to tell their health or illness story. The nurse is expected to follow their lead. In so doing, the nurse gets access to emic patient information and does not push for etic data or professional information alone. As the nurse assesses the patient, the goal is to enter the world of the patient rather than the world of the nurse. This allows the patient to tell his or her story and explain how health, illness, and care are known to him or her. This ethnonursing, people-centered approach has been developed to characterize transcultural nursing as an approach truly interested in discovering the person's worldview and other aspects influencing one's well-being (Leininger, 1985, 1991, 1995, 2006). It allows the nurse to discover the meaning and experiences of care and health and identify which factors are cultural facilitators or barriers to good health.

The ethno (people) nursing approach to health assessment requires that the nurse understand his or her own culture before trying to discover another culture. If the nurse is not first aware of his or her own culture, then cultural clashes, cultural imposition, and other problems may occur. With this people (ethno) approach, the nurse strives to get the emic or the patient's worldview. The nurse is an active observer of the patients or families in their homes or local environments. This natural context provides rich and accurate data that are usually different from data obtained in an unnatural or unfamiliar environment such as a hospital or clinic. As the nurse actively listens to the patient, he or she becomes attuned to the patient's ways of thinking and knowing. For example, if the patient wants to talk about family and health care, the nurse should pursue this focus because it is of interest to the patient. Gradually, with several visits, the nurse addresses the different dimensions in the sunrise model. If the patient did not address some areas, the nurse carefully asks the patient to "tell me about" these aspects. Initially, patients like to talk about what interests them most or what they are most comfortable talking about. Once a trusting relationship develops, patients will become more comfortable talking about topics that are more sensitive.

Nurses should try to obtain in-depth, rather than superficial, knowledge about patients and work to identify what care factors seem to have the most influence on their health and illness status. This process is done in a co-participant (nurse with patient) way to arrive at accurate assessments or research findings. By constantly reflecting on what is being stated and clarifying the patients' views and experiences using the different dimensions of the sunrise model, nurses

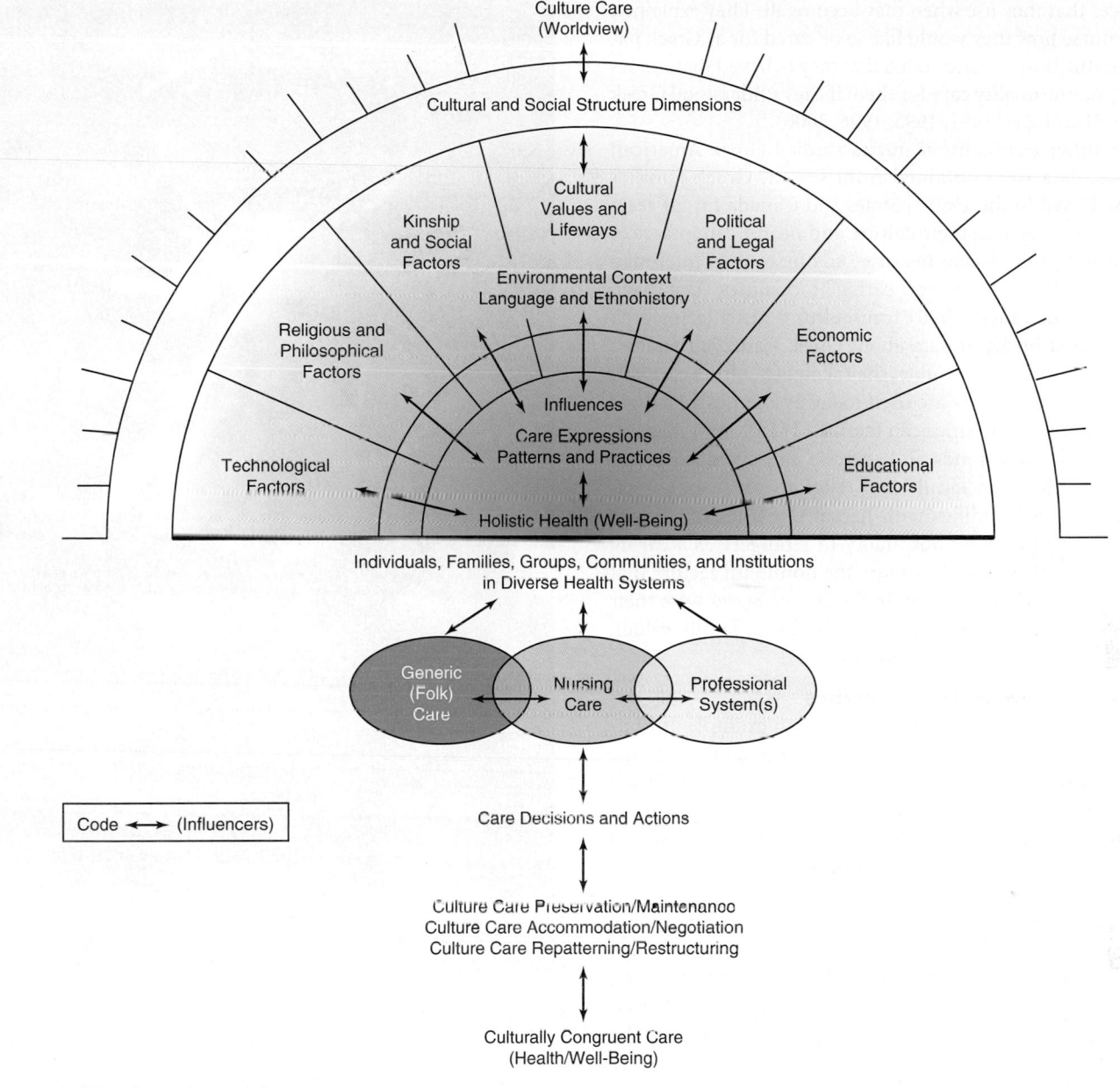

Culture Care
(Worldview)

Cultural and Social Structure Dimensions

Cultural Values and Lifeways

Kinship and Social Factors

Political and Legal Factors

Environmental Context
Language and Ethnohistory

Religious and Philosophical Factors

Economic Factors

Influences

Care Expressions Patterns and Practices

Technological Factors

Educational Factors

Holistic Health (Well-Being)

Individuals, Families, Groups, Communities, and Institutions
in Diverse Health Systems

Generic (Folk) Care

Nursing Care

Professional System(s)

Code ⟷ (Influencers)

Care Decisions and Actions

Culture Care Preservation/Maintenance
Culture Care Accommodation/Negotiation
Culture Care Repatterning/Restructuring

Culturally Congruent Care
(Health/Well-Being)

Leininger's sunrise model

usually discover some entirely new or different knowledge that has not been taught or addressed in nursing textbooks.

## ■ Application of the Theory and Model

### Greek American Families

A Greek American family was very pleased when visited by a nurse in their home because they could share many ideas about their generic herbs (folk practices) and how herbs were used to treat "little or big illnesses." They showed the nurse where the herbs grew in their home environment (backyard) and how and why they used herbs to "keep well." The Greek American family members talked about caring

practices at home (emic) and how different they were from hospital (etic) care. The family said, "We do not like to go to the hospital unless desperately ill because the hospital is a sick place and they use medicines and foods that are not good for us. They do not understand what Greek people need to keep them well." In their kitchen, they showed the nurse what foods they thought were good to eat and shared folk

❝ *Look around you! This is where the path of hatred has brought us.* ❞

—*Pocahontas*

practices that they use when they become ill. They explained to the nurse how they would like to be cared for as Greek patients in the hospital and stated that they believed that nurses could provide quality care for them if they understood Greek culture (Leininger, 1991, 1995, 1996, 2006).

As other transcultural nurses studied Greek American families, data were obtained from several Greek families who had lived in the United States and Canada for 20 years but had never shared their culture and health care practices with health professionals because "no one seemed interested in Greek beliefs, values, and caring" modalities (Leininger, 1991). Rosenbaum's (1990) transcultural nursing research has provided in-depth data about Greek Canadian widows and care. From several studies, the following culture care values were identified that are used today as a guide for nurses in the care of Greek American families: (1) Prevent illnesses with proper Greek foods and exercise and avoid hospitals, (2) keep active with family and religious services, (3) assist other Greek families with herbal remedies to prevent illnesses, and (4) show hospitality to strangers as a caring action. In all these Greek studies, the dominant factors that influenced the Greek families in the United States were their worldview, religion, kinship, specific cultural family values, generic care practices, and ethnohistory.

### Philippine American Families

To get a comparative cultural view, an example of Philippine Americans can be offered. Both Greek and Philippine cultures in the United States are good examples to teach nurses that cultural values and lifeways do not change readily. Nurse researchers studied several Philippine families in an urban context over a 2-year period and discovered culture care meanings and desired actions that should be considered by nurses and other health professionals. The Philippine families had lived in Midwestern, urban America for approximately 20 years, but their traditional cultural values, beliefs, and lifeways were still more apparent than Anglo-American values and lifeways. It was determined that the provision of culturally congruent care for Philippine families should include (1) maintaining smooth relationships with the family (*Pakikisama*), (2) remaining alert to "saving face" by avoiding shame and being demeaning in public talk, (3) showing respect for and deference to authority (especially elders), (4) showing mutual reciprocity by sharing between people (*Utang Na Loob*), (5) knowing how to provide holistic caring practices, (6) demonstrating gentle and tender ways of caring, and (7) remaining pleasant when caring for others, especially family members (Leininger, 1991).

These care meanings fit well with the dominant Philippine cultural values of (1) family unity and closeness, (2) respect for authority and elders, (3) leaving oneself to God (*Behala Na*), (4) use of hot/cold theory in care and health practices, (5) folk foods and care practices, (6) the importance of religion in caring practices (the majority are

This is a traditional Navajo medicine bag used to promote healing and well-being. Each bag is created specifically for the individual and often contains medicinal herbs, semiprecious stones, beading, and animal fetishes.

Roman Catholics), and (7) nurses showing an obligation to family members when caring for them.

Using the sunrise model as a guide, kinship (family and social) ties, religion, cultural values, environment, generic herbs and treatment, and historical factors all need to be considered to get a holistic care perspective. Although the research with the Greek American and Philippine American families identified distinct differences between the two cultures, there were many commonalities, such as an emphasis on religion, family ties, historical factors, generic care, and use of their home environment resources. In working with these two cultures, professional nursing and medical practices were not relied on entirely, but rather the inclusion of generic family care with folk care practices was important to maintain and preserve the families' well-being.

## ■■ CULTURAL CONNECTION

**❝** *I feel as if getting my skin painted gave me an identity; it was about fitting into my own skin. In our caring profession of nursing, will nursing accept me and my tattoos?* **❞**

—Serena Williamson, student nurse

Tattoos are simply symbols. They are along the same lines as stretch marks in childbirth, as reminders of a battle faced, an idea in time, and an immortalized piece of the past.

Barely two months into nursing school, I was warned by the main nurse recruiter of the bigger hospital in town that I would "never work in their facility." Next, a nursing faculty told me that with my visible tattoos, I would never have a job as a professional nurse. Ironically enough, I interviewed with the same recruiter and received a position in the "banned" facility the summer between my junior and senior years of nursing school.

So, I guess you could say I am used to the negative reaction that tattoos elicit. Nurses are not any different from the public; they just have the "professional image" hammer to use.

My professionalism is questioned and denied with one glance at my uncovered, tattooed arm. So I do what many people with tattoos do in these settings: I cover up. Asking people who are not tattooed about tattoos has elicited many interesting responses: "What are you going to do when your skin sags?" "What will your grandchildren think?" Then there are the gender-specific questions: "How do you handle the pain?", "What does your mother/father/boyfriend/aunt think?", and my favorite, "Tattoos on women—well, they are just loose women."

Social stigmas placed on tattoos are simply that—socially created and change as society changes. As we all know, we are taught certain things about certain "groups" and we can accept them without reservation or question, have experiences that confirm or refute the teachings, or never buy into them in the first place.

By the way, my tattoo artist told me he rarely tattoos a biker.

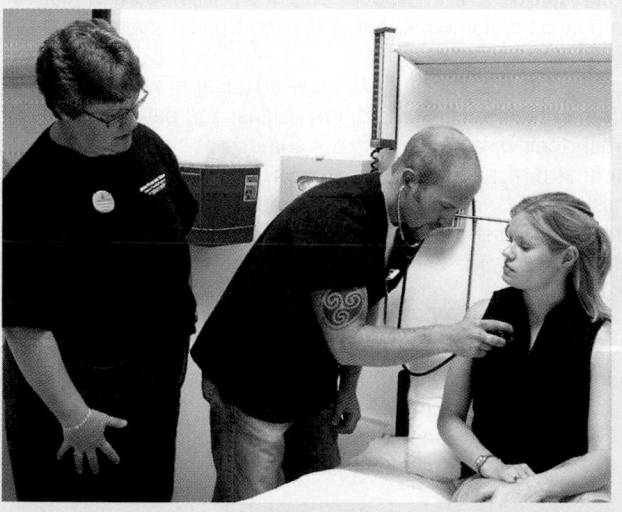

During my obstetrics clinical rotation, I observed in the antepartum clinic that, of the 15 patients we saw that day, 9 had visible tattoos. Maybe this was an atypical clinic, maybe not. Or just maybe, many, if not most, of our hospital patients of the future will have tattoos.

My tattoo symbolizes and is a metaphor of the many parts of my personal struggles and instrumental components of who I am today. The swan is how I see myself now, the ugly duckling who morphed into a "swan"—as a viable and productive member of society: The swan is black to represent my place in my family—forever the black sheep. Tiger lilies are the backdrop of the design: They represent my beloved deceased grandmother, who shaped my whole reality. I remember her yard being a gorgeous field of tiger lilies in the summer.

The most unexpected aspect of my tattoo experience was how it has changed the way I feel about my body. I met with my tattoo artist, Jeremy Justice, and gave him a brief idea of what I had in mind. He drew the tattoo especially for my body and told me that it would not look good on someone without curves. Now every time I look at my back and see how my waist curves in its natural state, I experience contentment. Using my skin as a canvas for the art of my life made me feel like I fit into it.

—Serena Williamson, senior nursing student,
University of Southern Mississippi School
of Nursing, Hattiesburg, Mississippi

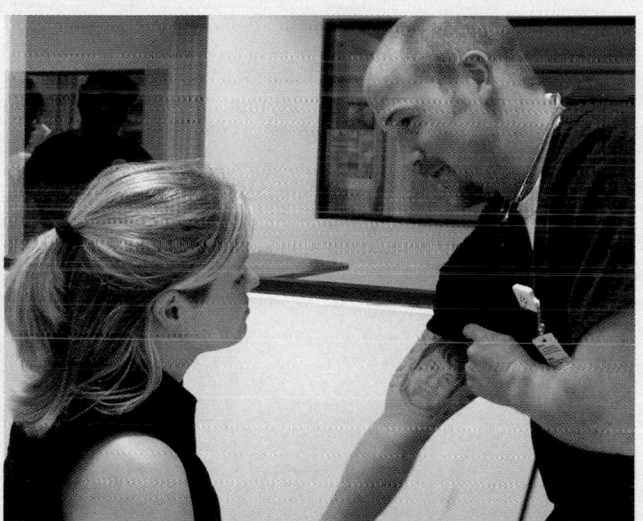

My older brother, Bhron, was 8 years older than me. He died on March 7, 2004, at the age of 29 from a toxic combination of Soma and alcohol, after a night on the town with me. I found him on the kitchen floor around eight the next morning at my parents' house in Meridian, Mississippi.

I was asleep on the couch, and my father awakened me, saying to "come in the kitchen—something is wrong." I walked into the kitchen to find my brother lying on the floor with one leg propped up and his hands over his chest as if he was asleep. My first thoughts were to laugh, because I thought he had just fallen asleep on the floor. However, within a few seconds,

■■ CULTURAL CONNECTION (CONT.)

I realized something was really wrong. His color was pale and his throat looked swollen and engorged. I quickly dropped to my knees and felt for a pulse. As I touched him, he seemed so cold and stiff . . . I knew then he had passed some hours before we found him. At this point, I knew there was nothing to do . . . I struggled with the idea of beginning CPR, but knew there was no point. I looked at my father as he stood next to the refrigerator showing a blank stare and said, "He's gone, Dad" . . . then I asked him to call an ambulance. He didn't respond, so I yelled it again . . . this time he ran to the phone and called 911. As my father dialed the number, he said to me "I've got to tell your mother. . . ."

I asked him not to, not yet . . . but he insisted, dropped the phone, and walked to my mother's bedroom. . . . I grabbed the phone, told the dispatcher the address and what had happened. She asked if I would like to perform CPR as she could instruct and help me to do so. . . . I explained to her that I knew how to perform CPR and that my brother had been dead for a while and that there was no point.

As I was on the phone, I could hear my mother come running up the hallway screaming frantically, "What's going on?" As she turned the corner to the kitchen and saw my brother, I heard the most blood-curdling scream in my life . . . I didn't know what to do. I found myself in a position in which I had to control the situation. My father didn't seem to know what to do; he just stood there with a blank stare. My mother was frantically crying and screaming.

I met the paramedics outside and informed them of the situation as they rushed into the house. Once they got inside to my brother and assessed him, I remember seeing one of the paramedics who had a disappointed and sad look on his face, as he made contact with the others. He shook his head. Soon the police showed up and had to conduct their work.

As all this was going on, I went to sit in another room just to try to calm myself . . . much of this event was a blur . . . family members began showing up . . . after a few hours of blur and

so much emotion and crying, I had to leave . . . and so I did . . . I got in my car and left for Hattiesburg to get away from everything and just sit alone at my apartment. . . .

I got the tattoo of my brother not only in memory, but also as a way for him to "live" through me . . . it has become a way for me to deal with it. I'm often approached about my tattoo and I am automatically inclined to tell the story of how he passed. Rather than carry a picture of my brother in my wallet or put one in my car or room, I have a permanent picture of my brother that is always with me and in a place I can always see.

Along with the portrait of my brother, I decided to expand the ideal of our brotherhood. Bhron and I had a favorite movie that we watched together many times, called the *Boondock Saints*. The movie is about two brothers with matching tattoos (which my brother and I have on our backs), who believe they are divinely obligated to rid their city and the world of sinners and evil.

With this movie in mind and my heritage of Scotch–Irish, I decided to use the first and last sentences of a prayer the two brothers would say to themselves often, after purging the sinners . . . "And shepherds we shall be, for thee my lord for thee . . . in nominee Patris, et Filii, et Spiritus Sancti," which translates to "in the name of the Father, the Son, and the Holy Spirit."

I also found a Celtic trinity symbol, which I thought was perfect with the quote, the movie, my heritage, and my brother. This symbol correlates with many other ancient symbols, including triskeles and mandalas, in which one continuous line forms the symbol and there are no closings to the design. . . . I drew the design with a few personal adjustments and added the quote around the symbol. . . . I also decided to put my brother's name on the back of my arm and add clouds around everything to "finish" the painting around my arm.

My tattoos have brought me praise as well as disapproval. I cannot think of a day that goes by that at least one person has not approached me or commented on my tattoo. Most of the people who make comments are younger and closer to my age. They ask me where I got it, what it means and usually compliment my tattoo. In contrast, I get strange or disappointing looks from members of the older generation. I sometimes feel like an outcast or someone that isn't to be trusted, based on these "disgusted looks."

In the hospital, I have received disapproving looks and comments from co-workers, physicians, and patients. I usually brush their disapproval off, but sometimes find myself taking them as direct and personal attacks. Maybe tattoos aren't what most people would do to commemorate a deceased relative, but to me it seems very appropriate. I try to cover my tattoos while at work or in clinicals for nursing school because I do not want my ideals to affect the persona of my professionalism in a clinical setting. My tattoos are a direct reflection of my life experiences; they are not a reflection of my abilities as a professional nurse. I am very proud of my tattoos—I would never go back and change a thing.

—Noah Seth Jordan, student nurse, University of Southern Mississippi School of Nursing

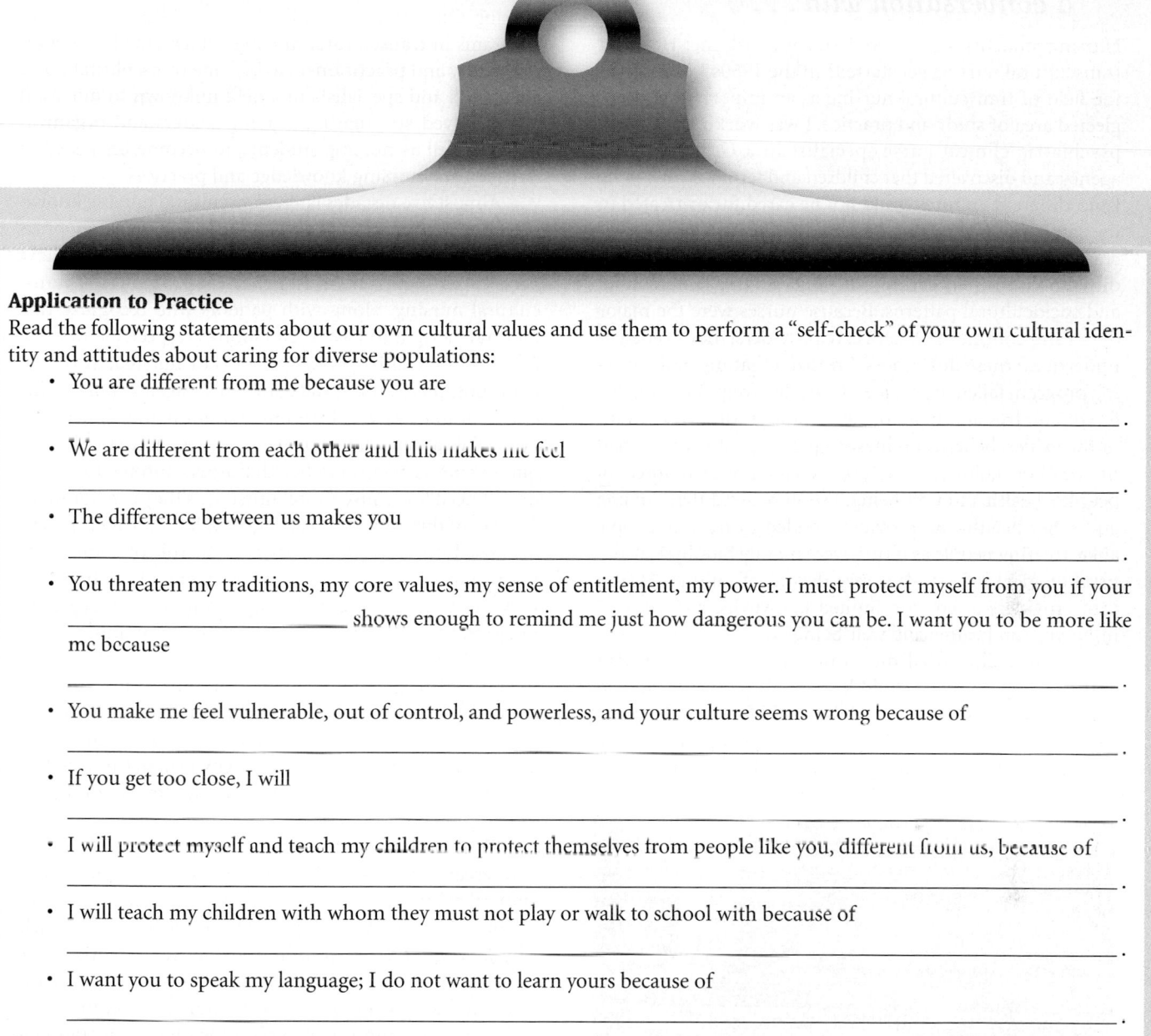

**Application to Practice**

Read the following statements about our own cultural values and use them to perform a "self-check" of your own cultural identity and attitudes about caring for diverse populations:

- You are different from me because you are

_____ .

- We are different from each other and this makes me feel

_____ .

- The difference between us makes you

_____ .

- You threaten my traditions, my core values, my sense of entitlement, my power. I must protect myself from you if your _____ shows enough to remind me just how dangerous you can be. I want you to be more like me because

_____ .

- You make me feel vulnerable, out of control, and powerless, and your culture seems wrong because of

_____ .

- If you get too close, I will

_____ .

- I will protect myself and teach my children to protect themselves from people like you, different from us, because of

_____ .

- I will teach my children with whom they must not play or walk to school with because of

_____ .

- I want you to speak my language; I do not want to learn yours because of

_____ .

*Source*: Davanaugh, G. F. (1991). *Psychiatric mental health nursing*. Philadelphia: Lippincott.

## Conclusion

As we enter the twenty-first century, the theory of culture care diversity and universality has become a major theory to guide nurses in arriving at community-based transcultural nursing. It is the only theory that has an explicit nursing research method designed to tease out relevant and appropriate culture care data. All too often, borrowed theories and methods from other disciplines fail to tap into nursing care phenomena, and the methods often prove to miss the cultural, environmental, and historical factors that hold special meaning and are stated in the people's language modes (Leininger, 1985, 1991, 1995, 2006). Moreover, in the past four decades, transcultural nursing researchers have found that qualitative research methods, such as ethnonursing, provide a wealth of rich culture and care data that are meaningful, specific, and appropriate in providing transcultural nursing care. It should be noted that research studies done in hospitals and clinics tend to reveal less opportunity for cultural informants to be heard or to get care that is culture specific and culturally congruent, unless the nurse is prepared in transcultural nursing and is a strong leader to support patients.

## " a conversation with . . . "

Nursing students and others frequently ask me: How did transcultural nursing get started? In the 1950s I envisioned the field of transcultural nursing as an important and neglected area of study and practice. I was working as a child psychiatric clinical nurse specialist in a child guidance agency and discovered that children and families who come from different cultures could not be cared for or treated in the same way. I observed that children of African, Appalachian, German, Jewish, and other cultures clearly revealed differences in their eating, sleeping, playing, interaction, and sociocultural patterns. Because nurses were the major direct and continuous health care providers, they needed to understand these differences. I realized that my basic nursing program failed to prepare me to effectively deal with different cultures and types of care. I was culturally ignorant of the values, beliefs, and lifestyle practices of people. I had no idea how cultures could exert such a powerful force on people's health and well-being. I soon realized that nursing and other health care providers tended to treat all people alike, treating people as if they were mainly biophysical and psychological beings who were devoid of culture. Health care providers acted with limited knowledge and cultural influences on healing and well-being.

These realities led me to pursue graduate study in anthropology so that I could learn from scholars who had been studying cultures around the world for over 100 years. After learning from the experts in anthropology, I faced the challenge of how to develop the new field of transcultural

nursing. One of the first tasks was to establish courses and programs in transcultural nursing, which entailed preparing faculty and practitioners to become transcultural nurse generalists and specialists in a field unknown to nurses. It also involved stimulating nursing leaders and organizations, as well as nursing students, to become interested in transcultural nursing knowledge and practices.

Almost five decades later, transcultural nursing knowledge is recognized as essential for teaching, research, practice, and consultation worldwide. Nursing students have been the strongest and most persistent promoters of transcultural nursing, along with patients who recognize that they have a right to have their cultures respected and given attention in health services. Schools of nursing, as well as many hospitals, clinics, and community agencies, are giving attention to diverse cultures in education and clinical services. This attention is necessary to meet accreditation requirements. Community health nurses continue to see the urgent need for transcultural nursing as they care for many families of different cultures. Since patients are increasingly dismissed from hospitals early, it is the role of community health nurses to maintain care services and relationships with cultural groups, including many new immigrants, refugees, and other newcomers to their communities.

In the early years there were nurses who were resistant to transcultural nursing. They were afraid to deal with cultural factors and wanted to protect themselves by not getting involved in areas they did not understand. Transcultural nursing education has helped many nurses face their fears and move forward to become more competent practitioners.

Transcultural nursing concepts, principles, theories, and research findings are guiding nurses to provide transcultural nursing services in the community, hospitals, clinics, hospices, and many other settings where nurses work. The *Journal of Transcultural Nursing* was established in 1988 and provides a rich source of transcultural nursing research findings and other information. In addition, many books, articles, and other publications focus on transcultural nursing to guide nurses in their practices.

The Transcultural Nursing Society, established in 1974, offers regional, national, and global conferences where nurses can meet with other transcultural nurses to share ideas and experiences and expand their worldview, in 1988 the Transcultural Nursing Society began to certify nurses to ensure that they could provide safe, competent, and effective care to people of diverse cultures. Today there are over 100 certified transcultural nurses (CTN), but many more are preparing themselves to meet the certification requirements. The Transcultural Nursing Society became the first organization to provide certification of nurses worldwide, which is a hallmark for future nursing directions.

—**Madeleine Leininger**

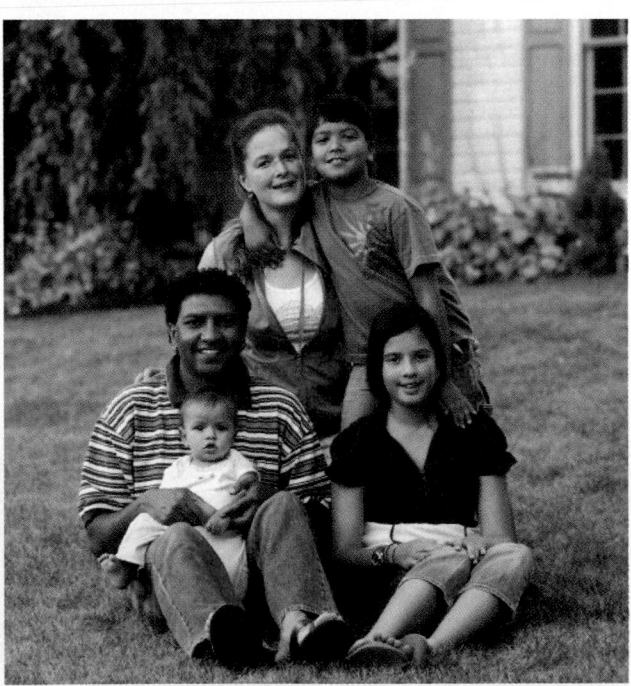

Mixed race families are becoming more common and accepted across the United States.

**Thanksgiving**

Leaves rain down
A thousand golden coins
And I remember

The smell of
New shoes and school books
And yellow buses
Filled with laughter

The first winter smoke
And talk of hog killin weather
To come
Children all

We lay upon the floor
Upon our bellies
Turning the pages
Filled with dreams
Of Christmas morning
A month away

Turkey in the oven
Jack-o-lantern pies,
The last of the gardens greens,
Sweet potatoes bake,
Dressing to "feed an army."

We
Gather together
This day
To give thanks.

I bow my head
And open my eyes to look upon the
Faces of all those I love.

*—Ann Lanier*

Explore Community Health Nursing on the Web!
To learn more about the topics in this chapter, use the passcode provided to access your exclusive website: **http://nursing.jbpub.com/ communityhealth.** If you do not have a passcode, you can obtain one at this site.

## ◼ CRITICAL THINKING ACTIVITIES

1. How many different cultural groups are there in your community? Who are they?
2. What are some of their traditions and values?
3. How are they different from you?
4. How are they like you?

## ◼ REFERENCES

Department of Health and Human Services, Public Health Services (DHHS). (2000). *Healthy People 2010.* [Conference Edition]. Washington, DC: U.S. Government Printing Office.

DeSantis, L. (1997). Building healthy communities with immigrants and refugees. *Journal of Transcultural Nursing, 9*(1), 20–31.

Horn, B. M. (1979). Transcultural nursing and child-rearing of the Muckleshoot people. In M. M. Leininger (Ed.), *Transcultural nursing: Proceedings from four transcultural nursing conferences* (pp. 57–69). New York: Masson.

Leininger, M. (1970). *Nursing and anthropology: Two worlds to blend.* New York: John Wiley & Sons. (Reprinted in 1994 by Greyden Press, Columbus, OH).

Leininger, M. (1978). *Transcultural nursing.* (Reprinted in 1994 by Greyden Press, Columbus, OH).

Leininger, M. (1981). *Care: An essential human need.* Thorofare, NJ: Charles B. Slack.

Leininger, M. (1985). *Qualitative research methods in nursing.* New York: Grune & Stratton.

Leininger, M. (1988). *Care: Discovery and uses in clinical and community nursing.* Detroit: Wayne State University Press.

Leininger, M. (1990). *Ethical and moral dimensions of care.* Detroit: Wayne State University Press.

Leininger, M. (1991). *Cultural care diversity and universality: A theory of nursing.* New York: National League for Nursing Press.

Leininger, M. (1995). *Transcultural nursing: Concepts, theories, research, and practice.* Columbus, OH: McGraw-Hill.

Leininger, M. (1996). Quality of life from a transcultural nursing perspective. *Nursing Science Quarterly, 9*(2), 71–78.

Leininger, M. (1997a). Cultural pain. *Images of Nursing* (Summer Edition), 19–20.

Leininger, M. (1997b). Future directions in transcultural nursing in the 21st century. *International Nursing Review, 44*(1), 19–23.

Leininger, M. (2006). Culture care diversity and universality theory and evolution of the ethnonursing method. In M. M. Leininger and M. R. McFarland (Eds.), *Culture care diversity and universality: A worldwide nursing theory* (2nd ed., pp. 1–41). Sudbury, MA: Jones and Bartlett Publishers.

Luna, L. (1998). Culturally competent health care: A challenge for nurses in Saudi Arabia. *Journal of Transcultural Nursing, 9*(2), 8–15.

Rosenbaum, J. (1990). Culture care of older Greek-Canadian widows within Leininger's theory of culture care. *Journal of Transcultural Nursing, 2*(1), 3–9.

Shapiro, M. L., Miller, J., & White, K. (2006). Community transformation through culturally competent nursing leadership: Application of theory of culture care diversity and universality and tri-dimensional leader effectiveness model. *Journal of Transcultural Nursing, 17*(2), 113–118.

# CHAPTER 11
# Ethics and Health

Pat Kurtz and Ronald L. Burr

Visit **http://nursing.jbpub.com/communityhealth** for interactive exercises, review questions, Web links, and more.

A different way of thinking about right and wrong actions may be needed in working with aggregate populations in the community. The situation becomes more complex when we attempt to weigh individual rights and privileges against what is best for the larger group.

It has become appallingly obvious that our technology has exceeded our humanity.

*—Albert Einstein*

A state legislature allotted its state health department $750,000 to match Ryan White federal funding for medication sufficient to treat 20 patients with acquired immune deficiency syndrome (AIDS). However, there were 100 patients who needed the help. Public health nurses in each district were asked to select patients for the medication program.

A terminally ill cancer patient who is in great pain begs the nurse for more medication than the physician has ordered. What should the nurse do?

A man was diagnosed and treated for a venereal infection by his family nurse practitioner. He agreed that his wife should also be treated but he did not want her to know that he acquired the disease from a prostitute and infected her. He asked the nurse practitioner if there was any way to avoid sharing this information.

When faced with situations like these, it sometimes feels like there are no "right" answers. What are your reactions to the three ethical dilemmas? What other information would be helpful to know about these situations to make a decision?

## CHAPTER FOCUS

**Virtue or Character Ethics**

**Principle-Based Ethics: Developing Moral Rules**
- Utilitarian Theories: Doing the Most Good for the Most People
- Deontological Theories: Balancing Rights and Obligations
- Justice in Health Care
- Values and Health Policy

**Ethics of Care**

**Ethical Problems Faced by Community Nurses: The Research**

**Ethical Decision Making**

**Service Learning: Discovering the Self and Developing Community Values**

## QUESTIONS TO CONSIDER

After reading this chapter, you will know the answers to the following questions:

1. What is bioethics, and how is it important to the community nurse?

2. What is the ethics of virtue, and what part do virtues play in the practice of nursing?

3. What is meant by principle-based ethics?

4. How does Kant's deontological approach differ from Mill's utilitarian approach?

5. What role does each of the four major ethical concepts—beneficence, nonmaleficence, autonomy, and justice—play in community nursing practice?

6. How can health care resources be distributed in a fair manner?

7. How does the ethical theory of care differ or agree with other theories?

8. What information does the nurse need to make ethically based decisions?

9. What is service learning, and how does it apply to community health?

## KEY TERMS

| | | | |
|---|---|---|---|
| Autonomy | Consequentialism | Ethical dilemma | Service learning |
| Benevolence | Deontological | Ethics | Trustworthiness |
| Bioethics | Discernment | Integrity | Utilitarianism |
| Casuistry | Ethic of caring | Justice | Virtue ethics |
| Compassion | Ethical decision making | Nonmaleficence | |

*❝One of the dilemmas of today's health care debate is that medical ethics, as currently structured and interpreted, is bad public policy and actually counterproductive to the total well-being of society.❞*

—Richard Lamm, Executive Director, Center for Public Policy and Contemporary Issues, and former governor of Colorado

THE SITUATIONS WE encounter as health care professionals may be complex and puzzling dealing with serious issues of well-being, life, and death. Our early experiences are usually of little help in guiding our actions in such complex situations. The philosophical discipline of **ethics** is the study of how we should behave, or how to determine the right thing to do in our interactions with others. **Bioethics** is the common name for the study of ethics as it relates to health and the moral problems that arise as a result of advances in health technologies and our increasing ability to do more to treat illness and prolong life. The theories resulting from ethical study provide a guide to examining ethical situations and to articulating preferred ways of living and behaving as health care practitioners. We must, however, remain aware that differences of opinion exist among those well versed in bioethics regarding which theories best fit which cases, as well as what kind of role character development plays in preparation for acting ethically in the community.

As our understanding of the universe, the nature of human behavior, and societal relationships has increased or changed, theories about ethical behavior have been modified and new theories developed. One essential difference in the various approaches to ethical decision making has to do with the target of the action. For whom or for what are we interested in doing the right thing—ourselves, a co-worker, an individual patient, a family, an organization, a community, a nation, or the world? Unfortunately, what may seem to be the right thing to do for one person or group may not be the right thing for another. A situation characterized by conflicting rights or obligations is known as an **ethical dilemma**.

Because of the variety of settings in which nurses practice and the philosophical assumption of the nursing community that nurses care for the whole person, nurses are often involved in all aspects of the patient's life as it relates to health. Bishop and Scudder (1990) point out that a major characteristic of nursing is that nurses practice "in-between." By this, they mean that in addition to giving direct care to the patient, nurses must manage and coordinate other aspects of the patient's care. This management includes advocating for the patient with the physician and other health care providers, interpreting the patient's needs to the agency, and interpreting agency policy and other constraints to patients and families. For a community health nurse, it may also mean advocating for agencies and policies in the political arena.

For the nurse practicing in the community, the community itself is another interested party in the patient's health care. Fry points out that in addition to their moral accountability for individual patients, community health nurses have a moral accountability for "how they provide health services to maximize total net health in population groups" (1996, p. 108).

A different way of thinking about right and wrong actions may be needed in working with aggregate populations. The situation becomes more complex when we attempt to weigh individual rights and privileges against assessments of what is best for a larger group. Horn (1999) suggests that considerations that compete in our conscientious ethical leanings and our ethical decision procedures include justice in distribution, the patient's comfort level or happiness, the patient's wishes, the expense of services, the patient's responsibility in acquiring a condition, and the social role of the patient.

One approach to increasing competence in dealing with ethical matters is to begin with clarification of your own values and identifying and understanding the values by which other people live. The cultural competence required for expert nursing care is a specific ethical demand on members of the profession to know and respect the values of others. Steele and Harmon (1983) and Uustal (1991) have developed strategies to aid in values clarification. The steps in the clarification process help people discover which values they hold and how strongly they hold them in relation to others. Values are often the result of years of consciously seeking information and weighing the importance of one point of view against another. However, they are also simply adopted from family tradition, religious teaching, or modeling people whom we admire without much reflection.

Over the millennia, philosophers, theologians, and others have attempted to formulate principles and rules that will guide us in ethical behavior. This chapter presents

*❝Everywhere, it appears, health care workers consider that the 'best' health care is one where everything known to medicine is applied to every individual by the highest trained medical scientist in the most specialized institutions.❞*

—M. Charlesworth, past director of the World Health Organization, 1993

Dr. Pat Kurtz, chapter author, counseling an elderly patient about a living will.

some of the basic principles of classical ethical theories (virtue ethics, deontology or formalism, and utilitarianism or consequentialism), as well as more recent formulations of biomedical ethics and care ethics. It includes a special focus on the justice issue of distribution of care and on the value systems that influence our national agendas for health care. Finally, research related to ethical dilemmas identified by community health nurses will be reviewed and frameworks for **ethical decision making** presented.

> **❝***The ultimate measure of a man is not where he stands in moments of comfort and convenience but where he stands at times of challenge and controversy.* **❞**

> **❝***Our lives begin to end the day we become silent about things that matter.* **❞**

> —Martin Luther King, Jr.

## Virtue or Character Ethics

One of the earliest philosophical approaches to correct behavior was that of **virtue ethics**. According to this approach, if a person has a "good" character, that person will behave ethically as a matter of course. Virtue ethics is based on the writings of the Greek philosopher Aristotle (384–382 BCE). Aristotle (1975) believed that there was general agreement that everyone has a "life goal" and that ultimate life goal was "happiness." Although each person has a different definition of happiness, Aristotle believed that happiness is achieved by what he called "excellence in performing rational activities" (thinking), which includes "excellence in choosing."

Behavioral choices lie on a continuum between ultimate extremes. Gluttony or self-denial might be the two extremes of a continuum representing eating or any other behavior relating to psychological or physiological needs. Foolhardiness and cowardice might be the extremes of a risk-taking continuum. Aristotle argued that the best choices lie between the two extremes, preferably somewhere in the middle, which he called the *golden mean*. The person who selects and acts on these middle-ground choices is virtuous. A person who does so with a pattern of consistency born of practice is thought to have good character.

Aristotle believed that becoming a virtuous person was a matter of habit and could be learned over time. The more one acts virtuously, the stronger the character trait becomes. In the throes of a crisis, character traits come to the fore and are more likely than relying on sudden decision making to result in good outcomes. From this standpoint, part of becoming a "good" nurse would require that students should practice a life of moderate choices based on those choices they believe an ethically ideal role model would make. Continuing to practice in this vein is believed to foster good habits that have the best likelihood of leading to right actions in professional practice. That is, the virtuous nurse would simply be disposed to do the ethically right thing, rather than having to reason to an ethical solution by some procedure. The word *ethics* actually stems from the Greek word *ethos*, which means "well-developed habits."

Like many other experiences in life, a given behavior may or may not be considered virtuous, depending on the culture of the individual. Honesty is often considered a virtue. However, if you belong to a criminal community or to a poverty-stricken family or community, honesty may not be valued in the same way it is in a community of middle-class property owners. Likewise, not all virtues are ethical in nature. Cheerfulness may be considered a virtuous social trait, but it is ethical only when displayed within an ethical situation. Even a right action is not ethical by itself, according to Aristotle, unless the action comes from ethical motivation. In other words, to be considered virtuous, not only must the behavior be the right action, purposefully done, but it must also come from an ethically appropriate inner urge to do the right thing. Box 11-1 describes characteristics of virtue ethics.

Characteristic of certain roles, occupations, and professions are expectations that its practitioners will have character and virtues beyond those of other people. In the case of nursing, it is expected that nurses will be (possess the virtue of) caring and will express that caring in all aspects of patient–nurse interaction. As a virtue, caring may be considered a mean between extremes on a continuum of attention to and feeling for others. At the one extreme would be rejection and callousness; at the other extreme would be over-involvement and indulgence. From a patient's point of view, caring includes or implies other virtues. For example, if nurses are caring, they are also trustworthy and can be relied upon to give fitting priority to the patient's welfare.

The Florence Nightingale Pledge identifies some virtues that were expected of nurses in the past. These virtues include purity, obedience, loyalty, and willingness to assume the handmaiden role to the physician (Davis & Aroskar, 1991). Changes in the societal expectations of the role of women in general and expectations from within nursing have devalued some of these historical virtues and replaced them with virtues of assertiveness, loyalty to and advocacy for the patient, and willingness to take appropriate risks.

---

**BOX 11-1**

**Virtue Ethics: Aristotle**

- The ultimate goal of life is to achieve happiness, which comes from excellence of thinking.
- An important aspect of excellence of thinking is excellence of choosing virtuous action—the golden mean.
- A virtuous action is moral only when it is done from a motivation to do the right thing.
- Virtue, for those of good character, is learned over time by the practice of acting in virtuous ways.
- Virtues are partly discerned from observing instances of sustained exemplary behavior by role models.

It is not uncommon for nurse educators and other nurses to question the virtuousness of today's nursing students and novice nurses. They complain that some nurses are joining the profession for its high salaries and security and do not show the ethical character traits of caring and the strict honesty that they believe are required of nurses.

Beauchamp and Childress (1994) have identified four virtues that they consider primary to the ethics of health professionals: compassion, discernment, trustworthiness, and integrity.

**Compassion**, a notion related to caring, includes a concern for others and an awareness of their pain or suffering. The compassionate person is disposed to respond with appropriate feelings of sympathy and mercy, as well as a desire to help decrease pain and other suffering. Ethically, being disposed to show these feelings also may be a critical factor in a patient's perception of being cared for.

While compassion has a strong emotional component, **discernment** is an intellectual trait. The discerning person is able to take decisive action based on insight resulting from a history of clear judgment and understanding. He or she is able to make ethical judgments without being unduly influenced by other personal or political factors. The person sees to the heart of the matter without the bias of personal involvement or personal feelings, without the common ethical flaw known as "conflict of interest." The discerning person is able to see what needs to be done, when, and in what way in situations involving ethical considerations.

**Trustworthiness** is a character trait that gives other people confidence that an individual will consistently do the right thing for the right (ethical) reasons. Beauchamp and Childress believe that the presence or lack of trustworthiness may be the most influential factor in whether a relationship continues between a patient and a caregiver. Importantly, in national polls, nurses have been consistently rated by the public as being the most trustworthy group among professionals.

**Integrity**, according to Beauchamp and Childress, exists when an individual habitually behaves in a way that is consistent with that individual's core values and beliefs. Persons of integrity, so to speak, "walk their virtuous talk." Integrity may be disturbed when the individual must compromise some beliefs and values. This compromising often results in a tension known as moral distress. People are said to have integrity when they are known not to compromise their ethical principles. We are more likely to trust people who we believe have integrity.

## Principle-Based Ethics: Developing Moral Rules

In principle-based approaches to ethics, the right or ethical action is determined not by the virtues (or habits) of individuals or authoritative tradition, but rather by the support of a set of beliefs developed by careful reasoning. Such beliefs include ideas about who has what kinds of rights and which rights or obligations have priority over other rights and ob-

ligations. For example, who has the right to make decisions about a patient's health care, and in what ways are health care providers obligated to support a decision with which they disagree? The two major principle-based approaches are utilitarianism and deontology.

### ■ Utilitarian Theories: Doing the Most Good for the Most People

The primary belief of people who have adopted the utilitarian position is that the most ethical action is the one that results in the greatest good (happiness) for the greatest number. A corollary to this notion would be that the best action is the one that causes the least harm to the fewest people. The philosopher cited most frequently as a proponent of **utilitarianism** is John Stuart Mill (1806–1873).

To a utilitarian, the important thing is not so much your good will toward others, but rather the consequences that result from your action. (Utilitarianism is also known as **consequentialism**.) Determining which action to take requires that all possible actions in the situation and the potential outcomes of each be examined for every person or group who may be involved. After the different outcomes are weighed and balanced, the action that leads to the best outcome for the most people is selected.

The utilitarian approach has obvious limitations. The first that may come to mind is the problem of how we can know what the outcomes will be for all the persons involved, because many factors beyond our control—or even beyond our knowledge—influence outcomes. Another problem arises when the preferred action and/or outcome is itself unethical. An example would be falsifying records in a home health agency so that the insurers will continue to pay for visits to otherwise ineligible patients. If the purpose of the falsification was to continue needed services to patients who would otherwise not receive them, the consequence is positive for the patient; however, the means are still unethical (as well as illegal). Recognizing this possible misuse of the theory as a rationalization for unethical behavior, Mill (1859/1871/1993) acknowledged that some behaviors were inherently unethical and could not be condoned, no matter what the favorable outcome. He specifically cited slavery as an example.

A more relevant issue in our time might be the use of migrant labor at pay rates below minimum wage and without decent provisions for living to produce cheaper food for the U.S. larger population. To avoid the misuse of this ethical approach, commonly expressed as "the ends justify the means," there must be general agreement about the ethical appropriateness of the proposed action and possible outcomes.

Another common criticism of the utilitarian approach is that it may not be practical for the average person. The principle of maximizing benefit for the greatest number may place the individuals making the decision in a position of always having to sacrifice their own preferences for the greater good. This self-sacrifice may be too difficult for the average person and raises questions about what the limits of our obligation to maximize benefit in that way are and whether it is even possible to make fair decisions in situations in which we may either be benefited or harmed. For example, suppose you are asked to support legislation that would provide increased health benefits for you and your family. After examining the proposed legislation, you realize that it will exclude many needy people who are benefiting from current legislation. In this instance, opposition to the proposed legislation would benefit more people, but at your expense.

The utilitarian approach is also criticized because it appears to give undue advantage to the majority population. For example, legislation that mandates increased health benefits (e.g., mammography) for participants in a health maintenance organization (HMO), Medicaid recipients, or those who have other private insurance will benefit a large number of people. At the same time, it excludes a minority who has no insurance and who may have more need for the services, but lacks the ability to pay for them. The criterion of justice (discussed in detail later)—so important in other approaches—may be missing from the utilitarian approach. Box 11-2 lists the major descriptors of utilitarianism/consequentialism.

A major area in which utilitarianism aids decision making is in public policy development, wherein it is often referred to as *cost–benefit analysis*. It is the presumed goal of policy makers that whatever money is appropriated or whatever regulations are adopted will further the general good of society. Developing public policy requires the careful examination of all possible options and the probable consequences of each. It is not uncommon that legislation is passed with good intentions, only to find later that a group of people has been left out, that the new legislation conflicts with other important practices, or that it encourages poor or fraudulent practices. It is important that nurses be at the

## BOX 11-2

**Utilitarianism/Consequentialism**
- The major determinant of ethical behavior is that it provides the most benefit to the most people or the least harm to the fewest people.
- The decision to act must be based on a careful examination of all possible actions in the situation and the possible consequences of each action.
- Regardless of consequences, actions themselves must be deemed to be ethical.

*A cynic is a man who, when he smells flowers, looks around for a coffin.*

—H. L. Mencken

### ETHICAL CONNECTION

Stason and Weinstein studied the cost-effectiveness of screening and treating hypertension using data from the Framingham longitudinal study and results of other hypertension studies. They projected various models of cost from initial screening to long-term treatment, considering such factors as dropout rates; nonadherence to medication; side effects; probability of more expensive events, such as stroke and myocardial infarction; and age. They found that it is more cost-effective to fund programs designed to increase adherence to the treatment regimen for those already in treatment than to institute screening for new cases. They also found that it is more cost-effective if hypertensive men start treatment when they are young, but women begin when they are older. The recommendation was that *if* screening is instituted, the focus should be on young men and older women.

What are the disadvantages to this utilitarian approach? Do you agree or disagree with this approach?

*Source:* Stason, W. B., & Weinstein, M. C. (1977). Public health rounds at the Harvard School of Public Health: Allocation of resources to manage hypertension. *New England Journal of Medicine, 296*(3), 732–739.

decision-making table to provide data about these options and consequences from their perspectives as caregivers and advocates. Further information about how to be effective in these activities is found in Chapter 8.

## ■ Deontological Theories: Balancing Rights and Obligations

Ethical theories categorized as **deontological** uphold the position that whether an action is ethical depends on the action itself—principally the motivational basis for the action. The word "deontological" was originally meant to differentiate an ethic of duty from the more utilitarian ethic of consequences. Today, the term includes any mixture of considerations that emphasizes other than consequences.

Immanuel Kant (1724–1804) is the philosopher who proposed the basis for our major theory of deontological ethics in his attempt to elaborate a rationale for ethical behavior based on pure reason, rather than tradition or authoritative pronouncement. Kant (1997) proposed two foundational principles, or rules, that he called "categorical imperatives" or unconditional "ethical laws." "Law" here means the generalized reason for an action, which would hold universally and which everyone must follow. If a rule meets that criterion, then it will always be true for every similar instance, and the individual is therefore obligated to follow the rule in every instance.

For example, you might want to determine whether it is ethical to lie to a patient about a diagnosis or prognosis. Is lying ethical? Based on Kant's procedures to determine the imperative, you would first determine whether lying could be an acceptable ethical behavior. Rationally, you would have to conclude that it could not; otherwise, no relationships that required trust could be developed. Therefore, lying is not ethical and is not acceptable in any situation. "Never lie" would be a categorical imperative. It could be argued, however, that some health care patients are special cases and that telling them the truth might cause psychological harm. Therefore, it is more ethical to lie than to risk causing harm. The imperative that one should never lie would have to be rejected or, at least restated, if this is thought to be true.

 ### Got an Alternative?

As more people seek out alternative health practices, nurses face a challenge. Nurses are often less familiar about these nontraditional treatments, so how can they practice in an ethical manner when their values are based on traditional medical treatment? ◢

Kant's second principle is that everyone should be treated as ends and not means to an end. Modern versions of deontological theory all include this second imperative in rules related to respect for individuals (the principle of autonomy). Box 11-3 describes deontological ethics according to Kant.

We have many examples of other approaches to this rule-based ethics. Of specific interest are theories of justice, notably those of Rawls and Nozick, which will be discussed later. Western civilization has had the Judeo-Christian ethic, which includes the Ten Commandments, which are universal rules proposed for adherents of those religions. Other religions have similar rules for behavior. Codes of ethics for professional groups are also examples of this approach.

Nurses rely to a large extent for guidance in ethical matters on the American Nurses Association *Code of Ethics* (ANA, 2001) and accompanying interpretive comments. This code focuses on professional responsibilities and on obligations of the nurse toward all patients. It clearly includes the community as a type of patient and the role of the nurse in the community. It does not go into detail about ethics with populations but is clearly consistent with the recently

> **"***A lie can travel halfway around the world while the truth is putting on its shoes.***"**
>
> —Mark Twain

published code of ethics for public health team members. The "Principles of the Ethical Practice of Public Health" are listed in the Cultural Connection feature.

Modern bioethics is another form of the deontological approach to ethics. Two events have influenced the development of modern bioethical theory: the medical experiments of German physicians during World War II (Davis & Aroskar, 1991) and the increasing development and use of technology in medicine (Beauchamp & Childress, 1994). In the first instance, interest in gaining new knowledge that would be helpful in the Nazi war effort, together with a disrespect for certain groups of people (e.g., Jews, Gypsies, mentally handicapped), motivated the Nazi doctors to perform experiments that were excruciatingly painful, degrading, and murderous. Revelation of these experiments at the Nuremberg trials following the war shocked the world community and increased awareness of humankind's capacity for inflicting harm. Further awareness and shock came with the revelation of inhumane research being conducted in the United States. Some, like the Tuskegee syphilis study being conducted on Southern African American men, was supported by the U.S. Public Health Service. The results of these and other revelations were a series of national and international codes of ethics for the conduct of research.

The introduction of increasingly more sophisticated technology over the last 40 years has enabled health care

---

### 🔨 ETHICAL CONNECTION

In 1932, the U.S. Public Health Service funded research to study the natural course of syphilis, a disease that at the time had no known, reliable treatment. Subjects for that study consisted of a group of 200 Black men who were infected with the disease and 100 Black men who were uninfected from the small area of Tuskegee, Alabama. The study continued for 40 years, during which time the infected population became more ill and had a much higher mortality rate than the uninfected control group. By the 1940s, it was found that penicillin was an effective treatment; however, none of the men were given the antibiotic. Many of the men did not know that they were subjects of a research study, were not told that penicillin would help them, and faithfully continued to appear for the periodic exams, believing that they were being treated. Articles reporting on the study were published in medical journals and, in addition to the nurse and physicians involved, many physicians from the Tuskegee medical center and around the state knew about the work. It was not until the project was exposed in 1972 in a Washington newspaper that the public became aware and expressed outrage about it. At this point the study was finally discontinued.

*Source*: Brandt, A. M. (1978). Racism and research: The case of the Tuskegee syphilis study. *Hastings Center Report, 8*(6), 21–29.

---

### BOX 11-3

**Deontological Ethics: Immanuel Kant**
- Individuals establish their own moral rules based on the criterion that the generalized intention of their action could apply to everyone—that is, could become a "law."
- The rules apply to every similar situation.
- People must be treated as ends and not means (given respect as autonomous persons).

providers to perform complicated surgical procedures, such as heart bypass and organ transplants; to keep premature infants alive; to identify genetic abnormalities in a fetus; and to maintain nutrition, hydration, and respiration in patients in irreversible coma. In the struggle to find the right actions in these and other situations, solutions for many ethical dilemmas were eventually sought from the courts.

 ENVIRONMENTAL CONNECTION

Toxic waste dumps and other contaminants that affect people's health are often located near impoverished and vulnerable populations. What are the ethical implications of this practice and how does it reflect government accountability for safeguarding the health of all its citizens?

❝ *An eye for an eye makes the whole world blind.* ❞

—*Mahatma Gandhi*

❝ *Be kind, for everyone you meet is fighting a hard battle.* ❞

—*Plato*

Beauchamp and Childress (1994) have identified four concepts they believe to be essential to a theory of modern bioethics: **autonomy** (respect for persons), **nonmaleficence** (refraining from harm), **benevolence** (doing good), and **justice** (fair distribution of burdens and benefits). Other principles, such as sanctity of life, truthfulness, confidentiality, and gratitude, are sometimes added to this list by other ethicists (Burkhardt & Nathaniel, 1988; Uustal, 1993). Some ethicists prioritize these principles by saying, for example, that when there is a conflict between principles, the principle of autonomy will take precedence. Others believe that none of the obligations that arise in the course of relationships is primary. Each principle may be overridden in a situation of conflict with another ethical obligation.

### Respect for the Autonomy of the Individual

Beauchamp and Childress define personal autonomy as "personal rule of the self that is free from both controlling interferences by others and from personal limitations that prevent meaningful choice, such as inadequate understanding" (1994, p. 121). Having respect for an individual's autonomy means understanding and acting on the belief that people have the right to make decisions and take actions based on their own beliefs and value systems.

The concept of autonomy is further elaborated by arguing that respect for autonomy is not just the negative action of not interfering, but also includes the obligation to take positive actions to promote the individual's capacity to be autonomous. An example of a positive action might be to provide care that will restore an individual's capacity to think clearly after a period of confusion. Working with family members to limit their pressure on the patient for a particular decision and providing information to an

### ■■ CULTURAL CONNECTION

**Principles of the Ethical Practice of Public Health, Version 2.2**

1. Public health should address principally the fundamental causes of disease and requirements for health, aiming to prevent adverse health outcomes.
2. Public health should achieve community health in a way that respects the rights of individuals in the community.
3. Public health policies, programs, and priorities should be developed and evaluated through processes that ensure an opportunity for input from community members.
4. Public health should advocate and work for the empowerment of disenfranchised community members, aiming to ensure that the basic resources and conditions necessary for health are accessible to all.
5. Public health should seek the information needed to implement effective policies and programs that protect and promote health.
6. Public health institutions should provide communities with the information they have that is needed for decisions on policies or programs and should obtain the community's consent for their implementation.
7. Public health institutions should act in a timely manner on the information they have within the resources and the mandate given to them by the public.
8. Public health programs and policies should incorporate a variety of approaches that anticipate and respect diverse values, beliefs, and cultures in the community.
9. Public health programs and policies should be implemented in a manner that most enhances the physical and social environment.
10. Public health institutions should protect the confidentiality of information that can bring harm to an individual or community if made public. Exceptions must be justified on the basis of the high likelihood of significant harm to the individual or others.
11. Public health institutions should ensure the professional competence of their employees.
12. Public health institutions and their employees should engage in collaborations and affiliations in ways that build the public's trust and the institution's effectiveness.

*The development and dissemination of the "Principles of the Ethical Practice of Public Health" is funded primarily by the Centers for Disease Control and Prevention through the Public Health Leadership Society (PHLS). The Center for Health Leadership and Practice, Public Health Institute, is acknowledged for its role in the initial development of the Principles. PHLS also acknowledges the work of the members of the original PHLS Ethics Work Group (responsible for drafting the code) and the current members of the PHLS Standing Committee on Ethics.*

individual or community group that needs to make a good decision regarding health care are other examples. Principles of privacy and confidentiality both are derived from respect for autonomy, as is the principle of informed consent, which refers to the patient's agreement to undergo a medical or nursing treatment or be a research subject.

### Nonmaleficence

"First, do no harm" has been part of the Hippocratic Oath taken by physicians for centuries and has been a cornerstone of ethical practice in medicine and nursing. For some (Frakena, 1973), the principles of nonmaleficence and beneficence are the ends of a continuum relating to harm and obligations to help. In this context, the principle with the highest priority of obligation is that of inflicting no harm. The second priority is that a person should prevent harm. The third priority is that of removing harm. The fourth priority is that of doing or promoting good. Rules that may be said to emerge from the nonmaleficence principle include not killing, not causing pain or suffering, not incapacitating others, not offending others, and not depriving others of the "goods of life." Major ethical issues related to nonmaleficence deal with treatments used to prolong life, such as intubation and artificial feeding.

❝*Don't go around saying the world owes you a living. The world owes you nothing. It was here first.*❞

—Mark Twain

## Communitarian Ethic*

❝*There is no power for change greater than a community discovering what it cares about.*❞

—Margaret Wheatley

Because of the relationships involved, a community has a "moral nature" as compared to the nature of a population. *Communitarian ethics* is based on the position that "everything fundamental in ethics derives from communal values, the common good, social goals, traditional practices, and cooperative virtues" (Beauchamp & Childress, 2001, p. 362). Communitarian ethics is applicable to moral relationships within any type of community, both large and small. As an ethical approach, it is distinguished because the epicenter of communitarian ethics is the community rather than beginning from the point of any one individual (Wildes, 2000). Populations in general, and moral communities in particular, are also the starting points for community nursing.

Some ethicists have tried to draw a strong distinction between ethical approaches that emphasize individualism and autonomy as differentiated from communitarian ethics, which emphasizes a common good. However, it is reasonable to assume that people can be interested in both their own well-being and the common good of the communities to which they belong. The value of considering communitarian ethics lies in the benefit that can be gained from illuminating and appreciating the relationships and in-

*This section was authored by Dr. Karen Rich and adapted from the following source: Rich, K. L. (2005). Community and public health nursing and leadership ethics. In J. B. Butts & K. L. Rich (Eds.), *Nursing ethics across the curriculum and into practice* (pp. 203–230). Sudbury, MA: Jones and Bartlett.

❝*The Buddhist Avatamsaka Sutra contains a story about how all perceiving, thinking beings are connected in a way that is similar to a universal community. The story is about the heavenly net of the god Indra. 'In the heaven of Indra, there is said to be a network of pearls, so arranged that if you look at one you see all the others reflected in it. In the same way each object in the world is not merely itself but involves every other object and in fact is everything else. In every particle of dust there is present Buddhas without number.*❞

—Sir Charles Eliot, as cited in F. Capra, *The Tao of Physics* (1999, p. 296)

terconnections between people that are often overlooked in everyday life. Although personal moral goals are significant, the importance of forming strong communities and identifying the moral goals of those communities must be appreciated for both individuals and communities to flourish.

An important point that distinguishes communitarian ethics from other ethical approaches, such as deontology or utilitarianism, is communitarians' acceptance that humans naturally favor the people with which they live and have frequent interactions. Deontologists, for example, base their ethics upon the existence of a more impartial stance toward the persons who are the receivers of their morally related actions.

Communitarians accept partiality as a way of relating to others but also believe that it is realistic to develop empathy and compassion toward people who are personally unknown to them. Nussbaum (2004) suggested that people often develop an "us versus them" mentality, especially when they are separated by significant cultural differences. People are able to generate sympathy when they hear about epidemics and disasters occurring on continents that are far away, but it is usually difficult for people to sustain that level of sympathy for more than a short period of time. People tend to stop and notice others' needs, but soon turn back to their own personal lives. According to Nussbaum, humanity will "achieve no lasting moral progress unless and until the daily unremarkable lives of people distant from us become real in the fabric of our own daily lives" (p. 958) and until people include others that they do not know personally within the important sphere of their lives. Nurses must broaden their scope of concern to include people affected by health care disparities, diseases, and epidemics all over the world.

❝*A human being is a part of the whole, called by us the 'universe,' a part limited in time and space. He experiences himself, his thoughts and feelings, as something separated from the rest, a kind of optical delusion of his consciousness. This delusion is a kind of prison for us, restricting us to our personal desires and to affection for a few persons nearest to us. Our task must be to free ourselves from this prison by widening our circle of compassion to embrace all living creatures and the whole of nature in its beauty.*❞

—Albert Einstein

"All communities have some organizing vision about the meaning of life and how one ought to conduct a good life" (Wildes, 2000, p. 129). Community nurses have an important role in bringing populations and communities together to work toward a common humanitarian good. Transforming communities from a "them versus us" mentality to one that seeks a common good is possible through education (Nussbaum, 2004). "Children [and people] at all ages must learn to recognize people in other countries as their fellows, and to sympathize with their plights. Not just their dramatic plights, in a cyclone or war, but their daily plights" (p. 959). This need for empathetic understanding also is important within one's own country, state, town, and neighborhood. Many people are suffering within the United States because they lack adequate health care, food, environmental sanitation, and housing.

The education of communities often occurs through role modeling (Wildes, 2000). Members of communities learn about what is and is not accepted as moral through personal and group interactions and dialogue within their communities. Narratives are told about the lives of exemplars, such as Florence Nightingale in nursing, to illustrate moral living. In Nightingale's efforts to improve social justice and health protection through environmental measures and her efforts to elevate the good character of nurses, she exhibited moral concern for her local society, the nursing profession, and people remote from her local community, such as people affected by the Crimean War. In learning from Nightingale's example, communitarian-minded nurses are in an excellent position to educate the public and other health care professionals about why they in many ways should assume the role of being their "brother's and sister's keeper."

### Beneficence

The principle of beneficence has to do with obligations to act in ways that would benefit or provide some good to others. Beauchamp and Childress (1994) focus on two aspects of beneficence: positive beneficence and utility. Positive beneficence provides the rationale for a number of specific moral rules generally accepted by our society (Box 11-4).

Theoretical arguments about beneficence have to do with the extent to which we are obligated to people who are not in a special relationship with us, the way in which children, parents, and friends are. Are we obligated to everyone, or only to special people? Formalized relationships between health care providers and patients have been identified as special relationships that do obligate the provider.

### Justice

Justice may be defined generally as "fair, equitable, and appropriate treatment in light of what is due or owed to persons" (Burkhardt & Nathaniel, 1998, p. 57). The major focus of ethical theories of justice in relation to health care is the concept of "right to health care," often meaning the right to government-subsidized health care for everyone. The arguments for or against the existence of such a right are consistent with the debaters' philosophical and political belief systems regarding the role of government in the lives of individuals.

In addition to being a major concept in the "principlest" approach to ethics, there are theories of distributive justice that "attempt to articulate, order, and justify principles that specify just distributions of benefits and burdens (other than punishments)" (Buchannan, 1992, p. 655). Buchannan identifies four major theories of justice: utilitarianism, Rawls' justice as fairness, rights-based egalitarianism, and Marxist egalitarianism.

> **"** *Although we can distinguish between ethics and politics, they are inseparable. For we cannot understand ethics without thinking through our political commitments and responsibilities. And there is no understanding of politics that does not bring us back to ethics. Ethics and politics as disciplines concerned with praxis are aspects of a unified, practical philosophy.* **"**
> —R. J. Bernstein. (1991). *The new constellation: The ethical-political horizons of modernity–postmodernity.* Cambridge, MA: MIT Press.

### A Good Read

# Ethics for the New Millennium (2001)
*By Dalai Lama, New York: Penguin Putnam.*

In a modern society characterized by insensitivity to violence, ambivalence to the suffering of others, and a high value placed on the profit motive, is talk of ethics anything more than a temporary salve for our collective conscience? The Dalai Lama thinks so. In his *Ethics for the New Millennium*, the exiled leader of the Tibetan people shows how the basic concerns of all people—happiness based in contentment, appeasement of suffering, forging meaningful relationships—can act as the foundation for a universal ethics.

---

## BOX 11-4

**Rules of Positive Beneficence**
- Protect and defend the rights of others.
- Prevent harm from occurring to others.
- Help persons with disabilities.
- Rescue persons in danger.

*Source:* Bauchamp, T., & Childress, J. (1994). *Principles of Biomedical Ethics* (4th ed.). New York: Oxford University Press.

According to Donaldson (1992), the philosopher David Hume (1711–1776) is credited with first identifying the circumstances under which justice is necessary:

- *Dependence.* Individuals are not self-sufficient. They require the cooperation of nature and of other humans to "achieve certain critical goods."
- *Moderate scarcity.* Some scarcity is required because if there is an overabundance, justice is not required; if there is severe scarcity, a decent life is impossible to achieve.
- *Restrained benevolence.* Humans are generous, but only to a point. They may frequently sacrifice at all levels (family–country), but over the long term, they show a deep-seated resilience to self-interest.
- *Individual vulnerability.* No matter what one's status, anyone can be subject to attack from others.

Utilitarianism and its criticisms were discussed earlier in this chapter. Rawls' "justice as fairness" theory was developed partly as a response to the shortcomings of utilitarianism. Rawls (1999) asks that we imagine an ideal situation in which the principles of justice for a democratic and free society are developed from an "original position" by a group of representative people who are unbiased, in a situation of equality. This "original position" is one where the framers work from a "veil of ignorance," where they do not know who they may be or what position they may hold within the society. Rawls believes that the group members would want to maximize their own positions, whatever those may turn out to be and so, through deliberative rationality, would agree to accept his two principles of justice. Box 11-5 presents these principles.

The "just savings principle" refers to Rawls' belief that every generation has an obligation to "save" for future generations. Thus each generation should pass on to the next generation an amount of capital (e.g., factories, infrastructure, and other resources) and those institutions that would ensure their liberty and well-being; these assets include ideas and culture. Although it is expected that a given generation will pass on the opportunity for a better life, it is not expected that the generation will unduly deprive itself to do so. Each generation receives from the previous one and gives to the next. What seems to be a reasonable savings depends on the circumstances of each generation.

The general rules are those that would be worked out from the "original position" in which the group members, working behind the "veil of ignorance," do not know which will be their generation. Current generational issues include our Social Security system, natural resource usage, transportation infrastructure, and educational systems.

Critics of Rawls say that his theory demands too much from those who are better off, even when those who are worse off would not suffer or their conditions could not be improved. He is also accused of being too optimistic about the general acceptance of the ideal situation. If too many of the citizens are alienated from the culture, consensus may not be attainable.

Adherents to the philosophy of radical libertarianism take the position that the role of the state is to enforce property rights—not redistribute wealth, except to rectify past violations of individual property rights. Nozick (1974) responded to Rawls' theory by asserting that enforced redistribution of goods violates individual rights requiring interference with individuals' lives, causing unacceptable disruption. In addition, the redistribution is intuitively unjust. According to Buchannan (1992), Nozick's critics respond that current tax laws provide redistribution with only minimal disruption, and we cannot assume that injustice doesn't arise after an accumulation of individual transactions that, by themselves, appear to be fair.

The original Marxist theories proposed that the need for redistribution would disappear after a class leveling occurred and a common control of the means of production was implemented. Clearly, that has not happened in communist systems, and more moderate Marxists now believe that there will always be a need for a principle of enforced distributive justice. They focus now on Marx's vision of a more rational and humane, post-capitalist society.

---

### BOX 11-5

**Rawls' Principles of Justice**

**First Principle**

Each person is to have an equal right to the most extensive total system of basic liberties possible in the society. These liberties can be restricted only for the sake of overall liberty. Liberty may be restricted in only two cases: (1) a less extensive than possible liberty must strengthen the total system of liberties for everyone and (2) a less than equal liberty must be accepted by those affected.

**Second Principle**

Social and economic inequalities are to be to the most benefit of the least advantaged, and offices and positions must be open to all under conditions of fairness of opportunity. Justice takes priority over efficiency and maximizing the sum of advantages. There are two exceptions: (1) any inequality of opportunity must be to the advantage of those with lesser opportunity and (2) an excessive rate of savings must generally decrease the burden of those who bear the hardship.

---

### ■ Justice in Health Care

Although Rawls' theory does not specify health care as a social good, Daniels (1985) believes that a theory of "just health care" was compatible as an extension of Rawls' general theory of justice and developed his theory based on assumptions of "rights to health care" in relation to individual needs. Daniels' composite list of rights is presented here:

- Society has the duty to its members to allocate an adequate share of its total resources to health-related needs, such as the protection of the environment and the provision of medical services.

### A Good Read

## Our Endangered Values: America's Moral Crisis (2006)

*By Jimmy Carter, New York: Simon and Schuster.*

President Jimmy Carter, Nobel Peace Prize Winner, is one of the most respected voices in the United States today in the areas of human rights, diplomacy, and good government.

In his book, *Our Endangered Values: America's Moral Crisis,* Carter presents a series of essays that outline his views about the key ethical and moral issues looming in the 21st century. Topics such as war, environmental negligence, the death penalty, civil liberties, moral responsibilities to the poor, and the separation of church and state are critically debated in the context of Carter's worldview and spiritual philosophy about our role as world citizens.

- Society has the duty to provide a just allocation of different types of health services, taking into account the competing claims of different types of health needs.
- Each person is entitled to a fair share of such services, where "fair share" includes an answer to the question, Who should pay for the services? (p. 8)

For Daniels, needs are defined as being "necessary to achieve or maintain species-typical functioning" (p. 26). If there is impairment of this functioning through either disease or disability, individuals are restricted in the expression of the normal range of opportunity their own talents and skills would otherwise allow them. Daniels proposed that the greater the impairment, the more important it is to prevent, cure, or compensate for the disease conditions.

In Daniels' theory, "normal range of opportunity" is defined for individuals as the reasonable life plans available to them in their particular society if they were healthy. This definition implies that there will still be differences among individuals (e.g., normal genetic endowment and cultural expectations and limitations). The emphasis is on fairness, meaning that society must refrain from imposing barriers to equal opportunity and must correct for interferences to equal opportunity. The assumption of the Rawlsian "veil of ignorance" should be applied here in regard to decisions about needs.

Allocation of societal resources among all social needs and among the various levels of health care needs (prevention, cure, restoration, and extended support) requires both moral judgment and extensive empirical knowledge about allocation consequences. Daniels also points out that protection of opportunity must not undermine a society's productive capacity.

In his analysis, Daniels deals with two related issues in the application of his theory: equitable access to health care and paternalism. Three general approaches may be taken in dealing with the issue of access. The first is utilization rates, by which differences and similarities in usage among groups are identified. For example, if a service is utilized equally between upper- and lower-class subgroups, equality of access is thought to exist. The second is the process approach, in which process variables are examined to determine whether some variable, such as geographic distance or waiting time, makes the process more burdensome for some. The third approach, the market approach, determines that access is equitable if there are no information, supply, or financial barriers that prevent access to what is referred to as a "reasonable" or "decent basic minimum" of service. Daniels asserts that the "decent minimum" in health care should reflect our ideas of "tolerable life prospects."

Daniels also proposed a "theory of justifiable paternalism," which relates to issues of equitable risk prevention in the prevention of disease. Reduction of disease risk may include general measures, such as mandatory water and waste treatment from which everyone benefits equally; alternatively, it may be specific, targeting workplace risks where only some individuals are affected. Regulating workplace risk by imposing standards and rules is said by some to be in conflict with an individual's freedom in lifestyle choices and the right to take risks voluntarily.

What needs to be considered is whether the workers (1) are truly informed of all risks to health, (2) are truly able to make a choice without depriving themselves of a reasonable living, and (3) are not subject to overt or covert coercion. Daniels states:

> In general we ought to preserve autonomy.... But we are not bound to preserve the illusion of autonomy. If unregulated worker "choices" about risk-taking must fail, or generally do fail, to be informed, competent, or truly voluntary, then we are not compromising autonomy by intervening. (p. 159)

### ■ Values and Health Policy

As Schlesinger (2002) explains, historically a market-based model for health care has had a variable level of support in the United States. Support has markedly increased since the beginning of the Reagan administration in the early 1990s. The market-based model views health care as a commodity similar to material goods, subject to the laws of supply and demand in relation to availability and cost. It has competed with two alternative models: the medical professionalism model and the societal rights model.

The medical professionalism model rejects the idea that consumers are competent to make good medical choices, arguing that medical care is too complex and still under development. Proponents of this model believe that medical providers should make health care decisions. The Great Depression of the 1930s saw the emergence of the "societal rights" framework. In the early 1940s, President Franklin Roosevelt called for the rights for all to medical care and the opportunity to achieve and enjoy good health.

The role of the government within the medical professional model is to promote scientific knowledge and the training of professionals. By contrast, in the social rights model, the role of government is to ensure a standard of equality and equal access to services. The then-dominant "rights" model during the 1960s and 1970s saw increases in the role of the government with the establishment and expansion of programs such as Medicare, Medicaid, and other health and social programs. The swing toward the market model was driven primarily by the marked increases in the costs of these health care programs. In the market model, the role of government is to support fair competition among providers.

Political conservatives have been among the entities most interested in cost reduction and in reduction of the role of government in health services. However, liberals were also supportive of "managed competition," believing it would transform medical care by breaking up the entrenched interests of the medical profession and make it more responsive to consumers—hence the support from the Clinton administration for expansion of managed care.

 THINK ABOUT THIS ·····················

Where, after all, do universal human rights begin? In small places, close to home—so close and so small that they cannot be seen on any map of the world. Yet they are the world of the individual person: the neighborhood he lives in; the school or college he attends; the factory, farm, or office where he works. Such are the places where every man, woman, and child seeks equal justice, equal opportunity, equal dignity without discrimination. Unless these rights have meaning there, they have little meaning anywhere. Without concerted citizen action to uphold them close to home, we shall look in vain for progress in the larger world.
—Eleanor Roosevelt (1884–1962),
U.S. author, diplomat, and First Lady,
statements at presentation of "In Your Hands: A Guide for Community Action for the Tenth Anniversary of the Universal Declaration of Human Rights," March 27, 1958

How has the United States changed since 1958 in regard to justice, as related to health care?

In spite of the support from both conservatives and liberals, there has been little real progress toward health care reform. Many proposals have been attempted, but until recently, at least, the reform has been limited. In an effort to understand these failures, Schlesinger (2002) carried out a series of research studies examining the values held by liberals and conservatives of both the "Washington elite" (congressional staff who had designated responsibility for health issues) and the general public. Table 11-1 shows the percentage of the "elites" identified as advocates for the market model who agreed with statements related to allocation of responsibility for care and health care issues. It can be

| Table 11-1 Percentage of Positive Responses of Policy Elites Who Advocate the Market Health Care Model by Self-Identified Political Ideology | | |
|---|---|---|
| **Fairness Measure** | **Conservative** | **Liberal** |
| ■ Individuals should be responsible for their own | | |
| Physician and hospital services | 87.0% | 4.2% |
| Nursing home and home health care services | 69.1% | 0.0% |
| Substance abuse treatment | 83.3% | 6.7% |
| ■ Norms for Health Care Equity | | |
| Most fair if individuals decide for themselves about health insurance and health care that matches how much they want to pay for it | 100% | 100% |
| The most productive people should make the most income and be offered the best fringe benefits | 40% | 11.1% |
| Equal treatment is the most important aspect of a just health care system | 0.0% | 55.6% |
| Health care should be based on needs, as determined by a medical expert, regardless of cost | 20% | 66.7% |

Elites who identified themselves as moderates are not included in this table.

*Source*: Adapted from Schlesinger (2002, p. 904).

**Table 11-2**    Percentage of Agreement with Ethical Norms Items Among Elites and the Public by Market Advocacy

| Ethical Norm Measure | Elites | | Public | |
|---|---|---|---|---|
| | Advocate | Non-advocate | Advocate | Non-advocate |
| ■ Most fair if individuals could decide for themselves about health insurance and health care that matches how much they want to pay for it | 85.7% | 20.6% | 79.4% | 46.4% |
| ■ Most productive people should make the most income and get the most fringe benefits | 23.8% | 12.9% | 31.8% | 27.8% |
| ■ Equal treatment is the most important aspect of a just health care system | 42.9% | 64.7% | 82.5% | 67.9% |
| ■ Health care should be based on needs as determined by medical experts, regardless of cost | 38.1% | 44.1% | 76.2% | 73.2% |

*Source:* Adapted from Schlesinger (2002, p. 907).

clearly seen from the data that although all respondents were supportive of a market model, they held very different views about issues of responsibility and equity in health care.

Schlesinger found that while 58% of congressional health staff supported the market model for health care reform, only 41% of the general public did so. When he compared the congressional staff with the general public on the responsibility measures, he found that market advocates among the elite were almost twice as likely as non-advocates to agree that individuals should be responsible for their own health care. By comparison, market advocates of the public were slightly less likely than non-advocates to support the personal responsibility statements. The differences between the groups were even more pronounced when Schlesinger considered the norms of fairness items; these responses are shown in Table 11-2. He concluded that these differences between the general public and the congressional elite may account for the problems that have emerged in trying to implement a market approach to health care reform.

❝ *In the end, we will remember not the words of our enemies but the silence of our friends.* ❞

—Martin Luther King, Jr.

## Ethics of Care

The previously discussed theories have in common the use of moral principles to guide behavior. These theories are concerned with the rights of individuals within a society and the obligations of individuals to others and to society. A more recently developed theory, known as the **ethic of caring,** takes a different position—namely, that relationships and responsibilities are more important than rights and obligations or outcomes. In this approach, the primary focus is on the well-being of the whole person. This means that the nurse

❝ *When nurses are attentive, efficient, and effective in their practice, they are being morally good persons, because they are fulfilling the moral sense of nursing by fostering the well-being of patients.* ❞

—A. Bishop & J. Scudder. (1990). *The practical, moral, and personal sense of nursing: A phenomenological philosophy of practice.* Albany, NY: State University of New York, p. 112.

is concerned with all aspects of the patient's well-being, not merely the disease process. Care is designed for needs in all realms—physical, psychological, social, and spiritual—with the understanding that each affects the others and the totality of health. The broader social environment that affects the patient is also of concern, such as the family. Nursing actions are deemed ethical when they take into consideration this whole person, who is labeled the "patient" or "patient." They are unethical when they focus on the disease process or disability.

There is also a component of compassion, which is a precursor to caring. The nurse who practices from this care approach will be concerned with developing personal characteristics and taking actions that will show caring. This ethical approach is still developing within nursing, where care has always been central. There are many barriers within the present health care system that interfere with care for the whole person, such as a technology focus, managed care, and specialization (Purtillo, 1999).

The ethic of care rings true for many nurses who believe it describes the context of and their feelings about their work. It is the connectedness and responsibility for having met the needs of individuals under their care that give satisfaction. Benner (1984) provides many examples from her interviews that support this view.

The person living a caring ethic bases his or her actions on the needs of those for whom the individual cares, either

---

### BOX 11-6

**The Ethics of Care**

- The focus is on the whole individual.
- The caregiver has a responsibility to meet the needs of those for whom the person is caring.
- There is an affective element of compassion in the relationship.

---

naturally or in a formal caring relationship. For the community health nurse, the focus changes from the individual to the population, but responding to needs at all levels remains the same (see Box 11-6).

## Ethical Problems Faced by Community Health Nurses: The Research

Several studies identifying the ethical problems related to community health nursing have been conducted by nurse researchers in both the United States and other countries. In one study, Aroskar (1989) sent questionnaires to more than 1,000 staff nurses who worked in community health and public health agencies in Minnesota. More than 300 nurses responded, listing the problems they had encountered. Aroskar categorized the problems according to the type of ethical conflict they represented. These categories and some examples are shown in Box 11-7.

---

### BOX 11-7

**Community Health Nursing Problems Categorized by Ethical Conflict**

**Conflict Between Autonomy and Beneficence**

- Getting patients to be responsible for their own care and well-being
- Wishes and rights of patients about living, dying, and refusing treatment
- Unnecessary treatment (use of narcotics)
- Apparent negligence of a child without evidence to report
- Refusal of treatment when the patient's condition is deteriorating

**Conflict Between Truth-Telling and Nonmaleficence**

- Stretching the truth or game-playing to satisfy criteria for treatment
- Withholding information or lying to the patient about diagnosis or treatment
- Nonbetrayal of colleagues to the patient and/or family about quality of care

**Distributive Justice**

- Unnecessary government subsidization for low-income families
- Lack of funds for medical care
- Struggle for equal care, regardless of race or finances

*Source*: Aroskar (1989).

---

### BOX 11-8

**Types of Ethical Conflict Reported by 40 Louisiana Public Health Nurses**

| Type | Frequency | Percentage |
|------|-----------|------------|
| Confidentiality | 21 | 53 |
| Privacy | 16 | 40 |
| Whistle blowing | 16 | 40 |
| Informed consent | 13 | 32 |
| Conflict of interest | 13 | 32 |
| Other discrimination | 9 | 23 |
| Truth-telling | 7 | 18 |
| Discrimination against patient | 6 | 15 |
| Disclosure | 2 | 5 |

*Source*: Folmar, Coughlin, Bessinger, & Sackoff (1997).

---

In a survey of 40 public health nurses in southern Louisiana, Folmar, Coughlin, Bessinger, and Sackoff (1997) found similar results to those uncovered by Aroskar. Those findings are shown in Box 11-8 in order of frequency of report.

In another study, using a list of 39 ethical problems, 745 hospital and community nurses were asked to indicate each one they had encountered in the last 12 months. The researchers (Wagner & Ronen, 1996) reported the 10 most frequently encountered dilemmas. Again, the major issues were similar to those found in previous studies. The percentages of nurses experiencing the most frequently encountered dilemmas are reported in Box 11-9 for the 239 community health nurses in the study. The community health nurses reported similar issues as the hospital nurses, but generally encountered them less frequently.

---

### BOX 11-9

**Issues Most Frequently Encountered by Israeli Community Health Nurses**

| Dilemma | Percentage |
|---------|------------|
| Need to care for offensive patient | 85 |
| Conflict between patient and family needs | 69 |
| Inability to treat—staff shortages | 61.2 |
| Reporting incompetence of nurses or physicians | 57.3 |
| Rude or offensive behavior toward patient by nurse | 48.9 |
| Giving treatment perceived as a mistake or wrong | 52 |
| Violence by patient or family toward caregiver | 48.7 |
| Withholding information from patient—family wishes | 45.2 |
| Giving treatment of questionable value | 49.8 |
| Pressuring a patient who refuses treatment | 48.2 |

*Source*: Wagner & Ronen (1996).

Gremmen (1999), using a grounded study method, interviewed 33 Dutch visiting (district) nurses, asking them about that they considered to be central to their work. This researcher was interested in the nurses' moral reasoning about their work. The theoretical focus of her study was on the apparent conflict between an ethic of care and an ethic of justice. The nurses described how they handled situations in which patients were resistant to treatment. Analysis of the interview data showed three parts to the process the nurses described, which Gremmen labeled "tuning in to the patients' lives," "convincing or even pushing patients while not forcing them," and "not withdrawing from patients while disagreeing with them." It was her conclusion that care and justice are both crucial to the work of public health nurses and can be complementary.

As part of a study of 30 community health nurses in British Columbia, Canada, Duncan (1992) asked them to report the clinical situations that created ethical dilemmas. One condition involved "patients' rights," specifically related to high-risk families, adults with mental health concerns, and adolescents who were at risk but didn't want their families involved. A second condition was described as "system interaction"—that is, problematic situations between nurses and consumers and problems with inadequate resources. "Allocation of resources" included problems about limiting resources for resistant patients, allocating visits, and effectiveness. "Nurses' rights" was the final condition. Employment contracts, high case loads, and limited resources jeopardized the nurses' rights to act according to their own values.

---

**⚒ ETHICAL CONNECTION**

It is not unusual that moral uncertainty is first experienced and escalates to moral distress as patients' rights are not respected or as institutional constraints are applied and nurses feel unable to act on their moral choices and judgments.
  —A. Hamrick. (2000). Moral distress in everyday ethics. *Nursing Outlook, 48,* 199.

---

Oberle and Tenova (2000) asked 22 Canadian public health nurses the following question: "Please describe a frequently recurring ethical problem (or problems) that you have experienced in practice—something that has been a common problem for you." Follow-up questions related to support and how they resolved the problems. The researchers identified five themes based on their analysis of the transcribed interviews:

*Theme 1: Relationships with health care professionals.* Relationships were ethical problems when they prevented the nurse from delivering optimal care—for example, the physician denigrating the nurses' advice, one-way communication only, and observing inferior care.

*Theme 2: Systems issues.* Systems issues included resource distribution, such as performance of quality care with inadequate resources; choices about offering programs, including how much and to whom; and too few resources.

*Theme 3: Patient relationships.* This theme encompassed issues such as the context and nature of the relationships, empowerment versus dependency, and boundary setting. The fact that the patient controlled the continued existence of the relationship challenged the nurses to find ways to establish working and trusting relationships. They had to decide between not intervening in some events to maintain the relationship and taking action to stop risky behavior (e.g., poor parenting). Professional versus personal relationship issues were more problematic in rural settings, when patients were encountered in social settings.

*Theme 4: Respect for persons.* Respecting autonomy was interlaced with all the themes and was seen as foundational to public health nursing. The issues in regard to autonomy were the questioning of whose rights (among family members) should be supported, deciding when someone was unable to make their own decisions, and learning how to be a confidante and still maintain confidentiality when the information was something that would be helpful to other providers.

*Theme 5: Putting self at risk.* Situations involving risks to the nurse's personal integrity and physical danger were the issues in this theme.

## Ethical Decision Making

Dozens of institutes and centers focus on the study of bioethics, most of these associated with universities. Some universities offer degree programs in ethics and in clinical ethics. More and more often, health care agencies use qualified ethicists on ethics committees as consultants to help them with ethical problems. In larger agencies, nurses are able to consult ethicists to help them with ethical decision making.

Often, however, nurses themselves must reason through the ethical problems they encounter. Several authors have presented decision-making models, most of which are based on a problem-solving format. The common steps in the process include these:

1. Determine how these problems affect the autonomy and quality of life of the individual. For example, is the person mentally competent? Is the health problem life-threatening? Is the individual able to communicate and relate to others? To what extent can the individual care for himself or herself? Is the problem likely to get worse? What kinds of treatments are available, proposed, and usual? Are the treatments likely to have positive outcomes? How painful or intrusive are they? What information does the person have about the problem?

2. Separate the ethical issues from those of a strictly medical nature and determine which individuals and groups will be affected by the decision. For example, what is

important for the patient? Which principles are involved: respecting the person, preventing harm, doing good, providing justice, maximizing outcomes for the greater number? Who are the stakeholders in this situation: family, hospital or agency administration, physicians, nurses, the community?

3. Identify and understand the values of those who will be affected, including those of the nurse. What do the individuals involved think about relevant issues, such as quality of life, prolonging life at all costs, autonomy in the face of increased risks, suffering, and the responsibilities of caring?

4. Develop alternative options and weigh them in the light of the rights and obligations of all concerned. What harms and benefits accrue to each of the stakeholders in relation to each option? If a patient refuses chemotherapy, for example, does this decision conflict with the physician's belief that such treatment will be beneficial? Will a family member feel guilty because "everything possible" wasn't done? Are there financial savings for third-party payers?

5. Decide on a course of action and later evaluate the outcome. Part of the decision includes determining who should make the decision.

This framework was designed primarily for use in situations involving individual or family care. Kass (2001) has developed a six-step framework for public health and aggregate populations that poses questions to be asked of program developers.

1. *What are the public health goals of the proposed program?* The goals should be related to reduction of morbidity or mortality. The goal may be an intermediary one, but there should be awareness of the relationship to the ultimate goal.

2. *How effective is the program in achieving its stated goals?* This step requires that assumptions about the effects of the program be identified and documented to the extent possible from previous research or program results.

3. *What are the known or potential burdens of the program?* There are usually three major burdens associated with public health programs: risks to privacy and confidentiality, risks to liberty, and risks to justice. Disease surveillance and vital statistics, communicable disease reporting, and contact tracing all have the risk of loss of confidentiality. The burdens of these programs are borne by the target groups for the benefit of all others, and there is a risk of biased reporting. Health education programs include the possibility that they may not work, may involve manipulation or coercion, and are potentially paternalistic. If findings from research studies are never implemented, there is potential harm to participants who have been misled about the goals of the project. Regulation and legislation constrain freedom of choice and often target some groups for the benefit of others (immunization, motorcycle helmets, smoking).

4. *Can burdens be minimized? Are there alternative approaches?* Programs must be modified to impose the least burden possible without decreasing effectiveness.

5. *Is the program implemented fairly?* Burdens and benefits must be distributed fairly and not solely to specific targeted populations without adequate justification.

6. *How can the benefits and burdens of a program be fairly balanced?* Health officials and professionals have a responsibility to promote programs that increase health benefits and to prevent programs that are unethical. Minority opinions must be taken into account; although dissent is not a reason not to implement a program. The greater the burden imposed by a program, the greater must be its benefits.

One time-honored approach to ethical decision making entails comparing the present case to those in the past. This process, known as **casuistry**, starts with identifying the relevant points and finding how this case is the same or different and which principles then apply. This approach has been foundational for developing church and judicial precedents.

## Service Learning: Discovering the Self and Developing Community Values*

One skill needed for developing ethical responses is what is called a *moral imagination*. In Kohlberg's terms, the imagination develops with moral growth. This imagination gives one the ability to see the moral dimensions of more situations and to empathize with more issues, sides, and sentiments. Such an active imagination is developed with experience and contact with events, situations, and others' ideas. What are your beliefs about the importance and effects of your own personal decisions and actions in the world of nursing and society? How might you find out? What are your values, positions, and beliefs about those people beyond your familiar community? How have you learned those values? Might they change? Do you really know your community? Who do you want to include or exclude from your personal community and why? What are the experiences of people who are different from you? The more these questions are asked and reflected on, the greater the moral imagination.

Even though learning by experience has always been a part of nursing through clinicals, practicums, and laboratory assignments, a new interest has grown in a different form of experiential learning called **service learning**. Service learning emphasizes needs and benefits to an actual group of persons or community rather than solely focusing on student academic and career learning. It is also distinguished by having an overt goal of developing a social consciousness, values, and skills regarding civic responsibility. In addition, to truly be service learning, it must include a strong emphasis on personal insight with planned methods and scheduled time for self-reflection and self-discovery.

*This section was written by Dr. Sherry Hartman, Associate Professor Emeritus, University of Southern Mississippi, School of Nursing.

The focus with this approach is on the lessons learned and insights gained from performing service work, not just clinical or professional intervention. The learner in performing a service is a "servant" to others. Many in nursing believe that service learning can help nursing develop and strengthen the legacy of values believed to underlie both nursing and public health. Service learning lets students face situations in which they foster intangible qualities and values such as empathy, self-awareness, self-confidence, a caring activism to advocate for health, a sense of democratic civic responsibility, a global ecological awareness, cultural competence, and social justice. These are learned in such a way as to become part of a student's life experiences; in turn, these experiences develop the moral imagination.

Even if your university does not have a service learning program, you can apply some of the methods yourself. When working in community centers, such as daycare centers, Meals on Wheels, senior centers, youth services, soup kitchens, drug education programs, and so on, think beyond the patients' immediate health concerns. Think also about what it feels like to see yourself "serving" them. Is "serving" a positive image for nurses? How can a group or community best be "served"? What is in their best interest? What gets in the way of meeting their needs? How can members of the group be empowered to help themselves? Which organizational, local, state, or federal policies need to be changed to assist them? How do you feel about the needy? What did you or anyone else do to contribute to their situation? What are your beliefs about them and their situations? Are justice and care present in their lives? How much are you influenced by the beliefs of your friends, family, church, and the dominant society? Do you have any obligations to the members of the group, beyond their physical health concerns? Would your personal beliefs and values ever make a difference?

## Conclusion

Because of the special relationship nurses have as care providers to their patients, they are frequent participants in ethical decision making relating to patients, families, and the community. Expectations of the community and the profession require that nurses possess certain virtues that will promote trust in all their professional relationships. Ethical decision making is based on the particular values individuals have acquired both as children and as thinking adults.

This chapter has presented the major thinking of philosophers, theologians, and other ethicists over the centuries. It should be clear that there is disagreement on both generalities and specifics. It is characteristic of the United States that there is wide variation in cultural, religious, educational, and ethnic backgrounds, and it is inevitable that values will also differ. We do, however, have many values in common. More recent philosophical approaches (post-modernism) present the view that there are no certainties and no foundational beliefs: We must each make our own way.

The value of understanding the principles of ethical theories is that it provides us with starting points for thinking through and developing our own set of beliefs, and our own frame of reference for the practice of nursing. For whether we like it or not, we are involved in situations that demand an ethical response almost daily in our work.

Explore Community Health Nursing on the Web! To learn more about the topics in this chapter, use the passcode provided to access your exclusive website: **http://nursing.jbpub.com/ communityhealth.** If you do not have a passcode, you can obtain one at this site.

## Application to Practice

### The Need for Home Care

Lila S., age 68, was referred to a home health agency after her discharge from an acute care agency, where she had been hospitalized for pneumonia and stabilization of her diabetes with insulin regulation. She lived with her six-year-old granddaughter in a small, grimy, cluttered trailer. The whereabouts of the girl's father were unknown, and her mother was in and out of drug treatment units.

Lila's poor eyesight from cataracts made it difficult for her to test her blood glucose or measure her insulin. Painful leg ulcers and arthritis made it difficult for her to walk.

Medicaid allowed four home visits by the nurse. This nurse had made home visits to Lila in the past and saw that her ability to care for herself had decreased and that she would need more help in the future. Lila S. has always been quite independent and does not agree that she is not taking care of herself well. She believes it is important that she maintain a home for her granddaughter.

### Medical Issues

- It is important that Lila S.'s glucose be monitored and that her insulin dosage be adjusted accordingly. Her diabetes is fairly stable but needs careful monitoring because of the severe episode of hyperglycemia that accompanied the pneumonia.
- Lila S.'s poor eyesight increases the probability that she will make errors in her diabetes regimen.
- The leg ulcers require care and should be monitored by a knowledgeable person.
- Lila S.'s diminished mobility increases her ability to go to sources of help.

Based on her assessment, the nurse decides that Lila S. needs a nurse to visit several times a week to monitor the glucose readings and help her adjust dosage and inject her insulin. Ideally, these visits should be done every day. An appeal made to the Medicaid reviewer for additional visits was denied, and the home health agency closed the case.

### Ethical Issues

The nurse understood that the agency must have reimbursement for the services it provides; however, she believed that she and the agency had an obligation to continue care that they had begun for this patient, who was obviously in need and whose lack of care might be life-threatening. Legally, no such obligation exists. Various possibilities were discussed with the patient, including trying to find someone she could live with or who could live with her, or going to a nursing home. Lila S. was insistent that she remain at home and care for her granddaughter. The ethical issues involved in this situation are as follows:

- The right of the patient to decide how she wants to live (autonomy)
- The responsibility of the nurse to do no harm or to prevent harm by not abandoning the patient (nonmaleficence) or causing harm to the granddaughter
- The responsibility of the nurse to provide competent care, directly or indirectly, to the patient (beneficence)
- The justice of a health care system that will not pay for needed health care that would be less expensive and likely prevent the otherwise high probability that the patient will need more expensive care later

### Utilitarian Approach

Utilitarians would start with the question, "Who would be affected by decisions in this instance?" The person most affected is the patient herself; next most affected is her granddaughter. The nurse and the home health agency also have some stake. Finally, society in general may be affected. In determining what would accomplish the most good for the most people, the effect of the decision on society would have the highest priority. Continuing home care to this patient might be expensive at the time, but the long-range projection is that without the immediate care, the patient will probably need much more expensive treatment and additional hospitalizations later. Based on concrete information about costs, utilitarians would most likely decide in favor of continuing visits. They may also attempt to change the laws or regulations that tend to prohibit the more cost-effective solution.

### Deontological Approach

The deontological, rule-based approach would examine the rights and obligations of the participants and determine which had higher priority. The foremost right is the right of the patient to make her own decisions based on her own values. The providers are obligated to determine whether the patient is competent to make rational decisions.

There is no reason to believe that Lila S. is incompetent, except for her unawareness that she is less able to care for herself. She values her independence and should be allowed to remain in her home. The providers are then obligated to allow and, preferably, support that choice by providing services to help her remain at home.

Another right of the individual is that of not being harmed by others. The health care providers must examine the medical and social information to determine whether the actions they take will be harmful in any way. Given the current situation, two alternatives present themselves. First, Lila S. remains in her home. It is probable that her diabetes will again go out of control. She will need hospitalization and may possibly need amputations. In this instance, she

### Application to Practice—cont'd

remains autonomous but incurs harm in the progression of her health problems. A second alternative is that Lila S. is persuaded to enter a nursing home, where she can get daily help with her medical and physical needs. The harm in this scenario is that her sense of self as an independent person may be damaged, and she may feel guilty for not taking care of her granddaughter. Whether the deontologist values autonomy or nonmaleficence most, the preferred solution for Lila S. would be continuing home visits.

Additional harm may be incurred by separating the granddaughter from her grandmother, who has provided a stable home and, presumably, love. If the granddaughter were older, she might be enlisted to help with the insulin injections, and perhaps the grandmother will not suffer any serious problems until the granddaughter is of an age to help.

The justice consideration is readily evident in this case: What would seem to be a decent minimum of care cannot be provided because the woman is poor. It is not clear that Lila S. was born disadvantaged, except that diabetes has a large genetic component. Being poor does mean you may not get the early health care you need and may suffer more negative consequences than others.

### Caring Approach

The major focus of the caring approach to this ethics problem will be the responsibilities of the nurse to the patient with whom she has a formal caring relationship. The legal contract for the relationship stipulates a certain number of visits, but the emotional contract has a broader scope. The patient will expect that the nurse will do everything possible to help her achieve her health goals. These expectations may include not abandoning the patient while she still needs help.

The nurse will respond to these expectations and try various avenues to enlist the help Lila S. needs to remain at home. If all else fails and the agency cannot continue visits; the Medicaid administration will not change the ruling; and no relatives, friends, or neighbors can be found to help; there is one last solution. The nurse may decide to utilize personal time, such as lunch hours to provide the needed nursing care. This kind of devotion is above and beyond what is expected legally or ethically, but the feeling of responsibility for some patients may generate that kind of behavior.

In all of the approaches described for this case, the issue of financial support is important. If finances were not a barrier, Lila would get all the help she needed to maintain herself and her granddaughter at home and satisfactorily manage her health needs. It is impossible to consider health care for individuals or groups without considering the benefits and cost to society. Even though a person may take a deontological or a caring approach to ethical decision making, most of the time the ultimate financial outcome must be considered.

## ■ CRITICAL THINKING ACTIVITIES

1. Some nursing students cheat on examinations. This implies an absence of virtue, and many believe that those individuals cannot then be trusted to be honest about the care they give to patients, because they may endanger patients by lying to protect themselves about errors or omissions of treatment. Should dishonest students be denied a license to practice nursing? What is the responsibility of other students who know about the cheating?

2. As a patient or as a family member of a patient, what virtues would you expect of a nurse? Is it reasonable to expect these virtues?

3. A 14-year-old girl revealed to the school nurse that she was sexually active and wanted contraceptive medications. She had seen many of her peers become pregnant, and she stated that she was not ready for a child, but planned to continue her sexual activity. What are the ethical considerations for the nurse in this situation?

4. John, age 32, is known to the public health clinic staff from his visits for intramuscular Haldol injections. He has spent time in the state hospital, where he was diagnosed with paranoid schizophrenia. John was stabilized on medication and discharged to live with his sister, who is married and has four children. He stayed with her only two weeks; he now lives under a bridge. He eats irregularly and has poor hygiene. The original plan was for John to be seen at the mental health clinic, but he refuses to go there. Most of the time his sister is able to persuade him to obtain his medication at the public health clinic. Recently, his sister reported that John is thin and appears ill. He refuses to return to her home and, when pressed, becomes angry and shouts that he wants to be left alone. The sister has appealed to the clinic staff to do something. What are the ethical considerations in this situation?

5. Select a local public health program you know about, or develop one you believe your community needs. Show how this program does or does not meet the ethical criteria proposed by Kass (2001).

6. In a large general hospital, many nurses and auxiliary personnel complain to the clinic staff about chronic back pain related to their jobs. The hospital administration has not been responsive to their complaints. Is this an instance in which regulation of ergonomic devices by OSHA should be required, or would this be unnecessary paternalism?

7. Develop a health care plan for your state that follows Daniels' justice theory. Start by identifying your values and goals.

## ■ REFERENCES

American Nurses Association (ANA). (2001). *Code of ethics for nurses with interpretive statements.* Washington, DC: Author.

Aristotle. (1975). *Aristotle's Nichomachean ethics,* trans. and ed. by H. Apostle. Grinnell, IA: Peripatetic Press.

Aroskar, M. (1989). Community health nurses: Their most significant ethical decision-making problems. *Nursing Clinics of North America, 24*(4), 967–975.

Beauchamp, T., & Childress, J. (1994). *Principles of biomedical ethics* (4th ed.). New York: Oxford University Press.

Benner, P. (1984). *From novice to expert: Excellence and power in clinical nursing practice.* Menlo Park, CA: Addison-Wesley.

Bishop, A. H., & Scudder, J. (1990). *The practical, moral, and personal sense of nursing: A phenomenological philosophy of practice.* Albany, NY: State University of New York Press.

Buchannan, A. (1992). Distributive justice. In L. Becker & C. Becker (Eds.), *Encyclopedia of ethics* (Vol. I, pp. 655–661). New York: Garland.

Burkhardt, M., & Nathaniel, A. (1998). *Ethics and issues in contemporary nursing.* Albany, NY: Delmar.

Daniels, N. (1985). *Just health care.* New York: Cambridge University Press.

Davis, A., & Aroskar, M. (1991). *Ethical dilemmas and nursing practice.* Norwalk, CT: Appleton & Lange.

Donaldson, T. (1992). Circumstances of justice. In L. Becker & C. Becker (Eds.), *Encyclopedia of ethics* (Vol. I, pp. 653–655). New York: Garland.

Duncan, S. (1992). Ethical challenges in community health nursing. *Journal of Advanced Nursing, 17,* 1035–1041.

Folmar, J., Coughlin, S., Bessinger, R., & Sackoff, D. (1997). Ethics in public health practice: A survey of public health nurses in southern Louisiana. *Public Health Nursing, 14*(3), 156–160.

Fry, S. (1996). Ethics in community health nursing practice. In M. Stanhope & J. Lancaster (Eds.), *Community health nursing practice. Health of aggregates, families, and individuals* (4th ed., pp. 93–116). St. Louis: Mosby.

Gremmen, I. (1999). Visiting nurses' situated ethics: Beyond care versus justice. *Nursing Ethics, 6*(6), 515–528.

Horn, P. (1999). *Clinical ethics casebook.* Belmont, CA: Wadsworth.

Kant, I. (1997). *Groundwork of the metaphysics of morals* (original work published 1785; trans. and ed. by M. Gregor.) Cambridge, UK: Cambridge University Press.

Kass, N. (2001). An ethics framework for public health. *American Journal of Public Health, 9*(11), 1776–1782.

Mill, J. (1993). *On liberty and utilitarianism.* New York: Bantam Books. (Original work published 1859/1871)

Nozick, R. (1974). *Anarchy, state, and utopia.* New York: Basic Books.

Oberle, K., & Tenora, S. (2000). Ethical issues in public health nursing. *Nursing Ethics, 7*(5), 425–439.

Purtillo, R. (1999). *Ethical dimensions in the health professions* (3rd ed.). Philadelphia: W. B. Saunders.

Rawls, J. (1999). *A theory of justice* (rev. ed.). Cambridge, MA: Belknap Press.

Schlesinger, M. (2002). On values and democratic policy making: The deceptively fragile consensus around market-oriented medical care. *Journal of Health Politics, Policy, and Law, 27*(6), 889–925.

Steele, S., & Harmon, V. (1983). *Values clarification in nursing* (2nd ed.). Norwalk, CT: Appleton-Century-Crofts.

Uustal, D. (1993). *Clinical and ethical values: Issues and insights.* East Greenwich, RI: Educational Resources in Health Care.

Wagner, N., & Ronen, I. (1996). Ethical dilemmas experienced by hospital and community nurses: An Israeli survey. *Nursing Ethics: An International Journal for Health Care Professionals, 3*(4), 294–304.

# CHAPTER 12
# Environmental Health

Carol J. Nyman, Patricia Butterfield, and Jean Shreffler-Grant

Visit **http://nursing.jbpub.com/communityhealth** for interactive exercises, review questions, Web links, and more.

"In the end, we must restore a balance within ourselves between who we are and what we are doing. Each of us must take a greater personal responsibility for this deteriorating global environment; each of us must take a hard look at the habits of mind and action that reflect—and have led to—this grave crisis."

—Al Gore

Only after the last tree has been cut down,
Only after the last river has been poisoned,
Only after the last fish has been caught,
Only then will you find that money cannot be eaten.

*—Cree Indian Philosophy*

There are five essential points in securing the health of houses:
1. Pure air
2. Pure water
3. Efficient drainage
4. Cleanliness
5. Light

*—Florence Nightingale, 1860*

The history of life on earth has been a history of interaction between living things and their surroundings.

*—Rachel Carson*

As you reflect on your personal relationship with the environment, how do these quotes reflect changes through the past century of humans and their environment? As nurses, do we consider environmental influences as we care for our patients?

## CHAPTER FOCUS

**Trends in Exposure and Disease**

**A World View**

**The Environment and Health**
- Environmental Health Policy: Historical Perspectives
- Recent Environmental Health Issues
- Historical Perspectives on Environment and Health
- Origins of Environmental Health Policy
- Environmental Policy: Government and Public Roles

**Nursing and the Environment**

**Roles of the Community Health Nurse**
- Identifying Risks
- Assessing Exposures
- Communicating Risks
- Assessing and Referring Patients

**Upstream Thinking: Making Connections Between Environmental and Human Health**

**Ethical Principles Addressing Environmental Health Nursing**

## QUESTIONS TO CONSIDER

After reading this chapter, you will know the answers to the following questions:

1. Which specific global environmental threats affect public health?
2. What are current trends in disease and exposure in the environment?
3. What is the history of environmental health in the United States?
4. What is environmental health policy?
5. How does environmental health policy evolve?
6. What is the government's role in environmental health policy?
7. What are the specific roles of the community health nurse in promoting a healthy environment?
8. What is an exposure assessment, and how is it conducted?
9. What is the role of effective communication in the education of community residents?
10. What is upstream thinking, and how is it related to environmental health?
11. What are the key ethical principles related to the environment?
12. How does a community health nurse develop a clinical practice in environmental health?

## KEY TERMS

| | | | |
|---|---|---|---|
| Environmental health | Risk assessment | Social justice | Toxins |
| Environmental justice | Risk management | Toxicology | Upstream thinking |

THE IMPACT OF environmental agents on human health is obvious when exposures are high and health effects are immediate. Nurses are most likely to see this type of situation in emergency rooms or poison control centers. Frantic parents might call to report that their 3-year-old daughter was found playing with a bag of fertilizer in the garage. A young father, stripping woodwork in a spare basement room, may be brought into the emergency room by his wife after being overcome by fumes from paint stripper. An elderly woman may be found unconscious in her home after using her gas stove burners to heat her small apartment. In each situation, nurses and other professionals organize a collective response to an immediate health crisis precipitated by an environmental agent. Detoxification procedures begin, and emergency efforts focus on protecting a person's target organ systems. In these scenarios, the link between an environment exposure and human health is clear. It is easy to see that harmful consequences can result from a single exposure to a toxic agent.

However, acute exposures represent only the tip of the iceberg in the domain of environmental health. In most situations, associations between exposures and disease are not easily traced; years or decades may have elapsed between exposure to the agent of concern and subsequent health effects. In addition, exposures may have occurred in small doses over time or may involve contact with a variety of compounds that interact with each other to cause small changes that ultimately lead to disease. An additional complicating factor is that, for many environmental factors, inconclusive science characterizes associations between exposure and the development of disease.

Because of these and other considerations, environmental health is one of the most challenging and rapidly developing parts of community health nursing. Fortunately, for many nurses, it is also one of the most rewarding areas of practice.

> **❝***I have therefore come to believe that the world's ecological balance depends on more than just our ability to restore a balance between civilization's ravenous appetite for resources and the fragile equilibrium of the earth's environment; it depends on more, even, than our ability to restore a balance between ourselves as individuals and the civilization we aspire to create and sustain. In the end, we must restore a balance within ourselves between who we are and what we are doing. Each of us must take a greater personal responsibility for this deteriorating global environment; each of us must take a hard look at the habits of mind and action that reflect—and have led to—this grave crisis.* **❞**
>
> —Al Gore, Earth in the Balance: Ecology and the Human Spirit, 1992

## Trends in Exposure and Disease

Health professionals and citizens are generally aware of the delicate balance that exists between the environment and global health. A goal of policy makers, both in the United States and elsewhere, has been to increase technology without compromising public health and safety. Unfortunately, despite our knowledge of the links between environmental contaminants and health problems, our society continues to manufacture, use, and dispose of many potentially hazardous chemicals. In 2003, U.S. industry reported the release of 4.44 billion pounds of potential toxic chemicals into the air, water, and soil (U.S. Environmental Protection Agency, 2005). The widespread use of chemicals with toxic effects (**toxins**) highlights the importance of educating nurses who can work to reduce exposures to those substances in homes, workplaces, and public areas. Many cases of environmentally induced illness can be prevented, but it requires actions that have not traditionally been a central part of community health nursing (Kleffel, 1996; Butterfield, 2002).

## A World View

Despite efforts to reduce industrial pollution and automobile emissions, increasing numbers of citizens the world over are facing health risks from environmental toxicants. Because of the rapid increase in the world's population, small changes in urbanization and agricultural production can have large consequences on global public health (Briggs, 2003). The health consequences of industrial globalization and planetary climate change are problems for the world that no single nation can hope to address alone (Kirk, 2002). The relationships of industrialization and deforestation to the emergence of new diseases and the reemergence of diseases previously thought to be under control (e.g., tuberculosis) are of special concern. Recent ecological changes associated with human health problems include the following:

- Population movements and the intrusion of humans into new habitats, particularly tropical forests
- Deforestation, with new forest–farmland margins that expose farmers to new vectors of disease (Daszak, Tabor, Kilpatrick, Epstein, & Plowright, 2004)
- Irrigation, especially primitive systems that serve as breeding areas of arthropods
- Rapidly expanding urbanization, with vector populations finding urban breeding grounds in standing water and sewage (Patz et al., 2004)
- Changes in agricultural practices, such as the use of antimicrobial-supplemented animal feeds and the crowding of animals in confined spaces (Thu, 2002)

It is apparent that these problems require a perspective that goes beyond national boundaries and mobilizes global concern and cooperation. Import policies in developed nations need to address the transfer of natural resources from developing countries, such as mineral wealth, oil, and exotic lumber. Environmentally sound practices in the mining, agriculture, and forestry industries need to be enhanced through cooperative efforts between industry and citizen groups. Several disease surveillance organizations have requested additional funding for the development of a system

Children play in contaminated water of the Ganges in India.

that could coordinate global reporting of disease surveillance and control efforts. Better diagnostic techniques, prevention strategies, and risk factor analysis must be taught to health care professionals worldwide. More funding for basic and applied research related to the environment and infectious diseases can yield significant improvements in public health. Education for a global perspective is needed to address the issue of infectious disease within the context of shared environmental responsibility. As our planet moves from a national to an international perspective on health problems, it is easy to see that environmentally destructive practices in one country can lead to health problems in many other parts of the world.

The Centers for Disease Control and Prevention (2004) analyzed the public health consequences from global heat waves—an increasingly common occurrence. Record high temperatures were reported in many European cities during the summer of 2003, and this analysis from *Morbidity and Mortality Weekly Report* provides evidence of excess mortality in the elderly during this time period. Many scientists have hypothesized that global changes in weather patterns will lead to critical changes in disease occurrence over the next few decades.

**❝** *I am I plus my surroundings; and if I do not preserve the latter, I do not preserve myself.* **❞**

—*Jose Ortega y Gasset*

## The Environment and Health

A healthy environment is one in which people—whether at home, in schools, at workplaces, or in their communities—have access to safe food and water, have adequate sanitation, and are protected from risks associated with chemical pollution, environmental degradation, and disasters (World Health Organization, 2008). The term **environmental health** refers to freedom from illness or injury related to toxic agents and other environmental conditions that are potentially detrimental to human health (Pope, Snyder, & Mood, 1995). Health care providers' roles in environmental health are expanding to include caring for people with exposures to hazards in their homes, workplaces, and communities through contaminated air, water, and soil.

Because "environment" is such a universal concept, it can be difficult to define the boundaries of environmental health. The application of environmental health in clinical practice ranges from descriptions of hospital rooms to international and global perspectives on the health of the planet. Although a hospital room differs from a global ecology perspective in complexity as well as along other dimensions, both views can provide insights into opportunities for health at the individual and collective levels. Just as the scope of clinical practice varies from individual emergencies to situations in which a health care provider is charged with the health assessment of populations, so too must the scope of environmental health assessment vary across situations.

Because of the rapid increase in chemical production and use since World War II, synthetically derived chemicals are often considered inherently dangerous. However, each environmental agent must be studied and understood; it is a big mistake to overgeneralize and say that all synthetic products are dangerous and that all natural products are inherently safe. Some of the biggest threats to human health throughout human history have come from "natural" substances such as lead, mercury, and arsenic. Furthermore, chemicals are often considered the only source of environmental health threats; however, physical agents (e.g., noise, vibration, ionizing radiation) and biological agents (e.g., bacterial contamination, fungal spores, viruses) also play significant roles in health problems of environmental etiology.

## CULTURAL CONNECTION

Some cultural and religious groups do not believe in the use of added minerals, such as fluoride, to drinking water. With current research providing evidence that fluoridated drinking water dramatically reduces tooth decay in children, how can these belief systems be respected while still preserving the health of the population?

## Environmental Health Policy: Historical Perspectives

In Europe and North America, early environmental health regulations focused exclusively on sanitation, water quality, and housing. The public health implications of these regulations cannot be overemphasized; mortality rates dropped significantly following the institutionalization of

quality standards for drinking water and sewage disposal (Kotchian, 1997). Following the publication of Rachel Carson's *Silent Spring* in 1962, citizen groups mobilized in support of more comprehensive legislation to protect the environment and endangered species. Examples of legislation passed during the 1960s and 1970s include clean air and water acts, occupational health and safety acts, toxic substances controls acts, and Poison Prevention Packaging Act. During these two decades, the Environmental Protection Agency (EPA), Occupational Safety and Health Administration, and Nuclear Regulation Commission were also established (Stevens & Hall, 1997).

Public and governmental actions addressing environmental health continue to this day, although some observers believe that responses have not been sufficient to reduce the health risks in the environment. Community right-to-know federal legislation, enacted in 1987, authorizes citizens' access to information addressing the presence, management, and release of hazardous chemicals in their community. Information addressing the storage and use of more than 300 chemicals was collected by the EPA, assembled into databases titled the Toxic Release Inventory, and made available to the public. The Pollution Prevention Act of 1990 authorized data collection activities addressing toxic chemicals that leave a community facility. These recent governmental efforts have greatly enhanced the ability of citizens to gain access to environmental data from their neighborhood. Such data can empower citizens to advocate on behalf of their community and hold government and private officials accountable for policy decisions.

**❝***They paved paradise and put up a parking lot.***❞**

—Joni Mitchell, 1970

## BOX 12-1

### An Outbreak of Hantavirus

In May 1993 a healthy, athletic 21-year-old Navajo woman living on the reservation in New Mexico died from a respiratory ailment of acute onset. Five days later, on the way to her funeral, her 19-year-old fiancé, who had been feeling ill for several days, went into respiratory failure and could not be resuscitated. In late May, the woman's brother, who lived in a trailer near one the couple had shared, died of acute onset of a similar illness, as did his wife 5 days later. By early June, 24 cases with similar symptoms, including 12 deaths, had been reported in the area. Alert Indian Health Service personnel and Department of Health officials took immediate action requesting assistance from the Centers for Disease Control and Prevention (CDC). Thanks in part to proactive epidemiology efforts and advances in molecular biology, within 4 weeks the CDC was able to identify the cause of death as pulmonary Hantavirus. This condition had not previously been seen in North America. The overall case fatality rate was 76%, with deaths in 13 of the first 17 confirmed cases (Duchin et al., 1994).

One of the strongest explanations for the appearance of this new and severe disease is environmental. The El Niño

weather pattern had brought unusually wet weather to the area in the early 1990s. For 5 years, there had been a severe drought in the area, but in the winter of 1992–1993, there had been record snowfall followed by a rainy spring, the piñon nut harvest was unusually large, as was the mouse population. The University of New Mexico had done an ecological survey of the area that spring and was impressed to note a sudden population explosion among the deer mice—a tenfold increase since the previous year. The CDC discovered that deer mice were carriers of the Hantavirus, passing it in their urine and feces. With their numbers greatly increased, the deer mice were making more contact with humans by invading their homes, establishing a lethal connection with a new disease. The epidemiologist who did a survey of the initial victims' home after their deaths reported the presence of numerous mouse droppings (Garrett, 1994). Hantavirus may have been present in North America before 1993, but notable environmental and weather changes that occurred that year created a situation that brought humans, mice, and virus together in a profound way, allowing for the disease's presentation in humans.

Despite recent advances in environmental information access, some environmental advocates point out that, although some environmental risks have been minimized or eliminated, new risks have been identified but not addressed. Citizen advocacy groups have observed that many health and safety regulations have not been uniformly implemented or enforced; loopholes exist in others. In addition, some policy makers and legislators believe that environmental initiatives and laws are not in the best interests of the economy; thus laws, standards, or initiatives have been canceled, weakened, or not given the funds they need to be effective.

 ENVIRONMENTAL CONNECTION

*What a man can be is born with him; what he becomes is a result of his environment.*

—North Dakota saying

## Recent Environmental Health Issues

In the second half of the twentieth century, awareness of the damage to the environment and its resulting effect on health grew dramatically. Population growth (see the following figures), urban spread, advanced technology, industrialization, and modern agricultural methods were the source of great progress, but they also led to the creation of environmental hazards that may not have been observed previously. It seems as if newspapers feature articles on the new threats almost daily, with citizens left to sort out the difference between hype and reality. Three trends that seem here to stay include: (1) the focus on the built environment, (2) an emphasis on children's environmental health, and (3) the environmental justice movement.

In regard to the built environment, many scientists are beginning to view cities and towns almost as ecosystems and to critically examine the placement of roads, sidewalks, and buildings. Using mapping and other research techniques, they can compare differences in obesity levels between neighborhoods with and without sidewalks (Booth, Pinkston, & Poston, 2005). Other scientists are examining the complex relationships among neighborhood factors such as walkability, grocery store access, and the availability of bike paths. Their studies are beginning to quantify what we already know intuitively: Depending on their attributes, "places" can promote or inhibit health in the same way that a poor diet can. In fact, the more we learn about built environment, the more scientists are beginning to see links between physical and mental health and automobile use (or overuse) (Pohanka & Fitzgerald, 2004).

Over the past five years, children's environmental health issues have also become the focus of greater scientific scrutiny. An increasing recognition that children absorb chemicals in different ways than adults has led to studies examining children's exposure to substances such as pesticides, mercury, and tobacco smoke (Reddy, Reddy, & Reddy, 2004). One big concern is the cumulative effect of exposure to multiple chemicals over a child's life. Historically, cancer studies have been conducted to examine links between a single agent (e.g., benzene) and a single type of cancer. Now, however, scientists are beginning to recognize the limitations of looking at just one agent at a time and are beginning to look at exposure to multiple chemicals in breast milk, in drinking water, and in school settings (Shendell, Barnett, & Boese, 2004).

The environmental justice movement has played a critical role in changing government policies addressing the placement and operation of factories and other industrial

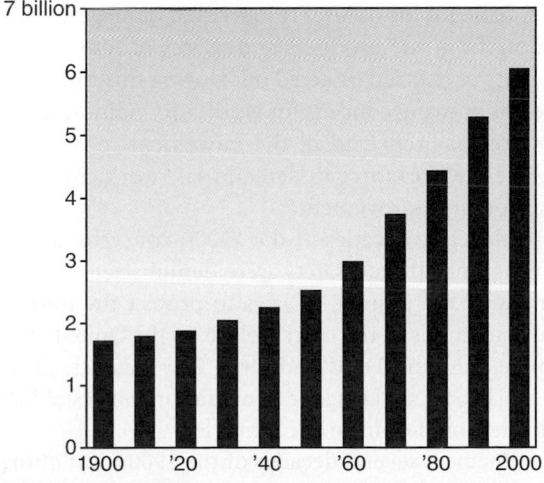

**World population**
One hundred years ago, 1.6 billion people lived on Earth.

Estimates of world population

*Source*: U.S. Department of Commerce; U.S. Census Bureau; United Nations; Worldwatch Institute.

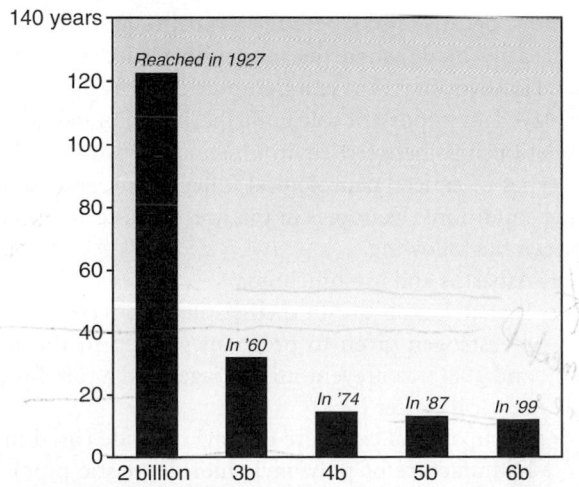

**Population growth**
There has been more population growth since 1950 than in the preceding 4 million years.

Years taken to reach one billion markers

*Source*: U.S. Department of Commerce; U.S. Census Bureau; United Nations; Worldwatch Institute.

facilities in the United States. When citizens began to protest the placement of factories in minority neighborhoods, state and local policy makers began to examine historical (and current) business and zoning regulations. What they found was a pattern of putting "dirty" businesses in poorer or minority communities, while higher-income neighborhoods remained free of such facilities (Frumkin, 2005). From these beginnings came the environmental justice movement, which sowed the seeds of activism across the nation. Today, environmental justice has come to be known as the fair treatment and meaningful involvement of all people, regardless of race, color, national origin, or income, with respect to the development, implementation, and enforcement of environmental laws, regulations, and policies (U.S. Environmental Protection Agency, 2008).

> *There is a unity of the body with the environment, as well as a unity of the body and souls into one person.*
>
> —Alfred North Whitehead

## Historical Perspectives on Environment and Health

The science of epidemiology has been closely linked to environmental health since the original work done by John Snow in 1854. The same deductive processes in inquiry that Snow used to link cholera deaths to contaminated Thames River water have been used countless times over the past century to link environmental agents with disease occurrence. Because the basic tenets of descriptive epidemiology (i.e., time, person, and place) have been so powerful a tool in establishing links between environmental agents and disease, this approach to scientific inquiry has stood the test of time for investigations of environmentally induced diseases at both local and global levels.

Some argue that epidemiological methods have been more effective in addressing infectious and acute diseases than chronic conditions. There may be some validity to this position, because links between exposure and disease are most easily made when the induction period is relatively brief. However, in recent years, chronic disease epidemiology has played an important role in furthering an understanding of relationships between environmental exposures and several types of cancer, neurological impairment, and autoimmune conditions. Examples in this area include associations between the following:

- Asbestos and mesothelioma
- Prenatal exposure to diethylstilbestrol (DES, a form of estrogen given to pregnant women in the 1950s and 1960s to prevent miscarriage) and a rare form of cervical cancer
- Occupational exposure to vinyl chloride (used in the manufacture of polyvinyl chloride plastic pipe) and the development of liver cancer

One of the biggest challenges in the area of chronic disease epidemiology is to establish evidence of exposure dose

for agents without biomarkers (i.e., physiological fingerprint of exposure). In these cases, exposure has most often been "estimated" using a questionnaire or interview guide. This method of estimating exposure can be problematic for exposures that may (or may not) have happened years or decades ago. Recently, the Centers for Disease Control and Prevention (CDC) has begun to test citizens for body burden levels of a variety of environmental chemicals. In 2003, CDC released findings that included citizens' blood and urine levels of 116 chemicals, including selected insecticides and herbicides, dioxins, phytoestrogens, and lead. Preliminary findings revealed that only 2.2% of children (ages 1–5) were found to have elevated blood lead levels—an improvement from the 4.4% rate seen in the 1990s. Other findings provided evidence that, on average, children had twice the blood level of chlorpyrifos, an organochlorine insecticide, than adults (CDC, 2008). The authors of this report noted that is it important to remember that there has been no baseline information available for most of these chemicals; therefore, one cannot say whether the levels found are safe or unsafe. The important gap that this study fills is in providing baseline information so that we can begin to understand what are "normal" ranges for these chemicals. There is good news on the horizon. The CDC is planning to release a new report every two years so that scientists can begin to understand trends in chemical exposures. Understanding these exposures will provide a scientifically accurate foundation for the development of U.S. chemical reduction policies (CDC, 2008).

## Origins of Environmental Health Policy

Although concerns for environmental risks to health and safety have existed to some extent for centuries, the current widespread awareness and concern about these risks among public and private sectors are relatively recent phenomena. With the Industrial Revolution in the 1800s, the developed world, including the United States, focused on modernization and rapid production of goods and services. Concerns about depletion of natural resources or damage and hazards resulting from the products and wastes of industrialization were not yet realized or acted on. During this time, however, there was growing concern for working conditions and safety of workers, as reflected in the movement to organize and unionize the workforce to demand safe work environments, among other improvements.

In the early decades of the 1900s, concerns about environmental health and safety were demonstrated by governments with the passage of laws to protect the public from hazardous goods in the marketplace. In the United States, for example, the Pure Food and Drug Law was passed in 1906 and the Food and Drug Administration was established in 1931 (Henson, Robinson, & Schmele, 1996).

In the next several decades of the 1900s, war efforts and postwar industrial rebuilding consumed the energies of governments and the public. Again, the international production of war and postwar goods and services took precedence,

## Application to Practice

### Health Policy Actions Result from Community Involvement

Pam and Steven are registered nurses practicing at a mobile clinic that provides health care for migrant farm workers and their families in a Midwestern state. They discuss the numerous children with skin and respiratory complaints that they have recently seen at the clinic. A review of clinic records reveals that more than twice the expected number of children had been seen in the clinic presenting with skin irritations, headaches, or abdominal cramping. The nurses begin to gather more detailed interview data from mothers who bring their children to the clinic with these symptoms. They learn that mothers are bringing their infants to the fields because there is no affordable day care available in this area. Older children work with their parents picking vegetables. They discuss their observations with the clinic's medical director and a toxicology consultant from the Migrant Council. They learn that the symptoms they have observed are common in pesticide exposure or poisoning.

A team from the clinic and Migrant Council visit the local vegetable fields and find multiple exposure risks for children. Some mothers carry infants into the fields in cloth carriers as they pick crops. Other infants are left at the edges of the crop rows in child carriers and strollers. Children as young as 4 years old pick vegetables next to their parents. Rubber gloves and other protective coverings are not available in sizes small enough for child workers. Some children are observed picking pesticide-dusted vegetable and eating them unwashed for lunch. On review of applicable federal and state laws, they find that while regulations protecting children from pesticides in foods are strict and clear, they are much less clear regarding protection of adults or children who harvest that food. Laws regulating or providing for safety for agricultural child workers are also not clear.

The team meets to examine the data collected and formulate an approach. They decide that an immediate priority is to reduce the potential pesticide exposures in this local area. They plan to work with farm owners to provide low-cost or no-cost day care and child-sized protective equipment. They also plan educational programs for migrant parents, offered after hours in their housing areas, focused on reducing exposures. Because migrant workers travel after harvest to other agricultural areas, reducing the problem in this area alone will not protect the children as they move to other areas. The team identifies informal leaders in the group of migrant workers and provides them with training in community development so that they will be better able to advocate for safe working conditions on behalf of their group wherever they work. The team also contacts legislators and policy makers to advocate for improved regulations to protect migrant workers and their families from pesticide exposures.

*Source*: Adapted from Crenson, 1997.

---

Recycling efforts have increased with significant environmental benefits.

and the lay public held a belief that their governments would protect them from environmental risks and hazards.

The birth of the consumer-driven environmental movement that continues today can be traced to the 1960s and 1970s. Multiple trends and events served to raise international consciousness that some aspects of the environment had become a growing risk to public health and safety. Disenchantment with postwar living conditions and the realization of the environmental effects of nuclear proliferation and war occurred after World War II. Public cynicism toward the government and other institutions occurred in the United States during and after the Vietnam War era. Several widely read exposés of environmental hazards also were published during this time. One influential publication, *Silent Spring* (Carson, 1962), predicted the poisoning and destruction of the natural environment in the name of progress with the use of pesticides. Rachel Carson's book was history making in its effect on thought and policy making following its publication. Consumerism gained momentum during this time as a result of the efforts of national leaders and consumer advocate groups. All of these trends and events resulted in public concern and activism followed by governmental responses to citizens' growing environmental awareness.

> **"** *The nation that destroys its soil destroys itself.* **"**
>
> —Franklin D. Roosevelt

## ■ Environmental Policy: Governmental and Public Roles

One of the primary purposes of government in a democratic society is to protect and safeguard the governed or the public. To fulfill this purpose, the government passes laws and enacts rules and regulations to prevent and reduce risks to the public. Government agencies and offices have been created to identify and monitor risks and hazards, monitor compliance with rules, and gather data to inform policy makers. Government initiatives have been implemented because of priorities of elected or appointed officials as well as in response to pressures from an environmentally conscious public.

Despite all of this governmental activity, our environment still poses hazards to the safety and health of the public. In many cases, the dangers are more complicated now than ever before. Reasons for that increased risk include the following:

- Environmental health has been addressed in a piecemeal fashion instead of in a potentially more effective comprehensive plan.
- Proposed policies and laws that improve the health of the environment are often perceived to be in conflict with what is in the best interest of business and the economy.
- Laws and policies cannot solve all environmental problems and risks without voluntary actions by individuals, groups, and organizations.
- Science has not been able to keep pace with potential environmental hazards and pollutants.
- In a world of finite resources, the costs of cleaning and protecting the environment are in competition with the costs of other desired and needed social programs.

At both the local and national levels, policy makers set national and state priorities among competing social programs, establish standards for environmental hazards and risks, take action against those who violate standards, and allocate billions of federal and state funds according to these established priorities. A broad set of population health goals to be achieved by the year 2000 was established by the U.S. Public Health Service 20 years ago and was reaffirmed with the publication of *Healthy People 2010* (U.S. Department of Health and Human Services, 2001). *Healthy People 2010*

objectives, which include environmental health as one of 28 priority areas, serve as the basis for federal and state policy formulation and action; selected objectives related to the environment are listed in the *Healthy People 2010* feature on page 277.

The public plays an important role in setting the stage for policy decisions by expressing its values and in the actions it takes as an electorate. Policy makes are also influenced by organized interest groups and elected and appointed officials who represent these interests. In the environmental health arena, these groups have traditionally been organized into two factions: (1) businesses and industries that depend on the environment for raw materials and/or disposal of waste and (2) citizen groups and voluntary organizations that have an interest in preventing or limiting the extraction of raw materials or disposal of waste. Nurses can work to foster health communication between groups and direct the dialogue to areas of common ground. In addition to participation of citizens, nurses can enlarge their role in environmental health policy making by increasing their political expertise and activity as professionals.

In the United States, policy makers and the public alike trust the nursing profession to be advocates for patients and to speak and act on behalf of the health of the population. Nurses are considered reliable and trustworthy sources of information about threats to health and also represent the largest group of health care professionals among the voting age population. By staying informed of current and accurate

Robert Kennedy, Jr., environmental activist, attorney, and author of *Crimes Against Nature*, with text author Dr. Karen Saucier Lundy.

**Objectives Related to Environmental Health**

*Outdoor Air Quality*

8.1 Reduce the proportion of persons exposed to air that does not meet the U.S. Environmental Protection Agency's (EPA's) health-based standards for harmful air pollutants.

8.4 Reduce air toxic emissions to decrease the risk of adverse health effects caused by airborne toxics.

*Water Quality*

8.5 Increase the proportion of persons served by community water systems who receive a supply of drinking water that meets the regulations of the Safe Drinking Water Act.

8.8 Increase the proportion of assessed rivers, lakes, and estuaries that are safe for fishing and recreational purposes.

*Toxins and Waste*

8.11 Eliminate elevated blood lead levels in children.

8.12 Minimize the risks to human health and the environment posed by hazardous sites.

*Healthy Homes and Healthy Communities*

8.16 Reduce indoor allergen levels.

8.20 Increase the proportion of the nation's primary and secondary schools that have official school policies ensuring the safety of students and staff from environmental hazards, such as chemicals in special classrooms, poor indoor air quality, asbestos, and exposure to pesticides.

*Infrastructure and Surveillance*

8.27 Increase or maintain the number of territories, tribes, and states, and the District of Columbia that monitor diseases or conditions that can be caused by exposure to environmental hazards.

*Global Environmental Health*

8.29 Reduce the global burden of disease due to poor water quality, sanitation, and personal and domestic hygiene.

*Source*: U.S. DHHS, 2001.

information on environmental risks, organizing and becoming actively involved with groups of nurses and others around environmental issues, and actively communicating with and lobbying policy makers as well as organized interest groups, nurses can effectively influence public policy. In the practice arena, nurses can also inform and mobilize citizen groups and other professionals to become actively involved in communicating with and lobbying policy makers about environmental issues of concern to themselves and their communities.

> 🔨 ETHICAL CONNECTION
>
> Attempts to ban smoking in bars have resulted in community divisiveness over public health and individual right to freedom of expression, especially in small, western U.S. towns. As a community health nurse, how can you provide advocacy for the entire population in this environmental health issue?

## Nursing and the Environment

Nursing's efforts to promote health by influencing environmental conditions predate the modern environmental movement by more than a century. Florence Nightingale, the founder of modern nursing, developed her theory of nursing with a strong emphasis on the individual's environment. Although the term "environment" did not appear in her published works, she addressed health using five environmental dimensions: (1) pure, fresh air; (2) pure water; (3) efficient drainage; (4) cleanliness; and (5) light—that is,

*"Within the last few years, a large part of London was in the daily habit of using water polluted by the drainage of its sewers and water closets. This has happily been remedied. But, in many parts of the country, well water of a very impure kind is used for domestic purposes. And when epidemic disease shows itself, persons using such water are almost sure to suffer."*

*Florence Nightingale, 1860*

direct sunlight (Nightingale, 1969/1860). To Nightingale, the environment was the surrounding context in which the individual lived: a person's health or illness was a direct result of environmental influences. Deficiencies in any of the five factors produced a health deficit. Nightingale also stressed the importance of a comfortably warm, noise-free environment and a good diet. Although originally intended to address a hospital environment, her concepts were broad enough to serve as a basis for public health nursing, and they remain integral parts of nursing and health care.

Nursing has long noted the influence of the environment on health and has assumed the role of managing the interaction between patients and their environments. Often, nursing's approach has been to assist the patient to adapt to the environment; thus the focus for intervention was changing the individual or community patient to facilitate a better match with the environment. An emerging role for nursing today is to intervene directly in environmental factors in an attempt to change unhealthy conditions and mobilize individuals or communities to do the same. Nurse scientists are conducting studies in environmental factors directly, such as water and air quality, policies, laws that influence health of the population, and conditions in workers' environments to improve understanding of healthful and unhealthful environmental conditions and the interventions that can improve them.

### Got an Alternative?

Using organic or nontoxic household products in the home is safer for the environment and for the residents of both the home and the community. One common concern is the high cost of these products. What can the community health nurse do in regard to educating families about reducing environmental toxins when the costs of these products limit their use among disadvantaged families?

Just as it is a challenge to draw a circle around the concept of environmental health, so, too, is it difficult to delineate the unique role of nursing in addressing environmental health issues. Many professional disciplines—from wildlife biologists to microbiologists to engineers—consider environmental health problems within their domain of expertise. Environmental health is an area in which many different professionals are needed to prevent, minimize, and improve environmental problems. Both basic and applied research efforts are required to understand all of the implications of environmental health problems. Professional nurses are well suited to participate in collaborative efforts because they have historically functioned at the center of the health care team. However, nursing efforts are focused exclusively on human health, in contrast to some professions, whose efforts are directed toward other species such as fish, large mammals, and plant life. Nursing interventions are directed toward preventing and minimizing the effects of environmental health problems on persons of all

The physical environment in which we live, such as the Colorado winter above, greatly affects a population's health.

ages. This focus does not mean, however, that concerns about animal and plant life are dismissed or that health connections between species are not recognized.

Community health and occupational health are the nursing practice specialties often associated with health hazards in the physical environment. In view of the universal presence of environmental hazards, it is critical that nurses in all practice specialties have an understanding of environmental health (Pope, Snyder, & Mood, 1995). As patient advocates, all nurses need to be concerned about health of the environment because it is a major determinant of their patients' health.

---

### MEDIA MOMENT

#### *Silkwood* (1983)

While working in a Kerr-McGee nuclear power plant in Oklahoma making nuclear reactors, Karen Silkwood (Meryl Streep) becomes exposed to radiation in this fact-based movie. Silkwood is a working-class mother who resides with a roommate (Cher) and boyfriend (Kurt Russell) and lives an ordinary working-class life, punching the time clock at the nuclear plant.

The nuclear plant in the film is behind on an important contract. People are working overtime and corners are being cut. A series of small incidents convinces Silkwood that the compromises are dangerous, that the health of the workers is being needlessly risked, and that the company is turning its back on the falsification of safety and workmanship tests. Silkwood sees the union as a way to address these complaints, but a meeting in Washington, D.C., yields little more than publicity for the union—and no real solution for the workers.

Silkwood died in a mysterious automobile accident, on her way to deliver some documents to a *New York Times* reporter when her car left the road. The documents were never found. The movie does not address whether the accident was actually a murder and, if so, by whom. The complications of being a "whistleblower" are examined, along with the many factions that may have wanted Silkwood out of the way. This is a thought-provoking movie about environmental threats and includes excellent performances by Streep, Cher, and Russell. The movie was nominated for multiple Academy Awards and Golden Globes and is based on a true story.

It is important to consider the depth of inquiry when addressing the role of nursing in environmental health. Which areas of inquiry contain the dimensions of environment that fall within the scope of nursing? Surely, given enough time and paper, one could generate a seemingly endless list of questions that relate human health to the environment. The challenge then lies in the ability to focus nursing assessment activities into areas that are most obvious to the clinical or research area of interest. One would expect to see overlapping areas of focus between environmental health, as it relates to professional nursing, and other professions such as **toxicology**, pharmacology, and the behavioral sciences. The goal in such a case is not to stake out a new specialty area for nursing practice, but rather to integrate knowledge from nursing and other disciplines and apply this knowledge to the patients' needs for health promotion or restoration.

Looking at the environment from a broad view, environmental factors are involved in almost all disease risks and include areas such as housing, nutrition, socioeconomic status, and lifestyle. Even the health of persons with genetic disorders can often be enhanced through nursing actions addressing personal and societal aspects of the environment. Environmental health includes a concern for not only the physical environment, but also the interrelated social, economic, psychological, and political environments. Such conditions as poverty, powerlessness, social injustice, and racism that arise from diverse environmental factors can reduce opportunities for health and contribute to illness just as certainly as do chemical or physical agents. A central goal of this chapter is to provide information that allows for a richer understanding of the connectedness among many features of the environment. Although information addressing physical agents predominates in this chapter, it is important to understand that aspects of the social and economic environment are also centrally linked to opportunities for health in civilizations throughout the world.

### 🖥 Research Alert

Amaya and colleagues have documented high rates of exposure to lead, trace elements, and pesticides in Hispanic persons residing in United States–Mexico border communities. As one part of a larger study examining the serum lead levels in pregnant Hispanic women, a case investigation of a family with two children with elevated lead levels was conducted. Dust samples were collected both inside and outside the residence; additional samples were taken from water, paint, and cookware in the home. The evidence supported a hypothesis that primary exposure occurred from battery recycling and burning of electrical wire conducted on the premises by the father and grandfather of the children. Steps to ameliorate exposure pathways were undertaken by community health nurses working with the family. Monthly lead levels taken on both children declined over the next 4 months. Unfortunately, the family moved away without notice and was lost to follow-up 9 months after the initial event.

Such investigations capitalize on the risk communication skills of nurses working in border communities. Nurses' abilities to locate and intervene effectively with disenfranchised families are unsurpassed among health professions. Case-series and case-control studies by nurse scientists can yield important findings at the local and national levels, while furthering the role of nursing and the environmental health sciences. Elevated blood lead levels have been reported in approximately 8% of low-income children in El Paso County, Texas. Nursing research addressing the areas of risk communication, health care access, and intervention strategies with families at risk for lead exposure can lead to a significant reduction of persons affected by this serious health problem. ◯

*Source*: Amaya, M. A., Ackall, G., Pingitore, N., Quiroga, M., & Ternazas-Ponce, B. (1997). Childhood lead poisoning on the US–Mexico border. A case study in environmental health nursing lead poisoning. *Public Health Nursing, 14*, 353–360.

## Roles of the Community Health Nurse

Nursing has a long history of identifying health risks and intervening directly on behalf of patient health. The role of the nurse in providing pure water, a restful setting, and a hygienic hospital environment was among the early environmental concerns of the nursing profession. By the late 1800s and early 1900s, nursing became concerned with identifying and resolving communicable disease outbreaks, improper food handling, inadequate disposal of wastes, and unsafe water supplies (Tiedje & Wood, 1995). During the growing environmental awareness of the 1960s and 1970s, nursing expanded its environmental concerns to include identification and interventions related to exposures to toxins and chemicals from the home and community environments. More recently, nursing has acknowledged that the environment relevant to our patients' health is larger and more multifaceted than was appreciated previously. Accordingly, nursing's concerns have expanded to regional, national, and global physical environmental hazards as well as influences arising from the social, economic, psychological, and political environments.

### ■ Identifying Risks

Community health nurses often emphasize primary prevention activities that address environmental health because many environmentally induced illnesses are preventable through risk management activities. In concert with other professionals, community health nurses often conduct a systematic review of risks known as a quantitative **risk**

## BOX 12-2

**Steps in an Environmental Risk Assessment**

1. Hazard identification: Does the agent cause the adverse effect?
2. Exposure assessment: Which exposures are currently experienced or anticipated?
3. Dose-response assessment: What is the relationship between the dose and incidence?
4. Risk characterization: What is the estimated incidence of the adverse effect in a given population?

 **THINK ABOUT THIS** ....................

After the damage inflicted by Hurricane Katrina and the resulting levee break in New Orleans in August 2005, the area's unprecedented environmental debris and hazards created the nation's greatest recycling challenge. The sheer volume of debris created by Katrina was staggering—about 25 million cubic yards of "green waste" (tree limbs, trunks, leaves, dead bushes), enough to fill up the Louisiana Superdome nearly twice. Some had to be incinerated; some was used as cover in landfills due to the time factor; and much is now being used as lawn and garden mulch and composting material. Flooded vehicles and hundreds of thousands of destroyed refrigerators, washing machines, and other appliances have yielded about 280,000 tons of steel, according to Louisiana state officials. Many builders, restoration experts, artists, and grass-roots organizations have recycled much of the debris into jewelry and for use in the restoration of homes.

**assessment**. Risk is the probability of injury, disease, or death for individuals or populations exposed to hazardous substances; it may be expressed numerically (e.g., "one in 1 million"), but this rate is often impossible to estimate. In such situations, risk may be expressed using terms such as high, medium, or low. The steps involved in a risk assessment are outlined in Box 12-2. **Risk management** involves developing and evaluating possible regulatory actions guided by the risk assessment plus other ethical, political, social, economic, and technological factors (U.S. Congress, Office of Technology Assessment, 1990).

### ■ Assessing Exposures

Community health nurses often participate in exposure assessments following the development of a case or suspected cluster of disease. Because of their methodical skills in home assessment, nurses are often called on to conduct comprehensive exposure assessments in homes or occupational settings. Strong interview, observation, and family assessment skills are needed by nurses to collect these data in a clear and systematic manner. Clues to potential solutions to environmental risks may occur during the course of community or home assessments, although the resolution of some risks may require the expertise of non-nursing professionals. Home visits often require follow-up conversations with toxicologists, industrial hygienists, or other scientists who have expertise with the exposures of interest.

Exposure assessments are much simpler when patients present with an acute illness, such as acute pesticide poisoning or inhalation fever. Assessments become much more complex when the specific types of agents have not been considered a priori or when the induction period between exposure and disease occurrence is unknown. The greatest challenges occur in persons with chronic disease or disease of unknown cause or when exposure to small doses of multiple agents has occurred over years or decades. In these types of clinical situations, it is very unusual to make a link between disease and a specific type of exposure with a high degree of confidence. Unusual conditions and rarer forms of cancer, such as the association between asbestos and development of mesothelioma, are the exception and can often be narrowed

down to a specific place and time in a one's life. Box 12-3 on page 281 includes basic information addressing the components of a home assessment and environmental exposure history. As one would expect, data collection is customized to address the unique aspects of the exposures, setting, and persons involved in the situation.

### ■ Communicating Risks

Often, the most successful strategies for responding to environmental risks affecting a community involve empowering citizens to address the problem. If successful, these strategies result not only in the resolution of the immediate problem but also in the creation of a group able to address future threats. Nurses should be encouraged to become familiar with the principles of environmental risk communication. An increased availability of information to the public increases the possibility that the community health nurse will be sought for advice and further information. Nurses are trusted in a community, and the public values their opinions. It is professionally responsible to share science-based information with persons most affected by that information. Nurses should understand the influence of the environment and environmental agents on human health based on knowledge of relevant epidemiological, toxicological, and exposure factors.

Basic principles of risk communication can be used in many environmental health situations, ranging from a toxic spill incident to a neighborhood meeting to discuss groundwater contamination. Overall, risk communication focuses on telling citizens what is known about a risk situation in a clear and forthright manner. In addition, it is important to directly explain what information is not currently known and the process by which additional information will be

## BOX 12-3

**Conducting a Home Assessment and Environmental Exposure History**

### Areas of Visual Inspection

Examine areas in the immediate vicinity of the home for the presence of the following:

- Water hazards
- Automobile, farm, or other large equipment
- Garbage/waste storage containers
- Garages, sheds, or other outbuildings for safety hazards
- Chemical storage areas
- Pets or livestock
- Areas where rats or mice could live around home or outbuildings
- General age and condition of home (e.g., presence of peeling paint, metal edges from siding)

   Consider whether any of the aforementioned items constitute a health threat to any family members or to the community in general.

### Questions to Consider in Assessing Environmental Agents in the Home

Ask family members about the following areas:

- Hobbies or crafts involving potential for lead exposure (e.g., stained glass, ceramic glazing)
- Potential for significant exposure to gasoline or diesel exhaust from car repair activities or from nearby traffic
- Safe storage of food (stored where vermin cannot contaminate food) and proper cooking and refrigeration facilities
- Storage and use of insecticides, lawn care products, fertilizers
- Home heating—type of furnace, use of wood stoves
- Use of cleaning products that are strong irritants
- Fumigants or other products used for tick or flea control in the home
- Storage of food in copper or brass containers (can contaminate food with copper or lead)
- Exposure to wood preservatives (e.g., pentachlorophenol) in log homes
- Potential for lead exposure through lead-based plumbing
- Source of water (municipal or private well)
- Any seasonal changes in water sources during the year (e.g., private well during the winter and water delivered to a cistern during the summer months)
- Recent home renovation activities such as sanding or stripping of old paint that could result in lead exposure to family members

### Questions Addressing Symptoms Related to Environmental Agents in the Home

Do any members of the family have symptoms that they attribute to an environmental exposure? If so, elicit the nature of symptoms, duration, fluctuations in symptoms over the day and from week to week, seasonal changes, related symptoms in other family members or others who spend extended time in the home.

### Ascertaining Agent-Specific Data from Individuals

#### *Exposures*

- Concurrent and past exposures to metal, dust, fibers, fumes, chemicals, biological hazards, radiation, noise, vibration
- Typical work day (job tasks, location, materials, agents used)
- Changes in routines or processes
- Other employees or household members similarly affected

#### *Health and Safety Practices at Work Site*

- Ventilation
- Medical and industrial hygiene surveillance
- Employment examinations
- Personal protective equipment (e.g., respirators, gloves, coveralls)
- Lockout devices, alarms, training, drills
- Personal habits (smoking, eating in the work area, handwashing with solvents)

#### *Work History*

- Description of all prior jobs, including short-term, seasonal, or part-time employment and military service
- Description of present job(s)

#### *Environmental History*

- Present and prior home locations
- Jobs of household members
- Home insulating, heating and cooling system
- Home cleaning agents
- Pesticide exposure (e.g., pet flea treatments, roach and ant sprays)
- Water supply
- Recent renovation/remodeling
- Air pollution, indoor and outdoor
- Hobbies: painting, sculpting, welding, woodworking, piloting, autos, firearms, stained glass, ceramics, gardening
- Hazardous wastes/spills exposure

#### *Medical History*

- Past and present medical problems
- Medications

*Source*: Adapted from Agency for Toxic Substance and Disease Registry, 2000.

communicated to all parties. Basic guidelines addressing the principles of risk communication are listed in Box 12-4. Infants and children have a unique vulnerability to being exposed to chemical agents.

Communicating a balanced view of these risks to parents is a challenge for nurses in the community. An example of this challenge involves the practice of breastfeeding. For many years, nurses have played a significant role in policies and clinical actions that support breastfeeding practices in new mothers. This advocacy role has been based on scientific findings that breast milk is the ideal infant food because of the easy digestibility of milk proteins, the presence of maternal antibodies, and safety from contamination through the use of improperly sanitized bottles.

Over the past two decades, scientists have become increasingly aware that human breast milk also carries a host of potentially serious risks to infant health. The greatest concern has been physiological evidence that many chemicals to which the mother has been exposed are transferred into breast milk. Of special interest are the findings from studies that examine the metabolism and fate of chemicals that have extremely long half-lives (i.e., years and decades)

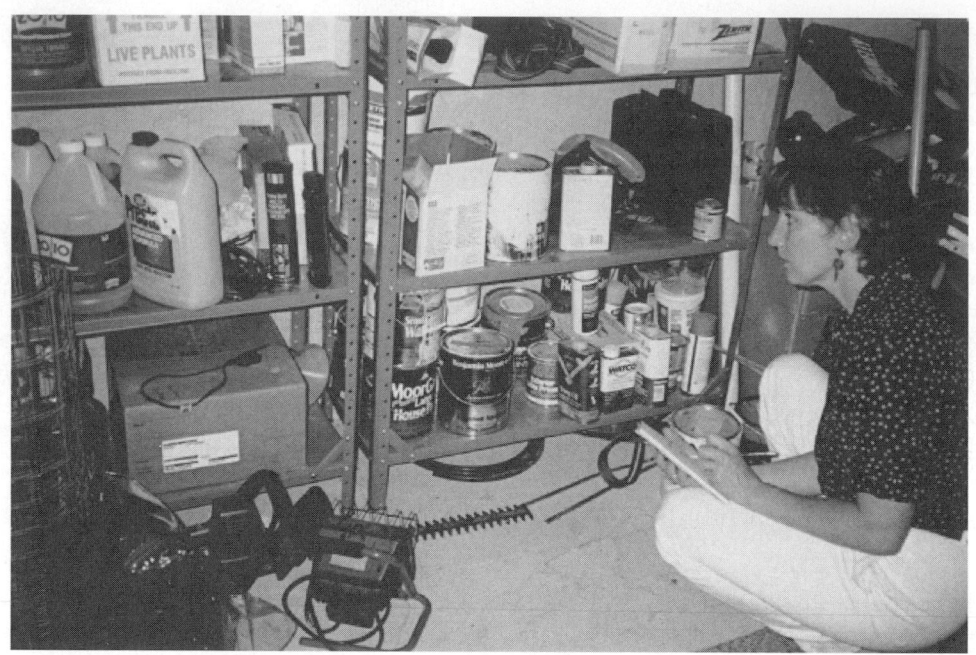

Chapter author Dr. Patricia Butterfield conducting a home environment exposure assessment.

## BOX 12-4

### Basic Guidelines for Risk Communication

Don't confuse people's understanding a risk with their acceptance of it—anger and resentment are often expressed when people are unwittingly exposed to an environmental hazard and feel that they have no control over the situation.

Avoid trivializing the risk or minimizing people's concerns. Frustration needs to be heard and acknowledged, not suppressed. It is important to listen attentively and respectfully to all concerns and respond in a clear manner with whatever information is currently available. Say what is known, also say what is not known. Gaining trust from the audience in a public meeting will not usually occur if people perceive that they are being patronized or placated. It is best to say what is currently known about the situation of concern and what is now known.

Often, health providers do not have all the information at hand or are waiting for additional information to come in (e.g., laboratory values or diagnostic tests from exposed persons). State clearly what information is not currently available and when that information will be available.

Respond to the different needs of different audiences. In an incident that involves a pesticide spill at a local school, the parents of schoolchildren will probably have different concerns than the janitor and physical facilities staff at the school. Think about your audience in advance—try to anticipate what questions you would have if you were in the audience and direct the discussion from that perspective.

Recognize that input from the public can help your agency make better decisions. Holding private meetings or trying to avoid public input is likely to fuel distrust in community members. By building in opportunities for affected persons to help remedy an environmental hazard situation, those persons gain a sense of control over the situation and feel like they are helping themselves and others. Think broadly about how to use citizens' help to get mailings out, set up phone trees, and form advocacy groups. If you do not allow citizens to work with you and your agency, they may begin to work against you.

*Source*: Adapted from Hance, B. J., C. Chess, and P. M. Sandman, "Improving dialogue with communities: A risk communication manual for government," 1990. Trenton: New Jersey Department of Environmental Protection. Used by permission.

within human populations. Such agents include polychlorinated organic pollutants, such as organochlorine pesticides, polychlorinated biphenyls (PCBs), and polychlorinated dibenzodioxins and dibenzofurans (PCDDs/PCDFs), as well as some forms of metals such as methylmercury. In most cases, persons ingest these agents in their diets, usually from contaminated fish and animal products such as meats, fats, cheese, and eggs. In large doses, many pesticide products and mercury compounds have affected neurobehavioral, neuromotor, and speech development (Kimbourgh, 1995). Unfortunately, much less is known about the long-term effects of low-dose exposure in breast milk. For a variety of feasibility and methodological reasons, scientific studies of low-dose and early-life exposures are extremely difficult to conduct. Such studies often help in the incremental advancement of scientific understanding but are not able to yield clear-cut answers to clinical questions (Gladen et al., 1999; Hooper, 1999).

Infants and children are particularly susceptible to the toxic effects of chemical exposure for a number of reasons. Pound for pound of body weight, a child eats much more food than an adult. Youngsters between the ages of 1 and 5 years eat and drink three to four times more food and water than do adults. In addition to this increased food intake, there is evidence that compared with adult bodies, the metabolic pathways of children have a diminished ability to metabolize or detoxify chemical agents effectively. Children's

Children are more vulnerable to environmental risks than adults due to greater time outdoors, immaturity of their immune systems, and other developmental differences.

daily activity patterns, such as playing on the ground and hand-to-mouth behavior, can also increase their exposure to some environmental toxicants. Because of incomplete scientific evidence about the long-term consequences of exposure to chemical agents, primary prevention activities that reduce the opportunity of exposure provide the first and most important line of defense on behalf of children's health (Schmidt, 1999).

## ■ Assessing and Referring Patients

A critical piece of comprehensive nursing practice is the identification of high-risk patients so that these individuals can be referred for further evaluation and follow-up. To provide such care for these patients, nurses must have a good understanding of the environmental health resources located within their geographic area. In many communities, professionals with environmental health expertise, such as industrial hygienists, physicians, and toxicologists, are located in the state health department. Other experts may be located in occupational health clinics in both hospital and community settings. For nurses working in agricultural communities, expertise in environmental health may often be found through contacts with county extension agents, pest management specialists, migrant and seasonal farm worker clinics, or agricultural medicine programs (Shreffler, 1996). It is essential that patients be referred to resources that are culturally and socioeconomically appropriate (Pope & Rall, 1995).

There is some evidence from applied research studies that both pediatric and adult patients are failing through the cracks of the health systems when they are in need of specialized environmental health services. In a review of children residing in New York City, Markowitz, Rosen, and Clemente (1999) estimated that only 60% of high-risk children were being screened for lead poisoning; of those children who were found to have elevated lead levels, nearly 60% were not receiving timely follow up by health care providers. In another recent study addressing the health consequences of lead exposure, elevated values were associated with an increased risk for hypertension later in life (Korrick, Hunter, Rotnitzky, Hu, & Speizer, 1999).

A third environmental health study focused on persons at increased risk of developing lung cancer caused by both household radon exposure and cigarette smoking. Researchers developed statistical models of risk and determined that the most effective strategy to reduce the risk of radon-related cancer was smoking cessation. Stopping smoking was more effective in reducing cancer risk than directly reducing the levels of radon in the home (Mendez, Warner, & Courant, 1998). Although it is always optimal to reduce disease risk through all possible means (e.g., smoking cessation as well as radon reduction interventions), this study demonstrates the importance of addressing both environmental and behavioral means to minimize disease risk in exposed persons.

Community health nurses are the health providers most familiar with their patients' home setting, lifestyle, work habits, and environmental exposures. Because of their unique presence in a variety of patient settings, nurses may become aware of patients' environmental health risks and work toward directing them to an appropriate source of evaluation and treatment. An Application to Practice feature addressing household environmental assessment and interventions for children with asthma is presented on page 285.

## Upstream Thinking: Making Connections Between Environmental and Human Health

One of the most challenging areas in environmental health is linking a past exposure from 10 to 20 years ago with the development of a current health problem. Even though we are intellectually aware that some agents have health consequences that may not be seen for years or decades, it can be difficult to take such a distant and uncertain threat seriously.

One conceptual approach that has been used in interdisciplinary public health efforts, referred to as **upstream thinking,** uses the analogy of a river to demonstrate connections between preceding exposures and later health consequences. This approach is based on an article by McKinlay (1979), who tells the story of a physician friend and his struggle to keep from feeling overwhelmed by the enormity of health problems that he encounters in clinical practice. The friend notes that he feels as if he is so caught up in rescuing individuals from the river that he has no time to look upstream to see who is pushing them in. In this analogy, the river represents illness and health providers' efforts to rescue people from illness. However, in this portrayal no one receives care until they are downstream in the river of illness, which precludes efforts to intervene before illness develops.

McKinlay challenges providers to look upstream, where the real problems lie. The river analogy includes many concepts in community health nursing, including the natural history of disease and levels of prevention. The power of the upstream conceptualization of health lies in its simplicity and the ease with which one can connect the causes of disease with their consequences.

Upstream thinking lends itself well to health problems of environmental origin and can be helpful in guiding practice decisions that have long- and short-term consequences for our patients. Examples of environmental upstream nursing actions include the following:

- Instructing a patient to wear a respirator when stripping paint from an old home
- Encouraging farmers who work with pesticides to refrain from wearing their work boots into the house
- Developing a school policy to establish waiting periods for children to be off the playground following applications of fertilizers and herbicides

In each situation, the nurse is acting from a primary prevention viewpoint to prevent or minimize the occurrence of an exposure. It is not even necessary to know the toxicology of all of the agents involved. Nurses can initiate an action and then seek guidance from experts in toxicology or other disciplines. The goal is to minimize the opportunity for

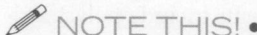 NOTE THIS!

A remarkable decrease in the incidence of many childhood communicable diseases has occurred during this and the last century in U.S. populations; these conditions include diphtheria, pertussis, and polio. Unfortunately, this progress against many communicable diseases has been offset by an equally remarkable increase in asthma occurrence in both pediatric and adult populations in industrialized nations throughout the world. Overall asthma prevalence has increased by 58% since 1980; the mortality rate has increased by 78%. Children from urban areas and racial/ethnic communities have experienced the greatest increases in both prevalence and mortality. Hospitalization and morbidity rates for nonwhite children are almost twice those for white children. Asthma symptoms are caused by hyperresponsiveness of the airway to a number of common environmental allergens, including dust mites, animal dander, cockroaches, fungal spores, and pollens. Exacerbation of asthma has also been associated with air quality problems such as increased levels of sulfur dioxide, nitrogen dioxide, and ozone. Cigarette smoking as well as exposure to secondhand smoke also contribute to exacerbation of several childhood conditions such as otitis media, pneumonia, bronchitis, and asthma. Currently, approximately 30% of American preschoolers are exposed to residential tobacco smoke. Just as the precipitating factors for asthma are multiple, so too must be prevention efforts by nurses and other health providers. These efforts need to address household and community-based patterns of exposure as well as continuity of care and ongoing management for affected persons.

*Source*: Eggleston, Buckley, Breysse, Wills-Karp, Kleeberger, & Jaakkola, 1999; Clark et al., 1999.

harm by linking an understanding of nursing actions today with the prevention of harmful health effects in the future (Butterfield, 1990).

## Ethical Principles Addressing Environmental Health Nursing

Nurses have a duty to safeguard patients from environmental hazards and risks regardless of patients' income, insurance status, or lack of access to care. The nurses' *Code of Ethics* addresses responsibilities to collaborate with other health professionals and citizens in promoting community and national efforts to meet the health needs of the public (American Nurses Association, 1985).

Justice is a highly valued ethical principle in most societies today and is one of the beliefs that guide the practice of nursing. The concept of fairness of opportunity is a value in the United States that is supported in laws that forbid discriminatory treatment that limits one's opportunities on the basis of unchangeable characteristics such as gender, race, or socioeconomic status. **Social justice** means fairness or equality in the distribution of the benefits and burdens of society. According to the principles of social justice, no one person or group should have a disproportionate share of the benefits available to a society nor of the burdens that are present.

Florence Nightingale believed in bringing nature into the hospital environment in the form of flowers to promote healing.

### Application to Practice

#### Asthma Management in a Young Girl

A public health nurse working in an urban area has been coordinating services with the school nurse practitioner at Northside Elementary, a primary school located in a low-income neighborhood. The nurse practitioner calls to request a home assessment for 7-year-old Lateesha. Lateesha is in the second grade, and the teacher notes that she has performed poorly in the classroom compared with her skill level during the previous year. In a phone interview, the mother states that she thinks the child's inattentiveness in the classroom results primarily from several recent colds that required Lateesha to miss school. The mother notes that Lateesha has missed 8 days of school so far this year and has had some difficulty with the make-up work following these absences.

When the nurse visits the home, she notes that Lateesha's mother, brother, sister, and grandmother live in a three-bedroom apartment near the school. When entering the home, the nurse notes that the room is very warm and sees an older model space heater in the kitchen area. The mother explains she wants to keep it warm for Lateesha's little sister, a 4-year-old who has complained that the apartment is too cool during winter. The nurse also notes several ashtrays in the living room and the presence of Tigger, the family cat. The mother informs the nurse that Lateesha has had four severe colds since October and that the last physician they saw at the clinic suggested that Lateesha has asthma. The mother received two types of inhalers for Lateesha following this clinic visit but notes that no one explained whether Lateesha is to use the inhalers every day or only after she develops a cold or breathing difficulties.

1. What should be the focus of the interventions of the community health nurse with this family?

When applied to environmental health, principles of social justice suggest that the ability to live in a healthy environment as part of the process for attaining or maintaining health should be available to all. Because health is of fundamental importance to having opportunities for life, liberty, and the pursuit of happiness, environmental risks that take place or are allowed to persist differentially that are based on gender, race, or socioeconomic status would not be consistent with justice or fairness of opportunity (Daniels, 1985). **Environmental justice** is not served when some persons or groups have disproportionate shares of the benefits of healthy environments and others have disproportionate shares of the burdens of contaminated ones.

Most environmental hazards do not pose uniform or equal risks to the health of an entire population. Some widespread hazards, such as global warming, acid rain, and air or water pollution, involve an entire region or country, but most environmental health concerns involve different exposures within the same population. Some exposures occur because of behaviors or practices that could be considered

### MEDIA MOMENT

#### A Civil Action (1998)

In this true story, John Travolta stars as a personal-injury lawyer who sues a major corporation when the drinking water in Woburn, Massachusetts, is found to contain high levels of industrial solvents. Believing the contamination is responsible for the large number of leukemia deaths among the town's children, the citizens—led by a woman (Kathleen Quinlan) whose child has died—hire a lawyer to take on the corporate polluters. Beatrice and Grace are the real-life companies represented in the movie. A Civil Action is based on Jonathan Harr's nonfiction best-seller, which won the National Book Award.

changeable as a result of choices the individual makes. The decision to not wear protective gear when applying pesticides is an example of choice that could easily be changed from health damaging to health protecting. Some exposures occur, however, because of unchangeable characteristics or circumstances of some individuals in the population, such as socioeconomic status, race, powerlessness, age, or gender. Lead exposure, for example, is most common in children who live in low-income housing. The disposal of toxic waste into sites located near low-income neighborhoods whose residents lack the financial resources and power to prevent it is another example of disproportionate exposure to environmental hazards (Bullard, 1990, 1993).

 **GLOBAL CONNECTION**

With 4% of the world's population, the United States accounts for about 25% of the earth's greenhouse gas emissions.

 NOTE THIS! •────────────────

In a nationwide survey more than 86,000 school children were asked what they worry about the most. Their answer? The environment!

*Source*: Environmental and Occupational Sciences Institute, Public Health and Risk Communication Division.

The distinction between changeable and unchangeable courses of action may not always be clear-cut. For example, the training one receives about pesticides safety and the availability of safety equipment may affect the use of safety measures more than personal choice. Many environmental risks occur from exposures to toxic substances on the job. Some individuals may have the ability to change occupations to reduce risks, but many others cannot reasonably entertain such an option. It also may be possible to alter some risks such as living in low-income housing with lead-based paint. In this example, although residents' incomes and ability to relocate may be unchangeable, they can work to improve the safety in their current housing and influence landlords to correct or reduce environmental hazards such as removal of lead-based paint.

Nurses play a role in promoting environmental justice in several ways. Educating individuals on ways to reduce exposure to toxic substances is important. Giving information about contacts in health departments or work safety committees is helpful to individuals and groups. Helping groups organize and present a united voice to industries and politicians is important to people who may otherwise have been powerless to protest. Community health nurses know the strengths of their communities and are able to identify the people who provide leadership to the group. Community

health nurses are also already sensitive to their community's cultural or ethnic attributes, which may affect the process of seeking environmental justice.

Activists concerned about environmental hazards and social justice have also begun to work with and for disadvantaged groups to increase their awareness of unequal environmental risks and possible strategies to improve them. Disadvantaged at-risk groups in a particular area may not be organized into a functioning community or have community or neighborhood organizations that can be readily mobilized for action. In this case, activists work with whatever organizations exist or form an informal group of concerned residents who may get others involved over time. An environmental hazard close to where people live is an issue that can be effective in organizing and mobilizing citizens to work together as a group.

## Conclusion

The role of community health nurses in environmental health is evolving in several ways:

- From illness treatment to illness recognition and prevention
- Toward a multidisciplinary foundation of basic and applied science
- Toward an emphasis on activities in which nursing excels, such as risk communication, community-based investigations, and patient advocacy strategies
- Toward an integration of environmental health principles into all domains of nursing practice and research

Knowledge of pollutants—whether physical, chemical, or biological—is characterized by incomplete science. The field is constantly changing, with the discovery of new hazards, but also innovative ways of minimizing hazard use and exposure. Nurses can participate in advancing environmental health science by participating in applied research activities on behalf of vulnerable groups or those disproportionately exposed to agents of concern. A list of Internet sites that provide scientifically sound environmental health information is provided in Table 12-1.

Nurses have functioned at the fringe of power and politics, which has often been detrimental to the nursing profession, perhaps even to health care. In the field of environmental health, nurses are capable of making great contributions to the social, political, and economic forces that presently guide environmental health care policy. By broadening nurses' understanding of the environment, new horizons in environmental health can be developed and expanded on behalf of the health of our patients, our nation, and our planet.

**Table 12-1**    Resources for Environmental Health Information

| Agency or Organization | Purpose | Internet Site Address |
|---|---|---|
| Agency for Toxic Substances and Disease Registry (ATSDR) | Part of the U.S. Department of Health and Human Services. Conducts public health assessments of waste sites, health consultations concerning specific hazardous substances, and applied research in support of public health assessments. Supports an environmental health nursing initiative. Also provides an exceptional list of fact sheets for specific toxics and a comprehensive group of case studies addressing specific exposures. | http://www.atsdr.cdc.gov/about.html |
| American Association of Occupational Health Nurses (AAOHN) | Professional organization for occupational and environmental health nurses. Provides information resources about nursing and environmental health. | http://www.aaohn.org/practice/environmental.cfm |
| Association of Occupational and Environmental Clinics | Conducts information sharing, education, and research through a network of clinics. Provides professional training, community education, exposure and risk assessment, clinical evaluations, and consultation services. | http://www.aoec.org/ |
| Environmental Protection Agency (EPA) | Employs 18,000 people across the United States, including in its headquarters offices in Washington, D.C., 10 regional offices, and more than a dozen labs. Develops and enforces regulations addressing environmental protection, performs research, and provides educational support throughout the country. | http://www.epa.gov/ |
| EnviRN | An information resource site operated by the University of Maryland School of Nursing. | http://envirn.umaryland.edu |
| National Center for Environmental Health (NCEH) | Part of the Centers for Disease Control and Prevention. Works to prevent illness from interactions between people and the environment. Especially committed to safeguarding the health of vulnerable populations. | http://www.cdc.gov/nceh/ |
| National Environmental Education and Training Foundation | An environmental education site with links to nursing and health education materials. | http://www.neetf.org/index.cfm |
| National Institute of Environmental Health Sciences (NIEHS) | Part of the National Institutes of Health. Works to reduce the burden of human illness from environmental causes by understanding each of these elements and how they interrelate. | http://www.niehs.nih.gov/ |
| RN No Harm | An American Nurses Association program focusing on the prevention of pollution and medical waste from hospitals and clinics. | http://www.nursingworld.org/rnnoharm/ |

## Application to Practice

### Broadening Nurses' Expertise in Environmental Health Clinical Practice: Thinking Upstream

Over the course of several years, a public health nurse was asked about water quality issues by patients attending the well-child clinic. These questions most commonly addressed parents' concerns about potable water contamination, and the nurse believed she was unqualified to answer these types of questions. After spending a few hours at home reviewing water quality information on the EPA's Internet home page, the nurse decided to seek some advice from the health department director about the lack of preparation to respond to patients' questions regarding environmental health. The director suggested that the nurse spend some time with a water quality specialist, who was located within another department, and authorized time for the nurse to work 1 week in that department. During her week with environmental health personnel, the nurse worked in the field when the environmental engineer inspected the installation of a private well west of town. She made a special effort to talk with all of the people in the environmental health department so that she had a better understanding of the full range of expertise within the department. After working in the field, she visited the laboratory to observe testing procedures for water quality and to learn about the different water tests available to the public.

When she returned to the well-child clinic the following week, the nurse decided to allocate at least half an hour per day to developing a resource library on water quality issues in the clinic. She obtained educational brochures from the environmental health department; in addition, she established a system where nurses could give interested patients a plastic bottle for water sampling and have them send it directly to the laboratory for analysis. The nurse also asked the environmental engineer to make his phone number available to respond to any questions from patients about their water and septic systems.

Over the next year, the nurse provided continuing education for the nursing staff until they became more comfortable providing patients with specific information about water quality and differentiating between questions they could answer and those that were best referred to the engineers and scientists in the other department. Nurses came to understand that the prevention of problems held the key to long-term sustainability of water quality in their community and ecosystem. Many of the same principles of prevention that were so familiar to them in public health nursing could be applied equally well to actions to reduce opportunities for water pollution.

During the next few months, the nursing staff reached beyond its original contacts with the environmental health department and extended further into partnerships with other environmental information and advocacy groups in the area. They worked with the local university's pollution prevention program to display and educate patients about the safe disposal of household products and solvents, to reduce solid waste, and to increase participation in recycling of paint and motor oil. Nurses found that they could often incorporate several minutes of "pollution prevention" instruction into many well-child visits and that parents were often appreciative of this information. The nurses worked to make other health departments aware of their efforts and presented a summary of their program at their annual public health association conference. As a culmination of their work, the nurses developed an Internet site to educate professional colleagues throughout the nation on their growing expertise in water quality and pollution prevention.

**Daffodils**

I gathered in the first of the daffodils this morning
And built a fire.
We always have one more cold day before the Easter
Out the window beyond the streaks of slow soft
    rain I see
The green netting of spring—high in the trees.
I remember how—on days like this— when I was
    very young
I fought to keep from running away
Such promises the yellow flowers made.

—*Ann Thedford Lanier*

Explore Community Health Nursing on the Web! To learn more about the topics in this chapter, use the passcode provided to access your exclusive website: **http://nursing.jbpub.com/ communityhealth.** If you do not have a passcode, you can obtain one at this site.

## ■ CRITICAL THINKING ACTIVITIES

1. Take a walk or a drive around your own neighborhood and identify any potential environmental health risks. What kind of prevention interventions can be done to minimize exposure to these hazards? As a nursing student, what role can you play?

## ■ REFERENCES

Agency for Toxic Substances and Disease Registry, U.S. Department of Health and Human Services. (2000). *Case studies in environmental medicine: Taking an exposure history.* Retrieved August 19, 2008, from http://www.atsdr.cdc.gov/CSEM/exphistory/ehcover_page.html

American Nurses Association (ANA). (1985). *Code of ethics for nurses with interpretive statements.* Kansas City, MO: Author.

Booth, K. M., Pinkston, M. M., & Poston, W. S. C. (2005). Obesity and the built environment. *Journal of the American Dietetic Association, 105*(5 suppl), 110–117.

Briggs, D. (2003). Environmental pollution and the global burden of disease. *British Medical Bulletin, 68,* 1–24.

Bullard, R. D. (1990). *Dumping in Dixie: Race, class, and environmental quality.* Boulder, CO: Westview Press.

Bullard, R. D. (1993). *Confronting environmental racism: Voices from the grassroots.* Boston: South End Press.

Butterfield, P. G. (1990). Thinking upstream: Nurturing a conceptual understanding of the societal context of health behavior. *ANS: Advances in Nursing Science, 12*(2), 1–8.

Butterfield, P. G. (2002). Upstream reflections on environmental health: An abbreviated history and framework for action. *ANS: Advances in Nursing Science, 25*(1), 32–50.

Carson, R. (1962). *Silent spring.* Boston: Houghton Mifflin.

Centers for Disease Control and Prevention. (2004). Impact of health waves on mortality—Rome, Italy, June–August 2003. *Morbidity and Mortality Weekly Report, 53*(17), 369–371.

Centers for Disease Control and Prevention, National Center for Environmental Health. (2008). *Third national report on human exposure to environmental chemicals* (NCEH Pub No. 03-0022). Retrieved October 23, 2008, from http://www.cdc.gov/exposurereport/pdf/thirdreport.pdf

Clark, N. M., Brosn, R. W., Parker, E., et al. (1999). Childhood asthma. *Environmental Health Perspective, 107*(suppl 3), 421–429.

Crenson, M. (1997, December 28). Kids at work in fields of unseen danger. *Missoulian,* p. A4.

Daniels, N. (1985). *Just health care.* Cambridge, UK: Cambridge University Press.

Daszak, P., Tabor, G. M., Kilpatrick, A. M., Epstein, J., & Plowright, R. (2004). Conservation medicine and a new agenda for emerging disease. *Annals of the NY Academy of Science, 1026,* 1–11.

Eggleston, P. A., Buckley, T. J., Breysse, P. N., Wills-Karp, M., Kleeberger, S. R., & Jaakkola, J. J. (1999). The environment and asthma in U.S. inner cities. *Environmental Health Perspectives, 107*(suppl 3), 439–450.

Frumkin, H. (2005). Health, equity, and the built environment (editorial). *Environmental Health Perspectives, 113*(5), A290–A291.

Garrett, L. (1994). *The coming plague: Newly emerging diseases in a world out of balance.* New York: Penguin Books

Gladen, B. C., Monaghan, S. C., Lukyanova, E. M., et al. (1999). Organochlorines in breast milk from two cities in Ukraine. *Environmental Health Perspectives, 107*(6), 459–462.

Henson, R. H., Robinson, W. L., & Schmele, J. A. (1996). Consumerism and quality management. In J. A. Schmele (Ed.), *Quality management in nursing and healthcare.* Albany, NY: Delmar.

Hooper, K. (1999). Breast milk monitoring programs (BMMPs): World-wide early warning systems for polyhalogenated POPs and for targeting studies in children's environmental health. *Environmental Health Perspectives, 107*(6), 429–430.

Kirk, M. (2002). The impact of globalization and climate change on health: Challenges for nursing education. *Nurse Education Today, 22*(1), 60–71.

Kleffel, D. (1996). Environmental paradigms: Moving toward an eccentric perspective. *ANS: Advances in Nursing Science, 18*(4), 1–10.

Korrick, S. A., Hunter, D. J., Rotnitzky, A., Hu, H., & Speizer, F. E. (1999). Lead and hypertension in a sample of middle-aged women. *American Journal of Public Health, 89*(3), 330–335.

Kotchian, S. (1997). Perspectives on the place of environmental health and protection in public health and public health agencies. *Annual Review of Public Health, 18,* 245–259.

Markowitz, M., Rosen, J. F., & Clemente, I. (1999). Clinician follow-up of children screened for lead poisoning. *American Journal of Public Health, 89*(7), 1088–1089.

McKinlay, J. B. (1979). A case for refocusing upstream: The political economy of illness. In E. G. Jaco (Ed.), *Patients, physicians, and illness* (3rd ed., pp. 9–25). New York: Free Press.

Mendez, D., Warner, K. E., & Courant, P. N. (1998). Effects of radon mitigation vs. smoking cessation in reducing radon-related risk of lung cancer. *American Journal of Public Health, 88*(5), 811–812.

New Jersey Department of Environmental Protection. (1990). *Improving dialogue with communities: A risk communication manual for government.* New Brunswick, NJ: Author.

Nightingale, F. (1969). *Notes on nursing.* New York: Dover. (Originally published by D. Appleton and Company, 1860)

Patz, J. A., Daszak, P., Tabor, G. M., et al. (2004). Unhealthy landscapes: Policy recommendations on land use change and infectious disease emergence. *Environmental Health Perspectives, 112*(10), 1092–1098.

Pohanka, M., & Fitzgerald, S. (2004). Urban sprawl and you: How sprawl adversely affects worker health. *AAOHN Journal, 52*(6), 242–246.

Pope, A. M., & Rall, D. P. (Eds.). (1995). *Environmental medicine: Integrating a missing element into medical education.* Washington, DC: National Academy Press.

Pope, A. M., Snyder, M. A., & Mood, L. H. (Eds.). (1995). *Nursing, health and the environment: Strengthening the relationship to improve the public's health.* Washington, DC: National Academy Press.

Reddy, M. M., Reddy, M. B., & Reddy, C. F. (2004). Scientific advances provide opportunities to improve pediatric environmental health. *Journal of Pediatrics, 145*(2), 153–156.

Schmidt, C. W. (1999). Poisoning young minds. *Environmental Health Perspectives, 107*(6), A302–307.

Shendell, D. G., Barnett, C., & Boese, S. (2004). Science-based recommendations to prevent or reduce potential exposure to biological, chemical, and physical agents in schools. *Journal of the School of Health, 74*(10), 390–396.

Shreffler, M. J. (1996). An ecological view of the rural environment: Levels of influence on access to health care. *Advanced Nursing Science, 18*(4), 48–59.

Stevens, P. E., & Hall, J. M. (1997). Environmental health. In J. M. Swanson & M. A. Nies (Eds.), *Community health nursing: Protecting the health of aggregates* (2nd ed., pp. 736–765). Philadelphia: W. B. Saunders.

Thu, K. M. (2002). Public health concerns for neighbors of large-scale swine production operations. *Journal of Agricultural Safety and Health, 8*(2), 175–184.

Tiedje, L. B., & Wood, J. (1995). Sensitizing nurses for a changing environmental health role. *Public Health Nursing, 12*(6), 356–365.

U.S. Congress, Office of Technology Assessment. (1990, April). *Neurotoxicity: Identifying and controlling poisons of the nervous system.* (Publication No. OTA-BA-436). Washington, DC: U.S. Government Printing Office.

U.S. Department of Health and Human Services, Public Health Service (DHHS). (2001). *Healthy People 2010.* Retrieved August 19, 2008 at http://www.healthypeople.gov/document/tableofcontents.htm

U.S. Environmental Protection Agency. (2005). *2003 TRI public data release e-report.* Retrieved August 19, 2008, from http://www.epa.gov/tri/tridata/tri03/pdr/2003eReport.pdf

U.S. Environmental Protection Agency. (2008). *Environmental justice.* Retrieved October 23, 2008, from http://www.epa.gov/compliance/environmentaljustice/

World Health Organization, Regional Office for South-East Asia. (2005). *Sustainable development and healthy environments.* Retrieved August 19, 2008, from http://www.searo.who.int/en/section23.htm

# APPENDIX

# Environmental Agents and Their Adverse Health Effects

Note: This table is not meant to be comprehensive, but to provide examples of several types of agents.

| Agent | Exposure | Route of Entry | System(s) Affected | Primary Manifestations | Aids in Diagnosis | Remarks |
|---|---|---|---|---|---|---|
| **METALS AND METALLIC COMPOUNDS** | | | | | | |
| ARSENIC | Alloyed with lead and copper for hardness, manufacturing of pigments, glass, pharmaceuticals; by-product in copper smelting; insecticides; fungicides; rodenticides; tanning | Inhalation and ingestion of dust and fumes | Neuromuscular | Peripheral neuropathy, sensory–motor | Arsenic in urine | |
| | | | Gastrointestinal | Nausea and vomiting, diarrhea, constipation | | |
| | | | Skin | Dermatitis, finger and toenail striations, skin cancer, nasal septum perforation | | |
| | | | Pulmonary | Lung cancer | | |
| ARSINE | Accidental by-product of reaction of arsenic with acid; used in semiconductor industry | Inhalation of gas | Hematopoietic | Intravascular hemolysis; hemoglobinuria, jaundice, oliguria or anuria | Arsenic in urine | |
| BERYLLIUM | Hardening agent in metal alloys; special use in nuclear energy production; metal refining or recovery | Inhalation of fumes or dust | Pulmonary (and other systems) | Granulomatosis and fibrosis | Beryllium in urine (acute); beryllium in tissue (chronic); chest x ray; immunological tests (such as lymphocyte transformation) may also be useful | Pulmonary changes virtually indistinguishable from sarcoid on chest x-ray |
| CADMIUM | Electroplating; solder for aluminum; metal alloys, process engraving; nickel–cadmium batteries | Inhalation or ingestion of fumes or dust | Pulmonary | Pulmonary edema (acute); emphysema (chronic) | | Also a respiratory tract carcinogen. |
| | | | Renal | Nephrosis | Urinary protein | |
| CHROMIUM | In stainless and heat-resistant steel and alloy steel; metal plating; chemical and pigment manufacturing; photography | Percutaneous absorption, inhalation, ingestion | Pulmonary | Lung cancer | Urinary chromate (questionable value) | |
| | | | Skin | Dermatitis, skin ulcers, nasal septum perforation | | |
| LEAD | Storage batteries; manufacturing of paint, enamel, ink, glass, rubber, ceramics, chemical industry | Ingestion of dust, inhalation of dust or fumes | Hematological | Anemia | Blood lead | Lead toxicity, unlike that of mercury, is believed to be reversible, with the exception of late renal and some CNS effects. |
| | | | Renal | Nephrotoxicity | Urinary ALA | |
| | | | Gastrointestinal | Abdominal pain ("colic") Palsy ("wrist drop") | Zinc protoporphyrin; free erythrocyte protoporphyrin | |
| | | | Neuromuscular | Encephalopathy, behavioral abnormalities | | |
| | | | Central nervous system (CNS) | Spontaneous abortion (?) | | |
| | | | Reproductive | | | |

*Source*: Tarcher, A. B. (Ed.). (1992). *Principles and practice of environmental medicine*. New York: Plenum Press.

| Agent | Exposure | Route of Entry | System(s) Affected | Primary Manifestations | Aids in Diagnosis | Remarks |
|---|---|---|---|---|---|---|
| **METALS AND METALLIC COMPOUNDS—cont'd** | | | | | | |
| MERCURY Elemental | Electronic equipment; paint; metal and textile production; catalyst in chemical manufacturing; pharmaceutical production | Inhalation of vapor; slight percutaneous absorption | Pulmonary CNS | Acute pneumonitis Neuropsychiatric changes (erethism); tremor | Urinary mercury | Mercury illustrates several principles. The chemical form has a profound effect on its toxicology, as is the case for many metals. Effects of mercury are highly variable. Though inorganic mercury poisoning is primarily renal, elemental and organic poisoning are primarily neurological. |
| MERCURY Inorganic | Agricultural and industrial poisons | Some inhalation and gastrointestinal (GI) and percutaneous absorption | Pulmonary Renal CNS | Acute pneumonitis Proteinuria Variable | Urinary mercury | The responses are difficult to quantify, so dose-response data are generally unavailable. |
| Organic | | Efficient GI absorption, percutaneous absorption, and inhalation | Skin CNS | Dermatitis Sensorimotor changes, visual field constriction, tremor | Blood and urine mercury (?sensitivity) | Classic tetrad of gingivitis, sialorrhea, irritability, and tremor is associated with both elemental and inorganic mercury poisoning; the four signs are not generally seen together. Many effects of mercury toxicity, especially those in CNS, are irreversible. |
| NICKEL | Corrosion-resistant alloys; electroplating; catalyst production; nickel–cadmium batteries | Inhalation of dust or fumes | Skin<br><br>Pulmonary | Sensitization dermatitis ("nickel itch") Lung and paranasal sinus cancer | | |
| ZINC OXIDE | Welding by-product; rubber manufacturing | Inhalation of dust or fumes that are freshly generated | | "Metal fume fever" (fever, chills, and other symptoms) | Urinary zinc (useful as an indicator of exposure, not for acute diagnosis) | A self-limiting syndrome of 24–48 hours with apparently no sequelae. |

| Agent | Exposure | Route of Entry | System(s) Affected | Primary Manifestations | Aids in Diagnosis | Remarks |
|-------|----------|----------------|--------------------|-----------------------|-------------------|---------|
| **HYDROCARBONS** | | | | | | |
| BENZENE | Manufacturing of organic chemicals, detergents, pesticides, solvents, paint removers; used as a solvent | Inhalation of vapor; slight percutaneous absorption | CNS<br><br>Hematopoietic<br><br>Skin | Acute CNS depression<br>Leukemia, aplastic anemia<br>Dermatitis | Urinary phenol | Note that benzene, as with toluene and other solvents, can be monitored via its principal metabolite. |
| TOLUENE | Organic chemical manufacturing; solvent; fuel component | Inhalation of vapor, percutaneous absorption of liquid | CNS<br><br><br><br>Skin | Acute CNS depression<br>Chronic CNS problems such as memory loss<br>Irritation dermatitis | Urinary hippuric acid | |
| XYLENE | A wide variety of uses as a solvent; an ingredient of paints, lacquers, varnishes, inks, dyes, adhesives, cements; an intermediate in chemical manufacturing | Inhalation of vapor; slight percutaneous absorption of liquid | Pulmonary<br><br><br><br>Eye, nose, throat<br>CNS | Irritation, pneumonitis, acute pulmonary edema (at high doses)<br>Irritation<br>Acute CNS depression | Methylhippuric acid in urine, xylene in expired air, xylene in blood | |
| KETONES<br>Acetone (methyl ethyl ketone—MEK, methyl N-propyl ketone—MPK, methyl N-butyl ketone—MBK, methyl iso-butyl ketone—MIBK) | A wide variety of uses as solvents and intermediates in chemical manufacturing | Inhalation of vapor, percutaneous absorption of liquid | CNS<br><br>Peripheral nervous system (PNS)<br>Skin | Acute CNS depression<br>MBK has been linked with peripheral neuropathy<br>Dermatitis | Acetone in blood, urine, expired air (used as an index for exposure, not for diagnosis) | The ketone family demonstrates how a pattern of toxic responses (i.e., CNS narcosis) may feature exceptions (i.e., MBK peripheral neuropathy). |
| FORMALDEHYDE | Widely used as a germicide and a disinfectant in embalming and histopathology, for example, and in the manufacture of textiles, resins, and other products | Inhalation | Skin<br><br>Eye<br>Pulmonary | Irritant and contact dermatitis<br>Eye irritant<br>Respiratory tract irritation, asthma | Patch testing may be useful for dermatitis | Recent animal tests have shown it to be a respiratory carcinogen. Confirmatory epidemiological studies are in progress. |
| TRICHLORO-ETHYLENE (TCE) | Solvent in metal degreasing, dry cleaning, food extraction; ingredient of paints, adhesives, varnishes, inks | Inhalation, percutaneous absorption | Nervous<br><br><br><br><br>Skin<br><br>Cardiovascular | Acute CNS depression<br>Peripheral and cranial neuropathy<br>Irritation, dermatitis<br>Dysrhythmias | Breath analysis for TCE | TCE is involved in an important pharmacological interaction. Within hours of ingesting alcoholic beverages, TCE workers experience flushing of the face, neck, shoulders, and back. Alcohol |

| Agent | Exposure | Route of Entry | System(s) Affected | Primary Manifestations | Aids in Diagnosis | Remarks |
|---|---|---|---|---|---|---|
| **HYDROCARBONS—cont'd** | | | | | | |
| TRICHLORO-ETHYLENE (TCE) cont'd | | | | | | may also potentiate the CNS effects of TCE. The probable mechanism is competition for metabolic enzyme. |
| CARBON TETRACHLORIDE | Solvent for oils, fats, lacquers, resins, varnishes, other materials; used as a degreasing and cleaning agent | Inhalation of vapor | Hepatic Renal CNS Skin | Toxic hepatitis Oliguria or anuria Acute CNS depression Dermatitis | Expired air and blood levels | Carbon tetrachloride is the prototype for a wide variety of solvents that cause hepatitis and renal damage. This solvent, like trichloroethylene, acts synergistically with ethanol. |
| CARBON DISULFIDE | Solvent for lipids, sulfur, halogens, rubber, phosphorus, oils, waxes, and resins; manufacturing of organic chemicals, paints, fuels, explosives, viscose rayon | Inhalation of vapor, percutaneous absorption of liquid or vapor | Nervous  Renal  Cardiovascular  Skin Reproductive | Parkinsonism, psychosis, suicide Peripheral neurophathies Chronic nephritic and nephrotic syndromes Acceleration or worsening of atherosclerosis; hypertension Irritation; dermatitis Menorrhagia and metrorrhagia | Iodine azide reaction with urine (nonspecific since other bivalent sulfur compounds give a positive test); $CS_2$ in expired air, blood, and urine | A solvent with unusual multisystem effects, especially noted for cardiovascular, renal, and nervous system actions. |
| STODDARD SOLVENT | Degreasing, paint thinning | Inhalation of vapor, percutaneous absorption of liquid | Skin  CNS | Dryness and scaling from defatting; dermatitis Dizziness, coma, collapse (at high levels) | A mixture of primarily alphatic hydrocarbons, with some benzene derivatives and naphthalenes | |
| ETHYLENE GLYCOL ETHERS Ethylene glycol monoethyl ether—Cellosolve, ethylene glycol monoethyl acetate—Cellosolve acetate, methyl- and butyl-substituted compounds such as ethylene glycol mono-methyl ether-methyl Cellosolve | The ethers are used as solvents for resins, paints, lacquers, varnishes, gum, perfume, dyes, and inks; the acetate derivatives are widely used as solvents and ingredients of lacquers, enamels, and adhesives. Exposure occurs in dry cleaning, plastic, ink, and lacquer manufacturing, and textile dying, among other processes | Inhalation of vapor, percutaneous absorption of liquid | Reproductive CNS Renal Liver | | | Ethylene glycol ethers, as a class of chemicals, have been shown in animals to have adverse effects including reduced sperm count and spontaneous abortion, as well as CNS, renal, and liver effects |

| Agent | Exposure | Route of Entry | System(s) Affected | Primary Manifestations | Aids in Diagnosis | Remarks |
|---|---|---|---|---|---|---|
| **HYDROCARBONS—cont'd** | | | | | | |
| ETHYLENE OXIDE | Used in the sterilization of medical equipment, in the fumigation of spices and other foodstuffs, as a chemical intermediate | Inhalation | Skin<br><br>Eye<br><br><br><br>Respiratory tract<br>Nervous system | Dermatitis and frostbite<br>Severe irritation; possibly cataracts with prolonged exposure<br>Irritation<br>Peripheral neuropathy | | Recent animal tests have shown it to be carcinogenic and to cause reproductive abnormalities. Epidemiologic studies indicate that it may cause leukemia in exposed workers. |
| DIOXANE | Used as a solvent for a variety of materials, including cellulose acetate, dyes, fats, greases, resins, polyvinyl polymers, varnishes, and waxes | Inhalation of vapor, percutaneous absorption of liquid | CNS<br><br><br><br><br>Renal<br>Liver | Drowsiness, dizziness, anorexia, headaches, nausea, vomiting, coma<br>Nephritis<br>Chemical hepatitis | | Dioxane has caused a variety of neoplasms in animals. |
| POLYCHLORINATED BIPHENYLS (PCBs) | Formerly used as dielectric fluid in electrical equipment and as a fire-retardant coating on tiles and other products. New uses were banned in 1976, but much of the electrical equipment currently used still contains PCBs | Inhalation, ingestion, skin absorption | Skin<br>Eye<br>Liver | Chloracne<br>Irritation<br>Toxic hepatitis | Serum PCB level for chronic exposure | Animal studies have demonstrated that PCBs are carcinogenic. Epidemiological studies of exposed workers are inconclusive. |
| **IRRITANT GASES** | | | | | | |
| AMMONIA | Refrigeration; petroleum refining; manufacturing of nitrogen-containing chemicals, synthetic fibers, dyes, and optics | Inhalation of gas | Upper respiratory tract<br>Eye<br>Moist skin | Upper respiratory irritation<br>Irritation<br>Irritation | | |
| HYDROCHLORIC ACID | Chemical manufacturing; electroplating; tanning; metal pickling; petroleum extraction; rubber, photographic, and textile industries | Inhalation of gas or mist | Upper respiratory tract<br>Eye<br>Mucous membrane, skin | Upper respiratory irritation<br>Strong irritant<br>Strong irritant | | |
| HYDROFLUORIC ACID | Chemical and plastic manufacturing; catalyst in petroleum refining; aqueous solution for frosting, etching, and polishing glass | Inhalation of gas or mist | Upper respiratory tract | Upper respiratory irritation | | In solution, causes severe and painful burns of skin and can be fatal. |

| Agent | Exposure | Route of Entry | System(s) Affected | Primary Manifestations | Aids in Diagnosis | Remarks |
|---|---|---|---|---|---|---|
| **IRRITANT GASES—cont'd** | | | | | | |
| SULFUR DIOXIDE | Manufacturing of sulfur-containing chemicals; food and textile bleach; tanning; metal casting | Inhalation of gas, direct contact of gas or liquid phase on skin or mucosa | Middle respiratory tract | Bronchospasm (pulmonary edema or chemical pneumonitis in high dose) | Chest x-ray, pulmonary function tests | Strong irritant of eye, mucous membranes, and skin. |
| CHLORINE | Paper and textile bleaching; water disinfection; chemical manufacturing, metal fluxing; detinning and dezincing iron | Inhalation of gas | Middle respiratory tract | Tracheobronchitis, pulmonary edema, pneumonitis | Chest x-ray, pulmonary function tests | Chlorine combines with body moisture to form acids, which irritate tissues from nose to alveoli. |
| OZONE | Inert gas-shielded arc welding; food, water, and air purification; food and textile bleaching; emitted around high-voltage electrical equipment | Inhalation of gas | Lower respiratory tract | Delayed pulmonary edema (generally 6–8 hours following exposure) | Chest x-ray pulmonary function tests | Ozone has a free-radical structure and can produce experimental chromosome aberrations; it may thus have carcinogenic potential. |
| NITROGEN OXIDES | Manufacturing of acids, nitrogen-containing chemicals, explosives, and more; by-product of many industrial processes | Inhalation of gas | Lower respiratory tract | Pulmonary irritation, bronchiolitis fibrosa obliterations ("silo filler's disease"), mixed obstructive–restrictive changes | Chest x-ray, pulmonary function tests | |
| PHOSGENE | Manufacturing and burning of isocyanates, and manufacturing of dyes and other organic chemicals; in metallurgy for one separation; burning or heat source near trichloroethylene | Inhalation of gas | Lower respiratory tract | Delayed pulmonary edema (delay seldom longer than 12 hours) | Chest x-ray, pulmonary function tests | |
| Isocyanates TDI (toluene diisocyanate) MDI (methylene diphenyldiiscyanate) Hexamethylene diisocyanate and others | Polyurethane manufacture; resin-binding systems in foundries; coating materials for wires; used in certain types of paint | Inhalation of vapor | Predominantly lower respiratory tract | Asthmatic reaction and accelerated loss of pulmonary function | Chest x-ray, pulmonary function tests | Isocyanates are both respiratory tract "sensitizers" and irritants in the conventional sense. |
| ASPHYXIANT GASES (simple asphyxiants: nitrogen, hydrogen, methane, and others) | Enclosed spaces in a variety of industrial settings | Inhalation of gas | CNS | Anoxia | $O_2$ in environment | No specific toxic effect; act by displacing $O_2$. |

| Agent | Exposure | Route of Entry | System(s) Affected | Primary Manifestations | Aids in Diagnosis | Remarks |
|---|---|---|---|---|---|---|
| **CHEMICAL ASPHYXIANTS** | | | | | | |
| CARBON MONOXIDE | Incomplete combustion in foundries, coke ovens, refineries, furnaces, and more | Inhalation of gas | Blood (hemoglobin) | Headache, dizziness, double vision | Carboxy-hemoglobin | |
| HYDROGEN SULFIDE | Used in manu-facturing of sulfur-contain-ing chemicals; produced in petro-leum product use; decay of organic matter | Inhalation of gas | CNS<br><br>Pulmonary | Respiratory center paralysis, hypoventilation<br>Respiratory tract irritation | PaO$_2$ | |
| CYANIDE | Metallurgy, electroplating | Inhalation of va-por, percutane-ous absorption, ingestion | Cellular meta-bolic enzymes (especially cytochrome oxidase) | Enzyme inhibition with metabolic as-phyxia and death | SCN in urine | |
| **PESTICIDES** | | | | | | |
| ORGANOPHOS-PHATES (malathion, parathion, and others) | | Inhalation, inges-tion, percutane-ous absorption | Neuromuscular | Cholinesterase inhi-bition, cholinergic symptoms: nausea and vomiting, salivation, diar-rhea, headache, sweating, meiosis, muscle fascicula-tions, seizures, unconsciousness, death | Refractoriness to atropine; plasma or red cell cholinesterase | As with many acute toxins, rapid treatment of organophos-phate toxicity is imperative. Thus diagnosis is often based on history and a high index of suspicion rather than biochemical tests. Treatment is atropine to block choliner-gic effects and 2-pyradine-alsoxine methio dide (2-PAM) to reactivate cholinesterase. |

*(continues)*

| Agent | Exposure | Route of Entry | System(s) Affected | Primary Manifestations | Aids in Diagnosis | Remarks |
|-------|----------|----------------|--------------------|------------------------|-------------------|---------|
| **PESTICIDES—cont'd** | | | | | | |
| CARBAMATES: (carbaryl [Sevin] and others) | | Inhalation, ingestion, percutaneous absorption | Neuromuscular | Cholinesterase inhibition, cholinergic symptoms: nausea and vomiting, salivation, diarrhea, headache, sweating, meiosis, muscle fasciculations, seizures, unconsciousness, death | Plasma cholinesterase; urinary 1-naphthol (index of exposure) | Treatment of carbamate poisoning is the same as that of organophosphate poisoning except that 2-PAM is contraindicated. |
| CHLORINATED HYDROCARBONS Chlordane DDT Heptachlor Chlordecone (Kepone) Aldrin Dieldrin Uridine | | Inhalation, ingestion, percutaneous absorption | CNS | Stimulation or depression | Urinary organic chlorine, or $p$-chlorophenol acetic acid | The chlorinated hydrocarbons may accumulate in body lipid stores in large amounts. |
| BIPYRIDYLS Paraquat Diquat | | Inhalation, ingestion, percutaneous absorption | Pulmonary | Rapid massive fibrosis, only following paraquat ingestion | | An interesting toxin in that the major toxicity, pulmonary fibrosis, apparently occurs only after ingestion. |

# UNIT 3

# Care of Communities and Populations

CHAPTER 13
Health Promotion and Wellness
*Joan H. Baldwin*
*Cynthia O'Neill Morgan*

CHAPTER 14
Nursing Informatics in Community Health
Nursing Practice
*Russell C. McGuire*
*Sandra L. Walker*

CHAPTER 15
Health Education in the Community
*Lucy Bradley-Springer*

CHAPTER 16
Complementary and Holistic Health
*Margaret A. Burkhardt*

CHAPTER 17
Global Health
*Sharyn Janes*

CHAPTER 18
Groups in the Community
*Peggy "Margaret" Hickman*
*Marilyn Givens King*
*Karen Saucier Lundy*

Joan H. Baldwin and Cynthia O'Neill Morgan

Visit **http://nursing.jbpub.com/communityhealth** for interactive exercises, review questions, Web links, and more.

"Of course, everyone wants to be healthy. The amusing thing is no one's really sure how to do it."

—Jerry Seinfeld

It is not stress that kills us, it is our reaction to it.

*—Hans Selye*

You have had the power to restore yourself all along.

*—Glinda, the Good Witch*, The Wizard of Oz

There is no need to go to India or anywhere else to find peace. You will find that deep place of silence right in your room, your garden, or even your bathtub.

*—Elisabeth Kübler-Ross*

At the end of the day, what do you do to remain healthy? What does being healthy mean to you? Has the meaning of health changed since you entered nursing school? Why do you think nursing is among the least healthy of all the helping professions?

## CHAPTER FOCUS

**Basic Concepts of Health and Health Promotion**
- Selected Definitions of Health Promotion and Wellness
- Community Health Promotion and Wellness

**Factors Influencing Health Promotion and Wellness**
- Changes in Societal Expectations
- Shifting Sands of the Health Care Delivery System
- U.S. Government Initiatives

- Public–Private Partnerships
- Growing Consumerism and Emphasis on Self-Care

**Models of Health Promotion and Wellness**
- Holistic Wellness: Self-Inventory of Personal Wellness Using the Medicine Wheel
- The 4+ Model of Wellness

## QUESTIONS TO CONSIDER

After reading this chapter, you will know the answers to the following questions:

1. What is the difference between health promotion and wellness?
2. What are levels of prevention?
3. What do health promotion and wellness look like?
4. Which factors influence health promotion and wellness?

5. What are the different models for health promotion?
6. How can community health nurses use these models in the promotion of health in their patients?
7. How can a nurse use these concepts to promote self-health?

## KEY TERMS

Health-promoting behaviors
Health promotion

High-level wellness
Levels of prevention

Personal health promotion
Professional health promotion

Wellness

HEALTH PROMOTION AND WELLNESS are important concepts throughout nursing education and practice in all settings. Nurses promote good health and wellness for themselves, their loved ones, and patients. Generally, the major steps to health and wellness include healthy eating, proper exercise, adequate sleep, and time to unwind and manage stress. Health promotion in this respect has always been a nursing focus. As the health care delivery system moves further into managed care, however, **health promotion** and **wellness** become still more important. Health promotion and disease prevention are the keys to managing health care costs. Promoting the health of individuals, families, populations, and communities is essential in nursing practice not only because it is the humane and ethical thing to do, but also because it has practical and economic benefits.

It may be surprising to learn that there are several different definitions for the terms *health promotion* and *wellness*. There are definitions of health promotion and wellness for self, for other individuals, and even for populations and communities.

What do nurses really mean when they say they promote good health and wellness? There are many aspects of health promotion and wellness that will be important to know as a professional nurse. In this chapter, we (1) briefly discuss basic concepts of health and health promotion as related to the concept of disease prevention, including definitions of *health promotion* and *wellness* as the terms are used in this chapter; (2) delineate factors influencing health promotion and wellness; (3) demonstrate some ways of looking at health promotion and wellness by discussing some models of health promotion, risk evaluation, and analysis tools, plus wellness guides that might be useful to know about to promote health and wellness; and (4) introduce two models of wellness.

## Basic Concepts of Health and Health Promotion

How people generally define health may influence how they define health promotion (Baldwin, 1995; Green & Raeburn, 1990; Raphael, 2000). For instance, if health is considered the absence of disease, the definition of health promotion would necessarily include the idea of disease prevention. However, if health is defined as a concept that expresses the positiveness of a full and joyful life, disease prevention is not a part of the definition. Edelman and Fain (1998) speak of this second characterization of health as "expanding consciousness, pattern or meaning recognition, personal transformation, and tentatively, self-actualization" (p. 9). One example is a woman living with a chronic disease such as diabetes, who still considers herself a healthy person; she may see herself being as far along toward self-actualization as she can be.

In 1983, Brubaker conducted a linguistic analysis of the term *health promotion* in nursing literature and found that it was rarely defined specifically and often used as though it had the same meaning as disease prevention. There continues to be debate about the definition of health promotion and whether the definition must necessarily include disease prevention.

Historically, health promotion as a concept has been linked with disease prevention. Clark and Leavell (1965) depicted three **levels of prevention**—primary, secondary, and tertiary—in a model. Primary prevention includes health promotion as part of the model. When primary prevention methods are used, the basic premise of the model is that health-promotion activities "serve to further general health and well-being" (Clark & Leavell, 1965, p. 20). Because this is a model describing disease prevention factors, it leads one to connect health promotion with disease prevention. In this particular model, primary prevention methods include **health-promoting behaviors** that are designed to improve general health and well-being, with the emphasis being on preventing a disease in the first place. For instance, brushing teeth after meals is one step in preventing tooth decay, which would also be good for general health.

As early as 1965, Clark and Leavell noted that "health promotion is not applied for specific disease and as yet is not widely utilized" (p. 24). Identifying health-promoting strategies for secondary and tertiary prevention still seems to be a bit difficult today, but health-promoting activities are important in these levels as well. *Secondary prevention* refers to the early detection of disease and prevention of disease sequelae—"abnormal conditions resulting from a previous disease" (*Webster's Encyclopedic Dictionary*, 1996, p. 1747). A health-promoting action for a woman who has a diagnosis of fibrocystic breast disease would be to avoid caffeine. Poe and O'Neill (1997) determined that caffeine slows the process of the body's natural defenses, which normally results in the elimination of precancerous cells. Therefore, the potential for proliferation of abnormal cells is increased with caffeine ingestion. Tertiary prevention focuses on the minimization of loss of function as a result of disease. Health-promoting activities in tertiary prevention might include training for a competition by a diabetic skier who has only one leg. Good and reasonable physical fitness promotes health.

Today there are also reasons for using health-promotion strategies, behaviors, or actions without necessarily having to consider prevention of disease. Someone may choose certain health-promoting actions just because the actions make the person feel good or healthy. For example, many people like to walk or run several times a week and comment that if they don't walk or run, they don't have as much energy during the day. In this example, these people are not specifically concerned about preventing disease; they just want to feel as good as they can.

GLOBAL CONNECTION

Why is the United States more associated with health promotion research and interventions than the rest of the world? Can other countries use health promotion strategies at the same time that they are still facing challenges in the form of basic public health problems as clean drinking water and infectious diseases?

## ■ Selected Definitions of Health Promotion and Wellness

For the purposes of this chapter, health promotion has two definitions depending on if the nurse is applying health-promotion strategies to other people or if the nurse is promoting his or her own health. The definition of **professional health promotion** on behalf of others reflects the "organized actions or efforts that enhance, support, or promote the well-being or health of individuals, families, groups, communities, or societies" (Kulbok, Baldwin, Cox, & Duffy, 1997, p. 17) An example of this definition is when a school nurse teaches elementary school children the importance of washing hands to eliminate germs and dirt. The nurse first coats the children's hands with an invisible product that can be washed away with soap and water. After handwashing, a special light is shined on the children's hands; areas not carefully washed clean of the product glow green, demonstrating to the children that if hands are not carefully washed, "germs" may remain, much like the green, glowing product. Health education programs and physical education activities, to name two possibilities, are also examples of professional health promotion on behalf of others.

**Personal health promotion** reflects more emphasis on self-actualization and taking care of oneself. This definition identifies what motivates people "to attain and maintain their highest state of wellness, overall fitness, and self-actualization" (Baldwin, 1992, p. 10). For instance, the school nurse may recognize that walking daily for 30 minutes after work maintains physical fitness, dissipates work stress, and provides a sense of renewal and joy as she or he appreciates the spring flowers blooming.

 *Got an Alternative?*

Nearly 38% of student nurses will experience a back injury during nursing school, according to *American Nurse* (September 2003). Back injuries are the most common occupational injury reported by nurses during their careers. Avoiding back injuries is more than proper body mechanics: New lifting technology in health care facilities and self-care exercise, such as yoga, tai-chi, and weight-bearing and strengthening exercises, are all important prevention strategies that nurses should use to avoid this chronic, often disabling condition.

Positive and nurturing relationships with friends and pets are associated with good health.

What is the relationship between health promotion and wellness? As defined in this chapter, health promotion relates to behaviors or activities that result in wellness. Dunn (1959/1980) describes **high-level wellness** as "an integrated method of functioning which is oriented toward maximizing the potential of which the individual is capable" (p. 447) The concept of high-level wellness is based on the assumption that every individual, regardless of personal challenges, has a potential for wellness within the limits placed by the challenge. In other words, high-level wellness is the highest level of well-being that a person can reach. To attain high-level wellness, there must be harmony in all aspects of a person's life. Box 13-1 lists two definitions of health promotion.

Health promotion and wellness, particularly when defined for one's own use, are closely related or even inter-related. In this chapter, *wellness* is a state of being; *health promotion* is how one gets there (Box 13-2). How one attains and maintains wellness is accomplished through various health-promoting behaviors. Examples of some health-promoting behaviors include (1) walking for at least 30 minutes

*Life is short, the art long, opportunity fleeting, experience treacherous, judgment difficult.*

—Hippocrates (460–377 BC)

6 days a week, preferably with some intensity as though a bit late for an appointment (Bach, 1998); (2) eating foods that have omega-3 or monounsaturated fats, limiting daily total fat intake to less than 25% of total calories (Simopoulos, 1999); (3) adapting traditionally high-calorie or high-fat recipes to today's healthier levels (Jones, 1999); (4) meditating or visualizing to increase well-being (Cohen, 1998); and (5) learning how to relax (Cohen, 1998). Researchers today are emphasizing health-promoting activities such as these for individuals, families, populations, and communities to attain and maintain states of wellness (McCarthy & Mandle, 1998; Sandhu, 1998).

A person can be sick and be moving toward wellness using health-promoting actions or behaviors or can have a chronic disease and actually be experiencing high-level wellness. Remember, high-level wellness means "maximizing the potential of which the individual is capable" (Dunn, 1959, p. 447). So, if the diabetic woman mentioned earlier in this chapter is maintaining a healthy lifestyle, has no difficulty managing her diabetes, is happy, and feels well balanced in her life, it could be said that the woman is likely to be experiencing high-level wellness. The woman is maximizing the potential of which she is capable.

The woman with diabetes is the one most likely to know what her maximum potential can be and how close she is to reaching it in her life. What high-level wellness is, using Dunn's (1959) definition, for any particular person is defined by that person and may change over time.

How can a 22-year-old student nurse who is in a car accident and becomes a paraplegic reach high-level wellness? According to the aforementioned definitions, the student nurse has a potential to be more or less well within the boundaries of the limits set by the condition. "Wellness is a bridge that takes people into realms far beyond treatment or therapy—into a domain of self-responsibility and self-empowerment" (Ryan & Travis, 1991, p. 3). The student nurse has choices. Relating to personal life, the student nurse has the choice to (1) do nothing about overcoming the physical, emotional, mental, and spiritual challenges of being a paraplegic; (2) learn to use a wheelchair to go to classes and elsewhere; or (3) perhaps even go so far as to become a gold medalist in the ParaOlympics. Professionally, the student nurse can bend to the pressure of the barriers and drop out of the nursing program or fight the system to remain, making adjustments as necessary. There is no reason that a full, satisfying, professional nursing career should be out of reach for this student.

It is important to note that nurses do not define high-level wellness for patients, but rather they assist patients in identifying what they are capable of reaching to maximize their potential for high-level wellness. Remember what was noted earlier in the chapter: High-level wellness is the highest level of well-being *that patients can reach*. An overweight, heavy-smoking, heavy-drinking person may think, and even state, the belief that he or she is healthy, but given Dunn's definition, it is unlikely that the person is experiencing high-level wellness and maximizing his or her potential to the best of his or her abilities. It is relatively easy to apply this concept to individuals, but how does high-level wellness translate to communities?

## ■ Community Health Promotion and Wellness

Communities have potential for high-level wellness, too. Communities can be defined within geographic boundaries or as population groups with special needs or interests (Baldwin, Conger, Abegglen, & Hill, 1998). Communities usually have systems in place, such as planning commissions or committees, to identify what is high-level wellness for that group. For example, one element of wellness identified in the motto for Sandy City, Utah, is support for family values. One way the community supports family values is by promoting healthy family activities. Toward this end, the community master plan establishes a network of neighborhood parks that will be developed as neighborhoods expand. This process maximizes the potential of the community to reach what it has defined as high-level wellness.

Some community interventions that support wellness are relatively easy to identify by community members. Others, especially related to population wellness, are more difficult for communities to pinpoint. Nurses often collaborate with community groups to identify these strengths, assets, problems, and needs.

People with chronic and even terminal diseases may live their lives in such a healthy and balanced manner that high-level wellness might be attained, at least for a time. A person can use health-promotion behaviors and activities even if ill or diseased "to become an active participant in the healing process instead of a passive recipient" (Ryan & Travis, 1991, p. 3).

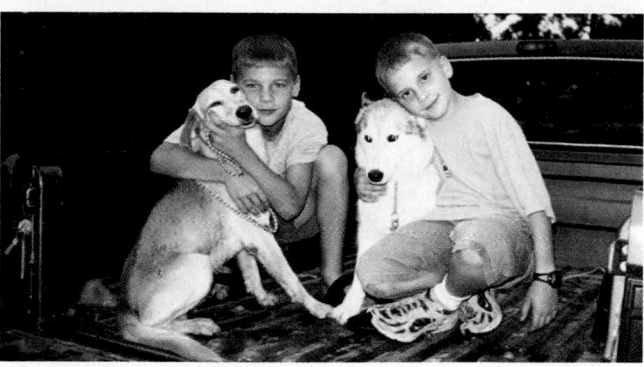

Learning to care for pets can promote health through teaching compassion and caring to children.

### CULTURAL CONNECTION

You have noticed that everything an Indian does is in a circle, and that is because the Power of the World always works in circles, and everything tries to be round. . . . The Sky is round, and I have heard that the earth is round like a ball, and so are all the stars. The wind, in its greatest power, whirls. Birds make their nests in circles, for theirs is the same religion as ours. . . . Even the seasons form a great circle in their changing, and always come back again to where they were. The life of a man is a circle from childhood, and so it is in everything where power moves.

—Black Elk, Oglala Sioux holy man, 1863

*"All of the information about exercise, eating right, and how my body works helped me change the physical me. The most important part is to understand that it is not as much about the weight as it is about making the connection. That means looking after yourself every day and putting forth your best effort to love yourself enough to do what is best for you. . . . The biggest change I've made is a spiritual one. It comes from the realization that taking care of my body and my health is really one of the greatest kinds of love I can give myself. . . . And there's no question I'm living a better life.*"

—Oprah Winfrey

## Factors Influencing Health Promotion and Wellness

Health care in the United States is finally experiencing a shift in focus from a rather one-sided emphasis on present and potential disease to a more balanced focus that includes an equal emphasis on health promotion, wellness, risk reduction, and disease prevention (Baldwin, Conger, Abegglen, & Hill, 1998). Educating patients, defined as individuals, families, populations, or communities, regarding their health requires information about health-promotion activities that the patients consider relevant to them. It is because of this shift in focus that we now are more strongly accentuating the importance of understanding the "why's" and "how-to's" of health promotion and wellness. Some of the factors influencing health promotion and wellness are the changes in societal expectations, shifting sands of the health care delivery system, U.S. government initiatives, public–private partnerships, and growing consumerism and emphasis on self-care.

### Changes in Societal Expectations

Over the years, people in the United States have vacillated as to what good health and wellness are all about. Some cultures had lifestyles that encompassed running and athletic feats, such as hunting, that sustained life; other groups were much more sedentary. Types of foods eaten varied, and little attention was paid to which foods were healthy and which

foods were not; the important thing was being able to eat. Prior to the 1960s, the social system was such that the majority of people spent more time worrying about food, shelter, and safety (lower levels of Maslow's hierarchy) than self-actualization (Maslow, 1970). The relationship of lifestyle and health had not been established scientifically. Health was primarily defined as the absence of disease, and health care delivery and research focused on controlling and trying to cure communicable diseases. The media played little or no role in sharing health-related information with the public other than reporting morbidity and mortality information.

Since the 1960s, societal expectations have changed. Increasing affluence has allowed the majority of society to move beyond a primary concern with food, shelter, and safety toward achieving self-esteem and self-actualization (Maslow, 1970). High-level wellness is a state of self-actualization, "maximizing the potential of which the individual is capable" (Dunn, 1959, p. 447). During the 1950s and 1960s, the leading causes of morbidity and mortality moved from communicable disease to chronic disease. With this shift, the health care profession had less success in controlling the causes of disease or in curing some of the diseases. Instead of cure, the focus became symptom management. It became more obvious that the method of control for chronic disease begins with health promotion and specific preventive measures.

**A Good Read**

## Gesundheit!: Bringing Good Health to You, the Medical System, and Society Through Physician Service, Complementary Therapies, Humor and Joy (1998)

*By Patch Adams and Maureen Mylander, Rochester, VT: Inner Traditions International.*

All those who loved the movie *Patch Adams* will want to read this enjoyable book to learn more about the revolutionary ideas of this fascinating physician and his successful practice at the Gesundheit Institute in Northern Virginia. Dr. Adams is a social revolutionary who presents his unique approach to "free medicine" through a collection of essays. Adams believes that today's high-tech medicine is too costly, impersonal, and boring. He demonstrates how healing can be a loving, creative, and humorous human-to-human experience between practitioner and patient, rather than a for-profit business. Through the efforts of Adams and his colleagues, the Gesundheit Institute was operated as a free health care service, without payment, malpractice insurance, or formal facilities.

Adams's book is an excellent example of the possibilities of how complementary and conventional medicine can be combined to deliver services to patients in a partnership based on mutual respect and a commitment to a vision of what good health can be.

---

Since the mid-1960s, there has been a proliferation of research relating health promotion and wellness to lifestyle practices. This information has become so popular that the media have developed an interest in reporting health-promotion strategies. Today, experts on morning television programs regularly report the latest in health-related research and health-promotion strategies. With these societal changes in perception and the increasing costs of health care, pressure came to bear to look for the most cost-effective methods to deliver health care.

### ■ Shifting Sands of the Health Care Delivery System

The health care delivery system, as a fee-for-service system, focused on the treatment of illness rather than on health promotion and prevention of disease (Butterfield, 1993). However, research has demonstrated that the causes of most chronic illness are the practice of health-depleting behaviors *and* social and environmental barriers that limit the choices individuals, families, populations, and communities have relating to health-promoting activities. In addition, in a seminal article by McGinnis and Foege (1993), the chief preventable causes of death are translated to lifestyle choices and social influences. These causes include tobacco use; poor diet and activity patterns; alcohol consumption; exposure to environmental microbial or toxic agents; inappropriate use of firearms; promiscuous, unprotected sexual behaviors; motor vehicle accidents; illicit drug use; and socioeconomic barriers.

There are many social barriers that limit the choices patients have in relationship to health-promoting activities. Prime examples are those who live in inner cities or who live in rural or frontier areas. Food choices are limited by distance to full-service grocery stores and availability of transportation. The stores that are available tend to be small family-owned markets or gas station mini-marts. Both provide limited choice of foods at prices higher than full-service chain stores. In addition, gas station mini-marts may not sell produce but do sell high-fat, high-calorie convenience foods.

With the move to managed care and other community-based services for individuals and families and the realization that chronic illness and even death are grounded, for the most part, in lifestyle choices and social barriers, the focus of health care is changing. The principles of managed care require that health-promotion and disease-prevention activities be included in practice at both individual and population levels to prevent the costly occurrence of chronic disease and disability. For managed care organizations to realize a profit, risk groups must be managed at both the individual and the aggregate levels (Baldwin, Conger, Abegglen, & Hill, 1998). Also, managed care organizations are becoming more involved in community activities such as community-based health centers, health fairs, Healthy Communities programs, and school-based clinics. Many managed care systems and other insurance companies encourage health-promotion education, activities, and behaviors for their members. In addition, industries have included wellness programs for employees, which may offer various types of reimbursement incentives, from lowering insurance premiums to giving bonuses to those members and employees who demonstrate health-promoting behaviors.

**ENVIRONMENTAL CONNECTION**

Tobacco companies have mounted extensive media campaigns targeting ethnic, lower-income urban areas while promoting their products. What are the possible environmental and ethical outcomes of these free-market-economy activities in regard to public health?

## ■ U.S. Government Initiatives

In the late 1970s, the Surgeon General of the United States, in a document titled *Healthy People*, reported to the nation about the expectations at that time regarding health promotion and disease prevention in this country (Baldwin, 1992, 1995; Kulbok & Baldwin, 1992; USPHS, 1979). The Surgeon General stated, "Let us make no mistake about the significance of this document, it represents an emerging consensus among scientists and the health community that the Nation's health strategy must be dramatically recast to emphasize the prevention of disease" (*Healthy People 2010*, 2008, p. 1).

In 1980, target outcomes, in the form of objectives for the year 1990, were given relating to the reduction of premature mortality in four age groups (Majese & Fox, 1998). At that time, prevention of disease was the main thrust, with health-protection factors addressed and health promotion mentioned. Revised and updated objectives, written in 1990 for the year 2000 (*Healthy People 2000: National Health Promotion and Disease Prevention Objectives*), changed the order of health priorities. Health promotion became the first consideration in the list of three important factors: health promotion, health protection, and preventive services (Baldwin, 1992; Kulbok & Baldwin, 1992). In 1998, the document *Healthy People 2010 Objectives: Draft for Public Comment* (DHHS) was published to elicit public and professional input into the developed national objectives for the year 2010. In November 2000, the second edition of *Healthy People 2010: Understanding and Improving Health* was published.

Nurses must be involved at all levels of policy development. They have been members of task forces developing the components of each *Healthy People* document, and with the availability of the Internet, nurses had opportunity to give input and feedback on the *Healthy People 2010* development. An interactive database system, *DATA 2010*, has been developed and contains the most recent national and state data related to all of the objectives and subgroups of *Healthy People 2010*. These data are updated quarterly (CDC, 2008). Health behaviors are also tracked by state with the Behavioral Risk Factor Surveillance System (BRFSS), which can be found at the CDC website, www.cdc.gov/nccdphp/aag/aag_brfss.htm.

The *Healthy People 2010* document provides a wonderful opportunity for nursing students to assess populations within their local regions related to progress toward one or more of the objectives. At Brigham Young University College of Nursing, beginning nursing students write a scholarly paper that is based on *Healthy People 2010* objectives. The students have 1 year, through several nursing courses, to complete the assignment. Students pick a topic such as immunizations or maternal–child issues, conduct a literature review, consider nursing implications, and assess what is being done in the local community for the population of interest. Recommendations are made as to additional approaches that might be taken, and these are shared with community agencies.

## ■ Public–Private Partnerships

Through a cooperative agreement between the American Public Health Association (APHA) and the Centers for Disease Control and Prevention (CDC), a major collaborative process resulted in another document, *Healthy Communities 2000 Model Standards: Guidelines for Community Attainment of the Year 2000 National Health Objectives* (APHA, 1991). The approach and document are considered valuable resources for communities wanting to explore and develop local health-promotion standards. The APHA built on the *Healthy People 2000* objectives, developing step-by-step criteria for each objective. Each objective had a measurable "goal" attached to it. For instance, the objective to reduce coronary heart disease deaths might have a measurable goal to reduce $x$ amount of these deaths per 100,000 people by some specific date. These guidelines for adapting measurable criteria to the national objectives have been adapted and used by leaders, including nurses and other health care professionals in many states, counties, regions, cities, and even some neighborhoods, who wish to facilitate more healthful lifestyles for the populations they serve.

The Healthy Cities program originated in 1985 with a presentation at an international meeting in Canada. The theme of the presentation was that health is the result of much more than medical care; people are healthy when they live in nurturing environments and are involved in the life of their community (Duhl, 1986). A recent publication, *Healthy People in Healthy Communities: A Guide for Community Leaders* (DHHS, 1998a), links healthy cities with healthy people to create a healthy community in a guide to how other cities and communities developed and implemented their healthy community initiatives.

There have been numerous partnerships and group efforts in which nurses have collaborated with Healthy Cities and Communities projects throughout the country. Flynn and other community health nurses began "Healthy Indiana," which was an early forerunner of ensuing Healthy Cities and Communities programs (Kellogg Foundation, 1988). Other examples include work with homeless populations (Moore, Neff, Smith, & Weber, 1999) and nurse managed care centers (Drapo & Woods, 1992). The growth of community nursing organizations demonstrates how nurses believe our focus should be on partnering and collaborating with

Health fairs are effective ways to reach specific populations for health promotion in communities.

communities and special populations in health-promoting efforts. Nurse educators and local public health nursing directors continue to forge collaborative bonds with cities, communities, and target population groups in developing community/population health-promotion needs and assets assessments (Baldwin, 1995; Raphael & Bryant, 2002).

The following is an example of nursing student involvement with community-level health promotion interventions. The Brigham Young University College of Nursing in Provo, Utah, offers a community/population assessment elective course to both nursing undergraduate students and university honor students. Various city and county health departments and local communities have requested assistance in assessing the needs of key population groups. For

### a conversation with . . .

**Janet Quinn**

A healing environment is one that facilitates the emergence of the Haelen effect, the synergistic, organismic, multidimensional response of whole persons in the direction of healing and wholeness. Healing, the emergence of right relationship at, between, and among all the levels of human being, is always accomplished by the one healing. No one and no thing can heal another human being. All healing is creative emergence, new birth, the manifestation of the powerful inner longing, at every level, to be whole. . . . We can remove barriers to the healing process. We can participate in creating environments that will support healing. We can become midwives to this process of healing, creating, and being a safe, sacred space into which the healing might emerge. We can literally become the healing environment.

—Janet F. Quinn, 1992, in "Holding Sacred Space: The Nurse as Healing Environment," *Holistic Nursing Practice*, 6(4), 26–36.

example, the members of the Healthy Taylorsville Project requested the class's help in assessing the needs and viewpoints of the youth of the community. The college students collaborated with the school superintendent, principals, teachers, counselors, and junior and senior high school students. They produced a document outlining the needs of the youth and their suggestions and ideas about health-promotion strategies for the city of Taylorsville (Browning, Huls, Rather, & Stout, 1997). One example of the Taylorsville youths' suggestions was to place stoplights at two of the busiest streets in the growing city so that students could safely cross those streets to get to and from school. The document will be a major guide toward anticipated changes for many of the needs stated by the youth (personal communication, J. I. Morgan, Director of Administrative Services, Taylorsville, Utah, March 1998).

### ■ Growing Consumerism and Emphasis on Self-Care

Since the late 1960s, consumers of health care have increasingly demanded information relating to their health care and to items that promote health. In the past, consumers almost complacently accepted what physicians and others in control of health care systems told them regarding their health care. Over the last 30 years, consumers have become better educated and more proactive in demanding their rights and insisting that health care professionals be accountable for their actions. Evidence can be seen in the proliferation of satisfaction surveys, opinion polls, and litigation, as well as in the nature of advertising. Information related to dietary management, such as lowering the fat content in recipes, and exercise activities that claim to be health promoting are seen throughout the media. People are requesting more information on labels so that they can discern whether the item contains anything that might be non-health promoting, especially something that might trigger an allergy or be too high in fat content. The health-promotion aspects of education have become a major focus for all age and ethnic groups.

Who is responsible for health? There is an expanding awareness that consumers must bear the responsibility for their own health. How can consumers do this? Self-care is the answer. Self-care is defined as those "activities initiated or performed by an individual, family, or community to achieve, maintain, or promote maximum health" (Steiger & Lipson, 1985, p. 12). Orem defines self-care as "the production of actions directed to self or to the environment in order to regulate one's functioning in the interest of one's life, integrated functioning, and well-being" (1985, p. 31).

**❝**Let us rise up and be thankful, for if we didn't learn a lot today, at least we learned a little; and if we didn't learn a little, at least we didn't get sick; and if we got sick, at least we didn't die; so let us all be thankful.**❞**

—Buddha (563–483 BC)

## Research Alert

The authors of a randomized controlled trial compared the outcomes of individuals chosen to participate in the 8-week People with Arthritis Can Exercise (PACE) program with those who did not receive the PACE intervention. The mean age of the 347 participants was 70, 90% were women, and all reported limitations due to arthritis. Patients completed a Health Assessment questionnaire and tests of physical function and physical activity. Researchers measured outcomes at baseline and 8 weeks, and the intervention group completed self-assessments at 3 and 6 months. Researchers adjusted the outcomes for possible confounding variables.

One-hour PACE program classes were conducted twice a week for 8 weeks. The mean number of classes attended by the intervention group was 9.4. After 8 weeks, patients in the intervention group had reduced pain and fatigue, and improved arthritis management. Program participants who continued the program for 6 months had better outcomes in pain, fatigue, and stiffness versus those in the control group.

*Source:* Barclay, L., & Vega, C. (2008). Eight-week exercise program may benefit elderly patients with arthritis. *Medscape Medical News.* Retrieved November 4, 2008, from http://www.medscape.com/viewarticle/568653

The impetus for the current interest in self-care began anew in the late 1970s and early 1980s. The U.S. Department of Health and Human Services (DHHS, 1982) published a document titled *Forward Plan for Health 1977–1981*. It seems remarkable to consider today, that for the first time ever, the authors of this report boldly suggested that lifestyle and psychosocial factors had a great impact on morbidity and mortality. A number of health-promotion elements such as nutrition, exercise, and fitness were mentioned.

In addition to the emphasis placed by government documents at that time, the popular press also supported the notion. In his book *Megatrends*, Naisbitt (1982, p. 131) forecast that self-care emphasizing health-promotion strategies would move health care out of the medical-institutional illness model into an era of self-responsibility for health and wellness. In 1999, the U.S. Public Health Service published a well-received book, *Promoting Physical Activity*: *A Guide for Community Action*. Shortly thereafter, several other exercise-motivation books appeared on the scene (Marcus & Forsyth, 2002).

The demand for self-care is currently coming from people themselves, private insurance carriers, managed care organizations, employers, and communities. In the past, individuals would never consider questioning the diagnoses or orders of their physicians. Insurance carriers now insist that there be at least two health care professionals' opinions before major surgery.

In addition, consumers are demanding information about complementary treatment options in addition to allopathic treatments suggested by physicians. Insurance and managed care companies are providing self-care books that

assist subscribers to self-diagnose and self-treat simple illnesses and injuries, as well as offer tips on health-promoting activities for all members of the family. Incentives include managed care organizations paying bonuses to members for smoking cessation, weight loss, and other health-promoting activities that move the members toward high-level wellness. At the workplace, large companies implement organizational wellness programs that assist employees to maximize personal wellness. Research has shown that an employee experiencing high-level wellness uses fewer sick days and is more productive on the job (National Institute for Occupational Safety and Health, 1996; DHHS, 1998b). At home or from a local library or other community establishment, patients can access numerous Internet sites on any subject relating to self-care.

Self-care and consumerism are processes that assist people to know about health-promoting items and activities. At the population and community levels, the Healthy Cities and Communities program depends heavily on people within communities to identify problems and assets and engage in problem solving and self-care to correct problems and promote maximal community wellness. The success of the *Healthy People 2010* objectives for the nation is equally dependent on patient education in health-promotion and self-care strategies as well as policy changes to improve social conditions allowing for the context within which personal choices about health are made. To make informed health promoting decisions, appropriate and correct health-promotion information must be available to patients, as well as to legislators who make the policies.

### NOTE THIS!

The percentage of Americans who walk to work dropped from 5.6% in 1980 to 3.9% in 1990 and 2.9% in 2000. Walking has been replaced by the automobile or mass transit. The change in residence for most Americans, from the city to the suburbs, has created the necessity for people to drive cars to their places of employment and has reduced the time that most people have at home. Urban sprawl has created fewer opportunities for employment in one's community, therefore increasing commute time and providing fewer chances for walking to work. Commute times are getting longer. The percentage of workers who reach their jobs in less than 20 minutes dropped to 47% in 2000 after hovering around 50% for decades.

—Alan Pisarski, *Commuting in America. III.* Transportation Research Board, National Research Council, October 16, 2006.

How does this trend affect the health of populations? What are ways that community health nurses can address this problem?

## Models of Health Promotion and Wellness

Numerous models of health promotion and wellness might be useful guides to assessing and promoting health and wellness in communities, populations, families, and individuals. Many models have been constructed to explain, assess, plan, or evaluate health-promotion education programs, states of health, wellness, and illness, and preventive measures.

As early as 1952, researchers expressed the need for a model to help explain and predict why certain at-risk populations took preventive actions and others did not, even when there was very little or nothing being charged for the preventive services (Rosenstock, 1974). The first popular model developed was the health belief model (Becker, 1974; Hochbaum, 1958; Padilla & Bulcavage, 1991; Rosenstock, 1974). In this model, "the individual's weighing of the positive and negative valences of the threats of illness was emphasized" (Baldwin, 1992, p. 27). How the individual perceived his or her susceptibility to an illness and what might be the perceived benefits and barriers to doing something about preventing the illness were important factors in the health belief model. Even when the individual decided it was in his or her best interest to take some action to prevent the illness, there needed to be a trigger or cue to action to motivate the person to carry out the action (Baldwin, 1992; Rosenstock, 1974).

Several other models have been developed that might be useful to the nurse of today. As researchers continue the quest to predict and explain which factors contributed to health-promoting and health-protecting behaviors, the multidimensionality of the process became clearer. Further developments of the predictors of preventive health behavior originating in the health belief model were instigated in later models. Cognitive factors such as patients' definitions of health and perceptions about health behaviors, including benefits, barriers, and control, were seen as important to patients' health-promoting behaviors. Modifying factors, ranging from demographic, biological, behavioral, and interpersonal factors to environmental issues, including access to care, as well as factors that might influence the initiating of health-promoting and health-protective behaviors, were explored. Many of these multidimensional factors can be seen in the health-promotion models constructed in the 1980s and early 1990s (Palank, 1991; Pender, 1987; Simmons, 1990) and in health-hazard risk evaluation and appraisal tools and wellness guides, which began appearing in the early 1970s and 1980s.

Health-hazard risk evaluation and appraisal tools are commonly designed in survey questionnaire form to provide quantitative data elicited from patients' responses regarding lifestyle and health habits. Questions regarding activities of daily living ranging from personal health habits, such as "How often do you brush your teeth?", "In what way and how often do you exercise?", and "Are you sexually active?" to questions about seatbelt use and consumption of caffeine products, are often asked. Often, information is required regarding family and personal medical histories and various demographic data. The information from these questionnaires can then be compared with known national and local health statistics to make predictions and health-promotion recommendations regarding morbidity and mortality risks for the patients. Wellness guides are generally in a question-

and-answer form, designed to appeal to consumers who may have a common health or wellness question or concern.

In the late 1980s, the *Guide to Clinical Preventive Services* (U.S. Preventive Services Task Force, 1989) was developed. In 1995, a second edition was published to help guide primary care health professionals providing preventive services. These tools and guides are used by physicians' and nurse practitioners' offices, hospitals, health departments, managed care systems, and other agencies to assist health care professionals in counseling patients about reducing potential risks and increasing health-promoting behaviors. Models, tools, and guides continue to be designed to help explore factors involved in health promotion and wellness decision making for individuals, families, populations, and communities.

Two recent models are described to demonstrate how these techniques might be used to assess and facilitate wellness interventions: (1) holistic wellness: self-inventory of personal wellness using the medicine wheel (McDonald, 1997) and (2) the 4+ model of wellness (Baldwin & Baldwin, 1998). These models are similar in some respects to earlier models and tools in the assessment of multidimensional variables affecting health and wellness, but they differ somewhat in the approaches. Both of these models may be used with any ethnic population, as may several of the earlier models. The holistic wellness model allows patients to identify aspects that determine wellness and to define what well and unhealthy states are for them. The 4+ model of wellness also encourages patient participation in the assessment of wellness and adds two other dimensions: the consideration of what might be the sources of nurture and depletion for a patient and ways that the nurse might facilitate interventions with the patient, focusing on those sources of nurture and depletion to promote health and wellness.

**ETHICAL CONNECTION**

What responsibilities do media personalities, such as actors and professional athletes, have in promoting healthy values about body image?

## ■ Holistic Wellness: Self-Inventory of Personal Wellness Using the Medicine Wheel

The medicine wheel is a sacred symbol that is common to almost all Native American tribes. Ivan McDonald, a member of the Blackfeet tribe and health educator for Indian Health Services in Browning, Montana, developed the holistic wellness model using the medicine wheel as a basis (see the figure that follows). Although the descriptors for this model are specific to the values and beliefs of the Blackfeet culture of Native Americans, the wheel can be used to assess wellness for any person of any culture. The descriptors of "healthy" states and "unhealthy" states for the spokes of the wheel should reflect the individuality of the person.

The holistic wellness model is grounded in the Native American understanding of existence. The medicine wheel, as a representation of this understanding, is depicted as a circle that comprises the four sacred directions. Each direction represents not only one of the basic elements necessary for survival, but also a human element.

The East is symbolic of the sun and fire and of one's own creative spirit. The South represents water and one's emotions. The West is the place of Mother Earth and one's intuition—the place of magic and dreams. The North represents air and minds filled with wisdom as one learns about the mystery of life.

Holistic wellness defines health in terms of the whole person, not only in terms of physical illness. The model represents how Native American people understand health as a balance within the person and between the person and everything around him or her—physical, vocational, psychological, social, emotional, environmental, spiritual, and intellectual. It focuses on optimal health, prevention of disease, and positive mental and emotional states (personal communication, I. McDonald, April 1998).

### Research Alert

Researchers used a computer simulation to determine the cost-effectiveness of lifestyle intervention or metformin for preventing type 2 diabetes. Data from published information was used to estimate how and at what cost diet and exercise counseling would affect patients with prediabetes versus the effect and cost of prescribing metformin. The researchers also estimated the costs of doing nothing for patients with prediabetes. They put the estimates into a computer model to calculate the cost of each strategy per year of life saved.

The results of the computer analysis indicated that both strategies—prescribing diet and exercise counseling and prescribing metformin—would delay diabetes, reduce complications, and improve survival rates. The effect of diet and exercise, however, was favorable for all adult ages, while metformin was not cost effective after age 65. Compared with no prevention, the cost estimate for diet and exercise counseling was about $8,800 and the cost estimate for metformin was about $29,000 per quality-adjusted life-year saved.

*Source*: Herman, W. H., Hoerger, T. J., Brandle, M., Hicks, K., Sorensen, S., Zhang, P. Hamman, R. F., Ackermann, R. T., Engelgau, M. M., & Ratner, R. E. (2005). The cost-effectiveness of lifestyle modification or metformin in preventing type 2 diabetes in adults with impaired glucose tolerance. *Annals of Internal Medicine* (pp. 323–332). Diabetes Prevention Program Research Group.

The spokes of the medicine wheel radiate from a center circle that represents wellness or "Healthy for Life." The spokes contain dimensions of the specific wellness (e.g., the Physical wellness spoke has the dimensions of unfit and fit), with the more positive part of the dimension being closest to the center Healthy for Life circle in the figure. The spokes are defined as follows:

- Physical wellness: maintenance of your body in good condition by eating right, exercising regularly, avoiding harmful habits, and making informed, responsible decisions about your health
- Vocational wellness: enjoyment of what you are doing to earn a living and/or to contribute to society
- Psychological wellness: maintenance of mental health or the ability to think reasonably clearly and to avoid wildly distorting reality
- Social wellness: ability to perform the expectations of social roles effectively, comfortably, and without harming others
- Emotional wellness: understanding emotions and knowing how to cope with problems that arise in everyday life; ability to endure stress
- Environmental wellness: minimizing personal and global risks to health, socioeconomic status, education, and various other environmental factors that affect health, such as noise pollution, radiation, air pollution, and water pollution
- Spiritual wellness: a state of balance and harmony with yourself and others; includes trust, integrity, principles, ethics, the purpose or drive in life, basic

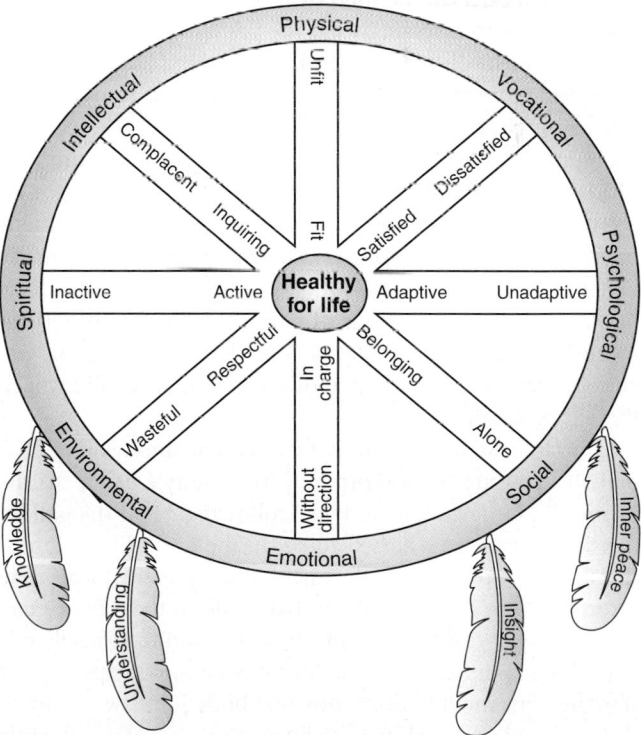

Holistic wellness: Self-Inventory of personal wellness using the medicine wheel survival instincts, feelings of selflessness, degree of pleasure-seeking qualities, commitment to some higher process or being, and the ability to believe in concepts that are not subject to a "state of the art" explanation

- Intellectual wellness: having a mind open to new ideas; covers such activities as speaking, writing, analyzing, critical thinking, and judgment

The eagle feathers at the bottom of the wheel represent the progression of personal development: knowledge, understanding, insight, and inner peace. Each element is a higher level than the one before. However, the element before must occur before one can aspire to the next level. The progression of the feathers is similar to the progression for each dimension reflected in the spokes of the wheel. As the patient develops inwardly toward Healthy for Life, there is progress from knowledge to inner peace.

The holistic wellness model includes social and environmental aspects as they relate to a person's wellness. From the perspectives of many cultures, a person's wellness depends on social relationships and harmony with the environment. For example, for some societies in Australia and Mexico, physical illness can be caused by breaches of social norm. Although this is not necessarily a common idea in many Western societies, from the worldview of most cultures, personal illness or wellness may be a result of social and environmental interactions.

### How to Use the Holistic Wellness Model

The nurse could use the holistic wellness model as an excellent visual depiction of a patient's self-defined wellness state. The model can be used by health professionals to help patients in both assessing what the patient's values are relating to the eight dimensions and determining how well he or she is functioning within each dimension. It is important to note, though, that if one dimension becomes the focus of changing behaviors, other dimensions may suffer from lack of attention. Therefore, facilitating interventions through the use of this model requires that the nurse and the patient together consider how to strengthen all of the dimensions as equally as possible. In addition, the holistic wellness model is handy for quick evaluations of progress. It is also important to understand that the balance may shift depending on circumstances and that, as symbolized by the medicine wheel, there is constant motion.

Several examples of how to intervene and facilitate the patient's considering a more healthful lifestyle using health-promoting behaviors include the following: (1) If the patient considers himself or herself to be on the unfit dimension of the Physical spoke, discuss ways for the patient to become more fit. What does the patient like to do in the way of exercise, and what can the patient physically and realistically do? If walking is difficult for an elderly person, perhaps suggest starting with moving every possible body joint two or three times during a television or radio commercial or a rest while reading. (2) If the patient believes he or she is inactive on the Spiritual spoke, review what spirituality means to the patient

Dr. Joan H. Baldwin, chapter author (center), works with nurse practitioner students in a wellness program on the Ute Indian reservation.

and see if he or she can discover ways to become more active in that realm. (3) If the patient sees that he or she is without direction on the Emotional spoke, address things that might be done by the patient to make him or her feel more in charge of life. The major issue here is what the patient believes he or she can realistically do to develop health-promoting behaviors that will lead to the patient being more healthy for life.

At a community level, the model could be applied by changing the names on the outer ring of the medicine wheel. For example, things such as public transportation, community pride, health care services, and so on could substitute for the physical, spiritual, and psychological elements. The spokes would translate similarly. For instance, public transportation might be present (meaning all possible modes of transportation are available) to absent (meaning there is no public transportation in the community). The feather could be redefined as knowledge to data, understanding to information, insight to creative solutions, and inner peace to harmony of factors.

### ■ The 4+ Model of Wellness

The 4+ model of wellness (Baldwin & Baldwin, 1998) is designed to assist critical thinking about things that might negatively deplete or positively nurture wellness in a patient. There are two layers, much like transparent plastic overlays, to this model: (1) the four domains of inner self and (2) the outer systems. When layer 2 is placed over layer 1, the total 4+ model of wellness appears.

The 4+ model of wellness begins with the inner self layer, depicting a sphere containing the four domains of inner self (see the following figure) of the patient. The patient might be oneself, another individual, a family, a population, or a community. The four domains of inner self are intellectual, physical, emotional, and spiritual (or spirit).

This portion of the 4+ model of wellness appears simple but is really quite complex. The intellectual component of the inner self relates to how the patient thinks. The physical is how the patient moves and senses things and includes all

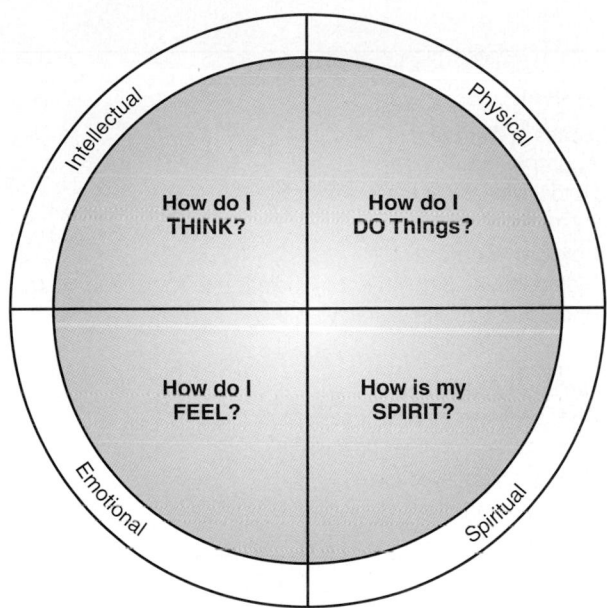

The 4+ model of wellness: The four domains of inner self

*Source*: Used by permission of Joan H. Baldwin.

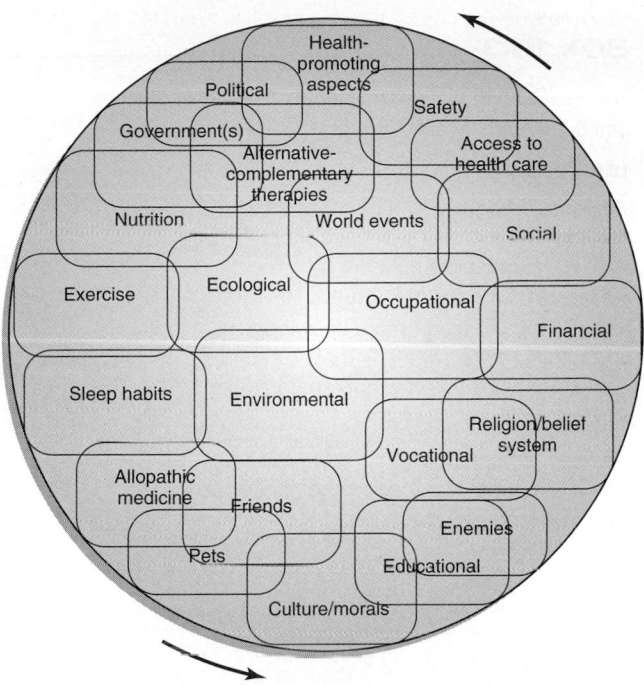

The 4+ model of wellness: The outer systems

*Source*: Used by permission of Joan H. Baldwin.

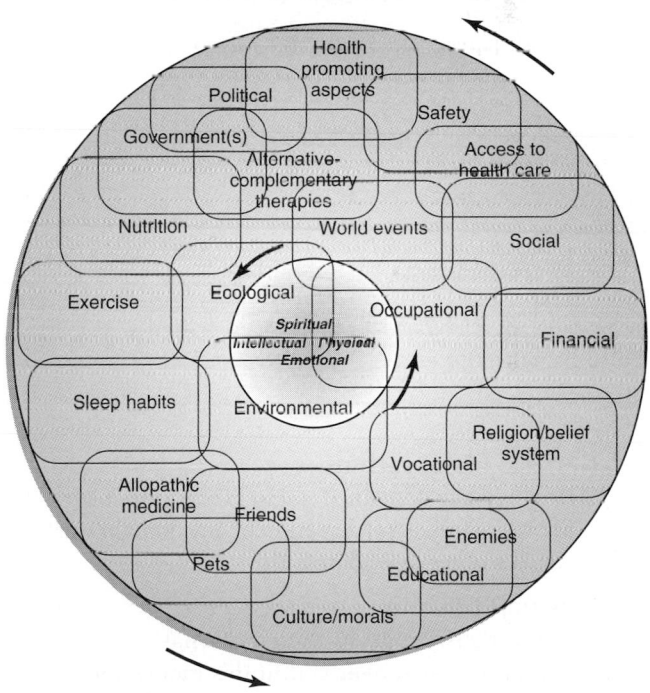

The 4+ model of wellness: The four domains of inner self plus the outer systems

*Source*: Used by permission of Joan H. Baldwin.

of the patient's physiological (or inner workings, as in the case of a community as patient) aspects. How a patient feels anger, excitement, and so on is reflected in the emotional aspect, and the spiritual denotes the fire that drives the engine that connects one to others and to a higher power. The spiritual domain also includes the capacity to give love. Thus the spiritual domain within each of us seems to have more than one role. This domain is likely to be the most complex and sometimes difficult to understand, although it is one of the most important to consider.

Achieving a holistic and harmonious state within the inner self is one part of the model. For example, think of the four domains of inner self as a tire. When all four of the domains—intellectual, physical, emotional, and spiritual—are "pumped up," the tire is rounded and rolls along evenly. This is what is meant by a holistic and harmonious state. This healthy state of harmony is further affected by interconnectedness and interaction with systems outside the inner self, which are depicted in the second overlay—the outer systems (see the figures above)—as facets of another sphere surrounding the sphere of the four domains of inner self. The outer systems portion of this model is similar to the tool known as an *Ecomap*, which is discussed in Chapter 2.

All of the elements of the outer systems sphere interact and interconnect with one another and with all the four domains of inner self. Imagine the two spheres constantly rotating about each other so that all components of each sphere interact with other elements within their own sphere and with one another at some time. The third figure depicts the idea of layering the spheres—the 4+ model of wellness: the four domains of inner self plus the outer systems.

Think of the total model as a patient system, one system with many moving components. Using the 4+ model of wellness, the nurse can look for things that might be deplet-

ing the elements of the inner self rather than nurturing the elements toward harmony. By working with the patient to consider things that might deplete any one or all of the four domains and thinking of ways to strengthen those things that nurture the patient, the nurse and patient may be able to identify health-promoting actions for the patient. Selected sources of nurture and depletion are listed in Box 13-3.

## BOX 13-3

**The 4+ Model of Wellness: Selected Sources of Nurture and Depletion**

### Intellectual

#### Sources of Nurture
- Books/intellectual media activities
- Observation/contemplation
- Experience/critical thinking
- Knowledge building more knowledge
- Practicing "brain work"—that is, children's play and games; children learn this way and so do adults
- Planning for the future

#### Sources of Depletion
- Brainwashing—imposed conditioned responses
- Mind-numbing repetition
- Boredom
- Noise
- Interruption
- Stresses/stressors
- Codependent behavior encouraged by a perpetrator—can lead to post-traumatic stress syndrome

### Emotional

#### Sources of Nurture
- Relief from stress
- Accomplishments
- Winning
- Physical well-being, exercise, diet
- Rest/relaxation
- Meditation/biofeedback, etc.
- Ability to "vent" appropriately

#### Sources of Depletion
- Physical illness
- Weak intelligence (inability to solve a problem)
- Isolation/noise/threats

### Physical

#### Sources of Nurture
- Appropriate nutrition
- Outdoor/indoor activities/exercise
- Rest/relaxation
- Physical "work"
- Biofeedback/complementary health therapies, and so on
- Appropriate physiological working
- Physical therapy

#### Sources of Depletion
- Disease/illness/prepathogenesis
- Toxins/environmental hazards
- Drug/substance abuse
- Poor nutrition/diet
- Lack of sleep
- Noise
- Stress/stressors/allergies
- Excessive exercise/exertion
- Trauma

### Spiritual

#### Sources of Nurture
- Giving love/connecting with others
- Being of service/loving animals
- Beauty/music/art
- Quiet/peace, meditation/prayer
- Physical exercise/cheering
- Being loved/hugs and pat-pats
- Intellectual stimulus/creating

#### Sources of Depletion
- Too much demand for support of others
- Failure to experience connectedness, love, belonging

*Source*: Baldwin & Baldwin, 1998. Used by permission of Joan H. Baldwin.

### General Observations

Strength in any domain, if not in excess, can nurture the other three domains. Also, depletion of any domain weakens and drains the other three domains.

### Spiritual Domain

On first consideration, the emotional and spiritual domains may appear similar, but in this model, these areas are quite different from each other. In this model, *spiritual* means the spirit or fire one has within. Excessive emotional highs may deplete the spirit. Of importance in this model is that *spiritual* does not mean religion or religious. Religion is actually a piece of the outer system that affects the inner self. Parts of a religion may, indeed, nurture the spirit, but sometimes, as in the case of overzealousness, depletion of the spirit may occur.

### Observations About Excesses

Excessive striving in any area can be destructive in all four domains. An illustration would be someone who ex-ercises to an extreme, to the detriment of personal relationships with others.

Excessive pain can be a depleting factor. For example, it is hard to think when you are suffering severe pain. One kind of severe pain is depression. Severely depressed people become so immobilized in several of the domains that they cannot move themselves toward strength in any of the areas through simple exercise or nutrition or even interaction with loving people. Serious disease or weakness (which can cause excessive physiological and other problems) can deplete several domains and can be a major factor in the patient suffering a downward spiral to total collapse and death.

Any excesses or "lacks" within any of the four domains throw the inner self sphere extremely "off balance or out of harmony." Think of the inner self sphere as being a tire; the difference in pressure on any portion of the tire will throw the tire off balance. People in various cultures speak of the tremendous importance of balance or harmony in a person's life.

Chapter author Dr. Joan Baldwin enjoying one of her favorite activities—long-distance bicycling.

Contemporary researchers and authors are proposing that changing and growing systems do not necessarily seek total equilibrium, that constant change alters the state of harmony or balance constantly (Coveney & Highfield, 1990; Prigogine & Stengers, 1984; Wheatley, 1994). This might explain how the assessment of a patient on one day may be far different from a similar assessment another day or even later in the same day. This is why it is important to observe the patient over time—to get a broader picture of what might be occurring within that patient system. There does not have to be "equilibrium" to have balance or harmony; in fact, a well-functioning system is always in a state of nonequilibrium because it constantly and inevitably changes focus. A system that is flexible and open can constantly move, changing and adjusting to regain harmony or a state as close to harmony as possible (Wheatley, 1994).

### ■ How to Use the 4+ Model of Wellness with Individuals, Families, Populations, and Communities

The nurse should begin by assessing the four domains of inner self for oneself or a patient. Then, the components of the outer systems, which encircle and move around the four domains of the inner self sphere, must be considered. By using the total 4+ model of wellness to assess the interactions and interconnectedness of the elements in the outer systems to all aspects of the inner self, the nurse will be able to critically assess and analyze much about himself or herself or others. The nurse and the patient may be able to determine which factors to work on strengthening or nurturing and which factors might be diminished or deleted to "pump up" the patient system's wellness. Remember that the patient can be a family, group, population, or community, as well as an individual.

### Individuals

Consider a grossly overweight, older man as an individual patient. The patient has been prescribed a diet that is nutritionally sound and, if followed, should help him lose weight. The patient could be thinking he is trying to follow his prescribed diet, and he is perplexed about not being successful in losing weight. The nurse could explore with the patient as many aspects as possible of his four domains of inner self, as well as the outer system components, to begin to figure out what interventions might facilitate health-promoting behaviors for this patient. After working with the patient to assess what might be sources of nurture and depletion for each of his four domains, the nurse (and, in some difficult cases, a team of health care professionals), along with the patient, would develop a wellness plan. Ideally, finding ways to nurture the patient's four domains and considering how the depleting sources could be diminished would constitute the initial part of the plan. For example, there might be work environment stressors (sources of depletion), such as the fact that doughnuts and other sweet, high-fat, and high-calorie foods are encouraged at break time at the workplace, which makes adhering to the prescribed diet difficult. Brainstorming with the patient about how he might discuss his need to be on the prescribed diet with his supervisor and how difficult it has been to not eat the doughnuts when they are in full view could be one step in the process.

There will be some sources of nurture that the patient could also strengthen. A source of nurture might be that the man has a dog as a pet. Possibly the man and his dog could work with children in a daycare center for developmentally disabled children. There have been many research articles relating the health-promoting aspects of the human–animal bond (Edney, 1992; National Institutes of Health, 1987). In addition, the process of connecting older people with younger people has many nurturing benefits (Piper, 1999). A service opportunity such as this could possibly nurture all four of the patient's domains, and certainly would nurture the children who are the recipients of this service (and maybe the dog, who might enjoy being with children).

## Application to Practice

### How Everything Affects Everything: A Saga of One Man's Life and the Negative Influences on Him and the Families Involved

Sam had a difficult childhood. His mother left the family when Sam was about 3 or 4 years old. His father probably was devastated, but Sam was too young to understand all that had happened. Sam's paternal grandparents raised Sam because Sam's father had to work long hours to even begin to make enough money to sustain himself, much less Sam. Sam's grandfather was strict and sometimes abusive to Sam's grandmother. No one in the family seemed to recognize that Sam believed that he was responsible in some way for his mother's leaving.

As Sam grew older, he became angry that his mother had left him although he seemed to appreciate the fact that his grandparents took reasonable care of him. He was certain his father had no real love for him. Sam was a fairly bright young boy and did well in school. Some time in the his teens, Sam began experimenting with marijuana. He managed to graduate from high school and began doing manual labor and odd jobs. He still lived with his grandparents.

Sam had several girlfriends over the next few years. The girls and many of his friends were younger than he was by several years. Sam was always the leader of the group. He and his friends abused alcohol and began taking many other kinds of "street drugs." Sam verbally abused his friends and girlfriends by telling them they were stupid and so on. Eventually he married one of the young women. After a time he was not only abusing her verbally, but also forcing her to start taking some of the drugs that he was taking.

Sam and his wife had a child. Amazingly the child was healthy. As the child grew, Sam insisted on having the child by his side when Sam wanted the child to be there. Otherwise, Sam ignored the child. Sam said he "loved" the child, yet burdened the young child (then about 3 or 4 years of age) with Sam's concerns about money and Sam's belief that the child's mother was no good. Sam also continued to have sexual liaisons with other women. Sam's wife made several attempts to leave Sam, especially after some fairly severe beatings. The child often observed these situations. After several years of abuse, Sam's wife left him and took the child with her to live elsewhere. Sam threatened to find her and kill her if the child was not returned. After almost 2 years of legal interventions, Sam's wife won a divorce and legal physical custody of the child (meaning that the child would live with her, but that Sam might have some input into the raising of the child). Sam tolerated this process for a short time before he began verbally harassing and threatening his ex-wife on the phone.

There were several more months of harassment and the involvement of police and other legal interventions. When Sam was finally arrested for selling drugs and being intoxicated, among other things, the court agreed that Sam would be denied contact with his son.

1. Using the 4+ model of wellness of Sam's four domains, how many were affected by his early life? by his high school adventures? by his adult life?

2. What additional information is needed in the scenario to assess Sam's wellness in the time before he went to jail? Consider what effect the outer systems components (e.g., social, vocational, environmental) may have had on Sam.

3. Which sources of nurture and/or depletion are recognizable? Which of Sam's domains may have been affected, given the sources of nurture and/or depletion noted?

4. Which health-promoting behaviors of Sam's family might have helped Sam during his early development? List Sam's family's possible sources of nurture and depletion.

5. While considering the 4+ model of wellness, which sources of nurture and/or depletion did the family of the ex-wife and child have? How might a nurse assist them to assess their own four quadrants individually and as a single-parent family?

6. How might a nurse help the ex-wife and child develop the health-promoting behaviors they might need individually and as a single-parent family?

7. Think about Sam's abuse of and involvement with substances. Consider his desire for drugs and Sam's early life and the life he was living as an adult. What view/attitudes might a nurse take as a logical and ethical approach toward Sam?

## Application to Practice

### A Target Population Within a Community

The Teen Mothers' High School Program, which was located in one of the local high schools in the town of Urbansville, was used by more than 100 young single women each year for 5 years. The City Council decided to participate in the formation of a community health-promotion program called "Healthy Urbansville." The council members wanted to improve the health-promoting aspects of their city. They called on leaders in the educational facilities in town, police/sheriff and fire departments, local business people, ecclesiastical representatives (e.g., of churches, temples, synagogues), and other local interested citizens, including representatives of the youth groups and senior citizens' centers, to be part of this community effort.

The city was fairly large and contained many community resource agencies and emergency funding processes to assist those in need. The city was located in an urban area of the western region of the country, with many parks and recreation areas. The city prided itself on the good relationships between its diverse populations, the cleanliness of the city, and the efforts toward appropriate city growth that had been in place for several years. There were several excellent libraries, theater and other media options, art and history museums, as well as restaurants of all kinds. Biomedical and complementary integrative health therapies co-existed. There were churches of many different denominations readily accessible by most of the populations. Transportation opportunities were well distributed throughout the city, although there were continuing construction projects at various times throughout the dry seasons. There were as in any large city varying socioeconomic groups including many homeless. Illicit drug dealing was being combatted daily by the police and others, but it was not out of hand. Violence was occasional, with robberies and burglaries being highest during the hotter months. Overall, the city considered itself a city with a future.

One of the major concerns of the Healthy Urbansville group that came forth after an in-depth community/population assessment process, which included the use of several surveys (plus the 4+ model of wellness), was that the rising numbers of teen pregnancies had a depleting effect on the community as a whole; families and resources within the community were hard hit. The age ranges of the teenage mothers was between 14 and 17, there were presently 1,000 young women in this age group, according to the most recent statistics. Statistically, teen pregnancies resulted in higher mortality rates than other age groupings. This concern became the main priority of the Healthy Urbansville group.

1. Using the 4+ model of wellness and given what this case study indicated, which assets (or sources of nurture) and which problems (sources of depletion) might exist in the community, Urbansville?

2. What might be the sources of nurture in the intellectual domain of the community? In the physical, emotional, and spiritual domains of the community?

3. Think of the teenage mothers in this community. What questions might you have regarding this target (at-risk) population? What are some of the sources of nurture (or assets) that might affect young women in the age group between 14 and 17 years of age? What are some of the potential sources of depletion (of problem areas) that might affect young women in this age group?

4. Given the sources of nurture (or assets) identified, which interventions might be made to strengthen these in the young women? Which potential things might be done to diminish or delete the depleting sources (or problems)?

5. List several interventions for both the community and target population that could facilitate health-promoting behaviors for those patients, either individually or by working to diminish a source of community depletion. ◓

## Research Alert

An exploration of the research in several disciplines related to the use of animals for therapy in health care demonstrated applicability of the findings to enhance health-promoting nursing interventions for patients. A selective historical tour of the literature regarding the human–animal bond and its therapeutic effect in health care is a segue to more recent research on the subject. Considerations about the pros and cons of having animals interact with hospitalized patients are developed. The link between the benefits of stress reduction and positive psychoneuroimmunology changes in patients as a result of human–animal bonding therapies emerges as the strongest health promotion possibility for the use of this animal-assisted therapy.

*Source*: Jorgenson, J. (1997). Therapeutic use of companion animals in health care. *Image*: *The Journal of Nursing Scholarship, 29*(3), 249–254.

Another important factor to remember when working with any patient is that the patient's goals or priorities in life may not be the same as what you might consider his, her, or its (in the case of a family, population, or community) goals or priorities "should" be. This is equally important to remember when establishing things that nurture or deplete a patient. These also are factors in why patients do not always do what a health care professional tells them to do. Too often, if patients choose not to do what the health care professional says, or cannot do something for some valid reason, health care professionals indicate that the patients are "noncompliant" or cannot figure out why patients do not do what

is "good" for them. These episodes sometimes create ethical concerns, especially concerning whose needs are being met. Building trust, rapport, and respect with patients often encourages the patients, in due time, to follow health care professionals' suggestions for health-promoting behaviors.

### Families

Using the 4+ model of wellness when assessing more than one individual becomes more complex than assessing an individual. Consider a family as a large patient system consisting of several smaller systems, or individual family members. Look for sources of nurture for the family. These sources might include things such as being broad-minded, being creative, having good problem-solving skills, being flexible, having family members who are interconnected with each other and the outer systems of the family, sharing spirituality, and being appropriately nurturing of the family's spirit and the spirits of others. A family that has developed these characteristics and continues to derive nurture from them among others demonstrates a fair amount of harmony, health, and wellness. In the family Application to Practice, look for potential sources of nurture and depletion in the various family patients.

### Populations and Communities

Now think about how the 4+ model of wellness might be used to examine a population or a community. If a family is a patient system, then a population or a community can also be a patient system; individuals within the population and individuals and target (or at-risk) populations within a community are the smaller systems within the larger patient system of population or community. Remember that your own goals, values, and priorities are not necessarily those

## MEDIA MOMENT

### *Life Is Beautiful* (1997)

This film is about the endurance of the human spirit and a sense of humor even in the worst of human conditions: a Nazi concentration camp. A Jewish Italian waiter named Guido (Roberto Benigni) is sent to a Nazi concentration camp during World War II, along with his wife (Nicoletta Braschi) and their young son (Giorgio Cantarini). Refusing to give up hope, Guido tries to protect his son's innocence by pretending that their imprisonment is an elaborate game and that everything is bearable with a great sense of humor, with the grand prize being a tank. Benigni also directed. Italian with English subtitles.

### *Patch Adams* (1998)

After committing himself to a mental institution, Hunter "Patch" Adams (Robin Williams) realizes that introducing his fellow patients to humor significantly improves their

quality of life. Upon leaving the institution, he decides to become a physician who cures people using laughter rather than cold, analytical processes. Although jeopardizing his future in medicine, Patch continues his unconventional, yet promising healing methods.

### *Amélie* (2001)

Amélie (Audrey Tautou) lives alone and works in a café. When she finds a box of toys hidden for 40 years behind a baseboard in her apartment, she is inspired to return the items to their entire rightful owner—no small or easy task. This journey and acts of anonymous generosity spark more benevolent acts. A celebration of life, *Amélie* reminds us of the small wonders that are all around us—if only we paused to look.

French with English subtitles. Nominated for multiple Academy Awards.

of populations or communities. These patient systems also have their own goals, values, and priorities that can create ethical dilemmas for the nurse.

Sources of nurture for populations and communities may be similar to those for a family. As the patient system becomes larger (as with more than one individual), the sources of nurture also become broader in many cases. Freedom from harassment, threats, or violence could be added to any level of patient system sources of nurture but seems to be often pertinent to an at-risk or target population or community. Sources of depletion for a population could be the reverse of the sources of nurture. For instance, an at-risk population of unwed pregnant teenagers might be depleted by harassment, ridicule, or shunning by others with extreme moral views against unmarried young women being sexually active. The target population and community Application to Practice on page 317 describes some of the things a nurse needs to consider when using the 4+ model of wellness.

## Conclusion

This chapter contains a discussion of basic concepts of health and health promotion as related to disease prevention, including definitions of *health promotion* and *wellness* as the terms are used in this chapter; delineation of factors influencing health promotion and wellness; a brief summary of some ways of looking at health promotion and wellness by describing some models, guides, and tools involved in health protection, health promotion, wellness and risk evaluation, analysis, and reduction; and introduction of two models of wellness. Key concepts, case studies, research alerts, and critical thinking activities are presented to reinforce concepts and assist in "pushing the envelope" and expanding ideas for health-promotion interventions.

Explore Community Health Nursing on the Web! To learn more about the topics in this chapter, use the passcode provided to access your exclusive website: **http://nursing.jbpub.com/communityhealth.** If you do not have a passcode, you can obtain one at this site.

## ■ CRITICAL THINKING ACTIVITIES

1. Can a person who has been diagnosed with bipolar disorder and who is appropriately and successfully being managed with medications achieve high-level wellness?

2. Can a community experiencing a severe gang problem achieve high-level wellness? If so, how might this be done?

3. How might the Jedi Women (a community action group consisting of single low-income mothers) define high-level wellness for their group? What activities might stimulate the group toward self-actualization?

4. Which social barriers might keep patients from exploring health-promoting activities, including healthy eating, exercising, and so forth?

5. Why is it that lifestyle choices and social limitations and barriers exist? Which situations might be lending themselves to building social barriers for patients?

6. Some population and community patients have noticeable limitations to their lifestyle choices, as noted in this chapter. Consider the populations that lived in major cities, as well as in rural and/or frontier areas, in the United States 50 years ago. Compare the positives and negatives of their lifestyle choices at that time to similar populations of today.

7. Discuss things a community or society could do to support an individual's self-care activities.

8. Describe how consumerism and self-care activities might encourage health-promotion and wellness behaviors.

9. Make a table with two columns. In the first, list self-care activities you engage in to nurture your wellness. In the second, list self-care activities you have not been doing but should. Plan interventions to include at least two new health-promoting behaviors in your daily life.

10. Identify two populations to which you belong. List five self-care, practices these populations engage in for the benefit and nurture of their members.

11. How can communities engage in self-care?

12. Redefine the descriptors "unhealthy" and "well" for each of the spokes of the holistic wellness model as they fit into your or your patient's cultural perspective.

13. Discuss the meaning of knowledge, understanding, insight, and inner peace, which are found on the eagle feathers on the bottom of the holistic wellness model, as they might fit your or your patient's culture.

14. With the patient, evaluate the patient's health at each spoke. Consider each spoke as having a weak or more negative dimension (e.g., on the Physical spoke, unfit would be the weak dimension and fit would be the healthy dimension). Have the patient place a dot on the spoke where the patient thinks he or she is at the time on that spoke's dimension. The closer the patient places the dot to the center of the wheel on any given spoke/dimension, the healthier the person considers himself or herself in regard to that dimension. Once a dot is placed on each spoke, the dots are connected to form a circle. The nurse and the patient can visually evaluate whether the circle is balanced and where the weak dimensions are.

15. Discuss potential interventions and/or changes the patient might decide to make to move himself or herself more toward the center of the holistic wellness wheel toward being "healthy for life."

16. For your own community, identify the system dimensions that would be important to assessing wellness.

17. Refer to Box 13-3. Which other items could be added to the box to describe sources of nurture and sources of depletion for each of the four domains for an individual, a family, a population, or a community?

18. From Box 13-3, choose a source of nurture in one of the domains and describe how that source of nurture might affect another domain in a patient.

19. How might an excess of any factor affect any (or all) of a patient's domains?

20. If a person has a physical injury, which of the other domains besides the physical one might be affected? In what way(s)?

21. Consider a woman who is the sole support of several children and must also be the caregiver for an elderly, ill parent. Which domains(s) in that person might be affected? How?

22. If that woman becomes totally depleted in several of her domains, how will the domains of the family she is caring for be affected? Describe.

## ■ REFERENCES

American Public Health Association (APHA). (1991). *Healthy communities 2000 model standards: Guidelines for community attainment of the year 2000 national health objectives* (3rd ed.). Washington, DC: Author.

Bach, M. L. (1998). *Shape walking.* Los Angeles: Heel to Toe Fitness Walking.

Baldwin, E. M., & Baldwin, J. H. (1998). *4+ model of wellness.* Unpublished manuscript.

Baldwin, J. H. (1992). Moving towards harmony: Types and meanings of cues that prompt health-promoting decisions in women in the middle years. Doctoral dissertation, Catholic University of America, Washington, DC. *UMI Dissertation Abstracts,* Order No. 9220772.

Baldwin, J. H. (1995). Are we implementing community health promotion in nursing? *Public Health Nursing, 12*(3), 159–164.

Baldwin, J. H., Conger, C. O., Abegglen, J. C., & Hill, E. M. (1998). Population-focused and community-based nursing—moving toward clarification of concepts. *Public Health Nursing, 15*(1), 12–18.

Becker, M. H. (Ed.). (1974). *The health belief model and personal health behavior.* Thorofare, NJ: Charles B. Slack.

Browning, B., Huls, J., Rather, R., & Stout, L. (1997). *Taylorsville youth assessment.* Unpublished manuscript. Provo, UT: Brigham Young University College of Nursing.

Brubaker, B. H. (1983, April). Health promotion: A linguistic analysis. *Advances in Nursing Science, 5,* 1–14.

Butterfield, P. G. (1993). Thinking upstream: Conceptualizing health from a population perspective. In J. M. Swanson & M. Albrecht (Eds.), *Community health nursing: Promoting the health of aggregates* (pp. 68–80). Philadelphia: W. B. Saunders.

Centers for Disease Control and Prevention (CDC). (2008). *Data2010: The Healthy People 2010 database.* Retrieved October 23, 2008, from http://wonder.cdc.gov/data2010

Clark, E. G., & Leavell, H. R. (1953/1965). Levels of application of preventive medicine. In H. R. Leavell & E. G. Clark (Eds.), *Preventive medicine for the doctor in his community: An epidemiologic approach* (3rd ed., pp. 14–38). New York: McGraw-Hill.

Cohen, J. (1998). Holistic health strategies. In C. L. Edelman & C. L. Mandle (Eds.), *Health promotion throughout the lifespan* (4th ed., pp. 333–356). St. Louis: Mosby.

Coveney, P., & Highfield, R. (1990). *The arrow of time: A voyage through science to solve time's greatest mystery.* New York: Fawcett Columbine.

Drapo, P. J., & Woods, E. (1992). Preparing community health nurses for the real world: Power, politics, and poverty. In *1991 Papers: State of the art in community health nursing education, research, and practice* (pp. 47–51). Lexington, KY: ACHNE.

Duhl, L. J. (1986). *Health planning and social change.* New York: Human Sciences Press.

Dunn, H. L. (1959). High-level wellness for man and society. *American Journal of Public Health, 49,* 789.

Dunn, H. L. (1980). *High level wellness.* Thorofare, NJ: Charles B. Slack.

Edelman, C. L., & Fain, J. A. (1998). Health defined: Objective for promotion and prevention. In C. L. Edleman & C. L. Mandle (Eds.), *Health promotion throughout the lifespan* (4th ed., pp. 3–24). St. Louis: Mosby.

Edney, A. T. B. (1992). Companion animals and human health. *Veterinary Record, 130*(4), 285–287.

Green, L. W., & Raeburn, J. (1990). Contemporary developments in health promotion: Definitions and challenges. In N. Bracht (Ed.), *Health promotion at the community level* (pp. 19–44). Newbury Park, CA: Sage.

Greene, B., & Winfrey, O. (1996). *Make the connection: Ten steps to a better body—and a better life.* New York: Hyperion.

Healthy People 2010. (2008). *Healthy People 2010.* Retrieved October 23, 2008, from http://www.wvdhhr.org/bph/hp2010

Hochbaum, G. M. (1958). *Public participation in medical screening programs: A socio-psychological study.* (Publication No. 572). Bethesda, MD: Public Health Service.

Jette, A. M., Lachman, M., Giorgetti, M. M., et al. (1999). Exercise—It's never too late: The strong-for-life program. *American Journal of Public Health, 89*(1), 66–72.

Jones, J. (1999). *Jeanne Jones' homestyle cooking made healthy.* Red Oak, IA: Rodale Press.

Kellogg Foundation funds 3-year "Healthy Cities Indiana" project. (1988). *American Journal of Public Health, 78*(12), 5.

Kulbok, P. A., & Baldwin, J. H. (1992). From preventive health behavior to health promotion: Advancing a positive construct of health. *Advances in Nursing Science, 14*(4), 50–64.

Kulbok, P. A., Baldwin, J. H., Cox, C. L., & Duffy, R. (1997). Advancing discourse on health promotion: Beyond mainstream thinking. *Advances in Nursing Science, 20*(1), 13–21.

Kulbok, P. A., Carter, K. F., Baldwin, J. H., Gilmartin, M. J., & Kirkwood, B. (1999). The multidimensional health behavior inventory. *Journal of Nursing Measurement, 7*(2), 177–195.

Maiese, D. R., & Fox, C. E. (1998). *Laying the foundation for Healthy People 2010—The first year of consultation. Public Health Reports, 113,* 92–95.

Marcus, B., & Forsyth, L. (2002, December). *Motivating people to be physically active.* Washington, DC: Human Kinetics.

Maslow, A. W. (1970). *Motivation and personality*. New York: Harper & Row.

McCarthy, N. C., & Mandle, C. L. (1998). Health promotion and the community. In C. L. Edleman & C. L. Mandle (Eds.), *Health promotion throughout the lifespan* (4th ed., pp. 171–192). St. Louis: Mosby.

McDonald, I. (1997). *Holistic wellness: Self inventory of personal wellness utilizing the medicine wheel*. Unpublished manuscript.

McGinnis, J. M., & Foege, W. H. (1993). Actual causes of death in the United States. *Journal of the American Medical Association, 270*(18).

Moore, V., Neff, D., Smith, G., & Weber, J. (1999). *The homeless in Utah County: Food & Care Coalition*. Unpublished manuscript. Provo, UT: Brigham Young University College of Nursing.

Naisbitt, J. (1982). *Megatrends*. New York: Warner Books.

National Institute for Occupational Safety and Health. (1996). *National Occupational Research Agenda*. (DHHS [NIOSH] Publication No. 96-115). Washington, DC: U.S. Government Printing Office.

National Institutes of Health. (1987). *The health benefits of pets*. (Publication No. 1998-216-107). Washington, DC: U.S. Government Printing Office.

Orem, D. E. (1985). *Nursing: Concepts of practice* (3rd ed.). New York: McGraw-Hill.

Padilla, G. V., & Bulcavage, L. M. (1991). Theories used in patient/health education. *Seminars in Oncological Nursing, 7*(2), 87–96.

Palank, C. L. (1991). Determinants of health-promotive behavior: A review of current research. *Nursing Clinics of North America, 26*(4), 815–832.

Pender, N. (1987). *Health promotion in nursing practice* (2nd ed.). East Norwalk, CT: Appleton & Lange.

Piper, M. (1999). *Another country: Navigating the emotional terrain of our elders*. Los Angeles: Riverhead Books.

Poe, B. S., & O'Neill, K. O. (1997). Caffeine modulates heat shock induced apoptosis in the human promyelocytic leukemia cell line HL-60. *Cancer Letters, 121*, 1–6.

Prigogine, I., & Stengers, I. (1984). *Order out of chaos*. New York: Bantam Books.

Raphael, D. (2000, December). The question of evidence in health promotion. *Health Promotion International, 15*(4), 355–367.

Raphael, D., & Bryant, T. (2002). The limitations of population health as a model for a new public health. *Health Promotion International, 17*(2), 189–199.

Rosenstock, I. M. (1974). Historical origins of the health belief model. In M. H. Becker (Ed.), *The health belief model and personal health behavior* (pp. 1–8). Thorofare, NJ: Charles B. Slack.

Ryan, R. S., & Travis, J. W. (1991). Introduction. In R. S. Ryan & J. W. Travis (Eds.), *Wellness: Small changes you can use to make a big difference* (p. 3). Berkeley, CA: Ten Speed Press.

Sandhu, G. K. (1998). Health promotion for the twenty-first century: Throughout the lifespan and throughout the world. In C. L. Edleman & C. L. Mandle (Eds.), *Health promotion throughout the lifespan* (4th ed., pp. 667–675). St. Louis: Mosby.

Segal, L., Dalton, A. C., & Richardson, J. (1998). Cost-effectiveness of the primary prevention of non-insulin dependent diabetes mellitus. *Health Promotion International, 13*(3), 197–211.

Simmons, S. J. (1990). The health-promoting self-care system model: Directions for nursing research and practice. *Journal of Advances in Nursing, 15*(10), 1162–1166.

Simopoulos, A. P. (1999). *The omega diet*. New York: HarperCollins.

Steiger, N. J., & Lipson, J. C. (1985). *Self-care nursing: Theory and practice*. Bowie, MD: Brady Communications.

U.S. Department of Health and Human Services (DHHS). (1982). *Forward plan for health 1977–1981*. Washington, DC: U.S. Government Printing Office.

U.S. Department of Health and Human Services (DHHS). (1998a). *Healthy people in healthy communities: A guide for community leaders*. Washington, DC: Office of Disease Prevention and Health Promotion.

U.S. Department of Health and Human Services (DHHS). (1998b). *Healthy People 2010 objectives: Draft for public comment*. Washington, DC: U.S. Government Printing Office.

U.S. Department of Health and Human Services (2000, November). *Healthy People 2010: Understanding and improving health* (2nd ed.). Washington, DC: U.S. Government Printing Office.

U.S. Preventive Services Task Force. (1989). *A guide to clinical preventive services: An assessment of the effectiveness of 169 interventions*. Baltimore, MD: Williams & Wilkins.

U.S. Public Health Service (USPHS). (1979). *Healthy people: The surgeon general's report on health promotion and disease prevention*. (DHEW Publication No. 79-55071) Washington, DC: U.S. Department of Health, Education, and Welfare.

U.S. Public Health Service (USPHS). (1980). *Promoting health/preventing disease: Objectives for the nation*. (DHHS Publication No. 0-349-256). Washington, DC: Department of Health and Human Services.

U.S. Public Health Service (USPHS). (1989). *Promoting health/preventing disease: Year 2000 objectives for the nation*. Washington, DC: U.S. Department of Health and Human Services.

U.S. Public Health Service (USPHS). (1990). *Healthy People 2000: National health promotion and disease prevention objectives*. Washington, DC: U.S. Department of Health and Human Services.

U.S. Public Health Service (USPHS). (1999). *Promoting physical activity: A guide for community action*. Washington, DC: Human Kinetics.

*Webster's encyclopedia unabridged dictionary of the English language*. (1996). New York: Gramercy Books/Random House.

Wheatley, J. (1994). *Leadership and the new science: Learning about organization from an orderly universe*. San Francisco, CA: Berrett-Koehler.

# CHAPTER 14
# Nursing Informatics in Community Health Nursing Practice

Russell C. McGuire and Sandra L. Walker

Visit **http://nursing.jbpub.com/communityhealth**
for interactive exercises, review questions,
Web links, and more.

The worlds of health care, communications, and information technologies are ever evolving, separately and together. As nurses in the community expand their practice definition to embrace new information technologies, opportunities for improved health care to populations seem endless. This evolution is seen as a merger of health care technology with information and communications technology, fostering the design and implementation of health care management information systems in a variety of clinical practice settings.

Computers are useless. They can only give you answers.

—*Pablo Picasso*

The purpose of computing is insight, not numbers.

—*R. Hamming*

Just because you have a computer doesn't mean you can't be stupid.

—*Beavis and Butthead*

Once an idea has stretched, the mind will never go back to the original state.

—*Oliver Wendell Holmes*

How has technology changed the way you communicate with others? Is the use of informatic technology in health care simply an advanced form of communication or will it revolutionize the way we care for patients?

## CHAPTER FOCUS

**The Science of Nursing Informatics**

**Community Health Nursing and Nursing Informatics**

**Benefits of Nursing Informatics for Community Health Nursing**
- Nursing Classification Systems

**Patient Information Management**
- Efficiency and Time Benefits

**Computer Applications in Community Health Nursing**
- Electronic Mail
- Databases
- Electronic Spreadsheets

**Internet Applications in Community-Based Nursing Practice**

**Health Care Delivery System Management Software**
- Networked Patient Care

**Communication Technology and Community Health Nursing**
- Telehealth Care Benefits
- Community Health Nursing Benefits of Telehealth Care

**The Future of Informatics and Telehealth**

## QUESTIONS TO CONSIDER

After reading this chapter, you will know the answers to the following questions:

1. What is nursing informatics?
2. How is the science of informatics used in nursing practice in the community?
3. What are the benefits of informatics?
4. How is patient information managed using informatics?
5. What are some computer applications used in community health nursing?
6. How are management and network systems used in community health nursing practice?
7. What are the community health nursing benefits to using telehealth?

## KEY TERMS

Database
Distributed data processing (DDP)
Electronic mail (e-mail)
Electronic spreadsheets

Health management information systems (HMIS)
Nursing classification systems

Nursing data
Nursing informatics
Nursing information

Nursing information systems
Nursing knowledge
Telemedicine/telehealth

THE CLINICAL PRACTICE settings in which the new technology of informatics is used include both the acute care and community-based practice environments. Organizations such as hospitals and community-based agencies such as public health departments and home health agencies use information and communications technologies to collect, store, retrieve, analyze, and present patient care data in the care delivery settings.

Health care continues to be a human endeavor that is necessarily complex in nature. Decisions related to patient care continue to increase in complexity, with the need for rapid, accurate information for clinical decision making as a priority for effective care. Clinical decisions are just as complex and critical in the community-based nursing settings. As a response to these informational needs, systems have been designed to meet the clinical information requirements of community-based practice. Public health, home health, hospice, and other providers of community-based nursing care have the opportunity to use information and communications technologies in the provision of nursing care. This chapter explores how information and communications technologies, coupled with nursing science, can provide answers to complex clinical scenarios in community health nursing.

## The Science of Nursing Informatics

The science of **nursing informatics** is a combination of information, communications, and nursing sciences. According to the American Nurses Association,

> Nursing informatics is a specialty that integrates nursing science, computer science, and information science to manage and communicate data, information, and knowledge in nursing practice. Nursing informatics facilitates the integration of data, information, and knowledge to support patients, nurses, and other providers in their decision making in all roles and settings. This support is accomplished through the use of information structures, information processes, and information technology. (2001, p. 17)

The emergence of the specialty known as nursing informatics is not a recent phenomenon. Nurses have been using computers since the 1950s, and nursing informatics emerged as an advanced specialty in the 1980s. In 1989, Graves and Corcoran devised a conceptual framework based on a definition of nursing informatics. This conceptual framework describes the relationship among computer science, information systems science, and nursing science. Graves and Corcoran believe information management processing of nursing data is achieved through the collection of data, the transformation of nursing data into nursing information, and finally into nursing knowledge. Nursing informatics came of age in the 1980s, and characteristics of what constitutes nursing data have emerged.

**"** *The best way to predict the future is to invent it.* **"**

*—Alan Kay*

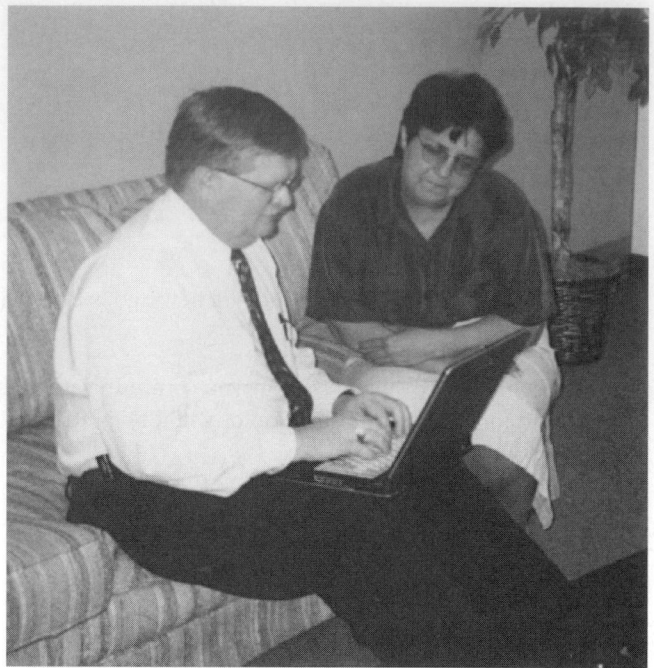

Chapter author Russell McGuire using a laptop computer during a home health visit.

Nursing informatics uses nursing science and computer and communications technologies to produce effective and efficient patient outcomes for individuals and communities. Through the collection of individual data elements, nursing as a professional discipline builds on its unique knowledge base. The transition from raw data to knowledge is a three-phase process.

**Nursing data** is the raw form of elements that make up nursing information. For example, patient name, gender, and diagnosis are each considered raw nursing data elements.

When a nurse forms relationships between the raw data elements, **nursing information** emerges as a more fully developed picture of the patient's clinical status is formulated. The nurse then acts on this information by formulating a set of interventions to deal with the particulars of a specific patient care situation. *Nursing information* is related data elements that now are in a form that can be subjected to analysis and interpretation.

Nursing information readily lends itself to archiving or storage in computer databases that allow for relational groupings of the data. Relational grouping of nursing information then allows for aggregation of information and the systematic study of nursing-related phenomena. Sets of nursing information that conform to theoretical and conceptual frameworks are known as **nursing knowledge.** When enough nursing information is collected, analyzed, and interpreted, aggregation of this information can be synthesized into nursing knowledge. It is nursing knowledge, when fitted to a logical, systematic set of standards, that provides the knowledge base of the discipline.

Computerized information systems used in the community health nursing practice setting can assist in the development of nursing knowledge through the automated process of collecting, storing, retrieving, analyzing, interpreting, and eventually presenting patient-related data. These data then can be used in an intervention effort to meet individual, family, and community health needs.

###  Research Alert

While research into the benefits and feasibility of mobile technology is ongoing, these authors sought to gain insights into the use of mobile computing (MC) by public health nurses in a school health program. The authors employed a descriptive, exploratory, qualitative study design to look at the change process of implementing MC into the nurses' practice and to examine the effects of the MC on the practice as well as the attitudes of the nurses after the MC practices were implemented. The study was conducted in Ontario, Canada, with a sample of eight unionized nurses with bachelor's degrees in nursing. The equipment cost for the program was approximately $12,000 (Canadian), and eventually a part-time IT support staff person was required. Data collection included participants' completion of a short survey, two 1.5-hour focus group interviews, and individual written reflections about using the MC in their practice.

Valaitis and O'Mara found that eight themes emerged from the data collected, and there were conflicts between each pair of themes. The themes included "*flexibility* afforded by the use of PDAs [personal digital assistants] versus *workplace rules, peer connectedness* versus *peer isolation, employer connectedness* versus *employer isolation*, and a *sense of increased status* versus a *widening gap in social status*" (p. 156). The participants indicated that the use of the PDAs made their practice more client-centered, and the participants' feelings about the technology improved over time. Advantages that were identified with using MC included increased efficiency and the ability to recruit and retain visiting nurses; disadvantages included the small screen size of the PDA, concerns about losing the PDA or having it stolen, and protecting patients' privacy.

*Source*: Valaitis, R. K., & O'Mara, L. M. (2005). Public health nurses' perceptions of mobile computing in a school program. *CIN: Computers, Informatics, Nursing, 23*(3), 153–160.

### GLOBAL CONNECTION

Only people in the most advanced industrialized countries have access to the Internet. The World Health Organization estimates that only 14% of the world's population has Internet access. Will the explosion of information technology further divide the most impoverished global populations from both primary health care and advanced health research discoveries?

**❝***Learning is what most adults will do for a living in the twenty-first century.***❞**

—Perelman

The accumulation of nursing data, information, and subsequently nursing knowledge in this fast-paced era of electronics has fostered the use of information systems throughout health care. **Health management information systems (HMIS)** are used to collect, store, and process health-related data in a health care facility. In a health care system such as the community health care setting, elements of care delivery such as nursing, medicine, laboratory, radiology, and administration use information systems to coordinate and manage care for achieving more efficient and better patient-related outcomes (Sebastian & Stanhope, 1999). **Nursing information systems,** which are a part of the health management information system, continue to evolve at a fast pace. This pace is accelerated because of the development of faster processing computer equipment, advances in data transmission, and increases in information systems' efficiency and data manipulation effectiveness.

Hassett and Thede (2003) describe characteristics of health care information systems and discuss the need for electronic patient records. Owing to restrictions mandated by the Joint Commission on Accreditation of Health Care Organizations (JCAHO) as well as the allocation of resources within health care systems, data from patient records needs to be available within a short amount of time with relative ease. Paper charts are cumbersome and often not formatted to different health care practitioners' needs in

###  Research Alert

This descriptive research study was conducted at a large magnet hospital in southwest Florida and sought to assess the needs, preferences, and perceptions of 100 nursing personnel regarding the electronic health record (EHR) documentation methods used in the hospital. The participating nurses completed five-point Likert scale surveys about the use of EHR and their perceived effects on patient care. More than one-third of the participants felt that the use of EHRs resulted in a decreased workload; almost two-thirds (64%) preferred bedside documentation of patient care. However, many stated that environmental and system barriers often prevented bedside documentation using the EHRs. Overall, approximately three-quarters of participating nurses thought that the use of EHRs had improved documentation quality as well as improved patient safety and patient care. Researchers also found that participating nurses who had expertise in computer use before the EHR implementation had a more favorable response to using the EHR in their nursing practice.

*Source*: Moody, L. E., Slocumb, E., Berg, B., & Jackson, D. (2004). Electronic health records documentation in nursing: Nurses' perceptions, attitudes, and preferences. *CIN: Computers, Informatics, Nursing, 22*(6), 337–344.

this age of collaboration. Thus health care systems should include an interface to assimilate the many types of information systems that are in place so that sharing of patient data is possible, yet the data remain protected to maintain the patient's privacy. The different types of health care information systems that may be used in a community health setting are listed in Box 14-1.

## Community Health Nursing and Nursing Informatics

In community-based nursing practice, the implementation of nursing information systems must be integrated with data systems that collect patient data for other disciplines. The profession of nursing leads the way in data collection, the use of standardized language classifications, and design support for automated systems that can assist in supporting the integration of other health care disciplines. This integration of nursing information is useful in community health nursing when multiple disciplines are responsible for the care of the patient and his or her caregivers and when coordination of care is paramount in achieving expedient and successful outcomes.

Nursing informatics deals with the collection, manipulation, analysis, and interpretation of several levels of data, information, and knowledge. Community-based nursing deals with the same levels of data for which computer technology, nursing informatics, and communications technology are used to transform data into knowledge.

The first level of data is related to patients and their caregivers. Data such as patient sociodemographic status, medical history, physical examination results, integrated health care assessments, and treatment plans are examples of patient-level data or information.

The second level of data is specific to the organization or agency. Examples of this level of data are an organization's productivity indicators, policies, and procedures, as well as the availability of community resources associated with a specific patient's or caregiver's health care needs.

The third level of data is domain specific. Domain-specific data are associated with care provided across the continuum of health care services delivery and are related to the patient and caregiver responses (outcomes) to community health nursing interventions. Domain-specific data include the medical diagnosis and subsequent nursing diagnosis, the efficiency and applicability of specific nursing interventions and the subsequent patient outcomes, and the data related to the specifics of providing care such as drug interactions with prescribed medications.

❝ *Technology: the invention, manufacture, and use of tools.* ❞

—*Arnold J. Toynbee, 1961*

 **Got an Alternative?**

The Internet provides unlimited information on over-the-counter herbs, vitamins, "miracle cures" for every ailment, and alternative, nontraditional health products. How does this plethora of information affect community health nurses and patient education, especially for those who are most vulnerable to untested and unreliable products, such as the elderly and patients with chronic, intractable pain and fatal conditions?

## Benefits of Nursing Informatics for Community Health Nursing

The combination of nursing and information systems management produces several benefits for nurses practicing in the community. These benefits include (1) the management of patient-level data; (2) the use of standardized nursing language to communicate what nurses do and how patients and their families respond to care; (3) provision of care in an efficient and productive manner; and (4) the use of information systems for research, health promotion, and illness prevention in the community.

### ■ Nursing Classification Systems

The different levels of data and subsequent levels of information and knowledge relevant to the practice of community-based nursing have been discussed thus far. To facilitate an understanding of how nursing languages are used to describe nursing practice and how standardized nursing languages are important in the context of automated nursing information systems, the discussion briefly turns to the evolution of **nursing classification systems.** It is important to remember that community health nurses use language as a medium for describing the patient's clinical status, the appropriateness of the clinical care environment, the support systems available to the patient, and the patient's level of response to nursing intervention. To facilitate the

**Table 14-1**    Summary of Nursing Classification System Features

| Name | Major Features |
|---|---|
| ■ NANDA: North American Nursing Diagnosis Association (Warren & Hoskins, 1995) | ■ Research-based nursing diagnosis system having nine different diagnosis patterns (exchanging, communicating, relating, valuing, choosing, moving, perceiving, knowing, and feeling). |
| ■ Visiting Nurses Association of Omaha Community Health Problem and Intervention System (Martin & Scheet, 1995) | ■ Three major components: (1) problems classification, (2) intervention scheme, (3) problem rating scale for outcomes. <br> ■ Developed for and researched in community-based nursing practice settings (home health, public health, school nursing, and clinic settings). |
| ■ HHCC: Home Health Care Classification (Saba & McCormick, 1996) | ■ Developed to provide a standardized language system for coding/categorizing the services provided by nurses in the home health practice setting. <br> ■ Coding scheme for nursing diagnosis, interventions, and outcomes that are easily coded for computer data collection and retrieval. |
| ■ NIC: Iowa Intervention Project: Nursing Intervention Classification (McCloskey & Bulechek, 1996) | ■ Large data set of research-based nursing interventions dealing with six domains (physiological basic and complex behavioral, safety, family, and health systems). <br> ■ Interventions have a specific label, are defined, and have a set of actions or activities performed by the nurse while providing client care. |
| ■ NOC. Iowa Outcomes Project: Nursing Outcomes Classification (Johnson, Maas, & Moorehead, 2000) | ■ The classification contains 260 outcomes, which are listed in alphabetical order. <br> ■ Each NOC outcome has a specific definition, a list of indicators that are used in the evaluation of client status, scale of measurement, and a list of references used in development of the outcome. Five-point Likert-type scales were developed for use with the outcomes to measure client status in relation to the outcome. |

use of language for communicating what nurses do, several professional nursing organizations have created initiatives to implement standardized nursing languages into clinical practice.

The American Nurses Association established the Steering Committee on Databases to Support Nursing Practice in 1990. The purpose of this committee was to develop policy to support the development of nursing classification systems, the uniformity of nursing data sets, and the implementation of a national data set. In 1992, the committee gave its support for the Unified Nursing Language System (UNLS). The UNLS is recognized by the National Library of Medicine for inclusion in the Unified Medical Language System. The Steering Committee on Databases to Support Nursing Practice currently recognizes five nursing taxonomies: (1) the North American Nursing Diagnosis Association (NANDA); (2) the Visiting Nurses Association of Omaha Community Health Problem and Intervention System; (3) the Home Health Care Classification (HHCC); (4) the Iowa Intervention Project: Nursing Intervention Classification (NIC); and (5) Iowa Outcomes Project: Nursing Outcomes Classification (NOC). A brief summary of each classification system is provided in Table 14-1.

The use of standardized nursing classification systems as described in Table 14-1 provides community health nurses with a uniform description of problems, interventions, and related outcomes while providing care to patients and their caregivers. In the community health nursing practice setting, the use of standardized nursing languages can (1) facilitate the appropriate selection of nursing interventions for cost-effective and clinically effective health care delivery; (2) assist in predicting patient and caregiver outcomes; (3) foster transdisciplinary communications; (4) assist community health nursing managers in appropriate allocation of financial and personnel resources; (5) promote reimbursement for nursing services; and (6) articulate community health nursing's worth to health care policy planners at the state, federal, and international levels (Grier & McGuire, 1999).

## ■■ CULTURAL CONNECTION

Consider how having a computer in a home might affect some cultural groups and their cultural values about privacy. Religious and cultural groups such as the Amish shun all technology. How will this practice affect their access to information and community health nursing care? How would a nurse caring for an Amish family explain his or her use of a computer for documentation? Should the nurse keep the laptop out of the home?

## Patient Information Management

Health care is data intensive. Much of the collection of patient-related clinical data takes a considerable amount of time and effort. The management of patient-level data provides the community health nurse with an accurate assessment of patients' and their caregivers' situation for the purpose of planning, implementing, and evaluating care. Information systems allow for the organization of myriad data collected during an individual's admission to a community health care facility. This information can be stored for future retrieval, and the aggregation of this information can be analyzed for the benefit of the community.

### ■ Efficiency and Time Benefits

The use of nursing information systems can provide community health nurse managers and staff with efficiencies in productivity. The collection of patient- and caregiver-centered information is often a time-consuming endeavor and uses financial and personnel resources. Savings in time are often demonstrated by the use of computer systems for communicating information over distance, over time, and to multiple users of the data. Clinical information can be shared with several users at the same time. An example is sharing laboratory results with a nurse practitioner at a remote community clinic at the same time the practitioner is consulting with a physician in a large tertiary center.

Information systems are beneficial to manage health care information for population groups. These benefits include (1) collecting data to demonstrate clinical effectiveness of community health nursing care delivery to a specific population, (2) analyzing the collected clinical data for statistical comparison, (3) determining the cost-effectiveness of community health nursing programs on the care of patients and caregivers, and (4) using cost-effective data collection for outcome measurement.

## Computer Applications in Community Health Nursing

Computer and communications technologies continue to grow rapidly in utilization with the community health care practice setting. This use will continue to grow in all segments of health care and will become more efficient and effective in meeting the goals of a community health care facility for information leading to sound clinical and financial decision making. Computer applications that support good communications and organization of clinically related data are available.

### ■ Electronic Mail

Computers have long been able to communicate with one another. In the past, communication between computer users had been an interactive endeavor; that is, both the sender and the receiver of the communication had to be at

their respective terminals for the communication to take place. With today's **electronic mail (e-mail)** applications, the sender and receiver need not be at their respective computer terminals because the message can be sent in a "store and forward" manner. Depending on the type of operating system and e-mail software package, the typical e-mail system sets up a computerized mailbox that receives the incoming message and stores it for viewing by the receiving computer user when it is convenient. The received message can be read on the computer's monitor, saved for future reference, or printed. Messages can be configured with an "attached" or inserted file such as a word processing document, presentations, animation, sound bites, or electronic spreadsheets. In the community-based practice setting, messages of a critical nature (e.g., patient status, critical laboratory reports, or case management information) can be sent to physicians or nurse practitioners from sources such as the laboratory, radiology department, health information systems departments, and remote sites such the public health department of home health agency.

### ■ Databases

Community-based health care delivery is data intensive. Patient charts contain massive amounts of data that individually are just single pieces of unrelated information. When data are used in this unrelated manner, analysis is difficult to perform. But when data are combined in a structure that demonstrates relationships between data elements, powerful

Example of database entry screen.

Example of electronic spreadsheet.

data analysis can begin. A **database** software package gives the computer user the ability to generate records that have data elements grouped together for relational value. These individual records can be grouped, and further delineation of the data elements can be achieved. For example, a public health nurse might want to construct a monthly report of all clinic pediatric patients of a certain age or age group, data related to their visits, the immunization status of each patient, and the type of health screenings that have been performed. If these data are first entered into a database program, age, dates of office visits, types of immunization, and types of health screening could be "queried" or selected by the nurse for the monthly report (see the preceding figure).

This type of database is known as *relational* because each data element in the database can be selected (or not selected) for report generation. Simple data analysis can then be performed on the individual and aggregate patient care level.

## Electronic Spreadsheets

**Electronic spreadsheets** assist the computer user with "crunching" or manipulating large amounts of numerical data. The software displays a series of rows and columns in a gridlike depiction of a spreadsheet. This grid is displayed on the computer's monitor. Each box created by the intersection of a row and column is known as a *cell*. Individual numbers or formulas can be entered into the cell to calculate results for a given problem. For example, a home health nursing manager may want to know the proportion of skilled nursing visits as a percentage of the total number of visits performed by all the professional staff in the agency. A column of cells is named "skilled nursing visits," and each of the registered nurses' monthly visits is entered in the cell next to their individual names. At the end of the column, the nurse manager designates one cell to enter a formula to (1) add all the cells that contain the registered nurses' monthly visits and (2) place the total number of professional visits for the agency into (3) a formula that would calculate a percentage (see the

figure above). Sophisticated statistical analysis, supported by user-defined formulas that are a part of the spreadsheet software, can generate reports with graphs of a meaningful nature. Spreadsheet data can also be "exported"—that is, moved from one type of computer application to another.

For example, a nurse manager may want to perform some sophisticated statistical analysis that involves comparisons between two groups of patients. After collecting the desired data and entering these data into an electronic spreadsheet, the nurse manager can export the spreadsheet data file to a statistical package such as SPSS (Statistical Package for Social Sciences) for complex statistical comparisons.

### Research Alert

Caring for the homeless has many issues, including accessing patient health records and information. Often, homeless patients are not the best health historians and family members are not available to provide patient information; also, fewer than 50% of the clients will see the same health care provider for a second visit (p. 250).

Healthcare for the Homeless–Houston (HHH) began a case study to determine the impact of clinicians using personal digital assistants (PDAs) for tracking patient information rather than the clinicians trying to carry around paper copies of patient records. Clinicians were provided with custom-designed software on Palm V handheld computers (palmOne, Inc., Milpitas, California). While there were some limitations to the new system (including storing and retrieving long-term data), preliminary evidence showed that by using the PDAs, clinicians were more focused on building relationships with their clients rather than completing cumbersome paper documentation of care provided.

*Source*: Buck, D. S., Rochon, D., & Turley, J. P. (2005). Taking it to the streets: Recording medical outreach data on personal digital assistants. *CIN: Computers, Informatics, Nursing, 23*(5), 250–255.

## Internet Applications in Community-Based Nursing Practice

As computer networks have become more established throughout the nation, and for that matter throughout the world, additional opportunities for sharing data, information, and knowledge have presented themselves to health care providers. The establishment of the Internet has enabled many health care practitioners to communicate and thus share community health–related data. The Internet is the product of a communications network known as the *ARPAnet,* a network of U.S. defense computers. This network was developed in the late 1960s to counter the detrimental effects of nuclear warfare on computer and communications technology. It was first used to link various major university academic computer centers where U.S. defense research was being conducted. As the academic centers proliferated and began to link to one another, the Internet became a conglomeration of academic, commercial, governmental, and personal websites used for the exchange of information, services, and research. The Internet affords the computer user the luxury of communicating with health care professionals from around the world. The Web has become a wonderful resource for communications, research, and education for community-based nurses and the patients and caregivers they serve. There are thousands of websites easily accessed by computer users throughout the world.

## Health Care Delivery System Management Software

Health care information systems software designers have developed many different financial and business solutions for various health care delivery settings. From the 1970s through the present, software developers focused most of their development on hospital software that dealt with financial issues such as cost, revenues, payer mix, and diagnosis-related group (DRG) identification and coding. Decision support systems were mostly aimed at answering business questions. Recently, an emphasis on clinical data collection and presentation has emerged in the development of software applications for health care. With the advent of managed care, prospective payment, managed care reimbursement, and increased competition in the health care industry, special health care application software has been and continues to be designed for the community-based practice setting.

Software applications and computer systems (as well as networks) are being developed from a clinical perspective. Outpatient clinics, public health departments, free-standing and hospital-based home health agencies, and schools are all excellent practice settings that have elements of information systems development. One example is the development of home health information systems. Sociodemographic data, patient assessments, visit notes, clinical pathways used for specific disease states, generation of Medicare forms for

 ENVIRONMENTAL CONNECTION

So many new technologies have appeared in the past half century that it is nearly impossible to list them all. Paul Boutin has identified the most significant technological advances that have revolutionized American life. Here is his list of the ten most life-changing technological advancements.

**10. Organ transplants**. The first organ transplants occurred when Dr. Joseph Murray removed the kidney from one human patient and implanted it in another. By using identical twins, the recipient accepted the kidney rather than rejecting it as a foreign body. Shortly thereafter, other researchers developed drugs that would suppress kidney transplants from unrelated donors. Fast forward to present day: Every year, some 25,000 Americans receive a new heart, kidney, liver, lung, pancreas, or intestine.

**9. Robots and artificial intelligence**. In 1920, Czechoslovakian playwright Karel Capek coined the term "robot"; "robata" is a Czech word for tedious labor. Many years later, George Devol built the actual industrial robot in 1954. In 1959, Massachusetts Institute of Technology established its Artificial Intelligence Laboratory in a quest to create the mechanical link between human minds and hands. Today, robots assemble products better, faster, and often cheaper than manual laborers can, while more than 8 million U.S. airline flights are scheduled, guided, and flown with the superhuman assistance of advanced software each year. While these technologically created human-like machines have been an economic boon, thousands of human workers have been displaced or lost jobs completely

due to their lack of education or training in the use of this technology. American author Kurt Vonnegut in his 1952 fictional story, "The Player Piano," visualized a future when machines might leave humans without any purpose or jobs.

**8. Electronic funds transfer (EFT)**. As early as 1972, the Federal Reserve Bank of San Francisco set up a paperless transfer system in its Los Angeles branch. By the late 1970s, instantaneous transfers of millions of dollars in value between banks, insurance companies, and other financial institutions had become common. How does this technology affect our lives today? We can get cash from our bank accounts or credit cards from anywhere in the world, making the traditional "wiring" of money almost obsolete. Personal bank checks have become the exception, as have cash payments, and their use is actually discouraged by many businesses. This has also created new threats on the Internet through stolen identity via the availability of personal financial information on the web.

**7. Nuclear power**. In 1956, when Queen Elizabeth II herself threw the switch on the world's first atomic power plant in England, nuclear reactors were seen as a source of cheap, pollution-free energy. The enthusiasm for this new energy source was dampened by a partial meltdown in 1979 at the Three Mile Island reactor in Pennsylvania, which caused the U.S. public to become cynical about the safety of nuclear energy. Today, only about 100 plants exist in the United States, but they generate 20% of the country's

## ENVIRONMENTAL CONNECTION (CONT.)

electricity, second only to coal as a source of power, and in recent years have been making a comeback.

6. **Mobile phones**. Cellular phone service has long existed in theory. Martin Cooper, a Motorola researcher, rang up his rival at AT&T Bell Labs to test the new phone as far back as 1947, but the first true call from the sidewalk outside the Manhattan Hilton was in 1973. Today, cell phones are used by more than 50% of all Americans; text messaging via cell phone by teens has eclipsed e-mail and voice phone calls. Many Americans use cellular phones exclusively, eliminating landline phones. These cellular networks are also making their way onto the Internet through broadband wireless networks. Skype technology has made talking through the Internet an easy matter: Not only is the service free when both parties download the Skype software, but video is easily available as well. This is a revolutionary change in the way calls are made, especially international calls, where phone-to-phone calls are especially expensive.

5. **Space flight.** Space travel has not completely met science's and the American public's expectations for interplanetary travel and discovery, with our only our trip being to the moon, where humans walked on the lunar surface. NASA has experienced financial and technological problems in the past several years, but the space race against the Russians in the 1960s and 1970s still led to the development of hundreds of enabling technologies, including synthetic fibers and integrated computer circuits, which are used by Americans every day. The early astronauts who flew to the moon did give us a broader sense of our place in the universe: "We saw the earth the size of a quarter, and we realized then that there is only one earth. We are all brothers."

4. **Personal computers**. The first personal-sized computers were the size of washing machines and required an air-conditioned room for their operation. IBM and Apple developed the desktop computer in the early 1980s, making the PC (personal computer) widely available to the public. This technological advancement cannot be overestimated in terms of how it has changed our lives. Today, thanks to the PC, many businesses have eliminated complete categories of occupations, such as secretaries and transcriptionists. We can do our own work, access the Internet with inexpensive technology and wireless networks, and keep "files" without a filing cabinet. As a result, our offices can be anywhere, at home, in cars, in cafés, or on the beach.

3. **Digital media**. With the development of Photoshop 1.0 in 1990, photos could be manipulated to create "unreal" images, those that could be easily changed by the average computer user. Digitized audio, pictures, movies, and text let even an amateur edit reality, or even create the image from scratch with no more than a keyboard and mouse. Just as important, digital media can be copied repeatedly nearly for free, stored permanently without fading, and sent around the world in seconds. This flexibility, Boutin says, "rightly worries the movie and music industries, but how do you put the genie back in the bottle if there's no bottle anymore?"

2. **Genetic engineering**. Watson and Crick unraveled the secret of DNA in 1953. Boyer and Cohen constructed the first organism with combined DNA from different species in 1973. Today, an estimated 70% of processed foods contain genetically modified ingredients. Of course, the much bigger potential, which has created perhaps the most passionate debate of all our technological advancements, lies in cloning or engineering humans. Such advancements can theoretically prevent serious birth defects and diseases from ever developing, thereby extending our life spans for years. Yet, the consequences of such possibilities are unknown, such as the results of testing the new cloning research on humans and the possibility of threats to the natural evolution of people. These ethical debates continue, with restrictions being placed on human cloning research in the United States, yet other countries move on with this research. Again, can the genie be put back in the bottle once such technology becomes available?

1. **The Internet**. The Internet has become the world's largest ever-changing library and the most unregulated information source the world has ever known. The "Net" has made news instantaneous, and turned communication, be it social or business, into a completely different cultural phenomenon. With an Internet connection, people can avoid shopping in physical locations, do business without stepping into a bank, and eliminate many travel costs by conference calling via the Net. It is easily the most affordable mass medium ever, as well as perhaps the most serious threat today to the privacy of information. As the Internet becomes more sophisticated, so do the "hackers," who have the potential to create havoc with major systems. Three-fifths of Americans now use the Net, but it remains to be seen how these instant connections and relationships will transform our culture.

*Source*: Adapted from Paul Boutin's 2004 article "10 Life-Changing Technologies." Boutin is a technology writer for *Wired* magazine and *Slate*. He has worked as a software engineer and manager at MIT and in Silicon Valley. Retrieved on October 23, 2008, from http://www.echeck2000.com/Life_changing_tech.asp

billing purposes, and agency financial management have been incorporated into the software.

## ■ Networked Patient Care

Computers used in a stand-alone configuration are powerful and productive business, academic, and clinical tools. The power of computers is enhanced or increased when they are linked together. When linked together, computer users can share application software and files, communicate, and thereby increase productivity. Community-based health care delivery systems use networks (the linking of computer and communications technologies) to transfer data, images, and video (medical video and health care teleconferencing).

For this transmission of data, networks have been designed and implemented in many health care settings. Wide area networks (WANs) are used by health care facilities for data transmission and data communications over a long distance. For example, WANs are used for data transmission

Home health nurses have almost instant access to a patient's health information through electronic databases and online patient records.

between several health care facilities and their central office. Local area networks (LANs) connect computer users who are generally within the confines of an office complex or the same building. Wireless networks use radio frequency or infrared technology for data transmission. This type of network allows for greater mobility in hardware use within a facility. An outgrowth of network development is patient–server computer architecture. As computer technology migrated from massive mainframe systems to smaller personal computers, the linkage of these personal computers to one another lead to patient–server technology. The server, a computer (either a powerful minicomputer, a large-capacity personal computer, or a mainframe) is connected to several personal computer workstations. These "patients" can use application software that resides on the server. An example of this relationship can be demonstrated by the use of a database that resides on the server. A computer user at a remote workstation queries the relational database, asking the server for specific records. Instead of the server sending all the records to the computer user, the server sends only those records that are specified by the patient workstation user.

Certain advantages are gained by using patient–server technology in the community-based nursing practice setting. First, the system configuration consists of several powerful machines that give the community health nurse a considerable amount of computer power at lower cost than traditional mainframe, centralized, "closed" computing systems. Second, the patient–server computer architecture is considered to be open systems technology. Community health care program planners can choose from among several hardware

and software vendors to configure their computer system based on specific organizational and clinical needs. Finally, the computer system can grow and be enhanced when the community health care organization's needs change. An example of this can be demonstrated in the community-based nursing practice setting.

Most community-based practice settings are influenced by external factors such as federal and state government health care reimbursement programs. As these programs change their reimbursement strategies and their regulations, different reporting and documentation requirements are generated for the service provider. When the community health care organization has an open systems architecture as a base for the computer system, new hardware (if needed) and software (for the new reporting requirements) can be installed easily with the existing system's configuration.

The advent of patient–server technology has led to more use of a network concept known as **distributed data processing (DDP).** In the DDP configuration, a community-based health care organization uses smaller computers as workstations at sites that can be situated within a single building or from off site, remote computing sites. These smaller competing sites are connected via telecommunications lines (POTS [plain old telephone service], T1 or T3, fiber-optic, or even satellite). The figure on page 333 depicts a DDP configuration.

The advantages of developing and maintaining distributed data processing configuration are numerous. The remote sites (e.g., off-site health department offices) can respond more quickly to service demands if data processing capabilities are available at the remote sites. Backup systems are more often available to the entire community health care organization, minimizing downtime caused by equipment or software failure. As health care service demands change within a community (as a result of external factors such as changes in Medicare, Medicaid, or managed care penetra-

*❝ a conversation with . . . ❞*

From the early days of creating the first computers for space travel, we knew that the technology would eventually change the world forever, that eventually data would be managed in ways never before possible, that computers would eventually make their way to the public. We just did not know that it would happen so quickly and that cybernetics would develop into such miniature phenomena. Werner Von Braun was the only person I worked with who seemed to understand this vision and its potential for changing forever the way persons would communicate with each other.

—**Marshall Wayne Saucier,** early computer researcher and mathematician for General Electric and the U.S. Space Program at NASA in Huntsville, Alabama, during the early 1960s, November 2005

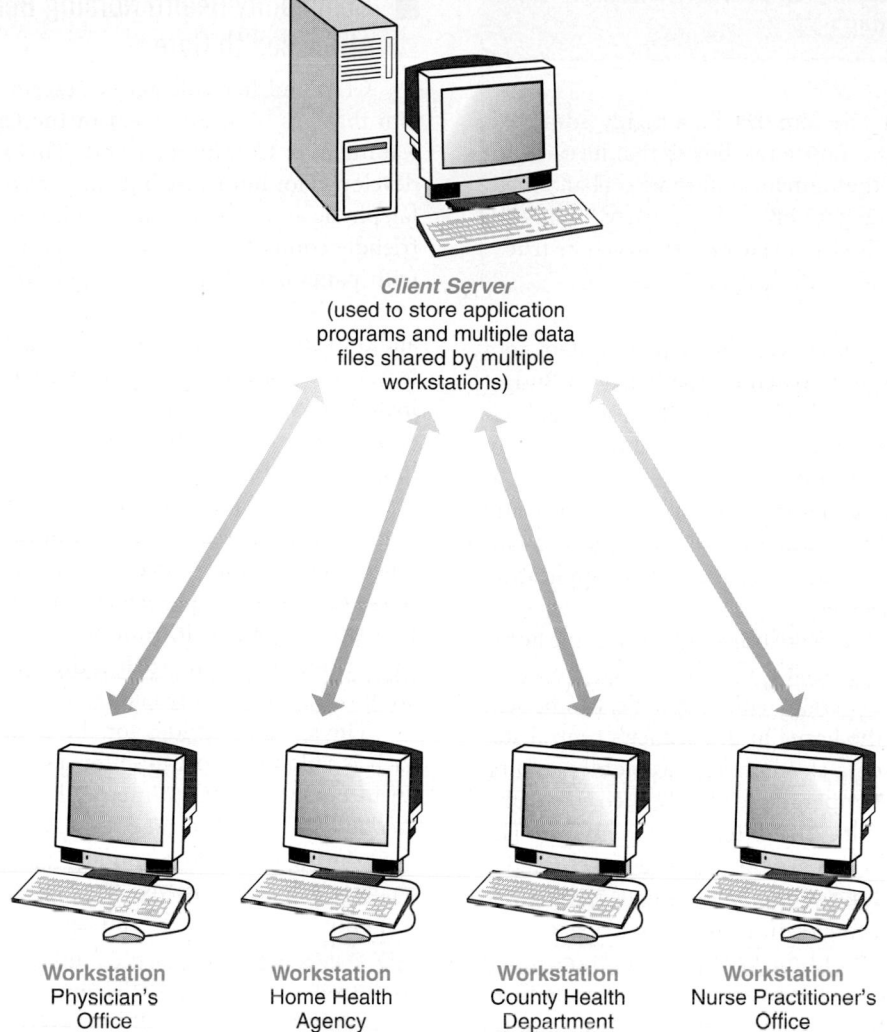

**Client Server**
(used to store application
programs and multiple data
files shared by multiple
workstations)

**Workstation**
Physician's
Office

**Workstation**
Home Health
Agency

**Workstation**
County Health
Department

**Workstation**
Nurse Practitioner's
Office

Distributed data processing

tion), a community-based organization can change the DDP configuration incrementally, often without great expense to the organization. Finally, the computing needs of nurse executives, managers, and staff can be tailored easily within the DDP configuration. Analysis of patient care data and more productivity at staff levels can be realized when a DDP system is developed, implemented, and maintained.

## Communication Technology and Community Health Nursing

Much of the United States is considered rural in geography, and thus there are inherent challenges to providing access to health care services. Lack of access to health care facilities and to limited numbers of health care providers tends to decrease opportunities for service provision. Distance to health care facilities and access to skilled health care providers are but two challenges to individuals seeking health care services in both rural and inner-city environments. **Telemedicine/**

**telehealth** is the delivery of medical services over telecommunications lines and is paving the way for providing specialized, skilled services in areas that would otherwise be without.

The following discussion demonstrates how current telehealth applications are being used in the community-based practice setting. As with all information and communications technology, these applications are evolving into faster, less expensive methods for delivering community-based health care services.

### ■ Telehealth Care Benefits

An example of the benefit that telehealth can provide can be demonstrated in home health care. Home health care is one of the fastest-growing industries in the United States. Along with this growth has come a certain amount of scrutiny with regard to reimbursement practices. In an effort to control costs, the federal government is in the process of

**◉ MEDIA MOMENT**

*Artificial Intelligence: A.I.* **(2001)**

In this futuristic fairy tale film, David, a highly advanced robotic boy, hopes to become a real boy so that he can win back the affection of the human mother who abandoned him. Like Pinocchio, he goes on a long journey hoping to find his "Blue Fairy," who can make his dreams come true.

converting from a cost-based reimbursement system to a prospective payment system based on the Balanced Budget Act of 1997. Managed care also is increasing in market penetration. As a response to the increased pressures to remain financially viable, home health care agencies are looking at many innovative technologies to supplement, enhance, and complement care. Crist, Kaufman, and Crampton (1996) discussed the advances of telemedicine and its application within home health agencies.

Three basic types of data are transmitted from the home setting to a central home health office via telecommunications. Data, which are generally patient specific, can be sent from a remote site to the home health agency's central station. This can include data elements such as blood pressure, blood oxygen, pulse, temperature, blood glucose, weight, electrocardiograph results, and other measurements. The second type of data that can be collected and transmitted is audio (e.g., heart and lung sounds). Voice data can include anything from voice conversation to stethoscope sounds and messages. The third and final type of data transmitted through telecommunication is image. It can take the form of still images (i.e., still-frame photographs) or full-motion video.

**☝ THINK ABOUT THIS** ·····························

Twenty-three percent of children in nursery school have gone online, and 32% have used the Internet, under adult supervision. Children use interactive stories and animated lessons that teach letters, numbers, and rhymes. Children today were born in the age of the Internet. They see it as part of the continuum of the way life is today. Students from elementary school through college write e-mail, instant-message one another, and have very little tolerance for waiting. Voice mail is too slow. By the time children enter first grade, more than 89% will have mastered beginning use of computers, including hand–eye coordination, the social component of working with classmates on computer exercises, and learning to take risks as they learn. While many older adults are still afraid that they are going to blow up the computer and lose all their data, children are more comfortable with this technology. ◢

*Source:* http://nces.edu.gov/publsearch

## ■ Community Health Nursing Benefits of Telehealth Care

Crist and her colleagues describe a telemedicine system that has been evaluated in the Cincinnati area (Crist, Kaufman, & Crampton, 1996). This system was primarily developed for home use but could also be used in the hospital, physician's office, or nursing home. The device is a user-friendly computer-based device used to communicate daily with patients and their caregivers to support their health care needs. The system was designed using touch screen and audio to coach patients through treatment protocols. Other features available from the unit are vital signs devices, which include thermometer, pulse oximetry, blood pressure cuff, and electrocardiograph; digital stethoscope to record heart, lung, and gastrointestinal sounds; a medication reminder system to increase patient compliance with medication administration; real-time telephone communication for scheduling activities; video transmission of patient to nurse, nurse to patient; and touch screens that allow for coaching to assist the patient in routine medical procedures, which can include procedures such as dressing changes, medication administration, and the taking of vital signs.

The system provides for the hookup of future devices such as a blood glucose monitor, a scale for obtaining weight, an intravenous (IV) pump, and a ventilator. The system can be customized to meet the particular needs of the patient during installation and also has an alarm function for changes in patient status. This system allows for 24-hour response to patient needs and care management with necessary skilled visits. The central nursing station accumulates health care data such as vital signs, request for medication, communication events, and requests for assistance on each patient for which a home-assisted nursing care (HANC) unit is installed. A unique feature of the system is the ability of the home health agency to change patient protocols as patient conditions change. The key factor to the successful application of the HANC network is the ability to customize the telecommunications systems for a particular patient needs.

## The Future of Informatics and Telehealth

The mainstreaming of telemedicine/telehealth brings a considerable amount of opportunity to community-based nursing practices. Patient monitoring, patient and caregiver education, transdisciplinary case conferences, and professional health care education are being achieved. Numerous researchers have examined the use of telehealth/telemedicine in home care and community-based health care.

Hebda, Czar, and Mascara (2005) write that many providers see that telehealth will change the way health care is delivered while providing new roles for health care providers. The World Wide Web (WWW) has already changed how health care providers interact with their patients, many of whom are not reticent to use the Internet to research health conditions and are now more likely to question their health

## MEDIA MOMENT

### *I, Robot* (2004)

It's the year 2035, and robots have been assimilated into the community to assist humans. Three laws are integrated into the robots' systems: they cannot harm a human being or allow harm to come to a human being if they can act to prevent it; they must comply with all orders from human beings unless the order violates law #1; and they have to defend themselves as long as the defense doesn't conflict with the first two laws. When the writer of the three laws, Alfred Lanning, falls from the tenth-floor of U.S. Robotics to his death, most of the Chicago Police Department believes it was a suicide. Detective Del Spooner, who hates robots, thinks he was murdered, and he suspects a Nestor Class-5 robot known as Sonny. If Sonny is guilty of murdering Alfred Lanning, he broke the three laws. Working with Dr. Susan Calvin, Detective Spooner must discover the truth before it's too late.

care practitioners regarding care and treatment. The Internet also provides new avenues for interactive examination and monitoring of patients in a home care setting. Additionally, health care providers can learn from and participate in continuing education offered through synchronous and asynchronous distance-learning offerings, enhancing their ability to provide care for their patients.

According to Hebda et al. (2005), the only hindrance to the growth of telehealth in the United States has been the lack of financial reimbursement, but the authors assert that the "demands for quality, patient safety, and more care options will help change the reimbursement picture" (p. 377). Although the Federal Communications Commission (FCC) has a telemedicine program, it has not been well utilized; however, in 2003, new rules were enacted that should improve access for rural health care providers. Since then, the FCC has been working with the National Rural Health Association and the HIMSS through a grant program to encourage rural health care providers to use the FCC telemedicine program (p. 377). After examining the growth of telemedicine/telehealth and nursing informatics over the past two decades, one can only imagine the numerous ways that information systems developments will continue to affect nursing practice, particularly in the home health and community health practice areas, in the future.

Nursing visits are conducted through telehealth systems. Warner (1996) states that some telehealth systems allow the nurse to remotely control camera functions to get a closer view of wound sites and infusion sites as well as scanning the patient's environment. Most systems will allow for an electronic capture of data elements necessary for a clinical record as well as still-frame photos and full-motion video.

According to Warner, quality-of-care issues will also be met through enhanced productivity by replacing the travel time that nurses have in making their daily caseload assignments. Telehealth systems would also allow nurses to make visits in adverse weather conditions and in high-risk neighborhoods where safety is often threatened.

The use of telehealth systems can provide a telecommunications information system that is interactive between the nurse and the patient, using text, video, audio, and/or graphics. Warner advocates a telehealth utilization by diagnosis, with less severe acuities being matched with technologies that are also less technical. She places the complexity of patient statuses on a continuum from less to more complex, more acute illnesses such as congestive heart failure, recovery after acute myocardial infarction, chronic obstructive pulmonary disease, and diabetes being on the higher end of the continuum and resulting in the need for more technical intervention. Warner discusses several factors that are related to determining when telehealth is appropriate for a particular patient. A primary consideration should be the stability of the individual's disease processes. It is also necessary that the patient possess sufficient cognitive ability, hearing, and vision to use the system or to have a caregiver to provide assistance. In addition, consideration must be made for the patient's and caregivers' feelings and beliefs with regard to allowing the system in their home (e.g., apprehension about technology, cost, or loss of privacy) (p. 794).

## Research Alert

As the population ages, more older people are accessing the Internet for health information. These researchers examined the usability of three websites specifically designed for use by older adults. The two-part study gained opinions of usability from both experts in web usability and gerontology as well as ten senior (age 55 or older) web users who met additional criteria (including being mentally intact). To test usability, the researchers developed tasks based on the three websites; participants were provided with worksheets to document their observations during the website testing. Also, a "Perceived Health Web Site Usability Questionnaire" (p. 328) including 15 items on a seven-point Likert scale was used.

Findings indicate that older adults prefer simple websites with clear directions, and that certain subpopulations of older adults have a great deal of interest in online health information. The findings' generalizability is limited, however, because a convenience sample was used. The researchers state that there is a need for future research for usability testing and older adults' use of websites for health care information.

*Source:* Nahm, E-S., Preece, J., Resnick, B., & Mills, M. E. (2004). Usability of health web sites for older adults: A preliminary study. *CIN: Computers, Informatics, Nursing, 22*(6), 326–334.

The future of nursing informatics will be based on supporting the individual practicing nurse's requirements for assessing, implementing, evaluating, and redefining care across all practice settings and teaching practicing clinicians how to use information and communication technologies. Gassert (1998), in her presentation to the American Medical Informatics Association, envisioned meeting these needs and those of patients and communities through a national nursing informatics agenda. Her two-part agenda includes (1) a strategic direction for preparing nurses in the use of information and communication technologies through the education of nursing students, practicing nurses, and nursing faculty and (2) strategies that affect patient care, including preparing nurses for information and communication use at the undergraduate, graduate, and continuing education levels; developing funding and programs for teaching specialized nursing informatic skills and, with other health care providers, developing collaborative programs in telecommunications that "will enhance the quality of clinical practice for populations at risk and contribute to the education of health providers" (p. 266); increasing nursing faculty exposure to information and communication technology use in nursing individual patients, communities, and caregivers; and developing the use of public and private resources such as the Internet to increase accessibility of health care knowledge resources for health care providers and the public (p. 267).

### Research Alert

The U.S. government is leading this charge into the medical information age based on technological record keeping and documentation for a simple reason: It pays for 46% of the nation's medical and health bills. The United States is number one in the world in terms of health care expenditures, a total of $1.8 trillion per year and rising at a rate more than twice as fast as our incomes, yet it ranked no better than sixteenth in a study of twenty-two industrialized countries in what medical professionals call outcomes. That is in part because so much unnecessary care is delivered (as much as one third) and in part because of the inefficiency of a system in which tens of thousands of patients die each year as a result of medical errors. Congress has passed legislation requiring a national registry by which medical and health care professionals can report errors anonymously as well as directives to move to a paperless patient documentation system.

## Conclusion

The use of information and communications technology in support of community nursing functions will continue to increase and offer community health nursing leaders and staff care for the patients and family caregivers they serve. The specialty of nursing informatics offers strategies for us-

### CULTURAL CONNECTION

All U.S. schools are now connected to the Internet, one computer for every five students. Most students are ahead of their teachers. Young students do not differentiate between the face-to-face world and the Internet world.

—Susan Patrick

You grew up with music in your blood; we have technology in our blood.

—Sean, high school student

Kids have a tremendous ability to expand their learning and a computer is just one tool.

—Mark Ginsberg, executive director of the National Association for the Education of Young Children

ing technologies such as those discussed in this chapter to (1) collect individual- and community-related data, (2) store and retrieve these data for clinical decision making (through the process of converting raw data into nursing information and ultimately into nursing knowledge), and (3) provide in-depth analysis of data for increasing productive service delivery while providing quality care.

Nursing informatics uses computer and communication technologies to collect information in a readily understandable format. To assist nurses in using computers to describe the care they render in a community-based practice setting, standardized nursing languages such as NANDA, NIC, NOC, HHCC, and Omaha were developed and continue to be added to through research efforts. Standardized languages in computer systems are used to assess patients and their communities, describe the care community health nurses perform, and are a basis for communications between community health nurses and other health care providers.

The use of computer applications such as e-mail, databases, and spreadsheets can provide community health nurses with tools to increase their productivity and knowledge. E-mail can be used to coordinate communications among health care providers in the community. Databases have been used to collect and organize massive amounts of patient- and community-related data to be used in research and business analysis. Spreadsheets can be used to perform complicated mathematical or statistical calculations that support clinical decision making. Information and communication systems continue to offer exciting new ways for community health nurses to maintain a cost-effective presence in the community even when distance is a challenge. The use of telemedicine/telehealth provides the community health nurse with several strategies for maintaining visual and/or audio contact with patients and family caregivers.

The future of nursing informatics and telehealth is bright and promising. Innovations in nursing science combined with advances in information and communication technologies will provide community health nurses and planners with tools that will increase their contact with the communities they serve.

Explore Community Health Nursing on the Web! To learn more about the topics in this chapter, use the passcode provided to access your exclusive website: **http://nursing.jbpub.com/ communityhealth.** If you do not have a passcode, you can obtain one at this site.

## ■ CRITICAL THINKING ACTIVITIES

1. You have been asked to prioritize the requirements of your public health nursing staff's documentation system. It has already been determined that ease, usability, and dependability are priorities. What else would you include in the system requirements?

2. Think about a typical day of practice and describe the setting. How many times would you, as a public health nurse, interact with information systems? How would you access the information systems? How does their location and ease of access impact nursing care?

## ■ REFERENCES

American Nurses Association. (2001). *Scope and standards of nursing informatics practice.* Washington, DC: Author.

Crist, T., Kaufman, S., & Crampton, K. (1996). Home telemedicine: A home health care agency's strategy for maximizing resources. *Home Health Care Management Practice, 8*(4), 1–9.

Gassert, C. (1998). The challenge of meeting patient's needs with a national nursing informatics agenda. *Journal of the American Medical Informatics Association, 5*(3), 263–286.

Graves, J., & Corcoran, S. (1989). The study of nursing informatics. *Image: The Journal of Nursing Scholarship, 21,* 227–231.

Grier, M., & McGuire, R. (1999). Nursing informatics: A means of change. In J. Lancaster (Ed.), *Nursing issues in leading and managing change* (pp. 533–553). St. Louis, MO: Mosby.

Hassett, M., & Thede, L. Q. (2003). Information in practice: Clinical information systems. In L. Q. Thede (Ed.), *Informatics and nursing: Opportunities and challenges* (2nd ed., pp. 222–239). Philadelphia: Lippincott Williams & Wilkins.

Hebda, T., Czar, P., & Mascara, C. (2005). *Handbook for informatics for nurses and health care professionals* (3rd ed.). Upper Saddle River, NJ: Pearson/Prentice Hall.

Johnson, M., & Maas, M., & Moorehead, S. (2000). *Iowa outcomes project: Nursing Outcomes Classification (NOC).* St. Louis, MO: Mosby.

Martin, K. S., & Scheet, N. J. (1995). The Omaha System: Nursing diagnosis, intervention, and patient outcomes. In *An Emerging framework: Data systems advances for clinical nursing practice* (pp. 105–113). Washington, DC: American Nursing Association Publication, June #NP-94.

McCloskey, J., & Bulechek, G. (1996). *Iowa intervention project: Nursing Intervention Classification (NIC)* (2nd ed.). St. Louis, MO: Mosby.

Saba, V., & McCormick, K. (1996). *Essentials of computers for nurses* (2nd ed.). New York: McGraw-Hill.

Sebastian, J., & Stanhope, M. (1999). Managing resources. In J. Lancaster (Ed.), *Nursing issues in leading and managing change* (pp. 505–531). St. Louis: Mosby.

Stallings, W., & Van Slyke, R. (1998). *Business data communications* (3rd ed.). Upper Saddle River, NJ: Prentice Hall.

Warner, I. (1996). Telehealth home care. *Home Health Care Nurse, 14*(10), 791–796.

Warren, J. J., & Hoskins, L. M. (1995). NANDA's nursing diagnosis taxonomy: A nursing database. In *An emerging framework: Data systems advances for clinical nursing practice* (pp. 49–59). Washington, DC: American Nurses Association Publication, June #NP-94.

# CHAPTER 15
# Health Education in the Community

Lucy Bradley-Springer

Visit **http://nursing.jbpub.com/communityhealth** for interactive exercises, review questions, Web links, and more.

All nurses, regardless of work site or specialty, are expected to teach individuals and their families about health-related matters. Nurses who work in the community have additional opportunities to help people change behaviors for the improved health of aggregate populations.

Be careful how you pronounce health promotion, lest the listener believe self-promotion to be your objective.

—*Mohan Singh*

Be careful of reading health books, you might die of a misprint.

—*Mark Twain*

You may ask, "Why should I teach? Why would I want to change people's behaviors? I went to nursing school to give patient care, not to teach. If I'd wanted to teach, I wouldn't have spent all this time learning to put catheters in and how to fill out care plans." The short answer is that **teaching** is an essential part of nursing. Nurses teach because it is a part of patient care. The longer answer is that teaching patients improves health care. Education positively influences health outcomes when patients experience fewer complications and faster recoveries; learn to care for themselves, increasing autonomy and self-confidence; and are better prepared to resume their lives. Think about your own experiences. Where you have learned best? Was it in a classroom or clinical setting? How did the teacher interact with the students?

## CHAPTER FOCUS

**Theoretical Bases**
- Concepts
- Learning Theory
- Behavior Change Theory

**The Health Education Process**
- Assessment
- Planning
- Implementation
- Evaluation

**Health Education in Communities**
- Individuals, Families, and Groups
- Community
- Beyond Community

**Ethical Issues in Health Education**

## QUESTIONS TO CONSIDER

After reading this chapter, you will know the answers to the following questions:

1. What is health education, and how does it differ in community settings?
2. What are behavioral concepts and theories in education?
3. How are behavioral concepts and theories used to provide direction for health education programs?
4. What are principles of education, and how can they be integrated into health education practice?
5. What are the various situations in community health nursing in which education for behavior change can be incorporated into nursing care at the individual, group, and community levels?
6. What are the ethical issues in health education that have emerged from the current healthcare environment?

## KEY TERMS

Absolutism
Adherence
Advocacy
Autonomy
Barriers
Behavior change

Behavior change theories
Benefits
Cognitive dissonance
Community-based teaching
Discharge teaching

Domains of learning
Empowerment
Health education
Learning goals and objectives
Learning theories

Motivation
Paternalism
Readiness
Self-efficacy
Teaching

**❝** *Wisdom is not a product of schooling, but the lifelong attempt to acquire it.* **❞**

—*Albert Einstein*

THE PURPOSE OF HEALTH education is to change behaviors that put people at risk for injury, disease, disability, or death. This may sound blunt, but whether you call it modifying behavior or influencing behavior (Rankin & Stallings, 2001), it all boils down to the same thing: Nurses teach patients, families, groups, and communities with the primary goal of getting people to change behaviors in ways that focus on disease prevention, illness intervention, and health promotion. The mission of health education is to "reduce current and future suffering" by addressing "individual and social factors that contribute to health problems" (Guttman, Kegler, & McLeroy, 1996, p. i). This chapter explores the topic of health education: its theoretical bases, its application, the problems associated with it, and the community heath nurse's role in health education.

Health education can also increase the knowledge, skills, and confidence needed to make decisions. It improves continuity of care, decreases the risk of problem recurrence, and uses resources more efficiently. Educated patients and their families are better able to cope and more likely to recognize problems before they become severe. All of these benefits help nurses do their jobs because knowledgeable patients have fewer complications and present with fewer of the acute emergencies that require more complex care (Hunt, 1997).

Initially, health education concentrated on crisis management ("What do you need to know now that you've got a colostomy?"). However, the healthcare system in the United States is evolving. The emphasis is now on cost containment, health maintenance, and managed care (Damrosch, 1991). Over the past decade, health education has had to adjust to support patient care in the midst of all these changes. Today health education includes disease prevention ("How do you keep from getting tuberculosis?" or "How can you decrease your risk of a stroke from hypertension?") and health pro-

**❝** *The fundamental conditions and resources for health are peace, shelter, education, food, income, a stable ecosystem, sustainable resources, social justice, and equity. Improvement in health requires a secure foundation in these basic prerequisites.* **❞**

—*World Health Organization, Ottawa Charter for Health Promotion, 1986*

motion ("How can you change to a healthier diet?") as well as continuing to deal with acute care issues. In addition, whether the focus is on reducing the rates of childhood infections or the deaths from cancer, health education and community-based programs are essential components of attaining every goal in the *Healthy People 2010* agenda (DHHS, 2000). Selected *Healthy People 2010* objectives related to health education are included in a box at the end of this chapter (page 358).

Although nurses are not the only healthcare professionals who have patient teaching responsibilities, their knowledge, skills, and access to patients, especially in the community, make them particularly well suited to this complex task (Spellbring, 1991).

## Theoretical Bases

When dealing with complex issues, it is wise to work from a theoretical base. Theories describe, explain, and predict behaviors within a functional framework (DiClemente, Crosby, & Kegler, 2002). Theories about health education and behavior change can help nurses understand behavior and thereby help them develop useful strategies that influence people's health.

---

■■ CULTURAL CONNECTION

I'm going to learn to relax—even if I have to work at it 24 hours a day, seven days a week.

—Author unknown

---

### ■ Concepts

Theories are based on concepts that are used to form the propositions that give structure to a theory. Some important concepts that support patient **autonomy** in health education are defined in Table 15-1. In addition, it would be helpful to discuss absolutism and paternalism, two concepts that have lost favor in health education not only because they tend to stifle autonomy, but also because they have not been found to be effective.

**Absolutism** is a tactic we have all used. When absolutism is used in health education, the teacher basically says, "This is what you must do." Absolutism requires absolute

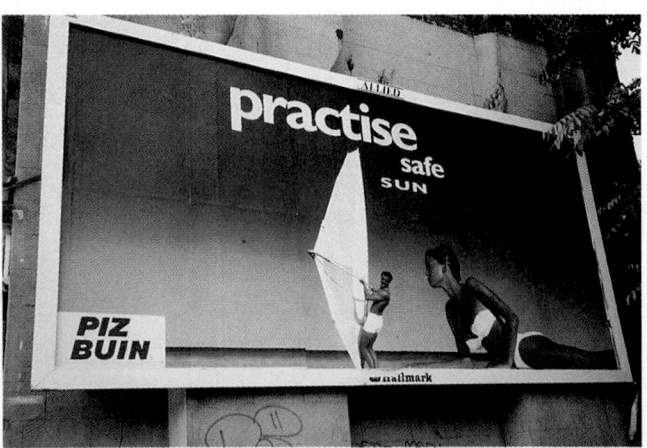

Public education campaign in Great Britain for prevention of skin cancer.

| Table 15-1 | Important Concepts for Health Education Theory |
| --- | --- |

| Concept | Definition |
| --- | --- |
| ■ **Advocacy** | Process in which patients are informed and supported so that they can make the best decisions possible (Spellbring, 1991); advocacy is a primary nursing function. |
| ■ **Barriers** | Those individually determined things that associate cost with a particular behavior (Palank, 1991); costs can be thought of in terms of money, time inconvenience, difficulty, risk, or interpersonal effort. Not having child care, for example, is a barrier for a mother who needs to attend a Narcotics Anonymous meeting. |
| ■ **Benefits** | Those individually determined things that reinforce or reward a particular behavior (Palank 1991); in other words, one person may see weight loss as a main benefit of exercise, but another may see meeting friends at the gym as the primary benefit. |
| ■ **Cognitive dissonance** | Tension or discomfort that accompanies actions that oppose personal beliefs (Rankin & Stallings, 2001); for example, a person who lectures co-workers about good nutrition eats chocolate cake and feels guilty about it. |
| ■ **Empowerment** | Process of helping people develop the abilities to understand and control their personal situations; can be applied at individual, group, and community levels (Israel, Checkoway, Schulz, & Zimmerman, 1994). |
| ■ **Motivation** | Complex concept that refers to those "forces acting on or within an organism that initiate, direct, and maintain behavior" (Redman, 1997, p. 7). |
| ■ **Readiness** | Motivation to perform a particular action at a particular time (Redman, 1997). |
| ■ **Self-efficacy** | Personal conviction of ability to carry out specific behaviors in order to achieve a desired end (Damrosch, 1991; Palank, 1991); the "I know I can do this" feeling. |

**adherence** to specific, prescribed strategies (Cates & Hinman, 1992). We have all done it because, as nurses, we know that smoking is not healthy and eating broccoli is. Absolute healthcare messages are usually well intentioned. They are based on evidence that, if used consistently and correctly, the prescribed methods will make people healthier. The problem is that complete adherence to any behavior is difficult. Think, for instance, about the last time you tried to lose weight or start exercising regularly. Were you always able to meet your goals? Did you always skip dessert? Did you show up at the gym every morning? Demanding absolute compliance with absolute behaviors is risky because most people cannot meet such high standards. When they fail to meet these standards, they can lose confidence in their abilities to change and give up (Strang, 1992). Maybe you have given up on some of your goals. Perhaps you knew that missing a workout session or eating a piece of chocolate cake did not spell disaster. Ideally, you chalked it up to experience and moved forward in your behavior change program. If you didn't, maybe it was because you believed an absolutist message: Do it right or don't do it at all. You can see how this would make health education and behavior change difficult.

Absolutism is perpetuated in an atmosphere of paternalism. **Paternalism** occurs when healthcare providers (or other "experts") decide what the patient should do (Rankin & Stallings, 2001; Yu et al., 2007). Although this also is usually done with altruistic motives, it runs counter to the concept of promoting patient autonomy. Paternalism and absolutism demand compliance (adherence). Compliance carries the expectation that patients will do exactly what providers tell them to do. If they don't, they are labeled "noncompliant," a term that implies patient responsibility for failure (Rankin & Stall-

ings, 2001). The nursing philosophy of holistic patient care supports individuals in their efforts to make health decisions and behavior changes. Absolutism, paternalism, and demands for strict compliance are all counter to this philosophy.

 ENVIRONMENTAL CONNECTION

How does the learning environment affect our ability to learn rather than simply "be taught"?

## ■ Learning Theory

Much health education is based on **learning theories** that have been developed over the past several decades. These theories are usually familiar to nurses, but some of the more important learning theory contributions to health education are briefly discussed here. The behavioral theorists, including Pavlov, Thorndike, and Skinner, showed how teachers could connect a stimulus to a desired response. This leads to a conditioned change in behavior that occurs every time the stimulus is presented. A patient could, for instance, learn that brushing her teeth in the morning is associated with taking her birth control pill. Developmental theories, by comparison, state that individuals need to acquire competence at one level of a developmental process before moving to the next level. Piaget showed that children go through specific developmental stages in their intellectual abilities, Erikson defined the psychosocial stages of growth and development, and Maslow explained a hierarchy of human needs where basic needs (e.g., food and shelter) must be met before working on higher level needs (e.g., social connections and self-actualization). In addition, Rogers contributed the concept of learner-centered care in which the patient learns to make decisions and solve problems (Hunt, 1997; Allender & Spradley, 2001).

Adult learning theory provides important information for health education. This theory holds that motivation to learn is based on four assumptions (Knowles, Holton, Swanson, 1998):

1. Adults perceive themselves to be self-directed: They want to have a say in what they learn.
2. Adults have a variety of life experiences and are insulted if these experiences are ignored: The wise teacher will build on these experiences.

3. Adults learn better when they see an immediate need: They are goal directed.
4. Timing education to coincide with an immediate need is more effective because the learner will see the immediate goal and be ready to learn.

### ■ Behavior Change Theory

Theories that specifically address behavior change and health education incorporate ideas from these learning theories. **Behavior change theories** provide direction for nurses who teach in a variety of situations. A brief overview of some of these theories is provided in Table 15-2.

---

**Table 15-2**    Overview of Selected Theories about Health Behavior

| Theory and Key Components | Case Study |
|---|---|
| **■ Health belief model:** Individuals are more likely to take action to improve health if:<br>  They perceive themselves to be at risk for a problem (susceptibility)<br>  The problem is seen as serious enough to warrant action (severity, perceived threat)<br>  The expected benefits of the action outweigh the anticipated costs (e.g., in terms of overcoming barriers related to time, effort, money)<br>  There is a personal sense of ability to perform the required actions (self-efficacy) (Mirotznik, Feldman, & Stein, 1995; Rosenstock, 1990) | Nina's mother and sister both died of breast cancer. Nina took care of her mother during the terminal phases of the disease, and she has told friends, "That was the most horrible thing I ever had to do." Nina was concerned about her own risk, so she talked to her nurse practitioner (NP). The NP gave Nina information about breast cancer, did a breast examination, scheduled Nina for a mammogram, and taught Nina how to do breast self-examination (BSE).<br>**Follow-up:** Nina sees breast cancer as a terrible disease, and she feels that she may be at risk. She is motivated to protect her health but has trouble remembering to do BSE. Doing it actually frightens her: What if she should find a lump? At her next clinic visit, her NP provides Nina with a chart, watches her do BSE in the office, and discusses her concerns about finding a lump. The NP is able to assure Nina that she is doing everything right. Nina establishes a habit of BSE that works for her. |
| **■ Harm reduction model:** Health risks can be decreased by having patients ask, What is healthier, safer, or less risky than what I am doing now? and Which steps am I willing and able to take to be healthier, safer, or less risky? Basic principles include the following:<br>  Most people are competent to make informed decisions about health behaviors; they are the only ones who know what will work for them in their specific situations.<br>  Needs are diverse and can be met in diverse ways; offering people a spectrum of potential behaviors is better than demanding that they adopt an absolute requirement.<br>  Incremental steps that provide chances for success work better than trying to make large, difficult changes where the risk of failure is high.<br>  People may need social support, education, referrals, and assistance to make changes (Bradley-Springer, 1996; Brocato & Wagner, 2003). | Bob, who smokes two packs of cigarettes a day, arrives at Occupational Health for his annual physical. He tells the nurse that he exercises regularly and feels "as healthy as a horse." He denies any smoking-related problems, saying, "Smoking is my only vice and I really like it. It relaxes me. I tried to stop smoking once and it was a disaster, so why bother? But I am worried about smoking around my kids—they've been sick a lot lately." The nurse asks, "What do you think would be healthier for your kids?" Bob lists ideas ranging from quitting smoking altogether to not smoking in the house. The nurse then asks, "Which of these things do you think would work best for you?" Bob decides to try smoking only in his office at home where "the kids can't come anyway."<br>**Follow-up:** The nurse helped Bob explore his options without taking over and telling him what to do. He was then able to choose a behavior that he thought would work in his situation. Bob sees the nurse several months later and says, "Hey, you know how we talked about smoking only in my office to protect my kids? Well, it's working real well. The kids haven't been sick as often and I'm not smoking as much either. I'm down to a pack and a half a day." By helping Bob see his options and by not demanding that he quit smoking, the nurse gave him the support he needed to make positive changes. Bob will now feel good about talking to the nurse if he wants to make further changes. |
| **■ Goal-setting theory:** Setting goals can help people change health-related behaviors by focusing effort, persistence, and concentration on the goal. The following steps are used:<br>  Determine the patient's commitment to change.<br>  Analyze the tasks required to make changes: Complex tasks need to be broken down into subgoals (strategic analysis); simple tasks can be motivated by a simple goal.<br>  Assess the patient's self-efficacy for performing required behaviors and help with skill development as needed.<br>  Goals should be difficult enough to require significant effort; they should be optimistic as well as realistic.<br>  Provide feedback on progress (Strecher et al., 1995). | At her last dental checkup, Ana's dentist pointed out that she had beginning gum disease and suggested that Ana start flossing. Ana said, "I know I should floss. I know how to do it. I floss for 2 to 3 days, but then I miss a day and I give up. I don't want to lose all my teeth like my mother did. I just can't keep it up." The dentist suggests that Ana set a goal of flossing every other day.<br>**Follow-up:** Ana was committed to making a change and already possessed the required skills. By suggesting a specific, attainable goal, the dentist provided additional motivation. At her next checkup Ana says, "It worked! I'm flossing almost every day now. When I miss a day it's not that big a deal because I know I will be able to floss the next day." During her oral examination, the dentist is able to tell Ana that her gums look much better. |

**Table 15-2    Overview of Selected Theories about Health Behavior—Cont'd**

| Theory and Key Components | Case Study |
|---|---|
| ■ **Theory of reasoned action:** Behavioral intention to act is based on a combination of the following:<br>  Personal beliefs and evaluations about what will happen if the behavior is used (perceived chance of success)<br>  Personal attitudes and values about the behavior<br>  Feelings about what key people (family, friends, healthcare providers) in the person's life think about the behavior<br>  Motivation to change behavior (Carter, 1990)<br>  All things being equal, people are expected to act in accordance with their intentions (Miller, Wikoff, & Hiatt, 1992). | Sue, a nursing student, has been dating Jack for 2 years. They plan to get married after she graduates. They have discussed having a family and agree that they do not want children for several years. Sue and Jack want to become sexually active. They visit the Student Health Center, where a nurse explains birth control options. Jack encourages Sue to use birth control pills (BCPs). Sue is worried because some of her friends have told her that BCPs caused them to gain weight.<br>**Follow-up:** Although Sue is worried about weight gain, she believes that BCPs are effective and easy to use. She is clear that she does not currently want a pregnancy. She has Jack's support. Sue rarely misses taking her vitamin pills, so she is sure that she can remember to take the pills every day. This model predicts that Sue is likely to use BCPs consistently and correctly. |
| ■ **Social learning theory:** Individual behavior, personal factors, and the environment create a triad of components that interact to influence health behaviors:<br>  A change in one component of the triad has an effect on all components (reciprocal determinism).<br>  Personal factors include behavioral capability, self-control, self-efficacy, internal reinforcements, emotional coping response, and a belief that performing a behavior will lead to expected outcomes.<br>  The environment (everything external to the individual) and the situation (the individual's perception of the environment) provide opportunities to observe behaviors performed by others in the environment (vicarious learning) (Perry, Baranowski, & Parcel, 1990). | Jose is a depressed 13-year-old who just entered a new school. He hasn't made any friends at the new school, a problem he blames on being 20 pounds overweight. The people Jose admires most at school all seem to be thin. He also notices that they are active in after-school activities. Jose's mother reminds him that he is a good swimmer and encourages him to join the swim team.<br>**Follow-up:** Jose's desire to lose weight is influenced by the rewards that he sees being given to slim people. His perception of weight and his emotional response to it create a desire to change that is supported by his mother and his swimming ability. Jose knows that swimming can help. He tries out for the team and discovers that he can do the butterfly stroke better than anyone else. He joins the team, and in addition to exercising regularly and losing weight, Jose makes new friends and develops a more optimistic outlook. |
| ■ **Diffusion theory:** New ideas, practices, or services (innovations) to improve health move from a resource (innovation developer) to the population (innovation users or adopters).<br>  Diffusion is more likely to occur if the innovation is cost-efficient, low risk, simple, flexible, and compatible with the social, economic, and value systems into which it is introduced. Innovations that are reversible (I can go back to where I was if I don't like it) and appear to be better than currently used methods have a better chance of being adopted.<br>  Diffusion can fail if the innovation does not work, if information about the innovation is not communicated well, if the potential user does not have the necessary resources for implementation, or if the innovation is in opposition to the user's value system. In addition, there may be a problem if components of the implementation process are abbreviated. An example of this would be when education about the innovation is omitted to save money. Maintenance of an innovation takes additional effort; without this, the adopted program can lose momentum and fade away (Orlandi, Landers, Weston, & Haley, 1990). | Injection drug users (IDUs) who do not share equipment to inject drugs are not at risk of infection with blood-borne diseases such as hepatitis B, hepatitis C, and human immunodeficiency virus (HIV). Activists in Metrotown, a community of 300,000, wanted to implement a needle and syringe exchange program (N/SEP) so that IDUs would have access to sterile injecting equipment. They gathered support from the city council, the health department, and law enforcement before setting up N/SEP sites around town. During the first week, only two IDUs brought in equipment to exchange.<br>**Follow-up:** Activists (resource) did a good job in Metrotown of involving the established power systems. No doubt they convinced all of these entities that N/SEPs would be cost-effective, simple, reversible, and better than allowing used injecting equipment to accumulate on the streets of the city. The activists were less effective in communicating the benefits of N/SEPs to the intended users of the program. IDUs need to know that obtaining sterile equipment will decrease the risk of disease, will be easily accessible, and will not put them at risk for being targeted by the police. Although Metrotown has made a difficult public health decision, it will not be successful unless the innovation diffuses to the intended users. |
| ■ **Social marketing theory:** Public acceptance of programs to improve health can be enhanced through marketing techniques. Marketing functions on a number of well-developed principles:<br>  Participants are offered benefits that are valued as being worth the cost (e.g., measured in effort, money, time). The consumer (patient) is the central concern. | Everyone at Russell High School (RHS) is shocked when three students, all with blood alcohol levels over the legal limit, are killed in a car accident. The principal forms a committee of students, teachers, and administrators to develop a program to decrease drunk driving. After assessing the situation at RHS, the committee proposes a plan to encourage the use of designated drivers. The program is kicked off at an assembly where student leaders (athletes, class officers, cheerleaders) describe the program. They all wear T-shirts that say, "I care about my friends. I'm a designated driver." Students are regularly reminded about the program in newspaper articles, intercom announcements, and student-lead discussions in homeroom classes. |

*(continues)*

**Table 15-2**   Overview of Selected Theories about Health Behavior—Cont'd

| Theory and Key Components | Case Study |
| --- | --- |
| Communication (in the form of advertising, public relations, direct marketing, promotion, and face-to-face encounters) is the key to getting information to the consumer.<br><br>The marketing process has six stages that occur in a cycle: (1) analysis; (2) planning; (3) development, testing, and refinement of the plan; (4) implementation; (5) assessment of effectiveness; and (6) feedback to analysis (completing the cycle).<br><br>Marketing strategies must be modified to function in situations in which social issues and health are the central concerns (Novelli, 1990). | **Follow-up:** RHS used marketing strategies focused on consumers (students) to develop a program that would meet the objective to decrease drunk driving. Although the adults on the planning committee had some reservations about a program that seemed to condone drinking, they paid attention to the analysis provided by student representatives and approved the program. A survey done 3 months later showed that 40% of RHS students had been designated drivers, resulting in a significant decrease in drunk driving rates. An additional, unforeseen benefit was a decrease in the overall rate of drinking, a direct result of designated driving being seen as "cool." |

The transtheoretical model, so called because it borrows from many other theories, provides new and helpful insights for health education. The central premise of the transtheoretical model is that people progress through a series of stages when they attempt to change behaviors. There are five stages of change: precontemplative, contemplative, preparation, action, and maintenance (Petty, Barden, & Wheeler, 2002). Progression through the stages is rarely linear. People will change their minds, will hesitate, and may relapse several times before behavior change is permanent. Ten different processes are used to enhance progression through the stages of change:

1. Consciousness raising (increasing the level of awareness)
2. Dramatic relief (experiencing and expressing feelings)
3. Environmental reevaluation (assessing how the environment affects the situation)
4. Self-reevaluation (assessing how a person thinks and feels about the situation)
5. Self-liberation (believing in the ability to change)
6. Helping relationships (caring and trusting relationships)
7. Social liberation (seeing social changes that support personal changes)
8. Counterconditioning (substituting more healthy behaviors for less healthy behaviors)
9. Stimulus control (restructuring the environment)
10. Reinforcement management (getting rewards)

MEDIA MOMENT

### *Good Will Hunting* (1997)
Will Hunting is a genius who's living a rough life in South Boston, while being employed at a prestigious college in Cambridge as a janitor. He's discovered by a Fields Medal–winning professor, who tries to get Will to turn his life around with the help of Sean Maguire, as Will begins to realize that there's more to himself than he thinks there is.

Table 15-3 gives an overview of the transtheoretical model, including examples of the 10 processes and interventions appropriate in each stage.

## The Health Education Process

**Health education** is a process of planned teaching and support activities that help people learn (Spellbring, 1991). The education process follows the format of the nursing process, including assessment, planning, implementation, and evaluation (Rankin & Stallings, 2001; Yu et al., 2007). While these steps are being taken, meticulous documentation should occur. The next section presents detailed information about each step in the education process, but before that, some important general points about education need to be made.

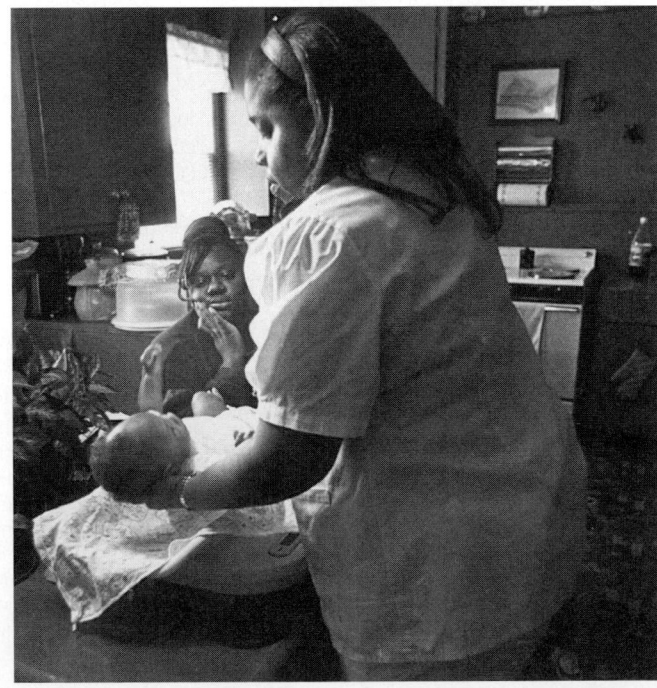

Nurse in the home setting educates new mother about newborn care.

**Table 15-3** Overview of the Transtheoretical Model (Also Known as the Stages of Change Theory)

| Stage: Patient's Perspective | Case Study and Interventions |
|---|---|
| ■ **Precontemplative:** Unaware of or unwilling to consider the problem; defensive about the change issue, resistant to information about the behavior, and reluctant to initiate a behavior change program; not considering change within the next 6 months; has little confidence in ability to change; sees many reasons not to change | During a routine physical, Sam, a 26-year-old lawyer, says, "You know, I was listening to the radio on the way over here and a woman was talking about having AIDS (consciousness raising). This whole thing scares me (dramatic relief). It's not just gay guys anymore. I know that I've had some risks, but the things I do are a part of my life and the people I hang with (environmental reevaluation)." <br> **Stage-specific interventions:** Raise awareness of the issue through community-appropriate public education and media programs. Provide information and feedback to increase individual awareness of physical, social, economic, and psychological problems related to the commission or omission of specific behaviors. Discuss the positive aspects of change. Do not spend time discussing details of specific change tactics or programs: You're wasting your time if it is clear that the patient is not ready to think about changing. |
| ■ **Contemplative:** Ambivalent; responds with "Yes, but . . ."; may see reasons to change as well as reasons to remain the same; indecisive, aware that a problem exists and more open to information, but still unsure of ability to change; intends to change behavior within next 6 months | Sam's nurse encourages him to continue talking about his concerns and those behaviors that make him think he has been at risk. He says, "Well, I have some crazy friends. I go out with them every Saturday. We compare notes on how much sex we get. We dare each other to do things like using a prostitute or having anal sex or coming on to a gay guy. I'm not proud of some of the things I've done. Maybe I'm getting too old for this (self-reevaluation)." <br> **Stage-specific interventions:** Tip the balance in favor of change. It is important to see this stage as the time when the patient will develop a commitment to change. It is still too early to look at strategies. The aim is to analyze risks and rewards of the behavior and to provide information. Clarify goals and discuss incentives to change. It is now time to emphasize negative aspects of not changing. A discussion of the risk for harm is appropriate. |
| ■ **Preparation:** Expresses desire to do something to initiate change; some experimentation with new behaviors may already be occurring; thinks change may be possible; seriously planning change within next 30 days but has not set specific goals | When asked how this makes him feel, Sam responds by saying, with a sigh, "I guess I should think about being more careful. I don't want to get anything bad, especially AIDS. I need to change my act (self-liberation)." <br> **Stage-specific interventions:** Now is the time to get down to details. Help the patient find change strategies that are acceptable, accessible, appropriate, and effective. Encourage the patient to experiment with a strategy: "Try it next time, see how you like it," or "Find out how your family/partner/friends react when you do it." Be available to the patient to discuss issues related to moving into the action stage. Help the patient establish specific objectives. In Sam's case, this could be limiting nights out with his friends to once a month. |
| ■ **Action:** Engages in action to create desired change; feels developing confidence in self-efficacy; thinks reasons to change outweigh reasons not to; behavior modified to meet goal(s) for 6 months | Over the course of the next 6 months, Sam and the nurse meet several times to discuss his progress. During this time, Sam says, "I've talked about this with my friend Mia. She just listens and never acts like I'm a bad person even when I tell her bad things I've done (helping relationship). Since I've started talking about it, I've had people tell me that I'm right to be concerned and that I should be more careful—even some of my buddies agree (social liberation)." Sam begins to take specific actions to decrease his risks. He begins to use condoms and decides to have sex only when he wants to and not "on a dare" (counterconditioning). <br> **Stage-specific interventions:** Be aware that this is not an easy process. Support change efforts. Patients will need continuing encouragement, help with problem solving, and a place to simply vent frustrations. |
| ■ **Maintenance:** Challenged to continue change; feels expanding self-efficacy; continues behavior change for more than 6 months | As Sam becomes comfortable with his new behaviors, he reports that other things are changing. He says, "I realized that my problems were related to my friends. They didn't understand why I wanted to change. They called me a wimp. So I decided to quit hanging out with them (stimulus control). The good thing is that I feel better about myself. Mia even told me that she's noticed that I seem happier (reinforcement management)." <br> **Stage-specific interventions:** Help the patient maintain change. Problem solving and unconditional support for the patient are extremely important during this stage. Relapse prevention efforts can include interactive discussions, role-playing, and "what if" sessions in which the patient identifies risks for relapse and develops workable strategies. |

*(continues)*

**Table 15-3** Overview of the Transtheoretical Model (Also Known as the Stages of Change Theory)—Cont'd

| Stage: Patient's Perspective | Case Study and Interventions |
|---|---|
| ■ **Relapse (not a stage):** An important event that can occur at any time in the change process; if relapse occurs, the patient may express anger and question ability to maintain change; may be embarrassed or ashamed; may blame self or others (including healthcare providers) for the relapse | Sam returns to clinic a year later. When asked about how he's doing, he blurts out, "I blew it. I ran into Jake a few weeks ago and we went for a drink. Before I knew it, we'd picked up a couple of women. I ended up in a strange apartment and no one ever thought about using condoms. I'm really embarrassed about this—especially after I made such a big deal out of being careful with my friends. Maybe I wasn't meant to be safe. Maybe I'm supposed to get the clap or HIV or something else that's just as bad. I can't even face Mia."  **Stage-specific interventions:** Patients may get "stuck" in relapse if they resort to self-incrimination or self-blame. Help the patient renew the change process at an earlier stage without getting demoralized. Explain that relapse is common and may occur many times before behavior change is permanent. Point out specific instances of success that show the patient's abilities to change. Provide referral to needed services. Sam, for instance, may need a work up for sexually transmitted disease.  Sam's nurse helps him understand the circumstance of his relapse: meeting Jake, having a drink, meeting the women, and so on. Sam and his nurse discuss the situation and role-play a similar situation so that he will feel better prepared if this should happen again. Sam also agrees to go to the STD clinic. |

*Source*: Adapted from Bradley-Springer, 1996.

Education is patient centered. An important question for the nurse to continually ask is, "How does *this* problem (e.g., diagnosis, stressor, need to change) affect *this* patient?" To truly make the process patient centered, nurses must remember that people live in complex social and culturally defined environments. Therefore, the involvement of family and significant others can help promote learning. In some cases, family involvement is essential, especially when health education is directed to children, patients with sensory deficits, or patients who are physically unable to perform the necessary skills (Yu et al., 2007). In general, involving others can provide social and emotional supports that help people make behavior changes (Rankin & Stallings, 2001). Unfortunately, patients do not always have healthy support structures, or they simply may not want others involved. In these cases, the nurse should not force the issue. Instead, referrals to community resources and support groups should be considered.

❝*It does not do to leave a live dragon out of your calculations if you live near him.*❞

—*J. R. R. Tolkien*

### ▮▮ CULTURAL CONNECTION

How are teaching and learning affected by our fast-paced culture? Has personal (one-to-one) teaching become less important with the rise of the Internet? How does this affect the educator role of the nurse?

### ■ Assessment

The task of assessment is to gather information. This can result in a huge amount of information that the nurse uses to determine needs and priorities. Obviously, educational needs cannot be determined without looking at the entire patient. Learning needs evolve from a knowledge of the patient's overall health problems (actual and potential). In most cases, some of the needs discovered through assessment will have a cognitive, skill, or attitudinal component that must be addressed through education (Rankin & Stallings, 2001).

Assessment requires active nurse–patient interaction. This can be time-consuming, but the nurse can use assessment time to develop rapport with the patient and significant others (Redman, 1997, 2008). Building a good working relationship during this phase will increase the amount of information the patient reveals and will make the rest of the education process more enjoyable for both the patient and the nurse. This is especially important in community health settings where nurses need to establish long-term relationships

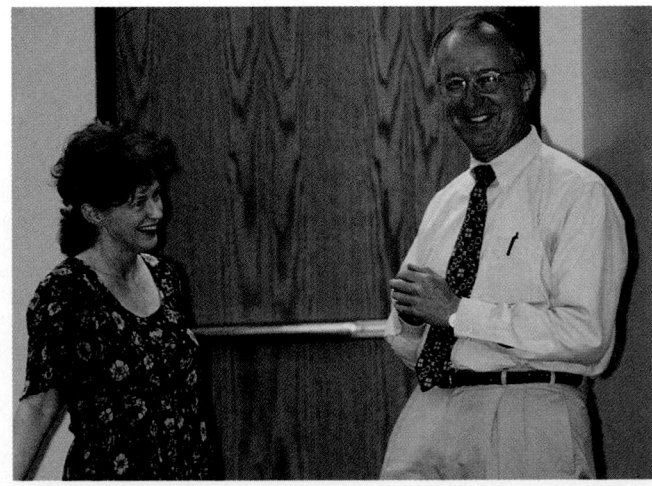

Chapter author Lucy Bradley-Springer and Kevin Morrisroe, RN, do a role-play on risk assessment at a class in New Mexico.

with individuals in the community. Table 15-4 lists some areas that need to be discussed during a health education assessment.

Data can be collected from a variety of sources, including direct observation, patient records, other members of the healthcare team, and professional literature. The best way to get the patient's point of view, however, is through an interactive interview. Patient disclosure of information is enhanced by the following tactics (Rankin & Stallings, 2001):

- *Establish an environment of trust.* This may require some time at the beginning of the conversation. Start by introducing yourself and telling who you are. ("Hi. I'm Faith Diaz, and I'm an RN from the home health agency.") Establish that you have experience in the area you will be addressing with the patient. ("I've been working with people who've had your kind of surgery for 2 years.") Describe the intention of the interview and make it clear that questions are asked to help the patient. As we all know, some of the questions that nurses need to ask can be embarrassing. Assure the patient that there are healthcare reasons for asking each question and that all answers are confidential.
- *Choose the right time.* Be sure that you have time to adequately assess the patient's needs. Ask if this is a good time for the patient. Be sure the patient is not in pain or anxious about an anticipated event. If you know that your time is short, introduce the assessment session by saying, "I know you are anxious about your wound care. I only have 15 minutes to spend with you right now, and I need to ask you a few questions. Your answers will help me plan how I will teach you about your wound. I'll come back this afternoon, and we'll go over everything in detail. Do you think that will work for you?"
- *Choose the right place.* The location of an interview should be comfortable and private. If it is not, the patient (and the nurse) may concentrate more on the room temperature or the hard chairs or the constant interruptions than on the interview. If possible, do the interview on the patient's "home turf." This can be in the patient's home or a private room at the clinic. Asking questions in a known environment helps the patient feel safe (Hunt, 1997).
- *Use open-ended questions.* Going through a list of "yes/no" questions does not provide the depth of information needed to develop effective, individualized teaching plans. Asking the patient to describe her problems doing exercises after a mastectomy, for example, will get a lot of those "yes/no" questions answered without your even asking them. The patient will also benefit from the experience of telling her story to an interested listener. Remember, patients (as adult learners) have unique perspectives that they need to share with you and that you should build into your teaching plan.
- *Use active listening skills.* Ask for clarification, summarize, and use open body language (nod and smile; do not act like you have to leave). These listening skills

## Table 15-4   Assessment Variables

| What to Assess | Assessment Questions |
|---|---|
| ■ Patient understanding of the problem in question | What do you think is the cause of this problem? |
| | Why do you think it is happening now? |
| ■ Patient perception of need to change | How does the problem affect you? |
| | Has this problem limited your activities in any way? |
| ■ Motivation to change: severity of problem and risks caused by the problem | How severe is the problem? Is it a short-term or a long-term problem? What harm could this problem cause you? |
| | What are the two to three main difficulties that you have because of this problem? |
| | What do you fear most about the problem? |
| | Why do you want to solve this problem? |
| ■ Readiness to change | What would you like to do about the problem in the next few days (weeks)? |
| | What are the most important things that you would like to have happen? |
| ■ Self-efficacy | How do you usually approach problems? |
| | How would you like to approach this problem? |
| | What do you think you can do about the problem? |
| | Have you tried to deal with this problem before? If so, what did you do and how did it turn out? |
| ■ Perceived benefits to change | How would you feel if you solved this problem? |
| | If you didn't have the problem, what would be better in your life? |
| ■ Perceived barriers to change | What has kept you from dealing with this problem in the past? |
| | Do you see things that may prevent your dealing with this problem? If so, what are they? |
| ■ Psychosocial issues | Who gives you the most support? Would you like her or him to be in on our teaching sessions? |
| | Also assess housing, economic status, educational background, community resources, cultural and religious contributions to health care, native language, and so on. |
| ■ Learning skills | How do you learn best? Would you like reading materials or videotapes or group sessions or private counseling or . . . ? |

*Source*: Adapted from Kreuter & Strecher, 1996; Palank, 1991; Rankin & Stallings, 2001; and Redman, 1997.

enhance interactions and ensure that you understand the patient's meanings.

- *Assess reading and literacy level of patient.* Include an evaluation of the patient's literacy level. Various tools are available, such as SMOG (Cutill, 2006; Demir, Ozsaker, & Ilce, 2008; McLaughlin, 1969).

When the interview is complete, summarize the main points and thank the patient for spending time with you. Tell the patient what you intend to do with the information and describe the next steps in the planning process. If you cannot continue the process at this time, tell the patient when you will return.

---

 **ETHICAL CONNECTION**

A high school student has requested information on pregnancy testing in the community. As a school nurse, you provide her with this information and educate her about the differences and quality of tests. The next day, the student's mother phones and tells you that she has found a pregnancy test kit in her daughter's room. The mother wants to know if you gave it to her daughter. How would you respond?

---

## ■ Planning

During planning, the nurse and patient discuss learning needs and potential goals. This is a negotiation process: The nurse provides input that the patient uses to make decisions about specific interventions. The result of this process is a list of learning objectives. In most cases, the list will not be too long, but some patients have many problems. In that case, it is best to prioritize the list by having the patient choose those problems (1) that are most pressing (cause the most discomfort for the patient) and (2) the patient is most willing to work on (an estimate of readiness). Limiting the teaching session to one or two objectives is less intimidating than trying to make a large number of changes at the same time (Kreuter & Strecher, 1996).

Based on the literacy assessment, the nurse should plan education appropriate for reading and comprehension level. For example, some patients may respond to visual materials presented according to reading level while others may prefer detailed explanations in written form. For example, reading materials can be assessed for readability using many word processing programs for word count and using the widely used and accepted SMOG (Simple Measure of Gobbledygook) assessment tool online (http://www.harrymclaughlin.com/SMOG.htm). McLaughlin developed the easy to use readability formula in 1969 and the tool is now available in an online version (McLaughlin, 1969). In health education materials, one size does not fit all (Cutill, 2006; Demir, Ozsaker, & Ilce, 2008; McLaughlin, 1969).

**Learning goals and objectives** are established in the initial part of the planning phase. Goals and objectives provide an agreed-upon direction for implementation and a guide for evaluation. Goals are broad statements of the desired outcome: "Jason will manage insulin administration to control his blood sugar," for example. Objectives are specific, detailed statements. They describe behaviors that will help meet a goal. They describe what the patient will do, define how it will be done, and prescribe time frames for task completion. Objectives for Jason could include the following:

1. Before he is discharged in 3 days, Jason will be able to list the signs and symptoms of high and low blood sugar.
2. By tomorrow, Jason will be able to test his blood for glucose with the equipment he will use at home.
3. By the day before discharge, Jason will be able to use a prescribed sliding scale to accurately draw up and inject insulin in the ordered doses at the ordered times.
4. Within a week after discharge, Jason will describe the benefits of controlling his blood sugar.

Notice that the objectives are specific and measurable. We will be able to tell when Jason accomplishes each objective (Rankin & Stallings, 2001).

Also notice that the objectives do not all look alike. That is because they address three different **domains of learning** (Redman, 1997). Some objectives refer to things that people need to know. These are called *cognitive objectives*. In Jason's case, the first objective asks him to know the signs of hyperglycemia and hypoglycemia. *Psychomotor objectives* refer to skills or behaviors. Jason will need to manipulate equipment (a skill) to meet the next two objectives. The final objective addresses an attitude: We want Jason to verbalize a positive outlook on his abilities. This objective occurs in the *affective* domain.

Knowing the type of objective helps the nurse and patient decide on teaching and learning methods. Jason may be able to learn the symptoms of hyperglycemia from a brochure, for instance, but he will need to practice drawing

---

 **A Good Read**

## The Alchemist (1993)

*By Paola Coelho, translated by Alan R. Clarke, New York: Harper Collins.*

This tale of Santiago, a shepherd boy who dreams of seeing the world, is compelling in its own right, but gains resonance through the many lessons Santiago learns during his adventures. He journeys from Spain to Morocco in search of worldly success. Eventually he makes his way to Egypt, where a fateful encounter with an alchemist brings Santiago at last to self-understanding and spiritual enlightenment. The story has the comic charm, dramatic tension, and psychological intensity of a fairy tale, but it's full of specific wisdom as well—about becoming self-empowered, overcoming depression, and believing in dreams.

**Table 15-5**    Domains of Learning

| Domain | Goals and Objectives | Teaching Methods | Application Case: Goal is to encourage breastfeeding in pregnant women who attend a low-income clinic |
|---|---|---|---|
| **COGNITIVE SUBDOMAINS** | | | |
| Knowledge (to know) | To state, to list, to define, to recall, to name, to repeat | Lecture, one-on-one instruction, programmed instruction, videos or audio tapes, reading materials, questions and answers | Display breastfeeding posters in prominent places around the clinic. Run a continuous video on breastfeeding in the waiting room. Leave brochures and printed materials in examination rooms. Plan a series of lectures at a convenient time for patients. |
| Comprehension (to understand) | To explain, to label, to describe, to interpret | Lecture, one-on-one instruction, programmed instruction, video program, reading materials, learning guides, study questions | Arrange face-to-face sessions during prenatal visits; ask if patient has questions or concerns. Follow up educational activities by asking, "What difference could breastfeeding make for your baby?" |
| Application (to use) | To illustrate, to apply, to give examples | Demonstration, group discussion, simulation exercises, games, role-play, clinical practice | Demonstrate breast care and the process of breastfeeding using a simulation model or a video. Encourage partner participation in education. |
| Analysis (to identify elements) | To compare, to contrast, to differentiate, to debate, to question | Group discussion, games, group interaction, simulation exercises, role-play, case studies | Arrange small group sessions where women can discuss concerns about breastfeeding. Role-play issues that emerge from group discussions. |
| Synthesis (to use in new ways) | To assemble, to prepare, to create, to design, to formulate | Group projects, group discussion, simulation exercises, games, role-play, case studies | Invite women from the community who are successfully breastfeeding to discuss the process in small groups of pregnant women. Support breastfeeding efforts after delivery. |
| Evaluation (to judge) | To assess, to justify, to measure, to choose | Group discussion, guided imagery, role-play, self-evaluation worksheet | Ask women to share success stories related to breastfeeding. Provide questionnaire that helps patient assess values and fears about breastfeeding; follow up with a one-on-one discussion. |
| Psychomotor (to perform) | To assemble, to demonstrate, to control, to manipulate | Demonstration, practice with supervision, independent practice, return demonstration, role-play, simulation, clinical experience | Demonstrate breast care and the process of breastfeeding using a simulation model or a video. Provide guidance and positive reinforcement to women after delivery as they initiate breastfeeding with newborn. |
| Affective (to feel) | To tolerate, to accept, to defend, to adopt, to appreciate, to value | Group discussion, group project, simulation exercises, games, role-play, life experience | Encourage patient involvement. Reinforce positive statements about breastfeeding. Encourage attendance at group sessions where breastfeeding is discussed. |

up insulin and injecting himself to really learn those skills. You cannot learn to give an injection by reading about it! Table 15-5 provides an in-depth overview of the domains of learning and teaching methods appropriate to each domain.

The planning stage is not complete until the patient agrees to the goals, objectives, and teaching methods. Although Jason's plan looks good on the surface, he may have a morbid fear of sticking himself. In that case, the objectives and plan would need to be changed to have someone in his household learn the "sticking" skills (injections and finger sticks), but Jason should be able to meet the other objectives and may eventually overcome his fears and learn the "sticking" skills himself.

MEDIA MOMENT

**Dead Poets Society (1989)**
Painfully shy Todd Anderson has been sent to the school where his popular older brother was valedictorian. His roommate, Neil, although exceedingly bright and popular, is very much under the thumb of his overbearing father. The two, along with their other friends, meet Professor Keating, their new English teacher, who tells them of the Dead Poets Society, and encourages them to go against the status quo. Each, in their own way, does so, and is changed for life. Robin Williams won an Academy Award for Best Actor in 1990 for his performance as Professor Keating.

## ■ Implementation

During implementation, the nurse and the patient use information from the assessment and planning stages to make decisions about learning activities. Learning activities must focus on the established objectives. Interventions are tailored to the patient's needs and abilities. Teaching plans are then put into action, but this is not a static process. The nurse continually observes and asks for feedback to track progress. The nurse should discuss any problems with the patient, modifying the plan as needs change. This is called *formative evaluation*: It helps the teacher adjust the format of the education as the teaching progresses. Box 15-1 provides some general pointers to guide teaching.

## ■ Evaluation

Evaluation is a process of gathering information to assess the extent to which learning objectives have been met—or not met. There are a number of ways to evaluate learning, but all evaluation methods should be based on the

Groups may come together for a specific purpose, such as child care.

---

### BOX 15-1

**Pointers for Health Education**

- Design teaching based on assessments of individual patients: needs, ability, knowledge base, learning styles, expectations, culture, language, readiness to learn, and so on.
- Develop educational objectives with input from the learner. Validate that the objectives are relevant to the learner's needs. Objectives serve as the basis for instruction and evaluation.
- Create a learning environment. It should be comfortable and free of distractions.
- Keep things simple.
- Focus on one issue at a time. Keep learning sessions short. Concentrate on outcomes that will be immediately obvious (e.g., feeling and looking better because of exercise rather than the more distant issue of preventing heart disease).
- Be sure written materials are appropriate. Keep sentences short. Use words a layperson can understand. Define medical words in simple terms. Use a font style and size that are easy to read. Use pictures and diagrams to clarify concepts.
- Be specific. "Lose weight," for instance, is not as effective as "Lose 2 pounds this week."
- Avoid threatening messages that generate fear. Mild anxiety enhances learning, but high fear levels can lead to denial, tuning out the message, or inability to concentrate.
- Explain what you will be teaching and why it is important. This provides an "advance organizer" to keep session centered on the topic.
- Provide for success. Divide learning tasks into sequential learning units that start with easier concepts and build to more difficult ones. Encourage success at each level before progressing to more difficult tasks. This enhances self-efficacy and personal satisfaction.

- Use a variety of teaching methods. People learn in different ways, and a combination of methods reinforces learning. Varying methods also keeps people involved.
- Provide visual learning materials. Seeing as well as hearing enhances retention.
- Show the patient what is expected. Model behaviors to demonstrate how things are done.
- Skills (both verbal and physical) require practice. (Examples: role-play communication skills, use a plastic model to teach self-catheterization techniques, use syringes to practice drawing up insulin.)
- Involve all the senses in practice sessions. This reinforces learning on several levels.
- Provide immediate feedback that praises or corrects specific details during practice sessions. Highlight successes and express honest confidence in the learner's abilities to accomplish learning objectives. If you have doubts about the learner's abilities, do not give false praise. Instead, reassess with the learner and develop a new teaching plan.
- Develop mechanisms for support. Include family and friends in education as possible and as acceptable to the patient. Support groups that focus on specific issues have been shown to enhance learning while encouraging positive change and maintenance of newly developed behaviors.
- Discuss resources for further information and/or practice.
- Review major points of each learning session. Discuss plans for follow-up, reinforcement, and expansion of learning experience.
- Keep learners involved: Ask for feedback and evaluation during teaching and learning.

*Source*: Adapted from Allender & Spradley, 2001; and Damrosch, 1991.

learning objectives. Objectives that are written with appropriate action verbs will tell you how to evaluate outcomes. An objective that says the learner will be able to list the steps in cardiopulmonary resuscitation (CPR), for instance, can be evaluated by asking her to write those steps on a piece of paper. If the objective states that the learner will be able to perform CPR, however, you will need to watch her perform the technique on a mannequin. Learning can be evaluated through quizzes, direct observation, physiological measures (Is the patient's blood pressure lower?), patient self-report and self-monitoring, or input from other healthcare team members (Redman, 1997, 2008).

The outcome of evaluation is a list of learning that has been accomplished as well as a list of those learning objectives that have not been met. *Summative evaluation* is a summary of what has occurred and is usually used as a summary of patient accomplishments when the nurse is closing out a case. More often, formative evaluation is used. As with the nursing process, information from formative evaluation feeds back to the assessment phase, and the teaching process repeats itself with new objectives, plans, and interventions until the patient and the nurse are satisfied with the final result (Rankin & Stallings, 2001).

## Health Education in Communities

All nurses, regardless of work site or specialty, are expected to teach individuals and their families about health-related matters. Nurses who work in the community have additional opportunities to help people change behaviors for the improved health of aggregate populations. The following section describes teaching efforts that can occur in community settings, including individual, group, and community education.

### ■ Individuals, Families, and Groups

People live in groups, and the family is the most basic social group. For purposes of this discussion, the *family* is what the patient says it is. For some, family members are related by blood or marriage. For others, family members include close social (and sometimes sexual) ties with people who are not otherwise related. Families may be supportive or not supportive. They may be healthy or unhealthy. They may be large and extended or small and nuclear. Some people have rejected or cannot identify a family; others have been rejected by their families. Regardless of family process or content, the individual is greatly influenced by this first social unit (see Chapters 30 and 31).

A *group*, by comparison, is defined as people who interact as individuals to reach a common goal (Rankin & Stallings, 2001). Groups may come together for short periods to address one purpose (e.g., a bereavement support group) or they may be more stable over time with larger purposes (e.g., a local unit of Alcoholics Anonymous) (see Chapter 18). Families and groups are important entities for community

health nurses to recognize. Families and groups may need direct education (e.g., the nurse teaches a parent group how to take an infant's temperature or how to recognize the signs of adolescent suicide), or they may need to be included as a support system for an individual patient (e.g., the nurse includes family members in a discussion of safe food preparation for an immune-suppressed child). This chapter looks at two specific issues related to community education of individuals, families, and groups: discharge teaching and community-based teaching.

 **GLOBAL CONNECTION**

As a travel nurse, you are assigned to a public health department in a developing country with a low literacy rate. How will you adjust your role as educator in this setting?

### Discharge Teaching

**Discharge teaching** happens in formal inpatient and outpatient care settings, but it provides a basis for community care. Discharge teaching has become more complex in recent years because of changes in the way health care is provided. People are now discharged from acute care settings earlier, with less recuperation time. More procedures, including some that are quite complicated, are being done in outpatient settings. Hospitalization after delivery is usually less than 48 hours. All of these changes have led to people going home with more complex medications, treatments, pain, and anxiety. In addition, because the patient spends less time in the formal care setting, there is less time for teaching. This is further complicated by the fact that teaching must often happen in the immediate aftermath of a procedure, a time when patients tend to be most anxious and least able to attend to educational messages (Hunt, 1997). Discharge teaching also occurs in community settings such as home health, occupational settings, and school settings as nurses educate individuals about managing their own care.

Nurses can overcome these barriers with careful assessment and planning. If possible, some teaching should take place in the clinic, home, or community before the acute event; preoperative education and prenatal classes are good examples of this. In addition, community resources need to be identified in advance: Is the family willing and able to provide care? Will home health services be required? Are there other options? Assessing these needs and establishing early contacts can ensure that the individual is well prepared. Bringing the needed supports (e.g., responsible family members or home care agencies) in early can decrease education time.

❝*To quit smoking is easy. I've done it hundreds of times.*❞
—*Mark Twain*

❝*Learning is what happens when what you thought would work doesn't.*❞

—*Unknown*

Education can then proceed through the teaching process as discussed earlier. Assessment should include a history of experiences that may influence this event, as well as individual and family coping mechanisms. Planning and implementation should be concise, clear, and supported by written information. Teaching should include demonstrations and return demonstrations for all treatments (e.g., dressing changes) and equipment (e.g., medication pumps). Follow-up telephone calls and referrals to community agencies for more intense follow-up should be scheduled (Hunt, 1997). The bottom line is that patients should not feel that they are on their own at the time of discharge. Ideally, they should feel secure in their own abilities to provide self-care. If this is not possible, patients should know how to arrange for the support they will need at home.

### Community-Based Teaching

Discharge teaching provides information for patients who have been treated in a formal healthcare setting. More and more often, however, people need health education as a part of their daily lives. **Community-based teaching** can be complicated by a number of variables. The home setting itself can be difficult. The nurse will be on the patient's "home turf," and there may be distractions from family members (especially if there are children in the house). In addition, teaching equipment will need to be brought into the house by the nurse, and the nurse may need to address learning needs for a wider range in individuals. Health education in the home must also be carefully coordinated among various care providers. To make matters even more difficult, all this must be done in a limited amount of time (Hunt, 1997). However, there are major advantages to teaching in the patient's home:

- The nurse can assess the patient's environment and make changes in the teaching plan to compensate for problems and to take advantage of strengths.
- The family can be more easily involved.
- The patient will usually be more comfortable in his or her own environment.
- The patient will be learning in the environment in which he or she will be using new information to perform new skills and behaviors.

Once again, application of the teaching process will help the nurse meet education goals. A most important step in community-based education is to keep the patient and significant others involved in the entire process from assessment to evaluation. This helps the nurse address those issues of highest concern, establish trust within the family setting, and provide the basis for further education. Nurses serve as case managers in the community: They are the professionals who are responsible for coordinating information between the patient and a variety of caregivers. In this process, nurses must cover objectives from each of the other care providers and integrate their orders with the needs of the patient and family. To accomplish this complex task, nurses need to be aware of community resources so that they can make appropriate referrals. The result should be that community-based patients feel comfortable with their self-care (or family-care) status. Patients should move toward independent care or toward the knowledge that care will be maintained by trusted family members and/or professional providers (Hunt, 1997).

Mural on the wall of a community shelter in Tallahassee, Florida.

*Got an Alternative?*

A nurse in the educator role will often be placed in situations where patients are more familiar with alternative and complementary therapies than the nurse is. How would you address this issue in a clinical setting?

## ■ Community

Community health learning occurs when knowledge, attitudes, and/or behaviors change within an entire community. Over the past decade, major changes have been made in communities in areas such as seatbelt use, limitations on smoking areas in public spaces, and decreased tolerance of drunk driving. All of these changes came about when individuals in communities stood up and demanded safer and more healthy environments. Changes such as these often require legislative action; at other times, a shift in the community norm is all that has to occur. Nurses have not often taken full advantage of their positions in communities to influence change, but they should. Education and political action are within the realm of what nurses should and can do to improve the health of communities and the individuals in those communities.

Communities consist of groups of people who identify membership in the community. These people share commonalities in language, tradition, ritual, and ceremony. They share values and norms and exert influence over one another. They have emotional connections, common needs, and a commitment to the community to meet those needs. Community may occur within a geographic location (as in a neighborhood or a town) or may be connected by something other than geography (as in ethnic or age-specific groups). Community is defined by all of these connections, so people who merely live in close proximity may not be a community (Israel et al., 1994). An individual may have membership in more than one community and may have to deal with conflicting values from those communities. As you can see, a community has power that can affect **behavior change**. Although community support can be a powerful contribution to individual behavior change, lack of community support may doom an intervention to failure (Bigbee & Jansa, 1991). Table 15-6 gives a case study to illustrate the process of community education.

### Community Assessment

As with individual health education, health education at the community level starts with community assessment. As in individual education, this assessment needs to take into

❝*There are some things you learn best in calm, and some in storm.*❞

—*Willa Cather*

The media is underutilized by health professionals as a way to communicate critical information about a community's health and well-being. In this photo, Governor Haley Barbour of Mississippi speaks to the press about the Hurricane Katrina disaster health problems and plans for recovery.

account the full spectrum of community variables. Individual behaviors take place within the context of community, and understanding this context can help nurses predict both barriers to and supports for behavior change (Israel et al., 1994). The nurse needs a clear idea of what the community is: How do people in the community define *health* and *health care*? What is the norm for nutrition, elimination, exercise, sleep, sexuality, reproduction, and coping with stress? How is intellect supported? How does the community perceive itself? How are roles and relationships established and supported? What does the community value? Which ethnic and cultural identities exist in the community? Which language(s) is(are) spoken? Which ceremonies occur? Which rituals are supported? How does the community share resources? Is there

a sense of shared responsibility (Krozy, 1996)? Nurses can gather this information from community leaders, written histories and records, observations, consultations, and other community members.

Communities, like individuals, experience stressors. These stressors range from daily hassles (as in ongoing arguments from businesses that want to limit government controls) to chronic problems (e.g., homelessness or air pollution) to major events (e.g., the closing of an industry) to cataclysmic events (e.g., an earthquake or food) (Israel et al., 1994). Other community problems can include poverty, overpopulation, social injustice, lack of social organization, overcrowding (Carr, Lhussier, Wilkinson, & Gleadhill, 2008; Krozy, 1996; Yu et al., 2007), a history of powerlessness, and

---

**Table 15-6   Community Education Process Case**

Kris works as a school nurse at Center High School in a moderately sized Midwestern city. At a weekly team meeting, she tells her friend Sam, "I am so frustrated—we have five pregnant girls already this semester." Sam, who works at two middle schools, says, "You think that's bad? I have a case of chlamydia in a sixth grader!" Others add their comments until one says, "We clearly have a problem. What should we do?" The nurses decide to "do something about the risks of teen sexual activity." Because they already know the community well, the nurses decide to assess the problem by listing positive and negative community factors related to the problem of teen sexual activity and to use those assessments to plan interventions.

| Assessment | Planning | Implementation | Evaluation |
|---|---|---|---|
| **Positive factors:** The community has a number of agencies that could be involved, including Planned Parenthood, Big Brothers/Big Sisters, the YMCA, churches, etc. Community schools have good reputations; most students graduate and many go to college. The state department of education supports a sex education curriculum based on harm reduction. School nurses have a ratio of 1:2,000 students. **Negative factors:** The school board (SB) supports and enforces an abstinence-only sex education curriculum as a result of pressure from a few vocal parents and one of the churches in the community. There are limited programs for students who are not succeeding in school and/or extracurricular activities. Most students come from families with working parents, and the majority have several hours of unsupervised time after school. Kris has had a number of students at her school tell her, "I want to get pregnant; it'd be cool." A survey of the nurses reveals 25 known teen pregnancies and 42 known cases of sexually transmitted diseases (STDs) in students over the past 24 months. | The nurses struggle with the question of what to do with the assessment information. After a long brainstorming session, they develop a plan. Each nurse will do the following: ■ Meet with his or her principal(s) to inform and educate about the problem ■ Attend the next two meetings of the SB and ask to have the topic of teen sexuality placed on the agenda ■ Encourage the use of the state's harm reduction curriculum ■ Volunteer to teach sexuality classes in the fifth to twelfth grades ■ Visit two to three community organizations (including churches) to discuss the problem, ask for support, and volunteer assistance to develop after-school programs | The nurses complete their assigned visits to the principals, SB, and local organizations. Each nurse reviews the state sex education curriculum and volunteers to teach classes at his or her assigned school(s). | **Summative evaluation:** All assignments are completed. **Formative evaluation:** All of the principals support the nurses' efforts. One principal asks about sexual abuse in students' families and peer relationships. The SB refuses to add the issue to the agenda. All of the nurses will teach sex education classes, but several principals and health teachers refuse to allow a harm reduction curriculum until approval by the SB. Two churches and the YMCA are interested in setting up sports, games, and homework assistance programs after school. Planned Parenthood wants to develop a peer education program to address pressures to have sex to be "cool." **Follow-up:** The nurses reassess the situation and plan for the next steps. The nurses will do the following: ■ Set up in-service programs for the nurses to learn about teaching a harm reduction curriculum ■ Set up nurse counseling services for any student who wants to discuss issues privately—available to all students, but especially for students in abusive relationships ■ Continue attending SB meetings; encourage principals, teachers, and parents to add their support at those meetings ■ Collaborate with agencies as new programs are developed and encourage other agencies to consider developing their own programs |

Community health nurses have limitless opportunities to educate parents about child care. Enlisting community lay volunteers in collaborative partnerships can be very effective in reaching specific populations.

**❝** *The illiterate of the twenty-first century will not be those who cannot read and write, but those who cannot learn, unlearn, and relearn.* **❞**

—*Alvin Toffler*

tensions created by inequity and discrimination (Israel et al., 1994). All of these contribute to community perceptions of powerlessness. Community empowerment, then, becomes a teaching strategy.

The good news is that communities also provide support for behavior change. The nurse should assess those things that enhance opportunities for education and change. These might include the emotional support given to community members who are trying to effect change. In addition, established agencies and services may already be available to support change. Information dissemination systems may be in place, and respected community members may be willing to sway opinion toward change (Israel et al., 1994).

### Planning for the Community

The main point that needs to be made about community planning should be obvious: Planning requires community involvement (Andrade & Doria-Ortiz, 1995). Shared decision making leads to better acceptance of change, support for the process, and commitment to programs that emerge from the process (Foran & Campanelli, 1995). Involving large portions of the community in planning can be difficult, but it is necessary. Representation should be sought from government, business, service, health care, and religious entities as well as from the individuals who will be targeted by the plan. Input can be gathered in community meetings, focus groups, and interviews with key informants. Opposing views must be sought, acknowledged, and considered in any planning activity (Krozy, 1996). Planning can then progress to setting educational goals and selecting an appropriate theory base, taking into account the strengths and weaknesses of the community.

Common broad-based goals for community health education are to (1) help people change unhealthy, unsafe, or risky behaviors; (2) equalize access to health and support services; and (3) decrease the incidence of preventable conditions that have negative effects on the community (Krozy, 1996). Goals and more specific objectives need to be established and agreed upon during the planning process. Consider using *Healthy People 2010* in this process. It delineates national goals for specific health issues targeted to at-risk populations (DHHS, 2000).

Foran and Campanelli (1995) identified the components of successful community health programs: They are flexible, they use ongoing evaluation to identify design problems as soon as possible, they use evaluation to guide change, they are valued by the community, and they evolve by incorporating new ideas and technologies as change occurs. Planners should understand all of these elements. And remember: Planning should develop teaching interventions as well as evaluation tools.

**❝** *You must learn from the mistakes of others. You can't possibly live long enough to make them all yourself.* **❞**

—*Sam Levenson*

### Implementing Community Plans

Andrade and Doria-Ortiz (1995) encourage an implementation process that helps a community meet its own needs. This requires empowerment of community organizations, adequate resources and services to meet the needs of at-risk community members, and sufficient resources in the healthcare system. Programs and services (especially those targeted to underserved populations) must be available, accessible, acceptable, and accountable. Programs that do not meet these criteria will not succeed.

It is important to remember that community education and change are long-term processes—they do not happen overnight. Even after programs are established, there must be commitment to a continuing process of assessment, planning, implementation, and evaluation. Implementation will be enhanced if the process is participatory (members of the

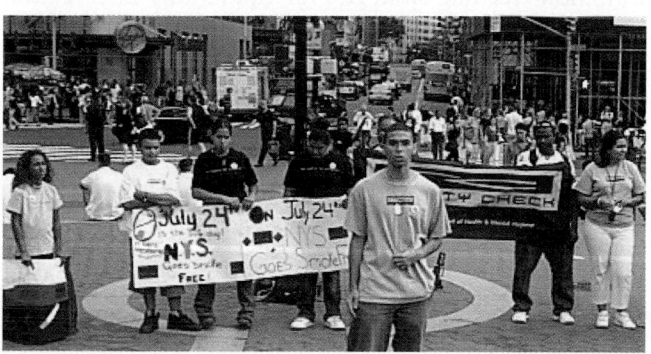

"Never underestimate that a small group of thoughtful, committed people can change the world; indeed, it's the only thing that ever has."
—Margaret Mead

## " a conversation with ... "

Education is less and less a preparation for life and more and more a part of it.

Our species thinks in metaphors and learns through stories.

Relying on competition as a way of motivating learning eventually subverts not only cooperation but also the willingness to learn.

—**Mary Catherine Bates**

community are involved), cooperative, collaborative, empowering, and balanced. At its best, the process will promote group identification, reinforcing the idea of a shared fate and the need to look at more global aspects of health (Carr et al., 2008; Israel et al., 1994).

The assessment and planning process will help nurses identify appropriate sites for community education. Where are the natural community networks? Are they centered on employment, recreational, religious, or commercial functions? Will organizations that are not viewed as healthcare agencies (e.g., schools and churches) get involved? Can early health-promotion programs be established in neighborhood elementary and middle schools? Are community colleges open to health education efforts? Will the justice system support health education for people who live in prisons, jails, and halfway houses? Establishing programs specific to people who congregate in these sites can promote education in ways that target at-risk individuals (Andrade & Doria-Ortiz, 1995; Carr et al., 2008).

How health education is implemented also depends on assessment and planning. It helps to have a theoretical base (see Tables 15-2 and 15-3), knowing that some models are better for community intervention than others. Diffusion theory and social marketing theory, for example, were developed from community-focused research. The transtheoretical model also includes components of community action. Common teaching strategies for community intervention include lectures, small group work, facilitated discussions, demonstrations, printed and audiovisual materials, simulation exercises, guided imagery, and social marketing (Krozy, 1996). The important thing to remember is that the teaching strategy needs to match the learning objective (see Table 15-5) as well as the developmental level of the audience.

### Evaluating Community Programs

As stated earlier, evaluation is an ongoing process in health education. Formal evaluation should be planned, and informal evaluation should be acknowledged and used in the process. Formative evaluation is used throughout the process. Summative evaluation occurs at a set point when goals are expected to have been met. Effective evaluation

" I know you told me there were side effects to the drugs...now is there a medication for the "SIDE EFFECTS"?

determines progress toward goals and identifies goals that have not yet been met. Data from evaluation are used to do the following:

- Determine whether unmet goals are still a priority
- Plan interventions to address unmet goals
- Assess the impact of goals that have been achieved
- Assess evolving needs
- Establish new community goals and objectives

The community health education process is much like the individual teaching process (it is cyclical and progressive in nature), but it is more complicated.

### ■ Beyond Community

Nurses who are involved in community education activities realize that some problems are too big to deal with on a community level. Sometimes, changes need to be made at the level of state and federal governments. Political advocacy then becomes a part of the health education agenda. Nurses can educate communities about the political process to encourage input into legislative activities, knowing that communities with identified needs can often influence legislative outcomes. Some examples of community needs that have been addressed through legislative intent include drunk driving laws, water fluoridation bills, motorcycle helmet requirements, and funding for various initiatives ranging from school-based health education programs to needle and syringe exchange programs. Andrade and Doria-Ortiz (1995) recommend the following legislative actions to support the health of the Mexican American community: provide national health insurance to cover the working poor, cooperate with Mexico to provide health care in border communities, address high-risk diseases (e.g., diabetes and tuberculosis) and conditions (e.g., teen pregnancy and violence), increase Hispanic access to health professions schools, and ensure input from Hispanic communities into federal policy and legislative planning activities. Nurses can help communities achieve goals such as these.

> ❝ *Self-love is the only weight-loss aid that really works in the long run.* ❞
>
> —*Jenny Craig*

## Ethical Issues in Health Education

Health education on the surface seems like an appropriate and ethical thing to do. After all, how ethical would it be to withhold information that could relieve suffering, prevent pain, and avert disease? But health education has its own controversies. Some of these are discussed next; others will become obvious to you as you educate individuals and communities.

A major problem occurs when there are unexpected, negative consequences because of health education. These can be the result of erroneous, poorly planned, or improperly implemented education efforts (Guttman et al., 1996). For instance, suppose you want to teach a group of people who are newly diagnosed with cancer that there is hope. You ask four or five people with cancer to speak to your group. Unfortunately, several of the presenters are dealing with anger and depression because of their disease, and they take this opportunity to share their pain and frustration with the healthcare system. At the end of the session, your audience is likely to be confused (at the least) or to feel complete despair (at the worst). They may lose confidence in the ability to survive cancer treatment; they may even decide to forgo therapy altogether and "get it over with." Although this example is quite blatant, problems can occur even under ideal circumstances.

One of the primary concerns that nurses have to address is the fact that, in many ways, health education manipulates patients to change behaviors. Granted, the changes we seek (based on our assessment of the latest scientific evidence) are for the patient's benefit, but we are nevertheless clearly trying to influence change (Redman, 1997, 2008). This may be difficult for nurses to accept. We have, after all, been taught to respect individual autonomy. Manipulation, no matter how subtle, is hard to justify. This is not a reason to stop teaching or to stop advocating for policies such as motorcycle helmet laws. Instead, it is something that each nurse must weigh carefully before, during, and after health education programs. It also helps to differentiate manipulation from information dissemination. Giving a pregnant adolescent information on options, including the whole spectrum of choices involved in either continuing or terminating her pregnancy, for instance, is information dissemination that

she can use to make an informed decision. Encouraging her to have an abortion, to give the infant up for adoption, or to have the baby and raise it herself is manipulation, especially if she makes her "informed" decision based on a lack of complete information that the nurse has failed to share.

Another issue is science itself and the rate at which knowledge expands (Redman, 1997). We have all heard patients say, "This is so confusing. How am I supposed to know what I should be doing? Last night there was a story on the news about how exercise can cause joint deterioration and here you are telling me that I need to exercise more!" Nurses have an obligation to keep up with advances in health care, but even nurses get confused. This all adds to the complex nature of education and reinforces the need to be able to read and critique research (see the following research alert for an example of a study about health education).

One of the real social issues in patient education has to do with the growing gap between socioeconomic classes (Guttman et al., 1996; Redman, 2008). People who are financially secure are better equipped to act on advice to improve their health. Those without economic resources, however, often see health behaviors (e.g., exercise and eating well) as things they simply cannot afford. Poverty affects individuals' health,

### 🖥 Research Alert

The primary objective of this study was to assess the suitability and readability level of publicly available educational print resources related to physical activity (PA). Educational print resources related to PA (n = 66) were requested from organizations (e.g., professional, commercial, government, and educational). The suitability assessment of materials (SAM) and the simple measure of gobbledygook (SMOG) readability measure were used to evaluate the suitability and readability of the PA resources. Of the 66 PA resources, suitability scores were superior in only 10 resources (15%), adequate in 36 resources (55%), and inadequate/not suitable in 20 resources (30%). The average reading grade level for the PA resources was a 10th grade level (S.D. = 1.82; Rg = 5th grade to 15th grade). Only 56.5% (n = 35) of PA resources depicted a primary PA recommendation that was consistent with the public health recommendation for PA. Results indicate that the majority of educational print resources related to PA have poor readability indices and inadequate to adequate suitability. Health educators developing educational print resources related to PA must ensure these resources conform to the highest suitability standards. This includes developing resources that contain information consistent with current public health recommendations and that can be utilized by all individuals regardless of health literacy status.

*Source:* Vallance, J., Taylor, L., & Lavallee, C. (2008). Suitability and readability assessment of educational print resources related to physical activity: Implications and recommendations for practice. *Patient Education & Counseling, 72*(2), 342–349.

## HEALTHY PEOPLE 2010

### OBJECTIVES RELATED TO HEALTH EDUCATION

#### Educational and Community-Based Programs

*School Setting*

7.2    Increase the proportion of middle, junior high, and senior high schools that provide comprehensive school health education to prevent health problems in the following areas: unintentional injury; violence; suicide; tobacco use and addiction; alcohol and other drug use; unintended pregnancy; HIV/AIDS and STD infection; unhealthy dietary patterns; inadequate physical activity; and environmental health.

7.3    Increase the proportion of college and university students who receive information from their institution on each of the six priority health-risk behavior areas.

*Healthcare Setting*

7.7    Increase the proportion of healthcare organizations that provide patient and family education.

7.8    Increase the proportion of patients who report that they are satisfied with the patient education they receive from their healthcare organization.

7.9    Increase the proportion of hospitals and managed care organizations that provide community disease prevention and health promotion activities that address the priority health needs identified by their community.

*Source:* DHHS, 2000.

---

which further decreases their ability to earn a living or to get ahead. Nurses need to recognize that poor health practices may be related to social and economic barriers as much as they are related to a lack of knowledge, motivation, or positive attitudes. When this is the case, social and community solutions need to be explored rather than falling into the trap of victim blaming (Marantz, 1990). How appropriate, for instance, is it to blame an alcoholic for her liver disease? What if she was raised in a house where alcohol was used to deal with stress? What if her life has been filled with loss, abuse, and trauma? And what if her only solace is to sink into an alcoholic daze? Is this situation her fault? Maybe. Maybe not. Is she beyond help? No, but help is not easy to give if you blame the patient for her disability. Repetitious, ineffective teaching will not help the situation either.

A final ethical issue that deserves attention has to do with community and cultural norms (Guttman et al., 1996; Redman, 1997). We each bring cultural biases into our social interactions. This is true of nurses as well as of patients. In addition to all of their other cultures, nurses bring the culture of health care and scientific bias into every encounter. This makes it difficult for nurses to deal with situations in which, for example, we know that fat infants grow up into fat adults, but the predominant culture believes that only fat babies are healthy. Nurses cannot ignore these conflicting values. They must instead use creative problem solving to develop acceptable solutions on a number of different levels. This can be a messy process with many trials and only a few successes. The alternative is to try to force the culture of science on people who are not going to accept it no matter how hard you try. So why not take some chances? The outcome could be that new messages or teaching methods or solutions emerge, and that could be the best possible conclusion to a difficult situation.

## Conclusion

Health education is an important intervention for nurses in all healthcare settings. The purpose of health education is to change behaviors and situations that put people at risk for injury, illness, disability, or death. It is a theory-based process that draws form learning theory as well as behavior change theory. The health education process is similar to the nursing process. It is appropriate in all clinical and community settings and can be applied to individuals, families, groups, and communities. Nurses may find that advocacy at the state and federal levels is required to make personal and community behavior change possible. Nurses must also be aware that health education poses some important ethical issues.

Explore Community Health Nursing on the Web! To learn more about the topics in this chapter, use the passcode provided to access your exclusive website: **http://nursing.jbpub.com/ communityhealth.** If you do not have a passcode, you can obtain one at this site.

One of the characteristics of early adolescence is the practice of eating fast food. In recent years, fast food consumption has skyrocketed, with some schools having a McDonald's on the school grounds. How can community health nurses educate teens to make healthier food choices, considering the cultural pressure of eating "fast and furiously"?

## ■ CRITICAL THINKING ACTIVITIES

1. Develop teaching plans for each of the following situations. Identify and use a theory base that can help guide the process. Discuss assessment, planning, implementation, and evaluation as a part of your process.
   - *Case 1:* Diane is a 48-year-old single mother who fractured her left wrist in a fall 3 weeks ago. The wrist was reduced in the hospital emergency room and set with a standard cast. Except for some pain and the need to modify a few of her activities, Diane has done well and feels that she will recover completely. Diane saw her nurse practitioner for a regular checkup 3 days ago. The nurse practitioner expressed concern about Diane's wrist and asked about the circumstances of the accident. When Diane described a situation that would not normally result in a fracture, the nurse

   practitioner ordered a scan to access bone density. The results show a 2.5% loss of bone mass. The nurse practitioner orders exercise and dietary changes. Diane and her provider agree to try these tactics for 6 months before considering medications. Diane's 14-year-old son lives with her. Her 20-year-old daughter recently married and moved out of state. The rest of Diane's family lives 350 miles away. She is the co-owner of a business that builds office complexes, and she typically works 10 to 12 hours a day. When you question her about her current diet and exercise routines, she shrugs and says, "To tell you the truth, I'm way too busy to worry about those things. They just take up too much time."
   - *Case 2:* Janet, the nurse at Allen Elementary School, has documented 12 cases of head lice during the past

week. Most of the affected students came from one third-grade class, but two cases came from a second-grade class, and one each came from a fifth-grade class and another third-grade class.

- *Case 3*: The nursing home in Sheridan County has a respite care center where families can leave elderly patients between the hours of 7 A.M. and 7 P.M. The program provides meals, organized activities, and nap facilities for 22 patients with various physical and cognitive disabilities. Families who use the service give positive feedback about improvements in their abilities to cope with the stresses of caring for elderly relatives in the home. Sheila is an 86-year-old woman with confusion and delusions who is a regular patient. Over the past week, Fred, the nurse manager, has noticed bruises around Sheila's wrists. Fred asks Sheila's daughter about the bruises, and she replies, "Oh, I guess she gets those from the restraints. She's started wandering around the house at night. I'm worried that she might fall and break a hip, so I talked

to some of the other families at our last group meeting and several of them suggested that I tie Mama into bed at night."

- *Case 4*: Community Care Center is a comprehensive outpatient healthcare facility that serves injection drug users. In addition to methadone treatment, the center provides counseling services, case management, first aid, and routine annual physical assessments. The physician who does the physicals is only in the center 2 days a week. She approaches Anita, the clinic nurse, and expresses concern about the number of chlamydia cases that she has diagnosed recently. She asks Anita, "What do you think we can do about this?" Although Anita agrees that the pattern the physician describes is an important concern, she worries about the ethical issues that could occur if the clinic takes any action. What ethical issues could develop? How can Anita address those issues for the clinic staff, patients, and surrounding community?

## ■ REFERENCES

Allender, J. A., & Spradley, B. W. (2001). *Community health nursing: Concepts and practice* (5th ed.). Philadelphia: Lippincott Williams & Wilkins.

Andrade, S. J., & Doria-Ortiz, C. (1995). *Nuestro bienestar*: A Mexican-American community-based definition of health promotion in the southwestern United States. *Drugs: Education, Prevention, and Policy, 2*, 129–145.

Bigbee, J. L., & Jansa, N. (1991). Strategies for promoting health protection. *Nursing Clinics of North America, 26*, 895–913.

Bradley-Springer, L. (1996). Patient education for behavior change: Help from the transtheoretical and harm reduction models. *Journal of the Association of Nurses in AIDS Care, 7* (Suppl.), 23–33.

Brocato, J., & Wagner, E. F. (2003). Harm reduction: A social work practice model and social justice agenda. *Health and Social Work, 28*(2), 117–125.

Carr, S., Lhussier, M., Wilkinson, J., & Gleadhill, S. (2008). Empowerment evaluation applied to public health practice. *Critical Public Health, 18*(2), 161–174.

Carter, W. B. (1990). Health behavior as a rational process: Theory of reasoned action and multiattribute utility theory. In K. Glanz, F. M. Lewis, & B. K. Rimer (Eds.), *Health behavior and health education: Theory, research, and practice* (pp. 63–91). San Francisco: Jossey-Bass.

Cates, W., Jr., & Hinman, A. (1992). AIDS and absolutism: The demand for perfection in prevention. *New England Journal of Medicine, 327*, 492–494.

Cutill, C. C. (2006). Do your patients understand? How to write effective healthcare information. *Orthopedic Nursing, 25*(1), 39–48.

Damrosch, S. (1991). General strategies for motivating people to change their behavior. *Nursing Clinics of North America, 26*, 833–843.

Demir, F., Ozsaker, E., & Ilce, A. O. (2008). The quality and suitability of written educational materials for patients. *Journal of Clinical Nursing, 17*(2), 259–265.

Department of Health and Human Services (DHHS). (2000). *Healthy people 2010: Conference edition*. Washington, DC: U.S. Government Printing Office.

DiClemente, R. J., Crosby, R. A., & Kegler, M. C. (Eds.). (2002). *Emerging theories in health promotion practice and research: Strategies for improving public health*. San Francisco: Jossey-Bass.

Foran, M., & Campanelli, L. C. (1995). Health promotion communications system: A model for a dispersed population. *AAOHN Journal, 43*, 564–569.

Guttman, N., Kegler, M., & McLeroy, K. R. (1996). Health promotion paradoxes, antimonies and conundrums. *Health Education Research, 11*(1), i–xiii.

Hunt, R. (1997). Teaching. In R. Hunt & E. L. Zurek (Eds.), *Introduction to community based nursing* (pp. 182–225). Philadelphia: Lippincott.

Israel, B. A., Checkoway, B., Schulz, A., & Zimmerman, M. (1994). Health education and community empowerment: Conceptualizing and measuring perceptions of individual, organizational, and community control. *Health Education Quarterly, 21*, 140–170.

Knowles, M. S., Holton, E. F., & Swanson, R. A. (1998). *The adult learner* (5th ed.). Woburn, MD: Butterworth-Heinemann.

Kreuter, M. W., & Strecher, V. J. (1996). Do tailored behavior change messages enhance the effectiveness of health risk appraisal? Results from a randomized trial. *Health Education Research, 11*, 97–105.

Krozy, R. E. (1996). Community health promotion: Assessment and intervention. In S. H. Rankin & K. D. Stallings (Eds.), *Patient education: Issues, principles, practices* (3rd ed., pp. 245–271). Philadelphia: Lippincott.

Marantz, P. R. (1990). Blaming the victim: The negative consequence of preventive medicine. *American Journal of Public Health, 80*(18), 186–187.

McLaughlin, G. H. (1969). SMOG grading: A new readability formula. *Journal of Reading, 12*(8), 639–646.

Miller, P., Wikoff, R., & Hiatt, A. (1992). Fishbein's model of reasoned action and compliance behavior of hypertensive patients. *Nursing Research, 41*, 104–109.

Mirotznik, J., Feldman, L., & Stein, R. (1995). The health belief model and adherence with a community center-based, supervised coronary heart disease program. *Journal of Community Health, 20*, 233–247.

Novelli, W. D. (1990). Applying social marketing to health promotion and disease prevention. In K. Glanz, F. M. Lewis, & B. K. Rimer (Eds.), *Health behavior and health education: Theory, research, and practice* (pp. 342–369). San Francisco: Jossey-Bass.

Orlandi, M. A., Landers, C., Weston, R., & Haley, N. (1990). Diffusion of health promotion innovations. In K. Glanz, F. M. Lewis, & B. K. Rimer (Eds.), *Health behavior and health education: Theory, research, and practice* (pp. 288–313). San Francisco: Jossey-Bass.

Palank, C. L. (1991). Determinants of health-promotive behavior: A review of current research. *Nursing Clinics of North America, 26*, 815–832.

Perry, C. L., Baranowski, T., & Parcel, G. S. (1990). How individuals, environments and health behavior interact: Social learning theory. In K. Glanz, F. M. Lewis, & B. K. Rimer (Eds.), *Health behavior and health education: Theory, research, and practice* (pp. 161–186). San Francisco: Jossey-Bass.

Petty, R. E., Barden, J., & Wheeler, S. C. (2002). The elaboration likelihood model of persuasion: Health promotions that yield sustained behavioral change. In R. J. DiClemente, R. A. Crosby, & M. C. Kegler (Eds.), *Emerging theories in health promotion practice and research: Strategies for improving public health* (pp. 71–99). San Francisco: Jossey-Bass.

Rankin, S. N., & Stallings, K. D. (2001). *Patient education: Principles and practice* (4th ed.). Philadelphia: Lippincott Williams & Wilkins.

Redman, B. K. (1997). *The practice of patient education*. St. Louis: Mosby.

Redman, B. (2008). When is patient education unethical? *Nursing Ethics, 15*(6), 813–820.

Rosenstock, I. M. (1990). The health belief model: Explaining health behavior through expectancies. In K. Glanz, F. M. Lewis, & B. K. Rimer (Eds.), *Health behavior and health education: Theory, research, and practice* (pp. 39–62). San Francisco: Jossey-Bass.

Spellbring, A. M. (1991). Nursing's role in health promotion: An overview. *Nursing Clinics of North America, 26*, 805–814.

Strang, J. (1992). Harm reduction for drug users: Exploring the dimensions of harm, their measurement, and strategies for reductions. *AIDS and Public Policy Journal, 7*, 145–152.

Strecher, V. J., Seijts, G. H., Kok, G. J., et al. (1995). Goal setting as a strategy for health behavior change. *Health Education Quarterly, 22*, 190–200.

Yu, M., Song, L., Seetoo, A., Cai, C., Smith, G., & Oakley, P. (2007). Culturally competent training program: A key to training lay health advisors for promoting breast cancer screening. *Health Education & Behavior, 34*(6), 928–941.

## CHAPTER 16

# Complementary and Holistic Health

Margaret A. Burkhardt

In recent years, healthcare professionals have become increasingly interested in therapies that lie outside the realm of conventional Western allopathic medicine. Many such therapies derive from folk wisdom, cultural perspectives, and healing practices of indigenous peoples and other ancient healing systems.

Health is wholeness, unfolding:
It is sharing, significantly, increasingly,
    in the varieties of human experience:
    physically, in the range of activities
      in which the human body can engage;
      not only aggression, but also conciliation,
      not only the proprieties, but also the singularities,
      not only to exhaustion, but also to the crest of vitality;
    sensually, in the possibilities of sensation;
      not confined to extremes:
        rage and excitement, passivity, suppression;
        not to pain:
        the pain of separation,
        the fear of aloneness;
      but knowing the quiet depths, the tenderness, the
        nuances flowing from tones, textures, odors,
        flavors;
        the joy of well-being, of union and reunion,
        the awesomeness of intimacy;
    culturally, socially, in the designs for living,
      across time and across the world:
    ways of talking, eating, dressing, pleasuring;
    ideas of beauty, of truth, of rightness.
It is growing in awareness:
    of sharing, significantly;

    of self;
    rising above existence, beyond time and space,
      the uniqueness of man.
And it is feeling good about it all, coming into Self-hood:
    expressing one's inner power,
    articulating one's reason-for-being,
    accepting one's sexuality,
      and interdependence:
      receiving and giving,
    holding on and letting go,
    following and guiding.
Toward wholeness:
    responding to the possibilities and limitations of
      human experience,
    reciprocating, resting, resurgent again;
    exploring, discovering
    opening, unfolding,
      from diffuseness toward coherence,
      simplicity toward complexity,
      disparity toward complementarity,
      vagueness toward decisiveness,
      confusion toward understanding,
      toward wholeness.

*—Nancy Milio*

After reading the poem, explain in your own words what "holistic" means to you. What has been your experience with complementary or alternative health practices?

## CHAPTER FOCUS

**Holistic Framework**

**Historical Influences**

**Complementary Modalities: What Are They?**
- Alternative Medical Systems
- Mind–Body Interventions
- Biologically Based Therapies
- Manipulative and Body-Based Methods
- Energy Therapies

**Complementary Health and Community Nursing Practice**
- The Right to Choose
- Nursing Assessment

**Potential Barriers to Use of Complementary Therapies**

**Integrating Complementary Therapies into Community Nursing Care**
- Spirituality
- Music Therapy
- Imagery
- Herbal Therapies
- Touch Therapy

## QUESTIONS TO CONSIDER

After reading this chapter, you will know the answers to the following questions:

1. What is complementary health?
2. How does a nurse know when to choose a complementary intervention?
3. What are barriers to using complementary therapy?
4. What are some of the most common complementary therapies?
5. How does the community health nurse evaluate the effectiveness of complementary therapy?

## KEY TERMS

| | | | |
|---|---|---|---|
| Complementary health | Herbal and natural therapies | Music therapy | Touch therapy |
| Healing | Mind–body interventions | Office of Alternative Medicine (OAM) | |

MORE PERSONS TODAY are using alternative or unconventional therapies, either instead of allopathic modalities or combined with other nonallopathic approaches. These approaches are often termed "complementary" when they are used in addition to conventional therapies. In this chapter, the term "complementary therapy" is used regardless of the pattern of use, recognizing that healthcare providers need to be open to exploring various approaches to health and healing to support the best possible outcomes for patients.

❝ *I begin to see that a man's got to be in his own heaven to be happy.* ❞

—Mark Twain

Nurses within the community need to be familiar with various healing modalities used by their patients and aware of complementary modalities that may promote health, enhance healing, or contribute to unhealthy outcomes with patients. This chapter discusses a holistic framework for the integration of complementary therapies into care, understanding of complementary modalities, and assessment processes and ethical issues regarding **complementary health**. Selected complementary modalities are discussed that can be incorporated into community nursing care.

❝ *Care and love are the most universal, the most tremendous, and the most mysterious of cosmic forces; they comprise the primal and universal psychic energy.* ❞

—Jean Watson

 ### Research Alert

This phenomenological study explored the meaning of spirituality among aging adults in Appalachia. Participants were adult volunteers ranging in age from 59 to 94 years old, in varying states of health, who lived independently in the community and at assisted living and skilled care facilities in an Appalachian community. Most of the participants were women. Data were collected through focus groups in which participants were asked open-ended questions about their perceptions of spirituality, spirituality and health, and the role of spirituality in helping them to cope. Data analysis revealed the themes of a conviction that God exists and acts in the lives of persons, calls them to action, and is a source of connection in times of loss. The data indicated that spirituality positively affects attitudes, especially as health declines, and that spirituality was of great importance in the lives of these elders. These participants expected empathetic and respectful health professionals who address both physical and spiritual concerns. Implications for nursing include the importance of incorporating spirituality into assessment and intervention with elderly and other patients. ◯

*Source*: Lowry, L. W., & Conco, D. (2002). Exploring the meaning of spirituality with aging adults in Appalachia. *Journal of Holistic Nursing, 20*(4), 388–402.

### MEDIA MOMENT

**Patch Adams**
After spending some time in a mental hospital, Patch Adams decides that he wants to use laughter to help people. He enrolls in medical school and is upset to find that students do not interact with patients until the third year. Determined to connect with patients, he starts entertaining children in the cancer clinic and eventually starts a clinic with the help of friends and fellow students.

Not everyone agrees with his methods though. The head of the medical school wants to expel Patch, and one of his fellow students, Corinne, disagrees with him, but eventually supports him and helps him in the clinic. Patch Adams prevailed and eventually founded the Gesundheit Institute.

"Dance is my therapy. Dance is my escape from real life. I can always forget my problems and be in a much better mood after ballet class. Dancing is fun. Dancing lets me express myself in a different way than words do."

—Tiffany, BSN, RN

## Holistic Framework

A holistic understanding of life that appreciates that each person is a bio-psycho-social-spiritual unity provides a framework for inclusion of complementary modalities into nursing care. Within a holistic framework, nurses are attentive to *healing* as well as to *curing* (Burkhardt, 1985; Burkhardt & Nagai-Jacobson, 2002; Quinn, 1989). Curing is a process that attends to disordered physical or psychological parts of a person, with a focus on disease processes and restoration of the integrity of a specific component (usually physiological) of a person. The allopathic approach focuses on curing by combating disease with techniques that produce effects different from those produced by the disease (Dossey & Guzzetta, 2005).

**Healing**, by contrast, acknowledges that disharmony in a whole person may be manifested as disease or illness and seeks to understand the totality of the lived experience for a person, taking into account the personal response to and meaning of the apparent disease or illness process (Burkhardt & Nagai-Jacobson, 1997b). Healing requires a relationship between the caregiver and care receiver that acknowledges common humanity and connectedness. Physical, emotional, and spiritual concerns are addressed within the healing relationship. Healing may be manifested as cure in one or more of the bio-psycho-emotional realms but can be present without a cure. Quinn (1989) aptly notes that, although diseases may be cured, people need healing. The desire to promote health, or the need for healing or curing, which is not being addressed by conventional approaches, often leads people to complementary modalities. Complementary or alternative therapies generally focus on body–mind–spirit integration through healing by an individual, healing between two individuals, or healing at a distance (Dossey & Guzzetta, 2005).

It is particularly important for nurses who work within the community to practice holistic nursing. Dealing with patients and families within their home environments enables nurses to appreciate cultural considerations in healing and to assess patients' use of complementary modalities. Because holistic nursing has the healing of the whole person as its goal, nurses work in therapeutic partnership with patients and families to integrate those modalities that best facilitate the patient's health and healing. Nurses also need to be aware of therapies that may be ineffective or cause potential harm when used alone or in combination with other modalities (Robison, 2004). The American Holistic Nurses Association's description of holistic nursing presented in Box 16-1 provides a frame of reference for holistic nursing practice based on sound academic principles incorporating both the art and science of nursing.

 Research Alert

The purpose of this study was to determine the effect of laughter on natural killer cell activity and self-reported stress. The study was conducted in a community health center in a Midwestern city. The sample consisted of 33 healthy women volunteers who met specific inclusion and exclusion criteria that controlled for as many immunoresponsive factors as possible. Subjects were randomly assigned to experimental (humor) or control (distraction) groups. Experimental subjects viewed a humorous video, whereas subjects in the control group viewed a tourism video. Pre- and post-tests measured self-reported stress and arousal (Stress Arousal Check List), mirthful laughter (Humor Response Scale), and immune function (chromium-release natural killer cell cytotoxicity assay).

Findings of the study included a decrease in stress for subjects in the humor group compared with those in the distraction group, correlation between the amount of mirthful (overt) laughter and post-intervention stress measures in the humor group, and increased immune function in post intervention subjects who scored greater than 25 on the Humor Response Scale. Although this study had some limitations, the findings suggest that mirthful laughter may reduce stress and improve natural killer cell activity, which is linked to enhanced immune response and, therefore, may be a useful cognitive behavioral intervention.

*Source*: Bennett, M. P., Zeller, J. M., Rosenberg, L., & McCann, J. (2003). The effect of mirthful laughter on stress and natural killer cell activity. *Alternative Therapies in Health and Medicine, 9*(2), 38–45.

**❝***The part can never be well unless the whole is well.***❞**

—*Plato*

## Historical Influences

Before discussing complementary healthcare modalities, let's take a brief look at the process through which allopathic or biomedical care became the accepted "conventional" approach to health care in the United States. The United States is often referred to as a "melting pot" of persons from many different cultures, educational and socioeconomic backgrounds, and experiences. Healthcare practices have evolved (and continue to do so) from the healing traditions of both native peoples and those who have immigrated to this country. Before the mid-1800s, practitioners from various healthcare systems, including allopathy, naturopathy, homeopathy, and botanics, were acknowledged as legitimate healers in the United States. Micozzi (1996) notes that the history of contemporary biomedicine as a scientific paradigm was as much influenced by social history as by scientific laws. Allopathic biomedicine began to predominate by the mid-1800s and gained further prominence by the late 1800s through state licensing laws sponsored by and lobbied for by the American Medical Association.

Dossey and Swyers (1994) note that the prominence of biomedicine was shaped in part by two important developments. One development was in the realm of scientific discoveries, such as the identification of specific organisms as the cause of particular disease states and the identification of substances and vaccines that ward off the effect of pathogens, which greatly influenced the direction of biomedicine. The other was the 1910 release of Abraham Flexner's report titled *Medical Education in the United States and Canada*, which was influential in upgrading medical education programs, enabling medical schools with a stronger biomedical orientation to receive more financial backing from philanthropic foundations. This, in turn, prompted the stifling of medical schools teaching theories other than biomedical regarding the origin of illness and appropriate therapies. What was considered scientific was defined by biomedicine's "way of knowing," which emphasized that knowledge about the world requires empiricism (Micozzi, 1996). Other paradigms were either relegated to the "fringe" or subsumed into the biomedical paradigm. Although biomedicine gained power and prestige and became the gold standard for health care, small numbers of naturopathic, homeopathic, chiropractic, and practitioners of other healing systems continued to provide care.

Over the past several decades, however, healthcare consumers have become more active in seeking care outside the biomedical system. Some of the factors that may have contributed to this phenomenon include the following:

- A shift away from infectious diseases as major causes of morbidity and mortality to health concerns that elude medical cure such as cancer, heart disease, hypertension, diabetes, and other chronic problems (Gordon, 1980)
- Increasingly depersonalized care and decreased personal control in healthcare decisions as a result of increased use of technology (Burkhardt & Nathaniel, 2002)
- A greater emphasis on self-care and personal responsibility for health
- A shrinking world that has allowed greater access to other cultures and their systems of healing
- Renewed appreciation that healing must address the whole body-mind-spirit person

Although people have been using complementary therapies for years, the landmark study conducted by Eisenberg, Kessler, Foster, Norlock, Calkins, and Delbanco (1993) documented an unexpected frequency of use of these therapies and caused the medical establishment to take note. The results of this national telephone survey of 1,539 adults indicated that one in three Americans of all sociodemographic groups used complementary therapies, and of those who used these therapies, 72% did so without informing their conventional healthcare provider. This study also indicated that people tended to use complementary modalities for chronic rather than life-threatening conditions. To identify trends in alternative medicine use in the United States, Eisenberg, Rogers, Ettner, Appel, Wilkey, Van Rompay, and Kessler (1998) conducted another national telephone survey of 2,055 English-speaking adults in 1997 asking about their use of 16 therapies. The therapies included relaxation techniques, herbal medicine, massage, chiropractic, prayer or spiritual healing by others, megavitamins, self-help groups, imagery, commercial diet, folk remedies, lifestyle diet, energy healing, homeopathy, hypnosis, biofeedback, and acupuncture. Results of this survey indicated that alternative therapy use increased from 33.8% in 1990 to 42.1% in 1997. Use of herbal medicine, massage, megavitamins, self-help groups, folk remedies, energy healing, and homeopathy increased the most.

In 2002, the National Health Interview Survey, conducted annually by the National Center for Health Statistics, included a detailed survey on complementary and alternative medicine (CAM) (Barnes, Powell-Griner, McFann, & Nahin, 2004). This survey of 31,044 adults documented that 75%

of American adults used some form of CAM at least once in their lives. The study also showed that 36% of respondents had used a CAM therapy within the past 12 months. This figure increased to 62% when prayer specifically for health reasons was included in the definition of CAM.

Keegan (1996) documented use of alternative therapies in 44% of Mexican Americans, noting that 66% of this population never report the use of alternatives to conventional healthcare providers. Through a self-reporting survey of the use of complementary therapies among people in rural West Virginia, Burkhardt, Nathaniel, Nemeth-Pyles, and Boyd (1999) found that 83% of respondents (*n* = 545) used at least one of the 17 listed therapies within the past year. In this study, 41% of respondents reported that they never discuss these therapies with their healthcare provider and 34% discuss them with their providers only sometimes.

In response to growing awareness and use of complementary therapies, the National Institutes of Health (NIH) created the **Office of Alternative Medicine (OAM)** in 1992. The OAM was established to facilitate scientific and fair evaluation of complementary modalities that can contribute to the health and well-being of many people and reduce barriers to awareness and availability of promising complementary therapies. In 1998, the OAM was elevated to the National Center for Complementary and Alternative Medicine (NCCAM), one of the 25 institutes and centers of NIH. The NCCAM's mission is to conduct and support basic and applied research and training and to disseminate information on complementary and alternative medicine to practitioners and the public. The congressional mandate for the NCCAM provides for research training programs and a public information clearinghouse; however, the center is not a referral agency. The importance of research on and reliable information about complementary therapies is reflected in the increase in budget for the NCCAM that supports research and education on CAM.

**❝** *What lies behind us and what lies before us are tiny matters compared to what lies within us.* **❞**

—Ralph Waldo Emerson

## Complementary Modalities: What Are They?

Although the terms "alternative," "complementary," and "unconventional" are often used interchangeably in reference to nonbiomedical interventions, the term "complementary" best reflects the awareness that these therapies need to be considered adjuncts to—not replacements for—medical and surgical treatments. The definition of complementary modalities that was developed at the NIH/OAM Second Conference on Research Methodology in April 1995 notes that the broad domain of CAM encompasses all health systems, modalities, and practices other than those intrinsic to the politically dominant health system of a particular society or culture. Currently the NCCAM defines CAM as a group of diverse medical and healthcare systems, practices,

### A Good Read

## Invitation to Holistic Health: A Guide to Living a Balanced Life (2004)
*By Charlotte Eliopoulos, Sudbury, MA: Jones and Bartlett.*

Dr. Eliopoulos provides an excellent overview to adopting a holistic lifestyle—for ourselves and our patients. This book is an extension of the American Holistic Nurses Association's commitment to teach consumers measures to promote optimal health and well-being of the body, mind, and spirit. Eliopoulos compiles the knowledge and practical wisdom of nurses for health promotion and holistic wellness. Authored by health professionals who have the closest, most frequent contact with consumers and understand consumers best, this book presents practical health promotion information in a unique manner, utilizing a holistic model. This book provides the practical "how to" information to enable consumers to safely and effectively use natural and complementary therapies. The public's skyrocketing interest and use of alternative and complementary therapies make this aspect of the book particularly timely and relevant. ◐

and products that are not presently considered to be part of conventional medicine (NCCAM, http://nccam.nih.gov). CAM includes all practices and ideas self-defined by their users as preventing or treating illness or promoting health and well-being.

Each healing system (including biomedicine) has its own explanatory model that "summarizes the perceptions, assumptions, beliefs, theories, and facts that guide the logic of health care delivery" (Cassidy, 1996, p. 20). Some important distinctions between complementary and conventional medicine include differences in philosophical underpinnings, types of therapies offered, ways in which therapies are administered, and interactions between practitioner and patient (Cassidy, 1996; Dossey & Swyers, 1994). For example, in the biomedical model, the practitioner has traditionally been considered the authoritative expert who determines and designs care based on standardized treatments in which the patient has variable involvement. With complementary systems, treatments are more often individualized and developed in collaboration with patients who are acknowledged as having responsibility for their own healing processes. Complementary systems generally appreciate that humans have natural, built-in recuperative powers and often focus on therapies that enhance the patient's natural healing processes. Unifying threads that are common to most complementary healing systems include emphasis on the following aspects:

- One's relationships, sense of values, place in society, and sense of self
- The role of spiritual values and religion in health

- The impact on health of consciousness manifested through thoughts, feelings, attitudes, emotions, values, and perceived meanings
- Diet, exercise, relaxation techniques, and modifications in lifestyle
- Utilization of whole foods and herbs rather than extracts (Dossey & Swyers, 1994)

Many of these threads are common parts of nursing practice as well, and conventional medicine is also beginning to pay more attention to them (Gordon, 2002; Sierpina, 2002).

NCCAM currently classifies complementary and alternative health practice into five categories or domains, each of which contains subcategories designated as *CAM* (practices that are not commonly used, accepted, or available in conventional medicine), *behavioral medicine* (practices that may fall within the domain of conventional medicine), and *overlapping* (practices that can be in either subcategory). The five categories with associated NCCAM classifications of alternative medicine practice are briefly summarized next. Given that the listing of specific modalities and therapies is updated and expanded on a regular basis, only a few selected examples are given here for each category. The reader is encouraged to visit the NCCAM website (http://nccam.nih.gov) for further information.

### ■ Alternative Medical Systems

Worldwide, only 10–30% of human health care is delivered by conventional biomedically oriented practitioners. The remaining 70–90% of care varies from self-care according to folk principles to care sought within an organized healthcare system derived from traditions or practices that flow from paradigms of health and healing different from those associated with biomedicine. Some of these explanatory models have sound bases that have been developed, tested, and practiced over thousands of years. Because they derive from a different worldview, however, the processes and modes of action of many of these modalities are not understood within the biomedical paradigm.

The NCCAM classification *Alternative Medical Systems* addresses complete systems of theory and practice other than the Western biomedical approach. Many of these systems evolved apart from and earlier than the conventional medical system that dominates Western cultures. Examples of such systems include these:

- Traditional Chinese medicine—includes acupuncture, herbal formulas, tai chi, diet
- Ayurvedic medicine and other traditional indigenous systems—include diet and herbal remedies, and emphasize body, mind, and spirit in both prevention and treatment
- Homeopathy—based on a belief that "like cures like" and uses highly diluted medicinal substances to treat symptoms
- Naturopathy—based on a belief that there is a natural healing power in the body that maintains and restores

health, and uses various means to support this power, such as nutrition, lifestyle counseling, dietary and herbal supplements, exercise, and treatments from modalities like homeopathy and traditional Chinese medicine

### ■ Mind–Body Interventions

**Mind–body interventions** focus on the mind's capacity to affect the body and explore healing systems that make use of the interconnectedness of mind, body, and spirit. Most traditional healing systems acknowledge and incorporate the interconnectedness of mind–body–spirit, recognizing the power of each to affect the other. In the past 30 years, biomedicine has become more open to the awareness of the impact of the mind on the body, although exploring the role of spirituality in healing is still in its infancy. Mind–body–spirit interventions often enable patients to experience and express their illnesses in new and clearer ways, and to explore the meaning of their illnesses, which can have direct consequences on their health. Scientific exploration suggests that there is a complex interaction among the mind, neurologic systems, and immune systems (psychoneuroimmunology) that can be affected by interventions in this category.

The NCCAM classification of mind–body interventions, which encompasses psychological, social, behavioral, and spiritual approaches to health, relates to this field of practice. Examples of CAM techniques and practices that are part of this category include these:

- Mind–body methods—specific modalities incorporating awareness of mind–body interaction in healing, such as yoga, tai chi, imagery, mental healing, and creative outlets such as music, art, and dance
- Religion and spirituality—the nonbehavioral aspects of religion and spirituality that relate to biologic function or clinical condition, such as nonlocality, meditation, prayer, forgiveness, and spiritual healing
- Social and contextual factors—interventions that are social, cultural, symbolic, or contextual in nature, such as caring-based approaches like holistic nursing, intuitive diagnosis, and community-based approaches like certain Native American rituals

### ■ Biologically Based Therapies

The CAM options classified as biologically based therapies use substances found in nature such as foods, vitamins, herbs, and other plants. Although these substances are considered natural, their efficacy is as yet scientifically unproven. This field includes a wide assortment of drugs, biologic products, dietary supplements, and nutritional interventions used to prevent illness, maintain health, and reverse the effects of chronic disease.

All cultures and healing traditions have included the use of plants and plant products. Many of today's drugs have herbal origins, and about 25% of drugs dispensed from pharmacies have at least one active ingredient derived from plants. According to the World Health Organization, an estimated 4 billion people (80% of the world's population) use herbal therapies for some aspect of their primary care. Herbal therapies are a major component of indigenous healing traditions. Because of federal Food and Drug Administration (FDA) regulations, herbal products can be marketed in the United States only as food supplements and cannot make any specific health claims.

The rise in chronic illnesses related to diet has prompted a shift in nutritional research in the United States toward dealing with the effects of nutritional excess and away from eliminating nutritional deficiency. Evidence indicates that inadequate intake of some micronutrients may increase risks of problems such as coronary artery disease, cancers, and birth defects, and that the required daily allowance for some minerals and vitamins may not be adequate to prevent chronic illnesses. Many alternative diets and dietary lifestyles that incorporate more fresh and freshly prepared fruits and vegetables and whole grains and legumes may offer greater resistance to illness.

Examples of interventions included in this category follow:

- Phytotherapy or herbalism—plant-derived preparations used for therapeutic and preventive purposes, such as gingko biloba, echinacea, and green tea
- Special diet therapies—dietary approaches used as alternative therapies for particular risk factors or for chronic disease in general, such as vegetarian, Pritikin, and macrobiotic diets
- Orthomolecular medicine—products not covered in other categories that are used (usually in combinations and at high doses) as nutritional and food supplements for preventive or therapeutic purposes, such as ascorbic acid, coenzyme Q10, and melatonin
- Cartilage products derived from sharks, chickens, and sheep, used for treating cancer; ethylene diamine tetraacetic acid (EDTA) chelation therapy, used for treating heart disease and preventing cancer; a liquid extract from mistletoe plants (Iscador), used to treat tumors

## Manipulative and Body-Based Methods

Touch or manipulation with the hands has been part of healing traditions as far back as one can explore. Although contemporary biomedical providers tend to be distanced from physical contact with patients because of attitudes of reliance on diagnostic equipment and tests, and legal and time constraints, at one time physicians' hands were considered their most important diagnostic and therapeutic tool. Manual healing methods derive from the understanding that dysfunction of one area of the body can affect the function of other discrete and not necessarily connected body parts. It is worth noting that osteopathic medicine was one of the earliest U.S. healthcare systems to use manual healing methods.

The NCCAM classification of manipulative and body-based methods focuses on therapies and systems that are based on movement or manipulation of one or more parts of the body. Examples of healing approaches found in this category include these:

- Chiropractic medicine—focuses on the relationship between the structure and function of the body and the effects of this relationship on preservation and restoration of health
- Osteopathic manipulation—emphasizes the musculoskeletal system as an important factor in health and illness and notes that all of the body's systems work together, with disturbances in one area affecting function elsewhere
- Massage and other body work such as Swedish massage, Chinese Tui Na massage and acupressure, and body psychotherapy

## Energy Therapies

The therapies in this category involve the use of energy fields, and are classified as either biofield therapies or bioelectromagnetic-based therapies. *Biofield* healing practices use subtle energy fields in and around the body for healing and health promotion. Examples of these therapies include healing touch, reiki, therapeutic touch, and external qi gong. *Bioelectromagnetics* includes the unconventional use of electromagnetic fields for healing and health promotion. It is an emerging science that studies how living organisms interact with electromagnetic fields.

The understanding that electrical phenomena are found in all living organisms and that electrical currents in the body can produce magnetic fields extending outside the body is basic to this field of study. Exploration suggests that changes in the body's natural fields can produce physical and behavioral changes and that certain frequencies have specific effects on body tissues. Examples of energy therapies include pulsed fields, magnetic fields, and alternating or direct current fields (Cuellar, 2005; Cuellar et al., 2007).

The national health goals established in *Healthy People 2010: Increasing the Span of Healthy Life for Americans, Reducing Health Disparities among Americans, and Achieving Access to Preventive Services for All Americans* are designed to help bring the people of the United States to their full potential. The opportunities or objectives designated for achieving these goals relate to health promotion, health protection, and preventive services. Although the document does not address complementary modalities per se, many people use complementary therapies as part of their efforts to promote health and prevent illness. Most complementary modalities included in the NCCAM classification system relate to the goal of increasing the span of healthy life for people in this country. Appropriate use of complementary therapies and their practitioners may ultimately contribute to the goals of reducing health disparities. Because many complementary therapies focus on health promotion and illness prevention, appropriately integrating them into health care may promote access to preventive services for people across the

United States. Although research on the role of many complementary modalities in health promotion and prevention has expanded in recent years, more validation of the efficacy of these therapies is needed. Because health promotion strategies relate to individual lifestyle choices, nurses need to be particularly aware of choices people make regarding the use of complementary therapies in dealing with health promotion and illness prevention.

## Complementary Health and Community Nursing Practice

Community health nurses must remember that decisions about health care are based on more than scientific expertise. Healthcare choices are influenced by a person's values, culture, and spiritual and other beliefs; evaluation of risks, benefits, and economic considerations; and effects on lifestyle and role. All of these areas must be considered in deliberations about health care. Cassidy writes that "cultural relativity is pivotal to the study of alternative medicine, because each alternative system of medicine provides a different set of ideas about the body, disease, and medical reality" (1996, p. 12). Community nurses need to be particularly attentive to the influence of culture because emotional, psychological, aesthetic, interpersonal, and other dimensions of health concerns differ across cultures and belief systems, impelling certain actions and constraining others (Cuellar, Aycock, Cahill, & Ford, 2003; Cuellar et al; 2003; O'Connor, 1996). Our culture teaches us the meaning of health; how to be sick; and when, how, and from whom to seek care.

Community nurses must be aware of the values, goals, and beliefs of personal culture (their own and that of their patients) as well as the culture of the biomedical system and of other healing systems as they develop healthcare plans with patients. With this awareness, nurses can be more alert for potential conflicts and negative value judgments that may interfere with integrating complementary modalities into care. Consider, for example, a situation in which a nurse learns that her patient with fibromyalgia is using herbs and vitamins recommended by a layperson who used kinesiology to determine what the patient needed. Recognizing that the culture of the biomedical system would find this process unscientific alerts the nurse to potential negative value judgments from the patient's biomedical practitioner regarding her choice and enables the nurse to consider ways to assist the patient in integrating the different modalities. Patients are more likely to discuss their complementary health practices with nurses who approach them with an openness to exploring and including different modalities in care than they are with nurses who place judgments on such modalities.

❝They may forget what you said, but they will never forget how you made them feel.❞

—Carl N. Buechner

## ■ The Right to Choose

Professional standards and codes of ethics direct nurses to respect each person and to value and support patient autonomy. Basic to autonomy are the ability to determine personal goals, the ability to decide on a plan of action, and the freedom to act on one's choice. Consequently, the principle of patient self-determination directs nurses to honor the right of persons to use modalities outside the realm of biomedicine in addressing their healthcare needs. When such choices are made, nurses may find it challenging to honor and respect the convictions derived from belief systems that underlie these choices, particularly when these beliefs are not understood or are contrary to their own. However, to deny such convictions in healthcare settings is "to deny the patient's very reality, sometimes risking serious psychological and emotional impact on patient and family alike, and always raising genuine ethical concerns about patient autonomy, provider beneficence, substituted judgment, and distributive justice" (O'Connor, 1996, p. 93). Attentiveness to patient values and desires for treatment options requires nurses to take seriously the patient's need for healing as well as curing, and the contributions to health offered by other explanatory models. When nurses do not understand the other modality or question the efficacy or safety of the choice, they must explore these considerations with the patient. A nonjudgmental approach that is respectful of differing values and beliefs and alert for ethnocentric bias on the part of the nurse enhances joint exploration (Burkhardt & Nathaniel, 1996, 2002; Robison, 2004).

## ■ Nursing Assessment

To have a broad picture of the many factors affecting a patient's health and healing, nurses need to be aware of the various therapies being considered or used by patients. Community nurses need to develop the ability to incorporate discussion of complementary therapies into their nursing assessment in an open way, because patients may be hesitant to bring up the subject. Discussion may be prompted through

### ⊚ MEDIA MOMENT

***The Fisher King*** (1991)

A talk DJ inadvertently convinces a psychotic man to blow away restaurant patrons and himself when the psychotic man calls in for advice. After 3 years of wallowing in his remorse, he is attacked and almost set on fire, but a street person rescues him. The DJ finds out the transient is on a mission to find the holy grail, and tries to repay his kindness with money. The transient has more hands-on assistance in mind, and tries to convince the DJ to help him in his quest for the grail.

open-ended questions such as "What do you do to take care of your health on your own?" "What other things have you tried (or thought about trying) for this health concern?" and "Sometimes people with your condition want to try other remedies, and I wonder if this is something that you have considered?" Another approach to opening a discussion of complementary therapies is to explore the use of specific modalities commonly used in your area with questions such as "Have you ever seen a (chiropractor, acupuncturist, herbalist, etc.) for that problem?" "Have you considered seeing the (*curandera*, medicine person, spiritual healer, etc.)?" or "Have you been using (special vitamins, a macrobiotic diet, herbal remedies, etc.) for your illness?"

Nurses must be knowledgeable about various modalities and therapies to effectively discuss their use with patients. Because of this, many nursing programs are now including courses on CAM and offering programs of study in holistic nursing (Fenton & Morris, 2003). Nurses need not subscribe to particular complementary therapies to effectively assess how patients use these therapies. Neither do nurses need to be practitioners of other modalities to discuss them with patients, any more than they need to be able to do surgery to discuss it. However, community nurses must be able to create an atmosphere that encourages a nonjudgmental assessment of all modalities being considered or used, with a goal of using whatever is beneficial for and will meet the needs of the patient and family (Cuellar, Rogers, & Hisghman, 2007).

Community nurses should become familiar with and develop at least a talking knowledge of complementary therapies that may be commonly used in their communities to be better able to discuss their use with their patients. Public education regarding CAM is essential to provide people with information on the risks and benefits of these therapies in the same way that risks and benefits of conventional therapies are discussed. Many therapies work as adjuncts to biomedical interventions, some may interact in unhealthy ways with particular biomedical treatments, and the efficacy of many modalities is not fully known.

When discussing choices with patients, nurses should draw on studies with which they are familiar in offering relevant information regarding particular therapies, allowing clinical and personal experience into the conversation in judicious ways, yet recognizing that the nurse never has all the pertinent information and that uncertainty is inherent in health choices (Hufford, 1996b). Based on their assessment and knowledge regarding particular therapies, nurses may find it appropriate to support or recommend some complementary modalities while discouraging the use of others.

Hufford (1996b) suggests that the patient has major responsibility for obtaining information regarding complementary therapies and making health choices in this regard. However, nurses need to have some knowledge about risks and benefits associated with these therapies. For example, although garlic may assist in lowering cholesterol, large doses can cause irritation to the digestive tract, which may result in some bleeding. Nurses should encourage patients to explore the validity of claims made about particular therapies and assist them in doing so, especially if the nurse perceives the therapy to be potentially harmful for the patient. However, complementary modalities should not be discounted merely because they are not understood within the Western biomedical framework. When patients are interested in complementary therapies, nurses should help determine whether risks are involved. When the potential for significant risks exists and the patient is committed to using the therapy, the nursing goal is to minimize risks while maximizing treatment. If the patient does not have a strong commitment to the complementary modality, nurses should encourage ongoing discussion of known risks and benefits related to various options (Hufford, 1996a). As part of their assessments, nurses need to determine the congruency between patient and nursing goals regarding healing and curing; they also should review options considered viable by each as a means of meeting these goals. Maintaining an openness to working with traditional systems and their healers facilitates more effective and culturally congruent nursing and health care.

## Potential Barriers to Use of Complementary Therapies

Professional integrity requires nurses to take an honest look at potential barriers that may limit availability of and access to complementary therapies for patients and that may hinder the research into complementary therapies. Dossey and Swyers (1994) suggest that barriers to use of complementary therapies can be structural in nature or can relate to regulatory, economic, and belief systems. Structural barriers include problems caused by a lack of common classification systems and definitions between biomedicine and complementary modalities, difficulty in obtaining original research on complementary therapies because they are not published in English in scientifically reviewed literature, and lack of understanding of culturally based explanatory models. For example, a family may wish to obtain more information about the efficacy of an herbal preparation that they heard may help with their mother's chronic illness, but the major research is published in Chinese or German. Regulatory and economic barriers include current federal mechanisms for regulating medical research, which do not favor the evaluation of many forms of complementary treatments; the cost of conducting the necessary laboratory and clinical trials of a product or procedure; and the existence of state medical practice acts that limit the practice of healing arts to holders of medical licenses. An example of this barrier is the limited access to naturopathic physicians because they are not licensed in most states.

Belief barriers include ideological skepticism flowing from comfort with the status quo, belief that high-technology interventions are more effective, and attitudes that any modality other than biomedicine is unscientific.

These barriers include attitudes of conventional practitioners that consider use of herbal preparations, for example, rather than a medical intervention to be a waste of money because they have not been "scientifically" studied, even when the patient is experiencing benefit from the preparations. Although the work of NCCAM and other organizations is helping reduce these barriers, nurses need to be alert for situations in which patients experience limited access to or availability of complementary modalities (Cuellar et al., 2003).

The power relationship between the nurse and the patient can present barriers to the patient's use of complementary therapies. The nurse is in a role of power and authority derived from professional knowledge and skills. Persisting paternalistic attitudes within healthcare settings, which foster the dependent role for patients, may manifest as attitudes indicating that approaches to managing health concerns other than those proposed by the nurse are unacceptable and without sound basis. Consider, for example, a nurse who is very willing to support the physician's recommendation of surgery or strong narcotics for the management of severe pain but who is unwilling to discuss the patient's interest in trying acupuncture, declaring that such approaches are unreliable. When nurses assume that a patient's values and thought processes are the same as their own, they may believe that the only reasonable courses of action are those that they as nurses would choose. Such attitudes may prompt nurses to question the decision-making capacity of patients who choose complementary therapies in lieu of or in addition to conventional therapies or label them as noncompliant, both of which can present barriers to the patient's use of therapies that may enhance the healing process.

❝ *There is no need to go to India or anywhere else to find peace. You will find that deep place of silence right in your room, your garden, or even your bathtub.* ❞

—*Elisabeth Kübler-Ross*

## Integrating Complementary Therapies into Community Nursing Care

As noted previously, holistic care should be the goal of all nursing practice. Although holistic care presumes attention to physical, mental, emotional, and spiritual concerns, many look upon spirituality as complementary therapy. The tendency to view body and spirit as separate and unrelated entities (which persists within contemporary healthcare settings) supports the view that physical concerns are the prime focus of biomedicine and that spirituality has little or no place in biomedical care. However, body–mind–spirit are inextricably intertwined, and spirituality cannot be separated from physical and emotional health.

This section briefly discusses ways of integrating spirituality and selected complementary modalities into nursing care. When considering integrating any modality into practice, nurses need to address two fundamental concerns:

(1) safety—the potential side effects and risks for harm when the therapy is used alone or in combination with other therapies, and (2) efficacy—the therapy's ability to produce the effect that it is intended to produce. The examples of complementary modalities presented here are chosen because they can be particularly valuable nursing interventions that clearly fall within nursing's domain of practice. Educational programs are available through which nurses can become certified practitioners of many of these therapies. Although it is within nursing's domain of practice to address diet, nutrition, and lifestyle changes, nurses must recognize that when such modalities are considered complementary or alternative, they are often based on nonorthodox systems of healing or are applied in unconventional ways. Nurses need to be aware that their patients are using these modalities, their reasons for using them, and potential risks and benefits.

The nursing role includes supporting that which promotes health and healing, advising caution where risks are involved, facilitating open communication about various options, and honoring the patient's right to choose. Nurses can become knowledgeable about and through training become practitioners of alternative healing modalities such as acupuncture, oriental medicine, homeopathy, and Ayurvedic medicine (Cuellar, 2005). Some aspects of other healing systems may be easily integrated into nursing care, such as use of particular acupressure points for relief of headaches or nausea. However, nurses need to be aware of the scope of

Complementary health research has consistently linked close human-pet relationships with improved health outcomes.

***What Dreams May Come*** **(1998)**
Physician Chris Nielson meets his true soulmate, Annie, marries her, and has two children. The children die in a car accident, and Chris dies 4 years later. Ending up in heaven, he is guided by friendly guardian angel Albert through the afterlife, where he is reunited with his dog and children. But when he finds out his wife has committed suicide, he desperately searches for her spirit, journeying through heaven and hell along the way.

practice stated in their state's nurse practice act and incorporate only those modalities that are within their scope of nursing practice.

## ■ Spirituality

Spirituality is the essence of who one is, a unifying or animating force that permeates all of one's life and being. This essence is expressed in and through connectedness with one's self, with others, with nature, and with a God or a Life Force. Although one's spirituality and relationship with God or Life Force is often nurtured and expressed through one's religious beliefs and practices, for many, spirituality transcends the boundaries of religion. Spirituality is connected to values and is vital to the process of discovering meaning and purpose in life. Spiritual issues are core life issues that are often related to mystery, suffering, forgiveness, grace, hope, and love (Burkhardt & Nagai-Jacobson, 1997a, 2002, 2005).

The nursing assessment of spirituality requires attentive listening, the ability to be fully present with the patient in this moment, and good communication skills. Assessment of spiritual concerns with patients includes exploration of issues of meaning and purpose; important values, beliefs, and practices; prayer or meditation styles; important relationships and their influence on the present circumstances; and desires for connection with religious groups or rituals. The process of assessment often is part of the intervention because merely providing the opportunity for patients to talk of their spiritual concerns enables them to become more aware of their spiritual journey and its impact on present life experiences. Because people often use story and metaphor in expressing their spirituality and spiritual concerns, nurses can approach spirituality by encouraging people to tell their stories. In this process, nurses can gain insight into those connections that support and inspire a patient, relationships in need of forgiveness and healing, sources of strength, experiences that have given life meaning, and ways in which the person questions the meaning of life. Nurses can help patients attune to their spirituality by exploring and incorporating meaningful rituals into care such as sacred readings, drumming, and music; facilitating processes focused on mindfulness such as relaxation exercises, imagery, and paying attention to physical sensations;

and fostering consideration of the place and meaning of prayer for patients and the ways they do or do not experience God or Life Force in their lives. Nurses need to be aware of their own spiritual perspectives to honor their own values and beliefs without imposing them on patients.

### Prayer

The experience of prayer or some form of connecting to the "beyond" is fundamental to human life and experience. The literature provides evidence indicating that prayer and religious devotion are associated with health outcomes (Burkhardt & Nagai-Jacobson, 2002; Dossey, L. 1993, 1996, 1997, 1998; Dunn & Horgas, 2000; Meisenhelder & Chandler, 2000; Walton &Sullivan, 2004). Dossey notes that research on intercessory prayer and distant intentionality indicate that open-ended, nondirective prayer such as "Thy will be done" or "Whatever is best for all concerned" is more efficacious than prayers for particular outcomes. He also reminds us that prayer does not require scientific evidence for validation. Prayer is an appropriate nursing intervention, whether the nurse prays for or with patients or arranges for patients to have the quiet and privacy needed for prayer or meditation. Nurses who include prayer as part of their patient care need to remember that prayer has many forms and expressions and is culturally conditioned.

When nurses incorporate prayer for patients into their personal spiritual practices, they should not presume to know what the patient needs; rather, they should express prayer in terms such as, "whatever is for the patient's highest good." Nurses who wish to pray with patients should do so with the patient's permission and encourage patients to use their own forms and expressions of prayer. Very often, patients in healthcare institutions need nurses to help them make sacred space within daily routines to attend to their own prayer, either alone or with others.

## ■ Music Therapy

Music has been a vital part of all cultures and societies and has been linked with healing throughout history. Guzzetta (1997, 2005) notes that **music therapy** complements conventional therapies by providing patients with integrated body–mind experiences and by facilitating relaxation, self-healing, and active participation in health and recovery. Music can promote relaxation and can produce changes in emotions, behavior, and physiology. Music can be used alone or in conjunction with prayer, meditation, relaxation exercises, and guided imagery. Musical vibrations can help restore or maintain the body's regulatory function; can help reduce pain, anxiety, isolation, and psychophysiological stress; can enhance the immune system; and can facilitate development of self-awareness and help improve memory (Guzzetta, 1997, 2005).

Guzzetta reminds us that, when considering using music therapy with patients, nurses need to assess patients' music preferences, the importance of music in their lives, and the

## *The Old Guitarist* by Pablo Picasso: Art and Nursing

*Jason Beasley*
*Senior BSN Nursing Student*
*The University of Southern Mississippi*

Art is a very powerful tool. It can express joy, hope, frustration, and many other human emotions in so many ways. Whether it is paint, crayon, clay, pencil, or charcoal, most people have a piece of art that they adore. *The Old Guitarist* by Pablo Picasso is the painting that I relate with health and grieving. The painting consists of an elderly man playing his guitar. The man's clothes are torn and dirty, but he plays. He looks like he does not have much longer to live, but he plays. His face tells a story of a hard life, but still he plays. To me, this painting symbolizes how people find ways to get through life. He looks as if he has nothing. I do not know what the history of the man was, but it looks as if he has endured his share of hardships. From what I see, he held on to his guitar—it is how he got through those hardships. He could have given up, just wasted away, but he has not. He is still playing—to play his guitar is to live.

My "guitar" is nature. There is nothing more enjoyable to me than going for a walk on a nature trail or through the woods. When my grandma died 3 years ago, I was torn apart. She was the first immediate family member of mine that passed away. I got very upset when I found out she had died. I left the house because I just did not want to be around anyone else at the time. I needed to be alone and process what was happening. I took a walk though the woods near our house as I had done so many times in my life. Walking through the woods, the trees, the birds, and the breeze . . . I just felt that everything had a reason. I am not a deeply religious person, but I am spiritual. I felt connected like I have never felt before. I reached one of the bigger pine trees, the one my niece had decided to decorate with ribbons. I sat down under the pine tree, and broke down into tears. How was I to deal with this, how was I supposed to deal with this? I did not understand death, was I supposed to understand death? I just did not understand why the physical body stopped and the spiritual soul was no longer here with me. I had so many questions that I knew nobody could answer. As I sat there, the breeze picked up again and I felt a sense of knowing. I knew that someone was out there keeping an eye on everything. I knew that my grandma was still with me, just not in physical form. And I knew that no matter what happened to me in the future or where I was, I could talk to her whenever I needed to. It was an awesome experience.

My grandpa passed away 2 weeks ago. Again, it was hard, but I knew how to deal with it a little better. It still was not easy, but my "guitar" this time was the Longleaf Trail. I rode my bicycle on the trail and just meditated on life. No, I did not find the secret to life, but I did find solace. I knew that I now had two people who truly loved me watching over me. That brought a peace to my soul that will never be replicated.

I feel that, like the guitarist in the painting, I need a "guitar" to hold on to. Everyone needs a "guitar" to support them through the tough times. Life is not fair or easy, but we must endure it. I cannot remember who said "the hardest thing in this world is to live in it," but the quote means more to me now. Rough things are going to come my way, as for us all, whether they are health, financial, or social problems. There is no way to avoid problems in life. You cannot just give up or pretend the problems are not there: Face the problems head on and keep your "guitar" close by. I hope that when I am older, I am still playing my "guitar." Not only to comfort myself, but to help others find their own "guitar."

---

types of music that make them happy, sad, relaxed, tense, and so forth. Nurses must be aware that no one selection or type of music is best for all people or in all situations and that the patient's mood and preferences determine the types of music used and the goals of each session. Nurses can introduce patients to music therapy, initially guide them through the process, and help them develop their own healing scripts and music libraries. Guzzetta (1997, 2005) offers guidelines for incorporating music therapy into clinical settings and provides a script that nurses can use with patients during a music therapy session. Research conducted through the music therapy program at the University of Miami indicated that music contributed to an increase in levels of melatonin and human growth hormone (leading to better sleep patterns and fewer aches and pains) in Alzheimer's patients and that the combined use of music and guided imagery in clinical trials contributed to lower liver enzymes in patients with chronic hepatitis B and lower levels of stress hormones in healthy persons (Simonton, Cohen, Kumar, McKinney, & Tims, 1997).

Music therapy may focus on listening to music, moving to music, or participating in making music, either alone or with others. Community recreational drumming circles—an example of the latter—can be a therapeutic intervention in many community settings. Drumming has been a part of healing rituals in many cultures across the ages. Recreational drumming can promote self-expression, provide group support, decrease stress, enhance the immune system, and improve mood states (Bittman et al., 2001; Stevens, 2003).

## ■ Imagery

Imagery is a way of using the imagination and connecting with the more subtle aspects of inner experiences that may involve all senses—vision, taste, smell, touch, and hearing. Images, which can be considered a bridge between conscious processing of information and physiological change, can be produced by conscious as well as subconscious acts and may precede or follow physiological change (Dossey, B. M., 1997;

## A Good Read

# Drumming On the Edge of Magic: A Journey Into the Spirit of Percussion (1990)

*By Mickey Hart, with Jay Stevens, New York: HarperCollins.*

Mickey Hart, former drummer of the Grateful Dead, has written an illuminating history of drums from an insightful journey through ethnic drumming. The book is well referenced and documented, with research on the connection between drumming and human survival. This book is illustrated with ample photos and artwork from around the world and throughout history, including images of drumming circles and the various objects used for drumming. In this important seminal book on our human need for rhythm, Hart studies the emotional, spiritual, and physical effects of drums, ancient and new, on the human species. Those interested in incorporating drumming into wellness and health promotion will find this book an invaluable, classic resource.

Shaub & Dossey, 2005). Imagery enables access to our emotions and to our spiritual or higher self. Dossey (1997) describes several types of imagery: receptive, active, symbolic, process, correct biological, end-state, general healing, packaged, customized, and interactive guided imagery. Although nurses can use any type with patients to enhance their healing processes, they need to appreciate individual variations of images, colors, shapes, symbols, and meanings related to cultural diversity. Nurses can use imagery to help promote a sense of well-being with patients; encourage healthy behaviors; and help them modify their perceptions about their diseases, strengths, treatments, and healing capacities. Relaxation exercises are a form of imagery.

An example of a situation in which imagery can be incorporated into nursing care is with bone or wound healing. Before the session, in terms the patient can understand, the nurse describes the basic biological process involved in the healing. The imagery process begins with a relaxation exercise. While the patient is in a relaxed state, the nurse instructs the patient to imagine the natural process of healing that is occurring, helping the patient by quietly describing the elements of the healing process, and ultimately imagining oneself as fully healed and back to normal activities.

Many resources are available for nurses who wish to develop skills in integrating imagery into nursing care (Achterberg, Dossey, & Kolkmeier, 1994; Dossey, B.M., 1997; Schaub-Dossey, 2005), including a nurses' certification program in interactive imagery sponsored by the American Holistic Nurses Association and the Academy for Guided Imagery.

## ■ Herbal Therapies

**Herbal and natural therapies**, which have been used for healing in all cultures from before the time of written history, are becoming more common and are available in grocery stores and regular pharmacies. Although many natural and herbal preparations can enhance health and contribute to the prevention of disease, they are not necessarily safe just because they are natural (Duke, 1997; Murray, 1995). Because plants cannot be patented, limited research has been done in the United States on plants as a medicinal agents and there is a lack of standardization regarding the amount of the active ingredient of the plant that is in any particular herbal preparation (Murray, 1995). Although research on plants as medicinal agents is still in its infancy in this country, there is research to support the efficacy of many herbal and natural preparations (e.g., St. John's wort and gingko biloba) that has been done in other countries (Murray & Pizzorno, 1998). Because many patients use herbs and other natural preparations, nurses need to become knowledgeable about common herbs, their uses, and potential interaction with pharmaceutical drugs.

For example, many people consider herbal supplements to be safe and without harmful effects because they are "natural." In reality, some herbal preparations can cause medical problems if they are used incorrectly, taken in large amounts, or taken with some pharmaceutical medications. Ephedra, for example, has been associated with increased blood pressure and stress to the circulatory system, causing sometimes fatal side effects. Because of this danger, dietary supplements containing ephedra have been banned by the FDA. Other supplements many have many health benefits and need to be used with careful consideration in only a few circumstances. For example, coenzyme Q10 (CoQ10) is made naturally by the body, helps cells produce energy, acts as an antioxidant, and stimulates the immune system. This dietary supplement can also reduce the body's response to the anticoagulant medication warfarin and can decrease insulin requirements for persons with diabetes (http://www.cancer.gov/cancertopics/pdq/cam/coenzymeQ10). People with these conditions who take CoQ10 must be carefully monitored.

Nurses need to ask about use of herbal and natural preparations in the same way they include discussion of other medications. Of particular importance is advising patients who take herbal preparations to read labels and buy only those that have standardized extracts of the active herb. Students are encouraged to explore the many good references available that discuss the healing benefits, side effects, and interactions of various herbal and natural preparations.

❝*All things share the same breath—the beast, the tree, the man . . . the air shares its spirit with all the life it supports.*❞

—*Chief Seattle*

### Aromatherapy

Aromatherapy refers to the therapeutic use of the essential (concentrated) oils extracted from different parts of aromatic plants. The oils, which are widely available, may be applied to the body through massage, inhaled as mists, used as a compress, or mixed into an ointment. Although research on the health benefits of aromatherapy is in its infancy, use of this therapy shows promise in promoting relaxation; relieving stress, anxiety, pain, discomfort, insomnia, and restlessness; promoting wound healing; enhancing self-esteem; and stimulating immune function (Stevensen, 1996). Although aromatic oils have been used for varied purposes for centuries, recent years have seen a resurgence in the use of aromatherapy among lay people as well as nurses. Robbins (1999) notes that aromatherapy is a safe therapy, with few adverse reactions reported in the literature, although its mechanisms of action and efficacy need further research. Robbins suggests that nurses who wish to consider using aromatherapy as an adjunct in nursing practice should have some formal training, use caution when using these oils with people with very sensitive skin or severe respiratory disorders, and be aware that most of these oils should not be ingested.

> **"** If you can walk, you can dance. If you can talk, you can sing. **"**
>
> —Zimbabwe proverb

### ■ Touch Therapy

Touch is essential for human survival and development. **Touch therapy** includes a broad range of hand techniques that a nurse can use on or near the body to support the patient's movement toward balance, wholeness, and optimal functioning (Shames, 1997; Keegan & Shames, 2005). Touch interventions used by nurses include both physical and energetic healing modalities such as therapeutic massage, therapeutic touch, healing touch, acupressure, shiatsu, and reflexology. Massage (particularly of the back) has long been considered an important nursing intervention used to promote relaxation, relieve muscle discomfort, and stimulate circulation. Many books and educational programs are available for nurses who want to expand their skills with therapeutic massage.

Therapeutic touch (TT), a noninvasive healing technique developed by a nurse, Dr. Delores Krieger (1979), involves touching with conscious intent to heal. In TT, the nurse works from a centered state using the natural sensitivity of the hands to assess the patient's energy fields and treat imbalances. Healing touch (HT) (Hover-Kramer, 2001) is a collection of energy-based healing techniques, which, like TT, are noninvasive. The HT practitioner also works from a centered state to assist in making energy available to patients through application of systemic and localized techniques. In addition to promoting relaxation, decreasing anxiety, and balancing energy, research suggests that these therapies can enhance immune functioning (Olson, Sneed, LaVia, Virella, Bonadonna, & Michel, 1997), promote wound healing (Wirth, 1992), and decrease pain sensation (Lin & Taylor, 1998; Smith, 2001). Continuing education workshops,

**" a conversation with . . . "**

In considering, reconsidering Caring in the Community, perhaps a case can be made for Pure Caring, in that it is noninstitutional, real-living situations, in the community where the most authentic, and yet demanding aspects of personal–professional caring become manifest. What the nurse offers first, by way of establishing relationship-centered care, is Self: by this I mean bring one's whole self into the present. It is from this professional and philosophical orientation that authentic caring can be witnessed and experienced at its finest.

—**Jean Watson, PhD, RN, FAAN, HNC**
Distinguished Professor of Nursing,
Endowed Chair in Caring Science,
University of Colorado Health Sciences Center,
Denver, Colorado

Dr. Margaret A. Burkhardt, chapter author, demonstrating healing touch with a patient.

academic courses, and certification programs are available for nurses who wish to develop skills in these modalities. Acupressure, shiatsu, and reflexology are systems that use the application of pressure (with fingers, thumbs, or a blunt instrument) to specific points along energy pathways (meridians) of the body (acupressure and shiatsu) or in the feet or hands (reflexology). Continuing education workshops and certification programs are also available for nurses who wish to study these modalities.

## Conclusion

This chapter has discussed the use of complementary therapies within a holistic nursing frame of reference. Nurses must be aware that many people use complementary therapies in addition to biomedical interventions but often do not disclose this fact to their biomedical practitioners. Complementary modalities encompass all health systems, modalities, and practices other than those intrinsic to the politically dominant health system of a particular society or culture. Such therapies include all practices and ideas self-defined by their users as preventing or treating illness or promoting health and well-being. Many complementary modalities are based in cultural healing practices, which derive from different explanatory models than that of biomedicine.

Nurses need to be attentive to patient values and desires for treatment options, taking seriously the patient's need for healing as well as curing and the contributions to health offered by other explanatory models. If nurses do not understand the other modality or question the efficacy or safety of the choice, they should explore these considerations with the patient. Nurses need to be aware of the various therapies being considered or used by patients so that they are aware of the many factors affecting a patient's health and healing. Community nurses need to develop the ability to incorporate discussion of complementary therapies into assessment in an open way and work toward integration of complementary therapies with conventional interventions. Holistic nursing care implies attentiveness to spiritual concerns as well as to physical and emotional concerns. Prayer, imagery, music therapy, and touch therapy are examples of complementary modalities that can be incorporated into health care with patients in the community.

Explore Community Health Nursing on the Web! To learn more about the topics in this chapter, use the passcode provided to access your exclusive website: **http://nursing.jbpub.com/ communityhealth.** If you do not have a passcode, you can obtain one at this site.

## ■ CRITICAL THINKING ACTIVITIES

1. Explore the history, current practice, and research of a selected healing system other than biomedical medicine.
   - Compare and contrast the selected healing system with biomedical modalities relative to the explanatory model.
   - How are practitioners of the selected healing system educated, trained, and/or certified?
   - What are the roles of the practitioner and the patient in the selected healing system?
   - Describe how the selected healing system focuses on healing and curing.
2. Shawn is an outpatient oncology nurse who has cared for 32-year-old Kim during her 4 years of living with breast cancer. Kim has endured surgery and radiation and is currently undergoing another course of chemotherapy for recently discovered metastasis. Kim tells Shawn that she thinks the medical therapies are only making her sicker and that she has been doing a lot of reading about other ways of dealing with cancer. Kim says she is seriously considering discontinuing chemotherapy treatments and seeking healing through prayer and herbal remedies. She also indicates that she knows God can heal, but that if she is to die, she would rather die with dignity than be stuck in a hospital at-

tached to machines. It is clear from what Kim says that she has thoughtfully considered the various options with their risks and benefits. Shawn tells the physician about Kim's plans; the physician exclaims that Kim is "out of her mind" and suggests that family members be enlisted to persuade Kim to continue with conventional interventions. What do you think of Kim's plan? What personal values are evident in Kim's decision? How do you think you would respond if you were in Kim's situation?
3. How can Shawn respond to Kim in a way that demonstrates respect for persons and supports her autonomy?
4. What perspective is reflected in the physician's response?
5. What ethical conflicts might occur? How might the nurse suspect that the family feels coerced?
6. How do you think a holistic nurse would approach Kim and her care?
7. Talk with someone who uses as complementary health modality on a regular basis and discuss why they use the modality, the benefits of the modality, whether they discuss the therapy with biomedical practitioners, the cost, and how they pay for the modality.

## ■ REFERENCES

Achterberg, J., Dossey, B. M., & Kolkmeier, L. (1994). *Rituals of healing*. New York: Bantam Books.

American Holistic Nurses Association. (2008). *What is holistic nursing?* Retrieved November 12, 2008, from http://www.ahna.org/AboutUs/WhatisHolisticNursing/tabid/1165/Default.aspx

Barnes, P., Powell-Griner, E., McFann, K., & Nahin, R. (2004). Complementary and alternative medicine use among adults: United States, 2002. *CDC Advance Data Report #343*. Retrieved October 25, 2008, from http://www.cdc.gov/nchs/data/ad/ad343.pdf

Bennett, M. P., Zeller, J. M., Rosenberg, L., & McCann, J. (2003). The effect of mirthful laughter on stress and natural killer cell activity. *Alternative Therapies in Health and Medicine, 9*(2), 38–45.

Bittman, B. B., Berk, L. S., Felton, D. L., et al. (2001). Composite effects of group drumming music therapy on modulation of neuroendocrine-immune parameters in normal subjects. *Alternative Therapies in Health and Medicine, 7*(1), 38–47.

Burkhardt, M. A. (1985). Nursing, health and wholeness. *Journal of Holistic Nursing, 3*(1), 35–36.

Burkhardt, M. A., & Nagai-Jacobson, M. G. (1997a). Psychospiritual care: A shared journey embracing life and wholeness. *Bioethics Forum, 13*(4), 34–41.

Burkhardt, M. A., & Nagai-Jacobson, M. G. (1997b). Spirituality and healing. In B. M. Dossey (Ed.), *Core curriculum for holistic nursing* (pp. 42–51). Gaithersburg, MD: Aspen.

Burkhardt, M. A., & Nagai-Jacobson, M. G. (2002). *Spirituality: Living our connectedness*. Albany, NY: Delmar.

Burkhardt, M. A., & Nagai-Jacobson, M. G. (2005). Spirituality and health. In B. M. Dossey, L. Keegan, & C. E. Guzzetta (Eds.), *Holistic nursing practice* (4th ed., pp. 137–172). Sudbury, MA: Jones and Bartlett.

Burkhardt, M. A., & Nathaniel, A. K. (1996). Patient self-determination and complementary care. *Bioethics Forum, 12*, 24–30.

Burkhardt, M. A., & Nathaniel, A. K. (2002). *Ethics and issues in contemporary nursing* (2nd ed.). Albany, NY: Delmar.

Burkhardt, M. A., Nathaniel, A. K., Nemeth-Pyles, M., & Boyd, J. (1999). Utilization of complementary health practices among people in southern West Virginia. Presentation at the 18th Annual American Holistic Nurses Association Conference: Holistic Nursing—Heritage to Vision. Phoenix, AZ, June 16–20.

Cassidy, C. M. (1996). Cultural context of complementary and alternative medicine systems. In M. S. Micozzi (Ed.), *Fundamentals of complementary and alternative medicine*. New York: Churchill Livingstone.

Cuellar, N. (2005). Hypnosis for pain management in the older adult. *Pain Management Nursing, 6*(3), 105–111.

Cuellar, N., Aycock, T., Cahill, B., & Ford, J. (2003). The use of complementary and alternative medicine by African American and Caucasian American elders in a rural setting: A descriptive, comparative study. *BMC Journal of Complementary and Alternative Medicine, 3*(8).

Cuellar, N., Cochran, S., Ladner, C., Mercier, B., Townsend, A., Harbaugh, B., et al. (2003). Depression and the use of conventional and non-conventional interventions of rural patients: A descriptive, comparative study. *Journal of the American Psychiatric Nurses Association, 9*(5), 151–158.

Cuellar, N. G., Rogers, A. E., & Hisghman, V. (2007). Sleep in the older adult: Evidenced-based research in complementary and alternative medicine (CAM). *Geriatric Nursing, 28*(1), 46–52.

Dossey, B. M. (1997). Imagery. In B. M. Dossey (Ed.), *Core curriculum for holistic nursing* (pp. 188–195). Gaithersburg, MD: Aspen.

Dossey, B. M., & Guzzetta, C. E. (2005). Holistic nursing practice. In B. M. Dossey, L. Keegan, & C. E. Guzzetta (Eds.), *Holistic nursing: A handbook for practice* (4th ed., pp. 5–37). Sudbury, MA: Jones and Bartlett.

Dossey, L. (1993). *Healing words*. New York: HarperCollins.

Dossey, L. (1996). *Prayer is good medicine*. San Francisco: HarperCollins.

Dossey, L. (1997). The return of prayer. *Alternative Therapies in Health and Medicine, 3*, 10–17, 113–120.

Dossey, L. (1998). *Be careful what you pray for . . . you just might get it*. San Francisco: HarperCollins.

Dossey, L., & Swyers, J. P. (1994). Introduction. In National Institutes of Health, *Alternative medicine: Expanding medical horizons* (NIH Publication No. 94-066). Washington, DC: U.S. Government Printing Office.

Duke, J. A. (1997). *The green pharmacy*. Emmaus, PA: Rodale.

Dunn, K. S., & Horgas, A. L. (2000). The prevalence of prayer as a spiritual self-care modality in elders. *Journal of Holistic Nursing, 18*, 337–351.

Eisenberg, D. M., Kessler, R. C., Foster, C., Norlock, F. E., Calkins, D. R., & Delbanco, T. L. (1993). Unconventional medicine in the United States. *New England Journal of Medicine, 328*, 246–252.

Eisenberg, D. M., Rogers, B. D., Ettner, S., et al. (1998). Trends in alternative medicine use in the United States, 1990–1997. *Journal of the American Medical Association, 280*(18), 1569–1575.

Fenton, M. V., & Morris, D. L. (2003). The integration of holistic nursing practices and complementary and alternative modalities into curricula of schools of nursing. *Alternative Therapies in Health and Medicine, 9*(4), 62–67.

Gordon, J. S. (1980). The paradigm of holistic medicine. In A. Hastings (Ed.), *Health for the whole person* (pp. 31–45). Boulder, CO: Westview.

Gordon, J. S. (2002). The White House Commission on Complementary and Alternative Medicine Policy: Final report and next steps. *Alternative Therapies in Health and Medicine, 8*(3), 28–31.

Guzzetta, C. E. (1997). Music therapy. In B. M. Dossey (Ed.), *Core curriculum for holistic nursing* (pp. 196–204). Gaithersburg, MD: Aspen.

Guzzetta, C. E. (2005). Music therapy. In B. M. Dossey, L. Keegan, & C. E. Guzzetta (Eds.), *Holistic nursing: A handbook for practice* (4th ed., pp. 617–640). Sudbury, MA: Jones and Bartlett.

Hover-Kramer, D. (2002). *Healing touch: A resource for health care professionals*. New York: Delmar.

Hufford, D. J. (1996a). Ethical dimensions of alternative medicine. Presentation at the First Annual Alternative Therapies Symposium: Creating Integrated Healthcare. San Diego, CA, January 18–21.

Hufford, D. J. (1996b). Informed consent and alternative medicine. *Alternative Therapies in Health and Medicine, 2*, 76–78.

Keegan, L., & Shames, K. H. (2005). Touch. In B. M. Dossey, L. Keegan, & C. E. Guzzetta (Eds.), *Holistic nursing: A handbook for practice* (4th ed., pp. 643–666). Sudbury, MA: Jones and Bartlett.

Krieger, D. (1979). *The therapeutic touch*. Englewood Cliffs, NJ: Prentice-Hall.

Lin, Y. S., & Taylor, A. G. (1998). Effects of therapeutic touch in reducing pain and anxiety in an elderly population. *Integrative Medicine, 1*(4), 155–162.

Lowry, L. W., & Conco, D. (2002). Exploring the meaning of spirituality with aging adults in Appalachia. *Journal of Holistic Nursing, 20*(4), 388–402.

Meisenhelder, J. B., & Chandler, E. N. (2000). Prayer and health outcomes in church members. *Alternative Therapies in Health and Medicine, 6*, 56–60.

Micozzi, M. S. (1996). *Fundamentals of alternative and complementary medicine*. New York: Churchill Livingston.

Murray, M. (1995). *The healing power of herbs* (2nd ed.). Rocklin, CA: Prima.

Murray, M., & Pizzorno, J. (1998). *The encyclopedia of natural medicine* (2nd ed.). Rocklin, CA: Prima.

O'Connor, B. B. (1996). Medical ethics and patient belief systems. *Alternative Therapies in Health and Medicine, 2,* 92–93.

Olson, M., Sneed, N., LaVia, M., Virella, G., Bonadonna, R., & Michel, Y. (1997). Stress-induced immunosuppression and therapeutic touch. *Alternative Therapies in Health and Medicine, 3*(2), 68–74.

Quinn, J. F. (1989). On healing, wholeness, and the Haelan effect. *Nursing and Health Care, 10,* 553–556.

Robbins, J. L. W. (1999). The science and art of aromatherapy. *Journal of Holistic Nursing, 17*(1), 5–17.

Robison, J., & Carrier, K. (2004). *Spirit and science of holistic health: More than broccoli, jogging, and bottled water. . . More than yoga, herbs, and meditation.* Bloomington, IN: AuthorHouse.

Schaub, B. G., & Dossey, B. M. (2005). Imagery. In B. M. Dossey, L. Keegan, & C. E. Guzzetta (Eds.), *Holistic nursing: A handbook for practice* (4th ed., pp. 567–614). Sudbury, MA: Jones and Bartlett.

Shames, K. H. (1997). Touch. In B. M. Dossey (Ed.), *Core curriculum for holistic nursing* (pp. 205–210). Gaithersburg, MD: Aspen.

Sierpina, V. S. (2002). Progress notes: A review of educational developments in CAM. *Alternative Therapies in Health and Medicine, 8*(8), 104–106.

Simonton, O. C., Cohen, D., Kumar, M., McKinney, C., & Tims, F. (1997). Music as a healing force. Presented at Second Annual Alternative Therapies Symposium: Creating Integrated Healthcare, Orlando, FL.

Smith, D. W. (2001). Pattern changes in people experiencing therapeutic touch, Phase II. Pandimensional pattern changes in healers and healees in a therapeutic touch series. *Rogerian Nursing Science News Online, 1*(1), 4–6.

Stevens, C. K. (2003). *The art and heart of drum circles.* Milwaukee, WI: Hal Leonard.

Stevensen, C. J. (1996). Aromatherapy. In M. S. Micozzi (Ed.), *Fundamentals of alternative and complementary medicine* (pp. 137–148). New York: Churchill Livingston.

Walton, J., & Sullivan, N. (2004). Men of prayer: Spirituality of men with prostate cancer. *Journal of Holistic Nursing, 22,* 133–151.

Wirth, D. (1992). The effect of non-contact therapeutic touch on the healing rate of full thickness dermal wounds. *Subtle Energies, 1,* 1–20.

Sharyn Janes

Visit **http://nursing.jbpub.com/communityhealth** for interactive exercises, review questions, Web links, and more.

In a world connected by supersonic transports and cyberspace, nurses need to be alert to developments in the changing world. Nurses need to continually update and modify their nursing practices in accordance with changing global political, social, economic, and cultural realities.

There are people in the world so hungry, that God cannot appear to them except in the form of bread.

—*Mahatma Gandhi (1869–1948)*

The issue will not be that we are diverse; it will be what we do with our diversity that is important.

—*Marie Farrell*

As community health nurses, we are often overwhelmed with the problems facing the communities around us. How can we extend our care to the international community while still keeping our focus on the community in which we live and work? Is it possible to "think globally" and "act locally" without ever leaving our home communities? As the largest and most advanced country in the world, what role should the United States play in helping global at-risk populations lead healthier lives?

## CHAPTER FOCUS

**Globalization and International Health**

**Role of International Agencies**
- United Nations
- United Nations Children's Fund
- World Health Organization
- World Bank
- Carter Center
- Bill and Melinda Gates Foundation

**Global Health Issues**
- Disease Burden
- Violence and War

- Poverty
- Women's Rights

**Global Initiatives**
- Declaration of Alma Ata
- Millennium Developmental Goals

**Global Nursing**
- Nursing Shortages
- International Council of Nurses
- Nursing and Human Rights

**Appendix 17–1**

## QUESTIONS TO CONSIDER

After reading this chapter, you will know the answers to the following questions:

1. How has globalization affected international health?
2. What roles do violence and war play in international health efforts?
3. How is world health influenced by women's rights issues?

4. What roles do nurses play in international health?
5. How do nongovernmental agencies contribute to global health efforts?
6. How does the International Council of Nurses collaborate with other organizations to improve health care and nursing worldwide?

## KEY TERMS

Bill and Melinda Gates Foundation
Carter Center
*Declaration of Alma Ata*
Global health
"Health for All by the Year 2000"

Millennium Developmental Goals
Non-governmental organizations (NGOs)
Poverty
Primary health care

United Nations (UN)
United Nations International Children's Emergency Fund (UNICEF)

Violence
War
World Bank
World Health Organization (WHO)

AT THE BEGINNING of the twenty-first century, we are living in a global society. The Internet provides instant contact with people from many parts of the world. Through e-mail and the World Wide Web there is immediate access to a wide variety of information in many different languages. Not only are we exposed to many cultures and ideologies, but, through rapid global transit, we are also exposed to many diseases and conditions only heard or read about in the past. Travel time has been reduced to hours to get to the other side of the world.

Globalization is not a new concept for nurses. "Travel nursing" dates back to the days of Florence Nightingale in the Crimea. Her influence was not only felt in her native England, but also throughout Europe, the Middle East, Australia, North America, and parts of Asia and Africa. Many of the healthcare challenges she faced in the mid-nineteenth century are similar to the healthcare challenges faced by nurses in the twenty-first century. Nightingale's systematic approach to nursing became the basis for modern nursing. In 1899, the nursing profession, realizing the importance of a global approach to nursing, established the International Council of Nurses (ICN), which was the first international organization for healthcare professionals. Today the ICN is a federation of 129 national nurses' associations, representing millions of nurses worldwide (ICN, 2008).

**❝**There were but two families in the world, Have-much and Have-little. **❞**

—Miguel de Cervantes

**❝**Go to the people. Live with them. Learn from them. . . . Start with what they know; build with what they have. But with the best leaders, when the work is done, the task is accomplished, the people will say, 'We have done this ourselves!'**❞**

—Lao Tzu (700 B.C.)

## Globalization and International Health

Health professionals, particularly nurses, have a duty to influence global health care from both preventive and restorative perspectives. Every nurse should consciously be involved with the business of **global health**, because health care is the business of nurses. The world is constantly changing, with poverty, epidemics, war, famine, rapid technological advances, environmental and natural disasters, and social injustice greatly influencing the health of the world's people (Basford, 2003).

Population demographics are shifting as the world's population expands. In 2006, the world population reached 6.6 billion, up from 6 billion in 1999, and it is expected to reach 8 billion by 2025. Ninety-nine percent of that growth is expected to occur in resource-poor countries. An estimated 4.3 people are born every second around the world (PRB, 2006). In many parts of the world the population is aging,

but in the countries affected by the HIV epidemic, life expectancy has dropped to 30–40 years. The current populations of these countries consist mostly of children and elders. The disappearance of the working-age population has greatly increased the levels of poverty for these regions in a world already overburdened by poverty.

**❝**Others say the human population level is okay and can continue to increase because science will meet our needs with new sources of energy and things like that. But even if we sustain 10 billion people, then as it goes it will become 15 billion, then 20 billion. Impossible!**❞**

—Dalai Lama

 CULTURAL CONNECTION

Do you consider poverty to be a cultural issue or an economic issue, especially as it relates to impoverished and underdeveloped countries?

As long as high birth rates and poverty continue to put pressure on populations, many people will see advantages in moving to countries believed to have more resources and greater opportunities. Each year, nearly 3 million migrants move from poor countries to wealthier ones. Increasingly, however, more of the migration is occurring between developing countries as the wealthier nations tighten immigration laws to protect themselves economically.

The population of the United States continues to diversify, with the number of foreign-born residents reaching an all-time high, even though the percentage of foreign-born individuals in the population is lower than it was in 1910. Even with this large number of immigrants, 60% of the U.S. population increase is attributable to natural increases (births minus deaths) in the native-born population. The United States is currently the world's third largest country and is expected to remain so through at least 2050 (see Box 17-1).

Most European nations and some industrialized Asian nations such as Japan are dealing with population declines that may have negative economic consequences for these countries in the future. These countries are challenged with raising their extremely low birth rates and/or developing immigration policies and social programs that benefit their own citizens while encouraging people from other countries to migrate (PRB, 2006).

## Role of International Agencies

### ■ United Nations

The **United Nations (UN)** was founded in 1945 when 51 nations came together after World War II to establish a commitment to world peace and security through international cooperation. Today, with a membership of 192 nations, the UN represents the interests of almost all countries of the world. When nations become members of the UN, they agree

## BOX 17-1

### The World's 10 Largest Countries by Population, 2006 and 2050

| 2006 | | 2050 | |
|---|---|---|---|
| Country | Population (millions) | Country | Population (millions) |
| China | 1,311 | India | 1,628 |
| India | 1,122 | China | 1,437 |
| United States | 299 | United States | 420 |
| Indonesia | 225 | Nigeria | 299 |
| Brazil | 187 | Pakistan | 295 |
| Pakistan | 166 | Indonesia | 285 |
| Bangladesh | 147 | Brazil | 260 |
| Russia | 142 | Bangladesh | 231 |
| Nigeria | 135 | Democratic Republic of the Congo | 183 |
| Japan | 128 | Ethiopia | 145 |

*Source*: Population Reference Bureau, 2006.

to accept the obligations of the UN Charter, which outlines the basic principles of international relations. However, the United Nations is not a form of world government. It does not make laws, but merely provides the means to help resolve global conflicts and formulate policies that affect all nations. All member nations, regardless of their size, wealth, or political system, have an equal vote in the decision-making process. While the UN cannot force any member nation to act on any recommendations made, its decisions reflect world opinion and represent the moral authority of the community of nations (United Nations, 2008).

The United Nations worked to combat all intolerance in all forms throughout the second half of the twentieth century and continues to do so in the twenty-first century. In 1948, the Universal Declaration of Human Rights was drafted by the General Assembly of the UN to outline the basic rights and freedoms to which all peoples of the world are entitled. Two International Covenants were developed, which most UN member nations consider to be legally binding. One addresses economic, social, and cultural rights; the other addresses civil and political rights. These two covenants, along with the Universal Declaration of Human

## ❝ *a conversation with . . .* ❞

Now I want to pass on five lessons I have learned during 10 years as Secretary-General of the United Nations, lessons I believe the community of nations needs to learn as it confronts the challenges of the twenty-first century.

Lesson One: In today's world, we are all responsible for each other's security. Against such threats as nuclear proliferation, climate change, global pandemics, or terrorists operating from safe havens in failed nations, no state can make itself secure by seeking supremacy over all others. Only by working to make each other secure can we hope to achieve lasting security for ourselves.

Lesson Two: We are responsible for each other's welfare. Without a measure of solidarity, no society can be truly stable. It is not realistic to think that some people can go on deriving great benefits from globalization while billions of others are left out or thrown into abject poverty. We have to give all our fellow human beings at least a chance to share in our prosperity.

Lesson Three: Both security and prosperity depend on respect for human rights and the rule of law. Throughout history, human life has been enriched by diversity, and different communities have learned from each other. But if our communities are to live in peace, we must stress what unites us: our common humanity and the need for our human dignity and rights to be protected by law.

Lesson Four: Governments must be accountable for their actions, in the international as well as the domestic arena. Every state owes some account to other states on which its actions have a decisive impact.

Lesson Five: How can states hold each other accountable? Only through multilateral institutions. Those institutions must be organized in a fair and democratic way, giving the poor and the weak some influences over the rich and the strong. Developing countries should have a stronger voice in international financial institutions, whose decisions can mean life or death for their people.

More than ever, Americans, like the rest of humanity, need a functioning global system. Experience has shown, time and again, that the system works poorly when the United States remains aloof but functions much better when there is far-sighted U.S. leadership. That gives American leaders of today and tomorrow a great responsibility. The American people must see that they live up to it.

—**Koffi A. Annan**, United Nations Secretary General, 1997–2006, and 2001 Nobel Peace Prize recipient, excerpt from a speech at the Truman Presidential Museum and Library, Independence, Missouri, December 11, 2006

Rights, constitute the International Bill of Human Rights (United Nations, 2002).

Through the years, the United Nations has established special organizations, such as the United Nations Children's Fund, to address various social and economic issues. Several independent intergovernmental organizations are also related to the UN through special agreements but are not under UN authority. They have their own memberships, charters, budgets, and staffs (see Box 17-2). Also working closely with the United Nations are many independent **non-governmental organizations (NGOs)**. The Carter Center and the Bill and Melinda Gates Foundation are just two of the many NGOs serving the vulnerable populations of the world.

Every day the UN and its family of organizations, collectively known as the UN system, work to promote respect for human rights, protect the environment, fight disease, and reduce poverty. In addition, the UN system leads international efforts to stop drug trafficking and terrorism, assist refugees, clear landmines, and increase food production and distribution (United Nations, 2008).

### ■ United Nations Children's Fund

The **United Nations International Children's Emergency Fund (UNICEF)** was created in 1946 to assist millions of sick and hungry children in war-torn Europe and China.

---

## BOX 17-2

**Global Agencies: Autonomous Organizations Linked to the United Nations through Special Agreements**

| | |
|---|---|
| Food and Agriculture Organization (FAO) | Works to improve agricultural productivity and food security, and to better the living standards of rural populations. |
| International Atomic Energy Agency (IAEA) | Works for the safe and peaceful uses of atomic energy. |
| International Civil Aviation Organization (ICAO) | Sets international standards for safety, security, and efficiency of air transport, and serves as the coordinator for international cooperation in all areas of civil aviation. |
| International Fund for Agricultural Development (IFAD) | Mobilizes financial resources to raise food production and nutrition levels among the poor in developing countries. |
| International Labor Organization (ILO) | Formulates policy and programs to improve working conditions and employment opportunities, and sets labor standards used by countries around the world. |
| International Maritime Organization (IMO) | Works to improve international shipping procedures, raise standards in marine safety, and reduce marine pollution by ships. |
| International Monetary Fund (IMF) | Facilitates international monetary cooperation and financial stability and provides a permanent forum for consultation, advice, and assistance on financial issues. |
| International Telecommunication Union (ITU) | Fosters international cooperation to improve telecommunications of all kinds, coordinates usage of radio and YV frequencies, promotes safety measures, and conducts research. |
| United Nations Educational, Scientific, and Cultural Organization (UNESCO) | Promotes education for all, cultural development, protection of the world's natural and cultural heritage, international cooperation in science, press freedom, and communication. |
| United Nations Industrial Development Organization (UNIDO) | Promotes the industrial advancement of developing countries through technical assistance, advisory services, and training. |
| Universal Postal Union (UPO) | Establishes international regulations for postal services, provides technical assistance, and promotes cooperation in postal matters. |
| World Bank Group (WBG) | Provides loans and technical assistance to developing countries to reduce poverty and advance sustainable economic growth. |
| World Health Organization (WHO) | Coordinates programs aimed at solving health problems and the attainment by all people of the highest possible level of health. Works in such areas as immunization, health education, and the provision of essential drugs. |
| World Intellectual Property Organization (WIPO) | Promotes international protection of intellectual property and fosters cooperation on copyrights, trademarks, industrial designs, and patents. |
| World Meteorological Organization (WMO) | Promotes scientific research on the Earth's atmosphere and on climate change, and facilitates the global exchange of meteorological data. |
| World Tourism Organization (WTO) | Serves as a global forum for tourism policy issues and a practical source of tourism know-how. |

*Source*: United Nations, 2008.

## ENVIRONMENTAL CONNECTION

You have noticed that everything an Indian does is in a circle, and that is because the Power of the World always works in circles, and everything tries to be round. . . . The Sky is round, and I have heard that the earth is round like a ball, and so are all the stars. The wind, in its greatest power, whirls. Birds make their nest in circles, for theirs is the same religion as ours. . . . Even the seasons form a great circle in their changing, and always come back again to where they were. The life of a man is a circle from childhood, and so it is in everything where power moves.

—Black Elk, Oglala Sioux holy man (1863–1950)

It soon became apparent that children all over the world needed help, so in 1950 its mandate was broadened to address the long-term needs of children and women in developing countries around the world. UNICEF became a permanent part of the UN system in 1953, when its name was shortened to the United Nations Children's Fund, though it retained UNICEF as its acronym (UNICEF, 2007a).

Today, UNICEF's primary objective is to provide economic and humanitarian relief for the world's most disadvantaged children without discrimination. The children in the countries with the greatest need receive the highest priority. Special protection is ensured to children who are victims of war, disasters, extreme poverty, and all forms of violence and exploitation, and to those with disabilities (UNICEF, 2007a).

UNICEF works to improve the lives of children in more than 190 countries around the world. Its programs and services are aimed at ending hunger and malnutrition, helping refugees, promoting the education of girls, controlling disease (primarily through immunization and HIV/AIDS programs), saving the environment, and securing human rights (UNICEF, 2007a).

### ■ World Health Organization

Organized efforts at providing a global health network date back to the 1830s, when an international alliance was formed to combat the cholera epidemic that was sweeping Europe. Sporadic efforts continued throughout the next hundred years until the **World Health Organization (WHO)** was founded in 1948 through a special agreement with the United Nations. Today WHO, as a partner in the UN system, is responsible for directing and coordinating international health. The focus of WHO's work is producing and disseminating global health standards and guidelines, helping countries to address public health issues, and supporting health research (WHO, 2007a). Its primary objective is for all people to attain the highest possible level of health (see Box 17-3). WHO defines health as "a state of complete physical, mental, and social well-being and not merely the absence of disease or infirmity."

---

### BOX 17-3

**Notable Achievements of the World Health Organization**

| | |
|---|---|
| **1948** | The World Health Organization's Constitution was founded on April 7—a date now celebrated every year as World Health Day. The first World Health Assembly established its top priorities as malaria, women's and children's health, tuberculosis, venereal disease, nutrition, and environmental sanitation. |
| **1952** | Dr. Jonas Salk (United States) developed the first successful polio vaccine. |
| **1952–1964** | The global yaws-control program used long-acting penicillin with one single injection to control yaws, a crippling, disfiguring disease. By 1965, the prevalence of yaws was reduced by more than 95%. |
| **1967** | Dr. Christian Bernard (South Africa) conducted the first heart transplant surgery. |
| **1974** | The World Health Assembly adopted a resolution to create the Expanded Program on Immunization to bring basic vaccines to all children in the world. |
| **1977** | The first Essential Medicines List was developed, 2 years after the World Health Assembly introduced the concepts of "essential drugs" and "national drug policy." |
| **1978** | The International Conference on Primary Health Care, in Alma Ata, Kazakhstan (former Soviet Union), set the historic goal of "Health for All." |
| **1979** | Smallpox—a disease that had maimed and killed millions—was eradicated. It was the first (and so far only) time that a major infectious disease has been eradicated and ranks as one of WHO's greatest achievements. |
| **1983** | Scientists at Pasteur Institute (France) identified HIV. |
| **1988** | The Global Polio Eradication Initiative was established. |
| **2003** | The first global public health treaty was adopted at the World Framework Convention on Tobacco Control. The treaty was designed to reduce tobacco-related deaths and diseases around the world. |
| **2004** | The Global Strategy on Diet, Physical Activity, and Health was adopted. |
| **2005** | The World Health Assembly revised the International Health Regulations. |

*Source:* WHO, 2007a.

---

The WHO membership consists of 193 countries and two associate members. Representatives from each of the member states meet every year at the World Health Assembly in Geneva, Switzerland, to set policy, approve the budget, and, every 5 years, to appoint a new Director-General. Their work is supported by the 34-member Executive Board, which is elected by the World Health Assembly (WHO, 2007b).

**BOX 17-4**

**World Health Organization Regional Offices**
African Region: Brazzaville, Congo
Eastern Mediterranean Region: Cairo, Egypt
European Region: Copenhagen, Denmark
Region of the Americas: Washington, D.C., United States
South-East Asia Region: New Dehli, India
Western Pacific Region: Manila, Philippines

*Source*: WHO, 2007a.

❝*Our success—WHO's and yours—will depend on shaping public opinion and stimulating public action through elected representatives and civil society—at local, national, regional, and global levels. The fundamental message we send is that health is a fundamental human right, enshrined in the Universal Declaration of Human Rights. This means more than universal access to care. It depends on the assurance of many other rights in the Declaration: access to education and information, the right to food in sufficient quantity and of good quality, the right to decent housing, and the right to live and work in an environment where known health risks are controlled.*❞

—Gro Harlem Brundtland, WHO Director-General,
Geneva, Switzerland, November 23, 1999

❝*The most sophisticated and effective health care in the world cannot produce results as good as simply remaining healthy in the first place.*❞

—Robert G. Evans

To better address the specific environmental, political, social, economic, and cultural needs associated with global healthcare issues in various parts of the world, WHO is divided into six major regions, each with its own regional office (see Box 17-4). More than 8,000 public health experts work in nearly 150 countries within these regions, as well as at WHO headquarters in Geneva, Switzerland. In addition to medical doctors, professional nurses and midwives, public health specialists, researchers, and epidemiologists, WHO staff include administrative, financial, and information systems specialists, as well as experts in the fields of health statistics, economics, and emergency relief (WHO, 2007a).

■ World Bank

Since its creation in 1944 as an international financial institution associated with the United Nations, the **World Bank** has attempted to meet the needs of a changing world economy. The World Bank, which was originally called the International Bank for Reconstruction and Development, began its operations in Washington, D.C., in 1946. Its primary function was to aid in the reconstruction of Europe after World War II. More than 60 years later, the World Bank's priorities have evolved from rebuilding war-damaged European nations to alleviating poverty in developing countries. Since the 1970s, this organization has

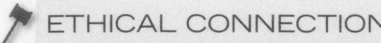 ETHICAL CONNECTION

Where, after all, do universal human rights begin? In small places, close to home—so close and so small that they cannot be seen on any map of the world. Yet they are the world of the individual person: the neighborhood he lives in; the school or college he attends; the factory, farm, or office where he works. Such are the places where every man, woman, and child seeks equal justice, equal opportunity, equal dignity without discrimination. Unless these rights have meaning there, they have little meaning anywhere. Without concerted citizen action to uphold them close to home, we shall look in vain for progress in the larger world.

—Eleanor Roosevelt (1884–1962), U.S. author,
diplomat, and First Lady, statements at presentation of
*In Your Hands: A Guide for Community Action
for the Tenth Anniversary of the Universal Declaration
of Human Rights* (March 27, 1958)

increasingly become more involved in health-related initiatives as a way to promote sustainable economic growth in its patient countries (Ruger, 2005).

Today the World Bank operates like a cooperative owned by 185 shareholder nations. The countries are represented by a board of governors, primarily consisting of ministers of finance or ministers of development from member nations, which meets once a year. The day-to-day work of the World Bank is conducted by 24 executive directors, who work at the World Bank headquarters. The five largest shareholder countries—France, Germany, Japan, the United Kingdom, and the United States—appoint an executive director from each, while other member countries are represented by 19 other executive directors. By tradition, the bank president is a citizen of the largest shareholder, the United States (World Bank, 2007a).

Over the past few decades, the World Bank has become increasingly instrumental in reducing poverty and raising the standard of living in many developing countries. Newly developed theories and evidence regarding successful economic development strategies have gradually changed the focus of the bank's lending policies. For example, in the 1950s and 1960s, promoting economic growth was viewed

 MEDIA MOMENT

***The Kite Runner*** (2007)
Based on the award-winning book by Khaled Hosseini, The Kite Runner tells the story of Amir, who is haunted by the guilt of betraying his childhood friend Hassan. The story is set against a backdrop of tumultuous events, from the fall of the monarchy in Afghanistan through the Soviet invasion, the mass exodus of refugees to Pakistan and the United States, and the rise of the Taliban regime. The movie is about redemption for past grievances and serves as a metaphor about the dismal past of a struggling country and its hopeful future.

as the key to development. At that time, the World Bank focused primarily on large investments in physical capital and government infrastructures. However, during the 1970s and 1980s, while still providing funding for economic growth and infrastructure support for governments, the World Bank began to focus some of its efforts on meeting basic human needs such as health care and education, recognizing them as important factors in development. Investment in government power sectors was reduced from 21% in 1980 to about 7% in 2007. By comparison direct funding for health, nutrition, education, pensions, and other social services increased from 5% to 22%. Table 17-1 lists some of the recent lending priorities for the World Bank.

While these successes are noteworthy, critics of the World Bank contend that more rapid progress is desperately needed. Major criticisms address the undemocratic governance and decision-making structures of the World Bank, which favor the elite interests within the wealthy nations. For example, the United States alone commands 16.4% of the World Bank's voting power. In its influential 1993 report *Investing in Health*, the World Bank stressed the importance of health to development while advocating for privatization of health services. In some situations, this approach has contributed to poor health outcomes by reducing access to health services for those who were unable to pay for such services. Many programs aimed at the poorest populations ignore structural deficiencies in social services (Birn & Dmitienko, 2005).

In 2003, the major international organizations representing nurses, teachers, and public-sector workers published serious criticisms of the World Bank's annual World

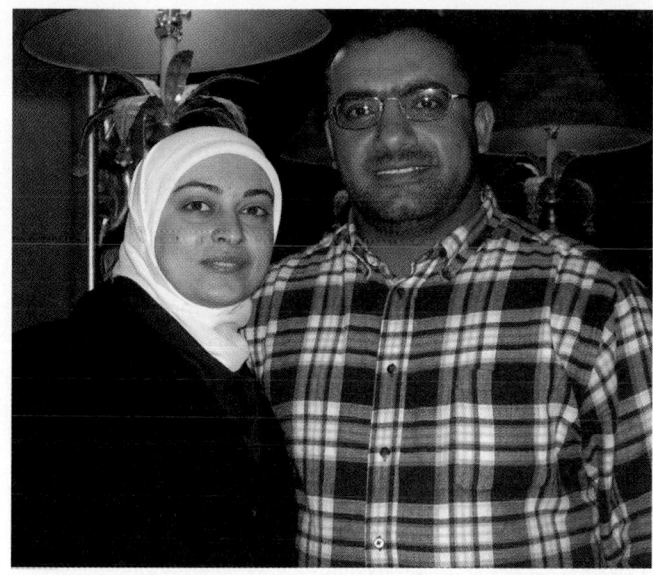

Muslim men and women vary considerably in their religious and cultural values. Community health nurses should avoid generalizations about this population regarding their health and religious practices.

Development Report (WDR). The ICN is the international federation for nurses' associations and unions, representing more than 12 million nurses in 129 countries; Education International (EI) is the global union federation for education unions, representing more than 26 million teachers in 155 countries; and Public Services International (PSI) is the global union federation for public-sector trade unions, representing more than 20 million workers in 149 countries (Communique, 2003). In a joint WHO communiqué, ICN,

| Table 17-1 | World Bank Development Projects |
|---|---|
| Education | ■ Provided $31 billion in loans and credits since 1963. |
| | ■ Currently funds 158 education projects in 83 countries. |
| | ■ Works closely with national governments, UN agencies, donors, NGOs, and other partners to help developing countries to provide primary education for all children—especially girls and disadvantaged children. |
| HIV/AIDS | ■ As a co-sponsor of UNAIDS, committed $1.7 billion to combat the spread of HIV/AIDS around the world. |
| | ■ Pledged that no country with an effective HIV/AIDS strategy will go without funding. |
| | ■ In partnership with African governments, launched the Multi-Country HIV/AIDS Program (MAP), which makes significant resources available to civil society organizations and communities. |
| Health | ■ Commits an average of $1 billion in new lending each year for health, nutrition, and population projects. The funds are helping to combat malaria in 46 countries and tuberculosis in 30 countries. |
| | ■ Helps provide iodized salt to more than 90% of households in China to significantly reduce miscarriages and stillbirths, physical deformity, and mental retardation caused by iodine deficiency. |
| Debt relief | ■ Launched the Heavily Indebted Poor Countries (HIPC) Initiative in 1996 to help reduce the external debt of the world's poorest, most indebted countries. Today, 26 countries are receiving debt relief projected to amount to $40 billion over time. |
| Biodiversity | ■ Since 1988, collaborated with Conservation International, the Global Environment Facility, the MacArthur Foundation, and the Japanese government in launching a fund for protecting biodiversity in developing countries. Because rural people in developing countries are most dependent on the environment for food, shelter, medicine, income, and cultural identity, more than $14 billion is being spent on environmental assessments and safeguard policies related to climate change, forests, and water resources. |
| Fight against corruption | ■ Since 1996, launched more than 600 anticorruption programs and governance initiatives in nearly 100 countries. |
| War/conflict | ■ Works in 40 conflict-affected countries supporting international efforts to assist war-torn populations, resume peaceful development, and prevent relapse into violence. |

*Source:* World Bank, 2007b.

EI, and PSI expressed concerns that the latest WDR inaccurately placed the blame for the failure of health, education, water, and other utility services in developing countries on the poor performance of providers—nurses, teachers, utility workers, and other public employees. They argued that the World Bank has failed to recognize that nurses, teachers, and utility workers in developing countries are poor themselves. The ICN Executive Officer, Judith Outon, stated that there were many cases where nurses and other healthcare workers produced positive outcomes by working together with the people. She also pointed out that the current state of public services in developing countries was largely a result of reforms initiated by the World Bank (Communique, 2003).

## ■ Carter Center

**❝**We believe good health is a basic human right, especially among poor people afflicted with disease who are isolated, forgotten, ignored, and often without hope.**❞**

*—Former U.S. President Jimmy Carter, founder and director of the Carter Center, Atlanta, Georgia*

The **Carter Center**, a nonprofit, non-governmental organization (NGO) located in Atlanta, was founded by Jimmy and Rosalynn Carter in 1982. This private, nonpartisan organization is associated with Emory University and governed by an independent board of trustees, which is chaired by former U.S. President Carter. Its many projects are supported by donations from individuals, foundations, corporations, and countries. Activities, directed by resident experts and scholars, are designed and implemented in cooperation with Jimmy and Rosalynn Carter, networks of world leaders, other NGOs, and partners in the United States and the rest of the world (Carter Center, 2006).

The Carter Center has been instrumental in alleviating global health problems through its commitment to promoting peace and fighting disease. Its work is guided by a fundamental commitment to human rights and the alleviation of human suffering. The Carter Center has three main objectives: (1) prevent and resolve conflicts, (2) enhance freedom and democracy, and (3) improve health. The belief that all three of these objectives work together to affect the prosperity and stability of entire nations is central to the work of the Carter Center in serving the needs of millions of forgotten people around the world (Carter Center, 2008).

## ■ Bill and Melinda Gates Foundation

The **Bill and Melinda Gates Foundation** is a nonprofit NGO that was founded in 2000 by Bill Gates, co-founder and CEO of Microsoft, and his wife Melinda French Gates. Bill Gates is one of the richest people in the world, with a net worth of more than $50 billion. Based in Seattle, Washington, the Gates Foundation is led by CEO Patty Stonesifer and co-chairs William H. Gates, Sr., Bill Gates, and Melinda French Gates. In developing countries, the foundation finances projects through its Global Development Programs and Global Health Programs that focus on reducing extreme poverty, improving health, and increasing access to public libraries. In the United States, programs are funded to ensure that all

## ❝❝ *a conversation with . . .* ❞❞

It is with a deep sense of gratitude that I accept this prize. I am grateful to my wife Rosalynn, to my colleagues at the Carter Center, and to many others who continue to seek an end to violence and suffering throughout the world. The scope and character of our Center's activities are perhaps unique, but in many other ways they are typical of the work being done by many hundreds of non-governmental organizations that strive for human rights and peace. . . .

I am not here as a public official, but as a citizen of a troubled world who finds hope in a growing consensus that the generally accepted goals of society are peace, freedom, human rights, environmental quality, the alleviation of suffering, and the rule of law. . . .

At the beginning of this millennium, I was asked to discuss, here in Oslo, the greatest challenge that the world faces. Among all the possible choices, I decided that the most serious and universal problem is the growing chasm between the richest and poorest people on earth . . . and the separation is increasing every year, not only between nations but also within them. The results of this disparity are root causes of the world's unresolved problems, including starvation, illiteracy, environmental degradation, violent conflict, and unnecessary illnesses that range from Guinea worm to HIV/AIDS.

Most of the work of the Carter Center is in remote villages in the poorest nations of Africa, and there I have witnessed the capacity of destitute people to persevere under heartbreaking conditions. I have come to admire their judgment and wisdom, their courage and faith, and their awesome accomplishments when given a chance to use their innate abilities. . . .

The bond of our common humanity is stronger than the divisiveness of our fears and prejudices. God gives us the capacity for choice. We can choose to alleviate suffering. We can choose to work together for peace. We can make these changes—and we must.

*—**Jimmy Carter**, former U.S. President, Carter Center founder and director and 2002 Nobel Peace Prize recipient, excerpts from Nobel Peace Lecture, Oslo, Norway, December 10, 2002*

people have access to a good education and to technology in the public libraries. In its local region around Seattle, the foundation funds projects that focus on improving the lives of low-income families (Gates Foundation, 2008).

## Global Health Issues

### ■ Disease Burden

#### Infectious Diseases

Throughout history, infectious diseases were the leading causes of death throughout the world. By the end of the twentieth century, however, medical science had developed successful prevention and treatment methods that greatly decreased the death rates from infectious diseases and raised the average life expectancy in middle- and higher-income countries by decades. Nevertheless, infectious diseases continue to kill more than 11 million people every year and cause disability and suffering for millions of others. The organisms that cause these diseases continue to evolve, often requiring the development of new drugs and methods to

Female children as young as 8 must take primary responsibility for younger children in many underdeveloped countries.

prevent and/or treat them. New pathogens are emerging or evolving from infecting animals to infecting humans. Recent estimates show that infectious diseases are responsible for one-third of all global mortality. Most of these deaths occur in low- and middle-income countries, emphasizing the fact that infectious diseases present a very different experience for the poor and the wealthy (Population Bulletin, 2006; Disease Control Priorities Project, 2006a).

In low- and middle-income countries, three infectious diseases are among the top causes of death for adults ages 15 to 59: HIV/AIDS causes more than 2 million deaths per year, tuberculosis (TB) causes approximately 1 million deaths per year, and lower respiratory infections kill approximately 330,000 people per year. In high-income countries, infectious diseases are not listed in the top 10 causes of death for adults. In low- and middle-income countries, 7 of the 10 leading causes of death for children younger than

### ❝ a conversation with . . . ❞

Every day, more than 1,000 children die because they didn't get a 15-cent measles vaccine. Almost 3 billion people around the world live on less than $2 per day. Here, in the United States, only one-third of students who start the ninth grade will graduate from high school with the skills they need to succeed in college and work. A disproportionate number of those who fall behind will be African American and Hispanic.

Our foundation and our partners are trying to solve these problems because we believe that all lives have equal value, no matter where they are being lived—in rich countries with high-quality health care or poor countries with almost none; in well-off suburbs with shiny new high schools or in disadvantaged communities where most kids drop out.

We also believe that from those to whom much is given, much is expected. We benefited from great schools, great health care, and a vibrant economic system. That is why we feel a tremendous responsibility to give back to society.

Some of the problems we work on already have solutions, and our focus needs to be on getting those solutions into the hands of the people who need them most. Other problems have never been given the attention they deserve, and we believe focused efforts can lead to amazing advances. The challenges we face are great, but so is the opportunity to improve people's lives.

—**Bill and Melinda Gates**, co-founders and co-chairs of the Bill and Melinda Gates Foundation, excerpts from a letter on the Gates Foundation website (http://www.gatesfoundation.org)

### ⑥ MEDIA MOMENT

#### *Rx for Survival: A Global Health Challenge* (2006)

From vaccines to antibiotics, clean water to nutrition, bio-terror threats to the HIV/AIDS pandemic, the six-part series *Rx for Survival* tells the tales of public health pioneers and captures the real-life drama of today's global struggle to overcome poor health and disease. Employing both historical dramatic sequences and current documentary stories, the series showcases milestones in public health history, such as the eradication of smallpox, alongside modern and future challenges, including SARS, a potential global flu pandemic, and recovery from the Asian tsunami catastrophe. The series can be previewed and ordered at http://www.pbs.org/wgbh/rxforsurvival/series/about/index.html.

14 years old are infectious diseases, which kill 6.5 million children each year. The leading infectious diseases causing high mortality rates in children are lower respiratory infections, diarrheal diseases, and malaria (Disease Control Priorities Project, 2006a).

### Chronic Diseases

In the twenty-first century, many developing countries are undergoing the same changes in the causes of morbidity and mortality that the developed countries experienced in the twentieth century. Because of changes in diet and lifestyle and increases in life expectancy, many developing countries are seeing increases in the incidence of chronic diseases such as cardiovascular diseases, cancers, diabetes, and chronic respiratory diseases. These diseases, which until recently were largely confined to wealthy nations, now account for more than half of all deaths in low- and middle-income countries (Disease Control Priorities Project, 2006b).

Obesity is fast becoming one of the world's leading risk factors for premature death. One in four people in the world is too fat. One-third of total deaths worldwide are directly linked to excessive weight, lack of exercise, and tobacco use. Most distressing is the rapid spread of obesity beyond wealthy developed nations to some of the poorest countries in the world (MSNBC, 2004). Because infectious diseases, malnutrition, and maternal mortality are still responsible for 40% of deaths in these countries, the rapid rise in chronic diseases is creating a dual burden of disease that many of the healthcare systems in these poor countries are ill equipped to handle (Disease Control Priorities Project, 2006b).

Cardiovascular disease is now the number one cause of death worldwide. Eighty percent of the world's 13 million cardiovascular disease deaths occur in low- and middle-income countries. Conventional risk factors such as tobacco

---

### Research Alert

To explore the state of reproductive health in Central and Eastern Europe since the dissolution of the Soviet Union, a study was conducted in two urban areas of the Ukraine. During a 19-month period between 1992 and 1994, 17,137 pregnancy outcomes were recorded. Sixty percent of the pregnancies were voluntarily terminated, generally before the 13th week. In pregnancies delivered after 20 weeks' gestation, fetal mortality was 29 per 1,000, nearly five times the rate among Caucasians in the United States. Perinatal mortality was estimated to be 35 per 1,000, about three times the U.S. rate. The data documented elevated reproductive risks in a former Soviet state. This study is believed to be the first to count and report pregnancy outcomes in the former Eastern bloc using World Health Organization definitions and research procedures.

*Source*: Little, R. E., Monaghan, S. S., Gladen, B. C., Shykryak-Nyzhnyk, Z., & Wilcox, A. J. (1999). Outcomes of 17,137 pregnancies in 2 urban areas of Ukraine. *American Journal of Public Health*, 89(12), 1832–1836.

---

### ✎ NOTE THIS! •

Of the 4.4 billion people in developing countries, nearly three-fifths lack access to safe sewers, a third have no access to clean water, a quarter do not have adequate housing, and a fifth have no access to modern health services of any kind.

More than 110 million active land mines are scattered in 68 countries, with an equal number stockpiled around the world. Every month more than 2,000 people are killed or maimed by mine explosions.

The three richest people in the world have assets that exceed the combined gross domestic product of the 48 least developed countries.

It is estimated that the additional cost of achieving and maintaining universal access to basic education for all, basic health care for all, reproductive health care for all women, adequate food for all, and clean water and safe sewers for all is roughly $40 billion a year—or less than 4% of the combined wealth of the 225 richest people in the world.

*Source*: UNDP, 1998.

---

use, high blood pressure, high blood glucose, lipid abnormalities, obesity, and physical inactivity contribute to the vast majority of cardiovascular disease mortality and morbidity. Even in sub-Saharan Africa, high blood pressure, high cholesterol, extensive tobacco and alcohol use, and low vegetable and food consumption are among the top risk factors for disease. More 13- to 15-year-olds around the world are smoking than ever before, and obesity levels in children are increasing not only in the United States and Europe, but also in countries as diverse as Brazil, China, India, and almost all island nations (Disease Control Priorities Project, 2006b).

Cancer is creating a quickly growing major global disease burden. The yearly incidence of cancer is projected to increase from 10 million to 15 million in 2020. Nine million cases are expected to occur in low- or middle-income countries. Cancer epidemiology differs between the developed and developing countries of the world, however. In Developed countries have relatively high rates of lung, colorectal, breast, and prostate cancer; in these countries there is a strong link between cancer and tobacco use, occupational carcinogens, diet, lifestyle, and obesity. By comparison, as many as 25% of cancers in developing countries are associated with chronic infections. Seven types of cancer account for 60% of all newly diagnosed cancer and cancer deaths in poorer countries: cervical, liver, stomach, esophageal, lung, colorectal, and breast (Disease Control Priorities Project, 2006b).

Diabetes is rapidly becoming a global pandemic with the unprecedented incidence and prevalence of type 2 diabetes. Type 2 diabetes, which until recently was an adult-onset disease, is being seen in more children, especially in the more developed nations. This trend is blamed on the epidemic increases in childhood obesity. In fact, today's youth are the first generation in history predicted to have a shorter life expectancy than their parents (Jain, 2004).

More than 141 million people with diabetes now live in low- and middle-income countries, which account for 72.5% of the world's total number of cases. These countries are spending between 2.5% and 15% of their annual health budgets on diabetic care. In 2025, it is predicted that more than 6% of the world's population will be diabetic, up 24% from 2003 levels (Disease Control Priorities Project, 2006b).

Chronic adult respiratory diseases, such as chronic obstructive pulmonary disease (COPD) and asthma, are major causes of the growing burden of chronic disease mortality and morbidity in the developing world. COPD, which includes emphysema, chronic bronchitis, and obstructive airway disease, is closely linked to cigarette smoking as well as to use of poorly vented, coal-burning cooking stoves. Asthma's prevalence worldwide is lower than the prevalence of other adult respiratory diseases, but studies done in some middle-income countries show that healthcare costs for asthma make up more than 1% of total healthcare costs (Disease Control Priorities Project, 2006b).

### GLOBAL CONNECTION

Bill Gates, founder of Microsoft, is the richest man in history, with an estimated fortune of $50–100 billion. Gates and his wife Melinda have also donated more money than anyone in history to projects designed to put computers in impoverished schools and created a foundation that pours millions of dollars into global health problems, such as HIV/AIDS in Africa and other countries.

## ■ Violence and War

### Levels of Violence

WHO defines **violence** as "the intentional use of force or power, threatened or actual, against oneself, another person, or against a group or community, that either results in or has a high likelihood of resulting in injury, death, psychological harm, maldevelopment, or deprivation" (WHO, 2002, p. 3). This definition includes all types of violence in all forms against individuals, families, and communities. *World Report on Violence and Health*, published by the World Health Organization in 2002, uses an ecological model to explore the biological, social, cultural, economic, and political factors that influence violent acts. The model categorizes violent behavior on four different levels—individual, relationship, community, and societal (WHO, 2002).

At the individual level, the model examines the biological and personal history that influence whether an individual may become a perpetrator or victim of violence. These factors may include not only demographic characteristics, such as age, education, and income, but also substance abuse, psychological or personality disorders, and a history of experiencing abuse or behaving aggressively. At the relationship level, the model looks at factors such as harsh physical punishment of children, lack of attention and bonding,

family dysfunction, association with delinquent peers, and marital or parental conflict to determine how relationships with families, friends, intimate partners, and peers influence violent behavior. The community level examines schools, workplaces, and neighborhoods in an attempt to identify characteristics that may increase the risk for violence, such as poverty, high population density, low social capital, transient residents, and the existence of gangs or drug cultures. The fourth level looks at societal factors that create an environment that encourages or inhibits violence. Health, economic, educational, and social policies that maintain economic or social inequalities between groups in society are all factors that encourage violent acts (WHO, 2002).

### Armed Conflict and War

Violent conflicts between nations and groups, acts of terrorism, rape as a weapon of war, the mass migration of people displaced from their homes, and gang warfare are occurring daily in many parts of the world. These acts of collective violence have devastating effects on physical and mental health, along with vast social, political, and economic consequences. During the last century, which was one of the most violent periods in human history, an estimated 191 million people lost their lives as a direct or indirect result of conflict. More than half of those fatalities were civilians. Besides the many thousands who are killed each year, there are huge numbers of people who are injured—including some who are mentally or physical disabled or physically mutilated. Torture and rape are used as methods to undermine communities, although exact numbers of people affected are not always known (WHO, 2002). Box 17-5 outlines some of the causes of death for civilians during violent conflict or **war**.

*Got an Alternative?*

Herbal remedies are commonly used in many countries, such as Cuba and Jamaica, as an integral part of their healthcare system and are not considered "alternative."

### BOX 17-5

#### The Consequences of Collective Violence

Increased civilian death rates during violent conflicts are usually due to the following causes:

- Injuries
- Decreased access to food
- Increased risk of communicable disease
- Decreased access to health services
- Decreased public health programs
- Poor environmental conditions
- Psychological distress

*Source*: WHO, 2002.

Armed conflicts disrupt trade and other business activities, diverting resources from vital services and programs to pay for defense. Food production and distribution are slowed or stopped as thousands of people are displaced from their homes. Famine related to war, other armed conflicts, or genocide killed an estimated 40 million people in the twentieth century (WHO, 2002).

## ■ Poverty

❝*There can be no peace as long as there is grinding poverty, social injustice, inequality, oppression, environmental degradation, and as long as the weak and small continue to be trodden by the mighty and powerful.*❞

—*Dalai Lama*

**Poverty** means powerlessness, lack of representation, and freedom. Almost half of the world's 6 billion people are poor. According to the World Bank, there are three levels of poverty: extreme, moderate, and relative. Extreme poverty, also known as absolute or abject poverty, is defined as living on less than $1 per day. At this income level, members of households are not able to meet basic needs for survival. They have chronic hunger, do not have access to health care, lack safe drinking water and sanitation, are uneducated and illiterate, and often do not have an adequate place to live or clothes to wear. Extreme poverty is the kind of poverty that kills. Moderate poverty is defined as living on less than $2 per day. At this income level, the basic survival needs of households are being met, but just barely. Relative poverty is defined as a household income below a given proportion of the national average. It means not having things that the middle class in countries take for granted (World Bank, 2007a; Sachs, 2005).

Extreme poverty now exists only in developing countries. In 2007, an estimated 1 billion people across the world lived in extreme poverty, down from 1.5 billion in 1981. While that decline indicates great global progress in poverty reduction, the progress has not been equal. Rapid economic growth in East Asia, especially China, and the Pacific regions has greatly reduced levels of poverty in those regions, although rapid population growth has kept Asia in the lead

 **MEDIA MOMENT**

### *The Last Emperor* (1997)

A dramatic history of Pu Yi, the last Emperor of China, from his lofty birth and brief reign in the Forbidden City, as the object of worship by half a billion people; through his abdication, his decline, and his dissolute lifestyle; to his exploitation by the invading Japanese; and finally to his obscure existence as just another peasant worker in the People's Republic.

American nursing students talk about nursing school experiences with nursing students in Jamaica.

with total numbers of poor people. South Asian countries have seen only moderate reductions in poverty levels, while poverty levels in the former Soviet Bloc countries in Eastern Europe and Central Asia increased in the last decade of the twentieth century before declining slightly. However, sub-Saharan Africa has the largest proportion of poor people, with almost half of the population living in extreme poverty. The overall per capita income of African nations decreased by 14% between 1981 and 2001, and poverty levels in that region rose from 41% to 46% over the same period (World Bank, 2007a; Sachs, 2005). Much of that increase is related directly to HIV/AIDS, drought, isolation, and civil wars (Sachs, 2005).

## ■ Women's Rights

❝*[As] the Millennium Declaration made clear, gender equality is not only a goal in its own right; it is critical to our ability to reach all the others.*❞

—*Kofi Annan, Secretary-General of the United Nations, 2004*

Every day, all over the world, girls are kept out of school, beaten, ignored, forced to marry and have sex, sold as slaves, made to fight in wars, and asked to sit silently while others make decisions affecting their lives (UNICEF, 2007b). In many countries of the world, women are not allowed to vote, own or inherit property, drive a car, get an education, or make any decisions about themselves or their children.

One woman dies from complications of pregnancy and childbirth every minute, accounting for more than half a million deaths worldwide each year. Ninety-nine percent of these deaths occur in the developing world, where the highest maternal mortality rates occur in sub-Saharan Africa, followed by South-Central Asia. According to recent findings by WHO, UNICEF, and the United Nations Population Fund (UNPF), a woman living in sub-Saharan Africa has a one in 16 chance of dying in pregnancy or childbirth during her lifetime, as compared with a one in 2,800 chance for a

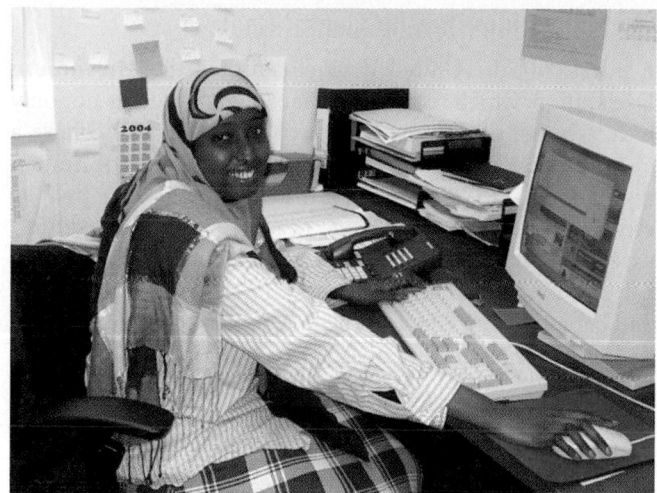

Women in many underdeveloped countries are making progress in careers previously restricted to men.

woman living in a developed country. Maternal mortality is both a human rights issue and an equity issue. Given that the vast majority of maternal deaths can be prevented with access to skilled prenatal, perinatal, and postnatal care, successful pregnancies and births should be a fundamental human right for all women (WHO, 2004).

Many women worldwide are victims of violence at all levels. Until recently, violence against women was considered to be a minor social problem by many governments and policy makers. This was especially true for women who were victims of violence perpetrated by their husbands or intimate partners. Beginning in the 1990s, however, the problem began to become more widely recognized as a serious human rights and public health issue. This rise in awareness

was spurred on by the efforts of women's organizations and governments, which were committed to eliminating violence against women under international human rights laws. It is believed that the only way to effectively eliminate violence against women is through political will and by legal action in all sectors of society (WHO, 2005).

In addition to violence, hunger, lack of education, and inferior legal status, HIV/AIDS and other infectious diseases disproportionately affect and further weaken the position of women in many of the world's poorest countries. Women typically have a more severe course of illness because of their lack of access to care, social inequalities, and restrictive cultural norms (Gerberding, 2004). In many cases the social, economic, and psychological effects of HIV are devastating. Fulfilling the traditional role of family caretaker means that women receive healthcare treatment only after the needs of their men and male children have been met. When their husbands or fathers die, the laws of many countries may allow women to lose their economic rights, which can leave them without property, without money, and without health care.

**"** *Women have an enhanced vulnerability to disease, especially if they are poor. Indeed, the health hazards of being female are widely underestimated. Economic and cultural factors can limit women's access to clinics and health workers. The World Health Organization reports that less is spent on health care for women and girls worldwide than for men and boys. As a result, women who become mothers and caretakers of children and husbands often do so at the expense of their own health. The leading causes of death among women are HIV/AIDS, malaria, complications of pregnancy and childbirth, and tuberculosis.* **"**

—*Carol Bellamy, United Nations Children's Fund, New York, 2004*

## Global Initiatives

### ■ Declaration of Alma Ata

In 1978, 164 countries and 67 international organizations met in Alma Ata, Kazakhstan, for the International Conference on Primary Health Care. The nations of the world came together to recognize the concept of **primary health care** as a strategy to reach the goal of "**Health for All by the Year 2000.**" The conference produced the document known as the ***Declaration of Alma Ata,*** which was a major milestone for public health in the twentieth century. The *Declaration* defined primary health care as "essential health care based on practical, scientifically sound, and socially acceptable methods and technology made universally accessible to individuals and families in the community through their full participation and at a cost that the community and country can afford to maintain of every stage of their development in the spirit of self-reliance and self determination" (PAHO, 2003).

The conference not only reaffirmed the WHO definition of health as a state of complete physical, mental, and

Although maternal mortality is still a significant problem for Nepalese women, it is being addressed by increases in postpartum care technology as Nepal struggles to improve the health status of women.

social well-being and not merely the absence of disease or infirmity, but also declared health to be a fundamental human right. The attainment of the highest possible level of health was identified as an important global social goal that will require the action of all nations and the collaboration of many social and economic government agencies within and among governments.

 THINK ABOUT THIS

The main health hazard in the world today is people who don't love themselves.

—Kinky Friedman

The *Declaration of Alma Ata* promoted the concept that governments have a responsibility to promote the health of their citizens by providing adequate health and social services. Governments, international organizations, and the entire world community were challenged to work toward attaining a level of health for all peoples of the world that will permit them to lead socially and economically productive lives by 2000. Primary health care, as part of economic development and social justice, was designated as the key to attaining the goal. Countries were encouraged to work together, in recognition of the fact that the attainment of health by the people in any one country directly concerns and benefits every other country. All governments were encouraged to develop national policies, strategies, and plans of action to include primary health care as part of a comprehensive healthcare system (PAHO, 2003). The United States, while not creating policy to address the goal of Health for All by the Year 2000, developed the *Healthy People 2000* objectives, which was updated to *Healthy People 2010* in 2000.

At the Fifty-Sixth World Health Assembly meeting in 2003, 25 years after the *Declaration of Alma Ata*, WHO reviewed the health status of the world's citizens and the progress made toward the attainment of the Health for All by the Year 2000 goal. Evaluations identified a genuine commitment within countries to the principles of primary health care. In those countries where the development of primary health care has not been successful, failures were attributed to a lack of practical guidance for implementation, poor leadership, insufficient political commitment, inadequate resources, and unrealistic expectations (WHO, 2003).

 MEDIA MOMENT

How do the images we view from other countries on television news shows, such as those broadcast by CNN and Fox News, shape our opinions about the U.S. role in global health?

## Millennium Developmental Goals

In 2000, the United Nations adopted the Millennium Declaration, which recognized that all governments not only have a responsibility to their own citizens, but also have a collective responsibility to uphold the principles of human dignity, equality, and equity for all of the world's people, especially the most vulnerable. Leaders from every country agreed on the importance of creating a world with less hunger, poverty, and disease; better survival rates for mothers and babies; better-educated people; equal rights for women; and healthier environments (United Nations, 2000, 2006).

The UN **Millennium Developmental Goals** were developed to coordinate and strengthen unprecedented global efforts to meet the needs of the world's poorest people. A target date of 2015 for meeting these goals was agreed on by all of the world's governments and the leading global developmental institutions. Box 17-6 lists the eight Millennium Developmental Goals.

## Global Nursing

### Nursing Shortages

WHO estimates it will take an additional 4.3 million healthcare workers (nurses, midwives, physicians, and support workers) to address the pandemic crisis of the shortage of global healthcare workers, which affects all countries of the world. Many developed nations are recruiting workers from less developed nations to alleviate their staffing shortages. This practice has resulted in a global redistribution of healthcare workers and has left the countries with the greatest needs with the greatest shortages. African nations carry 25% of the world's disease burden but have only 3% of the world's healthcare workforce. There are many reasons why nurses and physicians migrate. While higher incomes are a major consideration, safer working conditions and better resources to provide quality care are equally important (Emory University, 2006).

### International Council of Nurses

The ICN works to ensure quality nursing care for all, sound global health policies, the advancement of nursing knowledge, and the presence of a respected, competent, and satisfied global nursing workforce. Three goals and five core values guide all ICN programs and activities. ICN's goals are to bring nurses together worldwide, to advance nurses and nursing worldwide, and to influence health policy. Its five core values are visionary leadership, inclusiveness, flexibility, partnership, and achievement. The ICN Code for Nurses is the foundation for ethical nursing practice throughout the world (ICN, 2008).

### Nursing and Human Rights

Human rights are primarily concerned with the rights of individuals in relation to government. The goal of the global movement toward human rights is to ensure that all people

## BOX 17-6

**United Nations Millennium Developmental Goals**

| Goals | Target |
|---|---|
| 1. Eradicate extreme hunger and poverty | 1. Halve, between 1990 and 2015, the proportion of people whose income is less than $1 per day.<br>2. Halve, between 1990 and 2015, the proportion of people who suffer from hunger. |
| 2. Achieve universal primary education | Ensure that, by 2015, children everywhere, boys and girls alike, will be able to complete a full course of primary schooling. |
| 3. Promote gender equality and empower women | Eliminate gender disparity in primary and secondary education, preferably by 2005, and in all levels of education no later than 2015. |
| 4. Reduce child mortality | Reduce by two-thirds, between 1990 and 2015, the under-5 mortality rate. |
| 5. Improve maternal health | Reduce by three-fourths, between 1990 and 2015, the maternal mortality ratio. |
| 6. Combat HIV/AIDS, malaria, and other infectious diseases | 1. Have halted by 2015 and begun to reverse the spread of HIV/AIDS.<br>2. Have halted by 2015 and begun to reverse the incidence of malaria and other major infectious diseases. |
| 7. Ensure environmental sustainability | 1. Integrate the principles of sustainable development into country policies and programs and reverse the loss of environmental resources.<br>2. Halve, by 2015, the proportion of people without sustainable access to safe drinking water and sanitation.<br>3. By 2020, have achieved a significant improvement in the lives of at least 100 million slum-dwellers. |
| 8. Develop a global partnership for development | 1. Address the special needs of the least developed, landlocked countries and small-island developing states.<br>2. Develop further an open, rule-based, predictable, nondiscriminatory trading and financial system.<br>3. Deal comprehensively with developing countries' debt.<br>4. In cooperation with developing countries, develop and implement strategies for decent and productive work for youth.<br>5. In cooperation with pharmaceutical companies, provide access to affordable essential drugs in developing countries.<br>6. In cooperation with the private sector, make available the benefits of new technologies, especially information and communications. |

have an opportunity to survive to achieve their full potential. Safe water and food, adequate nutrition, protection against slavery or torture, access to education, health care, and basic freedoms are the foundation for human rights. The Universal Declaration of Human Rights, adopted by the United Nations in 1948, committed the international community to pursue a minimum standard of health care for all people (Williams, 2004).

Because the role and status of individuals in society strongly influence their health, human rights abuses contribute significantly to the disease development. Nurses must care about human rights because their presence or absence affects a nurse's ability to practice nursing. The fundamentals of nursing are rooted in the act of caring for other human beings. To provide the best nursing care, nurses must directly confront discrimination, poverty, and human rights abuses (Williams, 2004).

Explore Community Health Nursing on the Web! To learn more about the topics in this chapter, use the passcode provided to access your exclusive website: **http://nursing.jbpub.com/ communityhealth.** If you do not have a passcode, you can obtain one at this site.

## Application to Practice

### A Nursing Student's Story

Border issues affect everyone. During a clinical experience at a level 1 trauma center, another student and I were assigned to a room in the emergency room. A 16-year-old boy was brought in by the triage nurse. He was in obvious respiratory distress. He had renal failure, a Hickmann to right anterior chest wall, soiled dressings, bilateral rales, and +3 pitting edema. After assessment by the first-year resident, the chief resident was called and determined that this boy was not a candidate for emergency dialysis. An interpreter was called, and it was learned that the boy was from Honduras and had no medical coverage. He was admitted for observation. Following up on the patient's status the next day, we found the notation "illegal" recorded again and again in his medical record. Social Services could not help this young man. While we visited the patient, the chief nephrologist came to see him.

He wanted us to translate for him as he gave discharge instructions. There would be no dialysis, and the Hickmann would not be removed. He said, "Marry a U.S. citizen or go back to your country. You will be discharged today."

We told the patient we were sorry and asked for his phone number. We told him we would try to do something. We knew that there is no hemodialysis in Honduras and that Social Services could have attempted to make referrals. We did some research and found a hospital willing to treat our patient and referred our patient there. In this cultural experience, we were able to integrate respect for human rights, patient advocacy, and ethics with critical care skills to assist this patient. We hope that we empowered this patient to use available community resources to care for himself despite cultural differences.

—Jamy Josey, BSN Nursing Student

## CRITICAL THINKING ACTIVITIES

1. Which groups or organizations in your community are working locally to improve people's lives?

2. Are nurses actively involved with any of these groups? If so, in what capacity?

## REFERENCES

Basford, L. (2003). Global challenge: What if...? *Reflections on Nursing Leadership*, Fourth Quarter, 26–27.

Birn, A. E., & Dmitrienko, K. (2005). The World Bank: Global health or harm? *American Journal of Public Health, 95*(7), 1091–1092.

Carter Center. (2008). *About the Center*. Retrieved October 28, 2008, from http://www.cartercenter.org/about/index.html

Communique. (2003, September 22). *World Bank report lets down 58 million public service employees*. Geneva: World Health Organization.

Disease Control Priorities Project. (2006a). *Infectious diseases*. Retrieved October 28, 2008, from http://wwwdcp2.org/file/6/DCPP-InfectiousDiseases.pdf

Disease Control Priorities Project. (2006b). *Noncommunicable diseases*. Retrieved October 28, 2008, from http://wwwdcp2.org/file/58/DCPP-NCD.pdf

Emory University. (2006). Undelivered cures: 113 nations gather at Emory to tackle the global shortage of healthcare workers. *Emory and Global Health Magazine*.

Gates Foundation. (2008). *Foundation fact sheet*. Retrieved October 28, 2008, from http://www.gatesfoundation.org/about/Pages/foundation-fact-sheet.aspx

Gerberding, J. L. (2004). Women and infectious disease. *Emerging Infectious Diseases, 10*(11). http://www.cdc.ncidod/EID/vol10no11/04-0555.htm.

International Council of Nurses (ICN). (2008). *About ICN*. Retrieved October 28, 2008, from http://www.icn.ch/abouticn.htm

Jain, A. (2004). Fighting obesity. *British Medical Journal, 328*, 1327–1328.

MSNBC. (2004). *"Globesity" gains ground as leading killer*. Retrieved October 28, 2008, from http://www.msnbc.msn.com/id/4900095/?GTI-3391

Pan American Health Organization (PAHO). (2003). *Primary health care: 25 years of the Alma Ata declaration*. Retrieved October 28, 2008, from http://www.paho.org/English/dd/pin/alma-ata._declaration.htm

Population Bulletin. (2006). *Controlling infectious diseases*. Washington, DC: Population Reference Bureau.

Population Reference Bureau (PRB). (2006). *World population data sheet*. Retrieved October 28, 2008, from http://www.prb.org

Ruger, J. P. (2005). The changing role of the World Bank in global health. *American Journal of Public Health, 95*(1), 60–70.

Sachs, J. (2005, March 14). The end of poverty. *Time*, pp. 43–54.

UNDP. (1998). *Human development report*. New York: Author.

UNICEF. (2007a). *About UNICEF: Who we are*. Retrieved October 28, 2008, from http//www.unicef.org/about/who/index

UNICEF. (2007b). *Voices of youth: Stop discrimination and violence against girls*. Retrieved October 28, 2008, from http://www.unicef.org/voy/take action

United Nations. (2000). *Resolution adopted by the General Assembly: United Nations Millennium Declaration*. New York: Author.

United Nations. (2006). *The Millennium Development Goals report.* New York: Author.

United Nations. (2008). *The UN in brief.* Retrieved November 12, 2008, from http://un.org/Overview/uninbrief/

Williams, A. B. (2004). Nursing, health, and human rights: A framework for international collaboration. *Journal of the Association of Nurses in AIDS Care, 15*(3), 75–77.

World Bank. (2007a). *About us.* Retrieved October 28, 2008, from http://www.worldbank.org

World Bank. (2007b). *Ten things you never knew about the World Bank.* Washington, DC: Author.

World Health Organization (WHO). (2002). *World report on violence and health* [abstract]. Geneva: WHO Press.

World Health Organization (WHO). (2003). *International Conference on Primary Health Care, Alma-Ata: Twenty-fifth anniversary. Report by the Secretariat.* Geneva: WHO Press.

World Health Organization (WHO). (2004). *Press release: Making pregnancy safer.* Geneva: WHO Press.

World Health Organization (WHO). (2005). *Summary report: WHO multi-country study on women's health and domestic violence against women.* Geneva: WHO Press.

World Health Organization (WHO). (2007a). *Working for health: An introduction to the World Health Organization.* Geneva: WHO Press.

World Health Organization (WHO). (2007b). *About WHO.* Retrieved November 11, 2008, from http://www.who.int/about/en/

## APPENDIX

# Canada

Heather R. Sherry

Canada's healthcare system, commonly referred to as "Medicare," is designed to ensure reasonable access to healthcare services for all Canadian residents on a prepaid basis. It can be described as a series of 13 interlocking provincial and territorial health insurance plans and is funded predominantly through public tax dollars. Healthcare services are administered and delivered by the provincial and territorial governments, with funding assistance provided by the federal government. These services are provided to Canadian residents free of charge.

The *Canada Health Act (CHA)* is the federal legislation that governs the conditions under which provinces and territories may receive funding for the healthcare services they provide to Canadian residents. Provincial and territorial insurance plans must meet five specific criteria outlined in the CHA to be eligible for their full allocation of funding from the federal government:

- Public administration: The healthcare insurance plan of a province must be administered and operated on a nonprofit basis by a public authority appointed or designated by the government of the province. This public authority is accountable to the government and must be subject to audit.
- Comprehensiveness: The healthcare insurance plan of a province must insure all necessary health services including hospitals, physicians, and surgical dentists.
- Universality: All insured residents must be entitled to the same level of health care.
- Portability: Any resident who moves to a different province is guaranteed coverage from his or her home province during a minimum waiting period (also applies to residents who leave the country).
- Accessibility: All insured persons must have reasonable access to healthcare and healthcare providers must receive reasonable compensation for their services.

As stated in the CHA, the primary objective of Canadian healthcare policy is "to protect, promote, and restore the physical and mental well-being of residents of Canada and to facilitate reasonable access to health services without financial or other barriers" (Canada Health Act 1984, c.6,s.3). In support of this objective, primary care doctors, specialists, hospitals, and dental surgery are all covered under provincial insurance policies. More than half of all doctors in Canada are primary care physicians, and the remaining doctors are specialists who provide services outside the scope of primary care physicians.

Although most basic healthcare services are provided under the provincial insurance plans, some services are not covered. For example, prescription medications, vision, and dental (nonsurgical) services are covered only through private insurance plans, which can be used to supplement primary health coverage. Private insurance plans are typically used by individuals with specific needs that are not covered by the primary plan and are often offered as part of employee benefits packages. In addition, many private clinics exist in Canada that offer specialized services. By law, they are not allowed to duplicate services provided by the CHA, but many still do. Residents often use these clinics to reduce the wait times that they can experience in the public healthcare system. This is controversial because there is a sense that the existence of these clinics creates an imbalance in the healthcare system that favors individuals with higher incomes.

Over the years since public funding for healthcare began in Canada, the delivery of healthcare services has shifted away from hospitals and doctors and toward alternative care and public health interventions. Reforms have focused on primary healthcare delivery, which have included establishing 24-hour community healthcare centers; creating primary healthcare teams; emphasis on health promotion; prevention of illness and injury; management of chronic diseases; increased coordination and integration of comprehensive services; and improving the work environment of primary healthcare providers (Health Canada, 2007). Although there are some concerns about the efficiency of the Canadian healthcare system (which serves a population of more than 32 million people), Canadians as a whole continue to have a favorable health status. The average life expectancy in Canada is among the highest in the industrialized countries and the infant mortality rate is one of the lowest in the world.

## References

Canadian Health Care, http://www.canadian-health.org (accessed May 16, 2007).

Health Canada, http://www.hc-sc.gc.ca/hcs-sss/medi-assur/index _e.html (accessed May 15, 2007).

Health Canada Act, http://laws.justice.gc.ca/en/ShowFullDoc/cs/C-6///en (accessed May 16, 2007).

# Cuba

Juana Diasy Berdayes Martinez

Cuba, a Caribbean island nation with a population of more than 1 million, is located between the Caribbean Sea and the Atlantic Ocean, approximately 90 miles off the coast of the United States. After the Cuban Revolution in 1959, Cuba experienced many economic and social transformations, which led to the development of its current healthcare policy. The belief in the right to health care for all citizens and the duty of the state to guarantee it brought about the provision of free healthcare services for all Cuban citizens. A process of reorganization and expansion of the national healthcare system was initiated based on a primary care model. Several measures were taken to guarantee accessibility of healthcare services for all. For example, new hospitals were constructed in rural zones and mountain areas, greatly increasing the number of hospital beds nationwide. Health professionals no longer worked in private practices, but instead became a part of the government's primary care system (Jardnes, Ouvina, & Aneiro Riba, 1991).

From its beginnings, the Cuban public health system has included the participation of the community in its historic evolution. In 1964, the first polyclinic was created to deliver comprehensive health care to communities. Community participation in health care was reinforced in 1975 with the creation of health advisory committees. Health advisory committees consist of people in each community who participate in analyzing the health of the community and facilitating collaboration between the healthcare system and community residents. In 1984, the new Cuban primary care model was introduced with family physicians and nurses as essential components. Family practice physician offices, staffed by a physician and one or two nurses, began to spring up in every neighborhood. The principles of primary care proclaimed in Alma Ata in 1978 were applied in creative ways and adjusted to the economic and social conditions of Cuba. In this way, the truly humanistic dimensions of medicine and health care were applied to the care of people in their own communities. As a result, Cuba met the WHO's "Health for All" 2000 objectives in 1985.

Since 1989, with the collapse of the Soviet Union (with which Cuba conducted 85% of its economic trade), the living conditions of the Cuban population have deteriorated. In addition, the longstanding economic embargo of Cuba by

the United States has contributed significantly to the former country's economic depression. According to a 1997 study conducted by the American Association for World Health, the U.S. embargo has had a detrimental effect on the health and nutrition of large numbers of Cuban citizens. However, the negative impact has been offset by the commitment of the Cuban government to maintain a high level of budgetary support for the universal delivery of primary and preventive health care. The health services that have been affected most are organ transplant and other technology programs, surgical activity, the availability of medications, and the acquisition and maintenance of medical equipment. Despite these resource limitations, the goals of the Ministry of Public Health are focused on maintaining free and accessible health care for all citizens.

At present, Cuba has approximately 69,000 physicians and 150,000 nurses. Many of these physicians and nurses work in family practice settings in the community, with an emphasis on health promotion and illness prevention. Nurses working in communities are in privileged situations to identify and satisfy the needs of families. By interacting with individuals and families in the community on a daily basis, nurses are able to develop a holistic view of the health status of the community and its members.

Despite the difficulties encountered during recent years, Cuba offers a healthcare system that is highly developed and effective. Because of the focus on primary care in the community, Cuba's main health indicators (such as average life expectancy and infant mortality) are comparable to those of industrialized nations, placing Cuba far ahead of the rest of Latin America and other developing countries around the world. Cuban collaboration on health is currently present in 66 countries in Latin America, the Caribbean, Asia, and Africa. With more than 23,000 Cuban health collaborators at work internationally, their contributions have been noteworthy in the face of serious health problems in many developing nations.

## Reference

Jardnes, J. B., Ouviña, J., & Aneiro-Ribna, R. (1991). Education in the science of health in Cuba. *Public Health Cuban Magazine*, 25(4), 387–407.

# Jordan

## Waddah Demeh

Jordan, a country with a population of 5.5 million, is located in the heart of the politically volatile Middle East, between Iraq, Saudi Arabia, Syria, West Bank, and Israel. The first Ministry of Health (MOH) was established in 1950 and the first health insurance system was implemented among Force Army members in 1963. Health services are provided through five major sectors:

- Ministry of Health: hospitals, clinics, and mother–child health centers
- Royal Medical Services (Force Army)
- Private sector: hospitals and clinics
- United Nation Relief and Work Agency (UNRWA): clinics and mother–child health centers
- Medical services at governmental universities: Jordan University Hospital and the Hospital of King Abed Allah Ibn al-Hussein

Jordan has limited financial resources and is still considered to be a developing country. Since King Abdullah II took the throne in 1999, health care, education, and technology have advanced quickly. Under his leadership, emphasis was placed on industry and the importance of Jordanian social and economic development. Jordan has approached development from a holistic perspective, realizing that poverty, illiteracy, and health form a triangle and must be addressed together. Advances in the struggle against poverty and illiteracy, in addition to the spread of sanitation, clean water, adequate nutrition, and housing, have resulted in a healthier Jordanian citizenry. The main goal of Jordan's health strategy has been to provide adequate health coverage to all. Jordan's public health system has concentrated on primary health care (e.g., childhood immunization and prenatal care) in all parts of the country, while leaving tertiary health care mostly to the private sector. Jordan's healthcare system has improved dramatically in the last two decades, placing it among the top 10 countries of the world in reducing infant mortality.

Jordan's health needs are met by a high ratio of medical personnel per capita, with the only personnel shortage being in trained local nurses. The government is establishing new nursing colleges and encouraging students to specialize in nursing by offering incentives for trained nurses and giving priority in employment for both male and female Jordanian nurses. Five of eight public universities have nursing colleges that offer both bachelor's and master's degrees in nursing, and two other private universities offer a degree in nursing as well.

Jordan is taking the lead in the Middle East region in recognizing nursing as an independent profession. In 2002, the Jordanian Nursing Council (JNC) was established to regulate the nursing profession through the development of bylaws and credentials policies as well as strategies to protect the health, safety, and welfare of the public. Some accomplishments of JNC to date include the following developments:

- Revising the current law and suggesting amendments
- Laying down the strategic planning of the Council and the plan of action
- Forming committees to establish the clinical ladder
- Requesting institutions to participate in different committees that are defined in strategic planning (JNC, 2007)

Ninety-two percent of the population in Jordan are Muslim, and this plays a major role in individual and group perceptions about health. The purpose of Islam, as stated in the Qu'ran, is to foster beneficial relations between individuals and groups to weld mankind into a true brotherhood. Families are considered the primary social unit in the community, and it is mainly women within families who care for and maintain essential family functions. They determine the nutritional status of the family; they manage and budget the household income; they teach, educate, and care for their children; and they provide health care to the household and community (Mahasneh, 2001).

Women in Jordan have many freedoms. The majority of young women attend universities, have voting rights, drive, and cover themselves only by choice. In fact, many young feminist women in Jordan today are returning to traditional Islamic values (including traditional dress) through the original interpretation of the Qu'ran because they contend that the profit Muhammad defended the rights of women. These traditional religious beliefs influence their behavior on many levels, including teaching children to uphold the family honor in the name of God through maintaining virginity before marriage and not being seen alone with a man as a young girl. Shame brought on a family lasts generations and can influence family connections in the community. Men care for their families by protecting the women (Miller & Petro-Nustas, 2002).

## References

Jordanian Nursing Council (JNC). (2007). *JNC home.* Retrieved November 11, 2008, from http://www.jnc.gov.jo/english/home.htm

Mahasneh, S. (2001). Health perceptions and health behaviors of poor urban Jordanian women. *Journal of Advanced Nursing, 36*(1), 58–68.

Miller, J., & Petro-Nustas, W. (2002). Context of care for Jordanian women. *Journal of Transcultural Nursing, 13*(3), 228–236.

# CHAPTER 18
# Groups in the Community

Margaret J. Hickman, Marilyn Givens King, and
Karen Saucier Lundy

Visit **http://nursing.jbpub.com/communityhealth**
for interactive exercises, review questions,
Web links, and more.

As a nursing student, working in groups
will help you learn how to meet goals
through cooperation and collaboration.

Learn to lead in a nourishing manner.
Learn to lead without being possessive.
Learn to be helpful without taking the credit.
Learn to lead without coercion.

*—John Heider, The Tao of Leadership, 1985*

Nurses work most of their professional lives in groups, and yet student nurses most frequently cite group work as their least liked part of nursing school. Human beings would not have survived without the formation of groups. How do you feel about working with a successful group that meets its goals? What are the differences between a successful group and a group that is inefficient and a time waster?

## CHAPTER FOCUS

**Characteristics of Effective Groups**
- Collective Identity
- Shared Purpose
- Communication
- Group Norms
- Participation
- Shared Leadership
- Cohesion
- Shared Decision Making
- Conflict Management
- Problem Solving

**Stages of Group Development**
- Group Formation
- Group Maintenance: Cohesion, Norms, and Conflict Resolution

- Group Dissolution
- Group Stages and Formation

**Group Functions**
- Group Tasks
- Roles of Group Members
- Groups as Change Agents
- Concepts Related to Change

**Types of Groups**

**Working with Groups**
- Group Leadership
- Ethical Considerations
- Evaluating Groups

## QUESTIONS TO CONSIDER

After reading this chapter, you will know the answers to the following questions:

1. What are group characteristics?
2. What are the stages of group development?
3. What kinds of functions do groups perform?
4. What are the different types of groups in which community health nurses might be involved?
5. How is group process evaluated?
6. What is group leadership? How does it apply in community health nursing?

## KEY TERMS

Change
Coalitions
Cohesion
Decision making
Empowerment
Force field analysis
Goal attainment tasks
Group
Impact evaluation
Internal maintenance tasks
Leadership
Norms
Open communication
Outcome evaluation
Participation
Partnership
Process evaluation

LIVING IN GROUPS, working in groups, playing in groups, leaving in groups—all are critical to human survival. Community health nurses, perhaps more than others, achieve most of their success in meeting goals through the work of groups. In the course of their professional activities, nurses work with a wide variety of groups to achieve population health promotion and restoration goals. In addition, nurses are members of work-related groups focused on continuous improvement of health care, the healthcare system, and the nursing profession.

Working with groups in community settings is an essential component of public health and community health nursing practice. *Healthy People 2000, Healthy People 2010, and Healthy Communities 2000* indicate that national health objectives cannot be met effectively unless health professionals work in **partnership** with community and professional groups (APHA, 1991; DHHS, 1991, 2000) (Box 18-1). In a similar vein, professional nursing standards include repeated statements that the nurse is to practice *in partnership* with others to achieve desired health outcomes that are collectively held (ANA, 1986, 1991, 1996).

In many situations, nurses are able to work more effectively and efficiently when they work in groups than when they work individually. Some advantages of groups are as follows:

- Can accomplish tasks that may not be achievable by individuals
- Bring a wider range of resources, skills, and talents to bear on complex health issues
- Provide a means of decision making that allows for multiple and sometimes conflicting views to be evaluated and synthesized
- Have a synergy that surpasses the capacity of individuals to attain health goals

The Application to Practice feature on page 403 is an example of a clinical situation in which nurses working together form a community coalition to implement a teen health program that is much more comprehensive and effective than the services the nurses provided separately.

Working with groups requires a knowledge of group characteristics and dynamics, as well as a set of basic group facilita-

tion skills. Our understanding of groups and group behavior is based on a body of interdisciplinary research from fields such as sociology, anthropology, business, and health (Bracht, 1990). A variety of nursing theories, such as *Parse's Theory in Practice*, also help guide nursing practice with groups (Kelley, 1995). This chapter introduces the basic concepts, leadership skills, and ethical considerations needed for effective group development, maintenance, and evaluation.

 ## Research Alert

This article proposes that the two important forms of influence in focus groups occur (1) through the influence on people's beliefs about the substantive issues under discussion and (2) through the influence on self-efficacy beliefs. As a result of such influence, focus groups provide a learning context that may facilitate empowerment of participants through the development of communicative self-efficacy as they struggle over constructing and sharing understandings of controversial issues. A case study is presented that qualitatively analyzed transcripts of interaction and quantitative self-report measures into empirical conversation. The case study demonstrated that focus group participants were influenced in two important ways: Participation and interaction led to increased participant confidence and motivation toward participating in public.

*Source:* Zorn, T. E., Roper, J., Braodfoot, K., & Weaver, C. K. (2006). Focus groups as sites of influential interaction: Building communicative self-efficacy and effecting attitudinal change in discussing controversial topics. *Journal of Applied Communication Research, 34*(2), 115–140.

## BOX 18-1

### National Health Standards and Objectives

### Collective Responsibility for Change

*Healthy People 2000:* "While the responsibility for change lies with each of us, it also lies with all of us, and individuals cannot be expected to act alone" (DHHS, 1991, p. 85).

*Healthy People 2010:* "Community health is profoundly affected by the collective behaviors, attitudes, and beliefs of everyone who lives in the community" (DHHS, 2000; p. 3).

*Healthy Communities 2000:* "Improvements in public health require active community ownership and commitment" (APHA, 1991, p. xxiv).

### Practice Partnerships Among Healthcare Providers and Others

*Healthy People 2000:* "Practice can take the form of partnership with nonprofessionals in the pursuit of individual, family, and community health care. The effectiveness and efficiency of preventive services . . . will be enhanced by such partnership" (DHHS, 1991, p. 87).

*Healthy Communities 2000:* "Disease prevention is a shared partnership. . . . Cooperation among major community groups and organizations creates the foundation for communities to establish and achieve [health] goals and objectives" (APHA, 1991, p. xvii).

Student nurses often dislike working on group projects. Why is this a common "least favorite" part of nursing school?

## Application to Practice

### Working with Groups to Plan a Teen Health Clinic

J. C. Roberts, a school health nurse in an urban high school, runs a school-based education center targeting health problems affecting the student population. Lee Sorrel, a nurse in a nearby public health center, runs an after-school teen clinic to provide care for the same set of health problems. Although both nurses spent much time and energy implementing their respective programs, local teens are not using the services of either. After discussing their mutual frustration at a district nursing meeting, J. C. and Lee decide to work together. They form an advisory group made up of local teens to help them evaluate the two programs. The group learns the following:

- Students fear negative repercussions if teachers see them going into the health education center at school.
- Desired educational topics, such as safe sex and pregnancy prevention, cannot be offered by the health education center under existing school policy.
- Using a "problem-oriented" clinic has a negative social stigma among their peers.
- Many teens who might attend the health department clinic are working after school.

The group recommends a community-based program that includes social activities, health and education services, and job skills training. The nurse and advisory committee members initiate a coalition of community leaders and organizations that mobilizes resources for a comprehensive teen program at the local community center. The program is highly successful. Local teens are using a broader range of services than the school or health department were able to offer separately.

On a sheet of paper, list all the individuals (e.g., the two nurses, the teens), agencies, organizations, and community officials or representatives that should be part of the community coalition. Next to each, list examples of the knowledge, skills, and resources that each can potentially contribute to the pool of information that will be used as the basis for informed decision making.

1. Take a pencil and cover each entry, one at a time. What would be lost each time?
2. Look at each entry. What are the potential sources of power and influence for each?
3. Brainstorm a list of ground rules that would support shared leadership and decision making.

Look at the individuals, agencies, organizations, and community officials or representatives that you identified in the previous questions. Make a list of the potential sources and topics of conflict within this group.

1. Which, if any, detrimental effects to individuals and the group might result from these conflicts?
2. Which strengths might the group derive from these potential conflicts?
3. Brainstorm a list of ground rules that would support positive conflict management. ◉

Participation means that all group members listen and are listened to, share in decision making, and contribute to the achievement of the group's tasks and objectives.

### Research Alert

Quality of life is a concern for people living with diagnoses of persistent mental illness. This project explored the meaning of quality of life for a group of persons attending a community center for persons with mental illness. Parse's human becoming practice method was used to guide the group process for eight men who met weekly with a nurse for 75- to 90-minute sessions over 10 weeks. The nurse's commitment to live true presence with the group enabled their expressions about life and the meanings of living with their particular struggles and joys, sufferings and hopes. △

*Source*: Hee, N. C. (2004). Meaning of the quality of life for persons living with serious mental illness: Human becoming practice with groups. *Nursing Science Quarterly, 17*(3), 220–225.

## Characteristics of Effective Groups

A **group** is defined as two or more people who have a collective identity, communicate with each other regularly, and share a common purpose or goal. Although collective identity, shared goals, and open communication are defining characteristics of groups, additional characteristics associated with groups that can function effectively include group norms, cohesion, active participation, shared leadership, shared decision making, problem solving, and conflict resolution. To put this in simple terms: Group members are aware of being a part of "the group."

**❝***Doing more things faster is no substitute for doing the right things.* **❞**

—Stephen R. Covey

### ■ Collective Identity

Although groups are made up of unique individuals, effective groups develop a sense of collective identity. The group identity may be explicit and related to a shared characteristic of the group members. For example, "Bosom Buddies" groups are made up primarily of breast cancer survivors, and the "West End Neighborhood Association" denotes a group of people who define their collective identity based on shared geographic-political boundaries.

### ■ Shared Purpose

In addition to having a common identity, groups have a shared purpose or goal that transcends the individual goals of group members. Group goals must be clearly understood and relevant to all members of the group. Within effective groups, goals are determined cooperatively and clarified or modified to fit as closely as possible with individual goals (Berdahl & Craig, 1996).

### ■ Communication

Stable mechanisms of **open communication** in which each member of the group gives and receives information is a characteristic of effective groups. Mutual acceptance, trust, and understanding are basic to open communication patterns in which group members can freely share thoughts and feelings. Traditionally, a component of communication patterns in effective groups included regular face-to-face interaction. However, current health practice uses electronic means quite effectively to facilitate group communication. Electronic tools for collaboration have evolved into highly sophisticated Internet-based methods of communication and decision making in groups whose members are geographically dispersed (Dennis & Valacich, 1994; Laudon & Laudon, 1988; Preboth & Wright, 1999; Reagan-Cirincione, 1994; Sharf, 1997). For example, self-help groups such as Alcoholics Anonymous have been very successful in moving their 12-step programs to the Internet.

Health information clearinghouses provide extensive lists of health-related groups that meet and communicate online. Research about online groups that focus on illnesses such as cancer, diabetes, and alcoholism has found that the Internet actually strengthens group communication because there are no signs of age, gender, race, social status, dress, weight, disabilities, and other distinctions (Madara, 1997). However, a challenge for nurses and others using the Internet for group work is to develop ways of communicating thoughts and feelings in the absence of traditional visual cues.

### ■ Group Norms

**Norms** are the spoken and unspoken rules and politics that govern group behavior (Loomis, 1979). Because groups often bring together people with a variety of assumptions about acceptable group behavior, effective groups make implicit norms explicit by discussing and developing written rules for group conduct. If starting a new group, one may want to begin the first meeting by having the group identify some ground rules on which they agree and post this list where everyone can see it. The group may add additional rules as needed at subsequent meetings.

### ■ Participation

Groups are more effective when all members are active participants. **Participation** means that all group members listen and are listened to, share in decision making, and

Communication by all group members is a critical attribute of a successful work group.

contribute to the achievement of group tasks and objectives. Ground rules such as "Everyone will be given a chance to talk," "Only one person talks at a time," "No interrupting," "Everyone's ideas are important," and "Everyone has a vote" can help promote active participation in groups. Community development and organizational behavior research indicates that participation by all group members increases group motivation, leads to greater involvement in group activities, is associated with higher levels of commitment to group plans and objectives, and contributes to greater success in achievement of group goals (Cooke & Szumal, 1994; Minkler, 1997).

## ■ Shared Leadership

Although individuals within a group may exhibit a variety of **leadership** styles, effective groups distribute leadership among their members. As the need for formal leadership arises, various members of the group take turns in assuming leadership roles. As with participation, shared leadership is associated with higher levels of group motivation, involvement, commitment, and goal attainment (Hirokawa & Keyton, 1995; Schitterkate, 1996). One way to promote shared leadership is to end each meeting with the development of the agenda for the next meeting and have different group members volunteer to be discussion leaders for each item on the agenda.

## ■ Cohesion

Group **cohesion** refers to the ability of the group to "stick together"—that is, to retain members who can work together over a sufficient period of time to achieve group goals. Group cohesion is related to factors such as the following (Sampson & Marthas, 1981):
- Positive interpersonal relations among group members
- The desire of members to continue as part of the group
- The degree to which members like and are satisfied with the group's composition
- The level of acceptance, trust, and support among group members

### Research Alert

Cancer support groups are an important source of support for cancer patients. This research explored the views of 179 leaders of 184 cancer support groups in New South Wales, Australia. In the study, 416 members of 50 groups selected from the larger cohort completed questionnaires eliciting the importance of group processes, including leader qualities, and satisfaction with group leadership. Members of nine groups participated in focus groups regarding effective group processes. The importance of the leaders was emphasized in all stages of the research. Fifty-nine percent of group leaders were currently experiencing a difficulty, primarily related to infrastructure or group process. Three characteristics of effective leaders were identified: educational qualities, facilitation skills, and personal qualities. Leadership in these self-help groups can be an often overlooked aspect in the successful management of help for patients with cancer.

*Source*: Butow, P., Ussher, J., Kirsten, L., et al. (2006). Sustaining leaders of cancer support groups: The role, needs, and difficulties of leaders. *Social Work in Health Care*, 42(2), 39–55.

**❝** *There is nothing so useless as doing efficiently that which should not be done at all.* **❞**

—*Peter Drucker*

Cohesive groups put effort into team building and maintenance as well as task achievement. Setting ground rules that show respect for diversity and for the dignity and worth of each member of the group is an important part of ensuring group cohesion.

## ■ Shared Decision Making

In effective groups, power and influence within the group are shared relatively equally. All members are involved in setting goals, gathering information, identifying alternative ways to achieve goals, and deciding on the plan of action. An assumption underlying shared **decision making** is that each group member has information of value that will contribute to informed decision making (Ward, 2006). Input is based on a group member's knowledge, skills, and access to needed resources, rather than on the member's formal title or position in the organization or community. For shared decision making to be effective, all group members should understand the following (Ramey, 1993):
- The nature of the goal and task being undertaken
- Alternative approaches and strategies for achieving the goal or accomplishing the task
- Potential consequences (positive and negative) of each alternative being considered
- The social, economic, and environmental costs of each alternative to individuals, families, and organizations in the community, as well as to the community as a whole

A goal of groups should be to expand the knowledge and skills of its members in ways that will empower the group to make efficacious, informed decisions (Minkler, 1997; Ramey, 1993).

### Conflict Management

One of the strengths of a group lies in its ability to bring together individuals and organizations that have diverse views about an issue or problem. With diversity, the potential for conflict is high, so conflict management is critical. Conflict that is not managed effectively can be harmful to individuals and can destroy group cohesion and productivity; however, conflict also has a high potential for promoting involvement in a group and increasing the creativity and quality of decision making. Therefore, effective groups view conflict as a source of potential strength and develop productive ways of managing and resolving conflict (Antai-Otong, 1997).

### Problem Solving

Finally, groups must have the ability to solve problems collectively in ways that are long lasting and require minimal energy. Effective groups develop ways to identify problems early, provide opportunities for anticipatory problem solving, and develop mechanisms for evaluating the effect and quality of solutions (Ward, 2006).

## Stages of Group Development

Like individuals and families, groups go through several stages of growth and development. Many classic theories of group development (Table 18-1) reflect the belief that groups move by stages from a collection of unique, diverse individuals with conflicts to a cohesive group that maintains itself and achieves ongoing tasks and goals (Bion, 1961; Homans, 1950, 1961; Tuckman, 1965; Yalom, 1985). Others, including more recent theories, suggest that the life cycle of a group includes several stages of group formation, maintenance, and dissolution (Berman-Rossi, 1992; Feinberg, 1980).

### Group Formation

Group formation may take place in two phases: group initiation and group expansion. *Group initiation* is the phase

> ### ENVIRONMENTAL CONNECTION
>
> The environment in which the group meets is critical to the successful interactions of the members toward meeting group goals. How might a group for women who have experienced abuse be affected by meeting at someone's house compared to meeting at a church or hospital conference room?

in which the nurse and other members of a small planning body define the preliminary goal of the group and take care of arranging the first group meeting. *Group expansion* occurs as the larger group verifies and clarifies its purpose and begins the process of goal achievement.

Group formation begins with the planning group asking a series of critical questions: What is the purpose of the group? Why form a new group? What will this group do that is not already being done by other groups? How large should the group be? Who should be invited to join? How long should this group exist?

The answers to these questions will vary according to the type of group being developed. In general, groups should be kept small enough for all members of the group to interact with each other. Group membership and anticipated longevity will be closely related to the purpose of the group. For example, educational groups may be formed for a specified period of time and be open to all interested persons, whereas a support group may be ongoing and be open primarily to people affected by a specific health problem.

After the initial decisions about group membership and purpose have been made, someone must take responsibility for arranging a place and time for the initial group meeting, inviting prospective members to attend, and conducting the first meeting. The initial meeting is very important because it sets the stage for how well the group will develop and perform. At the initial meeting, invited participants should be involved in clarifying the group's purpose and goals and determining whether additional members are needed for the group to achieve its goals effectively and efficiently.

**❝***Murphy's Law: A meeting is an event at which the minutes are kept and the hours are lost.* **❞**

| Table 18-1 | Stages of Group Growth and Development: A Comparison of Theories | | | | |
|---|---|---|---|---|---|
| | **Stages of Group Development** | | | | |
| **Theorists** | **Initiation** | | **Maintenance** | | **Dissolution** |
| Bion (1961) | Flight | Fight | | Unite | |
| Tuckman (1965) | Forming | Storming | Norming | Performing | |
| Yalom (1985) | Orientation | Conflict | Harmony | Maturity | |
| Feinberg (1980) Berman-Rossi (1992) | Formation | Conflict resolution | Norms | Cohesion | Dissolution |

## Application to Practice

### *Health Needs of the Rural Elderly Population*

Darla Parker, RN, BSN, works with a small home health agency that is located in a rural Appalachian community. Population in the county is estimated to be 13,798, with 2,578 people between the ages of 55 and 64. Another 3,459 people are older than 65. Demographic data indicate that the elderly population will continue to grow, with the "graying of America" and young adults leaving the area to find work. Chronic health problems among the older population of this county include high rates of cancer, especially late-stage diagnosed uterine and breast cancers, chronic lung diseases (including a high rate of black lung disease), and high rates of cardiovascular diseases. The incidence of cigarette smoking, sedentary lifestyles, and obesity are also high for this community.

In consultation with Shirley Janeff, director of the regional office on aging, Darla learned that a recent assessment of the community had found that a number of elderly citizens with chronic health problems were having difficulty getting access to needed healthcare resources. Results of this survey also showed needs for transportation, for home caregivers, and for help with the purchase of medications. Janeff said, "I think the problem is complex, but some of the problems we are encountering are related to changes in Medicare reimbursement policies that limit access to home health and also that people are simply not informed about the many resources available to them in the community." Darla responded, "I know we can't solve the problems with reimbursement at this time, but maybe we can do something to inform people about resources." When Darla returned to her office she talked with her supervisor about setting up a task force to investigate some possible solutions to these issues. Her supervisor, Mary Jane, agreed with the need to work on this issue and suggested that Darla proceed.

Two weeks later Darla met with representatives of a variety of service agencies to develop some approaches to the documented needs of the elderly citizens of the community. After much discussion of the assessment data, the group decided to put on a health fair as one strategy to inform the community of the many resources in the area. At this first meeting, the group selected a date to coincide with Older Americans Month. They decided to hold it outdoors at the local county park, but they also identified another site in case of rain on the chosen date. The task force met two more times to complete planning for the event.

1. What are some factors Darla needs to consider when putting together a task force to plan this project? As you answer this question, think about the advantages and disadvantages of inviting various community and organizational representatives.

2. Once she has established the task force, what is Darla's role with the group? What are expected behaviors of the different possible roles she could assume?

3. At the first meeting, Darla is elected by the group to be the chairperson. What does is mean to be a leader? Describe leadership behaviors you would expect to see Darla exhibit.

4. Whenever a group of people come together to work on an issue or a project, conflict is a possibility. How could Darla intervene with the group to control conflict and keep them moving toward their goal? 

---

*Stakeholder analysis* is a technique often used to identify potential group members. In the example (planning teen health services) in the Application to Practice feature on page 403, two nurses initiated group development by inviting some teens from the local high school to come together to form an advisory group. At the first meeting, the nurses may have used the technique of stakeholder analysis to identify other teens who might represent segments of the student population not included in the first meeting. Similarly, when the group expanded and formed a community coalition, stakeholder analysis would have been a useful way to identify potential coalition members (Box 18-2).

## ■ Group Maintenance: Cohesion, Norms, and Conflict Resolution

As the expanded group moves into an active working phase, it must establish its rules of behavior (norms) and begin the process of developing group cohesion and conflict resolution. The success of this stage is related to sharing

**BOX 18-2**

**How to Conduct Stakeholder Analysis**

1. Identify the specific issue, health topic, or problem that is the intended focus of the group.
2. List all agencies, organizations, and/or individuals who affect or are affected by the issue, health topic, or problem that is the intended focus of the group.
3. Narrow the list to a workable size by asking two questions about each potential participant:
   - What can this person, agency, or organization contribute to achieving this group's goal?
   - What will be lost if this person, agency, or organization does not participate in the group?
4. Refine the initial list, based on the answers in step 2, adding names and addresses of each person, agency, or organization who will be invited.
5. Invite each stakeholder to participate in the next group meeting.

of leadership and participation and to the degree that goal achievement and group maintenance roles are fulfilled by group members.

### ■ Group Dissolution

When a group has achieved its stated purpose and goals, it is faced with the decision of whether to dissolve or continue with new goals and objectives (Keyton, 1993). The dissolution stage can be tricky if the group has developed tangible assets. In some cases, a group may decide to merge with another group having similar purposes. Consensus building and conflict resolution are essential if group dissolution is to be achieved in a positive manner.

### ■ Group Stages and Formation

Homans (1950, 1961) provided a framework for understanding the stages that a group moves through in the formation of group in the social structure. According to his framework, the three essential elements of a group system are activities, interactions, and attitudes, though the manager's leadership style and the organizational system certainly influence the development of group formation. Homans proposes that groups, both formal and informal, move through the following stages:

*Forming*: the initial stage of group development, in which individuals assemble into a well-defined cluster

*Storming*: the second stage of group development in which group members develop roles and relationships; competition and conflict generally occur

*Norming*: the third stage of group development, in which group members define goals and rules of behavior

*Performing*: the fourth stage of group development, in which group members agree on basic purposes and activities and carry out the work of the group

## Group Functions

Group functions may be divided into two categories: the activities that group members must perform if the group is to function effectively and efficiently and the role of groups themselves in creating the conditions that improved the health and quality of life of individuals and families in the community (change agent role).

### ■ Group Tasks

Groups must carry out two sets of tasks—internal maintenance tasks and goal attainment tasks—to function effectively. **Internal maintenance tasks** are the activities of group members that help the group move smoothly through the stages of development, such as formation and maintenance of a teen advisory board and community coalition. **Goal attainment tasks** are the activities that must be performed by members of the group so that the group can define and achieve its collective purposes and desired outcomes, such as establishment of comprehensive teen health services that are acceptable and accessible.

### ■ Roles of Group Members

Although the entire group shares responsibility for these tasks, there are many different roles that individual members can play in carrying out these tasks (Charns & Schaefer, 1983; Clark, 1994a, 1994b; Cole, 1998; Currat & Michel, 2006; Maznevski, 1994).

**Group Maintenance Roles**

Behaviors that ensure good relationships among group members are needed for groups to survive, grow, and function effectively. The roles related to group maintenance help the group spend its time and energy on goal achievement rather than on meeting the needs of the membership. While reading about each role, think about what you would do to carry out each role if you were one of the nurses involved in one of the groups planning teen health services.

*Gatekeeper*: The role of the gatekeeper is to ensure that everyone who wants to make a contribution to the group has an opportunity to do so. This includes finding ways of allowing and encouraging quieter group members to voice their opinions, as well as helping more vocal group members express themselves in ways that do not dominate others. In recent years, some groups have been exploring the use of computers and decision science technology to facilitate gatekeeping.

*Encourager*: The encourager complements the work of the gatekeeper by creating a climate of acceptance within the group so that members feel free to express themselves.

*Conflict manager*: As noted earlier, conflict is an inherent part of effective group functioning. The role of the conflict

**❝** *When you blame others, you give up your power to change.* **❞**

—*Robert Anthony*

## MEDIA MOMENT

*Survivor* (2000–present)

In this competition/reality television show, a diverse group of contestants is stranded in a remote location with little more than the clothes on their backs. The contestants start off divided into two teams that compete against each other, with the losing team being forced to vote a member off. When the number of contestants is reduced to 10, the teams merge and it's everyone for himself or herself.

manager is to facilitate a tone of harmony and compromise in which individuals with strongly held beliefs and opinions can modify their personal views in favor of the greater good of the group. A strategy that is often effective in reducing tension is the appropriate use of humor.

*Standard setter/tester*: When group relationships have broken down, the standard setter helps the group diagnose the situation and develop and implement standards of group behavior that will help correct the problem.

### Goal Attainment Roles

The roles of group members related to achievement of shared goals and objectives reflect behaviors that move the group through a process of planning and decision making. Continue to think about what you would do if you were one of the nurses in the teen health services project as you read about group attainment roles.

*Initiator*: The initiator is responsible for stating and clarifying the group's goals, defining or specifying the problem (if any) being addressed, and proposing how the group should proceed. At first, the initiating behaviors may come from the formal group leader, but as the group matures, the initiating role is shared. For example, one of the nurses may have been the initiator during the first teen advisory board meeting, but teen members of the group also would fulfill initiator roles in later meetings.

*Opinion and information seeker/giver*: For a group to move forward with developing activities and interventions, it is critical that a member of the group facilitate honest and open sharing of diverse opinions and a wide array of information.

*Clarification/elaboration builder*: A group member who accepts this role is responsible for clarifying ideas and proposals presented to the group and for helping the group develop the communication and synergy to combine and build on individual ideas.

*Summarizer*: Periodically, someone in the group needs to summarize what is taking place so that important ideas and decisions are not lost. In some groups, the person who takes minutes may perform this role.

*Decision-making facilitator*: The decision-making facilitator checks group progress toward decision making and readiness for closure. Premature closure tends to result in

decisions that are made with insufficient information or that lack member "buy in." Conversely, group members become bored and restless when closure is delayed too long. Both extremes have a negative impact on group cohesion.

*Consensus builder*: The consensus builder helps the group frame diverse ideas and opinions into proposals or decisions that reflect the corporate wishes of the group.

As a student nurse, you have learned communication skills that will help you perform group maintenance and goal attainment roles when working with face-to-face groups. If your nursing care involves working with groups, your care plan should include strategies for helping group members develop the skills and knowledge needed for shared leadership and task-related roles.

Researchers from a variety of disciplines are examining the tasks and roles needed for successful computer-mediated groups. Although the task-related roles and communication skills are similar to those of face-to-face groups, an additional set of technology-related skills and knowledge must be developed (Hollingshead & McGrath, 1995; Sosik, 1997).

### ■ Groups as Change Agents

Much of the current knowledge about group dynamics and groups as agents of **change** originates in the social psychology research conducted by Kurt Lewin in the 1930s and 1940s. Lewin found that the traditional methods of education, such as lecturing and individual instruction, were effective in transmitting units of information but did not result in

### A Good Read

## Lord of the Flies (1954)

*By William Golding, London: Faber and Faber, Ltd.*

William Golding's classic tale deals with a group of English schoolboys who are plane wrecked on a deserted island. At first, the stranded boys cooperate, attempting to gather food, make shelters, and maintain signal fires. Overseeing their efforts are Ralph, "the boy with fair hair," and Piggy, Ralph's chubby, wisdom-dispensing sidekick whose thick spectacles come in handy for lighting fires. Although Ralph tries to impose order and delegate responsibility, many in their number would rather swim, play, or hunt the island's wild pig population. Soon Ralph's rules are being ignored or challenged outright. His fiercest antagonist is Jack, the redheaded leader of the pig hunters, who manages to lure away many of the boys to join his band of painted savages. The situation deteriorates as the trappings of civilization continue to fall away, until Ralph discovers that, instead of being hunters, he and Piggy have become the hunted. This classic novel is an excellent example of a group's experiment to develop the perfect society from scratch.

**“** *Be sincere; be brief; be seated.* **”**
—Franklin Delano Roosevelt, advice on being an effective speaker

learning and behavior change. Instead, he found that people learn best in a social context through group discussion and decision-making approaches. Think about the various teaching/learning strategies you have encountered during your nursing education. Although you may have encountered copious amounts of information in lecture-based courses, it is likely that the courses using problem-based learning or group discussion focused on decision making have been more effective in helping you acquire the knowledge and skills that you use in the clinical setting.

Lewin also found that learning and behavior change were much greater in groups with democratic (participatory) leadership than in groups with autocratic (top-down) leadership (Lewin, 1949). Subsequent educational and health-related research not only has affirmed Lewin's findings but has also contributed to the development of the highly effective **empowerment** approaches to health promotion and restoration (Minkler, 1997; Moreland & Hogg, 1993; Sampson & Marthas, 1981). The shared leadership and shared decision-making approaches discussed earlier in this chapter are examples of how participatory leadership may be used in nursing practice with groups.

### 💻 Research Alert

This article explores contemporary women's perceptions of the experience of the menopausal process within the Western industrialized culture, describes and synthesizes the processes used by women to evaluate available information, and explores and facilitates processes used by women to envision and create change in their life world. An emancipatory group process was designed to facilitate dialogue between the investigator and nine women who met as a group eight times during a 10-week period in the home of one of the participants. Participants identified menses cessation as a time of change in all aspects of their lives. They employed decision making to cope with these changes and, as a result of the awareness that came through the research process, invited other women to celebrate the collective wisdom of women at all stages of life.

As demonstrated by this study, women experiencing menses cessation need information and time to process that information internally and in relation with others. Nurses can facilitate this process by providing knowledge, assisting women in decision making, and intervening in ways that contribute to a holistic quality of life for women. ◢

*Source*: Timmerman, G. M. (2005). Commentary on "Navigating the journey to menses cessation." *Journal of Holistic Nursing, 23*(1), 51–53.

### ■ Concepts Related to Change

Lewin's subsequent research on motivation, behavior change, and group dynamics led to the development of two concepts of change that serve as the foundation for many contemporary health promotion and disease prevention models. The first concept, known as **force field analysis**, states that behavior is strongly influenced by the forces in the social fields surrounding people. Forces that promote or support change are considered *driving forces*. Forces that oppose or inhibit change are *restraining forces*. To bring about individual or collective change, the practitioner must analyze the strength and direction of the forces that are preserving the status quo and develop action steps to strengthen the driving forces, while diminishing or changing the direction of the restraining forces (see the following three figures on this page and page 411). The analysis and action steps are group activities in which all members participate. For example, during the planning process, community coalition members may have identified individuals, groups, and social norms that were supportive of or opposed to each of the health services proposed for the teen health center. If the forces opposing the service outweighed support for the service, the group might ask, "Are there ways we help people feel more positive about this service? If not, is the opposition so strong that we should not offer this service at the teen center?" It is especially useful to conduct force field analysis on controversial areas, such as contraception education or services for teens.

Lewin's second concept is that change occurs in stages. During the first stage, unfreezing, the forces that preserve the status quo are analyzed and strategies targeting specific driving and restraining forces are developed. In the second stage, moving, the strategies are implemented. The modified

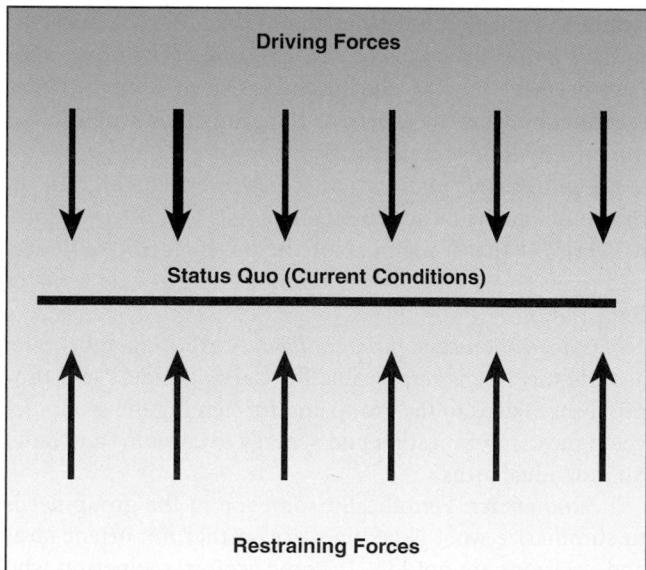

Stage 1 of Lewin's change process: unfreezing. Analyze the strength and direction of forces preserving status quo.

forces (e.g., new behaviors, policies, organizational structures) are tested and evaluated. In the third stage, refreezing, the changes that are to be adopted are reinforced by repetition, policy change, and other long-term change approaches (Lewin, 1951).

For example, nurses may be involved in groups that have a goal of reducing health problems related to tobacco use. During the unfreezing stage, group members would analyze

Stage 2 of Lewin's change process: moving. Change the strength or direction of forces.

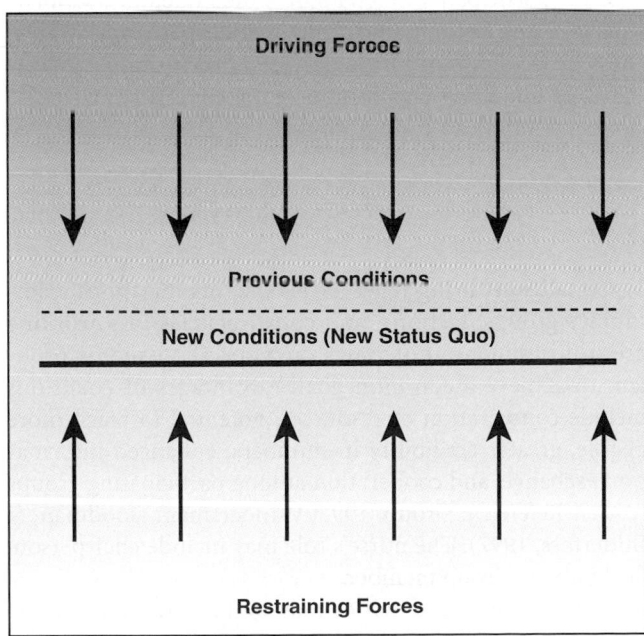

Stage 3 of Lewin's change process: refreezing. Reinforce and preserve changes.

a variety of physical, social, cultural, economic, educational, political, and environmental factors that provide positive or negative support for tobacco use by community members. One strategy might be to reduce the harmful effects of secondhand smoke in public places such as restaurants. The group might work with local restaurant owners to develop trial smoke-free nights and evaluate the impact of voluntary no-smoking policies on business (moving). If the trial period shows that business remains the same or increases, restaurant owners may adopt long-term smoke-free policies (refreezing). Furthermore, if restaurant owners develop positive opinions about smoke-free environments, they may be less of a restraining force (or may even become a driving force) if the group expands its strategies to include a local no-smoking ordinance.

**"** *I start with the premise that the function of leadership is to produce more leaders, not more followers.* **"**

—*Ralph Nader*

 GLOBAL CONNECTION

The Peace Corps works in groups in its efforts to improve the lives of residents of underdeveloped countries. The ability to work effectively as a group member under extreme conditions is a critical skill for selection as a Peace Corps volunteer.

## Types of Groups

So far the main type of group discussed has been a health planning coalition. In reality, groups have diverse goals and purposes. Groups that nurses may find themselves working with to achieve health goals include educational or learning groups, support groups, self-help groups, therapy groups, task groups, focus groups, and coalitions (Aspen Reference Group, 1997). A nurse's role within a group depends on the type of group with whom she or he is working.

*Educational* or *learning* groups are designed to provide members with knowledge and understanding regarding a specific issue or area of need. The nurse's role in these groups is to provide structure and focus for group learning. The nurse may also be the educational provider (Toseland, 1995). Examples of educational groups include Lamaze childbirth classes and diabetes education programs.

*Support* groups help members cope with situational crises, life transitions, and a variety of chronic health problems through the provision of emotional support, information, and guidance. The nurse's role with support groups

**"** *If I have seen farther than others, it is because I was standing on the shoulders of giants.* **"**

—*Sir Isaac Newton*

Parenting groups are an effective strategy for improving teen parenting skills.

is to facilitate group interaction and process and to serve as a role model of acceptance (Schopler & Galinsky, 1993; Sharf, 1997; Yates, 1995). Examples of support groups are Alzheimer's disease caregiver groups, hospice bereavement groups, and breast cancer support groups.

*Self-help* groups are defined by self-governance and a common concern or problem. Group members provide one another with emotional support, information, education, social advocacy, and sometimes material aid. High value is placed on experiential knowledge as a form of special understanding of a group member's experiences. Although nurses and other health professionals generally do not have a formal role in these groups, health professionals often make referrals to these groups (Humphreys, 1997; Ogborne, 1996; Schubert & Borkman, 1991; Social Policy Corporation, 1997; Stewart, 1990). Examples of self-help groups include Alcoholics Anonymous and Overeaters Anonymous.

*Therapy* groups provide treatment, most often professional, for people experiencing an emotional disturbance. The primary goal of these groups is to provide members with insight into themselves and help them change their behaviors. The nurse's role within these groups is therapeutic and involves role modeling acceptance and caring, encouraging group participation, helping members explore the reasons behind their feelings and behavior, and providing structure and maintenance of group process (Clark, 1994a; Corey & Corey, 1992). Examples might include therapy groups for people with depression, attention-deficit disorder, or schizophrenia. After the terrorist attacks of September 11, 2001, and the Hurricane Katrina disaster, nurses often found themselves in need of support and therapy groups as a way of coming to terms and working through the grief of losing colleagues in these disasters (Constantino & Smart, 2004).

*Task* groups have a primary goal of accomplishing some specified activity. Consequently, these groups are time limited and disband when the task is completed. The nurse's role within task groups, which is to facilitate progress toward goal accomplishment, is determined by the membership position of leader or group member (Bracht, 1990; Skvoretz & Fararo, 1996). Examples of task groups include a community group to establish a recreation center or a group of teachers, parents, and the school nurse planning a health fair.

*Focus* groups provide a forum for obtaining data through group interviews about a variety of issues of concern to nurses and other health professionals. Although these groups have primarily been used in the business arena for marketing purposes, nurses and other health professionals are now using the approach to obtain information from patients about health services and needs. The nurse's role within a focus group is to establish a nonthreatening and positive environment and to facilitate group process (Aspen Reference Group, 1997; Butterfoss, Houseman, Morrow, & Rosenthal, 1997; Quible, 1998).

 **Research Alert**

Focus groups were conducted in six Asian communities in Chicago to determine reasons for the downward trend in immunization rates among Asian American children. Participants ($n = 67$ [range 7–15]) were paid a $25 stipend. Results indicated that barriers to immunization include cost, language, information and records (lack of information, confusing immunization records, and uncertainty about records being up-to-date), difficulty in scheduling appointments and long waits to see doctors, and provider choice (participants weren't sure which doctors provided quality care). Recommendations include increasing awareness of free immunization services, decreasing language barriers, and providing immunization education materials to Asian American communities.

*Source*: Asian Health Coalition of Illinois. (2004). *Identifying immunization barriers among Asian American children: Results and recommendations.* Retrieved November 10, 2008, from http://www.cispiimmunize.org/resour/FAAP%20Presentations/Vickers.ppt

**Coalitions** bring together people, organizations, community groups, factions, and constituencies in a working group to influence outcomes on a specific issue or problem to achieve a common goal. Advantages of coalitions include conservation of resources, potential to reach more people, greater credibility in numbers, enhanced information exchange, and cooperation among participating groups (Aspen Reference Group, 1997; Wandersman, Goodman, & Butterfoss, 1997). The nurse's role may include chairperson, facilitator, or group member.

Team-building activities may be used to enhance the normal stages of group development and are an important aspect of managing groups. Team-building techniques may also be used when groups are experiencing conflict or failing to meet their goals.

Antai-Otong (1997) has identified four qualities that are present in successful teams:

- Open and effective communication
- Involved members who are committed to the team, understand team dynamics, and are emotionally invested in the team
- Clearly defined goals that identify member roles and responsibilities
- Trust and collegiality

## Working with Groups

This section focuses on general information about group leadership that can be adapted to a variety of settings. When working with specific types of groups, such as therapeutic or support groups, you should supplement the theory base you are using to guide your nursing care of groups with the research and theories specific to the specialty area linked to that type of group.

**❝** *If your actions inspire others to dream more, learn more, do more, and become more, you are a leader.* **❞**

—John Quincy Adams

### ■ Group Leadership

Two leadership styles—democratic and autocratic—were identified earlier in the chapter as part of the discussion about change. Although the democratic leadership style is most closely associated with long-term learning and change, both styles have utility (Hickman, 1990; VanOostrum & Rabbie, 1995).

Democratic leadership, more commonly known as *participatory leadership*, refers to the approach that involves group members in all levels of information gathering, discussion, analysis, decision making, and evaluation. In a more restrictive form of democratic leadership, group members are presented with information as a basis for informed decision making. Participatory leadership builds group cohesion and contributes to individual and collective empowerment.

> ### ● MEDIA MOMENT
>
> **CSI: Crime Scene Investigation (2000–present)**
> This television show follows the nights of the detectives working at the Las Vegas Police Department Crime Scene Investigations bureau. As members of the second busiest crime lab in the United States, CSI officers use the best scientific and technical methods to solve puzzles and catch criminals.

A strength of participatory/shared leadership is that it builds a broad base of support for long-term change. A corresponding reality is that the decision-making and change processes will take longer to achieve.

Autocratic leadership, also known as *authoritarian leadership*, is the "top-down" style of leadership found in many healthcare settings. The authoritarian leadership style also is reflected in the approach to teaching, planning, and behavior change used by many educators in the health professions. Two advantages of this approach are the volume of information that can be transmitted in a short time and the speed with which change can be made. On the negative side, knowledge does not necessarily lead to learning and growth, and changes made in this manner tend to be short-lived unless supported by major "selling" campaigns. Table 18-2 offers a comparison of different leadership styles.

Both styles of leadership have some usefulness. When a decision must be made quickly or rapid change is essential, then a shift toward a more authoritarian leadership style may be indicated. For example, an infection control nurse

**❝** *America would be a better place if leaders would do more long-term thinking. In Iroquois society, leaders are encouraged to remember seven generations in the past and consider seven generations in the future when making decisions that affect people.* **❞**

—Wilma Mankiller, principal chief, Cherokee Nation

| **Table 18-2** A Comparison of Leadership Styles | | |
|---|---|---|
| | **Participatory Leadership** | **Authoritarian Leadership** |
| ■ Nurse's roles | Facilitator | Director |
| | Partner with expertise | Expert information provider |
| ■ Group members' roles | Co-leaders | Recipients of information |
| | Partners with expertise | Providers of feedback |
| | Decision makers | Targets of change |
| ■ Leadership actions | Ask questions | Tell/lecture |
| | Stimulate/guide discussion | Lead discussion |
| | Link to resource providers | Arrange for resources |
| ■ Outcomes | Learning | Short-term change |
| | Empowerment | Knowledge expansion |
| | Sustained change | |

🖉 NOTE THIS! •
**Groupthink** is a sociological phenomenon characterized by decision-making processes that are driven by consensus. The group tends to reject information or alternatives that do not fit with group's original plan. ▲

might be working with a group of daycare center operators. During an outbreak of a communicable disease, the infection control nurse might *tell* the daycare operators what control measures they *must* adopt immediately to stop the outbreak (autocratic approach). However, in most group settings, the participatory leadership style is the preferred approach. For example, the infection control nurse might work with the group on a long-term basis to help the daycare operators develop and test the efficacy of a variety of strategies for preventing communicable diseases in their businesses (democratic approach). Furthermore, leadership style may be modified to fit with the capacities of group members. Factors such as age, physical or mental impairment, and physical disability may affect a group member's ability to engage in participatory or shared leadership (Cole, 1998; Seers & Woodruff, 1997; Toseland, 1995). Gender has also been demonstrated as a variable in leadership style. Men and woman may display different strategies in conflict resolution and consensus building (Currat & Michel, 2006).

❝When the best leader's work is done, the people say, 'We did it ourselves.'❞

—Lao-Tzu

## ■ Ethical Considerations

Group leadership brings with it some ethical considerations. Group leaders potentially have great power. Many of the world's belief systems warn of the corrupting effects of power that is not grounded in a set of higher moral values and a sense of responsibility. Furthermore, a skillful leader may be tempted to guide the group in the direction he or she believes is best for the group. Another consideration is that shared leadership, empowerment, and change will likely shift the existing balance of power. You also may face the dilemma of realizing that a group's actions or decisions may adversely affect individuals within the group or others in the community. Different approaches to ethical decision making will generate questions to guide reflective thinking. Some of these questions may include "How is my leadership style affecting the lives of the members of the group?" "Whose goals are being pursued?" "How is the balance of power being shifted?" "Who potentially benefits from this group's decisions and actions?" and "Who is potentially harmed?"

❝We must accept finite disappointment, but we must never lose infinite hope.❞

—Martin Luther King, Jr.

❝There cannot be a stressful crisis next week. My schedule is already full.❞

—Henry Kissinger

## ■ Evaluating Groups

Groups may be evaluated for process, impact, and outcome. **Process evaluation** often is focused on group dynamics and interactions. A useful tool for process evaluation is the *group interaction diagram*. The evaluator draws a circle that includes the initials of each member of the group. For each interaction, the evaluator draws an arrow from the person talking to the person being addressed. The direction and number of the arrows will show communication patterns within the group. In authoritarian groups, most of the interaction will be between the leaders and individual members of the group. In participatory groups, the direction of the arrows should be more evenly distributed. The diagram will also identify both nonparticipants and discussion dominators. It may be helpful to begin a new diagram when a new topic is introduced or after a major decision is made. Each diagram should be labeled clearly. (The following figures show examples of group interaction diagrams.)

**Impact evaluation** focuses on intermediate behavior changes among group members or by those whose behavior the group is attempting to change. **Outcome evaluation** is based on the degree to which the group's goal and objectives have been met.

🖉 NOTE THIS! •
Groups of up to about seven members can take part in the same conversation. Beyond that number it becomes progressively more likely that smaller groups will form and several conversations will take place. ▲

Beginning a process-recording diagram.

**Discussion primarily between leader and individual group members.**

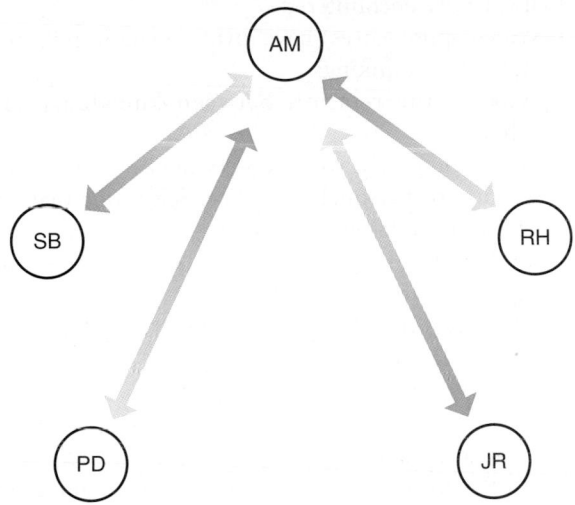

Process-recording pattern associated with authoritarian leadership.

**Discussion flows freely among all members of the group.**

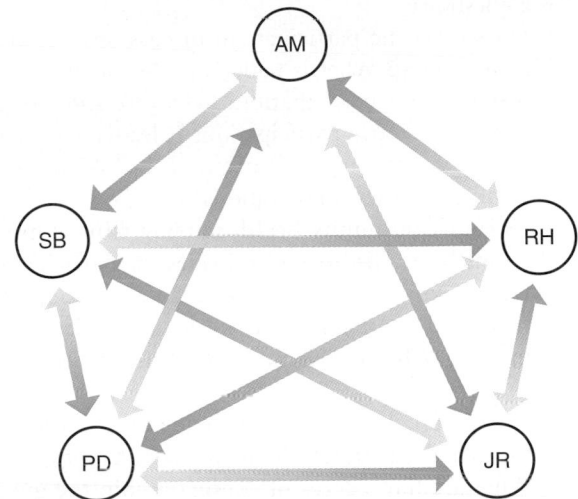

Process-recording pattern associated with democratic leadership.

 NOTE THIS!

Groups of more than 10 or 12 people have difficulty taking part in the same conversation unless one member assumes a leader role and regulates interaction so that everyone has a chance to contribute. Conversations directed to the group tend to become more formal at this size. Group members "address" the group rather than talk.

❝ *We are not retreating—we are advancing in another direction.* ❞

—*General Douglas MacArthur*

❝ *Treat people as if they were what they ought to be, and help them to become what they are capable of being.* ❞

—*Goethe*

## Conclusion

This chapter describes several types of groups encountered in nursing practice. Concepts, research, and strategies for effective nursing care of and with groups were discussed.

Although the focus of this chapter has been on working with small face-to-face groups, many of the concepts and skills are applicable to work with groups of all sizes, including community populations. For example, participatory leadership at the group level corresponds with the community development approach at the community level, and authoritarian leadership fits within the social planning model of community organization.

Explore Community Health Nursing on the Web! To learn more about the topics in this chapter, use the passcode provided to access your exclusive website: **http://nursing.jbpub.com/ communityhealth.** If you do not have a passcode, you can obtain one at this site.

## ■ CRITICAL THINKING ACTIVITIES

1. As a student nurse, you are probably involved in a variety of on-campus and clinical groups. Observe the next meeting of one of these groups and answer the following questions:
   - Does everyone participate in discussions and decision making? What is happening in the group that fosters active participation? What are some of the barriers to active participation? Is leadership shared among various members of the group? What do you think about these observations?
   - In your community health nursing clinical group, brainstorm a list of ground rules for participation. Decide which ones you will adopt as a group. Post them and try them out at your next clinical group meeting. What are the outcomes of using these group rules?
   - As a group, develop and implement some strategies for shared leadership. What are the outcomes?
   - What are the sources of conflict within the group? Is conflict viewed as a potential strength or as something to be avoided? How is conflict managed? In your clinical group, brainstorm some ground rules for positive conflict management. Try them out. Do they work? Why or why not?

2. Observe the different roles played by members of groups in which you are participating as a student nurse.
   - What are the goal achievement and group maintenance roles played by each person in the group? Does one person play more than one role? Do two or more people play the same role?
   - What are the different strategies that you might use to assist a group in goal achievement and group maintenance?

3. In your community health nursing clinical group, take turns fulfilling each of the goal achievement and task maintenance roles.
   - Discuss your reactions and feelings related to each role. Evaluate one another's role performance. Which roles are most comfortable for you? Which roles do your classmates observe you performing most in other group settings?
   - Develop a list of facilitating questions for each role.

4. Interview a nurse who is facilitating a group over the Internet. (*Hint*: Some of the members of the nursing faculty may be conducting classes and groups using the Internet.)
   - How does this person facilitate group maintenance and goal attainment using the Internet?
   - With your classmates, brainstorm how you would modify your behavior and questions for each group role if you were using the Internet.

5. Observe the various learning situations (formal and informal settings) that you have been in. Think about the various teaching/learning approaches and activities that you have encountered.
   - Which approach(es) have involved you in reflection and critical thinking?
   - What is the relation between knowledge and behavior?
   - List 10 things that you know about health promotion but do not personally practice. Select one that you would like to target for change.
     - What are the driving and restraining forces that preserve your current behavior?
     - How can you change these forces? Develop an action plan that includes the stages of unfreezing, moving, and refreezing.
     - How would a group approach fit with your proposed change?
   - List the groups in your community that fall into the category of groups that create or support change. How can you use these groups in nursing practice?
   - Make a list of health-related groups in your community. What is the purpose of each group? How does each group contribute to the health of individuals, families, or populations in your community?
   - Visit three of these groups. If possible, visit three different types of groups. Observe the behavior of group leaders. Which leadership styles are being used? How well do these leadership styles fit with the group's type and purpose? Which leadership style would you use with each group? Why?

6. There are many practical activities that must take place to ensure effective group meetings. Some of these activities may include arranging the time and place for the meeting, arranging the meeting room (e.g., lights, sound, seating, food, other resources, clean-up), inviting people to attend, setting the agenda, leading the meeting, taking minutes or notes (if appropriate), and evaluating outcomes. Select one type of group that might be found in one of your clinical settings. Make a table that has three columns. Label the first column "Practical Considerations." List all the specific activities that you can identify that would need to take place if your meeting is to be a success. Label the second and third columns "Participatory Leadership" and "Authoritarian Leadership." In the rows under each of these leadership styles, describe how you would ensure that the activities listed in the first column are carried out.
   - What are the similarities between the second and third columns? The differences?
   - What are the sets of skills needed for each of these leadership styles? Which of these skills do you

already possess? Which self-directed learning activities might help you expand your skills and knowledge base for effective group leadership?

- Which of these leadership styles are most comfortable for you? Why? What do you think about this?

7. You have been asked to develop an educational program about asthma for parents of elementary school-children. One step you plan to use in developing the program is to bring together a focus group of parents to identify what they need to know.

- Describe and explain the selection process you will use to identify participants for the focus group.
- What is your role as the group leader (before, during, and after the meeting)?
- How will you fulfill this role? What theories, concepts, and strategies will you use to guide your group leadership activities?

8. Observe the different ways that nurses work with groups in your community health clinical setting. Select one of these nurses and interview him or her.

- Which types of groups does he or she work with?
- What is his or her role with each group?

- Which skills does he or she think are needed to work with these groups effectively?
- What are the greatest challenges encountered when working with groups?
- What advice would he or she give to student nurses who will be working with groups in the community?
- Write a self-evaluation focused on working with groups. How effectively do you work in groups? Which group-related skills, knowledge, and experience do you already possess? How can you strengthen these during your remaining nursing education? after graduation?
- Which additional group-related skills, knowledge, and experience do you need to develop as part of your nursing education to increase your group work? after graduation?

## ■ REFERENCES

American Nurses Association (ANA). (1986). *Standards of community health nursing practice*. Washington, DC: Author.

American Nurses Association (ANA). (1991). *Standards of clinical nursing practice*. Washington, DC: Author.

American Nurses Association (ANA). (1996). *Scope and standards of advanced practice nursing practice*. Washington, DC: Author.

American Public Health Association (APHA). (1991). *Healthy communities 2000: Model standard* (3rd ed.). Washington, DC: Author.

Antai-Otong, D. (1997). Team building in a health care setting. *American Journal of Nursing, 97*(7), 48–51.

Aspen Reference Group. (1997). *Community health education and promotion: A guide to program design and evaluation*. Gaithersburg, MD: Aspen.

Berdahl, J., & Craig, K. (1996). Equality of participation and influence in groups: The effects of communication medium and sex composition. *Computer Supported Cooperative Work, 4*, 179–201.

Berman-Rossi, T. (1992). Empowering groups through understanding stages of group development. *Social Work with Groups, Special Issue, 5*(2–3), 239–255.

Bion, W. (1961). *Experiences in groups and other papers*. New York: Basic Books.

Bracht, N. (1990). *Health promotion at the community level*. Newbury Park, CA: Sage.

Butterfoss, F., Houseman, C., Morrow, A., & Rosenthal, J. (1997). Use of focus group data for strategic planning by a community-based immunization coalition. *Family and Community Health, 20*(3), 49–59.

Charns, M., & Schaefer, M. (1983). *Health care organizations: A model for management*. Englewood Cliffs, NJ: Prentice Hall.

Clark, N. (1994a). *The nurse as group leader*. New York: Springer.

Clark, N. (1994b). *Team building: A practical guide for trainers*. New York: McGraw-Hill.

Cole, M. (1998). *Group dynamics in occupational therapy*. Thorofare, NJ: Slack.

Constantino, J., & Smart, C. J. (2004). Death among us: Grieving the loss of a coworker is a group process. *American Journal of Nursing, 104*(6), 64.

Cooke, R., & Szumal, J. (1994). The impact of group interaction styles on problem-solving effectiveness. *Journal of Applied Behavioral Science, 30*(4), 415–437.

Corey, M., & Corey, G. (1992). *Groups: Process and practice*. Pacific Grove, CA: Brooks-Cole.

Currat, T., & Michel, L. (2006). Groups and gender: The effects of a masculine gender deficit. *Group Analysis, 39*(1), 133–142.

Dennis, A., & Valacich, J. (1994). Group, sub-group, and nominal group idea generation: New rules for a new media? *Journal of Management, 20*(4), 723–736.

Department of Health and Human Services (DHHS). (1991). *Healthy people 2000: National health promotion and disease prevention objectives. Full report with commentary*. Washington, DC: U.S. Government Printing Office.

Department of Health and Human Services (DHHS). (2000). *Healthy people 2010: Conference edition*. Washington, DC: U.S. Government Printing Office.

Feinberg, N. (1980). A study of group stages in a self-help setting. *Social Work with Groups, 3*(1), 41–50.

Hickman, P. (1990). Community health and development: Applying sociological concepts to practice. *Sociological Practice, 8*, 125–132.

Hirokawa, R., & Keyton, J. (1995). Perceived facilitators and inhibitors of effectiveness in organizational work teams. *Management Communication Quarterly, 8*(4), 424–446.

Hollingshead, A., & McGrath, J. (1995). Computer-assisted groups: A critical review of the empirical research. In R. Guzzo, E. Salas, & Associates (Eds.), *Team effectiveness and decision making in organizations*. San Francisco: Jossey-Bass.

Homans, G. (1950). *The human group.* New York: Harcourt Brace Jovanovich.

Homans, G. (1961). *Social behavior: Its elementary forms.* New York: Harcourt Brace.

Houseman, C., Butterfoss, F. D., Morrow, A. L., & Rosenthal, J. (1997). Focus groups among public, military, and private sector mothers: Insights to improve the immunization process. *Public Health Nursing, 14*(4), 235–243.

Humphreys, K. (1997). Individual and social benefits of self-help groups. *Social Policy, 27*(3), 12–19.

Kelley, L. (1995). Parse's theory in practice with a group in the community. *Nursing Science Quarterly, 8*(3), 127–132.

Keyton, J. (1993). Group termination: Completing the study of group development. *Small Groups Research, 24*(1), 84–100.

Laudon, K., & Laudon, J. (1988). *Management information systems: A contemporary perspective.* New York: Macmillan.

Lewin, K. (1949). Frontiers in group dynamics: Concept, method and reality in social science, social equilibrium, and social change. *Human Relations, 1*, 5–41.

Lewin, K. (1951). *Field theory in social science.* New York: Harper.

Loomis, M. E. (1979). *Group process for nurses.* St. Louis: Mosby.

Madara, E. (1997). The mutual-aid self-help online revolution. *Social Policy, 27*(3), 20–27.

Maznevski, M. (1994). Understanding our differences: Performance in decision-making groups with diverse members. *Human Relations, 47*(5), 531–550.

Minkler, M. (1997). *Community organizing & community building for health.* New Brunswick, NJ: Rutgers University Press.

Moreland, R., & Hogg, M. (1993). Theoretical perspectives on social processes in small groups. *British Journal of Social Psychology, 32*, 1–4.

Ogborne, A. (1996). Professional opinions and practices concerning Alcoholics Anonymous: A review of the literature and a research agenda. *Contemporary Drug Problems, 23*(1), 93–105.

Preboth, M., & Wright, S. (1999). Online support groups. *American Family Physician, 57*(6), 1379.

Ramey, J. (1993). Group empowerment through learning formal decision making processes. *Social Work with Groups, 16*(1–2), 171–185.

Reagan-Cirincione, P. (1994). Improving the accuracy of small group judgement: A process intervention combining group facilitation, social judgement analysis, and information technology. *Organizational Behavior and Human Decision Process, 58*(2), 246–270.

Sampson, E. E., & Marthas, M. (1981). *Group process for the health professions* (2nd ed.). New York: John Wiley and Sons.

Schitterkatte, M. (1996). Facilitating information exchange in small group decision-making groups. *European Journal of Social Psychology, 26*(4), 537–556.

Schopler, J. H., & Galinsky, M. J. (1993). Support groups as open systems: A model for practice and research. *Health and Social Work, 18*(3), 195–207.

Schubert, M. A., & Borkman, T. J. (1991). An organizational typology for self-help groups. *American Journal of Community Psychology, 19*(5), 769–787.

Seers, A., & Woodruff, S. (1997). Temporal pacing in task forces: Group development or deadline pressure? *Journal of Management, 23*(2), 169–186.

Sharf, B. (1997). Communicating breast cancer on-line: Support and empowerment on the Internet. *Women & Health, 26*(1), 65–84.

Skvoretz, J., & Fararo, T. (1996). Status and participation in task groups: A dynamic network model. *American Journal of Sociology, 101*(5), 1366–1414.

Social Policy Corporation. (1997). The future of self-help. *Social Policy, 27*(3), 2–3.

Sosik, J. (1997). Effects of transformational leadership and anonymity on idea generation in computer-mediated groups. *Group and Organization Management, 22*(4), 460–487.

Stewart, M. J. (1990). Professional interface with mutual-aid self-help groups: A review. *Social Science and Medicine, 31*(10), 1143–1158.

Toseland, R. (1995). *Group work with the elderly and family caregivers.* New York: Springer.

Tuckman, B. (1965). Developmental sequence in small groups. *Psychological Bulletin, 63*(6), 384–399.

VanOostrum, J., & Rabbie, J. (1995). Intergroup competition and cooperation within autocratic and democratic management regimes. *Small Group Research, 26*(2), 269–295.

Ward, D. E. (2006). Complexity in group work. *Journal for Specialists in Group Work, 31*(1), 1–3.

Yalom, I. (1985). *The theory and practice of group psychotherapy.* New York: Basic Books.

Yates, R. (1995). *Developing support groups for individuals with early-stage Alzheimer's disease.* Baltimore: Health Professions Press.

# UNIT 4

# Common Community Health Problems

CHAPTER 19
Communicable Disease
*Sharyn Janes*
*Gale A. Spencer*

CHAPTER 20
Sexually Transmitted Diseases and HIV/AIDS
*Sharyn Janes*
*Janet St. Lawrence*
*Julie B. St. Lawrence*

CHAPTER 21
Substance Abuse as a Community Health Problem
*Jean Haspeslagh*
*Judith A. Barton*

CHAPTER 22
Violence and Nursing's Response
*Sherry Hartman*
*Sharyn Janes*
*Anne Troy*

CHAPTER 23
Chronic Illness
*Edith Hilton*
*Kristin Ramsey*
*Linda Morris*

CHAPTER 24
Disasters in the Community
*Karen Saucier Lundy*
*Janie B. Butts*

# CHAPTER 19
# Communicable Disease

Sharyn Janes and Gale A. Spencer

CHEST X-RAY UNIT
MISSISSIPPI STATE BOARD
COOPERATING

Visit **http://nursing.jbpub.com/communityhealth** for interactive exercises, review questions, Web links, and more.

Throughout the world, the eruption and spread of new and old communicable diseases once again threaten the survival of our species.

The single biggest threat to man's continued dominance on the planet is the virus.

—*Joshua Lederberg, Nobel Laureate*

The microbe is nothing; the terrain is everything.

—*Louis Pasteur*

Many communicable diseases, such as tuberculosis, have made a "comeback" in the United States after many decades of dormancy. What has changed about the "terrain" of infectious diseases in recent years? What is the relationship between culture and communicable disease? How does the continued high rate of AIDS in Africa affect the health of U.S. populations? In this chapter you will learn about the importance of communicable disease prevention and treatment in community health.

## CHAPTER FOCUS

**The Problem of Communicable Disease**

**Transmission of Infectious Agents**
- Chain of Infection
- Routes of Infection
- Susceptibility Versus Immunity

**Communicable Disease Prevention**
- Primary Prevention
- Secondary Prevention
- Tertiary Prevention

**Control of Diseases**
- Vaccine-Preventable Diseases
- Routine Vaccinations Indicated for Adults

**Emerging and Reemerging Infectious Diseases**
- Health Care–Associated Infections
- Food-Borne Diseases
- Vector-Borne Diseases
- Zoonoses
- Parasitic Diseases
- Bioterrorism
- HIV/AIDS
- Tuberculosis
- The HIV/TB Connection

**Global Disease Eradication Efforts**

## QUESTIONS TO CONSIDER

After reading this chapter, you will know the answers to the following questions:

1. What is the current infectious disease threat both in the United States and worldwide?

2. What are the reasons for the emergence of new diseases and the reemergence of diseases previously under control?

3. What are the factors that make up the chain of infection?

4. What are the different types of immunity?

5. How do vaccines aid in the prevention of communicable disease?

6. What is the role of the community health nurse in the prevention and treatment of infectious disease?

## KEY TERMS

Acquired immunity
Active humoral immunity
Agent
Fomites
Herd immunity

Immunity
Incubation period
Isolation
Passive immunity
Pathogenicity

Period of infectivity
Personal surveillance
Quarantine
Reservoir

Segregation
Vector
Virulence
Zoonoses

# The Problem of Communicable Disease

Communicable disease, or infectious disease, has always been a focus of community health nursing practice. In fact, at the end of the nineteenth century, when public health nursing emerged as a nursing specialty, communicable diseases were the leading cause of illness and death. During the early years of the twentieth century, nurses continued to care for large numbers of adults and children who were sick or dying from a wide variety of infectious diseases. The typhoid epidemic in the early 1900s and the great influenza pandemic of 1918, which killed 20 million people worldwide (CDC, 1998), are just two examples of infectious diseases that caused enormous suffering and death. Tuberculosis (TB) was a leading killer until well into the 1930s and 1940s, when TB sanitariums were overflowing. Nursing students in

A home visit provided the public health nurse with an opportunity to assess a child with polio in familiar surroundings (circa 1951).

## CULTURAL CONNECTION

Think about how specific cultural groups define "hygiene." Can a culture's values about food preparation, personal hygiene, and child care practices influence a group's risk for communicable disease transmission? How can public health nurses intervene appropriately considering a patient's cultural values when teaching about infectious disease control and prevention?

hospital schools in bigger cities were routinely tested for antibodies against TB, and most of them who came from rural areas tested positive. After a year in the urban hospital wards of the 1930s and 1940s, it was almost a certainty that nursing students would test positive for TB (Garrett, 1994).

The development of antibiotics, particularly penicillin, in the mid-1940s curbed the spread of bacterial infections and significantly decreased the number of deaths from infectious diseases like TB and typhoid fever. Vaccinations against diseases such as polio, whooping cough, and diphtheria, along with urban sanitation efforts and improved water quality, dramatically lowered the incidence of infectious diseases (CDC, 1998). So although infectious disease still took an enormous toll in the rest of the world, a shift in leading causes of morbidity and mortality from infectious diseases to chronic diseases in industrialized nations like the United States caused attention to be focused on chronic conditions such as heart disease, cancer, and diabetes. Antibiotics became the "wonder drugs" of the latter half of the twentieth century, and modern medicine triumphed—or so we thought.

As early as the 1950s, penicillin began to lose its effectiveness against infections caused by *Staphylococcus aureus*. In 1957, and again in 1968, new strains of influenza originating in China rapidly spread throughout the world. During the 1970s, several new diseases were identified in the United States and elsewhere, including Legionnaires' disease, Lyme disease, toxic shock syndrome, and Ebola hemorrhagic fever. The 1980s brought human immunodeficiency virus/acquired immune deficiency syndrome (HIV/AIDS) and a resurgence of TB, which rapidly spread throughout the world. By the 1990s, it was apparent that the threat of infectious disease was again a global reality (CDC, 1998).

Now that we have entered the twenty-first century, we are again faced with infectious diseases that challenge medical and nursing practice. Some are old and familiar, like TB and influenza, and others are new and unfamiliar, like Ebola, SARS, avian flu, and hantavirus. Many of the new challenges are viral in origin, but the overuse and misuse of antibiotics over the last half century have also caused drug-resistant and often fatal strains of bacterial infections to emerge (Box 19-1).

The entire world is becoming much more vulnerable to the eruption and spread of both new and old infectious diseases. Infectious disease is a global problem brought about

**Facts About Antibiotics and Antibiotic Resistance**

- Alexander Fleming, a Scottish scientist, discovered the first antibiotic in 1928.
- Antibiotics became widely available in the 1940s.
- Two million pounds of antibiotics were produced in the United States in 1954. Today, more than 50 million pounds are produced.
- Antibiotics work by either killing bacteria or inhibiting their growth. They do not work on viral infections.
- People consume more than 235 million doses of antibiotics yearly. The Centers for Disease Control and Prevention estimates that 20% to 50% of that use is unnecessary.
- Antibiotic resistance occurs when bacteria causing a specific infection are not destroyed by the antibiotics taken to halt the infection. Unnecessary and improper use of antibiotics promotes the spread of antibiotic-resistant bacteria.

*Source:* Data from CDC, 1999a.

by recent dramatic increases in the worldwide movement of people, goods, and ideas. Not only are people traveling more, but they are traveling more rapidly and going to more places than ever before (Mann, 1994). Every day more than 2 billion people cross over national borders. Every year more than 1.5 billion people travel by air. At least 47 million people from around the world visit the United States each year. Currently more than 14 million people throughout the world die each year from infectious diseases (Drexler, 2002). Some of the contributing factors are the emergence of new

diseases, reemergence of diseases previously thought to have been contained, mass population shifts, and economic and social globalization. Control of many of these emerging and reemerging infectious diseases has become a global public health problem because of the lack of new effective vaccines and therapeutic drugs, or because drugs that offered successful treatment in the past have become resistant to new strains of existing microorganisms (Heymann, 2004).

*"In the old days, our neighbors were Canada and Mexico. Nowadays, with the frequency and speed of air travel, our neighbors are Sri Lanka and Paraguay, you name it."*
—Jeffrey Koplan, Former CDC Director

To address the increasing threat of infectious diseases, nurses must understand the problem from global and historical perspectives. There are many roles for nurses in the battle against infectious diseases. From a community health nursing perspective, primary and secondary prevention concepts must guide nursing practice. A holistic approach that includes health education, environmental health, political action, human rights, and cultural competency is the key. Communicable disease is, after all, not a new concept. Microbes have been an enemy of humans since ancient times. They did not disappear just because science developed drugs and vaccines or because Europeans and Americans cleaned up their cities and towns, and they certainly will not go away when humans choose to ignore or downplay their existence (Garrett, 1994). This chapter describes the present-day threat of infectious diseases and explores the role of community health nurses. Selected *Healthy People 2010* objectives related to communicable diseases are listed on this page.

## HEALTHY PEOPLE 2010

**Objectives Related to Communicable Diseases**

**Food Safety**
10.1 Reduce infections caused by food borne pathogens.
10.2 Prevent an increase in the proportion of isolates of *Salmonella* species from humans and from animals at slaughter that are resistant to antimicrobial drugs.
10.6 Improve food employee behaviors and food preparation practices that directly relate to food-borne illnesses in retail food establishments.

**Immunization and Infectious Diseases**
*Diseases Preventable through Universal Vaccination*
14.1 Reduce or eliminate indigenous cases of vaccine-preventable disease.
14.2 Reduce hepatitis B.
14.5 Reduce invasive pneumococcal infections.

*Diseases Preventable through Targeted Vaccination*
14.6 Reduce hepatitis A.
14.7 Reduce Lyme disease.

*Infectious Diseases and Emerging Antimicrobial Resistance*
14.9 Reduce hepatitis C.
14.11 Reduce tuberculosis.
14.15 Increase the proportion of international travelers who receive recommended preventive services when traveling in areas of risk for select infectious diseases: hepatitis A, malaria, typhoid.

*Vaccination Coverage and Strategies*
14.27 Increase routine vaccination coverage levels of adolescents.
14.29 Increase the proportion of adults who are vaccinated annually against influenza and ever vaccinated against pneumococcal disease.
14.30 Reduce vaccine-associated adverse events.

*Source:* DHHS, 2000.

ENVIRONMENTAL CONNECTION

*How* you travel can make you sick!

Infectious disease outbreaks aboard commercial cruise ships in the past few years led Centers for Disease Control and Prevention (CDC) to conduct a case-control epidemiological study of one cruise ship, which had five gastroenteritis outbreaks on five different cruises. The causative organism was determined to be norovirus (NoV). Passengers became ill with this virus on two consecutive cruises of ship X and continued to become sick on four subsequent cruises despite a one-week sanitization effort. The study documented transmission by food and person-to-person contact, as well as persistence of virus despite sanitization onboard, including introductions of new strains and seeding of an outbreak on land.

Noroviruses are the most common cause of infectious acute gastroenteritis and are transmitted feco-orally through food and water, directly from person to person, and by environmental contamination. These viruses are often responsible for protracted outbreaks in closed settings, such as cruise ships, nursing homes, and hospitals.

On November 20, 2002, cruise ship X recorded an elevated number of persons with acute gastroenteritis symptoms reporting to the ship's infirmary (84 [4%] of 2,318 passengers) during a seven-day vacation cruise from Florida to the Caribbean. According to federal regulations, when the incidence of acute gastroenteritis among passengers and crew exceeds 3%, an outbreak is declared and requires a formal investigation. The outbreak continued on the subsequent cruise (cruise 2), after which the vessel was removed from service for one week of aggressive sanitization. Despite cleaning, gastroenteritis also developed in 192 (8%) of 2,456 passengers and 23 (2.3%) of 999 crew on the following cruise (cruise 3).

Epidemiologists began an investigation on cruise 1 and collected stool specimens from persons with gastroenteritis on this cruise and the next five cruises. All 2,318 passengers on cruise 1 were surveyed to determine dates of illness onset, symptoms, cabin locations, activities, and food consumption. Additionally, a sanitary inspection of the ship was performed. A case-control design was used, and all passengers in whom illness developed early in the cruise (days 3 and 4) after embarkation (defined as day 1) and with passengers who became ill later (day 5) were included in the study. Controls were systematically selected among passengers who reported no symptoms of gastroenteritis throughout the entire cruise. The number of acute gastroenteritis cases on the subsequent five cruises were monitored, and researchers collected fecal specimens from ill persons on all six cruises. During the shipboard investigation, researchers also obtained stool specimens from ill persons in a long-term care facility affected by an outbreak of acute gastroenteritis, in which the index patient was a passenger who returned ill to the facility after disembarking from a cruise.

In this investigation, epidemiologic analysis suggested an initial food-borne source of infection with subsequent secondary spread from person to person, while molecular analysis provided several new insights into disease transmission. Application of genetic sequencing documented persistence of the same strain onboard between cruises by detecting identical sequences in stool samples from ill passengers before and after one week of the vessel's cleaning. Although these findings suggest that environmental contamination may have helped perpetuate the outbreak, infected crew members could have also been a reservoir of infection between cruises.

Molecular fingerprinting of detected viruses confirmed several introductions of new strains aboard, which underscores the difficulty in controlling outbreaks of NoV on cruise ships. Sequence analysis provided evidence that an outbreak of NoV in the care facility was caused by a person returning ill from an outbreak-affected cruise.

Like other outbreaks of viral gastroenteritis on cruise ships, this outbreak affected several hundred people, was transmitted by multiple modes, and recurred on subsequent cruises. Multiple routes of NoV transmission have been documented in other reports, such as that of an outbreak of gastroenteritis among football players, in which both initial food-borne transmission of virus and secondary person-to-person spread were demonstrated. Outbreaks of gastroenteritis aboard cruise ships are similar to those in other closed and crowded settings where identifying and interrupting multiple routes of transmission have proved particularly challenging.

This investigation suggested that efforts to control gastroenteritis outbreaks on cruise ships should address all possible modes of NoV transmission, including food-borne, environmental persistence, and person-to-person spread. Such measures should include extensive disinfection, good food-and-water-handling practices, isolating ill persons, providing paid sick leave for ill crew, and promoting handwashing with soap and water among passengers and crew. Developing strategies and incentives to dissuade symptomatic passengers from boarding may also minimize opportunities to introduce new strains aboard. Cruise ship outbreaks with less than 3% of passengers reporting ill should be considered for investigation because they may contribute substantial information on the transmission and epidemiologic characteristics of NoV, which could be used to develop control strategies and prevent future outbreaks on land and at sea.

*Source:* Isakbaeva, E. T., Widdowson, M.-A., Beard, R. S., et al. (January 2005). Norovirus transmission on cruise ship. *Emerging Infectious Disease.* Retrieved November 12, 2008, from http://www.cdc.gov/ncidod/EID/vol11no01/04-0434.htm

## Transmission of Infectious Agents

The role of nurses in the control of infectious disease prevention and treatment is based on an understanding of ways in which diseases are transmitted from one person to another. *Transmission* is "any mechanism by which an infectious agent is spread from a source or reservoir to a person" (Benenson, 1995, p. 544). There are three general modes of transmission: direct, indirect, and airborne.

### ■ Chain of Infection

The chain of infection is defined as the minimum requirements for an infectious or communicable disease to occur. Six factors make up the chain of infection: (1) an etiological agent or pathogen, (2) a source or reservoir of infection, (3) a means of escape from the source or reservoir (portal of exit), (4) a mode of transmission, (5) a portal of entry into the new host, and (6) a susceptible host.

The causative **agent** or pathogen is any substance or factor that can cause disease. Agents may be bacteria, virus particles, chemicals, or any other plant or animal substance that can cause illness, disease, disability, or death. Causative agents differ both in their ability to cause disease and in their ability to cause serious illness. **Pathogenicity** refers to the agent's capacity to cause disease in an infected host, whereas **virulence** defines the ability of the agent to produce serious illness. For example, both botulism and *Salmonella* are highly pathogenic agents (they can easily cause disease), but botulism is much more virulent (it causes more severe disease).

The source of infection, or **reservoir,** is the habitat or medium in which the agent lives and/or multiplies. Reservoirs can be living things (e.g., humans, animals, insects) or inanimate objects (e.g., food, intravenous [IV] fluids, feces, surgical instruments, stuffed animals) that are conducive to the maintenance or growth of the agent. Reservoirs of infection are human beings, animals, and environmental sources. Humans become reservoirs of infection when the infectious agent has entered the body and established itself. There are three levels of infection in humans: (1) colonization, (2) inapparent infection, and (3) clinically overt disease.

Colonization occurs when the agent is present on the surface of the body or in the nasopharynx and multiplies at a rate sufficient to maintain its numbers without producing any identifiable evidence of a reaction in the person. Inapparent infection (subclinical infection) occurs when the agent is not only present but multiplies in the human reservoir. In an inapparent infection, the agent causes a measurable reaction; however, it does not cause the human to have symptoms of illness. Inapparent infections are usually identified only through laboratory testing (Benenson, 1995; Merrill & Timmreck, 2006). Finally, clinical disease occurs when the agent is present in the human and causes physical symptoms. The time interval between initial contact with an infectious agent and the first appearance of disease symptoms is the **incubation period** (Benenson, 1995). The communicable period, or **period of infectivity,** is the time during which an infectious agent may be transferred directly or indirectly from an infected person to another person, from an infected animal to humans, or from an infected person to animals. All infected persons, including those with colonization, are reservoirs for the agent. Animal reservoirs are mainly domestic animals and rodents.

**Zoonoses** are animal diseases that are transmissible to humans under natural conditions. Animals transmit the disease directly to humans, but these diseases usually are not transmitted from human to human. Examples of zoonoses are bovine TB, rabies (although theoretically it can be transmitted by humans), and anthrax. Environmental reservoirs also transmit directly to humans. An example of an environmental reservoir is hookworm in soil. Inanimate objects such as food, surgical instruments, and human feces can also be reservoirs for diseases.

The agent leaves the reservoir through a portal of exit. Portals of exit and portals of entrance are similar. They include the following: respiratory, oral, gastrointestinal, reproductive, IV, urinary, skin, conjunctival, and transplacental (Merrill & Timmreck, 2006).

The last factor in the chain of infection is a susceptible host. The agent must enter a human host who is vulnerable to the specific disease agent. Susceptibility can be related to factors such as age, immunological status, lifestyle habits, or the presence of other infectious diseases or chronic illnesses.

### ETHICAL CONNECTION

Public health nurses are often faced with ethical conflicts when patients diagnosed with sexually transmitted diseases refuse to name possible contacts. Most states have some type of mandatory reporting of specific STDs, including notification of possible contacts of the patient. How can the nurse provide responsible care for the patient as well as fulfill legal obligations to report these diseases and possible contacts?

### ■ Routes of Infection

The agent then must be transmitted to the next susceptible host through a mode of transmission. Transmission can be direct, indirect, or airborne. (See Table 19-1.)

Direct transmission consists of the direct and immediate transfer of an infectious agent from one infected host or reservoir to a portal of entry in the new host. This may be through direct contact that occurs through biting, kissing, or sexual intercourse or by direct projection of droplet spray into the conjunctiva of the eye or mucous membranes of the eye, nose, or mouth. The projection of droplet spray occurs with sneezing, coughing, talking, singing, or spitting and is usually limited to a distance of approximately 1 meter (Benenson, 1995; Merrill & Timmreck, 2006).

Indirect transmission usually occurs through a vector or by a vehicle. A vector is some form of living organism, usually an animal or an arthropod. Arthropods are insects such as flies and mosquitoes. Flies often carry organisms that are picked up on their feet or proboscis and transferred to food or water. When the organism is carried in this manner, it is called *mechanical vector-borne transmission* because the organism (or agent) does not multiply in the carrier. Mosquitoes, however, are often carriers of *biological vector-borne transmission* as multiplication and development of the organism occurs in the mosquito before the organism is transmitted to the new host through a bite (or inoculation). An example of this type of vector-borne disease is the transmission of malaria by the bite of a mosquito.

*Vehicle-borne transmission* is defined as contaminated inanimate objects, called **fomites,** which serve as an intermediate means by which an infectious agent is transported and

**Table 19-1**   Classification of Major Infectious Diseases by Mode of Transmission

| Airborne Respiratory Diseases | Intestinal Discharge Diseases | Open Sores or Lesion Diseases | Zoonoses or Vectorborne Diseases | Fomiteborne Diseases |
|---|---|---|---|---|
| Chickenpox | Amebic dysentery | AIDS | African sleeping | Anthrax |
| Common colds | Bacterial dysentery | Anthrax | sickness | Chickenpox |
| Diphtheria | (shigellosis) | Erysipelas | Encephalitis | Common colds |
| Influenza | (staphylococcal) | Gonorrhea | Lyme disease | Diphtheria |
| Measles | Cholera | Scarlet fever | Malaria | Influenza |
| Meningitis | Giardiasis | Smallpox | Rocky Mountain | Meningitis |
| Pneumonia | Hookworm | Syphilis | spotted fever | Poliomyelitis |
| Poliomyelitis | Poliomyelitis | Tuberculosis | Tularemia | Rubella |
| Rubella | Salmonellosis | Tularemia | Typhus fever | Scarlet fever |
| Scarlet fever | Typhoid fever | | Yellow fever | Streptococcal |
| Smallpox | Hepatitis | | | throat |
| Throat infections | | | | infections |
| Tuberculosis | | | | Tuberculosis |
| Whooping cough | | | | |

*Source:* Merrill, R. M., & Timmreck, T. C. (2006). *Introduction to epidemiology* (4th ed.). Sudbury, MA: Jones and Bartlett.

introduced into a susceptible host through an appropriate portal of entry (Benenson, 1995; Merrill & Timmreck, 2006). Examples of fomites are toys, bedding, soiled clothes, surgical instruments, and contaminated IV fluids. An example of a vehicle-borne disease is *Salmonella,* which can be transmitted from a kitchen countertop contaminated while thawing raw chicken for dinner.

Airborne transmission occurs through droplet nuclei and dust, which are particles suspended in the air in which microorganisms may be present. Droplet nuclei result from the evaporation of fluid from droplets disseminated by coughing, talking, or sneezing between one infected person and another host. Droplet nuclei can remain suspended in the air for long periods in a dry state. During this time, some droplet nuclei retain their infectivity, while others lose their infectivity or virulence. The particles are very small and are easily breathed into the lungs, where they are retained. When these particles reach the terminal air passages, they begin to multiply and an infection begins in the new host (Benenson, 1995; Merrill & Timmreck, 2006). Pulmonary TB and legionellosis (Legionnaires' disease) are two illnesses that are transmitted by droplet nuclei.

Dust particles in which microorganisms may be present can also become airborne and thus can be breathed into the lungs and cause infection. Contaminated bedding and clothes are examples of objects that can create dust that may carry infectious microorganisms from one infected person to another host. Dust particles contaminated with deer mouse feces may be one way to transmit hantavirus to human hosts.

The cycle of transmission can be broken by breaking the chain of infection—by eliminating the agent, eliminating the reservoir of infection, eliminating transmission at the portal of exit or the portal of entry, or eliminating susceptible hosts.

## ■ Susceptibility Versus Immunity

For a disease to be transmitted, the new host must be susceptible to that disease. The concept of immunity forms the basis of understanding host resistance to disease. **Immunity** is the increased resistance on the part of the host to a specific infectious agent (Valanis, 1999). There are two types of acquired immunity found in humans: active and passive (Atkinson & Wolfe, 2003).

**Acquired immunity** can occur after having had the disease or through vaccination. If a person is infected with the disease (with or without clinical signs and symptoms), the disease agent stimulates the body's natural immune system. However, if the person is inoculated with the agent (in a killed, modified, or variant form), the vaccination artificially stimulates the immune system (see Box 19-2 for a list of vaccine-preventable diseases). Both methods of acquired immunity result in active humoral immunity because the

---

**BOX 19-2**

**Vaccine-Preventable Diseases**

| | |
|---|---|
| Adenovirus | Mumps |
| Anthrax | Pertussis |
| Cholera | Plague |
| Chickenpox (varicella) | Pneumococcal pneumonia |
| Diphtheria | Polio |
| Hepatitis A | Rabies |
| Hepatitis B | Rubella |
| *Haemophilus influenzae* | Smallpox |
| Influenza | Tetanus |
| Japanese encephalitis | Typhoid |
| Measles | Yellow fever |
| Meningococcal infections | |

*Source:* CDC, 1994, 2003.

human body produces its own antibodies when the immune system is stimulated. **Active humoral immunity** is based on a B-lymphocyte response, which results in immunity that lasts for several years with diseases such as tetanus or a lifetime with diseases such as measles or mumps (Atkinson & Wolfe, 2003; Benenson, 1995). **Passive immunity** can be acquired either through the transplacental transfer of the mother's immunity to a disease to her unborn child or from the transfer of already-produced antibodies into a susceptible person (such as the use of immune serum globulin for persons exposed to hepatitis A). Passive immunity is based on a cellular, T-lymphocyte sensitization. Passive immunity is of short duration, lasting from days to months (Benenson, 1995; Merrill & Timmreck, 2006).

**Herd immunity** is the resistance of a population or group to the invasion and spread of an infectious agent (Benenson, 1995; Merrill & Timmreck, 2006). Herd immunity is based on the level of resistance a population has to a communicable disease because of the high proportion of group members in the population who cannot get the disease because they have been previously vaccinated or have previously had the disease. Jonas Salk, one of the developers of the polio vaccine, suggested that if 85% of the population were immunized against polio (the herd immunity level), a polio epidemic would not occur (Timmreck, 1998). Herd immunity provides barriers to the direct transmission of infection through a group or population because the lack of susceptible individuals in the population stops the spread of infection.

## Communicable Disease Prevention

One of the foundations of public health is the prevention and control of communicable disease. Timmreck (1998) states that the three key factors in the control of communicable disease are as follows:

1. The removal, elimination, or containment of the cause or source of infection
2. The disruption and blockage of the chain of disease transmission
3. The protection of the susceptible population from infection and disease

Approaches to the control of communicable disease should be based on the levels of prevention—primary, secondary, and tertiary.

### ■ Primary Prevention

Primary prevention activities are targeted at intervening before the agent enters the host and causes pathological changes. This level of prevention attempts to increase the host's resistance, inactivate the agent (source of infection), or interrupt the chain of infection.

A major focus of primary prevention is on increasing the resistance of the host. This can be accomplished through health education and/or immunization. Health education

can target many subjects to increase the resistance of the host. It can identify a variety of activities that will improve the host's resistance, such as frequent hand washing, proper nutrition, adequate rest, and proper attire. Immunization is another method of primary prevention that increases the host's resistance. Immunization uses vaccines that are obtained either from the agent in a killed, modified, or variant form or from fractions or products of the agent (Merrill & Timmreck, 2006; Valanis, 1999). Vaccines are available for many common infectious diseases. See Box 19-2 for a list of vaccine-preventable diseases.

Inactivating the agent involves stopping the agent by chemical or physical means. The protection of food has become particularly important in the last few years, with frequent food-borne illness outbreaks occurring as a result of improper storage, preparation, and handling. Proper temperatures must be maintained to inactivate the agent when storing, preparing, and cooking food. Proper food handling, which includes hand washing during preparation, is also important. Many bacterial agents (e.g., staphylococci, salmonellae, and *Escherichia coli*) can contaminate food and make the consumers of the food extremely sick. Irradiation of food (particularly beef and vegetables) has been suggested as a method of control, but this continues to be vigorously debated. Chemical methods are also used to inactivate agents. Chemical methods are used to chlorinate water supplies and to treat sewage, as well as to disinfect infectious or potentially infectious materials.

A common method of breaking the chain of infection is environmental control. Environmental control is aimed at providing clean and safe air, food, milk, and water; managing solid waste (garbage) and liquid waste (sewage); and controlling vectors (insects and rodents). Environmental control may target the reservoir, such as chlorination of a water supply. Environmental control may also be aimed at destroying the vector that transports the agent. One way a community may target the vector is to spray swamp areas (known to serve as reservoirs) with an insecticide to prevent mosquito-borne viral encephalitis. However, when this method is used, care must be taken to preserve the ecosystem as much as possible. Another method of breaking the chain of transmission is to encourage good personal hygiene and use of protective clothing. Methicillin-resistant *S. aureus* (MRSA) is an increasingly difficult nosocomial infection seen on medical and surgical floors in hospitals and in nursing homes. Healthcare providers must protect themselves and their patients by using proper hygiene and standard precautions when caring for all patients.

Primary prevention also includes restricting the spread of infection to human reservoirs and preventing the spread to other susceptible human hosts (Valanis, 1999). The four most commonly used methods are isolation, quarantine, segregation, and personal surveillance.

**Isolation** is the separation of infected persons during the period of communicability (Benenson, 1995; Merrill & Timmreck, 2006; Valanis, 1999). These infected persons may be under one of several different types of isolation (strict isolation, contact isolation, respiratory isolation, tuberculosis isolation, enteric precautions, and drainage/secretion precautions).

**Quarantine** is the restriction of healthy persons who have been exposed to a person with a communicable disease during the period of communicability. These persons are considered contacts of the infected human host. Quarantine prevents further transmission of the disease during the incubation period if the healthy contacts should become infected. Quarantine usually occurs for the longest usual incubation period of the disease. Quarantine is rarely if ever used today; however, before vaccination for diphtheria, it was often used in the United States.

**Segregation** is another method to control the spread of communicable disease. It is used to separate and observe a group of people who are infected with a specific disease. Segregation has been used in some countries to separate HIV-infected individuals from the general public in an effort to control the spread of AIDS. The United States still has public health laws that allow the segregation of persons with TB; however, those laws are rarely enforced, although in the early part of the twentieth century, persons with TB were segregated from the general public in hospitals known as *sanitariums*. With the advent of new drug therapies and treatment, these sanitariums are no longer necessary.

**Personal surveillance** is close medical or other supervision of contacts and identified carriers of a specific disease without restricting their personal movement (Benenson, 1995). For example, public health officials continue to require personal surveillance of persons known to have had TB and to be carriers of typhoid.

As distinct from personal surveillance, disease surveillance is the continuing investigation of all incidence and spread of a disease that are relevant to effective control (Benenson, 1995). Public health surveillance is the systematic collection, analysis, interpretation, dissemination, and use of health information. Surveillance and data systems provide information on morbidity, mortality, and disability. Surveillance information is used to plan, implement, and evaluate public health programs to control communicable disease. To provide maximum benefits, surveillance data must be accurate, timely, and available in useful form (DHHS, 1991; Merrill & Timmreck, 2006).

Although successful disease surveillance involves collaboration among federal, state, and local agencies, the U.S. Public Health Service (PHS) takes a leading role. PHS activities include collecting and analyzing health information at the national, regional, and when possible, state and local levels; providing data to federal, state, and local agencies for further analysis or use; assisting states and local agencies in conducting public health surveillance and evaluating data; and coordinating a network of federal, state, and local public health surveillance for diseases of public health importance (DHHS, 1991). Since 1961, the CDC has been collecting and publishing data on nationally reportable diseases. While reporting of communicable diseases at the national level is voluntary, reporting communicable diseases at the state level is required. Each state health department determines which diseases are reportable in order to address state-specific issues (Merrill & Timmreck, 2006). Infectious diseases that are currently reported by most states are presented in Table 19-2. State health departments require physicians, dentists, nurses, allied health practitioners, and medical examiners to report any disease listed as reportable by their specific state. Some states may require that any reportable diseases also be reported by laboratory directors and administrators of hospitals, clinics, nursing homes, schools, and nurseries.

## ■ Secondary Prevention

Secondary prevention activities are targeted at detecting disease at the earliest possible time to begin treatment, stop progression, and initiate primary prevention activities to protect others in the community (Merrill & Timmreck, 2006). Secondary prevention in infectious disease contributes to primary prevention because it restricts the infection to the human reservoir and prevents its spread to other susceptible individuals. Case finding and health screening are common activities used to accomplish this task. An example of case finding is following up on food handlers who may be infected during an outbreak of hepatitis. Screening for new cases of diseases can significantly decrease the spread of infection. Examples include screening for TB, through tuberculin testing, to detect and treat cases of TB among new immigrants; screening for herpes simplex virus type 2 in pregnant women to prevent infection of the infant during

 **GLOBAL CONNECTION**

An influenza pandemic of the type that ravaged the globe in 1918 and 1919 could kill as many as 62 million people today, with 96% of the deaths occurring in developing countries, according to the World Health Organization. The illness caused by the 1918 virus was largely untreatable. There were no antiviral drugs, no mechanical ventilators to help people breathe, and no antibiotics to treat bacterial pneumonias that often set in after the viral infection. All are available now and would reduce the death toll, although some interventions would be in short supply during a pandemic.

Historical accounts suggest that what became known as Spanish flu emerged at an Army camp in Kansas in early March 1918 and was carried to Europe by American troops. The infection circulated in Europe before undergoing a change early the next fall that made it unusually lethal. It spread around the world and was brought back to the United States, where it killed hundreds of thousands of Americans in October and November 1919. The disease continued to circulate until early 1920, with virtually everyone on Earth eventually being exposed to the virus.

The global death toll from the pandemic is unknown, though rough estimates put mortality in the range of 50 to 100 million.

*Sources*: Barry, J. (2004). *The great influenza: The epic story of the 1918 pandemic*. New York: Viking Publications; *Influenza 1918*. (1998). PBS film series: The American experience. Retrieved August 21, 2008 from http://www.pbs.org/wgbh/amex/influenza/

| Table 19-2 | Nationally Notifiable Infectious Diseases in the United States, 2005 | | |
|---|---|---|---|
| Acquired immunodeficiency syndrome (AIDS) | HIV infection | | Streptococcal disease, invasive, Group A |
| Anthrax | Influenza-associated pediatric mortality | | Streptococcal toxic shock syndrome |
| Arboviral neuroinvasive and nonneuroinvasive diseases | Legionellosis | | *Streptococcus pneumoniae,* drug resistant, invasive disease |
| Botulism (food-borne infant, wound, and unspecified) | Listeriosis | | *S. pneumoniae,* invasive in children younger than 5 years |
| Brucellosis | Lyme disease | | Syphilis, primary and secondary |
| Chancroid | Malaria | | Syphilis, congenital |
| *Chlamydia trachomatis,* genital infections | Measles | | Tetanus |
| Cholera | Meningococcal disease | | Toxic shock syndrome |
| Coccidioidomycosis | Mumps | | Trichinellosis (trichinosis) |
| Cryptosporidiosis | Pertussis | | Tuberculosis |
| Cyclosporiasis | Plague | | Tularemia |
| Diphtheria | Poliomyelitis, paralytic | | Typhoid fever |
| Ehrlichiosis | Psittacosis | | Vancomycin-intermediate *S. aureus* |
| *Escherichia coli* infections | Q fever | | Vancomycin-resistant *S. aureus* |
| Giardiasis | Rabies | | Varicella (morbidity) |
| Gonorrhea | Rocky Mountain spotted fever | | Varicella (deaths only) |
| *Haemophilus influenzae* invasive disease | Rubella | | Yellow fever |
| Hansen's disease (leprosy) | Rubella, congenital syndrome | | |
| Hantavirus pulmonary syndrome | Salmonellosis | | |
| Hemolytic uremic syndrome, post-diarrheal | Severe acute respiratory syndrome-associated coronavirus (SARS-CoV) disease | | |
| Hepatitis, viral, acute | Shigellosis | | |
| Hepatitis, viral, chronic | Smallpox | | |

*Source:* Merrill, R. M., & Timmreck, T. C. (2006). *Introduction to epidemiology* (4th ed). Sudbury, MA: Jones and Bartlett.

Nurses and physician administering Salk polio vaccine to a child (circa 1955).

the birth process; screening for venereal diseases as a requirement for marriage licenses in some states; and administering gamma-globulin or immune serum after exposure to hepatitis.

Health education also plays a significant role in secondary prevention because it provides education about signs and symptoms, which enables individuals to identify illness and seek care early. Knowledge of health risk behaviors that contribute to the spread of disease may influence infected individuals to modify their behavior and thus assist in the prevention of the spread of disease.

## Tertiary Prevention

Tertiary prevention limits the progression of disability (Merrill & Timmreck, 2006; Timmreck, 1998). Hearing impairment from frequent ear infections, paralyzed limbs from polio, impaired vision from severe conjunctivitis, and shingles are just a few of the possible disabilities resulting from infectious disease. Treatment of symptoms and rehabilitation vary with each specific disease.

## Control of Diseases

### Vaccine-Preventable Diseases

Immunization is one of the most accepted and cost-effective preventive health practices in the United States. In the last 50 years, vaccines have prevented countless days of illness and hundreds of thousands of deaths. Most healthcare providers take for granted the rarity of vaccine-preventable diseases; many healthcare providers will never see a child with diphtheria, measles, or polio. Childhood immunization needs and practices are discussed in Chapter 34. Therefore, this chapter focuses on the vaccine-preventable diseases of adults and the need for adults to be immunized against them.

Adult immunization is extremely important. Each year in the United States alone, at least 45,000 adults die from complications resulting from influenza, pneumonia, or hepatitis B, despite the availability of safe and effective vaccines to prevent these diseases. In 2002, only 56% of adults in the

## SABIN ORAL SUNDAY
### POLIO PREVENTION PROGRAM
This Certifies That

*Ruth Saucier*

(NAME)

HAS RECEIVED SABIN ORAL POLIO VACCINE TYPE:

(1)     (3)     (2)

BRING THIS CARD FOR NEXT IMMUNIZATION. AFTER THIRD IMMUNIZATION, GIVE CARD TO YOUR FAMILY DOCTOR.

## SABIN ORAL SUNDAY
### POLIO PREVENTION PROGRAM
This Certifies That

*Marshall Saucier*

(NAME)

HAS RECEIVED SABIN ORAL POLIO VACCINE TYPE:

(1)     (3)     (2)

BRING THIS CARD FOR NEXT IMMUNIZATION. AFTER THIRD IMMUNIZATION, GIVE CARD TO YOUR FAMILY DOCTOR.

Vaccination cards from polio prevention program (circa 1956).

United States were immunized, compared to 75% of children (PreventionInfo.org, 2004).

### Hepatitis

Viral hepatitis encompasses several distinct infections. All are hepatatrophic and have similar clinical presentations. However, they differ in their cause and in some clinical, pathological, immunological, and epidemiological characteristics. Their prevention and control also vary (Benenson, 1995; Heymann, 2004).

### Hepatitis A

Hepatitis A is a highly contagious viral infection of the liver. Since 1990, an average of 27,000 cases annually have been reported in the United States (Atkinson &

## " a conversation with . . . "

As informed providers, nurses are in a unique position to educate health planners, legislators, and community leaders about immunizations and preventive care. Nurses can serve as advocates for immunizations personally and through professional organizations.

At a time when costs are skyrocketing, it is encouraging to know how much can be accomplished with relatively low-cost prevention. Nurses need to be in the forefront to inform our citizens about health promotion and prevention activities as important aspects of personal health care.

—**Hillary Rodham Clinton** (1993)

Wolfe, 2003). Hepatitis A is the most common vaccine-preventable disease in travelers (National Foundation for Infectious Diseases, 2002b). The hepatitis A virus (HAV) is found in the stool of infected people. The mode of transmission is person to person by the fecal–oral route. The infection is passed on by infected persons who do not wash their hands after having a bowel movement and contaminate everything they touch. Outbreaks have been related to contaminated water and to food prepared by food handlers who are infected with the hepatitis A virus. People are also infected with hepatitis A by eating contaminated raw shellfish, fruits, or vegetables (Heymann, 2004).

People at risk for being infected with hepatitis A include the following individuals (*Hepatitis learning guide,* 1998):

- Those who share a household with someone who is infected with hepatitis A
- Individuals in a daycare center (adult employees or children) where a child or employee is infected with hepatitis A
- Those who travel to countries such as Africa, Asia (other than Japan), the Caribbean, Central and South America, Eastern Europe, the Mediterranean basin, and the Middle East
- Residents or staff of custodial institutions
- Men who have sex with men (MSM)

The symptoms of hepatitis A differ from person to person. Although many people infected with hepatitis A have no symptoms (particularly children), those with symptoms usually have an identifiable pattern. These symptoms include fever, nausea, vomiting, jaundice, diarrhea, fatigue, abdominal pain, dark urine, and loss of appetite. Respiratory symptoms, joint pain, and rash occasionally occur (CDC, 2004a; *Facts about hepatitis A for adults*, 1996).

The incubation period is from 15 to 50 days, with the average time being approximately 28 days. The period of infectivity is during the last half of the incubation period, up to and including a few days after the onset of jaundice (Benenson, 1995; Heymann, 2004).

Hepatitis A is prevented through the following means (Benenson, 1995; Heymann, 2004):

- Vaccination with the hepatitis A vaccine (with an initial injection providing protection for up to 1 year, with a booster dose [6 to 12 months after the first dose] providing prolonged protection)
- Education of the public about good sanitation and proper hygiene, with careful emphasis on hand washing
- Proper water and sewage treatment
- Education of employees in child daycare centers about the need for thorough hand washing after every diaper change and before feeding children or eating
- Immunization of child daycare employees
- Cooking shellfish to the proper temperature (85–90°C, or 185–190°F)
- Immunization with the hepatitis A vaccine of all travelers going to developing countries

## Hepatitis B

Hepatitis B is also a highly contagious virus that infects the liver. It is caused by the hepatitis B virus (HBV), which infects approximately 300,000 Americans annually. In the United States, more than 1 million people are chronically infected with HBV. Globally, there are an estimated 350 million chronic HBV carriers (*Hepatitis learning guide,* 1998). The World Health Organization estimates that more than 2 billion people have been infected with HBV worldwide. Each year about 1 million people die from HBV and more than 4 million new cases occur (Heymann, 2004).

The virus is found in the blood and body fluids of infected people. All persons who test positive for the hepatitis B antigen are potentially infectious. The mode of transmission can be person to person through sexual contact as well as through direct contact with blood or blood products resulting from sharing of needles or razors and from infected mother to infant during the birthing process. Hepatitis B is often described as a silent disease because it infects many people without making them feel ill. Infants are usually asymptomatic, and small children usually have a milder case of the disease. When symptoms do occur, the infected person will often complain of flulike symptoms, with loss of appetite, nausea and vomiting, stomach cramps, and extreme fatigue, which may progress to jaundice. Hepatitis B can progress to fulminating hepatic necrosis and death (Atkinson & Wolfe, 2003; CDC, 2004b; Heymann, 2004).

The incubation period for hepatitis B is 45 to 180 days, with an average of 60 to 90 days. This disease occurs worldwide with little seasonal variation. Hepatitis B is prevented by the hepatitis B vaccine, which consists of a series of three intramuscular (IM) injections of the hepatitis B vaccine over 6 months. This vaccine is used to protect everyone, from newborn infants to older adults (National Foundation for Infectious Diseases, 2002c; Heymann, 2004).

## Hepatitis C

Hepatitis C is also a viral infection of the liver. It has been referred to as *parenterally transmitted hepatitis,* and before blood donor screening, it was the most common cause of post-transfusion hepatitis worldwide. Ninety percent of hepatitis C occurrence in Japan, the United States, and Western Europe is a result of exposure to blood or other body fluids (*Hepatitis C,* 1997).

Hepatitis C virus (HCV) is found worldwide. The World Health Organization (WHO) estimates that up to 3% of the world's population is infected with HCV (*Hepatitis learning guide,* 1998; Heymann, 2004). In the United States, hepatitis C has infected an estimated 3.9 million people (1.8% of the U.S. population). Its occurrence is highest in IV drug users and hemophilia patients; moderate in hemodialysis patients; low in heterosexuals with multiple partners, homosexual men, healthcare workers, and family members of HCV patients; and lowest in volunteer blood donors (Benenson, 1995; CDC, 2004c). The reservoir for the virus is in humans. The mode of transmission is indirect, spread through contaminated needles and syringes; however, this accounts for fewer than 50% of the infected cases in the United States. Transmission rates through household contact and sexual activity appear to be low, and perinatal transmission is uncommon. The route of transmission cannot be identified in more than 40% of infected patients (Benenson, 1995).

The incubation period of hepatitis C is from 2 weeks to 6 months, with most cases occurring within 6 to 9 weeks after infection. Most infected individuals with hepatitis C are asymptomatic (up to 90%); this includes even those with chronic disease (*Hepatitis C,* 1997; Heymann, 2004). The most common symptoms are fatigue, nausea, vague abdominal discomfort, and jaundice. Severity ranges from inapparent cases (approximately 75%) to rare fulminating, fatal cases (Benenson, 1995).

Ribavirin has been shown to be somewhat effective as an antiviral agent against hepatitis C when used in combination with interferon (*Hepatitis C,* 1997; Heymann, 2004).

Prevention measures for hepatitis C include the following (CDC, 2004c; *Hepatitis C,* 1997; *Hepatitis learning guide,* 1998):

- Universal screening of blood and blood products
- Effective use of standard precautions and barrier techniques
- Sterilization of reusable equipment and destruction of disposable equipment
- Public health education regarding the risks of using unsterilized equipment

Because there is no vaccine against hepatitis C, prevention is the primary strategy against the virus.

## Hepatitis D

Hepatitis D virus (HDV) is a defective, single-stranded RNA virus that requires the helper function of HBV to replicate. HDV is found worldwide, but its prevalence varies. Because it requires the HBV to replicate and to infect cells, it occurs either epidemically or endemically in populations with high rates of HBV infection (Benenson, 1995; Heymann, 2004). Places where HDV is found to be endemic are Africa, southern Italy, Romania, parts of Russia, and South America. Populations that have high rates of hepatitis D include hemophiliacs, drug addicts, people with frequent blood exposures, residents in homes for the developmentally disabled, and male homosexuals.

Humans serve as the reservoir for hepatitis D. The modes of transmission are similar to those of hepatitis B, with direct contact with blood or blood products the most efficient. Sexual transmission is less efficient than that of hepatitis B, and perinatal transmission is rare.

The onset of hepatitis D is usually abrupt, with signs and symptoms similar to those of hepatitis B. Hepatitis D varies from being self-limiting to progressing to chronic hepatitis. It can be acquired either as a co-infection with hepatitis B or as a superinfection in persons with chronic HBV infection (CDC, 2004d). When it is acquired as a co-infection, the person has a greater risk of severe acute disease, with a 2% to 20% chance of fulminant hepatitis. Chronic HBV carriers who acquire hepatitis D as a superinfection have a greater chance of developing chronic HDV infection. The superinfection with HDV has been found to increase the development of chronic liver disease with cirrhosis 70% to 80% compared with 15% to 30% of patients with HBV alone (*Hepatitis learning guide,* 1998).

The incubation period is approximately 2 to 8 weeks. Peak infectivity is thought to occur just before the onset of the illness. Symptoms are similar to those of hepatitis B and are identified as joint pain, abdominal pain, loss of appetite, nausea and vomiting, fatigue, and jaundice. No vaccine exists for HDV. The method of control is immunization with the hepatitis B vaccine; however, this is effective only in persons who are not already infected with HBV. For those infected with HBV, avoidance of any possible exposure to HDV is the only preventive measure (*Hepatitis learning guide,* 1998; Heymann, 2004).

### Hepatitis E

Hepatitis E is similar to hepatitis A in that there is no evidence of a chronic form. The fatality rate for hepatitis E is also similar to that of hepatitis A, except in pregnant women during the third trimester, when the fatality rate may reach 20%. Hepatitis E virus (HEV) is transmitted by the fecal–oral route. Contaminated water from feces of infected humans is the most commonly documented vehicle of transmission. Person-to-person transmission (seen in hepatitis A) does not appear to be a mode of transmission in hepatitis E, because secondary household cases are not common during outbreaks. The attack rate is highest in young adults; cases are uncommon in children and the elderly (Benenson, 1995; CDC, 2004e).

The reservoir is human beings, although an animal reservoir is possible. In the United States, as well as in most other industrialized countries, hepatitis E cases have been documented only among travelers returning from HEV-endemic areas (Benenson, 1995). HEV is endemic in Mexico, Central America, Asia, North Africa, the Middle East, and a few sub-Saharan African countries along the western coast (*Hepatitis learning guide,* 1998).

The incubation period is 15 to 64 days, with the mean incubation period ranging between 26 and 42 days (Benenson, 1995; Heymann, 2004). Symptoms of hepatitis E include loss of appetite, nausea and vomiting, fever, fatigue, and abdominal pain. Many people who contract HEV have no symptoms. Prevention of hepatitis E relies primarily on the provision of clean water. Hygiene practice must be strict among travelers to prevent contracting hepatitis E when traveling in developing countries, such as avoiding drinking water and beverages with ice, uncooked shellfish, and uncooked fruits and vegetables (CDC, 2004e; *Hepatitis learning guide,* 1998). There is no vaccine and no identified treatment at this time; thus, prevention is very important.

### Influenza

Influenza is another vaccine-preventable disease important in adults. "The flu" is an extremely contagious viral infection of the nose, throat, and lungs. In temperate zones, epidemics occur in the winter season, and in tropical zones, they occur during the rainy season. Influenza derives its importance from the rapidity with which epidemics occur, the high morbidity rate, and the severity of the complications that result from the infection. Annual influenza epidemics account for 3 to 5 million cases of severe illness and 250,000 to 500,000 deaths worldwide each year (InfluenZone, 2005). During major epidemics, the most severe illnesses and deaths occur in the elderly population and in those with debilitating diseases.

In fact, influenza deaths in the United States increased substantially in the last two decades partly because of the general aging of the population (Thompson et al., 2003). On average, 114,000 people are hospitalized and 36,000

**Application to Practice**
You are a nurse in a neighborhood-based clinic. In October, Mrs. Clark, a 75-year-old woman, comes into the clinic for her regular yearly physical examination. Mrs. Clark is in good health overall, with relatively few minor complaints. Last year, as part of her yearly visit, Mrs. Clark had been given an influenza vaccination. During this visit, however, Mrs. Clark tells you that she does not need to be vaccinated against influenza because she had gotten her "flu shot" last year. She also said, "I don't want the flu shot this year because I know somebody who got sick from it. I don't want to get sick."

1. Should you convince Mrs. Clark to get the influenza vaccination this year? Why or why not?
2. What other vaccines should you consider offering to Mrs. Clark?
3. What are the patient education considerations for Mrs. Clark? ◯

deaths occur from influenza annually in the United States (Goldrick, 2004).

There are three types of influenza viruses: A, B, and C. Type A, associated with widespread epidemics and pandemics, causes moderate to severe illness and affects all age groups; type B, associated with regional or widespread epidemics, generally causes milder disease than type A and primarily affects children; and type C, associated with sporadic and minor localized outbreaks, is rare and has not been associated with epidemic disease (Atkinson & Wolfe, 2003; Benenson, 1995). Occurrence is worldwide. The United States has an epidemic almost every year with type A, type B, or sometimes with both A and B.

Influenza symptoms are fever, myalgia, headache, sore throat, dry cough, and some gastrointestinal symptoms, such as nausea, vomiting, and diarrhea. Humans are the primary reservoir, with swine and avian reservoirs as likely breeding grounds for new strains. Avian influenza is discussed further under zoonoses on page 440. The mode of transmission is airborne, which is aerosolized or droplet material from the respiratory tract. The incubation period is very short, ranging from 1 to 3 days. People are infectious from 1 to 2 days before onset of symptoms to 4 to 5 days after onset (CDC, 1995; Heymann, 2004).

Most cases of influenza are preventable through a vaccine. Because the virus changes from year to year, it is necessary to be vaccinated yearly. The following people should receive a yearly vaccine: people 65 years and older, people with chronic disease (cardiac and/or respiratory), people who are immunocompromised, pregnant women who will be in their second or third trimester during the flu season, residents in long-term care facilities, healthcare workers, and adolescents receiving long-term aspirin therapy (who are at risk for Reye's syndrome) (National Foundation for Infectious Disease, 2002d).

---

### GLOBAL CONNECTION

Although clean water is taken for granted in the United States, most of the world's population does not have access to sanitary water. This poses a formidable challenge in the control of water-borne diseases—especially dysentery, which is a major cause of high morbidity and mortality rates throughout the world.

### Pneumococcal Disease

Pneumococcal disease is an acute bacterial infection. It is characterized by a rapid onset with shaking chills, fever, pleural pain, a productive cough, dyspnea, tachycardia, anorexia, malaise, and extreme weakness. Its onset is not as rapid in the elderly, and the first evidence is usually by x-ray examination. In infants and young children, the onset may be characterized by fever, vomiting, and convulsions. Pneumococcal disease is most severe in infants and elders, with higher death rates in both groups. The mortality rate is 5% to 10% with antibiotic therapy but can be as high as 60% for infants in developing countries where antibiotics are unavailable. The infectious agent is *Streptococcus pneumoniae* (pneumococcus). Its occurrence is worldwide, with peaks in the winter and early spring in temperate zones. However, it occurs in all climates and in all seasons (Benenson, 1995; Heymann, 2004).

The reservoir for pneumococcal disease is humans, and pneumoncocci are often found in the lungs of healthy people worldwide. The mode of transmission is airborne through droplets spread either by direct transfer or by indirect transfer when droplets have recently contaminated articles of clothes or bedding with discharge from the respiratory track. Person-to-person transmission is common. The incubation period may be as short as 1 to 3 days.

Pneumococcal disease can be prevented in children and adults through vaccination with polyvalent vaccine. One immunization lasts most adults a lifetime against almost all the bacteria that cause pneumococcal disease. The following adults should be vaccinated: people 65 and older, because risk of infection and fatality rates increase with age; people with chronic diseases; people who are immunosuppressed; and residents of long-term care facilities.

### ■ Routine Vaccines Indicated for Adults

All adults should be protected against many of the same diseases as adolescents and children. The tetanus and diphtheria (Td) vaccine should be given to all adults (Table 19-3). It is important for adults to be immunized against diphtheria and tetanus because 1 of every 10 people who get diphtheria will die from it (Heymann, 2004), and 40 to 60 cases of tetanus occur each year, resulting in at least 10 deaths. Almost all reported cases of tetanus occur in people who are inadequately immunized (Atkinson & Wolfe, 2003).

Adults born before 1957 do not usually require the measles, mumps, and rubella vaccine because most of these adults have acquired immunity as a result of having the diseases during childhood. However, all adults born after 1957 should be immunized (see Table 19-3). Women of childbearing age should be given the rubella vaccine unless they have documentation of immunization after their first birthday. Currently, approximately 12 million women of childbearing age are susceptible to rubella. If rubella occurs during pregnancy, severe birth defects, miscarriages, and still-births can result (Atkinson & Wolfe, 2003; National Foundation for Infectious Diseases, 2002a). Although laboratory evidence of rubella immunity is acceptable, a stated previous history of rubella is unreliable and should not be accepted as proof of immunity. Before giving rubella immunization, the nurse should determine the likelihood of pregnancy during the next 3 months. The nurse should discuss with the woman her plans for reliable birth control during the following 3 months. Although there is no evidence that the rubella vaccine or other live viruses cause birth defects, the possibility exists. Thus, healthcare providers should not give any live vaccine to women known to be pregnant (Atkinson & Wolfe, 2003).

**Table 19-3    Recommended Adult Immunization Schedule, by Vaccine and Age Group**

| Vaccine ▼    Age Group ▶ | 19–49 Years | 50–64 Years | ≥65 Years |
|---|---|---|---|
| Tetanus, diptheria, pertussis (Td/Tdap) | One-dose Td booster every 10 years / Substitute one dose of Tdap for Td | | |
| Human papillomavirus (HPV) | Three doses (females) | | |
| Measles, mumps, rubella (MMR) | One or two doses | | One dose |
| Varicella | Two doses (0, 4–8 weeks) | Two doses (0, 4–8 weeks) | |
| Influenza | One dose annually | One dose annually | |
| Pneumococcal (polysaccharide) | One to two doses | | One dose |
| Hepatitis A | Two doses (0, 6–12 months, or 0, 6–18 months) | | |
| Hepatitis B | Three doses (0, 1–2, 4–6 months) | | |
| Meningococcal | One or more doses | | |

All adults without a reliable history of varicella disease (chickenpox) should receive the varicella vaccine. Adults who are either at highest risk for susceptibility or at high risk for exposing people to varicella should be targeted for varicella immunization (see Table 19-3). These adults include teachers, college students, military personnel, healthcare workers, and family members of immunocompromised persons. Although varicella is not considered a serious disease of childhood, adults are 25 times more likely to die from the disease. Adolescents and adults who develop varicella are 10 times more likely to require hospitalization and/or develop pneumonia, bacterial infections, and encephalitis (Atkinson & Wolfe, 2003; *Facts about adult immunizations,* 1997).

### Got an Alternative?

Many complementary health practices, such as yoga and meditation, can reduce stress and anxiety, thereby enhancing the immune system and reducing the risk of contracting an infectious disease.

Mississippi nurses discuss immunization rates in their state with Captain Joyce Goff, RN (U.S. Public Health Service), Nurse Epidemiologist, at the Centers for Disease Control and Prevention, Atlanta.

## Emerging and Reemerging Infectious Diseases

Infectious diseases continue to be a problem for all people, regardless of age, gender, lifestyle, ethnicity, or socioeconomic status. New and mutated infectious diseases that have the potential to cause suffering and death and impose an enormous financial burden on individuals and society are always emerging. Two examples occurred in 1997, when a new strain of influenza that had never been seen in humans began to kill previously healthy people in Hong Kong and strains of *S. aureus* with diminished susceptibility to vancomycin were reported in both Japan and the United States. If scientists cannot replace antibiotics that are losing their effectiveness, some diseases may become untreatable, as they were in the pre-antibiotic era (CDC, 1998).

**❝** *Everybody knows that pestilences have a way of recurring in the world; yet somehow we find it hard to believe in ones that crash down on our heads from a blue sky.* **❞**

—*Albert Camus, 1948, The Plague*

Emerging infectious diseases are diseases that have appeared for the first time or that have occurred before but are appearing in populations where they had not previously been reported. Reemerging infectious diseases are familiar diseases caused by well-understood organisms that were once under control or declining but are now resistant to common antimicrobial drugs or are gaining new footholds in the population and increasing in incidence (AAWH, 1997; Dzenowagis, 1997).

Concern about emerging and reemerging infectious diseases prompted a 1992 report issued by the Institute of Medicine (IOM) of the National Academy of Sciences. The report, *Emerging Infections: Microbial Threats to Health in the United States,* concluded that emerging and reemerging infectious diseases are a major threat to the health of Americans and challenged the U.S. government to take action. The IOM report (1992) defined emerging or reemerging infectious diseases as those diseases whose incidence had increased within the last two decades of the twentieth century or threatened to increase in the near future. Modern conditions that favor the spread of disease are listed in the Environmental Connection on the following page.

## ENVIRONMENTAL CONNECTION

### Modern Demographic and Environmental Conditions That Favor the Spread of Infectious Diseases

- Global travel
- Globalization of the food supply and centralized processing of food
- Population growth and increased urbanization and over-crowding
- Migration due to wars, famines, and other artificial or natural disasters
- Irrigation, deforestation, and reforestation projects that alter the habitats of disease-carrying insects and animals
- Human behaviors, such as intravenous drug use and risky sexual behavior
- Increased use of antimicrobial agents and pesticides, hastening the development of resistance
- Increased human contact with tropical rain forests and other wilderness habitats that are reservoirs for insects and animals that harbor unknown infectious agents

*Source:* CDC, 1998.

 THINK ABOUT THIS

Don't get sick on cruise ships: Protect yourself. Over the past couple of years, outbreaks of gastroenteritis or Norwalk-like viruses have afflicted hundreds of people, especially aboard cruise ships where confined living conditions allow the virus to spread rapidly.

Whether you're at home or traveling, you can fend off the Norwalk virus with these tips offered by the Johns Hopkins University *Health After 50* medical letter:

- Wash your hands frequently with soap and water, particularly before and after meals, and keep your hands away from your face and mouth.
- Every so often, use alcohol-based hand sanitizers.
- Don't share eating utensils or drinking glasses.
- Avoid eating uncooked food.
- If you're traveling, drink only bottled water.
- If you're planning a trip and are older than 65 or have a weakened immune system, your healthcare provider can suggest additional precautions.

*I think the weakest point in the United States is our false security that there will be no problems . . . we still have this feeling in the United States that we don't need to worry, that it's someone else's problem . . . but these diseases don't respect barriers. They don't respect borders.*

—Dr. David Heymann, Director of the Office of Emerging Infectious Diseases at the World Health Organization, 1997

As a result of the IOM report, in 1994 the Centers for Disease Control and Prevention (CDC) and other healthcare groups launched a national effort to support public health efforts to control the negative impact of infectious diseases.

*a conversation with . . .*

With all our experience, we have not gone far on the road to eradicating disease. This knowledge keeps us humble. We have trouble out-thinking a virus. Even smallpox humbled us until the very end. That virus seemed to have a better understanding of nature, human behavior, and ways to achieve immortality than the entire smallpox eradication team. The emergence and reemergence of infections must be approached with humility.

**—William Foege, MD,**
former director of the CDC and the
Carter Center, Emory University, Atlanta

As funds became available the CDC, in partnership with the IOM, state and local health departments, medical and public health professional associations, and international organizations, implemented a plan titled "Addressing Emerging Infectious Disease Threats: A Prevention Strategy for the United States." The four major goals of the plan and the implications for nursing are described in Table 19-4.

### ■ Health Care–Associated Infections

Health care–associated infections (HAIs), also known as nosocomial infections, are acquired by patients while being treated for other conditions in a healthcare setting. According to the CDC, an estimated 2 million HAIs occur annually, resulting in 90,000 deaths. The number of HAIs is steadily increasing with a financial burden of $4.5 billion per year (Kestel, 2006).

*Staphylococcus aureus,* often referred to as "staph," is one of the leading causes of nosocomial (hospital-acquired) infections and is the most common cause of skin infections in the United States. Most of these skin infections are minor and can often be treated without antibiotics. Staph bacteria are commonly carried on the skin or in the noses of healthy people. At any given time 25–30% of the population can be colonized with *Staphylococcus aureus* without showing any signs of illness. However, staph bacteria can also cause severe illness (such as surgical wound infections, bloodstream infections, catheter-associated urinary tract infections, and pneumonia) in people who have weakened immune systems (CDC, 2007h).

#### MRSA

Methicillin-resistant *Staphylococcus aureus* (MRSA) is a type of staph that is resistant to antibiotics called beta-lactam, which include methicillin and other more common antibiotics such as oxacillin, penicillin, and amoxicillin. Over the years the number of staph infections caused by MRSA has grown steadily from 2% in 1974 to 63% in 2004 (CDC, 2007h) making it one of the most common nosocomial infections. Vancomycin has been successful in treating MRSA

**Table 19-4** Goals of CDC Plan Outlined in *Addressing Emerging Infectious Disease Threats: A Prevention Strategy for the United States*

| Goals of CDC Plan (CDC, 1994) | Rule of Nurses in CDC Plan (Cohen & Larson, 1996) |
| --- | --- |
| **GOAL I SURVEILLANCE**<br>Detect, promptly investigate, and monitor emerging pathogens, the diseases they cause, and the factors influencing their emergence. | **GOAL I SURVEILLANCE**<br>Support, explain, and circulate to the nursing community any recommendations made by CDC and partner agencies focusing on the implications for nursing. |
| **GOAL II APPLIED RESEARCH**<br>Integrate laboratory science and epidemiology to optimize public health practice. | **GOAL II APPLIED RESEARCH**<br>Promote a population-based, epidemiological, systems approach for nursing practice and research. |
| **GOAL III PREVENTION AND CONTROL**<br>Enhance communication of public health information about emerging diseases and ensure prompt implementation of prevention strategies. | **GOAL III PREVENTION AND CONTROL**<br>1. Collaborate with other professions and policy-making groups to support, endorse, and evaluate global strategies to prevent or reduce the threat of emerging infectious diseases.<br>2. Communicate with other nursing groups and recommend that they develop and disseminate policies and standards to prevent the spread of emerging infections.<br>3. Identify mechanisms to promote the appropriate prescription and use of antibiotics.<br>4. Address strategies to enhance host resistance and immunity.<br>5. Take a leadership role in initiatives to promote preventive strategies.<br>6. Take an active role in promoting science education for students in grades K through 12. |
| **GOAL IV INFRASTRUCTURE**<br>Strengthen local, state, and federal public health infrastructures to support surveillance and implement prevention and control programs. | **GOAL IV INFRASTRUCTURE**<br>Serve as a clear voice to policy makers for support of public health, public education, public health infrastructure, and policies that protect the environment and promote ecological balance. |

until the last few years, in which eight cases of vancomycin-intermediate Staph aureus (VISA) with partial resistance to vancomycin and three cases of vancomycin-resistant Staph aureus (VRSA) have been reported. Before the advent of antibiotics, *Staphylococcus aureus* infections were often fatal. Healthcare providers are concerned that increasing antibiotic resistance may again make staph a leading cause of death (Todd, 2006).

Until the late 1990s, MRSA was confined to patients with weakened immune systems who were being treated for other illnesses in hospitals or other healthcare settings. A new form of MRSA, known as community-acquired MRSA, began occurring in otherwise healthy people in the community (CDC, 2007h; Krisberg, 2006). Community-acquired MRSA, genetically different from hospital-acquired MRSA, accounts for about 10% of all MRSA infections and is still treatable with a variety of antibiotics, although antibiotic-resistant strains are being identified (Gorwitz et al., 2006). While most community-acquired MRSA infections are mild, severe invasive conditions such as necrotizing pneumonia and empyema, osteomyelitis, and necrotizing fasciitis have occurred (Gorwitz et al., 2006; Krisberg, 2006). Community-acquired MRSA has been reported in a variety of populations groups and environmental settings. Its genetic distinction indicates that the organism is mutating and evolving rapidly (Krisberg, 2006), which may make it more virulent, more able to affect people with healthy immune systems, and more easily transmitted (CDC, 2007h).

Primary prevention is the best form of defense against all forms of MRSA. Good handwashing is critical in both hospital and community settings. As always, nurses in all healthcare settings should use standard precautions when exposed to any open skin lesions or wounds. People in the community with skin infections need to be monitored for MRSA and all community members should be informed of the potential risk for MRSA and taught proper handwashing techniques and good general hygiene (CDC, 2007h).

## ■ Food-Borne Diseases

Infections caused by food-borne parasites or viruses are common. Each year in the United States, 76 million people get sick from food-borne diseases and more than 5,000 of them die. In recent years, food-borne illness has become one of the fastest growing threats to community health in the United States (Foodborne illness, 1998; Hoffman et al., 2005; Mahon et al., 1999; NAS, 2005). Much of the reason for this is that enormous quantities of food are being produced in central locations and then being widely distributed to all parts of the country (Mahon et al., 1999). There have also been sharp increases in the number and types of food being imported from other countries (NAS, 2005). In response to these factors, the National Food Safety Initiative (NFSI) was created in 1997 to improve the safety of the nation's food supply (CDC, 1998; "Foodborne illness," 1998). The NFSI ended in 2001, but the CDC has institutionalized its funding and activities as an ongoing food safety program (Hoffman et al., 2005). The health care for people with food-borne illnesses can be very expensive. The yearly cost for food-borne illnesses in the United States is $6.9 billion in medical costs and lost productivity (NAS, 2005).

Foods can serve as a medium for growing bacterial pathogens or as a passive vehicle for transferring parasitic or viral pathogens. Although most food-borne infections are directly related to foods of animal origin such as meat, fish, shellfish, poultry, eggs, and dairy products (Kaferstein & Meslin, 1998), foods of plant origin can also be contaminated. Many food-borne bacterial diseases have emerged or increased during the last two decades. Some of the factors that bring about the multiplication and distribution of these bacteria in food are poor hygienic practices at the animal husbandry, slaughterhouse, and food processing levels as well as poor food preparation practices.

## Prevention

There are three measures of protection against food-borne pathogens (Kaferstein & Meslin, 1998):

1. Prevention of contamination of food
2. Prevention of growth of pathogens
3. Prevention of the spread and survival of pathogens

First, the quality of food at the production level must be improved. The environmental conditions under which food animals are raised and the use of fertilizers and pesticides for food plants must be monitored and controlled.

Second, food processing technology must be improved and used to prevent the survival and spread of food pathogens. Pasteurization, sterilization, and irradiation contribute significantly to food safety by reducing or eliminating disease-causing organisms.

Third, all food handlers must be educated in the principles of safe food preparation. This is probably the most critical line of defense, because most food-borne diseases are a result of one or more of the following (Kaferstein & Meslin, 1998):

- Insufficient cooking of food
- Preparation of food too many hours before it is eaten, along with improper storage
- Use of contaminated raw food
- Cross-contamination where food is prepared
- Food preparation by infected persons

### Nurses' Roles in Prevention

Because many cases of food-borne diseases are a result of mishandling food in the home, community health nurses who visit families in their homes are in an excellent position to provide education for the persons in a family who are responsible for food handling and preparation (Kaferstein & Meslin, 1998). It is important to stress safety in all stages of food handling. This includes: (1) what to look for when purchasing food at the store or market, (2) how to store food in the home, (3) the importance of good handwashing and clean utensils and surfaces for food preparation, and (4) proper cooking techniques (Dols, Bowers, & Copfer, 2001).

School nurses can be successful in reducing the incidence of food-borne infections by educating children in the schools about the concepts of food safety. Educating children is not only an effective way to communicate safe food handling procedures to parents, but also a way to implant the principles of safe food preparation in the minds of future adults (Kaferstein & Meslin, 1998). School nurses should monitor school food programs and educate school food services personnel about proper handling and storage of foods. Educational programs should also be provided for teachers because of the amount of "food treats" that are served in the classrooms, especially in elementary schools.

## Common Food-Borne Diseases in the United States

### Campylobacteriosis

Campylobacteriosis, caused by bacteria of the genus *Campylobacter,* is one of the most common diarrheal diseases in the United States. The symptoms (diarrhea, abdominal pain, fever, nausea, and vomiting) usually develop within 2 to 5 days after exposure and typically last 1 week. Most people infected with *Campylobacter* will recover with no treatment except for drinking plenty of fluids for the diarrhea. However, in more severe cases, an antibiotic such as erythromycin can be used. Most cases of campylobacteriosis are a result of handling or eating raw or undercooked poultry. Most cases occur as isolated, sporadic events, although small outbreaks have been reported. More than 10,000 cases are reported to the CDC each year. However, because many cases are undiagnosed or unreported, campylobacteriosis is estimated to affect more than 2 million people every year (CDC, 2008a; Potter, Kaneene, & Hall, 2003).

### Listeriosis

Listeriosis, caused by the bacterium *Listeria monocytogenes,* has been recognized as a serious public health problem in the United States. The symptoms are fever, muscle aches, and sometimes nausea or diarrhea. If the infection spreads to the nervous system, headache, stiff neck, confusion, loss of balance, or seizures can occur. *L. monocytogenes* is found in a variety of raw food, such as uncooked meats and vegetables, as well as in processed foods that become contaminated after processing. The disease primarily affects pregnant women, newborns, and adults with weakened immune systems. An estimated 2,500 people become ill from listeriosis each year, and 500 of them die. Most deaths occur among immunocompromised and elderly patients. Infected persons are treated with antibiotics. However, even with prompt treatment some infections can result in death (CDC, 2008f).

### Salmonellosis

Salmonellosis, caused by many different kinds of *Salmonella* bacteria, is a diarrheal disease that has been known for more than 100 years. The symptoms (diarrhea, fever, and abdominal cramps) usually develop within 12 to 72 hours after exposure and usually last 4 to 7 days. Salmonellosis usually does not require any treatment, but if the patient becomes severely dehydrated or the infection spreads from the intestines to other body parts, rehydration with IV fluids and antibiotic therapy may be necessary. *Salmonella* can be transmitted to humans by eating foods contaminated with animal feces. Many raw foods of animal origin are frequently contaminated, but fortunately, thorough cooking kills *Salmonella*. Foods may also be contaminated by the unwashed hands of an infected food handler. Approximately 40,000 cases of salmonellosis are reported in the United States each year, but the actual number of cases may be 30 or more times greater (CDC, 2008b).

### *Escherichia coli* O157:H7

*Escherichia coli* O157:H7 is a leading cause of food-borne illness. *E. coli* O157:H7 is one of the hundreds of strains of the bacterium *E. coli*. Most strains of *E. coli* are harmless and live in the intestines of healthy humans and animals, but *E. coli* O157:H7 produces a powerful toxin that can cause severe illness. The combination of letters and numbers in the name refers to specific markers on the surface of the bacterium that distinguish it from other types of *E. coli*. The symptoms of *E. coli* O157:H7 are bloody diarrhea and abdominal cramps, although sometimes there are no symptoms. Most people recover in 5 to 10 days without antibiotics or other specific treatment. In about 8% of infections, particularly among young children and elders, hemolytic uremic syndrome develops. This complication causes destruction of the red blood cells and kidney failure. Hemolytic uremic syndrome is a life-threatening condition usually treated with blood transfusions and kidney dialysis. With intensive care treatment, the death rate for hemolytic uremic syndrome is 3% to 5%. Many persons with hemolytic uremic syndrome have permanent abnormal kidney function and may require long-term dialysis. Most cases of *E. coli* O157:H7 are associated with eating undercooked, contaminated ground beef; drinking raw milk; or swimming in or drinking sewage-contaminated water (CDC, 2006b, 2008g).

## ■ Vector-Borne Diseases

A **vector** is an "animal, particularly an insect, that transmits a disease-producing organism from a host to a non-infected animal" (Agnus, 2004). Vector-borne diseases were responsible for more human disease and death from the seventeenth century through the early twentieth century than all other causes combined (Gubler, 1998). In the late 1800s, mosquitoes were discovered to transmit such diseases as malaria, yellow fever, and dengue from human to human. By 1910, other major vector-borne diseases, such as African sleeping sickness, plague, Rocky Mountain spotted fever, Chagas's disease, sandfly fever, and louse-borne typhus, all had been shown to be transmitted by blood-sucking arthropods (Gubler, 1998).

Most prevention programs have centered on vector control. Through a global effort during the twentieth century, most of the vector-borne diseases in the world had been effectively controlled, primarily by the elimination of arthropod breeding sites and limited use of chemical insecticides.

However, the benefits of vector-borne disease control programs were short-lived. Vector-borne diseases such as Lyme disease and malaria began to emerge and reemerge in different parts of the world during the 1970s, and the numbers of cases have greatly increased over the last three decades. Although the reasons for the resurgence are complex and poorly understood, two factors have been identified: (1) the diversion of financial support and subsequent loss of public health infrastructure and (2) reliance on quick-fix solutions such as insecticides and drugs (Gubler, 1998).

### Lyme Disease

In the 1990s, Lyme disease was listed as the most important emerging infection in the United States, accounting for 90% of vector-borne illness (Herrington et al., 1997). First identified in 1975, when unusually high numbers of children living in Lyme, Connecticut, were diagnosed with juvenile arthritis, the annual number of reported cases of Lyme disease increased to 23,305 cases reported in 2005 for a national average of 7.9 cases per 100,000 population. In the 10 states where Lyme disease is most common, the average was 31.6 per 100,000 (CDC, 2007a).

The disease is caused by infection with the spirochete *Borrelia burgdorferi*, transmitted by infected *Ixodes scapularis* ticks in Northeastern, Midwestern, and Southern states and *I. pacificus* on the West Coast (CDC, 2007a). (See Box 19-3.) These ticks generally feed on white-tailed deer and the white-footed mouse. Most cases of human illness occur in late spring and summer when ticks are most active and people spend more time outdoors (CDC, 2007a).

The symptoms of Lyme disease are multistage and multisystem. Early disease symptoms include a red rash resembling a bull's-eye forming over the tick bite and systemic flulike symptoms such as headache, muscular aches and pains, and fatigue. If untreated, symptoms can progress to include heart problems such as an irregular heart rate, shortness of breath, or dizziness; neurological problems such as meningitis, Bell's palsy, numbness, pain, or weakness in the limbs, or poor muscle coordination; and arthritis that shifts

---

### BOX 19-3

**States with the Highest Incidence of Lyme Disease, 2005**

|  | Cases per 100,000 |
| --- | --- |
| Delaware | 76.6 |
| Connecticut | 51.6 |
| New Jersey | 38.6 |
| Massachusetts | 36.5 |
| Pennsylvania | 34.5 |
| New York | 28.9 |
| Wisconsin | 26.4 |
| Maryland | 22.1 |
| New Hampshire | 20.2 |
| Maine | 18.7 |

Source: CDC, 2007a.

from joint to joint, with the knee being most commonly affected. About 60% of untreated patients develop chronic arthritis (CDC, 2007a).

Most cases of Lyme disease can be treated with antibiotic therapy. The earlier the treatment is begun, the more successful the treatment will be. However, early diagnosis is difficult because many of the disease symptoms mimic those of other disorders, and the distinctive bull's-eye rash is absent in 20–30% of those infected (CDC, 2007a). It is important for the nurse to interview patients presenting with flu symptoms thoroughly to determine whether possible exposure to deer ticks could have occurred, particularly in warm weather months.

### Malaria

Malaria is one of the oldest known diseases, with the first recorded case appearing in 1700 B.C. in China. In ancient Chinese, it was called "the mother of fevers" ("The mother of fevers," 1998). Malaria is the most important of all vector-borne diseases because of its global distribution, the numbers of people affected, and the large numbers of deaths (CDC, 2007d; Gubler, 1998). Worldwide, 8% of all deaths of children younger than 5 years of age are attributed to malaria. Each year, approximately 350–500 million people are infected by it, and as many as 1 million children (WHO, 2005).

Today, cases of malaria are reported in 107 countries throughout the world. Although more than 60% of cases and 80% of deaths occur in sub-Saharan Africa, the disease is also found in parts of Asia, the western Pacific, and Central and South America. At the end of 2004, 3.2 billion people lived in areas at risk of malaria transmission (CDC, 2007b). Air travel has brought the disease to the doorsteps of industrialized countries, resulting in increased illness and death among travelers to areas with endemic disease (Nchinda, 1998). (See Box 19-4.) Although malaria is not endemic to the United States, it is the most common imported disease in the United States. Although malaria is not a widespread problem in the United States, nurses should be alert for imported malaria infection in their patients who travel abroad. Of the 1,337 malaria cases reported in the United States in 2002, all but five were imported by travelers infected while visiting malaria-endemic countries (CDC, 2007b).

Malaria in humans is caused by a protozoon of the genus *Plasmodium* and the four subspecies, *falciparum, vivax, malariae,* and *ovale* (Nchinda, 1998). *P. falciparum* causes the most severe form of the disease in humans (Molyneux, 1998; Yin, 2006). The disease is transmitted through the bite of *Anopheles* mosquitoes (CDC, 2007b; Marsh & Waruiru, 1998; Nchinda, 1998). Once inside the human host, the malaria organism enters the bloodstream and travels directly to the liver, where it hides and multiplies. After about 2 weeks, the newly produced organisms burst out of the liver into the bloodstream, where they attack red blood cells. These new malaria organisms rapidly reproduce in the bloodstream over the next few days until there are tens of millions of them. It is at this point that the human host begins to feel symptoms of illness (CDC, 2007b; Marsh & Waruiru, 1998).

 **Research Alert**

*Campylobacter jejuni* is one of the most common causes of bacterial gastroenteritis in the United States. Including undiagnosed and unreported cases, it is estimated to affect more than 2 million people annually, with its costs estimated to be between $1.3 billion and $6.2 billion.

This prospective, matched case-control study was implemented to determine the risk factors for *C. jejuni* enteritis in rural communities. It was hypothesized that exposure to food animals is a major risk and that the odds of infection change with exposure to different species. Study participants were selected from among all new cases of *C. jejuni* reported to the Michigan Department of Community Health during the one-year period from October 2000 to October 2001. Each case subject was matched with two control subjects according to specified criteria. All participants completed a self-administered postal questionnaire.

The results of the data analysis indicated that contact with farm animals was a significant risk factor. Specifically, the caring for and raising of poultry increased the odds for the disease seven times more than the odds associated with husbandry of other species known to be reservoirs of *C. jejuni*. The study concluded that an estimated 18% of *C. jejuni* cases occurring in rural areas are attributable to poultry husbandry.

*Source:* Potter, R. C., Kaneene, J. B., & Hall, W. N. (December 2003). Risk factors for sporadic *Campylobacter jejuni* infections in rural Michigan: A prospective case-control study. *American Journal of Public Health, 93*(12), 2118–2123.

---

### BOX 19-4

#### Factors Contributing to the Resurgence of Malaria

- Increased resistance of malaria organisms to drugs currently used for treatment
- Civil wars in many countries, forcing large populations to relocate to different geographic regions
- Changing rainfall patterns and water development projects (e.g., dams, irrigation systems), which create new mosquito breeding places
- Poor economic conditions resulting in reduced health budgets and inadequate funding for drugs
- Changes in mosquito biting patterns, from indoor to outdoor biters

*Source:* Nchinda, 1998.

---

The first signs of illness are usually fever and malaise, often accompanied by a severe headache. At this stage of the illness, many people think they are experiencing the flu. Other malaria symptoms, such as vomiting, diarrhea, or coughing, might lead nurses or other healthcare providers to suspect gastric upset or respiratory infection. Malaria is a great imitator, making it important for nurses to suspect any fever as a potential case of malaria for patients who have recently traveled to a country where the disease is known to exist. Early diagnosis and rapid treatment are the keys to the secondary prevention efforts necessary to keep the disease from progressing to a complicated or severe state (CDC, 2007b; Marsh & Waruiru, 1998).

### West Nile Virus

West Nile virus is a flavivirus commonly found in Africa, West Asia, and the Middle East. The first case of West Nile virus was discovered in the West Nile District of Uganda, Africa, in 1937. It appeared in Egypt and Israel in the 1950s where it was recognized as a cause of severe human meningoencephalitis. In recent years it has emerged in the temperate regions of Europe and North America with the first case in the United States occurring in 1999. In 2005, there were 3,000 cases of West Nile virus reported in the United States with 119 deaths. The virus is spread by infected mosquitoes and can infect humans, horses, many types of birds, and a few other kinds of animals (CDC, 2007c).

Humans generally experience a mild form of the disease, characterized by flu-like symptoms that generally last only a few days and do not appear to cause any long-term negative effects. However, in less than 1% of cases, humans can develop severe neurological diseases—West Nile encephalitis, West Nile meningitis, or West Nile meningoencephalitis. Among those with severe illness, case fatality rates range between 3% and 15% and are highest among elderly patients (CDC, 2007c; Petersen & Marfin, 2002).

### ■ Zoonoses

Many of the infectious diseases that have emerged or re-emerged in the past few years have been zoonotic. Zoonoses are diseases that are caused by infectious agents that can jump from species to species—jumping from vertebrate animals to humans (Agnus, 2004; Murphy, 1998). Vector-borne diseases can also be considered zoonotic because they are indirectly transmitted from animal reservoirs to human reservoirs via another living source, usually insects. Throughout time, humans have interacted with the other animals that share this earth. Whether domesticated work animals, animals raised or hunted for food, family pets, or unwanted household pests, animals and their products are an integral part of our daily lives (Meslin & Stohr, 1998). A variety of both domestic and wild animals carries viruses, bacteria, or parasites that can be transferred to humans either through direct contact with the animals and their waste products or through food products of animal origin (Heymann, 1998). About half of all microorganisms known to infect humans come from animals. In the past three decades, scientists have identified more than 30 new infectious diseases, most of which have come from animals (Drexler, 2002). Zoonotic diseases seem to be increasing at a rapid pace for several reasons: Global human populations are increasingly bringing people into closer contact with animal populations; modern air travel has made it possible to travel to the other side of the world in a matter of hours; enormous environmental changes have been brought about by human activity; and bioterroristic activities are increasing, and the infectious agents of choice are usually zoonotic (CDC, 2007d; Murphy, 1998).

### Hantavirus

Hantavirus pulmonary syndrome was first recognized in the southwestern United States in 1993 when several deaths occurred from acute respiratory distress syndrome (CDC, 2007e; "Hantavirus infection," 1993).

Initial symptoms include fever plus muscle aches and pains, and may include gastrointestinal upset and headache. Late symptoms occur 4–10 days after initial symptoms and include respiratory difficulty as the lungs fill with fluid. As of January 2007, 460 cases were reported in 30 states, with 35% of cases resulting in death (CDC, 2007e).

Deer mice are the primary reservoir hosts for the southwestern states, along with cotton rats and rice rats in the Southeast and white-footed mice in the Northeast. Infection can occur when saliva or feces particles are inhaled in aerosol form during direct contact with the rodents or when dried materials contaminated by rodent excreta are loosened, directly introduced into open wounds or eyes, or ingested in contaminated food or water. Humans can also become infected through rodent bites (CDC, 2007e; "Hantavirus infection," 1993). Avoidance of contact with most rodent populations is the best way to prevent infection and control disease. Risks can be controlled through environmental hygiene practices that deter rodents from inhabiting home and work environments (CDC, 2007e; "Hantavirus infection," 1993).

There is no specific treatment, cure, or vaccine for hantavirus. If infected individuals are diagnosed early, they can be intubated and receive oxygen therapy. However, if the individual experiences full respiratory distress without being treated, it is too late to begin oxygen therapy and the infected person usually dies (CDC, 2007e).

### Avian Influenza

Since 2003, the World Health Organization has been monitoring the progress of avian influenza (H5N1), also known as bird flu, a highly pathogenic influenza virus found in parts of eastern Asia that has the potential to cause a major pandemic. As of early 2007 only a few cases had been reported in humans, with transmission occurring primarily from birds to humans. However, the high mortality rate and lack of effective treatment or vaccines for avian influenza have health professionals concerned that the virus could mutate and become transmissible from human to human. As more and more migratory birds carry the infection to western Asia, Africa, and other parts of the world, it could prove to be a serious threat to human health and wreak the kind of worldwide devastation caused by the 1918 Spanish influenza epidemic that killed more than 50 million people and created social, economic, and political havoc (InfluenZone, 2005; Schwartz, 2006).

### Pet Diseases

Pets, especially cats and dogs, are considered members of the family by many people worldwide. People give their pets names, share their food, and sometimes even share their beds with them, all in exchange for unconditional love (De Menezes Brandao & Anselmo Viana da Silva Berzins, 1998). Unfortunately, pets can be a source for zoonotic diseases. However, if pets are well nourished, properly vaccinated, and

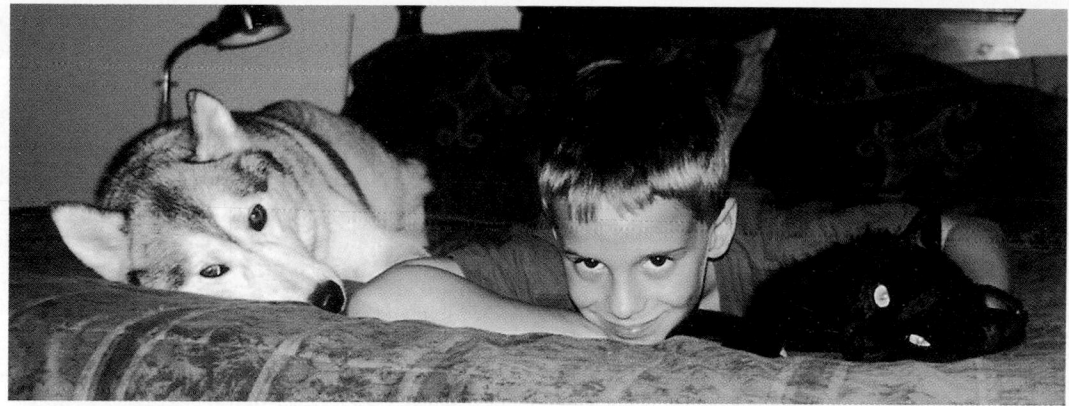

In American households, pets are members of the family. Children are especially vulnerable for exposure to infectious agents carried by pets.

regularly examined by a veterinarian, there is little to fear (CDC, 2007f; Chomel, 1998).

Cat-scratch fever, caused by *Bartonella henselae,* is generally a benign local inflammation of the lymph nodes transmitted through a break in the skin caused by a cat scratch. However, in people with weakened immune systems, it causes bacillary angiomatosis, a life-threatening vascular disease in which tumors are formed from blood cells. The organism is transmitted from cat to cat primarily by fleas (CDC, 2007f; Chomel, 1998).

In countries where plague is endemic, cats can become infected or carry fleas from infected rodents they may have killed. Several cases of bubonic and pneumonic plague in humans in the United States have been associated with pet cats (CDC, 2007f; Chomel, 1998).

Pets can carry infectious agents such as *Campylobacter* or *Salmonella,* which can cause diarrheal and gastrointestinal illness. Puppies and kittens with diarrhea pose the greatest risk. Reptiles are also carriers of a wide variety of *Salmonella* species. Pet turtles and iguanas have been linked to several severe, and even fatal, cases of *Salmonella* among young children worldwide. It is easy to see why hand washing is extremely important after handling pets and before eating (CDC, 2007f; Chomel, 1998).

### Rabies

Rabies is probably the best known and most feared of the zoonoses because the disease is almost always fatal in humans once symptoms occur. WHO estimates that more than 55,000 deaths from rabies occur a year, but the figure may actually be higher because of the large number of deaths worldwide that go unreported. In the United States, the number of rabies-related deaths has declined from more than 100 annually in 1900 to only one or two per year in the 1990s. Modern prevention efforts have proven almost 100% effective, with U.S. deaths occurring only in people who do not recognize their risk and fail to seek medical treatment (CDC, 2007g).

The virus is usually transmitted through bites from infected animals, but in rare cases, it can also be transmitted through infected licks on mucous membranes, inhaled infected bat secretions, and corneal transplants from undiagnosed human donors. Reservoirs for infection are domestic dogs and cats as well as many wild animals such as skunks, raccoons, foxes, wolves, and bats (Wilde & Mitmoonpitak, 1998). Before 1960, most rabies cases were in domestic animals, but now, more than 90% of cases occur in wild animals (CDC, 2007g). Efforts by U.S. wildlife agencies have helped control rabies in wild animal populations in recent years.

Although human rabies deaths in the United States are rare, the public health costs to prevent and control rabies exceed $300 million a year. These costs include vaccinations for pets and other domestic animals, animal control programs, maintenance of rabies laboratories, and medical costs related to Rabies Exposure Prophylaxis (PEP) treatment for humans bitten by at-risk animals (CDC, 2007g).

 NOTE THIS!

### Rabies and the Vampire Legend

The vampire legend began in Hungary around 1721 to 1728, at approximately the same time that a major rabies epidemic was occurring in dogs and other animals. Neurologist Juan Gomez-Alonso of Xeral Hospital in Vigo, Spain, said that patients with rabies often have a tendency to bite others and cannot tolerate mirrors or strong smells. When exposed to mirrors or garlic, they will often have spasms of the facial and vocal muscles causing hoarse sounds, bared teeth, and frothing at the mouth of bloody fluid.

Rabies occurs in men seven times more frequently than in women, and most vampire legends involve male vampires. Men with rabies suffer from insomnia and tend to wander at night, and because the disease affects the limbic system, which regulates emotions and behavior, they also become hypersexual.

In the 1700s, corpses were often exhumed to see if the person was a vampire. The signs of being a vampire included a lifelike appearance and blood flowing from the mouth. However, rabies can leave bloody liquid draining from the mouth long after death, and burial in the cold, humid climate of Eastern Europe preserved corpses for months or years.

*Read More!*

- Gomez-Alonso, J. (1998). Rabies: A possible explanation for the vampire legend. *Neurology, 51,* 856–859.

- Stoker, B. (1897). *Dracula.* London: Constable Publishers.

*Source:* Adapted from IntelliHealth News, 1998.

After entering the host, the rabies virus multiplies slowly at the portal of entry. It then invades the surrounding nerve tissue and slowly migrates to the spinal cord and brain. Once there, it multiplies, causing a rapid death. The incubation period can range from a few days to many years (CDC, 2007g; Wilde & Mitmoonpitak, 1998). Rabies in humans is preventable by immediately cleansing all animal bites with soap and water and using rabies immune globulin and vaccine as indicated (Benenson, 1995; Heymann, 2004; Wilde & Mitmoonpitak, 1998). Current rabies vaccinations are the best protection for pets and other domestic animals, thus significantly reducing the risk of exposure for humans.

## ■ Parasitic Diseases

Parasitic diseases, although more common in developing countries, have been on the rise in recent years in the United States. According to *Webster's Dictionary* (Agnus, 2004), a *parasite* is an animal that lives on or in an organism of another species, from which it derives sustenance or protection without benefit to, and usually with harmful effects on, the host. The most common parasites are helminths (worms and flukes) and one-celled protozoans.

### Helminths

Pinworm infection (enterobiasis) occurs worldwide and is the most common helminth intestinal infection in the United States, with the highest prevalence in school-aged children, followed by preschoolers. The prevalence is low in adults except for mothers of infected children. Pinworm infection often results in no symptoms, but in some persons, there may be perianal itching and disturbed sleep. Diagnosis can be made by applying cellophane tape to the perianal region early in the morning before bathing or defecating. Transmission occurs by direct transfer of infective eggs from the anus to the mouth or indirect transfer through contaminated clothing, bedding, food, or other fomites. Treatment with oral vermicides and disinfection of clothing and bedding is usually effective (Benenson, 1995; Heymann, 2004).

Roundworm infection (ascariasis) occurs worldwide, with the highest prevalence in children between 3 and 8 years of age living in moist, tropical countries. Typically, no symptoms occur. Live worms, passed in stools or occasionally through the mouth or nose, are often the first sign of roundworm infection. Transmission occurs by ingestion of infective eggs from soil contaminated with human feces or from uncooked produce contaminated with soil containing infective eggs; it is not transmitted directly from person to person. Treatment with oral vermicides is usually effective (Benenson, 1995; Heymann, 2004).

Hookworm infection (ancylostomiasis) is widely endemic in tropical and subtropical climates but can also occur in temperate climates. Approximately 1 billion people (about one-fifth of the world's population) are estimated to be infected with hookworms. In persons with heavy infections, there is severe iron deficiency, which leads to severe anemia. Children with heavy, long-term infection may have hypoproteinemia and may be delayed in physical and mental development. Light hookworm infections generally produce no clinical symptoms. Diagnosis is made by finding hookworm eggs in feces. Transmission occurs by larvae in the soil penetrating the skin, usually of the foot. The larvae then enter the bloodstream and travel to the lungs, where they enter the alveoli and migrate up the trachea to the pharynx. They are swallowed and reach the small intestine, where they develop into mature half-inch worms in 6 to 7 weeks. They attach to the intestinal wall and suck blood. Treatment with vermicides is usually effective (Benenson, 1995; CDC, 2008c; Heymann, 2004).

### 💻 Research Alert

Recent government-sponsored research (2006) has found that the mutated, drug-resistant "superbugs" that are causing an increasing number of hospital infections and deaths can live for weeks on bed linens, on computer keyboard covers, and under acrylic fingernails. *Staphylococcus aureus,* a methicillin-resistant strain, is usually harmless and very common, found on skin or in the noses of about 30% of all people. In hospitals, methicillin-resistant *S. aureus* (MRSA) can cause serious and sometimes deadly infections, including necrotizing fasciitis or "flesh-eating" disease. Only vancomycin administered intravenously can treat MRSA. Computer keyboards can contaminate the fingers, bare or gloved, of a nurse or physician, who could then transfer bacteria to patients.

*Source*: Centers for Disease Control and Prevention. (2007). *MRSA in healthcare settings.* Retrieved August 21, 2008 from http://www.cdc.gov/ncidod/dhgp/ar_mrsa_spotlight_2006.html

### Protozoans
#### Giardiasis

Giardiasis is a disease caused by *Giardia lamblia,* a microscopic, one-celled parasite that lives in the intestines of humans and animals. This parasite is found in every part of the United States and every region of the world. In recent years, giardiasis has become one of the most common waterborne diseases in the United States. Transmission is through the fecal–oral route or through ingestion of contaminated food or water from swimming pools, lakes, rivers, springs, ponds, or streams. The most common symptoms of giardiasis are diarrhea, abdominal cramps, nausea, fatigue, and weight loss. Symptoms usually appear within 1 to 2 weeks after exposure and generally last 2 to 6 weeks, but they can last longer (CDC, 2008d; Heymann, 2004).

Persons at risk for giardiasis are child care workers, children in diapers who attend daycare centers, international travelers, hikers, campers, or anyone who drinks untreated water from a contaminated source. Because chlorine does not kill *G. lamblia,* several community outbreaks have been linked to contaminated community water supplies (CDC, 2008d; Heymann, 2004).

Giardiasis is difficult to diagnose and may require examination of several stool specimens over several days. The pharmacological treatment for giardiasis is metronidazole

(Flagyl). Nurses can help prevent giardiasis outbreaks in their communities by teaching patients in community settings to wash their hands after using the bathroom and before handling food, to wash and peel all raw vegetables and fruits, and to avoid drinking water from any source unless it has been filtered or chemically treated (Benenson, 1995; CDC, 2008d; Heymann, 2004).

### Cryptosporidiosis

Cryptosporidiosis, often called *crypto,* is a disease caused by *Cryptosporidium parvum,* a microscopic, one-celled parasite. Although not a new disease in the developing world, cryptosporidiosis made its first major appearance in the United States in 1993, when 400,000 people became ill with diarrhea after drinking contaminated water. Today, crypto is still a major threat to the U.S. water supply. Transmission is through the fecal–oral route or through ingestion of food or water contaminated with stool, including water in recreational parks or swimming pools (CDC, 2008e; Heymann, 2004).

Immunocompromised persons are most at risk for crypto infection, particularly HIV-positive persons or persons receiving chemotherapy for cancer treatment. Other persons at risk for infection are child care workers, children in diapers who attend daycare centers, persons exposed to human feces by sexual contact, and caregivers of persons infected with crypto. The most common symptoms are watery diarrhea and cramps, which in some cases can be severe. Weight loss, nausea, vomiting, and fever may also occur (CDC, 2008e; Guerrant, 1997; Heymann, 2004).

Currently, no cure exists for crypto, but some drugs (e.g., paromomycin) may reduce the severity of the symptoms. Oral rehydration powders and sports drinks can help prevent dehydration. Nurses can help at-risk populations reduce their risk by teaching them to wash their hands often with soap and water; to avoid sex that involves contact with stool; to avoid touching farm animals; to avoid touching the stool of pets; to wash and/or cook food; to be careful when swimming in lakes, rivers, pools, or hot tubs; to drink safe water; and to take extra precautions when traveling, particularly to developing countries (CDC, 2008e; Heymann, 2004).

## ■ Bioterrorism

A bioterrorism attack occurs when viruses, bacteria, and other infectious agents are used to deliberately cause illness or death in people, animals, or plants. Infectious agents make perfect instruments of destruction. They self-propagate, adapt easily, jump international borders effortlessly, and it only takes a small amount to wreak havoc on a nation's healthcare system. Agents used for biowarfare are living organisms or toxins secreted by living organisms (Drexler, 2002). The anthrax outbreaks in the United States during the fall of 2001 proved that bioterrorism could be a significant threat to public health (CDC, 2006c).

Many infectious agents found in nature can be used even more effectively as biological weapons when altered to increase their ability to cause disease, resist current medications, and spread more rapidly in the environment (CDC, 2006c). In a bioterrorist attack, health officials might not notice until too late. Pathogens require an incubation period to multiply in the body before triggering symptoms. It could be days or weeks before the first signs of disease are apparent and even longer to identify outbreaks as an epidemic. By the time an epidemic situation is established, it may be impossible to determine the triggering event or events (Drexler, 2002).

Bioterrorism agents kill by causing suffocating pneumonia, septic shock, massive bleeding, or paralysis. At the CDC bioterrorism agents are divided into three categories, depending on how easily they can spread and the severity of the illness they can cause. Category A agents include organisms or toxins that are considered the highest risk to public and national security because they can be easily spread or transmitted from person to person and result in high death rates. They have the greatest potential for major public health impact because they can cause public panic and social disruption and require special action for public health preparedness (Drexler, 2004; CDC, 2006c). Category B agents are the second highest priority because they are moderately easy to spread, result in moderate illness and low death rates, and require specific enhancements of the CDC's laboratory capacity and enhanced disease monitoring. Category C agents are the third highest priority because they are easily available, easily produced and spread, and have the potential for high morbidity and mortality rates and major public health impact. The agents include emerging pathogens that could be engineered for mass spread in the future (CDC, 2006c). See Box 19-5 for the diseases listed under each category.

Response to a bioterrorism event will require a rapid deployment of limited public health resources. The health of America's communities will depend on the nation's public health workforce. This workforce includes physicians, nurses, environmental health scientists, health educators, laboratory personnel, and managers, supplemented by other professionals, first responders, and volunteers that will form the public health frontline of defense. Preparation in the core competencies of bioterrorism and emergency preparedness is essential for agencies and, communities to respond appropriately. Extensive partnerships are required among federal, state, and local agencies, educational institutions, and professional organizations to ensure a systematic approach to education and training (CDC, 2002). The nurse's role in bioterrorism response is described in Chapter 24.

## ■ HIV/AIDS

The most significant emerging disease in the world during the last 30 years is HIV/AIDS (see Chapter 20). AIDS is the life-threatening, late clinical stage of infection with HIV. The disease was first recognized as a distinct syndrome in 1981, and the virus was first isolated in 1983 (Benenson, 1995; Heymann, 2004).

## BOX 19-5

**Categories of Bioterrorism Agents/Diseases**

**Category A**
- Anthrax (*Bacillus anthracis*)
- Botulism (*Clostridium botulinum* toxin)
- Plague (*Yersinia pestis*)
- Smallpox (variola major)
- Tularemia (*Francisella tularensis*)
- Viral hemorrhagic fevers (filoviruses [e.g., Ebola, Marburg] and arenaviruses [e.g., Lassa, Machupo])

**Category B**
- Brucellosis (*Brucella* species)
- Epsilon (toxin of *Clostridium perfringens*)
- Food safety threats (e.g., *Salmonella* species, *Escherichia coli* O157:H7, *Shigella*)
- Glanders (*Burkholderia mallei*)
- Melioidosis (*Burkholderia pseudomallei*)
- Psittacosis (*Chlamydia psittaci*)
- Q fever (*Coxiella burnetii*)
- Ricin toxin (from *Ricinus communis* [castor beans])
- Staphylococcal enterotoxin B
- Typhus fever (*Rickettsia prowazekii*)
- Viral encephalitis (alphaviruses [e.g., Venezuelan equine encephalitis, eastern equine encephalitis, western equine encephalitis])
- Water safety threats (e.g., *Vibrio cholerae, Cryptosporidium parvum*)

**Category C**
- Emerging infectious diseases such as Nipah virus and hantavirus

*Source:* CDC, 2007. http://bt.cdc.gov/agentlist.

 THINK ABOUT THIS ·····································

Avoidance of AIDS is in our hands—inform yourself, protect yourself.
—AIDS Sanatorium Santiago de las Vegas, Havana, Cuba

" *If I were going to imagine a real terror it would be a deadly virus that kills 100% of its victims, but incubates so slowly, say a decade, that millions of people are infected before they know it. It would be a virus that is transmitted sexually, attacking young adults while it takes advantage of our social inhibitions and bigotry about sex.* "

—Dr. Joe McCormick, Chairman,
Community Health Sciences Department,
Aga Khan University, Pakistan

As of December 2005, the cumulative number of AIDS cases in the United States was 988,376. Total number of deaths from AIDS in the United States was 550,394 (CDC, 2006b). As of December 2006, there were 1.4 million people estimated to be living with HIV in the United States. Worldwide, the number of adults and children estimated to be living with HIV was 39.5 million. During 2006, the World Health Organization and UNAIDS estimated that about 4.3 adults and children were newly infected with HIV and an estimated 2.9 million deaths occurred (UNAIDS, 2006).

HIV can be transmitted from person to person through unprotected sexual contact, through direct contact with blood or blood products through sharing needles or razors, and from mother to baby during gestation or the birthing process (Benenson, 1995; Heymann, 2004). HIV/AIDS is addressed further in Chapter 20.

## Tuberculosis

TB is one of the leading causes of death worldwide from an infectious agent. Approximately 2 billion people, one-third of the world's population, are infected with TB, with about 2 million deaths occurring annually (AAWH, 1998; WHO, 2006a; Ziv, Daley, & Blower, 2004).

Historically, TB has been one of the great scourges of humankind. It was a leading killer in the United States until the advent of antibiotics in the 1950s. For the next 30 years, TB was on a steady decline, at least in the developed countries (AAWH, 1998; CDC, 2005). The 1980s, however, saw a sharp increase in TB cases, which has been primarily the result of the development of multidrug-resistant strains of the disease (AAWH, 1998; CDC, 2005). Other reasons for the upsurge include the spread of TB in institutional living facilities such as shelters and correctional facilities, a declining public health infrastructure, increased immigration from regions where TB is endemic, and the HIV/AIDS pandemic (Clark, Cegielski, & Hassell, 1997).

Although the incidence of TB has declined since 1992, TB continues to be a major health problem in the United States, where more than 14,000 cases were reported in 2005 (CDC, 2007i). The number of reported TB cases in the United States has shown a steady decline, but the rate of decline has been slowing each year since 2000. Cases are still high among high-risk groups such as the incarcerated, the homeless, elders, and HIV-infected persons, as well as underrepresented racial and ethnic groups and immigrants from countries with high TB rates and inadequate control measures (AAWH, 1998; CDC, 2007i).

TB is caused by *Mycobacterium tuberculosis* and is transmitted by droplets in the air. It usually affects the lungs (pulmonary), which accounts for 75% of all cases, although other body organs may be involved (extrapulmonary) about 25% of the time. TB can live in an infected person's body and not cause illness. This is called *inactive* TB or latent TB. Approximately 5% of people with inactive TB develop active TB or TB disease later in life. Only about 10% of all persons infected with TB actually develop active TB. Symptoms of active TB include fatigue, weight loss, fever, chills, and night sweats. Symptoms of pulmonary TB also include a persistent cough, chest pain, and bloody sputum (CDC, 2005).

TB is both preventable and curable. Prevention is focused on treating persons with inactive TB infection prophylactically with anti-TB medications such as isoniazid (INH) for 6 to 12 months. It is extremely important for infected persons to complete the preventive therapy treatment both to prevent progression to active disease and to prevent the development of drug-resistant organisms (CDC, 2005).

Treatment for persons with active TB disease commonly includes such drugs as INH, rifampin, pyrazinamide, ethambutol, and streptomycin. These drugs are usually prescribed in various combinations. It is important that persons with active TB take the medication therapy prescribed for at least 6 months (CDC, 2005).

Multidrug-resistant TB disease (MDR-TB) may occur when medications are not taken consistently for the 6 to 12 months necessary to completely destroy the *M. tuberculosis* organism. In some U.S. cities, more than 50% of TB patients fail to complete their prescribed course of therapy. Many of these patients are homeless persons, drug addicts, or other persons living in poverty, who may not be reliable about taking their medications. Many individuals with TB may feel better after only a few weeks of therapy and stop taking their medications because of unpleasant side effects. MDR-TB is difficult and complicated to treat. Inappropriate treatment can have life-threatening results. Depending on the combination of alternative drugs needed, treatment can last as long as 2 years and be very costly (CDC, 2005).

The best method of treatment for persons in high-risk circumstances is direct observed therapy (DOT). DOT is a community-based prevention program in which a nurse or other healthcare provider is paired with a person infected with TB to ensure that the patient follows the prescribed treatment plan. DOT programs have been successful in curing 95% of patients with pulmonary TB (Torres, 1998) and have the potential to save millions of lives worldwide over the next few years ("DOTS: A breakthrough," 1998).

### ■ The HIV/TB Connection

WHO estimates that 13 million people worldwide are co-infected with HIV and TB. In countries with high HIV prevalence, up to 80% of people with TB test positive for HIV (WHO, 2007). Worldwide, TB is the leading killer among people infected with HIV. TB is listed as an AIDS-defining opportunistic infection for people who are infected with HIV. TB often occurs early in the course of HIV infection and may be the first indication that a person has HIV (HIV-related conditions, 1999; CDC, 2007j; WHO, 2007).

Early diagnosis and treatment of TB are critical for HIV-infected patients because the risk for drug-resistant TB is higher among people with HIV infection compared with other groups (Moore, McCray, & Onorato, 1999; "Prevention and treatment of tuberculosis," 1998; WHO, 2007). For people with HIV infection, the death rate for MDR-TB is as high as 80%. Because TB symptoms are the same as the symptoms for many other HIV-related opportunistic infections, TB is easy to overlook initially. HIV-infected patients may not react to tuberculin skin testing because their immune systems are suppressed ("HIV-related conditions," 1999). A comprehensive health history is an essential tool for assisting nurses and other healthcare providers to identify TB exposure risks in HIV-infected patients.

## Global Disease Eradication Efforts

Despite the emergence and reemergence of infectious diseases in recent years, significant advancements in the elimination or eradication of some diseases that have existed for centuries have occurred through a united global effort. The eradication of smallpox by 1979 is thought to be the greatest triumph of modern public health (Garrett, 1994). WHO, in collaboration with other international public and private health organizations, has targeted six other communicable diseases for eradication in the beginning of the twenty-first century. These diseases are polio, maternal and neonatal tetanus, measles, leprosy, guinea worm disease, and lymphatic filariasis. According to WHO, these crippling and sometimes deadly diseases can be eliminated in parts of the world and even completely eradicated worldwide within a generation. The methods being used to accomplish this goal are immunization and vaccination, drug therapy, community training, health education, and national disease surveillance efforts (WHO, 2006a; Wittenberg, 1998).

## Conclusion

Community health nurses have played a significant role in the prevention, control, and treatment of communicable diseases throughout recent history. Nurses' skills and knowledge will continue to be a vital part of global eradication efforts well into the twenty-first century.

Explore Community Health Nursing on the Web! To learn more about the topics in this chapter, use the passcode provided to access your exclusive website: **http://nursing.jbpub.com/ communityhealth.** If you do not have a passcode, you can obtain one at this site.

## ■ CRITICAL THINKING ACTIVITIES

1. As a nurse working with WHO, what actions would you take to eliminate the reservoir for a vector-borne diseases such as malaria? What kind of actions would you take to eliminate the reservoir for an airborne disease such as legionellosis?

2. Discuss the differences between active immunity and passive immunity. Give two examples of each kind of immunity. How long does immunity last for each example?

3. Identify one infectious disease and discuss primary, secondary, and tertiary prevention methods appropriate for that disease on the community level.

4. Compare and contrast the five viral types of hepatitis. Identify similarities and differences regarding the following:
   • Occurrence in the world
   • Infectious agent
   • Reservoir
   • Incubation period
   • Methods of control

## ■ REFERENCES

Agnus, M. E. (2004). *Webster's new world college dictionary* (4th ed.). New York: Macmillan.

American Association for World Health (AAWH). (1997). *Emerging infectious diseases: Reduce the risk.* Washington, DC: Author.

American Association for World Health (AAWH). (1998). *TB alert.* Washington, DC: Author.

Atkinson, W., & Wolfe, C. (Eds.). (2003). *Epidemiology and prevention of vaccine-preventable diseases* (7th ed.). Atlanta: DHHS, Centers for Disease Control and Prevention.

Benenson, A. S. (Ed.). (1995). *Control of communicable diseases manual* (15th ed.). Washington, DC: American Public Health Association.

Centers for Disease Control and Prevention (CDC). (1994). *Addressing emerging disease threats: A prevention strategy for the United States.* Atlanta: U.S. Department of Health and Human Services.

Centers for Disease Control and Prevention (CDC). (1995). *Epidemiology and prevention of vaccine-preventable diseases.* Atlanta: U.S. Department of Health and Human Services.

Centers for Disease Control and Prevention (CDC). (1998). *Preventing infectious diseases: A strategy for the twenty-first century.* Atlanta: U.S. Department of Health and Human Services.

Centers for Disease Control and Prevention (CDC). (1999a). *Antibiotic resistance. A new threat to your and your family's health.* Atlanta: U.S. Department of Health and Human Services.

Centers for Disease Control and Prevention (CDC). (1999b). *Listeriosis.* Atlanta: U.S. Department of Health and Human Services.

Centers for Disease Control and Prevention (CDC). (1999c). *HIV/AIDS prevention.* Atlanta: U.S. Department of Health and Human Services.

Centers for Disease Control and Prevention (CDC). (2002). *Centers for Public Health preparedness.* Atlanta: U.S. Department of Health and Human Services. http://www.cdc.gov/programs.

Centers for Disease Control and Prevention (CDC). (2004a). *Viral hepatitis: A fact sheet.* Atlanta: U.S. Department of Health and Human Services.

Centers for Disease Control and Prevention (CDC). (2004b). *Viral hepatitis B fact sheet.* Atlanta: U.S. Department of Health and Human Services.

Centers for Disease Control and Prevention (CDC). (2004c). *Viral hepatitis C fact sheet.* Atlanta: U.S. Department of Health and Human Services.

Centers for Disease Control and Prevention (CDC). (2004d). *Viral hepatitis D fact sheet.* Atlanta: U.S. Department of Health and Human Services.

Centers for Disease Control and Prevention (CDC). (2004e). *Viral hepatitis E fact sheet.* Atlanta: U.S. Department of Health and Human Services.

Centers for Disease Control and Prevention (CDC). (2005). *Questions and answers about TB.* Atlanta: U.S. Department of Health and Human Services.

Centers for Disease Control and Prevention (CDC), Division of Bacterial and Mycotic Diseases. (2006a). *Escherichia coli 0157: H7.* Atlanta: U.S. Department of Health and Human Services.

Centers for Disease Control and Prevention (CDC). (2006b). *HIV/AIDS surveillance report, 2005.* Atlanta: U.S. Department of Health and Human Services.

Centers for Disease Control and Prevention (CDC). (2006c). *Bioterrorism.* Atlanta: U.S. Department of Health and Human Services.

Centers for Disease Control and Prevention (CDC). (2007a). *Learn about Lyme disease.* Atlanta: U.S. Department of Health and Human Services.

Centers for Disease Control and Prevention (CDC). (2007b). *Malaria.* Atlanta: U.S. Department of Health and Human Services.

Centers for Disease Control and Prevention (CDC). (2007c). *West Nile virus*. Atlanta: U.S. Department of Health and Human Services.

Centers for Disease Control and Prevention (CDC). (2007d). *Division of Vector-Borne Infectious Diseases*. Atlanta: U.S. Department of Health and Human Services.

Centers for Disease Control and Prevention (CDC). (2007e). *All about hantaviruses*. Atlanta: U.S. Department of Health and Human Services.

Centers for Disease Control and Prevention (CDC). (2007f). *Healthy pets, healthy people*. Atlanta: U.S. Department of Health and Human Services.

Centers for Disease Control and Prevention (CDC). (2007g). *Rabies*. Atlanta: U.S. Department of Health and Human Services.

Centers for Disease Control and Prevention (CDC). (2007h). *MRSA*. Atlanta: U.S. Department of Health and Human Services.

Centers for Disease Control and Prevention (CDC). (2007i). *Division of Tuberculosis Elimination: Fact sheets*. Atlanta: U.S. Department of Health and Human Services.

Centers for Disease Control and Prevention (CDC). (2007j). *TB and HIV/AIDS*. Retrieved October 28, 2008, from http://www.cdc.gov/.hiv/resources/factsheets/hivtb.htm

Centers for Disease Control and Prevention (CDC). (2008a). *Campylobacter*. Retrieved October 28, 2008, from http://www.cdc.gov/nczved/dfbmd/disease_listing/campylobacter_gi.html

Centers for Disease Control and Prevention (CDC). (2008b). *Salmonellosis*. Retrieved October 28, 2008, from http://www.cdc.gov/nczved/dfbmd/disease_listing/salmonellosis_gi.html

Centers for Disease Control and Prevention (CDC). (2008c). *Hookworm infection*. Retrieved October 28, from http://www.cdc.gov/ncidod/dpd/parasites/hookworm/factsht_hookworm.htm

Centers for Disease Control and Prevention (CDC). (2008d). *Giardiasis*. Retrieved October 28, 2008, from http://www.cdc.gov/ncidod/dpd/parasites/giardiasis/factsht_giardia.htm

Centers for Disease Control and Prevention (CDC). (2008e). You can prevent *cryptosporidiosis*. Retrieved October 28, 2008, from http://www.cdc.gov/hiv/resources/brochures/crypto.htm

Centers for Disease Control and Prevention (CDC). (2008f). *Listeriosis*. Retrieved October 28, 2008, from http://www.cdc.gov/nczved/dfbmd/disease_listing/listeriosis_gi.html

Centers for Disease Control and Prevention (CDC). (2008g). *Escherichia coli*. Retrieved October 28, 2008, from.http://www.cdc.gov/nczved/dfbmd/disease_listing/stec_gi.html

Chomel, B. B. (1998). Diseases transmitted by pets. *World Health, 51*(4), 24–25.

Clark. P. A., Cegielski. J. P., & Hassell, W. (1997). TB or not TB? Increasing door-to-door response to screening. *Public Health Nursing, 14*(5), 268–271.

Clinton, H. R. (1993). Nurses in the front lines. *Nursing & Health Care, 14*(6), 286–288.

De Menezes Brandao, M., & Anselmo Viana da Silva Berzins, M. (1998). When does a pet become a health hazard? *World Health, 51*(4), 20–21.

Department of Health and Human Services (DHHS). (1991). *Healthy People 2000: National health program and disease prevention objectives*. Washington, DC: U.S. Government Printing Office.

Department of Health and Human Services (DHHS). (2000). *Healthy People 2010: Conference edition*. Washington, DC: U.S. Government Printing Office.

Dols, C. L., Bowers, J. M., & Copfer, A. E. (2001). Preventing food- and water-borne illnesses. *American Journal of Nursing, 101*(6), 24AA–24HH.

DOTS: A breakthrough in TB control. (1998). *World Health, 51*(2), 14–15.

Drexler, M. (2002). *Secret agents: The menace of emerging infections*. Washington, DC: Joseph Henry Press.

Dzenowagis, J. (1997). Using electronic links for monitoring diseases. *World Health, 50*(6), 8–9.

*Facts about adult immunization*. (1997). Bethesda, MD: National Coalition for Adult Immunization. http://www.nfid.org/factsheets/adultfact.html.

*Facts about hepatitis A for adults*. (1996). Bethesda, MD: National Coalition for Adult Immunization. http://www.nfid.org/factsheets/hepaadult.html.

*Facts about hepatitis B for adults*. (1997). Bethesda, MD: National Coalition for Adult Immunization. http://www.nfid.org/factsheets/hepbadult.html.

*Facts about influenza for adults*. (1997). Bethesda, MD: National Coalition for Adult Immunization. http://www.nfid.org/factsheets/influadult.html.

Foodborne illness. (1998, July/December). *AAWH Quarterly, 12*(3–4), 8.

Garrett, L. (1994). *The coming plague. Newly emerging diseases in a world out of balance*. New York: Farrar, Straus, and Giroux.

Goldbrick, B. A. (2004). Influenza 2004–2005. What's new with the flu? *American Journal of Nursing, 104*(10), 34–38.

Gorwitz, R. J., Jernigan, D. B., Powers, J. H., Jernigan, J. A., & Participants in the CDC Convened Experts Meeting on Management of MRSA in the Community. (2006). Strategies for clinical management of MRSA in the community: Summary of an experts meeting convened by the Centers of Disease Control and Prevention. http://www.cdc.gov.ncidod/dhqp/ar_mrsa_ca.html.

Gubler, D. J. (1998). Resurgent vector-borne diseases as a global health problem. *Emerging Infectious Diseases, 4*(3), 442–449.

Guerrant, R. L. (1997). Cryptosporidiosis: An emerging, highly infectious threat. *Emerging Infectious Diseases, 3*(1).

Hantavirus infection—Southwestern United States: Interim recommendations for risk reduction. (1993, July 30). *Morbidity and Mortality Weekly Report, 42*, 1–13.

*Hepatitis C*. (1997). Geneva: World Health Organization.

*Hepatitis learning guide*. (1998). Abbott Park, IL: Abbott Diagnostics.

Herrington, J. E., Campbell, G. L., Bailey, R. E., Cartter, M. L., Adams, M., Frazier, E. L., Damrow, T. A., & Gensheimer, K. F. (1997). Predisposing factors for individuals' Lyme disease prevention practices: Connecticut, Maine, and Montana. *American Journal of Public Health, 87*(12), 2035–2038.

Heymann, D. L. (1998). Zoonoses—disease passed from animals to humans. *World Health, 51*(4), 4.

Heymann, D. L. (2004). *Control of communicable diseases manual* (18th ed.). Washington, DC: American Public Health Association.

HIV-related conditions. Focus on: Tuberculosis (1999, June/July). *HIV Frontline. A Newsletter for Professionals Who Counsel People Living with HIV, 37,* 6.

Hoffman, R. E., Greenblatt, J., Matyas, B. T., et al. (2005, January). Capacity of state and territorial health agencies to prevent foodborne illness. *Emerging Infectious Diseases.* Retrieved October 28, 2008, from http://www.cdc .gov/ncidod/eid/vol11no01/04-0334.htm

InfluenZone. (2005). *Medscape Resource Center.* http://www .medscape.com.

Institute of Medicine. (1992). *Emerging infections: Microbial threats to health in the United States.* Washington, DC: National Academy Press.

IntelliHealth news. (1998, September 21). Rabies may explain the vampire legend. *The PointCast Network.*

Kaferstein, F. K., & Meslin, F. X. (1998, July/August). Keeping foods of animal origin safe. *World Health, 51*(4), 28–29.

Kestel, F. (2006). Preventing HAIs. *Advance for Nurses* (Florida ed.), *7*(16), 25–26.

Krisberg, K. (2006, September). Public health responding to new threat of staph infections. *The Nation's Health: The Official Newspaper of the American Public Health Association,* pp. 1, 12.

Mahon, B. E., Slutsker, L., Hutwagner, L., et al. (1999). Consequences in Georgia of a nationwide outbreak of *Salmonella* infections: What you don't know might hurt you. *American Journal of Public Health, 89*(1), 31–35.

Mann, J. M. (1994). Preface. In L. Garrett (Ed.), *The coming plague. Newly emerging diseases in a world out of balance.* New York: Farrar, Straus, and Giroux.

Marsh, K., & Waruiru, C. (1998). What is malaria? *World Health, 51*(3), 6–7.

Merrill, R. M., & Timmreck, T. C. (2006). *Introduction to epidemiology* (4th ed.). Sudbury, MA: Jones and Bartlett.

Meslin, F. X., & Stohr, K. (1998). Animals that infect humans. *World Health, 51*(4), 5.

Molyneux, M. (1998). Severe malaria. *World Health, 51*(3), 8–9.

Moore, M., McCray, E., & Onorato, I. M. (1999). Cross-matching TB and AIDS registries: TB patients with HIV co-infection, United States, 1993–1994. *Public Health Reports, 114,* 269–277.

The mother of fevers. (1998, March/April). *World Health, 51*(2), 12–13.

Murphy, F. A. (1998). Emerging zoonoses. *Emerging Infectious Diseases, 4*(3), 429–435.

National Academy of Sciences (NAS). (2005). *Addressing foodborne threats to health: Policies, practices, and global coordination: Workshop summary.* Available from http://www.nap.edu/catalog/11745 .html

National Foundation for Infectious Diseases (2002a). *Facts about adult immunization.* Retrieved October 28, 2008, from http:// www.nfid.org/_old/factsheets/adultfact.html

National Foundation for Infectious Diseases (2002b). Facts for Hepatits A for adults. Retrieved October 28, 2008, *from* http:// nfid.org/_old/factsheets/he;aadult.html

National Foundation for Infectious Diseases (2002c). *Facts about hepatitis B for adults.* Retrieved October 28, 2008, from http:// www.nfid.org/_old/factsheets/hepbadult.html

National Foundation for Infectious Diseases (2002d). *Facts about influenza for adults.* Retrieved October 28, 2008, from http:// www.nfid.org/_old/factsheets/influadult.html

Nchinda, T. C. (1998). Malaria: A reemerging disease in Africa. *Emerging Infectious Diseases, 4*(3), 398–403.

Petersen, L. R., & Marfin, A. A. (2002). West Nile virus: A primer for the clinician. *Annals of Internal Medicine, 137*(3), 173–179.

Potter, R. C., Kaneene, J. B., & Hall, W. N. (2003). Risk factors for sporadic *Campylobacter jejuni* infections in rural Michigan: A prospective case-control study. *American Journal of Public Health, 93*(12), 2118–2123.

PreventionInfo.org. (2004). *Health trends: Immunizations.* Retrieved October 28, 2008, from http://Preventioninfo.org/trends_ immunization.htm

Prevention and treatment of tuberculosis among patients infected with human immunodeficiency virus: Principles of therapy and revised recommendations. (1998, October 30). *Morbidity and Mortality Weekly Report, 47*(RR-20), 5.

Schwartz, R. D. (2006, October/November). Pandemic flu preparedness and response in corrections facilities. *Infectious Diseases in Corrections Report.* http://www.idcronline.org.

Thompson, W. W., Shay, D. K., Weintraub, E., et al. (2003). Mortality associated with influenza and respiratory syncytial virus in the United States. *Journal of the American Medical Association, 289*(2), 179–186.

Timmreck, T. C. (1998). *An introduction to epidemiology.* (2nd ed.). Boston: Jones and Bartlett.

Todd, B. (2006). Beyond MRSA: VISA and VRSA. *American Journal of Nursing, 106*(4), 28–30.

Torres, M. (1998, July). Tuberculosis update. *National Council of La Raza Center for Health Promotion Fact Sheet.*

UNAIDS. (2006). *AIDS epidemic update: December 2006.* Geneva, Switzerland: UNAIDS & WHO.

Valanis, B. (1999). *Epidemiology in health care.* (3rd ed.). Stamford, CT: Appleton & Lange.

World Health Organization (WHO). (2005). World malarial report 2005. http://rbm.who.int/wmr2005/.

World Health Organization (WHO). (2006a). Tuberculosis fact sheet. http://www.who.int/mediacentre/factsheets.html

World Health Organization (WHO). (2006b). *Division of Communicable Disease Newsletter, 8.* Regional Office for the Eastern Mediterranean.

World Health Organization (WHO). (2007). Tuberculosis and HIV. http://www.who.int/tb/hiv/faq/en/index.html.

Wilde, H., & Mitmoonpitak, C. (1998). Canine rabies in Thailand. *World Health, 51*(4), 10–11.

Wittenberg, R. L. (1998). From the president. Efforts toward eliminating seven diseases from the globe. *American Association for World Health Quarterly, 12*(2), 2.

Yin, S. (2006). Special section: Malaria. In M. M. Kent & S. Yin, *Population Bulletin: Controlling Infectious Diseases, 61*(2), 14–16. Washington, DC: Population Reference Bureau.

Ziv, E., Daley, C. L., & Blower, S. (2004). Potential public health impact of new tuberculosis vaccines. *Emerging Infectious Diseases, 10*(9). http://cdc.gov/ncidod/EID/vol10no9/03-0921.htm.

# Sexually Transmitted Diseases and HIV/AIDS

Sharyn Janes, Janet St. Lawrence, and Julia B. St. Lawrence

Visit **http://nursing.jbpub.com/communityhealth** for interactive exercises, review questions, Web links, and more.

Sexual activity is a way to express intimacy and positive emotions, enable reproduction, and provide physical pleasure, but it also can be associated with potentially harmful consequences. The undesired outcomes from sexual activity include unintended pregnancies and sexually transmitted diseases (STDs), including infection with the human immunodeficiency virus (HIV), which can lead to acquired immune deficiency syndrome (AIDS). STDs have been described as America's "hidden epidemic" because the rates of some STDs are now higher than they were three decades ago and the United States has the highest rates of STDs in the industrialized world.

Nonetheless, he knew that the tale he had to tell could not be one of final victory. It could only be the record of what had had to be done, and what assuredly would have to be done again in the neverending fight against terror and its relentless on-slaughts, despite their personal afflictions, by all who, while unable to be saints but refusing to bow down to pestilences, strive their utmost to be healers.

*—Albert Camus, The Plague*

Camus wrote these words long before the appearance of HIV/AIDS. Does it have meaning for the HIV epidemic? What does it say to you as a nurse? Can you refuse to bow down and strive to be a healer in an epidemic that has so many moral, political, and ethical undertones?

## CHAPTER FOCUS

**Scope of the Problem**

**Common STDs**
- Syphilis
- Chlamydia
- Gonorrhea
- Herpes Simplex Virus
- Human Papillomavirus

**Health Consequences of STDs**
- Cancers
- Reproductive Health Problems
- Health Consequences for Pregnant Women and Infants
- Health Consequences for Men

**HIV/AIDS**
- Scope of the Problem
- Populations at Risk for HIV/AIDS
- Nursing Care of Families with HIV

**STDs and the U.S. Healthcare System**
- Problems of Access
- Health Services
- Screening and Prevention

**The Role of Community Health Nurses**

## QUESTIONS TO CONSIDER

After reading this chapter, you will know the answers to the following questions:

1. How are STDs affecting global health?
2. What are some of the most common STDs in the United States?
3. What are some of the major health consequences of STDs?
4. How is the HIV/AIDS pandemic affecting global health?
5. What are some of the populations at risk for HIV in the United States and why?
6. How is the U.S. healthcare system handling the overload of sexually transmitted diseases and HIV/AIDS?
7. What is the role of the nurse in the diagnosis and treatment of STDs and HIV/AIDS?
8. What are some of the prevention efforts being done by communities?
9. What is the role of the community health nurse in prevention efforts?

## KEY TERMS

Acquired immune deficiency syndrome (AIDS)
Chlamydia

Gonorrhea
Herpes simplex
Human immunodeficiency virus (HIV)

Human papillomavirus
Ryan White CARE Act
Sexually transmitted diseases (STDs)

Syphilis
Transtheoretical model of behavior change

## Scope of the Problem

There is no such thing as a "typical" STD patient. **Sexually transmitted diseases (STDs)** affect people of all socioeconomic levels, races, ethnicities, genders, ages, and religions. STDs are almost always transmitted from one person to another during sexual intercourse. They are transmitted most efficiently during anal or vaginal intercourse and less efficiently during oral intercourse. Some STDs, such as hepatitis B and HIV, can also be transmitted parenterally and are particularly problematic among intravenous drug users who share injection equipment. In some cases, a pregnant woman can transmit an STD to her infant prenatally, during birth, or postnatally during breastfeeding, as happens with HIV, for example.

Against this backdrop of high STD rates, some subpopulations have higher STD incidences than average. In most parts of the United States, sexually active adolescents have high rates of STDs, particularly chlamydia, regardless of their race or socioeconomic status. In addition, men who have sex with other men, especially young men, generally have higher rates of STDs. STDs are also common among persons who use illicit drugs, including both injection drug users (IDUs) and non-IDUs. The presence of an STD greatly increases the risk of HIV transmission during sexual activity.

## Common STDs

The term *STD* refers to infectious organisms that can be transmitted during sexual contact and cause dozens of different clinical presentations (see Box 20-1). Five of the most common STDs are described briefly in the following sections. HIV/AIDS is discussed separately in a later section.

### ■ Syphilis

**Syphilis** is a systemic disease caused by *Treponema pallidum*. The disease progresses through three stages, with different clinical presentations at each stage. The three stages, with some of the most common clinical symptoms, are

1. Primary infection: ulcer or chancre at the infection site
2. Secondary infection: rash, mucocutaneous lesions, and adenopathy
3. Tertiary infection: cardiac, neurological, ophthalmic, auditory, liver, or bone damage

Latent syphilis is defined as the periods when patients are seropositive but have no signs or symptoms. Treatment of latent syphilis is important to halt the progression of the disease. Although most associated with tertiary infection, central nervous system disease can occur at any stage of syphilis. Persons diagnosed with syphilis showing any neurological symptoms such as ophthalmic or auditory symptoms, cranial nerve palsies, and signs and symptoms of meningitis should have a cerebrospinal fluid examination. Severe dementia can occur if syphilis infection is left untreated (CDC, 2007a; Heymann, 2004).

Pregnant women should be screened for syphilis in the early stages of pregnancy because early treatment of the mother's syphilis infection has a high success rate in preventing the baby from acquiring congenital syphilis. In communities in which the prevalence of syphilis is high or for patients at high risk, serological testing should also be done at 28 weeks and 32 weeks gestation and at delivery. No infant should leave the hospital or birthing center without the mother having been screened for syphilis at least once during pregnancy. Children born with congenital syphilis can have birth defects affecting all systems, including severe neurological abnormalities ("Sexually transmitted diseases," 2006).

Penicillin G, given intramuscularly, has been an effective treatment for syphilis for many years. It is a cure in the early stages of syphilis and helps slow disease progression and prevent complications in later stages. Dosage and duration of treatment depend on the stage and severity of the disease. For nonpregnant patients with penicillin allergies,

---

### BOX 20-1

**Clinical Presentations of Sexually Transmitted Diseases**

In the case of sexually transmitted diseases (STDs), one organism does not cause one identifiable syndrome. Instead, similar presentations can be caused by different STDs. For example, pelvic inflammatory disease (PID) can be caused by gonorrhea, chlamydia, or other bacteria. Genital ulcers can be caused by herpes, chancroid, or syphilis, as well as by other infections. Some STDs, such as syphilis or HIV/AIDS, have many different clinical presentations and mimic many other health problems. Some diseases that were at one time not perceived as being particularly serious now are known to lead to very serious outcomes. For example, human papillomavirus infection (HPV) was widely associated with genital warts but not regarded as a serious condition until after it was discovered that HPV also causes several types of cancers.

---

### BOX 20-2

**Basic STD Facts**
- More than half of all people will have an STD at some point in their lifetimes.
- The estimated number of people in the United States with a viral STD is more than 65 million.
- More than $8 billion is spent each year to diagnose and treat STDs and their complications.
- Each year, one in four teens contracts an STD, and one in four Americans has genital herpes.
- More than 6 million people are infected with human papillomavirus (HPV) each year. Most have no symptoms.
- HPV causes about 70% of all diagnosed cervical cancers.
- Every year, there are 3 million new cases of chlamydia.

doxycycline or tetracycline can be used. However, patients with poor treatment compliance histories or those who are pregnant should be desensitized and treated with penicillin. All sexual partners should be identified and treated (CDC, 2007a; "Sexually transmitted diseases," 2006).

After remaining at a steady level through the 1970s and into the 1980s, syphilis increased substantially from 1987 to 1990, then began to decrease once again (CDC, 2006a). By 2000, the incidence and prevalence rates of primary and secondary syphilis were the lowest since reporting began in 1941. Since then, however, syphilis rates have steadily increased. Between 2004 and 2005 alone, the national rates were increased by 11.1%, from 2.7 to 3.0 cases per 100,000 population. The highest increases were seen primarily in males, with a rate increase of 8.5%, up from 4.7 per 100,000 in 2004 to 5.1 per 100,000 in 2005. The rate of reported cases for females also increased for the first time in more than 10 years. Additionally, the syphilis rates for African Americans have increased steadily since 2004 after a decade of steady decline (CDC, 2007b).

## Chlamydia

**Chlamydia,** caused by *Chlamydia trachomatis,* is the most common bacterial STD in the United States. It is estimated that as many as 2.5 million Americans are infected each year. Because many infections are asymptomatic, however, it is difficult to determine exact infection rates. The prevalence is higher in women younger than 25 years of age. Women are frequently reinfected if their sex partners are not treated (CDC, 2006b, 2007b; "Sexually transmitted diseases," 2006).

If symptoms occur, they usually appear within 1 to 3 weeks after exposure. Early signs of chlamydia include abnormal genital discharge or painful urination. However, these symptoms often are ignored because they are so mild. Chlamydia can be transmitted during vaginal, anal, or oral sex with an infected partner. Pregnant women may pass the infection to their newborns during delivery, leading to neonatal eye infections or pneumonia (CDC, 2006b, 2007b; "Sexually transmitted diseases," 2006).

Chlamydia is completely curable if diagnosed before complications occur. The antibiotics most commonly used are a 1-day course of azithromycin or a 7-day course of doxycycline. Other antibiotics such as erythromycin or ofloxacin are also effective. Pregnant women are treated with azithromycin, erythromycin, or amoxicillin (CDC, 2007b; "Sexually transmitted diseases," 2006).

## Gonorrhea

**Gonorrhea,** a bacterial infection caused by *Neisseria gonorrhoeae,* is spread through vaginal, anal, or oral sexual activity with an infected partner. Pregnant women can pass the infection to their newborns during delivery, leading to eye infections or life-threatening blood infections in their babies. The early symptoms are often mild, and many women never develop symptoms. If symptoms occur, they usually appear within 2 to 10 days after exposure. Initial symptoms in women include pain or burning with urination and yellow or bloody vaginal discharge. Men usually experience a penile discharge and burning with urination that may be severe. Symptoms of rectal infection include anal itching, discharge, or painful bowel movements (CDC, 2007c; "Sexually transmitted diseases," 2006).

Gonorrhea is becoming increasingly resistant to antibiotics, resulting in more expensive treatment because the usual options are no longer effective. As recently as 1976, almost all gonorrhea infections could be cured with penicillin

| **Table 20-1** | The Five Ps Approach to Effective Clinical Interviewing to Identify STD Risk Factors |
|---|---|
| Partners | • Do you have sex with men, women, or both? <br> • In the past few months, how many sex partners have you had? <br> • In the past 12 months, how many sex partners have you had? |
| Prevention of pregnancy | Are you or your partner trying to get pregnant? If no, what are you doing to prevent pregnancy? |
| Protection from STDs | What do you do to protect yourself from STDs and HIV? |
| Practices | To understand your risks for STDs, I need to understand the kind of sex you have had recently. <br> • Have you had vaginal sex, meaning penis in vagina? <br> • If yes, do you use condoms never, sometimes, or always? <br> • Have you had anal sex, meaning penis into rectum/anus? <br> • If yes, do you use condoms never, sometimes, or always? <br> • Have you had oral sex, meaning mouth on penis or vagina? <br> For condom answers: <br> • If never, why don't you use condoms? <br> • If sometimes, in which situations or with whom, do you not use condoms? |
| Past history of STDs | • Have you ever had an STD? <br> • Have any of your sex partners had an STD? |
| Additional questions to identify HIV and hepatitis risk | • Have you or any of your sex partners ever injected drugs? <br> • Have you or any of your sex partners ever exchanged money for sex? <br> • Is there anything else about your sexual practices that I need to know about? |

*Source:* Sexually transmitted diseases treatment guidelines, 2006. (2006). *Morbidity and Mortality Weekly Report, 55*(RR-11). Atlanta: Centers for Disease Control and Prevention.

(Aral & Holmes, 1991). Currently, one of the most effective treatments for gonorrhea is ceftriaxone, which can be given in a single dose. Other effective antibiotics include cefixime, ciprofloxacin, or ofloxacin. Because gonorrhea often occurs simultaneously with a chlamydial infection, combination therapy with ceftriaxone and doxycycline or azithromycin is often effective. Since dual therapy for gonorrhea and chlamydia was initiated, the incidence of chlamydia has decreased significantly in some populations. Routine co-treatment many possibly help to hinder the development of microbial-resistant strains of gonorrheal infections ("Sexually transmitted diseases," 2006). As more antimicrobial strains continue to evolve, the CDC may run out of treatment options.

## ■ Herpes Simplex Virus

Sexually transmitted **herpes simplex** virus (HSV) infection is widespread and produces intermittent painful ulcers. Although the ulcers can be treated, the underlying infection persists and ulcers recur. This is of concern because HSV can be transmitted to a sex partner even in the absence of a genital ulcer and can also be passed from an infected mother to her newborn during childbirth. Approximately 200,000 to 500,000 new cases of HSV occur each year in the United States, and it is estimated that 45 million individuals are currently infected. This prevalence estimate means that one of every four women and one of every five men in the United States will become infected with HSV during their lifetimes (CDC, 1997, 2007e; "Sexually transmitted diseases," 2006).

There are two types of HSV, both of which can cause genital herpes. HSV type 1 most often causes fever blisters and cold sores around the mouth area, but it can cause genital herpes as well. HSV type 2 generally causes genital lesions, but it can also cause sores around the mouth. Eighty percent of people with genital herpes never develop symptoms or do not recognize them. If symptoms do occur, they will usually appear within 2 weeks after exposure. The first episode of ulcers usually lasts 2 to 4 weeks. Early symptoms include genital itching or burning; pain in the legs, buttocks, or genital area; and vaginal discharge. Later symptoms include lesions inside the vagina or in the urinary tract. Small red bumps occur first, followed by blisters, and then painful sores. However, as already mentioned, many people with HSV type 2 infections are unaware of the infection because they never develop symptoms, or the symptoms are mild and may be mistaken for a rash or other skin condition (CDC 2007e; "Sexually transmitted diseases," 2006).

Genital herpes cannot be cured, but it can be controlled with acyclovir. Treatment with acyclovir also reduces the risk of transmission to sexual partners. A baby born with herpes can develop encephalitis, severe rashes, and eye problems. Early treatment with acyclovir greatly reduces serious complications in infants. Delivery by cesarean section also greatly reduces the risk of newborn infection ("Sexually transmitted diseases," 2006).

**Morning Ghost**

In dream I awoke without turning on the lights as I so often do at the first pink of dawn. In robe and house shoes I step into the kitchen to grind the coffee.

Rob slips in beside me, hair a mess, night eyes still heavy with sleep and mouth still unwilling for voice.

There he stood all six foot three child of my womb. Christmas pajamas in need of replacement, robe open, sash dangling, bare feet on that cold stone floor.

He reaches for his favorite cup—the big blue bowl. So much like his grandfather. He half fills with hot milk—shoves it toward me for the steaming black brew.

He complains softly about the color . . . how can I drink it that strong, he asks . . . I suggest he add hot water or more milk . . . he starts to explain the subtleties of brewing "good coffee." I listen and fill my own cup . . . stack a tray with saucers, bread, butter, and jam.

Without talking we climb the stairs and out onto the deck to watch the pinking of the sky over the waters . . . mumbling softly he continuous on about different grinds and different roasts and different cafes and different mornings.

Just as the dream came—returning that beautiful to me—the dream slipped away and I awake to the sounds of my husband's soft breath and the visit of that beloved ghost still holding near.

I wrap the warmth of my robe close, slip into my worn house shoes and go to the kitchen to grind the coffee and look forward to another morning dream.

I think strange thoughts of growing old and senile and finding that the thought does not frighten me if it means that the dreams will come of those I love. Of having tea in the garden with my aunt, or playing under the oak tree with my sister, or having coffee with my son, or making love with my husband. I would only wish that I will not awake to find them gone or worse yet, as old as I.

—*Ann Thedford Lanier, written about her son after his death at age 27 from AIDS.*

## ■ Human Papillomavirus

**Human papillomavirus** (HPV) is one of the most common STDs in the world, occurring across all socioeconomic levels. An estimated 6.2 million Americans are infected each year. At least 50% of sexually active people will have HPV at some time in their lives. Almost half of all HPV infections in the United States occur in women between 15 and 25 years old. Of the more than 100 known types of HPV, 40 are spread through sexual contact. Low-risk types of HPV cause genital warts (condylomata acuminata). High-risk types of HPV can cause vaginal, cervical, and anal cancers ("Quadrivalent human papillomavirus," 2007).

Genital warts are very contagious. Approximately two-thirds of people who have sexual contact with a person with genital warts will develop warts, usually within 3 months of exposure. In women, warts can occur inside and outside the vagina, on the cervix, or around the anus. In men, warts can occur on the tip or shaft of the penis, on the scrotum, or around the anus. Left untreated, genital warts may disappear or may grow into a raised fleshy growth with a cauliflower-like appearance. Because there is no way to predict whether warts will disappear or grow, people who suspect that they have genital warts should seek treatment ("Quadrivalent human papillomavirus," 2007; "Sexually transmitted diseases," 2006).

The primary goal of treatment is removal of the warts. Although there is no cure for HPV, treatment can induce wart-free periods. Treatment varies with each individual case and is guided by the preference of the patient, the experience of the healthcare provider, and the available resources. Available treatment include patient-applied therapies (e.g., podofilox, imiquimod) and provider-applied therapies (e.g., cryotherapy, podophyllin resin, trichloroacetic acid, bichloracetic acid, interferon, surgery). Like many other STDs, HPV often has no visible symptoms. It is estimated that nearly 50% of people infected with HPV are unaware of their infection and the risk of transmission to others.

Examination of sex partners is not necessary because chance of reinfection is minimal, and in the absence of a cure, treatment to reduce transmission is not realistic. However, sex partners should be counseled about the implications of having a partner who has HPV. Because there is no cure for HPV, patients and sex partners should be aware that the patient might remain infectious after the warts are gone. Condom use may decrease the risk of infection but does not eliminate it ("Sexually transmitted diseases," 2006).

## Health Consequences of STDs

Most people are not aware of the long-term health consequences of STDs other than HIV/AIDS. There are several reasons why STDs rarely command attention or concern. Many STDs are without symptoms and go undetected until years after infection, when serious sequelae appear. Many of the major adverse outcomes that do occur from STD infections arise years after the initial infection, so the connection is not made between the original infection and the later consequence, except for the awareness that HIV infection leads to AIDS. Viral STDs, in particular, often result in lifelong infection for which there is no cure at present. Public discourse is also hampered by the stigma of STDs. Finally, many people—including health providers—find it difficult to discuss sexual behavior openly and comfortably. This can make it difficult for a health provider to take a patient's sexual history or to counsel a patient effectively about his or her sexual health.

### ■ Cancers

The relationship between sexually transmitted diseases and several types of cancers has only recently been recognized by the public. Some cancer-related STDs include HPV, hepatitis B, and human herpes virus type 8. In fact, human

### ■ CULTURAL CONNECTION

**Pan American Health Organization HIV/STD Policy Positions for Countries in the Americas**

PAHO supports the implementation of the following national level policies:

1. Universal access to comprehensive HIV/STD prevention and treatment, including HAART and other necessary care options, free of cost at the point of service delivery.
2. Evidence-based health promotion and HIV/STD programs for and with members of affected groups or other relevant populations whose quality of life can be improved by reducing their vulnerability and eliminating risk.
3. Gender-sensitive policies and programs focusing on reducing inequalities that arise from the different roles of men and women arising from unequal levels of legal, economic, political, and social power.
4. Revitalized commitment to STD prevention and control because of the important role the presence of STD plays in HIV transmission.
5. Recognition of health as a human right and addressing the broader social and political determinants of health. National policies should reflect the values of equity, excellence, solidarity, respect, integrity, efficiency, participation, and autonomy.

*Source:* Adapted from Pan American Health Organization. (2005). The Regional HIV/STI Plan for the Health Sector, 2006–2015.

papillomaviruses are now recognized as the major cause of cervical cancer. An estimated 10,000 women in the United States are diagnosed with cervical cancer every year, and approximately 4,000 die from it. Worldwide, nearly half a million women develop cervical cancer each year, with nearly 250,000 dying from the disease. Studies show that HPV may also be involved in cancers of the anus, vulva, and vagina. A few types of oropharyngeal and penile cancer have been linked to certain types of high-risk HPV infections as well (NCI, 2007).

In 2006, the U.S. Food and Drug Administration (FDA) approved a vaccine for HPV for females 9 to 26 years of age for the prevention of cervical cancer. The vaccine is highly effective in preventing the high-risk HPV infections that cause 70% of cervical cancers and 90% of genital warts. The HPV vaccine is recommended for 11- to 12-year-old girls and can be given to girls as young as 9 because it is most effective in females who have not yet been infected with any of the types of HPV covered by the vaccine. Because the vaccine has been widely tested in 9- to 26-year-old females, it is only approved for use with that group. Studies are being done with women older than 26 and with males to determine if the vaccine can prevent HPV infection in these populations as well (CDC, 2007f).

### ■ Reproductive Health Problems

Many reproductive health problems are the consequence of unrecognized or untreated STD infections. Such reproductive health problems may be short term, as is the case for PID, pregnancy complications, or epididimitis, or long term, such as infertility.

Gonorrhea and chlamydia infections are the most common causes of pelvic inflammatory disease (PID) in women. PID occurs when bacteria move upward from the vagina or cervix into the uterus, fallopian tubes, and other reproductive organs. If left untreated, PID can lead to serious complications that may include infertility, ectopic pregnancy, internal abscesses, and chronic pelvic pain. More than 50% of all preventable infertility in women is a result of sexually transmitted diseases (CDC, 2004). Each year in the United States, more than 1 million women develop PID, with 100,000 becoming infertile and more than 150 dying. A large proportion of ectopic pregnancies are believed to be due to PID.

Prompt and appropriate treatment of PID can help prevent complications. Because of the difficulty in identifying the agent infecting the internal reproductive organs, PID is usually treated with at least two antibiotics that are effective against a wide range of microorganisms. Treating STDs early can prevent PID. Yearly chlamydia screening is recommended for all sexually active women younger than age 25 and for all older women with risk factors such as new or multiple sex partners (CDC, 2007d; "Sexually transmitted diseases," 2006).

### ■ Health Consequences for Pregnant Women and Infants

STDs create many complications for pregnant women and their infants. Pregnant women with STDs can transmit the infections prenatally, during birth, or after birth (see Table 20-2). Common STDs that are known to create adverse outcomes in pregnant women and their babies include chlamydia, gonorrhea, syphilis, cytomegalovirus, genital herpes, and HIV (CDC, 2007g).

The harmful effects for babies include stillbirth, low birth weight, conjunctivitis, pneumonia, neonatal sepsis, neurological impairments, blindness, deafness, acute hepatitis, meningitis, chronic liver disease, and cirrhosis. To prevent many of these problems, pregnant women should be screened for STDs starting early in the pregnancy, with testing being repeated close to delivery, if necessary. Pregnant women should be treated for STDs occurring in pregnancy and infants can be treated if infection is found at birth (CDC, 2007g).

### ■ Health Consequences for Men

The consequences of some STDs are similar in both men and women. HPV, for example, is associated with penile and anal cancers in men, although both are less common than cervical cancer among women. Most people are not aware that STDs produce long-term problems such as infertility for men, but the health burden of chancroid, chlamydia, gonorrhea, HIV, and syphilis is high among men as well as among women.

## HIV/AIDS

By impairing and eventually destroying the immune system, **human immunodeficiency virus (HIV)** progressively eliminates the body's ability to fight infections and certain cancers. A badly weakened immune system is unable to fight off microbes that would not cause illness in a healthy person. These life-threatening diseases are called *opportunistic infections* and are generally the first sign that an HIV-infected person has progressed to **acquired immune deficiency syndrome (AIDS)**. AIDS is the end stage of HIV disease, which includes the whole spectrum of HIV infection, from initial infection with the virus to clinical AIDS and eventual death. HIV is found in semen, vaginal secretions, blood, and breast milk. This virus does not live outside the body and can be transmitted only through unprotected anal, vaginal, or oral sex; contaminated needles for injection drug use; contaminated blood products; or from an infected mother to her infant during pregnancy or delivery or through breastfeeding. The most common route of transmission is sexual contact (Heymann, 2004).

In 1993, the criteria for an AIDS diagnosis were amended to include three additional opportunistic infections (invasive

| Table 20-2 | Estimated Number of Pregnant Women Infected with Specific STDs Each Year in the United States | |
| --- | --- |
| **STD** | **Number of Pregnant Women** |
| Bacterial vaginosis | 800,000 |
| Herpes simplex | 800,000 |
| Chlamydia | 200,000 |
| Trichomoniasis | 80,000 |
| Gonorrhea | 40,000 |
| Hepatitis B | 40,000 |
| HIV | 8,000 |
| Syphilis | 8,0000 |

*Source:* CDC, 2007g.

## Objectives Related to Sexually Transmitted Diseases

### Bacterial STD Illness and Disability

25.1 Reduce the proportion of adolescents and young adults with *Chlamydia trachomatis* infections.

25.2 Reduce gonorrhea.

25.3 Eliminate sustained domestic transmission of primary and secondary syphilis.

### Viral STD Illness and Disability

25.4 Reduce the proportion of adults with genital herpes infection.

25.5 Reduce the proportion of persons with human papillomavirus.

### STD Complications Affecting Females

25.6 Reduce the proportion of females who have ever required treatment for pelvic inflammatory disease.

25.7 Reduce the proportion of childless females with fertility problems who have had a sexually transmitted disease or who have required treatment for pelvic inflammatory disease.

25.8 Reduce HIV infections in adolescent and young females aged 13 to 24 years that are associated with heterosexual contact.

### STD Complications Affecting the Fetus and Newborn

25.9 Reduce congenital syphilis.

25.10 Reduce neonatal consequences from maternal sexually transmitted diseases, including chlamydial pneumonia, gonococcal and chlamydial ophthalmia neonatorum, laryngeal papillomatosis (from human papillomavirus infection), neonatal herpes, and preterm birth and low birth weight associated with bacterial vaginosis.

### Personal Behaviors

25.11 Increase the proportion of adolescents who abstain from sexual intercourse or use condoms if currently sexually active.

25.12 Increase the number of positive messages related to responsible sexual behavior during weekday and nightly prime-time television programming.

### Community Protection Infrastructure

25.13 Increase the proportion of tribal, state, and local sexually transmitted disease programs that routinely offer hepatitis B vaccines to all STD patients.

25.14 Increase the proportion of youth detention facilities and adult city or county jails that screen for common bacterial sexually transmitted diseases within 24 hours of admission and treat STDs (when necessary) before persons are released.

25.15 Increase the proportion of all local health departments that have contracts with managed care providers for the treatment of nonplan partners of patients with bacterial sexually transmitted diseases (gonorrhea, syphilis, and chlamydia).

### Personal Health Services

25.16 Increase the proportion of sexually active females aged 25 years and younger who are screened annually for genital chlamydia infections.

25.17 Increase the proportion of pregnant females screened for sexually transmitted diseases (including HIV infection and bacterial vaginosis) during prenatal health care visits, according to recognized standards.

25.18 Increase the proportion of primary care providers who treat patients with sexually transmitted diseases and who manage cases according to recognized standards.

25.19 Increase the proportion of all sexually transmitted disease clinic patients who are being treated for bacterial STDs (chlamydia, gonorrhea, and syphilis) and who are offered provider referral services for their sex partners.

*Source:* DHHS, 2000.

---

cervical cancer, tuberculosis, and recurrent pneumonia) with a positive HIV antibody test and/or a CD4 blood cell count of 200 cells/mm³. Before 1993, a positive HIV antibody test and a diagnosis of 1 of 23 specific opportunistic infections were the only criteria for an AIDS diagnosis. As a result, AIDS cases were undercounted before 1993.

## ■ Scope of the Problem

Since its discovery in 1981, HIV/AIDS has had a devastating effect in the United States and throughout the world. In 2006, an estimated 1.6 million people were living with HIV in the United States, including almost 1 million with AIDS. The cumulative AIDS deaths reached more than 500,000 (CDC, 2007h, 2007i). AIDS death rates increased during the first 15 years of the epidemic and were highest in the mid-1990s. Since then, the death rates have dropped significantly, primarily due to the standardized treatment with highly active antiretroviral therapy (HAART). HIV prevalence is currently at its highest level and continues to rise each year. The only exception to the steady rise in prevalence occurred in the mid-1990s, before the introduction of HAART, when the annual number of deaths exceeded the number of new HIV infections. The increasing prevalence of HIV/AIDS is due not only to the availability of effective treatment options, which has reduced HIV-related morbidity and mortality, but also to the continuing number of new infections each year, estimated at 40,000 (CDC, 2007h; Kaiser Foundation, 2006).

An overview of HIV/AIDS in other parts of the world is even more serious. It is estimated that there were more than 39.5 million people worldwide living with HIV by 2006.

### MEDIA MOMENT

***And the Band Played On*** (1993)
This is the story of the discovery of HIV. The film relives events from the early days in 1978, when numerous homosexuals in San Francisco began dying from unknown causes, to the identification of the human immunodeficiency virus by French and U.S. scientists in 1984. It is based on the book by Randy Shilts.

*And that was the day that we knew, oh! In the world there is a new disease called AIDS. I thought surely this will be the greatest war we ever fought. Surely many will die. And surely we will be frustrated, unable to help. But I also thought the Americans will find a treatment soon. This will not be forever.*
—Dr. Jayo Kidenya, Bukoba, Tanzania, 1985

More than 95% of them live in developing countries, where social, economic, cultural, and political conditions that contribute to the spread of the virus are more prevalent (see the following figures). In 2006 alone, more than 4.3 million new HIV infections occurred around the world. The most frightening concern for worldwide prevention and treatment efforts is the fact that more than half of all HIV-infected people, especially in developing countries, do not know they are infected. Sadly, in the absence of an affordable cure, most of the people in the world living with HIV will die within a decade (Johnson, 2007; UNAIDS, 2006).

The introduction of the "triple-drug cocktails" (various combinations of antiretroviral drugs and protease inhibitors in 1996 caused a significant drop in new AIDS cases and AIDS deaths in the United States. The new drug therapies, referred to as *highly active antiretroviral therapies* (HAART), have enabled persons infected with HIV to live longer, more healthful lives by slowing the progression of HIV infection

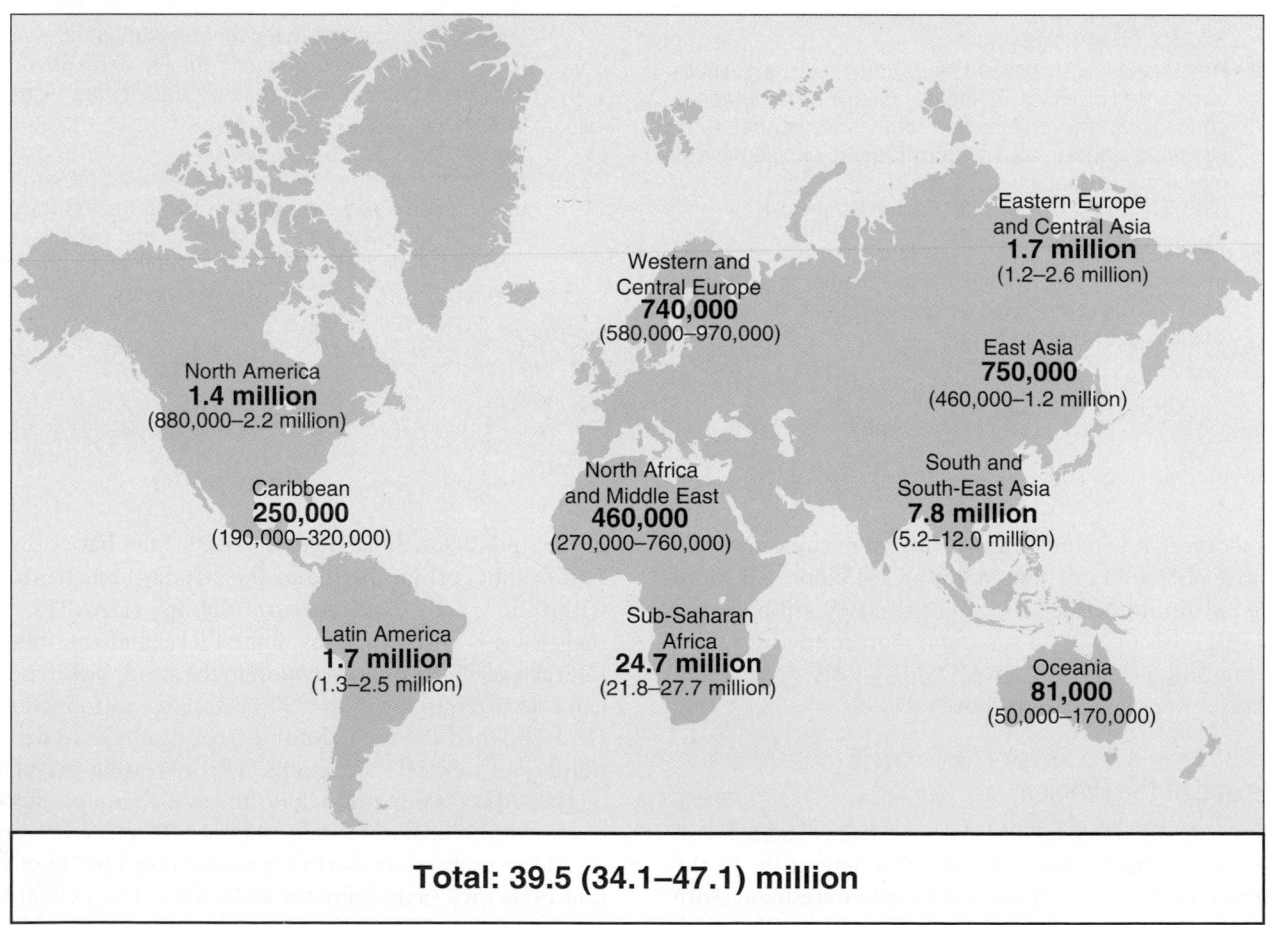

Adults and children estimated to be living with HIV in 2006.

*Source*: Reprinted by kind permission of UNAIDS. www.unaids.org

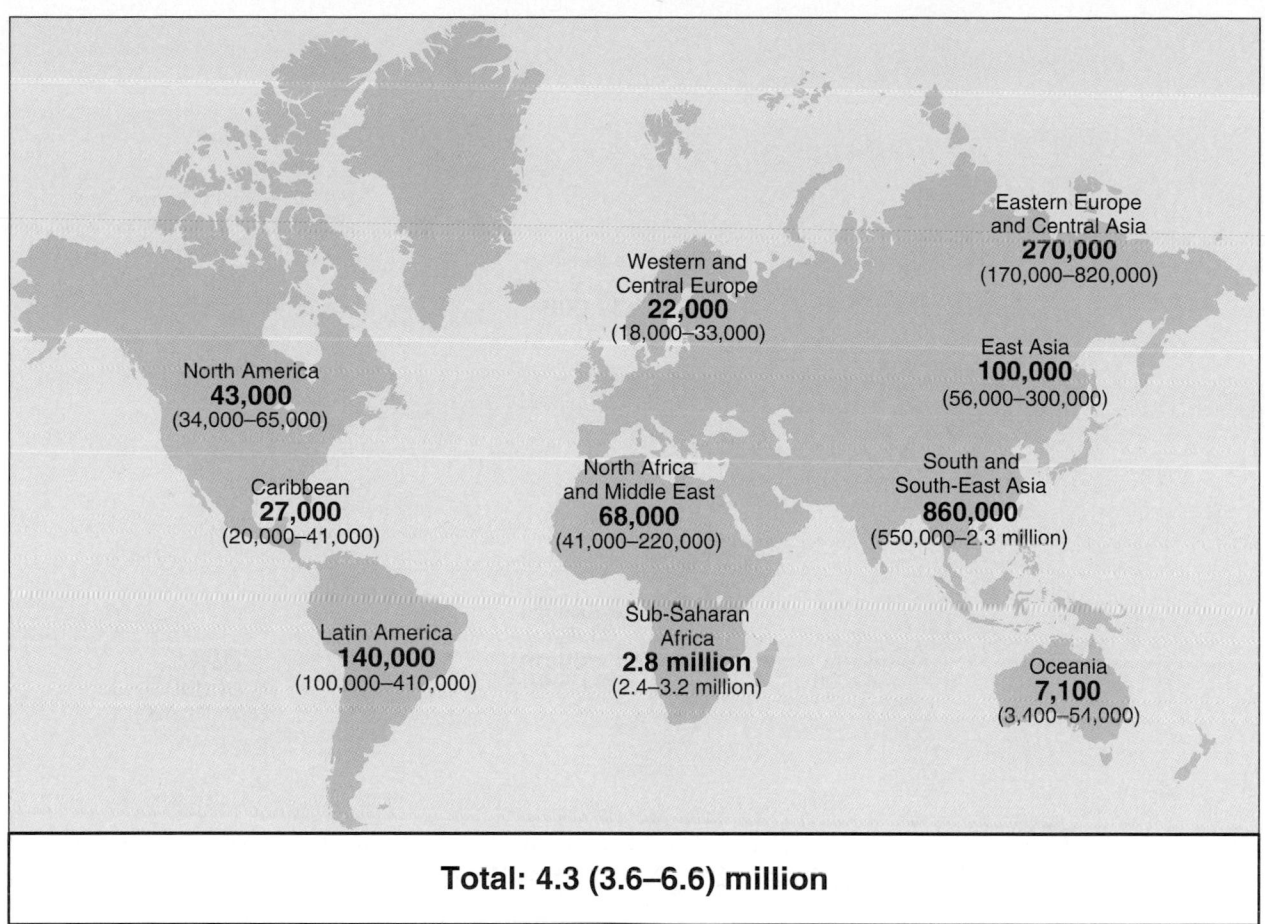

**Total: 4.3 (3.6–6.6) million**

Estimated number of adults and children newly infected with HIV during 2006.

*Source*: Reprinted by kind permission of UNAIDS. www.unaids.org

| Table 20-3 | PAHO Regional HIV/STI Plan for the Health Sector |
|---|---|

| Overall Objective | Critical Lines of Action, Targets, and Milestones |
|---|---|
| By 2015, halt and begin to reverse the spread of HIV/AIDS as well as STDs in the region of the Americas by providing universal access to prevention, care, and treatment. | To achieve the overall objective of the regional plan and to respond to countries' needs, five critical lines of action have been identified. |
| **Target 1:** By 2010, there will be a 50% reduction in the estimated number of new HIV infections, followed by a further 50% reduction in new infections by 2015. | 1. Strengthening health sector leadership and stewardship and fostering the engagement of civil society. |
| **Target 2:** By 2010, there will be universal access to comprehensive programs, and building human resources capacity. | 2. Designing and implementing effective, sustainable HIV/AIDS/STD care including prevention, care, and antiretroviral treatment. |
| **Target 3:** By 2015, incidence of mother-to-child transmission will be less than 5% and incidence of congenital syphilis will be less than 0.5 case per 1,000 live births. | 3. Strengthening, expanding, and reorienting health services. |
| | 4. Improving access to medicines, diagnostics, and other commodities. |
| | 5. Improving information and knowledge management, including surveillance, monitoring and evaluation, and dissemination. |

*Source*: Reproduced with the permission of the Pan American Health Organization. PAHO Regional HIV/STI Plan for the Health Sector Overall Objective and Proposed Lines of Action, 2005. To obtain information about PAHO publications visit their website at: http://publications.paho.org

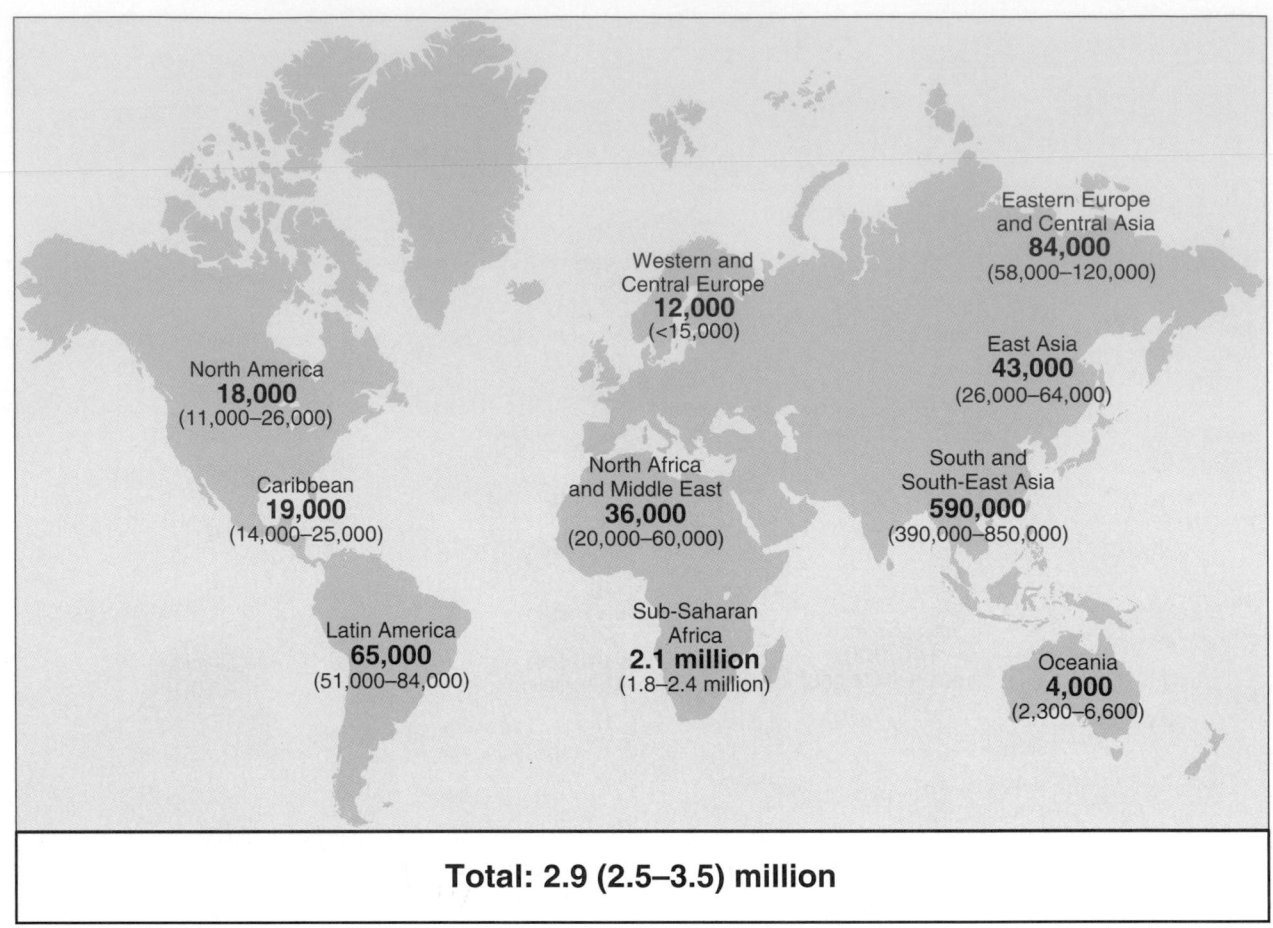

North America
**18,000**
(11,000–26,000)

Western and
Central Europe
**12,000**
(<15,000)

Eastern Europe
and Central Asia
**84,000**
(58,000–120,000)

East Asia
**43,000**
(26,000–64,000)

Caribbean
**19,000**
(14,000–25,000)

North Africa
and Middle East
**36,000**
(20,000–60,000)

South and
South-East Asia
**590,000**
(390,000–850,000)

Latin America
**65,000**
(51,000–84,000)

Sub-Saharan
Africa
**2.1 million**
(1.8–2.4 million)

Oceania
**4,000**
(2,300–6,600)

**Total: 2.9 (2.5–3.5) million**

Estimated adult and child deaths from AIDS during 2006.

*Source*: Reprinted by kind permission of UNAIDS. www.unaids.org

into AIDS and lowering the death rate from AIDS complications. Combination drug therapy can improve the ability of the drugs to control HIV so well that in many cases the viral load becomes so low that HIV cannot be detected in the blood. HAART may also significantly decrease the incidence of drug resistance in HIV patients when strict compliance to drug treatment regimes is maintained (Goodroad, 2003).

Unfortunately, HAART, which has been very effective in controlling the HIV disease progression in the United States, is not available to most of the people infected with HIV in the rest of the world. The high cost of the drugs exceeds the healthcare budgets of developing countries, where the majority of HIV-infected persons live. The number of people receiving HAART in low- and middle-income countries has tripled since 2001. However, even with these substantial increases, only one person in 10 in Africa and one in 7 in Asia who needs HAART was receiving it in 2005 (UNAIDS, 2005).

Treatment is problematic in the United States as well. The cost of HAART is prohibitive for many uninsured and underinsured patients. **Ryan White CARE Act** funding (Box 20-3), which was enacted in 1990 and reauthorized in

### 🖉 NOTE THIS! ●——

Rock icon, Nobel Peace Prize nominee, and fashion mogul Bono challenged the corporate world to start an AIDS-themed product line called Product Red, an offshoot of his own global AIDS conglomerate called Debt, AIDS, Trade, Africa (DATA). Companies such as American Express, Converse, Gap, and Giorgio Armani are releasing products with the Red label and sending part of the profits to the Global Fund to Fight AIDS, Malaria, and TB. Bono says, "I think doing the Red thing, doing good, will turn out to be good business for them."

*Source:* POZ, May 2006.

1996 and 2000, is providing the necessary drugs for some, but the number of patients needing treatment is increasing while funding is not. Also, while progression to clinical AIDS and eventual death has been slowed, the number of people with HIV remains high and continues to rise in certain populations. In 2006, the Ryan White CARE Act was reauthorized again. The new law includes expanded resources for women, children, and ethnic minorities (HRSA, 2006a).

## BOX 20-3

### Ryan White Comprehensive AIDS Resources Emergency CARE Act

. . . signed into law by the U.S. Congress on August 18, 1990, to improve the quality and availability of care for people with HIV/AIDS and their families.

. . . managed by the Health Resources and Services Administration (HRSA), an agency of the U.S. Department of Health and Human Services.

. . . HRSA's HIV/AIDS Bureau administers programs under four titles and Part F.

1. Title I—provides grants to metropolitan areas that are disproportionately affected by the HIV epidemic. Grants are awarded to the chief elected official and are used to fund services such as outpatient health care; support services like case management, home health and hospice care, housing and transportation assistance, nutrition services, and day care and respite care; and inpatient case management services that expedite discharge and prevent unnecessary hospitalization.

2. Title II—provides grants to the states and territories to provide services for people living with HIV/AIDS. Some of these services include home and community-based health care and support services; continuation of health insurance coverage; pharmaceutical treatments through an AIDS Drug Assistance Program; local organizations that assess needs and organize and deliver HIV services in collaboration with healthcare providers; and direct health services.

3. Title III—supports outpatient HIV early-intervention services for low-income, medically underserved people in existing primary care systems. Educational, clinical, and psychological services are provided for prevention, treatment, and support through community and migrant health centers, homeless programs, local health departments, family planning centers, and so on. Small time-limited grants are also available to prepare organizations to plan for the development of HIV early-intervention services or to provide capacity building for organizations to develop, enhance, or expand their capabilities to provide HIV primary care services.

4. Title IV—provides comprehensive, community-based, family-centered services for women, children, adolescents, and families. A special focus for Title IV is to help identify HIV-positive pregnant women and connect them to health care. A large percentage of the people served are from poor, minority families with limited access to housing and transportation.

5. Part F—provides funding for special programs and services related to HIV/AIDS. Examples include:
   - Special Projects of National Significance (SPNS) Program—supports the development of innovative models of HIV/AIDS care designed to address minority and hard to reach populations.
   - AIDS Education and Training Center Program—a national network of 15 centers that provide HIV/AIDS education and training for healthcare professionals.
   - HIV Dental Programs—(1) The Dental Reimbursement Program assists institutions with accredited dental or dental hygiene programs by defraying their unreimbursed costs associated with providing oral health care to people with HIV. (2) The Community-Based Dental Partnership Plan provides increased access to oral health services for HIV-positive individuals while providing education and clinical training for dental care providers, especially those located in community-based dental practices and clinics.

*Source:* HRSA, 2006a.

## ■ Populations at Risk for HIV/AIDS

The HIV/AIDS pandemic has affected different populations in different ways around the world. In the United States and Europe, HIV/AIDS has been primarily a male disease, with high rates of infection among homosexual and bisexual men, IDUs, and their sexual partners. In the early years of the U.S. epidemic, hemophiliacs were also infected at high rates because of contaminated blood products used in the production of factor VIII. However, after April 1985, when testing of the blood supply for HIV antibodies was initiated, the incidence of HIV in this population greatly declined and has remained low. In the rest of the world, however, the male/female HIV infection ratio has always been nearly equal, with transmission primarily through heterosexual contact (Vuylsteke, Sunkutu, & Laga, 1996). In recent years, we have seen new trends in HIV/AIDS infection in industrialized nations like the United States. Although infection rates remain high among homosexual and bisexual men, IDUs, and their sexual partners, the numbers of women, adolescents, and members of underrepresented ethnic groups, particularly African Americans and Latinos, have risen at alarming rates (HRSA, 2006a).

### Men Who Have Sex with Men

The fact that AIDS was first identified in 1981 in the American homosexual, Caucasian, male population, and was, in fact, called *gay-related immune deficiency syndrome* (GRID) for a short time, greatly affected the way it was perceived worldwide (Coxon, 1996; Shilts, 1987).

Because homosexual behavior is stigmatized in most societies, efforts aimed at prevention or treatment were limited early in the pandemic. However, gay organizations such as the Gay Men's Health Crisis Center in New York City and

ACT UP (AIDS Coalition to Unleash Power) were formed at the beginning of the U.S. epidemic and were instrumental in providing information and influencing HIV/AIDS policy.

The efforts of the gay population to spread the prevention message resulted in reported behavioral changes among gay, white males, with a subsequent drop in HIV/AIDS diagnoses during the late 1980s and 1990s. However, recent surveillance data show an increase in HIV/AIDS incidence for this group. Men who have sex with men (MSM) still continue to account for the largest number of people living with AIDS by risk group. It would be a mistake to think that high-risk behaviors are no longer a problem for MSM. Young men who have never lived in a world without HIV and who are possibly motivated by the success of HAART, which has minimized negative perceptions of HIV infection, are engaging in unprotected intercourse with greater frequency. This may be partly due to their misguided perceptions that HIV/AIDS is a disease of older gay men or that their peers are not practicing safer sex (CDC, 2007j).

Men of color account for and represent more than half of reported AIDS cases related to the MSM HIV exposure category. Many ethnic minority men have poor access to health care because of poverty and lack of health insurance. In addition, MSM of color must cope with many different types of stigma—for being a minority, for engaging in sexual activity with other men, and for being HIV positive. As a consequence, many ethnic minority MSM fear condemnation from their families, communities, and service providers. Men of color become infected at earlier ages than whites and are more likely to be diagnosed later in the disease process. Many minority MSM do not self-identify as gay or bisexual, meaning that prevention messages aimed at the gay community are often ineffective. They are often reluctant to seek services at organizations perceived to be gay oriented (HRSA, 2006b).

Community prevention programs must continue to address the needs of MSM, particularly young gay and bisexual men and gay and bisexual men of color. The involvement of social and political leaders in the community is important to be able to overcome cultural barriers related to homophobia and stigmatization. Prevention efforts must be geared to both uninfected and infected MSM, because research shows that HIV-infected MSM are continuing to practice high-risk sexual behavior. Treatment and prevention of other STDs are critical for this population because studies of MSM who are treated in STD clinics have shown consistently high rates of HIV infection (CDC, 2007j).

### Ethnic Minority Populations

In recent years, HIV/AIDS has disproportionately affected the African American and Hispanic/Latino communities in the United States. In fact, AIDS is the number one killer of African Americans and other blacks. Blacks account for more than 50% of new AIDS cases in the United States. This is particularly significant considering that African Americans make up only 13% of the total U.S. population (Arias, 2007; CDC, 2007k).

Although the statistics in Tables 20-4 and 20-5 reflect the fact that African American and Hispanic/Latino populations are disproportionately affected by HIV/AIDS, they are not meant to suggest that individuals are at high risk for HIV/AIDS just because they are members of ethnic minority groups. Community prevention efforts for HIV/AIDS must consider not only the multicultural nature of our U.S. society, but also social and economic factors such as poverty, unemployment, and poor access to health care that disproportionately affect ethnic minority populations.

Social barriers also play a significant role in blocking HIV/AIDS education efforts in ethnic communities, especially in African American and Hispanic communities,

**Table 20-4** Estimated Numbers of Cases and Rates (per 100,000 Population) of AIDS, by Race/Ethnicity, Age Category, and Sex, 2005—50 States and the District of Columbia

| | Adults or Adolescents | | | | | | Children (<13 years) | | Total* | |
| | Males | | Females | | Total* | | | | | |
| Race/Ethnicity | Number | Rate | Number | Rate | Number | Rate | Number | Rate | Number | Rate |
|---|---|---|---|---|---|---|---|---|---|---|
| White, not Hispanic | 10,852 | 13.1 | 1,830 | 2.1 | 12,681 | 7.5 | 8 | 0.0 | 12,689 | 6.3 |
| Black, not Hispanic | 14,216 | 103.6 | 7,776 | 49.9 | 21,992 | 75.0 | 39 | 0.5 | 22,030 | 59.0 |
| Hispanic | 6,558 | 39.7 | 1,865 | 12.2 | 8,423 | 26.4 | 9 | 0.1 | 8,432 | 19.8 |
| Asian/Pacific Islander | 444 | 8.2 | 104 | 1.8 | 547 | 4.9 | 1 | 0.1 | 549 | 4.0 |
| American Indian/ Alaska Native | 152 | 15.9 | 44 | 4.4 | 196 | 10.0 | 0 | 0.0 | 196 | 8.0 |
| **Total†** | **32,430** | **27.2** | **11,710** | **9.4** | **44,140** | **18.1** | **58** | **0.1** | **44,198‡** | **14.9** |

These numbers do not represent reported case counts. Rather, these numbers are point estimates, which result from adjustments of reported case counts. The reported case counts have been adjusted for reporting delays, but not for incomplete reporting.

Data exclude cases in persons whose state or area of residence is unknown, as well as cases from U.S. dependent areas, for which census information about race and age categories is lacking.

*Because row totals were calculated independently of values for the subpopulations, the values in each row may not sum to the row total.

†Includes person of unknown race or multiple races. Because column totals were calculated independently of the values for the subpopulations, the values in each column may not sum to the column total.

‡Includes 302 persons of unknown race or multiple races.

*Source:* CDC, 2006c.

**Table 20-5**  Estimated Numbers of Cases and Rates (per 100,000 Population) of HIV/AIDS, by Race/Ethnicity, Age Category, and Sex, 2005—33 States with Confidential Name-Based HIV Infection Reporting

| | Adults or Adolescents | | | | | | Children (<13 years) | | Total* | |
| | Males | | Females | | Total* | | | | | |
| Race/Ethnicity | Number | Rate | Number | Rate | Number | Rate | Number | Rate | Number | Rate |
|---|---|---|---|---|---|---|---|---|---|---|
| White, not Hispanic | 10,018 | 18.5 | 1,711 | 3.0 | 11,729 | 10.6 | 29 | 0.1 | 11,758 | 9.0 |
| Black, not Hispanic | 11,891 | 127.6 | 6,515 | 61.4 | 18,406 | 92.3 | 104 | 1.9 | 18,510 | 72.8 |
| Hispanic | 5,487 | 57.6 | 1,432 | 16.1 | 6,919 | 37.6 | 25 | 0.4 | 6,944 | 28.5 |
| Asian/Pacific Islander | 333 | 14.9 | 91 | 3.9 | 425 | 9.2 | 5 | 0.4 | 429 | 7.6 |
| American Indian/ Alaska Native | 141 | 19.5 | 57 | 7.6 | 198 | 13.4 | 0 | 0.0 | 198 | 10.6 |
| Total† | 28,037 | 37.0 | 9,893 | 12.4 | 37,930 | 24.4 | 166 | 0.5 | 38,096‡ | 20.2 |

These numbers do not represent reported case counts. Rather, these numbers are point estimates, which result from adjustments of reported case counts. The reported case counts have been adjusted for reporting delays, but not for incomplete reporting.

Data include persons with a diagnosis of HIV infection (not AIDS), a diagnosis of HIV infection and a later diagnosis of AIDS, or concurrent diagnoses of HIV infection and AIDS.

*Because row totals were calculated independently of values for the subpopulations, the values in each row may not sum to the row total.

†Includes person of unknown race or multiple races. Because column totals were calculated independently of the values for the subpopulations, the values in each column may not sum to the column total.

‡Includes 257 persons of unknown race or multiple races.

*Source:* CDC, 2006c.

where HIV/AIDS is still identified with homosexuality and drug use. Until HIV/AIDS prevention and treatment efforts gain support from the community, including churches and political leaders, HIV/AIDS will continue to affect ethnic minority groups in disproportionate numbers (CDC, 2007k).

### Illicit Drug Users

Although the estimated number of new HIV/AIDS cases among injection drug users (IDUs) has steadily decreased since 2001, injection drug use continues to contribute to the spread of HIV disease in significant proportions. Its impact on HIV transmission goes far beyond the circle of those who inject drugs. Sexual partners of IDUs are at high risk for HIV infection, as well as babies born to mothers who are IDUs or who have had sex with IDUs. Use of non-injection drugs, such as "crack" cocaine, also contributes to the spread of HIV/AIDS when drug users trade sex for drugs or money, or when they engage in risky sexual behavior that they would not engage in if not under the influence of drugs (CDC, 2002).

Substance abuse prevention is strongly related to HIV prevention, so comprehensive community-based programs must provide information, skills, and support for reducing risks for both. Community HIV/AIDS prevention programs require a wide range of approaches, including the following (NIDA, 2008):

- Initial drug use prevention
- Street outreach programs
- Access to high-quality substance abuse treatment programs
- HIV prevention programs in correctional facilities
- Comprehensive health care for HIV-infected drug users
- HIV risk-reduction counseling for drug users and their sex partners

Effective substance abuse treatment programs that assist people to eliminate drug use not only eliminate the risk of HIV transmission through contaminated needles, but also reduce the risk of engaging in behaviors that contribute to the risk for sexual transmission. Unfortunately, the need for substance abuse treatment in the United States greatly outweighs the ability to provide it. There is a long waiting list for admission to available drug treatment programs and U.S. laws exist that restrict the possession, distribution, or sale of any drug injection equipment. The U.S. government bans the use of federal funds for needle exchange programs that allow IDUs to exchange dirty needles for clean ones to reduce the transmission of HIV. Scientific studies have provided sufficient evidence that needle exchange programs, when combined with a comprehensive prevention program, reduce HIV transmission without increasing drug use (NIDA, 2008).

The absence of needle exchange programs and insufficient numbers of substance abuse treatment programs make efforts aimed at HIV prevention for IDUs even more critical. IDUs should be taught to use sterile needles and to never reuse needles. But if using sterile needles is not always possible, IDUs should be taught to clean their needles with a chlorine bleach and water solution between uses. However, it should be noted that cleaning needles with bleach is not as safe as using sterile needles (NIDA, 2008).

### Adolescents

Worldwide, greater and greater numbers of adolescents are infected with HIV. More than half of all new infections occur in those 15 to 24 years of age, with approximately 7,000 young people becoming infected each day (WHO, 2007). Adolescents in developing countries are most affected, but the risk is high for teens in industrialized countries, too.

In the United States and Canada, HIV is spreading, with 13% of all new infections in the United States occurring in young people between the ages of 13 and 24. Since the beginning of the epidemic, more than 40,000 young people in the United States have received a diagnosis of AIDS and more than 10,000 have died. They account for about 4% of all AIDS cases and 2% of total AIDS deaths in this country. During 2001–2004, in the states with long-term, confidential name-based HIV reporting, 62% of 13- to 24-year-olds with an HIV/AIDS diagnosis were males and 38% were females (CDC, 2006d).

Sexual exposure accounts for the majority of adolescent HIV infections. For young men, the biggest sexual risk is homosexual contact; for young women, it is heterosexual contact. Adolescents engage in multiple high-risk behaviors, often associated with drug and alcohol use. Alcohol and other drug use is common among high school students, often leading to high-risk sexual behavior. The 1995 CDC Youth Risk Behavior Surveillance shows that nearly 50% of all high school students have had sexual intercourse. By the time teens reach twelfth grade, more than 60% have had sexual intercourse. Nearly one in four sexually active twelfth graders have had four or more sex partners, yet only 50% of them report consistent condom use ("Youth Risk Behavioral Surveillance," 2006).

Adolescents are difficult to engage in the care needed for the diagnosis and treatment of HIV disease. They often believe they are invincible and tend to deny they are at risk. This belief may cause them to engage in high-risk behavior, delay HIV testing, or delay or refuse treatment when they have tested positive for HIV. When adolescents are treated by healthcare providers for other reasons, HIV risk is seldom discussed. Recent studies show that fewer than half of adolescents with histories of "survival sex" (sex to earn money to live on the street), injection drug use, same-gender sexual behavior, or prior STD infection seek treatment or help for these HIV-related issues. Thus prevention is the key weapon in reducing the incidence of adolescent HIV/AIDS (CDC, 2006b).

Behavioral science has shown that young people respond best to a balance of different approaches to prevention. To be effective, a wide range of activities must be implemented in communities. For example, school-based programs must include kindergarten through twelfth-grade education programs that address not only HIV prevention but also prevention of STDs, unintended pregnancy, and tobacco and drug use and programs that encourage healthy eating and physical exercise. School programs should address social norms that regulate gender roles, develop good decision-making skills, and increase self-esteem and self-efficacy. Other community-based programs to reach teens not in school are needed for homeless and runaway youth, juvenile offenders, or school dropouts (CDC, 2007).

### Women

Women are the fastest-growing group of people living with HIV/AIDS. Women account for 50% of cumulative AIDS cases worldwide. Globally, about half of the estimated 12,000 people ages 15 to 49 infected daily are women. The numbers are larger for younger women, who make up 62% of all people between the ages of 15 and 24 who are living with HIV/AIDS (Auerbach, 2004).

The "feminization of AIDS" is a result of many different factors—biological, social, economic, and political—that interact differently for women and men. More than a quarter century into the epidemic, gender inequality and the low status of women remain two of the major forces driving the spread of HIV/AIDS. Global responses to HIV have only just begun to address the social, cultural, legal, and economic factors that put women at risk for HIV infection and make treatment efforts more difficult. Women and girls traditionally have had less access to education and HIV information, have experienced inequality in marriage and sexual relationships, and have been the primary caregivers in their families and communities. Poverty is highly correlated with high rates of HIV. Worldwide, women are more likely than men to be poor with no source of personal income and no legal rights to property or inheritance (UNAIDS, 2007; WHO, 2004).

Violence is also a significant risk factor for women. Domestic violence is considered private—even normal—in many cultures. Laws protecting women in these societies are nonexistent, weak, or poorly enforced (Auerbach, 2004; UNAIDS, 2007). Rape is often used as a weapon for subjugation in war and armed conflict situations, especially in relation to "ethnic cleansing." International commitments are being made to

---

### ⚖ ETHICAL CONNECTION

In a study of HIV-risk behaviors, sexual orientation, and sexual abuse, surveys were used from five school-based cohorts in Seattle, Washington, and British Columbia. Secondary analyses were done on surveys of more than 800,000 adolescents conducted between 1992 and 2003. An HIV-risk scale of seven items assessed risky sexual behaviors and injection drug use. Self-identified sexual orientations included heterosexual, bisexual, and gay/lesbian. Analyses of co-variance were conducted separately by gender and were adjusted for age and sexual abuse when comparing means.

Gay/lesbian and bisexual adolescents had higher mean age-adjusted risk scores compared with heterosexual adolescents. When controlled for sexual abuse history, mean scores were 2 to 4 times higher among abused students than among nonabused students in each sexual orientation group. The study concluded that sexual minority adolescents reported higher HIV-risk behaviors, and higher prevalence of sexual victimization may partially explain these risks.

What are the ethical implications for community health nurses when working with high school students in at-risk, abusive relationships? ◯

*Source:* Saewyc, E., Skay, C., Richens, K., Reis, E., Poon, C., & Murphy, A. (2006). Sexual orientation, sexual abuse, and HIV-risk behavior among adolescents in the Pacific Northwest. *American Journal of Public Health, 96*(6), 1104–1110.

improve the status of women, but in many areas of the world efforts have been small scale and haphazard (UNAIDS, 2007).

Worldwide, most women are infected with HIV through heterosexual contact. Women are more biologically vulnerable to HIV than men, because the physiology of the female reproductive tract makes women two to four times as likely as men to acquire HIV during heterosexual sexual intercourse. In addition, cultural, legal, religious, and economic factors often limit the amount of control many women have over their own bodies, putting them at increased risk for HIV infection. For example, condom requests by women are often misinterpreted by male partners as an indication of mistrust or infidelity, leading to loss of the male partner or domestic violence. Women with minimal education and job skills are often unable to negotiate safer sex practices because of economic dependence on their partners for both themselves and their children (Auerbach, 2004; HRSA, 2006c; UNAIDS, 2007).

In the United States, HIV is taking an increasing toll on women. The proportion of all reported AIDS cases among adult and adolescent women more than tripled from 1985 to 2004, from 8% to 27% (Kaiser Foundation, 2006). For most of these women, heterosexual sex (70%) or injection drug use (28%) are the primary means of HIV transmission. HIV infection rates are highest among women of color. In fact, the rate of HIV/AIDS among African American women is 23 times higher and the rate among Hispanic women is 5 times higher than the rate among Caucasian women. African American women account for two-thirds of the female HIV/AIDS cases in the United States, even though they account for only 13% of the total female population. Latina women account for almost 17% of the female HIV/AIDS and 14% of the total female population. In 2002, HIV/AIDS was the leading cause of death in women of color aged 25 to 44, but the sixth leading cause of death for women in that age group overall (Kaiser Foundation, 2006).

Cultural and economic factors also mean that many women do not have access to preventive care and early treatment, resulting in their later diagnosis and earlier death from HIV/AIDS. Research, prevention, and care activities for women have been slow to develop, even though the number of women infected in the developing world has been equal to the number of men infected since the beginning of the pandemic. Much of this may be related to the unequal role and status of women worldwide. Another factor may be that, until recently, the proportion of cases of AIDS in women in the industrialized world, where most of the research is conducted, was much lower than for men.

Because most women with HIV/AIDS are of childbearing age, most of the research involving women with HIV has centered on reproduction, with an emphasis on the fetus or infant. HAART has been the standard treatment for HIV-infected pregnant women in the United States since 1992, an approach that has reduced perinatal HIV infection from a high of 30% to approximately 2%. Although it is a positive breakthrough that fewer children are becoming infected with HIV, a small number of perinatal infections continue to oc-

cur each year, primarily among African Americans (Kaiser Foundation, 2006). Parents with HIV/AIDS—and particularly mothers, because they are often single parents—are often confronted with difficult decisions about what and how to tell their children about their illness and who will care for their orphaned children if they die.

As a result of the emphasis on the maternal role, many women living with HIV have been stigmatized as a potential source of infection, instead of being regarded as people with their own healthcare needs. HIV/AIDS is often associated with guilt or blame because becoming infected with HIV implies failure in the traditional and expected role of women as caregivers and moral guardians who are responsible for the next generation (Aranda-Naranjo, Barini-Garcia, Pounds, & Davis, 2005).

Currently, the female condom is the only female-initiated HIV prevention method available. It is bulkier and more expensive than male condoms and has been poorly marketed. Its obvious presence makes it more likely to be rejected by male partners during intercourse. An effective microbicide would be a big breakthrough in the search for female-controlled HIV prevention not detectable by males. "First-generation" candidate microbiocides are currently being tested in large-scale efficacy trials in Africa and Asia. A microbiocide that is only 60% effective could potentially prevent as many as 1 million new HIV infections per year. Research is under way to develop "second-generation" microbiocides with higher efficacy rates for future testing (UNAIDS, 2007).

With an effective microbiocide still years in the future, community HIV-prevention efforts need to emphasize interventions aimed at women. Conventional education programs that address male and female condom negotiation and use, routine HIV testing, and drug abuse still need to be implemented, but programs that address domestic abuse, self-esteem, and self-efficacy need to be developed and implemented as well. In addition, more community-supported domestic crisis centers, daycare facilities, educational and job training programs, and support groups specifically for women at risk need to be established. High-quality care for women living with HIV must address not only their medical and physical needs, but also their economic needs, their relationships, their culture, their emotional needs, and their spiritual needs. In other words, a systems approach is needed to address all aspects of a woman's life (Aranda-Naranjo et al., 2005).

---

☞ THINK ABOUT THIS ·····················

Ninety-two percent of women carry lip protection. Ten percent of women carry HIV prevention.
—American Foundation for AIDS Research (AmFAR), public service slogan, 2004

---

**❝***The stigma about AIDS comes from machismo. There's a lack of communication in the home and everywhere else—women are taught that men are in charge of sex.* **❞**

—*Amelia Vega, Miss Universe 2003*

### Children

UNAIDS and WHO estimate that, throughout the world, approximately 4 million children younger than 15 years of age have been infected with HIV since the epidemic began in 1981. More than 90% of them were infants born to HIV-positive mothers. Because HIV infection progresses quickly in children, most HIV-infected children younger than age 15 have progressed to AIDS, and most of these have died. In several African countries, the under-5 mortality rate rose from 2% in 1990 to 6.5% in 2003, adding another devastating consequence to the HIV epidemic (CAH, 2005; UNAIDS, 2005).

Although the numbers of people receiving HAART in low- and middle-income countries has more than tripled since the end of 2001, the fact remains than only one person in 10 in Africa and one in seven in Asia in need of treatment received it in 2005. While international efforts to provide adequate treatment and prevention programs are moving faster, the HIV infection rate is still sprinting far ahead of providers' efforts. Worldwide, fewer than one in five people at risk for HIV infection has access to basic prevention services and only one in 10 people living with HIV has been tested and is aware that he or she is infected (UNAIDS, 2005). Without HAART, the infection rate for children born to mothers with HIV is between 25% and 30%; with HAART, the infection rate for children born to mothers with HIV is less than 2%. It is obvious that comprehensive prevention, treatment, and support programs have nearly eliminated HIV transmission from mothers to their babies in industrialized countries. Some healthcare professionals say that having a life-saving treatment that is available only to a privileged few is the highest form of human cruelty.

In addition to bringing suffering and death for those infected, the HIV/AIDS epidemic has had another devastating consequence: 13 million children around the world have lost their mothers or both parents to HIV/AIDS. AIDS orphans have become a major problem in the developing world. In parts of Africa, grandparents whose adult children have succumbed to HIV/AIDS are raising as many as 30 grandchildren with very few resources. In other families, children younger than 12 are struggling to care for dying parents and to raise younger siblings after their parents have died. With the family wage-earners dead or dying, these fragmented families are sinking further into abysmal poverty. The intense psychological stress already experienced from dealing with poverty and illness is intensified by the stigma associated with HIV/AIDS. Increasingly, these children must withdraw from school, losing any opportunities for acquiring the knowledge and skills needed to create sound families and living environments for the future (CAH, 2005).

In the United States, almost all new HIV/AIDS infections diagnosed in children are a result of perinatal transmission. In 2004, an estimated 48 AIDS cases were diagnosed among children younger than 13, a 61.3% decrease from 2000. In the 25 states with confidential name-based HIV reporting, the number of perinatally infected infants dropped by 75.5% between 1994 and 2004 (HRSA, 2006d). Although new HIV infections among infants have dropped dramatically, some infections still occur, often because HIV-positive pregnant women do not always get appropriate prenatal care with HIV counseling, testing, or treatment. In 2004, of the children living with AIDS, 63% were black and 21.6% were Hispanic (CDC, 2007). Babies infected at birth are living longer than ever because of treatment measures, with many reaching adolescence or young adulthood; however, they remain at risk for the physical and psychosocial complications related to HIV infection, such as mental illness, body image problems related to delayed development, chronic skin conditions, or lipdystrophy (HRSA, 2006d).

### Older People

The number of older people (older than 50 years) with HIV or AIDS is growing rapidly. Between 10% and 15% of people with AIDS in the United States are more than 50 years old. In some cities, as many as 25% of AIDS cases involve older people. Making an initial AIDS diagnosis in older people is common, with half of all people older than 50 with AIDS having been infected for less than a year. Older adults are infected through the same high-risk behaviors as young adults, though they many not be aware that they are at risk for HIV/AIDS. Unfortunately, few HIV education campaigns target older Americans (AIDS InfoNet, 2008; Gottesman, 2005; NAHOF, 2007).

The older population is steadily growing larger with the maturing of the "baby-boomer" generation. Social norms about divorce, sex, and dating are changing, and drugs such as Viagra are facilitating a more active sex life for older adults (NAHOF, 2007). Heterosexual women age 50 and older are most in need of the HIV-prevention message. Most stop using protection because pregnancy is no longer a concern. After menopause, however, decreased lubrication and thinning vaginal walls put them at higher risk for HIV transmission (Gottesman, 2005).

Rates of HIV infection (not AIDS) are difficult to determine in the older population because older people are not routinely tested, early misdiagnosis is common, and the immune system naturally weakens with age (NAHOF, 2007). Healthcare and service providers—and often older people themselves—do not realize that elders have many of the same risk factors as other populations, including having unprotected sex (homosexual and heterosexual) and using illicit drugs. Healthcare providers are often reluctant to initiate discussions related to sexuality with their older patients (AIDS InfoNet, 2008; NAHOF, 2007).

HAART seems to work as well in older people as it does in younger people in controlling viral loads, for both newly infected people and people who were diagnosed and began treatment before age 50 and then got older. However, T-cell levels do not recover as quickly in older people and treatment side effects may be more frequent. Older people

## Application to Practice

### *Providence Home and Family Services, Inc.*

In 1989, the University of Texas Health Science Center in San Antonio, Texas, established the South Texas AIDS Center for Children and Families, a Ryan White Title IV-funded demonstration project, with John Mangos, MD, as director and Barbara Aranda-Naranjo, RN, as assistant director. The mission of the project was to provide comprehensive health services to children and their families infected and affected by HIV disease.

During the first year of the project, many children experienced the death and/or debilitation of one or both parents. Many of the children were being left orphans or needed a safe place to stay while their parents were hospitalized. After observing this phenomenon, nurse Barbara Aranda-Naranjo saw a need for a residential/respite care for children. After discussion with Dr. Mangos and other community leaders, she approached another nurse colleague, Sr. Barbara Hyzak, RN, and began exploring the idea of a respite center. Sr. Barbara Hyzak was a member of the Sisters of Divine Providence, a Catholic order of nuns, and the director of the Stella Maris Clinic. The clinic, located in the west side of San Antonio, served the poor and migrants that had worked in the area for more than 30 years. As a result of changes in migrant employment and the establishment of other for-profit and non-profit clinics, the sisters were looking for a new mission for the clinic.

After discussion about the needs of the children and families living with HIV infection, a proposal was developed to present to the clinic board of directors. The proposal included the description of the needs of the population and the link with the South Texas AIDS Center. In addition, the primary goal of the proposal was to set up a residential care center and day care in place of the Stella Maris clinic. The development of the proposal was a joint effort with the University of Texas Health Science Center, the Sisters of Divine Providence, and other community-based organizations such as Project ABC.

Providence Home was established in 1990 as a non-profit agency to serve the needs of women, children, and their families infected and affected by AIDS. The Texas Department of Health granted Providence Home a license as a special care facility. The home offers services to infants and children from birth to 13 years of age. The services included residential as well as respite care for children. The first director was Sister Barbara Hyzak, RN.

In 1993, the home opened the Providence Home Learning Center as a therapeutic daycare center. The learning center is open five days a week from 9 A.M. to 3 P.M. The capacity of the learning center is 30 children. Providence Home is staffed with full-time and part-time employees. The University of Texas Health Science Center, the South Texas AIDS Center, and the University of the Incarnate Word Nursing School provide nursing, medical, and psychological support. A vast number of volunteers and nursing students also make contributions to Providence Home's quality of health services. The current director of Providence Home is Carol Bova-Rice; the Sisters of Divine Providence continue to sponsor the home.

Applying the nursing assessment of the environment, two nurses in this case study were able to observe a need in the community, develop a proposal, and create a home from an existing health center. The collaboration by these two nurses assisted in the creation of both a residential and respite center that has met the needs of many families living with HIV infection in South Texas. More than 100 families have benefited from the services of Providence Home, which continues to serve the changing needs of families living with HIV infection.

---

generally have other chronic health conditions that require medications that may adversely interact with HAART (AIDS InfoNet, 2008; NAHOF, 2007).

## ■ Nursing Care of Families with HIV

Nursing care for families with HIV-infected children requires an in-depth assessment of the needs of all members of the family. The nurse should initially ask the primary caregiver, usually the mother, but sometimes the father or grandparent, who is considered to be family and who in the family knows about the HIV status.

This analysis should include the physical, psychological, social, and spiritual needs of every member of the family. It is also helpful to draw a family genogram to determine the relationships and lines of communication in the family. The assessment cannot be done in one visit, and the nurse should be sensitive to the emotional stress of the primary caregiver and plan accordingly for a series of visits to complete the assessment.

A multidisciplinary family care plan may be developed based on the initial assessment and the input of team members such as the psychologist, physician, or social worker. The primary caregiver can give input into the care plan and may be provided with a copy. The care plan should be updated at least quarterly, especially for families with three or more infected members.

Educational sessions for every member of the family may be established based on the initial and subsequent assessments and recorded as goals and objectives on the care plan. Educational sessions may also include addressing social, emotional, or spiritual issues. The nurse must consider that there will be episodic failures for the caregiver in achieving objectives and must be prepared to help the family through these normal episodes (Crespo-Fierro, 1997).

The entire plan of care and the coordination for meeting the multiple needs of any family must take place using a sensitive and compassionate approach. Many women and children feel isolated, depressed, and overwhelmed by their HIV infection. The nurse and the multidisciplinary staff can give anticipatory guidance and thereby increase the quality of life for the entire family.

## STDs and the U.S. Healthcare System

### ■ Problems of Access

Most of the disease burden produced by sexually transmitted infections, including HIV/AIDS, could be prevented or treated with increased access to services, expanded screening and treatment, and behavior changes that lower STD risk. Clearly, a widespread availability of high-quality STD care is necessary to ensure that infections are detected and treated in a timely and appropriate manner. Despite increased media efforts to inform the public, many Americans still believe

> **"***Yes, it's true life can be scary, but life can also be exciting, thrilling, and fabulous. And to be honest with you, I would much rather have life than the alternative. I don't regret this disease. It's taught me some valuable lessons—helped me face some exciting and new challenges and introduced me to some charming people. All of which never would have happened had it not been for this disease. It's true I may die tomorrow. But if I do die, I'm going to die happy, without regrets. If I had to live my life all over again, I wouldn't change a thing. I'd take it all—AIDS included. I don't have HIV, I have AIDS and I am proud of who I am. And I am proud of the person I am going to become. My name is Rob Lanier and I have AIDS and I am alive. I am alive! I am alive!***"*
>
> *—Rob Lanier died in 1995, at the age of 28*

that all STDs are curable, and many more are not aware that having an STD facilitates HIV transmission. STDs that cause genital lesions can create a portal of entry for HIV. Even without lesions, STDs increase the number of CD4 target cells in cervical secretions, thereby increasing HIV susceptibility in women. In fact, people who are already infected with an STD are two to five times more likely to become infected with HIV. Yet only half the public health departments in this country provide STD services, compared with 97% that provide immunizations (AAWH, 1999; Landry & Forrest, 1996).

### ■ Health Services

STD care is often lacking outside of dedicated STD clinics. Community outreach for STD prevention programs

---

### 🏛 HEALTHY PEOPLE 2010

**Objectives Related to HIV**

13.1 Reduce AIDS among adolescents and adults.

13.2 Reduce the number of new AIDS cases among adolescent and adult men who have sex with men.

13.3 Reduce the number of new AIDS cases among females and males who inject drugs.

13.4 Reduce the number of new AIDS cases among adolescent and adult men who have sex with men and inject drugs.

13.5 Reduce the number of cases of HIV infection among adolescents and adults.

13.6 Increase the proportion of sexually active persons who use condoms.

13.7 Increase the number of HIV-positive persons who know their serostatus.

13.8 Increase the proportion of substance abuse treatment facilities that offer HIV/AIDS education, counseling, and support.

13.9 Increase the number of state prison systems that provide comprehensive HIV/AIDS, sexually transmitted diseases, and tuberculosis (TB) education.

13.10 Increase the proportion of inmates in state prison systems who receive voluntary HIV counseling and testing during incarceration.

13.11 Increase the proportion of adults with tuberculosis (TB) who have been tested for HIV.

13.12 Increase the proportion of adults in publicly funded HIV counseling and testing sites who are screened for common bacterial sexually transmitted diseases (STDs) (chlamydia, gonorrhea, and syphilis) and are immunized against hepatitis B virus.

13.13 Increase the proportion of HIV-infected adolescents and adults who receive testing, treatment, and prophylaxis consistent with current Public Health Service guidelines.

13.14 Reduce deaths from HIV infection.

13.15 Extend the interval of time between an initial diagnosis of HIV infection and AIDS diagnosis in order to increase years of life of an individual infected with HIV.

13.16 Increase years of life of an HIV-infected person by extending the interval of time between an AIDS diagnosis and death.

13.17 Reduce new cases of perinatally acquired HIV infection.

*Source:* DHHS, 2000.

## *a conversation with . . .*

Dr. Ann Lanier congratulates her son, Rob, on his one-man stage play. New York City, 1994.

On Saturday, February 18, 1995, we held a memorial for Rob at the Ridiculous Theater in New York City—among his friends and family—among stage props and red gels and sound equipment and fading velvet curtains—among wigs and green eyeliner—among photographs of him in a multitude of silly costumes—with him in his laughing face and somber mood. Among 200 daffodils and hundreds of daffodil bulbs tied up in yellow tulle and small green ribbons, we ate his favorite food and listened to his collection of music. We shared a moment of love with friends and family who played tribute to him by playing the flute, dancing, reading poetry, and performing dramatic readings. We told stories of his generosity, his silliness, his love of living—and among all the daffodils and all the promises of spring and life, we said good-bye to his physical presence on earth.

Such a strong and loving spirit will stay with us. As his mother, I will always see the boy who organized a production of *Candide* using the children who lived on his mountainside in Colorado. The little boy in Texas who talked his rough-and-tumble cousins into putting on a musical production

for all the relatives in his grandfather's barn among the bales of hay. The young man trying out for the role of the older "young prince" in the summer production of *Richard III* in Boulder. When called back for the fourth time, the director said, "I'd love to cast you as the young prince, but you're three inches taller than the lead." The young man who lied about his age so he could go to work to help his single mother. The young man, who in his free time, spent long hours directing the senior citizens group in their production of *Blithe Spirit.* The young man who played the role of the father in *What's the Matter with Father?* because it had a special meaning to him that he never explained. The young man who walked 4 miles in the Colorado winter to take his SATs. The young man who tried out for NYU's Tisch School of the Arts by performing a piece he wrote, *Gorilla Warfare in Texas.* The young college student who worked double shifts and tried to pawn his watch to get the money to go to Paris for all the love and adventure it promised.

We, as his family, will always see the man who lived and worked among people he loved, in all the tears and laughter of the theater. We will see the man with our family on the Chesapeake Bay that he loved, with the red and gold of fall leaves, the dogs, and the boats. And with the family that came much later in life than it should have, with whom he felt loved and accepted for being "Rob" and was always chosen first for a game of Trivial Pursuit. Above all we remember his last play, *Mortality Waltz,* that taught us about coming of age, about life, and about living with AIDS.

Until his last breath, Rob did just as he promised in his play. He lived every moment of his life. He said, "I will not discuss dying. I will only talk of living." He did just that. He never spoke of dying again. His energy—his sense of love and life—stayed with him as it will always stay with each of us who loved him. Family and friends were with him and held his hands long after that beautiful spirit left his body and wrapped around us like a cloak. We cry now because we must reach back into our memories to pull out his laughter—to see his smile—to hear him tell us stories—to feel his arms around us—or to see him wink. We desperately miss the touch, feel, and smell of that wonderful person, and the world will miss so many more gifts he had to offer.

—**Dr. Ann Thedford Lanier,**
Mother of Rob Lanier

Chapter author Dr. Sharyn Janes (center) plans a statewide HIV education program for healthcare providers with Craig Thompson (left), Director of the STD/HIV Division of the Mississippi State Department of Health, and Cheryl Hamill, RN, Director of the Resource Center of the Delta Region AIDS Education and Training Center at the University of Mississippi Medical Center.

have increased, but cuts in funding have limited many of the services offered. Public health clinics cannot reach all of the people who need STD care, and greater effort is needed to stimulate and encourage private providers to take sexual histories, screen for asymptomatic infections, and provide a range of STD services in their practices. More recently, managed care organizations have emerged as a dominant organizational framework for medical care across much of the United States, particularly for the more disadvantaged segments of the population, and could serve many individuals at risk for STDs. However, STD and HIV prevention and testing are not generally included in routine services.

## ■ Screening and Prevention

People often do not know they are infected with STDs because they do not have or do not recognize symptoms. Studies of STD screening outside of healthcare settings (e.g., in jails, workplaces, and other community-based settings) reveal that a large number of persons with gonorrhea and chlamydia have no symptoms or signs of infection (CDC, 2006b, 2007b, 2007c).

The fact that gonorrhea and chlamydia so often do not produce any symptoms has many implications for community health nursing because no matter how effectively access to healthcare is enhanced, many of these silent infections will go undetected and untreated unless screening and treatment are provided in nontraditional settings. Even though asymptomatic individuals will not access health care specifically for STD testing or treatment, they do visit a variety of healthcare settings for other purposes. There are many opportunities to identify and treat asymptomatic but infected persons in healthcare settings when they present for other unrelated problems (e.g., in emergency rooms, in family planning clinics, during routine or sports physicals, during immunization visits) and in nonhealthcare settings such as schools and jails.

## The Role of Community Health Nurses

To prevent the spread of STDs, it is not enough to screen for and treat infections; community nurses also need to be able to help individuals change their behavior by counseling about how to prevent infections and reinfections. It is not who one is but what one does that determines whether a person becomes infected or reinfected with an STD. Screening and treating infection are effective for a current infection, but unless individuals can be helped to change their behavior, they may continue to behave in ways that put them at risk for further infections.

A number of different behaviors can be targeted to reduce infections: increasing the seeking of appropriate health care, improving patients' adherence to medication and cooperation with efforts to notify their partners of possible infection, reducing the rate of partner change, and lowering the number of sex partners. Increasing consistent and correct condom use can prevent some infections, such as gonorrhea and HIV, but is less effective with other STDs such as HPV. The most effective counseling interventions are those that are directed at a specific behavior. Perhaps the most difficult task facing community health nurses is identifying the behaviors that warrant change for specific patients and matching their intervention to the patients' readiness to change behavior.

Decisions about the behaviors in need of change should be based on a careful assessment of the patient's sexual and drug-use history. Although many nurses are uncomfortable taking such histories, most patients view sexual and drug histories as an expected part of a medical examination. At the very least, information should be gathered about the number and type of sexual partners (regular and occasional partners), types of sex practiced, condom use (with regular and occasional partners), use of both injected and noninjected drugs, and in the case of IDUs, information about their use of sterile syringes and disinfection of shared injection paraphernalia. It is only by taking such histories that behaviors that are placing the patient at risk can be identified. These behaviors should then be the target of the nursing intervention ("Sexually transmitted diseases," 2006).

All too often, however, the goals of an intervention are vague (e.g., staying healthy, losing weight, preventing an STD), rather than focusing on a specific changeable behavior (e.g., always using a condom with every partner, telling one's partner to always use a condom). It is the latter type of intervention that is most likely to produce successful behavior changes. The distinction between overly broad goals and specific behaviors is not always obvious. For example, "using condoms" is not a specific behavior but a broad goal. Condoms are used for specific sexual activities with specific partners, and the factors that influence condom use for

## Research Alert

This study examined the effects of an HIV prevention intervention on women's condom-use behaviors. The community-level intervention targeted sexually active women of child-bearing age in four different inner-city communities. At the beginning of the study, nearly 70% of the participants did not intend to use condoms with their sexual partners. After 2 years of theory-based and culturally specific intervention activities, increases in talking with partners about condoms and attempting to use condoms with partners were significantly larger in the intervention communities than in comparison communities. The results of this study show that (1) large-scale community interventions can be implemented successfully in low-income, inner-city neighborhoods; (2) many women were still not using condoms, which confirms the necessity for relevant, effective prevention interventions that target women; and (3) a community-level intervention can affect women's condom-use behavior. To be successful in low-income neighborhoods, interventions must address social, economic, and cultural issues that affect the target population's access to information and its ability to focus on health-related behaviors.

*Source:* Lauby, J. L., Smith, P. J., Stark, M., Person, B., & Adams, J. (2000). A community-level HIV prevention intervention for inner-city women: Results of the women and infants demonstration projects. *American Journal of Public Health, 90*(2), 216–222.

vaginal sex with a spouse are different from those that can influence condom use with an occasional partner. Furthermore, while using a male condom is a behavior for men, for women, the goal may be a behavior that influences the partner's behavior.

People also differ in their readiness for change. The type of counseling a nurse provides is more effective when it is matched to the individual's readiness to make changes. The **transtheoretical model of behavior change** is a helpful framework for understanding individual differences and for identifying appropriate interventions (Prochaska, Redding, Harlow, Rossi, & Velicer, 1994). Some individuals who are engaging in risky behaviors will have no intention of changing their behavior or adopting more healthful behaviors (precontemplative stage). Any one of several strategies (e.g., recognizing that the behavior is putting them at risk) may help those individuals to consider change, whether immediately or in the future (contemplative stage). After deciding to change the behavior, initial attempts to adopt new behaviors may follow (preparation or ready for action stage). Eventually, a new behavior is adopted (action stage) and will become a routine part of the person's life (maintenance stage). Movement through these stages may be sequential, or the person may skip some stages or relapse back to an earlier stage, and then cycle back through the stages several times

before he or she successfully reaches long-term maintenance of a new behavior.

To help people change behavior, the nurse should first determine where each person is on this continuum of behavior change and then develop an intervention to help him or her move toward the next stage. Generally speaking, if the person has decided to make a change, has the skills to be able to perform the new behavior, and does not face environmental barriers that will prevent him or her from making the change, it is almost certain that the new behavior will be performed.

Once the risk assessment has been completed and a decision reached about what behavior needs to be the first target of an intervention, the next step is to assess the person's readiness and capability to perform that behavior. This can easily be evaluated by asking the patient if he or she plans on starting (or continuing) to practice the risk-reducing behavior. For example, "Do you plan to use condoms every time you have sex with your boyfriend? How sure are you about this?" If the person wants to perform the behavior but has not been able to do so, it is important to determine whether this is because he or she does not have the skills to act on the good intentions or whether environmental constraints are preventing him or her from doing so. Depending on which of these is operating, the intervention can be directed at increasing the person's skill or at helping the individual to overcome the perceived barriers. If the person has no intention of performing the safer behavior, the intervention can be directed at helping to motivate the person to make a change. This may involve helping the person to change his or her attitudes about the behavior, addressing social pressures to perform or not perform the behavior, or reinforcing beliefs that the person can do so successfully (self-efficacy).

For example, let's assume that a sexual history indicated that a young woman was at risk for acquiring an STD because she had no intention whatsoever of using a condom for vaginal sex with her boyfriend. The following questions provide an example of how to elicit information that would help guide counseling for her:

- Do you feel mostly positive or mostly negative about always using a condom for vaginal sex with your boyfriend?
- Do people who are important to you think you should or should not always use a condom when you have vaginal sex with your boyfriend?
- Considering all of the things that can make it difficult to always use a condom, how certain are you that you could always use a condom for vaginal sex with your boyfriend?

If the first question reveals that the person has negative attitudes toward using condoms, the next step is to try to understand the person's beliefs about using condoms. For example, she can be asked to describe what she thinks will happen if condoms are always used for vaginal sex with her boyfriend. More specifically, she can be asked to describe what she thinks are the advantages and the disadvantages. Counseling can then be directed at disputing counterproductive beliefs that lead to negative outcomes and at increasing or strengthening beliefs that will lead to positive outcomes.

If her answers to the second question indicate that important others are opposed to consistent condom use, then it becomes important to understand which of the people in her social network support and oppose condom use. She can be asked about specific individuals in her social network who would oppose consistent condom use and to describe who would think consistent condom use for vaginal sex with her boyfriend was a good thing to do. The interaction can then be directed at clarifying misperceptions or pointing out others in her life who would be supportive.

Finally, if the young woman was positively predisposed to using condoms and had supportive social relationships but little sense of self-efficacy with respect to condom use, then a more careful examination of the reasons for her low self-efficacy need to be examined. She can be asked to describe the things that make it hard to consistently use condoms with her boyfriend (barriers) and to describe things that would make it easier to consistently use condoms (facilitators). The intervention can then be directed at helping her to overcome barriers or find ways to facilitate condom use. It is also essential to pay attention to whether the person has the skills to be able to carry out the behavior. This may involve demonstrating how to use a condom correctly and having the patient practice the behavior several times using

## " a conversation with . . . "

I am on the road to AIDS. I knew it first in 1991. I had just survived a bitter divorce. I was not ready to have a 3- and a 1-year-old, no husband, and AIDS. If I offered a prayer those days, it might have been, "Why me, O Lord? Why me?" Over time, whatever my complaints had been gave way to something better and more useful. I began to see AIDS as less than a curse in my life, and more as a call to speak out, to show courage to my children, and to ask others to consider healing instead of indifference and compassion instead of judgment. I was not a victim, I was a pilgrim, called by God to walk humbly and obediently with other pilgrims on the road to AIDS. I didn't know what I could do that might make a difference. But I decided to speak out. For gay men who had been rejected by their families, I spoke out. For women who were isolated, and frightened, and powerless, I spoke out. From the echoing halls of the United States Senate to the whisper-quiet corridors of hospitals, I spoke out—believing that by speaking out, I could make a difference.

And then I looked around to see what difference I had made. I was still a pilgrim walking down the road to AIDS. Those who had lined the pilgrims' road still called out judgments, still rejected those who were sick and dying, still hurled insults and discrimination at pilgrims as we marched by. That had not changed. The only change I saw was that the pilgrim band grew larger every year. The number of women first doubled, then tripled, then went beyond counting. And the pilgrims were increasingly drawn from communities of color. The hard, plain truth was that I couldn't change it. Only God could do that. And so with Carvin Winans and a few friends, the idea of Gospel Against AIDS was born, conceived in the belief that we need to reach into our neighborhoods—into the apartments and the alleyways, the gas stations and the beauty shops.

And that's why we're here. To tell the nation's policy makers that our children are growing sick and dying, to insist that power and money support compassion and hope. To remind the nation that we need forgiveness. To remember when AIDS was a "gay disease," we did not care, as if those who were gay were less than God's children; and to confess that now as our women and children become infected, we do care—that's why we seek forgiveness. Once we were a part of the crowd that said, "They do not matter. Let them go. . . ." But we are here to say that they do matter, that they are not less than God's other children.

Because AIDS is creating orphans who need parents, who need community, who need love and comfort that only flows from God's children—that's why we're here. We are here for the "good news" of the gospel. It is a gospel of oneness. Jews and Gentiles, blacks and whites, gays and straights, men and women—all are God's children, all are welcome in God's house.

I am now a veteran pilgrim on the road to AIDS. I've learned that pilgrims sometimes lose hope. The virus wears us down. The medications wear us out. The sleeplessness, the lesions, and the cancers—like a faucet dripping in the dark, they take away our hope drop by drop. We read happy headlines about promised cures, but it isn't a cure that we experience—it's fever, sores, and family members who grow angry at our anger and hopeless at our hopelessness. Some of us have given up hope that even God could love us.

God's family needs to show others that the gospel is not about judgment, but about grace. It is a gospel not of death, but of life—a hopeful gospel, a healing gospel. What science cannot heal, God's family can embrace. And what life itself cannot sustain, the gospel can heal. That is why we're here and that is why there is a Gospel Against AIDS.

—**Mary Fisher,**
Gospel Against AIDS, December 6, 1997

a model to gain both comfort and familiarity with using a condom. It may involve helping her practice how to negotiate with her boyfriend for condom use.

When nurses understand their patients' behavioral skills, beliefs, and attitudes, it becomes possible to tailor an appropriate, brief, and practical intervention strategy for each person, helping them move along the continuum of change described earlier. Changing behavior can be difficult, and it is a good idea to check with the patient at the next visit to see if any difficulties arose. If so, the nurse can help with problem solving to overcome these impediments.

At the community level, successful population interventions often take the form of media campaigns, peer counseling, diverse educational strategies, and partnerships with community-based organizations. Community health nurses should be directly involved with policy development as related to the prevention and treatment of STDs and HIV/AIDS.

## Conclusion

STDs are a hidden epidemic with enormous health and economic consequences in this country. They remain hidden because so many Americans are unable to address sexual health issues openly and because of the biological and social characteristics of these diseases.

All Americans have a vested interest in STD prevention because every community is affected by STDs and everyone directly or indirectly pays for the costs of these diseases.

STDs are public health problems that lack easy solutions because they are rooted in fundamental human behavioral and social problems. Despite the barriers to open discussion of sexuality, there are prevention programs that are effective and that can be implemented on a local level.

Ultimately, multifaceted approaches are needed at both the individual and community levels to produce the best results. Although no intervention is perfect, together they can have a synergistic and positive impact on lowering the disease burden in this country. Subpopulations such as adolescents and disenfranchised adults will need special attention and outreach efforts.

To develop more effective STD treatment and prevention in the United States will require full participation by the public and private sectors. Community health nurses can be key stakeholders in modifying how STD services are provided and by accepting new responsibilities to ensure that the hidden epidemic of STDs in this country is addressed.

Explore Community Health Nursing on the Web! To learn more about the topics in this chapter, use the passcode provided to access your exclusive website: **http://nursing.jbpub.com/ communityhealth.** If you do not have a passcode, you can obtain one at this site.

## ■ CRITICAL THINKING ACTIVITIES

1. What are some of the reasons the United States has vastly higher rates of STDs compared with other developed countries?

2. How can you, as a community health nurse, play an important role in changing the STD burden in the United States?

3. How comfortable are you in talking about sexual health and sexual behavior with your family? with your friends? with your patients?

## ■ REFERENCES

AIDS InfoNet. (2008). Older people and HIV fact sheet. Retrieved October 28, 2008, from http://www.aidsinfonet.org/fact_sheets/new/616

American Association of World Health (AAWH). (199). *AIDS—end the silence.* Washington, DC: Author.

Aral, S. O., & Holmes, K. K. (1991). Sexually transmitted diseases in the AIDS era. *Scientific American, 264,* 62–69.

Aranda-Naranjo, B., Barini-Garcia, M., Pounds, M. B., & Davis, R. (2005). Addressing cultural issues to improve quality of care. In J. R. Anderson (Ed.), *A guide to clinical care of women with HIV.* Washington, DC: Health Resources and Services Administration.

Arias, D. C. (2007). HIV continues to inflict harder toll on black Americans. *The Nation's Health: The Official Newspaper of the American Public Health Association,* December 2006/January 2007, p. 12.

Auerbach, J. D. (2004). The overlooked victims of AIDS. *Washington Post,* October 14, 2004.

Centers for Disease Control and Prevention (CDC). (1997). *Sexually transmitted disease surveillance 1996: US Department of*

*Health and Human Services, Public Health Service.* Atlanta: Author.

Centers for Disease Control and Prevention (CDC). (2002). *Drug-associated HIV transmission continues in the United States.* Atlanta: Author.

Centers for Disease Control and Prevention (CDC). (2004). *Report to Congress: Infertility and prevention of sexually transmitted diseases 2000–2003.* Atlanta: Author.

Centers for Disease Control and Prevention (CDC). (2006a). *Sexually Transmitted Disease Surveillance 2005 supplement: Syphilis surveillance report.* Atlanta: Author.

Centers for Disease Control and Prevention (CDC). (2006b). *Trends in reported sexually transmitted diseases in the United States, 2005: National surveillance data for chlamydia, gonorrhea, and syphilis.* Atlanta: Author.

Centers for Disease Control and Prevention (CDC). (2006c). *HIV/AIDS surveillance report, 2005. Vol. 17.* Atlanta: Author.

Centers for Disease Control and Prevention (CDC). (2006d). *HIV/AIDS among youth: CDC HIV/AIDS fact sheet.* Atlanta: Author.

Centers for Disease Control and Prevention (CDC). (2007a). Syphilis fact sheet. Retrieved October 28, 2008, from http://www.cdc.gov/std/syphilis/STDFact-syphilis.htm

Centers for Disease Control and Prevention (CDC). (2007b). Chlamydia fact sheet. Retrieved October 28, 2008, from http://www.cdc.gov/std/chlamydia/STDFact-chlamydia.htm

Centers for Disease Control and Prevention (CDC). (2007c). Gonorrhea fact sheet. Retrieved October 28, 2008, from http://www.cdc.gov/std/gonorrhea/STDFact-gonorrhea.htm

Centers for Disease Control and Prevention (CDC). (2007d). Pelvic inflammatory disease fact sheet. Retrieved October 28, 2008, from http://www.cdc.gov/std/PID/STDFact-PID.htm

Centers for Disease Control and Prevention (CDC). (2007e). Genital herpes fact sheet. Retrieved October 28, 2008, from http://www.cdc.gov/std/herpes/STDFact-herpes.htm

Centers for Disease Control and Prevention (CDC). (2007f). HPV vaccine questions and answers. http://www.cdc.gov/std/healthcomm/fact_sheets.htm.

Centers for Disease Control and Prevention (CDC). (2007g). STDs and pregnancy. Retrieved October 28, 2008, from http://www.cdc.gov/std/STDFact-STDs&pregnancy.htm

Centers for Disease Control and Prevention (CDC). (2007h). *A glance at the HIV/AIDS epidemic: CDC HIV/AIDS fact sheet.* Atlanta: Author.

Centers for Disease Control and Prevention (CDC). (2007i). Basic statistics. Retrieved October 28, 2008, from http://www.cdc.gov/hiv/topics/surveillance/print/basic.htm

Centers for Disease Control and Prevention (CDC). (2007j). *HIV/AIDS among men who have sex with men: CDC HIV/AIDS fact sheet.* Atlanta: Author.

Centers for Disease Control and Prevention (CDC). (2007k). HIV/AIDS and African Americans. Retrieved October 28, 2008, from http://www.cdc.gov/hiv/topics/aa/print/index.htm

Centers for Disease Control and Prevention (CDC). (2007l). Pregnancy and childbirth. Retrieved October 28, 2008, from http://www.cdc.gov/hiv/topics/prenatal

Child and Adolescent Health and Development (CAH), World Health Organization. (2005). HIV/AIDS. Retrieved October 28, 2008, from http://www.who.int/child-adolescent-health/hiv.htm.

Coxon, A. P. M. (1996). Male homosexuality and HIV. Section I: Behavior changes among homosexual men. In J. Mann & D. Tarantola (Eds.), *AIDS in the world II* (pp. 252–254). New York: Oxford University Press.

Crespo-Fierro, M. (1997). Compliance/adherence and care management in HIV disease. *Journal of the Association of Nurses in AIDS Care, 8*(4), 43–54.

Department of Health and Human Services (DHHS). (2000). *Healthy People 2000: Conference edition.* Washington, DC: U.S. Government Printing Office.

Goodroad, B. K. (2003). Managing antiretroviral therapy. In C. Kirton (Ed.), *ANAC's core curriculum for HIV/AIDS nursing* (2nd ed., pp. 51–63). Thousand Oaks, CA: Sage.

Gottesman, N. (2005, July/August). HIV over 50. *AARP Magazine.* Available from http://www.aarpmagazine.org/

Health Resources and Services Administration (HRSA), HIV/AIDS Bureau. (2006a). Ryan White Care Act. Available from http://www.hab.hrsa.gov

Health Resources and Services Administration (HRSA), HIV/AIDS Bureau. (2006b). Men of color who have sex with men and HIV/AIDS in the United States. Available from http://www.hab.hrsa.gov

Health Resources and Services Administration (HRSA), HIV/AIDS Bureau. (2006c). Women and HIV/AIDS in the United States. Available from http://www.hab.hrsa.gov

Health Resources and Services Administration (HRSA), HIV/AIDS Bureau. (2006d). Pediatric HIV/AIDS in the United States. Available from http://www.hab.hrsa.gov

Heymann, D. L. (2004). *Control of communicable diseases manual* (18th ed.). Washington, DC: American Public Health Association.

Johnson, T. D. (2007). Millions around world observe, pay respects on World AIDS Day. *The Nation's Health: The Official Newspaper of the American Public Health Association,* December 2006/January 2007, p. 22.

Kaiser Foundation. (2006). *AIDS at 25: An overview of major trends in the U.S. epidemic.* Washington, DC: Kaiser Family Foundation.

Landry, D. J., & Forrest, J. D. (1996). Public health departments providing STD services. *Family Planning Perspectives, 25,* 261–266.

National Association of HIV Over Fifty (NAHOF). (2007). HIV and older adults educational tip sheet. Available from http://www.hivoverfifty.org/tip.html

National Cancer Institute (NCI). (2007). Human papillomaviruses and cancer: National Cancer Institute fact sheet. Retrieved October 28, 2008, from http://www.cancer.gov/cancertopics/factsheet

National Institute on Drug Abuse (NIDA). (2008). Principles of HIV prevention in drug-using populations. Retrieved October 28, 2008, from http://drugabuse.gov/POHP/FAQ_1.html

Pan American Health Organization (PAHO). (2005). Regional HIV/STI plan for the health sector: 2006–2015. Washington, DC: Author.

Prochaska. J. O., Redding, C. A., Harlow, L. L., Rossi, J. S., & Velicer, W. F. (1994). The transtheoretical model of change and HIV prevention: A review. *Health Education Quarterly, 481*–486.

Quadrivalent human papillomavirus. (2007). *Morbidity and Mortality Weekly Report. 56*(RR-02), 1–24. Atlanta: Centers for Disease Control and Prevention.

Saewyc, E., Skay, C., Richens, K., Reis, E., Poon, C., & Murphy, A. (2006). Sexual orientation, sexual abuse, and HIV-risk behavior among adolescents in the Pacific Northwest. *American Journal of Public Health, 96*(6), 1104–1110.

Sexually transmitted diseases treatment guidelines, 2006. (2006). *Morbidity and Mortality Weekly Report, 55*(RR-11). Atlanta: Centers for Disease Control and Prevention.

Shilts, R. (1987). *And the band played on: Politics, people, and the AIDS epidemic.* New York: Penguin.

UNAIDS. (2005). *AIDS epidemic update: December 2005.* Geneva, Switzerland: UNAIDS & WHO.

UNAIDS. (2006). *AIDS epidemic update: December 2006.* Geneva, Switzerland: UNAIDS & WHO.

Vuylsteke, B., Sunkutu, R., & Laga, M. (1996). Epidemiology of HIV and sexually transmitted infections in women. In J. Mann & D. Tarantola (Eds.), *AIDS in the World II* (pp. 97–109). New York: Oxford University Press.

World Health Organization (WHO). (2004). Combating gender inequality crucial in fight against HIV/AIDS, says WHO [Press release, March 5, 2004]. Geneva: Author. http://www.who.int/.

World Health Organization (WHO). (2007). HIV/AIDS and adolescents. Retrieved October 28, 2008, from http://www.who.int/child-adolescent-health/HIV/HIV_adolescents.htm

Youth Risk Behavioral Surveillance—United States, 2005. (2006). *Morbidity and Mortality Weekly Report, 55*(SS-5). Atlanta: Centers for Disease Control and Prevention.

## CHAPTER 21

# Substance Abuse as a Community Health Problem

Jean Haspeslagh and Judith A. Barton

COMMUNITY
SUBSTANCE
ABUSE CENTER
═ 9-11 ═

Visit **http://nursing.jbpub.com/communityhealth** for interactive exercises, review questions, Web links, and more.

The top public health problems in the United States are linked with substance abuse. Research about the risks for substance abuse (such as age, gender, and culture) can guide community health nurses in developing effective prevention interventions for vulnerable populations.

Macduff: What three things does drink especially provoke?

Porter: Marry, sir, nose-painting, sleep and urine. Lechery, sir, it provokes and unprovokes. It provokes the desire, but it takes away the performance; therefore, much drink may be said to be an equivocator with lechery; it makes him and it mars him; it sets him on, and it takes him off, it persuades him, and disheartens him, makes him stand to and not stand to, in conclusion, equivocates him in a sleep, and, giving him the lie, leaves him.

*—Macbeth, Act 2, Scene 3*

After reading the quote from *Macbeth*, how would you interpret Shakesphere's "picture" of how alcohol affects a person? Would you identify this description as abuse or overuse of alcohol? Why or why not?

## CHAPTER FOCUS

**The Nature of Substance Abuse as a Community Health Problem**
- Definitions of Substance Abuse
- Scope of Substance Abuse
- Impact of Substance Abuse on Society
- Impact of Substance Abuse on the Individual

**Risk Factors for Substance Abuse**
- Society's Influence
- The Family's Influence
- The Workplace's Influence
- Personal Factors

**Nursing Assessment**
- Nurses' Attitude Self-Assessment
- Drug History
- Recognizing the Signs of Substance Abuse

**Interventions**
- Society's Response
- Interventions with Special Populations

## QUESTIONS TO CONSIDER

After reading this chapter, answer the following questions:

1. What is the scope of substance abuse in the community?
2. What are the most commonly abused drugs?
3. What are the community health consequences of substance abuse?
4. What are the risk factors associated with substance abuse?
5. How does a nurse's self-awareness relate to addressing the problem of substance abuse in the community?
6. How are primary, secondary, and tertiary prevention strategies implemented in the community?
7. What are specific intervention strategies for various age groups in the prevention of substance abuse?
8. Which specific population groups are most at risk for substance abuse?
9. What is the role of the community health nurse in substance abuse prevention in schools and in the workplace?

## KEY TERMS

Addiction
Alcoholism
Comprehensive school health
Dependence

Interdiction
Primary prevention
Return to work contract

Secondary prevention
Social control
Social modeling theory

Substance abuse
Supply
Tertiary prevention

SUBSTANCE ABUSE AS A MAJOR public health problem in the United States affects society on multiple levels. All of us know someone who has been affected by substance abuse. Directly or indirectly, every community is affected by drug abuse and addiction, as is every family. The abuse of drugs in all forms takes a tremendous toll on societies and communities. This includes healthcare expenditures, lost earnings, and costs associated with crime and accidents. Community health nurses are faced with the costs and consequences of substance abuse from homelessness to child and family abuse. The top health problems of the community can often be directly linked to substance abuse: cancer, cardiovascular disease, HIV/AIDS, drug abuse, accidents, and violence. Drug addiction and substance abuse are preventable. Effective primary prevention efforts in the community involve families, schools, communities, and the media. Although many events and cultural factors affect drug and substance abuse trends, research consistently demonstrates that drug education can be effective to help youth and the public to understand the risks of drug abuse. The community health nurse is in an ideal position to assist communities in efforts to enhance protective factors and reverse or reduce risk factors in the population. In this chapter, risks associated with substance abuse and addictions are explored and protective factors that affect all populations are identified. Variables, such as age, gender, ethnicity, culture, and environment, are examined in the context of the role of the community health nurse.

 THINK ABOUT THIS ·············

> Every form of addiction is bad, no matter whether the narcotic be alcohol or morphine or idealism.
>
> —Carl Gustav Jung

## The Nature of Substance Abuse as a Community Health Problem

### ■ Definitions of Substance Abuse

When speaking of substance abuse, one finds a number of terms used in the literature, including *substance abuse, chemical dependence,* and *addiction.* In this chapter, *substance abuse* is used to cover the broad spectrum of abuse of alcohol and other drugs, including dependence and addiction. **Substance abuse** is the use of any drug (alcohol, street drugs, or prescription and over-the-counter medications) that results in a loss of control over the amount taken and when it is taken. It also includes continuation of drug use regardless of the consequences (physical, social, and psychological). Misuse of prescription drugs as well as over-the-counter drugs is a form of substance abuse often encountered in the community. Box 21-1 lists the major classes of abused drugs.

**BOX 21-1**

**Major Classes of Abused Drugs**

**Sedative-Hypnotics**
Central nervous system depressants
Benzodiazepines
Barbiturates
Alcohol

**Stimulants**
Amphetamines and methamphetamines
Cocaine

**Opioids/Opiates**
Codeine
Heroin
Morphine

**Hallucinogens**
LSD (acid) and LSD-like drugs (mescaline, psilocybin)
MDMA (ecstasy) and MDMA-like drugs

**Inhalants**
Glue
Solvents
Aerosols
Nitrous oxide
Gasoline

**Cannabinoids**
Marijuana
Hash
THC

**Nicotine**
Tobacco
Smokeless tobacco

**Phencyclidine (PCP)**

**Dependence** or **addiction** is present when there are physiological symptoms that occur with withdrawal of the substance. However, the important thing to remember is that, whether the individual is experiencing dependence or is "merely" overusing or misusing drugs, the effects on the person and the community are similar.

> **❝** *There was a time when all I cared about was the next game, the next party, the next tee time. I've come to a crossroads. I can't think of one thing that drinking has done that's been good for me or my family. I'm not saying everyone in the world should quit drinking, but I wasn't the best drinker in the world, so I'm quitting it.* **❞**
>
> —Brett Favre, Green Bay Packers Quarterback, 1999

 ETHICAL CONNECTION

Addiction should never be treated as a crime. It has to be treated as a health problem. We do not send alcoholics to jail in this country. Over 500,000 people are in our jails who are nonviolent drug users.

—Ralph Nader

## BOX 21-2

### Most Drug Users Are in the Workforce

"The typical drug user is not poor and unemployed," Barry McCaffrey, the White House drug policy director, said in a statement. "He or she can be a co-worker, a husband or wife, a parent."

A report issued by the U.S. Department of Health and Human Services (DHHS) found that 7.7% of workers ages 18 to 49 had used illegal drugs in the past month. (The report was based on research conducted by the Substance Abuse and Mental Health Services Administration.) Nationwide, 7 in 10 drug users were full-time workers in 1997.

The report also found that 19% of restaurant workers, 14% of construction workers, and 10% of transportation and material-moving workers used illegal drugs.

*Source:* Associated Press, 1999.

## ■ Scope of Substance Abuse

The use and abuse of alcohol and other drugs contribute to one of the major public health problems facing society today. The use and abuse of alcohol and other drugs are widespread across all races and ethnic groups in society; furthermore, someone you know at work could be using drugs (Box 21-2). Alcohol use and abuse are occurring at a younger age, making the need for prevention programs in schools essential. For young people going off to college, the military, or first jobs, their newly found independence also includes new peer pressures to drink, smoke, or use recreational drugs. In addition, as persons live longer and experience more chronic health problems, they are faced with an existence that includes the use of multiple drugs. Along with the benefits associated with improved pharmacological management of chronic conditions, it is necessary to acknowledge the problems associated with the misuse of these same agents.

### Illicit Drug Users

An estimated 19.5 million Americans used some form of illicit drugs in 2003. This number indicates that 8.7% of the population 12 years and older used an illicit drug in the month prior to the National Survey on Drug Use and Health

### MEDIA MOMENT

### *Tender Mercies* (1983)

Alcoholic drifter Mac Sledge (Robert Duvall) comes into the life of a lonely widow (Tess Harper) and her young son (Allan Hubbard) in the barren flatlands of Texas. When Mac is revealed as a once-famous country singer, he must face a painful past, and an uncertain future, including an addiction to alcohol—but the new relationships he forges inspire him to revive his career. The cast also includes Wilford Brimley, Betty Buckley, and Ellen Barkin.

(NSDUH) conducted by the Substance Abuse and Mental Health Service Administration (SAMHSA, 2004). By comparison, the number is greatly reduced from its highest level in 1979, when the estimate was that 25 million or 14.1% of Americans used illicit drugs.

Marijuana continues to be the most commonly used illicit drug in the United States. In 2003, 14.6 million people were current users of marijuana. By contrast, two million people used cocaine, hallucinogens were used by 1.2 million persons, and heroin by 166,000 persons (SAMHSA, 2004). Volkow (2000) indicated there has been an increased number of teens and adults abusing prescription drugs with 10.5% of twelfth graders using Vicodin and 4.5% using Oxycotin without a prescription. Men continue to have higher rates of illicit drug use than women do. The rates of illicit drug use in metropolitan areas are higher than in nonmetropolitan areas. Illicit drug use rates remain highly correlated with educational status. Among young adults 26 to 34 years old, those who had not completed high school had the highest rates of current use, whereas college graduates had the lower rate. Illicit drug use for African Americans (9.7%) was similar to that for whites (8.5%) and Hispanics (7.2%) (SAMHSA, 2004).

### Use of Alcohol

Alcohol use is a part of American culture. Approximately 61% of adults (21–14 years of age) report having drunk alcohol in the past year. (See Box 21-3.) Thirty-two percent of current drinkers report having five or more drinks on at least 1 day in the past year, according to the National Center for Health Statistics annual 2007 survey. Alcohol use tends to be more moderate among African Americans than among other racial/ethnic groups. Men's use of alcohol was greater than women's use. Although the overall rate of alcohol use is lower in rural areas than in metropolitan areas, the rates of binge drinking (5 or more drinks on the same occasion in the past month) and heavy alcohol use in rural areas were similar to the rates in nonrural areas. In contrast to the

## BOX 21-3

### Age and Alcohol Use by Youth

| Age | Percent Users |
|---|---|
| 12 years | 2.0 |
| 13 years | 6.5 |
| 14 years | 13.4 |
| 15 years | 17.9 |
| 16 years | 29 |
| 17 years | 36.2 |
| 18 years | 29 |

*Binge drinkers, ages 18–20:*
7.2 million (19.3%)
*Heavy drinking, ages 18–20:*
2.3 million (6.2%)
*Youth driving under the influence of alcohol and drugs:*
alcohol, 14.3%; drugs, 4.2%

*Source:* Substance Abuse and Mental Health Services Administration. (2002). National survey on drug use and health (NSDUH).

pattern for illicit drugs, the higher the level of education, the more likely the current use of alcohol (National Center for Health Statistics, 2007).

### Use of Tobacco

Tobacco use continues to be a major public health concern, with 70 million current smokers in the United States. This actual number of tobacco smokers represents a smoking rate of 29.2% for those 12 and older. Current smokers were more likely than nonsmokers to be heavy drinkers and illicit drug users. In addition, an estimated 3% of the population are current users of smokeless tobacco (SAMHSA 2004).

The current smoking rate among young adults ages 18 to 25 continues to move upward from 34.6% in 1994 to 39.5% in 2003. The smoking rate among 12- to 17-year-olds was 11.9%, declining in use from recent years. Smoking rates are similar among different races and ethnic groups. Males had higher rates of smoking than females (27.7% versus 22.3%). Lower educational attainment was correlated with higher tobacco use (SAMHSA, 2004).

### Youthful Illicit Drug Users

The Monitoring the Future study (National Institute on Drug Abuse, 2007) concluded that illicit drug use by middle and high school students continues to decline. Past year prevalence of illicit drug use has fallen by 44% among eighth graders since the peak year of 1996. From 2006 to 2007, the percentage of eighth graders reporting lifetime use of any illicit drug declined from 20.9% to 19.0%. Past year prevalence fell 27% among tenth graders and 15% among twelfth graders since the peak year of 1997.

Marijuana is still the most widely used illicit drug among the nation's youth, although its use continues to decline. Although there was evidence of some decline in alcohol use at all three grade levels, 29% of all high school seniors reported being drunk at least once in the 30-day interval preceding the survey (National Institute on Drug Abuse, 2007).

Overall, the conclusions of the 1998 survey of illicit drug use among youth were promising. The study points out that behaviors change very slowly, and often only after there has been some reassessment by young people about

> **❝** *If we hear somebody's sniffing something, we're not shocked—it's an everyday occurrence.* **❞**
> —Sophomore high school student, Newark, Delaware

---

## ENVIRONMENTAL CONNECTION

### The Poor Man's Cocaine: Methamphetamine as a Growing Public Health Threat

#### The Drug

Methamphetamine (in all of its forms—powder, crystal, or pills) is a powerfully addictive stimulant that affects the central nervous system. It is easy to make using inexpensive materials such as pseudoephedrine, paint thinner, kerosene, battery acid, brake cleaner, and Red Devil lye. The final product may or may not be a "pure" methamphetamine. Because of its stimulant effects, other drugs such as cocaine, marijuana, heroin, and alcohol are often used to bring the person down from the stimulant effects.

#### The User

Methamphetamine (meth) use has increased from 1% of substance abusers in 1999 to 7% in 2004 (SAMHSA, 2005), and that rate continues to rise. Notable populations in which methamphetamine use is growing include white- and blue-collar workers, prostitutes, long-haul truckers, and runaway youth.

Methamphetamine users can be identified by signs such as agitation, rapid speech, decreased appetite, and insomnia. Physical manifestations include dilated pupils, elevated blood pressure, irregular pulse, chest pain, shortness of breath, and elevated temperature. Users may exhibit sudden episodes of violent behavior, intense paranoia, and hallucinations. Drug exposure doesn't readily wear off and is highly addictive from first use.

#### The Environment

Manufacturing of methamphetamine is not limited to urban areas. There has been a rapid increase in use of this drug in rural areas of the South, Southwest, and Midwest. Clandestine laboratories routinely dump waste materials into fields, streams, and sewage systems. Waste materials include ignitable, corrosive, and reactive toxic chemicals that present a high risk for explosions, fires, and toxic fumes. Toxic fumes make houses and buildings uninhabitable. Estimates for cleanup are approximately $2,000 to $4,000 per site. Meth labs produce materials that are toxic by-products (lye, sulfur with acid, camping fuel, ether), and these toxins are dumped outside in rural areas where pets and wild animals—as well as children—may happen upon them.

Strict control of at least some of the ingredients used to "cook" meth has occurred at both national and state levels. Medications including the ingredient pseudoephedrine (which is found in over-the-counter allergy and cold medications) are now sold behind the counter, and limited in supply for individual purchase. In 2005, Congress passed the Combat Methamphetamine Epidemic Act, which states that purchasers of these products must present identification and can be tracked by signature.

#### Implications

Users of methamphetamine are at increased risk of engaging in behaviors that place them at greater risk for HIV/AIDS and sexually transmitted diseases. Research has also indicated that the use of methamphetamine slows the user's response time (21% slower than nonusers), a phenomenon that is especially evident in tasks requiring working memory, immediate storage of information, and mental calculations (Swan, 2003).

Neglect of children is also an issue when methamphetamine enters the picture. Authorities have found that 20% of meth labs had children present when the makers were manufacturing the drug ("Meth Alert," 2004).

the dangers of drugs and how acceptable they are in the peer group. Other effects include more attention being paid to drug issues by community groups, parents, government, and the media.

## Impact of Substance Abuse on Society

A 2005 report issued by the Department of Health and Human Services indicated that alcohol was associated with 100,000 preventable deaths each year and that alcohol cost taxpayers nearly $185 billion annually. Healthcare costs related to smoking are estimated at $75 billion (Goodman, 2004). The annual financial losses to victims of alcohol-related violence (approximately 500,000 persons annually) total more than $400 million, while the average victim of such violence paid $1,500 out of pocket for related medical expenses (Goodman 2004).

The U.S. Department of Transportation (2007) reported that alcohol was involved in all 1998 fatalities. The Drug Enforcement Administration of the U.S. Department of Justice (2005) reported that alcohol abuse was a factor in 4 in 10 violent crimes and that approximately 4 in 10 criminal offenders reported using alcohol at the time they committed their offense. The National Justice Institute asserts that abuse of alcohol and other drugs by criminal offenders, parolees, and probationers contributes to 80% of crime in the United States. In incidents of spouse abuse, alcohol use by the offender was documented in 75% of reported cases.

## Impact of Substance Abuse on the Individual

The effects of substance abuse on the individual are many and range from loss of a job and loss of relationships to major health problems. Substance abusers find themselves at greater risk for death as a result of auto accidents and violence (suicide and homicide), and numerous health problems. They are also more likely to develop chronic health problems such as central nervous system neuropathy, impaired cognition, cardiovascular disease, hypertension, and chronic gastrointestinal problems, including gastritis. Acute and chronic pancreatitis and liver disease are often associated with alcohol abuse. Nutritional deficiencies and anemia are often identified and are a result of not only poor dietary habits but more importantly the physiological changes that result from abuse of alcohol and other drugs.

Although low self-esteem is a common characteristic exhibited by the person who abuses substances, no personality factors or other behaviors have reliably differentiated substance abusers from other individuals. It would appear that low self-esteem appears to be more a result of the substance abuse rather than a causative factor (West & Kinney, 1996, p. 28). After reviewing psychological theories related to substance abuse, Goldsmith (1997, p. 6) concluded that the idea that there is an addictive personality is a myth. It appears that the depression, anxiety, and lack of self-esteem are as much a result of the substance use as they are causative factors. Zwickler (2004) indicates childhood sexual abuse increases the risk for drug dependence in adult women.

Participation in high-risk behaviors such as intravenous drug use and promiscuous sexual activity put the substance abuser at greater risk for acquiring sexually transmitted diseases. There are associated high rates of positive tests for human immunodeficiency virus (HIV) in high-risk groups, which include intravenous drug users, "sex workers" (i.e., prostitutes), and those who have multiple sex partners. Individuals who are using illicit drugs and need to find ways to pay for their drugs often turn to prostitution to help support their habit, placing them in this high-risk group.

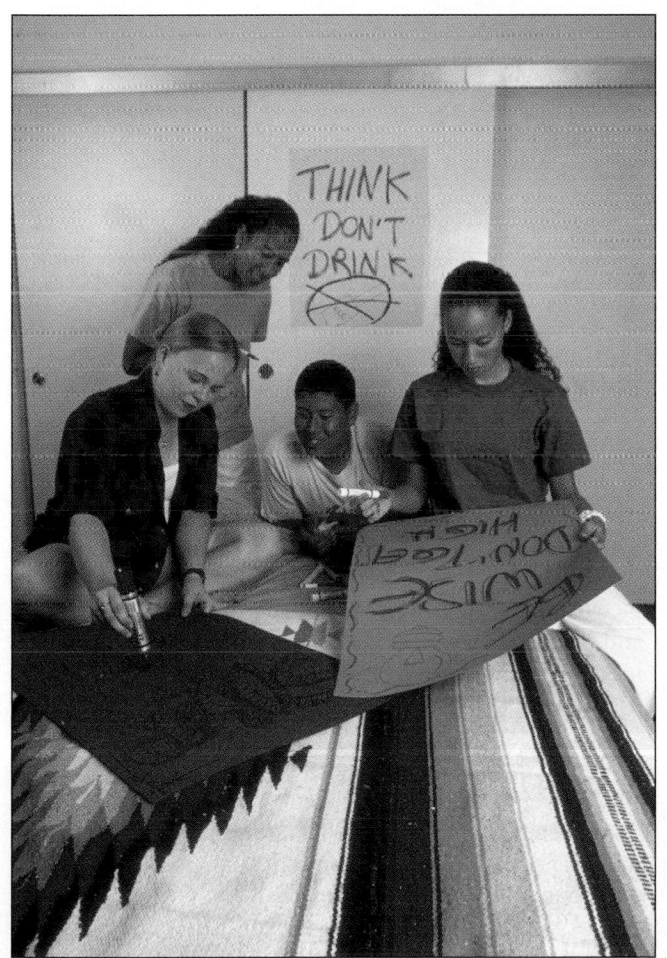

Students participate in a campaign to prevent substance abuse.

### ETHICAL CONNECTION

Teens who are 14 or younger who use alcohol are twice as likely to have sex as those in the same age group who don't. The risk is four times as great for those who use drugs as for those who don't. What are the ethical implications of informing teens about having sex and using drugs without "moralizing" and complicating their decision making?

# Risk Factors for Substance Abuse

## ■ Society's Influence

### Media Influences

Societal factors that influence the use and abuse of alcohol and other drugs are all around us. Television and movies present the use of alcohol and tobacco as glamorous, a rite of passage, something the sophisticated person does. The Research Alerts on pages 482 and 483 highlight recent studies on the potential influence of the media on substance use in our society.

Advertisements tell us we need a break, we need to relax and unwind, and what better way than by having a drink or smoke? We live in a fast-paced world where people are encouraged not to feel. Ads remind us that if it hurts, take something; if you are stressed, have a drink, take a pill, smoke another cigarette.

> ❝*I admire addicts. In a world where everybody is waiting for some blind, random disaster, or some sudden disease, the addict has the comfort of knowing what will most likely wait for him down the road. He's taken some control over his ultimate fate, and his addiction keeps the cause of death from being a total surprise.*❞
>
> —Chuck Palahniuk

### Societal Attitudes

Attitudes toward legal and illegal substances, abuse of substances, and interventions and treatment for drug-addicted individuals vary according to society, community, ethnicity, social status, gender, and time. In other words, substance abuse is a socially constructed concept. Sometimes drug use is considered okay, and other times it is not okay. For example, the use of amphetamines or tranquilizers by a businessperson might be considered a matter of personal judgment, but the use of the same drugs by a young person who wishes to experience their effects produces much more emotion. Society's influence can again be seen when one looks at alcohol, which was actually prohibited in the United States through a constitutional amendment—the Eighteenth Amendment, passed by the U.S. Congress in 1920. After 13 years of unsuccessful efforts to enforce the law, Prohibition was repealed. Currently, tobacco use is increasingly being viewed as deviant, and those individuals and groups who use tobacco are experiencing stigmatization and subsequent discrimination.

 **Research Alert**

### Portrayal of Substance Use in the Media

This study examined the frequency and nature of substance use in the most popular movie rentals and songs of 1996 and 1997. The intent was to determine the accuracy of public perceptions about extensive substance use in media popular among youth. Because teenagers are major

 **ENVIRONMENTAL CONNECTION**

Children are often present in meth labs while the drug is being cooked; thousands are being exposed to the highly addictive drug and its toxic by-products. The drug's ingredients—acids, bases, metals, solvents, and salts—soak into fabrics and porous surfaces and produce toxic gases that find their way into ventilation systems. People, pets, and toys may all become contaminated in these "home meth labs." Following are some of the toxic substances often used in the preparation of methamphetamines:

Acetone, acetic acid, vinegar
Alcohol, isopropyl
Ammonia, anhydrous, farm fertilizer
Benzene, dye, varnish
Ether, starter fluid
Ethyl ether, computer dust-off
Freon
Hydrochloric acid/muriatic acid, iron ore processing, concrete cleaner
Iodine crystals, antiseptic
Lithium metal, batteries
Red phosphorus, match striker plates
Sulfuric acid battery acid
Toluene brake cleaner fluid
Trichloroethane gun scrubber

consumers of movies and music, there is concern about the potential for media depictions of tobacco, alcohol, and illicit drugs to encourage use.

The study examined the 200 most popular movie rentals and 1,000 of the most popular songs from 1996 and 1997. Substances included in the study were illicit drugs, alcohol, tobacco, and over-the-counter and prescription medicines. The researchers examined what was used, by whom, how often, under what circumstances, and with what consequences.

Findings revealed that 98% of the movies studied depicted illicit drugs, alcohol, tobacco, or over-the-counter and prescription medicines. Fewer than half (49%) of the movies portrayed short-term consequences of substance use, and only 12% depicted long-term consequences.

The major finding from the song analysis was the dramatic difference among music categories (country, alternative rock, hot 100, rap, and heavy metal), with substance references being most common in rap. Illicit drugs were mentioned in 63% of rap songs versus about 10% of the lyrics in all other categories.

*Source:* Kelly, K., & Donohew, L. (1999). Media and primary socialization theory. *Substance Use and Misuse, 34*(7), 1033–1045.

Research Alert

### Study Links Television Viewing Time with High School Student Drinking

A Stanford University study of 1,533 ninth graders found that high school students who watch lots of television and music videos are more likely to start drinking than other youngsters. Youngsters who rented movies were less likely to start drinking, while playing video and computer games had no effect. Watching TV and music videos made no difference in the drinking habits of those who had already begun to drink alcohol.

*Source:* Robinson, T. N., Chen, H. L., & Killen, J. D. (1998). Television and music video exposure and risk of adolescent alcohol use. *Pediatrics, 102*(5), 1202–1209.

 Research Alert

### Substance Abuse Policies Related to Societal Attitudes

Although public health policies and practices are making slow but sure progress toward improving the health of particular groups of Americans (e.g., children with infectious diseases, cancer patients) through insurance coverage, screening, and treatment, the prevention and treatment of substance use has not kept up.

The federal government's continued policy of spending nearly double the amount on supply reduction (interdiction) as on demand reduction (prevention and treatment) is considered perplexing by public health professionals because of the large treatment gap for substance abuse.

It is estimated that although more than 5.3 million persons in the United States are in severe need of substance abuse treatment, only 37% receive such treatment. It is estimated that providing treatment to all in need could save more than $150 billion over the next 15 years, at a price tag of just $21 billion. In other words, funding treatment for persons addicted to drugs is good fiscal policy because every dollar invested in drug treatment generates $7 in savings of future costs!

*Source:* Amaro, H. (1999). An expensive policy: The impact of inadequate funding for substance abuse treatment. *American Journal of Public Health, 89*(5), 657–659.

### Substance abuse as a criminal activity or as a disease

**Alcoholism** in American culture has been defined as a chronic disease manifested by repeated drinking causing injury to the drinker's health and/or social or economic functioning. Alcohol for individuals 21 years of age and older is legal in the United States, and being defined as a chronic disease has shifted alcohol-related problems from the category of sin or crime to the category of sickness. Nevertheless, many in our society tend to stereotype the alcoholic as a skid row derelict. Consequently, many persons who regularly drink to excess do not seek treatment because they do not

### *a conversation with . . .*

Alcoholism and other drug addiction is an equal-opportunity disease—women and men, young and old, all walks of life are affected. It is a complex disease of mind, body, and soul.

The chronic nature of alcoholism and other drug addiction is often what gets in the way of understanding and awareness. There continues to be many myths about this illness and much stigma attached to alcoholics and addicts.

The Betty Ford Center, in addition to having over 38,000 women, men, and their families participate in our treatment programs, offers unique training opportunities. Licensed professionals and students take part in the Professional in Residence Program, which is an experiential, hands-on program. Nurses, in particular, who are often on the frontline of intervention and treatment, have been eager participants in this training experience.

There is no question that our national drug policy is failing. I believe that is because the majority of emphasis continues on interdiction rather than treatment and prevention. This failure has even led to calls of legalization. Legalization would be an invitation to young people to use drugs. This would be a disaster. We need to change the emphasis of our national programs.

—**Betty Ford,**
founder of the Betty Ford Center
*Source:* Betty Ford, personal communication, October 25, 1999.

see themselves as fitting that stereotype. Although excessive use of alcohol has been viewed as a disease, the excessive use of other psychoactive drugs in our society has not (Carroll, 1996).

Currently, there is some movement toward defining alcohol and drug addiction as meeting the criteria for a disability under the Americans with Disabilities Act (ADA). The medical community is taking leadership in this movement. The American Medical Association (AMA) and the American Society of Addiction Medicine (ASAM) are particularly concerned about managed care denials for individuals with drug addictions. Although it appears that our society is far from decriminalization of illicit drug use or the legalization of drugs, there is a growing concern about the prevention and treatment of drug addiction. The Research Alert on this page discusses current substance abuse treatment policy, which is based on the attitude that substance abuse is a criminal activity to deter rather than a disease to treat. The conversation with Betty Ford, former President Ford's wife, contributed especially for this nursing textbook discusses addictions and the need for more emphasis on treatment of addictions as a disease.

### Cultural Influences

Research has demonstrated that peer pressure, particularly for youth, is highly correlated with the use of illicit substances. If peer pressure to use substances is joined with other cultural influences, the risk of use becomes even stronger. For example, Goldsmith (1997) found that first use of alcohol and drugs often occurs in a social setting, suggesting that peer pressure and positive social/group attitudes about using substances, availability of the drugs, and pro-use norms in the community contribute to substance abuse.

Think about the many cultural influences for and against the use and potential abuse of drugs in the United States. Will the restriction of billboards promoting the glamour of cigarette smoking reduce the use of tobacco? Will smoking rates continue to decline as more and more public facilities restrict use? Are the current movement by the National Organization for the Reform of Marijuana Laws and the resurgence of the use of marijuana in Hollywood movies going to have an influence on the use of marijuana in our society?

❝ *Vodka is tasteless going down, but it is memorable coming up.* ❞

—*Garrison Keillor*

### ■ The Family's Influence

Although in modern society many of the socialization functions of the family have been taken over by other institutions such as schools, churches, or the media, the family remains a significant agent of socialization. Parents normally take care to monitor their offspring's behavior and pass on the language, values, norms, and beliefs of their culture. Research in the area of adolescent substance abuse has demonstrated that the family can have a positive effect in reducing the risk of initiation into alcohol, tobacco, and other drug use among children and youth (Hahn, 1993; Hahn & Rado, 1996; Hahn, Simpson, & Kidd, 1996; Goodman, 2004). For example, a young man who is raised in a family where all the male role models drink heavily will most often follow their lead. The opposite is also true—the person who is raised in a

family or culture where there are strong prohibitions against drinking may be more inclined to experiment with alcohol at a later time, hopefully when he or she is more mature and will not end up abusing alcohol. Research continues to indicate that young people surveyed indicated parental disapproval of drug use was a very important factor influencing their decision to abstain from drug use (Hawkins, 2002; Bauman et al., 2001; Kosterman et al., 2001; Kelly et al., 2004).

The family can play a role in either maintaining a family member's escalation into substance abuse or their recovery from substance abuse. Non-substance-abusing family members initially experience emotions such as anger, fear, resentment, guilt, and shame when they first recognize that a spouse or child is a substance abuser. Because many people in our society view substance abuse as a character weakness, non-substance-abusing family members often share in the stigma (i.e., discrediting and discrimination) imposed on the substance abuser. Literature indicates spouses and parents most likely have inaccurate knowledge about the extent of their spouse's or child's substance abuse activities and therefore are inclined to show a great deal of tolerance of untoward behavior among family members, often taking a long time to acknowledge that a problem exists. In most cases, families attempt to cope with the abuser's problem; however, in some cases, the problem is dealt with by means of divorce or ejection of the adolescent (Barton, 1991; Weinberg & Vogel, 1990; Kelly 2004).

A family history of alcoholism or addiction as well as biochemical and genetic factors also make certain family members more sensitive to the effects of substances. Research in this area, although not totally confirming, is becoming more definitive as to the correlation between familial alcoholism and offspring alcoholism (Hill, 1998). In addition, the problem of drug dependence during pregnancy is known to lead to babies who show withdrawal symptoms (Schneider et al., 1996) and the concern could be that these children will exhibit tendencies toward substance abuse in their youthful and adult lives.

### ■ The Workplace's Influence

Substance abuse in the workplace is a concern for both employers and consumers of products and services. Only 14.4% of persons who use drugs are unemployed, while 74.6% are employed either full-time or part-time (NSDOH, 2002). The cost in lost work time alone accounts for $10 billion per year (SAMHSA 2004). This does not include such things as the cost of intervention, treatment, and reduced productivity. How substance abuse is viewed in the workplace is important. Does management send a message that drinking and using drugs in the workplace are unacceptable? Does management simply avoid confronting the issue of substance abuse with the stand that "We don't have anyone on our staff who does that"? Failure to acknowledge that substance abuse can be a problem in the work environment is itself a problem that can lead to further risk for employees.

## MEDIA MOMENT

**"Warning Labels," Doug Stone (1992)**
They oughta put warning labels on those sad country
  songs:
Harmful, to your heart when you're left all alone
And if you're drinkin' you'll start thinkin' 'bout love that
  went wrong
They oughta put warning labels on those sad country
  songs:
They warn me 'bout cigarettes, whiskey, and beer
No one ever warned me about the music I hear
I don't guess I would listen to what they said anyway
But at least I'd been ready when the first sad song played

Acknowledgment that substance abuse can be a problem for many workers, creation of health promotion and prevention programs, and policies related to treatment for workers will put all workers on alert that the demands of work require workers to deal with their substance abuse problem.

## ■ Personal Factors

Substance abuse affects people of all ages, socioeconomic groups, and occupations. Box 21-4 lists populations vulnerable to substance abuse. Young people remain the most vulnerable to substance abuse, with the highest rate of illicit drug use occurring in those younger than 20 years of age, while only a small portion of illicit drug use occurs in the over-50 group. There appears to be little difference between whether the individual lives in an urban or rural setting.

According to the 2003 household survey (SAMHSA, 2004), the use of illicit drugs appears to be higher in young people who have dropped out of high school and is lowest in college graduates. Similarly, although 60% of individuals use alcohol, the group most likely to binge or fall into the heavy drinking category tends to be individuals between 18 and 35 years of age who have not completed high school. Alcohol use is also strongly associated with illicit drug use.

When looking at risk factors for alcoholism and addiction, it is essential to consider such things as the biochemical and genetic factors that make one individual more sensitive

## BOX 21-4

**Vulnerable Populations**
- Children and adolescents
- High school dropouts
- People with dual diagnoses
- People with family history of alcoholism/addiction
- Unemployed individuals
- College students

## BOX 21-5

**Individual Risk Factors**
- Family history of substance abuse
- Genetic/biochemical factors
- Prenatal exposure
- Psychiatric disorders

to the effects of drugs, prenatal exposure to drugs, and preexisting or coexisting psychiatric disorders. Box 21-5 provides a list of individual risk factors nurses should be alert to during any assessment.

Research has indicated that there is no one clear-cut cause for substance abuse disorders. It has been found that for many people, a family history of alcoholism or addiction is a red flag indicating that the risk of becoming addicted or dependent on alcohol and/or other drugs is greater. It would stand to reason, then, that babies who were born addicted because of maternal drug abuse will be at a higher risk for developing substance abuse problems should they experiment with alcohol or other drugs when they are older.

The existence of preexisting or coexisting psychiatric disorders may also contribute to substance abuse. Anthenelli (1997) and Waller (1997) found evidence that persons with both a psychiatric diagnosis and a substance abuse problem are not uncommon. Persons with antisocial personality disorders, schizophrenia, and bipolar disorders are at greater risk for developing a substance abuse disorder. Goldsmith (1997) emphasized that "alcohol exaggerates both mood disorders and anxiety and that alcohol and drugs cause organic mood and organic anxiety disorders" (p. 6).

In an age when families are often scattered and talking with a neighbor appears to be a lost art, the sharing and receiving of emotional support is difficult for many people in our society. The image of rugged individualism, self-reliance, and high achievement often discourages people from allowing others to see their vulnerability and leads them to seek other ways of dealing with emotional pain. For some individuals, using alcohol or other drugs becomes their way of coping with their emotional pain. What results is a vicious cycle in which the person experiences emotional pain, uses alcohol or drugs to relieve that pain, experiences emotional pain related to consequences of substance abuse, and turns back to the substance to dull the emotional pain.

 GLOBAL CONNECTION

Opium production in Afghanistan rose 60% in 2006, after the U.S. invasion of Iraq. According to the United Nations, 6,100 tons of opium is enough to make 610 tons of heroin. The supply of heroin is outstripping heroin users' demands by one-third.

## Nursing Assessment

### ■ Nurses' Attitude Self-Assessment

For community health nurses to work effectively with substance abusers, it is important that they develop an awareness of their own issues and attitudes about substance abuse. The nurse's attitudes regarding use of legal and illicit drugs, about those people who use or abuse drugs, and past experiences with substance abuse/abusers need to be assessed.

One of the first areas of self-awareness that needs to be addressed is what feeling the nurse has about the use of alcohol, tobacco, and recreational drugs. Questions to ask oneself include the following:

- What do I believe about the use of alcohol, tobacco, and recreational drugs? Is it morally wrong?
- Is it okay to use alcohol and tobacco but not marijuana or other recreational drugs? Marijuana but not any other illegal drugs?
- Is the use of any mind-altering substance up to the individual's freedom of choice?

The second area that one needs to examine is one's attitude about the substance abuser.

- How do I feel about the person who uses and abuses alcohol, tobacco, or other drugs?
- Is that person just weak-willed, immoral, or undisciplined or ill and in need of treatment?
- Is the answer to the substance abuse problem punishment and incarceration?

Third, the community health nurse must look carefully at how past experiences with substance abuse/abusers may have influenced attitudes toward those individuals who abuse substances. Nurses should ask themselves the following questions:

- Have I known someone who abused alcohol or other drugs? How did their substance abuse affect me and my relationship with them?
- Was I raised in an alcoholic or addicted family? What did this mean to me? Have I received any assistance in dealing with my own issues?
- Have I ever lost someone who was important to me as a result of substance use?
- Have I ever been physically, sexually, or emotionally abused by someone who was abusing alcohol or other drugs?

For some people, asking and answering these questions may bring up uncomfortable, painful feelings. If this occurs, it is important that available resources be used to work through those feelings. For those individuals who have never shared their experiences, working with substance abusers may be difficult unless those unresolved issues are addressed. Failure to do so may result in the nurse's unconsciously avoiding interactions, being judgmental, and failing to be therapeutic when working with this population.

### ■ Drug History

One of the nurse's critical tasks when substance abuse is suspected is to conduct a drug history, taking note of the

---

> **BOX 21-6**
>
> **Key Elements in a Drug History**
> - Which drug/drugs have been taken? In what combination?
> - Which route was used to administer the drug (e.g., injection, intravenous, oral, sniffed, smoked)?
> - How much of the drug was taken?
> - What is the frequency of drug use?
> - When was the drug last taken?
> - At what age did drug use begin?

❝ *Just 'cause you got the monkey off your back doesn't mean the circus has left town.* ❞

—*George Carlin, on addiction and recovery*

drugs of choice, the route of administration, the amount used, the frequency of use, and polysubstance use. Box 21-6 summarizes key elements to address in a drug history. Information regarding the initiation of drug use, including the age and drugs first used, is important. Drug histories may need to be repeated to get a more accurate picture of what drugs have been used and how often. The substance abuser may give inaccurate information initially for a number of reasons: confusion because of drugs, fear, lack of trust, and uncertainty regarding what drugs were taken. The latter is often a problem with street drugs because the purity of these substances is often questionable.

### ■ Recognizing the Signs of Substance Abuse

To address substance abuse issues, it is essential that the nurse recognize that abuse of drugs is multifaceted, with a variety of substances being used either singularly or in combination (see Box 21-1 for a listing of major classes of abused drugs). The community health nurse needs to be aware of those major drug groups that are subject to abuse. In addition, for community health nurses, knowledge regarding the signs of substance abuse is essential if they are to recognize such abuse early so that intervention can be planned. Efforts must be made to detect the problem as soon as possible. Common signs indicative that an individual may be abusing one or more substances are found in Boxes 21-7 and 21-8.

---

> **BOX 21-7**
>
> **Indicators of Possible Substance Abuse: Common Signs Across Categories**
> - Changes in attendance patterns (school or work)
> - Change in mood or attitude (e.g., self-discipline, work habits, efficiency)
> - Poor physical appearance
> - Association with known substance abusers
> - Heightened secrecy
> - Borrowing of money
>
> *Source:* Adapted from Carroll, 1996.

## BOX 21-8

### Specific Indicators of Possible Substance Abuse Across Categories of Psychoactive Drugs

**Narcotics**
- Lethargic, drowsy behavior
- Restlessness
- Constricted pupils and red, watery eyes
- Loss of normal appetite
- Equipment such as syringes and bent spoons as well as "track" marks on arms, hands, or legs

**Depressants**
- Behavior similar to alcohol intoxication
- Headaches, irritability, and anxiety
- Confusion and memory impairment
- Insomnia
- Impaired motor skills
- Faulty judgment, moody

**Stimulants**
- Extended wakefulness, irritability, hostility
- Dilated pupils
- Flushed skin, palpitations, increased sweating
- Chronic runny nose

**Marijuana**
- Intoxicated-type behavior
- Dulling of attention, lethargy
- Distorted sense of time and distance
- Seeds and shreds of plant material in pockets

**Psychedelic (Hallucinogens)**
- Difficulty in communicating
- Profound changes in thinking patterns or mood
- Trancelike states or fearful behavior
- Nausea, chills, flushing, and sweating

**Phencyclidine (PCP)**
- Amnesia
- Noncommunicative with blank staring eyes
- Increased insensitivity to pain
- Profound changes in thinking and mood

*Source:* Adapted from Carroll, 1996.

---

## MEDIA MOMENT

### Days of Wine and Roses (1962)
While this film is dated, it provides an outstanding portrayal of alcoholism and its consequences for a married couple, both of whom are trying to outdrink the other.

---

Becoming familiar with the indicators of potential substance abuse is important for nurses, particularly those who work in primary care or community settings because it is at these nonstigmatizing medical settings (as opposed to drug abuse treatment centers) that the substance abuser may first make contact with healthcare professionals.

The assessment process, however, is not always straightforward. The early stages can be difficult to recognize. The psychological, social, and physical manifestations vary widely, depending on the particular substance or substances used, the amount used or the frequency of use, and factors such as age and the physical health of the user (Grant & Hodgson, 1991).

## Interventions

### ◼ Society's Response

Society today is increasingly responding to the problems associated with substance abuse in a two-pronged approach: politically and as a healthcare issue. In the past, the political response to substance abuse was focused on punishment for the use or supplying of illicit drugs. Indeed, the acquisition and sales of illicit drugs continues to be the focus, with emphasis on law enforcement and punishment. However, the National Drug Control Strategy (NCADI, 2006) speaks to the importance of prevention. It indicates the need for a "balanced" program that addresses not only the **supply** (i.e., support to developing countries to put an end to their drug market) and **interdiction** (i.e., to stop drug trafficking at U.S. borders) issues, but also prevention, education, and treatment. The strategies recognize substance abuse problems as being international and long term, and as such they must be addressed with realistic programs that support families, schools, and communities and that include the international aspects of drug control.

These strategies do recognize that persons who are addicted need assistance. They hold individuals accountable for their negative behaviors but offer treatment that can help change those self-defeating destructive behaviors.

*Healthy People 2010* has recognized the seriousness of substance abuse and has identified 25 objectives related to alcohol and other drugs and 21 specifically focused on tobacco. Much of the emphasis in the objectives is placed on youth and decreasing the use and abuse of alcohol, tobacco, and other drugs within this group. One of the biggest needs identified in *Healthy People 2010* is access to culturally, linguistically, and age-appropriate service, education, and research necessary to meet the objectives. In addition, it is recognized that ongoing research must be undertaken to identify changes, evaluate the effectiveness of interventions and programs, and determine where further emphasis is needed. See the box on this page for selected *Healthy People 2010* objectives.

### Primary Prevention

**Primary prevention** involves the *prevention* of diseases or conditions through protective factors as well as through health-*promotion* activities. In the case of substance abuse, the first level of intervention pertains to activities that are begun before drug abuse occurs. Typical primary prevention techniques include education for responsible decision making, knowledge of risk factors, legislation and law enforcement, interdiction activities, and programs to strengthen resistance to substance abuse (Carroll, 1996).

One example of a primary prevention program conducted on a community level is the Kansas City comprehensive community program for drug abuse prevention with high- and low-risk adolescents. The program targeted early adolescent children within the community because research has demonstrated that this is the first risk period for onset of drug use. The program targeted multiple agencies within the community—schools, parents, community leaders, and mass media. Drug use resistance skills training took place for adolescents in grades six or seven, parent–school organizations set agendas to review school prevention policies, and parents were trained in positive parent–child communication; community leaders were organized into a drug abuse prevention task force; and considerable media coverage was given to the program. Research on the outcomes of the program indicates that the community-based prevention program was effective in reducing cigarette smoking and marijuana use at the ninth- and tenth-grade levels (3 full years after delivery of the

---

### ▥ HEALTHY PEOPLE 2010

#### Objectives Related to Substance Abuse and Tobacco Use

#### Substance Abuse

##### Adverse Consequences of Substance Use and Abuse

26.1 Reduce deaths and injuries caused by alcohol- and drug-related motor vehicle crashes.

26.3 Reduce drug-induced deaths.

26.4 Reduce drug-related hospital emergency department visits.

26.5 Reduce alcohol-related hospital emergency department visits.

26.7 Reduce intentional injuries resulting from alcohol- and illicit drug-related violence.

26.8 Reduce the cost of lost productivity in the workplace due to alcohol and drug use.

##### Substance Use and Abuse

26.9 Increase the age and proportion of adolescents who remain alcohol and drug free.

26.12 Reduce average annual alcohol consumption.

26.15 Reduce the proportion of adolescents who use inhalants.

##### Risk of Substance Use and Abuse

26.17 Increase the proportion of adolescents who perceive great risk associated with substance abuse.

##### Treatment for Substance Abuse

26.18 Reduce the treatment gap for illicit drugs in the general population.

26.20 Increase the number of admissions to substance abuse treatment for injection drug use.

26.21 Reduce the treatment gap for alcohol problems.

##### State and Local Efforts

26.23 Increase the number of communities using partnerships or coalition models to conduct comprehensive substance abuse prevention efforts.

26.24 Extend administrative license revocation laws, or programs of equal effectiveness, for persons who drive under the influence of intoxicants.

26.25 Extend legal requirements for maximum blood alcohol concentration levels of 0.08% for motor vehicle drivers aged 21 years and older.

#### Tobacco Use

##### Tobacco Use in Population Groups

27.1 Reduce tobacco use by adults.

27.2 Reduce tobacco use by adolescents.

27.3 Reduce initiation of tobacco use among children and adolescents.

##### Cessation and Treatment

27.5 Increase smoking cessation attempts by adult smokers.

27.6 Increase smoking cessation during pregnancy.

27.7 Increase tobacco use cessation attempts by adolescent smokers.

##### Exposure to Secondhand Smoke

27.9 Reduce the proportion of children who are regularly exposed to tobacco smoke at home.

27.11 Increase smoke-free and tobacco-free environments in schools, including all school facilities, property, vehicles, and school events.

27.12 Increase the proportion of worksites with formal smoking policies that prohibit smoking or limit it to separately ventilated areas.

##### Social and Environmental Changes

27.14 Reduce the illegal buy rate among minors through enforcement of laws prohibiting the sale of tobacco products to minors.

27.16 Eliminate tobacco advertising and promotions that influence adolescents and young adults.

27.18 Increase the number of tribes, territories, and states and the District of Columbia with comprehensive, evidence-based tobacco control programs.

*Source:* DHHS, 2000.

Public education involves the entire community.

school-based program). The program did not demonstrate a significant reduction in the use of alcohol by ninth and tenth graders who had participated in the program. However, the program was equally effective with both high- and low-risk adolescents. Overall, the program suggests that social/behavioral approaches to prevention that are addressed to whole populations can be effective and that prevention effects can be enduring (Johnson et al., 1990).

Programs that involve students in the design of a prevention campaign have two advantages. First, students are mobilized to become involved in the prevention of substance abuse among peers; second, the messages in health educational materials will be relevant to the population. For example, at the University of Colorado at Boulder, students in journalism classes had a unique assignment: create an ad

ETHICAL CONNECTION

Campaigns featuring slogans such as "Drug-Free Zones" and "We are a drug-free school" have been common for the past several years in U.S. schools—and yet teens are more likely to abuse nonprescribed and over-the-counter drugs and marijuana than alcohol today. Recent research shows an alarming trend among teens involving the use of caffeinated "energy" drinks such as Volt mixed with cough syrup or other high-alcohol drinks. While alcohol use is down in general among teens, use of prescription drugs, marijuana, and methamphetamine is up. Are we sending the right message to teenagers that drugs—even those that preserve and save lives—are bad and wrong? What are alternatives to this approach?

**Application to Practice**

A nurse at a university health services clinic has noticed a high number of females from sororities coming into the clinic complaining of "hangover" symptoms during the rush season. She begins to compare the numbers with the year before and finds a 200% increase in the number of females who have presented with alcohol-related symptoms. The nurse would like to do a population assessment of the sororities at the university and plan educational programs and interventions related to responsible and safe alcohol use.

1. Who should the nurse contact first to begin the assessment process?
2. What kind of demographic information would the nurse need to know in the planning of appropriate interventions?
3. Are there other professionals and laypersons who need to be involved in educational interventions for this population group?
4. How should the sororities be involved with the assessment, planning, and intervention related to safe alcohol use?
5. What kinds of evaluation measures could the nurse use to determine intervention effectiveness?

campaign aimed at college students that emphasizes responsible drinking. Students in the class knew that their peers would not respond to fear tactics because college-age youth still have a tendency to think that nothing tragic will happen to them. The class decided it would be best to focus on social issues like sexually transmitted diseases and poor sexual performance. The students created six print and voice ads that appeared in newspapers, buses, and movie theaters as well as on a local radio station ("Drinking—get real," 1998). See the figure on page 490 for an example of a relevant health education message developed by students themselves.

Community health nurses can and will be more involved in participating in population-focused intervention such as the previously mentioned programs. In addition, preventing the initial use of illicit substances or intervening to prevent further escalation of illicit substance use by our nation's youth before they move into adulthood should be a goal for all community health nurses who work with youth and their families. This goal is especially true for school health nurses, public health nurses, and nurses working in

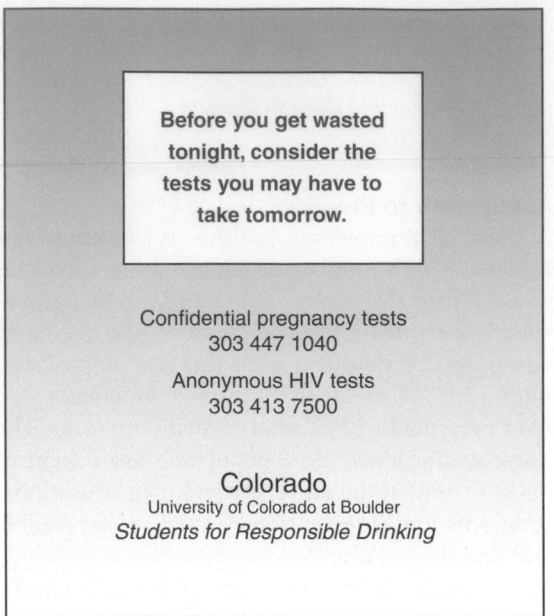

Before you get wasted tonight, consider the tests you may have to take tomorrow.

Confidential pregnancy tests
303 447 1040

Anonymous HIV tests
303 413 7500

Colorado
University of Colorado at Boulder
*Students for Responsible Drinking*

A focus on prevention: an advertisement campaign designed by University of Colorado college students for college students.

*Source:* "Before you get wasted tonight, consider the tests you may have to take tomorrow" from an ad campaign designed by the University of Colorado, Students for Responsible Drinking. Used by permission.

 *If they took all the drugs, nicotine, alcohol, and caffeine off the market for six days, they'd have to bring out the tanks to control you.* **"**

—*Dick Gregory*

community-based primary care settings. Efforts to prevent a public health problem before it begins or arresting it quickly in the early stages is far more effective than waiting until a substance abuse problem is firmly established. Remember, always include prevention strategies and keep substance abuse assessment criteria in mind whenever you are working with youth.

### Secondary Prevention

**Secondary prevention** efforts are focused on the early stages of substance abuse. The goal of secondary prevention is *to detect and arrest substance abuse* before the individual becomes physically addicted and the problem becomes a chronic condition.

Efforts are made to detect the problem as soon as possible and to begin treatment so that the condition does not progress. Health professionals need training in substance abuse as a significant health problem. Nurses and other health professionals need knowledge of high-risk populations and indicators of possible substance abuse, skills in assessment for the problem, and knowledge of interventions at the individual, family, and community levels. The primary aims of the assessment are outlined in Box 21-9.

After early detection and a beginning willingness on the part of the individual and his or her family to break the silence of denial, the next task involves getting the substance

abuser into treatment to prevent physiological addiction. Perhaps the entire family is in a crisis state. The nurse would be involved, along with a healthcare team, in crisis intervention with the family. It is no longer wise or necessary to assume that the individual needs to "hit bottom" before he or she can be helped. Indeed, it is detrimental for the individual and the family to receive help only after the loss of physical and mental health, family and friends, job, and self-respect. The substance-abusing individual needs to initiate treatment. Persuading the individual to do so at an early stage in substance abuse is difficult but can be accomplished. If possible, intervention is best implemented through a coalition of a healthcare team and family members of the substance abuser. Planning for an actual confrontation is often the best way to "shock" the individual into seeking treatment. Depending on the circumstances, the best time for confrontation is when the substance abuser's defenses are low—for example, shortly after the loss of a job, a drunk-driving arrest, a warning from a physician about a health problem, or the threat of a divorce (Carroll, 1996).

---

### BOX 21-9

**Secondary Prevention: Primary Aims of Substance Abuse Assessment**
- To meet the goal of secondary prevention with early detection and referral
- To obtain as much accurate information as possible about the individual's substance(s) use (frequency, amounts)
- To identify the factors associated with substance abuse, such as physical illnesses and social and psychological problems
- To identify the strengths and weaknesses of the individual and his or her family and ability to cope with and assist in the management of the problem

*Source:* Adapted from Grant & Hodgson, 1991.

---

 THINK ABOUT THIS

Caffeine is the most used drug in the world, followed by alcohol. Cigarette smoking and misuse of over-the-counter and prescribed drugs are common drug abuse issues. As a society, why do we focus on illegal drug use more than on the most commonly abused drugs? How do the media affect our ideas concerning drug use and abuse? What are your own opinions about drug use, misuse, and abuse?

---

### CULTURAL CONNECTION

Many European countries do not have an age limit for purchasing or using alcohol. They sanction the use of alcohol (usually wine and beer) with meals and allow children to drink small amounts of diluted alcohol as they age. These countries often have lower alcoholism rates than the United States. What do you think of these liberal values in regard to alcohol use?

## Tertiary Prevention

The third level of prevention, **tertiary prevention,** is initiated during later or advanced stages of substance abuse. Tertiary interventions include physical, mental, and social treatment procedures; detoxification; institutionalization; or outpatient drug-maintenance programs. You will find community health nurses working in all aspects of tertiary care. Many hospitals have drug treatment units. County mental health services sponsor detoxification centers where nurses are needed to do medical assessments, counseling, and referral. A major role for community health nurses in tertiary care is case or care management involving ongoing assessment and care coordination among the various services a chronic substance abuser may need in order to slowly move toward a potential recovery.

The primary goal of tertiary prevention is *to prevent reactivation* of substance-abusing behaviors (Carroll, 1996). Many health authorities now view dependence on alcohol or other drugs as a chronic relapsing disease. As such, drug dependence is often marked by a return of the substance abuse problem. Some professionals believe that it is more reasonable to think in terms of remissions (a lessening or reduction of the problem and its associative symptoms) rather than a cure (NIDA, 1998). Box 21-10 is a partial listing of potential tertiary treatment programs.

Although treatment is the focus of tertiary prevention, it is essential that common barriers to treatment be removed or reduced. Emotional support must be available. This is a primary intervention area for community health nurses because all nurses receive education and experience in interpersonal interaction with caring as a philosophical base. Financial support must be ensured through social policies that promote workplace drug assistance programs or through job counseling, job training, and a return to employment. Child care may also be an important treatment enhancer.

### BOX 21-10

**Tertiary Prevention: Partial Listing of Substance Abuse Treatment Options**

**Drug-Free Treatments**
- Therapeutic community
- Self-help groups such as Alcoholics Anonymous and Narcotics Anonymous
- Psychotherapy, including cognitive, behavioral, supportive-expressive, and family therapy
- Behavioral therapy specifically aimed at prevention of relapse

**Drug-Based Treatments**
- Methadone maintenance for heroin addicts
- Naltrexone (nonaddicting narcotic antagonist, also used in treating alcoholism)
- Antabuse (blocks alcohol metabolism)
- Psychoactive medication when indicated

*Source:* Carroll, 1996.

## ■ Interventions with Special Populations

### Children and Adolescents

#### Youthful deaths and substance abuse

Three-quarters of all deaths among school-age youth and young adults in the United States result from four causes: auto accidents, other unintentional injuries, homicide, and suicide. Research has also shown that Native Americans, African Americans, males, and those youths with the least education and income are at greater risk of both overall and injury-specific youth mortality (SAMSA 2005). Furthermore, many of these unintentional injury deaths are associated with substance abuse (Mezzich, Giancola, Tarter, Lu, Parks, & Barrett, 1997; U.S. Department of Transportation, 2007). It is particularly disturbing that U.S. suicide rates are highest among persons 15 to 24 years of age and in those older than 65 years of age. The association between suicide and the abuse of alcohol and other drugs is also a significant problem as highlighted in data gathered from the Drug Abuse Warning Network (DAWN), a large-scale drug abuse data collection system sponsored by the National Institute on Drug Abuse. DAWN records substances linked with emergency department admissions in various metropolitan areas of the United States. According to the DAWN report on annual trends in total drug-related episodes in emergency departments (SAMHSA, 2005), the most commonly reported motive for taking a substance was suicide.

### MEDIA MOMENT

***28 Days* (2000)**
Sandra Bullock stars in this movie about a 28-day rehab center and her struggles to stay sober.

#### Specific prevention programs for children and adolescents

The type of substance abuse prevention program most often used in schools has been either the presentation of factual information about the dangers of substance use (fear-arousal) or "affective" education to enhance self-esteem, responsible decision making, and social development. One program that is very popular in school districts and communities is the Drug Abuse Resistance Education (DARE) program. The DARE curriculum is organized into classroom sessions conducted by a police officer, coupled with activities taught by the regular classroom teacher. DARE combines the fear-arousal approach with the affective educational approached just described.

Despite the long tradition of these two approaches to prevention of substance abuse among youth, it is abundantly clear from scientific research that these approaches have only a short-term effect (Botvin & Botvin, 1992; Resnicow & Botvin, 1993). Why do these approaches fail to prevent substance abuse among youth? First, they fail to address the psychosocial factors promoting substance use, particularly peer pressure. Second, although the affective programs attempt to reduce the intrapsychic motivations to engage in substance use, the methods used are inadequate in that they do not place enough emphasis on skills training using behavior-change techniques (Botvin & Botvin, 1992).

Literature in the area of substance abuse prevention is abundant. However, there is a consensus in the literature that substance use prevention must begin early and that drug use resistance programs (in particular programs that use peer influences) are far superior to programs that focus on information and general affective programs involving self-esteem enhancement and problem-solving skills (Bukoski, 1997; U.S. Department of Transportation, 2007).

**❝** *Alcohol was beginning to compete with my affections for my wife and my family. It was beginning to crowd out my energy. And I decided to quit.* **❞**

—*President George W. Bush, September 19, 2000*

### Families

Many of the studies on families and illicit substance use by youths within the family are based on **social modeling theory.** Using this perspective, Fleming, Brewer, Gainey, Haggerty, and Catalano (1997) examined the relationship among parental drug use, bonding to parents, and child substance use. The families in this study were headed by substance abusers in methadone treatment for opiate addiction. The results of this study support the social development model and suggest that family interventions for preventing substance use in children of substance abusers should focus on reducing parental drug use and promoting bonding to parents who are abstinent.

**Social control** through parental involvement with youth is a second area of research that has been conducted on families as a risk factor in substance abuse in youth. In a study of male narcotic addicts, Nurco and Lerner (1996) found that an

---

**BOX 21-11**

**HELP! What Do I Do When I Get the Call That My Daughter or Friend Has Been Arrested on Drug Charges?**

1. Don't panic—stay calm.
2. Talk with the authorities and find out the charges and the details of what occurred.
3. Don't argue, challenge, or become defensive—it won't help.
4. Talk with an attorney about options. If you can't afford one, the court will appoint one.
5. If you need to get a bail bonds person, pick one carefully. Don't use the first one who approaches you. Ask others to recommend an honest reliable bail bonds person.
6. Take a friend with you to the hearings so you have moral support.
7. Don't attempt to talk with the person being charged until you have permission from the authorities/court.
8. Don't panic—stay calm.

---

 Research Alert

In an analysis of family structure and substance abuse risk, the Center on Addiction and Substance Abuse found that children living in two-parent families who have a fair or poor relationship with their father are at 68% higher risk of smoking, drinking, and using drugs compared with all teens living in two-parent households. The average teen living in a household headed by a single mother is at 30% higher risk compared with all teens in two-parent households. The results of this survey emphasized that "parent power" is the key to preventing drug use by children and youth. ●

*Source:* Center on Addiction and Substance Abuse. (1999). *CASA survey: Many dads AWOL in the battle against teen substance abuse.* Available from http://www.casacolumbia.org

---

intact family structure and parental disapproval of misbehavior by subjects were identified as significant deterrents to later addiction. Aseltine (1995) studied the reciprocal associations of family and peer relations and adolescent drug use over time. In this study, parental social control (e.g., being alert, having rules) was found to be stronger at the initiation stages of drug use but weaker than peers at maintenance. Parents may also indirectly help in the prevention of adolescent drug use by acting as friendship "gatekeepers," thereby preventing youths from associating with other youths who are using drugs.

A third area of research on family and risk factors for substance abuse is the influence of family functioning and drug use. Researchers at Arizona State University followed 179 adolescents, ages 11 to 15, over a 3-year measurement period. All youth entered into the study as nonusers of illicit drugs. Over the 3-year measurement period, 88 initial abstainers began to use substances. Results showed that older adolescents and adolescents from disorganized home environments were more likely to initiate substance use than younger adolescents and those from homes high in family organization that exhibited good communication and good problem solving (Hussong & Chassin, 1996). The Research Alert above highlights the importance of having fathers involved in family functioning.

#### Family-focused interventions

The family has been viewed as a target of nursing care since the time of Florence Nightingale. The practice of nursing in the United States began in family homes. There is a return to the importance of family nursing in the twenty-first century as healthcare finance reform is moving health care back into community settings. How do nurses intervene with families in which one or more members of the family has a substance abuse problem? Craft and Willadsen's (1992) investigation into nursing interventions related to family provides a taxonomy of general nursing interventions that are appropriate to use with substance-abusing families. Table 21-1 provides a list of generalized family-focused interventions to use when caring for a family in which one or more members has a substance abuse problem. It is

**Table 21-1**    Family Nursing Interventions and Their Defining Activites

| Nursing Intervention | Defining Activities |
| --- | --- |
| ■ Family support | Promotion of family interest and goals |
| ■ Family process maintenance | Minimization of disruption in family environment |
| ■ Family integrity promotion | Promotion of family cohesion and unity |
| ■ Family involvement | Promoting all family members in problem solving their situation of having one or more family members with a substance abuse problem |
| ■ Family mobilization | Utilization of family strengths to influence substance-abusing member(s) in positive direction |
| ■ Caregiver support | Provision of necessary information, advocacy, and emotional support |
| ■ Family therapy | Interaction with the family as a change agent to move family toward a more productive way of living |
| ■ Sibling support | Helping family understand the need to provide support (and attention) to nonabusing sibling whenanother sibling is the substance-abusing family member |
| ■ Parent education | Assistance to parents to understand effects of different substances and theories on causes of substance abuse |

*Source:* Adapted from Craft & Willadsen, 1992.

---

 NOTE THIS! •────────────────

What does the "proof" mean in regard to alcoholic content of beverages?

Proof comes from the process of unloading cargo of whiskey when merchants had only one way to tell the strength of the liquior they were carrying. They mixed a spoonful of whiskey with a pinch of gunpowder. When a lighted match was dropped into the mixture, it ignited with an audible "proof." This would only happen if alcohol mixture was 50% or more by volume. Today proof is defined as twice the alcohol content by volume. Whiskey with 100 proof is 50% alcohol.

---

important to note that these interventions fall within the practice domain of nursing. Often, nurses feel that they do not have the practice skills to deal with a family in which one or more members has a substance abuse problem. Nurses do have skills in family support, education, facilitation of problem solving, and so on, which should be and are effective nursing interventions to be used when a family needs nursing care for a substance abuse problem.

### Schools

Although there has been a downward trend in adolescent substance use since 1996, schools are definitely a target for substance abuse prevention. Indeed, the critical period for initial experimentation with one or more drugs and the subsequent development of regular patterns of use typically spans the beginning to middle adolescent years (SAMSA, 2005).

The movement known as **comprehensive school health** is a broad strategy for improving student health. This movement views education and health as highly integrated. The movement proposes that healthy children learn better and cautions that no curriculum can compensate for deficiencies in student health status (Kann, Collins, Pateman, Small, Ross, & Kolbe, 1995). The goal of the movement is to improve student risk behaviors in the areas of alcohol and other drugs, unintentional injuries, tobacco, diet, physical activity, and sexual intercourse (Symons, Cinelli, James, & Groff, 1997). Despite growing support for the movement

among parents, communities, and the federal government, local school leaders, who are under tremendous pressure to improve academic achievement, and other political stakeholders often remain unconvinced that improving student health represents a means to achieve improved academic outcomes. Instead, the current primary approach toward students with substance abuse behaviors is to discipline the offenders—suspending or expelling students, thus putting the youth at more risk for academic failure and future life difficulties. Adults working with children need to teach them how to identify and express their feelings. Provide a healthy adult–child relationship, especially with children of substance-abusing parents (SAMHSA, 2002).

### Workplace

Substance abuse in the workplace is a concern for both employers and consumers of products and services. Failure to address substance abuse in the workplace affects not only the person abusing substances, but also co-workers. It has been found to be a frequent factor in workplace violence (SAMHSA, 2005). In communities without occupational health nurses, the community health nurse is sometimes called on to provide employers with assistance in the development of programs to address workplace substance abuse problems. In addition to the signs of substance abuse found in Boxes 21-7 and 21-8, signs specifically found in the workplace are listed in Box 21-12.

---

### BOX 21-12

**Workplace Signs of Potential Substance Abuse**
- Decreased productivity or work fall off
- Decreased quality of job performance
- Increased work-related injuries, accidents, or illness
- Increased absenteeism, especially just before or after days off (e.g., holidays or vacations)
- Increasingly longer breaks and meal times

To deal effectively with substance-abusing employees, it is necessary to take some proactive measures. For this to occur, it is important to consider not only the needs of the company but also the legal issues, equal employment opportunity laws, the National Labor Relations Act, drug-free workforce rules and regulations, the ADA, Department of Transportation drug testing rules and regulations, and just-cause dismissal regulations (Naegle, 1993).

It is important to develop policies and processes for dealing with substance use and abuse in the workplace. Many times, nurses will be asked to participate in committees that develop these policies, particularly policies that are being developed by their own employers. These policies should be provided to new employees and periodically reviewed with all employees to ensure that they fully understand the policies and how the policies affect them. Any substance abuse policy needs to include a statement regarding drug testing. This statement needs to include when drug testing will be done (e.g., on employment, randomly). It should also include how the testing will take place, who will do it, how the security of the specimen will be maintained, who will pay for the testing, and how confidentiality of results will be handled.

For any drug policy to be effective, the employers, management personnel, and supervisory personnel should become familiar with what alcoholism, addiction, and substance abuse are; how to recognize them; and how to handle an employee experiencing such problems. Often, it is the community health nurse who is called on to assist in providing educational programs regarding substance abuse.

Many employers turn to community-based employee assistance programs (EAPs) to address the issue of substance-abusing employees. For EAPs to be effective, it is essential that any service, counseling, or intervention be kept separate from supervision of employees, with maintenance of confidentiality critical. The nurse working in a community-based EAP needs to be sure that policies and procedures regarding follow-up with supervisors who refer employees for assistance are handled in such a way that the employee's confidentiality is maintained. Reviewing policies and procedures regularly and being sure that they are in compliance with governmental rules and regulations are essential, and the nurse will often be actively involved in this process.

### Rural

Approximately one-quarter of all Americans and of the total elderly population live in rural areas. Farm foreclosures and the declining farm economy are stressors faced by those living in rural communities. In addition, rural communities are aging, with all of the health concerns associated with getting older.

Limited income, unemployment, and poverty are added stressors for rural families. Although illicit drug use does not appear to be as much of a problem in rural communities, high alcohol consumption and tobacco use, especially smokeless tobacco, are concerns. Attempts at establishing and carrying out prevention programs in rural communities

---

**BOX 21-13**

**Factors to Consider When Planning Rural Substance Abuse Intervention Programs**
- Geographic distance
- Transportation
- Rural economy
- Shortage of healthcare providers
- Shrinking tax base
- Isolation
- Access
- Issues of stigmatization

---

are directly related to the rural nature of these communities. Key factors that the community health nurse needs to consider in planning for this population include the following: a shortage of healthcare providers, geographic distance, isolation, transportation, access, rural economy, a shrinking tax base, and issues of stigmatization (Box 21-13).

For substance abuse prevention programs to be effective in rural communities, they must be accessible and available at neutral sites such as schools, churches, and community centers. Prevention efforts need to target those groups at greatest risk. Smoking and the use of smokeless tobacco are of particular concern in rural communities. Information about the health effects of smokeless tobacco should be made available and included in any drug prevention program. Potential users need to be made aware of not only the addictive nature of smokeless tobacco but also the long-term health effects. Box 21-14 is a summary of the health effects of dipping and chewing smokeless tobacco, which is a particular problem in rural communities.

Because depression and alcohol abuse can be coexisting conditions in rural communities, programs that provide for self-esteem building, decreased negative self-talk, building of support networks, and identification of accessible resources are needed. The community health nurse is often the person who is called on to plan, develop, and sometimes conduct these programs. The nurse may also become involved in planning and implementing groups for rural women conducted through the church, planning and implementing men's groups at the volunteer fire department hall, or arranging support groups for all substance abuse prevention efforts.

---

**BOX 21-14**

**Health Effects of Smokeless Tobacco**
- Oral cancer
- Gum problems
- Loss of teeth
- Heart problems

> **❝***I know folks all have a tizzy about it, but I like a little bourbon of an evening. It helps me sleep. I don't much care what they say about it.* **❞**
>
> —Lillian Carter, RN, mother of President Jimmy Carter

### Neighborhoods

The communities and neighborhoods where people live, work, play, and raise their families are important areas for addressing the problems associated with substance abuse. Interventions that are focused on the substances (drugs) are often aimed at eliminating the accessibility of drugs, limiting the sale of alcohol and tobacco, and providing education regarding the health effects of tobacco and drug use. Efforts to discourage and prevent substance abuse in neighborhoods have been found to be effective means of providing intervention to people where they live. See Box 21-15 regarding community action for addressing youth.

For many individuals, the idea of using official agencies (e.g., hospitals, clinics, health departments, social welfare agencies) is unpleasant. Fears of authority and prior experiences that might have been embarrassing or upsetting often discourage the use of such agencies, making it difficult to accept intervention and treatment.

People prefer contacts with community health nurses in their own neighborhoods. Neighborhood programs that actively involve residents have been shown to be highly effective in drug prevention efforts. The community health nurse is often asked to assist in the development of such a program. The first step the nurse needs to take is to assess the neighborhood. Six questions need to be asked (Office of Substance Abuse Prevention, 2004):

1. Do convenience stores, liquor stores, and gas station minimarts in your neighborhood check identification of people purchasing alcohol and tobacco? Do they sell beer in six-packs, not singles?
2. Do bars and restaurants in the neighborhood refuse service to intoxicated patrons? Make sure intoxicated patrons get rides home? Promote nonalcoholic drinks during happy hours?
3. Do employers in your neighborhood have a policy on alcohol use? Do they require nonalcoholic beverages to be served at social events they sponsor? Do they refuse to pay for alcoholic drinks at business meals? Do they provide for transportation, if needed, after social events where alcohol is served?
4. Can you find health messages about alcohol and tobacco use on local radio and TV stations?
5. Is there a communitywide policy that prevents alcohol- and drug-related problems at sporting events, rock concerts, and other large community gatherings?
6. Do local schools, universities, and sports centers accept advertising for alcoholic beverages or tobacco that is displayed at the sports arenas or in program?

It is important that community health nurses not only assume a role in promoting neighborhood involvement, but also become actively involved themselves. The community health nurse can assist with as well as encourage others to take the following six steps:

1. Write letters to support legislation on alcohol and drug policy.
2. Join a coalition of organizations involved with alcohol and drug policy.
3. Organize educational programs about alcohol- and drug-related programs.
4. Work with the media on developing health messages regarding alcohol, tobacco, and drug use.
5. Work with community organizations to implement alcohol-safe policies for large community events.
6. Set up programs to monitor the granting of new alcohol licenses.

The community health nurse is seen as a leader and role model within the community. As a role model, it is important that residents see nurses taking proactive roles in drug prevention efforts. When issues related to substance abuse arise, nurses should take the lead in informing elected officials about the need to support legislation and programs for prevention and treatment. Write and call your political leaders urging action. Ask others to also contact their elected officials. It is also important to activate supporters of prevention programs regarding legislation about substance abuse prevention, especially if there is a threat to such programs. Meet with elected officials and speak about your concerns. If necessary, mobilize the community to take action regarding substance abuse through letter writing, petitions, and other positive actions to make the neighborhood needs known.

### Women

Walton-Moss and Becker report 45% of women they surveyed used alcohol, 26% used tobacco, and 13% used drugs. Use of drugs (illicit or prescription) and alcohol by women is not a new phenomenon, but the response to women who are substance abusers is often different than it is for their male counterparts. In the 1980s, it was reported that women who were alcoholic were considered sicker, wives of

---

## BOX 21-15

**Community Action**

**Parents**
- Talk with children
- Provide boundaries before problems occur
- Set family rules

**Educators**
- Address early aggressive behavior and poor conduct
- Provide support for the learner who is struggling

**Community**
- Assess community risks
- Plan for prevention services, early intervention, and family counseling

*Source*: NIDA, 2003.

👆 THINK ABOUT THIS ·······················

I learned more about myself by being an RN than anything else I have ever done.
—Naomi Judd, RN, award winning country music singer, founding member of the Judds, and mother of actress Ashley Judd and country music singer Wynonna Judd

Florence Nightingale first published information about an association between health and music. Country music portrays human emotions in the rawest and most vivid of terms and has been described as a "three-minute soap opera." Watch the music video "Little Rock" by Collin Raye, which depicts alcohol and family abuse and provides a visual resource for Al-Anon at the end of the video.

"Little Rock" by Collin Raye, written by Tom Douglas (1994)

Think about the concepts that are explored in this song: abuse, child trauma, family dysfunction, violence, alcoholism, and recovery.

- Explore the issue of alcoholism, recovery, and relationships as depicted in this song and music video.
- How did you feel about the man's situation? Is he likely to maintain sobriety? Why or why not?
- How did you feel the child experienced the abuse?
- What role does religion play in this song?
- Is there a nurse's role in this scenario?

💻 Research Alert

In-depth interviews were conducted with 60 pregnant or postpartum women who were crack cocaine users to better understand the issues and problems these women face. Findings suggested fears about bearing a drug-dependent baby and/or concerns about losing custody were very real. Guilt, fear, and pressure to take action were common feelings. The women initially dealt with the threats to their self-esteem by delaying acknowledging the pregnancy and seeking care. However, once they did acknowledge the pregnancy, they attempted to make the best of the situation by decreasing drug use, trying to improve their diet, and trying to avoid conflict and worry. When healthcare providers were perceived as threatening custody of the child, they tried to avoid the healthcare system and "relied on their own self-care to optimize pregnancy outcomes" (p. 212).

For the community health nurse, it is essential that the nurse recognize the fears and concerns of the substance-abusing pregnant woman and provide avenues for entry into care that support the mother-to-be and foster trust and safety rather than fear and distrust.

*Source:* Kearney, M., Murphy, S., Irwin, K., & Rosenbaum, M. (1996). Salvaging self: A grounded theory of pregnancy on crack cocaine. *Nursing Research, 44*(4), 208–213.

alcoholics were considered enablers, and husbands of alcoholic wives were looked at with respect for putting up with their wives' problem (Sandelowski, 1981). Things are beginning to change, but some issues still need to be addressed when working with the problems associated with substance abuse in women. Women's drug use differs from men's in that they often use prescription drugs in combination, are less likely to have a stable relationship/marriage, and most often have children living with them. Zwickler (2004) reported a study from the Medical College of Virginia Commonwealth

🌀 MEDIA MOMENT

***Passion Fish*** (1992)

A movie about recovery, redemption, and two women who form an unlikely friendship because of their common losses and addictions. The film features a former daytime soap-opera star who becomes addicted to alcohol after a disabling accident. She returns to her home in the bayous of southern Louisiana, where she employs a nurse as her caregiver who also is recovering from a serious addiction problem.

University in which there was a high incidence of childhood sexual abuse in women who are drug dependent. How these women view themselves is an important factor in addressing issues of their substance abuse. The Research Alert addresses the issue of pregnant women and substance abuse.

Most treatment programs use a model that was developed when the majority of persons receiving treatment were men. Women tend to be hesitant about entering treatment programs that use confrontation and mixed-sex groups. For substance-abusing women, who often have experienced abuse (physical and verbal) from men, verbalizing their vulnerability in a mixed group is difficult if not impossible. Low self-esteem is an issue for this population. Snow and Anderson (2000) found depression to be a common factor among women with substance abuse problems, often resulting in relapse. A second contributor was related to the effects of "violent relationships and inability of the women to recognize this area as a contributor to their alcohol/drug abuse." Providing same-sex groups where the women feel safe and supported and are received in a nonjudgmental manner is helpful in facilitating the treatment process. The same-sex groups also provide the opportunity for women to openly discuss relationship issues. Williams (2004) found intervention with women is often more successful if they are first treated with one-on-one sessions before moving into group therapy.

Treatment issues related to the pregnant woman and to women with children need to be addressed. The highest incidence of substance abuse in pregnant women is found in women younger than 25 years of age, with a large percentage of these women being unmarried. A major problem is the lack of treatment programs geared to caring for women who are pregnant and using drugs or for women with children who are using drugs.

Community health nurses need to focus their attention on two areas when addressing the problems associated with substance abuse in women: education and advocacy. First, educating women about the effects of alcohol and drug use is essential, especially with young women who are of childbearing age. Knowledge about the effects of drug use on the unborn child is essential for young women to make informed decisions (Kinney, 1996). Second, it is essential that the community health nurse take an advocacy position and lobby for treatment programs that adequately provide for women with young children, addressing such issues as child care, treatment for the pregnant woman, and physical and sexual abuse. Community health nurses have an obligation to keep informed about which programs are most effective in treatment and prevention of substance abuse and its associated problems if they are to meet the needs of this special population. Williams (2004) indicated women prefer community-based programs that use a holistic approach that addresses women's multiple social roles and needs such as clothing, food, and daycare. These programs need to be convenient and "comfortable."

### Elders

Substance abuse in the elderly population is often a hidden problem. It has been estimated that by the year 2030, the fastest-growing segment of the population will be persons older than 85 years of age. Fewer than 50% of elders live in institutions, and at least half of older people have some health problems. According to the 2002 National Survey on Drug Use and Health, this group has the lowest rate of illicit drug use and the highest use of over-the-counter drugs. Prescription medication use is also a reality for 60% to 78% of the older population. Nelson (1998) indicated that one of the major concerns with this population results from the adverse effects of drug–drug and drug–alcohol interaction, leading to an increased risk for illness, injury, and death (Table 21-2).

Adams and Kinney (1996) suggest that even minimal alcohol use/abuse can be a problem for the older person. The problem in part is due to alcohol interaction with other prescription drugs, as well as the physiological changes that are associated with aging, such as impaired absorption and excretion of those substances (Meiner, 1997). For example, alcohol use by an older person who is taking a nonsteroidal anti-inflammatory agent increases the likelihood of gastrointestinal bleeding. Problems such as these are further complicated by the movement of former prescription medications into the over-the-counter category.

It is essential that the community health nurse recognize the potential for problems because it is often the nurse who must sort out the elder's shoebox of prescription and over-the-counter-medications and make sense of what that individual is really taking. Therefore, it is important that the nurse recognize the possibility that alcohol use/abuse could be a complicating factor.

For the elderly population with multiple chronic health problems, additional factors that may contribute to alcohol and drug abuse are limited income, inadequate instructions

Chapter author Dr. Jean Haspeslagh assists an elder patient with understanding multiple drug interactions.

| Table 21-2 | Common Alcohol–Drug Interactions to Look for in the Elderly |

| Drug Category | Interaction/Effect |
| --- | --- |
| ▪ Antibiotics | Nausea, vomiting, headache, possible seizures, reduced effectiveness of the medication |
| ▪ Anticoagulants | Acute alcohol consumption = increased risk of hemorrhage |
| | Chronic alcohol consumption = reduced blood thinning effect and potential for blood disorder |
| ▪ Antidepressants | Increased sedative effects, elevated blood pressure |
| ▪ Antidiabetic medications | Nausea, headache |
| | Acute alcohol consumption = prolonged effect |
| | Chronic alcohol consumption = decreased effect |
| ▪ Cardiovascular medications | Dizziness, fainting, reduced effectiveness of some antihypertensives |

regarding their medications and alcohol interaction, and poor follow-up. Community health nurses must carefully assess the older person's medication regimen and determine how well it is being followed.

When attempting to determine whether there is a substance abuse problem, the family and friends of the elder are often the first to identify the potential problem. Nelson (1998) reported that the elderly most at risk for a substance abuse problem are those who are "widowed, single, living in disadvantaged areas, blue-collar workers, and those with criminal records" (p. 28). Nelson also indicated that older women have the potential to develop drinking problems later in life as a result of such factors as outliving their spouses and having a higher poverty rate. Community health nurses, especially those who work with the elderly in their homes, need to be aware of the potential for a substance abuse problem and provide necessary referral should the problem be identified. An effective treatment program must take into consideration the health problems and necessary medications to treat those problems when planning care. When working with the elder who has a substance abuse problem, it is important for the community health nurse to recognize that this person is a survivor and to build on that strength when planning care. Any intervention planned by the community health nurse must include contact for the elder with other people and assistance in identifying ways to provide meaningful activity for the elder.

Primary prevention efforts should focus on teaching about age-specific dangers of alcohol use, particularly in relation to medications that are being taken. The Council on Scientific Affairs of the AMA indicated that there are no safe guidelines for drinking for older adults. Prevention programs need to include content that reviews medications and their appropriate use, problems associated with mixing medications and alcohol, mixing prescription and over-the-counter medications, and proper disposal of medications (see Box 21-16). The Office of Substance Abuse Prevention suggests that programs encouraging responsible use of medications be implemented. It encourages having "dumping contests" (i.e., a contest for throwing away outdated and no longer used medications). We need to remember that prevention efforts are not just for the young and that our elderly also need our assistance if they are to avoid problems with substance misuse and abuse.

### NOTE THIS!

Bhutan became the first country in the world to ban the sale of tobacco.

### Nurses and Other Healthcare Professionals

Nurses and other healthcare professionals are another group at risk for substance abuse problems. Accurate reports of substance abuse in the general population of nurses and healthcare providers is difficult to determine because denial is a key component of alcoholism and substance abuse, related to these issues, lessening the likelihood of accurate

---

**BOX 21-16**

**Need to Knows for Elders**

1. Some medications don't mix well with other medications, including over-the-counter (OTC) medications and herbal remedies.
2. Many medications do not mix well with alcohol.
3. Medications for sleep, pain, or depression make use of alcohol unsafe.
4. If there is no history of a drinking problem, one drink a day is the recommended limit (12 ounces of beer, 1.5 ounces of distilled spirits [hard liquor], or 5 ounces of wine).
5. Keep lists of all medications from all doctors. Include all regularly used OTC drugs and herbal remedies. Update as doses or medications change.
6. Have your doctor review all of your medications once a year.

*Sources:* Center for Substance Abuse Treatment (CSAT). (2001). *Aging, medicine and alcohol;* U.S. Department of Health and Human Services (USDHHS). (2004). *As you age: A guide to aging, medicine, and alcohol.*

---

self-reporting in surveys. The American Nurses Association has estimated that approximately 6% to 8% of nurses have a substance abuse problem (Kinney, 1996). In addition, there is a high rate of smoking among nurses (see Table 21-3).

Because substance abuse in nurses affects not only the nurse but also those who receive health care and those who work with the nurse, it is important that community health nurses recognize the issues associated with nurses who abuse substances. Community health nurses will encounter substance-abusing nurses and other healthcare professionals in the community both as patients and as colleagues. Factors influencing how you may respond can be found in Box 21-17.

As with any chronic condition, recognition that the condition exists is the first step toward rehabilitation. Signs of substance abuse in nurses range from mood swings to blackouts. Box 21-18 presents a list of indicators of substance abuse that may be noticed in a nurse's job performance. Deteriorating work performance is often one of the later signs of the problem. One recovering nurse reported that even at the peak of her active drug use, she continued to receive good

---

### MEDIA MOMENT

Philip Morris, the largest cigarette maker in the United States, began running advertisements in 2006 discouraging Hollywood from using its products on the big screen, citing studies that have shown cinematic portrayals of tobacco use can entice children to smoke.

Richmond-based Philip Morris USA ran advertisements in *Daily Variety, Hollywood Reporter,* and other trade publications imploring moviemakers: "Please Don't Give Our Cigarette Brands a Part in Your Movie."

## BOX 21-17

### Factors Influencing Responses to Substance-Abusing Nurses

- Prior experience with someone else who is a substance abuser
- Hold a view that a nurse is a "superhuman being" who should be able to avoid such behavior
- Hold a strong moralistic view of substance abuse as being morally wrong
- Feel anger at anyone who would "steal" medication from patients
- Feel fear and anxiety that this could easily happen to themselves

## BOX 21-18

### Indicators of Possible Substance Abuse in Nurses

#### Any Substance

- Frequent medication errors
- Poor documentation—illogical, sloppy, illegible
- Patient complaints
- Withdrawal, isolation—removing self from professional committees and organizations
- Signs out more controlled substances than others
- Volunteers to work extra hours or assignments that provide access to drugs

#### Narcotics

- Incorrect counts of controlled substances
- Large amounts of drugs wasted
- Significant variation in quantity of drugs required on the unit when that nurse is working
- Discrepancies between patient's and nurse's reports of pain
- Patient reports of ineffective pain medication only when suspected nurse gives the medication
- Patient complaints of pain or restlessness only when the suspected nurse is working

*Sources:* Crosby & Bissell, 1989; Sullivan, Bissell, & Williams, 1988; Haspeslagh, 1990.

## BOX 21-19

### Resources for Return to Work Contract Requirements

Crosby, L., & Bissell, L. (1989). *To care enough* (pp. 255–260). Minneapolis: Johnson Institute.

Durburg, S., & Werner, J. (1989). Re-entering the professional practice environment. In M. R. Haack & T. L. Hughs (Eds.), *Addiction in the nursing profession* (pp. 119–171). New York: Springer.

Maher-Brisen, P. (2007). Addiction: An occupational hazard in nursing. *American Journal of Nursing,* 107, 8, 78–79.

Naegle, M. (1993). *Substance abuse education in nursing* (vol. 3, pp. 231–235). New York: National League for Nursing.

### MEDIA MOMENT

**"Drunker Than Me," Trent Tomlinson (2005)**

'Cause I ain't worryin' about who's drivin' home,
Who's got the keys, who's got the 'phone,
Who'll pay the bill, call a cab.
I don't mean to make you mad,
But I don't want that responsibility,
An' I can't be with a woman, baby, who gets drunker than me.

performance evaluations from her supervisor. During that time, she was never confronted about her performance even though she was experiencing blackouts (periods when she was unable to recall what happened).

A number of programs have been developed to address the needs of substance-abusing nurses. In addition to community treatment programs and employee assistance programs, programs specially designed for the recovering nurse have been developed to assist the nurse toward recovery and to monitor the nurse's progress. There are two types of programs: those sponsored by state nurses associations and those associated with state boards of nursing. The latter programs have legal power, provide oversight to the nurse, and have power to grant permission to work with certain stipulations (requirements) that must be met to retain a

nursing license. Such programs ensure that the substance abusing nurse is meeting those requirements placed on the license to practice.

Nurses returning to active nursing must have a **return to work contract.** This contract protects the nurse and the agency employing the nurse, and ultimately the patients. This contract should include the stipulations for returning to work, the length of time for the stipulations, frequency of random drug screens, restrictions on license, required group and individual counseling sessions, and written reports. Box 21-19 is a list of resources that provide information on return to work contract requirements.

| Table 21-3 | Profile of Registered Nurses Who Smoke |
|---|---|

- 15% of RNs smoke.
- 10–14% of nursing students smoke.
  By specialty:

| | |
|---|---|
| Mental health/psychiatry | 23% |
| Gerontology | 18% |
| Emergency room | 18% |
| Pediatrics | 8% |
| Oncology | 7% |

*Source:* www.tobaccofreenurses.org.

Haspeslagh (1990) found that returning to work was a process during which the recovering nurse could either cope successfully or relapse. The time when nurses are most vulnerable for relapse is between 3 months and 1 year after treatment. There are three factors that put recovering nurses at risk for relapse: not working their aftercare program, not going to aftercare/support groups, and only doing what is required for their license or family, not for themselves. She also found that nurses who had the support of colleagues and supervisors who were knowledgeable about substance abuse and relapse were more likely to not relapse. For community health nurses, it is important to be able to recognize issues associated with substance abuse in nurses and other healthcare professionals. It is essential for the nurse to understand the importance of confronting substance abuse in nurses and to provide support for the returning recovering nurse. It is imperative that the community health nurse be cognizant of the signs of relapse and the proper steps to take if a co-worker begins to take that walk down the path to relapse.

## Conclusion

Substance abuse is a major public health concern. Community health nurses have a responsibility to address this problem as both healthcare professionals and private citizens. Looking at yourself and identifying your own issues and biases regarding the substance abuser is the first step to developing and providing appropriate care for those populations affected by substance abuse. The nurse must take an active role in assessment and early identification of persons at risk for substance abuse. Planning and implementing prevention programs is a primary role for community health nursing practice. Working with community leaders in the planning and implementation of programs that address the issues of drugs and youth, programs for women and children, drug-related crime, and community-focused prevention programs must be addressed if the *Healthy People 2010* objectives are to be achieved.

Explore Community Health Nursing on the Web! To learn more about the topics in this chapter, use the passcode provided to access your exclusive website: **http://nursing.jbpub.com/ communityhealth.** If you do not have a passcode, you can obtain one at this site.

# ■ CRITICAL THINKING ACTIVITIES

1. In the 1998 legislative session, the state legislature passed three bills related to alcoholic beverages. One bill set a zero tolerance level (when tested, no level of alcohol can be present) for intoxicated adolescents picked up by authorities. The second bill raised the alcohol level allowed in beer sold in the state, thus allowing for a stronger beverage. The third bill permitted the establishment of microbreweries in the state.
   - What kind of message do these three bills send?
   - If you were a resident of this state, how would you react?
   - What do you see as the major issue(s) related to the passage of these three bills?
   - Which moral and ethical dilemmas can you identify?
   - Which options are available to address these issues?
2. You are a community health nurse working in home health. One day your patient's daughter tells you the following about one of the agency's home health aides:

   I really like Mrs. Green—she is a good person and has so many responsibilities, but I need to tell you she does tend to fall asleep when she is staying with dad. Last week he said that he thought he smelled alcohol on her breath but couldn't be sure. I've noticed she has been late coming to work more and more. Monday, when she came, she had a number of bruises and looked like she might have fallen down. I hate to complain, but I'm concerned about dad's safety. I also like Mrs. Green and am concerned about her.

   - How would you respond to the daughter?
   - What should the agency do about Mrs. Green? Why?
   - What is your responsibility?
   - How would you feel in this situation?

# ■ REFERENCES

Adams, W., & Kinney, J. (1996). The elders. In J. Kinney (Ed.), *Clinical manual of substance abuse* (2nd ed.). St. Louis: Mosby.

Agency for Health Care Policy and Research (AHCPR). (1996). *Clinical practice guidelines on smoking cessation.* Washington, DC: Department of Health and Human Services.

Amaro, H. (1999). An expensive policy: The impact of inadequate funding for substance abuse treatment. *American Journal of Public Health, 89*(5), 657–659.

Anthenelli, R. (1997). A basic clinical approach to diagnosis in patients with comorbid psychiatric and substance use disorders. In N. Miller (Ed.), *The principles and practice of addictions in psychiatry* (pp. 119–126). Philadelphia: W. B. Saunders.

Aseltine, R. H. (1995). A reconsideration of parental and peer influences on adolescent deviance. *Journal of Health Social Behavior, 36*(2), 103–121.

Associated Press. (1999, September 8). Seven in ten drug users work full time, report says. *Hattisburg American,* p. 4A.

Barton, J. A. (1991). Parental adaptation to adolescent drug abuse: An ethnographic study of role formulation in response to courtesy stigma. *Public Health Nursing, 8*(1), 39–45.

Bauman, K. E., Foshee, V. A., Ennett, S. T., Pemberton, M., Hicks, K. A., King, T. S., et al. (2001). The influence of a family program on adolescent tobacco and alcohol. *American Journal of Public Health, 91*(4), 604–610.

Borvin, G. J., & Botvin, E. M. (1992). Adolescent tobacco, alcohol, and drug abuse: Prevention strategies, empirical findings, and assessment issues. *Developmental and Behavioral Pediatrics, 13*(4), 290–301.

Bukoski. W. J. (Ed.). (1997). Meta-analysis of drug abuse prevention programs. *NIDA Research Monograph, 170.*

Bull, C. (1998). Aging in rural communities. *National Forum, 18*(2), 34–41.

Carroll, C. (1996). *Drugs in modern society* (4th ed.). Dubuque, IA: Brown and Benchmark.

Center on Addiction and Substance Abuse. (1999). *CASA survey: Many dads AWOL in the battle against teen substance abuse.* Available from http://www.casacolumbia.org

Center for Substance Abuse Treatment (CSAT). (2001). *Aging, medicines and alcohol* [Brochure]. Rockville, MD: Author.

Craft, M. J., & Willadsen, J. A. (1992). Interventions related to family. *Nursing Clinics of North America, 27*(2), 517–531.

Crosby, L., & Bissell, L. (1989). *To care enough.* Minneapolis: Johnson Institute.

Department of Health and Human Services (DHHS). (2000). *Healthy People 2010: Conference edition.* Washington, DC: U.S. Government Printing Office.

Department of Health and Human Services (DHHS). (2004). *As you age: A guide to aging, medicine, and alcohol* [Brochure]. Rockville, MD: Author.

Drinking—get real. (1998, December). *The Coloradan,* p. 2.

Durburg, S., & Werner, J. (1989). Re-entering the professional practice arena. In M. Haack & T. Hughs (Eds.), *Addiction in the nursing profession* (pp. 119–171). New York: Springer.

Fleming, C. B., Brewer, D. D., Gainey, R. R., Haggerty, K. P., & Catalano, R. F. (1997). Parent drug use and bonding to parents as predictors of substance use in children of substance abusers. *Journal of Child and Adolescent Substance Abuse, 6*(4), 75–86.

Goldsmith, R. J. (1997) The integrated psychology for addiction psychiatry. In N. Miller (Ed.), *The principles and practice of addictions in psychiatry* (pp. 3–10). Philadelphia: W. B. Saunders.

Goodman, A. (2004). Passive smokers unite. *Cure. 3*(1), 64–67.

Grant, M., & Hodgson, R. (Eds.). (1991). *Responding to drug and alcohol problems in the community.* Geneva: World Health Organization.

Haack, M. R., & Hughes, T. L. (Eds.). (1989). *Addiction in the nursing profession.* New York: Springer.

Hahn, E. J. (1993). Parental alcohol and other drug (AOD) use and health beliefs about parent involvement in AOD prevention. *Issues in Mental Health Nursing, 14,* 237–247.

Hahn, E. J., & Rado, M. (1996). African American head start parent involvement in drug prevention. *American Journal of School Health, 20*(1), 41–51.

Hahn, E. J., Simpson, M. R., & Kidd, P. (1996). Cues to parent involvement in drug prevention and school activities. *Journal of School Health, 66*(5), 165–170.

Haspeslagh, J. (1990). Recovering nurses' perceptions of job re-entry. Unpublished Ph.D. dissertation. Louisiana State University Medical Center, New Orleans.

Hawkins, J. D., Catalano, R. F., & Arthur, M. (2002). Promoting science-based prevention in communities. *Addictive Behaviors, 90*(5), 1–26.

Hill, S. Y. (1998). Alternative strategies for uncovering genes contributing to alcoholism risk: Unpredictable findings in a genetic wonderland. *Alcohol, 16*(1), 53–59.

Hussong, A., & Chassin, L. (1996). Substance use initiation among adolescent children of alcoholics: Testing protective factors. *Journal of Studies on Alcohol, 58*(3), 272–279.

Johnson, C. A., Pentz, M., Weber, M., et al. (1990). Relative effectiveness of comprehensive community programming for drug abuse prevention with high-risk and low-risk adolescents. *Journal of Consulting and Clinical Psychology, 58*(4), 447–456.

Johnston, L. D., O'Malley, P. M., & Bachman, J. G. (1998). *Drug use by American young people begins to turn downward.* Retrieved November 2, 2008, from http://www.nih.gov/news/pr/dec98/nida-18.htm

Kann, L., Collins, J. L., Pateman, B. C., Small, M. L., Ross, J. G., Kolbe, L. J. (1995). The School Health Policies and Programs (SHPPS): Rationale for a nationwide status report on school health programs. *Journal of School Health, 65*(8), 291–294.

Kann, L., Warren, C. W., Harris, W. A., et al. (1996). Youth risk behavior surveillance United States 1995. *Mortality and Morbidity Weekly Report CDC Surveillance Summary, 45*(4), 1–84.

Kearney, M. H., Murphy, S., Irwin, K., & Rosenbaum, M. (1995). Salvaging self: A grounded theory of pregnancy on crack cocaine. *Research, 44*(4), 208–213.

Kelly, E., Darke, S., & Ross, J. (2004). A review of drug use and driving: Epidemiology impairment, risk factors, and risk perceptions. *Drug Alcohol Review, 23*(3), 319–344.

Kelly, K., & Donohew, L. (1999). Media and primary socialization theory. *Substance Use and Misuse, 34*(7), 1033–1045.

Kimball, A., Beckley, S., & Ngugi, E. (1998). International aspect of the AIDS/HIV epidemic. In P. Lee & C. Estes (Eds.), *The national health* (5th ed., pp. 114–136). Sudbury, MA: Jones and Bartlett.

Kinney, J. (1996). *Clinical manual of substance abuse* (2nd ed.). St. Louis: Mosby.

Kosterman, R. Hawkins, J. D., Haggerty, K. P., Spoth, R., & Redmond, C. (2001). Preparing for the drug free years: Session-specific effects of a universal parent-training intervention with rural families. *Journal of Drug Education, 31*(1), 47–68,

Kosterman, R., Hawkins, J. D., Spoth, R., Haggerty, K. P., & Zhu, K. (1997). Effects of a preventive parent-training intervention on observed family interactions: Proximal outcomes from *Preparing for the Drug Free Years. Journal of Community Psychology, 25*(4), 337–352.

MacKinnon, D. P., Johnson, C. A., Pentz, M. A., Dwyer, J. H., Hansen, W. B., Flay, B. R., & Wang, E. Y. (1991). Mediating mechanisms: A school-based drug prevention program: First-year effects of the Midwestern Prevention Project. *Health Psychology, 10*(3), 164–172.

Maher-Brisen, P. (2007). Addiction: An occupational hazard in nursing. *American Journal of Nursing, 107*(8) 78–79.

Meiner, S. (1997, July). Polypharmacy in the elderly. *Advance for Nurse Practitioners,* 29–33.

Methamphetamine. (1998). In *Community Drug Abuse Bulletin* (NIDA, National Institute of Health).

Mezzich, A. C., Giancola, P. R., Tarter, R. E., Lu, S., Parks, S. M., & Barrett, C. M. (1997). Violence, suicidality, and alcohol/drug use involvement in adolescent females with a pyschoactive substance use disorder and controls. *Alcoholism Clinical and Experimental Research, 21*(7), 1300–1307.

Naegle, M. (1993). *Substance abuse education in nursing* (vol 3). New York: National League for Nursing.

National Center for Health Statistics. (2007). *Health: With chartbook on trends of the health of Americans.* Hyattsville, MD: Author.

National Clearinghouse for Alcohol and Drug Information (NCADI). (1998). *Drug control strategy: An overview.* Available from http://www.health.org

National Highway Traffic Safety Administration. (2007). *Traffic Safety Facts Research Note.* U.S. Department of Transportation Report No. DOT HS 810 821. Washington, DC.

National Institute on Drug Abuse (NIDA). (1998). *Monitoring the future—1998.* Rockville, MD: Department of Health and Human Services.

National Institute on Drug Abuse (NIDA). (2003). NIDA-funded research drives revision of guide to prevention programming. Retrieved August 22, 2008, from http://www.drugabuse.gov/NIDA_Notes/NNVol18N4/tearoff.html

National Institute on Drug Abuse. (2007). *Monitoring the future: National survey results on drug use, overview of key findings.* Bethesda, MD: Author.

National Institute on Drug Abuse & Drug Enforcement Administration. (2008). *Methamphetamine (Meth).* Retrieved August 22, 2008, from http://www.drugfree.org/Portal/drug-guide/methamphetamine

National survey on drug use and health (NSDUH). (2002). Substance Abuse and Mental Health Services Administration. *National treatment improvement study.* (1997). Available from http://www.health.org

Nelson, M. (1998). Alcohol use in the older adult. *American Journal for Nurse Practitioners, 2*(6), 24–32.

Nurco, D., & Lerner, M. (1996). Vulnerability to narcotic addiction: Family structure and functioning. *Journal of Drug Issues, 26*(4), 1007–1025.

Office of Substance Abuse Prevention. (2004). *Prevention Plus: Tools for creating and sustaining drug-free communities.* Rockville, MD: Department of Health and Human Services.

Resnicow, K., & Borvin, G. (1993). School based substance use prevention programs: Why do effects decay? *Preventive Medicine, 22,* 484–490.

Robinson, T. N., Chen, H. L., & Killen, J. D. (1998). Television and music video exposure and risk of adolescent alcohol use. *Pediatrics, 102*(5), 1201–1209.

Sandelowski, M. (1981). *Women, health, and choice.* Englewood Cliffs, NJ: Prentice Hall.

Schneider, C., Fischer, G., Diamant, K., et al. (1996). Pregnancy and drug dependence. *Wiener Klinisch Wochenschrift, 108*(19), 611–614.

Singh, G. K., & Yu, S. M. (1996). Trends and differentials in adolescent and young mortality in the United States, 1950–1993. *American Journal of Public Health, 86*(4), 560–564.

Snow, D., & Anderson, C. (2000). Exploring factors influencing relapse and recovery among alcohol and drug addicted women. *Journal of Psychosocial Nursing, 38*(7), 8–18.

Substance Abuse and Mental Health Services Administration (SAMHSA). (1996). *Annual trends in annual drug-related episodes.* Available from http://www.health.org

Substance Abuse and Mental Health Services Administration (SAMHSA). (1998). *Discussion of results from the 1997 national household survey on drug abuse.* Available from http://www.health.org/pubs/nhsda/98hhs/findings/12results.htm

Substance Abuse and Mental Health Services Administration (SAMHSA). (2002). You can help: A guide for caring adults working with young people experiencing addiction in the family. Available from http://neadistore.samhsa.gov/catalog/ProductDetails.aspx?ProductID=16052

Substance Abuse and Mental Health Services Administration (SAMHSA). (2004). *Overview of findings from the 2003 national survey drug use and health* (Office of Applied Studies, NHSDA Series H-24, DHHS Publication No. SMA 04-3963). Rockville, MD: Author.

Substance Abuse and Mental Health Services Administration (SAMHSA). (2007). *2006 national survey on drug use and health.* Rockville, MD: Author.

Sullivan, E., Bissell, L., & Williams, E. (1988). *Chemical dependency in nursing.* Menlo Park, CA: Addison-Wesley.

Symons, C., Cinelli, B., James, T. C., & Groff, P. (1997). Bridging student health risks and academic achievement through comprehensive school health programs. *Journal of School Health, 67*(6), 220–227.

U.S. Department of Justice, Drug Enforcement Administration (DEA). (2005). *Drugs of abuse.* Retrieved November 2, 2008, from http://www.usdoj.gov/dea/pubs/abuse

Walton-Moss, B., & Becker, K. (2000). Women and substance use disorders. *Primary Care Practitioner, 4,* 290–302.

Weinberg, T. S., & Vogel, C. (1990). Wives of alcoholics: Stigma management and adjustments to husband–wife interaction. *Deviant Behavior, 11,* 331–343.

West, D., & Kinney, J. (1996). Overview of substance use and abuse. In J. Kinney (Ed.), *Clinical manual of substance abuse.* St. Louis, MO: Mosby. (pp. 17–39).

Williams, J. S. (2004). Researchers adopt HIV risk prevention program for African American Women. *NIDA News, 19*(1).

Zwickler, P. (2004). Childhood sexual abuse increases risk for drug dependence in adult women. Retrieved November 2, 2008, from http://www.drugabuse.gov/NIDA_Notes/NN Vol17N1/Childhood.html

Sherry Hartman, Sharyn James, and Anne Troy

Visit **http://nursing.jbpub.com/communityhealth** for interactive exercises, review questions, Web links, and more.

Nearly two million people worldwide lose their lives to violence each year, making violence a leading cause of death for people between the ages of 15 and 44.

When there is light in the soul, there is beauty in the person
When there is beauty in the person, there is harmony within the home
When there is harmony within the home, there is order in the nation
When there is order in the nation, there is peace in the world.

—*Lau Tzu*

I Have Been Thinking

I have been thinking about violence. I have been thinking about an airplane full of terrified women and men and children smashing into a tower full of unsuspecting women and men who were just sipping their morning coffee. I have been thinking of the burning people jumping from the 100th floor, jumping for their lives. I have been thinking about the hundreds of firefighters and police officers who were lost, crushed under a collapsing tower. I have been thinking about a husband waiting in his office for 14 hours for his wife who worked on the 104th floor, his wife who had not called, who was probably never going to call, and yet he was still waiting. I was thinking of the man who called his mother from the hijacked plane to tell her he loved her, to remember he loved her. I have been thinking about the debris and the dust on New Yorkers' shoes and how shocked we are here in America, how protected we have been. I have been thinking about all the war torn countries I have been to, Bosnia, Kosova, Israel, Afghanistan, and the dust on the peoples' shoes and the debris. I have been thinking about the people who were driven to hijack airplanes with knives and box cutters and fly them through buildings, who were ready, eager to lose their lives to hurt other people. I have been thinking about why, what would make people want to do that. I have been thinking about the words "retaliation" and "punishment" and "act of war." I have been thinking about violence, what it feels like to be nothing to someone else. What it feels like to be a consequence of someone else's disassociated rage, disconnected fury. I have been thinking about the cycle of hurt for hurt, nation against nation, tit for tat. I have been thinking about how deeply something else is required. I have been thinking about the courage it requires to think about something other than violence as a response to violence. I am thinking about the complexity of this and the loneliness of this and the helplessness and the sorrow that would be felt in the space where violence once was and the grief. I have been thinking that for those of us who are living on the planet right here, right now, we must live in this dangerous space, allowing the helplessness, the grief, the sorrow to create new wisdom that can and will and must free us from this terrible prison of violence. I urge you, each one of you—fall into this space, weep, be lost, let go, die into the grief—inside the emptiness and the pain it will be revealed.

—*Eve Ensler, playwright, author of The Vagina Monologues, "Stop the Violence. Spread the Word. Join Us,"
September 12, 2001, http://www.vday.org/contents/vday/press/alertsandpressrel/amessagefromevee*

How has violence touched your life? Where were you on September 11, 2001? Have you or someone close to you ever been the victim of violence? After reading Eve Ensler's "I've Been Thinking," can you imagine "feeling the consequence of someone else's disassociated rage"? Do you think that we can ever think about "something other than violence as a response to violence"? How can nurses lead communities to nonviolent solutions—in schools, in churches, in the workplace?

## CHAPTER FOCUS

**From Criminal Justice to Public Health**

**Defining and Explaining Violence**

**Types of Violence in U.S. Society**
- Violence in the Family
- Youth Violence
- Workplace Violence
- Mass Violence and War

**Interventions to Prevent Violence**
- Microlevel Interventions with Individuals and Families
- Mesolevel Interventions: Community Structures
- Macrolevel Interventions: Society and Culture

## QUESTIONS TO CONSIDER

After reading this chapter, answer the following questions:

1. How does a public health approach to violence differ from a criminal justice approach?
2. What are the forms of behavioral violence?
3. What are the forms of structural violence?
4. What are the factors that contribute to violent behavior?
5. Which populations are at greater risk for violence?
6. What is the typical pattern of abuse episodes in family violence?
7. What are the forms of violence among youths?
8. Which factors contribute to youth violence?
9. What roles do nurses have in relation to the global issue of the violence of war?
10. Which primary, secondary, and tertiary interventions contribute to the prevention of violence?

Abuse
Behavioral violence

Intimate partner violence
Learned helplessness

Learned hopefulness
Structural violence

Survivors

VIOLENCE ACCOUNTS FOR 14% of global deaths among males and 7% of deaths among females. Additionally, for every individual who dies because of an act of violence, there are many more who are injured and who suffer a wide range of physical, mental, sexual, and reproductive health problems. Violence places major economic burdens on national governments worldwide, costing countries billions of US dollars each year to pay for health care, law enforcement, and lost productivity (WHO, 2002).

Various forms of violence, such as torture, human trafficking, violence against women, violence against children, and harmful traditional cultural practices, have been long recognized as human rights issues. But only recently have we begun to realize that, when human rights are respected, protected, and fulfilled, the underlying societal conditions that foster violent behavior are controlled. Many of the risk factors common to many forms of violence, such as poverty, unemployment, gender inequality, racial discrimination, and weak economic and social safety nets are closely linked to human rights such as the right to equality and freedom from discrimination, the right to education, the right to an adequate standard of living, and the right to social security (WHO, 2008).

> **"**Real success for new health agendas will depend on researchers involving themselves in finding ways to help reduce community violence. **"**
>
> —Sr. Rosemary Donley, past president of
> Sigma Theta Tau International,
> Reflections, Fall 1996

## From Criminal Justice to Public Health

Violence has been a part of humankind's world at least since recorded history. Our oldest texts are rife with tales of violence at individual and collective levels. In more recent history, violent behavior has been regarded as a social problem having moral overtones, with prevention efforts focused on tertiary prevention through imprisonment, capital punishment, and sometimes, psychosocial rehabilitation. Violence had remained primarily a criminal justice issue of deviant and antisocial behavior (WHO, 2002). In discussing interpersonal violence, Hawkins (1999) commented that "one of the widely noted developments of the past decade is the trend toward viewing interpersonal aggression and

## MEDIA MOMENT

**"Independence Day," Martina McBride (1993)**

Well she seemed all right by dawn's early light though she looked a little worried and weak.
She tried to pretend he wasn't drinking again but daddy left the proof on her cheek.
I was only eight years old that summer and I always seemed to be in the way so I took myself down to the fair in town on Independence Day.

Well word gets around in a small, small town.
They said he was a dangerous man.
But momma was proud and she stood her ground, she knew she was on the losing end.
Some folks whispered, some folks talked but everybody looked the other way.
and when time ran out there was no one about on Independence Day.

Let freedom ring, let the white dove sing.
Let the whole world know that today is a day of reckoning.
Let the weak be strong, let the right be wrong
Roll the stone away, let the guilty pay, it's Independence Day.
Now I ain't saying that it's right or it's wrong
But maybe it's the only way.
Talk about your revolution,
It's Independence Day.

Written by Gretchen Peters
Country Music Association Award—1994 Music Video of the Year
Country Music Television (CMT) Europe's number 1
1994 Video of the Year
Martina McBride was the recipient of the
Grand Ole Opry's Minnie Pearl Humanitarian
Award for domestic violence efforts.

violence as a public health concern rather than as a matter to be handled exclusively by the criminal justice system" (p. 87). It was in the 1980s that the Centers for Disease Control and Prevention (CDC) initiated efforts to prevent injuries from violence by using a public health approach. Both a rapid rise in homicide rates in the United States and a growing acceptance by public health workers of the importance of behavioral factors in the etiology of disease and injury encouraged the efforts. Violence was becoming a "behavior-based epidemic that kills and injures as certainly as a disease of the flesh" (Jones, 1993, p. 9). It became accepted that the nation needed to have more than a criminal justice approach to violence.

Criminal justice approaches, however, continue to attend to violence with secondary and tertiary interventions after violence has occurred. A public health approach does not imply that violence is only or mainly a problem of health or that responsibility for solutions lies with health professionals. It provides a multidisciplinary, scientific approach that brings the methods of epidemiology to study how primary prevention strategies can reduce violence (CDC, 2008a; Mercy, Rosenberg, Powell, Broome, & Roper, 1993). A public health approach implies the belief that violence is a learned behavior and, therefore, can be changed and prevented. Describing the scope of the problem, identifying risk and protective factors, evaluating interventions, and implementing promising community programs are the components of the CDC approach to prevention.

Nurses have long played a role in addressing the trauma of violence and its health consequences and continue to be highly involved. In 1991, the American Nurses Association (ANA) issued a statement about physical violence against women that reflected the important nursing research that had been done in the area. In recognition of the magnitude of the health problems related to violence, several other nursing organizations have since issued position statements on violence. Violence against women, children, and elders in familial or intimate relationships was given special emphasis as a form of violence with high incidence and prevalence resulting in morbidity and mortality and requiring healthcare interventions.

This chapter provides a public health approach to violence and examines many varieties of its expression. Some forms will be more common and will be familiar from

### THINK ABOUT THIS

Many believe that violence is an innate feature of society. What do you think? How does violence on a personal level compare to societal violence? As a nurse, what is your idea of violence? How have your ideas been influenced by your family, personal experiences, and violence in the media? Can community health nurses use primary prevention efforts to affect violence, on both a personal level and a societal level?

courses focusing on women's health, children's health, and mental health. The emphasis here is on populations at risk and interventions directed to communities and populations. The broader context within which violence occurs and the complex interplay of individuals with their larger community and with society need to be understood in order to take on the task of reducing harm from violence.

## Defining and Explaining Violence

Depending on the discipline and purposes of inquiry, conceptualizations and explanations of violence vary. The most common and narrow definition of violence is of physical harm at an interpersonal level. Barash (1991) defines the more traditional meaning, which suggests that violence is physical and readily apparent through direct injury or the infliction of pain. Gilligan (1997) distinguishes one form of violence as **behavioral violence,** which refers to "the non-natural deaths and injuries caused by individuals against individuals, such as the deaths we attribute to homicide, suicide, soldiers in warfare, capital punishment, and so on" (p. 192). Such violence is related to interpersonal interactions.

Proposed explanations of individual behavioral violence include biological causes such as instinct, heredity, lesions of the brain, drugs and alcohol, and various neurochemical causes such as increased testosterone or lowered serotonin. In psychological theories, violent behavior is sometimes further distinguished as "emotive" aggression, as seen in crimes of passion, and "instrumental" aggression governed by rewards and punishments stimulated by a number of personal or material gains such as power, status, money, and sex. Developmental approaches look to early life experiences and parental relationships that develop violence potential. Related to this is the belief that violence is learned in the family from the social role models, which may sanction physical punishment and the privacy of family interactions.

Personality or character disorders in which the person is inadequate in coping and communications is another perspective. In the cases of child and elder abuse, stress, inadequacy, and frustration from the dependency of the child or elder influence the abuser's choice in using violence.

A more comprehensive look at violence comes from the World Health Organization (WHO). WHO (2002) defines violence as:

The intentional use of physical force or power, threatened or actual, against oneself, another person, or against a group or community, that either results in or has a high likelihood of resulting in injury, death, psychological harm, maldevelopment, or deprivation. (p. 3)

This definition includes a wide range of behaviors and acts, not only physical actions, but also physical and psychological threats and intimidation. Violence in any form compromises the well-being of individuals, families, and communities (WHO, 2002).

Broader definitions are congruent with both the public health approach and nursing's holistic approach to individuals, which recognizes the need to view the individual as part of a greater whole. Systems theory, multivariate theories, and ecological theories applied to violence recognize this need for a comprehensive approach to explanation (O'Neil & Harway, 1997; Van Soest, 1997).

**Structural violence** is indirect and insidious and often built into the foundations of political, social, and cultural institutions without being recognized. Gilligan (1997) describes it as "the increased rates of death and disability suffered by those who occupy the bottom rungs of society, as contrasted with the relatively lower rates experienced by those above them" (p. 192). Structural violence is a product of society's collective human choices and values, such as how to distribute available resources and services.

 GLOBAL CONNECTION

### The Other Victims of War: A Nurse's Experience in a Refugee Camp

As a new graduate, I felt unprepared for my role as a nurse in Thailand, working with Cambodian refugees. We carried walkie-talkies and knew the warning signal to leave the camp, if the North Vietnamese were entering the area. The very thought of deserting these gentle people, after spending months with them, seemed impossible. Equally impossible was the task of screening the recipients for food, by age. Only women and children under 6 were to be fed. Man's inhumanity to man was everywhere. I looked into the face of children who had survived hell. How could I say they were too old to eat? A photographer for a U.S. magazine asked me if I wanted to come along into the jungle for pictures. I started to follow, only to have a still small voice remind me that I wasn't in New Jersey anymore and that those paths led to places no one should have to see.

—Anne Troy, RN, FNP,
refugee relief worker, Cambodia, 1982

The figure on the right shows the relationship of behavioral and structural violence. There are several implications of the model for understanding violence. First, there are reciprocal effects of the micro, meso, and macro system levels on each other. Individual behavior is affected by all levels: personal characteristics and the environment of institutions and culture. The top level is the most obvious overt form of violence that we can see and assess. The second two levels refer to the unseen, covert forces that guide thoughts, words, and actions. These can be forces or situations that in subtle ways hinder health, growth, and development of individuals or certain groups of individuals. For example, at the institutional or mesosystem level, policies for reporting domestic violence have the potential to put the victim at greater harm from retaliation by the abuser. Because there are no required assessment, training, or screening policies, women often remain undiagnosed for domestic violence. Until recently,

No matter where we are from or what our philosophy of life, to a greater or lesser extent, we are all sorry to hear of other's suffering. . . . Wars, crime, violence of every sort, corruption, poverty, deception, fraud, and social, political, and economic injustice are each the consequence of negative human behavior. And who is responsible for such behavior? We are. . . . There is not a single class or sector of society which does not contribute to our daily diet of unhappy news.

. . . These human problems, because they are all essentially ethical problems, can be overcome. The fact that there are so many people, again from every sector and level of society, working to do so is a reflection of this intuition: There are those who join political parties to fight for a fairer constitution; those who become lawyers to fight for justice; those who care, both on a professional and on a voluntary basis, for the victims of harm. Indeed, we are all, according to our own understanding and in our own way, trying to make the world—or at least our bit of it—a better place for us to live in.

—**His Holiness the Dalai Lama**
*Source:* His Holiness the Dalai Lama. (1999).
*Ethics for the new millennium* (pp. 24–25).
New York: Riverhead Books.

Relationship of behavioral and structural violence.
*Source:* Adapted from Potter, 1999; Van Soest, 1997.

# The Work of Forensics: The Care of the SANE Nurse

*Anne Troy, RN, LNC, SANE*

A thirty-minute response time was required, from the first beep, to arrival at the ER outpatient unit. Thirty minutes to steal oneself against vicarious trauma. Bridging a victim's journey from attack through treatment required empathy, courage, and spiritual fortitude. Sometimes it was barely enough time to pray and will those qualities into action before pushing open the exam door. This night, I faced a frail woman, barely twenty, with tears drenching the exam table. "He made me do those things," she whispered as the detective left to give us privacy. Her own rape was not the source of her agony. He had made her perform fellatio on her three-year-old son. I found myself shocked and overwhelmed as she retold the horror of their abduction into a city park.

We were to learn this was not his first rape. As DNA provided the evidence, the circumstantial facts solidified into a sordid history of serial raping. He would drop his girlfriend off at a local college and use her car to abduct, by gunpoint, women as they walked from bus stops or shopped for their families. If he had applied for nursing school, there would have been nothing to warn of his deviant behavior by his social presentation. Well spoken and well loved by a courtroom full of family, who still believe him innocent, he gave no indication of his intent by his appearance.

As this woman consented to a forensic exam, I ensured the chain of evidence was maintained and vaginal swab samples were dried before boxing and taping. As I reviewed the prophylactic medications we could provide, I anticipated her despair as I offered the HIV medication. Instead, as her mother came screaming into the exam room, she stood and whispered in my ear, "I'm HIV positive; don't tell my mom. I hope he got it from me." I couldn't share her sense of retaliation as I sorted through my reeling emotions. Most rapists are known to their victims, so he didn't fit the statistical profile. However, all rapists repeat the act and I feared for his future victims, should he have acquired HIV from his present attack.

I offered her new clothing, as we bagged hers for collection of leaves and possible fiber evidence. I talked to her several times prior to going to court. She did not want to return to the hospital for any follow-up appointments. I focused on her guilt about her son and provided for their follow-up counseling.

As I entered the court, I was ushered into a room with the three victims waiting to testify. I was an expert witness and planned on testifying about the chain of evidence. Two of the victims sat alone with sweatshirts pulled to cover their faces. They had not acknowledged each other. Their shame and fear was still haunting them. I told them all quietly how much I and every woman in our city, thanked them for their bravery in facing this perpetrator. I told them that because of what they were about to do in court, my daughter was safer on the street. I reminded them not to allow the rape to define them or their life. I was proud that, as women, they were strong in spite of the personal cost. Slowly, the sweatshirts came down and we talked instead of whispered. I was proud of the role of nursing in helping women find their way back. Our voices united and he received three consecutive life sentences. There wasn't joy, as his family collapsed in agony. Our work of prevention has just begun. The time, before the beeper goes off again, is the time I am desperately working in to stop the insanity. ⬣

---

in many states, it was legal for a husband to rape his wife. Many of the barriers to access to health care are the result of bureaucracy and oppressive social policy and are examples of structural violence at the institutional level.

Like the young fish who asks the wise, old fish, "So what is this 'ocean' I hear others talking about?", individuals live their lives surrounded and affected by the forces represented by the macrosystem. This desensitization is reflected in our youth culture. Today's young people struggle to even identify their exposure to violence as they are bombarded daily with misogynist messages in music and videos. This is also shown in unconscious acceptance of inequalities and deprivations such as differential infant mortality rates, premature death, or lack of political representation. These indicate the excess suffering of some groups over others. Seldom, however, are the forces leading to this type of suffering referred to as *violence*.

According to Van Soest (1997), the pattern of thinking that is most revealing is the continued easy acceptance of threat or use of violence as a method of social control and an appropriate method of problem solving.

One example of the cultural propensity to use force and attack to solve problems is the frequent characterization of health and social problems as an enemy that becomes an opponent to engage in battle, as "war" is waged against drugs and violence. Just as the child who experiences violence is thought to learn to respond with violence, some believe that

## BOX 22-1

### Risk Factors Related to Violent Behavior

**Microsystem**

*Individual*

- Prenatal and perinatal factors
- Neurobiology and genetics
- Substance abuse
- Hormones—cortisol, testosterone, serotonin
- Premature, special-needs children
- Male sex
- Temperament
- Low IQ
- Slow language development
- Processing and attributing hostile intent
- Attention deficit/hyperactive disorder
- Conduct disorder
- Poor social skills
- Lack of sympathy/empathy
- Low self-esteem
- High stress levels
- Alcohol and/or drug use
- Younger than 30 years of age
- Head trauma

*Family, peers, school, and religious communities*

- Physical and/or sexual abuse or neglect
- Witness of violence in home
- Rejection by peers
- Witness peer fighting/homicides
- Free access to weapons
- Inadequate coercive posting
- Single female head of household
- Disadvantaged schools
- Bullied
- School dropout
- Gang activity
- Spiritual alienation

**Mesosystem**

- Collective powerlessness in neighborhood/community
- Collective sense of confusion in transient neighborhoods
- Gentrification of neighborhoods
- Overcrowding/demolition of housing projects
- Substandard high cost rental units
- White flight to suburbs
- Poor economy with joblessness
- Oppressive work environment
- Lack of access to health care in general, and substance abuse rehabilitation and mental health therapy in particular

**Macrosystem**

- Poverty
- Income inequality—minimum wage is not a living wage
- Community instability—political corruption
- Exposure to dramatic violence in media (TV, music, film)
- Economic activities supporting violence such as gun and drug trafficking and prostitution
- Declining public assistance programs
- Denigration of minorities, gays, ethnic groups, refugees, and people with disabilities
- Organizational structures that maintain and tacitly support violence against women
- Pornography of women legal and considered erotica
- Changes in gender roles that produce fear of power loss in males
- Tacit acceptance of violence to resolve conflict: war and weapons, child punishment, and death penalty
- Rigid stereotypes of roles of men and women
- Correctional facilities as economic base to communities
- Inequity of justice for poor and people of color

---

meeting violence with violence at the structural and cultural levels also breeds a cycle of violence. Gilligan (1997) explains how the horrific violence committed by the prisoners he worked with may seem senseless if studied in isolation. Combining the insights of psychiatry with a public health approach to violence, he believes their violent acts have a logic when seen as a response to structural violence of social conditions that stimulate shame and guilt. He details how these emotions lead to violent acts that are counterviolence to the social conditions of structural violence. He lists poverty, race, age discrimination, and gender asymmetry as the most important of these.

Box 22-1 is based on work of Potter (1999), who reviewed the research on violence and classified influences based on an ecological model. In public health terms, these can be viewed as factors associated with the risk of violent behaviors. From this perspective, the presence or absence of certain factors or circumstances determines the likelihood of instigating violence. This compilation is not an exhaustive list of the various influences that have been studied related to violence, nor do the influences always lead to violence. A complex interaction between individuals, their varied environments, and existing social ills combine to lead to violence.

# Types of Violence in U.S. Society

## ■ Violence in the Family

❝ *War, to sane men at the present day, begins to look like an epidemic insanity, breaking out here and there like the cholera or influenza, infecting men's brains instead of their bowels.* ❞
—Ralph Waldo Emerson, Miscellanies, 1884

Family violence is a pervasive and often lethal problem of epidemic proportions, with far-reaching challenges and consequences for all members of society. Family violence is often silent and hidden from view—a family secret. It physically, emotionally, financially, and spiritually devastates victims and their children. It threatens the stability of the family and violates communities' safety and economies by costing billions of dollars annually in medical expenses, sick leave, absenteeism, and nonproductivity (Davey & Davey, 1998; Waters et al., 2004).

---

### ■■ CULTURAL CONNECTION

Retail gun outlets outnumber McDonald's restaurants in the United States and the ratio of guns to people is almost one to one. What does this say about American cultural values?

---

There is growing recognition that family violence is a major health problem for women and children in the United States as well as around the world. Family violence presents unique challenges and opportunities for healthcare providers. Because victims of family violence and their children are found across healthcare services, as are nurses, nurses are in unique positions to assess and identify those affected by family violence. As such, nurses, and especially community health nurses, have the opportunity to be leaders in the prevention of family violence. Nursing approaches to domestic violence have an advocacy orientation that can be absent from other healthcare professionals. Research has shown that healthcare professionals can contribute to further subjugation of domestic violence victims. In many cases, those victimized by violence are viewed as a deviant group. Those victimized are often members of disenfranchised groups, minority or ethnic groups, and/or women and children. Professionals may try to distance themselves from such groups and their problems by holding the belief that it is the problem of an "other" or deviant group. Many nurses who work and research in this area are believed by some to have avoided the victim blaming that is characteristic of some disciplines. Their research has grown out of clinical, grassroots concerns that have developed an activist agenda and a recognition of **survivors'** needs for empowerment (Campbell, Harris, & Lee, 1995; Donovan & Vlais, 2005; UNIFEM, 2003).

❝ *The right to swing my fist ends where the other man's nose begins.* ❞
—Oliver Wendell Holmes

❝ *Throughout history, the leading causes of premature death have been infectious diseases and violence. For two centuries, the world has made gains against infectious diseases and despite the problems of emerging infections, as well as the development of resistance to antibiotics and insecticides, the world is a much safer place when it comes to microorganisms than ever before in history. The same is not true of violence. The age of science has provided more efficient means of inflicting violence, and it has changed the ethic of violence. People can now kill and maim without confronting the effects of their actions due to the distance, time, and filters placed between them and the victims. Many forces in society have made it possible for arms to be acquired by almost anyone, regardless of age, wealth, or propensity for violence. What is the cost of this situation and is there real hope for changing the equation?* ❞
—W. Foege, 1997

According to Campbell, Harris, and Lee (1995), there are three main theories useful for exploring family violence. The first emphasizes the abuser and the possible behavioral or psychopathological causes, such as mental illness, developmental disability, or substance abuse. In the family violence model, "the cycle of violence," with its use of force, is created when violence is learned in childhood and transmitted across generations. The third theory speculates that stressful situations precipitate violence. For example, violence arises when adults are unable to cope appropriately with the stress of unemployment or caring for a dependent elder. Children with special needs can increase stress and potential abuse (DHHS, 2008).

❝ *The invention of nuclear weapons has changed everything—except the way we think....We shall require a substantially new manner of thinking if mankind is to survive.* ❞
—Albert Einstein

---

###  MEDIA MOMENT

**"Goodbye Earl," Dixie Chicks (1999)**
Well it wasn't two weeks after she got married that
Wanda started gettin' abused
She put on dark glasses and long-sleeved blouses
And make-up to cover a bruise
Well she finally got the nerve to file for divorce
She let the law take it from there
But Earl walked right through that restraining order
And put her in intensive care.

Written by Dennis Linde.

## " a conversation with . . . "

Nurses historically have been in a key position to assess and prevent domestic violence. We typically spend more time with patients and their families than any other health care professional. We are with people at all the important times in their lives and can see how patients and families interact with each other. National surveys also have shown that patients trust nurses and are likely to confide in us.

. . . We cannot let another year go by without having a strong, nationwide educational and assessment program to educate health care professionals to assess for domestic violence and work with women to promote their health and safety.

After all, asking the right questions won't hurt women. Not asking those questions, certainly will. ◉

—Patricia Underwood, PhD, RN
Secretary of the American
Nurses Association, 1999

### Violence Against Women

Violence against women is known by many names: *spouse abuse, wife abuse, wife beating, battering, marital assault, woman battery, domestic violence,* and *intimate partner abuse.* These terms are sometimes used interchangeably, and occasionally, a term is used to refer to a specific problem (e.g., *family violence* to indicate wife and children are being battered). There are also many behavioral and legal definitions of violence against women, which sometimes makes it unclear what is meant by the term. This lack of clarity can lead to inconsistencies in healthcare providers' identification and interventions as well as differences in research terminology.

In 1995, the Fourth World Conference on Women, held in Beijing, developed a platform for action on violence against women and defined it as follows: "Violence against women: any act of gender-based violence that results in, or is likely to result in, physical, sexual, or psychological harm or suffering to women, including threats of such acts, coercion, or arbitrary deprivation of liberty, whether occurring in public or private life" (United Nations Division for the Advancement of Women, 1995).

The Centers for Disease Control and Prevention (2006) uses the term **intimate partner violence** (IPV) to define abuse that occurs between two people in a close relationship. The term *intimate partner* includes current and former spouses and dating partners. IPV includes four types of behavior:

1. Physical abuse is when a person hits, kicks, burns, or uses other forms of physical force to hurt or try to hurt a partner.
2. Sexual abuse is forcing a partner to participate in a sexual act when the partner does not consent.
3. Threats of physical or sexual abuse include the use of words, gestures, weapons, or other means to communicate the intent to cause harm.
4. Emotional abuse is threatening a partner or his or her possessions or loved ones, or harming a person's sense of self-worth. Stalking, name-calling, intimidation, and isolation are some examples.

Most abusive relationships are male batterers of female victims; however, the reverse may be true. Intimate partner violence also occurs in gay and lesbian relationships. It cuts across all of society, all ethnic and cultural groups, and all educational and socioeconomic levels. Three types of batterers have been described based on the severity of their violence, who they direct violence toward, and their degree of personality disorder. Some batter with less severity and only within the family; others use more violence, mostly in the family, and show some signs of distress and emotional instability; and the most severe batterers are violent outside the family and often demonstrate criminal activity, alcohol and drug abuse, and antisocial personality disorder (Hotzworth-Monroe & Stuart, 1994). More attention has been given to the characteristics of male batterers than to abused women because these characteristics have been found to be more helpful in assessing risk of partner violence. Batterers are not a homogenous group and vary greatly in their profiles. However, there are some generalities (CDC, 2007; Hampton, Vandergriff-Avery, & Kim, 1999). Batterers often suffer from low self-esteem and have a need to use power and control tactics over victims. They usually minimize their own behavior and blame the victim for the violence. They tend to be more jealous, abusive to children, and sexually aggressive toward partners. After battering episodes, batterers manipulate by offering remorse, loving words, and promises to change—anything to gain control over the partner. Alcohol often is involved in partner violence.

For some women, IPV can lead to **learned helplessness.** Women are viewed as helpless, passive victims who restrict their behaviors because they lose the ability to predict whether their actions will be effective. What is viewed as helplessness is just the reality of a situation in which resources to enable escape are inadequate. As isolation from support continues, abuse escalates, leaving a previously confident woman struggling to not believe it is partly her fault. Women logically try to protect themselves and their children, but police response, child care, shelter, education and employment opportunities, and community support are lacking or are already overwhelmed.

An approach that counters learned helplessness in women draws on the societal expectation that women must be responsible for maintaining relationships. Relationship hope is present in women in general, and **learned hopefulness** in battered women is their belief that the perpetrator will change behavior or personality. The concept explains why women stay with or return to abusers, especially if the abusers enroll in treatment programs. Box 22-2 outlines the signs that may indicate a women is the victim of intimate partner violence.

The prevalence statistics found in Box 22-3 have been obtained from numerous studies. There are few national sources

## BOX 22-2

**Indicators of Occurrence of Intimate Partner Violence**
- Recurrent trauma history
- Proximal injuries, such as to head, neck, torso, breast, abdomen, or genitals
- Patterned, multiple, or bilateral injury
- Poor explanations or no explanations for injuries
- Concealing or acting ashamed of injuries
- Delay in seeking treatment for injury with wounds in various stages of healing
- Physical injury during pregnancy, especially to abdomen or breasts
- Signs of depression: flat affect, failure to make eye contact, mood swings, poor hygiene
- Other psychological cues such as suicidal thoughts, anxiety, difficulty sleeping, panic attacks
- Alcohol or substance abuse symptoms
- Chronic pain with no known cause
- Seeking medical care for minor problems to maintain contact with professional
- Missing scheduled appointments or only coming for acute care
- Overly protective, controlling partner who visits professionals with patient and refuses to leave his or her side

*Sources:* Cassidy, 1999; Scott-Tilley, 1999; CDC, 2006.

## BOX 22-3

**Facts About Intimate Partner Violence**
- About 4.8 million intimate partner victimizations occur each year among U.S. women age 18 and older. Men are the victims of about 2.9 million intimate partner assaults (CDC, 2006).
- Intimate partner violence resulted in nearly 1,600 deaths in 2004. Of these deaths, 75% were female and 25% were male (CDC, 2006).
- Intimate partner violence costs billions of dollars every year in medical care, mental health services, and lost productivity (CDC, 2006).
- Intimate partner violence occurs across all populations, irrespective of social, economic, religious, or cultural group. However, young women and those below the poverty line are disproportionately affected (Heise & Garcia-Moreno, 2002).
- As many as 324,000 women each year experience intimate partner violence during pregnancy (Gazmarian, Peterson, Spitz, Goodwin, Saltzman, & Marks, 2000).
- Forty-four percent of women murdered by an intimate partner had visited an emergency department within 2 years of the homicide, 93% of whom had at least one injury visit (Crandall, Walters, Kernic, Holt, & Rivara, 2004).

of epidemiological data on intimate partner violence. Most states collect data from law enforcement agencies. Although these sources provide information on trends, it is generally believed that domestic violence is seriously underreported and severely underdiagnosed by healthcare providers.

 **Got an Alternative?**

"All we are saying is give peace a chance."
—*John Lennon*

What complementary health practices can promote a sense of peace?

### Child Maltreatment

Child maltreatment includes all types of abuse and neglect resulting in harm to children younger than 18 years of age. There are four common types of abuse:

1. Physical abuse occurs when a child's body is injured by hitting, kicking, shaking, burning, or other forms of physical force.
2. Sexual abuse involves engaging a child in sexual acts such as fondling, rape, and exposing a child to any sexual activity.
3. Emotional abuse refers to any behavior that harms a child's self-worth or emotional well-being. Examples include name calling, shaming, rejection, withholding love, and threatening.
4. Neglect is the failure to meet a child's basic needs, which include housing, food, clothing, education, and access to health care (CDC, 2008b).

Although families living in poverty and single parent families are at increased risk, all socioeconomic levels and family patterns experience child maltreatment. Box 22-4 shows some of the risk factors associated with child abuse.

#### Incidence of child abuse

In 2006, U.S. state and local child protective services (CPS) investigated 3.6 million reports of children being abused or neglected. CPS classified more than 900,000 of these children as victims. Nearly 75% of them had no prior history of abuse or neglect. A non-CPS study reported that 14% of U.S. children experienced some form of maltreatment. Overall, girls (52%) were more likely than boys (48%) to experience all forms of child maltreatment (CDC, 2008c).

More than 1,500 children ages 0–17 died from abuse and neglect (2.04 per 100,000 children). Almost 80% of these deaths occurred among children younger than age 4 (CDC, 2008b, 2008c). In fact, infants during their first day of life are most at risk for homicide (Paulozzi, 2002). Shaken-baby syndrome is a leading cause of brain injury, with as many as 25% of the victims dying from their injuries (Committee of Child Abuse and Neglect, 2001).

Consequences of abuse for survivors vary depending on the nature of the act, the child's age, and the general environment. Physical harm can include disability or disfigurement, sexually transmitted diseases, and pregnancy in older children. Extreme stress can disrupt early brain development

---

**BOX 22-4**

**Key Facts About Child Physical and Sexual Abuse**
- Girls are sexually abused 3 times more often than boys.
- Surveys show at least 20% of women and 5% to 16% of men experienced sexual abuse as children.
- Two percent of all forms of confirmed abuse occurred in daycare or foster care settings.
- The most vulnerable age for sexual abuse is 7 to 13 years.
- Children are mostly abused by adult related to them or known to their families; however, as many as 30% may be by strangers.
- Children are more likely to be physically abused by their fathers than by their mothers, and more severe abuse is committed by men.

- Mothers who are victims of domestic violence are more likely to abuse their children.
- There is a dramatic increase in adolescents who commit sexual aggression against other children.
- Single-parent families and families in poverty are at increased risk of abuse.
- Younger and less educated parents are at greater risk to abuse their children than older or more educated parents.
- Families in which prenatal care was absent or inadequate or in which the mother is depressed are at greater risk.

*Sources:* Aron & Olsen, 1997; Tjaden & Thoennes, 2000.

---

**Application to Practice**

Childhood sexual abuse is a particularly heinous form of violence, with implications for all healthcare workers, especially nurses. Research cited in Bal et al. (2003) reveals that the negative symptomatology associated with sexual abuse, such as borderline pathology, behavior problems, depression, suicidal ideation, drug abuse, sexual problems, and self-mutilation attempts, are more frequently reported in sexually than physically abused adolescents.

As nurses, we are in a unique situation not only to report cases of suspected sexual abuse, but also to assist in the treatment of these children. This may include accurate assessment of the victim and family, provision of a safe environment, support of positive coping strategies, as well as monitoring of symptomatology and implementation treatment protocols. In this manner, nurses have an opportunity to be a positive and dynamic force in a potentially devastating situation.

*—Susan Rick, DNS, RN, CNS*

> **❝***I know not with what weapons World War III will be fought but World War IV will be fought with sticks and stones.* **❞**
>
> *—Albert Einstein*

> **❝***If we have no peace, it is because we have forgotten that we belong to each other.* **❞**
>
> *—Mother Teresa*

Table 22-1 lists both behavioral and physical signs of child maltreatment. Box 22-5 provides information for educating parents on protecting their children from abuse. The enactment of "Megan's Law" requires sex offenders to register and notify the community they are residing in, to allow parents the opportunity to protect their children. Some experts are concerned that there is no consistent tool used to establish the perpetrator's risk of re-offending. Each state has the discretion to determine which offenders are subject to registration and notification (Zevitz & Faikas, 2000).

### Elder Maltreatment

Elder maltreatment can be compared with child maltreatment regarding the dependent situation of the victim. Elders who are abused are frail and often mentally or physically impaired. They have a special relationship with and are dependent on a family member or caregiver. Federal definitions of elder abuse, neglect, and exploitation were first used in the 1987 amendments to the Older Americans Act. Categories of abuse include domestic abuse, institutional abuse, self-abuse, and neglect. State statutes define these with various degrees of specificity. As with children, abuse takes the forms of physical, sexual, and emotional abuse; neglect; and abandonment. Elders are also at risk for financial or material exploitation. Abuse can be both unintentional and extensional. Perpetrators are most often family members.

Caring for frail elders can be difficult and stressful. Elders who are mentally or physically impaired are especially needy of special care that the family or caregiver is ill equipped to provide. Both skills and resources in the form of family or

and can negatively affect the development of the nervous and immune systems. Children who are abused are at much higher risk for health problems as adults. These problems may include alcoholism, depression, drug abuse, eating disorders, obesity, sexual promiscuity, smoking, suicide, and certain chronic diseases (CDC, 2008b).

**Table 22-1** Physical and Behavioral Indicators of Child Maltreatment

| | Physical Indicators | Behavioral Indicators |
|---|---|---|
| ■ Physical abuse | Unexplained bruises (in various stages of healing)<br>Unexplained burns, especially cigarette burns or immersion burns<br>Unexplained fractures, lacerations, or abrasions<br>Swollen areas<br>Evidence of delayed or inappropriate treatment for injuries | Self-destructive<br>Withdrawn and/or aggressive, behavioral extremes<br>Arrives at school early or stays late as if afraid to be at home<br>Chronic runaway (adolescents)<br>Complains of soreness or moves uncomfortably<br>Wears clothing inappropriate to weather to cover body<br>Bizarre explanation of injuries<br>Apprehensive when other children cry |
| ■ Physical neglect | Abandonment<br>Unattended medical needs<br>Consistent lack of supervision<br>Consistent hunger, inappropriate dress, poor hygiene<br>Lice, distended stomach, emaciated<br>Inadequate nutrition | Regularly displays fatigue or listlessness, falls asleep in class<br>Steals food, begs from classmates<br>Reports that no caretaker is at home<br>Frequently absent or tardy<br>Self-destructive<br>School dropout (adolescents)<br>Extreme loneliness and need for affection |
| ■ Sexual abuse | Sexual abuse may be *nontouching*: obscene language, pornography, exposure; or *touching*: fondling, molesting, oral sex, intercourse<br>Torn, stained, or bloody underclothing<br>Pain, swelling, or itching in genital area<br>Difficulty walking or sitting<br>Bruises or bleeding in genital area<br>Venereal disease<br>Frequent urinary or yeast infections | Withdrawn, chronic depression<br>Excessive seductiveness<br>Role reversal, overly concerned for siblings<br>Poor self-esteem, self-devaluation, lack of confidence<br>Peer problems, lack of involvement<br>Massive weight change<br>Suicide attempts (especially adolescents)<br>Hysteria, lack of emotional control<br>Inappropriate sex play or premature understanding of sex<br>Threatened by physical contact, closeness<br>Unwilling to change clothes in front of anyone<br>Exhibits fantasy or babylike behavior<br>Frequent nightmares<br>High level of unexplained anxiety |
| ■ Emotional abuse | Emotional abuse may be name-calling, insults, put-downs, etc., or may be terrorization, isolation, humiliation, rejection, corruption, ignoring<br>Speech disorders<br>Delayed physical development<br>Substance abuse<br>Ulcers, asthma, severe allergies | Habit disorder (sucking, rocking, biting)<br>Antisocial, destructive<br>Neurotic traits (sleep disorders, inhibition of play)<br>Passive and aggressive, behavioral extremes<br>Delinquent behavior (especially adolescents)<br>Developmentally delayed<br>Fire setting<br>Cruelty to animals |

*Sources:* National Children's Advocacy Center, 1998; Miller & Knutson, 1997; DHHS, 2006.

 MEDIA MOMENT

**Anger Management (2003)**

Overworked and undervalued Dave Buznik is a businessman whose life practically seems stuck in second gear. He's got a boss who would just as well step on him as acknowledge the fact that Dave does all the work while the boss gets the credit. He's got a pacifist nature that always gets the best of him, causing him to avoid conflict whenever possible. But matters only seems to get worse for Dave when he can't take action and lets everything just sit. When a misunderstanding aboard an airplane lands Dave in court, the only way out is through the therapy of Dr. Buddy Rydell, a psychiatrist and anger management expert. While the unconventional Buddy seems harmful and psychotic, he might just be Dave's only solution to a problem that seriously needs to be addressed. Adam Sandler (Buznik) and Jack Nicholson (Rydell) star in this film.

## BOX 22-5

**Intervention with Parents: Teaching Tips for Child Safety**

Know everything you can about your children's activities and friends. Monitor children's activities and participate with them. Do not allow children to play alone in fields, on playgrounds, or in other dangerous or isolated areas.

Teach your children about strangers.

Teach your children to refuse anything from strangers, including money, gifts, and rides. Know where new items come from.

Teach your children how to safely enter home alone. Teach them how to pretend you are home and how to answer the phone if they are alone.

Teach your children to keep a safe distance from strangers and not to give strangers directions or help. Adults need to get help from other adults.

Use secret codes with your children (for use when they may need to positively identify each other or ask for help).

Do not let your children go to public places, especially restrooms, alone. Develop a family plan stressing where to meet if lost, when you are away from home. Do not have children meet you in the parking lot.

Do not place your children's names on their clothing or on the outside of their possessions.

Teach your children to say NO to "touches" on the part(s) of their bodies covered by a swimming suit.

Teach your children to say NO, to TELL SOMEONE, and to GET AWAY if someone bothers them.

Join with other concerned parents to set up safety systems for your neighborhood.

Teach your children about secrets and that some "secrets" have to be told if children and their parents are to be kept safe.

*Source:* Project SAFE, HISD, and the Child Abuse Prevention Network, Houston, TX.

---

financial support may be lacking. Increased stress and poor coping combine to lead to stress. The more impaired and dependent the elder, the greater the likelihood of maltreatment. Adult children who abuse are often dependent on the parent themselves because of their own mental, social, emotional, or financial problems. Abuse signals their response to their own inadequacies. As with other forms of abuse, the learned behavior is passed through the generations as children who were abused learn and reciprocate when a parent becomes vulnerable. Often, caregivers are themselves elderly and are unable to care for another.

There are no federal laws providing protective services and shelters for elderly victims, but all 50 states have such legislation. These laws establish guidelines for reporting and investigating suspected abuse and vary widely in terms of age and circumstances for eligibility. In many states, separate laws exist to cover long-term care and other institutions. All states have laws authorizing a long-term care ombudsman program, which is a requirement for receiving federal funds. They are advocates for those residing in long-term care.

### Definitions and types of elder abuse

The lack of a standard definition and consistent terminology is a major difficulty in reporting and responding to

 **CULTURAL CONNECTION**

Some religious faiths believe that parenting includes physical punishment based on biblical support of "Spare the rod and spoil the child." As a community health nurse, how would you work with a family whose values differ from yours and that employs physical punishment based on biblical interpretation that leaves physical marks on their young children?

elder abuse. A white paper done for the National Center on Elder Abuse (Wood, 2006) reports that while various agency records offer some information related to the incidence and prevalence of the problem, policymakers and healthcare providers cannot mount an effective public health response without clear and standardized data. Comparing the definitions and terminology used by the World Health Organization (WHO), the National Center on Elder Abuse (NCEA), and the National Research Council (NRC) illustrates the problem.

The WHO (2006) states that elder abuse is:

a single or repeated act, or lack of appropriate action occurring within any relationship where there is an expectation of trust, which causes harm or distress to an older person. Elder abuse can take many forms including physical, psychological, and sexual abuse, financial exploitation, neglect and self-neglect, medication abuse, abandonment, scapegoating, and marginalization of older people in institutions or social and economic policies. (p. 1)

According to the NCEA:

Elder abuse is a term referring to any knowing, intentional, or negligent act by a caregiver or any other person that causes harm or a serious risk of harm to a vulnerable adult. The specificity of laws varies from state to state, but broadly defined, abuse may be physical abuse, emotional abuse, sexual abuse, exploitation, neglect, or abandonment. (Wood, 2006, p. 22)

The NRC uses the term "elder mistreatment" defined as:

(a) intentional actions that cause harm or create a serious risk of harm (whether or not harm is intended) to a vulnerable elder by a caregiver or other person who stands in a trust relationship to the elder, or (b) failure by a caregiver to satisfy the elder's basic needs or to protect the elder from harm. (Wood, 2006, p. 22)

The 2004 Survey of State Adult Protective Services (NCEA, 2006) reported that only 21 U.S. states or territories (40.4%) maintain an abuse registry or database of alleged perpetrators, while 31 (59.6%) do not. Using data reported by the states, the survey found that self-neglect was the most common category of substantiated reports (37.2%), followed by caregiver neglect (20.4%) and financial exploitation (14.7%). States reported that 65.7% of elder abuse victims were female and 52.7% of the alleged perpetrators were also female. Of the victims over age 60, 42.8% were over age 80, while 75.1% of the alleged perpetrators were under age 60. The most common relationships of victims to alleged perpetrators were adult offspring (32.6%) and other family member (21.5%). The majority of the victims were Caucasian (77.1%) and the vast majority (89.3%) of elder abuse occurred in domestic settings. Only four states (Colorado, Connecticut, Louisiana, and Massachusetts) and

one territory (Guam) provided information on outcomes of Adult Protective Services involvement. These survey results outline the need for:

- Accurate and uniform data at both state and national levels so that abuse trends can be tracked and studied.
- Uniform definitions of abuse and standard measures for reporting.
- Training on the identification of abuse for potential reporters of abuse such as municipal agents, postal service workers, utility workers, and hospital discharge planners.
- Increased numbers of reports, investigations, and substantiation that may lead to increased local, state, and national intervention and education efforts targeted toward the abuse of older adults.

Box 22-6 outlines the indicators for various forms of elder abuse.

## BOX 22-6

### Indicators of Elder Abuse

#### Physical Abuse
- Bruises, black eyes, lacerations, and rope marks
- Bone fractures
- Open wounds, and punctures, untreated injuries in various stages of healing
- Sprains, dislocations, and internal injuries/bleeding
- Broken eyeglasses/frames
- Physical signs of being subjected to punishment—flinching when approached
- Laboratory findings of medication overdose or underutilization of prescribed drugs
- An elder's report of being hit, slapped, kicked, or mistreated
- An elder's sudden change in behavior
- Caregiver's refusal to allow visitors to see an elder alone

#### Sexual Abuse
- Bruises around the breasts or genital area
- Unexplained venereal disease or genital infections
- Unexplained vaginal or anal bleeding
- Torn, stained, or bloody underclothing
- An elder's report of being sexually assaulted or raped

#### Emotional Psychological Abuse
- Being emotionally upset or agitated
- Being extremely withdrawn and uncommunicative or nonresponsive
- Unusual behavior usually attributed to dementia (e.g., sucking, biting, rocking)
- An elder's report of being verbally or emotionally mistreated

#### Neglect
- Dehydration, malnutrition, untreated bed sores, or poor personal hygiene
- Unattended or untreated health problems
- Hazardous or unsafe living condition/arrangements (e.g., improper wiring, no heat, or no running water)

- Unsanitary and unclean living conditions (e.g., dirt, fleas, lice on person, soiled bedding, fecal/urine smell, inadequate clothing)
- An elder's report of being mistreated

#### Abandonment
- The desertion of an elder at a hospital, nursing facility, or other similar institution
- The desertion of an elder at a shopping center or other public location
- An elder's report of being abandoned

#### Financial or Material Exploitation
- Sudden changes in bank account or banking practice, including an unexplained withdrawal of large sums of money by a person accompanying the elder
- The inclusion of additional names on an elder's bank signature card
- Unauthorized withdrawal of the elder's funds using the elder's ATM card
- Abrupt changes in a will or other financial documents
- Unexplained disappearance of funds or valuable possessions
- Substandard care being provided or bills unpaid despite the availability of adequate financial resources
- Discovery of an elder's signature being forged for financial transactions or for the titles of his/her possessions
- Sudden appearance of previously uninvolved relatives claiming their rights to an elder's affairs and possessions
- Unexplained sudden transfer of assets to a family member or someone outside the family
- The provision of services that are not necessary
- An elder's report of financial exploitation

*Source:* National Center for Elder Abuse (2008). http://www.ncea.aoa.gov

### Patterns of Behavior in Family Violence

Many individuals who use violence in their intimate relationships grew up in homes where they saw violence between adults and were abused themselves. Many saw frequent drug abuse by adults. They themselves often abuse alcohol and other drugs. They have little experience with

men and women dealing successfully with each other to solve problems nonviolently. They tend to have rigid ideas about men's and women's roles. Many do not use violence outside of the home, and some have no criminal record before a family violence incident. They find approval for their behavior in daily life through media, entertainment, and sports events, as well as from peers.

For batterers, family violence is often a pattern of behaviors directed at a victim. It is not an isolated event. It is a pattern of multiple episodes of a variety of abusive acts, which occur over the course of the familial relationship. In each episode, there is often a buildup of tension, followed by a violent episode, followed by remorse, gifts, and attention. Each episode builds on the last and sets the stage for future events. Some perpetrators use a particular set of abusive behaviors repeatedly, whereas others use a wide variety of behaviors randomly. These abusive and coercive behaviors take several different forms, including physical, sexual, psychological, and economic. Box 22-7 gives examples of abusive behaviors occurring in families.

## ENVIRONMENTAL CONNECTION

"Let us reform our schools and we shall find little need of reform in our prisons."

—John Ruskin

How does the physical environment of schools either promote or decrease violence in school children? What are ways that school nurses can implement primary health strategies in school health programs to decrease the "culture of violence" in today's school system?

---

## BOX 22-7

### Examples of Abusive Behaviors Occurring in Families

**Physical Abuse: Inflicting injury or illness, withholding necessities of health**
- Spitting
- Scratching
- Biting
- Grabbing
- Shaking
- Choking
- Twisting
- Slapping
- Pushing
- Restraining
- Burning
- Punching
- Using weapons
- Inappropriate use of drugs
- Inappropriate use of physical restraint
- Force feeding
- Withholding food, medications, assistive devices

**Sexual Abuse: Coercing any sexual contact without consent, undermining sexual identity**
- Coerced sex
- Unwanted touching
- Sexual assault or battery
- Rape
- Sodomy
- Coerced nudity
- Sexually explicit photographing
- Forced prostitution
- Undermining sexuality by criticizing desirability

**Psychological Abuse: Instilling fear, isolating, undermining sense of self-worth**
- Verbal assaults
- Insults
- Threats
- Destruction of pets or property—punching holes in walls
- Intimidation
- Humiliation
- Harassment
- Isolation from family or friends
- Withholding transportation and/or phone access
- Isolation from regular activities
- Silent treatment
- Ongoing accompaniment
- Constant "checking up"
- Restricting entry or exit from home
- Spiritual designation
- Threatening to take the children
- Jealousy

**Economic Abuse: Taking funds making financially dependent**
- Cashing checks without authorization
- Forging signature on checks
- Stealing money or possessions
- Deceiving into signing any financial documents
- Improper conservatorship, guardianship, or power of attorney
- Controlling financial resources
- Accumulating bills for which victim is responsible
- Preventing concentration at work by visits or phone calls

## Youth Violence

### Scope of the Problem

For public healthcare providers, there is growing concern over the victimization and violent behavior of children and youth. Despite a decrease in overall violent crime rates and indications that there are declines in fighting and weapon carrying among U.S. adolescents (USDHHS, 2007), violent injury and death disproportionately affect youth in the United States.

Youth violence is described as harmful behaviors that can start early and continue into young adulthood. The young people involved can be victims, offenders, or witnesses to the violence. Youth violence includes a wide range of behaviors and actions. Some behaviors, such as bullying, slapping, or hitting, often cause more emotional harm than physical harm. Other violent acts, such as robbery, assault, or rape can lead to serious injury or even death. Many young people seek medical care for violence-related injuries. Some injuries, like gunshot or stab wounds, can lead to lasting disabilities. Violence can have a powerful effect on the health and well-being of entire communities by increasing healthcare costs, decreasing property values, and disrupting social services. The cost of youth violence exceeds $158 billion dollars each year (CDC, 2008e). Box 22-8 presents further evidence on the problem of youth violence.

### School Violence

In the United States, an estimated 55 million students are enrolled in pre-kindergarten through twelfth grade. Although less than 1% of all homicides among school-age children (5 to 19 years of age) occur in or around school grounds or on the way to and from school, violent events against youths at school are an increasing health concern (CDC, 2008F). Whether children turn their aggression against others or toward themselves, the increasing climate of violence is evident. As the baseline of violence rises, the chance of deadly incidents increases. Society demands that our schools be safe for our children, yet as the NOTE THIS! feature shows, schools are not always safe places.

In recent years, bullying has become a major problem associated with violence in schools. Though universal, bullying behavior did not become a research or policy issue until the late 1990s. The fact that bullied children became revenge killers brought to light the need to address this form of violence (Mc-Ghee & DeBernardo, 1999). The CDC (2008f) reports that:

- Young people who bully are more likely to smoke, drink alcohol, get into fights, vandalize property, skip school, and drop out of school.
- Sixty percent of boys who were bullies in middle school had at least one criminal conviction by the age of 24.
- Among the student perpetrators of school-associated homicides, 20% were known to have been victims of bullying.
- 160,000 students go home from school early on any given day because they are afraid of being bullied.

Box 22-9 on page 522 outlines the risk factors for youth or school violence.

**MEDIA MOMENT**

*The Upside of Anger* (2005)

Sharp-witted suburban wife Terry Wolfmeyer is left to raise her four headstrong daughters when her husband unexpectedly disappears. Things get even more hectic when she falls for her neighbor Denny, a once-great baseball star turned radio disk jockey. This relationship leaves her daughters out on a limb. They are forced to juggle their mother's romantic dilemmas as well as their own.

**NOTE THIS!**

**Facts About School Violence In the United States**

A nationwide survey during the 2005–2006 school year reported:

- 38% of public schools reported at least one incident of violence to police.
- 24% of students reported gangs at their schools.
- 10% of teachers in urban schools, 6% of teachers in suburban schools, and 5% of teachers in rural schools reported being threatened with injury by students.
- 6.5% of students carried a weapon on school property in the 30 days preceding the survey. Weapons included guns, knives, or clubs.
- 7.9% of students were threatened or injured on school property in the 12 months preceding the survey.
- 13.6% of students were involved in a physical fight on school property in the 12 months preceding the survey.
- 8.4% of students attempted suicide one or more times in the 12 months preceding the survey.
- 25.4% of students were offered, sold, or given an illegal drug on school property in the 12 months preceding the survey.
- 30% of students reported moderate or frequent bullying. This included 13% as a bully, 10.6% as a victim, and 6.3% as both.

*Source:* CDC, 2008f.

---

### BOX 22-8

**Facts About Youth Violence in the United States**

- In 2005, 5,686 young people ages 10 to 24 were murdered—an average of 16 each day.
- Of these homicide victims, 86% were male and 14% were female.
- Homicide is the second leading cause of death for young people ages 10 to 24 years old.
- Of these deaths, 82% involved a firearm.
- Homicide rates among non-Hispanic African American males 10 to 24 years of age (58.3 per 100,000) exceed those of Hispanic males (20.9 per 100,000) and non-Hispanic white males (3.3 per 100,000) in the same age group.
- In 2006, more than 720,000 young people ages 10 to 24 were treated in emergency departments for injuries sustained from violence.

*Source:* CDC, 2008d.

THINK ABOUT THIS

**What women have to say about war...**

All wars are wars among thieves who are too cowardly to fight and who therefore induce the young manhood of the whole world to do the fighting for them.

—Emma Goldman, "Address to the Jury,"
*Mother Earth,* July 1917

It is the people who have no say in making wars who suffer most from the consequences of them.

—Philippa Carr, *The Gossamer Cord,* 1992

History more often records the brilliant successes and spectacular defeats of contending forces than the effect of war on the common people.

—Mildred Cable, with Francesca French,
*The Gobi Desert,* 1942

The calamity of war, wherever, whenever and upon whomever it descends, is a tragedy for the whole of humanity.

—Raisa M. Gorbachev, *I Hope,* 1991

You can no more win a war than you can win an earthquake.

—Jeannette Rankin, in Hannah Josephson,
*Jeannette Rankin,* 1974

All of the horror of the twentieth century should surely teach us that war feeds on itself and that armed violence reflects, not an extension of politics by other means, but the failure of politics; not the defense of civilization, but the breakdown of civilization.

—Rosalind P. Petchesky, "Phantom Towers," in *Ms.,* 2002

Wars produce warlike societies, which in turn make the world more dangerous for other societies, which are thus recruited into being war-prone themselves.

—Barbara Ehrenreich, in *Los Angeles Times,* 2003

The practice of violence, like all action, changes the world, but the most probable change is to a more violent world.

—Hannah Arendt, "On Violence,"
*Crises of the Republic,* 1972

One is left with the horrible feeling now that war settles nothing; that to win a war is as disastrous as to lose one!

—Agatha Christie, *An Autobiography,* 1977

No war can end war except a total war which leaves no human creature on earth. Each war creates the causes of war: hate, desire for revenge and have-nots, desperate with need.

—Zelda Popkin, *Open Every Door,* 1956

War brutalizes all whom it touches; if it did not do so it could not be endured.

—Agnes Newton Keith, *Three Came Home,* 1947

The worst barbarity of war is that it forces men collectively to commit acts against which individually they would revolt with their whole being.

—Ellen Key, *War, Peace, and the Future,* 1916

There's a consensus out that it's OK to kill when your government decides who to kill. If you kill inside the country you get in trouble. If you kill outside the country, right time, right season, latest enemy, you get a medal.

—Joan Baez, *Daybreak,* 1968

Everything you do in a war is crime in peace.

—Helen McCloy, *A Change of Heart,* 1973

If you are required to kill someone today, on the promise of a political leader that someone else shall live in peace tomorrow, believe me, you are not only a double murderer, you are a suicide, too.

—Katherine Anne Porter, "The Situation in American Writing" (1939), *The Days Before,* 1952

I don't believe that the big men, the politicians and the capitalists alone, are guilty of the war. Oh no, the little man is just as guilty, otherwise the peoples of the world would have risen in revolt long ago!

—Anne Frank, *The Diary of a Young Girl,* 1952

There never was a war that was
not inward; I must
fight till I have conquered in myself what
causes war.

—Marianne Moore, "In Distrust of Merits,"
*Nevertheless,* 1944

War is bestowed like electroshock on the depressive nation: thousands of volts jolting the system, an artificial galvanizing, one effect of which is loss of memory. War comes at the end of the twentieth century as absolute failure of imagination, scientific and political.

—Adrienne Rich, *What Is Found There,* 1993

All wars are in reality money squabbles.

—Margaret Mitchell, *Gone with the Wind,* 1936

The first casualty in every war is truth.

—Muriel Lester, *It Occurred to Me,* 1937

It isn't enough to talk about peace; one must believe in it. And it isn't enough to believe in it; one must work at it.

—Eleanor Roosevelt, Voice of America radio,
November 11, 1951

Marx was wrong: It is not only the "means of production" that shape societies, but the means of destruction. In our own time, the costs of war, or just war readiness, are daunting.... The resulting cost squeeze has led to a new type of society, perhaps best termed a "depleted" state, in which the military has drained resources from all other social functions.

—Barbara Ehrenreich, in *Los Angeles Times,* 2003

I do not want to see mothers and fathers digging graves for their children.

—Audrey Hepburn, on her work for UNICEF,
in Warren G. Harris, *Audrey Hepburn,* 1994

I dream of giving birth to a child who will ask, "Mother, what was war?"

—Eve Merriam, in *Peacemaking: Day by Day,* 1989

THINK ABOUT THIS ·······················································································

**Hate Crimes: Can Community Health Nurses Really Do Anything to Prevent the Damage?**

The effects of hate crime on any particular community are not limited to bleeding victims in the emergency department of the hospital or scenes from school shootings. Why hate crimes? Why now? And what can nurses possibly do to prevent it from occurring?

The significance of hate crimes to the community goes beyond the physical injuries of the victims. If you do not believe that hate crimes affect you and your community, consider the following questions: Did your perception of safety in your school change after the first time you heard about shootings at school? Did it the second? What about the third and all the times after that? Have you ever changed your behavior in an effort to avoid potential harm that might come to you based on some personal characteristic of yours? Is there anywhere in your community that you avoid because you do not "belong there" and fear that harm would come to you if you went there? These are just a few of the ways that hate crime shapes our perceptions of safety, the ways in which we interact, and our actions toward each other.

Is there anything about you that someone else might not like? Anything about your physical nature, the color of your skin, your gender, any disability? What about your sexual orientation or practices, your ethnic or national origin or that of your family, or your religious practices? Remember, this is not asking about your tolerance of others; this is asking about the potential tolerance of others toward you.

In short, the answer is that there are always people out there who will react negatively toward you based on some personal characteristic of yours. It does not have to be logical, it does not have to be justified, and it does not have to be out in the open.

It is human nature to reject what makes us uncomfortable or what we do not understand and seek the company of others like ourselves. The more positive expression of this tendency is demonstrated within social circles: With common interests or shared characteristics, more can be accomplished as a group. People of the same religious faith gather together to practice that faith and celebrate its tenets; those who share fondness for a sport find others to play with or observe with; and those who share characteristics such as being parents of small children or having the same disability find support and advice in each other's company. Nurses are always being reminded that there is strength in numbers; by joining together, nurses can influence legislation and make changes in the way things are done. People are more powerful in groups.

Neutrality is also possible. An individual may "agree to disagree" with someone else on some point of difference, if there are other points they share. An example of this would be friendship between people of different religious faiths. Neither person is expected to relinquish his or her beliefs; neither one is "right" or "wrong." If they are willing to seek out points of sharing and commonality rather than focus on differences, people from widely differing groups can also share strength and enrich each other's experience. This is a true expression of tolerance: acceptance of others based not on their similarity to oneself, but on the merits of their own characteristics.

The dark side of this aspect of human nature emerges when the characteristics of one's own group are considered the only correct ones. It is not enough to associate with others like oneself. Those who are different are less trustworthy, dangerous, less human. The discomfort felt when in the presence of someone different from this "norm" leads to action against that individual. Those who are different must be kept out, moved away, eliminated. There are untold millions of examples of this intolerance in human history; all people, of all cultures, share in this inheritance.

This is the origin of hate crimes. One of the aphorisms of Hippocrates is, "Of two pains existing at the same time, but not in the same place, the stronger obscures the other." Hatred in this case is the stronger pain, drawing attention from its quieter companions, fear of the other, fear of the unknown, fear of what is different.

This fear is intolerable, and the reaction of the individual is hatred for the thing that has caused this discomfort. The hatred is louder, obscuring the existence of the fear, but the fear is there.

At present, the federal statute regarding hate crimes is 18 U.S.C. §245, which covers the threat, attempt to use, or use of force to injure, intimidate, or interfere with "any person because of his race, color, religion, or national origin" who is participating in one of six federally protected activities. These are (1) enrolling in or attending a public school or public college; (2) participating in or enjoying a service, program, facility, or activity provided or administered by any state or local government; (3) applying for or enjoying employment; (4) serving in a state court as a grand or petit juror; (5) traveling in or using a facility of interstate commerce; and (6) enjoying the goods or services of certain places of public accommodation.

The Hate Crimes Prevention Act of 1999 eliminates the "federally protected activities" requirement because some cases that have satisfied juries as to bias motivation had to be dismissed because the victims were not involved in one of the six protected activities. This act also adds gender, perceived or actual sexual orientation, and disability to the list of bias motivations. Other attempts at legislation with similar intent were the Violent Crime Control and Law Enforcement Act of 1994 and the Bias Crimes Compensation Act of 1993, neither of which made it into law.

Are you surprised? Many members of the public assume that any crime motivated by bias can be prosecuted as a hate crime; with a vague sense that there are "hate crime laws," they believe the issue to be closed. There are also misperceptions of the purpose of hate crimes legislation.

If bias against a certain religion is the motivation for killing someone, is the victim any less dead than if the action had taken place during a robbery? Aren't they both murder, which is against laws that already exist? Is it less heinous if the victim was at home rather than participating in one of the six federally protected activities? Is it more wrong to kill someone who is in one group than someone who is in another? Why should the motivation for the act or the identity of the victim make any difference in the prosecution? Then answers are: no, yes, no, no, and please pay attention, because that comes next.

*(continues)*

THINK ABOUT THIS (continued) ·····················································

### Hate Crimes: Can Community Health Nurses Really Do Anything to Prevent the Damage?—cont'd

Burt Neuborne, the John Norton Pomeroy Professor of Law at the New York University School of Law, testified before the Senate on May 11, 1999, in support of the Hate Crimes Prevention Act of 1999 (S. 622). He stated, "The First Amendment does not protect violence merely because it is motivated by hatred. No principle of First Amendment law shields a violent offender against increased punishment because the crime was motivated by group hatred." The two things to note here are "increased punishment" and "group hatred." Remember the nature of prejudice: Another group of people is perceived as a threat. Neuborne contended that the heavier penalties for hate crimes would act as a deterrent against activities of hate and that hate crimes legislation would have "educational value" because it singles out the unacceptability of organized bias crimes. Murder is a crime; the perpetrator should be punished. But if the murder is part of the program of a hate group, should that group not also be punished? What if the murderer is not a member of a hate group but singles out victims with certain characteristics?

The victims of random crime are no less valuable than the victims of hate crime; that is not the reason different penalties are sought. The reason that hate crimes are different from other crimes: Existing laws punish random actions, while hate crime laws seek to punish organized activities of hate, whether they are the actions of hate groups or of individuals.

Nurses can have an effect on hate crimes and the communities they damage. The politics of difference can have a chilling effect on the pursuit of justice; by authoring or monitoring legislation, nurses can promote politics of equity. The 104th Congress asked the Library of Congress to make federal legislative information available via the Internet. Beginning in January 1995, this information has been available through Thomas, a service of the Library of Congress. This is one online source that should remain current for many years to come; the URL is http://thomas.loc.gov. By using this resource, nurses can follow the progress of federal legislation.

Nurses can also work to promote tolerance in their communities. If fear is the basis for prejudice, then understanding and information are the countermeasures. This is not something that can be imposed from outside. Peace comes from partnering with the community. It is important to respect the concerns of the members of the community and help them to move toward their own acceptance and tolerance of others. To that end, I offer this quotation from C. S. Lewis:

> For every one pupil who needs to be guarded from a weak excess of sensibility there are three who need to be awakened from the slumber of cold vulgarity. The task of the modern educator is not to cut down jungles but to irrigate deserts. The right defence [sic] against false sentiments is to inculcate just sentiments. By starving the sensibility of our pupils we only make them easier prey to the propagandist when he comes. For famished nature will be avenged and a hard heart is no infallible protection against a soft head (p. 27, The Abolition of Man).

Written for educators in 1944, this is relevant for nurses working with the community now; fear and mistrust have created deserts that separate people from each other, and the apathy that grips the population must be akin to the slumber of which Lewis wrote. Promoting tolerance of diversity and providing learning opportunities form the best protection against hard hearts; the "soft heads" will never be any less soft until efforts are made to improve the situation.

**—Regina Hood Posey, RN, MSN**

---

## BOX 22-9

### Risk Factors for Perpetrators of Youth Violence

#### Individual
- History of violent victimization
- Attention deficit, hyperactivity, or learning disorders
- History of early aggressive behavior
- Association with delinquent peers
- Involvement in gangs
- Involvement with drugs, alcohol, or tobacco
- Low IQ
- Poor academic performance
- Low commitment to school or school failure
- Poor behavioral control
- Deficits in social, cognitive, or information processing abilities
- High emotional stress
- Antisocial beliefs and attitudes
- Social rejection by peers
- Exposure to violence and conflict in the family
- Lack of involvement in conventional activities

#### Relationship
- Harsh, lax, or inconsistent disciplinary practices
- Low parental involvement
- Low emotional attachment to parents or caregivers
- Low parental education and income
- Parental substance abuse or criminality
- Poor family functioning (e.g., communication)
- Poor monitoring and supervision of children

#### Community/Societal
- Diminished economic opportunities
- High concentration of poor residents
- High level of transiency
- High level of family disruption
- Low levels of community participation
- Socially disorganized neighborhoods

*Source:* CDC, 2008f.

### Gangs

The growth of youth gangs in the past decades is a major concern, especially with the expansion of gang activity in rural and suburban communities and in cities where gangs did not previously exist (U.S. Department of Justice, 2000). As gangs migrate across the country, they bring with them drugs, weapons, and criminal activity. In recent years, gangs have become more sophisticated and aggressive in their use of violence and intimidation practices. They threaten our schools, our children, and our homes. As gang members relocate they establish new branches of their gang in the new locale, bringing gang activity to areas without previous gang activity or entering into deadly conflict with local gangs (Bureau of Justice Assistance, 2005).

Gangs are the primary distributors of illicit drugs throughout the United States and around the world. Gang members have become efficient in their use of computers and technology. Devices such as cell phones, navigation systems (e.g., GPS), and laptop computers, are being used to communicate, facilitate criminal activity, and avoid detection by law enforcement. In some communities colors, tattoos, and outward acknowledgment of gang membership are less visible as gangs try to hide from law enforcement. In other communities, gang affiliation is flaunted as an intimidation weapon or gangs are uniting to facilitate stronger networks for criminal activity. Often, community leaders refuse to acknowledge that gang activity exists. Community denial of gang activity is a gang's greatest ally (Bureau of Justice Assistance, 2005).

New immigrant populations in the United States are vulnerable to gang formation because immigrants are often isolated in communities because of language and employment difficulties. Hispanic gangs flourish as a means of providing their communities with support and protection. Asian gangs, however, often victimize Asian communities, as the community members may be less likely to report crimes to police (Bureau of Justice Assistance, 2005). For a better understanding of the dynamics associated with gangs, gang members, and violent activity see the Cultural Connection feature.

---

 ## CULTURAL CONNECTION

### Violence in the Community Setting: Understanding Gangs, Cults, and Other Deviant Groups

Gangs and cults are about power, fear, intimidation, crime, and very often extreme forms of violence, including murder. Gang and cult activities cut across all socioeconomic, racial/ethnic, and gender boundaries and exist in rural, inner-city, suburban, and other community configurations where an opportunity for power, revenge, and rewards associated with crime (especially drug sales) exists. Preadolescence and adolescence are times in which youngsters experiment, rebel, and often feel very insecure (a feeling that is commonly generated by their own subculture) during this critical transition period. Thus youngsters are susceptible to gang/cult activity and the trappings associated with this subculture.

*Gang* and *cult* are terms referring to specific types of groups but here are used to also represent similar deviant groups that may operate within a community setting. The term *gang* or *cult* is defined as a group composed of three or more individuals who have a common identity and who have committed at least one crime, whether the crime is a felony or misdemeanor. There are other groups of individuals who have created ganglike organizations with a central focus of providing for their membership and/or immediate community needs; however, they have not (nor do they intend to) committed any crimes.

Within the "street setting," gangs will generally refer to themselves as an "organization." In fact, many gangs will admit to being an organization but will vehemently deny being a gang. Gangs will even go as far as to say they do not "jump in" their members, but "bless" or "invite" them into the organization. "Jumping in" is when gang members beat a new recruit; if the new member happens to be a female, she is "sexed in" (has sex with male members of the gang) as part of her initiation into the gang. These activities prove a new member's worth, loyalty, and desirability for membership. When female members choose to be beat in to a gang, rather than to be sexed in, they are generally more respected by the membership.

There are differences between gangs and cults. A gang tends to focus more on economic and personal or interpersonal needs of its membership, whereas a cult tends to focus on some religious or spiritual belief system, along with an individual's need to belong and identify with a group. Although there are gangs that almost totally focus on economics, which are most often associated with the drug trade, other gangs thrive on racial and/or ethnic hate. Within this context, the difference between an occult and a cult warrants a brief discussion. An occult is a nontraditional religious belief system in which a group tends to believe; however, there is no emphasis on manipulating and controlling its members (or others) for deviant means. By contrast, cults will often have the same beliefs as an occult, but their focus will be to control and manipulate their membership and others for deviant and criminal purposes. In addition, the typical cult tends to focus more on its leader's desire for power, whims, and fantasies rather than improving the lives of its members. Last, there is a gang/cult category called a "hybrid" that tends to be a combination of belief systems that may include traditional or nontraditional religious beliefs in combination with ethnic/racial hate, along with various criminal activities.

The question often asked is, "Why would an individual join a deviant group?" Affiliations with deviant groups tend to focus around a person's real or perceived needs and/or wants, which are often associated with concepts such as identity, low self-esteem, recognition, protection, drug habit, revenge, reward, power, desire for structure and discipline, respect, sex, understanding, excitement, hate, acceptance, and love; however, the bottom line for joining deviant groups is most often focused on economics, and the economics of gang activity is correlated with crime and violence.

*(continues)*

CULTURAL CONNECTION (CONT.)

### Violence in the Community Setting: Understanding Gangs, Cults, and Other Deviant Groups—cont'd

#### Warning Signs of Gang/Cult Membership

- Unexplained wealth in the form of large amounts of cash
- Unexplained change in types and designs of jewelry
- Lack of participation in typical family activities such as church, school, family outings, and attention to chores
- Unexplained and atypical music being honored
- Habitual lying or distorting the truth
- Aggressive or violent behavior toward family or former friends
- Drug/alcohol use
- Defiance of authority
- Blaming others for his or her troubles and concerns
- Unexplained tattoos
- Denial of a problem
- Refurbishing or reorganizing his or her room and fixtures
- Expressing feelings of rejection
- Association with youngsters of similar styles of dress, grooming, writing, and language

Although some items may not necessarily be gang related, a combination of items may point to an association.

#### Crimes and Violent Behavior Associated with Gangs/Cults

- Criminal exploits associated with joining
- Criminal adventures connected with moving up in rank or position within the gang/cult structure
- Protecting turf
- Saving face or protecting one's honor
- Drug sales
- Use of weapons, especially firearms and knives
- Stealing and robbery
- Home invasions
- Extortion
- Intimidation, harassment
- Sexual offenses, both heterosexual and homosexual
- Animal abuse and mutilation
- Drive-by shootings
- Homicides
- Vandalism
- Graffiti
- Maiming to prove a point or intimidate
- Abduction of both children and adults
- Ritual abuse

Levels of gang involvement in membership roles will often vary according to the type of gang and peculiarities associated with individual gangs. These include (1) wannabes—potential members who are trying to prove themselves and are very often the most dangerous of all membership levels; (2) peripheral—those youngsters who are not in, but not out, and at times participate in gang-related activities; (3) regulars—youngsters who are members and participate regularly in gang-affiliated activities; (4) leaders—hard-core members who direct gang-affiliated endeavors and who are in contact with upper level leadership within a geographical region; and (5) imitators—those individuals who are not (and most likely would never be) gang members but "talk the talk" and "walk the walk," wear the clothing, and try to impress others through being "cool." Any of these five levels of gang involvement or affiliation can be dangerous for both participants and those that come into contact with them in the community setting.

#### Gang Associated Signs and Symbols

##### *Blood/People and Vice Lord Gangs*

- Left orientation
- Color red
- Five-point star
- Pyramid
- Cane

##### *White Supremacists*

- Skull and crossbones
- Rebel flag
- Swastika
- Anarchy symbol

##### *Folks/Crips and Gangsters Gangs*

- Right orientation
- Color blue
- Six-point star
- Pitchfork
- Three-point crown

##### *Cults*

- Pentagrams
- Inverted pentagrams
- Circles
- Candles (red, white, black)
- Celtic crosses
- Ankhs

#### Response to Gang/Cult Activity

The response to gang and cult activity should focus on strategies associated with prevention, intervention, and suppression. Prevention tactics are those strategies that the home/school/community select to prevent gangs/cults from forming and/or exploiting others. Intervention focuses on those techniques that are employed in the home/school/community setting that respond to youngsters who are on the fringes of gang/cult involvement or are actually participants. Suppression is more associated with enforcement, prosecution, and incarceration of members who have committed a crime within the community and/or suspension/expulsion for violating school district policy. To adequately combat gang/cult activities the home/school/community has to work together and employ all three strategies or the youngsters will manipulate the system and take advantage of the structural void that is created. The two most important issues that must be overcome before an effective gang/cult response is possible are for all entities within a community to admit that a problem exists and to overcome agency and individual jurisdictional issues (turf issues). There is no single solution to cult- or gang-related violence within our communities; however, there is hope especially when a community is aware of what is happening around them, admits that a problem exists, and collectively responds through strategies associated with prevention, intervention, and suppression. ◯

—Johnny R. Purvis, PhD

### Gun Control

Firearms are the second leading cause of traumatic death in the United States and the second leading cause of death overall for Americans ages 15 to 24. For every gun-related death there are nearly three nonfatal gun injuries treated in emergency departments each year (Violence Policy Center, 2008). In addition to smoking and drinking, owning and using firearms have become a part of youthful experimentation. Firearm-related crime dropped significantly between 1993 and 2004 but began increasing again in 2005 (U.S. Department of Justice, 2008). Ease of access has contributed to the situation, and interest in public policy on gun control has become more intense.

America is losing too many children to gun violence. Each year, more children and teens die from gunfire than from cancer, pneumonia, influenza, asthma, and HIV/AIDS combined. In a single year, at least 3,000 children and teens are killed by gunfire in the United States. That is one child every 3 hours, eight children every day, and more than 50 children every week. In addition, four to five times as many children and teens suffer from nonfatal firearm injuries each year. American children are more at risk from firearms than the children of any other industrialized nation. In one year, firearms killed no children in Japan, 19 in Great Britain, 57 in Germany, 109 in France, 153 in Canada, and 5,285 in the United States. American children are 16 times more likely to be murdered with a gun, 11 times more likely to commit suicide with a gun, and 9 times more likely to die from a gun accident than children in 25 other industrialized nations combined (National Education Association, 2005).

When a gun is present in a home the risk of homicide and suicide is greatly increased for those residing there. In 2001, 55% of suicides were committed with a firearm (Anderson & Smith, 2003). Some studies indicate that increased concentration of firearms (indicated by permits issued, new sales, or surveys of ownership) is associated with increased firearm robbery, assault, and homicide. Both the American Nurses Association and the American Public Health Association have been long-time advocates for policy proposals to decrease access to guns.

**❝**_A sad soul can kill you quicker than a germ._**❞**

—*John Steinbeck*

### Dating Violence

Dating violence is defined as physical, sexual, or psychological violence within a dating relationship (CDC, 2006b, 2006c). Dating violence is a serious problem in the United States because 72% of teens are already dating by the time they are in the eighth and ninth grades. Many adolescents do not report dating violence because they are afraid to tell friends and family. But the fact is that teens experience dating abuse more often than other age groups. According to the CDC, 1 in 4 adolescents experience verbal, physical, emotional, or sexual abuse each year, and 1 in 11 have been physically hurt by someone they were dating. Among teens,

⚖ ETHICAL CONNECTION

How would you react to the prospect of caring for a male patient in a home health setting who has had a prior history of spousal abuse?

boys often start the violence and use greater force. Girls are more likely than boys to be victims of sexual abuse. Studies show that teens who abuse their dating partners are more depressed, have lower self-esteem, and are more aggressive than peers (CDC, 2006d).

Dating violence has a negative effect on health throughout life. Teens who experience dating violence are more likely to do poorly in school and often engage in unhealthy behaviors like drug and alcohol use. The anger and stress that victims feel may lead to depression, eating disorders, and even suicide. Abused high school students are three times more likely than their nonabused peers to experience dating violence later in college or the workplace. In adulthood, they are more likely to be involved in intimate partner violence (CDC, 2006d).

Teens need to understand that we can only change what we can acknowledge. A forum is needed where teens can learn facts about dating violence and practice resistance skills. The idea that oral sex is not sex has influenced the decision-making skills as young as in middle school. Both sexes need to have knowledge of the deleterious consequences resulting from the present culture of permissiveness. Studies have shown that early maturation can place women at risk because they become targets for older youth (Weisner & Attel, 2002). Nurses can support parents in their pivotal role in helping their teen-aged children postpone sexual activity and decrease their risk of rape by making wise choices about alcohol and drugs and avoiding intimacy with dating or friendly acquaintances.

### Suicide

Suicide is the eleventh leading cause of death in the United States. Although suicide occurs in all age groups, it is the second leading cause of death among 25–34 year olds and the third leading cause of death among 15–24 year olds (CDC, 2007b). More than 90% of suicides in the United States are among whites. Gay and lesbian youth are two to three times more likely to commit suicide, pointing to issues of sexual identity and experienced abuse as risk factors for suicide (Van Wormer, Wells, & Boes, 2000). Males take their own lives at nearly four times the rate of females, although women attempt suicide two to three times as often as men (Levay & Valente, 2003). Suicide is the eighth leading cause of death for males and the 16th leading cause of death for females. Among males, adults age 75 and older have the overall highest rate of suicide (Lubell, Swahn, Crosby, & Kegler, 2004) and among females, those in their 40s and 50s have the highest rates. Firearms are the most commonly used method of suicide among males, while poisoning is the most common method for women (CDC, 2007b).

> **❝***It is no measure of health to be well adjusted to a profoundly sick society.***❞**
>
> —*Krishnamurti*

In addition to prevention efforts to screen and counsel those at risk for suicide, nurses will be involved with the families and friends of those who both succeed and fail at suicide attempts. Families and friends experience anger and guilt over the suicide event and often are unable to discuss it. Nurses intervene during the immediate shock phase and assist with the eventual integration of the event into the survivors' lives.

### Causes of Youth Violence

The theories on causation of youth violence are similar to those cited earlier for violence in general and to family violence. The focus with youth is on the early development of aggressive behavior and the tendencies for it to exhibit at earlier ages. The escalation of violence may, as proposed earlier, be due to societal factors that have made youth aggression more destructive than in the past (see Box 22-9, page 524). Easy access to handguns is also a factor. A second strong social factor is the increasing violence in the media. Television, movies, and video games have been declared

**MEDIA MOMENT**

***Gandhi*** **(1982)**

This film describes the life and times of Mahatma Gandhi, the Indian political leader who managed to free his country from British rule using peaceful means, giving hope and inspiration for generations to come. This epic won eight Academy Awards.

culprits. Technology such as the Internet and satellite and cable television gives children greater access to a wide range of violent images.

Research studies indicate a strong correlation between television violence and violent behavior both immediately and long term (Aronson, 2000). The critical period for lasting harm is childhood. Research suggests that parents limit television watching to one or two hours daily and keep televisions out of children's bedrooms. Exposure to violent video games is associated with a decrease in empathy (Funk, Baldacci, Pasold, & Baumgardner, 2004). Cultural norms, group norms, and family charcteristics also are important in determining the effects of media violence on children's

 **THINK ABOUT THIS** ·············································

**Gun Control**

Nurses debate the question: Are tighter gun control restrictions the answer to the epidemic of violence in schools, workplaces, and communities?

**Yes**

There is some truth in the slogan "Guns don't kill people, people kill people"; nevertheless, people without access to guns are more often than not stymied in their murderous impulses, whether those impulses arise from a distorted perception of reality or from evil. Of course, a substantive cure for the epidemic of violence in our country includes meaningful employment for all, better mental health programs, warm and welcoming families for all children, improved educational systems, increased serenity, and the uprooting of all forms of bigotry. But while we as people are struggling to bring all these about, ought we not, at the very least, do what is within our immediate grasp? It is within our current legislative and enforcement power to (1) make illegal the sale and possession of those particular guns for which the purpose is to kill lots of people quickly; (2) make the ownership of all guns as traceable as that of the automobile; and (3) disqualify for gun ownership persons who have committed felonies or given evidence of potential harm to themselves or to others. For reasons of public health and the common good we restrict entry into school for children who have not been immunized. It seems only common sense that we also restrict the possession of firearms in an effort to control the public health menace of easy killing.

**—Mary Margaret Mooney, DNSc, ARNP, FAAN**
Dubuque, Iowa

**No**

I do not believe that tighter gun control restriction is the answer to the epidemic of violence in our schools, workplaces, and communities. I do not believe the answer is that simple. Violence in our society is a multilevel problem. We need to start with education at an early age to help our children deal with anger. Our children today are taught to handle their anger with violence, as evidenced in modern television, movies, and video games. The average child lacks the skills to deal with his or her frustrations. Television and movies show adults being rude and nasty to others, and this is perceived as being funny. Hitting and fighting back (getting revenge) are displayed as the right thing to do. We need to educate our children to respect others. Parents of today are often overwhelmed with material concerns and lack the energy to teach their children respect of others. Other concerns are seen as more important. Education regarding respect for others is needed at a young age, as well as how to deal with one's anger. Proper channeling of one's frustration will help prevent some of the violence in our society today. We, as health care providers, should stress the importance of stress management for our patients. We should also write our legislators to give our opinion of the violence on television and in the movies. We need to change the way our society views aggression and seek ways to help the public deal with it.

**—Daria Napierkowski, MSN, RN**
Stanhope, New Jersey

*Source*: Kaleidoscope. (1999). *The American Nurse*, 31(5), 4.

aggressive behavior. Violent portrayals most likely to influence behavior are those that show social approval, result in reward, are perceived as real, and are fast paced (Jason, Hanaway, & Brackshaw, 1999). The industry has taken steps to solve some of these issues, with rating of media and blocking options. These steps, however, only regulate content; they do not improve the material viewed by children. Parents must still play a large role and need assistance in understanding the industry classifications of films and videos and obtaining information on film and game content. They must be encouraged to monitor both the time spent and the content of viewing by children (Jason et al., 1999).

### ■ Workplace Violence

Although concerned about those who are victims of violence, nurses are increasingly aware of their own vulnerability in the workplace. Workplace violence, like domestic violence, is not new but has been hidden by much denial. It is an emerging field of study. Workplace violence exists on a continuum from verbal abuse to physical assault to homicide. It includes homicide, beatings, rape, assault, battery, theft, robbery, threats, harassment, and intimidation (McClure, 1999; OSHA, 2002).

Perpetrators of violence can be frustrated or threatened coworkers, a random thief, or disgruntled patients. An average of 20 workers a week are murdered while working, and it is estimated that 2 million more are assaulted annually. Retail establishments open at night have the highest rates of homicide. According to the estimates of the Bureau of Labor Statistics, nonfatal assaults on hospital workers in 1999 occurred at a rate of 8.3 per 10,000 workers. This rate is much higher than the rate of 2 per 10,000 nonfatal assaults for all private-sector industries workers (OSHA, 2002). Patients are most often responsible for these assaults, but their friends and family members can also be violent. Jobs in health care, education, and social services are the settings at highest risk of violence for women. The leading cause of occupational

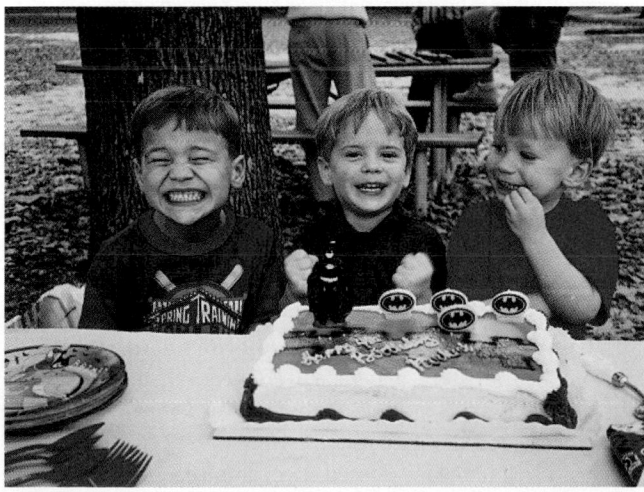

Male children raised in the United States embrace action figures who often use violence to triumph over their foes.

*a conversation with . . .*

Nurses care for victims of violence, perpetrators and witnesses to violent acts. The experiences of nurses who care for those affected by violence in many parts of the world point out the pervasive nature of violence. In addition, nurses themselves are at risk for violence in their personal lives, in their communities and, unfortunately, in their places of work. Violence in nursing is seldom discussed and if it is, it is in hushed tones and with a 'thank goodness it is not me' sentiment. Nurses care for and about others. It's why you are a nurse; it's why I am a nurse. We are courageous, but we don't have to suffer indignities or harm to do our jobs. All we need is respect for our professional work and to be safe. It is little enough to ask.

—**Eleanor J. Sullivan**
**RN, PhD, FAAN**
President, Sigma Theta Tau, International Nursing
Honor Society of Nursing, 1999–2000
*Source:* Sullivan, E. J. (1999).
President's message, *Reflections, 25*(3), 4.

death for women is violence. These statistics show that nurses are a population at particular risk for workplace violence.

Some risk factors are the same for all work settings and include an increasingly violent society, availability of handguns and other weapons, and high crime neighborhoods. Also included for all work settings are organizational characteristics such as negative management practices; a culture at work that creates pressure for performance; poor staffing, hiring, and retention practices; and increased diversity in the workforce, which can create conflict over differences (McClure, 1999, OSHA, 2002). Parents should monitor the workplaces of their children, as certain jobs such as convenience store clerks may be subject to robbery or even murder.

Risk factors specific to nursing situations include the presence of money and drugs, working alone as well as on nights and holidays, poorly lit parking lots, and open exits and entrances. Untrained security guards can add to escalating interactions or fail to respond in a timely manner. Emergency departments and psychiatric units are two of the highest risk work areas for nurses. Also, reduced staffing levels and sicker patients with shorter lengths of stay increase

✎ NOTE THIS! ●———————————————

The United States leads the industrialized world in the number of homicides per capita. Compared with the country with the next highest homicide rate, Italy, the U.S. rate is eight times higher. The U.S. homicide rate is 20 times higher than Canada's rate and 40 times higher than Japan's rate. As a result of this high violent crime rate, the United States has a higher percentage of its population in prison than any other industrialized nation.

*Sources:* National Center for Health Statistics, *Vita Statistics,* 1990; World Health Organization, *Statistical Annuals,* 1990.

the frustration levels of patients and families. The release of more acutely and chronically ill patients has increased the number of potentially dangerous patients in community health settings and emergency rooms.

On October 28, 2002, three nursing professors at the University of Arizona were murdered in full view of their students, by a nursing student. Subsequently, protocols for identifying and intervening with at risk for violence students were developed (Stauffer, 2002).

## Mass Violence and War

Modern nursing was born in the battlefields of the Crimean War when Florence Nightingale revolutionized the care of the soldiers in that battle. The history since that time has been marked by continuous instances in which nurses have served the wounded in battle. Nursing also has a history of peace activism among its historical leaders (Temkin, 1997). It has only been in the very recent past that public health professionals, including nurses, have begun to view the violence of war as a proper social ill to address in the public health model of prevention. Less than 25 years ago, when violence was recognized as a public health issue, very little was written in public health literature on the violence of war. Groups of health professionals did have divisions of professional organizations or independent groups that had a special interest in peace, but war was not brought to the forefront until most recently.

Levy and Sidel (1997) introduced the first comprehensive examination of the relationship between war and public health. They documented the public health consequences of war, roles of health professionals, and prevention interventions. There have been cautions in social science literature about the overextension of preventive health measures to inappropriate areas, or the inappropriate role of health sciences (usually referring to medicine) as the "social guardian of morality." However, there seems to be a growing number who believe that identifying risks, developing interventions to lower risk, and implementing the interventions are pos-

## *a conversation with . . .*

Killings in Kosovo, shootings in schools, bombings in Belgrade—all extreme acts that have become the expression of our differences. Violence has invaded our homes, workplaces, communities, and countries as we continue to document increases in homicide, suicide, and sexual, physical, and domestic abuse. Is it not time for our society to look into its soul and ask what has gone so terribly wrong?

It seems to me there is this common theme that runs through all these acts of violence: an all-too-frequent willingness on the part of people to resort to violence when they disagree with someone or find another person's lifestyle or skin color objectionable. . . . Many nurses are not turning away from this problem. . . . While they recognize no one will provide answers or be perfect, they are taking positive, effective action. In this way they are preserving human dignity, tending to the health of populations and protecting basic societal principles while respecting differences.

—**Nancy Dickenson-Hazard**
**RN, MSN, CPNP, FAAN**
Executive Director, Sigma Theta Tau
International Honor Society of Nursing

### A Good Read

# Beware of Crumb Snatchers

A man was placed in a cage.
He was surrounded by men who had none.
A conflict was enraged when
other men wanted some
of his crumbs.
Violence swept the floor.
Men fell to cold graves.
Those who gained, wanted more.
The battle lasted for days.
Finally, one man arose yelling
and screaming
"Yes, I've won!
But he was still locked in a cage with
slain companions
and a crumb.

—Imani Abdul-Haqq

### MEDIA MOMENT

*A History of Violence* **(2005)**
In Millowbrook, Indiana, mild-mannered Tom Stall owns a diner and has a calm life with his beloved wife Edie Stall, his teenager son Jack, and his little daughter Sarah. His life turns upside-down when he kills two cold-blooded killers in his diner to protect his waitress, becoming a local hero and being shown on the front page of the newspaper and on TV. The mobster Carl Fogarty comes to the town calling him "Joey Cusack" and telling that he was a former hitman. When Carl and his men threaten his family, Tom defends them, and violence is released in a chain reaction.

sible for war. Conscious steps can be taken to measure and reduce the risk of arms, mass violence, and conflict (Foege, 1997). Mass violence of war can be claimed as a legitimate inclusion on community health prevention agendas. Amnesty International and Human Rights Watch, for example, investigate and monitor for suffering and abuse in people across the world.

### Epidemiology of War

The health consequences of war are both direct and indirect. Box 22-10 details major health consequences of warfare. Nightingale is recognized as the first to do statistical analyses on the management of mass casualties during war (Nightingale, 1954). In recent decades, rates of mortality attributable to war have risen. World War II caused the death of 3% of the world's population of the time. The former Soviet Union lost 10% of its population in that war and the United States lost 0.3%. The number of civilian deaths in war has risen such that in 1990 civilian deaths accounted for 90% of all deaths in war. The rate of wounding during combat has decreased from 97 per 1,000 troops in the Civil War to 27 per 1,000 in World War II. Indirect effects indicate that more deaths follow from wars than occur during war itself. These deaths result from breakdown of the normal systems of sanitation, food, and other supplies and the lack of available medical care. One measure of the burden of disease, disability adjusted life years (DALYs) combines both death and suffering. In looking at the global burden of disease, violence ranked second only to respiratory disease in DALYs lost, representing its disease burden on the world (World Bank, 1993).

Nursing adopted a resolution in 2001 at the American Academy of Nurses meeting addressing the issue of torture. After the Abu Ghraib prison incident, it became apparent that the profession must make a contribution in preventing inhumane treatment of prisoners (Glittenberg, 2003). No torture is justified. Presently, the United States, Israel, Russia, and other nations are on the front line in the war on terrorism. The suicide bombers who attacked on September 11, 2001, left the United States with anticipation of future attacks (Lee, 2004). Nursing assumed a role of caring for the survivors and the caregivers at Ground Zero. In military branches across the United States, nurses are activated and essential to the present effort in the war on terrorism.

### Roles of Nurses Related to War

Levy and Sidel (1997) list the following war-related activities for nurses: surveillance and documentation of the health effects of war and factors causing war; education and awareness-raising programs on the health effects of war; advocation of preventive policies and actions; and direct action to prevent war and its consequences, such as participation in nonviolent conflict resolution and building trust. The last role requires skills that many expert community health nurses develop. These skills include refinement of interpersonal communication skills; knowledge of conflict processes

---

**BOX 22-10**

**Mass Violence and War: Scope of the Health Problem**

**Physical Health**
- Increased mortality from direct violence, famine, disease
- Malnutrition from lowered food production, poverty, displacement
- Physical trauma of wounded, maimed, disfigured
- Epidemics from lowered vaccination rates and overcrowding
- Increased human immunodeficiency virus (HIV) rates from soldiers' sexual abuse and rape

**Psychological Health**
- Persistent threat of attack
- Grief from loss of family, homes, land, possessions
- Witnessing of atrocities
- Capture and torture
- Forced to perform violence and condone violence

**Soldiers' Postcombat Health**
- Interpersonal and family violence
- Suicide
- Addiction
- Post-traumatic stress
- Alienation
- Psychic disintegration

**Impact on Health Determinants**
- Flight from homes creates displaced persons, abandoned and orphaned children
- Economic crisis—national resources spent on defense—no money for food, required health services, infrastructures
- Diminished health care—costs prohibitive, delivery systems destroyed, access to remaining healthcare system is reduced or dangerous
- Limited time and focus on parenting, caregiving as safety, basic needs, and avoidance of attack predominate
- Schools destroyed—access to education decreased and illiteracy increased, compromising both personal health education and future health manpower systems
- Health workers' morale and income decreased, thus lowering quality of health care
- Massive environmental destruction and increased hazards

---

at the individual, group, and community levels; understanding and using theories of conflict and conflict resolution; clarification of the history and origins of a conflict situation; and a humanitarian commitment to the pursuit of just, peaceful conflict resolution.

The Research Alert on page 530 illustrates the work of nurses that focuses on the experiences of war refugees. Care is provided by nurses to war refugees either by traveling to serve in relief missions or through contact with refugees who come to the United States. Refugees present unique health problems related both to previous traumatic experiences and to marginalization from the mainstream society (Allotey, 1998).

## Research Alert

The purpose of this study was to investigate the ways in which children ages 10 to 17 who have grown up amid violence "make sense" of their experiences. The interpretive methods used gave voice to individual experiences but placed them within the socially constructed political, economic, and cultural context in which violence is allowed. The children's exposure to violence was conceptualized, then, not as a private or individual problem, but as a public problem demanding social change.

Dialogue, reflection, and critique—methods of critical research—guided the data collection and analysis of data from 16 children of war and 16 children of battered women. All had witnessed violence but were no longer living with violence.

It was typical for the children of battered women to have no warm memories or happy moments to hold on to. Violence for them had been an everyday part of their lives in subtle and not so subtle ways. In contrast, for the children of war, the violence marked a temporary disruption in their previously happy lives.

Both groups had profound feelings of betrayal. For those who suffered war, the betrayal was from outside the home by those previously viewed as friends. The children of battered women felt betrayed from within their homes by those who were to protect them. Similar emotions of sadness, anger, and confusion were felt by both groups, but those of battered women also experienced shame and embarrassment.

Their experiences of suffering revealed the distinct ways in which war and woman abuse are socially and politically constructed. Both were in battlefields, but the battlefields of war were publicly declared and fought. They were justified, rationalized, and given legitimacy in the world. International bodies set up rules for the regulation of war. These are rules for all to abide by. In contrast, the violence directed toward women and children was conducted in secrecy, the privacy of their homes, and without rules of fair play. Rules were set by the perpetrators.

The stories of the children showed their capacity to find surprising resources. They had self-confidence, hope, and optimism for things to be better. Their "escapes" made them feel lucky, but they felt they were unlikely to forget what had happened to them.

The author concluded that although the children showed remarkable insight and strength, they faced many challenges. In spite of common conceptions that children cannot talk about deeply troubling experiences, the research demonstrated that children want to discuss their experiences and welcome the opportunity.

*Source:* Berman, H. (1999). Stories of growing up amid violence by refugee children of war and children of battered women living in Canada. *Image: Journal of Nursing Scholarship, 31*(1), 57–63.

Community health nurses who work with refugee populations must manage feelings of anger, frustration, guilt, and loneliness; sleeplessness; and recurring images of suffering. Following resettlement in countries that grant asylum, refugees often experience depression symptoms related to both premigration and postmigration experiences. Interventions for these symptoms and other health-related problems are particularly sensitive to the need for culturally congruent care (ICN, 2008).

## Interventions to Prevent Violence

Recognition of violence as a public health issue is a relatively recent development. Those who practice or do research in the field readily admit that knowledge of both causes and risk factors, and thus of prevention, are only beginning to be developed. Interventions related to violence can be directed to all three system levels—micro, meso, and macro—that were shown in the figure on page 508. In addition, such interventions can be representative of the three areas of prevention: primary, secondary, and tertiary. Following the public health approach to the problem, interventions are efforts to break the causal chain between potential violence and actual violence. Although much more needs to be known about the complicated interplay of causes of violence, the factors identified in Box 22-1 and discussed throughout the chapter represent a summary of those factors that guide current intervention strategies. At the microlevel, characteristics that put individuals at risk for perpetration (e.g., use of alcohol by batterers) or victimization (e.g., children in unstable homes) can be targeted for screening and group prevention activities. Similarly, as we know more about

### HEALTHY PEOPLE 2010

**Objectives Related to Injury and Violence Prevention**

*Injury Prevention*

15.3 Reduce firearm-related deaths.

15.4 Reduce the proportion of persons living in homes with firearms that are loaded and unlocked.

15.5 Reduce nonfatal firearm-related injuries.

*Violence and Abuse Prevention*

15.32 Reduce homicides.

15.33 Reduce maltreatment and maltreatment fatalities of children.

15.34 Reduce the rate of physical assault by current or former intimate partners.

15.35 Reduce the annual rate of rape or attempted rape.

15.36 Reduce sexual assault other than rape.

15.37 Reduce physical assaults.

15.38 Reduce physical fighting among adolescents.

15.39 Reduce weapon carrying by adolescents on school property.

societal influences on development and expression of violence, macrolevel interventions directed toward laws, education, and media images are implemented. See the *Healthy People 2010* box for selected objectives related to violence.

Currently, healthcare practitioners' response to violence is sometimes criticized. This is related to the fairly recent recognition of violence as not just a criminal justice problem, but as a health behavior problem as well. It was just in 1999 that the membership of the American Association of Colleges of Nursing approved their position statement on domestic violence and delineated necessary competencies for nurses to provide high-quality care to victims of violence (AACN, 1999). Education efforts are prevalent among all healthcare workers to raise their awareness and increase assessment and screening for abuse. Studies have indicated that physicians and nurses seldom routinely inquire about abuse. Even when treating the injuries of abused patients, psychosocial assessment or safety issues are most frequently not addressed. Although the healthcare response needs to be improved, there are many ways in which community health nurses do currently initiate and collaborate in violence interventions. These are described in the following sections, according to level of intervention.

❝ *Peace cannot be achieved by violence; it can only be achieved by understanding.* ❞

—*Albert Einstein*

## Microlevel Interventions with Individuals and Families

Community health nurses are confronted with individuals who have experienced violence in all of the many community based settings in which they live and work. Nurses in home health, schools, clinics, religious communities, homeless shelters, and other community sites will encounter victims and potential victims of violence. Those who work in institutional settings also design protective programs for individuals who are members of populations at risk such as frail and vulnerable nursing home residents, daycare residents, and co-workers at risk for workplace violence.

### Primary Prevention
Primary intervention strategies focus on strengthening the resistance of vulnerable individuals. Such efforts, including encouraging interest and involvement in school, can be successful and should begin as early as possible before young people adopt violent beliefs and behaviors (Hawkins, 1999). The general population of youth can be targeted and outreach to high-risk youth can also be extended to those who engage in physical fights, those with criminal records or history of inflicting or receiving violent injuries, drug users, gang members, and school dropouts. Relocated youth from immigrant, refugee, and mobile communities, as well as those with emotional or mental problems, are also at risk (CDC, 2008f; ICN, 2008).

Collaborative interventions by nurses in schools, daycare settings, after-school programs, and community youth organizations include nonviolent conflict resolution training, mediation training, coping and stress management training, life and social skills training, self-esteem and ethnic pride enhancement, mentoring programs, parenting classes, and personal safety classes that include gun safety (Jones & Selder, 1996). As part of the team that is implementing programs, nurses can ensure that gender-specific issues of power and control in male–female relationships, date rape, other dating violence, and attitudes toward women are added to the often gender-neutral and male-male focus of programs.

Young people should be taught the risk factors or "red flags" that warn of potential abusive relationships. Programs such as "Safe Dates" can offer a countercultural message of self-respect and protect against tolerance of abuse (Foshee, Bauman, & Everett, 2004).

Nurses in New Orleans have posted notices in bars during Mardi Gras warning that sex with an intoxicated person is sex with someone incapable of consent, or rape. Young people should realize that the number one date rape drug is alcohol and they are giving it to themselves. Instruction is also needed regarding the long-term consequences of so-called harmless drugs like ecstasy (McGuire, 2000; Morgan, 2000).

Although early intervention with youth is an optimal time for prevention, the same factors are the target for modification when working with those who are older and in situations of potential violence. Other developmental periods such as marriage, pregnancy, and retirement present opportunities for prevention by service providers. An elder's registration for Medicare could provide an opportunity for health and social service interventions to support healthy family adapting (Institute of Medicine, 1999). Further primary prevention strategies include coping, self-esteem development, early drug and mental illness treatment, realistic parenting expectations, enhanced family bonding, and development of alternatives to the use of violence for conflict resolution. The nurse should also encourage avoidance and/or protection in situations conducive to violence such as bars, high-crime areas, presence of guns in homes, lone work situations, or use of alcohol in dating situations. Individual and family counseling and referral are appropriate.

Some programs have screening protocols to assess for the potential for abuse among pregnant mothers in overburdened families and to initiate home visits for those at high risk (Southern Regional Children's Advocacy Center, 1998). Hawaii's Healthy Start program of home-based services is targeted to families at risk for child abuse and neglect and uses lay home visitors trained and supervised by professional health providers. Parental attitudes toward children and parent–child interaction patterns show measurable benefits. Programs to prevent elder abuse include efforts to reduce caregiver stress by ensuring respite care, daycare, and homemaker and aid services to the family.

*Got an Alternative?*

Anger management classes have effectively used meditation, yoga, biofeedback, and other self-management techniques that teach men and women how to mediate anger before violence occurs.

### Secondary Prevention

Secondary prevention involves actions that are taken when violence and abuse are present. Goals include identifying the fact of abuse and intervening to aid the victim. Often, the only, or the first, practitioners to come into contact with victims are healthcare providers. One pressing issue is the need to increase the recognition, diagnosis, and assessment of violence by these professionals. Support for such assessment was provided when the Joint Commission on Accreditation of Healthcare Organizations set standards, in 1992 and 1994, for assessment protocols in emergency departments, alcohol abuse centers, ambulatory care centers, and all inpatient and outpatient facilities accredited by the organization. Such protocols have been developed and implemented by nurses for specific organizations (Campbell & Dienemann, 1999). General guidelines for routine screening that were released by the Family Violence Prevention Fund (FVPF) have had the support of the ANA (Family Violence Prevention Fund, 1999). The FVPF guidelines recommend routine screening of all women older than 14 years of age, whether or not symptoms or signs are present and whether or not the provider suspects abuse has occurred. Examples of questions for screening are shown in Box 22-11.

In cases of sexual assault, increasing numbers of nurses are becoming specialized as Sexual Assault Nurse Examiners (SANEs). Their work is specialty work in forensic nursing. They work closely with law enforcement in collecting and preserving evidence of crimes. Their role is special in that they are trained to perform the necessary technical procedures during examinations, and at the same time, they can counsel and provide support in a patient's time of crisis. SANEs provide consistency as they follow up with victims of assault at monthly intervals to review lab results and assess psychological and spiritual healing. SANEs have qualified as expert witnesses in court and have been instrumental in the conviction of perpetrators.

Reporting of abuse to authorities is a mandated task of healthcare providers on behalf of victims. Healthcare providers in all 50 states and in the District of Columbia are required to report confirmed or suspected instances of child abuse. Most states require reporting of suspected abuse of the elderly, and state laws and procedures should be known. Mandatory reporting in the case of adults who have injuries due to domestic violence is an ongoing legal issue. At present, most states have some type of reporting of all patients who have injuries as a result of domestic violence. Some states have mandatory reporting by healthcare providers in instances in which the patient has an injury that appears to have been caused by a gun, knife, firearm, or other deadly weapon. Some states require reporting when there is reason to believe the patient's injury may have resulted from an illegal act. Other states mandate reporting when the health provider believes injuries resulted from an act of violence. Still other states require mandatory reporting when domestic violence or adult abuse is suspected (DHHS, 2006; NCEA, 2006).

Laws such as those described in the previous paragraph are somewhat controversial. Some contend more harm is done than good. Ethically, there are those who argue that such mandates violate patient autonomy. The stereotype of a passive/helpless victim is perpetuated. It is argued that partner abuse is not considered the same as elder abuse (cases in which there are vulnerable victims). Another potential harm is to the healthcare provider–patient relationship by violating confidentiality and overriding informed consent of patients. There are also arguments that such reporting affects women's safety by discouraging care. Women fear risk of retaliation to themselves or their children by perpetrators, or perpetrators may restrain women from seeking care. Also, until better resources in the form of shelters, counseling, and even effective law enforcement of policy and procedures are, in fact, in place, reporting gives women false hopes of help and assistance. Nurses need to deliberate carefully and consider the patients' best interests when making a decision to report abuse. The decision should be made jointly.

Victims of abuse need to be protected from further abuse, and this may require placement of children in foster care and of victims of domestic violence in shelters or safe houses. Box 22-12 outlines interventions that may be needed

---

## BOX 22-11

### Recommended Questions to Screen Women for Family Violence

**Framing questions**
- Because violence is so common in many people's lives, I've begun to ask all of my patients about it.
- I'm concerned that your symptoms may have been caused by someone hurting you.

**Direct questions**
- Are you in a direct relationship with a person who physically hurts or threatens you?
- Did someone cause these injuries? Was it your partner/husband?
- Has your partner or ex-partner ever hit you or physically hurt you?
- Has your partner or ex-partner ever threatened to hurt you or someone close to you?

*Source:* Family Violence Prevention Fund, 1999; CDC, 2006a. Used by permission of Family Violence Prevention Fund. Used by permission of Family Violence Prevention Fund.

---

**❝** *Testosterone may be the most dangerous substance on earth.* **❞**

—*William H. Foege, MD, former Director of the Centers for Disease Control and Prevention*

## BOX 22-12

**Domestic Violence Assistance Programs**
- Safety planning for women and children
- Help obtaining protection orders
- Support and advocacy during interviews with law enforcement, medical personnel, and legal representation
- Someone to go to court with victims
- Pretrial services
- Assistance with crime victim compensation claims
- Services for children
- Transitional housing
- Assistance and advocacy with employers regarding safety in the workplace and retention of employment
- Supportive services of clothing, food, shelter, transportation, education
- Job training or job relocation
- Counseling
- Child care
- Safety planning and other daily living needs

## BOX 22-13

**Interventions to Raise Awareness About Domestic Violence in the Community**
- Organize a bumper-sticker slogan contest for the community reflecting the needs of that area.
- Ask men in the community to speak out against domestic violence and use their influence as workers and community members to let other men know that violence against women and children is wrong and will not be tolerated.
- Challenge radio stations' disparaging remarks about women. Offer to speak on violence issues to the public.
- Personally speak out about domestic violence and refuse to listen to anyone make derogatory jokes or comments about women.
- Review your community's newspaper for articles on domestic violence and determine whether there is victim-blaming language included in the articles. Speak with the newspaper editor periodically to discuss your findings and offer solutions.
- Organize a fund-raising effort for your local family violence shelter.
- Assess businesses' employee assistance programs and determine if community businesses offer help and referrals for employees who are victims of domestic violence. If not, offer information detailing options for referrals.
- Spearhead multidisciplinary coalitions in the community to address primary prevention issues with adolescents.

by victims of domestic violence and their children. For reasons discussed previously, some victims may choose not to leave the abusive situation. The nurse should support and assist the patient in decision making. Contingency plans and shelter information should be provided. Interventions can also be directed to treatment for the perpetrators of abuse. Nurses can act as facilitators in group treatment sessions or make referrals to group programs or couples counseling. It must be taken into account that couples counseling may increase the woman's danger in the relationship. Often, such counseling may be court ordered. Approaches to content vary, but usually address at least anger management, skill building, and resocialization. Dropout and resistance are common in such programs. Assessment protocols for male batteres exist currently (Kropp & Hart, 2000).

### Tertiary Prevention

Many of the same strategies that help build resistance to the use of violence are also used to rehabilitate and prevent further incidences of abuse. Education, counseling, skill building, modification of unsafe situations, stress reduction, support, and guidance are all part of the rehabilitative efforts directed toward victims and abusers. Research has shown that women can predict their risk of injury at a 96% accuracy rate. A woman's predictions should be given serious attention (Wiesz, Tolman, & Saunders, 2000).

## ■ Mesolevel Interventions: Community Structures

Prevention at this level is focused on broader factors in the larger community that contribute to violence or encourage the presence of violence. Such interventions recognize the general belief that violence prevention will not be successful unless coordinated, comprehensive, multidisciplinary, community-based approaches are initiated. These efforts must address the broader service system issues and move away from fragmented efforts. One term often used to describe such interventions is *community development*, which is action to enhance the ability of communities to meet the needs of its members. Communities are characterized as having more or less community efficacy or competence. Structures and programs must be coordinated.

One step that is needed to motivate coordinated action toward a community problem is the recognition that the problem exists. Box 22-13 outlines steps nurses can take to raise community awareness of the problem of domestic violence. Nurses working with the community often must become involved in outreach activities to promote healthier communities through partnerships with other groups, including citizens. Such work is long term, and results are often not immediate. To optimize community resources, all residents, organizations, agencies, institutions, and other components of the community must be included in the response. This makes the community response prevention and intervention oriented, not just crisis oriented.

Because each community is unique, they have different needs and resources, which means the ways to access a communitywide response to violence will be varied. What works in one community might very well not work in another. Also, consider that often there are communities within communities. For example, a neighborhood might have a Jewish ethnic group and an Italian ethnic group, each with their own traditions and sense of community. There are also self-contained communities such as Native American reservations (see the following Research Alert), prisons, religious neighborhoods, community colleges, and senior universities. Self-contained communities may have different governing principles, needs, and resources than the community-at-large.

Collaboration and partnership of community citizens, institutions, and organizations are essential in establishing a communitywide response to domestic violence. Citizens must have ownership of the response and see themselves as playing a significant role in articulation and attainment of the response vision. Support of the members includes the support of the key leaders (both formal and informal) in the community. These are the people who are highly regarded for their knowledge and contributions to the community. Nurses can identify these leaders by doing the following:

- Getting to know the community before any decisions are made that will impact citizens
- Finding out where women in the community go for help when needed
- Asking for advice and support from co-workers who live in the community
- Asking for advice and support from others who provide direct and supportive services to individuals living in the community
- Volunteering in a community-based organization

After community leaders are identified, meetings and ongoing communication are necessary to develop a common definition of violence and common goals. This step will prevent the development of conflicting interventions and thus tension between participants. For instance, traditional services for battered women and their abused children have not been coordinated and are often in conflict regarding the goals of their interventions. There is a wide range of interventions, initiatives, and cooperative effort possible, limited only by the imagination and commitment of the nurse and community participants.

### 🖥 Research Alert

Both of these studies sought to determine the extent of domestic violence (physical only) experienced in Native American populations. Outcomes were improved documentation of the severity and high prevalence of domestic violence in the communities. In the Apache group, depression and post-traumatic stress disorder symptoms were highly associated with domestic violence. Among the Navajo, receipt of government assistance (low socioeconomic status) was associated with greater rates of domestic violence. ◉

*Sources:* Fairchild, D. G., Fairchild, M. W., & Stoner, S. (1998). Prevalence of adult domestic violence among women seeking routine care at a Native American health care facility. *American Journal of Public Health, 88*(10), 1514–1517.

Hamby, S. L., & Skupien, M. B. (1998). Domestic violence on the San Carlos Apache reservation. *The IHS Primary Care Provider, 23*(8), 102–105.

One outcome of awareness interventions in the community may be an increase in the demand for individual advocacy and supportive services of violence programs. Work has been suggested, for example, to improve such areas as police response, enforcement of present laws, and safer situations for reporting of cases of abuse. Community services need to be in place that increase social and psychiatric services for at-risk youth, expand alcohol and drug treatment services for pregnant and parenting women, and increase educational and employment opportunities. Child protective agencies need an increased capacity to assist patients through the provision of training, funding, and appropriate caseload assignments. Safe environments need to be created through increased surveillance, such as metal detectors at schools, and increased policing in high crime neighborhoods. Recreational facilities and programs for youth need to be available. Research supports a direct relationship between neighborhood characteristics and adolescent outcomes. Living in a high-risk neighborhood can double the incidence of behavioral and academic problems (Halpern-Felsher et al., 1997; Kalil & Eccles, 1998).

### ■ Macrolevel Interventions: Society and Culture

Policy issues dominate the types of interventions that nurses undertake at the macrosystem level of intervention. These interventions go far beyond reducing the virulence of the perpetrator (agent) or strengthening the victim (host) to recognize the preconditions (environment) underlying events of violence. Action at this level is directed at large-scale efforts to address poverty, income disparity, prejudice, sexism, ageism, media violence, handgun control, and the culture of violence. These prevention efforts are attempts to change society's norms and values related to those factors that contribute to and allow violence to occur.

Risk factors for violence, such as binge drinking, can be mitigated by increasing alcohol taxes, maintaining and enforcing the minimum drinking age, and implementing education programs routinely (Cook & Moore, 2002; Holder et al., 2000). Faith-based connections in a community are found to be successful in helping to curtail neighborhood violence (Lee & Bartkowski, 2004; Osgood & Chambers, 2000). Religious involvement promotes civic volunteerism and a social justice mentality that benefits the entire community (Becker & Dhingia, 2001).

Policy can be promoted and legislated that moves change in the right direction. Nurses, nursing organizations, and coalitions of other healthcare providers lobbied successfully for the comprehensive Violence Against Women Act passed in 1994 that promotes protection of women in many areas. Global history reflects the suffering that can be inflicted on entire populations if good citizens remain complacent. Jews in Europe during the Holocaust, large groups of people in Bosnia and Cambodia who endured ethnic cleansing, African Americans under Jim Crow laws in the

Southern United States, and blacks under apartheid in South Africa are some examples of the groups who have suffered in the twentieth century. These groups, among others, should serve as reminders of the need for constant vigilance against hatred and violence.

## Conclusion

Community health nursing can seem daunting to some because of the broad perspective that community health nurses must address in taking on a population focus. Community health nurses, by virtue of their cooperative work with many disciplines, need to develop multiperspectival and multilingual skills. They learn to understand and communicate in many different ways (Diekemper, SmithBattle, & Drake, 1999). All public health problems challenge nursing, but the problem of violence by its very nature may be the most challenging. Alleviating all of the many forms of violence to have health, well-being, and peace for individuals in communities may be the ultimate prevention project. The challenge has been compared with the biblical task of "taking on Goliath" because of how large it looms (Hartman, Lundy, & Janes,

1997). The following thoughts by the leader of the peaceful "Velvet Revolution" in the former Czechoslovakia, Vaclav Havel, give encouragement:

> *Hope,* in this deep and powerful sense, is not the same as joy that things are going well, or willingness to invest in enterprises that are obviously headed for success, but rather an ability to work for something because it is good, not just because it stands a chance to succeed . . . definitely not the same thing as optimism. It is not the conviction that something will turn out well, but the certainty that something makes sense, regardless of how it turns out. (Havel, 1991, p. 181)

Explore Community Health Nursing on the Web! To learn more about the topics in this chapter, use the passcode provided to access your exclusive website: **http://nursing.jbpub.com/ communityhealth.** If you do not have a passcode, you can obtain one at this site.

## ■ CRITICAL THINKING ACTIVITIES

1. Consider the following quotes from two famous people. How do you interpret them and how are they related?

   "The deadliest form of violence is poverty."

   —Mohandas Ghandi

   "The most violent element in society is ignorance."

   —Emma Goldman

2. Consider the quote below. Should war properly be considered an "ailment" of humankind, and if so, is it "curable"? How would you put military action into a prevention framework? Or could you?

   Those worthy gentlemen who look upon war, if successful, as a cause of opulence and prosperity might with equal justice . . . look upon the loss of a leg as a cause of swiftness (Jeremy Bentham, 1987).

3. For reference for questions 3 and 4, read Sidel, 1997. Potential ethical conflicts exist when health professionals and war intersect:
   • Conflict between caring for personnel of their own military force versus opposing forces or civilians who may need their care
   • Conflict between combatant and noncombatant roles for health personnel
   • Conflict between obligation to serve one's country in the military and broader obligation to prevent war
   *Discuss these dilemmas with a military nurse and ask how they resolve their obligations.*

4. Discuss the criticism of caring for victims of war as making war more tolerable.

## ■ REFERENCES

Allotey, P. (1998). Traveling with "excess baggage": Health problems of refugee women in Western Australia. *Women and Health, 28*(1), 63–81.

American Association of Colleges of Nursing. (1999). *Violence as a public health issue.* Washington, DC: Author.

American Nurses Association (ANA). (1991). *Position statement: Physical violence against women.* Washington, DC: Author.

Anderson, R. N., & Smith, B. L. (2003). Deaths: Leading causes for 2001. *National Vital Statistics Report, 52*(9), 1–86.

Aron, L. Y., & Olsen, K. K. (1997). Efforts by child welfare agencies to address domestic violence. *Public Welfare* (Summer), 4–13.

Aronson, E. (2000). *Nobody left to hate.* New York: Worth.

Barash, D. P. (1991). *Introduction to peace studies.* Belmont, CA: Wadsworth.

Becker, P. E., & Dhingia, P. W. (2001). Religious involvement and volunteering: Implications for civil society. *Sociology of Religion, 62,* 315–335.

Bentham, J. (1987). A plan for a universal and perpetual peace. In H. P. Kainz (Ed.), *Philosophical perspectives on peace* (pp. 128–136). Athens: Ohio University Press. (Originally published in 1843).

Bureau of Justice Assistance. (2005). *2005 National gang threat assessment.* Washington, DC: Author.

Campbell, J. C., & Dienemann, J. (1999, June). *Symposium on violence against women.* Presentation at Sigma Theta Tau International Research Conference, London, England.

Cassidy, K. (1999). How to assess and intervene in domestic violence situations. *Home Healthcare Nurse, 17,* 665–671.

Centers for Disease Control and Prevention. (2002). *Violence. Occupational hazards in hospitals.* Atlanta: Author.

Centers for Disease Control and Prevention. (2006a). *Understanding intimate partner violence fact sheet.* Retrieved July 7, 2008, from http://www.cdc.gov/injury.

Centers for Disease Control and Prevention. (2006b). Physical dating violence among high school students—United States, 2003. *MMWR, 55,* 532–535.

Centers for Disease Control and Prevention. (2006c). *Dating abuse fact sheet.* Retrieved July 7, 2008, from http://www.cdc.gov/ncipc/dvp/DatingViolence.htm.

Centers for Disease Control and Prevention. (2006d). *Understanding teen dating abuse fact sheet.* Retrieved July 7, 2008, from http://www.cdc.gov/injury.

Centers for Disease Control and Prevention. (2007a). *Understanding sexual violence fact sheet.* Retrieved July 7, 2008, from http://www.cdc.gov/injury.

Centers for Disease Control and Prevention. (2007b). *Suicide facts at a glance.* Retrieved July 7, 2008, from http://www.cdc.gov/injury.

Centers for Disease Control and Prevention. (2008a). *Violence prevention.* Retrieved July 7, 2008, from http://cdc.gov/ncipc/dvp/prevention_at_CDC.htm.

Centers for Disease Control and Prevention. (2008b). *Understanding child maltreatment fact sheet.* Retrieved July 7, 2008, from http://www.cdc.gov/injury.

Centers for Disease Control and Prevention. (2008c). *Child maltreatment facts at a glance.* Retrieved July 7, 2008, from http://www.cdc.gov/injury.

Centers for Disease Control and Prevention. (2008d). *Youth violence facts at a glance.* Retrieved July 7, 2008, from http://www.cdc.gov/injury.

Centers for Disease Control and Prevention. (2008e). *Understanding youth violence fact sheet.* Retrieved July 7, 2008, from http://www.cdc.gov/injury.

Centers for Disease Control and Prevention. (2008f). *Understanding school violence fact sheet.* Retrieved July 7, 2008, from http://www.cdc.gov/injury.

Committee on Child Abuse and Neglect. (2001). Shaken baby syndrome: Rotational cranial injuries technical support. *Pediatrics, 108,* 206–210.

Cook, P. J., & Moore, M. J. (2002). The economics of alcohol abuse and alcohol control policies: Price levels, including excise taxes, are effective at controlling alcohol consumption. *Health Affairs, 21,* 120–133.

Crandall, M., Walters, A. B., Kernic, M. A., Holt, U. L., & Rivara, F. P. (2004). Predicting future injury among women in abusive relationships. *Journal of Trauma, Injury Infection, and Critical Care, 56*(4), 906–912.

Davey, D. B., & Davey, P. A. (1998, Nov/Dec). Domestic violence today. What nursing students should know. *Imprint,* 41–43.

Department of Health and Human Services (DHHS). (2000). *Healthy People 2010.* Washington, DC: U.S. Government Printing Office.

Diekemper, M., Smith-Battle, L., & Drake, M. A. (1999). Bringing the population into focus. A natural development in community health nursing practice: Part I. *Journal of Public Health Nursing, 16*(1), 3–9.

Donovan, R. J., & Vlais, R. (2005). *VicHealth review of communication components of social marketing/public education campaigns focusing on violence against women.* Melbourne: Victorian Health Promotion Foundation.

Family Violence Prevention Fund (FVPF). (1999). *Preventing domestic violence: Clinical guidelines on routine screening.* San Francisco, CA: Author.

Foege, W. (1997). Arms and public health. In B. Levy & V. Sidel (Eds.), *War and public health.* New York: Oxford University Press.

Foshee, V. A., Bauman, K., & Everett, S. (2004). Assessing the long-term effects of the safe dates program. *American Journal of Public Health, 94*(4), 619–624.

Funk, J. B., Baldacci, B. H., Pasold, T., & Baumgarner, J. (2004). Violence exposure in real life, video games, television, movies, and the Internet: Is there desensitization? *Journal of Adolescence, 27,* 23–39.

Gazmarian, J. A., Peterson, R., Spiz, A. M., Goodwin, M. M., Saltzman, L. E., & Marks, J. S. (2000). Violence and reproductive health: Current knowledge and future research directions. *Maternal and Child Health Journal, 4*(2), 79–84.

Gilligan, J. (1997). *Violence. Reflections on a national epidemic.* New York: Vintage Books.

Glittenberg, J. (2003). The tragedy of torture: A global concern for mental health nursing. *Issues of Mental Health Nursing, 24*(6–7), 627–638.

Halpern-Felsher, B. L., Connell, J. P., Spencer, M. B., et al. (1997). Neighborhood and family factors predicting educational risk and attainment in African American and White children and adults. In T. Brooks-Gunn, G. J. Duncan, & J. L. Avet (Eds.), *Neighborhood Poverty: Context and consequences for children,* (Vol. 1, pp.146–173). New York: Russell Sage Foundation.

Hartman, S., Lundy, K. S., & Janes, S. (1997, June). *Taking on Goliath: Nursing's response to violence.* Paper presented at Association of Community Health Nursing Educators' Annual Spring Institute, Vancouver, British Columbia, Canada.

Havel, V. (1991). *Disturbing the peace.* New York: Random House.

Hawkins, D. (1999). Preventing adolescent health-risk behaviors by strengthening protection during childhood. *Archives of Pediatrics and Adolescent Medicine, 153,* 226–234.

Heise, L., & Garcia-Moreno, C. (2002). *Violence by intimate partners: World report on violence and health.* Geneva: World Health Organization.

Holden, H. A., Gruenwold, P. J., Ponicki, W. R., et al. (2000). Effect of community-based interventions on high risk drinking and alcohol-related injuries. *Journal of the American Medical Association, 284,* 2341–2347.

Hotzworth-Monroe, A., & Stuart, G. L. (1994). Typologies of male batterers: Three subtypes and the differences among them. *Psychological Bulletin, 116*(3), 476–497.

Institute of Medicine. (1999). *Violence and the American family; Report of a workshop. Next steps: A guide to effective action.* Washington, DC: National Academics Press.

International Council of Nurses. (2008). *Nursing matters. ICN on displaced persons: A global challenge.* Retrieved July 7, 2008, from http://www.icn.ch/matters_displacedpersons_print.htm.

Jason, L. A., Hanaway, L. K., & Brackshaw, E. (1999). Television violence and children problems and solutions. In T. P. Gullotta & S. J. McElhaney (Eds.), *Violence in homes and communities: Prevention, intervention, and treatment* (pp. 133–156). Thousand Oaks, CA: Sage.

Jones, F. C., & Selder, F. (1996). Pyschoeducational groups to promote effective coping in school-aged children living in violent communities. *Issues in Mental Health Nursing, 17,* 559–571.

Jones, L. (1993, November 26–28). Can a doctor stop the violence? *USA Weekend,* p. 9.

Kalil, A., & Eccles, J. S. (1998). Does welfare affect family process and adolescent adjustment? *Child Development, 69,* 1597–1613.

Kropp, P. R., & Hart, S. (2000). The spousal assault risk assessment (SARA) guide: Reliability and validity in adult male offenders. *Law and Human Behavior, 24,* 101–118.

Lee, C. (2004, April). Most say they are less safe since 9/11. *Washington Post,* p. A3.

Lee, M. R., & Bartkowski, J. P. (2004). Civic participation, regional subcultures and violence: The differential effects of secular and religious participation on adult juvenile homicide. *Homicide Studies, 7,* 1–35.

Levay, S., & Valente, S. (2003). *Human sexuality.* Sunderland, MA: Sinaurer.

Levy, B. S., & Sidel, V. W. (1997). *War and public health.* New York: Oxford University Press.

Lubell, K. M., Swahn, M. H., Crosby, A. E., & Kegler, S. R. (2004). Methods of suicide among persons aged 10–19 years—U.S. 1992–2001. *Morbidity and Mortality Weekly Report, 53,* 471–473.

McClure, L. F. (1999). Origins and incidence of workplace violence in North America. In T. P. Gullotta & S. J. McElhaney (Eds.), *Violence in homes and communities: Prevention, intervention, and treatment* (pp. 71–99). Thousand Oaks, CA: Sage.

McGee, T. P., & DeBernardo, C. R. (1999). The classroom avenger: A behavioral profile of school based shootings. *Forensic Examiner, 8,* 16–18.

McGuire, P. (2000). Long-term psychiatric and cognitive effects of MDMA use. *Toxicology Letters, 112,* 153–156.

Mercy, J. A., Rosenberg, M. L., Powell, K. E., Broome, C. V., & Roper, W. L. (1993). Public health policy for preventing violence. *Health Affairs, 12*(4), 7–29.

Miller, K., & Knutson, T. (1997). Reports of severe physical punishment and exposure to animal cruelty by inmates convicted of felonies and by university students. *Child Abuse and Neglect, 21,* 59–82.

Morgan, M. J. (2000). Ecstacy (MDMA): A review of possible persistent psychological effects. *Psychopharmacology, 152,* 230–248.

National Center on Elder Abuse. (2006). *The 2004 survey of state adult protective services: Abuse of adults 60 years of age and older.* Washington, DC: Author.

National Center on Elder Abuse. (2008). *Frequently asked questions.* Retrieved July 7, 2008, from http://www.ncea.aoa.gov/NCEA-root/Main_Site/FAQ/Questions.aspx.

National Education Association. (2005). *NEA Health Information Network statistics: Gun violence in our communities.* Retrieved July 7, 2008, from http://www.neahin.org/programs/schoolsafety/gunsafety/statistics.htm.

Nightingale, F. (1954). Notes on matters affecting the health of the British army. In F. Nightingale. *Selected Writings, 1820–1910.* New York: Macmillan.

Occupational Safety and Health Administration. (2002). *OSHA fact sheet: Workplace violence.* Washington, DC: U.S. Department of Labor.

O'Neill, J. M., & Harway, M. (1997). A multivariate model explaining men's violence toward women: Predisposing and triggering hypotheses. *Violence against Women, 3*(2), 182–203.

Osgood, D. W., & Chambers, J. M. (2000). Social disorganization outside the metropolis: An analysis of rural youth violence. *Criminology, 38,* 81–115.

Paulozzi, J. (2002). Variations in homicide risk during infancy—U.S. 1989–1998. *Morbidity and Mortality Weekly Report, 51*(9), 187–189.

Potter, L. B. (1999). Understanding the incidence and origin of community violence: Toward a comprehensive perspective on violence prevention. In T. P. Gullotta & S. J. McElhaney (Eds.), *Violence in homes and communities: Prevention, intervention, and treatment.* Thousand Oaks, CA: Sage.

Scott-Tilley, D. (1999). Nursing interventions to prevent domestic violence. *American Journal of Nursing, 99*(10), 24–27.

Sidel, V. W. (1997). The roles and ethics of health professionals in war. In B. S. Levy & V. W. Sidel (Eds.), *War and public health.* New York: Oxford University Press.

Southern Regional Children's Advocacy Center. (1998). *Healthy families—North America.* Retrieved July 7, 2008, from http://www.ncac-hsv.org/hfl.html.

Stauffer, T. (2002 November 3). University of Arizona tries to limit student threats. *Arizona Daily Star.* Retrieved July 7, 2008, from http://www.AZstarnet.com.

Temkin, E. (1997). Nurses and the prevention of war: Public health nurses and the peace movement in World War I. In B. S. Levy & V. W. Sidel (Eds.), *War and public health.* New York: Oxford University Press.

Tjaden, P., & Thoennes, N. (2000, November). *Full report of the prevalence, incidence, and consequences of violence against women: Findings from the National Violence Against Women Survey* (NJC 183721). Washington, DC: National Institute of Justice.

UNIFEM. (2003). *Making a difference: Strategic communications to end violence against women.* New York: United Nations Development Fund for Women.

United Nations Division for the Advancement of Women. (1995). *Bejing declaration and platform for action: Strategic objectives and actions: Violence against women.* Retrieved July 7, 2008, from http://www.un.org.womenwatch/daw/beijing/platform.

U.S. Department of Health and Human Services. (2007). *Fact sheet at a glance: Messages.* Retrieved July 7, 2008, from http://www.surgeongeneral.gov/library/youthviolence/messages.htm.

U.S. Department of Health and Human Services. (2008). *Child maltreatment 2006.* Washington, DC: Government Printing Office.

U.S. Department of Justice. (2000, September). Preventing adolescent gang involvement. *Juvenile Justice Bulletin,* pp. 1–11.

U.S. Department of Justice. (2008). *Firearms and crime statistics.* Retrieved July 7, 2008, from http://www.ojp.usdoj.gov/bjs/guns.htm.

Van Soest, D. (1997). *The global crisis of violence: Common problems, universal causes, shared solutions.* Washington, DC: National Association of Social Workers.

Van Wormer, K., Wells, J., & Boes, M. (2000). *Social work with lesbians, gays, and bisexuals: A strengths perspective.* Boston: Allyn and Bacon.

Violence Policy Center. (2008). *National Rifle Association information. Gun violence in America.* Retrieved July 7, 2008, from http://www.vpc.org/nrainfo/phil.html.

Waters, H., Hyder, A., Rajkotia, Y., Basu, S., Rehwinkel, J. A., & Butchart, A. (2004). *The economic dimensions of interpersonal violence.* Geneva: World Health Organization.

Wiesner, M., & Attel, A. (2002). Relations of pubertal timing and depressive symptoms to substance use in early adolescence. *Journal of Early Adolescence, 22,* 5–23.

Wiesz, A., Tolman, R., & Saunders, D. (2000). Assessing the risk of severe domestic violence: The importance of survivors' predictions. *Journal of Interpersonal Violence, 15,* 75–90.

Wood, E. F. (2006). *The availability and utility of interdisciplinary data on elder abuse: A white paper for the National Center on Elder Abuse.* Washington, DC: American Bar Association Commission on Law and Aging.

World Bank. (1993). *World development report, 1993.* New York: Oxford University Press.

World Health Organization. (2002). *World report on violence and health.* Geneva: Author.

World Health Organization. (2006). *Elder abuse and alcohol.* Geneva: Author.

World Health Organization. (2008). *Violence, health, and human rights.* Retrieved July 7, 2008, from http://www.who.int/violence_injury_prevention/violence/activities/human_rights/en/print.

Zevitz, R. G., & Faikas, M. (2000). *Sex offender community notification: Assessing the impact in Wisconsin.* Washington, DC: Institute of Justice.

## APPENDIX A

# A Day in the Life of a Nurse Who Faces Violence: Prison Nursing

Miriam Cabana, RN, MSN

The nurse supervisor turned on to the blacktop road that ribboned through the 22,000-acre southern prison. As the expansive horizon of flat delta land passed on her short drive to the prison hospital, she recalled the conversation with her husband earlier in the day. He was the warden of the prison and had mused that the full moon usually means some form of violence would erupt within the prison units and that it was an "ideal" time for an escape attempt. She knew he was diligent in his efforts to protect the community as well as to maintain a safe environment for those incarcerated, which often included protecting them from violence inflicted on each other; and he shared her strong opinion about society's obligation to provide inmates with access to safe, competent health care. At the very least, there would be more physical altercations among the inmates or increased somatic complaints screened by phone from the emergency department. She instinctively knew her evening shift would be busy. Oh, for the days in her nursing career that the "full moon" myths were associated only with increased birth rates!

The transition between shifts for both nursing and security personnel was smooth. Predictably, several inmates remained in the large holding room with barred windows and door waiting their turn to see the physician. They were the last patients of the scheduled sick call. Once their assessment, diagnostic tests, or treatments were completed, the hospital correctional officers assigned to transportation would return them in handcuffs and a secured van to their respective housing units. The phone rang constantly and required the nursing supervisor and a second RN to screen the calls from officers in the housing units who reported the inmate complaints, requests for medications, refills, accidents, or any unusual behavior or symptoms observed by the officers. The nurses made the decision that required assessment in the emergency room, and two hospital officers would pick up the inmate and bring him to the hospital. The LPN and two EMTs assisted the physician. Finally, at around 8 P.M., the nursing supervisor realized that the phone calls were becoming less frequent. She always felt like she was playing Russian roulette, hoping she and her staff asked the right questions or were receiving accurate replies for accurate phone assessments.

The loud ring from the "red" emergency phone jarred everyone into a state of readiness. The phone was connected to the warden's office, the central security office, and the hospital emergency department, so that all key personnel were alerted with the dialing of a single number. The ominous sound always meant an emergency of some description. As nursing and security staff gathered at the doorway to listen, the nursing supervisor quickly picked up the receiver. The excitable, stuttering voice on the other end was barely intelligible. It was obvious the officer was in trouble and had to be coaxed by the security chief to report the housing unit

number. The nursing supervisor had heard the word "stabbing" and the unit number. Suddenly she heard the quivering male voice on the other end cry out, "Oh my God, he's gonna kill all of us!" before the line went dead. She immediately dispatched one of the two life-support ambulances. The second ambulance was on its way to another far-flung maximum security housing unit so the RN, a former critical care unit nurse, could assess an inmate complaining of severe chest pain. The supervisor instructed the transportation officer and RN to report to the scene of the stabbing as soon as the assessment was completed unless the inmate required further monitoring in the emergency department. She and the remaining nursing and security personnel then put into action the plan they had developed as a team shortly after her arrival. The two major trauma rooms and the staff were ready to receive victims of violence within minutes after the departure of the ambulance. The physician on call was on her way to the hospital to await their arrival.

The radio was crackling with orders and the relaying of information from security. The ambulance crew was unable to enter the housing unit until the violent rampage had been quelled and the drug-crazed inmate had been subdued by the E-squad, officers who received continuous training in confronting violence within the prison and searching for escaped felons. She could hear and feel the palpable fear and chaos; the number of victims could not be immediately determined and could not be reached because the perpetrator wielded a homemade knife, daring the officers to come near him or the victims. She had never been so close to violence. The ambulance crew described the horror of the scene to her as they arrived with the first victim removed from the unit: a young male with multiple stab wounds to the chest. A second physician was called for assistance because two other victims were reportedly arriving. She and the physician worked quickly to start IVs, insert chest tubes, and stabilize the first victim for transport to a hospital intensive care unit 30 miles away. The second victim arrived with cardiopulmonary resuscitation (CPR) in progress; he had been stabbed in the back repeatedly, then literally picked up and flipped over and stabbed in the face, chest, and abdomen. Each time his chest was compressed, blood gushed from the multiple wounds, which totaled more than 50. After a grueling hour, the inmate, in his early twenties, was pronounced dead. She had never seen so much blood. Linens were soaked with the warm, moist liquid that continued to drip from the sides of the stretcher on which the inmate lay, and one could not avoid the pools of blood on the floor.

She silently wondered what could provoke such a hideous act of violence. She choked back the tears of anger, fear, and bewilderment. There were no family or friends to mourn or

CHAPTER 22 Violence and Nursing's Response

to console, since the family would be notified by phone. Her past experiences and education had not prepared her for the little value placed on life within prison and the potential for raw violence within human beings. She gently covered him with a clean sheet as she remembered her husband's frequent rebuttal to her complaints about late-night phone calls from inmates' parents: Everybody here is some mother's baby.

She entered the corridor and knew the pounding of her heart could be heard over the din of the animated conversations between officers and healthcare personnel. She managed to assign staff to transport the first victim to the hospital and to prepare the body of the deceased victim for the funeral home before she retreated into the quiet conference room. She could not control the violent shaking of her entire body or the feeling of revulsion that manifested as an overwhelming nausea. She knew what she had to do; but for the first time since she had become a nurse, she doubted her ability to be nonjudgmental. How could she provide care for someone who had committed such a senseless act of violence? The respect for the individuality of patients and human worth had been the foundation of her 20-year nursing career; yet, for the first time, she questioned her own ability to follow these beliefs. She also had to confront her paralyzing fear for the safety of her family as well as her own safety in her world of nursing. Finally she was able to leave the conference room and enter the noisy clinical area. Still shaking, she took a deep breath and picked up the chart of the next patient to be assessed: the inmate who had stabbed the first two patients and had brought violence into her world that night.

---

## APPENDIX B
# Letter to the Newspaper Editor from Concerned Community Faculty

If a woman gets murdered in Louisiana and nobody hears her cries for help, is there sound? The silence in this city is deafening. Last week the *Times Picayune* published statistics that screamed out the fact that Louisiana was the most dangerous place for women to live, as only Alaska had a greater number of deaths of women at the hands of men. Despite this outrageous fact, the noise in the city was the usual traffic, garnished with the morning DJ's encouraging young girls on cell phones, on their way to school, to ponder the question of whether they would trap a man with pregnancy if the price were right. Condemning such "trifling ho's" on the air, the morning show echoed a culture where no moral lines are drawn and no topic taboo, if a laugh can be had. If you listened closely, you could hear the women talk about the "wife beater" their boyfriend wore to the mall. How did abuse become so inevitable, that we have named clothing after a false stereotype of perpetrator clothing?

Last night, he stood staring at some half-naked girl trying to imitate the Hollywood stars. He told nobody in particular, "I'd like to hit that," to suggest his sexual intentions, if not forewarn of his already-learned interpersonal techniques of power and control.

Bombarded by commercials that suggest that consequences don't apply to them, our "what happens in Vegas, stays in Vegas" generation feels immune to STDs, pregnancies, and heartache, as they buy into the belief that sexualized behavior is a rite of passage. A world of *Girls Gone Wild* followed by women found dead. The majority are not found dead by the frightening hand of a serial killer, but a trusted known hand of an intimate, someone dropping red flags all over their dating landscape.

Are we blind and deaf? The warning signs of potential violence, such as isolating a partner and jealousy, cannot be articulated with ease by those most at risk. Why are we failing to counter the "anything goes" propaganda with nurturing protective facts? The number one date rape drug is alcohol. Verbal abuse can be more devastating than physical abuse. No one deserves to be emotionally, sexually, or physically abused. You cannot defend yourself from something you do not recognize. We are the worst state in the continental United States at preventing interpersonal violence. We value driver's education but spend no time teaching anger management and interpersonal skills. We *could* equip a generation to withstand the music, media, and history of abuse that surrounds them. Where is the outrage over the direction we are going? Am I the only one bothered by the silence?

—Anne Troy, RN, LNC, SANE

## CHAPTER 23

# Chronic Illness

Edith Hilton, Kristin Ramsey, and Linda Morris

Visit **http://nursing.jbpub.com/communityhealth** for interactive exercises, review questions, Web links, and more.

Chronic illness has become one of the most important issues within our health-care system in the twenty-first century. With the population of the United States growing older, combined with advances in care, more people are living longer with chronic conditions. Nurses must understand all related implications of this trend.

When suffering knocks at your door and you say there is no seat for him, he tells you not to worry because he has brought his own.

—*Chinualumogu Achebe, Nigerian author and scholar, 1964*

For illness runs like a thread through every life; in some it is a thin gossamer, barely discernable filament; in others it is like a heavy line which, as it grows with time, loops, bends, and strangles.

—*Goldfarb, 1976*

How do these quotes connect suffering and chronic illness? We often associate chronic illness with advanced age, but as you will see in this chapter, many people have chronic conditions that occur early in life. As you read this chapter, think about what it means for a patient to have an "illness for life."

## CHAPTER FOCUS

**Chronic Illness in the United States**

**Caregivers for Individuals with Chronic Conditions**
- Prevention Measures

**Vulnerable Populations**
- Disability
- Disability versus Chronic Illness
- Experiences of Chronic Illness

**Caring for Persons with Long-Term Health Problems**

**Quality of Life in Disability and Chronic Illness**

**The Chronic Care Model**

**Roles for Community Health Nurses**
- Change Agent
- Advocate
- Professional Caregiver

**Role Models**
- Interdisciplinary Roles and Responsibilities

**Financing Costs of Chronic Illness**

**Self-Determination: The Patient as Partner**

**Sensitivity in Community-Based Caring**
- Gender-Specific Considerations

**Issues Community Health Nurses Encounter**
- Supporting Community-Based Caregivers
- The Advanced Practice Nurse with a Community Health Focus
- Palliative and Hospice Care
- Institutionalization
- Health Promotion in Chronic Illness and Disability

**The Future Role of Community Health in Chronic Illness and Disability**

## QUESTIONS TO CONSIDER

After reading this chapter, you will know the answers to the following questions:

1. What are the reasons for the increase in chronic illness in the United States?

2. Which population groups are most vulnerable in regard to chronic illness?

3. How do chronic illness and disability differ?

4. How do the concepts of paradox and loss relate to the experience of chronic illness?

5. What are current and future roles of the community health nurse in caring for persons with chronic illness?

6. How does the financing of chronic illness affect persons with chronic illness?

7. What are specific challenges in caring for diverse groups with chronic illness?

8. How are the health issues of caregivers of the chronically ill related to nursing management?

9. What is hospice care?

10. What role do institutions play in the management of chronically ill individuals?

## KEY TERMS

| | | | |
|---|---|---|---|
| Chronic care model | Congregate housing | Handicap | Power |
| Chronic illness | Disability | Impairment | Sick role |
| Chronic sorrow | Geriatric depression | | |

CHRONIC ILLNESS IS ONE of the present day's most pressing challenges. In 2005, 133 million people, almost half of all Americans, lived with at least one chronic illness. Chronic disease accounts for 70% of all deaths in the United States (CDC, 2008a). As our society ages and the number of individuals with chronic illness increases, growing demands on existing healthcare infrastructures and resources will challenge long-standing values that have been shifting during the past century. The magnitude of human suffering that chronic illness and disability cause is difficult to grasp or describe. Because of the complexity of the experiential component of living with an incurable state or condition, and because recent medical and technological advances have extended the life expectancy of many persons with these conditions, research into chronic illness and disability is drawing broader interest. In the past decade, there has been an upsurge in interdisciplinary research focused on quality of life. Much attention is currently directed at improving the life quality of individuals with chronic conditions and helping others to modify current health practices that contribute to the onset of chronic illness and disability. Once these conditions develop, they require daily self-care and management (ICIC, 2008). The number of individuals with chronic conditions and disability is projected to increase substantially during the next five decades.

More than 50 years ago, chronic illness was identified as the major challenge of the era (Mayo, 1956). Now, at the beginning of the twenty-first century, new challenges are confronting society and community health nurses. In great measure, new immigration patterns, sophisticated emerging technological applications, utilization of increasingly scarce healthcare resources, and increases in healthcare knowledge are all affecting the outcomes of those with chronic illness and disability. Increased public awareness of and interest in quality-of-life research provide affected individuals with reference points wherein they can make informed decisions about treatment options that reflect their experiences as both patient and consumer.

Changing societal expectations of chronic illnesses and disability have provided the impetus for the broad expansion of community health nursing services during the past decade. Since 2000, new populations have developed from survivor groups—that is, groups comprising those who lived through previously untreatable illnesses. The driving forces for this change include social, technological, economic, political, and environmental factors (Wilson & Satterfield, 2007). The prevalence of chronic illness will only increase as the population ages. In response to the Americans with Disabilities Act (ADA), the American public has fewer reservations and clearer expectations about chronically ill or disabled individuals remaining at or returning to employment, given that the ability to manage symptoms associated with chronic processes improves constantly. Disease management including "broad, long-term approaches that encompass a diverse array of programs and services designed to promote the well-being of individuals, families, and communities" is a clearly articulated goal in 18 states (Klein, Cruz, O'Donnell, Scully, & Birkhead, 2005).

One example of this emerging trend is HIV and AIDS, which are now considered chronic diseases. Health departments are intensely involved in prevention efforts aimed at limiting the spread of HIV and AIDS; they are also involved in extensive management of human services including hospice care, nursing homes, AIDS adult day care, and home health care for those affected by HIV/AIDS (Klein et al., 2005). Currently, the public's concern about HIV/AIDS is falling due in part to the powerful multi-drug regimens of antiretroviral therapies (Jaffe, 2004). Disease management is increasingly important to community health nurses who are focusing their efforts on outcomes, maintenance, and reinforcing the importance of individuals knowing their HIV status.

Local and global efforts to address preventive, acute, and chronic health problems are facing increasing scrutiny from many quarters. Old ways of thinking are being discarded, while more workable solutions to conditions not previously identified are increasingly sought. Researchers from various continents face both similar and different issues that urgently demand their attention, consideration, and resolution. Old, unresolved health problems such as malnutrition, contagious diseases such as tuberculosis and pertussis, and newer diseases including severe acute respiratory syndrome (SARS) pose challenges for globally scattered populations as well as those found locally. Paradoxically, existing travel has opened the world to far-reaching advances and has fostered information sharing but, because of numerous sources of contagion worldwide, has catapulted the traveling public into harm's way.

When considering the present and future health needs of the public, chronic diseases are of utmost importance. Many stem from acute processes, others from lifestyle choices, and still others from genetic disorders or entrenched poverty, both in the United States and globally. Nurses working in the community are in prime positions to positively affect the quality of life of those whom they serve. Nurses working in the local and global communities must be aware of problems whose solutions lie within the environment and existing systems. They must also be aware of their important role as advocates for the nation's health and equip themselves with reliable information and critical thinking abilities. To

---

■■ CULTURAL CONNECTION

Cultural differences exist regarding the family's role in managing chronic disease. For example, some Native American tribes seek the authority of the tribal healer prior to using Western medications or interventions. The community health nurse should determine how these influences will affect the patient's management of his or her chronic disease based on the totality of the patient's life and family.

identify barriers to change that affect access to health care and disparities within and among various racial, ethnic, gender, and age-specific groups, community health nurses must think in different ways and seek new solutions to persistent problems.

This chapter considers chronic illness and disability with a global lens that highlights individuals and groups for the purpose of improving health and health care and identifying areas of future research. Roles and activities of community health nurses are explored in this context as well.

> **ff** *The world is full of suffering. Birth is suffering, decrepitude is suffering, sickness and death are sufferings. To face a man of hatred is suffering, to be separated from a beloved one is suffering, to be vainly struggling to satisfy one's needs is suffering. In fact, life that is not free from desire and passion is always involved with suffering.* **JJ**
>
> —Buddha

## Chronic Illness in the United States

Chronic diseases form the cornerstone of anticipated healthcare needs for this century. Until prevention becomes universally accepted and incorporated into the daily practices of all, nursing practice in the community will continue to involve caring for those in whom chronic diseases developed from unresolved acute processes. The health burden of chronic disease is staggering (see Table 23-1), not only in physical and emotional loss, but also in its economic costs. Chronic diseases account for more than three-fourths of all healthcare expenditures, or in excess of $1 trillion annually.

Chronic diseases have replaced many of the devastating epidemics of the eighteenth, nineteenth, and twentieth centuries. Because contagion and disease transmission routes and vectors for many illnesses are known, the mystery of their occurrence is diminished. However, epidemics persist; tropical, viral, bacterial, and parasitic infections continue to affect destitute populations in poorly developed countries. Worldwide, HIV/AIDS, malaria, and tuberculosis are acknowledged as paramount health concerns and have been aggressively attacked on many fronts with sustained efforts (Molyneux, 2004). SARS, which has killed more than 800 people in 30 countries, and bird flu, which has affected 10 Asian nations, demonstrate that health emergencies may arise without warning (Manila Times, 2004). Most of these conditions produce chronic illness or disabled states after the acute phase is past, so the long-term consequences of present-day contagion are enduringly evident and, in many cases, catastrophic.

### ■■ CULTURAL CONNECTION

A patient's culture and meaning of pain can influence the management of chronic illness. Think of how different cultures express pain or discomfort and how these variations will affect the community health nurse's interventions. ◉

### ☞ THINK ABOUT THIS

Migraine headaches affect an estimated 6 million Americans and are believed to afflict from 5% to 10% of the world's population. The Greek physician Hippocrates (460–357 B.C.) described the pains of a migraine episode. Pliny the Elder (A.D. 23–79), the Roman medical writer, refers to the symptoms we now know as migraine. The term *migraine* is originally derived from the Greek word *hemicrania,* which means "half of the head." The head pains of migraine are attributed to biochemical changes causing nausea, vomiting, irritability, visual impairment, and unsteady gait.

Millions of dollars are wasted and needless suffering is experienced by patients who are misdiagnosed or who resort to jaw reconstruction, neck surgery, hormonal manipulation, and sinus surgery in an effort to "cure" the migraine headache. Too often migraine headaches are lumped together with other forms of head pain. Also, patients often seek relief from nontraditional forms of intervention.

Migraine headaches are often labeled as psychological disorders; in actuality, they are the result of a chronic condition that can be controlled and effectively treated when considered the result of a chronic neurological disorder, influenced by hereditary factors, hormones, and particular "trigger" influences in diet and the environment. Although migraine is one of the most painful and frustrating disorders known, it is relatively benign and not life-threatening. Most migraineurs (migraine sufferers) function well even while the symptoms are coming on. Not until they are overcome by the fatigue, head pain, and nausea do they become functionally "disabled."

Effective prevention and early intervention, non-narcotic treatments are available now that allow the migraine sufferer to live a normal life. Complementary and self-care environmental management focusing on a holistic approach to migraine prevention offers the best control for this debilitating chronic condition.

Among those who have been tormented by the disorder in history are Joan of Arc, Charles Darwin, Sigmund Freud, Thomas Jefferson, Frederic Chopin, Saint Paul, Julius Caesar, Immanuel Kant, Lewis Carroll, Ulysses S. Grant, Edgar Allan Poe, Leo Tolstoy, Lewis Carroll, Charles Dickens, Virginia Woolf, and Peter Ilich Tchaikovsky. More contemporary personalities with this problem include Whoopi Goldberg, Star Jones, Lisa Kudrow, Carly Simon, Loretta Lynn, Scotty Pippin, and Kareem Abdul-Jabbar. ◉

Other global challenges including hunger, weather-related phenomena such as devastating hurricanes and earthquakes, military conflicts in many regions of the Middle East and Africa, disease control, education, financial instability in underdeveloped countries, widespread corruption within the global business community, migration, trade barriers, and access to water are putting pressures on the resources of both communities and the world as a whole. Domestic violence, also a widespread phenomenon, is so prevalent in the United States that its burden exceeds the toll

| Table 23-1 | Quick Facts: Economic and Health Burden of Chronic Disease | | |
| --- | --- | --- | --- |
| **Disease/Risk Factors** | **Morbidity (Illness)** | **Mortality (Death)** | **Direct Cost/Indirect Cost** |
| ■ Arthritis | Arthritis affects 1 in 5, or 26 million adults, making it one of the most common chronic conditions. Over 40% of (nearly 19 million) adults with arthritis are limited in their activities because of their arthritis. By 2030, nearly 67 million (25%) of U.S. adults will have doctor-diagnosed arthritis. In addition, adults with arthritis-attributed activity limitations are projected to increase from 16.9 million (7.9%) to 25 million (9.3% of the U.S. adult population). | From 1979–1998, the annual number of arthritis and other related rheumatic conditions (AORC) deaths rose from 5,537 to 9,367. In 1998, the crude death rate from AORC was 3.48 per 100,000 population. | The total costs attributable to arthritis and other rheumatic conditions (AORC) in the United States was approximately $128 billion ($80.8 billion in medical care and $47 billion in earnings losses). This equaled 1.2% of the 2003 U.S. gross domestic product. |
| ■ Cancer | About 1.3 million people in the United States are diagnosed with cancer each year. | Cancer is the second leading cause of death in the United States. In 2004, an estimated 553,000 people died of cancer. | NIH estimates that the overall costs for cancer in the year 2007 at $219 billion: of this amount, $89 billion for direct medical costs and $130 billion for indirect costs such as lost productivity. |
| ■ Diabetes | More than 2.8 million Americans have diabetes, and about 6.2 million don't know that they have the disease. | Diabetes is the sixth leading cause of death. Over 200,000 people die each year of diabetes-related complications. | The estimated economic cost of diabetes in 2007 was $174 billion. Of this amount, $116 billion was due to direct medical costs and $58 billion to indirect costs such as lost workdays, restricted activity, and disability. |
| ■ Heart Disease and Stroke | More than 80 million Americans currently live with a cardiovascular disease. | More than 870,000 Americans die of heart disease and stroke each year, which is about 2,400 people dying every day. | The cost of heart disease and stroke in the United States in 2008 was more than $440 billion, including direct and indirect costs. |
| ■ Overweight/Obesity | In 2005–2006 more than 34% of adults aged 20 years or older were obese. Over 125 million or 17.1% of children and adolescents 2–19 years of age were overweight. | A recent study from CDC scientists estimated that about 112,000 deaths are associated with obesity each year in the United States. | Direct health costs attributable to obesity were estimated at $52 billion in 1995 and $75 billion in 2003. Among children and adolescents, annual hospital costs related to overweight and obesity more than tripled in 20 years. |
| ■ Tobacco | An estimated 45.3 million adults in the United States smoke cigarettes even though this single behavior will result in death or disability for all regular users. | Tobacco use is responsible for approximately 483,000 deaths each year. | The economic burden of tobacco use is enormous: more than $96 billion in medical expenditures and another $97 billion in indirect costs. |

*Source*: CDC, 2008. http://www.cdc.gov/print.do?url=http://cdc.gov/nccdphp/press/

of some epidemics caused by contagion and adversely affects 1.5 million individuals (mostly women) annually (Sorenson & Wiebe, 2004).

Individuals with chronic illnesses whose lives are affected by these overarching issues may find fewer resources available to them to address their health problems and to provide preventive care aimed at increasing their life span and quality of life. It is increasingly important that community health nurses become involved in future planning for management of chronic illness care so they are able to advocate for those affected by changing local and global resource allocation. Age has long been recognized as a source of stigma in health care. The aged, chronically ill, or disabled are frequently unwelcome consumers in the current healthcare system, which has been designed around the episodic, acute care needs of middle-aged and younger persons. In many cases, caring for these individuals has been relegated to the least experienced, least educated, and, occasionally, least desirable segments of the healthcare community. Historically, those who focused their nursing activities in geriatrics,

## Research Alert

Many home health agencies are actively recruiting new home health nurses while trying to retain qualified home health nurses. According to a survey of home health administrators, 82% of them reported difficulty attracting nurses, and 63% reported difficulty retaining nurses. Due to rising healthcare costs and the desire of patients and families to receive care in their home environment, more and more healthcare is being provided outside the typical acute care setting. Because of the unique demands of the home healthcare setting, nurses must have a strong clinical background, usually with at least one year of acute care experience. Home care nurses need a wide variety of clinical and technical skills to provide care safely in a patient's home. Nurses with a high degree of self-efficacy and varied clinical experience tend to be more successful and satisfied in home care positions. Nurse autonomy and control over the practice environment are two factors attracting and retaining home care nurses. Nurses go into community health nursing (CHN) because of the level of the independence and autonomy that CHNs have in their career, and because of the flexibility associated with the community setting.

Although healthcare delivery is moving away from institutions toward a variety of community settings, nursing education continues to concentrate on acute care settings, and most prelicensure BSN students do not perceive themselves as pursuing a career in community or public health nursing.

In one study, students' attitudes changed somewhat after they had a positive clinical experience in CHN, although CHN did not rank as the students' first choice for a career in nursing. This may have been due to the students' awareness that nurses are required to have at least one year of experience before being employed in community health nursing.

*Source:* Prestia, Mindy (2008). Nursing students' attitudes about home health nursing. *Home Healthcare Nurse, 20*(0), 496.

---

## BOX 23-1

### Janet Reno: A Public Experience with Parkinson's Disease

From 1993–2001, Janet Reno served as the Attorney General, the United States' top law enforcer, with the longest tenure in the history of the office. Since 1995, she has also lived with Parkinson's disease, with little self-acknowledgment of the affects it had on her demanding professional role as U.S. Attorney General. Reno made no effort to hide her tremors and continued to embrace her responsibility with the same vigor and tenacity. By being public with a disease that has in the past been hidden and restrictive, she moved forward for all persons who have such a chronic illness.

rehabilitation, or hospice were cast in an unfavorable light (Lubkin & Larsen, 2002). However, aging baby boomers and their predicted healthcare needs are bringing these nursing specialty areas to the forefront.

## ENVIRONMENTAL CONNECTION

Long-term care facilities provide essential services to some chronically ill persons. Injuries and the resulting increased morbidity and mortality from falls are among the greatest environmental risks for residents of these facilities. In recent years, the use of physical restraints in such settings has decreased; these measures led to undesirable results such as reduced mobility, inhibited communication, and prevention of socialization. With increased availability of technology, such as cameras, alarm systems, movement sensors, and staff surveillance, the safety of residents has been enhanced while patient autonomy is preserved.

Ethnic and racial disparities in health constitute a persistent and formidable challenge to those in the United States with chronic illnesses and disability. Cardiovascular disease, in particular, is problematic in this regard. Despite the fact that it is the most frequent killer worldwide, this disease affects some groups more frequently than others. Rates of death from diseases of the heart are 30% higher among African Americans than among whites, and mortality resulting from stroke is 41% higher in African Americans (National Center for Chronic Disease Prevention and Health Promotion, 2008). It is well recognized that the proportion of African Americans who are hypertensive exceeds the proportions of other population groups with high blood pressure (Peters, 2004). Diabetes disproportionately affects American Indians and Alaska Natives, who develop this disease 2.3 times more frequently than do whites. African Americans experience diabetes 1.6 times more frequently than whites, and Hispanic Americans are 1.5 times more likely to have diagnosed diabetes. HIV/AIDS disproportionately affects these groups, which account for 75% of both AIDS and new HIV infections among U.S. adults and 62% of all people living with HIV/AIDS in the United States. Rates of pediatric AIDS cases are similarly disproportionate in the United States, with such cases being composed of 82% minority individuals.

Activities aimed at eliminating the health-related gap between racial and ethnic groups represent tests of the effectiveness of programs under the umbrella Racial and Ethnic Approaches to Community Health (REACH) project. This important initiative of the Centers for Disease Control and Prevention (CDC) is designed to eliminate disparities in health and represents new and innovative partnerships among government, business, faith-based organizations, and communities. Examples of the programs supported by REACH include those targeting cervical cancer screening among Asian Americans and those targeting cardiovascular disease among African Americans.

We have learned a great deal about infectious disease epidemics globally during the past two centuries. The burden of chronic illness has been less well documented, because large numbers of those persons with acute diseases perished before their diseases became chronic. During the nineteenth century, immigration from Europe taxed sanitation and housing resources in many East Coast cities in the United

States. With repeated epidemics, poor health conditions among established and relocated populations dwindled. Chronic conditions such as heart disease, diabetes, neurological problems, and blood disorders are identified in literature of that time. Because drugs and therapeutic regimens were scarce, overall survival rates for these diseases were poor in those eras, especially in vulnerable populations.

Major inroads into treatment, management, and prevention were made worldwide during the twentieth century. Because of improved sanitation, widespread use of antibiotics and technology, rapid advances in research and communication, and comprehensive, nurse-driven health initiatives and education, the standard of living for many Americans has improved. However, these relatively recent developments have fostered trends of developing chronic illnesses that have become more prevalent in the twenty-first century in the United States.

An example of this trend can be seen with chronic renal failure. Until dialysis became available in the 1960s, renal failure was essentially untreatable and, therefore, fatal. Dialysis is now a common intervention for both acute and chronic phases of treatment. Additionally, organ transplantation is now considered a routine surgical procedure aimed at restoring renal function and improving the associated quality of life. Because of improved medical and postoperative management, renal transplantation now may avoid steroid-induced immunosuppression and reduce postoperative healing time through use of minimally invasive laproscopic procedures (Powelson, 2005). This consideration is especially important to community health nurses, because they are often involved with encouraging follow-up appointments and monitoring patients who experience uremic symptoms. Chronic renal insufficiency may present early in the disease trajectory with symptoms of sleep disturbance, muscle spasms/stiffness, excessive fatigue, and bone pain in addition to altered lab values (Pugh-Clarke, 2004). In this predialysis phase, patients often report that the intrusiveness of disease symptoms adversely affects their quality of life.

Another example of the development of a chronic condition from a formerly fatal condition is HIV/AIDS. Initially, few patients survived the opportunistic invaders that manifested with disease progression. Although it is still an extremely serious condition, HIV/AIDS is no longer synonymous with rapid progression, unmitigated suffering, and certain death (Mitchell & Linsk, 2004).

 THINK ABOUT THIS ·········································

> The truth is, if you asked me to choose between winning the Tour de France and cancer, odd as it sounds, I would rather have the title of cancer survivor because of what it has done for me as a human being, a man, a husband.
>
> —Lance Armstrong

Many infected individuals now survive for years with HIV and AIDS thanks to newly formulated medications and combination antiretroviral drug regimens. They are living highly productive and satisfying lives for many years. With effective prophylaxis and treatment, many are able to return to their jobs on a full-time basis and remain largely self-sufficient and autonomous. As a chronic, long-term illness, HIV/AIDS can affect patients, families, and communities in numerous and complex ways. Understanding the context in which those individuals are living with the condition will assist community health nurses to assess and intervene by supporting their initiation of medical treatment, suggesting coping strategies, and teaching and reinforcing understanding of the complex and challenging medical regimen.

## Caregivers for Individuals with Chronic Conditions

Because increasing numbers of those with chronic illness and disability remain in community-based care settings, including their homes, swelling numbers of caregivers—many of them unpaid family members—face a new role for which they are poorly prepared. In particular, caregivers for those with neurological impairments, including Parkinson's disease, multiple sclerosis, neuropathy, spinal

### 🖥 Research Alert

Chronically ill persons in communities may include those with chemical dependency, chronic mental illness, tuberculosis, and hepatitis C. Stable chronic conditions, affecting as many as 30% of the U.S. adult population, include cardiovascular disease, neurological diseases including Alzheimer's disease, some slow-developing forms of cancer, emphysema, diabetes, fetal alcohol syndrome, learning disability, adjustment disorders, genetically linked diseases including Down syndrome (trisomy 18 and 21), sickle cell disease, cystic fibrosis, Tay-Sachs, and schizophrenia. New medications are enabling individuals with these and other chronic diseases to live longer than ever before. Many chronically ill individuals remain in community settings and depend on others to render all or part of their physical and/or mental care. Despite our attention to the acute outbreak of SARS, the continuing threat of bioterrorism, and the effect of the war in Iraq, the most costly health problems in the United States are still the result of chronic diseases. We have come a long way, yet sadly, we also have not gone far. Attacking the problem of chronic illness in the United States presents us with a set of challenges that is complex and difficult to disentangle, especially when we focus on improving outcomes for populations. Chronic health problems provide ample opportunity to engage in primary, secondary, and tertiary preventive measures that use our nursing strengths.

*Source*: Abrams, S.E. (2003). Chronic illness: "Chronic" boredom. *Public Health Nursing, 20*(4), 250.

cord diseases, amyotropic lateral sclerosis, cerebrovascular disease, Alzheimer's disease, and chronic pain from arthritis, osteoporosis, or back problems, may experience problems with their own health associated with caregiving activities (Hilton & Henderson, 2003). Osteoporosis, in particular, is of great concern because the volume of cases is increasing at an astonishing pace; 29% of all women older than age 65 are estimated to have this painful and debilitating disease (Gelbach, Fournier, & Bigelow, 2002). This condition of bone demineralization places those affected at increased risk for vertebral, pelvic, and hip fractures. For those who are family caregivers, osteoporosis adds a component of silent deterioration that may be aggravated by the lifting, turning, bending, stooping, and walking that are inherent in many caregiving activities.

Care of individuals in the United States with the previously mentioned neurological diagnoses may include activities such as supervision, assistance with the execution of various tasks, and decision making about aspects of care (Lopes, Piementa, Kurita, & Oliveira, 2003). Caregivers for individuals with such diagnoses may feel the care they provide constitutes a burden. Because caregivers may have few or no resources to share the tasks and responsibility necessary to maintain or restore the chronically ill or disabled individual, and because caring activities may persist for an undetermined length of time, caregivers may experience fatigue, depression, emotional distress, sadness, loss of leisure activities, difficulties in their sexual activities, future planning, personal grooming, and disrupted family relationships.

Perhaps not unexpectedly, caregivers in Japan and in Brazil experience nearly identical issues while in the caregiving role, suggesting caregiver role strain is not unique to the U.S. population. Cultural differences may affect the perceived value of the caregiving role in which the individual is dependent upon a caregiver while sick, however. In the case of chronicity for an indeterminate interval, this caregiving role is recognized as essential in both Japan and Brazil. For those individuals experiencing chronic pain, caregivers may provide extensive psychological support aimed at promoting successful coping and restoring the locus of control for analgesic modalities and relaxation interventions. This type of care may be extremely taxing to caregivers because of the frequency of interventions required and because of the in-

herent discouragement that may accompany the recurrence of symptoms as the patient and the caregiver seek to establish order out of chaos (Bullington, Nordemar, Nordemar, & Sjöström-Flanagan, 2003).

The importance of family caregiver issues related to the challenging and difficult work of caring for an individual with chronic conditions cannot be overemphasized (Grey, Knaft, & McCorkle, 2006). Supports including respite care services and social workers are useful and important in providing long-term care. In caring for the caregivers, however, it is also important to recognize the nurse and his or her contributions to the therapeutic relationship (Hickey, 2003). Both conscious and unconscious responses of the community health nurse should be considered. Nurses may also experience caregiver burden if they go unrelieved in dealing with the consistent demands of care necessitated by individuals with disabilities and chronic illnesses. If possible, this problem should be anticipated and addressed by a "break" in the assignments of this population so the nurse is able to attend to his or her own self-care and spiritual renewal.

## Prevention Measures

Recent data indicate that increasing numbers of Americans believe their physical and mental health-related quality of life is deteriorating and that they are less able to engage in their usual activities (Zack, Moriarity, Stroup, Ford, & Mokdad, 2004). Given that disability and chronic illness contribute overwhelmingly to these factors, prevention and management are increasingly important to individuals and health agencies.

According to the U.S. Department of Health and Human Services (2000), chronic health conditions affect both individuals and the larger society. U.S. healthcare costs are greatly affected by chronic illness (see Table 23-2).

## Vulnerable Populations

Some populations are more likely than others to develop chronic illnesses. Chronic illnesses affect various ethnic and racial groups, and some disease processes are gender preferential. Examples of this relate to all types of cancer. Cancer incidence rates for men are highest among blacks, followed by whites, Hispanics, Asian/Pacific Islanders, and American Indian/Alaska Natives. However, the cancer incidence rates for women are highest among whites, followed by blacks, Hispanics, Asian/Pacific Islanders, and American Indian/Alaska Natives. Cancer death rates for men are highest among blacks, followed by whites, Hispanics, American/Indians/Alaska Natives, and Asian/Pacific Islanders. Among women, the cancer death rates are highest among blacks, followed by whites, American Indian/Alaska Natives, Hispanics, and Asian/Pacific Islanders. Cancer incidence rates and cancer death rates do not match according to gender and ethnicity. American Indian/Alaska Native men have the lowest incidence rates of cancer; however, Asian/Pacific Islander men have the lowest death rates. White women have

**Table 23-2** Costs of Chronic Disease

The United States cannot effectively address escalating healthcare costs without addressing the problem of chronic diseases:

- In 2005, 133 million people—almost half of all Americans—lived with at least one chronic condition.
- Chronic diseases account for 70% of all deaths in the United States.
- The medical care costs of people with chronic diseases account for more than 75% of the nation's $2 trillion medical care costs.
- Chronic diseases account for one-third of the years of potential life lost before age 65.
- Hospitalizations for pregnancy-related complications occurring before delivery account for more than $1 billion annually.
- The direct and indirect costs of diabetes is $174 billion a year.
- Each year, arthritis results in estimated medical care costs of nearly $81 billion, and estimated total costs (medical care and lost productivity) of $128 billion.
- The estimated direct and indirect costs associated with smoking exceed $193 billion annually.
- In 2008, the cost of heart disease and stroke in the U.S. is projected to be $448 billion.
- The estimated total cost of obesity was nearly $117 billion in 2000.
- Cancer costs the nation an estimated $89 billion annually in direct medical costs.
- Nearly $98.6 billion is spent on dental services each year.

*Source*: CDC, 2008.

 MEDIA MOMENT

**Lorenzo's Oil (1992)**

Lorenzo's Oil is a true story, based on the struggles of parents to find a cure for their young child's terminal illness. Not satisfied with modern medicine, they research the disease and turn to a controversial remedy for help. The parents' actions illustrate the very different ways in which people respond to chronic illness: Lorenzo's mother (played by Susan Sarandon) reacts with an obsessive, laser-like focus on his daily care, firing caregivers and managing his environment with the skill of a CEO; Lorenzo's father (played by Nick Nolte) approaches his son's illness with his scientific objectivity, focusing his time and passion on understanding the etiology of the illness, creating a method that systematically controls the deadly symptoms. This movie is an excellent look at the various ways that families and society as a whole respond to diseases without cures, those that the medical establishment chooses to treat only symptomatically.

the highest incidence rates of cancer; however, black women have the highest death rates. American Indian/Alaska Native women have the lowest incidence rates of cancer and the third highest death rates (U.S. Cancer Statistics Working Group, 2007). Population-specific vulnerability is especially important to consider when projecting needs for development of community resources.

Because of their limited defense mechanisms, such as diminished, or slowed, reflexes, people with chronic illness are more susceptible to environmental sources of pollution. The destruction of the World Trade Center on September 11, 2001, created the largest acute environmental disaster that ever has befallen New York (Landrigan et al., 2004). In addition to experiencing severe post-traumatic stress disorder, those individuals with asthma and emphysema living in the area most closely affected by the buildings' collapse experienced exposure-related exacerbations of their diseases.

## ■ Disability

The composition of disability is intricate. It is embedded in societal values of mind–body functioning that separate mental and physical impairments (Imrie, 2004). According to Kaplan (2008), disability policy scholars identify four distinctive social and historical models of disability: a moral model that regards disability as the result of sin; a medical model that considers disability as a sickness or defect that must

be cured; a rehabilitation model that regards disability as a deficiency that must be fixed; and the disability model under which the problem is defined as a dominating attitude toward the person with a disability by professionals and others.

The World Health Organization's International Classification of Functioning, Disability, and Health (2001) employs performance-based contexts as a vehicle for delimiting disabilities based on individual attributes and societal values ascribed to limitations. The WHO defines **disability** as any restriction or lack (resulting from an impairment) of ability to perform an activity in the manner or within the range considered normal for a human being. **Impairment** is defined as any loss or abnormality of psychological or anatomical structure or function; **handicap** is defined as a disadvantage for a given individual, resulting from an impairment or disability that limits or prevents the fulfillment of a role that is normal, depending on age, sex, social and cultural factors, for that individual (WHO, 2001).

The original purpose of the Americans with Disabilities Act was to protect individuals from discrimination. Current thinking reflects a trend in public policy to regard disability as a functional status, not a list of physical impairments. Unfortunately, stigmatization and stereotyping accompany the delineation of disabled, so many choose not to identify themselves as disabled (Kaplan, 2008). Disability is viewed

ETHICAL CONNECTION

Chronic illness is not typically a focus of public health services in a community. This bias may result in persons with chronic illnesses having few resources for drug and medical expenses. Why do you think chronic illness has not typically been considered a public health "problem" until very recently?

**Objectives Related to Chronic Illness**

## Access to Quality Health Services

### Primary Care
1.9 Reduce hospitalization rates for three ambulatory care–sensitive conditions—pediatric asthma, uncontrolled diabetes, and immunization-preventable pneumonia and influenza in older adults.

### Long-Term Care and Rehabilitative Services
1.15 Increase the proportion of persons with long-term care needs who have access to the continuum of long-term care services.

## Arthritis, Osteoporosis, and Chronic Back Conditions

### Arthritis and Other Rheumatic Conditions
2.1 Increase the mean number of days without severe pain among adults who have chronic joint symptoms.

2.2 Reduce the proportion of adults with chronic joint symptoms who experience a limitation in activity due to arthritis.

2.5 Increase the employment rate among adults with arthritis in the working-age population.

2.7 Increase the proportion of adults who have seen a health care provider for their chronic joint symptoms.

### Osteoporosis
2.9 Reduce the overall number of cases of osteoporosis.

2.10 Reduce the proportion of adults who are hospitalized for vertebral fractures associated with osteoporosis.

### Chronic Back Conditions
2.11 Reduce activity limitation due to chronic back conditions.

## Cancer
3.15 Increase the proportion of cancer survivors who are living 5 years or longer after diagnosis.

## Chronic Kidney Disease
4.1 Reduce the rate of new cases of end-stage renal disease (ESRD).

4.3 Increase the proportion of treated chronic kidney failure patients who have received counseling on nutrition, treatment choices, and cardiovascular care 12 months before the start of renal replacement therapy.

4.7 Reduce kidney failure due to diabetes.

## Diabetes
5.1 Increase the proportion of persons with diabetes who receive formal diabetes education.

5.2 Prevent diabetes.

5.3 Reduce the overall rate of diabetes that is clinically diagnosed.

## Heart Disease and Stroke

### Blood Pressure
12.9 Reduce the proportion of adults with high blood pressure.

12.10 Increase the proportion of adults with high blood pressure whose blood pressure is under control.

### Cholesterol
12.13 Reduce the mean total blood cholesterol levels among adults.

12.14 Reduce the proportion of adults with high total blood cholesterol levels.

## Medical Product Safety
17.3 Increase the proportion of primary care providers, pharmacists, and other health care professionals who routinely review with their patients all new prescribed and over-the-counter medicines.

## Nutrition and Overweight

### Weight Status and Growth
19.2 Reduce the proportion of adults who are obese.

19.3 Reduce the proportion of children and adolescents who are overweight or obese.

### Schools, Worksites, and Nutrition Counseling
19.7 Increase the proportion of physician office visits made by patients with a diagnosis of cardiovascular disease, diabetes, or hyperlipidemia that include counseling or education related to diet and nutrition.

## Respiratory Diseases

### Asthma
24.2 Reduce hospitalizations for asthma.

24.3 Reduce hospital emergency department visits for asthma.

24.4 Reduce activity limitations among persons with asthma.

### Chronic Obstructive Pulmonary Disease
24.9 Reduce the proportion of adults whose activity is limited due to chronic lung and breathing problems.

*Source*: DHHS, 2000.

---

by some as social prejudice, and by others as a physical condition affecting life quality (Koch, 2001). The nature of disability may be linked to social variables such as class, ethnicity, gender, and geographical location (Morgan, 1996). According to Hurst (2000), disability may be construed as "something that happens to you, not something you have."

As defined in 1956 by the Commission on Chronic Illness (cited in Strauss, 1975), impairments or deviations from normal have one or more of the following characteristics: (1) are permanent; (2) leave residual disability; (3) are caused by nonreversible pathological alterations; (4) require special training of the patient for rehabilitation; and (5) may be expected to require a long period of supervision, observation, or care. In addition to chronic illness, multiple chronic conditions in the same person are frequently noted (Strauss, 1975). For example, diabetes may affect nerve tissue, causing damage to sensory nerve pathways; leading to diabetic-induced visual loss from retinal disease; and coexisting with hypertension.

Acute illness is defined as a disease (or process) with a sudden, dynamic onset with signs and symptoms related to the disease process itself, which either resolves shortly with complete recovery or results in death. Differences between acute and chronic illness are notable in terms of their treatment, duration, and perceived significance. Another important difference between acute and chronic illness relates to coping abilities taxed during severe and sustained illness.

Acute and chronic illnesses also occur together. Examples of this phenomenon include asthma and diabetes, in which acute manifestations emerge from chronic problems in regulating the diseases. One challenge presented by chronic illness is that of keeping patients motivated to achieve and maintain optimal levels of health. Supporting patients' efforts to learn to manage their chronic illness requires skill, creativity, and persistence to keep each patient's entire life pattern in focus.

## ■ Disability versus Chronic Illness

Disabled individuals are generally unable to initiate or complete self-care activities alone because of physical impairments. To achieve independence or optimal levels of self-care, focused rehabilitative efforts are usually required. In some cases, rehabilitation is also useful in maintaining established progress in self-care activities. Likewise, rehabilitation is employed in conditions of disability associated with chronic health problems and degenerative diseases such as epilepsy and multiple sclerosis (Hickey, 2003).

The terms *disability* and *disabled* are not used to diminish or label persons or groups for the purpose of undermining their individual rights or freedoms; rather, they are meant only to provide a context in which needs may be addressed from a position of specificity. An example of this notion may be found in professional literature discussing and describing assistive devices and equipment that are fabricated to meet specific needs and possess specific functions (Dewsbury, Clarke, Randall, Rouncefield, & Somerville, 2004).

**Chronic illness** differs from disability in the following manner: Disability does not necessarily imply sickness or less than optimal health, whereas chronic illness is always related to a permanent decrease in health status that will not, in all likelihood, result in restoration of former or normal health status. Chronic illness is contrasted to disability in the following three examples: (1) chronic renal failure may result in chronic illness but not disability in every individual (Klang & Clyne, 1997); (2) a hip fracture may result in disability but not necessarily in chronic illness; and (3) a spinal cord injury may result in both conditions, because disability immediately develops as a consequence of spinal cord damage, and chronic illness may ensue if prolonged immobility causes development of decubitus ulcers, urinary tract infections, or muscle spasms unrelieved by medications. Disability resulting from spinal cord injury may, for example, cause numerous problems of chronic illness that relate to development of decubitus ulcers: Patients may require surgical interventions to enable healing. Because of inadequate sensory innervation, necessary position changes may be overlooked while individuals are in wheelchair-sitting positions.

Patients with chronic disability often define themselves in terms of their illness role and diagnosis. Definitions of this type may be limiting. When individuals with disabilities are viewed as striving toward higher-level wellness, they may be supported by interacting with their environment in an integrated manner, thereby promoting their personhood and emphasizing their human qualities, instead of their disabilities (Davidhizar & Shearer, 1997).

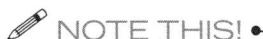

**MEDIA MOMENT**

### First, Do No Harm (1997)
Based on a true story, *First, Do No Harm* details the challenges of a mother (played by Meryl Streep) who goes to extraordinary lengths to help find a cure for her son who suffers from epilepsy. When the family's insurance runs out, the mother immerses herself in medical research and seeks alternative treatments. The film offers a critical assessment of the healthcare system and explores the lengths to which families go to find answers when health professionals no longer respond to their concerns.

✏ NOTE THIS! •————————————————

Stable, chronic conditions affect as much as 30% of the U.S. adult population.

## ■ Experiences of Chronic Illness

Chronic illness may assume many forms. Psychiatric and mental illness including dysthymia, major depression, and unipolar depression are typically considered more chronic than other forms of depression (Antai-Otong, 1995). Women's health was studied across the United States, and the results were reported in the *American Journal of Public Health* (Bromberger et al., 2004). Data indicated that 22% of middle-age women residing in the community reported clinically significant depressive symptoms. Furthermore, women who had previous depressive episodes were at increased risk for recurrences. Middle-age women were examined for racial/ethnic differences in significant depressive symptoms. The researchers reported Hispanic and African American women had the highest risk of developing severe symptoms, and Chinese and Japanese women the lowest. Contributing factors included low socioeconomic status, financial strain, physical inactivity, low social support, stress, and poor physical health. Social support is of particular importance to individuals whose chronic illness waxes and wanes, such as is seen in depression.

### Paradox and Loss

In each chronic illness, disease forms a path through lives that is not always apparent at outset and may not be clearly understood. Wellness and optimal health are subjectively described by each person experiencing those conditions, and chronic illness is best described and experienced by those living the phenomenon. A seeming contradiction associated with chronic illness is that they often present with minor or mysterious symptoms. An example of this paradox is described by a woman with chronic asthma:

> I didn't have a fever and my doctor said all my blood tests and x-rays were fine. At first my friends were sympathetic, but then they began asking whether I was really taking care of myself. Even my doctor seemed exasperated, and so I began to think I was crazy and had made all this up. Little did I know when this happened two years ago that I was heading for chronic asthma. My asthma finally got so bad that I had to stop teaching. (Wilson, 1992, p. 42)

Paradox is present in many chronic disease processes and contributes to feelings of loss, fear, and frustration. Johnson (1991, p. 33) explains the paradoxical nature of myocardial infarction:

> The signs and symptoms of a heart attack often begin insidiously and escalate over a period of hours. Heart attacks have a paradoxical nature. Although potentially fatal, the early signs of a heart attack mimic minor and trivial complaints. Unless the heart attack is extensive, the early symptoms may be interpreted as indigestion, the flu, a pulled muscle, or food poisoning. The irony of delaying treatment is caused in part by the mixed messages given to the public. On the one hand, the signs and symptoms of heart attack are well publicized because it is assumed that people will . . . seek help early. On the other hand, people are reluctant to go to the hospital emergency room or "bother" their physicians with seemingly minor complaints.

Losses may be the first awareness of chronic disease processes "taking hold." Fear of loss sets in quickly, and is accompanied by awareness and understanding of chronic disease processes (Schaefer, 1995). Losses associated with chronic illness may include fear, social status, self-concept, self-esteem, role, family support, recognition by the healthcare community, and loss of independence related to financial and personal issues. Losses may also relate to insufficiency of status or stigmatization by feelings of imperfection; by being different, some feel as though they fall short of cultural norms relating to identity (Scambler, 2004).

This perception of loss is especially important in hidden conditions in which no visual validation is apparent. The paradox of lived disability that presents with no outward signs may compel the individual to conceal the disabling condition in an effort to preserve social acceptance. Secondary gains may enhance the "invisible" sick role such as that seen in diabetes, in which marginal control of blood glucose may prompt individuals to abandon their careers. Children may experience paradox when their developmental tasks conflict with limitations imposed by their chronic illness. For example, a child with asthma may find his or her medication regimen leaves the child unprepared to engage in the rigorous activities of many of his or her peers unless medications are adjusted (Agius, 2003).

Uncertainty coupled with numerous losses makes chronic illness particularly devastating for patients who also face challenges of an evolving disease process. Those with chronic heart failure, for example, describe feelings of physical incapacity that adversely affect the whole life situation. Those with chronicity identify with feelings of fear, anxiety, fatigue, pain, grief, astonishment, anger, dependence, hope, and hopelessness. A diagnosis of heart failure is associated with high morbidity and mortality and is increasingly identified in the aging population (Dosh, 2004). Despite well-recognized symptom manifestation of heart failure, onset of progressive changes heralds a downward spiral that results in mortality in 59% of men and 45% of women at five years. Losses associated with heart failure include uncertainty and lessened endurance, because symptoms may be silent yet contribute to overall fatigue related to an inability of the heart to deliver sufficient oxygenated blood to meet the needs of organs and tissues during rest or exercise. Fatigue associated with activities of daily living (ADLs) may promote discouragement, depression, and contribute to social isolation.

Individuals with chronic kidney disease face some similar challenges in that the disease process unfolds in a predictable manner and is associated with significant mortality and morbidity. However, the disease differs from heart failure in several important ways. Most notably, early in the disease process, renal disease (which currently affects nearly 20 million Americans) involves nearly all body systems. The incidence and prevalence of renal failure have doubled during the past decade, and associated causal conditions of renal failure—including diabetes mellitus, hypertension, ischemia, increased susceptibility to infections, obstructions, toxins, and autoimmune and infiltrative diseases—are also on the rise (Snively & Gutierrez, 2004). The prospects of additional numbers of aging individuals developing this disease, and the implications of such a trend, are staggering.

Disease progression is frequently discussed in terms of treatment response. However, actions to slow progression of the disease—maintaining glycemic control, in particular—can slow the progression of associated nephropathy and, therefore, enhance quality of life. Maintaining excellent glycemic control is a daily struggle for many with chronic renal disease. The renal diet is generally low in protein, and many patients find this and other stringent dietary restrictions burdensome to comply with and difficult to remember. Frequently, renal disease leads to malnutrition and hypoalbuminemia. These conditions may result in fatigue, decreased endurance, and poor stamina, all of which may worsen as the disease inevitably progresses. Community health nurses can play a major role in helping patients to understand the effects of their behaviors. Assistance with dietary planning to better suit the tastes and budgets of patients can have a great influence on compliance with dietary restrictions and improved outcomes for diabetes management.

In chronic hepatitis C, diagnostic testing sensitivity and specificity are as high as 99%, yet diagnosis remains elusive in those who are not screened or tested for previous exposure or current, active infection. Because the symptoms of fatigue and nausea are commonly seen in other chronic processes, carriers may not seek or receive appropriate treatment until symptoms of cirrhosis develop (Ward, Kugelmas, & Libsch, 2004). Although 2.7 million persons in the United States are estimated to have this condition, most remain undiagnosed. Highly successful treatment modalities exist and afford relief in 50% to 80% of all persons who receive medications for hepatitis C. Disease progression is of great concern, because cirrhosis is essentially irreversible and progression accelerates in the presence of increased age, male gender, and use of alcohol. Nurses can make a huge difference in hepatitis C outcomes by encouraging high-risk patients to be tested so that hepatitis C infection can be diagnosed early and treated before cirrhosis develops.

In the United States, back pain accounts for nearly 25% of all workers' compensation claims and is the most frequent type of claim filed (Strunin & Boden, 2004). The social and personal aspects of back pain are substantial and interfere with personal integrity and role functioning. The following statements reflect these concerns: "You feel a lot of times that you are half a person," "I don't think I'm as good as I was," and "It kind of made me feel like an invalid." Family responsibilities may have to be assumed by others if back pain persists and becomes chronic.

Because the etiology of back pain is often unclear and damage is obscure in many cases, persons with back pain may have no defined path to symptom relief or cure. They may visit a variety of healthcare providers seeking both validation and relief of their symptoms. "Individuals who experience bodily suffering but who fail to gain acceptance for this suffering find themselves with illness but without sickness and can be described as inhabiting a liminal space, being both well and sick, and being neither" (Dumit, 1998). This statement tacitly refers to the importance of the sick role in which individuals seek relief from particular duties in acknowledgment of their suffering for a stipulated period of time. In the **sick role** in Western society, the physician functions as a "gatekeeper" and is responsible for monitoring signs of disease, worsening of the condition, or improvement. The patient is expected to "act sick," cooperate with physicians and their designees, and be cared for until able to resume his or her productive place in society. Because of the nature of back pain and the current state of the science and its limited ability to provide relief, individuals may experience loss and burden related to the chronic pain experience. However, because the individual is increasingly responsible for his or her improvement and ultimate recovery, the person may be challenged to use support groups, alternative and complementary strategies, and coping behaviors including

courage, empowerment, and partnership with the healthcare community to master this situation.

Losses and resulting sorrow may lead to development of **chronic sorrow** that develops from grief emerging from continual loss during the trajectory of an illness or disability. For example, persons with Parkinson's disease—a slowly developing, progressive, neurological disorder—and their spouses often experience chronic sorrow. Losses triggering sorrow include loss of future plans, restrictions on social life, inability to travel, and decreased ability to participate in hobbies (Lindgren, 1996).

The meaning of chronic illness to individuals and to society varies widely. Individuals may undertake to control chronic physical or psychiatric illnesses using strict adherence to treatment regimens, or they may eschew traditional healthcare practices in favor of nontraditional methods. Control of healthcare behaviors, however, does not always relate to successful outcomes, and some chronic diseases remain difficult to manage with current therapy options.

Adjustment to losses becomes a recurrent theme in many chronic illnesses, but each loss may represent a singular and significant experience that must be grieved. Diagnosis of chronic illness may result in releases of powerful emotions, including denial, shock, depression, and suicidal ideation. Consider the following example of a woman with chronic illness:

> I wanted to go jump in front of a car, and I can remember one day staying home. I was just so depressed that my husband got very alarmed and took off a day of work to stay with me because he was concerned about what I might do. As I thought about jumping in front of a car, I thought it would be my luck just to be maimed. (Wolf, 1994, p. 372)

By trying to protect herself from facing the reality that something is wrong, this woman pretends not to be ill and hopes that people will not notice her intrusive symptoms (Wolf, 1994).

### Suffering

The socialization process ensures that adults will be able to assume roles in society recognized as necessary for members of society and for continuation of society. Socialization in children and adolescents with chronic illness can also present problems. Adolescents with cancer, for example, believe that hopefulness is essential to their successful coping with the cancer experience (Hinds, 2004). Celiac disease and the ensuing dietary control essential for maintenance of health have many far-reaching effects on both the ill child and family. Children with asthma or bronchitis related to environmental sources experience interference with socialization and with developmental tasks. Children who spend more time outdoors and who engage in team sports in areas

**❝** *We are healed of a suffering only by experiencing it in full.* **❞**

—*Marcel Proust, 1871–1922*

with excessive ozone levels associated with automobile exhaust have more respiratory symptoms, including increased respiratory rate, persistent mucus production, increased respiratory illness, and decreased endurance. Long-term consequences of these problems are being identified with increasing frequency in urban areas.

Not all chronic illnesses are physical in nature. For instance, abilities and determinations that are aspects of personality may also be compromised in cases of chronic mental illness. Additionally, mental illness carries a social stigma that is not commonly encountered with physical problems, such that supports that are readily available to some chronically ill persons are not universally available to individuals with mental illness. **Geriatric depression**—a frequently noted condition in elders with chronic illness—is associated with lower quality of life (Small, Birkett, Meyers, Loran, Bystrick, & Nemeroff, 1996). Geriatric depression has been found to respond well to treatment, when it is instituted. Specifically, medication provided relief to elders with depression as frequently as younger patients in a comparison group without chronic illness (Small et al., 1996).

Younger individuals also face stigma with chronic physical or mental illness. A woman with asthma shares the following story:

> I was really embarrassed so I was trying to pretend that I wasn't short of breath. So I'd get up and turn around for a minute so that they wouldn't see. When I finally caught my breath, I'd start lecturing again. . . . I hid the inhaler in my pocket and went to the ladies room; I always hid it from my employer and my teachers. (Wolf, 1994)

Another woman with ulcerative colitis recalls her feelings:

> I never wanted to be stigmatized as someone who has a chronic problem or who is labeled as a chronic disease-type person. I've known people who just call out sick. I've never wanted to be stigmatized as one who abused sick time in that way. (Wolf, 1994)

### Power and Powerlessness

**Power** can be equated to individual possession of adequate resources enabling chronically ill people to be in control of their lives, or in substantial control of important aspects of their lives (Miller, 1992). Resources include perceptions of power that unfold with other inner attributes and coping strategies that emerge as a consequence of diminished health capacity and confronting of adversity (Miller, 1992).

Powerlessness is a nonadaptive coping mechanism resulting from loss of self, loss of self-esteem, loss of autonomy, and loss of hope. Chronic illness may result in additional losses without appropriate healthcare interventions that are sensitive to needs of individuals with ongoing challenges, uncertainly, and suffering for prolonged intervals. During illness, it is the fear of loss of the whole or a part of the body that is a focus of great psychological concern (Smith, 1974).

Survival of chronically ill individuals depends, in some measure, on individual ability and determination to endure aspects of suffering for long periods of time that must be endured if they cannot be altered or avoided. Community nurses may help to alleviate powerlessness by providing both physical and emotional support and by providing education related to self-care skills and the availability of community resources.

## Caring for Persons with Long-Term Health Problems

Knowledge of patient perceptions of care is essential to community health nurses who plan, coordinate, manage, and evaluate community-based care. Maintaining an optimal quality of life becomes a paramount consideration when the future is uncertain and when limitations are both recognized and anticipated. Limitations and permanent disability can be daunting prospects to those who never considered themselves to be vulnerable to long-term health issues.

Facing devastating physical limitations may cause individuals to question their future and to wonder if they will be able to tolerate rigors of chronicity (Johnson, 1991). A challenging example is chronic pain resulting from development or deterioration of many conditions related to aging. Management of chronic pain is essential to avoid debilitating physical limitations. Another common problem is hypertension, which is a major risk factor for heart disease, stroke, and renal failure, among other serious conditions. Because this condition is "silent," many affected individuals do not seek care from their primary providers or adhere to necessary regimens once the condition has been diagnosed. Given that the risk of cardiovascular disease increases substantially in women after menopause, follow-up with community health nurses is essential to optimal blood pressure management and will result in decreased mortality and morbidity, especially in women who are age 50 or older (Hirao-Try, 2003).

Nurses can be instrumental in facilitating adaptation to chronic disease processes and promote optimal health within a framework of disease-imposed limitations. Nurses can also support patient-generated activities that sustain endurance and alleviate suffering. Community-based nurses are in an optimal position to identify and promote adaptation to chronic disease processes resulting in diminished limitations.

### MEDIA MOMENT

Persons with chronic health conditions are seldom portrayed on network television and in movies. Conversely, many advertisements for products and drugs to treat chronic illnesses appear on a daily basis. How would you explain this dichotomy?

### Application to Practice

#### *Osteoporosis*

Mrs. A. was discharged to her home 3 weeks after having her right hip replaced. She was in a long-term care facility for 2 weeks after she was released from the hospital and was happy to be home again, among familiar surroundings. Mrs. A. had just passed her 77th birthday when she fell getting out of her bathtub at home. She managed to reach the telephone and called a neighbor, who came over and helped get Mrs. A. to the hospital in an ambulance. Although always ambulatory, Mrs. A. spent the next week recovering in bed from hip replacement surgery. She had physical therapy twice daily and ambulated with assistance in her room. She was surprised to learn from her physician that she had experienced a significant overall loss of bone.

Factors contributing to loss of bone density include small bones, smoking, low calcium intake, early menopause without estrogen replacement, amenorrhea, lack of exercise, and a familial history of osteoporosis. Other factors related to osteoporosis include chronic diseases, excessive alcohol consumption, and eating disorders (Dowd & Cavalieri, 1999).

After sustaining the fracture, suspicions that Mrs. A. had weakened and fragile bones were confirmed by bone densitometry that was arranged by her community health nurse. Medicare recently added bone mass measurements to its benefits for those fitting risk criteria, so Mrs. A.'s bone density scan was covered. Her osteoporosis could have been diagnosed much earlier if she had known the risks associated with its development. Her community health nurse explained symptoms and factors contributing to development of osteoporosis. Looking back, Mrs. A. recalled one symptom in particular: losing her height. She had been 5'5" and was now just over 5'1". The community health nurse also explained how to prevent falls and directed Mrs. A. to an equipment supply store, where she ordered a metal grab-bar for her bathtub, which would reduce the possibility of future falls while bathing. Now home, Mrs. A. continued the calcium and Vitamin D supplements and bisphosphonates therapy initiated in the hospital and planned to start a walking program at the senior center near her house. Her progress will be monitored for the next few weeks by her community health nurse.

*Source*: Adapted from Dowd & Cavalieri, 1999.

## Quality of Life in Disability and Chronic Illness

Acute phases of many chronic illnesses are managed in a hospital or nursing home by healthcare professionals, but the majority of ongoing care takes place in the home. Because the needs of chronically ill persons often outstrip the resources available to them, community health nurses must seek out solutions to care for chronically ill individuals in the most cost-effective manner using available resources of the extended family. This situation is especially relevant in elderly populations in which increased longevity and aging of the baby boomers will result in not only a larger population of elderly, but also a higher prevalence of disability (Spillman, 2004). Medical interventions must be designed and implemented not only to prolong life, but also to promote health and independence.

Many times, chronic illnesses are not immediately fatal but are disabling by virtue of their progression and side effects of social isolation and fatigue. Despite the nonfatal nature of some chronic diseases, they erode quality of life and diminish individual, family, and community resources. Part of the suffering that accompanies chronic health problems is increased by uncertainty, by remissions and exacerbations, by depleted or inadequate coping mechanisms, and by fatigue, which is a factor to consider while planning appropriate activities. The most predictable outcome of chronic

### Research Alert

The study described community-dwelling women's knowledge of heredity, familial, and sporadic breast cancer risk factors and identified characteristics associated with this knowledge. Using a descriptive, cross-sectional design and survey methods, women between 30 and 85 years of age ($n = 184$) from diverse racial and ethnic backgrounds and with no previous diagnoses of cancer were included in the study sample. Findings of the study indicated that most women recognized heredity as a risk factor but did not recognize the impact of paternal family history on risk. Some women did not identify the importance of aging in terms of risk factors, or were unfamiliar with known relationships between breast and ovarian cancers. Education was identified as the most important characteristic associated with knowledge of risk factors.

Interestingly, 49% of those surveyed in the study were college graduates. Despite this demographic, knowledge of breast cancer risk factors was incomplete. Implications for nursing relate to the need for women to receive education about the three types of breast cancer: hereditary, familiar, and sporadic. Additionally, advanced practice nurses should provide individualized counseling to women seeking information about their risk factors.

*Source*: Katapodi, M. C., & Aouizerat, B. E. (2005). Do women in the community recognize heredity and sporadic breast cancer risk factors? *Oncology Nursing Forum*, 32(3), 617–623.

### Research Alert

This study sought to assess patterns of medical consultation, diagnosis, and medication use in representative samples of adults with migraine in England and the United States. Validated computer-assisted telephone interviews were conducted in the United Kingdom ($n = 4,007$) and the United States ($n = 4,376$). Individuals who reported six or more headaches per year meeting the criteria for migraine were interviewed.

Patients with migraine in the United Kingdom were more likely to have consulted a doctor for headache at least once in their lifetime (86% versus 69%, $p < 0.0001$), but also were more likely to have lapsed from medical care (37% versus 21%, $p < 0.001$). In the United States, patients with migraine who had consulted physicians made more office visits for headache and were more likely to see a specialist. In the United States but not in the United Kingdom, women with migraine were more likely than men to consult doctors for headache. Patients with migraine in the United Kingdom were more likely to receive a medical diagnosis of migraine (United Kingdom, 67%; United States, 56%; $p < 0.05$). Patterns of medication use were similar in both countries, with most people treating the headaches with over-the-counter (OTC) medications. Substantial disability occurred in a high proportion of those who never consulted physicians (United Kingdom, 60%; United States, 68%), never received a correct medical diagnosis (United Kingdom, 64%; United States, 77%), and treated only with OTC medication (United Kingdom, 72%; United States, 70%).

Implications for community health nurses are that medically unrecognized migraine remains an important health problem both in the United States and the United Kingdom. Furthermore, there may be barriers to consultation for men in the United States that do not operate in the United Kingdom. While effective treatment exists for preventing and treating migraines, patterns of OTC treatment and lack of follow-up exist in both countries, which indicates a need for greater emphasis on population-focused education.

*Source*: Lipton, R. B., Scher, A. I., et al. (2003). Patterns of health care utilization for migraine in England and in the United States. *Neurology, 60*(3), 441–448.

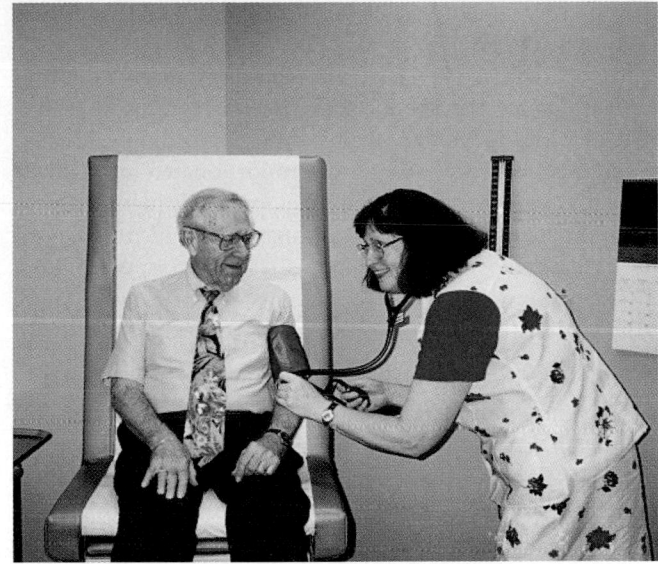

Chapter author Dr. Edith Hilton conducts an assessment of an elder patient with heart disease.

bers of adult cancer survivors have indicated to the healthcare community that, when it comes to treatment choice, quality of life is as important as overall therapeutic effect. Patients are concerned with the impact of cancer therapy on their daily lives. Chemotherapy-induced nausea and vomiting is one of the most devastating adverse effects of cancer treatment and adversely affects quality of life (Wickham, Goodin, & Lynch, 2004). Abandonment of chemotherapy owing to this problem is common. Improving control of this distressing side effect of cancer treatment greatly enhances the patient's ability to tolerate the full dose of chemotherapy. Serotonin-receptor antagonists, neurokinin, and steroids are part of current treatment protocols that accomplish this useful goal (Wickham et al., 2004). By mitigating side effects, chemotherapies are more easily tolerated; hence improved outcomes become possible.

Age alone is not the sole determinant of enhanced or diminished quality of life. The specific condition or disease process may adversely affect individuals differently at different points during their lives. Consider the chronic illness and disability associated with Parkinson's disease. Although related to age, Parkinson's disease also affects some persons who are younger (21–40 years) and may alter their quality of life because of the earlier onset of motor complications and disease progression (Jung, 2004). As expected, older adults with Parkinson's disease also face issues related to quality of life. They may encounter daily issues associated with disease onset and progression including tremor, bradykinesia, postural instability, cognitive changes, and depression (Whitney, 2004). Worsening symptoms that indicate deterioration, although more gradual than in younger adults, may adversely affect quality of life. Maintaining their usual activities, modifying their physical environment to enable maximal autonomy, accepting their limitations, and modifying the daily routine to make the most of their functional capabilities

illness is unpredictability (Schaefer, 1995). Patient autonomy characterizes the current era of health care, which is safeguarded by nursing (Miller, 1991). Patient quality of life is an appropriate consideration in chronic illness. Assessment of quality of life is directly related to the goals of nursing care, including promotion of health and restoration of maximal functioning of the patient.

These nursing goals become increasingly important when thinking about cancer as an acute event shifts to consideration of cancer as a chronic condition. Increasing numhelp preserve quality of life for individuals with this disease (Whitney, 2004).

Not surprisingly, racial and ethnic variations in household dynamics may produce differing perceptions of health-related issues including quality of life. Accordingly, because older African Americans are disproportionately more likely to acquire caregiving responsibilities for family members with chronic illness or disability, they may distinguish quality of life in different ways than whites with similar responsibilities.

## The Chronic Care Model

Broadly defined, models are illustrative representations of the interrelations that exist within a system or process (*Mosby's Dictionary*, 2007). They are frequently used in nursing to explain phenomena and to make predictions about patients or outcomes. Prediction and control of outcomes are highly desirable when managing chronic illness and disability on a case-by-case basis and in contemplating future needs and settings. The model of chronic care discussed here was developed by E. H. Wagner and refined and further developed by a group supported by the Robert Wood Johnson Foundation. The model was tested nationally and revised accordingly. Discussion of this model provides information about advancements in chronic care gleaned from research and numerous clinical applications and offers insights into innovative programs that have been identified by leading experts in the United States (ICIC, 2008).

The **chronic care model** identifies the essential elements of a healthcare system that promotes high-quality chronic disease care. High-quality chronic disease care encompasses several interrelated elements, including the community, the health system, self-management support, delivery system design, decision support, and clinical information systems (ICIC, 2008). When informed patients interact with these elements and have access to providers with resources and expertise, the result is healthier patients, more satisfied providers, and cost savings.

According to this model (ICIC, 2008), community resources must be mobilized to meet the needs of patients and avoid costly duplication of services. Shared services such as mobile clinics or meals-on-wheels programs are examples of

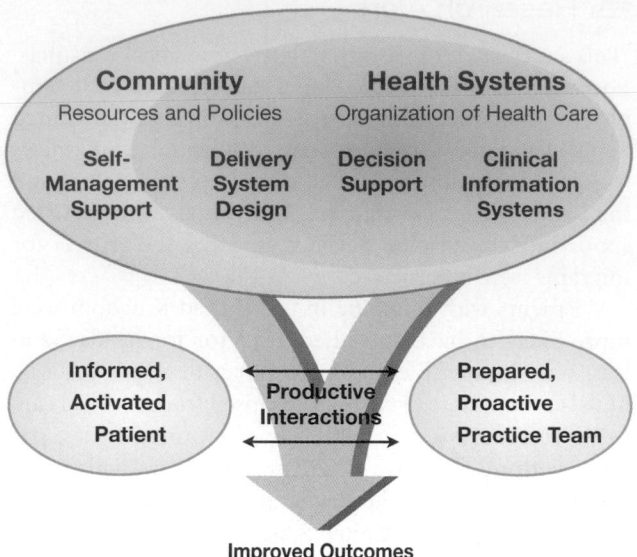

**THE CHRONIC CARE MODEL**

*Source*: Chronic Care Model: Edward H. Wagner, MD, MPH, Chronic Disease Management: What Will It Take to Improve Care for Chronic Illness? *Effective Clinical Practice*, Aug/Sept 1998, Vol 1, Figure 1. Used with permission.

this idea. Self-help strategies may be promoted by partnering with national patient organizations such as the American Diabetes Association. Additionally, local and state health policies, insurance benefits, and civil rights for those with disabilities should be emphasized by patient advocates.

A culture, organization, and mechanisms that promote safe, high-quality treatment must be created if chronic illness care is to be improved. According to the ICIC (2008), care improvement goals must be clearly articulated by senior management and implemented through the use of incentives. Prevention of errors through reporting mechanisms and analysis of problems areas with corrective action must be incorporated into the working plans of system management. Communication should be facilitated and data sharing should be optimized as patients navigate across settings and providers.

The ICIC (2008) model emphasizes empowerment of patients to enable them to effectively manage their own health and health care. By acknowledging the central role of the patient in chronic illness care, self-management support strategies provided by the community health nurse and others lay the foundation for better disease control and desirable outcomes. By fostering a sense of responsibility for their individual health, patients and providers work collaboratively to prioritize goals, define problems, and monitor for progress throughout the process.

In the chronic care model, the delivery of effective and efficient clinical care and self-management support is essential. Because the current healthcare system is reactive and responds primarily to those who are ill, it provides few

 GLOBAL CONNECTION

In addition to the immediate devastating effects of war, chronic disease and disabilities are long-term consequences that persist for decades in countries where conflicts occur. Conditions such as cancer from chemical warfare, stress-related illnesses, and injuries to the musculoskeletal system are just a few of the chronic, debilitating conditions that plague countries even after war ends.

*Got an Alternative?*

Persons with chronic illness are more likely to embrace nontraditional interventions than other patients. Why do you think this is true? What is the role of the community health nurse in educating persons with chronic illness related to complementary and alternative health choices?

opportunities for keeping people healthy. The chronic care model emphasizes the importance of keeping in close communication with all patients to facilitate aftercare and proposes the implementation of case management or care management, depending on the complexity of each case. To facilitate efforts to reach this goal, tasks and responsibilities should be distributed among community-based health team members. The role of prevention is especially emphasized to enable optimal health for chronically ill individuals. Intensive management of those with complicated or multiple chronic processes is articulated. Finally, the model stresses the need for cultural sensitivity and health literacy in the health professionals who support those with chronic illnesses.

The model supports the use of evidenced-based care and consideration of patient preferences. Treatments should be based solely on explicit proven guidelines that are supported by clinical research. Providers must stay up-to-date on trends, and supportive specialists are considered an essential part of the treatment team that provides expert guidance. Changes to the treatment plan should result from the application of timely reminders, feedback, and standing orders. Finally, the performance of the practice team and care system should be monitored.

The model of chronic care has unique utility for community health nurses in that it can be applied to a broad, diverse cross-section of patients. Those who are permanently disabled *and* chronically ill, in particular, may identify strengths in the enduring nature of the evaluation component and note the ongoing advocacy built into the model. A further strength of this model is its ability to adapt to changing needs and changing characteristics of specific disease states as progression or improvement of symptoms develops. Finally, the use of functional and clinical outcomes ensures standard measures are applied to persons with disabilities and chronic, progressive diseases.

## Roles for Community Health Nurses

Community health nurses caring for individuals with chronic illness attempt to mitigate effects of chronic, disabling conditions for individuals and communities by functioning in many roles in established and nontraditional settings. Settings in which they work include free-standing clinics, homeless shelters, shopping malls, schools, apartments, hospitals, churches, rural settings, urban residences, and wherever healthcare needs occur.

Nurses identify risk factors associated with chronic diseases, and they anticipate complications arising from acute illnesses superimposed on chronicity. Further, nurses provide direction for modification of current health policy to reflect changing priorities and identify silent and underserved groups of chronically ill persons.

Community health nurses may intervene to facilitate use of adaptive coping mechanisms. Coping enhancement involves incorporation of social support—for example—which is believed to mediate and buffer effects of stressors associated with chronic illness. Another coping mechanism that may mitigate feelings of hopelessness and loss is spiritual support, which is also identified as a helpful mechanism of coping by chronically ill populations (Miller, 1992). Use of spiritual support may provide comfort and alleviate prolonged grieving.

Nurses function as change agents, advocates, professional caregivers, and role models. The role of prevention grows more important every year. Nursing interventions help delineate areas in which nurses have specialty knowledge and expertise. Some nursing interventions that have had limited applications in research may be explicated further in future clinical investigations, thereby providing additional support for practice.

## ■ Change Agent

As the number of nurse practitioners and family practice physicians entering primary care within the community multiply, community health nurses will have increasing opportunities to identify changing needs that require immediate attention. Long waiting periods to access primary care will be shortened, and turnaround times for maintenance care activities will decrease. Nurses will be an important source of support, facilitating better and faster follow-up care, and more in-depth prevention activities for all disabled and chronically ill.

> **❝** *Every time I think that I'm getting old, and gradually going to the grave, something else happens.* **❞**
>
> —Lillian Carter, nurse and mother of President Jimmy Carter

## ■ Advocate

Advocating for chronically ill patients may result in provision and expansion of services where they are either currently unavailable or are of limited availability. By increasing necessary services, additional supports and effective interventions may be identified in the future that capitalize on use of extended familial caregivers and community-based volunteers. Political activity associated with enabling increased access to health-promoting activities may be of increasing importance in the future, as populations of chronically ill increase in the new millennium.

### ■ Professional Caregiver

An area of great need will be that of professional caregivers who assist chronically ill persons to cope over the long term. Coping with chronic illness may mean development of personal and societal resources as a means of enhancing quality of life and survival. Development of personal resources may include increasing coping abilities so as to endure painful or prolonged aspects of disease. Adjustment to losses associated with chronic diseases becomes essential. Adjustment entails coping with physical symptoms and uncertainty. Facilitating adjustment may include use of nursing interventions such as family integrity promotion, decision-making support, and mutual goal setting (Luckmann, 1997).

## Role Models

Role-modeling behaviors of the community health nurse will include smoking cessation, weight control, and physical fitness to encourage preventive behaviors in the chronically ill. Health teaching will increase in importance, and nurses in community settings will be sought to initiate effective educational programs specifically designed to address the needs of the chronically ill population.

### ■ Interdisciplinary Roles and Responsibilities

As care providers, change agents, and advocates, community health nurses work as an integral part of interdisciplinary healthcare teams. Other team members include both paraprofessional and professional individuals. Some of these individuals will have no direct contact with, or knowledge of, the chronically ill patient. Others will have day-to-day contact with the patient and will depend on the community health nurse for essential information and opinions.

Use of the rehabilitation interdisciplinary model frequently adds to the team concept of care that has long been in place and effectively used by healthcare personnel (Hickey, 2003). Rehabilitative treatments of patients depend on the efforts of many healthcare specialists and demand that patients be actively engaged in their treatment protocols. Community health nurses will continue to have an active role in supporting rehabilitation efforts in chronically ill populations to optimize these patients' functional independence and self-reliance.

## Financing Costs of Chronic Illness

By 2020, nearly 157 million Americans are expected to have a chronic condition. Direct medical costs for these conditions are expected to be more than $10 trillion, accounting for more than 80% of total U.S. healthcare spending (Partnership for Solutions, 2001). In the current political and economic climate, record numbers of Americans and immigrants residing in the United States have no health insurance; this situation is a source of grave concern to 89% of surveyed adults (Partnership for Solutions, 2001).

Fees for health care are generally set by formulas put forth by federal and state governments (Hickey, 2003). Medicare, Medicaid, and third-party payers are involved in both establishment of fee schedules and cost-management efforts that determine "who gets what" in terms of services. Both direct and indirect healthcare costs are considered when estimating the magnitude of chronic illness. Chronic illness costs society millions of dollars annually and results in massive productivity losses. Treatments for chronic illnesses are rising in cost as more people survive longer because of earlier and more accurate diagnostics. Cancer and heart disease are examples of these phenomena, with heart disease alone affecting an estimated 80 million people in the United States (CDC, 2008).

Age and chronic illness are positively related. Persons older than age 65 represent a rapidly growing segment of the world's population. Elderly have the highest rates of hospitalizations and visits to physicians in the United States, even though they experience the lowest rates of acute illnesses (CDC, 2008a, 2008b). The cost of caring for such individuals is a substantial concern, as chronically ill elders may experience a long-term financial burden related to their needed care.

Funding initiatives for community-based supports vary. Some private funds are available through service organizations, religious, and secular groups. Public funds for community supports for home-based caregivers vary widely from region to region. Use and availability of supports affect the indirect costs of caring for chronically ill persons. Additional or indirect costs of caring for the chronically ill population include time lost from work in the case of home-based caregivers, resulting in lost productivity. The cost of hospitalizations secondary to exacerbations of symptoms and medications, supplies, and treatments are other indirect costs. For example, diabetic supplies can cost hundreds of dollars monthly; this cost is often offset, at least in part, by federal tax dollars. Prioritizing these issues has engendered fierce debate in political arenas, as rising healthcare costs and increasing numbers of chronically ill require new funding sources.

Planning for U.S. healthcare reform given the current numbers of chronically ill persons is a complex matter. Recent discoveries in technology, pharmacology, and professional research are changing the outlook for chronicity. The number of chronically ill persons is anticipated to rise because of increasingly effective symptom control resulting in longer life expectancy for these individuals.

Many Americans lack basic health insurance, and their inability to anticipate improved health care may result in additional numbers of chronically ill persons joining the ranks because of neglected preventive and maintenance measures. Health care is currently fragmented, and despite ongoing efforts to fund essential healthcare services, many people with chronic disease will likely continue to be uninsured and underinsured (National Coalition on Health Care, 2008).

Chronically ill individuals are particularly vulnerable to reforms in healthcare policy that decrease or eliminate essential services, including home-based nursing care, needed to improve and maintain their health status. These patients are often unable to effectively advocate for themselves, so they rely on healthcare professionals to secure needed services for them. If fragmentation of health care continues, the chronically ill population will experience increased difficulties in accessing adequate health care.

## Self-Determination: The Patient as Partner

Chronically ill patients frequently experience perceptions of life quality that are not shared by physicians. Elderly, chronically ill outpatients may perceive their lives to have acceptable quality, despite the physician's perceptions to the contrary. Research suggests patients' perceived emotional, socioeconomic, intellectual, and physical functioning affect their perceptions of quality of life (Wilson & Satterfield, 2007). Quality of care may directly affect quality of life. Those who experience adequate management of symptoms and undesirable side effects may rate their quality of life as acceptable or better. In cases characterized by uncontrolled relief from chronic symptoms that result in reduced or unbearable daily symptoms, quality of life will decrease markedly.

## " a conversation with . . . "

Rose is an 87-year old woman who has been dependent on others for many years for her daily care. She is unable to ambulate and is in a wheelchair. She lives in a long-term care facility and experiences chronic pain from arthritis in nearly all her joints. She has been in arthritic pain for many years and has used different drugs at intervals, but she continues to experience severe pain that interrupts all other activities. She grimaces as she moves in her wheelchair, and speaks about her pain:

"The pain is always there. I would like to be without it just for a day, now and then. I've really forgotten how it is to just get up and do for yourself. I never wanted to have to ask other people to help me all the time, but lately, that's how it is. I'm so tired all the time. The pain keeps me awake, and when I fall asleep, if I try to turn over, it reminds me right away by waking me up! I have the pain all the time, more or less. I take some of the arthritis medicine for it, and it helps a good bit, but it always wears off, and then it feels like the pain comes back real strong. Either sittin' or standin' it bothers me, and I can't walk any distance at all. My niece comes to take me out some, but I don't always feel like going. 'Course, it's real nice to have her come, it's just that I can't go like I used to. We both miss getting out together, but then, at my age, I'm expecting to have pain. They all tell me you don't die from it, but it sure keeps you from doing like you want to."

—Rose

## Sensitivity in Community-Based Caring

More than 50 million Americans are currently involved in assisting chronically ill or elderly persons with either personal or household management issues (National Family Caregivers Association, 2008). All ethnic, racial, and gender groups are involved in caring for chronically ill individuals. Community health nurses are in the unique position of entering private homes to render or assist in care provision. Each of these groups and each individual has issues and expectations that may present unique challenges to healthcare workers in provision of gender-, ethnic-, and racially sensitive care. Care rendered in ethnic- and culturally sensitive ways will enhance the nurse's efforts to individualize important interventions.

### ■ Gender-Specific Considerations

Overall, women live longer than men. In addition, women tend to rely more on daughters, sisters, mothers, and female friends than on male children or spouses when chronic illnesses occur. Men tend to rely on these same groups of caregivers but most often rely on female spouses. Consequently, there are many more women functioning as caregivers than men. For many reasons, including societal expectations, women tend to put the needs of others before their own needs. Many women, especially older women, may have difficulty articulating their needs and preferences in aspects of care, and need to be reassured, offered options, and consulted about all aspects of care as both patients and caregivers.

Chronically ill women may use a variety of coping strategies to handle the effects of their disease or illness. Effective coping strategies will underscore their desire to maintain normalcy to the greatest extent possible. Women with early-onset disability may strive to prevent secondary complications from developing (Goodwin & Compton, 2004). Consequently, many more women are invested in health promotion to improve their day-to-day experiences and to extend their life expectancy. An example of this idea is controlling the fatigue associated with cancer: Scheduled exercises may be carefully planned around levels of least fatigue in an effort to promote a sense of normalcy and encourage women to take control of their physical symptoms (Coon & Coleman, 2004). The role of motivation and engagement in rehabilitation makes a strong case for those with disability to achieve and maintain high-level wellness.

One issue of increasing concern is women's increasing mortality rate compared to men. An example of this problem is the rapidly rising rate of lung cancer from cigarette smoking in women. Nicotine addiction, in particular, has increased among women during the past two decades, and greatly hampers their ability to achieve high-level wellness. This particular form of addiction results from a distinct, routine, and harmful social behavior that reflects the changing role and status of women (Pampel, 2003). This disturbing trend has been documented in nine high-income industrialized nations—the United States, the United Kingdom,

Ireland, Australia, Austria, Canada, Denmark, New Zealand, and Sweden. Not surprisingly, the United Kingdom and the United States have the highest rates of mortality from smoking and lung cancer in women (Pampel, 2003). Activities of the community health nurse should include leading by example, repeatedly encouraging patients to quit smoking, and discouraging women from starting smoking with the knowledge that prevention is far easier to promote than cessation.

## Issues Community Health Nurses Encounter

Professional issues encountered in providing and managing community-based care for chronically ill individuals include understanding long- and short-term goals, patterns of disease progression, resource allocation, development of support systems, education, and home-based caregiver roles. In daily care, routines provide a framework and format for use of the nursing process. Continuous supervision by nurses is generally not needed by all chronically ill individuals, but activities of daily living may be supported by home-based caregivers. These caregivers, who are frequently relatives or close friends of the individual with chronic illness, provide valuable services that enable chronically ill persons to retain autonomy in their homes. Paraprofessional caregivers who work in the community and function with a great deal of autonomy include nurse aides, therapy assistants, and transport staff, all of whom facilitate activities of daily living, maximal independence, and travel within the community. The home setting is desirable for many chronically ill patients and supports self-identity and self-determination, whereas institutional settings may depersonalize and socially isolate some chronically ill individuals from familiar surroundings, personal belongings, and cherished supports. Institutional settings may be desirable in situations in which home-based caregiving is not realistic.

### Research Alert

A qualitative study was undertaken to detect differences in the way caregivers in three ethnic groups (African American, Puerto Rican, and Caucasian) describe their reactions to caregiving. An ethnographic method was appropriately used to focus on scientific descriptions of cultural groups. The stratified, random sample consisted of 18 caregivers who were selected from a sample of 409 caregivers. All interviews were conducted in informants' homes, with one exception. Informed consent was ensured, and data were collected through use of CES-D and guided, unstructured conversations. Data were analyzed using content analysis to discover themes and meanings expressed by caregivers.

Findings revealed differences in expression of burden, both by ethnicity and gender within ethnicity groups. Generally, caregiving was associated with negative feelings and situations. Almost all Caucasians described their

situations negatively. African Americans described their situations as demanding and time-consuming. Puerto Rican caregivers reported that it was difficult to meet the demands of the care required. Several reported caregiving to be a rewarding and satisfying experience. These individuals had an extended network of support in which there were other people involved in the care and assistance of the disabled. Level of outside support was key in decreasing caregiver burden. The authors state that their findings can assist practitioners to better understand the cultural idiosyncrasies that are important in developing a culturally sensitive plan. ◗

*Source*: Calderon, V., & Tennstedt, S. L. (1998). Ethnic differences in the expression of caregiver burden: Results of a qualitative study. *Journal of Gerontological Social Work, 30*(1–2), 159–178.

### ■ Supporting Community-Based Caregivers

In addition to provision and direction of care, another additional role of importance for community health nurses is providing support to home-based caregivers. Daily provision of care to chronically ill persons can be both challenging and rewarding for home-based caregivers, and support systems, both formal and informal, may be necessary for a positive experience. Their anticipation of needs and understanding of disease progression make nurses invaluable assets to home-based caregivers who may have unrealistic or unachievable goals. For example, home-based caregivers for persons with COPD need to understand that perceived quality of life and use of coping mechanisms may contribute more to comfort and adaptation than does use of oxygen and medications (Herbert & Gregor, 1997).

Respite services are urgently needed by family caregivers who provide care to home-bound elders with chronic illness and/or disability. Because of the nature of chronic illness and disability, home care may be provided for extended periods and may challenge the resources of the caregiver. Respite involves four elements: (1) purpose, (2) time, (3) activities, and (4) place; it may occur in the home or elsewhere (Lubkin & Larsen, 2002). In addition to home-based care, sites of respite care include senior centers, daycare centers, long-term care facilities, and group living facilities. Respite care has the unique purpose of relieving caregivers so as to provide them with time for themselves so they are able to resume their caregiving role. The community health nurse may underscore these efforts by devising flexible schedules and interventions to address the needs of both care recipient and caregiver.

Support groups have become popular during the past decade as a means of facilitating coping with illness and/or disability. They may offer concrete assistance with adjustment to illness and associated role changes in addition to providing a neutral "sounding board" and informational services. Larger cities tend to have more support groups for specific needs, but since the Internet has eliminated many communication barriers, numerous support groups may be accessed online. Group leaders are frequently health professionals who have expertise in topical areas related to disabilities identified by potential group members. Some groups may be particularly helpful to individuals who are returning home from a hospitalization or who are working through illness-related issues. By taking advantage of the link to an empathetic community, individuals may feel better connected to others with similar issues and will reintegrate more easily. For those who live in rural areas, an Internet group may be especially useful if social contacts are limited by distance.

In addition to the Internet, the postal service and the telephone are excellent tools to encourage connectedness and engagement. Handwritten letters may provide a continuing source of enjoyment to the recipient. Those with memory loss are often comforted and reassured by "hardcopy" or tangible reminders of others. Similarly, phone calls are frequently welcome reminders of social connections and common interests. Each of these modalities may provide indispensable links and social support that is instrumental in preventing social isolation and loneliness.

Non-nursing caregivers provide care and services for chronically ill individuals in numerous community and institutional settings. Familial caretakers most frequently include women in the roles of wife, mother, daughter, sibling, or grandparent. Often, these female caregivers have chronic or unmet health needs themselves, and must subordinate their own needs to render care to their relative on a continuing basis. Continuing care can be extremely demanding and exhausting, if the familial caregiver is unrelieved. Neglect of self may develop in these circumstances, and depression, decreased overall health, and exhaustion may follow.

It is important to anticipate caregiver burnout and to suggest alternatives to prevent it from developing. Community-based programs and resources have been developed in some areas to help familial caregivers to take care of themselves. Respite and episodic care of chronically ill programs enable these caregivers to receive physical and psychological support at periodic intervals, while nurses and other members of the healthcare team assume responsibility for care of the chronically ill individual. Both of these options are available through some Veterans Administration (VA) hospitals, nursing homes, public hospitals, and community health agencies. These services are available only to provide temporary relief to community-based, familial caregivers. If the burdens of giving full-time care exceed the abilities and resources of the familial or home-based caregiver over the long term, institutionalization becomes the primary source of care.

Issues encountered by familial caregivers include other family commitments, personal physical health, recreational needs, fear of using needed equipment, stress, loss of independence, role change, loss of privacy, decreased well-being, depression, negative feelings, physical strain, anxiety, anger,

guilt, loss of self, and caregiver burnout. Effects of chronic illness on families are a major problem for some parental caregivers of children, who often attempt to cope with illness by adapting. Parental caregivers who lack professional help and support in care of their children may feel burdened and overwhelmed. These feelings may lead to development of abusive behaviors. Home-based caregivers of chronically ill children and adults may perpetrate abuse because of feelings of overwhelming frustration, social isolation, and powerlessness. Some family systems may have characteristics that promote abuse, including lack of family support, familial caregiver reluctance, overcrowding, isolation, family burdens, marital conflict, or differing opinions about institutionalization (Lubkin & Larson, 2002).

In chronic illness, abuse may be obvious or covert. If neglect, self-neglect, exploitation, and coercion are not readily apparent, the community health nurse needs to be sensitive to suspected cases of abuse (Luckmann, 1997). Use of several familial caregivers may relieve the frustration and feelings of isolation that underlie abuse. Another important factor in diminishing burdens of familial caregiving is engagement in social interaction, fun, and recreation, which may enhance the caregiver's sense of well-being (Thompson, Futterman, Gallagher-Thompson, Rose, & Lovett, 1993). Caregiver burnout has been linked with lack of assistance in day-to-day activities and should be examined proactively to incorporate supports necessary to benefit both the familial or home-based caregiver and the patient.

## ■ The Advanced Practice Nurse with a Community Health Focus

The role of the advanced practice nurse (APN) in the community has expanded substantially during the past decade. Fundamental to this role expansion is the moral commitment of caring that is foundational in nursing practice (Sumner, 2005). An APN has a master's or doctoral degree that is clinically focused within a specialized area; such professionals include nurse midwives, nurse anesthetists, clinical nurse specialists, and nurse practitioners. In addition to filling the valuable role of the community health nurse, APNs are able to provide a higher level of advanced nursing skills, such as a detailed health history and physical examination, screening evaluations, education, counseling, psychotherapy, coordination of services, symptom management, prevention of complications, diagnosis, and prescriptive ability (Health Resources and Services Administration, 2002; Ingersoll, McIntosh, & Williams, 2000).

The American Nurses Association (1995) identifies three characteristics that distinguish advanced nursing practice from basic nursing practice: (1) specialization or provision of care for a specific population with complex needs; (2) expansion or acquisition of new knowledge; and (3) role autonomy extending beyond the scope of traditional nursing practice. These characteristics allow the APN to function more independently than the traditional nursing role.

To the outsider, the role of the APN may appear to coincide with that of the primary care physician; however, APNs are indeed nurses first, and, as such, they are focused on the caring model. Several preliminary studies have attempted to quantify outcome measures of APNs, and most have demonstrated comparable or superior outcomes when compared to physician care (Ingersoll et al., 2000). Many of these nurses address patient education, counseling, and coordination of services, so their work cannot be directly compared to that in a physician model because these behaviors are more commonly associated with nursing care (McCorkle, Robinson, Nuamah, Lev, & Benoliel, 1998; McCorkle et al., 2000; Ingersoll et al., 2000). Some of the outcomes that seem to be most sensitive to advanced practice nursing are satisfaction with care delivery, symptom resolution or reduction, perception of being well cared for, compliance or adherence with treatment plan, knowledge of patients and families, and quality of life (Ingersoll et al., 2000).

Advanced practice nurses have an important role to play in the management of chronic illnesses and disability. Because many persons with chronic illness have more than one concurrent process, and many patients have four or more, increased numbers of chronic conditions expand the likelihood of developing complications and activity limitations (Crumbie, Conley, & Burman, 2004). Use of regular preventive care by community-based APNs will lessen this inevitability and enable patients to collaborate effectively with their primary providers to decrease onset of complications.

APNs employed in community health settings have the potential to significantly affect the health outcomes and satisfaction of patients and families. The roles most often identified for these nurses in community settings emphasize health promotion and disease prevention (Sumner, 2005). Additionally, APNs have a role in policy making, leadership, and responsibility at the organizational level. They are also excellent resources for community health nurses and other professionals involved in the care of patients with chronic illness. Advanced practice nurses are changing the nature of health care in the community for those with chronic illnesses and disability, and are providing new options and better outcomes.

## ■ Palliative and Hospice Care

Hospice or palliative services provide care and support to terminally ill individuals and their families in the final stages of life, and support death with respect and dignity. For those with chronic illnesses, great comfort may be obtained by having hospice services provided within the home. This allows the familial caregiver to have a rest from caring activities and to have an opportunity to consider relevant quality-of-life issues. The role of community health nurses in hospice care varies, but usually includes referral through the attending physician, facilitation of transfer of care of the chronically ill patient, and consultation as needed. Community-based hospice nurses may also provide education, coordination, and support services. Although palliative

and hospice services had their roots in oncology, the principles underlying that field have been applied to care for those with other diseases such as HIV/AIDS. Since the advent of highly effective antiretroviral therapies, the disease trajectory of HIV/AIDS has been altered, such that it is not always predictable. Community health nurses may be involved in caring for HIV/AIDS patients who have an uncertain future and who may not fit in the traditional paradigm of palliative or hospice care (Cochrane, 2003).

**Congregate housing** is another option for care that maximizes resources while carefully considering quality of life. *Congregate housing* and *assisted living* are considered interchangeable terms. Those who qualify for this type of living arrangement characteristically have a stable chronic condition and require assistance with three or more functional activities of daily living. Bringing needed services into individuals' homes, whether private or congregate, is an effective way to reduce institutionalization in those with chronic conditions (Sheehan & Oakes, 2003). Congregate housing services typically include the following core services: three meals daily, housekeeping and laundry services, transportation, social programs, and 24-hour security. Additionally, nursing supervision is available 20 hours per week, and emergency services are always available. Community health nurses may be involved with planning and supervision of care in these dwellings, which emphasize autonomy.

THINK ABOUT THIS

Sometimes I look at the sarcoidosis as a mean monkey on my back. In a way, I tried to mourn for the person who I was and figure out who I am now. I did as much research as I could and I took ownership of this illness, because if you don't take care of your body, where are you going to live?

—Karen Duffy

## ■ Institutionalization

Chronically ill persons who elect to receive institutional-based care are relatively few in number; however, they may be frail and require care that is not available in the community. The population requiring institutional provision of care, which currently includes fewer than 2 million individuals in the United States, is expected to increase rapidly over the next 40 years as baby boomers age and experience health problems.

Long-term care facilities provide essential services to some chronically ill persons, but there are several drawbacks to the current system. One of the most well-known and least desirable practices in long-term care facilities is use of physical restraints; use increases with age and degree of cognitive impairment of the patient. Both physical restraints and bed rails have been employed in the interest of safety and to prevent patients from wandering away to unsupervised areas. Although recent evidence suggests that restraints may actually increase injuries. Restraints also have the effect of reducing mobility, inhibiting communication, preventing individual reorientation, and restricting patterns of socialization within and without the facility. In facilities with decreased use of physical restraints, security and safety of residents may be enhanced by use of cameras, alarm systems, and staff surveillance. Unfortunately, falls and patient injuries continue to be a major problem encountered in institutional settings due to staffing levels and the age and physical condition of patients. Many are frail and require frequent assistance with all activities of daily living. Other problematic issues related to long-term care include loss of privacy, decreased choices in routines, diminished autonomy, and adverse relocation consequences.

Facility selection is an important decision, and community health nurses should support consultation of the chronically ill patient with family members who may assist in the process. The physical environment, accessibility, nurse-to-patient ratio, friendliness of the staff, availability of medical and support services, cost, and location will all be of concern to patients and families considering placement.

Both private and publicly funded facilities for long-term care of chronically ill patients exist. Long-term care facilities with religious affiliations are available in many geographic areas and may be Medicare certified for reimbursement purposes. Nonsectarian facilities are also available and may be affiliated with state or local governments. Both public and private institutions must adhere to standards of care that are put forth and monitored by local, state, and federal agencies. Areas subject to regulation in all long-term care facilities include resident rights; admission, transfer, and discharge rights, resident behavior and facility practice; administration; physical environment; infection control; quality of life; resident assessment; quality of care; nursing; rehabilitation; and medical services.

Nursing home selection may cause emotional distress to chronically ill individuals, who may have decreased coping skills and decreased endurance to withstand a major lifestyle change. Often, the community health nurse is aware of plans to move an individual to a nursing home. Elderly persons with chronic health problems may experience severe adjustment issues related to perceived and actual losses, feelings of powerlessness, and despair. Coping with these changes will require sensitive support and time to process changes. Rapid adjustment to lifestyle changes should not be expected.

## Research Alert

This epidemiological study examined the association between exposure to environmental tobacco smoke (ETS) and demographic, lifestyle, and occupational characteristics and self-reported health conditions. The cross-sectional study, using data from multiphasic health checkups between 1979 and 1985, examined 16,524 men aged 15–89 years and 26,197 women aged 15–105 years who never smoked and who were enrolled in a health plan in Northern California. Results indicated that 68% of men and 64% of women reported current ETS exposure (at home, in small spaces other than home, or in large indoor areas) with an exposure time from all three sources of ETS correlating negatively with age. Men and women reporting high-level ETS exposure were more likely to be black, to be never married or separated/divorced, to have no college or partial college education, to consume three alcoholic drinks per day or more, and to report exposure to several occupational hazards.

Consistent correlations (chi square, analysis of covariance) were found between exposure to ETS and a positive history of hay fever/asthma (odds ratio [OR] = 1.22 in men, 1.14 in women), hearing loss (OR = 1.30 in men, 1.27 in women), severe headache (OR = 1.22 in men, 1.17 in women), and cold/flu symptoms (OR = 1.52 in men, 1.57 in women). Any current ETS exposure was also associated with chronic cough (OR = 1.22) in men and with heart disease (OR = 1.10) in women. Self-reported stroke was not associated with any current ETS exposure in men (OR = 0.27). No associations were noted for cancer or tumor and for migraine.

Implications for community health nursing are a need for increased education in households that have ETS risks and other multiple risk factors that compound health risks. ETS exposure is associated with several self-reported acute and chronic medical conditions and should be part of all patient screening in primary care settings, regardless of the patient's chief health concerns.

*Source*: Iribarren, C., Friedman, G. D., Klatsky, A. L., & Eisner, M. D. (2001). Exposure to environmental tobacco smoke: Association with personal characteristics and self-reported health conditions. *Journal of Epidemiology and Community Health*, 55(10), 721–728.

## Health Promotion in Chronic Illness and Disability

Health promotion activities that focus on improving function across a spectrum of diagnoses and a range of age groups are effective in reducing secondary conditions experienced by, and outpatient physician visits made by, people with disabilities. Health promotion strategies for persons with chronic illnesses and/or disability may be adapted from those activities already identified for the mainstream population. An example of this idea is maintenance of normal weight. Obesity—once stigmatized as an unfortunate and undesirable condition—has dramatically increased in frequency and now adversely affects American adults and children in record numbers. Considered the worst health problem in the United States, obesity affects those living in poverty much more frequently than the affluent (Colvin, 2004). Obesity is associated with a 50% to 100% increased risk of death from all causes. Persons with chronic conditions are at even greater risk for mortality and increased morbidity if they develop obesity.

Health promotion strategies, including encouragement of a regular exercise program and patient education teaching healthy eating practices, will benefit both healthy and chronically ill populations. Those with disabilities also must strive to achieve or maintain normal weight. Those with mobility or endurance challenges will be adversely affected if they develop obesity, so prevention is a top priority with this population. Meal replacements may warrant consideration for those with difficulty in limiting portions, managing food preparation, or maintaining weight in a normal range (Noakes, Foster, Keogh, & Clifton, 2004).

Indeed, health promotion activities for all groups are increasingly important. Preventing the development of secondary complications related to risk behaviors is essential. Complications are far more costly to treat than health-promoting behaviors are to adopt. This is surely the case for chronically ill and disabled. Many persons with disability have no additional health problems and are well; these individuals may benefit substantially from health promotion activities. Structural changes associated with normal aging may also be mitigated by health-promoting behaviors. With the projected growth in the number of aging individuals worldwide, health promotion must soon move to the top of the health agenda for all providers as resources are stretched to accommodate greater-than-ever-numbers. Complications associated with preventable cardiovascular disease alone consume astonishing quantities of resources that could be beneficially directed in numerous other ways. Historically, nurses have optimized all available resources to promote healing and health (Phillips, 2005). Because of their proximity to the patient base, community health nurses are ideally positioned to provide leadership in the area of health promotion for their disabled and chronically ill patients.

## The Future Role of Community Health in Chronic Illness and Disability

❝*Folks, I'm telling you,*
*Birthing is hard*
*And dying is mean—*
*So get yourself*
*A little loving*
*In between.*❞

—Langston Hughes, from the poem Advice, 1946

Customarily, public health departments have not been closely involved in activities relating to prevention of chronic diseases and disability because these conditions are generally not communicable in nature. Because these conditions account for nearly 80% of all mortalities in the United States, and because caring for the health of the public is the concern of public health departments, their future efforts may well focus on prevention and control of chronic diseases and conditions. According to Friedan (2004), use of traditional public health strategies may be particularly helpful in helping to control chronic diseases. Activities routinely used by

public health staff include surveillance (including mandatory reporting), environmental modifications, regulation, clinical care and monitoring of care provided by others, outbreak detection, case management, immunization, and health education.

Surveillance in chronic disease may monitor the current epidemics of diabetes and obesity, the array of cardiovascular diseases, and smoking cessation. Cancer surveillance may be aimed at tracking prevention efforts, stage at diagnosis, and treatment effectiveness community-wide, not merely detailing occurrences. Surveillance is currently being used to monitor chronic disease development in communities with the highest acuity of smoking, diabetes, hypertension, hypercholesterolemia, depression, and obesity (Friedan, 2004). In communities in which this type of monitoring is ongoing, definitive, community-specific data are being generated to guide local action. Disease registries and those used to track local treatment progress and outcomes have great potential to improve chronic disease management.

Environmental interventions might be used to encourage and promote more active lifestyles and to eliminate architectural barriers. Preventive services may be placed at points of contact to encourage their use.

Clinical care efforts may lead to provision of smoking cessation clinics and cancer screening areas as well as supplement local efforts in hypertension control, diabetes management, and cholesterol monitoring. These initiatives will extend local efforts aimed at achieving optimal control, not eliminating primary care sites. Use of public health efforts will require increased funding but will result in improved chronic disease prevention and control (Friedan, 2004).

## Conclusion

Traditionally, community health nurses have cared for many chronically ill patients. By assessing the severity of the illness as well as the person's barriers, resources, self-efficacy, acceptance, current health-promoting behaviors, and current quality of life, the community health nurse will formulate a plan of care that will enable achievement of both long- and short-term wellness goals (Secrest, 2005). The current climate in healthcare services and distribution of healthcare resources make continued provision of care to chronically ill members of the community a challenge. As advocates and leaders in health care, community health nurses must ensure that appropriate and effective provision of services to chronically ill individuals expands by engaging in education, participating in political activity, and becoming involved in healthcare policy and research.

Explore Community Health Nursing on the Web! To learn more about the topics in this chapter, use the passcode provided to access your exclusive website: **http://nursing.jbpub.com/ communityhealth.** If you do not have a passcode, you can obtain one at this site.

## ■ CRITICAL THINKING ACTIVITIES

1. Discuss power and powerlessness. What aspects of each are essential to consider in planning care for the chronically ill? Consider how the same chronic disease may affect perceptions of power and powerlessness differently in children and adults.

2. Think of an image that would help you forget about the unpleasant sensation of nausea. Describe an image that might help you to focus on positive thoughts about disease outcomes like gaining strength or taking control.

3. Analyze health teaching strategies that enhance retention of new material. Think of two specific techniques you can use to involve chronically ill children in prevention activities. Contrast these activities with those of an elderly adult. Develop a teaching plan that incorporates use of visual aids for each population.

## ■ REFERENCES

Agius, R. (2003). *Airborne environmental pollutants and asthma.* Retrieved October 21, 2004 from http://www.agius.com/hew/resource/asthma.htm

Antai-Otong, D. (1995). *Psychiatric nursing biological and behavioral concepts.* Philadelphia: W. B. Saunders.

Bromberger, J. T., Harlow, S. A., Kravitz, H. M., & Cordal, A. (2004). Racial/ethnic differences in the prevalence of depressive symptoms among middle-aged women: The study of women's health across the nation (SWAN). *American Journal of Public Health, 94*(8), 1378–1385.

Bullington, J., Nordemar, K., & Sjostrom-Flanagan, C. (2003). Meaning out of chaos: A way to understand chronic pain. *Scandinavian Journal of Caring Sciences, 17*(4), 325–331.

Centers for Disease Control and Prevention. (2008a). *Chronic disease overview.* Retrieved November 8, 2008, from http://www.cdc.gov/nccdphp/overview.htm

Centers for Disease Control and Prevention. (2008b). *Death rates by age and age-adjusted death rates for the 15 leading causes of death in 2005: United States, 1999–2005.* Retrieved November 8, 2008, from http://www.disastercenter.com/cdc/Leading%20Cause%20of%20Death%201999-2005.html

Cochrane, J. (2003). The experience of uncertainty for individuals with HIV/AIDS and the palliative care paradigm. *International Journal of Palliative Nursing, 9,* 9.

Colvin, G. (2004). Get ready for a life and death battle over obesity. *Fortune, 150*(1), 64.

Coon, S. K., & Coleman, E. A. (2004). Keep moving: Patients with myeloma talk about exercise and fatigue. *Oncology Nursing Forum, 31*(6), 1127–1135.

Crumbie, S. A., Conley, V. M., & Burman, M. E. (2004). Advanced practice nursing model for comprehensive care with chronic illness. *Advanced Nursing Science, 27,* 1.

Davidhizar, R., & Shearer, R. (1997). Helping the patient with disability achieve high-level wellness. *Rehabilitation Nursing, 22,* 3.

Department of Health and Human Services (DHHS). (2000). *Healthy people 2010.* Washington, DC: U.S. Government Printing Office.

Dewesbury, G., Clarke, K., Randall, D., Rouncefield, M., & Somerville, I. (2004). The anti-social model of disability. *Disability and Society, 19*(2).

Dosh, S. A. (2004). Diagnosis of heart failure in adults. *American Academy of Family Physicians.* Retrieved November 8, 2008, from http://www.aafp.org/afp/20041201/2145.html

Dumit, J. (1998). Symptomatic, ill, and structurally damned: Notes on liminal creativity and social movements. Unpublished work.

Friedan, T. R. (2004). Asleep at the switch: Local public health and chronic disease. [Editorial]. *American Journal of Public Health, 94*(12), 2059–2061.

Gelbach, S. H., Fournier, M., & Bigelow, C. (2002). Recognition of osteoporosis by primary care physicians. *American Journal of Public Health, 92*(2), 292–295.

Goodwin, D. L., & Compton, S. G. (2004). Physical activity experiences of women aging with disabilities. *Adapted Physical Activity Quarterly, 21,* 2.

Grey, M., Knafl, K., & McCorkle, R. (2006). A framework for the study of self and family management of chronic conditions. *Nursing Outlook, 54,* 278–286.

Health Resources and Services Administration. (2002). *Nurse practitioner primary care competencies in specialty areas: Adult, family, gerontological, pediatric, and women's health.* Washington, DC: U.S. Department of Health and Human Services, Health Resources and Services Administration, Bureau of Health Professions, Division of Nursing.

Herbert, R., & Gregor, S. (1997). Quality of life and coping strategies of patients with COPD. *Rehabilitation Nursing, 22,* 4.

Hickey, J. V. (2003). *The clinical practice of neurological and neurosurgical nursing.* Philadelphia: Lippincott Williams & Wilkins.

Hilton, E. L., & Henderson, L. J. (2003). The nature, meanings, and dynamics of lived experiences of syringomyelia in a middle-aged man: A phenomenological case study. *SCI Nursing, 20,* 1.

Hinds, P. S. (2004). The hopes and wishes of adolescents with cancer and the nursing care that helps. *Oncology Nursing Forum, 31*(5), 927–944.

Hirao-Try, Y. (2003). Hypertension and women: Gender specific differences. *Clinical Excellence for Nurse Practitioners, 7*(1–2), 4–8.

Hurst, R. (2000). To revise or not to revise. *Disability and Society, 12*(3), 325–340.

ICIC. (2008). *The chronic care model elements: Delivery system design.* Retrieved November 8, 2008, from http://www.improvingchroniccare.org/index.php?p=The_Chronic_Care_Model&s=2

Imrie, R. (2004). Demystifying disability: A review of the International Classification of Functioning, Disability, and Health. *Sociology of Health and Illness, 26*(3), 287–305.

Ingersoll, G. L., McIntosh, E., & Williams, M. (2000). Nurse-sensitive outcomes of advanced practice. *Journal of Advanced Nursing, 32,* 1272–1281.

Jaffe, H. (2004). Whatever happened to the U.S. AIDS epidemic? *Science, 305,* 5688.

Johnson, J. (1991). Adjustment following a heart attack. In J. M. Morse & J. I. Johnson (Eds.), *The illness experience* (pp. 13–88). Newbury Park, CA: Sage.

Jung, S. K. (2004). A young onset Parkinson's patient: A case study. *Journal of Neuroscience Nursing, 36*(5), 273–277.

Kaplan, D. (2008). *The definition of disability.* The Center for an Accessible Society. Retrieved November 8, 2008, from http://www.accessiblesociety.org/topics/demographics-identity/dkaplanpaper.htm

Klang, B., & Clyne, N. (1997). Well-being and functional ability in uremic patients before and after having started dialysis treatment. *Scandinavian Journal of Caring Science, 11*, 3.

Klein, S. J., Cruz, H., O'Connell, D., Scully, M. A., & Birkhead, G. (2005). A public health approach to "prevention with positives": The New York State HIV/AIDS Service Delivery System. *Journal of Health Management Practice, 11*(1), 7–17.

Koch, T. (2001). Disability and difference: Balancing social and physical constructions. *Journal of Medical Ethics, 27*(6), 370–376.

Landrigan, P. J., Lioy, G., Thurston, G., et al. (2004). Health and environmental consequences of the World Trade Center disaster. *Environmental Health Perspectives, 112*, 6.

Lindgren, C. L. (1996). Chronic sorrow in persons with Parkinson's disease and their spouses. *Scholarly Inquiry for Nursing Practice, 10*, 4.

Lopes, D., Piementa, C., Kurita, A., & Oliveira, A. C. (2003). Caregivers of patients with chronic pain: Responses to care. *International Journal of Nursing Terminologies and Classifications, 15*(1), 5–14.

Lubkin, I. M., & Larsen, P. D. (2002). *Chronic illness impact and interventions* (5th ed.) Sudbury, MA: Jones and Bartlett.

Luckman, J. (1997). *Saunders manual of nursing care.* Philadelphia: W. B. Saunders.

Manila Times. (2004, April 23). *Health epidemics top agenda of Asian health ministers' meeting.* Retrieved January 9, 2005, from http://www.manilatimes.net/national/2004/apr/23/yehey/world/2004423wor3.html

Mayo, L. (1956). *Chronic illness.* Paper presented at the meeting of the Commission on Chronic Illness, Washington, DC.

McCorkle, R., Robinson, L., Nuamah, I., Lev, E., & Benoliel, J. Q. (1998). The effects of home nursing care for patients during terminal illness on the bereaved psychological distress. *Nursing Research, 47*, 2–10.

McCorkle, R., Strumpf, N., Nuamah, I. F., et al. (2000). A specialized home care intervention improves surgical care among older post-surgical cancer patients. *Journal of the American Geriatric Society, 48*, 1701–1713.

Miller, J. F. (1992). *Coping with chronic illness: Overcoming powerlessness* (2nd ed.) Philadelphia: F. A. Davis.

Mitchell, C., & Linsk, N. L. (2004). A multidimensional conceptual framework for understanding HIV/AIDS as a chronic long-term illness. *Social Work, 49*(3), 469–477.

Molyneux, D. H. (2004, July 24). Neglected diseases but unrecognized successes—challenges and opportunities for infectious disease control. *Lancet, 364.*

Morgan, M. (1996). The meaning of high blood pressure among Afro-Caribbean and white patients. In D. Kelleher & S. Hillier (Eds.), *Researching cultural differences in health.* London: Routledge.

Mosby. (2007). *Mosby's Dictionary of medicine, nursing, and health professionals* (8th ed.). St. Louis: Elsevier Health Sciences.

National Center for Chronic Disease Prevention. (2008). *Racial and ethnic approaches to community health: Finding solutions to health disparities: At a glance 2008.* Retrieved November 8, 2008, from http://www.cdc.gov/nccdphp/publications/aag/reach.htm

National Coalition on Health Care. (2008). *Health insurance coverage.* Retrieved September 15, 2008, from http://www.nchc.org/facts/coverage.shtml

National Family Caregivers Association. (2008). *About NFCA.* Retrieved September 15, 2008, from http://www.thefamilycaregiver.org/about_nfca/

Noakes, M., Foster, P., Keogh, J. B., & Clifton, P. M. (2004). Meal replacements as effective as weight-loss diets for treating obesity in adults with features of metabolic syndrome 1, 2. *Journal of Nutrition, 134*(8), 1894–1899.

Pampel, F. (2003). Declining sex differences in mortality from lung cancer in high-income nations. *Demography, 40*, 1.

Partnership for Solutions. (2001). *Statistics & research: Prevalance.* Retrieved November 8, 2008, from http://www.partnershipforsolutions.org/statistics/prevalence.html

Peters, R. M. (2004). Racism and hypertension among African Americans. *Western Journal of Nursing Research, 26*(6), 612–631.

Phillips, L. J. (2005). Analysis of the explanatory model of health promotion and quality of life in chronic disabling conditions. *Rehabilitation Nursing, 30*(1), 18–24.

Powelson, J. (2004). New protocols in kidney transplantation. *Fact Sheet: Brigham and Women's Hospital.*

Pugh-Clarke, K. (2004). Quality of life and symptomatology in chronic renal insufficiency. *Nephrology Nursing Journal, 31*, 2.

Scambler, G. (2004). Re-framing stigma: Felt and enacted stigma and challenges to the sociology of chronic and disabling conditions. *Social Theory and Health, 2*, 29–46.

Schaefer, K. M. (1995). Women living in paradox: Loss and discovery in chronic illness. *Holistic Nursing Practice, 9*, 3.

Secrest, J. (2005). Commentary. *Rehabilitation Nursing, 30*(1), 24.

Sheehan, N. W., & Oakes, C. E. (2003). Bringing assisted living services into congregate housing: Residents' perspectives. *Gerontologist, 43*, 5.

Small, G. W., Birkett, M., Meyers, B. S., Loran, L. M., Bystricky, A., & Nemeroff, C. B. (1996). Impact of physical illness on quality of life and antidepressant response in geriatric major depression. *Journal of the American Geriatric Society, 44*, 10.

Smith, S. (1974). The psychology of illness. In V. A. Christopherson, P. P. Coulter, & M. O. Wolanin (Eds.), *Rehabilitation nursing.* New York: McGraw-Hill.

Snively, C. S., & Gutierrez, C. (2004). Chronic kidney disease: Prevention and treatment of common complications. *American Family Physician.* Retrieved January 3, 2005, from http://www.aafp.org/afp

Sorenson, S. B., & Wiebe, D. J. (2004). Weapons in the lives of battered women. *American Journal of Public Health, 94*(8), 1412–1417.

Spillman, B. C. (2004). Changes in elderly disability rates and the implications for health care utilization and cost. *Milbank Quarterly, 82*(1), 157–194.

Strauss, A. L. (1975). *Chronic illness and the quality of life.* St. Louis: Mosby.

Strunin, L., & Boden, L. I. (2004). Family consequences of chronic back pain. *Social Science and Medicine, 58*, 1385–1393.

Sumner, J. F. (2005). Caring—The foundation of advanced practice nursing. *Topics in Advanced Practice Nursing eJournal.* Available from http://www.medscape.com

Thompson, S. C., Futterman, A. M., Galagher-Thomas, D., Rose, J. J., & Lovett, S. B. (1993). Social support and care-giving burden in families of frail elders. *Journal of Gerontology: Social Sciences, 48*, 5.

U.S. Cancer Statistics Working Group. (2007). *United States cancer statistics: 2004 incidence and mortality.* Atlanta, GA: Department of Health and Human Service, Centers for Disease Control and Prevention, and National Cancer Institute.

Ward, R. P., Kugelmas, M., & Libsch, K. D. (2004). Management of hepatitis C: Evaluating suitability for drug therapy. *American Family Physician, 69,* 6.

Whitney, C. M. (2004). Maintaining the square: How older adults with Parkinson's disease sustain quality in their lives. *Journal of Gerontological Nursing, 30*(1), 28.

Wickham, R. S., Goodin, S., & Lynch, K. (2004). Demystifying CINV control in the complex aging patient: Assessing the complexities of the aging oncology pt. *Spotlight on Symposia, ONS News, 19,* 9.

Wilson, J. S. (1992). Our nation's walking wounded: The chronically ill. *Home Healthcare Nurse, 5,* 5.

Wilson, K. M., & Satterfield, D. W. (2007, July). Where are we to be in these times? The place of chronic disease prevention in community health promotion. *Preventing Chronic Disease* [serial online], *4*(3). Available at http://www.cdc.gov/pcd/issues/2007/jul/07_0014.htm

Wolf, Z. R. (1994). Seeking harmony. Chronic physical illness. In P. Munhall (Ed.), *In women's experience.* New York: National League for Nursing.

World Health Organization (WHO). (2001). *International classification of functioning, disability, and health.* Geneva: Author.

Zack, M. M., Moriarity, D. G., Stroup, D. F., Ford, E. S., & Mokdad, A. H. (2004, August). *Adult Americans health-related quality of life has recently gotten worse.* Retrieved November 8, 2008, from http//www.cdc.gov/nccdphp/press/trends.htm

# CHAPTER 24
# Disasters in the Community

Karen Saucier Lundy and Janie B. Butts

Visit **http://nursing.jbpub.com/communityhealth** for interactive exercises, review questions, Web links, and more.

Nurses are some of the first to respond during times of disaster. Think of recent events in New York City and New Orleans—do you know nurses who gave of themselves?

Today our fellow citizens, our way of life, our very freedom came under attack in a series of deliberate and deadly terrorist acts.

—*President George W. Bush, following the September 11, 2001, terrorist attacks*

Crises, such as Hurricane Katrina and the unprecedented "disaster of disasters" in New Orleans, show society speeded up, its evolution compressed into a moment in time. The poor and dispossessed, the weak and the sick, always suffer disproportionately. And how society responds—or doesn't—is a reflection of its values, its way of organizing and caring for people.

—*Professor Jennifer Leaning, Harvard University, School of Public Health*

If I don't know my options, I don't have any.

—*Diana Korte*

Noble souls, through dust and heat,
Rise from disaster and defeat
The stronger.

—*Henry Wadsworth Longfellow, "The Sifting of Peter," 1880*

Hurricane Katrina resulted in human loss that exceeded our imagination. The losses go beyond counting, as numbers of deaths, homes destroyed, and jobs and businesses lost cannot count the irreplaceable: lives cut short, health and quality of life compromised, a way of life permanently lost and cultures permanently altered. Individual stories capture these losses, but not the magnitude of the challenges that face us.

—*Betsy Foxman, 2006*

Think about the last time that you saw a television report on a terrorist event or saw the devastation of Hurricane Katrina. What went through your mind? If the context of the event were outside the United States, would you have viewed it differently? If you had a personal experience with either of these disasters, did it change your view of the events? How can community health nurses help communities heal after a disaster? What are ways that we can all protect ourselves and our families and communities from the catastrophic health damage from disasters?

## CHAPTER FOCUS

**The Nature of Disasters**
- Definitions and Types of Disasters
- NA-TECH
- Disaster Characteristics
- Global Disaster Issues
- Natural Disaster Reduction
- Disaster as a Global Public Health Problem
- Populations at Risk in Disasters

**Stages of Disaster**

**Disaster Planning**
- Steps in the Disaster Process
- The Disaster Plan
- Disaster Management

**Disaster Response**
- Response and Recovery
- Levels of Disaster Response
- National Disaster Medical System

- Federal Emergency Management Agency and Disaster Responsiveness and Recovery
- Other Disaster Agencies
- Evacuation
- Rescue
- Triage
- Disaster Shelters

**Role of the Community Health Nurse in Disasters**
- General Functions of the Community Health Nurse
- Specific Nursing Approaches
- Shelter Management and Care

**Disaster Recovery**
- Effects on Survivors
- Special Survivor Populations: Elders and Children
- Collective Trauma: The Loss of Community
- Nurses' Reactions to Disasters
- Prevention Strategies for Nurses

## QUESTIONS TO CONSIDER

After reading this chapter, you will know the answers to the following questions:

1. What are the categories and types of disasters community health nurses might deal with?
2. What are the variables by which disasters can be understood?
3. What is a global disaster?
4. Who are the populations most at risk in a disaster? Why?
5. What are the stages of disaster, and how does each stage affect both the disaster workers and the affected population?
6. What are the steps in the disaster process?
7. What are the characteristics of a disaster plan?
8. What are the common elements of a disaster plan?
9. What is disaster response? What are the different levels of response?
10. What is disaster triage? Why and how should it be implemented?
11. What is the role of the community health nurse in the disaster relief process?
12. Which specific approaches should a community health nurse use to mitigate human and material losses in a disaster?
13. What happens to the survivors in a disaster? How can a community health nurse promote recovery after a disaster?
14. Which factors can place individuals in a vulnerable position?
15. Why are children and elderly at greater risk during a disaster? What can be done to intervene?
16. What are the sources of stress for the disaster workers, and how can they be managed?

## KEY TERMS

Department of Homeland Security (DHS)
Disaster
Disaster planning
Disaster triage
Emergency
Emergency stage

Federal Emergency Management Agency (FEMA)
Human-generated (human-made) disasters
Impact stage
Interdisaster stage
Level I response

Level II response
Level III response
Level IV response
Major disaster
National Disaster Medical System (NDMS)
Natural disasters

Post-traumatic stress disorder (PTSD)
Predisaster stage
Reconstruction (rehabilitation) stage
Recovery
Response

DISASTER! THE VERY WORD can evoke fear, panic, and a pounding heart. A major disaster occurs almost daily somewhere in the world: plane crashes, floods, hurricanes, tornadoes, fires, earthquakes, acts of terrorism, droughts, famines, and wars. Who among us can ever forget the images of the elderly and others dying in the New Orleans Superdome and Convention Center, following Hurricane Katrina, people sitting on rooftops and on highways pleading to be rescued, Herculean rescues of patients from area hospitals, and bodies floating in the putrid water that literally covered the entire city of New Orleans. We will most likely never know the full impact on people's lives of dealing with the loss of those who died as a result of the flooding and coping with being transported to other states and shelters.

The community health nurse can assist communities in preparing for disasters such as Hurricane Katrina and limiting their damage in the aftermath. Communities can become stronger and healthier as a result. But what are the real threats of disaster? How can community health nurses be better prepared to strengthen communities in their responses to disasters? This chapter will help you answer these questions as you develop a better understanding of the nature of disasters and learn about the various levels of disaster preparedness in which community health nurses are involved. Start by reading the feature about the familiar *Titanic* disaster of 1912 (Box 24-1) as an illustration of the role of preparedness in mediating the harmful effects of both natural and human-generated disasters.

When Hurricane Katrina made landfall on the Mississippi Gulf Coast and near New Orleans, Louisiana, in August 2005, Americans became keenly aware of how a natural disaster can threaten the health of an entire population. Through the images on television of people stranded on rooftops, trapped in the New Orleans Superdome in a makeshift disaster shelter, and facing the total destruction of the Mississippi Gulf Coast, we were all affected in some way from the ravages of this "disaster of disasters." More than 1,300 people died, many because of levee failures in New Orleans, and Hurricane Katrina earned the dubious distinction of being the worst natural disaster in U.S. history. Since the September 11, 2001, terrorist attacks on the World Trade Center, in Pennsylvania, and at the Pentagon, the U.S. public has become much more aware of the devastating national and global effects of terrorism as a current disaster threat. The United States has experienced a string of unprecedented disasters since the late 1980s, including major earthquakes, hurricanes, tropical storms, floods, landslides, volcanic eruptions, severe winter storms, and wildfires.

Outside the United States, the Indian Ocean tsunami occurred on December 26, 2004, following a 9.1-magnitude earthquake; it killed more than 200,000 people in Indonesia, India, Sri Lanka, Thailand, and many other countries as far away as South Africa. Entire towns and villages were swept away. In South Asia, more than 73,000 people died and tens of thousands were injured when an earthquake measuring 7.6 on the Richter scale struck Pakistan and other parts of

## BOX 24-1

### The Making of a Disaster: The Sinking of the "Unsinkable" *Titanic*

#### Nondisaster or Interdisaster Phase

The *Titanic* was on its maiden voyage when it sank on April 14, 1912. This ship was the crown jewel of the White Star Line, a mammoth 46-ton British liner of incomparable luxury, three football fields long and eleven stories high, which was the world's largest and purportedly safest vessel on the water. On this maiden voyage, the *Titanic* had as its passengers both British and American aristocracy, along with immigrants coming to the "New World" with promises of a new life. The boat deck and bridge were 70 feet above water. According to White Star Line documentation, a "trial test" of 6 to 7 hours total was conducted 1 month before leaving Great Britain. This trial consisted of turning circles and compass adjustment; also, the ship sailed "a short time" at full steam, but never at full speed before passengers boarded.

The crew and officers of the *Titanic* (numbering 899) joined the ship a few hours before the passengers and went through only one drill: They lowered two lifeboats on starboard side into water. No evidence of crew duties being delineated as to task or role in event of disaster were noted by Congress. Congressional hearings found that the crew did not know their "proper stations" or assignment until after passengers had already boarded in Queenstown, Ireland.

There were 1,324 passengers on board the ship, and together with 899 crew members, a total of 2,223 persons were on the maiden voyage of the *Titanic*. Congress found no evidence of passengers having any orientation in disaster procedures. There were 1,176 lifeboats and life jackets for all persons on board. The *Titanic* was considered "unsinkable," having been constructed with special watertight bulkhead compartments that could be sealed off if the ship took on water. There was no evidence of a disaster plan or safety instructions posted or provided to passengers, nor were crew members prepared for their roles in the event of a disaster. The crew staffed the *Titanic* round the clock and had lookouts posted in the crow's nest for any water-related hazards.

#### Predisaster or Warning Phase

The *Titanic* had received several ice warnings on the third day of the voyage, and the captain noted them. On the day of the disaster, a warning message cited icebergs within 5 miles of the track that the *Titanic* was following, very near the place where the accident occurred. Congressional hearings revealed that despite repeated warnings, no general discussion took place among the officers, no conference was called to consider these warnings, and no heed was given to them. The speed was not reduced, the lookout was not increased, and the only extra vigilance noted was from the officer of the watch, who gave instructions to the lookouts to "keep a sharp lookout for ice." The speed of the ship had been gradually increased, and just before the collision, the ship was making her maximum speed of the voyage. Passengers had no advance knowledge of any possible risks of the ship related to the icebergs.

#### Impact Phase

At 10:13 P.M. on Sunday, April 14, the lookout signaled the bridge and telephoned the officer of the watch with this message: "Iceberg right ahead." The officer of the watch immediately ordered the quartermaster at the wheel to put the helm "hard astarboard" and reverse the engines. The *Titanic* immediately struck the ice, and the impact caused the vessel to roll slightly. The impact, which ripped a hole in the steel plating of the ship, was not violent enough to disturb the crew or passengers. During this time, the damage was reported by crew members from the boiler room related to water coming in; the captain began inspecting the ship for damage. Passengers were still not aware of the accident.

#### Emergency Phase

The reports by the captain after various inspections of the ship revealed that the compartments were rapidly filling with water and that the bow of the ship was sinking deeper and deeper. Through the open hatches, water promptly began overflowing into the other bulkheads and decks. No emergency alarm was sounded, no whistles were blown, and no systematic warning was given the passengers.

Within approximately 15 minutes after his inspection, the captain issued a distress call to ships in the area. The call was heard by several ships in the vicinity. The *Carpathia*, which was 58 miles away, responded to the distress signal by turning immediately toward the sinking ship. Other ships also attempted to sail toward the sinking ship but were too far away to be of any reasonable assistance. The closest ship, the *Californian*, was only 19 miles north of the *Titanic* but did not attempt to rescue the ailing ship. Proceedings indicate that the crew of the *Titanic* began firing distress rockets at frequent intervals and that the crew of the *Californian* saw them. The captain of the *Californian* failed to heed the warning signals and was chastised by Congress for "indifference or carelessness" and for not responding to the *Titanic*'s distress calls in accordance with the dictates of international usage and law.

The captain immediately gave the signal to retrieve the lifeboats, with the order to put women and children in the boats first. The proceedings report that the lack of preparation at this time was most noticeable. There was general chaos as passengers learned of the accident from each other, from some crew members who knocked on cabin doors, and from being awakened by the movement of people running on the ship.

"There was no system adopted for loading the boats; there was great indecision as to the deck from which boats were to be loaded; there was wide diversity of opinion as to the number of crew necessary to man each boat; there was no direction whatever to the number of passengers to be carried by each boat, and no uniformity in loading them" (p. 548). In some boats, there would be only women and children; in others there would be an equal proportion of men and women. Only a

*(continues)*

**BOX 24-1**

**The Making of a Disaster: The Sinking of the "Unsinkable" *Titanic*—cont'd**

few of the lifeboats were loaded to capacity; most were only partially loaded, which resulted in needless losses. If all of the lifeboats had been fully loaded at capacity for 1,176 persons, more than the 706 persons could have reasonably survived.

Furthermore, the proceedings noted that if the sea had been rough (which it wasn't), it is questionable whether any of the lifeboats would have reached the water without being damaged or destroyed. The lifeboats were suspended 70 feet above the water, and in the event of the ship's rolling (with a rough sea), the boats would have swung out from the side of the ship and then crashed back into the ship as it was being lowered. Also, had the survivors been concentrated in fewer boats once on the water, the staff could have returned and rescued more passengers.

Once the ship sank at 12:47 A.M., it broke in half and people died from drowning, exposure, and trauma; 1,517 persons died, 706 survived. Survivors of the *Titanic* reported rowing toward the lights of a ship in the distance, which has now been established as those of the *Californian*. There were questions about the way passengers were evacuated relative to whether they were in first-, second-, or third-class accommodation. Sixty percent of first-class passengers survived, 42% of second-class passengers survived, and only 25% of third-class passengers survived. These statistics suggest that there may have been a distinction in the warning and evacuation based on class accommodation. Twenty-five percent of the crew were saved.

The rescue of survivors came from the *Carpathia* crew and eventually from the crew of the *Californian*. After a thorough search, ships returned to New York and Nova Scotia with the survivors. A brief burial prayer service for the dead was held at 8:30 A.M. by the captain of the *Carpathia*. Public media notification occurred the evening of April 15, 1912.

**Reconstruction or Rehabilitation Phase**

The wreck of the *Titanic* represents in myth and reality a disaster beyond human comprehension at a time when technological advances were seen as our defense against the disasters of nature. Because of lack of preparedness and lack of planning for ship disasters, technology could not have saved the passengers on the *Titanic*.

The recommendations that evolved from the *Titanic* hearings held by Congress in May 1912 were no less than revolutionary in terms of safety preparedness. One was that inspection certificates would be contingent on sufficient lifeboats to accommodate every passenger and every member of the crew. Inspection certificates that mandate these requirements would apply to all boats who carry passengers from ports of the United States. Lifeboats should be positioned in such a way that they would not be subject to damage from height related to water level. There would be no fewer than four members of the crew, trained in handling boats, on each lifeboat. All crew members assigned to this duty would be drilled in lowering and rowing the lifeboats not less than twice per month and the "fact of such drill or practice should be noted in the log." Recommendations also included assigning passengers to lifeboats before sailing and posting the shortest route to the lifeboats in each room. Two electric searchlights were to be present on boats carrying more than 100 passengers. A radio operator must be on duty at all times, 24 hours a day. And finally, all ships from that point on would be required to meet construction standards related to watertight compartments and hulls.

*Source:* Kuntz, T. (Ed.). *The Titanic disaster hearings: The official transcripts of the 1912 Senate investigation.* New York: Pocket Books.

---

the region in October 2004. The thousands who remained homeless continued to suffer disease and exposure to the elements from the aftermath of these two disasters, and the death toll continued to climb 2 years later (Burnham & Abdallah, 2008; Garheld & Hamid, 2006; Hassmiller, 2007; Telford & Cosgrave, 2007).

From 1991 to 2005, almost 1 million people were killed worldwide from natural disasters alone. In the last two decades, natural disasters such as earthquakes, tsunamis, hurricanes, floods, and volcanic eruptions have adversely affected the lives of at least 800 million more people. Floods continue to be the most common natural disaster in the world.

Natural disasters result in more deaths and property destruction in developing and least-developed countries. During 2005, natural disasters cost the world a record $150 billion. Most of the increase in natural disaster damage was due to a combination of deforestation and climate change, including global warming (EM-DAT: The OFDA/CRED International Disaster Database, 2006).

🖉 NOTE THIS! •————

Two-thirds of families still do not have basic emergency plans, even after 9/11 and Hurricane Katrina in 2005. The report sponsored by the Council for Excellence in Government also found:

- People 65 and older were less likely to be prepared than younger people.

- People with higher education and income levels were likely to be better prepared than others.

- Hispanics are less prepared than whites and African Americans.

- Parents of schoolchildren who know about their school's emergency plans are likely to be much better prepared, but most parents did not know details of the school emergency plans.

- Full-time employees who know about and have practiced company disaster plans are better prepared.

What are the implications of these findings for community health nurses? ⊙

*Source:* Peter D. Hart Research, & Public Opinion Strategies. (2005). *The aftershock of Katrina and Rita: People not moved to prepare.* Washington, DC: The Council for Excellence in Government and the American Red Cross.

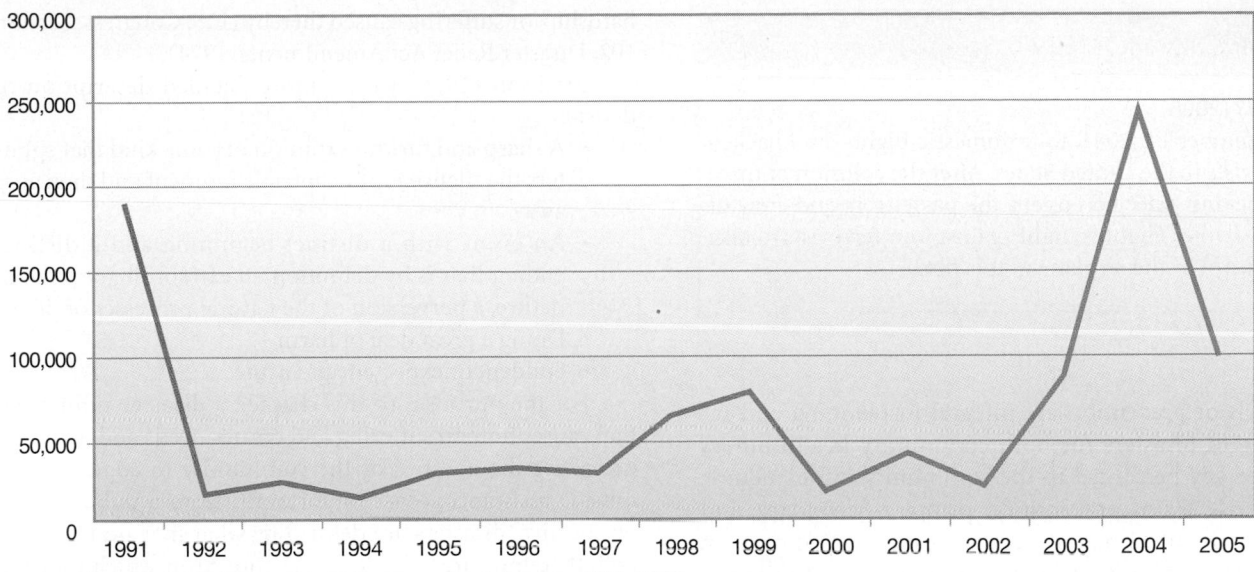

Number of people worldwide reported killed by natural disasters 1991–2005

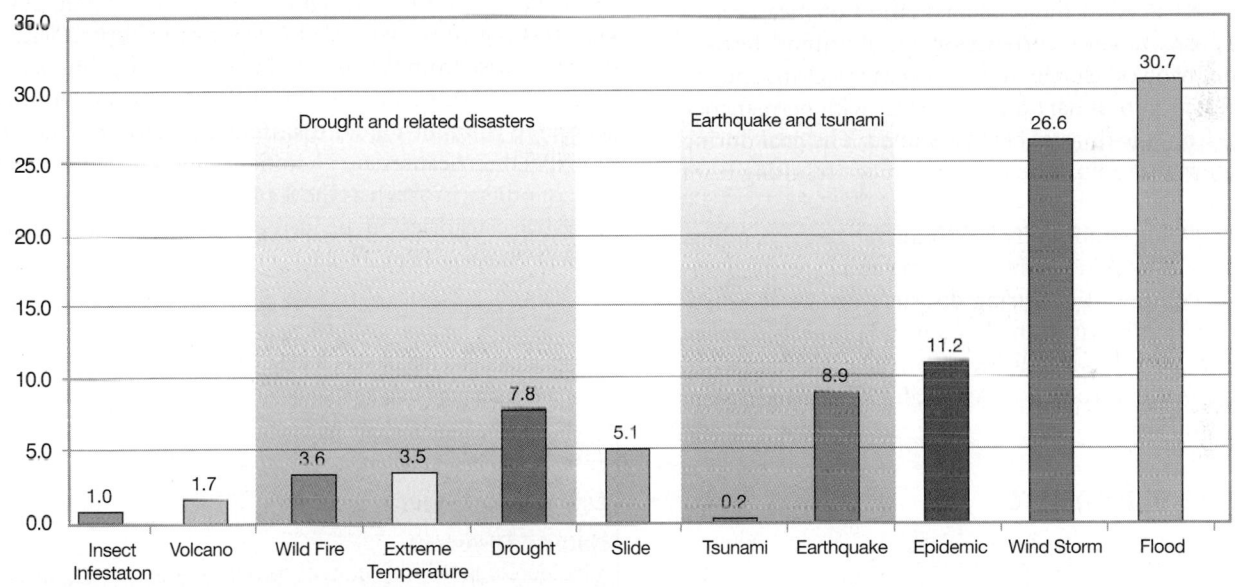

Distribution in percentage of natural disasters by type 1991–2005
International Strategy of Disaster Reduction

*Source of data*: EM-DAT: The OFDA/CRED International Disaster Database—www.emdat.net—Université Catholique de Louvain—Brussels—Belgium. Reprinted by permission.

Community health nurses sometimes feel unprepared to react competently in a community disaster situation. For most practicing nurses, formal disaster education or training is not comprehensive. Therefore, the training that is received by nurses does not include the whole picture on levels of preparedness, which range from the basic emergency department response to the highest level of response from the community infrastructure. The disaster training that pertains to nurses' agency positions is usually the only training received, which often limits their understanding of the community's perspective on preparedness and response (Burnham & Abdallah, 2008; Salama et al., 2004).

Although the training delivered may not be comprehensive in many institutions, an important goal for community health nurses is for them to feel a greater sense of disaster preparedness. When community health nurses are prepared for disaster, research has indicated that communities benefit. Research has revealed that improved organization in delivering nursing care, planning the disaster response, and understanding the effects of disasters on families, communities, health professionals, and, ultimately, society can prevent or reduce the detrimental short- and long-term effects of disasters (Noji, 1997; Landesman et al., 2005; Salama, 2004).

Levels of prevention are integral in planning and responding to disasters for both community health nurses and other key personnel in the community infrastructure. The three levels of prevention—primary, secondary, and tertiary—are integrated at certain points in this chapter. Primary prevention is aimed at reducing the probability of disease, death, and disability resulting from a disaster. Secondary prevention includes the immediate identification of disaster problems and the implementation of measures to treat and prevent their recurrence or complications. Tertiary prevention involves rehabilitation of disaster victims and the community to an optimal functional level, with permanency of change from the disaster being assumed. The goal during rehabilitation is to minimize further damage resulting from the disaster.

By increasing community health nurses' understanding, confidence, and skill in disaster planning and care, the damage to our communities during disasters can be lessened. Not only can lives be saved and human and property damage reduced, but also the overall health of the community can be strengthened (Burnham & Abdellah, 2008; Landesman, 2005; Garcia, 1985).

## The Nature of Disasters

### Definitions and Types of Disasters

Some of the many distinctions made between disasters include the definitions of an emergency and a major disaster. An **emergency** is any hurricane, tornado, storm, flood, high water, wind-driven water, tidal wave, earthquake, volcanic eruption, landslide, mudslide, snowstorm, drought, fire, explosion, or other catastrophe in any part of the United States that requires federal emergency assistance to supplement state and local efforts to save lives and protect property, public health, and safety or to avert or lessen the threat of a disaster (U.S. Congress, Section 102, Disaster Relief Act Amendments, 1974). A **major disaster** may be any of the events listed as an emergency in any part of the United States that, in the determination of the U.S. president, causes damage of sufficient severity above and beyond emergency services by the federal government to supplement the efforts and available resources of states, local governments, and disaster relief organizations in alleviating the damage, loss,

hardship, or suffering caused thereby (U.S. Congress, Section 102, Disaster Relief Act Amendments, 1974).

Erickson (1976) gave a more detailed description of disaster:

- A sharp and furious eruption of some kind that splinters the silence for one terrible moment and then goes away
- An event with a distinct beginning and a distinct ending that is by definition an extraordinary freak of nature, a perversion of the natural processes of life
- Doing a great deal of harm
- Sudden, unexpected, and acute

For the purposes of this chapter, a **disaster** is an event that causes human suffering and creates needs and demands exceeding the abilities of the community to cope without outside assistance. Most importantly, from a public health perspective, disasters are defined by what they do to people and, therefore, are relative to the context in which they occur. What results in a disaster in one community might not necessarily be considered a disaster in a different community (Noji, 1997; Telford & Cosgrave, 2007; Landesman, 2005). Disasters fall into two broad categories or types: **Natural disasters** arise from the forces of nature, such as hurricanes, tornadoes, earthquakes, and volcanic eruptions; **human-generated (human-made) disasters** are those in which the principal direct causes are identifiable human actions, deliberate or otherwise, such as the September 11 terrorist attacks. These two categories can be further subdivided into different types of disasters (Box 24-2).

---

**BOX 24-2**

**Categories and Types of Disasters**

**Natural Disasters**
- Meteorological: hurricanes, tornados, hailstorms, snowstorms, and droughts
- Topological: landslides, avalanches, mudslides, and floods
- Disasters that originate underground: earthquakes, volcanic eruptions, and tidal waves
- Bacteriological: communicable disease epidemics (e.g., *Ebola* virus) and insect swarms (e.g., locusts)

**Human-Generated Disasters**
- Warfare: conventional warfare (bombardment, blockage, and siege) and nonconventional warfare (nuclear, chemical, and biological; acts of terrorism)
- Civil disasters: riots and demonstrations
- Accidents: transportation (planes, trucks, automobiles, trains, and ships); structural collapse (buildings, dams, bridges, mines, and other structures); explosion; fire; chemical (toxic waste and pollution); and biological (sanitation)

*Sources*: Modified from Garcia, 1985; Noji, 1997.

### ■ NA-TECH

Although disasters can be grouped according to the stated definitions, in reality the distinction between natural and human-generated disasters is often blurred, because a natural disaster can trigger secondary disasters, such as explosions, fires, floods, and toxins released into the air after an earthquake. Such combination-type synergistic disasters are referred to as NA-TECH disasters, a NA-TECH disaster is a technological accident triggered by a natural event. (Natural-technological = NA-TECH). An example of a NA-TECH disaster occurred in the former Soviet Union when windstorms spread radioactive materials across the country, increasing by up to 50% the land area contaminated in an earlier nuclear disaster at Chernobyl (see Box 24-10). Hurricane Katrina and the flooding of New Orleans, after levee failure following landfall in Mississippi, is also an example of an NA-TECH disaster (Noji, 1997; Norwalk, 2007).

**❝** *There can be no winners in a world of man-made epidemics.* **❞**

— *King Hussein, 1996*

As noted on page 573, floods are the most common natural disaster in the world, accounting for more than one-third of all disasters in the past 10 years. The number of floods worldwide increased 57% in 2005 as compared to the previous 5 years (ISDR, 2006). One example of a horrendous flood, although not necessarily a typical disaster, was the Mississippi River Flood of 1927, which has been cited as one of the worst natural disasters in U.S. history. In 1927, the Mississippi River swept across a geographic area larger than Massachusetts, Connecticut, New Hampshire, and Vermont combined and resulted in water as deep as 30 feet on the land, stretching from Illinois and Missouri south to the Gulf of Mexico and New Orleans. This flood forced almost 1 million people from their homes and resulted in thousands of deaths.

Many of the dead were still being pulled out of the Mississippi River at New Orleans even months after the flood. When more than 40,000 homes were destroyed close to where the dam broke in Mississippi, camps were set up in the Confederate National Park in Vicksburg. American Red Cross nurses (Box 24-3), nurses from the Mississippi State Department of Health, and nurses from other states were assigned to relief efforts for several months in the spring of 1927. A total of 383 nurses worked in the Mississippi flood disaster. Nurses worked in these refugee camps, battling typhoid and nutritional deficiencies such as pellagra. The waters from the Mississippi did not recede for 3 months (Barry, 1997; Sabin, 1998).

Of course, a more recent flooding disaster occurred after Hurricane Katrina, when thousands of persons in New Orleans were left stranded after the levees broke, flooding the entire city with several feet of water. This unprecedented flooding left a major American city underwater for more

than 4 weeks after the hurricane (Nigg, Barnshaw, & Torres, 2006). The major levee breaches in the city included breaches at the 17th Street Canal levee, the London Avenue Canal, and the wide, navigable Industrial Canal, which left approximately 80% of the city flooded. Flooding from the breaches put the majority of the city under water for days, in many places for weeks (Boyer, 2005; Norwalk, 2007). Electricity and water were still not functioning in many of the hardest-hit parts of the city as of 2007.

### ■ Disaster Characteristics

Disasters have different characteristics. Knowledge of these variables is necessary in disaster management and planning. Dynes, Quarentelli, and Kreps (1972) identified six variables by which disasters can be understood: predictability,

Public health nurse in disaster recovery during one of the worst natural disasters in the United States—the Mississippi River Flood of 1927.

## " *a conversation with . . .* "

**David Lyon, nursing student who lost his family home on Mississippi Gulf Coast**

The storm came on a Monday morning but we were not able to cross over the railroad tracks to see the destruction until 4 days later. It was a Friday and the first time the hospital allowed my mother, a nurse who rode out Katrina in a local hospital, to leave work. She had stayed during Katrina in her position as manager of nursing services at Memorial Behavioral Health in Gulfport, Mississippi. Although my family had evacuated, my mother worked during the entire hurricane and for 4 days afterwards. Mother said she wanted to try to get across the tracks and find our house. The guards were not officially allowing people to access their property at that point. The entire coast looked like a war zone and we feared the worst. We parked near the railroad crossing at the corner of Railroad St. and Cleveland Ave. I walked with my mother up to the armed National Guard posted at the road access. A HumVee was parked to block traffic. My mother started talking to one of the soldiers, but wasn't able to get more than three words out before she lost her voice and began sobbing uncontrollably. She choked up, unable to talk through her grief, as she looked past the guards toward the destruction of our neighborhood. Our house was a full five blocks south of the tracks and I guess we had held out hope that we had been spared. I finally had to step in and speak for my mother, attempted to explain the situation and asked what we had to do to get down there. I think it was probably my mother's sobbing more than my words that influenced the guard to let us through the barricade. He told us that we had 30 minutes to drive to our house, look at the wreckage, and drive back out. We drove down and spent about an hour there. The images of our neighborhood will always be imprinted on my brain; no words are adequate to describe the scene. When I think about that fated afternoon, all I can recall was my mother crying at the railroad crossing and having to be her voice, speaking for her. I cannot recall a time when I had seen my mother cry. I have seen her get misty over a sad ending to a movie, but never actually sob. This photo here is of our tragic discovery, the debris of our lives and what was lost forever.

—David Lyon, senior BSN nursing student
The University of Southern Mississippi College of Nursing

David Lyon, RN, BSN, sifts through the remains of his home after Hurricane Katrina.

### ☝ THINK ABOUT THIS

I helped rebuild communities in my home state of Gujarat after an earthquake in 2000, which killed 15,000 people and destroyed over a million homes. In India, one year after the earthquake in Gujarat, much of the affected areas had been rebuilt and the Indian government had given 100,000INR (roughly US$2,250) to every family who had lost a loved one. That large sum is about two-thirds the average yearly income in India, the U.S. equivalent would be almost $30,000. The families of those who died during Hurricane Katrina have received nothing from their government.

When Martin Luther King, Jr., traveled to India he was introduced to an audience he was about to address as "a fellow untouchable from the United States of America." He initially took great offense, but then thought about "twenty million of my brothers and sisters still smothering in an airtight cage of poverty in an affluent society" and realized that, "Yes, I am untouchable" because he was African American. Many years after Martin Luther King's visit in New Orleans, I saw my "untouchable" brothers and sisters still living in these conditions.

Less than a year after the earthquake, Gujarat was back to normal, with people living in their own villages and cities. Here I stood on the land of the super power, the wealthiest nation in the world, where the debris of almost 40,000 homes remained unmoved nearly a year later. Ironically, FEMA offered to sell its systems and services to India to aid in Gujarat after the earthquake. Seeing their results in New Orleans I was glad India declined. The Indian government is far from perfect, but at least it recognized that it had a responsibility towards its people.

*Martin Macwan is an advocate for the human rights of the people in India, founder of the Nasvarjan Trust, and 2000 winner of the Robert F. Kennedy Human Rights Award.*

*Source*: Macwan, M. (2006). *Human Rights Day and Hurricane Katrina: "Untouchable" New Orleans*. BBSNews Special 2006. Retrieved December 10, 2006, from http://bbsnews.net/index.php?topic=katrina

controllability, speed of onset, length of forewarning, duration of impact, and scope and intensity of impact.

*Predictability* is influenced by the type of disaster. A hurricane has a high degree of predictability in industrialized countries, but earthquakes are considerably less foreseeable than floods. Although we often assume that disasters are rare occurrences, certain areas of the globe are clearly more prone to disasters, such as the flood plains of the Ohio River

Valley or low-lying areas in Louisiana swamps. The Gulf Coast of Mississippi, Texas, Louisiana, Florida, and Alabama is vulnerable to the threat of hurricanes born from the warm waters of the Caribbean. Tornadoes are more common in Kansas, Texas, and Mississippi and less common in North Dakota and Idaho.

*Controllability* refers to the degree to which interventions can be used to control the disaster, such as using dams for flood control. Earthquakes, for example, have very little controllability.

*Speed of onset* is quick with floods and tornadoes, whereas hurricanes generally are slow to develop.

*Length of forewarning* is the period between warning and impact. Communities in the path of a hurricane may have the luxury of a 24-hour warning, whereas a tornado warning may provide only a few minutes of preparation.

*Duration of impact* also varies. A tornado may be on the ground for only a few minutes, whereas a flood's impact usually lasts for days. The worst combination of variables from the viewpoint of damage is the disaster that is rapid in onset, gives no warning, and lasts a long time. An earthquake with strong aftershocks is such a disaster.

*Scope and intensity of impact* refers to geographic and social space dimension. A disaster such as a tornado may be limited to a mile or two, whereas a flood may involve hundreds of miles. The population density of an area influences this variable and can lead to widespread consequences. An example of the effect of density can be seen in the Oklahoma City bombing, which was limited to a few city blocks but affected a large, dense population. The structure of New Orleans—also a densely populated urban area that is essentially trapped in a geographical "bowl"—led to devastating consequences when Hurricane Katrina struck, including the loss of thousands of lives and destruction of property that will take years to repair. A disaster in a densely affected area can also result in disruption of community functions, depending on the number of persons involved and the geographic impact (Norwalk, 2007).

The World Trade Center and Pentagon attacks of 2001 have had global consequences, including U.S. military action. Although the July 7, 2005, terrorist attacks on the London subway and buses were geographically limited, the population of the area was dense. Some 52 persons were killed and more than 700 injured in the deadliest attack in Great Britain since World War II; as with the 2001 U.S. attacks, the U.K. bombings resulted in significant global political consequences (Ingram, Franco, Rio, & Khazai, 2006).

From a global perspective, the 2004 Indian Ocean tsunami killed more than 200,000 people across South and Southeast Asia, including parts of Indonesia, Sri Lanka, India, and Thailand. This great undersea earthquake's epicenter, off the west coast of Sumatra, Indonesia, was the second largest earthquake ever recorded on a seismograph at (9.1 on the Richter scale) and was the longest duration of faulting ever observed, lasting between 8 and 10 minutes. It was large enough that it caused the entire planet to vibrate as much

## THINK ABOUT THIS

### Hurricane Katrina: The Perfect Disaster?
Hurricane Katrina is one of the costliest and deadliest storms in U.S. history. Katrina was part of an unprecedented (and record-breaking) hurricane season, with 28 named storms (of which 15 became hurricanes), surpassing the previous record of 21 set in 1933. For the first time ever, the National Weather Service ran through an entire list of alphabetized proper names and resorted to naming hurricanes after Greek letters.

Levees failed in the city of New Orleans following Katrina's landfall on the Mississippi Gulf Coast, causing massive postdisaster flooding of the city of New Orleans. New Orleans was inundated with floodwaters for weeks in many areas after the storm. More than 1,300 people died in four states.

Katrina also exposed the nation's inadequate preparation for a disaster of this magnitude. Elders were left to die in nursing homes while they waited for transport, even though each nursing home was required by law to have transportation in place for evacuation. No one had counted how many transport companies existed or if the system might be easily overloaded. Disaster relief officials at the local, state, and federal levels were apparently unaware of the existence of frail and ill persons trapped in nursing homes and hospitals, so they focused their efforts on transporting the generally healthier, more visible group taking refuge in the Superdome. The number of elderly receiving in-home care, those who lived alone, and those with mental illness who lived on the street and were left stranded will probably never be accurately known.

*Source:* Boyer, 2005; Knabb et al., 2005; Bourne, 2004; Waltham, 2005; Baum, 2006; Foxman et al., 2006; Kiewra, 2006.

*These terrorists kill not merely to end lives, but to disrupt and end a way of life. . . . From this day forward, any nation that continues to harbor or support terrorism will be regarded by the United States as a hostile regime. Our nation has been put on notice: We are not immune from attack. We will take defensive measures against terrorism to protect Americans. . . . Great harm has come to us. We have suffered great loss. And in our grief and anger we have found our mission and our moment. Freedom and fear are at war. . . . We will rally the world to this cause, by our efforts and by our course. We will not tire, we will not falter, and we will not fail.*

—President George W. Bush in address to Congress on terrorism, September 20, 2002

as half an inch and to minutely "wobble" on its axis by as much as 1 inch. The total energy released by this earthquake was equivalent to the explosion of 250 megatons of TNT. The shift of mass and massive release of energy very slightly altered the earth's rotation. Although the exact amount is yet undetermined, theoretical models suggest the earthquake shortened the length of a day by 2.68 microseconds. It also triggered earthquakes in other locations as far away as Africa and Alaska in the United States (Telford & Cosgrave, 2007; Ingram et al., 2006; Stein & Okal, 2005).

## ■ Global Disaster Issues

As humans continue to migrate throughout the globe and population densities continue to increase in flood plains, along vulnerable coastal areas, and near faults in the earth's crust, we can expect natural disasters to worsen and affect more people. The global community continues to witness complex emergencies resulting from the breakdown of traditional state structures, armed conflict, and the upsurge of ethnicity and micronationalism (Noji, 1997; Hayes, 2005; Rowitz, 2005; Stein & Okal, 2005; Garheld & Hamid, 2006; Telford & Cosgrave, 2007). One need look no further than today's newspaper headlines or watch CNN to find these political and cultural conflicts as they play out on a daily basis, such as in Bosnia, Darfur, Somalia, Rwanda, Chechnya, and Iraq, to name but a few of the disaster areas. Because of these political and cultural upheavals, refugees have become a large and vulnerable population with complex health problems. Between 1965 and 2006, 90% of all natural disaster victims lived in Asia and Africa. The number of people affected (killed, injured, or displaced) by disasters worldwide rose from 100 million in 1980 to 157 million in 2005. By the mid-1990s, the number of refugees affected by a combination of natural and human-made disasters increased to an estimated 17 million throughout the world (ISDR, 2006; Bradt, 2002).

Earthquakes are global incidents that have been cited as causing the greatest number of deaths and the largest monetary loss of any type of natural disaster. The tragic earthquake that occurred in the 2004 Indian Ocean and the ensuing tsunami caused the deaths of more than 200,000 people, and the restoration of that area may take decades. This has further added to the poverty of these countries as well as adding to the already strained burden of immigration to other countries (Kumar, Murhekar, Hutin, Subramanian, Ramachandran, & Gupte, 2007; Telford & Cosgrave, 2007; Berz, 1984).

Not only are these displaced vulnerable populations at risk for serious health consequences, the economic costs for their care are also devastating (Noji, 1997). As former United Nations Secretary General Boutros Boutros Ghali stated:

> There is no hard-and-fast division in terms of their [disasters'] effects on civilian populations between conflicts and wars, and natural disasters. Droughts, floods, earthquakes, and cyclones are just as destructive for communities and settlements as wars and civil confrontation. Just as preventive diplomacy can foresee and prevent the outbreak of war, so the effects of natural disasters can be foreseen and contained. (cited in Noji, 1997, p. xv)

Much of the destruction caused by natural disasters can be avoided. For almost every natural disaster in the world in the 1990s, an ounce of prevention or preparedness would have made a significant difference in terms of damage to persons and property (Noji, 1997, p. 7). Natural hazards, such as weather, earthquakes, and floods, are, in fact, only natural agents that transform a vulnerable condition into a disaster (Noji, 1997, p. 11).

People often do not know their limitations until they reach them. As technology has advanced and provided humans with opportunities to live in and explore the world without the territorial constraints of our ancestors, the probabilities that the future will be marked by periodic disasters are certainly increased. In many cases in recent disasters, building codes were ignored, communities were located in dangerous areas, warnings were not issued or followed, or plans were unknown to all community residents or were ignored (Noji, 1997).

We know much about the cause and nature of disasters, populations at risk, and the inevitable outcome when communities are not prepared for disasters. Such knowledge assists us in anticipating some of the effects that a disaster may have on the health of communities. Knowing how people are injured and killed in disasters is critical prerequisite knowledge for preventing or reducing injuries and deaths during future disasters (Noji, 1997). For example, although none of the advances in science and technology have done much to arrest the force of natural disasters, we often see them coming a few hours earlier and can measure their destructiveness with greater precision afterward. Yet those very advances have rendered us in many ways even more vulnerable to potential catastrophes, because persons often feel a false sense of security regarding the likelihood of serious threat from a disaster (Erickson, 1976). Persons in the New Orleans area hardest hit by Hurricane Katrina live below sea level and are certainly accustomed to hurricane warnings, for example.

### 🖥 Research Alert

**Indian Ocean Tsunami, December 26, 2004**

The 9.0 undersea earthquake occurred December 26, 2004. The earthquake generated a tsunami that was among the deadliest disasters in modern history. The tsunami wreaked devastation along the shores of Indonesia, Sri Lanka, South India, Thailand, Maldives, and other countries where waves of up to 30 meters hit the coast. Even areas as far as the coast of East Africa sustained damage and recorded fatalities. The World Health Organization (WHO) estimates that between 228,000 to 310,000 people died as a result of the tsunami although an accurate count will never be known due to the number missing and destruction of the public health infrastructure in affected areas.

*Sources*: Garheld, R., & Hamid, A. Y. (2006). Tsunami response: A year later. *American Journal of Nursing, 106*(1), 76–79; Hassmiller, S. (2007). The 2004 tsunami. *American Journal of Nursing, 107*(2), 74–77; Kumar, M. S., Murhekar, M. V., Hutin, Y., Subramanian, T., Ramachandran, V., & Gupte, M. D. (2007). Prevalence of post-traumatic stress disorder in a coastal fishing village in Tamil Nadu, India, after the December 2004 tsunami. *American Journal of Public Health, 97*(1), 99–101; Telford, J., & Cosgrave, J. (2007). The international humanitarian system and the 2004 Indian Ocean earthquake and tsunamis. *Disasters, 31*(1), 1–28.

THINK ABOUT THIS ·······························

> Healthcare needs of people in developing and underdeveloped countries experiencing violent conflict and disaster are similar. In such cases, nurses can play key roles in disease detection and control, social support, and rehabilitation. Nurses already provide much of the care in these situations because they are present on a daily basis, have key clinical and organizational skills, and have a high level of popular trust.
>
> This commentary recommends that we can do more with systems training, disaster skill development, and participation in policy and research related to preventing and reducing the effects of disaster. Nurses are usually invisible, serving without discipline-specific orientation. The reasons for the lack of nursing's presence during disasters include unresolved ethical and political issues among nursing leaders regarding the role and image of nursing, humanist values, and relations between the profession and government. We are always the first on the scene and the last to leave, but rarely is our presence acknowledged in the press or official accounts of the disaster. Nightingale knew that better organization, autonomy, and recognition of the unique contribution that nurses make in times of war and disaster could do much to prevent further harm to damaged populations.

*Source:* Garfield, R., Dresden, E., & Rafferty A. (2003) Commentary: The evolving role of nurses in terrorism and war, *American Journal of Infection Control, 31*(3), 163–167.

**❝** *There's a lot of loss going on. There's a lot of mourning going on. Only through storytelling can you heal.* **❞**

—Douglas Brinkley

## Natural Disaster Reduction

The United Nations General Assembly declared the 1990s to be the International Decade for Natural Disaster Reduction (IDNDR) and led the way in calling for a global, scientific, technical, and political effort to reduce the impact of catastrophic acts of nature (Advisory Committee IDNDR, 1987). The IDNDR was later renamed the International Strategy for Disaster Reduction (ISDR). This declaration came about because both disasters and the number of their victims have increased in recent decades (Pickens, 1992; Rowitz, 2005). The United Nations (UN) has continued to meet yearly on this issue and, in June 2006, launched the 2006–2007 "Disaster Risk Reduction Begins at School" campaign.

When a natural disaster strikes, children are among the most vulnerable groups, especially those attending school in times of disaster. Disasters such as the October 2005 earthquake in Pakistan, in which more than 16,000 children died in schools that collapsed, or the 2006 mudslide on Leyte Island in the Philippines, where more than 200 school children were buried alive, are just a few tragic examples of why more needs to be done to protect our children during catastrophic events. The UN/ISDR secretariat and its partners have made disaster risk education and safer school facilities the two key

themes of the 2006–2007 World Disaster Reduction campaign. The "Disaster Risk Reduction Begins at School" initiative aims to inform and mobilize governments, communities, and individuals to ensure that disaster risk reduction is fully integrated into school curricula in high-risk countries and that school buildings are built or retrofitted to withstand natural hazards. In all societies, children represent hope for the future. Because of their direct link to youths, schools are universally regarded as institutions of learning, for instilling cultural values, and for passing on both traditional and conventional knowledge to younger generations. Protecting our children during natural disasters, therefore, requires two distinct yet inseparable priorities for action: disaster risk education and school safety (ISDR, 2006)

The massive adverse impacts on the health of global populations resulting from disaster have now been recognized as a significant public health problem. Sudden-impact disasters, such as earthquakes and tornadoes, may result in large numbers of people killed, injured, or disabled for life; health facilities damaged or destroyed; and national healthcare development efforts in underdeveloped countries set back for years. As human societies have become denser owing to the twin forces of urban migration and population growth, more people are now exposed and vulnerable to the hazards of disaster than ever before. Their increasingly sophisticated and technical physical infrastructure make more developed countries, such as the United States, even more vulnerable to destruction than in past generations. For instance, a major disaster could disrupt the computer networks of the federal government or some other large organization. Damage from both natural and technological disasters tends to be more and more extensive when proper planning and precautions are not taken. In the past 50 years, much has been learned about disasters and their after-effects. Disaster preparedness involving careful and methodical planning does make a difference in mediating the destructive nature of disasters (Noji, 1997).

THINK ABOUT THIS ·······························

> "Begin at the beginning" the King said, gravely, "and go till you come to the end; then stop."
> —*Lewis Caroll's* Alice's Adventures in Wonderland, *1865*

## Disaster as a Global Public Health Problem

The Centers for Disease Control and Prevention (CDC) has led the way and has major responsibilities to prepare for and respond to public emergencies such as disasters. The CDC is also responsible for conducting investigations into the health effects and health consequences of disaster. The first major comprehensive research study of disasters was published in 1962 by Baker and Chapman in their book *Man and Society in Disaster*. Since then, many research centers have been established to study the health effects of disaster;

> *Will you be a hero in your daily work? . . . We may give you an institution to learn in, but it is you who must furnish the heroic feelings of doing your duty, doing your best, without which no institution is safe.*
>
> —Florence Nightingale

among them are collaborative centers under the guidance and sponsorship of the World Health Organization (WHO) and the Pan American Health Organization. The major aim of these research efforts is to assess risk for death and injury and to develop strategies for preventing or mitigating the impact of future disasters.

Disasters affect communities in myriad ways. Most effects of a disaster affect health, directly or indirectly (Noji, 1997). Communication lines, such as telephones, television, and computer links, may be disrupted, as well as transportation links, such as roads and methods of transportation. Public utilities (electricity, water, gas, and sewer) are often disrupted early in a massive disaster. A substantial number of persons may be without homes. Casualties may require medical and nursing care. Damage to food, damage to food preparation and sources, and lack of sanitation resources may create serious public health threats. A long-term effect is the community's possible destruction of its industrial or economic base. A detailed summary of disasters and public health can be found in Box 24-4 and the health effects of disasters in Box 24-5.

---

**BOX 24-4**

**Public Health Problems That May Result from Disasters**

- Excessive deaths and injuries can tax the local health services and therapeutic capabilities, which may require external assistance.
- Destruction or disruption of acute care health facilities, such as clinics and hospitals, may leave services and resources unable to provide care to the injured from the disaster and predisaster patient population needs.
- Disruption of routine health services and preventive activities can lead to long-term consequences in terms of morbidity and mortality.
- Environmental hazards can lead to increased risks for communicable disease and injury from a damaged ecosystem.
- Psychological and social behavioral stressors, including panic, anxiety, neuroses, and depression, can be exacerbated.
- A shortage of safe, nutritional food sources may lead to severe nutritional deficiencies and sequelae in the very young and the very old.
- Displaced populations to overcrowded hospitals and shelter facilities may increase the dangers of communicable disease.

*Sources*: Adapted from Logue, Melick, & Hansen, 1981; Noji, 1997.

---

**BOX 24-5**

**Health Effects of Disasters**

**Physical**
Sleep disturbance
Poor concentration
Back pain
Tachycardia
Poor diet

**Psychological**
Loss of self and relationships
Emotional pain
Brooding
Aggressive thoughts
Depression

**Sociocultural**
Loss of intimacy
Loss of sense of belonging to once-claimed culture

*Source*: From Nurses' Role in World Catastrophic Events: War and Dislocation Effects on Serbian Australians by N. Procter and J. Cheek. In B. Neuman (Ed.) *The Neuman Systems Model* (3rd Int. ed.) pp. 119–131, 1995. Reproduced by permission.

---

### ■ Populations at Risk in Disasters

Not all persons in the world are equal regarding the probability of disaster occurrence or severity of consequences. The more vulnerable a population to a disaster, the more serious the outcomes of injury and damage to persons and property (Mizutani & Nakano, 1989; Garheld & Hamid, 2006; Telford & Cograve, 2007). As far as individual health characteristics, persons with conditions that put them at risk, such as those with chronic diseases, elder persons, pregnant women, the disabled, homebound persons, or children, are among the most vulnerable in any society concerning impact of disaster (FEMA, 2007). Industrialized countries are buffered from disasters by characteristics and abilities that are summarized in Box 24-6.

---

**BOX 24-6**

**Resources for Industrialized Countries**

- Sophisticated technology to forecast storms
- Development and strict enforcement of codes for earthquake-resistant and fireproof buildings
- Widespread mandatory use of communications networks to broadcast disaster warnings, alerts, and information about disaster preparedness
- Resources to provide timely and high-quality emergency health services and accommodation
- Contingency planning to prepare the population and public agencies for possible disasters
- Shelters for evacuation widely available and used by population

*Source*: Adapted from Garcia, 1985.

The low death rate associated with recent disasters in the United States, such as hurricanes Katrina and Rita (2005), Hugo (1989), Andrew (1992), and Georges (1998), and earthquakes in San Francisco (1989) and Los Angeles (1994), are evidence of the success of the United States's devotion of resources in disaster warning and recovery, which reduces the death risks to vulnerable populations (Noji, 1997; Rowitz, 2005). The following major factors contribute to the degree of vulnerability of populations:

- Human vulnerability resulting from poverty and social inequality
- Environmental degradation resulting from poor land use
- Rapid population growth, especially among the poor

It is estimated that 95% of the deaths that result from natural disasters occur among 66% of the world's poorest population. The poor are most at risk for greatest damage for the following reasons (EM-DAT, 2006):

- They are likely to live in substandard housing with little structural protection.
- They often live in coastal locations that are at high risk for disasters.
- They are likely to live in flood plains and other less desirable land.
- They are likely to live in substandard housing built on unstable geographic slopes.
- They are likely to live near hazardous industrial sites.
- They are not usually well educated about safe and appropriate life-saving behaviors.
- They are more dependent on others for transportation.

## Stages of Disaster

Disasters can be divided into five chronological stages that require specific levels of prevention and levels of response at various points during each stage. Knowing the disaster stages will assist in the development of the disaster plan, role responsibilities, and the setting of priorities in each phase of the disaster plan. Refer to Box 24-1 as an illustration of the stages of disaster. The stages of a disaster are as follows:

1. Nondisaster, or interdisaster, stage
2. Predisaster, or warning, stage
3. Impact stage
4. Emergency stage
5. Reconstruction, or rehabilitation, stage

Disaster planning should begin before the disaster event. During the nondisaster stage (**interdisaster stage**), planning and preparation for a disaster include the two critical elements of disaster preparedness: (1) disaster training and education programs for the community and (2) the development of a disaster plan for all involved in the mitigation of a potential disaster (Noji, 1997; Rowitz, 2005). Mitigation is preventive in nature and is defined as action taken; to prevent or reduce the harmful effects of a disaster on human health and property (Malilay, 1997; Langan & James, 2004). Included in this critical phase of primary prevention are assessment of hazards and risks, vulnerability analysis, inventory of existing resources for coping with a disaster (human, communication, and material), and the establishment of a disaster plan. Disaster planning is discussed in more detail in a later section.

A disaster is imminent during the warning stage (**predisaster stage**). The disaster plan, when available, is implemented, which includes early warnings based on predictions of impending disaster and mobilization as well as implementation of protective measures for the affected communities and populations (Garcia, 1985). Because primary prevention is the focus during this stage, disaster team members, officials, and emergency personnel prepare the population for disaster by providing information via multiple communication routes. Advisories and warnings are issued, and evacuation measures are taken where indicated. Mobilization can occur in the form of evacuation to shelters, preparation such as using sandbags around riverbanks to divert floodwaters, boarding up windows and tying down boats when a hurricane is forecast, moving to the basements or inner halls of homes and schools in the event of a tornado, or evacuating geographically vulnerable persons after volcano warnings. Healthcare workers may be placed on alert call for health facility staffing and disaster shelter management. The effectiveness of these protective measures will depend largely on the community's preparedness and contingency plans developed in the nondisaster phase (Noji, 1997).

Problems associated with such warnings include the fact that the communication systems may be inadequate in transmission and/or reception, or there may not be enough time to send warnings; in addition, the community must recognize the warning threat as serious and legitimate. Nevertheless, some people in the targeted community may deny the need for taking action based on previous experience with the specific disaster (e.g., persons who live on a fault line or on a coastline), and the presence of false alarms in the past can desensitize persons to appropriate reaction (Bozeman, 2003; Bradt, 2002; Garcia, 1985; Janis & Mann, 1977; Rosenkoetter et al., 2007).

The **impact stage** involves "holding on" and enduring the impact of the disaster. This stage may last from minutes (as in earthquakes, plane crashes, tornadoes, and bomb blasts) to days or weeks (hurricanes, floods, fire, and drought). People who are directly experiencing the disaster may be unable to comprehend the scope of the disaster (Garcia, 1985). If possible, disaster team members during the impact phase or immediately afterward should conduct a preliminary assessment and inventory of injuries and property damage so that the implementation of secondary prevention strategies of setting priorities can be set in motion. How much the impact affects community members depends on several factors: population density, the extent of

## ENVIRONMENTAL CONNECTION

### Why was New Orleans a "disaster waiting to happen"?

The city of New Orleans sits below sea level. Why is this so? According to Tidwell, author of *Bayou Farewell*, the answer is the levees. The huge earthen river dikes that have kept the city dry and inhabitable for 300 years have also resulted in a virtual giant bathtub. Every great river delta in the world is shaped by two defining geological phenomena: One feature involves the flooding resulting from overflow, in this case, of the sediment-rich Mississippi River. This has created over the past 7,000 years a vast deltaic coast from the water borne deposits composed of sediments and nutrients flowing from two-thirds of the United States. The second feature is subsidence, or sinking. The deposits of alluvial soil are extremely fine and unstable. Over time, they tend to compact, shrink in volume, and sink. This natural process of sediment deposit counterbalanced the sinking and resulted in net land building. By corseting the river with levees right out to the Gulf of Mexico's Continental Shelf, we are left with a sinking "bowl."

When French colonists first settled in Louisiana 300 years ago, vast dense hardwood forests lay between what is now New Orleans and the Gulf of Mexico. There were fresh water marshes, endless saltwater wetlands, and a strong network of strong barrier islands. Today all that land is essentially gone. Because of the levees and the "law of unintended consequences," New Orleans is a sunken, walled city, essentially jutting out exposed to the hurricane-prone Gulf of Mexico. Had Katrina struck 50 or 100 years ago, the destruction would not have been the same. In 2005 there were simply no land structures left to slow Katrina's deadly blow.

Every day, even without hurricanes, 50 acres of land in coastal Louisiana turns to water. Every 10 months, an area of land equal to Manhattan joins the Gulf of Mexico. It is the fastest disappearing land mass on Earth. This is why Katrina happened, why people drowned, lost their homes.

The entire coat of Louisiana including New Orleans began rapidly sinking, dropping 2–3 feet in the 20th century alone:

It would be criminally irresponsible of us to fix a single broken window in New Orleans, pick up a single piece of debris, or fix a single cubic foot of levee without simultaneously committing as a nation to the massive plan to rebuild the entire Louisiana coast. To do one without the other is to simply set the table for the next nightmare hurricane.

—Mike Tidwell, author of *Bayou Farewell:
The Rich Life and Tragic Death of
Louisiana's Cajun Coast* (Pantheon, 2003)

the damage, the preparedness of the community, the extent of community resiliency, and response to the consequences of the damage.

During the **emergency stage,** the community faces the consequences of the disaster's impact. This stage begins during the actual impact and continues until the immediate threat of additional hazards has passed (Garcia, 1985; Bozeman, 2003; Bradt, 2002). Secondary prevention strategies are used to minimize damage and prevent further complications. This stage is divided into three parts—isolation, rescue, and remedy.

*Isolation* of the affected population can occur as a result of limited access (as a result of disaster damage, such as closed roads, downed trees, or building obstruction). The

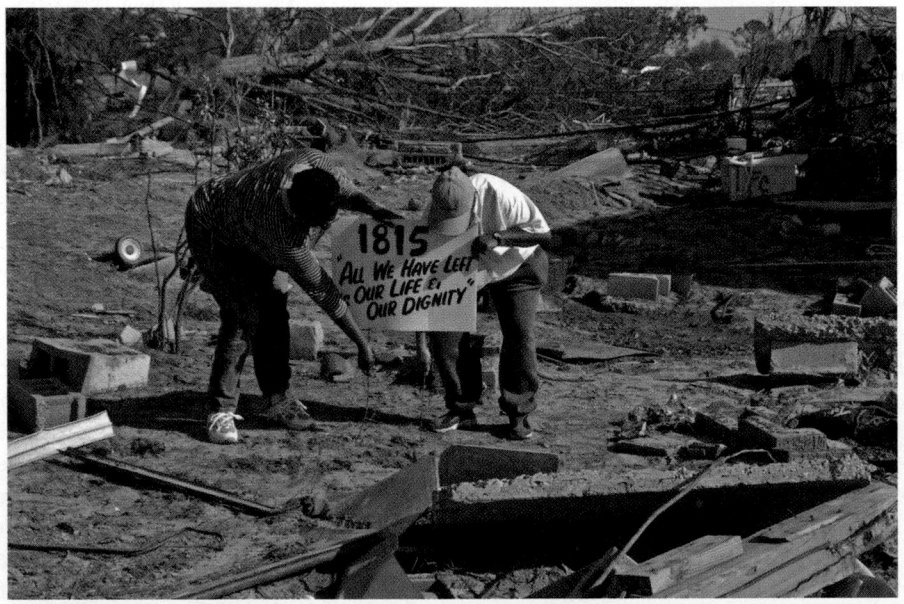

After a disaster, communities must come to terms with rebuilding their entire lives from the ground up. After Hurricane Katrina, these residents illustrate the shock of such devastation and the resilience of the human spirit.

community members themselves must assume responsibility for their own needs relative to the disaster until outside help arrives.

*Rescue* begins when outside resources arrive and provide search-and-rescue operations. Community members are often harried, stressed, and nonproductive in this early stage. First aid, emergency medical assistance, and a command post for disaster management are established. Restoration of means of communication begins, and regional, state, federal, and voluntary organizations and agencies converge to meet the needs of the community.

*Remedy* begins with the establishment of organized, professional, and voluntary relief operations and organization. The panic and confusion of the earlier phases tend to subside. Community members, disaster workers, and volunteers "get on with the task" of providing appropriate medical aid, clothing, food, and shelter to the affected population. The injured and ill are triaged, transportation becomes more organized, morgue facilities are established, reunions of family members become organized, and communication networks are established to provide early data of the disaster damage (Garcia, 1985). Later in the emergency stage, surveillance of public health effects (e.g., infectious disease, sanitation issues, safety concerns, and environmental fallout, such as flood debris and air pollutants) is put in place and interventions are developed (Wilson, 2006). When communities are well prepared and disaster plans are in place to help people know the "what, when, and how" of disasters for their population, both self-reliance and the effectiveness of early assistance can save lives and reduce injury during this critical period (Bozeman, 2003; Noji, 1997; Rowitz, 2005; Langan & James, 2004).

The **reconstruction (rehabilitation) stage** begins when communities start the process of healing. Reconstruction or rehabilitation optimally restores the community to predisaster conditions (Noji, 1997). Health services are restored to normal. Damaged homes, facilities, and buildings are repaired and reconstructed. This period is also the time for evaluation and reflection by the community and disaster team members, community officials, and voluntary agencies, as lessons learned from the disaster are shared and documented (Noji, 1997). This period, which may combine secondary and tertiary prevention, may take days, months, or years, depending on the nature of the disaster, the response of the community, and the extent of the damages. For persons in the impact area, the recovery can be a long course and, in some cases, can be a lifelong readjustment to life and community living after the disaster (Garcia, 1985; Wilson, 2006; Norwalk, 2007; Cardoza et al., 2004).

In the wake of the September 11 disasters, people in New York City have reconstructed their lives in varied ways. Memorials have been held, artwork has been created, and a new community ethic of connectedness seems to have emerged. There appeared to be a need to invest in the future, to define

---

## ■■ CULTURAL CONNECTION

### Redefining "Normal" After 9/11 from a Manhattan Nurse

"The word 'normal' has taken on a whole new meaning for me. It is now normal for my heart to race when I hear a fire alarm or a siren, or to stop and look at the sky if I hear the engine of a plane that is loud. It is now normal for me to keep supplies in a closet at home for another possible attack; I have become familiar with anthrax, smallpox, and other diseases. I am not afraid to travel, but I am afraid that if I travel and another attack occurs I won't be able to get back to the people and things I love. For me, nothing will ever be the same."

Peter J. Ungvarski, MS, RN, FAAN, was a clinical nurse specialist in HIV infection and director of quality assessment and regulatory compliance at the Visiting Nurse Service (VNS) of New York at the time of the 9/11 terrorist attacks. Ungvarski was in his VNA office in Manhattan at 8:47 A.M. when the first plane, American Airlines Flight 111, crashed into Tower One of the World Trade Center.

*Source:* Ungvarski, P. J. (2002). 9/11: Redefining the word "normal" in Manhattan. *Association of Nurses in AIDS Care, 13*(5), 21–24.

---

and reach for goals, and to invest energy in plans to rebuild both the city and individual lives that had been personally touched by the trauma and loss. Klagsbrun (2002) suggests that by moving on in our personal lives, as well as in our communal lives, we are attempting to regain control over our destiny. Each person often reviews his or her own history and recognizes how the individual has overcome losses, difficulties of all kinds, pain, and failure and has succeeded in being able to go on. The crises managed in the past then become healthy patterns of coping with the present unthinkable disaster (Silove, 1999; Cardoza et al., 2004).

It is during the rehabilitative phase that victims often suffer from post-traumatic stress disorder. **Post-traumatic stress disorder (PTSD)** is recognized by the American Psychiatric Association (APA) with the following symptoms and circumstances: The sufferer is a victim of an extremely distressing event who persistently reexperiences the event after it is over (compulsive and obsessive thoughts and details about the event), persistently avoids stimuli that remind the victim of the event, and experiences numbing of responsiveness and persistent symptoms of arousal not present before the trauma (APA, 2006; Galea et al., 2003). In conjunction with disaster, other symptoms include flashbacks, depression, inability to form close personal relationships, and sleep disturbances (Barker, 1989; Rhoads, Mitchell, & Rick, 2006). Florence Nightingale is thought to have suffered from PTSD after the Crimean War. This condition, once diagnosed, requires professional mental health intervention and follow-up (Waters, Selander, & Stuart, 1992; Rhoads et al., 2006; Adams, 2007; Hyre, Ompad, & Menke 2007).

## Research Alert

This study surveyed workers, truck drivers, heavy equipment operators, laborers, and carpenters about their work-related exposures and somatic and mental health symptoms. Respondents reported debilitating consequences of their work, being poorly prepared to work in a disaster, lacking protective equipment and training, and being overwhelmed by the devastation at the World Trade Center site.

*Source:* Johnson, S. B., Langlieb, A. M., Teret, S. P., Gross, R., Schwab, M., Massa, J., Ashwell, L., & Geyh, A. S. (2005). Rethinking first response: Effects of the cleanup and recovery effort on workers at the World Trade Center disaster site. *Journal of Occupational and Environmental Medicine, 47*(4), 386–391.

## Disaster Planning

A planned response to disasters must occur to lessen the terror of a disaster, to cushion the impact by providing care for the greatest number of potential survivors, and to increase society's ability to survive disasters and grow more self-sufficient and self-reliant in the process (Waeckerle, 1991; Henderson, Thomas, Inglesby, & O'Toole, 2002). Clearly, the benefits of disaster planning for society today are more significant than ever as widespread disasters become more common and more costly, in both human and property terms.

Anticipating a disaster and planning for the possibility of multiple outcomes from disasters strengthen a community's adaptability. Consequently, the disaster team develops the ability to respond more quickly and more effectively in the face of disaster (Muench, 1996; Levy & Sidel, 2002). Another benefit to planning is the delineation of roles and responsibilities of the players in disaster preparedness. The result is less confusion over who does what and the roles of the multitude of organizations and volunteers once resources become available.

Once a disaster is imminent, it is too late to plan a response. Knowledgeable and experienced leaders and officials in the community should coordinate a clear community disaster plan for all contingencies. Such a plan must be as inclusive as possible, including input from health professionals; voluntary agencies; policy makers; officials from local, state, and federal levels, such as the civil defense and the Federal Emergency Management Agency (FEMA); emergency response system personnel; and all other components of the healthcare delivery system from acute care to home health to residential care, including medical and nursing schools (Waeckerle, 1991; Langan & James, 2004; FEMA, 2007; Burnham & Abdallah, 2008).

## ■ Steps in the Disaster Process

When a major disaster has occurred, such as Hurricane Katrina in 2005, the president of the United States intervenes after the governor of the affected state requests the president to declare the area a major disaster. However, all major disaster declarations must follow certain steps (FEMA, 2006).

First, local government agencies, such as the mayor and civil defense, which includes neighboring communities and volunteer agencies, must respond. Second, if the local agencies become overwhelmed, the state responds at the governor's request through state agencies and the National Guard. Third, local, state, federal, and volunteer organizations make a damage assessment.

Fourth, when state resources have been exhausted, the governor of the state makes a request to the president for a declaration of a major disaster. The governor bases this request on the already-completed damage assessment collected by the civil defense team and commits a certain amount of state funds and resources to the long-term recovery from the disaster.

Fifth, FEMA evaluates the request and recommends action to the White House. Sixth, either the president gives the executive order for the declaration or FEMA informs the

Tornados often leave a path of severe destruction, especially in densely populated urban areas.

## ENVIRONMENTAL CONNECTION

"I'm a strong proponent of the restoration of the wetlands, for a lot of reasons. There's a practical reason, though, when it comes to hurricanes: The stronger the wetlands, the more likely the damage of the hurricane."

— President George W. Bush, discussing post-Katrina wetland improvements, New Orleans, March 1, 2007

A new report on environmental effects of Hurricane Katrina in 2007 indicates that the Louisiana gulf coast is sinking. Findings a year after Katrina indicate that the coastline in southern Louisiana is gradually shifting, sliding ever so slowly into the Gulf of Mexico. The implication of this for future disaster risks is significant as engineers repairing the levees around New Orleans must now reconsider how this will affect previous plans to rebuild the levees. This lateral movement of land into the Gulf indicates that the bedrock under southern Louisiana southward has been triggered by deep underground faults that are slipping under the enormous weight of the sediment from the disaster as well as from the Mississippi River.

*Source:* Tidwell, M. (2006). Exporting calamity: Katrinas for everyone. *World Watch,* *19*(5), 13–45.

Chapter author Dr. Karen Saucier Lundy (left) at an American Red Cross shelter after Hurricane Allen in Galveston, Texas.

governor the request has been denied. The whole process may take only a few days. If the executive order is given, federal and financial resources are mobilized through FEMA for search and rescue and for the provision of basic human needs. Long-term federal programs are mobilized during this time.

## The Disaster Plan

The purpose of **disaster planning** is to reduce a community's vulnerability to the tremendous consequences of disasters and to prevent or minimize problems resulting from system damage associated with the disaster. Community health nurses are involved in disaster planning, as are other healthcare professionals in the community. Specific ways that a nurse can be more prepared for a disaster in his or her community are described in the next section (Burnham & Abdallah, 2008; Langan & James, 2004; Drabek, 1986).

In a disaster, the usual strategies and process for providing care may not work. Deviating from a routine plan of care may present a few problems for nurses and other healthcare professionals when disaster occurs. Disaster health care is very different from daily nursing practice; it is not routine (even compared with emergency department services), and the philosophy of care is based on providing the greatest good for the greatest number. Abiding by this standard of care is often difficult for healthcare professionals, especially for those in routine practice settings who practice holistic care and provide optimal care to all who need services. The disaster plan is fundamental in the preparation of healthcare professionals (Waeckerle, 1991). Drabek (1986) identified general principles that can guide community health nurses who take part in disaster planning. These principles are listed in Box 24-7.

### BOX 24-7

**Principles to Guide Disaster Preparedness for All Persons Involved in Planning**

Measures used for everyday emergencies generally do not work in major disasters.

- Disasters are more uncertain, less predictable, with more unknowns, and citizens have little consensus on what needs to be done in a disaster.
- Laypersons are most likely to jump in and provide aid without direction and knowledge of prioritization and triage.

Plan for specific population needs and consider "disaster planning" as a verb, which is ongoing, rather than as a noun, such as the limits of a written plan.

Provide information regularly to the community to correct misconceptions.

- Widespread looting and theft are actually quite uncommon.
- People should be given information and details about the extent of the disaster to enable them to take appropriate action, in contrast to the long-held belief of health workers that people will panic if they "know too much."

Involve the entire community in the planning process, not just officials and emergency personnel.

- Such inclusion limits confusion about who does what and where the lines of authority are.

Use routine working methods and procedures in the disaster plan, which will eliminate the need to learn new procedures and prevents confusion at the disaster site.

Disaster plans should be flexible.

Roles and responsibilities of team members should be identified by position or title, not by names of individuals, to avoid having to revise the plan when people change positions.

As Waeckerle has stated, "Disaster planning is an enormous undertaking" (1991, p. 815). As in other areas of health care, enormous amounts of money are spent in the United States on disaster relief during the recovery period, yet few funds are made available for communities to use in disaster preparedness and disaster planning. This emphasis poses challenges in the development of a disaster plan. Although the disaster plan is usually developed from guidelines set forth by local, state, and federal officials, communities are often on their own and must rely on local officials and volunteers to do much of the work when organizing a disaster plan and evaluating its validity through mock disaster drills (Burnham & Abdallah, 2008).

Since the 2001 anthrax attacks on U.S. mail facilities and the emergence of the threat of smallpox bioterrorism, disaster plans must include much more detail on protocols for managing communicable diseases and chemical agents, most of which current healthcare professionals have never seen. Bioterrorism, germ warfare, and disaster/bioterrorism preparation have become common terms on news shows and in the vocabulary of the American public since September 11, 2001 (Porche, 2002). As the terrorist attacks in which anthrax spores were distributed through the U.S. Postal Service demonstrated, these threats are a means to produce fear and could potentially target unsuspecting individuals, but most citizens are unclear as to how to protect themselves. In addition to being prepared and educated about bioterrorist agents such as anthrax and smallpox, disaster planners need to prepare for even rarer infectious diseases that could be used in bioterrorism, such as *Brucellosis,* plague, tularemia, Q fever, and botulism. Additionally, chemical agents are substances that can injure and kill through a variety of mechanisms. Choking, blood, blister, or neural agents are the ones most likely to be used in a terrorist attack, as they will cause the highest rates of morbidity and mortality (Porche, 2002; Smith, 2000).

Garrett (2000) warns that the collapse of the public health infrastructure in the United States leaves us particularly vulnerable to such epidemics. Public health is the only viable protection against epidemics, whether natural or human-made, and public health is responsible in most states

for disaster planning. Through the last two decades, health departments have been chronically underfunded, according to Garrett (2000; see also Colias, 2005), because of their successes in the past century at keeping children immunized, the air breathable, factories safer, and citizens better educated about self-care. Disaster plans, however, must change as threats to the public's health evolve.

### Characteristics of Disaster Plans

Through research into past disasters and the presence or absence of disaster plans, disaster specialists have determined common characteristics of effective disaster plans (Drabek, 1986; Noji, 1997; Waeckerle, 1991; Ingram et al., 2006):

- The disaster plan is based on a realistic assessment of potential problems that can happen, such as destruction to property, material, and utilities; impairment of communication; and geographic isolation.
- Estimates of types of injuries that would result from the disasters most likely to occur in the area and the possible destruction of health facilities and alternative agency use are included in the plan.

 NOTE THIS!

**Online Resources for Disaster Preparedness**

*Pets and Disaster: Get Prepared*
Developed with Humane Society of the United States, this resource provides recommendations and specific suggestions on having a pet disaster plan: pet disaster supplies, what to do when a disaster threatens, and alternatives since pets are not allowed in shelters.

For more information, visit http://www.redcross.org/services/disaster/0,1082,0_604_,00.html

*Disaster Preparedness for People with Disabilities*
This 46-page booklet is designed for use by anyone who has a disability or who works with, lives with, or assists a person with a disability. It has information on possible disaster effects, assessing personal needs and abilities, suggestions about forming a personal support network, and fill-in-the-blank checklists.

For more information, visit http://www.redcross.org/services/disaster/0,1082,0_603_,00.html

*Facing Fear: Helping Young People Deal with Terrorism and Tragic Events*
This curriculum supplement for teachers will help deal with children's concerns, fears, anger, and feelings when human-caused events occur. It is aligned with national standards in social studies, health, and language arts and available in four complete sets for teachers of grades K–2, 3–5, 6–8, and 9–12.

*Terrorism, Preparing for the Unexpected*
This is a brochure for the general public providing information about how to prepare for disasters of any type. It includes fundamental family disaster preparedness tips, what to do when disaster strikes, instructions on how to shelter in place and evacuation, and an abbreviated first aid primer.

*Your Family Disaster Plan*
This 4-page brochure describes four steps to disaster safety—finding out what can happen, planning, preparing, and practicing. ⬤

👆 THINK ABOUT THIS ·····················

**Children and Disasters: Protecting Our Future**

*How to teach children about disasters and their role in saving lives and livelihoods: An online game*
The secretariat of the United Nations (UN) International Strategy for Disaster Reduction has created an online game aimed at teaching children how to build safer villages and cities against disasters. This initiative comes within the 2006–2007 World Disaster Reduction Campaign "Disaster Risk Reduction Begins at School." ⬤

To access the game, go to www.stopdisastersgame.org.

- The plan is brief, concise, and inclusive of all who can provide disaster aid.
- The plan is organized by a timeline; it details the stages of a disaster, who must be involved, what must occur, and how each stage unfolds throughout the disaster process.
- The plan is approved by all agencies that provide authority endorsement, as well as sanctioned by those who have the most power to see that the plan is updated periodically and carried out when disaster strikes.
- The plan is regularly tested through mock drills and revised based on drill results.
- The plan is always considered a work in progress because needs and resources in a community relative to disaster preparedness change constantly.

### Common Elements of Disaster Plans

Although disaster plans should be targeted for the specific community, certain components should be included in all disaster plans. Each component may have more or less elaboration, detail, and specifics according to the needs of the community to which it applies. These components consist of authority; communication; supplies; equipment; human resources (health professionals, both acute and public health); emergency and disaster specialists; officials of government and voluntary agencies; engineers; weather specialists; community leaders, both lay and official; team coordination; transportation; documentation; record keeping; evacuation; rescue; acute care; supportive care; recovery; and evaluation. Details of these components are summarized in Box 24-8.

### ■ Disaster Management

The goal of disaster management is to prevent or minimize death, injury, suffering, and destruction (Taggert, 1982). Disaster management by nature is an interdisciplinary, collaborative team effort (Sullivan, 1998); however, community health nurses are integral in planning for and responding to disasters. Specific community officials, such as those in civil defense, usually coordinate disaster management.

Once the civil defense efforts are begun, individuals overseeing these agencies carry out coordination of the many networks in the community disaster infrastructure. Some

---

### BOX 24-8

**Common Elements of a Disaster Plan**

**Authority:** Issues warnings and official responses and is the central authority for disaster declarations and delegation

**Communication:** Warnings to public and how communicated, whether by weather sirens, television, radio, police loudspeakers; includes chain of notification, rumor control, and restriction and access to the press in the disaster area

**Equipment and supplies:** Sources and where located, usual and special needs, staging areas, and controlled access to supplies; dissemination of donated food, clothing, and storage

**Human resources:** Health professionals, both acute and public health; emergency and disaster specialists; utility officials; officials of government and voluntary agencies; engineers; weather specialists; community leaders, both lay and official

**Team coordination:** Central operations, staging area, chain of command

**Transportation:** Traffic control, access and escape routes, control of risk to victims and rescuers related to transportation

**Documentation:** Details of disaster plan, how and where disseminated; procedures for managing records of injuries, deaths, supplies, and agency reporting responsibilities; development of brief forms with minimal duplication

**Evacuation:** Logistics and procedures, destiny of evacuees, and routes of escape

**Rescue:** Search-and-rescue operations; details the removal of victims and immediate first aid, who is responsible, and what equipment is needed

**Acute care:** Casualty collection points, triage, and detailed role descriptions of healthcare workers for immediate emergency care

**Supportive care:** Shelter management

**Recovery:** Postdisaster team meeting, debriefing, critical incident stress debriefing, press conferences, and reports to media

**Evaluation:** Mock disaster drills and revision of disaster plan based on results

---

### ETHICAL CONNECTION

After the greatest natural disaster in American history, the U.S. government was often accused of being too slow in its response to the plight of abandoned residents in New Orleans after Hurricane Katrina in 2005. Often referred to as "an epic failure of the imagination," did the federal government, specifically FEMA, fulfill its mission, "to lead America to prepare for, prevent, respond to, and recover from disasters with a vision of 'A Nation Prepared'" to protect U.S. residents after disasters?

---

examples include the mayor, chief executive officer(s) of the local hospital(s), executive officer of the local American Red Cross chapter, the emergency medical system manager, and the emergency/triage physicians and nurses. Other agencies or resources and staff persons who make up the disaster team include local, state, and federal disaster management agencies; private relief organizations, such as churches and the Salvation Army; fire and police departments; political leaders who function under the mayor's administration; engineers, geologists, and meteorologists; sociologists, epidemiologists, and other researchers; community volunteers; and the media, including television news reporters, cable weather broadcasters, and radio communication persons (e.g., short-wave radio, HAM radio).

# Disaster Response

Disaster response is a complex plan that is sometimes difficult to coordinate and carry out. All healthcare and other personnel should become knowledgeable about the disaster plan and their anticipated roles. As pointed out previously, regularly evaluating the performance of all involved personnel through mock disaster drills is an important function of community health nurses and other personnel involved in coordinating disaster response (Dixon, 1986; Neff & Kidd, 1993).

## ■ Response and Recovery

The disaster team's **response** is initiated during and after the impact stage of the disaster. Local, state, regional, national, federal, and volunteer agencies assist communities in need (FEMA, 2006). **Recovery** is a long-term process that occurs during the rehabilitation stage of the disaster. Sometimes, severe financial strain is placed on the local or state government during this time.

## ■ Levels of Disaster Response

Disasters are usually defined in terms of severity and levels of response required. Neff and Kidd (1993) identified four levels of disaster response, which are explained in the following paragraphs.

A **level I response** is limited to emergencies that require medical resources from the local hospital and community, such as minor injuries incurred in a local disaster, but also may include severe injuries incurred in multicar accidents or a plane crash. Occasionally, level I responses may include state and federal agency involvement (Neff & Kidd, 1993). In general, hospital and community resources are adequate to provide field and hospital triage, medical treatment, and stabilization for multiple casualties.

All hospitals maintain a written disaster plan that corresponds to the local civil defense and community disaster plan. Fundamental to all written level I hospital disaster plans is the assurance that a command post and chain of command will be established. Usually, the chief executive officer or a senior administrator of the hospital will be in command. Communication via telephones, cellular systems, and portable radios is limited to the commander, security, and other authorized personnel. Water conservation and backup generators are important considerations just in case they are needed. A smooth flow of patients depends on an efficient triage system in the field and within the hospital.

A **level II response** involves multiple casualties that require the use of multijurisdiction healthcare personnel and medical facilities across a specified region (Auf der Heide, 1989; Neff & Kidd, 1993; Boseman, 2003; Bradt, 2002). When more than one geographic jurisdiction is involved or required, the chain of command structure becomes unified for the sake of clarity, information flow, and minimization of duplications. Coordination and communication efforts among the agencies are emphasized at this response level.

When a mass-casualty disaster occurs, a **level III response** is required (Auf der Heide, 1989; Neff & Kidd, 1993). This level of disaster, such as occurred with Hurricane Andrew in South Florida in 1992 and the attacks on the World Trade Center and Pentagon in 2001, is so overwhelming that medical resources at the local and regional levels are exhausted. Consequently, state and federal agencies intervene.

A **level IV response** occurs when FEMA intervenes by providing financial and oversight assistance. FEMA is an independent agency that reports to the president of the United States. Level IV response efforts sometimes require an executive order from the president to declare the disaster a major disaster. (Discussion of the presidential response to FEMA was discussed in the section "Disaster Planning.") From 1953 to early 2007, 1,688 disasters (an average of 30 per year) were declared by the president of the United States as level IV disasters (FEMA, 2005).

## ■ National Disaster Medical System

The **National Disaster Medical System (NDMS)** is a federally coordinated system that augments the United States' medical response capability. The overall purpose of the NDMS is to establish a single, integrated national medical response capability for assisting state and local authorities in dealing with the medical impacts of major peacetime disasters and to provide support to the military and the Department of Veterans Affairs medical systems in caring for casualties evacuated back to the United States from overseas armed conventional conflicts. The NDMS's efforts, such as recommendations and guidelines for disaster planning and response, filter down to state and local governments and officials, such as the civil defense office and the emergency medical services in the community (NDMS, 2006).

The National Response Plan utilizes the NDMS as part of the Department of Health and Human Services, Office of Preparedness and Response, under Emergency Support Function #8 (ESF #8), Health and Medical Care, to support federal agencies in the management and coordination of the federal medical response to major emergencies and federally declared disasters. These events may include any of the following situations.

- Natural disasters
- Technological disasters
- Major transportation accidents
- Acts of terrorism including weapons of mass destruction events

Nurses are involved on every level of the NDMS. Some of the functions of community health and other nurses include serving on the NDMS's national-level task force and board; decision making regarding guidelines and policies; disaster planning on the state and local levels; collaborating with other disaster team members on plans, procedures, and tasks; coordinating the disaster team at various locations within the community; triaging victims at community and hospital locations; and managing the care of victims.

**New Orleans Residents and the "Katrina Cough": Respiratory Problems After the Disaster**

People returning to New Orleans and other flood-ravaged areas in 2005 exhibited a constellation of symptoms—coughs, sore throats, runny noses, and respiratory trouble—that health officials have named the "Katrina cough." The Centers for Disease Control and Prevention (CDC) attributes it mainly to the mold and contaminated dust left behind by the floodwaters that have been stirred up by cleanup and demolition work.

Although "Katrina cough" has not been associated with significant negative effects for the general population in New Orleans, it can be serious for people with asthma, respiratory illness, or compromised immune systems. In previous research studies of New York City residents in the aftermath of 9/11, early symptoms like coughs can exacerbate chronic health problems among people who are not protected from ongoing hazards. If Katrina cough follows the 9/11 pattern, more people are likely to become sick years after the disaster incident.

Following 9/11, numerous research studies have found that residents and workers at Ground Zero were exposed to asbestos, lead, glass fibers, concrete dust, and other toxins. The damage was caused not by a few days of rescue work, but by weeks and months of cleaning up the site or living nearby.

The aftermath of Katrina differs from 9/11 in the specific toxins that have been released into the environment. Residents who returned to their homes in New Orleans following Katrina were exposed to petroleum products, arsenic, lead, mercury, bacteria, and rampant mold. More than 16% of New Orleans children suffered from asthma, for example, according to the American Lung Association. They are at particularly high risk in mold-infested houses.

Although the U.S. Environmental Protection Agency (EPA) recommended that people who were involved in repairing homes in the post-Katrina New Orleans area wear protective equipment, like respirators, many were unable to purchase such equipment. Few retail businesses were open during the first 6 months following the disaster, which resulted in a severe shortage of the needed respirator mask model, called an N95, which filters about 95% of particulate matter and costs about $18 for a box of 20. Painters' masks offer no protection and can actually be worse than no mask at all since the material traps the debris inside the mask.

Links between post-disaster exposure, cancer rates, and other serious illnesses will not be known for years regarding exposed populations after 9/11 and Hurricane Katrina.

*Sources*: Schaffer, A. (2005). Katrina cough: The health problems of 9/11 are back. *Slate*. Retrieved July 18, 2008, from http://www.slate.com/id/2130421; EMS wire service. (2006, January). "Katrina cough" besets residents. *Emergency Medical Services, 35*(1), 16.

## Federal Emergency Management Agency and Disaster Responsiveness and Recovery

The **Federal Emergency Management Agency (FEMA)** is a formerly independent agency that became part of the Department of Homeland Security in March 2003. FEMA is tasked with responding to, planning for, recovering from, and mitigating against disasters.

FEMA can trace its roots to the Congressional Act of 1803. This act, which is generally considered the first piece of disaster legislation, provided assistance to a New Hampshire town following an extensive fire. In the century that followed, ad hoc legislation was passed more than 100 times in response to hurricanes, earthquakes, floods, and other natural disasters. In 1934, Congress passed the Flood Control Act, which gave the U.S. Army Corps of Engineers greater authority to implement flood control projects. The piecemeal approach to disaster assistance throughout these decades was problematic and required little cooperation between federal and state disaster response agencies and the American Red Cross.

The 1960s and early 1970s brought massive disasters requiring major federal response and recovery operations by the Federal Disaster Assistance Administration, established within the Department of Housing and Urban Development (HUD). Hurricane Carla struck in 1962, Hurricane Betsy in 1965, Hurricane Camille in 1969, and Hurricane Agnes in 1972. The Alaskan earthquake hit in 1964, and the San Fernando earthquake rocked Southern California in 1971. These events served to focus attention on the issue of natural disasters and brought about increased legislation. In 1968, the National Flood Insurance Act offered new flood protection to homeowners; in 1974, the Disaster Relief Act firmly established the process of presidential disaster declarations. Although coordination improved, emergency and disaster activities remained fragmented. When hazards associated with nuclear power plants and the transportation of hazardous substances were added to natural disasters, more than 100 federal agencies were involved in some aspect of disasters, hazards, and emergencies. Many parallel programs and policies existed at the state and local levels, compounding the complexity of federal disaster relief efforts (Burnham & Abdallah 2008).

President Jimmy Carter's 1979 executive order merged many of these separate disaster-related responsibilities into FEMA. Among other agencies, FEMA absorbed the Federal Insurance Administration, the National Fire Prevention and Control Administration, the National Weather Service Community Preparedness Program, the Federal Preparedness Agency of the General Services Administration, and the Federal Disaster Assistance Administration activities from HUD. Civil defense responsibilities were also transferred to the new agency from the Defense Department's Defense Civil Preparedness Agency. John Macy, FEMA's first director, emphasized the similarities between natural hazards preparedness and the civil defense activities. To respond to this issue, FEMA began development of an Integrated Emergency Management System with an all-hazards approach that included "direction, control, and warning systems which are common to the full range of emergencies from small isolated events to the ultimate emergency—war."

Research Alert

A new journal for disaster research . . .
*The Journal of Homeland Security and Emergency Management* (JHSEM)

Available online at http://www.bepress.com/jhsem

*The Journal of Homeland Security and Emergency Management* (JHSEM) was created 3 years ago to meet the needs of emerging issues on public health and disaster management. The journal features articles and important research on public health in the context of homeland security and emergency management. Issues have featured topics on diverse subjects, such as the effects of mass public outbreaks (e.g., pandemic flu and SARS) and secondary disasters, such as the flooding of New Orleans. By bridging health issues and homeland security and emergency management, *JHSEM* offers a forum where various fields can find common ground.

The new agency faced many unusual challenges in its first few years that emphasized how complex emergency management can be. Early disasters and emergencies included the contamination of Love Canal, New York; the Cuban refugee crisis; and the accident at the Three Mile Island nuclear power plant in Pennsylvania. Later, the Loma Prieta earthquake in 1989 and Hurricane Andrew in 1992 focused major national attention on FEMA. In 1993, President Bill Clinton nominated James L. Witt as the new FEMA director. Witt became the first agency director with experience as a state emergency manager. He initiated sweeping reforms that streamlined disaster relief and recovery operations, and insisted on a new emphasis regarding preparedness and mitigation. The end of the Cold War also allowed Witt to redirect more of FEMA's limited resources from civil defense into disaster relief, recovery, and mitigation programs.

In 2001, the months after the terrorist attacks of September 11 saw FEMA's efforts being refocused on issues of national preparedness and homeland security, and tested the agency in unprecedented ways. The agency coordinated its activities with the newly formed Office of Homeland Security, and FEMA's Office of National Preparedness was given responsibility for helping to ensure that the nation's first responders were trained and equipped to deal with weapons of mass destruction.

Billions of dollars of new funding were directed to FEMA to help communities face the threat of terrorism. Just a few years past its twentieth anniversary, FEMA was actively directing its "all-hazards" approach to disasters toward homeland security issues. In March 2003, FEMA joined 22 other federal agencies, programs, and offices in becoming the **Department of Homeland Security (DHS)**. The new department brought a coordinated approach to national security issues stemming from emergencies and disasters, both natural and human-made. FEMA is one of four major branches of DHS. More than 5,000 stand-by disaster reservists supplement about 2,500 full-time employees in the Emergency Preparedness and Response Directorate. FEMA's mission remains to lead the United States to prepare for, prevent, respond to, and recover from disasters with a vision of "A Nation Prepared" (FEMA, 2005).

FEMA may respond during the impact stage or the rehabilitation stage of the disaster, or both. It may respond early, during impact, to increase mobilization of personnel and supplies. During recovery or rehabilitation, FEMA responds as the result of an executive order (FEMA, 2005). In the recovery process, FEMA assists in rebuilding communities so that communities and agencies can return to a functional status.

✎ NOTE THIS! ●————————————

Top U.S. States for Federal Declaration of Disaster

| | |
|---|---|
| Texas | Alabama |
| California | Kentucky |
| Florida | Pennsylvania |
| New York | Ohio |
| Louisiana | Mississippi |
| Oklahoma | |

*Source*: http://www.fema.gov/news/disaster_totals_annual.fema

## ■ Other Disaster Agencies

### American and International Red Cross Disaster Services

The American Red Cross (ARC) is a humanitarian organization led by volunteers and guided by the Congressional Charter and the Fundamental Principles of the International Red Cross Movement (ARC, 2008). The ARC provides relief to victims of disasters and helps people prevent, prepare for, and respond to emergencies.

On May 21, 1881, Clara Barton and a group of her friends founded the ARC because of her commitment to and hard work with the mass casualties of yellow fever, dysentery, and many other infections during the Spanish–American War (ARC, 1990; Frantz, 1998). In gratitude for the efforts of the Red Cross nurses during the Spanish–American War, Cuba communicated the committed efforts of Clara Barton to important officials. A former schoolteacher and government worker from Massachusetts, Barton was not actually a nurse. Nevertheless, her organizational skills were exceptional.

The unique contribution that Barton made to the worldwide Red Cross movement was her organization of volunteers to help disaster victims (ARC, 1990). America became the thirty-second nation to support the Red Cross international treaty at the Geneva Convention in 1882. In 1900, the U.S. Congress granted the ARC its charter. The Red Cross nurses of the Spanish–American War were also responsible for the congressional decision of 1901 to establish the Army Nurse Corps.

The ARC is composed of more than 1.2 million adult and youth volunteers. Many nurses are considered disaster volunteers. Community health nurses, for example, should take a voluntary leadership role in the ARC's disaster preparedness, response, and shelter management. Increasingly, ARC volunteers are being trained for technological disasters, such as those involving toxic chemicals, explosive materials, radiation, bioterrorism, and chemicals.

### Salvation Army

William Booth founded the Salvation Army in London in 1865 (Salvation Army, 2008). The Salvation Army was founded on Christian principles. The Salvation Army Act of 1980 described this organization's mission; "the advancement of Christian religion . . . of education, the relief of poverty, and other charitable objects beneficial to society of the community of humanity as a whole" (Salvation Army, 2008).

During a disaster, the Salvation Army provides food, water, shelter, and clothing and helps trace families. With the goal of carrying out God's mission, Salvationists reach out to suffering and needy people by providing the word of God and basic human physical needs (Salvation Army, 2008).

## Evacuation

Community health nurses, among many other health-care personnel, need to realize that wild panic reactions are different from fleeing from a threat (Auf der Heide, 1989; Weeks, 2007). Mileti, Drabek, and Haas (1975) have noted that panic might occur but usually arises only when at least one of three conditions is present: (1) a perception of immediate danger, (2) an encounter with blocked escape routes, and/or (3) a feeling of being isolated. When panic occurs, it is usually of short duration and not contagious, depending on the response from the media (Bransma et al., 2007; Auf der Heide, 1989).

### ENVIRONMENTAL CONNECTION

What can we do to evacuate large numbers of people in advance of a major natural disaster?

After Hurricane Katrina, one of the primary problems cited by planning commissions was the inability to evacuate vulnerable populations. One of the solutions proposed by the state of Mississippi is the use of school buses and cafeterias. What solutions other than these might make mass evacuation more effective and save lives in natural disasters?

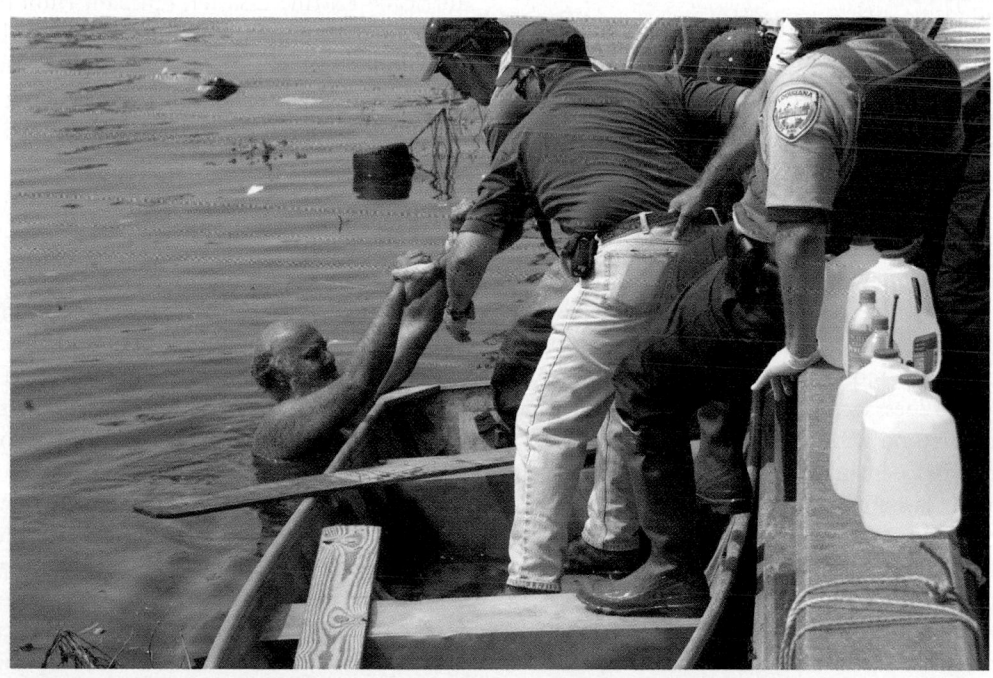

Hurricane Katrina created massive flooding after the storm when the levees failed. Residents were trapped in their homes or left alone in the water; many suffered and died as a result of the rising waters.

Disaster planning includes the rapid evacuation of large populations via U.S. interstate highways.

Evacuation traditionally has been a difficult task to carry out because of people's reluctance to evacuate (Quarantelli & Dynes, 1972; Wenger, James, & Faupel, 1985; Langan & James, 2004). Several reasons explain this reluctance. The primary reason for hesitancy is that some people do not believe that they are in danger. Another reason is that some people want to remain at the site to protect their property. Not wanting to evacuate until the family can be removed as a unit is another reason for hesitancy. The head of the household or another member may refuse to leave until other family members, who may also include dogs or other pets, are safe (Landesman, 2005; Saunders, 2007).

Besides demonstrating concern for human lives, FEMA is concerned for the lives of animals and, more specifically, the human–animal bond (Lockwood, 1997; FEMA, 2005; Rosenkoetter et al., 2007). Many owners of pets have developed close relationships with their pets. Lockwood (1997) has explored why animal owners will risk danger to themselves and not evacuate disaster areas without assurance of their animals' well-being; the most common responses are that people love their animals and treat them as part of the family.

The key to motivating people to evacuate is to improve warning effectiveness, which relies on several strategies (Auf der Heide, 1989; Saunders, 2007; Rosenkoetter et al., 2007). The credibility of the present warning and the validity of past evacuation warnings, for example, both influence a person's decision about whether to evacuate. Consistency and repetition of the warning by different sources of the evacuation command always increase the chance that a person will heed the warning. Commands to evacuate by agency and community officials are taken more seriously, which promotes the believability of the message. A clear, specific message to evacuate that is understood will yield better results. Finally, an effective strategy is to ensure a full range of protective actions, such as ample law enforcement officers on duty, for those people evacuating.

A significant problem in the evacuation of New Orleans residents prior to and during Hurricane Katrina was rooted in the Louisiana State Evacuation Plan. The plan left the means of evacuation up to individual citizens, parish governments, and private caretakers. Unfortunately, many private caretaking facilities relied on the same bus companies and ambulance services for evacuation and so were unable to function for this purpose. Fuel and rental cars were in short supply, and most forms of public transportation had been shut down well before the storm struck (United States Congress, 2006; Hayes, 2005; Balinsky, 2003; Kiewra, 2006; Burnham & Abdallah, 2008; Bransma et al., 2007).

## Role of the Media

The mass media can be either a friend or a foe in the management of disasters (Dwyer & Drew, 2005; United States Congress, 2006). To enhance disaster response, the media can provide accurate information, convey instructions to the public, and stimulate donations from parts of the country not affected by the disaster. Conversely, the media may complicate the operations by putting a "feeding frenzy" spin on the facts (Haygood & Tyson, 2005). Reporters may make unreasonable demands on resources, facilities, and officials (Auf der Heide, 1989). Distortion of the facts, overreaction, and perpetuation of disaster myths are other factors that may interfere with the disaster response operations (Haygood & Tyson, 2005). For example, during the Hurricane Katrina disaster, rampant rumors about looting, homicides, mass uprisings, and deaths in the New Orleans Superdome proved to be unfounded, yet they dramatically affected both the communities experiencing the disaster and the general public's perceptions about the disaster.

---

**MEDIA MOMENT**

**When the Levees Broke: A Requiem in Four Acts** (2007)
Spike Lee commemorates the people of New Orleans with a 4-hour epic documentary about the destruction of the city of New Orleans from Hurricane Katrina and ill-fated disaster relief efforts. Lee doesn't just recount the events of late August 2005, but rather asks *why* they unfolded the way they did. Weaving interviews with news footage and amateur video, Lee uses the film to give meaningful voice to the people who were left behind. With a detached, unsentimental eye, he delivers a poignant account of a major moment in recent U.S. history. While offering no simple answers, you will be left with even more questions, such as "How could this unprecedented disaster involving a major U.S. city have happened in the United States?"

Good communication is vital during the evacuation operations (Yellowlees & MacKenzie, 2003; Norwalk, 2007). The Weather Bureau, radio stations, television announcements, local sirens and announcements, and computers should be used to alert the public of the impending threat. Another key medium is the Emergency Broadcast System, where officials provide local, state, or national information and warnings. When the evacuation is in process, a large volume of requests place overwhelming demands on the media as well as on public officials of the city and county. One of the major findings of the 2006 U.S. Congress report on Hurricane Katrina, entitled *A Failure of Initiative: Final Report of the Select Bipartisan Committee to Investigate the Preparation for and Response to Hurricane Katrina,* was the critical problems in rescue efforts related to communication technology breakdown, such as the destruction of cellular and relay towers, radio and television station destruction, and a lack of alternatives with such failure.

## Rescue

The search-and-rescue mission is the most challenging part of the disaster operations (Silverstein, 1984; Waeckerle, 1983, 1991; Hayes, 2005; Saunders, 2007). Searching for and rescuing disaster victims tax the physical capabilities and emotions of rescuers. Emotional demands can also be extremely traumatic to the rescuers, who may require psychosocial debriefing (Rhoads et al., 2006). Teams of healthcare personnel, fire and security officials, and volunteers comb the designated area many times in search of casualties. Once the casualties are located, quick triage actions are necessary. After the victims are categorized by way of triage, rescue workers need to continue to search the area for undiscovered injured people or dead bodies.

## Triage

The triage system normally practiced in emergency departments across the country is not the same triage system used during a disaster (Kitt, Selfridge-Thomas, Proehl, & Kaiser, 1995; Norwalk, 2007; Waltham, 2005). Field (disaster) triage is used when mass casualties result from disaster. The initial triage that takes place in the field is called the primary triage. Secondary triage occurs at the point of entry into the medical facility. Tertiary triage occurs in the specified area where the patient is located, such as the emergency department, pediatrics, and so on.

**Disaster triage** allows healthcare personnel to identify the most salvageable patients so that treatment can be initiated immediately. Colored tags with symbols are attached to disaster victims so that healthcare personnel (Burnham & Abdallah 2008) can readily see level of triage (Kitt et al., 1995).

Several factors may affect the triage system (Dixon, 1986), such as the patient's general state of health. For example, an elderly person may have a poor cardiovascular status, which may decrease the person's survival expectation.

Another factor that may affect the outcome of triage is the healthcare worker's experience (or lack thereof) in triage and assessment. Lack of supplies or equipment is another factor. Not having proper supplies and equipment in sufficient quantities can adversely influence the disaster victim's triage status (Neff & Kidd, 1993; Balinsky, 2003; Langan & James, 2004; Weeks, 2007).

## Disaster Shelters

Trained volunteers and/or ARC nurses manage shelters. When help is needed, the executive director of the affected local chapter of the ARC calls upon nurses and other volunteers. Shelters are opened by volunteers in the community through coordinated efforts of the ARC, the mayor, civil defense, and other officials of the community. Churches, schools, civic centers, and community centers may all be used as shelters.

**Application to Practice**

*Thinking Critically . . . an Ethical and Management Nightmare from "Ground Zero" during Hurricane Katrina*
Imagine you are the top nurse administrator at a large mental hospital in New Orleans after Hurricane Katrina hit. All hospitals in the metro area have evacuated and closed, with only your hospital remaining open. Nurses are having difficulty deciding which patients to care for, with a severe shortage of nurses and hundreds of patients pouring into the emergency room needing hospitalization. As a mental health facility, you do not have the resources for medical problems. Nurses are having ethical conflict over making decisions about which patients should be transferred via FEMA air lifts. They fear that their patients will be more at risk due to their fragile mental state if transferred. Food and water begins to run out after 2 days and the morgue cannot take any more bodies. Rationing of basic supplies, food, and water has begun. Ice has run out and water from the flood remains in the halls and most patient rooms. A local television station is broadcasting from the hospital ER and has requested to enter the hospital for patient and nurse interviews. What actions should you take? Can you ask the station to stop broadcasting? Can you force them to do so? List the things that would be priority for you as nurse manager?

It is sometimes difficult to determine or anticipate shelter needs during disasters. The local ARC chapter depends on other ARC chapters, the mayor, and civil defense teams to report anticipated numbers of persons who are evacuating their premises and reporting to a shelter. In widespread disasters, shelters are opened in a number of areas that house local residents as well as victims who have traveled a long distance to escape more immediate danger. An example of a widespread disaster was Hurricane Camille in 1969, which traveled from the Mississippi Gulf Coast to North Mississippi and beyond. Persons in the most danger were on the Mississippi Gulf Coast, so they evacuated to cities and towns north of the coast, while the local residents of those areas also were evacuating their premises and relocating to the same shelters. In instances, anticipating the correct number of shelter residents is difficult.

By the time Hurricane Katrina hit in 2005, 26 years later, ARC officials were better able to plan the evacuation route and anticipate how and when evacuees would most likely relocate. Even with mock disaster drills and extensive planning for facilitating disaster shelter triage of residents, the extensiveness of the affected disaster area (over many miles) meant that the system was ill prepared to handle the number and risk level of the evacuees from the New Orleans area (Nigg et al., 2006).

Good communication between city officials and remote areas regarding evacuation numbers must be a priority prior to the disaster, because communication is often hampered by the destruction of electricity, phone lines, and cell phone relay towers (Balinsky, 2003; Langan & James, 2004; Weeks, 2007). For each shelter, there is one team manager, at least one nurse volunteer, multiple people to keep records, and numerous volunteers trained to assist victims. Activities include keeping thorough records; coordinating meals; providing snacks, cots, blankets, and other essentials; providing health care, such as first-aid treatment and over-the-counter medications that have been authorized by a physician; acting as a liaison between victims and resource agencies and their families; and protecting the victims from harm by keeping alert to possible fire outbreaks, accidents, and other mishaps. When help is needed, the ARC coordinates mass recruitment of supplies, equipment, food, and shelter. For example, after the summer Midwest floods in 1993, Wal-Mart loaned the ARC a large warehouse, forklifts, and staff to expedite distribution of urgently needed supplies to the shelters (ARC, 1995). Other retail stores and pharmaceutical companies offered many supplies and a large amount of monetary assistance.

### 🖉 NOTE THIS!

**Hurricane Camille**

Hurricane Camille was a category 5 hurricane that hit the coasts of Mississippi, Alabama, and Louisiana with winds in excess of 200 mph. Hurricane Camille resulted in the deaths of 141 persons, 9,472 injuries, property loss and damage for 74,000 families, and more than $1 billion total damage. At the 30-year anniversary of the storm, the scars and influence of Camille still exist on the Mississippi Gulf Coast, where the most severe damage occurred. The storm produced 24-foot tidal waves in August 1969 and remains one of the deadliest storms of the twentieth century.

**Comments from Survivors**

"Afterwards, it looked like we had been bombed. My house was 'caddy whompas' on its foundation. All you could hear were helicopters and people crying. It was the most horrible experience I have ever had."

"The thing that I remember were the dead cows on the beach."

"The beach looked like a holocaust. A woman slipping and sliding through mud and muck clutching a lifeless child to her chest."

*Source: Hattiesburg American*, August 14, 1994, p. 7A.

## Role of the Community Health Nurse in Disasters

Why should community health nurses be involved in disasters? Aren't trauma and hospital nurses better qualified to work in disasters than nurses in the community?

Good questions—ones that many student nurses and practicing nurses alike may ask. Our ideas about disasters, including what happens and who is involved—both victims and rescuers—are often shaped by the media. The disaster movie formula developed as a major box office draw in the 1970s with such movies as the *Airport* series about jet liner crashes; *The Towering Inferno* (1974), about a burning skyscraper; *The Hindenburg* (1975), about the real-life zeppelin airship disaster of 1937; and *The China Syndrome* (1979), about a fictitious nuclear power plant accident, which became an eerie prelude to the actual Three Mile Island nuclear accident that same year. During the past 30 years, U.S. and international moviegoers have been fascinated by disasters and continue to line up for movies such as *Armageddon* (1998), *Deep Impact* (1998), *The Day After Tomorrow* (2004), *Independence Day* (1996), and *Titanic* (1997), the biggest movie money-maker of all time.

These movies, as well as television programs such as *ER*, portray disasters as a backdrop for story lines and romances, heroes and villains, and greatly influence the way we visualize disasters. As a result, disaster planning and disaster prepared-

### ☞ THINK ABOUT THIS

What would you do in a terrorist biological attack?

Assume you are a nurse administrator responsible for a large urban hospital when a biological terrorist attack occurs in your city. What precautions would you need to take? Think about things like quarantining patients, protecting the staff, decontaminating rooms and equipment, obtaining and securing antidotes, and monitoring the spread of disease. Do you think the same techniques would be applicable in a chemical or nuclear attack? What additional actions would you take in these circumstances?

ness are given very little attention. In truth, the most recent terrorist attacks on the World Trade Center and the Pentagon provided more specific details about actual recovery and effects of aftermath for the public through extensive media coverage. At least temporarily, the American public appears to be more aware about the need for preparedness for disaster.

Community health nurses are much better prepared than most other healthcare professionals are to manage disasters in the community, because emergency treatment and triage are but two of many activities that help people cope with disaster. Successful strategies often pair a community health nurse with a trauma nurse in the disaster setting. Among the major determinants of how effectively a disaster is managed are not only how well we carry out our individual roles in a disaster, but also how well we allow others to carry out their roles (Suserud & Haljamae, 1997; Weeks, 2007).

## General Functions of the Community Health Nurse

Community health nurses, as well as other nurses, are involved in emergency treatment and triage during the impact stage of the disaster. Good physical assessment skills are vital for success. Only healthcare personnel highly skilled in assessment should perform the triage function. Most healthcare personnel are not trained in advanced assessment skills and cannot make acuity judgments proficiently.

Nursing is specialized, as are most health professions. As a result, community health nurses often are more knowledgeable about teamwork and interdisciplinary effort than nurses in other specialties are because they rely on group efforts daily in community health nursing practice. Community health nurses are experts in program planning, community assessment, and group dynamics—all skills that are critical to the effective management of a disaster crisis. Because community health nurses are population focused, assessing and intervening with vulnerable populations are second nature to them.

Other functions that enable community health nurses to work effectively in disasters include working with the media to inform and educate, the use of public health interventions to minimize risks from communicable diseases, and the securing of community resources for victims. These functions are accomplished while coordinating multiagency efforts in the mediation of health risks at the disaster site. The background work of disaster management, for which community health nurses are perfectly suited, may not make it to the big screen, but such activities are what ultimately influence how well a community survives and heals from disaster.

## Specific Nursing Approaches

A major goal of community health nurses is to be an asset to the community, not a burden. Specific approaches that community health nurses should take to mitigate human and material losses in a community disaster include the following strategies:

### Got an Alternative?

The Role of Art in Healing After the 9/11 Disaster

"Americans need the solace of art, along with their other diverse cultural, spiritual, and religious practices, now more than ever."

—Karen VanMeenen

Art is created and viewed for pleasure, for distraction, to tell stories, to emote, for documentation purposes, as an educational tool, to channel creative energies, for the processing of personal experience and for healing. Artists have always responded to personal and political challenges with their own outpourings of creative practice—documenting their illnesses, celebrating their survival, working through their difficulties, calling for change. Artists and health professionals have long known the beneficial effects of creating and viewing artwork on an individual and a communal level (e.g., the success of the AIDS Quilt). Art can tell personal truths as well as allow viewers access to universal truths, universal experience.

*Source*: Vanmeenen, K. (2001, November/December). Media art AS/IN therapy [special issue]. *Afterimage, 29*(3).

**Personal Preparedness**
- Be disaster-prepared and disaster-aware.
- Maintain your own emergency equipment, supplies, and skills.
- Be certain that your family knows what to do during a disaster, when to do it, who to call, and where to go.
- Use caution and prudence when selecting the location of your home.

**Community Involvement**
- Become familiar with local disaster plans and emergency evacuation procedures.
- Get involved in the political issues in your community that relate to disaster preparedness and recovery.
- Support leaders who choose long-term, focused solutions in loss reduction and emergency preparedness rather than those who choose short-sighted, politically expedient solutions.
- Help modify land use and develop ordinances that reflect the best knowledge of geography and water hazards.
- Support local emergency assistance organizations by serving on advisory boards.
- Assist in the education of the public in personal disaster preparedness.
- Visit schools to help prepare children for assuming the lifetime responsibility of being prepared for disasters in the community.

**Professional Preparedness**
- Become trained and certified in professional disaster nursing by the local ARC chapter.

- Get involved in the development of agency and community disaster plans.
- Attend continuing education classes and disaster skills updates to keep current in disaster management skills.
- Be supportive of administrative efforts to increase disaster preparedness.
- Write news stories, volunteer to speak at community meetings, write letters to the editor of local newspapers, and publish articles in nursing journals about the nursing role in disaster preparedness (Garcia, 1985; Burnham & Abdallah, 2008).

## Shelter Management and Care

Roles played by healthcare workers in disasters are critical to community recovery. Community health nurses play a vital role in disaster preparedness and response. In fact, the leadership administered by community health nurses may greatly affect the public's reception and comprehension of disaster education and warnings. See the Application to Practice feature on page 603 for examples of successful shelter management.

Neither the public nor many nurses realize the impact that nurses have before, during, and after a disaster (Burnham & Abdallah, 2008; Landesman et al., 2005). The leadership role that community health nurses can take may prevent deaths and property damage.

Red Cross disaster nurses and other volunteers are often trained to coordinate and manage shelters, conduct tertiary triage within the shelter, and administer first aid to sick or wounded people. Currently, the Red Cross has a pool of more than 15,000 trained disaster volunteers, many of whom are nurses (ARC, 2006). With Hurricane Katrina, the number of disaster-trained nurses proved inadequate, and the ARC sought all RNs who could assist with the overwhelming number of shelters opened in the disaster area. These nurses were trained "on the spot" and were often asked to be on duty for much longer times owing to the magnitude of the disaster. Additionally, because of the large numbers of persons left homeless by Katrina, shelters in many areas remained open for months after the disaster.

Volunteers are ready for immediate assignment for damage assessment, case management, and shelter management at a moment's notice. The ARC shelter manager, often a community health nurse, organizes and manages the shelter operations by fulfilling the roles of administrator, leader, and supervisor (Garcia, 1985; Saunders, 2007). The way the manager conducts operations affects the flow of operations and activities within the shelter. Functions of the manager include allocating space, obtaining supplies and equipment, scheduling staff, completing reports and records, and attending to problems. If the community health nurse volunteer happens to be the manager and the nurse on duty, the dual roles and functions can become overwhelming. Care should be coordinated by application of the nursing process. Good

## *a conversation with . . .*

### Toni D. Frioux

Because of the tremendous response from caring volunteers at the Oklahoma City bombing disaster, the first critical step was to establish a centralized system to manage the number of individuals calling to report to the emergency site. Once established, we were able to schedule, validate licenses, and orient volunteers from the Oklahoma State Medical Association, Oklahoma Nurses Association, American Red Cross, hospitals, and other entities to the expectations and limitations of the bomb site.

There was tremendous generosity from everyone. Medical supplies, equipment, and medication were immediately available and continued to be delivered at the site for many days. Public health was responsible for centralizing and assuring that these supplies were used appropriately and responsibly by licensed providers. It was important to assure that the appropriate practice guidelines were in place.

Providing disaster services as a public health function doesn't end with just providing emergency services. Public health is also responsible for ensuring that volunteers that provide ongoing emergency health services are competent and properly licensed. It is important to be familiar with your state's nurse practice act and knowledgeable regarding any actions that might be needed to invoke licensure reciprocity in the event that the disaster is of such magnitude that volunteers arrive from other states or countries to assist.

Planning and ongoing networking with all players in the emergency response team are very important. While personnel may change, the fundamental needs in an emergency generally do not. Having a public health work force that is prepared in disaster response is very beneficial.

Any coordination and networking that can be in place with state and local American Red Cross chapters prior to a disaster benefits both the public health agency and the American Red Cross.

—Toni D. Frioux, MS, CNS, ARNP, Chief, Nursing Service, Oklahoma State Department of Health

assessment and planning skills are among the most important functions of the community health nurse volunteer. Interventions in this setting include preventing disease and illness, providing emotional support, protecting health, and providing intermittent, temporary care to this vulnerable population. With Hurricane Katrina, residents were often displaced from their homes and family, which made the housing issue much more challenging. Many residents in these shelters did not know if they had a home to return to, nor did they know where their families were. Because of the rapid evacuation of survivors from the New Orleans and Mississippi Gulf Coast, many had nothing except the

## NOTE THIS!

**What is the American Red Cross?**

The American Red Cross is a voluntary, nonprofit organization that responds to all disasters, regardless of size and scope. The Federal Emergency Management Agency (FEMA) is a federal agency under the Department of Homeland Security. FEMA responds when a disaster has received a presidential declaration. FEMA is involved with community recovery, such as repairing and building bridges and public buildings and assisting in security of disaster areas; ARC provides humanitarian aid to individuals. Nurses have always been a cornerstone for the provision of services by the American Red Cross. Historically, Red Cross nurses have provided their assistance during times of disaster and conflict beginning with the 1889 Johnstown floods and the 1888 Yellow Fever epidemic. Jane Delano formally established the Red Cross Nursing Service in 1909. Red Cross nursing has also had a major role in the historical evolution of nursing and nursing leadership in the United States with many Red Cross nurses, including Jane Delano, Clara Noyes, Julia Stimson, and others, playing strategic roles in the development of American nursing.

Today more than 30,000 nurses continue to be involved in paid and volunteer capacities at all levels and in all service areas throughout the American Red Cross. These activities consist of:

- Providing direct services such as local disaster action teams, health fairs, volunteering in military clinics and hospitals, blood collection teams, and first aid stations
- Teaching and developing courses in CPR/First Aid, automatic emergency defibrillator (AED), disaster health services, nurse assistant training, babysitting, and family care giving
- Acting in management and supervisory roles including chapter and blood services region executives
- Functioning in governance roles such as local board member to national board of governors

*Source*: American Red Cross. (2008). *Disaster services*. Retrieved July 22, 2008, from http://www.redcross.org/services/disaster

American Red Cross nursing pin.

***Then and now . . . perspectives on disaster***

"*The detection and control of saboteurs are the responsibilities of the FBI, but the recognition of epidemics caused by sabotage is particularly an epidemiologic function. . . . therefore any plan of defense against biological warfare sabotage requires trained epidemiologists alert to all possibilities and available for call at a moment's notice, anywhere in the country.*"
—*Alexander Langmuir, 1952, Founder of the Centers for Disease Control and Prevention (CDC) Epidemiological Investigation Service (EIS) Program*

"*It is public health's job to train rapid-response teams [in a disaster] that can go out and gather data early on. Without statistically meaningful numbers, you cannot know where the greatest needs are. Resources must be distributed based on need, not who gets there first. When that standard crumbles, there is community outrage.*"
—*Professor Jennifer Leaning, 2006, Harvard School of Public Health*

clothes on their back, no medication, and few necessities for self-care. As in most disasters of this severity, elders, patients with chronic physical and mental problems, and children accounted for a large number of the evacuees (Garcia, 1985; Burnham & Abdallah, 2008).

Anticipation of certain problems will facilitate the operations and care of the community health nurse volunteer. For instance, in the shelter population, the nurse should expect some everyday, normal occurrences, which will include chronically ill people who are dependent on medications and equipment, normal episodes of illness and infection, communicable disease, and emotional stress reactions. Evaluation of the shelter population should be ongoing, including one-on-one conferences with shelter families and staff members. In the Hurricane Katrina example, the ARC was able to use advanced technology to keep up-to-date shelter resident rosters all over the affected area, which assisted nurses in helping residents locate their families in shelters located throughout the United States.

## Disaster Recovery

Toffler, in his classic study *Future Shock*, described future shock as "the response to overstimulation" (1970, p. 344). He described numerous examples of stress in situations requiring constant change; among them are persons in disasters. Toffler described persons who experienced a disaster as being trapped in environments that are rapidly changing, unfamiliar, and unpredictable. Results of such situations can be devastating, even for the most stable and well-prepared person. Victims of disasters may be hurled into antiadaptive states and be incapable of the most elementary decision making (Toffler, 1970). Evidence of this reaction can be seen in pictures of a woman, after a destructive earthquake, strolling down a dangerous, debris-filled road with a dead or wounded baby in her arms, her face blank and numb, appearing impervious to the danger around her. Persons can be overwhelmed and become paralyzed as familiar objects and relationships are transformed. Where a person's house once stood, a tornado can within minutes change the environment into an unrecognizable pile of rubble and gushing water pipes. The Oklahoma City bombing destroyed life and property within minutes, replacing familiar landmarks with images of unimaginable horror and destruction.

Simple acts taken for granted hours before, such as making a telephone call or pouring a cup of coffee, are no longer appropriate or possible. Signs, sounds, and other psychological and cultural cues surround disaster victims without meaning, without recognition during and immediately after the impact. Every word, every action, every movement is characterized by uncertainty. Even in a crowd, victims often experience a sense of isolation and loneliness, abandonment, and an overwhelming sense of loss of the world as they know it. Confusion, disorientation, and distortion of reality occur spontaneously; fatigue, anxiety, tenseness, and extreme irritability follow. Apathy, emotional withdrawal, and pessimism result when victims develop a sense of little hope for the future or when they see themselves as never being safe or stable again (Toffler, 1970).

After a major disaster, such as Hurricane Andrew in Homestead, Florida, and Hurricane Katrina on the Mississippi Gulf Coast and New Orleans, Louisiana, healthcare facilities are often disabled or destroyed. Recovery may take years and the community is often faced with inadequate or nonexistent health services. This is often referred to as the "disaster after the disaster"—catastrophic community changes that can hamper recovery efforts and further damage a community's health. The havoc wrought by a major disaster affects the lives of healthcare facilities' staff, patients, and the community for many years after the initial disaster.

For example, a year after Hurricane Andrew struck Homestead, Homestead Hospital had lost 70% of its employees, many of whom had worked tirelessly through the disaster. Charity care spiked from 11% of patients to 26%. The hospital went from years of profitability to an $8 million loss. Additionally, demographic shifts in the community created challenges for the hospital. Many senior citizens left the community, never to return; replacing them were young families attracted by the affordable, federally funded housing market. These demographic changes are common after a hurricane, especially in coastal areas that attract large numbers of retirees. In addition to losing Medicare dollars and adding more Medicaid-insured families, hospitals often have to completely reorganize their services to meet the needs of the post-disaster community (Colias, 2005).

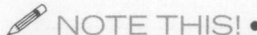

### NOTE THIS!

**Children, Terrorism, and Disasters: Web Resources**

Society's most vulnerable population, children, is at a greater risk for developing health problems as a result of terrorism and disasters. Additionally, exposure to media coverage about disasters and other catastrophic events can have adverse emotional and psychological effects for children. The American Academy of Pediatrics (AAP) has an area on its website dedicated to children, terrorism, and disasters. The website helps pediatricians, parents, community leaders, and others prepare for and meet children's needs during a disaster. Examples of information available include the following:

- Family Readiness Kit: Preparing to Handle Disasters
- The Youngest Victims: Disaster Preparedness to Meet Children's Needs
- AAP resources, federal resources, and medical journal and report information on topics such as biological, chemical, and nuclear agents
- How to communicate with children in the wake of a disaster

See http://www.aap.org/terrorism

**In Their Own Words: 9/11 Parents Help Other Parents and Schools with Lessons Learned**

Through the constructive advice of experienced parents, this publication discusses emergency planning for schools. The events of September 11 and its aftermath have challenged health, environment, and education agencies to understand how children are different from adults in relation to environmental hazards, and how schools are different from offices in terms of their responsibilities for the occupants and the demands on the facilities.

See http://www.healthyschools.org/documents/INTHEIROWNWORDS .pdf

**School Nurse Role in Bioterrorism Emergency Preparedness and Response**

It is the position of the National Association of School Nurses that school nurses should be designated and recognized as first responders to mass casualty emergencies, including those resulting from bioterrorist events. School nurses should be trained in protection, detection, and treatment of victims of such events and in the command and control management techniques of the logistics of such a situation. The strategic position of well-prepared nurses within the school environment has significant potential for minimizing the effects of a bioterrorist attack in school settings and, subsequently, in the community at large.

See http://www.nasn.org/Portals/0/positions/2005psbioterrorism.pdf

**How Schools Can Become More Disaster Resistant: Resources for Parents and Teachers**

FEMA recommends the following actions for all school officials: (1) Identify hazards likely to happen to your schools; (2) mitigate against the hazards; (3) develop a response plan, including evacuation route; (4) plan for coping after a disaster; and (5) implement drills and family education.

See http://www.fema.gov/kids/schdizr.htm

Fuel shortages often accompany major disasters and add to the stress of recovery.

 NOTE THIS!

**The Bush–Clinton Fund for Hurricane Katrina recovery**
"I just went the first time I saw New Orleans. My mother went to nursing school here. I have been coming here since I was three years old."

—President Bill Clinton, upon his first visit to New Orleans after Hurricane Katrina, Interview May 18, 2006

Former Presidents Bill Clinton and George H. W. Bush have paired up to raise funds for the hurricane disasters via the Bush–Clinton Fund and had raised $100 million as of 2006.

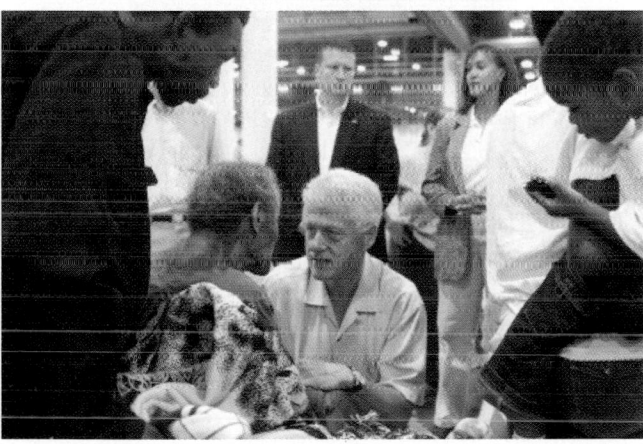

The Bush–Clinton Katrina Fund is made possible by contributions received from donors throughout the nation and the world in response to Hurricane Katrina. The fund was set up to provide grants for medium- to long-term recovery needs in the affected areas. In December 2005, Presidents George H. W. Bush and William J. Clinton allocated $20 million from the Bush–Clinton Katrina Fund (BCKF) for local and regional faith-based organizations located in the affected areas prior to Hurricane Katrina in Alabama, Louisiana, and Mississippi. The fund sought applications from religious organizations to assist in rebuilding houses of worship and to cover costs for temporary relocation. The BCKF seeks to make a distinct impact on the unmet needs of the affected region in the following areas: financial self-sufficiency, economic opportunity, and quality of life.

Visit www.bushclintonkatrinafund.org

Hurricane Katrina was a "wake-up" call for hospitals throughout the Gulf Coast region, according to Brian Keeley, CEO of Baptist Health South Florida in Coral Gables, Florida. "My conclusion is that it's beyond the capability of the municipal or state government to adequately respond to a disaster of that magnitude. It has to be a federal effort, and we've seen firsthand that it takes a long time to get them in here" (cited in Colias, 2005, p. 44). Baptist Health is spending millions to ensure that all of its hospitals in the Gulf Coast area can withstand a Category 5 hurricane—that is, have diesel storage, backup water and air-conditioning systems, reinforced windows, hurricane shutters, and the ability to turn on generator power for 2 weeks.

In the classic study *Everything in Its Path,* sociologist Kai Erickson (1976) described the 1972 Buffalo Creek flood and its aftermath in terms of disaster impact and the destruction of community. This study provided a detailed and analyzed view of a disaster and the resulting conflict between individualism and dependency, self-assertion and resignation, and self-centeredness and community orientation. The results of this devastating disaster included loss of community connection, declining morality, rise in crime, and the rise in out-migration from the sudden loss of neighborhood and community. Organized disaster activity was largely provided by outsiders.

Collective deaths, like those in a disaster, do not permit persons to set up the usual barriers between the living and the dead, as is customary in the deaths of the hospital, where "death is screened from view, sanitized, muffled, tidied up" (Erickson, 1976, p. 169). In disaster, "death lies out there at its inescapable worst. There are no wreckers to rush the crushed vehicle away, no physicians to shroud death in a crisp white sheet or to give it a clean medical name, no undertakers to wash away the evidence of death and to knead out the creases of pain or fear . . . and the sight does not go away easily" (Erickson, 1976, p. 169).

## ■ Effects on Survivors

When death is experienced on a wide scale, such as in a disaster, survivors often experience guilt as a result of their own survival (Erickson, 1976). They may even come

One of the consequences of a major disaster, such as Hurricane Katrina, is the challenge of keeping families together.

---

✏️ NOTE THIS! •————————————————

Four years after 9/11, thousands of people who worked at Ground Zero or lived in lower Manhattan were still sick with respiratory problems and other illnesses because of the contaminants they were exposed to. Some do not respond to standard medications and are unable to work. The total impact on the population from these toxins will most likely remain unknown for years.

---

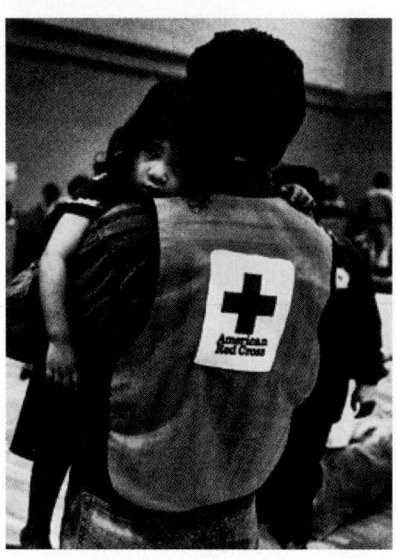

to regret their own survival, when others around them were killed in what seems like a meaningless and capricious way, in part because "they cannot understand by what logic they came to be spared" (p. 170). Survivor guilt has often been described in disaster research literature. Lifton (1967), in his classic study of the psychological effects of the atomic bomb in Hiroshima, found that survivors described the open eyes of corpses as evoking guilt: It was as if the eyes were saying, "Why me, why not you?"

Lifton and Olson (1976) identified five major elements that may be found in some type of combination in all disasters. Psychological difficulty or maladaptive response is more likely to occur if all five elements are found in a single disaster, as in the Buffalo Creek flood. The five elements are suddenness of the event, human callousness in causation (human-made rather than natural causation), continuing relationship of survivors to the disaster, isolation of the community, and totality of destruction.

The experience of the disaster can have both short- and long-term effects on mental health and functioning, such as dissociation, depression, and PTSD (Gerrity & Flynn, 1997). Refer to Box 24-5 for other health effects associated with disasters. Meichenbaum (1994) has compiled from disaster research a list of factors that can place individuals in a vulnerable position for developing psychological problems when all five of Lifton and Olson's (1976) elements are present in a disaster:

- Objective and subjective characteristics of the disaster, such as proximity of the victim to the disaster site, the duration, the degree of physical injury, and the witnessing of grotesque, graphic scenes
- The characteristics in the community of the postdisaster response and recovery environment, such as cohesiveness of community and disruption of social support systems
- The characteristics of the individual or group—for example, elders, unemployed persons, single parents, children, those with previous history of mental disorders, and those with marital conflict before the disaster

## Research Alert

Those who lived through Hurricane Katrina in August 2005, especially residents of New Orleans and the Mississippi Gulf Coast, were at risk for developing post-traumatic stress disorder (PTSD) and most suffered some degree of emotional distress from trauma and loss. People who watched the disaster unfold on television have also reported symptoms of emotional distress, even if they did not experience the disaster personally. This article provides an extensive review of previous studies about PTSD in disaster survivors, and the etiology of traumatic stress disorders. The authors provide specific guidance for all nurses in the identification of PTSD and appropriate nursing interventions to promote healing from the horror of disaster.

*Source:* Rhoads, J., Mitchell, F. A., & Rick, S. (2006). Posttraumatic stress disorder after Hurricane Katrina. *Journal for Nurse Practitioners, 2*(1), 18–26.

 **NOTE THIS!**

An estimated 35,000 workers—who responded from all across the country after the worst terrorist attacks on U.S. soil—were exposed to concrete dust that may have contained asbestos, lead, fiberglass, and other particles released when the twin towers collapsed after being hit by two hijacked aircraft.

Most studies on the aftermath of disasters have reported that the first reaction of survivors is a state of dazed shock and numbness. The "disaster syndrome" consists of classic symptoms of mourning and bereavement on a communitywide scale: grief for lost community members and homes and grief for lost culture and familiar surroundings (which will never be the same again, no matter what form the recovery takes). To make this reaction worse, government and rescue workers often control access to the disaster area, keeping residents from their own homes and cleaning up wreckage without consulting the community members. Often, such work by disaster workers, although necessary, further distances the survivors from their need to be a part of the recovery process and exacerbates feelings of loss of control caused by the disaster itself. People may experience symptoms of PTSD, such as intense fear, helplessness, and horror. Research has found that many persons who survived Hurricane Katrina as well as those who watched the disaster unfold on television experienced one or more common stress reactions for several days and possibly weeks. Affected individuals may experience temporary psychological reactions, cognitive responses, physical complaints, or changes in psychosocial behavior that cause them to avoid large crowds or social activities where they might have to recall the event. While PTSD is always a risk, most persons affected by Hurricane Katrina will most likely experience only mild, normal stress reactions (Adams, 2007; Hyre et al., 2007; Rhoads et al., 2006).

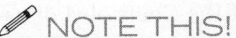 **NOTE THIS!**

More than 5 million people's livelihoods were affected during Hurricane Katrina in 2005. Fifty percent experienced moderate to severe psychological distress.

Among the symptoms of extreme trauma that can affect an entire society (such as the Oklahoma City bombing, the September 11 terrorist attacks, and Hurricane Katrina) is a sense of vulnerability, a feeling that one has lost a certain natural immunity to misfortune, a growing conviction that the world is no longer a safe place to be (see Box 24-9 and the Application to Practice feature on page 603). A lingering thought grows into a prediction of sorts: If this can happen, something even more terrible is bound to happen—the line has been crossed (Erickson, 1976). Box 24-10 describes an

### BOX 24-9

**Words of Wisdom from Nurses Working the Oklahoma City Bombing**

I realized that in the midst of the organized chaos, I had found the focus which nurses have had since Florence Nightingale, when she attended wounded soldiers of the Crimean War. I found that my degree of specialization no longer mattered. I had become a trauma nurse for one patient when he needed me.

—Melissa Craft, RN

These memories are hard to forget. But I will remember the strength and goodness that could not be extinguished even by such devastation. For its part, nursing as a caring profession was made manifest during this time.

—Karen Bradford, RN

*Source:* Top: Used by permission of Melissa Craft, RN, PLO, AOCN. Bottom: From "The many graces of Oklahoma City nurses" (1996), *Reflections, 22,* (1), 10–12. Reproduced by permission.

### BOX 24-10

**The Chernobyl Nuclear Disaster: Will It Ever Be Over?**

On April 26, 1986, a reactor blew up in Chernobyl in the former Soviet Union, resulting in an explosion that threw out 100 million curies of dangerous radionuclides to surrounding areas of the Ukraine, Belarus, and Russia. The World Health Organization estimates that 4.9 million persons were affected, making it the largest nuclear disaster in history. The results: Livestock, vegetables, grains, the soil, and the environment continue to be hazardous for human existence, although a large population still inhabits these areas. Cancer, rare pediatric cancers, leukemia, chromosomal damage, and stress-related disorders plague the region and result in premature death and disability among all age groups. Scientists even now do not know how long the nuclear danger will remain or if ever again the region will be safe to live in.

*Source:* Edwards, 1994. Michael W. Edwards/National Geographic Image Collection.

example of the far-reaching effects of the Chernobyl disaster, which continues to threaten the well-being of affected communities.

### Special Survivor Populations: Elders and Children

Children are at special risk during a disaster because of their immaturity—they have not yet developed adult coping strategies and do not yet have the life experiences to help them understand what has happened to them. In addition, we know that children rely on routine and consistency in their environment, relationships, and home life for a sense of security and identity. These areas are often disrupted in a disaster. Problems can emerge at school and last for much longer periods when compared with adults (Gerrity & Flynn, 1997; Dugan, 2007). Children may suffer from fears, phobias, sleep disorders, nightmares, excessive dependence, fear of being alone, hypersensitivity to noise and weather conditions, and regression, such as thumbsucking, bedwetting, and "baby talk" or stuttering (Laube & Murphy, 1985; Kumar et al., 2007; Salama et al., 2004; Galea, 2003).

Elders often experience significant depression and despair from losing homes and being uprooted from familiar surroundings. Many of the elderly will have already lost primary family members and friends before the disaster. Among their valuables are family photos and mementos, Bibles, and keepsakes. Loss of this sort has a considerably greater effect on elders than others. There are also the compounded problems of more chronic diseases and health problems among this population, making them more vulnerable to disaster stress (Gerrity & Flynn, 1997). Disorientation and memory disturbances have also been noted in this population (Laube & Murphy, 1985). Refer to Box 24-5 to review health effects in disasters.

Simple intervention methods, such as group work for children and elders and short-term counseling immediately after the disaster, have proven quite effective in helping the recovery process. Community health nurses are in an excellent position to intervene with these vulnerable populations. Community health nurses must be able to locate children and elders so that immediate action can be taken. The most likely place to find these populations is in community shelters.

Recovery teams to assist the community in looking within for healing energy have also used traditional healers and informal community resource persons effectively. Women's associations, community development schemes, family welfare workers, and church volunteers have all had significant success in mobilizing community resources to promote community healing and recovery. Such strategies reduce the need for outside resources and help the community regain its stability using its own assets of solidarity (Richman, 1993).

**A Good Read**

## The 9/11 Terrorist Attacks from a Child's Perspective

*My Country Fights Terrorism: The Terror Begins*

On September 11, 2001, four American planes on their way to California were hijacked by 14 terrorists. The terrorists flew two of the planes into the World Trade Center Twin Towers in New York City and the sound of two 110-story buildings thundering down filled the city. One of the planes flew into the Pentagon and the last one crashed in Pennsylvania that officials think was headed for the White House. Over 5,000 people were killed when the Twin Towers fell. Children lost their mothers and fathers in a split second on that horrible day. Firefighters were killed finding and rescuing people and many bodies are still missing. Many people still need our help in donating blood to the hospitals in New York City and they need our prayers to help them get well again and to never forget this horrible day.

> September 30, 2001
> Parker Lundy, Age 10
> Fifth Grade
> Excerpt from an essay for Mrs. Kim Watts Evans
> English composition class
> Purvis Middle School
> Purvis, Mississippi

### Collective Trauma: The Loss of Community

Erickson (1976) detailed not only the loss of the sense of community, which occurs in a mass disaster, but also the loss of communality, which consists of a network of relationships that make up their general human surround. Communality can be described as a "state of mind shared among a particular gathering of people" (p. 189). In a sense, this community is one that cushions the pain, provides a context for intimacy, represents morality, and serves as the repository of old traditions and culture.

When a disaster demolishes a community, people find that they no longer have the collective reservoir of pooled resources, both physical and emotional, from which to draw. Communities act as a "cluster of people acting in concert and moving to the same collective rhythms who allocate their personal resources in such a way that the whole comes to have more humanity than its constituent parts. In effect, people put their own individual resources at the disposal of

## Application to Practice

### The Oklahoma City Bombing, April 19, 1995

On the morning of April 19, 1995, the Alfred P. Murrah Federal Building in Oklahoma City was the site of a devastating terrorist bomb. In addition to federal employees and other government workers, the building was the site of a daycare center. Because of the effectiveness of the city's disaster plan, rescue and recovery began within minutes after the explosion. Oklahoma experiences frequent, deadly tornadoes throughout the state and consequently maintains a highly organized disaster planning response. Initial priorities the morning of the bombing included getting people out of the building, triaging injuries, and transporting the injured to six nearby hospitals. Nurses in hospitals, home health agencies, and public health and other facilities in the community quickly responded to the needs of the victims. By midafternoon of that day, the four trauma departments had seen 40 to 80 persons each. Victims were transported by ambulances, private vehicles, cabs, and vans. A family communication center was quickly set up at a local church, 5 miles from the bomb site, by the American Red Cross and FEMA. This center, which "wrapped its arms around the families of the victims of the blast," provided mental health professionals, hospice nurses, psychiatric nurses, and counselors 24 hours a day for 2 weeks after the bombing. The medical examiner's office communicated with the families of the victims there, and rescue workers from the bomb site frequently reported back to the families concerning the progress of the search teams.

A play area for children was set up, and the Salvation Army provided comfort services, including food and cloth-ing. Pets were brought by local groups to provide solace for the victims. A Native American healer was present for tribal members. Toll-free numbers were provided by the state mental health department for direct and indirect victims' use to prevent and treat post-traumatic stress disorder. Support groups were set up, television talk shows featured survivors and disaster workers, and articles were printed in the local newspapers, all directed toward giving the people of Oklahoma a chance to talk through the horror of their collective experiences. The city's convention center became a huge hostel that fed, clothed, and housed thousands of rescue workers during this period. Roses and chocolates appeared on the pillows of disaster workers, stress management was available, massages were provided for sore muscles, and there was "always a listening ear for sore souls."

Nurses were involved at all levels of the disaster, including triage at the command center, accompanying surgeons as they removed the legs of a child in the bombed building, providing grief counseling for the families of victims and for the disaster workers themselves, providing direct care at hospitals to the injured, and visiting the families of victims in their homes for forensic identification and later on as follow-up.

According to Wilson (1996), an "important reason why the people here worked so well was because of disaster planning. When people live in an area that is nicknamed 'tornado alley,' they plan for disaster" (p. 24). "Though we will never rectify the loss of life incurred in a disaster by planning ahead, we can be ready to mobilize the resources to make all of us a little less vulnerable" (p. 25). ◯

*Source:* Wilson, 1996.

---

the group—placing them in the communal store and then drawing on that reserve supply for the demands of everyday life" (p. 194).

When a community is destroyed, people find themselves without the reservoir of support on which they have relied in the past. They find that they are almost empty of feeling, empty of affection, and empty of confidence and assurance. Residents feel abandoned, often expressing feelings of fear, apathy, and demoralization. Comments from survivors often reflect despair: "I thought this was the end of the world" or "It looked like Dooms Day" (Erickson, 1976, p. 199).

> **❝** *Whoever fights monsters should see to it that in the process he does not become the monster. And when you look into the abyss, the abyss looks into you.* **❞**
>
> —Nietzsche

## ■ Nurses' Reactions to Disasters

Nurses should attend to the needs of the disaster workers themselves during and after a disaster to reduce the possibility of producing secondary victims. Rescue personnel are often reluctant to take breaks to replenish food, water, and rest when time is of essence in the search and recovery phase when they are needed. Nevertheless, nurses should be firm in reminding workers that, to remain useful, they must not exhaust themselves in the process. Seeing that workers are rotated and providing rest, nourishment, and relaxation for the rescuers should be considered essential responsibilities of the community health nurse.

Nurses often experience the same disturbing, and sometimes dramatic, emotional problems as those found in their patients who were victims. Nurses may experience difficulty concentrating, fatigue, irritability, insomnia, and other unique symptoms of stress. These unique symptoms may include depersonalization of the victim, a macabre sense of dark humor, hypervigilance, and excessive unwillingness to disengage or leave the disaster scene or the helping role (e.g., refusal to leave after the arrival of a relief shift) (Ger-

Residents in New Orleans sought refuge and disaster rescue on interstate highways after Hurricane Katrina.

## Research Alert

This study examined associations between alcohol use and PTSD symptoms among Red Cross workers who responded to the 9/11/2001 attacks. Seven hundred seventy-nine Red Cross paid and volunteer staff who responded during the first 3 months to the September 11, 2001, attacks against the United States were randomly assigned to receive one of four questionnaire packets. Women made up 64% of the sample. The sample was chosen from an American Red Cross mailing list of all paid and volunteer staff ($N = 6,055$ with valid addresses) who participated in the disaster relief operations in response to the 9/11 attacks. This study is based on the fourth group, which received the alcohol questionnaires. The researchers found that overall, traumatic stress symptoms and alcohol use were low. Hyperarousal and intrusion symptoms on the Impact of Events Scale-Revised (IES-R) were associated with alcohol consumption, hazardous alcohol consumption, and change in alcohol consumption when controlling for age, gender, and worksite. Positive associations between intrusion and avoidance scores and hazardous consumption were stronger for younger participants. Individuals who reported increasing or decreasing alcohol use had higher IES-R scores than did those who maintained their normal rate of alcohol consumption, though effects were stronger for increasing alcohol use. Associations between alcohol variables and avoidance symptoms were minimal. The results suggest that there is a functional relation between posttraumatic stress symptoms and alcohol consumption. The study suggests that efforts to cope with traumatic stress symptoms may manifest in either increases or decreases in alcohol consumption.

*Source:* Gaher, R., Jacobs, G., Meyer, D., & Johnson-Jimenez, E. (2005). Associations between alcohol use and PTSD symptoms among American Red Cross disaster relief workers responding to the 9/11/2001 attacks. *American Journal of Drug & Alcohol Abuse, 31*(2), 285–295.

rity & Flynn, 1997; Rhoads et al., 2006; O'Boyle, Robertson, & Secor-Turner, 2006). Reactions of nurses are magnified when the nurse is a member of the affected community and when the nurse may have endured property and community damage, as well as stress related to family well-being. According to Laube-Morgan, nurses should be considered "normal persons reacting in a very normal manner to an abnormal condition" (1992, p. 19).

A qualitative study conducted in 2003 by O'Boyle, Robertson, and Secor-Turner (2006) found that nurses who work in hospitals that are designated as receiving sites during public health emergencies continue to express a "fear of abandonment" regarding their work assignments during a major disaster. The nurses in the study reported concerns about their own safety, fear of nursing colleagues refusing to work, failure to have a clear chain of command, and the stress of working in a chaotic environment without adequate preparation. Clearly, there is much work to be done on a national basis to involve all nurses in all healthcare settings with disaster planning and preparedness—not just the administrative staff in selected facilities.

Sources of stress for the disaster nurse can be generally classified into three categories:

- Event stressors—the trauma and fatigue associated with the extreme intensity of the disaster event, of the highest intensity if the nurse lives in the affected community and has family who are potential victims
- Occupational stress—stress related to role conflict, role overload, and role confusion
- Organizational stressors—factors that emerge from the organizational response itself, multiagency demands, and the complex tangle of bureaucracy that emerges in a major disaster (Hartsough & Myers, 1985)

With every disaster victim treated, nurses often experience an unconscious fear that the victim could just as easily have been one of their loved ones.

Nurses are educated to maintain professional composure in any type of stressful situation, even in the face of grief, suffering, and death. This composure has been termed "de-

## ■■ CULTURAL CONNECTION

"I guess the pain of the hurricane (Katrina) is yesterday's news in Washington"
—Comments made by Louisiana Governor Kathleen Blanco after President George W. Bush failed to mention Hurricane Katrina in his January 2007 State of the Union Address

Did the failure of President Bush to mention Hurricane Katrina reflect what some call "disaster amnesia" regarding past disasters? What do you think about Governor Blanco's comment?

tached concern" by Coombs and Goldman (1973). Detached concern is the adaptive ability to care for critically ill and injured patients while maintaining an acceptable emotional detachment. Research has revealed that nurses function effectively in disasters, and very few have long-term emotional difficulties after the disaster. Chubon's (1992) study of nurses who worked during the Hurricane Hugo disaster in Florida supported the findings of previous studies—namely, nurses continued to function effectively in their work roles despite their emotional responses. In this research study, nurses' functioning was generally consistent with their predisaster work patterns. Sources of stress consistently related to the safety of their own loved ones and family. Suggested interventions were (1) to bring outside nurses from other home health agencies to care for assigned patients until the local nurses stabilize their own family situations and (2) to make mental health resources available in the immediate postrecovery period for the nurses in the agency.

In Laube's (1973) study of the Hurricane Celia disaster, the majority of nurses functioned in their role without impairment from anxiety. Researchers into excessive physical demands have identified major stressors that nurses may experience during disasters, such as concerns for personal safety, inadequate supplies, seeing people suffer and not being able to meet basic needs of all, hurt children, disorganization, and concern for their own family's welfare (Waters et al., 1992).

Family roles seem to play a critical part in the nurse's response to disaster. Healthcare workers who are from the disaster area experience exceptional stress; not only must they work through their own reactions to and losses of the community from the disaster, but they also must resolve the family/community role conflict (Waters et al., 1992; Adams, 2007; Hyre et al., 2007; Rhoads et al., 2006; Weeks, 2007). In other words, when the well-being of the nurse's family is jeopardized, professional effectiveness decreases and stress becomes more likely to affect the nurse's role. This finding means that relying on outside disaster workers is indicated early in the course of disasters and should continue until the local healthcare providers can be assured of their own family's safety (Laube & Murphy, 1985).

## " a conversation with . . . "

### Dr. Jerri Laube

### How did you become interested in disaster research?

In 1970 I was fresh out of my master's program at the University of Colorado and was asked by the local American Red Cross Chapter in Dallas to give a talk to their nurses on the psychological effects of disaster. I thought they wanted me to talk about the psychological effects of disaster on nurses (later learned that they just wanted the effects in general). I had no experience so I went to the library to research the subject and found only one reference specific to the effect on nurses—Jeannette Rayner's article written in 1958. By generalizing from publications about army nursing, plus Rayner's article, I managed to meet my assignment but felt a great need for an in-depth study of the psychological effects of disaster on nurses. I later wrote a small grant to the American Red Cross for funding to survey nurses' reactions in a recent tornado close to home. While waiting on that response, Hurricane Celia hit the coast of Texas. I immediately called and requested that I be sent to that area. This was granted and I was on site within 24 hours of the disaster. That study was published in *Nursing Research*. I later broadened my area of study to cover all health care providers in disaster. Not long after my first study I was invited to be a part of a task force to revise the Disaster Act to include assistance for psychological aspects of disaster. That was completed and has been carried forth ever since.

### Should BSN nurses be prepared in disaster response and recovery?

Students in baccalaureate programs should have classes and simulated experience in reducing the impact of disaster. If available, collaboration with the local Red Cross chapter is ideal. Nursing students who take their courses can earn hours toward Red Cross certification, thus shortening the time after graduation to become a Red Cross nurse.

### Why do you believe BSN nurses should be prepared in disaster nursing?

Nurses are uniquely qualified by the nature or their education and experience. Nurses are prepared to work with the whole patient—physically and psychologically. They work both in crisis and chronic conditions which is necessary because a disaster victim, definitely in crisis, may also have a chronic illness. Thus they have the basic qualifications. Updating their knowledge and skills should continue through workshops and disaster drills sponsored by/through their place of work.

—Jerri Laube, RN, PhD, FAAN
Dr. Jerri Laube is co-author, with Dr. Shirley A. Murphy, of *Perspectives on Disaster Recovery* (1985, Appleton-Century-Crofts).

❝*It's when Mother Nature gets so angry at man and his arrogance that she whips up a little humble pie.*❞
—Jimmy Buffett, 1998, on a tornado in Brookings, South Dakota

Stuhlmiller (1996) suggests that, because nurses are typically involved with suffering and disruption of lives of their patients, they may actually be in a better position than other disaster workers to mediate the effects of the disaster. By participating in debriefings, nurses begin healing themselves even as they help others begin their own process of healing. Stuhlmiller contends that we often assume that workers are at risk for post-traumatic stress and proceed with negative assumptions about how they should react. By doing so, we unwittingly hamper their "natural restorative capacities" (p. 19). In other words, looking for the negative effects may overshadow the positive outcomes on which nurses tend to focus—the positive outcomes that come from helping people in extreme need.

"Disasters challenge self-understanding and meanings just as illness does . . . what the rescuers need most then is what nurses are particularly good at providing. Nurses can foster emotional recovery and growth by attending to what approaches work best and by acknowledging the validity of the person's expressed pain, fear, and grief" (p. 19). Such a view is consistent with Laube's (1973) conclusion that, even with all of the possible stressors nurses face during disasters, studies consistently reveal that nurses' responses to disaster do not interfere with their effectiveness as professionals (Laube, 1973).

Because of these findings, it can be concluded that nurses are extremely vulnerable to PTSD in the aftermath of a disaster. The Research Alert feature describes nurses' reactions and feelings during and after Hurricane Hugo. Box 24-9 consists of actual quotes from nurses who expressed their feelings about their work in a disaster.

## ▪ Prevention Strategies for Nurses

By becoming prepared for a disaster through specialized training and anticipatory stress counseling, nurses can reduce the damage of a disaster to self. Simple measures such as appreciating the intensity of emotions and dealing with them; taking breaks; eating nutritious foods in the form of smaller, more frequent meals; avoiding drinking large amounts of caffeine and alcohol; exercising; and sleeping as much as possible have given nurses the added strength to not only survive but actually flourish in a disaster. Seldom can as much attention be given to the victims as the nurse believes is necessary (Weeks, 2007).

Although nurses seem to be effective in mediating stressors in the disaster setting, they are certainly not immune to possible ill effects. Based on her research into the

 **Research Alert**

Chubon was in the midst of an ethnographic study of home care nurses' job stress when Hurricane Hugo struck the South Carolina coast in 1989. The home health agency was heavily damaged by wind and water and was uninhabitable for more than a week. Because the nurse researcher had observed the nurses for 10 weeks before the hurricane, she was able to collect data about their response to the disaster in the context of their usual role of home health nurse. The nurses in the agency were simultaneously victims and caregivers for their home health patients. They experienced grief, anger, and frustration about their losses, as well as conflict between family responsibilities and work responsibilities. Chubon's work supported the findings of previous studies in which nurses continued to function effectively in their work roles despite their emotional responses. Because baseline data were available before the hurricane struck, this study indicated that the nurses' functioning was generally consistent with their predisaster work patterns. Sources of stress consistently related to the safety of their own loved ones and family. Suggested interventions were (1) to bring outside nurses from other home health agencies to care for assigned patients until the local nurses stabilize their own family situations and (2) to make mental health resources available in the immediate postrecovery period for the nurses in the agency. ◗

*Source*: Chubon, S. J. (1992). Home care during the aftermath of Hurricane Hugo. *Public Health Nursing, 9*(2), 97–102.

1989 Loma Prieta earthquake in California, Laube (1992) has suggested that prevention programs for disaster workers should be included in disaster preparedness. For primary-level prevention, a crisis team should work with the disaster staff before a disaster strikes. This crisis team should include a social worker, minister, psychiatric nurse, and other mental health professionals as available. It should have input into the disaster plan and be included in disaster drill critiques and debriefing. At a secondary level of prevention, the same team should be highly visible during the impact of the disaster. Its members could provide emotional support and monitor the emotional stability of workers, intervening as necessary. At the tertiary level of prevention, after the disaster, the team should take an active role in organizing and conducting mandatory disaster debriefing sessions. Counseling referrals should be made at this time, and nurses should have input into the critique of the disaster plan's effectiveness related to worker response and recovery (Laube, 1992). Such strategic interventions can prevent burnout and emotional casualties of the healthcare provider.

## Conclusion

Disasters are increasing in number and severity each year, so community health nurses need to be adequately prepared to deal with them. Lillian Wald, a famous nursing theorist and community activist, responded to her societal needs by developing the Henry Street Settlement House in 1893. At the time, Wald stated, "Nurses not only serve the individual but also promote the interest of a collective society" (as cited in Kippenbrock, 1991, p. 209). This statement also applies today, especially in the face of disasters.

Being prepared for future disasters means that community health nurses must plan disaster care for multicultural populations. The hallmark of American society is multiculturalism (Sobier, 1995). The major disaster goal for nurses now and in the future is to retain maximum wellness of individuals and populations in communities (Procter & Cheek, 1995). Learning to work with appropriate resources and placing emphasis on specific approaches to enhance individuals, families, and communities are integral to protection and healing from a disaster.

Melanie Dreher, past president of Sigma Theta Tau International (1996), pointed out that nurses are very resilient and can be called everyday heroes. Numerous nurses have performed heroic acts, such as Nightingale, Alcott, and Cavell. Dreher contended that nurses with "heroine" status are recognizable by traits and actions: "They define their life's work not in terms of paychecks, working conditions, and employment benefits, but in terms of the number of lives saved, families in crisis who were counseled, and patients comforted" (p. 5).

Explore Community Health Nursing on the Web! To learn more about the topics in this chapter, use the passcode provided to access your exclusive website: **http://nursing.jbpub.com/ communityhealth.** If you do not have a passcode, you can obtain one at this site.

## ■ CRITICAL THINKING ACTIVITIES

1. Based on the Application to Practice feature on page 603, answer the following questions:
   - What were the primary, secondary, and tertiary prevention disaster interventions carried out by nurses during the Oklahoma City bombing?
   - Identify activities in each of the stages of disaster recovery.

   - Give examples of the three categories of stressors that disaster nurses faced in Oklahoma.
   - Identify the components of the Oklahoma City disaster plan. What would be your recommendations for the disaster team?

2. How can community health nurses better prepare individuals for the present and future threat of bioterrorism and terrorism?

## ■ REFERENCES

Adams, L. M. (2007). Mental health needs of disaster volunteers: A plea for awareness. *Perspectives in Psychiatric Care, 43*(1), 52–54.

Advisory Committee on the International Decade for Natural Hazard Reduction. (1987). *Confronting natural disasters: An international decade for natural hazard reduction.* Washington, DC: National Academy Press.

American Psychiatric Association (APA). (1987). *Diagnostic and statistical manual of mental disorders* (3rd ed. rev.). Washington, DC: Author.

American Red Cross (ARC). (1990). *A history of helping others* (ARC Publication No. 4627). Washington, DC: ARC National Headquarters.

American Red Cross (ARC). (1995). *Disaster is everybody's business* (ARC Publication No. 5061). Washington, DC: ARC National Headquarters.

American Red Cross (ARC). (2008). *About Us.* Retrieved November 8, 2008, from http://www.redcross.org/aboutus/

American Red Cross (ARC). (2006). *A year of healing: The American Red Cross response to Hurricanes Katrina, Rita and Wilma—One year report.* Washington, DC: Author.

Anderson, M. B. (1991). Which costs more: Prevention or recovery? In A. Kreimer & M. Munasinghe (Eds.), *Managing natural disasters and the environment.* Washington, DC: World Bank.

The anniversary of Hurricane Camille. (1994, August 14). *Hattiesburg American*, p. 7a.

Auf der Heide, E. (1989). *Disaster response: Principles of preparation and coordination*. St. Louis: Mosby.

Baker, G., & Chapman, R. (1962). *Man and society in disaster*. New York: Basic Books.

Balinsky, W. (2003). The home care emergency response to the September 11 tragedy. *Caring, 22*(9), 38–40.

Barker, E. (1989). Care givers as casualties. *Western Journal of Nursing Research, 11*, 5.

Barry, J. M. (1997). *Rising tide: The great Mississippi flood of 1927 and how it changed America*. New York: Simon & Schuster.

Baum, D. (2006, August 16). Letter from New Orleans: The lost year. *The New Yorker*.

Berz, G. (1984). Research and statistics on natural disasters in insurance and reinsurance companies. *Geneva Papers on Risk and Insurance, 9*, 135–157.

Bourne, J. K. (2004, October). Gone with the water. *National Geographic*.

Boyer, P. J. (2005, September 26). Letter from Mississippi: Gone with the surge. *The New Yorker*.

Chubon, S. J. (1992). Home care during the aftermath of Hurricane Hugo. *Public Health Nursing, 9*(2), 97–102.

Colias, M. (2005, October). The disaster after the disaster. *Hospitals and Health Networks*, 36–44. Available from http://www.hhnmag.com

Coombs, R. H., & Goldman, L. J. (1973). Maintenance and discontinuity of coping mechanisms in an intensive care unit. *Social Problems, 20*, 3.

Demi, A. S., & Miles, M. S. (1984). *An examination of nursing leadership following a disaster. Topics in clinical nursing*. Rockville, MD: Aspen Publishing.

Dixon, M. (1986). Disaster planning—Medical response: Organization and preparation. *American Association of Occupational Health Nurses, 34*(12), 580–584.

Drabek, T. E. (1986). *Human system response to disaster: An inventory of sociological findings*. New York: Springer-Verlag.

Dreher, M. C. (1996, First Quarter). Heroism. *Reflections*, 4–5.

Dugan, B. (2007). Loss of identity in disaster: How do you say goodbye to home? *Perspectives in Psychiatric Care, 43*(1), 41–46.

Dynes, R. R., Quarantelli, E. L., & Kreps, G. A. (1972, December). *A perspective on disaster planning, TR-77* (pp. 6–8). Washington, DC: Defense Civil Preparedness Agency.

Dwyer, J., & Drew, C. (2005, September 29). Fear exceeded crime's reality in New Orleans. *New York Times*.

Edwards, M. (1994, August). Living with the monster—Chernobyl. *National Geographic, 186*, 2.

EM-DAT: The OFDA/CRED International Disaster Database. (2006). Brussels, Belgium: UCL. Available from http://www.em-dat.net

Erickson, K. (1976). *Everything in its path: Destruction of community in the Buffalo Creek flood*. New York: Simon & Schuster.

Federal Emergency Management Agency (FEMA). (2006). *The federal disaster declaration process and disaster aid programs: Response and recovery*. Retrieved November 8, 2008, from http://www.fema.gov/hazard/dproc.shtm

Federal Emergency Management Agency (FEMA). (2005). *History of Federal Emergency Management System*. Washington, DC: Government Printing Office. Retrieved March 6, 2007, from http://www.fema.gov.

Foxman, B., Camargo, C. A., Lillienfeld, D., et al. (2006). Looking back at Hurricane Katrina: Lessons for 2006 and beyond. *Annals of Epidemiology, 16*(8), 652–653.

Frantz, A. K. (1998). Nursing pride: Clara Barton in the Spanish–American War. *American Journal of Nursing, 98*(10), 39–41.

Garcia, L. M. (1985). *Disaster nursing: Planning, assessment, and intervention*. Rockville, MD: Aspen.

Garheld, R., & Hamid, A. Y. (2006). Tsunami response: A year later. *American Journal of Nursing, 106*(1), 76–79

Garrett, L. (2000). *Betrayal of trust: The collapse of global public health*. New York: Hyperion.

Gerrity, E. T., & Flynn, B. W. (1997). Mental health consequences of disasters. In E. K. Noji (Ed.), *The public health consequences of disasters* (pp. 101–121). New York: Oxford University Press.

Guha-Sapir, D., & Lechat, M. F. (1986). Reducing the impact of natural disasters: Why aren't we better prepared? *Health Policy and Planning, 1*, 118–126.

Hartsough, D. M., & Myers, D. G. (1985). *Disaster work and mental health: Prevention and control of stress among workers*. Rockville, MD: National Institute of Mental Health.

Hassmiller, S. (2007). The 2004 tsunami. *American Journal of Nursing, 107*(2), 74–77.

Hayes, B. (2005). Natural and unnatural disasters. *American Scientist, 93*(6), 496–499.

Haygood, W., & Tyson, A. S. (2005, September 15). It was as if all of us were already pronounced dead. *Washington Post*.

Henderson, D. A., Inglesby, T. V., & O'Toole, T. (2002). *Bioterrorism: Guidelines for medical and public health management*. Chicago: American Medical Association Press.

Hyre, A., Ompad, D., & Menke, A. (2007). Symptoms of posttraumatic stress disorder in a New Orleans workforce following Hurricane Katrina. *Journal of Urban Health, 84*(2), 142–152.

Ingram, J. C., Franco, G., Rio, C. R., & Khazai, B. (2006). Postdisaster recovery dilemmas: Challenges in balancing short-term and long-term needs for vulnerability reduction. *Environmental Science & Policy, (7/8)*, 607–613.

International Strategy for Disaster Reduction (ISDR). (2006). *2006–2007 World Disaster Risk Reduction Campaign: Disaster Reduction Begins at School*. Geneva, Switzerland: United Nations Inter-agency Secretariat for the International Strategy for Risk Reduction.

Janis, I. L., & Mann, L. (1977, June). Emergency decision making: A theoretical analysis of responses to disaster warnings. *Journal of Human Stress*, 35–48.

Kiewra, K. (2006, Winter). The eye of the storm: What lessons do Katrina and other humanitarian crises teach us about managing calamity? *Harvard Public Health Review*. Retrieved November 8, 2008, from http://www.hsph.harvard.edu/review/rvwwinter06_katrinaeye.html

Kippenbrock, T. A. (1991). Wishing I'd been there. *Nursing and Health Care, 12*(4), 209.

Kitt, S., Selfridge-Thomas, J., Proehl, J. A., & Kaiser, J. (1995). *Emergency nursing: A physiologic and clinical perspective* (2nd ed.). Philadelphia: W. B. Saunders.

Klagsbrun, S. C. (2002). A mental health perspective on 9/11. *Journal of the Association of Nurses in AIDS Care, 3*(5), 67.

Knabb, R. D., Rhome, J. R., & Brown, D. P. (2005, December 20). *Tropical cyclone report: Hurricane Katrina*. Miami, FL: National Hurricane Center.

Kumar, M. S., Murhekar, M. V., Hutin, Y., Subramanian, T., Ramachandran, V., & Gupte, M. D. (2007). Prevalence of posttraumatic stress disorder in a coastal fishing village in Tamil Nadu, India, after the December 2004 tsunami. *American Journal of Public Health, 97*(1), 99–101.

Landesman, L. Y. (2005). *Public health management of disasters: The practice guide* (2nd ed). Washington, DC: American Public Health Association.

Langan, J. C., & James, D. C. (2004). *Preparing nurses for disaster management.* Upper Saddle River, NJ: Prentice Hall.

Levy, B. S., & Sidel, V. W. (2002). *Terrorism and public health: A balanced approach to strengthening systems and protecting people.* New York: Oxford University Press.

Laube, J. (1973). Psychological reactions to nurses in disaster. *Nursing Research, 22*, 343–347.

Laube, J., & Murphy, S. A. (1985). *Perspectives on disaster recovery.* Norwalk, CT: Appleton-Century-Crofts.

Laube, J. (1992). The professional's psychological response in disaster: Implications for practice. *Journal of Psychosocial Nursing, 30*(2), 17–22.

Lifton, R. J. (1967), *Death in life; Survivors in Hiroshima.* New York: Random House.

Lifton, R. J., & Olson, E. (1976). The human meaning of disaster. *Psychiatry, 39*, 1–7.

Lockwood, R. (1997). *FEMA: Through hell and high water: Disasters and the human–animal bond.* Washington, DC: FEMA and the Humane Society of the United States.

Logue, J. N., Melick, M. E., & Hansen, H. (1981). Research issues and directions in the epidemiology of health effects of disasters. *Epidemiological Review, 3*, 140–162.

Malilay, J. (1997). Floods. In E. K. Noji (Ed.), *The public health consequences of disasters* (pp. 287–301). New York: Oxford University Press.

The many graces of Oklahoma City nurses. (1996). *Reflections, 22*(1), 10–12.

Mileti, D. S., Drabek, T. E., & Haas, J. E. (1975). *Human systems in extreme environments: A sociological perspective* (Monograph No. 21). Boulder, CO: Program on Technology, Environment, and Man, Institute of Behavioral Science, University of Colorado.

Mizutani, T., & Nakano, T. (1989). The impact of natural disasters on the population of Japan. In J. I. Clarke, P. Curson, S. L. Kayastha, & P. Nag (Eds.), *Population and disaster.* Cambridge, MA: Basil Blackwell.

Muench, J. (1996). Disaster training pays off for Juneau nurses. *Alaska Nurse, 46*(5), 1.

National Disaster Medical System (NDMS). (2006). *Department of Health and Human Services, Office of Preparedness and Response.* Washington, DC: U.S. Government Printing Office. Retrieved February 2007 from http://www.oep-ndms.dhhs.gov/index.html

Neff, J. A., & Kidd, P. S. (1993). *Trauma nursing: The art and science.* St. Louis: Mosby.

Nigg, J. M., Barnshaw, J., & Torres, M. R. (2006). Hurricane Katrina and the flooding of New Orleans: Emergent issues in sheltering and temporary housing. *Annals of the American Academy of Political & Social Science, 604*, 113–128.

Noji, E. K. (1997). *The public health consequences of disasters.* New York: Oxford University Press.

O'Boyle, C., Robertson, C., & Secor-Turner, M. (2006). Nurses' beliefs about public health emergencies: Fear of abandonment. *American Journal of Infection Control, 34*(6), 351–357.

Pickens, S. (1992). The decade for natural disaster reduction. *Nursing & Health Care, 13*, 192–195.

Porche, D. J. (2002). Biological and chemical bioterrorism agents. *Journal of the Association of Nurses in AIDS Care, 13*(5), 57–64.

Pretto, E. A., & Safar, P. (1991). National medical response to mass disaster in the United States: Are we prepared? *Journal of the American Medical Association, 266*, 1259–1262.

Procter, N. G., & Cheek, J. (1995). Nurses' role in world catastrophic events: War dislocation effects on Serbian Australians. In B. Neuman (Ed.), *The Neuman systems model* (3rd ed., pp. 48–70). Norwalk, CT: Appleton & Lange.

Quarantelli, E. L., & Dynes, R. R. (1972, February). When disaster strikes (it isn't much like what you've heard about or read about). *Psychology Today, 72.*

Rhoads, J., Mitchell, F. A., & Rick, S. (2006). Posttraumatic stress disorder after Hurricane Katrina. *Journal for Nurse Practitioners, 2*(1), 18–26.

Richman, N. (1993). After the flood. *American Journal of Public Health, 83*(11), 1522–1524.

Rosenkoetter, M. M., Covan, E. K., Cobb, B. K., Bunting, S., & Weinrich, M. (2007). Perceptions of older adults regarding evacuation in the event of a natural disaster. *Public Health Nursing, 24*(2), 160–168.

Rowitz, L. (2005). *Public health for the 21st century: The prepared leader.* Sudbury, MA: Jones and Bartlett.

Sabin, L. (1998). *Struggles and triumphs: The story of Mississippi nurses.* Jackson, MS: Mississippi Hospital Association Foundation.

Salvation Army. (2008). *About us: What is the Salvation Army?* Retrieved November 8, 2008, from http://salvationarmy.org/ing/www_sa.nsf/vw-dynamic-index/5F1804ED9ED2270 FF80256D480044DBA2?openDocument

Saunders, J. M. (2007). Vulnerable populations in an American Red Cross shelter after Hurricane Katrina. *Perspectives in Psychiatric Care, 43*(1), 30–37.

Silverstein, M. E. (1984). *Triage decision trees and triage protocols.* Washington, DC: FEMA Headquarters.

Smith, P. (2000). Terrorism awareness: Weapons of mass destruction: Part I, Chemical agents. *Internet Journal of Rescue and Disaster Medicine, 2*(1). Retrieved October 10, 2002, from http://www.icaap.org/iuicode?86.2.1.6

Sobier, R. (1995). Nursing care for the people of a small planet: Culture and the Neuman systems model. In B. Neuman (Ed.), *The Neuman systems model* (3rd ed.). Norwalk, CT: Appleton & Lange.

Stein, S., & Okal, E. A. (2005). Speed and size of the Sumatra earthquake. *Nature, 434*, 581.

Stuhlmiller, C. M. (1996, First Quarter). Studying the rescuers. *Reflections*, 18–19.

Sullivan, T. J. (1998). *Collaboration: A health care imperative.* New York: McGraw-Hill.

Suserud, B., & Haljamae, H. (1997). Acting at a disaster site: Experiences expressed by Swedish nurses. *Journal of Advanced Nursing, 25*(1), 155–162.

Taggert, S. D. (1982). *Emergency preparedness manual.* Salt Lake City: University of Utah.

Telford, J., & Cosgrave, J. (2007). The international humanitarian system and the 2004 Indian Ocean earthquake and tsunamis. *Disasters, 31*(1), 1–28.

Toffler, A. (1970). *Future shock.* New York: Random House.

United States Congress. (2006). *A failure of initiative: Final report of the Select Bipartisan Committee to Investigate the Preparation for and Response to Hurricane Katrina.* Washington, DC: U.S. Government Printing Office.

Waeckerle, J. F. (1983). The skywalk collapse: A personal response. *Annals of Emergency Medicine, 12,* 651.

Waeckerle, J. F. (1991). Disaster planning and response. *New England Journal of Medicine, 324,* 815–821.

Waltham, R. (2005). The flooding of New Orleans. *Geology Today, 21*(6), 225–231.

Waters, K. A., Selander, J., & Stuart, G. W. (1992). Psychological adaptation of nurses post-disaster. *Issues in Mental Health Nursing, 13,* 177–190.

Weeks, S. M. (2007). Mobilization of a nursing community after a disaster. *Perspectives in Psychiatric Care, 43*(1), 22–29.

Wenger, D. E., James, T. F., & Faupel, C. E. (1985). *Disaster beliefs and emergency planning.* New York: Irving.

Wilson, J. F. (2006). Health and the environment after Hurricane Katrina. *Annals of Internal Medicine, 144*(2), 153–156.

Wilson, J. S. (1996). Healing Oklahoma's wounds. *Home Healthcare Nurse, 14*(1), 23–25.

Yellowlees, P., & MacKenzie, J. (2003). Telehealth responses to bioterrorism and emerging infections. *Journal of Telemedicine & Telecare, 9*(suppl 2), S80–S82.

# UNIT 5

# Vulnerable Populations

CHAPTER 25
Vulnerability: An Overview
*Angeline Bushy*

CHAPTER 26
Urban and Homeless Populations
*Janie B. Butts*
*Karen Saucier Lundy*

CHAPTER 27
Rural Populations
*Gale A. Spencer*
*Lindsay Lake Morgan*

CHAPTER 28
Adolescent Pregnancy
*Loretta Sweet Jemmott*
*Michelle Cousins Mott*
*Susan Oliver Dodds*
*Karen Saucier Lundy*
*Lynn Reynolds Stabler*

CHAPTER 29
Disabilities and Health
*Valerie M. Rachal*
*Linda G. McDowell*

# Vulnerability: An Overview

Angeline Bushy

Visit **http://nursing.jbpub.com/communityhealth** for interactive exercises, review questions, Web links, and more.

Community health nurses traditionally have been recognized as crusaders and advocates for populations described as vulnerable and at risk. Compared with the general population, persons in these groups experience disparities in access and uneven quality of care, which contributes to poorer health outcomes.

What a devil art thou, Poverty! How many desires—how many aspirations after goodness and truth—how many noble thoughts, loving wishes toward our fellows, beautiful imaginings thou hast crushed under thy heel, without remorse or pause!

—*Walt Whitman*

To be shelterless and alone in the open country, hearing the wind moan and watching for day through the whole long weary night; to listen to the falling rain, and crouch for warmth beneath the lee of some old barn or rick, or in the hollow of a tree; are dismal things—but not so dismal as the wandering up and down where shelter is, and beds and sleepers are by thousands; a houseless rejected creature.

—*Charles Dickens*

Loneliness and the feeling of being unwanted is the most terrible poverty.

—*Mother Teresa*

When the rich wage war it is the poor who die.

—*Jean-Paul Sartre*

America is an enormous frosted cupcake in the middle of millions of starving people.

—*Gloria Steinem*

What does it mean to feel vulnerable? Have you experienced times in your life when things seemed hopeless? How did this affect your health? Vulnerability is a complex concept and related to health and social risks of specific populations. As a student nurse, how do you view those who are poor, disenfranchised, and stigmatized by society?

## CHAPTER FOCUS

**Basic Concepts Related to Risk and Vulnerability**
- Risk
- Vulnerability
- Persons with Special Needs
- Vulnerable Populations

**Web of Causation: The Interrelationship of Risk and Vulnerability**

**Poverty: Impact on Risk and Vulnerability**
- Historical Perspectives
- Cultural Perspectives
- Policy Perspectives
- Health-Related Perspectives
- Community Perspectives

**Vulnerable Populations with Special Needs**
- Children and Adolescents
- Elders

- Underrepresented Ethnic Groups
- Women
- Disenfranchised Populations
- Uninsured and Underinsured Populations

**Nursing Considerations**
- Limited Access to Care
- Ethical and Legal Considerations
- Patients' Strengths and Resources

**Nursing Roles**
- Advocate and Activist
- Case Manager
- Educator and Counselor
- Collaborator and Partner
- Researcher

## QUESTIONS TO CONSIDER

After reading this chapter, you will know the answers to the following questions:

1. What is vulnerability?
2. What are the risk factors that contribute to vulnerability and poor health?
3. What is the relationship between poverty and vulnerability?
4. What are some examples of vulnerable populations?
5. What are some characteristics of specific vulnerable populations?
6. How can nurses intervene to bring about positive health outcomes for vulnerable populations?

## KEY TERMS

| | | | |
|---|---|---|---|
| Access to care | Hardiness | Risk | Vulnerable families |
| At risk | Medically indigent | Underinsured | Vulnerable populations |
| Disadvantaged | Near poor | Uninsured | Working poor |
| Disenfranchised | Poverty index | Vulnerability | |

HEALTHY PEOPLE 2010 (DHHS, 2000) lists specific objectives for illness prevention and health promotion that target populations described by some as at risk and vulnerable. Specifically cited are the poor, homeless, very young, elderly, adolescents who are pregnant, severely mentally ill persons, substance abusers, victims of abuse, and the disabled. Also targeted in this policy-guiding document are persons at risk for, or who already have, communicable diseases, specifically human immunodeficiency virus (HIV), hepatitis B virus (HBV), and other sexually transmitted diseases. The interaction effect of multiple risk factors results in comorbidity among people who are vulnerable. Therefore, the epidemiological web of causation model is useful for nurses to understand the interrelationship of risks and vulnerability. Poverty is a recurring theme and an important intervening factor in health status but surely not the only one. Furthermore, nurses must examine patients' hardiness and level of resilience, their strengths, access to community resources, and social support systems because these can counterbalance other risk factors that promote vulnerability.

## Basic Concepts Related to Risk and Vulnerability

The concepts of **risk** and **vulnerability** are sometimes difficult for nurses to fully understand because of the multiple factors that contribute to them. Moreover, not all people experience these factors in the same way. While one person may thrive after experiencing certain risks, for example, another individual may have less favorable outcomes. Essentially, understanding the interrelationship of the two concepts is influenced by personal beliefs, cultural values, and societal attitudes about dependency. The terms *risk* and *vulnerability* often are interchanged in health policy discussions and in the nursing literature. Even though the two concepts are closely related, there are some differences in their meanings and what the words refer to (Fitzpatrick, Villarruel, & Porter, 2004; Sebastian & Bushy, 1999).

### ■ Risk

The term *risk* emerges from writings on the natural history of diseases. In epidemiological models, *risk* refers to health conditions that result from the interaction of many factors, including a person's genetic makeup, lifestyle, and the physical and social environments in which he or she lives and works. The effect of the integration of multiple factors subsequently makes it more or less likely that a person will develop a particular health problem (Sebastian, 2004).

### ■ Vulnerability

The term *vulnerability* has it origins in the Latin word *vulnerare*, which means "to wound." Broad definitions of the term include the notion of susceptibility to injury and lack of protection from danger—that is, a potential for physical attack and being insufficiently defended; being liable to censure and criticism; or being more liable to succumb to persuasion and temptation. More specifically, in reference to health policy and community health nursing, *vulnerability* refers to a person or group that is more likely to develop a health-related problem and have more serious outcomes stemming from their exposure to multiple risks (Smedley, Stith, & Nelson, 2002).

### ■ Persons with Special Needs

The notion of special needs is used in reference to individuals, groups, families, and communities who manifest social service and healthcare needs that are distinct, exceptional, and different from what is considered "ordinary" or "usual" (National Center for Health Statistics, 1999). These individuals often are forgotten, discounted, or misunderstood and may or may not be **at risk,** vulnerable, or disenfranchised. In most cases, the community and families of persons with special needs have additional challenges in meeting their healthcare needs, which may be emotional, economic, physical, or social in nature (Aday, 1993, 1994).

### ■ Vulnerable Populations

It is important to stress that the vulnerable are not a homogenous group, but rather represent all segments of society. **Vulnerable populations** are a (sub)group that shares common risks or combinations of risk factors; one that is pervasive is poverty or low socioeconomic status (DHHS, 2000, 2008). Vulnerability implies that, compared with the general population, some people are more sensitive to risk factors; this can affect their health, usually for the worse. Those who are vulnerable are particularly sensitive to risks that originate from economic, physical, social, biological, and genetic factors, along with their lifestyle behaviors.

Rarely does one risk factor act in isolation, as shown in the web of causation model (see the figure on page 615). For example, a person with a chronic mental illness or a physical disability, such as a seizure disorder or respiratory condition that is difficult to manage, may not be able to maintain a full-time job. Therefore, the person probably will not have a regular or adequate salary. In turn, this has an impact on his or her ability to secure adequate and/or safe housing, essential health care, and pharmacological services, and may prevent the person from pursuing further education to seek

THINK ABOUT THIS

> If a free society cannot help the many who are poor, it cannot save the few who are rich.
>
> —John F. Kennedy
>
> In a country well governed poverty is something to be ashamed of. In a country badly governed wealth is something to be ashamed of.
>
> —Confucius

The web of causation model

a job that will pay a higher wage. Associated with chronic symptoms and the inability to be financially self-sufficient, the person may experience chronic depression and lowered self-esteem. To deal with the seemingly overwhelming emotional issues, and in an effort to self-manage the physical symptoms, the person may resort to using over-the-counter medications or alcohol or increase the dosage of prescribed medications. The interaction of these multiple risks results in the person becoming even more susceptible (vulnerable) to additional factors that can negatively impact his or her health status (Sebastian & Bushy, 1999).

**Vulnerable families** is another phrase often found in the health policy literature. These families are at particular risk because of the intensity or clustering of multiple stressors associated with unanticipated life events and normal maturational changes. Examples of families at high risk and who are particularly vulnerable to future health problems include those who have a member who is chronically ill or disabled, has a chronic mental illness, or abuses alcohol or other mind-altering substances. Families with a pregnant teenager also are considered vulnerable. Special or unexpected events can promote vulnerability, too, such as a family member receiving a diagnosis of a fatal disease, the sudden death of a child, unemployment, and natural or manmade disasters such as a devastating fire, flood, hurricane, tornado, or earthquake. Trauma-related events such as auto accidents, domestic violence, sexual abuse, and violent crimes also predispose a family, as well as a community, to subsequent physical, emotional, and social problems. An increasing combination of intense and multiple stressors (risks) coupled with the depletion of resources can push the family or a community beyond its ability to cope, hence intensifying vulnerability.

Therefore, nurses in community health practice must closely listen to patients to learn about their personal stories. What words are used to describe a health problem in relation to their lifestyle and activities of daily living? Understanding the patient's perspective is essential for instructing, counseling, advocating, developing, and evaluating nursing interventions that are deemed appropriate and acceptable by a targeted population (Fitzpatrick et al., 2004; Leininger, 1997).

## Web of Causation: The Interrelationship of Risk and Vulnerability

From the preceding discussion it becomes obvious that numerous antecedents (risks) contribute to vulnerability. It also fits the web of causation model that is used in epidemiology to understand and approach health and illness (O'Connor, 1994; Sebastian & Bushy, 1999). This schematic model can assist nurses in the community to understand the interrelationship among multiple factors that contribute to the choices made by individuals, families, and communities that ultimately affect their health status. Factors commonly associated with vulnerability that could be included in a web of causation model include disadvantaged socioeconomic status, lifestyle behaviors, low self-esteem, feelings of powerlessness, and disenfranchisement. Consistent with the web of causation model, the interaction between individual assets, social assets, and demographic factors contributes to a higher likelihood of poorer versus better health. Moreover, age, race, ethnicity, and gender are demographic variables associated with variations in health outcomes. Even more noteworthy is the role that social, economic, and cultural factors play in developing vulnerability or resilience. The web of causation can be useful in determining areas where nursing interventions can most effectively be focused to prevent or manage particular risks that predispose a person, family, or even a community to a particular health risk.

For example, a variation that results from genetic predisposition is breast cancer. Or, for instance, race and ethnicity are associated with an intricate set of socioeconomic variables that correlate to chronic illnesses such as hypertension, diabetes, and cardiovascular diseases (Gaines, 2004). Health disparities are examined in greater detail later in this chapter. Individual assets include skills and resources that contribute to one's ability to be economically self-sufficient, such as education and employment. Social assets are characteristics of one's social network that provide emotional and instrumental support, such as family structure, friendship ties, neighborhood connections, and religious organizations. These are but a few of the many risk factors and intervening variables that contribute to vulnerability and resilience.

In applying the web of causation model to teenage pregnancy, for example, nurses in community health settings are able to reflect on the multiple factors that contribute to this costly public health problem (Sebastian & Bushy, 1999). It is important to emphasize that this problem cannot be viewed from an isolated perspective such as not using birth control or the lack of morals of teenage girls. The risk factor of **disadvantaged** status partly is attributable to adolescents' lack of physical and emotional maturity, which predisposes them to impulsive lifestyle choices and poorer pregnancy outcomes than women who are several years older. Low self-esteem is another characteristic shared by many adolescents, resulting in some emulating peers to feel accepted. Unprotected sex is a risky lifestyle behavior that often is fostered by the use of mind-altering substances such as alcohol and street drugs. These behaviors increase the risk of exposure to communicable infections such as HIV, hepatitis, and other sexually transmitted disease, all of which contribute to less than optimal pregnancy outcomes.

Risky lifestyle behaviors are reinforced or discouraged by community as well as family attitudes regarding sex education and family planning in school curricula. Low socioeconomic status is closely related to level of education and employment opportunities, characteristics that are common themes among adolescent parents. Poverty persists because a young, single mother cannot get a job that provides an adequate salary to support herself, much less a family. As for political and social factors, these are reflected in policies related to public assistance programs (welfare) and child care programs. Ultimately, these can enable, or deter, an adolescent from obtaining the necessary skills to secure a job that can provide an adequate wage to support a family (DHHS, 2008; NRHA, 2001).

In brief, adolescent pregnancy is a complex problem involving many risk factors that makes a highly susceptible group even more vulnerable. Moreover, it has a direct impact on the children of adolescent parents, who are the adults of the future. The interaction of these factors, as well as many others, are determinants in the rate of adolescent pregnancies in a particular community. Other vulnerable groups similarly are caught up in a web of causation composed of many risk factors.

## Poverty: Impact on Risk and Vulnerability

Poverty is closely associated with risk, even though it is not the only contributing factor to vulnerability. Being poor affects the health and well-being of individuals of all ages as well as families and communities. Although it often is hidden in a community, poverty exists even within areas that seem affluent. Poverty significantly contributes to other health risk factors, thereby increasing the vulnerability of all community residents, especially other poor residents (DHHS, 2000, 2004, 2008).

Most health professionals and policy makers contend that poverty is associated with poorer health. Yet one of the greatest obstacles in addressing the problem is the multitude of definitions and individual perspectives about poverty and who truly is "poor." Almost everyone has an idea about poverty; however, it tends to be a relative concept based on personal experiences and cultural values (Sebastian & Bushy, 1999). To understand the meaning of poverty and its impact on the daily lives of families, community health nurses should first examine their own perspectives about the issues as well as their personal beliefs in relation to others' views. The self-appraisal process can be an effective approach to glean insights on what being poor can mean to others, especially vulnerable patients and their families. In addition, the self-appraisal should reflect on social, cultural, and environmental factors and consider how they contribute to poverty for a particular at-risk group, such as the homeless, single

 THINK ABOUT THIS

I used to think I was poor. Then they told me I wasn't poor, I was needy. Then they told me it was self-defeating to think of myself as needy. I was deprived. (Oh not deprived but rather underprivileged.) Then they told me that underprivileged was overused. I was disadvantaged. I still don't have a dime. But I have a great vocabulary.

—Jules Feiffer

The poverty of our century is unlike that of any other. It is not, as poverty was before, the result of natural scarcity, but of a set of priorities imposed upon the rest of the world by the rich. Consequently, the modern poor are not pitied but written off as trash. The twentieth-century consumer economy has produced the first culture for which a beggar is a reminder of nothing.

—John Berger

How do changing labels and language influence community nurses and care for vulnerable populations, such as those in poverty?

parents, elderly, children, or persons infected with a communicable disease. Insights about another's life situation can go a long way to helping nurses become more accepting and nonjudgmental when working with patients whose personal choices and life situations are different from their own.

## ■ Historical Perspectives

It also can be useful for nurses to understand the historical evolution of society's attitudes about poverty and people who are poor and dependent (Sebastian, 2004). Historically, people in the United States have been rather ambivalent in their views on the topic. Over the centuries, two common themes consistently emerge: a strong work ethic and religious/moral beliefs. When our nation was first established, the view of poverty held by some groups was that it was a temporary condition that could and would be overcome with commitment and hard work. Then, citizens believed that poor people were worthy of assistance and displayed a sense of responsibility to help the needy. The notion that poverty could be a permanent state did not fit with the ideals of our founding fathers, however, who embraced self-sufficiency and individual achievement. Therefore, people were willing to help others who were afflicted with poverty, but it was assumed that persons in need would be on their own, sooner rather than later.

> ❝ *Poverty is the parent of revolution and crime.* ❞
>
> —Aristotle

With the Industrial Revolution at the end of the nineteenth century, the public's frame of reference changed about poverty and assisting those in financial need. At that time, the prevailing attitude was that poor and dependent persons were deserving of their plight in life. Affluence was seen as a moral issue. In other words, it was a just reward for hardworking individuals and a punishment for those who did not work hard. This perspective corresponded with the lack of public assistance programs for the poor and disadvantaged in our nation. In fact, it was not until the mid-1930s, after the Great Depression, that the Social Security program went into effect in the United States. The Medicare program, which focused on the health care of the elderly, went into effect about 30 years after that.

Ambivalence toward the poor and dependent continues even today (Sebastian, 2004). Persons who are seen as "temporarily" poor are considered to be worthy of public assistance. This view became a central theme in the 1995 debates leading to the enactment of U.S. welfare reform legislation in 1996. Since then, eligibility criteria have become quite stringent as to who does and who does not qualify for public assistance, and for how long. Greater financial responsibility

> ❝ *We are not concerned with the very poor. They are unthinkable, and only to be approached by the statistician or the poet.* ❞
>
> —Edward M. Forster

in caring for the poor has shifted from the federal government to the state governments and the private sector. The long-term effect of the welfare-to-work legislation has been mixed. On the one hand, the actual number of recipients of welfare has dropped in most states in the short term. On the other hand, there has been an increase in the number of families that are classified as "near-poor" and children living in poverty, many of whom are single mothers with children.

In addition, educational and job opportunities in small towns and rural areas often are limited. In turn, this means that persons receiving public assistance may need to move out of their community to develop the necessary work skills and to obtain employment, often part-time and at the minimum wage. For some, it means leaving behind family and other support systems. The situation can become even more complicated because child care in many instances is nonexistent or inadequate for women who must work outside of the home. Another approach to help reduce the cost of public assistance to single mothers with children has been a concerted effort to ensure that child support is paid by fathers who are not present in the home. In brief, long-range consequences for vulnerable families of the welfare-to-work program remain to be seen. Current public sentiment for the most part is to reduce financial entitlements to people who are perceived as not wanting to help themselves (Fletcher, Winter, & Shih, 2008).

> ❝ *Anyone who has struggled with poverty knows how extremely expensive it is to be poor.* ❞
>
> —James Baldwin

## ■ Cultural Perspectives

The meaning of poverty and the approaches taken to deal with it are culturally based and vary widely among societies and individuals. Often, the cultural beliefs of a particular subgroup or community may conflict or even contradict public sentiment. For example, some people give poverty spiritual relevance by believing that poor people on earth will earn riches in heaven. Still others view most aspects of poverty quite negatively and believe that if poor people would get motivated and work for a living they would be better off and others wouldn't have to support them and their children for the rest of their lives (Leininger, 1997).

Professional groups describe poverty in terms related to the culture of their various disciplines. For instance, social scientists often use the term *impoverished* to describe a variety of conditions related to the lack of a home, relationships, or material possessions. This term also can refer to limited educational, occupational, and financial resources. Healthcare providers tend to define poverty in terms of not having sufficient financial resources to meet basic living expenses such as food, clothing, shelter, transportation, and health care. Therefore, adequate or inadequate financial resources can either counterbalance or intensify other risk factors that contribute to vulnerability.

Roessel is a Navajo writer and photographer and author of *Kinaalda: A Navajo Girl Grows Up*. Although this is a children's book, it provides insights for all adolescents about the importance of ritual in the milestones of womanhood. The main character, Celinda McKelvey, looks like a typical 13-year-old American, and most of the time she lives like one, but her roots are deep in the Navajo nation. With her family, she returns to the reservation to solemnize and celebrate her change from girl to woman. The ceremony, called Kinaalda (Dine or Navajo for "puberty"), marks the coming-of-age for a Navajo girl and is usually held once a Navajo girl has her first menstrual period. Celebrated outdoors and in the family hogan, it is composed of 2 days of prayer, ritual, feasting, running, and rejoicing. Celinda mixes the traditional (a hand woven dress) with the new (store bought clothing) while avoiding processed foods, such as sugar. She blesses her relatives and is blessed by them. She mixes a huge cake, made in part from cornmeal she has ground herself, dedicated to the sun god, and shared with all who attend the Kinaalda. Roessel's text describes Celinda's preparations and the ceremony itself and relates the ancient myth of Changing Woman, the most honored of all Navajo Holy People.

Think about how the Kinaalda ritual honors adolescent fertility, in contrast to the negative societal views about teen sexuality and pregnancy. What are implications for community health nurses in caring for adolescent females as a vulnerable population?

*Source*: Roessel, M. (1993). *Kinaalda: A Navajo girl grows up*. Minneapolis, MN: Lerner Publishing Group.

> **❝***Poverty is an anomaly to rich people. It is very difficult to make out why people who want dinner do not ring the bell.***❞**
>
> —Walter Bagehot

below this standard are considered poor; hence, they qualify for public assistance programs. This standard is referred to as the **poverty index,** which is determined by calculating the cost of specific goods and services within a given time frame. The federal poverty index takes into consideration the cost of food for a minimum/adequate diet for an individual. This rate is then adjusted for the number (size) and ages of members in a household and place of residence. In 2004, for example, the poverty threshold for a family of four was $18,850. In other words, a family of four whose income falls below this economic index is considered poor; those above the threshold are not. Families who have a slightly higher income sometimes are referred to as the **near poor.** Poverty guidelines are issued by the U.S. Department of Health and Human Services and revised annually based on the consumer price index. Subsequently, the guidelines are used to determine whether a person or family qualifies for assistance or services under a particular federal or state entitlement program, such as Medicaid, WIC, Head Start, Welfare-to-Work Program, Children's Health Insurance Program (CHIP), and Pell educational grants. The U.S. Bureau of the Census uses this index for statistical purposes to compare national, state, and county socioeconomic and other quality-of-life factors (National Center for Health Statistics, 2004).

There is some question as to the adequacy of the federal poverty index as a tool used in determining services for poor families. Standards that are used to derive the index are disputed, in particular by health professionals (Sebastian & Bushy, 1999). Criticism centers on conceptual and measurement approaches that are used to calculate the index, specifically the diet plan and substance indicators. These are proposed to be an adequate measure of poverty. A broader measure is recommended by advocates for the poor, because the standard of living that is offered by the financial resources of the poverty index is far from adequate. Others suggest that reluctance to revise the poverty index has political implications. In other words, if new measures are adopted or higher inflation adjustments are used, substantially more people would be added to the national poverty rolls. No one in federal and state governments, particularly elected officials, wants to be held responsible for an increase in the number of people receiving public assistance. Regardless, community health nurses will often encounter the poverty index and poverty thresholds, because these have implications for planning, coordinating, and evaluating services for at-risk patients who are vulnerable and also poor.

Economists and policy developers use the phrase *persistent poverty* to categorize individuals, families, communities, and counties that are very poor for an extended time. For instance, a number of rural counties across the United States have been classified as having persistent poverty for nearly half a century. In persistent poverty families, poverty is transmitted from one generation to another. Community planners talk about *neighborhood poverty,* which refers to geographically defined urban areas that characteristically are poor, with substandard housing and high levels of unemployment. *Underclass poverty* refers to the display of negative attitudes and behaviors that are associated with poverty and indicate a deviance from social norms. Essentially, each person, family, community, and professional discipline has a perspective on the definition, cause, and cure of poverty. A community health nurse may find these frames of reference useful in examining personal attitudes and biases about poverty, people who are poor, and the risks that promote and sustain vulnerability (NRHA, 2001).

## ■ Policy Perspectives

The federal and state governments use an absolute economic standard to delineate poverty based on the criteria of an "adequate living wage" for a family with a certain number of members (U.S. Department of State, 2004). People who fall

## ■ Health-Related Perspectives

Compared with those with a higher socioeconomic status, health care generally is less available and accessible to the poor, as evidenced by wide health disparities, especially among underrepresented ethnic groups (DHHS, 2008; NRHA, 2001). For example, the poor have higher rates of infant mortality, complex health problems, and physical limitations resulting from chronic illness. Furthermore, they are hospitalized three times more often than people in higher income brackets. Common hospital admission diagnoses for the poor are asthma, diabetes, hypertension, and other chronic illnesses that in many instances could be better managed with education and routine health care.

Low socioeconomic status can have an impact on the health of people in other ways, too. For example, some types of cancer have significantly higher morbidity and mortality rates among people who are poor, especially if they are members of an underrepresented ethnic group. Likewise, poor people are more vulnerable to trauma-induced injuries and death by violence. Injuries to children in poor families most often are associated with fires, drowning, and suffocation. In impoverished communities, infant mortality rates create additional acute and chronic health concern. Also, there is a higher incidence of adolescents who become parents. Patterns of risk exposure that contribute to vulnerability continue throughout adulthood, as evidenced by a higher incidence of chronic diseases that are not managed, trauma-related injuries, and early death. Even though low socioeconomic status is not a direct cause of vulnerability, it certainly is a stressor that can intensify the impact of other risk factors.

**"***A poor man with nothing in his belly needs hope, illusion, more than bread.***"**

—Georges Bernanos

### ■ Community Perspectives

Rural and urban communities of all sizes and cultures have poor people in their midst. Poor communities and neighborhoods share several commonalties, including a higher proportion of underrepresented ethnic groups and single mothers, higher rates of unemployment, and lower wages for those who are employed. In poor communities, children in single-parent households are poorer in income and other resources compared with counterparts in communities with higher average family incomes (National Center for Health Statistics, 2004). People of color who also are poor are more likely to experience violence, discrimination, and police brutality than more affluent counterparts. Other correlates of poverty include increased rates of communicable disease (especially tuberculosis and HIV), premature death, occupational hazards, unsafe housing, and homelessness. Especially unfortunate correlates for impoverished children include delayed development, depression, anxiety with increased incidences of separation from families, and placement in foster care. Using the web of causation model, nurses can visualize how poverty intensifies other risk factors that contribute to and sustain vulnerability in an individual, family, and community.

**"***Whoever shuts his ears at the cry of the poor, they also shall cry themselves, but not be heard.***"**

—Bible

**"***Poverty is the worst form of violence.***"**

—Mahatma Gandhi

Poor neighborhoods have higher rates of crime and substance abuse with lower-quality levels of education. Housing often is less than adequate—sometimes even deplorable. Community health nurses should not be surprised to find poor individuals and families living in condemned buildings, on the street, in cardboard boxes, under highway viaducts, in stalled vehicles, or in storage sheds. It is not unusual for poor families to be intermittently homeless (DHHS, 2008). Substandard living conditions result in residents being exposed to a range of environmental hazards (risks), including inadequate heating, sanitation, and bathing facilities; vermin and other pests; and unsafe drinking water. Poor neighborhoods are more likely to be situated near highly industrialized areas, landfills, and toxic waste sites and have gang-related activity. Thus living in a poor neighborhood poses an additional risk that contributes to increased morbidity and mortality independent of an individual's lifestyle, behaviors, and occupation.

Living in a resource-depleted environment affects vulnerability in other ways, too. Poor people continually are faced with multiple risks associated with chronic stressors such as frustration over employment options, inadequate and unsafe housing conditions, repeated exposure to violence and crime, inadequate child care assistance, and the insensitive attitudes of health and social service agencies. Bombardment of stressful situations on an already vulnerable patient, family, or community perpetuates feelings of powerlessness, hopelessness, and helplessness; poor self-esteem; anxiety; chronic depression; and physical illness. It is not unusual for an individual, family, neighborhood, or community to become immobilized. In other words, they do not have the ability to effectively respond to even the routine activities of daily living. They go from crisis to crisis and try to cope as best they can. As coping abilities are strained by unpredictable and unrelenting events, vulnerable individuals, families, and communities lose their ability to master multiple stress-producing situations, which can be a detriment to their health.

## Vulnerable Populations with Special Needs

There are many at-risk vulnerable populations with special needs in this nation. The needs of the vulnerable populations that are receiving the most public attention are discussed here—specifically, children, elders, underrepresented ethnic groups, women, the **disenfranchised,** and the **uninsured** and **underinsured** (Fitzpatrick et al., 2004). As mentioned earlier, at-risk individuals usually experience comorbidity and fall into more than one of these groups, thereby intensifying their degree of vulnerability. Other chapters in this text offer greater detail for some of these groups.

## ■ Children and Adolescents

Compared with adults, nearly twice as many children live in poverty. In recent years, the number of adults and elderly living in poverty has decreased, while the number of children living in poverty has increased dramatically. Of all persons in the United States who are poor, nearly 40% are younger than 18 years of age, and about 11% are older than 65. One in five American children younger than 6 years of age and one in four children younger than 18 is poor. Children in single-parent households are twice as likely to be poor as those who live in two-parent homes. Of all children who are poor, about one-third are African American. In recent years, poverty among Latinos has increased more than any other group. Native American children, however, probably are the poorest and the most likely to be in substandard living conditions, especially those who live on Indian Reservations (DHHS, 2000; National Center for Health Statistics, 2004; U.S. Bureau of the Census, 2008). Despite these statistics, many Americans do not see poverty as a major problem for children.

Dr. Jocelyn Elders, a former U.S. Surgeon General, has stated that many of these children are members of the 5-H Club; that is, they are hungry, homeless, hugless, hopeless, and without health care. Furthermore, low income, low educational level, and low-wage occupations correlate with infant mortality, low birth weight, birth defects, and infant deaths (DHHS, 2000, 2008). Poverty also increases the risk in young children for developing chronic diseases, trauma-induced injuries and death, developmental delays, poor nutrition, inadequate immunizations, iron deficiency anemia, and elevated serum lead levels. Compared with nonpoor children, their poor counterparts are more likely to go hungry and suffer from fatigue, dizziness, irritability, headache, and ear infections. Poor children have a higher incidence of

upper respiratory infections, weight loss, inability to concentrate, and absenteeism from school. The youngest are at the greatest risk and are more vulnerable to developmental delays associated with inadequate nutrition and lack of routine preventive health care.

As for disadvantaged adolescents, usually they do not have the opportunity to acquire the skills and knowledge that are associated with success in adulthood. Correspondingly, they lack a sense of personal mastery and self-esteem. Compared with more affluent teens, those who are poor are more likely to have below-average academic skills and subsequently to drop out of school (National Center for Health Statistics, 2004).

**❝** *Poverty is uncomfortable; but 9 times out of 10 the best thing that can happen to a young man is to be tossed overboard and be compelled to sink or swim.* **❞**

—James A. Garfield, U.S. President

**❝** *You're braver than you believe. Stronger than you seem. And smarter than you think.* **❞**

—Christopher Robin in Pooh's Grand Adventure

### ◉ MEDIA MOMENT

**To Kill a Mockingbird (1962)**
Based on the Pulitzer Prize–winning novel by Harper Lee published in 1960, the film won numerous awards and is considered one of the most important films of the twentieth century. The film and novel are loosely based on Lee's observations of her family and neighbors, as well as an event that occurred near her hometown in 1936, when she was 10 years old. The story takes place in a small Southern town and was one of the first to deal with the serious social issues of rape and racial inequality.

**ATL (2006)**
Chronicles the lives of teenagers in Atlanta and the challenges of inner-city living. The film presents a rare portrait of male parents raising their children alone under harsh conditions with hope for the future.

**A Boy's Life (HBO Films 2004)**
Documentary by award-winning filmmaker Rory Kennedy, this film presents a dramatic and unflinching portrait of the disturbing family and social forces that have influenced the life of a 7-year-old boy from the Mississippi delta. From his grandmother and single mother (who conceived Robert as a result of a rape at age 16) along with his therapist and school officials, viewers are presented with various opinions of the boy's destructive behavior. Social, cultural, family, and environmental influences emerge as contributing variables in this excellent film about a vulnerable family, hope, and possibility in the face of seemingly insurmountable conditions. http://www.hbo.com/docs/programs/boys_life/index.html.

Elders and children have greater risks for many diseases.

## Research Alert

A primary goal of welfare reform was to overcome welfare dependency through the promotion of work and the setting of lifetime limits. While at first glance this goal may have appeared reasonable for young recipients, it does not address the needs of older recipients, particularly women. Based on in-depth interviews with welfare recipients in four impoverished rural Appalachian counties over a 4-year time span (1999–2001; 2004), this article evaluates the experiences of older women as they confront the changes brought on by welfare reform legislation. Findings suggest that impoverished older women in isolated rural communities experience multiple crises as they attempt to negotiate the "new" welfare system. As a result of spatial inequality, limited social capital, and the effects of ageism, they have tremendous difficulty meeting even their most basic needs.

*Source:* Henderson, D., & Tickamyer, A. (2008). Lost in Appalachia: The unexpected impact of welfare reform on older women in rural communities. *Journal of Sociology & Social Welfare, 35*(3), 153–171.

Regardless of their race, poor adolescents are about six times more likely to have children than their nonpoor counterparts. A number of reasons are cited for this demographic variance, including lack of knowledge about sexual development and practicing safe sex, limited access to family planning services, and lack of responsible adult role models. With welfare reform (e.g., welfare-to-work programs), there are restrictions on the length of time that one can receive public assistance. During this time frame, the welfare recipient is expected to make significant life changes that will lead to financial independence. Most often, this entails the person's completing the necessary education to obtain a job. Usually, these are entry-level positions in the service industry offering the minimum hourly wage. Many times, it is only a part-time job that does not provide health insurance benefits. Although single-parent women may eventually be removed from states' welfare rolls, they often do not make an adequate living wage to support themselves and their children. Community health nurses should be aware that poor money management skills, along with the costs of child care, contribute to the problem of sustained poverty among single-parent families. A variety of innovative programs are being implemented across the nation to help address the special needs of vulnerable children and adolescents, such as after-school recreational programs and employer-sponsored child care services. Community health nurses have an important role in health promotion, anticipatory guidance, and illness prevention strategies in these initiatives.

## ■ Elders

Elderly persons constitute another vulnerable group who are at risk (DHHS, 2000, 2008). Many of them live on fixed incomes, have chronic health problems, live alone, and are unable to manage their own affairs. For example, elders in many instances do not have transportation because they do not own a vehicle, cannot drive, and have no access to public transportation or anyone to transport them. The elderly who are in long-term care or extended care facilities are particularly vulnerable because of the additional stress (risk) of being displaced from their home and family. Even though the poverty rate among elders has decreased in the last two decades, many experience numerous risks that predispose them to health problems, including environmental, nutritional, and sociocultural factors. The decline in poverty is partly attributable to changes in Social Security benefits, coupled with the increased availability of other federal and state entitlement programs that focus on the elderly population. A few elders, even though they are eligible for entitlement benefits, are not aware that these programs exist, and others may not know how to access these services. This phenomenon occurs most often in rural areas, where a person may be socially or geographically isolated, and among individuals who cannot speak or read English or for whom English is their second language. Elderly people who are members of underrepresented ethnic groups, particularly African Americans, Latinos, and Native Americans, tend to experience higher rates of chronic illness, which contributes to the health disparities that have been identified within these groups.

## ■ Underrepresented Ethnic Groups

Race and ethnicity are related to risk and vulnerability (DHHS, 2000, 2004, 2008). Similar to poverty, the factors of race and ethnicity do not operate in isolation. People of color who are also poor are more likely to be exposed to other risk factors, which interact negatively to affect the health status of their communities. (The predominant underrepresented ethnic groups in the United States are African Americans, Latinos/Hispanics, Asian Americans, Native Americans, and Alaska Natives.) Although health status in the United States improved throughout the twentieth century, disparities still exist across various segments of the population. Health

### GLOBAL CONNECTION

"Keep, ancient lands, your storied pomp!" cries she
With silent lips. "Give me your tired, your poor,
Your huddled masses yearning to breathe free,
The wretched refuse of your teeming shore.
Send these, the homeless, tempest-tossed, to me;
I lift my lamp beside the golden door."
                    —Emma Lazarus (1849–1887), U.S. poet.

Written for inscription on the Statue of Liberty.

Based on Bushy's definition of vulnerable and marginalized populations, why are the immigrants in the above poem by Lazarus vulnerable?

disparities among underrepresented ethnic groups are rooted in economic, environmental, and socioeconomic circumstances (National Center for Health Statistics, 2004).

Essentially, those having a low socioeconomic status and fewer years of education do not fare as well in terms of morbidity, mortality, injuries, exposure to environmental hazards, and access to health care as do people with more financial resources and higher educational backgrounds. For example, the overall infant mortality rate in the United States in 2004 was 6.78 infant deaths per 1,000 live births, not significantly different from the rate of 6.84 in 2003. There continue to be racial/ethnic disparities in infant mortality rates. Non-Hispanic black women had the highest infant mortality rate in the United States in 2004—13.60 per 1,000 live births compared to 5.66 per 1,000 births among non-Hispanic white women. Women of Cuban ethnicity in the United States had the lowest infant mortality rate of 4.55 per 1,000 live births. Other infant mortality rates in the United States broken down by race and Hispanic origin include American Indian (8.45), Puerto Rican (7.82), Mexican (5.47), Asian/Pacific Islander (4.67), and Central/South American (4.65). The overall infant mortality rate has declined by 10 percent since 1995, when the rate was 7.57 per 1,000 live births. However, the rate has not declined much since 2000 when it was 6.89 (National Center for Health Statistics, 2004).

Studies have shown that it is not race or ethnicity that is the primary contributor to these poor outcomes, but lower socioeconomic status. In comparing the gap in life expectancies between African Americans and Caucasians in the United States, gaps (disparities) have been associated with socioeconomic status rather than race. Thus members of certain subsets of the population are at higher risk or are more vulnerable to poor health than the population as a whole, and these vulnerabilities have much to do with economic and social circumstances. The view that health is an outcome of both personal assets, such as heredity and lifestyle, and social and environmental context (e.g., access to health care, healthy living and working environments, access to nutritious foods) is not a new one but is receiving increasing attention in policy and research arenas (Sebastian & Bushy, 1999).

The goal for the United States is elimination of "the disparities in six areas of health status experienced by racial and ethnic minority populations while continuing the progress we have made in improving the overall health of the American people." These six areas are infant mortality, cancer screening and management, cardiovascular disease, diabetes, HIV and acquired immune deficiency syndrome (AIDS), and immunizations. *Healthy People 2010* (DHHS, 2000) calls for a reduction in health disparities between the majority population and special populations in the United States, particularly for people of color. Communities that are particularly vulnerable are those in persistent poverty counties, especially Native Americans living on reservations, African Americans living in the rural South, and migrating farm workers of Latino origin. Many in these communities

**A Good Read**

## Rachel and Her Children: Homeless Families in America (1988)

*By Jonathan Kozol, New York: Fawcett Columbine.*

Kozol writes in extraordinary detail about the lives of urban homeless families in a poor inner-city neighborhood.

experience living standards and health outcomes that compare with those in Third World countries (NRHA, 2001).

### ■ Women

Another highly vulnerable group is women who are poor. The term *triple jeopardy* is used in reference to poor women of color. Another risk factor that could be added to those three is age (DHHS, 2000; National Center for Health Statistics, 2004). Women tend to outlive their spouses, often by more than a decade. This further contributes to the increase in poverty and isolation, especially among women of color.

Poverty has particularly serious negative consequences for women of childbearing age. Poor women are more likely than nonpoor women to receive late or no prenatal care, resulting in poorer pregnancy outcomes. More precisely, a significant indicator of the health of a nation is infant mortality and morbidity rates. The health status of women has a direct effect on perinatal outcomes and an indirect effect on the health and well-being of their families. Women who are

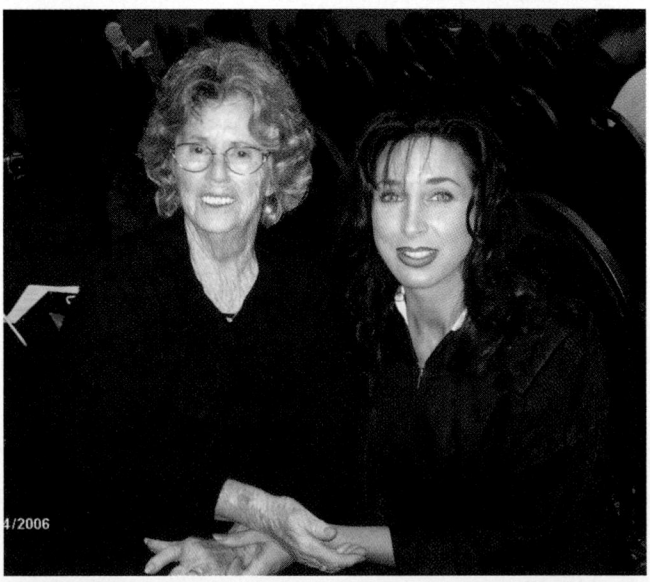

Young and elder women may share the same health issues that make them more vulnerable than men. Can you identify any possible health risks that these two women share?

## ENVIRONMENTAL CONNECTION

**The Year After the Perfect Disaster**

A year after Hurricane Katrina devastated the city of New Orleans, the Brookings Institution tracked reconstruction efforts with a "Katrina Index." The 1-year report by the Brookings Institution found some signs of life and hope in the metropolitan area of New Orleans. The housing market was making slow gains, with home rehabilitation and demolition proceeding and rentals on the rise; many hospitals and schools had reopened and there was some indication that tourists were slowly returning to the French Quarter. Yet, fewer than half of all bus and streetcar routes were running, only a third of the region's restaurants and grocers had reopened, as had fewer than a quarter of child care centers. Gas and electricity were flowing into 40% and 60%, respectively, of homes and businesses that received those services before the hurricane struck in August of 2005. Six months after the hurricane, the city's labor force had dropped by a third, from 633,759 to 429,469. As of August 2006, it stood at just 444,153, and the unemployment rate was rising faster than the growth of the labor force.

Hurricane Katrina posed a special threat to vulnerable populations, such as the poor, elders, children, and people with disabilities. How can the lessons learned from this disaster help community health nurses better reduce the environmental risks for vulnerable populations in U.S. urban areas such as New Orleans?

*Source:* Liu, A. (2006). *Building a better New Orleans: A review of and plan for progress one year after Hurricane Katrina,* Brookings Institution, August 6, 2006. Retrieved November 8, 2008, from http://www.brookings.edu/metro/pubs/200608_katrinareview.htm

mothers tend to be the primary caregivers and decision makers regarding healthcare choices. In addition, women play a very important role in transmitting health information from professional sources to their families. Community health nurses may find that interventions that focus on women provide the greatest potential for success in changing health behaviors of a vulnerable population.

## Disenfranchised Populations

Some people who are disenfranchised may be vulnerable, but that is not necessarily true in all cases. Disenfranchisement refers to feelings of separation from mainstream society (Sebastian, 2004). When this phenomenon occurs, an individual or group does not experience an emotional connection with the rest of society. The disenfranchised include the chronic mentally ill, the homeless, prisoners, persons with HIV/AIDS, refugees, and immigrants.

Some veterans of the war in Iraq and Afghanistan, for example, are disenfranchised as a result of serving in the military for a war that is not supported by a majority of the American public. The current conflicting political environment, exacerbated by post-traumatic stress disorders that often develop as a result of intense combat experiences, contribute to their feelings of isolation from society. Some believe that no one else understands their plight. Interestingly, veterans make up a significant proportion of the homeless population in the United States.

Disenfranchisement also suggests that a person or group may not have the necessary support systems to effectively cope with stress or to manage a healthful lifestyle. In part, this can be attributed to the reality that some vulnerable people do not have well-established links with formal organizations in their community such as social service agencies, churches, or schools. Sometimes, they have fewer informal sources of support, too, such as family, friends, or neighbors. For example, homeless people often have few people whom they can call on for assistance. However, all vulnerable people are not without social support or other kinds of resources. In fact, many families report that they have reliable and even consistent support from churches, extended families, neighbors, and the community even though they may feel disenfranchised from society as a whole. Coupled with the perceived disenfranchisement, certain vulnerable groups, such as poor children, older women, the homeless, and migrant farm workers, are hidden and essentially remain invisible to society. Hence, these groups may be disregarded and often are forgotten by health professionals and in social planning initiatives. Nurses in community health settings often are the principal contact for many of these individuals.

## Uninsured and Underinsured Populations

Even though vulnerable populations are more likely to need healthcare services, many are not able to access them (U.S. Bureau of the Census, 2008). A number of reasons are cited for this phenomenon (Box 25-1), but one of the most problematic is the lack of healthcare insurance. More precisely, in 2007 more than 45 million people in the United States did not have health insurance benefits. Three groups are particularly affected by escalating healthcare costs and reductions in service within a community—the elderly, poor children, and growing numbers of individuals who do not

### BOX 25-1

**Select Dimensions of Limited Access to Care**

- Lack of adequate healthcare insurance
- Inability to pay for services
- Language and cultural carriers
- Inequitable distribution of healthcare providers (more often in inner cities and remote rural counties)
- Geographic and social isolation
- Challenges associated with transportation and communication infrastructures (great distances to providers, poor travel conditions, lack of telephone services)
- No public transportation
- Inconvenient hours to see patients at clinic or health center
- Insensitive attitudes by healthcare providers toward patients who are poor or of another racial/ethnic/cultural background

have health insurance or do not receive public assistance, specifically Medicaid. Of these, some may qualify for public assistance, but the family does not have the ability to apply or lacks the motivation to do so. Some of the **medically indigent** fall in the category of **working poor** or near poor. That is, there are working adults in the family, but they do not have enough money to purchase healthcare insurance, yet their income is too high (above the federal poverty index), so they are disqualified from obtaining public assistance. A number of families have health insurance but do not have adequate coverage (underinsured) with low reimbursement rates, high copayments, or prohibitive clauses in their contracts for preexisting medical conditions.

Although the elderly, poor children, and the near poor have been in the public spotlight, other populations are also affected. As cost-containment strategies are implemented by employers, many employees find that their insurance benefits have been reduced or eliminated. Families often assume they have adequate coverage until a family member experiences a catastrophic illness or chronic disability, and subsequently they are confronted with excessive medical expenses. Community health nurses should also be sensitive to the fact that the working poor/near poor are likely to underuse preventive services. For many of them, illnesses often go untreated until there is an acute manifestation of symptoms or an emergency. This behavior has implications for designing, implementing, and evaluating nursing services that target at-risk vulnerable groups and populations with special needs.

## Nursing Considerations

### ■ Limited Access to Care

At-risk and vulnerable individuals, families, and populations tend to have numerous nursing care needs. For example, poor health conditions often are exacerbated because the vulnerable, especially those who also are poor, have limited access to healthcare professionals and primary healthcare services (DHHS, 2000, 2008). **Access to care** means more than having health services available in a neighborhood or a community. Existing health care or social services must fit with the needs and preferences of the population for these to be deemed as acceptable and appropriate. Achieving "fit of service" implies that community health nurses must partner and work with the community. The following strategies have been found useful in designing appropriate and acceptable services for vulnerable patients in diverse settings.

- Getting to know the community and working with residents to identify what services are needed and the best way to provide those services
- Scheduling clinic visits for patients at times that are convenient for vulnerable populations, such as after finishing field work or at times when public transportation is operational
- Having bilingual nurses available in the healthcare facility for the convenience of patients who do not speak English

- Having staff members who reflect the cultural, racial, and ethnic background of the patients who use the healthcare facility
- Ensuring that all employees are sensitive to the plight of others, especially the poor and those having other belief systems. This may involve offering sensitivity programs for employees
- Demonstrating a nonjudgmental attitude when working with people who are poor and of another culture

### ■ Ethical and Legal Considerations

There are innumerable ethical and legal issues accompanying poverty and providing care to vulnerable and at-risk populations (Fitzpatrick et al., 2004; Gaines, 2004; Sebastian, 2004). Community health nurses often find themselves in key positions to advocate for vulnerable populations and help them effectively solve their problems and become contributing members of society. Associated with this responsibility are ethical and legal considerations that must be understood. One of the most common ethical issues encountered is the allocation of scarce resources. At the core of this value-laden issue are a number of questions. For example, who is most needy, worthy, or deserving to receive scarce resources? Who decides? Where does enabling dependent behavior end? Where does helping the needy to become more self-sufficient start? As resources become scarcer, grappling with ethical issues will become paramount in our society, especially when

---

### ⚖ ETHICAL CONNECTION

"Here the melting pot stands open—if you're willing to get bleached first."

—Buffy Sainte-Marie

"This country was founded by slave owners who wanted to be free. Am I right? A group of slave owners who wanted to be free, so they killed a lot of white English people in order to continue owning their black African people, so they could wipe out the rest of the red Indian people and move west and steal the rest of the land from the brown Mexican people, giving them a place to take off and drop their nuclear weapons on the yellow Japanese people. You know what the motto of this country ought to be? You give us a color, we'll wipe it out."

—George Carlin

"When I gave food to the poor, they called me a saint. When I asked why the poor were hungry, they called me a communist."

—Dom H. Camara

The current debate about immigrants, refugees, and undocumented workers in the United States involves passionate and conflicting views among U.S. citizens. Political debates often result in few solutions that are acceptable to the public, regardless of people's beliefs and values. What ethical implications do our ideas about who deserves health care and other social services affect our ability to provide care for all?

designing nursing services for vulnerable populations in medically underserved regions.

There also is an array of corresponding legal issues associated with poverty. For instance, poor neighborhoods often experience more violence and crime. Consequently, legal situations may arise related to maintaining confidentiality versus reporting criminal activity that nurses may encounter, such as domestic abuse, child neglect, and gang- and drug-related activities. Community health nurses are encouraged to become familiar with ethical and legal issues related to their nursing practice and to reflect on approaches to prevent and deal with such situations in an appropriate manner.

## ■ Patients' Strengths and Resources

Successful nursing interventions build on resources that are available to and acknowledged by the patient. Moreover, health promotion research focuses on factors that contribute to health and maintain long-term well-being. Specifically, negative risk factors must be balanced against health-enhancing factors such as hardiness and support systems. The concepts of hardiness and support systems are best understood as interfacing catalysts, one enhancing the effects of the other.

### Hardiness

**Hardiness** is a term used to describe aspects of human resilience (Low, 1996). Theoretically, hardiness alludes to a combination of factors that keep some people from developing a problem, even with exposure to a health risk. It is identified as a potential intervening factor in individuals and families (perhaps communities, too) who seem to overcome the most adverse conditions and still lead meaningful lives. For example, hardiness may be a factor in why some persons with HIV infections survive for decades, whereas others become very ill or even die within a short time after becoming infected. Dimensions of the concept of hardiness include control, commitment, and challenge. The interrelationship among the three dimensions is the essence of hardiness. Essentially, faced with stressful life events, the hardy person will attempt to change or modify the event (control) into something that is consistent with his or her life purpose (commitment), which will result in learning and personal growth (challenge). There may be additional aspects related to all three dimensions that are relevant to community health nursing, in particular that of "control," or the lack of it, among at-risk and vulnerable groups.

**❝** *I want there to be no peasant in my kingdom so poor that he cannot have a chicken in his pot every Sunday.* **❞**

—Henry IV

### Support Networks

Support networks also can be counterbalancing and mediating forces to risk factors that contribute to vulnerability. Support can be formal or informal in nature. Furthermore, there is no prescription as to who should be included in the individual's network or the family's or community's circle of support (Fitzpatrick et al., 2004; Sebastian & Bushy, 1999).

Women and children are often identified as vulnerable groups in society. Do you agree? Why or why not? What are variables that contribute to their degree of vulnerability?

Preference and use of support varies by individuals, families, and communities and is culturally defined. For instance, some cultures have extensive social support networks, as is the case for many Native American, African American, and Latino families. The extent of these networks often becomes evident when a patient visits the clinic or is hospitalized, accompanied by a contingent of relatives representing several generations. Such an extensive network is not the case for everyone, however. Community health nurses will find that some patients are unable to identify even one person in their support network. For these people, the healthcare system becomes even more significant.

For example, a middle-aged homeless man, recently released from prison after being incarcerated for several decades, lost all contact with his family. In another case, a 25-year-old homosexual man was diagnosed with HIV/AIDS in a large city located in another state. Upon visiting his parents in a very small town, he told them about his diagnosis and how the infection probably was acquired. They responded by asking him never to come back to their home or their town. Their religious belief system does not condone homosexuality. More than likely they would be extremely ashamed if the community found out about their son's diagnosis or sexual orientation. Increasingly, many faith communities are identifying and supporting vulnerable congregation members. Parish nurses, along with other community health nurses, assume a variety of roles in developing and sustaining support networks for the most vulnerable individuals, families, and populations.

## Nursing Roles

Nurses in community health settings assume a variety of roles in coordinating services and developing interventions for at-risk and vulnerable individuals, families, and communities. When developing a plan of care, it is important for nurses not only to assess the multiple risk factors, but also to identify mediating resources, such as the individual's, family's, or community's resiliency and the quantity and quality of their support networks. Assessment goes beyond helping to identify formal and informal resources, however. It implies the use of specific nursing roles, including advocate, activist, case manager, educator, counselor, partner, collaborator, and researcher. The roles change when developing, implementing, and evaluating interventions to fit vulnerable patients' particular needs and preferences (Sebastian, 2004).

### ■ Advocate and Activist

In the role of advocate, the nurse must first be sensitive to the healthcare needs of the vulnerable individual, family, or community, in addition to having a broad knowledge of community resources and how to access them. The nurse also must possess the ability to communicate in a professional manner with and for a patient to coordinate a continuum of services. Persistence is needed on the part of the nurse when acting on behalf of a vulnerable patient. Time and patience often are necessary to maintain contact with these patients and direct them to the appropriate resources. Political activism at the local, state, and national levels is another aspect of the advocacy role. Nurses can make a difference in the lives of those who are vulnerable and poor by getting involved in the policy arena and by working with elected officials. Community health nurses are in positions to work with public and private entities to provide the necessary resources for new or more comprehensive services (CityNet Healthy Cities, 2008; Flynn, 1996, 1997; Flynn & Dennis, 2004). An example of this is using formal and informal opportunities to discuss issues relevant to public health with legislators and policy makers. Remember, during these interactions the nurse is seen first and foremost as a professional role model having expert power. Nurses in community health practice are in a unique position to advocate for improving the economic and

---

**┃ ETHICAL CONNECTION**

The Digital Divide . . . are the poor part of the technology revolution?

Ninety-three percent of children whose family income is $75,000 or more per year have computers in their homes. Only 32% of children have computers at home when the family income is less than $20,000 per year. A white child in a poor family is four times more likely to have Internet access than black or Latino children in poor families (Statistical Abstracts, 2002).

If information is power and the poor have limited access to the vast resources available online through the Internet, what are the ethical issues related to resource allocation and technology? How does this influence community health nursing care of vulnerable populations?

---

health status of vulnerable populations and for those having special needs.

Advocacy involves representing special consumer groups to regulatory organizations and even local health commissions. The nurse advocate publicly supports and sometimes opposes federal and state initiatives. Advocacy may entail grassroots lobbying for legislation that provides a financial safety net for people with catastrophic costs that are not covered by Medicare or health insurance. Sometimes, it involves a nurse testifying against the views of an elected official who does not support a safe house for abused women, or a residential home for the mentally challenged, or a halfway house for youth offenders. The overall goal of a nurse advocate is to represent vulnerable populations and help these patients solve problems and develop appropriate solutions for their concerns. Advocacy and activism do not mean taking care of, enabling, or promoting long-term dependency. It means teaching people how to help themselves by developing greater resilience and more effective coping skills to deal with their concerns (Sebastian & Bushy, 1999).

### ■ Case Manager

A case manager is another role for nurses who work with patients having special needs. This role usually involves the nurse in partnership with an individual patient. Case management is a process in which services are organized and coordinated to meet a patient's particular needs and to use scarce resources more effectively. In community health nursing centers, case management for a patient can extend over a very long period, sometimes months or even years. Moreover, case managers will find that the need for formal and informal services often increases in intensity and complexity as patients are exposed to other health risks and stressful situations. Nurses in the role of case manager, especially those working with vulnerable patients who experience multiple risks, must ensure that needed services are used and care plans are modified to reflect changes. Effective case management requires a broad knowledge base of nursing roles, formal resources, and informal community support networks and an innate ability to integrate all three. Case managers are crucial in preventing and resolving confusion that can arise when patients have multiple members on their healthcare teams. Confusion is especially problematic among patients in very large agencies. Inherent in case management are the activist and advocacy roles described earlier, along with the nurse educator and counselor roles (Sebastian & Bushy, 1999).

### ■ Educator and Counselor

Two other important, often overlapping roles for nurses are teacher and counselor. People might change risky lifestyle behaviors if they learn about the detrimental impact on their health. Education can be one of the most cost-effective and noninvasive interventions to inform consumers, regardless of their socioeconomic status, about pharmacotherapy protocols, health promotion, stress management, developmental

### Got an Alternative?

Models, such as the Eden Alternative, have presented a theoretical basis for attempting to create a therapeutic environment by bringing live-in animals and plants into the nursing home. This research article reports on the implementation and assessment of an intervention termed the "Living Habitat," which applies concepts from the Eden Alternative model. Implemented on a 32-bed unit of a large urban nursing home, the Living Habitat offered numerous plants, a parakeet to any resident who requested one, and two cats and a dog for the unit. A baseline assessment of residents (N = 26) was conducted prior to the introduction of the animals and plants, and follow-up data were obtained 6 months after the intervention began. Results indicate that, following the introduction of the Living Habitat, residents higher in cognitive status became more positively engaged with their environment but reported a decreased sense of control. Residents who had greater affinity for pets also became more positively engaged with their environment. System interventions for implementing the "Living Habitat" project are discussed.

What are specific ways that community health nurses can use this research in working with vulnerable populations, such as homebound elders?

*Source:* Ruckdeschel, K., & Van Haitsma, K. (2001). The impact of live in animals and plants on nursing home residents: A pilot longitudinal investigation. *Alzheimer's Care Quarterly, 2*(4), 17–28.

changes, and symptom management of chronic health problems. Education, accompanied by counseling interventions, can be used by nurses in supporting patients through the grief process; in adjusting to anticipated, and unanticipated, life events; and for improving communication skills between family members and with health professionals. Education and counseling, in some instances, can be used to teach high-risk patients to ask appropriate questions of investigating agencies they encounter. The educator and counselor roles are important to enable patients to locate and access community resources. However, nurses cannot do it all alone. Community-focused interventions must be developed to expand a nurse's span of effectiveness using resources that are available and acceptable to the patient (Sebastian & Bushy, 1999).

### ■ Collaborator and Partner

Nurses can collaborate with providers from community-based agencies and citizen groups to address the particular concerns of vulnerable and at-risk populations with special needs to create a seamless continuum of care. Nurses in community health settings must learn to partner with administrators and others from institutions outside the healthcare system, specifically education, housing, and employment bureaus. Collaboration can be useful to extend and enhance scarce resources, especially in medically underserved and

**Application to Practice**

*Partnership Exemplar: Fighting Violence with Knowledge*

The following exemplar highlights two vulnerable groups: adolescents and Vietnam veterans, that formed a partnership in one community to address the problem of violence.

Shortly after finding two pipe bombs in a locker at a junior high school in Massachusetts, school officials looked for assistance from a local nonprofit group, the Veterans Education Project (VEP). This group was organized in 1982 by several veterans of the Vietnam War who were concerned about the glamorous and inaccurate portrayal of war in the media, especially in movies. The overall mission of VEP was to give young people an accurate portrayal of war and its impact on people. Subsequently, members of VEP were invited by the school to address the students, and now they speak regularly to the student body on a subject with which they were are all too familiar—violence and its consequences. One of the VEP speakers, a former U.S. Marine, said, "War is an extreme example of violence. By talking about it we try to draw some parallels between the violence of war and violence in the street." In 1990, VEP started addressing the growing epidemic of teenage brutality and violence in the United States. According to the Children's Defense Fund, more than 60,000 children have died from gunshot wounds since 1979. This is more than the number of American soldiers who died in the conflicts in Vietnam, the Persian Gulf, Haiti, Somalia, and Bosnia combined. Members of VEP know they cannot completely stop violence by talking about it; however, by describing how violence adversely affected them and the people they love, members of VEP believe they can give vulnerable kids hope.

1. As a school nurse, what could be your role in this partnership?
2. What kind of community activities could this group organize to promote their message of nonviolence?

*Source:* Wexler, 1998.

Research Alert

**Driving while distracted: Teens with attention deficit/ hyperactivity disorder (ADD/HA) and auto accidents**

This research provides compelling evidence that ADHD is associated with significantly increased risks for various adverse outcomes while driving, including increased traffic citations (particularly speeding), motor vehicle crashes for which the driver is at fault, repeated crash occurrences, and more severe crashes as determined from dollar damage and likelihood of bodily injuries from the crash. Teens with ADHD are more likely to have their licenses suspended and even fully revoked. Research further suggests that these driving risks cannot be accounted for by the comorbid disorders likely to be associated with ADHD, such as ODD, conduct disorder (CD), depression, or anxiety, or by lower than normal levels of intelligence. Teens diagnosed with attention deficit/hyperactivity disorder (ADD/HA) have almost four times more auto accidents as those without the disorder. They receive three times more speeding violations than those without ADD/HA and are more likely to have auto accidents resulting in bodily injury. The authors offer some explanation of how the disorder conveys such increased risks. The findings of studies indicate that ADHD interferes with the basic operational components of driving by means of the impairments it produces in attention, resistance to distraction, response inhibition, slower and more variable reaction time, and the capacity to follow rules that may compete with ongoing sensory information. Those with ADD/HA are more easily distracted and when placed in situations that require critical moment-to-moment concentration, such as driving a car, may be a greater risk for accidents involving driving. Added to the risk of driving is the use of mp3 players and cell phones, which has moved these "tools of distraction" from the home to the car. Parents of teens with ADHD should be advised about these heightened risks and encouraged to take steps that may reduce them, including the consideration of more graduated licensing for adolescents with ADHD and the possible use of stimulant medication in teens with ADHD while they are operating a motor vehicle.

How can the community health nurse apply this research to practice with this vulnerable population?

*Source*: Barkley, R. (2004). Driving impairments in teens and adults with attention-deficit/hyperactivity disorder. *Psychiatric Clinics of North America, 27*(2), 233–260.

persistent poverty communities. Nurses should also learn to collaborate with private and not-for-profit entities on community projects that focus on the needs of groups who are at risk for poor health outcomes. Even if community health nurses are not involved directly in partnerships, they can serve as liaisons or facilitators to promote collaboration between community groups (see the Application to Practice feature). The challenge for community health nurses is to become as proficient in partnering/collaborating roles as in direct caregiving skills (Sebastian & Bushy, 1999).

■ **Researcher**

The role of the nurse as a researcher has become very important in recent years. The needs of vulnerable and at-risk populations can be significant, and there are no easy answers to meet them, especially in communities with seemingly few resources. There is an urgent need for nursing research on implementing and evaluating interventions that can be used with vulnerable and medically underserved segments of society. In many instances, vulnerable populations with special needs must first be identified, because they may be hidden or forgotten. In addition, outcome studies are needed to measure the health-related effects of existing community-based nursing interventions within a targeted population. Nurse scholars report that the sky is the limit for studying health concerns of particular populations that experience multiple risk factors that promote vulnerability. Likewise, there is a need for evidence-based and cost-effective nursing practice models that target selected at-risk groups and lead to favorable health outcomes (Fitzpatrick et al., 2004; Sebastian & Bushy, 1999).

## Conclusion

This chapter examined the issues surrounding risk and vulnerability and its impact on health. Definitions were examined as well as risk factors that contribute to vulnerability and poor health status. *Healthy People 2010* objectives (DHHS, 2000) specifically address the factors that contribute to health disparities among vulnerable groups, including the homeless, children, elders, pregnant adolescents, the chronic mentally ill, substance abusers, victims of abuse, and those with disabilities. Community health nurses should be aware that vulnerability is precipitated by a multitude of interrelated risk factors. Perhaps the one risk that most exacerbates the effect of others is poverty. In other words, not having enough money to procure safe housing, adequate nutrition, preventive health care, and the education to develop the skills to work in a job that provides a living wage all can contribute to level of vulnerability. Community health nurses must learn to accept, respect, and understand how these risk factors contribute to vulnerability and influence a patient's lifestyle and healthcare behaviors. Sensitivity entails recognizing health risks as well as the person's, family's, or community's strengths and resources when designing a holistic nursing care plan.

**❝***It is increasingly evident that violations of dignity are pervasive events with potential severe and sustained negative effects on physical, mental, and social well-being.***❞**

—Jonathon Mann

Explore Community Health Nursing on the Web! To learn more about the topics in this chapter, use the passcode provided to access your exclusive website: **http://nursing.jbpub.com/ communityhealth.** If you do not have a passcode, you can obtain one at this site.

# ■ CRITICAL THINKING ACTIVITIES

1. How do you define poverty? Which words are used in your family when talking about poor or dependent families and individuals?

2. Which characteristics or attributes do you associate with a family or individual who is poor? On which experiences or situations do you base your ideas? Family? Friends? Classmates? Personal experience?

3. Which sorts of resources are available in your community to address the needs of the poor or vulnerable? Make a list of formal and informal resources to refer to when referring patients. If possible, contact one or two agencies or providers to discuss the criteria that are used to determine who can receive entitlements.

4. Interview an elderly person or a single mother who is on a fixed income that is provided by an entitlement program, such as Social Security or a welfare-to-work program. Ask the person to share personal insights on what it means to be dependent, with very limited financial resources. What at-risk or vulnerable group does the person fall into? Is this group cited in *Healthy People 2010*? How does the person/family feel about public services that they are enrolled in, and how do they describe healthcare providers' attitudes toward them or their family?

5. Ask someone you know to share his or her life story with you. Identify risk factors that contribute to vulnerability. Which strengths and resources are used to cope with those risk factors? Describe the person's health care-seeking behaviors when he or she needs professional care for a health problem. What suggestions does the person have to make healthcare services more accessible? Reflect on potential ethical and legal implications that contribute to vulnerability in this person's lifestyle. How can these best be addressed?

6. The Application to Practice feature on page 627 is an example of collaboration among two vulnerable groups. Learn about partnership models in your community. Ask local school officials, the ministerial association, law enforcement, and public safety officials if similar initiatives exist. Describe these and share your findings with peers. Develop strategies to give credit to the partners, and encourage other groups to assume a proactive role in dealing with the special populations who are at risk in your area; for instance, interview participants for the school newspaper or invite them to speak to peers.

# ■ REFERENCES

Aday, L. A. (1993). *At risk in America: The health and health care needs of vulnerable populations in the United States.* San Francisco: Jossey Bass.

Aday, L. (1994). Health status of vulnerable populations in the United States. *Annual Review of Public Health, 15,* 457–509.

CityNet Healthy Cities. (2008). WHO Collaborating Center in Healthy Cities. Retrieved November 8, 2008, from http://www.iupui.edu/~citynet/citynet.htm

Department of Health and Human Services. (DHHS). (2000). *Healthy people: 2010.* Hyattsville, MD: Author. Retrieved November 8, 2008, from http://www.healthypeople.gov

Department of Health and Human Services (DHHS). (2004). *2004 poverty guidelines.* Retrieved November 8, 2008, from http://aspe.os.dhhs.gov/poverty/04poverty.shtml

Department of Health and Human Services (DHHS). (2008). *Health United States: 2007.* Hyattsville, MD: Author. Retrieved November 8, 2008, from http://www.cdc.gov/nchs/hus.htm

Fitzpatrick, J., Villarruel, A., & Porter, C. (2004). *Annual review of nursing research: Eliminating health disparities among racial and ethnic minorities in the United States.* New York: Springer.

Fletcher, C., Winter, M., & Shih, A. (2008). Tracking the transition from welfare to work. *Journal of Sociology & Social Welfare, 35*(3), 115–132.

Flynn, B. (1996). Healthy cities: Toward worldwide health promotion. *Annual Review of Public Health, 17,* 299–309.

Flynn, B. (1997). Partnerships in healthy cities and communities: A social commitment for advanced practice nurses. *Advanced Practice Nursing Quarterly, 2*(4), 1–6.

Flynn, B., & Dennis, L. (2004). Health promotion through Healthy Cities. In M. Stanhope & J. Lancaster (Eds.), *Community and public health nursing* (6th ed., pp. 333–342). St. Louis: Mosby-Yearbook.

Gaines, A. (2004). The ethics of research on vulnerable populations. Retrieved July 1, 2004, from Online Ethics Center for Engineering and Science at Case Western University, http://onlineethics.org/reseth/mod/vulnres.html

Leininger, M. (1997). Transcultural nursing research to transform nursing education and practice: 40 years. *Image: Journal of Nursing Scholarship, 29*(4), 341–347.

Low, J. (1996). The concept of hardiness: A brief but critical commentary. *Journal of Advances in Nursing, 24*(3), 588–590.

National Center for Health Statistics. (2007). *About NCHS.* Retrieved September 15, 2008, from http://www.cdc.gov/nchs/about.htm

National Rural Health Association (NRHA). (2001). *Rural minority health resource book.* Kansas City, MO: Author.

O'Connor, F. (1994). A vulnerability-stress framework for evaluating interventions in schizophrenia. *Journal of Nursing Scholarship, 26,* 231–237.

Sebastian, J. (2004). Vulnerability and vulnerable populations: An introduction. In M. Stanhope & J. Lancaster (Eds.), *Community and public health nursing* (6th ed., pp. 623–646). St. Louis, MO: Mosby.

Sebastian, J., & Bushy, A. (Eds.). (1999). *Health issues of special populations.* Gaithersberg, MD: Aspen.

Smedley, B., Stith, A., & Nelson, A. (Eds.). (2002). *Institute of Medicine: Unequal treatment: Confronting racial and ethnic disparities in health care.* Washington DC: National Academy Press.

U.S. Bureau of the Census. (2008). Washington, DC: Government Printing Office. Available from http://www.census.gov/

U.S. Department of State. (2004). *2004 poverty guidelines.* Retrieved June 26, 2004, from http://travel.state.gov/povert.html

Wexler, M. (1998). Front line—F.Y.I.: Fighting violence with knowledge. *Modern Maturity, 41R*(1), 68.

# CHAPTER 26
# Urban and Homeless Populations

Janie B. Butts and Karen Saucier Lundy

Visit **http://nursing.jbpub.com/communityhealth** for interactive exercises, review questions, Web links, and more.

Living in urban areas often means "living in one's car." Poverty in urban populations has been the source of many problems that have developed in cities, especially, stress, hunger, communicable diseases due to overcrowding, violence and crime, homelessness, and inadequate housing.

Who could deny that privacy is a jewel? It has always been the mark of privilege, the distinguishing feature of a truly urbane culture. Out of the cave, the tribal tepee, the pueblo, the community fortress, man emerged to build himself a house of his own with a shelter in it for himself and his diversions. Every age has seen it so. The poor might have to huddle together in cities for need's sake, and the frontiersman cling to his neighbors for the sake of protection. But in each civilization, as it advanced, those who could afford it chose the luxury of a withdrawing-place.

*—Phyllis McGinley, 1959*

Beggars ought to be abolished; for one is vexed at giving to them and vexed at not giving to them.

*—Frederich Nietzsche, 1881*

City life is millions of people being lonesome together.

*—Henry David Thoreau*

If you have lived in or visited an urban area, what have you observed about the culture, people's behavior, and those who find themselves homeless?

Based on the preceding quote, what does McGinley mean by a "withdrawing-place" and how does this relate to the homeless? How does Nietzsche's quote apply to our reaction to the homeless more than 2,000 years later?

Most people reading this chapter will have never experienced being "homeless." What are your impressions of those who are on the streets begging for change, rummaging through garbage cans, or talking to themselves? Why as nurses do we avoid taking jobs that involve the homeless?

## CHAPTER FOCUS

**Urban Populations**
- Health and Social Problems
- Programs for Healthier Urban People
- Urban Sprawl and Health

**The Homeless Population**
- Scope of the Problem
- Definitions of Homeless People
- Historical Perspective
- The Health Problems of Homeless People

**Nursing Care of Urban and Homeless People**
- Be Committed
- Use Leadership Skills
- Use Available Resources
- Be an Advocate
- Foster Communication and Trust
- Assess the Problem
- Plan and Give Care

## QUESTIONS TO CONSIDER

After reading this chapter, you will know the answers to the following questions:

1. What are the major factors contributing to homelessness today?
2. How is poverty related to homelessness?
3. What is the Healthy Cities movement?
4. What is the Federal Emergency Relief Administration?
5. What was the first federal legislation specifically passed to aid the homeless?
6. What are barriers to health care for the homeless?
7. What are some of the most common health problems of the homeless?
8. What is the role of the community health nurse in addressing the needs of urban homeless persons?

## KEY TERMS

Federal Emergency Relief Administration (FERA)
Ghetto counterculture

Healthy Cities
Homeless

Stewart B. McKinney
Homeless Assistance

Act of 1987
Urban population

# Urban Populations

People who live in urban areas are under siege. Community health nurses traditionally have been accustomed to solving difficult health and social problems in various populations. Today, problems associated with urban and homeless people pose challenges requiring every skill that can be mustered by community health nurses. Strong community leadership for dealing with these problems is essential. Community health nurses can be the leaders on the forefront in preventing and managing these problems. Urban communities are exposed to diseases, health disorders, violence, crime, hunger, poverty, drug abuse, and homelessness at alarming rates. Although homelessness is a problem in both rural and urban areas, most homeless people exist in urban areas.

An **urban population** is at least 50,000 people in an incorporated or unincorporated area (United States Conference of Mayors 2006; U.S. Department of Commerce, 2002). Cities have continued to increase in population as people—especially young adults—have migrated to cities from rural areas in hopes of fulfilling their dreams of success. With the promise of wealth and a new way of life, young people are charmed, sometimes only to find disappointment in their careers, poverty, and stress (Darbyshire, Muir-Cochrane, Fereday, Jureidini, & Drummond, 2006; Goldstein & Kickbusch, 1996; Salomonsen-Sautel et al., 2008; Wehler et al., 2004). Some have been unable to find jobs. Not only do many people migrate to the city, but many people are born and remain in the city for the duration of their lives.

Low income and unemployment perpetuate urban poverty and its problems. With a rapidly growing population, urban officials cannot keep pace with the needs of the people. A majority of urban problems are associated with rapid growth, such as diminishing supplies of clean water, air pollution, crime and violence, poverty, diseases, overcrowding, racial discrimination, and inadequate housing.

## ◼ Health and Social Problems

People in urban areas face many stressors that are different from those in rural areas. Although some of the same problems exist in rural areas, the health and social problems associated with living in urban areas usually are more pronounced.

Poverty in urban populations has been the source of many problems that have developed in cities, especially hunger, health problems, communicable diseases because of overcrowded conditions, violence and crime, homelessness, and inadequate housing.

Lack of steady employment is a major problem. However, many Americans continue to view government support for the poor as the main cause of the social problems in the United States. As a result, the public, as well as many governmental policy makers, increasingly rejects such programs. The consequence of these attitudes has been a deterioration of health and welfare programs for poor people (Jones, 2006).

Racial discrimination remains an unsettling issue. A "color line," described by Lewis (1993, p. 251), has caused whites and nonwhites to remain segregated. Major in-

---

### ⚒ ETHICAL CONNECTION

Historically, the nursing metaparadigm has been used to describe four concepts of nursing knowledge (person, environment, health, and nursing) that reflect beliefs held by the profession about nursing's context and content. The authors offer an assessment of the metaparadigm as it applies to community and public health nursing in urban settings and offer an amendment of the metaparadigm to include the central concept of social justice. Each of the metaparadigm concepts and the central concept of social justice are discussed as they apply to a model of urban health nursing teaching, research, and practice. ◯

*Source:* Schim, S. M., Benkert, R., Bell, S. E., Walker, D. S., & Danford, C. A. (2007). Social justice: Added metaparadigm concept for urban health nursing. *Public Health Nursing, 24*(1), 73–80.

come and healthcare differences exist between whites and nonwhites overall. Poverty and overcrowding in nonwhite populations have been linked to the exacerbation of communicable diseases (Jones, 2006).

Poverty in inner cities is also linked to a poor quality of life and increased health problems among adults of all ages (Jones, 2006; Polednak, 1997; U.S. Conference of Mayors, 2006). A substantially higher infant mortality rate among nonwhites has been found in metropolitan areas (Corburn, 2004; Gamst et al., 2006; Polednak, 1997; Wehler et al., 2004). Lack of access to health care, poor prenatal care, adolescent pregnancy, substance abuse, and an overall poor quality of life are consequences of poverty. Causes of mortality among African Americans and other nonwhites in urban areas included cardiovascular diseases, renal diseases, and homicides at higher rates than whites (Cheung & Hwang, 2004; Salomonsen-Sautel et al., 2008; Wenzel, Tucker, Elliott, & Hambarsoomians, 2007).

In the latter part of the twentieth century, the movement of people to the suburbs has contributed to higher rates of obesity, less community cohesiveness, and higher stress due to greater driving commutes, less time for exercise, and greater isolation of families.

**Ghetto counterculture** is a term that has been used to label a phenomenon in urban America (Massey & Denton, 1993, p. 48). Ghetto counterculture is used to describe the racial segregation that has taken place in residential areas. This residential segregation has created nonwhite urban underclass communities, producing "concentration" effects in these areas (p. 48). The concentration of nonwhites in high-poverty areas, such as inner cities, has resulted in a spiraling decline in the human condition. Rap music has evolved as a musical expression of ghetto life. Concentration effects lead to increased social problems such as crime and drugs, physical deterioration of buildings, poor access to healthcare facilities and other services, and fewer quality educational opportunities. Respiratory infections, tuberculosis (TB), skin infections, and many other illnesses occur in concentrated areas. The Research Alert on page 633 highlights the public health threat of adult pertussis in urban people.

## Research Alert

The efficacy of a nurse case-managed intervention was evaluated in subsamples of participants with one of the following characteristics: female gender, African American, recruited from a homeless shelter, a history of military service, lifetime injection drug use, daily alcohol and drug use, poor physical health, and a history of poor mental health. The purpose of this study was to determine whether a nurse case-managed intervention with incentives and tracking would improve adherence to latent tuberculosis infection treatment in subsamples of homeless persons with characteristics previously identified as predictive of nonadherence. A study was conducted with 520 homeless adults residing in 12 homeless shelters and residential recovery sites in the Skid Row region of Los Angeles from 1998 to 2003. Study results revealed that daily drug users, participants with a history of injection drug use, daily alcohol users, and persons who were not of African American race had particularly poor completion rates, even in the nurse case-managed intervention program (48%, 55%, 54%, and 50%, respectively). However, the intervention achieved a 91% completion rate for homeless shelter residents and significantly improved latent tuberculosis infection treatment adherence in 9 of 12 subgroups tested, including daily alcohol and drug users, when potential confounders were controlled using logistic regression analysis.

Nyamathi, A., Nahid, P., Berg, J., Burrage, J., Christiani, A., Aqtash, S., et al. (2008). Efficacy of nurse case-managed intervention for latent tuberculosis among homeless subsamples. *Nursing Research, 57*(1), 33–39.

Another health problem associated with urban living in the United States is the reemergence of communicable diseases, such as measles. The Centers for Disease Control and Prevention (CDC) (2005) has documented a 20-fold increase in measles in the last 15 years, which is largely attributed to failure to vaccinate children in accordance with established public health guidelines. The CDC recently found that only 50% of all children living in the inner cities were vaccinated by their second birthday (CDC, 2005).

Other health problems have emerged in the last decade. Contamination of community water supplies has contributed to many outbreaks of infectious diseases in urban areas, such as the *Cryptosporidium* infection in Milwaukee (MacKenzie et al., 1994). There has been the reappearance of plague, cholera, and dengue fever in many parts of the world, especially in the "mega-cities" of 10 million or more people (*United Nations Statistical Yearbook,* 2005).

## ■ Programs for Healthier Urban People

*Healthy People 2010* specifies two major goals to improve the health of Americans (DHHS, 2000). Although the goals do not specifically mention urban populations, they can be applied to urban populations. One goal is to eliminate health disparities. A large percentage of the population in inner cities is nonwhite. Mortality, morbidity, and lack of healthcare access and utilization continue to soar among nonwhites, especially in inner cities (DHHS, 2000). As a result, several national health programs have been targeted for African Americans and other underrepresented ethnic groups. Many of the national programs have stemmed from the Public Health Service. Community health nurses are in an excellent position to help manage these health programs or coordinate the health care.

The **Healthy Cities** movement was initiated by the World Health Organization (WHO) in Europe in 1984. It was brought about by a speech given at an international meeting in Canada with a theme that "health is much more than medical care" (IHCF, 2002). Soon after the initiation of Europe's Healthy Cities project, others followed, including programs in Canada, the United States, Latin America, Africa, and Asia.

The International Healthy Cities Foundation (IHCF) was established in August 1994 (IHCF, 2002). From the beginning, this organization was envisioned by global advisory boards as a dynamic interconnection of people, organizations, and networks involving many disciplines and interest groups. The goal of IHCF and the WHO is to increase the level of health for all citizens of the world.

IHCF's mission is to facilitate linkages among people, issues, and resources to support the development of the Healthy Cities movement (IHCF, 2002). With this mission in mind, IHCF developed an infrastructure of three programs: communications, resource tools, and training and advisory services. Many people at various levels are involved in IHCF, including partners from public health and safety; educators; religious groups; alcohol and drug programs; and community groups focusing on civil and human rights, volunteerism, housing, labor, business, environment, occupation, and many others. Virtually every discipline on the global front has a voice in IHCF.

WHO recognized that urban cities held almost half the world's population. Through the Healthy Cities program, local individuals and local resources are recruited to work together to identify and help resolve health problems in their community. There are numerous participating cities throughout the United States and the world. In the Healthy Cities program, attention is given to modifying the physical, social, and economic environment of the community to improve the health of individuals.

## MEDIA MOMENT

### *Dark Days* (2000)

Documentarian Marc Singer focuses his camera on a group of homeless people who live deep underground in an abandoned New York City railroad tunnel. By day, they scavenge for food on the mean streets of Manhattan. At night, they retreat to the tunnel, where they have built huts out of scrap metal, plastic, and plywood, which are equipped with electricity, furniture, working kitchens, and a sense of community.

One of the first major United States cities to launch a Healthy Cities project was Boston. Since its inception in 1992, Boston has served as a leader of the Healthy Cities movement in the United States. After an extensive evaluation of the Healthy Boston project, the Office of Community Partnerships realized that the project had been very successful in reaching its goals, which were to create a collective community voice, serve as a catalyst to optimize services, create new partnerships, embrace multicultural and collaborative values, embrace health issues, and create healthy communities. Only four recommendations for improvement came from the evaluation. One of those recommendations was for the improvement of leadership development and more support for coalitions. Community health nurses could fill this role by becoming leaders and providing support and coordination of health and political coalitions. Community health nurses need to realize the potential healthy outcomes for urban populations when a Healthy Cities project has been successfully undertaken.

At the International Healthy Cities Conference in Athens, Greece, in June 1998, the third phase of the Healthy Cities movement was launched. Jo Asvall, WHO's Regional Director for Europe, stated at this conference, "WHO is emphasizing the diversity and seriousness of urban health issues and the need for action at the local level" (WHO, 1998, p. 1). At this conference, the members evaluated outcomes and the impact of the movement for the previous 10 years.

Several other programs have been specially targeted at the African American population in inner cities, such as the Harlem Health Connection and the Safe Kids/Healthy Neighborhoods Injury Prevention Program in Harlem (Polednak, 1997). African American inner-city churches and community groups have also been committed to improving living conditions in urban areas.

Urban development projects across U.S. cities have provided health opportunities for urban populations. Improving the health outcomes of these people through better access to health care with an emphasis on health promotion and prevention of disease is a result of urban development efforts. Many problems still exist, but the urban development efforts of communities are becoming beneficial to the urban residents. Many of these projects start at the grass-roots level and are coordinated and managed by city officials and community leaders.

One urban development project that began at the local level and has spread rapidly throughout the United States is the Atlanta Project, which has now become the America Project (TAP, 1995; Berger, 2007; Biven, 2002). This project was developed by former President Jimmy Carter in an effort to promote hope and healing and to unite the Atlanta people to improve the quality of life in neighborhoods. The success of the project spread quickly throughout the United States and has been adopted by many major city officials. The project's mission required several elements for success, which included having a vision, planning well, empowering the community, collaborating, volunteering, and communicating effectively.

West (1994) emphasized that young African American urban people are faced with despair and are fighting the forces of death, destruction, and disease. With consistent efforts, programs such as the Healthy Cities movement and other urban development programs can provide the resources for health promotion and healing. Community health nurses have a responsibility to become involved in urban policy making, urban development projects, and urban health care (Corburn, 2004; Lowe, 2008).

### ◼ Urban Sprawl and Health

Urban health efforts in the late 1990s and into the twenty-first century have initiated research and programs that focus on the "built environment"—such as architecture and locations of stores, schools, and community services. One such example is the study of urban sprawl and its connection to physical activity, obesity, stress, and mental health issues. Urban sprawl occurs as large numbers of urban residents move to the suburbs. These suburbs are characterized as decentralized, automobile-dependent neighborhoods, often called "bedroom communities."

The built environment most associated with urban areas includes the inferior air quality of workplaces, street layout, presence or absence of sidewalks, walkable streets, and population density. When populations move out of the central city, fewer businesses, such as local grocery stores, are within walking distances for this already vulnerable population. Given that many urban poor are dependent on mass transit, health is affected through poorer nutrition, obesity, and less attention to preventive care (Lopez & Welker-Hood, 2007; Corburn, 2004).

Urban sprawl affects nurses as well. Long hours at work and long commutes decrease exercise possibilities and contribute to greater stress and poor nutritional choices (Lopez & Welker-Hood, 2007).

## The Homeless Population

Today the United States is faced with overwhelming social problems, including the tragedy of the homeless. We even have difficulty defining homelessness or knowing how many people in the United States are homeless on a daily basis. Interwoven throughout the homeless population are the social problems of substance abuse, racism, violence, limited education, crime, and poverty (Gamst et al., 2006; North, Eyrich, Pollio, & Spitznagel, 2004; Washington, 2002; Wehler et al., 2004).

A new culture of homeless people has emerged. The number and composition of homeless people during the last two decades of the twentieth century have grasped the attention of the American people and have continued to plague us as a society. We exhibit attitudes ranging from "blaming the victim" to feeling helpless in doing anything about this serious social problem. The individuals comprising the homeless populations are no longer the "skid row bums," "hobos," and "tramps" found years ago. Now women, adolescents,

**Rescue Mission**

> They'll sit like that for hours
> for a ticket away from
> their hunger rack ribs
> with their shirts off
> in summer lined up
> as if waiting on
> Buck Rogers' next
> scuffle
> those racks look
> like evil fingers
> closing around
> empty innards
> when the bell chimes
> Jesus saves
> and the door flings open
> they file in like boys
> returning from an
> exhausting recess
> it's bread that saves now
> as they sit quietly
> almost broken of old habits
> although a few
> (perhaps toothless?)
> still neatly trim
> the crust away

—*James A. Lopresti, Denver, Colorado, 1977*

families with children, and elderly people represent a large portion of the homeless population (Baum & Burnes, 1993; Gamst et al., 2006; Wenzel et al., 2007).

The homeless lifestyle is a barrier to good health practices and thus leads to more prevalent health problems (Meadows-Oliver, 2006; Galea & Vlahov, 2002). Community health nurses play a vital role in breaking down the barriers that prevent positive health practices in this new culture of homeless women, men, and children. As we will see later, outreach to nontraditional service locations and case management are key strategies on which community health nurses can focus (Bolland & Callum, 2002; Cousineau, Wittenberg, & Pollatsek, 1995; Rosenblum, Magura, Kayman, & Fong, 2005). Although the *Healthy People 2010* objectives do not specifically address the issue of homelessness, they address all of the conditions, problems, and population groups affected.

## ■ Scope of the Problem

Cities all across the United States have unmet needs for shelter and food. Actually, homelessness is a global problem. The homeless population is located in both urban and rural areas, although the largest number are in urban areas. Women, adolescents, substance abusers, families with children, and people with mental illness or who are deinstitutionalized make up the homeless population (Interagency Council on the Homeless, 2000; Lezak & Edgar, 1996; DHHS, 2003). The estimate of homeless children is 100,000 at any

given day or night (Institute of Medicine, 1988). Still more astounding are the facts that each year 30% to 50% of all homeless people are families with children and 7% of all homeless people are children (see Table 26-1) (Darbyshire, Muir-Cochrane, Fereday, Jureidini, & Drummond, 2006).

A problem exists in counting accurate numbers of homeless people because of the "one point in time" reference. The group of homeless persons may be different people and different numbers from one night to another. During a 7-day period in March 1987, statistics revealed that more than 600,000 homeless people sought shelter from the outside environment (Burt & Cohen, 1989). During the 2000 Census, the U.S. Department of Commerce (2002) attempted to gather statistics on numbers of homeless people. The department was unable to obtain specific numbers across the country but gathered data in certain cities over a specific number of days and nights. Currently, the U.S. Conference of Mayors studies specific U.S. cities every year to draw conclusions about the scope of the problem and characteristics of the population of homeless people.

Researchers have estimated the number of homeless people across the United States, suggesting that the number of individuals experiencing homelessness is even greater than previously expected. In the latter part of the 1980s, as many as 9.32 million persons were believed to have been homeless at least once (Culhane, Dejowski, Ibanex, Needham, & Macchia, 1993; Interagency Council on the Homeless, 2000;

*✎ NOTE THIS!* •————————

In 1996, a survey found that homeless individuals reported an average income of $348 per year.

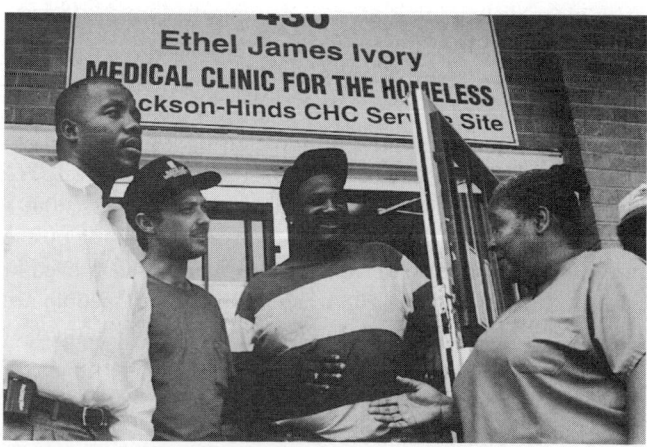

Homeless clinics in inner-city locations can provide essential care for the homeless population.

**Table 26-1** Characteristics of Homeless People in 2000

| Characteristics | Findings in the Homeless Population |
|---|---|
| ▪ Family status | 44% are single men |
| | 36% are families with children; of these families, 76% are headed by a single parent, and 7% are unaccompanied minors |
| | 13% are single women |
| ▪ Race and ethnicity | 50% are African American |
| | 35% are Caucasian |
| | 12% are Hispanic |
| | 2% are Native American |
| | 1% are Asian American |
| ▪ Institutional history | 66% have problems with alcohol and drug abuse, or mental illness |
| | 9% have AIDS or HIV-related illness |
| ▪ Employment | 44% are employed in full- or part-time jobs |
| ▪ Homeless veterans | 22% are veterans |
| ▪ Financial status | 28% report not having enough to eat |
| | 21% have received money from family or friends |
| ▪ Crime | 27% have been physically assaulted |
| | 7% have been sexually assaulted |
| | 38% report theft of their personal possessions |
| | 30% have been homeless for more than 2 years |

*Source*: U.S. Conference of Mayors, 2000.

---

### BOX 26-1

**Who Are the New Homeless People?**
- Single adults unaccompanied by children
- Single mothers with children
- Families with children
- Individuals who have been deinstitutionalized
- Persons who are diagnosed with mental illness
- Runaway and throwaway youths
- Abandoned children
- Unemployed, impoverished adults
- Immigrants
- Veterans—both women and men
- Elderly people

---

 CULTURAL CONNECTION

Urban poverty rates are about twice as high as suburban poverty rates—16.4% versus 8.0%, respectively, in 1999.

African Americans have been effectively frozen out of suburbs by racial covenants, discriminatory mortgage practices, and racial bias since the 1950s. Whites have benefited from access to low-cost suburban homes, low interest rates on government-subsidized home mortgages, and publicly funded transportation projects linking their suburban homes to unemployment recreation and commercial centers.

I don't think Dr. King helped racial harmony, I think he helped racial justice. What I profess to do is help the oppressed, and if I cause a load of discomfort in the white community and the black community, that in my opinion means I'm being effective, because I'm not trying to make them comfortable. The job of an activist is to make people tense and cause social change.

—The Reverend Al Sharpton

---

Link, Phelan, Breshan, Stueve, Moore, & Susser, 1995). Even more disturbing is the fact that families are the fastest-growing segment of the homeless population (U.S. Conference of Mayors, 2000). Box 26-1 delineates the composition of homeless people.

The estimated number of homeless people does not include the growing segment of people who are on the verge of homelessness (Interagency Council on the Homeless, 2000). More than 1 million families are on waiting lists for public housing at any given time. Many more people have moved in with friends or relatives. Increasing numbers of people are paying more than half their income for rent, making them at risk for homelessness at any time.

### ■ Definitions of Homeless People

An official definition of **homeless** was offered by the federal government in the Stewart B. McKinney Homeless Assistance Act of 1987 (U.S. Congress, House, 1987). Any individual lacking a fixed, regular, and adequate night-time residence is defined as a homeless person. The definition includes any individual with a primary night-time residence at shelters, missions, welfare hotels, and public or private places not designated for sleeping quarters. Any person needing institutionalization but instead residing in an institution providing only temporary residence for homeless people is also considered homeless. Box 26-2 provides an insight into the way the term *homeless* has been used in the past.

Other definitions of homeless include individuals with no mailing address or place to sleep; people who sleep outdoors on streets or in parks, at train stations, at subways, underground, or in cars; and people on the verge of home-

## " *a conversation with . . .* "

### Donald, a Homeless Man in Gulfport, Mississippi

*"You never know, it could be your brother . . . out there needing your help."*

Nurse: Donald, you told me you were from New York and that you came here. Do you have any family down here?

Donald: No, no family at all. Like a bird I fly south for the warm weather. This time in New York right now it's freezing and it's really crowded in the line of business I'm in.

Nurse: What line of business is that?

Donald: I do a little everything. I am over here now a couple of days 'cause people give me a lot of yard work over here, and they feed me, give me a little change of clothes. I sprinkle a little water on myself.

Nurse: You don't find this weather cold down here right now? It's like 40 something degrees out here.

Donald: Yeah, it's like 40-something degrees here and maybe 20-something degrees in New York City. I'm pretty well prepared: I got about four layers of clothing on. Most of the time down here, I have to strip some of this off.

Nurse: Well, let me ask you something, Donald. Like I explained to you, I'm a nurse and I'm studying health care. Where do you go when you get sick—how do you go about getting some help, about seeing a doctor?

Donald: Well, most of the hospitals here, they've been all right, they direct me to the emergency room . . . they'll fix you up, say if I just have a cold.

Nurse: Well you look fairly young anyway . . .

Donald: Yeah, I am in pretty good health.

Nurse: Well, I see that you got some stuff with you.

Donald: This is just basic essentials, you know—sneakers, a little change of clothes. I have my blanket; I have been running into some cold nights. I have some utensils, and things, nothing much, just everyday homeless persons' things. People give me this, I go to shelters. I have been lucky to catch a few shelters down here, but you know last night it was a little crowded and I had to stay outside, but I am pretty much prepared for it.

Nurse: How long do you plan to stay down here?

Donald: As long as business is good. I say that as long as I can make a meal, work somewhere, and make a meal, I'll stay.

Nurse: You say you don't have any family down here, but do you have any family up in New York?

Donald: I have a sister, last address unknown. I don't bother anybody; I am self-sufficient; I try to take care of myself; I don't ask for much; I lead a simple life.

Nurse: Like I said before, if I ask you anything personal and you don't want to answer, you don't have to. Do you drink any alcohol?

Donald: Very little, very little . . . like my sign reads here "Will work for food," it doesn't say, "for alcohol." . . . Now occasionally I have been known to take a good sip—it warms the innards.

Nurse: How about the people who you meet at the shelters: Do you notice that they drink much alcohol?

Donald: The majority of them are heavy wine drinkers. Well, they drink whatever they can get a hold of, anything that's over 1% alcohol they drink it.

I am basically a loner. I travel alone. I've been all over this country. I've been by myself, I've been making it.

Nurse: You're not scared out on the roads . . . the violence?

Donald: Yeah, there's times I'm scared, but, you know, luckily people know I don't have anything. They don't bother me. I have run into a lot of good people. They just don't bother me ever.

Nurse: Was there anything you think would be helpful for me to know about people who live on the roads?

Donald: Yes, if you could get to talk to some more people or if more people would talk openly, I think that you would find that the homeless situation is really bad and people who could lend a hand in any kind of way, just donating some old clothes to Salvation Army or Goodwill, they should really look into it. I think the states should look more into the homeless situation 'cause it's really out there and it's really bad. It could be your brother, one of your relatives—out there needing your help.

**—Interviewer: James Ryan, RN, MSN, ANP**
Ryan found Donald under a freeway underpass in Mississippi holding a sign that said "Will work for food."
Interview used with permission.

lessness (Bean, Stefl, & Howe, 1987; Benda & Dattalo, 1988; Phillips, Pauley, & Rudolph, 1997; Interagency Council on the Homeless, 2000; Rivilin, 1986; Stark, 1987).

Homelessness has also been described in terms of three stages (Belcher, Scholler-Jaquish, & Drummond, 1991). *Episodic homelessness* characterizes people who live below the poverty line and who are on the verge of homelessness or may actually experience one or more episodes of homelessness for short periods. *Temporary homelessness* describes people who have recently become homeless but still view themselves as part of their community. *Chronic homelessness* describes people who have adopted their state of being as a

way of life and have declined in social status, financial status, and interpersonal and family connections.

## ■ Historical Perspective

### The Beginning of Homelessness in America

As long as can be remembered, homeless people have been inhabitants of America (Institute of Medicine, 1988). English people who settled on North American soil segregated themselves by classes. The workers and the more affluent people gave assistance to poor people (Trattner, 1984). During the 1600s, colonists adopted England's ideology

## BOX 26-2

### Use of the Term "Homeless"

In the latter part of the 1970s, the term "homeless" became a trendy way to refer to individuals living on the streets or in shelters (Interagency Council on the Homeless, 2000). At that time, homeless individuals were predominantly males who had been deinstitutionalized. The term was popularized by proponents as a way to describe homeless people in a nonstigmatizing, nonjudgmental way. However, the term became synonymous with "bums." A new kind of homelessness has placed a strain on the use of the term. In the last two decades, poverty has brought families, women, and children in record numbers to face homelessness.

and many principles of England's law, which was written to protect the welfare of families and communities. Therefore, adult white men, "free" African Americans, and Indians were left to wander aimlessly and beg for food, clothing, and other assistance. The only individuals who warranted assistance at that time were white women, children, and disabled people.

As the mid-1800s approached, a new generation of poor people surfaced in the United States during the industrialization and farming era. Sporadic and transient labor became essential (Hoch & Slayton, 1989). Most of the homeless populations consisted of men because they were the providers and often had to leave home to find work. Some who traveled the land by railways to look for transient work were labeled as "hobos." Other men who sought transient work on foot were labeled as "tramps." Then there were "bums," who usually traveled by railways, stole from others, and begged for money and food. The Civil War and migration to the West created another mass of homeless people, who were labeled "cowboys," "Indian scouts," and "gold seekers" (Hoffman, 1953).

Not long after the turn of the twentieth century, "skid rows" surfaced in major cities, where homeless and indigent people gathered for food, assistance, and word-of-mouth information at diners, bars, mission homes, and old hotels. Most of these people were older white men. The skid row population fluctuated with the status of the U.S. economy (Momeni & Wiegand, 1989). Shantytowns, where homeless

 GLOBAL CONNECTION

The primary factor that influences a country's growth is industrialization. The more industrialized the country, the greater the urban growth.

In 1800, only 3% of the world's population lived in cities. Today, half of the world's population lives in cities, and 75% of people in the world's industrialized nations live in cities. Without the Industrial Revolution, this urbanization of the world could not have taken place.

**A Good Read**

# Ironweed (1983)

*by William J. Kennedy, New York: Penguin.*

Winner of the 1984 Pulitzer Prize for Literature, *Ironweed* follows Francis Phelan during the Great Depression during his years of living on the streets. Phelan had a promising baseball career when a series of bad decisions and unfortunate events, including accidentally killing his infant son, drives him to refuge in alcohol and a homeless life. Francis and his other friends on the street, specially Helen Archer and Rudy, move forward, day by day, despite or until mental and physical difficulties impede them. While the reader will sympathize with their dismal existence, the characters maintain their pragmatic sensibility of their plight, without whining and complaining. Although a dismal topic and book, the richness of Phelan's life "as a bum" is revealed in possibilities, hope, and redemption. Both Phelan and Archer know that they have chosen their lives and do not blame others or life for their plight, which perhaps is the greatest accomplishment of this book: portraying the eternal hope of the human condition. Kennedy writes without sentimentality, depicting the harsh lives lived by those without families and homes while giving them virtues shared by the rest of society. The book is a wonderful read, filled with humor, realistic dialogue, and rich details of the stories of those invisible to most of society.

people colonized, sprang up across the United States after the crash of the stock market in 1929. The skid row population continued to increase until World War II brought new jobs.

### Societal and Governmental Influences Through the 1970s

Because manifestations of mental illness place persons at high risk for homelessness, a large proportion of the homeless population was believed to be mentally ill in the 1800s. In 1890, New York was the first state to enact a law allowing the state government to assume full responsibility for individuals classified as the "insane poor" (Anderson, 1934).

A federal plan was not initiated until 1933, when the **Federal Emergency Relief Administration (FERA)** supplied food, shelter, clothing, money, jobs, and health care to homeless individuals (Anderson, 1940). In 1935, FERA was replaced by the Works Progress Administration (WPA) federal program, which was aimed at creating jobs only for people who could meet strict residency standards. Because a residence was required to receive assistance, homeless people were not included in this plan.

## Research Alert

Links between homelessness and ill health are well established. However, homeless people are less likely to access traditional health care owing to administrative barriers and the hostility of healthcare professionals. For this reason, more flexible modes of healthcare delivery, including nurse-led care, have been explored. There has been a rapid increase in innovative nursing roles over the last two decades, and the literature suggests that a clear role definition, good interprofessional working relationships, and supportive cultures are some of the features that ensure role effectiveness.

A large study exploring new roles in nursing and midwifery in Northern Ireland identified an innovative nurse-led approach in meeting the needs of single homeless people. The aim of this paper was to explore the effectiveness of this role using a public health framework. A case study design was used that incorporated semi-structured interviews with analysis of secondary sources and a period of observation. Results demonstrated that the role fitted within a public health framework in that it involved assessment of needs, skills to meet those needs, facilitation of access to care, partnership working, health promotion, health protection and influencing policy, and strategy development. The conclusion is that the role met the set criteria for innovative nursing roles. Furthermore, such a practitioner meets the criteria for advanced nursing practice, providing evidence of effective nurse-led care that meets the health agenda of targeting inequalities in health. ◁

*Source*: Poulton, B., McKenna, H., Keeney, S., Hasson, F., & Sinclair, M. (2006). The role of the public health nurse in meeting the primary health care needs of single homeless people: A case study report. *Primary Health Care Research & Development*, 7(2), 135–146.

The 1940s and World War II created new jobs and decreased poverty and homelessness for a few years, but the 1960s brought a substantial increase in the homeless population. In 1963, the Community Health Centers Act was enacted, which deinstitutionalized approximately 430,000 people with mental illness (Rossi, 1989). These people were released from the institutions in which they lived, and many of them had nowhere to live and no job. Deinstitutionalizing thousands of people was cited as a humane act but detrimentally expanded the homeless population.

The combination of deinstitutionalization and the declining economy in the 1970s forced courts to rule on homelessness for the first time. In 1972, the U.S. Supreme Court ruled that vagrancy was no longer a crime (Cook, 1979). The Court also declared that governmental assistance provided only to people who claimed a permanent residence was unconstitutional. In the same decade, the New York Supreme Court ruled that homeless people should be provided a clean place to sleep, nutritious food, supervision, and security. Efforts were made to comply with the court ruling. Many, but not all, homeless people in New York were given assistance.

### Societal and Governmental Influences in the 1980s

The state of New York's move toward improving homeless conditions contributed to the federal government's actions toward homeless programs. Several other major events occurred in the United States during the 1980s that drove the federal government into action to provide federal assistance (Interagency Council on the Homeless, 2000). A dramatic increase in poverty and the shrinking of affordable housing were major forces that led to the homeless epidemic.

Racial discrimination in the job market presented another concern. By 1985, less than 45% of African American men ages 16 to 24 were able to find employment, compared with 70% of white men of the same age range (Interagency Council on the Homeless, 2000). Other situations that contributed to homelessness and poverty were substance abuse, disabilities, chronic health problems, and changes in the family structure that led to a shift toward female-headed households.

Also in the 1980s, a shift in the labor market from a focus on goods production to a focus on services caused plants to relocate or close and farms to shrink or cease to operate. Laborers were no longer in high demand. Rather, the demand was for highly skilled and educated people. A way of life had disappeared; jobs were gone; a new culture of homeless people existed.

The combined tensions created by all of these problems placed at-risk people at serious disadvantages and thus strained many households to the point of homelessness.

Table 26-2 provides a list of governmental activities during the 1980s. Historically, the assistance offered by government programs and local groups has provided only immediate relief and has failed to address the long-term problems of homelessness (Fuchs & McAllister, 1996). The **Stewart B. McKinney Homeless Assistance Act of 1987** and the grass-roots efforts of local relief groups were instrumental in prompting the federal government to make a commitment to reduce homelessness (Interagency Council on the Homeless, 2000).

**❝***There is nothing new about poverty. What is new is that we now have the techniques and the resources to get rid of poverty. The real question is whether we have the will.* **❞**

—*Martin Luther King, Jr., 1968*

### Societal and Governmental Influences in the Late 1990s and Early Twenty-First Century

Many programs were born during the 1990s. Once the initial Stewart B. McKinney Homeless Assistance Act of

**Table 26-2** Governmental Activities for Homeless People in the 1980s

| Date | Activities of the 1980s |
|---|---|
| ■ 1982 | The Community for Creative Non-Violence in Washington, D.C., estimated that 2.2 million Americans lacked shelter. |
| ■ 1982 | The U.S. Conference of Mayors reported that the demand for emergency services for the homeless far outweighed the capabilities to provide services. In fact, only 43% of the demand was met. |
| ■ 1983 | The Emergency Food and Shelter (EFS) Program of the Federal Emergency Management Agency (FEMA) allocated $100 million to the U.S. Department of Agriculture's Temporary Emergency Food Assistance Program (TEFAP) to reduce the impact of the homeless crisis. |
| ■ 1984 to 1987 | FEMA allocated $325 million for continued relief. Other agencies that allocated money for relief efforts included the Health and Human Services Emergency Assistance Program and the HUD Community Development Block Grant Program. |
| ■ 1987 | The Stewart B. McKinney Homeless Assistance Act was enacted to provide emergency shelters, job training, and other assistance to homeless people providing $490 million. |
| ■ 1988 | The National Resource Center on Homelessness and Mental Illness was established by the Policy Research Associates (PSA) to provide on-site technical assistance, targeted workshops, publications, databases, and instant access to homeless people with mental illness. |

1987 was developed, the program branched into numerous programs throughout the federal government (Interagency Council on the Homeless, 2000). Table 26-3 outlines a few of those programs. By 1994, the McKinney programs had expanded to $1.2 billion. Numerous non-McKinney programs also were created. Today almost a dozen of these non-McKinney programs target homeless people. Many federal programs, although not targeted to the homeless, provide indirect assistance to homeless people. The McKinney Act has been the major federal vehicle to assist homeless people (Interagency Council on the Homeless, 2000).

The 1990s brought about unprecedented growth and complexity in the homeless population. As a result, nurses, so-cial workers, agencies, and others have gained rich, abundant experiences in trying to manage homelessness. The same social problems leading to homelessness persist: declining wages, poor education, persistent illiteracy, racial discrimination, chronic health problems, violence, crime, and poverty.

Americans must face that even as new programs have sprung up, the problem of homelessness has grown because economical, health, and social forces are ever-present. Organizations have historically looked for easy solutions to seemingly unresolvable problems. Homelessness remains a problem without an easy solution, just as it has always been. The United States is now faced with even more complex human problems: newer, stronger, and more addictive drugs, such as heroin and

 THINK ABOUT THIS

**How Could a Nurse Ever End Up Homeless?**

What if you, as a nurse, were laid off and could not find a position that accommodates your small children? Eventually, child support disappears or never existed. You are living from month to month and eventually are evicted from your apartment. Through an unfortunate turn of events, you end up without relatives or friends who can take you in for more than a few days.

Now imagine yourself on the streets or living out of your car. Your car breaks down; you do not have the money to repair it. You are essentially living on the streets, putting the children in the car at night. The area around you becomes unsafe for the children but you cannot move the car. Soon, you are bathing your children in public bathrooms, such as those in subway stations, gas stations, and McDonald's restaurants. As the children grow dirtier and their clothes more worn, these options seem to close down due to the owners' reactions and denial of your use of their facilities.

Your days are spent looking for work. Even with an RN license, the work history interruption and your unkempt appearance (no professional clothes and lack of bath facilities) leave you with few or no options. You have to leave your children alone while job hunting, which exposes them to violence and sexual abuse. Your days begin to run together. You and the children spend hours each day looking for food, in garbage cans and McDonald's trash.

You find homeless shelters, but they are often riskier for yourself and your children than being on the streets owing to the risk of theft and the shelters' limited hours. You find yourself trusting no one, having no friends, and living in constant fear that you or your children will be attacked or raped. People pass you on the street and make disparaging remarks, such as "Get a job," turn their eyes away, or run you off from the place where you are sleeping. Police ticket you for vagrancy. You cease to care about what others think of you.

*This could not happen to you, you think, right? Neither did the nurse.*

*Source*: This is based on an actual case from Dr. Karen Saucier Lundy's personal experience in an urban homeless shelter. The nurse had a master's degree and three children ranging in age from 6 to 12 and was interviewed in a homeless shelter. The nurses in that shelter never saw her again.

| **Table 26-3** | Governmental Activities for Homeless People in the 1990s and Early Twenty-First Century |

| Date | Activities of the 1990s and Early Twenty-First Century |
|------|--------------------------------------------------------|
| ■ 1992 | Funding was set aside to provide rental assistance to 4,750 disabled homeless households annually for 3 years. |
| ■ 1993 | President Clinton committed to make homelessness a top priority in the White House. |
| ■ 1994 | The Interagency Council on the Homeless published a proposal to reduce the homeless population. The main objective was to find "a decent home and a suitable living environment" for every American, which would become known as the "continuum of care." The reality was that the council hoped to reduce homelessness by one-third. |
| ■ 1995 | President Clinton proposed a reorganization of the HUD McKinney programs under a single account. Homeless projects continued as a high priority in the Oval Office. |
| ■ 1995 | President Clinton vetoed the balanced budget bill, which would have cut federal welfare by $81.5 billion and virtually eliminated homeless assistance programs provided by the McKinney Act. The President's budget proposed consolidating three runaway and homeless programs. The budget also focused on disadvantaged groups, including veterans and other homeless people. |
| ■ 1995 | The National Law Center on Homelessness and Poverty published a report that evaluated NIMBY (not in my backyard) opposition to services for homeless people in 36 jurisdictions across the United States. |
| ■ 1995 | Funding was set aside to provide rental assistance to 15,000 homeless households annually for 5 years. |
| ■ 2003 | U.S. Department of Health and Human Services published *Ending Chronic Homelessness: Strategies for Action* with specific ways that the federal and state governments can increase flexibility and limit restrictions on health and social services to the homeless. |

## BOX 26-3

### Why Are People Homeless?

- Poverty
- Changes in the labor market from focus on goods production to services
- Lack of affordable housing
- Devaluation of the dollar and devaluation of federal income assistance
- Unemployment
- Street violence, domestic violence, and crime
- Crisis in families; abuse, neglect, and incestuous relationships
- Lack of kin support
- Mental illness
- Deinstitutionalization
- Substance abuse
- Socially stigmatizing infectious diseases (e.g., HIV, tuberculosis)

*Sources:* Interagency Council on the Homeless, 2000; Jahiel, 1992; Sumerlin & Bundrick, 1997; Susser, Struening, & Conover, 1997.

cocaine; socially stigmatizing infections such as tuberculosis, sexually transmitted diseases, and human immunodeficiency virus (HIV); and decline of family support, which means that relatives often do not take in family members needing assistance anymore. Box 26-3 delineates several factors that may contribute to an individual's homelessness.

## ■ The Health Problems of Homeless People

### Common Health Problems

Homelessness in the United States translates into major health problems. People who are homeless are faced with myriad health problems, which fall into three basic categories: health problems that contribute to a state of homelessness, health problems that are the consequence of

homelessness, and treatment of health problems that is complicated by homelessness (Institute of Medicine, 1988).

The first category involves health problems that contribute to a state of homelessness. Most people with chronic health problems that lead to a state of homelessness suffer from lack of employment because of their disabling state of health (Berne, Dato, Mason, & Rafferty, 1993; Corburn, 2004; Institute of Medicine, 1988; Wehler et al., 2003). These homeless persons usually do not have a support network of family members and friends. Chronic schizophrenia, dementia, and personality disorders are examples of mental illnesses that may actually contribute to a state of homelessness and financial insecurity. Relationships with family and friends may become excessively strained when an individual's ability to cope with everyday life situations diminishes. Family members may become so stressed trying to deal with everyday problems that they abandon or throw out the mentally ill family member into the streets.

Individuals with acquired immune deficiency syndrome (AIDS) may become homeless when they are no longer able to work because of illness and opportunistic infections (Institute of Medicine, 1988). They often lose their houses or

### ◉ MEDIA MOMENT

#### *Children Underground* (2001)

Director Edet Belzberg explores the tragic policy decision by Romanian dictator Nicolei Ceaucescu to outlaw contraceptives and encourage his impoverished populace to have more children. Thousands of children were born to broken or dysfunctional families in a nation steeped in political and economic instability, resulting in a large and rapidly growing population of homeless children (estimated at more than 20,000) in the city of Bucharest. Nominated for Academy Award Best Documentary in 2002.

apartments and face overwhelming medical expenses. Living on the street or in a shelter becomes a way of life for them. Alcoholism, drug dependency, and other disabling health problems (e.g., accidental injuries or degenerative diseases) may lead to similar life situations. In 15 studies on alcoholism in the homeless population (as cited in Rossi, 1989), 33% of homeless people abused alcohol and were homeless as a result of alcoholism (Rosenblum et al., 2005; Salazar et al., 2007; Salomonsen-Sautel, 2008).

The second category includes many disorders and illnesses that result from living on the streets or in shelters. Examples of physical problems include skin and blood vessel diseases, respiratory disorders and infections, malnutrition, parasitic infestations, foot and lower extremity problems, physical assault, rape, trauma, periodontal disease, tooth decay, degenerative joint disease, sexually transmitted diseases, cirrhosis, and hepatitis (Institute of Medicine, 1988). Psychological and social problems that may be triggered include personality disorders, alcohol and drug dependence, prostitution,

poor oral and body hygiene, hunger, adolescent pregnancy, developmental and learning delays in children, violence, criminal convictions, depression, low self-esteem, and other mental illnesses (Institute of Medicine, 1988; Interagency Council on the Homeless, 2000; Rossi, 1989). Table 26-4 reflects specific health problems associated with homelessness.

Skin, blood vessel, and traumatic problems that homeless people experience are often related to strenuous walking and wandering, inadequate clothing, improper fitting of shoes, and exposure to infections and parasites. Some of these problems include venous stasis, varicose veins, peripheral vascular disease, cellulitis, skin ulcerations, skin infestations, bruises, contusions, lacerations, abrasions, abscesses, and burns of all severities (Cheung & Hwang, 2004; Gamst et al., 2006; Rossi, 1989).

Communicable diseases affect scores of homeless people and are cause for a major public health concern (Rossi, 1989). Living on the streetzs or in shelters subjects homeless people to poor sanitary conditions, poor hygiene, and inadequate, if

**Table 26-4**   Common Health Problems of Homeless People

| Classification | Specific Health Problems |
|---|---|
| ■ Skin and traumatic disorders | Skin ulcerations |
| | Skin infestations (e.g., lice, scabies, worms) |
| | Peripheral vascular disease, varicose veins |
| | Cellulitis |
| | Carbuncles |
| | Bunions, corns |
| | Abrasions, lacerations |
| | Wounds |
| | Bruises, contusions |
| | Sprains, strains |
| | Burns |
| ■ Acute disorders/diseases | Tuberculosis, pneumonia, influenza, asthma |
| | Bladder and renal infections |
| | Female-specific genitourinary infections |
| | Male-specific genitourinary infections |
| | Diabetes mellitus complications |
| ■ Chronic disorders/diseases | Psychosocial disorders/problems |
| | Cancer of all types |
| | Endocrine disorders (e.g., diabetes mellitus) |
| | Anemia and other nutritional deficiencies |
| | Eye, ear, mouth, and dental disorders |
| | Cardiovascular disorders (hypertension, heart, and circulatory disorders) |
| | Arthritis and other musculoskeletal disorders |
| | Pregnancy |
| | HIV/AIDS and other sexually transmitted diseases |
| | Seizures and other neurological disorders |
| | Obstructive pulmonary disease |
| | Gastrointestinal disorders |
| ■ Mental illnesses | Personality disorders |
| | Criminal convictions |
| | Jail, prison, or detention sentencing |
| | Drug and alcohol abuse |
| | Lack of family or friends support system |
| | Poverty |

*Source*: From *Down and Out in America: The Origin of Homelessness*, by Rossi, 1989. Used by permission.

any, sleeping quarters. Communicable diseases (e.g., tuberculosis) are easily transmitted in these living conditions.

The third category results from complications associated with the treatment of acute or chronic health problems in homeless people (Institute of Medicine, 1988). One major chronic disease that is complicated by inadequate treatment is diabetes mellitus. Daily injections and a diabetic exchange diet are difficult, if not impossible, to maintain while homeless. Protecting syringes from theft or contamination, for example, is challenging. Hypertension, renal disease, liver disease, peripheral vascular disease, and schizophrenia are other chronic problems that are complicated by homelessness. Inability to follow the prescribed medical regimen, lack of money to cover medical and health expenses, or inability to follow the prescribed dietary regimen complicate these health problems.

Homeless families have similar acute and chronic physical and mental problems. Homeless children also are at risk for developing chronic physical disorders (Forchuk, Russell, Kingston-MacClure, Turner, & Dill, 2006). In a study conducted by Wright and Weber (1987), 16% of the homeless children were reported to have a variety of chronic physical disorders. Some of the most common disorders included asthma, anemia, and malnutrition. Some other disorders reported at high rates were various types of respiratory infections, skin infections, ear and eye infections, dental problems, and gastrointestinal problems.

In another study of homelessness in New York City in 1985 (Chavkin, Kristal, Seabron, & Guigli, 1987), the infant mortality rate of the homeless population (24.9 per 1,000 live births) was more than twice the overall infant mortality rate in New York City (12 per 1,000 live births). In the same study, the researchers found that homeless pregnant women were more likely to give birth to infants of low weight than nonhomeless pregnant women.

HIV transmission is a primary concern for all homeless people, especially homeless adult and adolescent women. In a survey of homeless adults who were entering a storefront medical clinic, 69% were found to be at risk for acquiring HIV

infection because of several at-risk behaviors: unprotected sex with multiple partners, injection drug use, sex with a partner who injects drugs, or exchanging sex for money or drugs, primarily crack (St. Lawrence & Brasfield, 1995). Safe, intimate relationships may be difficult, if not impossible, for homeless people to maintain because of drug use, mental illness (Darbyshire et al., 2006), violence, survival sex (sex in exchange

---

### Rescue Mission 2

They gather themselves in groups of twelve
around shakey cardtables
some unvarnished wood
and others metal and formica

they're here for another supper
for some the last one
before they lean slowly
toward another side of town

here they all gather at the Riverside mission
apostles of the alleys
sheltered in boxes and
doorways opened onto the
promised streets and rails

lord, are these bones hungry
these tweeds and wools shine
but not with grace from the father
a dull halo of wear

in the seat where a man
can rub thin with contact
from concrete and unpainted benches
and still turn the other cheek

some bring their own wine
refusing the coffee or tea
and milk can no longer faithfully
support these crumbling bones

no one will be betrayed here
though some have thought of a sellout
at times for thirty cents to luck
onto more wine or cigarettes

the bread is passed around again
wholly for the sake of one's almighty health
a man's got to eat to save himself
though the word wasn't made flesh
enough to bless them with a small
taste of steak

after supper they file out on
the thin soles of unpolished shoes

the moon rests like a large stone
rolled to close a room where a brother
waits with a good steak, new tweed
a cigarette and a rousing story of
how when he was hungry there was always
someone to share their bread

—*James A. Lopresti, Denver, Colorado, 1977*

---

✍ THINK ABOUT THIS ............................

The urban giants: Population of the ten largest megacities (more than 10 million residents) in the world by ranking
1. Tokyo, Japan
2. Mexico City, Mexico
3. Bombay, India
4. São Paulo, Brazil
5. New York City, United States
6. Lagos, Nigeria, Africa
7. Los Angeles, California, United States
8. Calcutta, India
9. Shanghai, China
10. Buenos Aires, Argentina

*Source*: United Nations, 2000.

for food, money, or drugs), and transient living conditions. In their survey, Fisher, Hovell, and Hofstetter (1995) found that 91% of homeless women experienced battery and 56% experienced sexual assault. Cheung and Hwang (2004) found that homeless women younger than age 45 had higher death rates than older women. Deaths among younger women often approach or are equal to those of homeless men.

Homeless mothers have been a forgotten population in terms of research or published literature. Berne, Dato, Mason, and Rafferty (1993) noted that homeless mothers traditionally have waited to seek health care until their conditions developed into emergency situations. Chronic stressors, physical and sexual abuse, lack of family ties, poverty, lack of coping abilities, domestic violence, street violence, overcrowded conditions, poor hygiene, and poor nutrition predispose homeless mothers to chronic physical, social, and mental problems. Tuberculosis, depression, sexually transmitted diseases, HIV/AIDS, drug abuse, prostitution for money or drugs, and poor parenting skills often result (Austin, Anderson, & Gelberg, 2008; Cooke, 2004; Wehler et al., 2004).

Adolescents are also vulnerable to a variety of social and health problems, including violence, prostitution, drug abuse, and physical and mental disorders (Meadows-Oliver, 2006). The following Research Alert summarizes research findings about homeless youth and their exposure to and involvement in violence while living on the streets.

A study of women veterans indicates an alarming overrepresentation of women among homeless veterans. This trend has been attributed to the increasing numbers of women serving in military conflicts, such as in Iraq (Gamache, Rosenheck, & Tessier, 2003).

The accumulation of problems that homeless people experience is overwhelming to say the least. Reducing or alleviating homelessness is critical to the general health and human condition in our society. Public policies are needed to meet two goals: to reduce or combat the short-term problems of pain and suffering in homeless individuals and to address the long-term problems by reducing the risk of becoming homeless. By becoming a political advocate for the basic rights and health of the homeless population, community health nurses can help create or change public policies involving homelessness.

### Barriers to Health Care

Researchers have indicated that lack of access is a major barrier to health care for homeless people (Corburn, 2004; Hunter, Getty, Kemsley, & Skelly, 1991; Snowden & Yamada,

---

 **ETHICAL CONNECTION**

As community health nurses, do we have an ethical responsibility to care for the homeless as part of the public's health? Such individuals are difficult to locate, they are transient, and their problems are deep-seated and complex. Should we instead concentrate on those populations where preventive health care can be more effective?

---

## MEDIA MOMENT

### *The Fisher King* (1991)

Robin Williams stars as a homeless man who is well educated and shares his philosophy about life and his choice to remain homeless. He believes himself to be the "fisher king," the person who is guarding the "Holy Grail." His plight as a homeless man resulted from watching his wife be brutally murdered. Jeff Bridges also stars in this excellent movie that presents the viewer with complex choices, defies homeless stereotypes, and gives a glimpse into the culture of the homeless. Grace and forgiveness are major themes. This entertaining movie ends with hope and more understanding of who becomes homeless and how mental illness is socially defined.

---

2005; Wood & Valdez, 1991). Homeless people cannot afford health insurance and, not surprisingly, homeless people experience even more problems in accessing health care than nonhomeless people with or without insurance. Homeless people typically do not have a regular family practitioner. They seek care from emergency departments more often than poor people who are not homeless. Homeless people may also be discouraged from obtaining healthcare services or even turned away by healthcare personnel from private clinics (Freeman, Blendon, Aiken, Sudman, Mullinix, & Corey, 1987). Other barriers to health care include the following (Flynn, 1997; Hatton, 1997; Institute of Medicine, 1988; Nyamathi, Flaskerud, & Leake, 1997; Percy, 1995; Forchuk et al., 2006):

- Lack of systematic communication with healthcare professionals
- Lack of transportation to a healthcare facility
- Lack of social and family support
- Psychological depression; hard-to-reach homeless people
- Lack of motivation by the homeless person to seek health care

---

 ## Research Alert

A survey of 432 youth between the ages of 13 and 23 years old, who were homeless or at imminent risk for homelessness, revealed that males and females were exposed to equally high levels of violence on the streets. Females were more likely to have been sexually assaulted but less likely to report it or report any other violent acts. Ethnic identity was not a significant predictor of exposure to violence. The overall findings revealed that these youth were exposed to violence at a significantly higher level than other youth in national surveys.

*Source:* Kipke, M. D., Simon, T. R., Montgomery, S. B., Unger, J. B., & Iversen, E. F. (1997). Homeless youth and their exposure to and involvement in violence while living on the streets. *Journal of Adolescent Health, 20*, 360–367.

## Nursing Care of Urban and Homeless People

Community health nurses function on all three levels of prevention—primary, secondary, and tertiary—regarding the care of urban and homeless aggregate populations. Homeless people have generated a culture all their own, enriched with diverse customs and backgrounds that should be taken into consideration when managing care for them (Acosta & Torro, 2008; Corburn, 2004; Family and Youth Services Bureau, 1994; Lowe, 2008). Managing health and social problems for urban and homeless individuals and populations is among the most challenging functions of the community health nurse.

Homeless people suffer from myriad emotional and physical ups and downs. The Research Alert below reflects a summary of research findings on the experiences of homeless female-headed families.

Both young and old homeless people need what everyone needs—opportunities, advantages, and services that help them live healthier lives. Ed DeBerri, Assistant Director at the National Resource Center on Homelessness and Mental Illness (1997), has stated that the most effective programs and policies have human dignity as their guiding principle. Through hands-on experience with homeless individuals, DeBerri (1997) learned five important principles about homeless people and their needs.

First and foremost, DeBerri found that homeless people have talents, needs, and desires. They want to be shown respect for who they are and what they know. Second, shelters and case management traditionally have not been sufficient to prevent the problems of homelessness or to end homelessness. Housing, financial support, and social and family support are needed to improve the conditions. Third, providing comprehensive health care, social services, and housing can reduce homelessness. Fourth, helping to find work for homeless individuals is essential. Homeless people need to feel productive and useful, just like all people. Fifth, new resources need to be developed and used creatively; then the successes of these programs need to be publicized.

### Research Alert

Homeless families are at high risk for severe physical, emotional, and social health problems. Eighty-five percent of all homeless families are headed by single women. Sixteen of these women were asked to describe their experiences of being the head of the homeless family. The themes that emerged were loss of freedom, a sense of being different, feeling down, maternal survival (motherhood), and living under pressure. They described being homeless as a nightmare, not knowing what will happen to them or where they will be from day to day.

*Source*: Menke, E. M., & Wagner, J. D. (1997). The experience of homeless female-headed families. *Issues in Mental Health Nursing, 18*, 315–330.

**If I'm Lucky**

Buddy, can you spare me a quarter?
I've got an important call to make.
And maybe if I bum enough quarters
A little drink will help me heal my heartache.
You see, I'm drowning
In a river of liquor.
I'm going down for the last time.
I'm a loser . . .
I'm a boozer . . .
On lower Broadway.
If I'm lucky
I won't see the sun rise.
Years ago, I hopped a Greyhound to Nashville.
A big country star would I be.
And if I must confess
I met with some success
But success got the better of me.
So tonight I'll wrap my arms around my bottle
In an old cardboard box
We will lie.
I'm a loser . . .
I'm a boozer . . .
On lower Broadway.
If I'm lucky
I won't see the sun rise.
So don't preach to me
About Jesus.
Cause Jesus don't live on the streets.
He lives in a white ivory tower
in the heart of someplace
called Belle Meade.
You see, there's one thing in life
I've got faith in,
Is this warm toasty feeling inside.
I'm a loser . . .
I'm a boozer . . .
On lower Broadway.
If I'm lucky
I won't see the sun rise.
If I'm lucky
I won't see the sun rise.

—*Music and lyrics by Felton Keyes, BSN, RN, 1985*
*Used with permission.*

These five principles also can be applied to the care of urban populations. Drawing on the strengths of urban or homeless individuals and the resources available in the community will enable community health nurses to implement appropriate interventions that can actually work. An example of drawing on the strength of a homeless person would be to find a homeless person who can sew and asking him or her to teach a group of people in the shelter how to mend their clothes. Another example is to recruit a person from the shelter to teach good hygiene and hand washing

"Most Americans want the homeless off the streets, but no one wants them next door."

—C. Jencks, 1994

techniques to the children in the shelter. The community health nurse's interventions will help create social and economic viability, build diversity in skills and resources, strengthen the community, and contribute to healthier people in the community.

However, improving the conditions of urban people and reducing the rate of homelessness are outcomes that need a collaborative effort among multidisciplinary agencies in the community. Without communitywide participation, poor conditions among the urban and homeless populations and increased incidence of homelessness will persist. Furthermore, without communitywide efforts to eliminate poverty, prejudice, violence, and discrimination, the nurse's attempts to improve the health and human conditions among urban and homeless populations will be fruitless (Jones, 2006).

Specific interventions that the community health nurse should implement are described in the following sections. The interventions are aimed at managing health and social problems of urban and homeless populations.

### ■ Be Committed

Be committed to make a difference in the community. To properly intervene, community health nurses first need to be committed enough to help make a difference in the community. A high level of commitment will facilitate nurses' care of urban and homeless patients in the community. In fact, all three levels of prevention interventions will follow more easily if commitment to make a difference in the community has already been established. Commitment from community health nurses translates to hope and healing among the urban and homeless populations.

A paramount example of one person's commitment to make a difference is former President Jimmy Carter. The Atlanta Project (TAP) was initiated by Carter in 1991 (TAP, 1995). The central mission of this project was to bring the "two Atlantas" (the affluent and poverty groups) together to improve the quality of life in Atlanta's neighborhoods, especially urban areas. TAP has been somewhat successful since its induction in decreasing the gap between the rich and the poor. In fact, Carter became committed to spreading TAP to all of America, thus becoming The America Project. By 1995, more than 100 official delegations from numerous cities across America had begun modeling their urban enhancement and development programs after TAP (Berger, 2007; Biven, 2002).

### ■ Use Leadership Skills

Become an enthusiastic leader and an encourager. Being committed to enthusiastically leading the way in solving problems for urban and homeless people will help others catch on, pitch in, and follow. Once others start contributing their time and efforts into this mission, specialized expertise areas will start to develop among the workers. Acting as a leader and encourager can be used at all three levels of prevention. One example of using excellent leadership skills is when, upon recognizing the need for a community health center, the community health nurse promotes and sells the idea to key people in the community and political officials, leads the way in planning and organizing, and then coordinates the activities. Before long, the nurse's dream will be realized through hard work and commitment.

Good, effective leadership provides the glue to pull everything together (TAP, 1995). Community health nurses are in a position to become leaders of the community. However, they need a vision, effective communication, effective delegation, and commitment to follow through to the end of the project.

Another effective leadership characteristic involves recognizing the talents of those populations being served. Urban and homeless people are people with numerous talents. Caring, concern, and good communication skills may be talents that urban and homeless people can contribute. Other talents include artistic and musical talents. The community health nurse needs to recognize and use those talents to expand available resources. Also, by recognizing value in others' contributions, self-esteem among the people will be increased and an atmosphere of team effort will be established. One example of using a person's strengths is to ask a homeless person, who has been recognized as having a team attitude and leadership abilities, to help plan and coordinate an activity or event at a homeless shelter.

## Use Available Resources

Draw on every federal and community resource available to you. Community health nurses should realize that to make a difference, they need to network with other agencies and draw on existing community and federal resources. The management of care involved in this level of intervention is secondary prevention. Drawing on federal and community resources to provide outreach programs mandates that the community health nurse maximize the use of collaborative partnerships with disciplines and agencies within the community.

One of the fundamental elements that contributed to the success of TAP was its personnel's realizing that everything and every resource needed to make a difference in Atlanta was within reach. Mark O'Connell, president of the United Way of Metro Atlanta, speaking about one solution for improving urban life, stated, "The answer is in how we use the resources we already have and in how we value people" (TAP, 1995). In this regard, community health nurses can equate O'Connell's statement about valuing people to caring about urban and homeless people, which takes a high level of commitment to help with improving the community.

Local resources can help supply meals, hygiene products, clothing, and even health care. Food missions, local free clinics, churches, Salvation Army, and American Red Cross are valuable resources that the community health nurse can use. State and federal resources can be drawn upon for financial, health, education, and shelter programs, as well as other types of programs. Medicare, welfare, Medicaid, Head Start, and food stamps include a variety of state and federal programs that can be used.

## Be an Advocate

Become a political advocate for preventing homelessness and the problems associated with the urban population. Intervention at this level is primary prevention, which involves taking political action. Talking to politicians and speaking out in favor of prevention of homelessness and the problems associated with urban populations are essential to effecting change

*Even Fuji is without beauty to one who is hungry and cold.*

—Japanese saying

in the community. Even more important is for community health nurses to speak out in numbers through their professional organizations, such as the American Nurses Association and the American Public Health Association, and encourage new public policies to be adopted. Being a united voice through large numbers of community health nurses is powerful and grabs the attention of politicians across the country.

In becoming politically involved, community health nurses need to remember not to become overwhelmed or take on too many issues at one time. It is more effective to concentrate on one or two problems at a time. Promoting ideas and attitudes and selling a political viewpoint or solution can go a long way toward reducing the problems associated with homelessness or the urban poverty population. Writing letters to local, state, and federal officials and congressional members is an effective way to capture attention. Other ways include presenting concerns at public meetings, getting elected as a lobbyist through organizations, interacting with members of Congress on a one-on-one basis, and publicizing the needs and concerns of these populations through brochures, newspapers, radio, and television.

To better persuade policy makers and city officials of specific needed interventions, community health nurses should learn exactly what needs and concerns exist in their community. The National Law Center on Homelessness and Poverty (1999a) has stated that permanent solutions to homelessness must address the fundamental cause—that homeless people cannot pay for housing. The Law Center notes that permanent solutions to prevent homelessness include ensuring affordable housing, adequate income, and social services, as well as prohibiting discrimination. These solutions are issues that community health nurses can address when speaking out politically.

The National Law Center on Homelessness and Poverty (1999b) has also listed selected rights of homeless people. Community health nurses should become familiar with the rights of homeless people to detect violations of these rights

 MEDIA MOMENT

### *Home Alone II: Lost in New York* (1992)

Often thought of as a comedic child's movie, this film finds Kevin once again left "home alone" while his parents take a plane to Florida and he takes the wrong plane to New York City. A homeless woman, the "Pigeon Lady," becomes part of Kevin's life, cares for him, and opens his eyes to the wisdom of her world. Look carefully for this underlying theme, which is overlooked due to the antics and comedy involving the 11-year-old boy "lost in New York."

**Vagrant**

he floated like a guppy once
didn't need to care
didn't care to need

it's all there in the sac
the warmth and cushion
the belly always filled first

but he still had to let go
though stubborn; a caesarian
and make his way in the world

there was a breast for a spell
and he grew into a plump little
pear on buttermilk bisquits and gravy

he stole apples and squash
sneaking in and hiding the plunder
in the crowded cupboards

it doesn't take long for years
to rot and ripe and rot again
and jobs came and went

why, once not long back he even
sold carnations—fullblown white ones—
on street corners for change

he's shrunk and wrinkled like a
sunbaked codfish now
wandering from mission to mission

turning up on doorsteps like some
crazy orphaned bouquet of lillies-of-the-valley

not caring to need
not needing to care

—*James A. Lopresti, 1977*

 **Got an Alternative?**

One of the threats to health for the homeless is related to their feet, due to standing for long periods of time, poor footwear, and exposure to adverse environmental conditions. One successful strategy that homeless shelter clinics have utilized in the past to promote their services has been to offer whirlpool footbaths. Once in the clinic, the community health nurse can use the time with the patient to assess and offer assistance in other health areas.

by certain groups, organizations, or individuals. Preserving the rights of homeless people through political advocacy is an important intervention for community health nurses. The rights include but are not limited to the following (National Law Center on Homelessness and Poverty, 1999b, pp. 1–2):

- Homeless children have a right to attend school.
- Homeless children have the right to participate in mainstream federal, state, and local programs.
- Homeless people have the right to apply for the Earned Income Tax Credit.

***House of Sand and Fog* (2003)**

This film is about the concept of "home" and the lengths to which people will go to preserve it. An alcoholic woman who has been dumped by her husband, Kathy Nicolo (Jennifer Connelly) finds her family house in the California hills seized in foreclosure and put up for public auction by a local sheriff deputy (Ron Eldard). An exiled Iranian Air Force colonel (Ben Kingsley) sees Nicolo's house as his family's dream home and quickly snaps it up. Trouble is, Nicolo is obsessed with getting the house back and goes to extreme measures to reclaim it. This film is about family, cultural issues, alcoholism, and redemption. An emotional rollercoaster, this outstanding movie covers the full range of human reactions to isolation and fear of homelessness.

- Homeless people have the right to vote.
- Homeless people have the right to sleep in public if there is nowhere else to sleep.
- Homeless people have the right to apply for food stamps, Medicaid, and Supplemental Security Income.

Purposefully exposing themselves to urban and homeless people by placing themselves in strategic locations within the community is an excellent way for community health nurses to learn about the needs of urban and homeless people. Meeting these individuals face to face and interacting with them will help community health nurses to see individualized problems. The broad picture of health and social problems among these people also will become more focused. Ultimately, the community health nurse can communicate these health and social problems and prevention strategies to policy makers at all levels of government.

## Foster Communication and Trust

Develop open communication and trust among the urban and homeless populations. A climate of open communication and trust is pivotal to developing an environment of security and support. Violations of trust and conveying a false sense of security have serious consequences and should be avoided when interacting with urban and homeless people. Nurses need to remember not to make promises of hope that will never be met. Trust is built on truth, reliability, and open communication. For a leader to be effective, trustworthiness is critical. Following through on a project or goal and being dependable are ways that the community health nurse can establish trust and open communication.

## Assess the Problem

Develop and practice good assessment skills. For primary prevention, assessment is aimed at identifying factors that play a role in the problems of urban living and problems that contribute to homelessness. At this level of prevention, community health nurses need to assess the political structure of

## Application to Practice

### Descent of a Woman: From Rags to Riches to Rags

*"You're about to enter a secret world, hidden from thousands carrying on the business of the day just steps away. It's a dark world of broken lives and shattered dreams. And if you don't think you could wind up there, wait until you meet the woman about to guide you through this twilight zone. . . . What could possibly make a woman who had it all leave her home, her life, her children, for a terrifying existence underground?" (Phillips, Pauley, & Rudolph, 1997, p. 8).*

By age 26, Nadine had a husband, three healthy sons, a prosperous clothing boutique in New York's trendy Soho district, and a lifestyle she had always wanted. Her life as a child was saddened by the abandonment of her mother, who turned to drugs and prostitution. Nadine, by age 8, was herself experiencing the effects of alcohol. Later, she turned to marijuana and cocaine, often smoking marijuana with her father.

She temporarily cleaned up her life. But taking care of a family and attending to a business with all its financial demands resulted in too much pressure for Nadine. Nadine and her husband sometimes experimented with cocaine as they celebrated their newfound success. The drugs, the money, and the success pushed Nadine and her husband to vicious fights. Soon the money was gone. Nadine left her family. Nadine's drug use became excessive—from pot and cocaine to, finally, a powerful addiction to heroin. The drug had so much power over her that she turned to prostitution to support a $100-a-day habit.

When she had exhausted all of her resources, her boyfriend (a drug pusher) introduced her to "the condo," an underground subway escape in New York where thousands of homeless people live to stay high on drugs and to escape life, family, and the law. People refer to the underground people as the "mole people." After unsuccessfully trying drug rehabilitation 20 times, Nadine felt she had hit rock bottom. She had even been pronounced clinically dead once in an emergency department in New York.

"She joined a band of drug addicts descending under an iron plate literally into the bowels of New York city, down 13 metal steps, then around and around a grimy concrete staircase . . . just a few blocks and a world away from her old life. Instead of a bathroom . . . the subway tracks were her toilet.

The kitchen? Whatever they could beg, borrow, or steal. And this soot-filled platform right next to the roaring train, her bedroom. [Under New York] there's another city. . . . This one has about 45,000 people in it . . . the homeless who are sleeping underground" (Phillips, Pauley, & Rudolph, 1997, p. 16).

After a long time living homeless and like a mole underground, Nadine's break came. She crossed paths with Renny Chun, a journalist. Chun pushed Nadine, through numerous contacts, to rehabilitation. Nadine wanted help but was afraid of being sober and of failure. She desperately wanted to see her sons, which provided her the strength she needed to kick the habit cold turkey. Now Nadine lives one day at a time and hopes to never be in the condo again. She reunited for a short while with her sons. *Dateline NBC* reported that she was seeking legal visiting rights for the future. Nadine's courage has helped her to be clean and sober today and hopefully tomorrow.

Underground living is a reality for homeless people in major cities where subway escapes exist. Rudolph (Phillips, Pauley, & Rudolph, 1997) discussed the nightmare that Nadine experienced and related the magnitude of the problem of the underground. Nadine took Rudolph and the television viewers to "the condo" to see the drug addicts lying with the rats, the human waste, the garbage, and the sewer. She noticed that the same people she had previously known were still underground.

1. What are some factors, psychological and external, that led Nadine to homelessness? As you answer this question, think about her life as a child and as an adult.
2. What health problems/infections would you anticipate Nadine to have while exposed to underground living? As a prostitute? As a homeless person? If Nadine had been homeless in your city, list resources that would have been available to her.
3. How would you, as a community health nurse, help Nadine? Include how you could intervene using a holistic approach. Include as many physical, psychosocial, cultural, developmental, and spiritual factors that you should take into consideration when planning Nadine's care.

*Source*: Phillips, Pauley, & Rudolph, 1997.

·······················

Can our cities be saved? Here are 25 ways to improve urban health:

1. Reclaim dangerous neighborhoods.
2. Discover the effects of stress in the lived environment.
3. Build learning communities.
4. Understand the local culture.
5. Reach out to immigrants.
6. Target cancer prevention efforts.
7. Keep on the offensive.
8. Use community health workers.
9. Eliminate disparities in health.
10. Broaden diabetes treatment.
11. Unleash positive peer pressure.
12. Nurture connectedness.
13. Anticipate expanding needs.
14. Understand HIV-risk behaviors.
15. Take aim at illegal gun sales.
16. Highlight stores' healthy foods.
17. Give back to cities.
18. Train mental health mentors.
19. Start a school of science.
20. Undo the trauma of violence.
21. Rebuild aging infrastructure.
22. Clear the air.
23. Roll out injury prevention.
24. Prepare for home emergencies.
25. Share your insights.

   Read the article from the publication below for more detail about successful research-based urban health interventions. Select one of the preceding options and identify one way that community health nurses can influence a city's health. Who would you involve in your efforts?

*Source: John Hopkins Public Health* (Magazine of the Johns Hopkins Bloomberg School of Public Health), Fall 2006, pp. 14–53.

·····························································

the city and state and resources available in the community at all levels of government.

Secondary prevention assessment involves evaluating the health and social problems associated with urban poverty and homelessness. A good understanding of these problems will help the community health nurse to develop a strong and purposeful plan for outreach. Also involved at this level is an assessment of access to health care, screening programs, food missions, and other resources (Darbyshire et al., 2006).

Tertiary prevention assessment is aimed at evaluating available resources to help people cope with the chronic problems associated with urban poverty and homelessness. Healthcare, mental health, and social services that take referrals for indigent people are important resources to assess. A significant problem among the homeless is that of hospice or care of the dying. These people often end up without access to pain medication and palliative care; after death, they are often left nameless in a city morgue (Kushel & Miaskowski, 2006). Identifying the needs of urban and homeless people is also considered assessment at the tertiary prevention level. Free clinic access, alcohol and drug detoxification programs, protection from communicable

*Homeless* as a term was first used in 1981 by Mitch Snyder and Robert Hayes to describe the growing number of persons living in boxes and eating out of garbage cans in urban areas as a result of the worst recession in half a century.

*Source:* Jencks, 1994.

diseases, and care of chronic mental and physical problems are some specific needs that will be identified. Social needs that will be identified include protection from violence and sexual assault, literacy programs, job training programs, and housing/shelter programs (Forchuk et al., 2006).

### ■ Plan and Give Care

Develop and implement an effective plan of care. Planning care for urban and homeless populations means that community health nurses will need to focus on basic life care needs as well as population needs. First, short-term and long-term goals need to be identified at the primary, secondary, and tertiary levels. Needs should also be prioritized from most urgent human needs to least urgent.

However, an effective plan of care is futile if the plan does not lead to action on the part of the community health nurse and other community resource providers. Actually following through with an effective plan goes back to maintaining a high level of commitment. Resource agencies and people are available and ready to help. The community health nurse must be committed to finding these resources and then using them. Although referral agencies are critical to good outcomes for homeless people, community health nurses need to realize the importance of the nursing role. The community health nurse provides a continuity of care that no other discipline offers. While providing continuity, the nurse's quality of care has an excellent chance to improve health and holistic outcomes for the person.

## Conclusion

Inner cities cannot keep pace with the needs of the rapidly growing population. Many problems existing in inner cities are the result of the rapid increase in population, not necessarily the result of poverty. Poverty remains the culprit for many problems in urbanized areas, including hunger, homelessness, health problems, communicable diseases, overcrowded living conditions, violence and crime, and inadequate housing. Poverty in inner cities is directly related

---

**◉ MEDIA MOMENT**

***Brother, Can You Spare a Dime***
Once I built a railroad, made it run.
Made it race against time.
Once I built a railroad, now it's done
Brother, can you spare a dime?

—E. Y. "Yip" Harburg (1896–1981)

to higher infant mortality rates among African Americans, a poor quality of life, and increased health problems among all adults in inner cities. Several massive efforts have been under way to help improve the quality of life in urbanized areas. Many of the programs have been the result of *Healthy People 2000* and *Healthy People 2010*. Some specific programs include the Healthy Cities movement, urban development projects, and the America Project. Several other programs have been targeted for African American urban populations.

Today, the United States is faced with an overwhelming problem of homelessness. A new culture of homeless people has emerged—whole families, single mothers with children, teens, and veterans. Families are the fastest-growing segment of homeless people in the United States.

Barriers to health care of homeless individuals include poverty, lack of access to health care, lack of communication with healthcare professionals, lack of transportation to a healthcare facility, lack of family and social support, psychological depression, lack of motivation to seek health care, and difficulty in locating homeless people for follow-up care. The homeless population experiences many health and social problems, some of which include communicable diseases, foot and leg ulcerations, arthritis, poor hygiene, malnutrition, respiratory and cardiovascular problems, substance abuse, chronic health problems that are poorly managed, HIV/AIDS, mental illness, prostitution because of sex-for-drug swaps, violence, crime, and assault.

Community health nurses need to function at all three level of prevention—primary, secondary, and tertiary—to be effective in managing care of urban and homeless people.

All urban and homeless people need what everyone else needs—opportunities, advantages, and services that help them live more healthful lives.

Explore Community Health Nursing on the Web! To learn more about the topics in this chapter, use the passcode provided to access your exclusive website: **http://nursing.jbpub.com/communityhealth.** If you do not have a passcode, you can obtain one at this site.

## ■ CRITICAL THINKING ACTIVITIES

1. Think about Nadine's state of homelessness as described in the Application to Practice feature on page 649. Consider her desire for drugs and the life she was living during her period of homelessness. What views/attitudes should you, a community health nurse, take as a logical and ethical approach toward Nadine?

2. Discuss the way each of the following six ethical principles might apply to Nadine, her situation, and her health care. See Chapter 11 for ethical issues in community health nursing.

   | | |
   |---|---|
   | Autonomy | Privacy |
   | Freedom | Beneficence |
   | Veracity | Fidelity |

3. John, 36 years old, is a homeless man with a history of intravenous drug use and AIDS. He is wasting away and has multidrug-resistant tuberculosis. He went to the free neighborhood health clinic where you work, presenting with fever, cough, and purulent blood-tinged sputum. As a community health nurse, discuss four health outcomes that John and you would plan for his care. Give the rationale for each.

4. Discuss some therapeutic communication strategies the community health nurse might use with a single mother with two children, all of whom are homeless. The mother has a crack addiction, and you have reason to believe that she swaps sex for drugs while the children, ages 2 and 8, are left alone on the street.

5. Select nursing interventions at the primary, secondary, and tertiary levels for an elderly homeless female with a history of congestive heart failure and insulin-dependent diabetes mellitus. Include interventions that address the holistic nature of the individual.

6. Yolanda, a homeless African American adolescent, 16 years old, has presented to a shelter for food, clothing, and sleep. You are the community health nurse assisting her. You learned through your assessment that she has had morning sickness and has been very sick, to the point that she slept on the streets for 7 nights because she did not have the strength to walk 2 miles to the shelter. She had become dehydrated and weak. She admitted to using crack cocaine on a regular basis and stated that she could not control her desire to use the drug. She has not seen a family practitioner for her morning sickness and dehydration or to receive a pregnancy test. She thinks that she is at least 3 months pregnant by a young man she met on the streets. He has since been imprisoned for selling drugs. She ran away from home several months ago to escape a poor family relationship with her mother.

   - Based on what you have learned about Yolanda, list the risk factors that may have contributed to Yolanda's homelessness and her situation.

   - Knowing that shelter care would not be enough for Yolanda, what would be your plan of care for her? Include resources, social support, family, and other agencies you may use.

   - Yolanda receives medical attention and is stabilized for now. What can you do in the first few days at the shelter to instill in Yolanda a sense of competence, a sense of usefulness, a sense of belonging, and a sense of power and control? Include cultural considerations and values.

   - What barriers will Yolanda face when she makes any decisions concerning her well-being? Obtaining a primary practitioner? Returning to her environment? Returning to school?

# ■ REFERENCES

Acosta, O., & Toro, P. A. (2000). Let's ask the homeless people themselves: A needs assessment based on a probability sample of adults. *American Journal of Community Psychology, 28,* 343–366

Anderson, N. (1934). *Homeless in New York City.* New York: Board of Charity.

Anderson, N. (1940). Highlights of the migrant problem today. *Proceedings of the National Conference of Social Work.* New York: National Conference of Social Work.

Austin, E., Andersen, R., & Gelberg, L. (2008). Ethnic differences in the correlates of mental distress among homeless women. *Women's Health Issues, 18*(1), 26–34

Baker, S. G. (1994). Gender, ethnicity, and homelessness: Accounting for demographic diversity on the streets. *American Behavioral Scientist, 37,* 476–504.

Baum, A. S., & Burnes, D. W. (1993). *A nation in denial: The truth about homelessness.* Boulder, CO: Westview Press.

Bean, G., Stefl, M., & Howe, S. (1987). Mental health and homelessness: Issues and findings. *Social Work, 32,* 411–416.

Belcher, J. R., Scholler-Jaquish A., & Drummond, M. (1991). Three stages of homelessness: A conceptual model for social workers in health care. *Health and Social Work, 16*(2), 87–93.

Benda, B. B., & Dattalo, P. (1988). Homelessness: Consequence of a crisis or long-term process? *Hospital and Community Psychiatry, 39,* 884–886.

Berger J. (2007). "There is tragedy on both sides of the layoffs:" Privatization and the urban crisis in Baltimore. *International Labor & Working-Class History, 71,* 29–49.

Berne, A. S., Dato, C., Mason, D. J., & Rafferty, M. (1993). A nursing model for addressing the health needs of homeless families. In G. D. Wegner & R. J. Alexander (Eds.), *Readings in family nursing.* Philadelphia: J. B. Lippincott.

Biven, W. C. (2002). *Jimmy Carter's economy: Policy in an age of limits.* Chapel Hill, NC: University of North Carolina Press.

Bolland, J. M., & McCallum, D. M. (2002). Touched by homelessness: An examination of hospitality for the down and out. *American Journal of Public Health, 92,* 116–118.

Burt, M., & Cohen, B. (1989). *America's homeless: Numbers, characteristics, and the numbers that serve them.* Washington, DC: Urban Institute.

Centers for Disease Control and Prevention (CDC). (2005). *National Immunization Survey: A User's Guide for the 2005. Public-Use Data File.* Retrieved August 25, 2008, from http://www.cdc.gov/nis/pdfs/nispuf05_dug.pdf

Chavkin, W., Kristal, A., Seabron, C., & Guigli, P. (1987). The reproductive experience of women living in hotels for the homeless in New York City. *New York State Journal of Medicine, 371,* 10–13.

Cheung, A. M., & Hwang, S. W. (2004). Risk of death among homeless women: A cohort study and review of the literature. *Canadian Medical Assessment Journal, 170*(8), 1243–1247.

Cook, T. (Ed.). (1979). *Vagrancy: Some new perspectives.* New York: Academic Press.

Cooke, C. L. (2004). Joblessness and homelessness as precursors of health problems in formerly incarcerated African American men. *Journal of Nursing Scholarship, 36*(2), 155–160.

Corburn, J. (2004). Confronting the challenges in reconnecting urban planning and public health. *American Journal of Public Health, 94*(4), 541–545.

Cousineau, M. R., Wittenberg, E., & Pollatsek, J. (1995). *Study of the health care for the homeless program.* (HV 4505). Bethesda, MD: Department of Health and Human Services, Bureau of Primary Health Care.

Culhane, D. P., Dejowski, E. F., Ibanex, J., Needham, E., & Macchia, I. (1993). *Public shelter admission rates in Philadelphia and New York City: The implications of turnover for sheltered population counts.* Washington, DC: Fannie Mae Office of Housing Research.

Darbyshire, P., Muir-Cochrane, E., Fereday, J., Jureidini, J., & Drummond, A. (2006). Engagement with health and social care services: Perceptions of homeless young people with mental health problems. *Health & Social Care in the Community, 14*(6), 553–562.

DeBerri, E. (1997). Listening to the voice of homelessness. *Access, 9*(1), 2.

Department of Health and Human Services (DHHS). (2000). *Healthy People 2010: Conference edition.* Washington, DC: U.S. Government Printing Office.

Department of Health and Human Services (DHHS). (2003). *Strengthening homeless families: An annotated resource guide for homeless shelters.* Washington, DC: U.S. Government Printing Office.

Family and Youth Services Bureau. (1994). *A guide to enhancing the cultural competence of runaway and homeless youth programs.* (DHHS Contract No. 105-92-1709). Silver Spring, MD: U.S. Government Printing Office.

Fisher, B., Hovell, M., & Hofstetter, C. R. (1995). Risks associated with long-term homelessness among women: Battery, rape, and HIV infection. *International Journal of Health Services, 25,* 351–369.

Flynn, L. (1997). The health practices of homeless women: A causal model. *Nursing Research, 46*(2), 72–77.

Forchuk, C., Russell, G., Kingston-MacClure, S., Turner, K., & Dill, S. (2006). From psychiatric ward to the streets and shelters. *Journal of Psychiatric & Mental Health Nursing, 13*(3), 301–308.

Freeman, H. E., Blendon, R. J., Aiken, L. H., Sudman, S., Mullinix, C. F., & Corey, C. R. (1987). Americans report on their access to care. *Health Affairs, 6*(1), 6–18.

Fuchs, E., & McAllister, W. (1996). *A continuum of care: A report on the new federal policy to address homelessness* (HUD Contract No. DU100C000018360). Washington, DC: Department of Housing and Urban Development, Center for Urban Policy.

Galea, S., & Vlahou, D. (2002). Social determinants and the health of drug users: Socioeconomic status, homelessness and incarceration. *Public Health Reports, 117*(1), 5135–5145.

Gamache, G., Rosenheck, R., & Tessier, R. (2003). Over representation of women veterans among homeless women. *American Journal of Public Health, 93*(7), 1132–1135.

Gamst, G., Herdina, A., Mondragon, E., Munguia, F., Pleitez, A., Stephens, H., et al. (2006). Relationship among respondent ethnicity, ethnic identity, acculturation, and homeless status on a homeless population's functional status. *Journal of Clinical Psychology, 62*(12), 1485–1501.

Goldstein, G., & Kickbusch, I. (1996). *A healthy city is a better city. World Health Organization.* Geneva, Switzerland: World Health Organization.

Hatton, D. C. (1997). Managing health problems among homeless women with children in a transitional shelter. *Image: Journal of Nursing Scholarship, 29*(1), 33–37.

Hoch, C., & Slayton, R. A. (1989). *New homeless and old: Community and the skid row.* Philadelphia: Temple University Press.

Hoffman, V. F. (1953). *The American tramp, 1870–1900.* Unpublished master's thesis, University of Chicago, Chicago, IL.

Hunter, J. K., Getty, C., Kemsley, M., & Skelly, A. H. (1991). Barriers to providing health care to homeless persons: A survey of providers' perceptions. *Health Values, 15*(5), 3–11.

Institute of Medicine. (1988). *Homelessness, health and human needs.* Washington, DC: National Academy Press.

Interagency Council on the Homeless. (2000). *The federal plan to break the cycle of homelessness.* Washington, DC: Department of Housing and Urban Development.

International Healthy Cities Foundation (IHCF). (2002). *What is the Healthy Cities movement?* Retrieved November 13, 2008, from http://www.healthycities.org/overview.html

Jahiel, R. I. (Ed.). (1992). *Homelessness: A prevention-oriented approach.* Baltimore, MD: Johns Hopkins University Press.

Jencks, C. (1994). *The homeless.* Cambridge, MA: Harvard University Press.

Jones, T. (2006). Resilience in homeless adults: A review of literature. *Journal of the National Black Nurses Association, 17*(1), 36–44.

Kipke, M. D., Simon, T. R., Montgomery, S. B., Unger, J. B., & Iversen, E. F. (1997). Homeless youth and their exposure to and involvement in violence while living on the streets. *Journal of Adolescent Health, 20*, 360–367.

Kushel, M. B., & Miaskowski, C. (2006). End-of-life care for homeless patients. *Journal of the American Medical Association, 296*(24), 2959–2966.

Lewis, D. L. (1993). *W. E. B. DuBois: Biography of a race, 1868–1919.* New York: Henry Holt.

Lezak, A. D., & Edgar, E. (1996). *Preventing homelessness among people with serious mental illnesses: A guide for states.* (DHHS Publication No. 3106). Rockville, MD: Department of Health and Human Services, Center for Mental Health Services.

Link, B., Phelan, J., Breshan, M., Stueve, A., Moore, R., & Susser, E. (1995). Lifetime and five-year prevalence of homelessness in the United States: New evidence on an old debate. *American Journal of Orthopsychiatry, 65*, 347–354.

Lopez, R., & Welker-Hood, K. (2007, January). Environment, health, and safety: Urban sprawl and the built environment. *American Nurse Today.*

Lowe, S. (2008). It's all one big circle: Welfare discourse and the everyday lives of urban adolescents. *Journal of Sociology & Social Welfare, 35*(3), 173–194.

MacKenzie, W. R., et al. (1994). A massive outbreak in Milwaukee of cryptosporidium infection transmitted through the public water supply. *New England Journal of Medicine, 331*(3), 161–167.

Massey, D. S., & Denton, N. A. (1993). *American apartheid: Segregation and the making of the underclass.* Cambridge, MA: Harvard University Press.

Meadows-Oliver, M. (2006). Homeless adolescent mothers: A metasynthesis of their life experiences. *Journal of Pediatric Nursing, 21*(5), 340–349.

Menke, E. M., & Wagner, J. D. (1997). The experience of homeless female-headed families. *Issues in Mental Health Nursing, 18*, 315–330.

Momeni, J. A., & Wiegand, G. (1989). *Homelessness in the United States.* New York: Greenwood Press.

National Law Center on Homelessness and Poverty. (1999a). *Solutions to homelessness in America.* Available from http://www.nlchp.org

National Law Center on Homelessness and Poverty. (1999b). *Selected rights of homeless persons.* Available from http://www.nlchp.org/

Nennig, M. E., Shinefield, H. R., Edwards, K. M., Black, S. B., & Fireman, B. H. (1998). Prevalence and incidence of adult pertussis in an urban population. *Journal of the American Medical Association, 275*, 1672–1674.

North, C. S., Eyrich, K. M., Pollio, D. E., & Spitznagel, E. L. (2004). Are rates of psychiatric disorders in the homeless population changing? *American Journal of Public Health, 94*, 103–108.

Nyamathi, A., Flaskerud, J., & Leake, B. (1997). HIV-risk behaviors and mental health characteristics among homeless or drug-recovering women and their closest sources of social support. *Nursing Research, 46*, 133–137.

Percy, M. S. (1995). Children from homeless families describe what is special in their lives. *Holistic Nursing Practice Journal, 9*(4), 24–33.

Phillips, S. (Announcer), Pauley, J. (Announcer), & Rudolph, L. (Reporter). (1997, August 19). *Dateline NBC.* New York: National Broadcasting System. Transcript from Burrelle Publishing, Livingston, NJ.

Polednak, A. P. (1997). *Segregation, poverty, and mortality in urban African Americans.* New York: Oxford University Press.

Rivilin, L. G. (1986). A new look at the homeless. *Social Policy, 16*(4), 3–10.

Rosenblum, A., Magura, S., Kayman, D., & Fong, C. (2005). Motivationally enhanced group counseling for substance users in a soup kitchen: A randomized clinical trial. *Drug & Alcohol Dependence, 80*(1), 91–103.

Rossi, P. H. (1989). *Down and out in America: The origin of homelessness.* Chicago: University of Chicago Press.

St. Lawrence, J. S., & Brasfield, T. L. (1995). HIV risk behavior among homeless adults. *AIDS Education and Prevention, 7*, 22–31.

Salazar, L., Crosby, R., Holtgrave, D., Head, S., Hadsock, B., Todd, J., et al. (2007). Homelessness and HIV-associated risk behavior among African American men who inject drugs and reside in the urban south of the United States. *AIDS & Behavior, 11*, S70–77.

Salomonsen-Sautel, S., Van Leeuwen, J., Gilroy, C., Boyle, S., Malberg, D., & Hopfer, C. (2008). Correlates of substance use among homeless youths in eight cities. *American Journal on Addictions, 17*(3), 224–234.

Snowden, L. R., & Yamada, A.-M. (2005). Cultural differences in access to care. *Annual Review of Clinical Psychology, 1*, 143–166.

Stark, L. (1987). A century of alcohol and homelessness: Demographics and stereotypes. *Alcohol, Health and Research, 11*, 8–13.

Sumerlin, J. R., & Bundrick, C. M. (1997). Research on homeless men and women: Existential-humanistic and clinical thinking. *Psychological Reports, 80*, 1303–1314.

Susser, E., Struening, E., & Conover, S. (1987). Childhood experiences of homeless men. *American Journal of Psychiatry, 144*, 1599–1601.

The America Project (TAP). (1995). *Because there is hope: Gearing up to renew urban America.* Atlanta: Carter Collaboration Center.

Trattner, W. I. (1984). *From poor law to welfare state: A history of social welfare in America* (3rd ed.). New York: Free Press.

United Nations. (2005). *United Nations Statistical Yearbook.* New York, NY: United Nations Publication.

United States Conference of Mayors (2006). *Hunger and homelessness survey: A status report on hunger and homelessness in America's cities.* Retrieved August 26, 2008, from http://www.usmayors.org/hungersurvey/2005/HH2005FINAL.pdf

U.S. Congress, House. (1987). *Stewart B. McKinney Homeless Assistance Act, conference report to accompany H.R. 558.* Washington, DC: 100th Congress, First Session.

U.S. Department of Commerce. (2002). *2000 census of population: General population characteristics, United States.* Washington, DC: Department of Health and Human Services, U.S. Government Printing Office.

Vladeck, B. C. (1990). Health care and the homeless: A political parable for our time. *Journal of Health Politics, Policy, and Law, 15*, 305–317.

Washington, T. A. (2002). The homeless need more than just a pillow, they need a pillar: An evaluation of a transitional housing program. *Families in Society, 83*, 183–188.

Wehler, C., Weinreb, L. F., Huntington, N., Scot, R., Hosmer, D., Fletcher, K., et al. (2004). Risk and protective factors for adult and child hunger among low-income housed and homeless female-headed families. *American Journal of Public Health, 94*, 109–115.

Wenzel, S., Tucker, J., Elliott, M., & Hambarsoomians, K. (2007). Sexual risk among impoverished women: Understanding the role of housing status. *AIDS And Behavior, 11*(6 Suppl), 9–20.

West, C. (1994). *Race matters.* New York: Vintage.

Wood, D., & Valdez, R. B. (1991). Barriers to medical care for homeless families compared with housed poor families. *American Journal of Diseases of Children, 145*, 1109–1115.

World Health Organization Regional Office for Europe (WHO). (1998). *International healthy cities conference: Athens, 20–23 June 1998.* http://www.who.dk/cpa/pr98/pr9806e.htm.

Wright, J. D., & Weber, E. (1987). *Homelessness and health.* New York: McGraw-Hill.

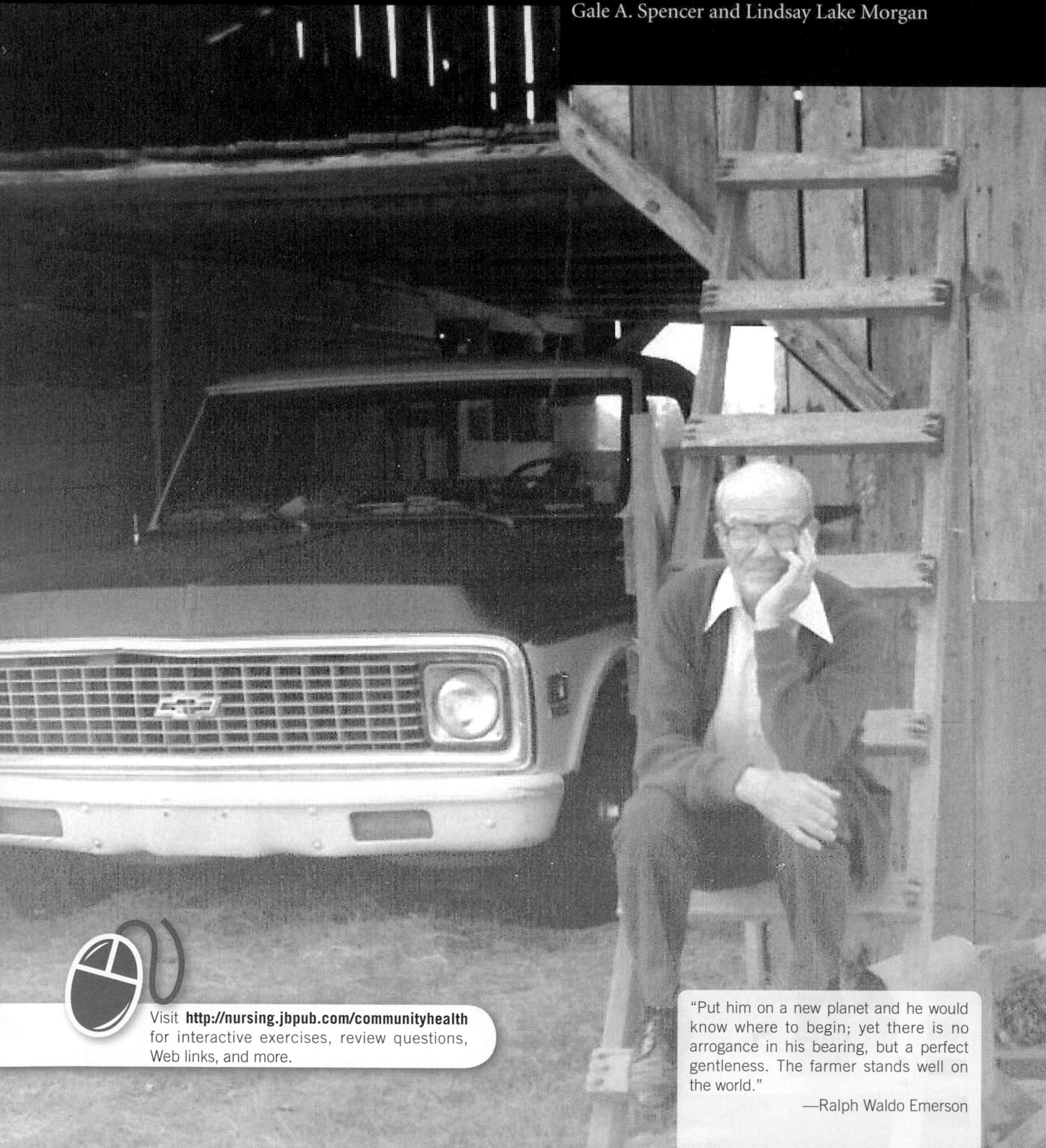

Gale A. Spencer and Lindsay Lake Morgan

Visit **http://nursing.jbpub.com/communityhealth** for interactive exercises, review questions, Web links, and more.

"Put him on a new planet and he would know where to begin; yet there is no arrogance in his bearing, but a perfect gentleness. The farmer stands well on the world."

—Ralph Waldo Emerson

The farmer is a hoarded capital of health, as the farm is the capital of wealth; and it is from him that the health and power, moral and intellectual, of the cities came.

He stands close to Nature; he obtains from the earth the bread and the meat. The food which was not, he causes to be. The city is always recruited from the country.

The men in cities who are the centers of energy, the driving-wheels of trade, politics or practical arts, and the women of beauty and genius, are the children or grandchildren of farmers, and are spending the energies which their fathers' hardy, silent life accumulated in frosty furrows, in poverty, necessity and darkness.

Put him on a new planet and he would know where to begin; yet there is no arrogance in his bearing, but a perfect gentleness. The farmer stands well on the world.

The first farmer was the first man, and all historic nobility rests on possession and use of land.

—*Ralph Waldo Emerson, Chapter VI, "The Farmer," in The Complete Works of Ralph Waldo Emerson, ed. Edward Waldo Emerson. Boston: Houghton Mifflin, 1903–1904*

What is your image of farming and rural communities? We often associate rural areas with stereotypical images of unsophisticated people without the advantages and resources of their more fortunate and affluent urban counterparts. How does this perspective influence the way nurses care for this population? What does Emerson mean that the farmer "was the first man" and that "it is from him that the health and power, moral and intellectual, of the cities came"?

## CHAPTER FOCUS

**Definitions of Rural**

**Rural Population Characteristics**

**Perspectives and Stereotypes**

**Issues, Concepts, and Populations**
- Lifestyle: Adolescents
- Isolation: Rural Elders

- Culture: Migrant Farm Workers
- Housing: Homeless People
- Confidentiality: Persons with HIV/AIDS
- Access to Health Care: Agricultural Workers

## QUESTIONS TO CONSIDER

After reading this chapter, you will know the answers to the following questions:

1. What are the various definitions of rural health?
2. How do rural populations differ from urban populations?
3. Which lifestyles and behaviors of rural adolescent populations put them at risk for illness or injury?
4. Which specific characteristics of rural life increase isolation for rural elders?
5. Which specific cultural characteristics of migrant workers provide a challenge for community health nurses?
6. What are the differences between rural and urban homeless populations?

## KEY TERMS

Access to health care
Agricultural hazards
Confidentiality
Culture

Housing
Intentional injury
Isolation
Lifestyle

Metropolitan statistical areas
Migrant farm workers
Rural–urban continuum

Sexual activity
Substance use and abuse
Unintentional injury

## Definitions of Rural

Definitions of *rural* are based on geographic, demographic, sociological, and economic perspectives. A simple definition of rural is "country." If you don't see many houses or buildings but you do see nature—mountains, plains, forests, or other scenery—you are in a rural area. This definition is based on geography and the environment. It is the most subjective definition. Eighty-four percent of the land area in the United States is considered rural, but only 25% of the total U.S. population lives in those rural areas. Although this is a small percentage of the population, people living in these areas have many special health needs. Community health nurses are a significant source of health care for rural people.

When the characteristics of a place are taken into consideration, sociological ideas are applied to the definition. The availability of services such as libraries, colleges,

**❝** *Welcome to Lake Wobegon, where all the women are strong, all the men are good-looking, and all the children are above average.* **❞**

—Garrison Keillor, Prarie Home Companion

newspapers, transportation, and health care affect people's perceptions regarding how urban or rural life seems. One commonly used definition of rural combines demographics and proximity to services. Proximity to services is assumed when a place is near an urbanized center. The **rural–urban continuum** (USDA, 2003) describes counties by both population and proximity to services. The continuum identifies **metropolitan statistical areas** (MSAs) as one or more counties that are considered metropolitan. Counties that are not in MSAs are either micropolitan or non metropolitan, but they range on a continuum based on their urbanization, population, and adjacency to an MSA (see the figure below). Counties are described as follows (North Carolina Rural Health Research and Policy Analysis Center, 1998):

- Urbanized, adjacent to MSA (4)
- Urbanized, not adjacent to MSA (5)
- Less urbanized, adjacent to MSA (6)
- Less urbanized, not adjacent to MSA (7)
- Thinly populated, adjacent to MSA (8)
- Thinly populated, not adjacent to MSA (9)

Examples of rural counties are seen in the schematic drawing and are given numbers according to their urbanization and adjacency to an MSA. There are three categories of

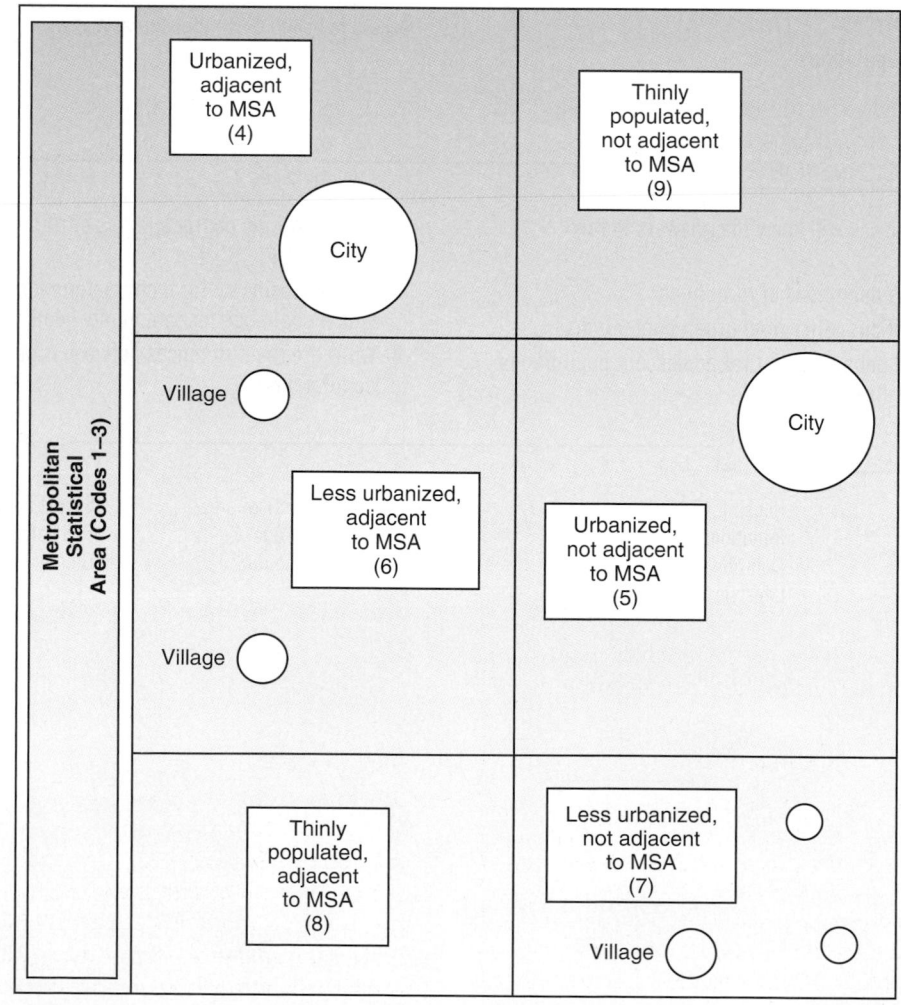

Schematic of rural counties

metro counties; they are included in the MSA and are numbered in the schematic as 1–3 (USDA, 2003).

Economists have defined rural counties in terms of their economic base. This way of defining a rural area helps in predicting the impact of events. For example, if an area is dependent on farming and the weather interferes with crop growth, economists can project earnings and losses for the region. When the major income of an area declines, it can be expected that services (e.g., car sales, new construction) in that area will also suffer. Some types of counties defined by their economic base include the following:

- Farming-dependent counties (440 total, 403 nonmetro): remotely located, sparsely populated, geographically concentrated in the Midwest
- Mining-dependent counties (128 total, 113 nonmetro): most are in the South or West
- Manufacturing-dependent counties (905 total, 585 nonmetro): account for 31% of the nonmetropolitan population; three-fifths are in the Southeast, with a more urban orientation
- Government-dependent counties (381 total, 222 nonmetro): approximately 75% are state and local government jobs, whereas 25% are federal; evenly distributed across the country
- Services-dependent counties (340 total, 114 nonmetro): serve as centers for trade, services, or recreation; evenly distributed across the country
- Nonspecialized counties (948 total, 615 nonmetro): may have economic activities such as construction, agricultural services, forestry, or fisheries; found across the country, but most are in the South (Cook & Mizer, 1994; USDA, 2005a)

Using all of the definitions together will help community health nurses get the most complete picture of the area. Combining the concepts of population density, resources, access and distance to services, and predominant economic base guides the nurse in identifying the barriers to health and health care.

In general, rural areas are sparsely populated, isolated from services, and have limited services from which to choose. Rural people sometimes have multiple roles such as farmer, judge, rotary president, and church elder. This is because there are fewer people to fulfill all the necessary functions of a community.

There are many other ways to define rural, depending on the professional discipline and the purpose of the defini-

### CULTURAL CONNECTION

Immigrants have traditionally migrated to urban areas in the United States. These trends have shown signs of changing over the past decade as more foreign-born residents have settled in rural areas, particularly in the Southeastern part of the United States. Because these immigrant populations often have different and greater healthcare needs than U.S.-born residents, the strain on rural healthcare systems and resources is being felt in many new areas.

### Research Alert

This research study used a convenience sample of 100 migrant farm workers living temporarily in a migrant worker center in El Paso, Texas, to determine the use of complementary herbal remedies for health and illness. A structured interview instrument was designed to elicit information about reasons for medicinal herb use, forms in which herbs were ingested, serious side effects experienced, location of purchase, effectiveness of treatment, and use of allopathic medications. The majority of workers used herbal remedies or other natural products because they believed them to be more effective than pharmaceuticals and because of tradition. Most learned about herbal remedies from a relative—primarily from their mother—and the majority who used herbal remedies believed them to be very helpful in treating specific illnesses. No adverse reactions to any herbal remedy were reported. The majority of participants did not inform their physicians about their use of herbal remedies.

Implications for community health nurses include the need to maintain up-to-date knowledge about the use of herbal remedies among migrant farm workers, research about these remedies' use, and interactions with traditional interventions. By showing an understanding of and sensitivity to the use of these remedies, healthcare providers will be able to conduct more comprehensive health assessments of migrant workers and their families and provide them with more culturally competent care.

*Source*: Poss, J., Pierce, R., & Prieto, V. (2005). Herbal remedies used by selected migrant farmworkers in El Paso, Texas. *Journal of Rural Health, 21*(2), 187–191.

tion. Twenty-six different definitions of *rural* were used by authors who published articles in *The Journal of Rural Health* between 1993 and 1995 (Ricketts & Johnson-Webb, 1997). It is important to know what definition is being used when evaluating literature or programs. An area that an author defines as rural may have more services available than the community for which you are planning interventions.

## Rural Population Characteristics

In 2002, the Census Bureau found that 25% of the U.S. population resided in rural areas, while the Office of Management and Budget (OMB) classified 23% as nonmetro. (USDA, 2008). The introduction of the new definitions resulted in major shifts in rural geography and population. The Census Bureau estimates that a net of approximately 5 million people have been added to the urban population by the new definitions and that the rural population has been decreased by 3 million; see Table 27-1 (USDA, 2003).

Rural populations differ demographically from urban populations in the following ways. Elders make up a larger proportion of rural populations. In 2001, 20% of the rural

| Table 27-1 | Regional Population Change 1990–2000 | | |
|---|---|---|---|
| | **Population per Thousand** | | |
| **Region** | **1990** | **2000** | **% Change** |
| ▪ United States | 248,765 | 281,422 | 13.1% |
| ▪ Rural (nonmetro) | 50,904 | 28,954 | −43.1% |
| ▪ Urban (metro) | 197,861 | 232,581 | 17.5% |

*Source*: Adapted from USDA, 2003.

population was composed of people 65 years and older compared with 15% of the urban population (Rogers, 2002, p. 30).

Although rural counties have had a slower growth in elderly populations from 1990 to 2000, elders continue to make up a larger proportion of the population. Rural elders have characteristics and needs that differ from their urban counterparts. Health and social services are deficient for 25% of all older persons living in rural areas. Nearly 6% of rural elders are age 75 or older compared with 5% of urban elders. The older population found in rural areas is predominately white (Table 27-2). The older population is concentrated in the rural South (45%), with a substantial older population also found in the rural Midwest (31%). Rural elders are more likely to be married than their urban counterparts (61% rural to 57% urban). However, widowhood increases with age, and by age 75, 41% of rural women are likely to be widowed. Rural elders are also more likely to assess their health as fair or poor, with 37% of rural elders reporting health problems compared to 32% of urban elders (Rogers, 2002, p. 31).

There are also key ethnic differences in elder populations living in rural and urban areas. The following are just a few of these differences (USDA, 1999, p. 35):

- Elders who are members of underrepresented ethnic groups make up a smaller proportion of the elderly population living in rural than in urban areas.
- Rural African American elders are more likely to be widowed and live alone than their urban counterparts.
- Elders who are members of underrepresented ethnic groups in rural areas are less educated and less healthy than white elders living in both rural and urban areas.
- Elders who are members of underrepresented ethnic groups living in rural areas tend to be poorer than their urban counterparts.

The rural population of the United States is predominately non-Hispanic white, which represents 81.5% of the rural population and 73% of the urban population. Hispanics represent 12% of the urban population and 6.3% of the rural population (USDA, 2005b). Although African Americans make up approximately 14% of the urban population, they account for only 8.4% of the rural population (Klein et al., 2002; USDA, 2005b).

Poverty is more extensive in rural areas. In 2002, the poverty rate was 14% in rural areas and 12% in urban areas (USDA, 2004). The poverty gap of 2 to 3 percentage points between rural and urban areas remained quite stable and is also evident when poverty is analyzed by family structure, ethnicity, race, and age (USDA, 2004). However, in rural areas, 26% of the residents live in households with income just above the poverty guideline (Box 27-1), compared with 18% of urban households (USDA, 2004; Connor et al., 2007). This fact makes rural residents vulnerable to downturns in the national or regional economies, as well as to personal or family economic setbacks.

Based on the 2000 Census, ethnic and racial minorities make up 17% of the urban (nonmetro) U.S. population. The rural (nonmetro) ethnic and racial minority populations are growing in all 50 states. The U.S. poverty rates are higher for rural minority populations than for non-Hispanic whites.

Rural children also live in poverty at higher rates than do urban children. In 2002, 2.6 million children living in rural nonmetro areas were poor, constituting 36% of the rural poverty population in the United States. One out of every five children living in a nonmetro area was poor. Forty-six

| Table 27-2 | Persons Age 60 and Older by Race-Ethnicity and Residence, 2001 | |
|---|---|---|
| | **Rural/Nonmetro** | **Urban/Metro** |
| ▪ White/non-Hispanic | 92% | 84% |
| ▪ Hispanic | 2% | 6% |
| ▪ African American | 6% | 10% |

*Source*: March 2006 Current Population Survey (CPS) data file.

**BOX 27-1**

**What Does the Poverty Guideline Mean?**
Poverty guidelines are the minimum income level needed by a family or individual to meet basic needs of food, shelter, clothing, and other essential goods and services. The official poverty guidelines are adjusted for family size and are set by the Department of Health and Human Services for use by all federal agencies. They are adjusted every year for inflation. In 2008, the poverty guideline was $21,200 for a family of four, $14,000 for a family of two, and $10,400 for a single individual.

*Source:* DHHS. (2008). 2008 HHS poverty guidelines. *Federal Register, 73*(15), 3971–3972.

 THINK ABOUT THIS

**The Farmer**
He bends to the order of the seasons, the weather, the soils and crops, as the sails of a ship bend to the wind. He represents continuous hard labor, year in, year out, and small gains. He is a slow person, timed to Nature, and not to city watch.

—Ralph Waldo Emerson

percent of all non-Hispanic black children were poor, and 43% of nonmetro Native American children were poor (USDA, 2004, p. 3).

The majority (62%) of rural poor children lived in single-parent families, and females headed 55% of these families (USDA, 1999, p. 83).

Rural elders also have a substantially higher poverty rate than urban elders (13% rural to 9% urban). This rate essentially was the same as that of working adults. Poverty is more pronounced among older women, elders living alone, and the oldest old. Women 60 years and older living in rural areas in 2000 were more likely to be poor than older men (15% of women versus 11% men). Rural elders living alone are more likely to be poor (28%) than their counterparts living with a spouse or another family member (6%); by age 85, one-third of rural elders living alone were poor. Underrepresented ethnic groups also make up a larger share of poor elders than would be expected based on their smaller percentage of the population. Sixteen percent of older

women are poor; 14% of them are white, 40% are African American, and 34% are Hispanic (USDA, 2000). This population is more likely to be less healthy and to have less access to good housing, adequate nutrition, transportation, and support services than their healthier and wealthier urban counterparts (USDA, 1999, p. 40).

## Perspectives and Stereotypes

The word *rural* means many different things to people. It may bring to mind a place where a person can be close to nature and a place where people rely on honesty and hard work. To others, *rural* may be a place where tiny trailers surrounded by rusting automobiles express the poverty of country life.

Learning about our personal biases and preexisting ideas is a lifelong process. We learn as professional nurses to put aside our impressions to give the best care possible to our patients. Even when we try to overcome our biases about people, however, these thoughts may still underlie our behaviors. Constantly confronting what we think and asking where these beliefs come from will always enlighten our behaviors. Recognizing the power of the media and the biases expressed in them helps us stay alert to subtle influences in our lives.

## Issues, Concepts, and Populations

Rural life is associated with certain issues and concepts that nurses need to be aware of when caring for rural populations. Because rural populations are diverse, it is difficult to find similarities for discussion. For example, elderly Amish people present very different health needs than elderly coal miners. For this reason, special at-risk populations are discussed in relation to more broad issues and concepts found in rural life. See page 670 for selected *Healthy People 2010* objectives related to rural life. Some of the more important issues and concepts identified in rural health care are **lifestyle, isolation, culture, housing, confidentiality,** and **access to health care.** These concepts serve as the framework for the following discussion of at-risk populations in rural areas. Each concept is identified and related to a selected at-risk population. These are examples upon which to add your own experience and study of issues, concepts, and populations in rural areas.

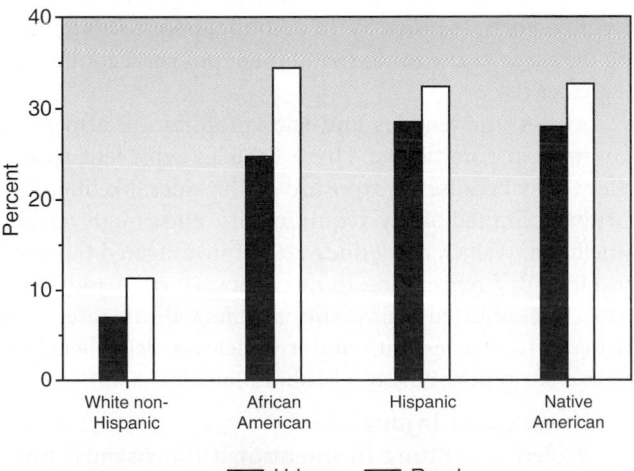

Comparison of rural–urban poverty rates by race/ethnicity.

*Sources:* Adapted from U.S. Department of Agriculture, 2000; Annual Social-Economics Supplement to the current population survey.

### ENVIRONMENTAL CONNECTION

Rural residents are often exposed to more pesticides and other chemical toxins than are urban residents due to agricultural and farming activities. Which kinds of preventive strategies can community health nurses include as part of routine physical examinations that take into account these higher risks?

## ◼ Lifestyle: Adolescents

Health behaviors and lifestyle profoundly affect the health of all people. Rural people especially lack opportunities for health promotion and health education because of limited access to healthcare providers. Although rural adolescents face many of the same health problems as adolescents in urban areas, they also face unique barriers to health promotion, which include limited access to appropriate health services (DHHS, 1991, 2000a; Connor et al., 2007) There is a limited amount of ressearch specifically on the health status of rural adolescents; however, the risks that have been identified for all adolescents will be discussed as they relate to rural adolescents and rural lifestyle. These risks include **unintentional injury** from bicycles and automobiles, particularly in combination with alcohol consumption; **intentional injury,** including homicide, suicide, and dating violence; **substance use and abuse** and its related consequences of delinquency and human immunodeficiency virus (HIV) disease; and **sexual activity,** with the risks of sexually transmitted diseases and unintended pregnancy (Fahs et al., 1999; Foster & Frazier, 2008; Johnson et al., 2008; Spencer & Bryant, 2000). One additional risk for rural adolescents that is not identified for urban adolescents is that of **agricultural hazards** (Harvey, 2008).

### Unintentional Injury

Unintentional injuries are responsible for more deaths in children than from any other cause. In addition, a substantial proportion of childhood hospitalizations and emergency department visits are attributable to unintentional injury (Grossman, 2000). The age-adjusted death rate for unintentional injury in the most rural counties is 86% higher than the corresponding rate in suburban or metropolitan areas (Eberhart & Pamuk, 2004).

Unintentional injuries are found to occur most often when driving or riding in a moving vehicle, whether it be a bicycle, all-terrain vehicle, snowmobile, or automobile. Bicycle helmets have been proven to be effective in preventing head injuries, but many adolescents still are not using helmets. In rural areas, bicycles may be the only source of transportation because of poverty, isolation, or multiple roles of family members who must share one car (Bureau of Labor Statistics, 2008). Thus bicycle safety issues are of great importance. There may also be more hazards in the rural areas because there are no designated bicycle paths, which results in riding on country roads. The roads are often rough and have no shoulders to allow the rider to get out of the way of automobile and truck traffic.

An example of rural housing.

Automobile driving behaviors of adolescents have always been of concern in rural areas. Studies by Kidd and Holton (1998) and Grossman (2000) found that risky driving practices in rural areas were correlated with alcohol use, risk-taking motivations, a low grade-point average in school, age of 15 to 19 years, and male gender. Rural adolescents often drive all types of vehicles at a much younger age than in urban areas because they can drive without a license on private property. In addition, poor roads and using the car to cruise for entertainment put rural adolescents at greater risk.

All-terrain vehicles and snowmobiles are also more common in rural areas. These vehicles represent special safety risks because of exposure of the rider, likelihood of turnover, limited safety requirements, and rough terrain. Muellman, Walker, and Edney (1993) investigated the magnitude of difference in death rates between rural and urban areas. Age-adjusted unintentional injury death rates were higher in rural areas, with motor vehicle accidents being the main contributor (Bureau of Labor Statistics, 2008).

### Intentional Injury

Violence resulting in intentional injury most often results from the use of firearms. Intentional injuries can be against oneself or against others. In a study by Brent, Perper, Moritz, Baugher, Schweers, and Roth (1993), access

Research Alert

All-terrain vehicles (ATVs) are a popular form of transportation and recreation for youth, especially for farm-related activities. This study was developed to determine differences in ATV-related behaviors, exposures, risk factors, and injuries between farm youth and their non-farm peers. A cross-sectional study design was used, and a survey was administered to 652 youths in agricultural education programs throughout the state of Arkansas. A majority (60%) of students had operated ATVs within the past month. Cross-tabulations found that farm youth who rode ATVs were more likely to be white and male, to own a three-wheel ATV, and to ride more often with a single rider. Risk factors for sustaining an ATV-related injury were related to frequency of use, number of persons on the ATV, and use of a helmet. Farm youth were less likely to use a helmet and to ride on a road.

*Source:* Jones, C. S., & Bleeker, J. (2005). A comparison of ATV-related behaviors, exposures, and injuries between farm youth and nonfarm youth. *Journal of Rural Health, 21*(1), 70–73.

Families in rural settings during the early part of the twentieth century experienced a high infant and maternal mortality rate.

to a gun by an adolescent was associated with suicide, thus increasing the risk of intentional injury to oneself. In another study by Rausch, Sanddal, Sanddal, and Esposito (1998), the researchers found that deaths in a rural pediatric practice have changed from the 1980s to the 1990s. Deaths related to suicide and homicide have increased; injuries related to firearms have also increased. Eberhardt and Pamuk's (2004) study found the age-adjusted suicide rate among rural residents 15 years and older is 37% higher than that for suburban residents.

Alcohol and other risk behaviors such as carrying weapons have been correlated with violence against others. In a study by Spencer and Bryant (2000), high school students in rural school districts were found to carry a weapon to school and in the community more often than students in urban or suburban school districts. It might be expected that the rural students would carry guns in the community more often because hunting is an acceptable sport in rural areas. The significant differences found between rural, urban, and suburban students carrying weapons to school is of concern, particularly in light of the 1998 and 1999 school shootings in small rural communities.

Dating violence is most frequently studied in college populations; however, a study by Symons, Groer, Kepler-Youngblood, and Slater (1993) examined self-reported

incidence of dating violence in rural adolescents. This study found that most of the students had been involved in at least one incident of dating violence, and one-fourth of the students had been involved in dating violence two or more times. Dating violence, including date rape, occurs more often than expected in high school students. However, most adolescents are not able to accurately label date rape even when they can clearly report the incident (Fahs et al., 1999). Violent behavior was found in the reported studies to be correlated with adolescents who took more drug risks, carried weapons, were involved in fights, and who were more likely to be victimized (Johnson et al., 2008; Spencer & Bryant, 2000).

### Substance Use

*Substance use* and *abuse* are terms often used to discuss tobacco, alcohol, and other drugs. Most available research has found that smoking cessation is much more successful among those who started smoking after the age of 13. Few differences were found between urban and rural adolescents in rates of smoking. However, in a study of upstate New York adolescents, smoking was found to be significantly higher in rural adolescents than in their urban counterparts, with 58% of the rural adolescents indicating use of tobacco, compared with 43% of the urban adolescents (Atav & Spencer, 2002). From the data collected in this study, the parents of the rural adolescents were not as well educated, and many smoked themselves, making the behavior more acceptable (Atav & Spencer, 2002; Hartley, 2004). These adolescents also spent more time without parental supervision, which would also allow them to smoke without parental censure.

### ETHICAL CONNECTION

Home health nurses in rural areas often visit patients who know one another. How should the home health nurse respond when a patient asks about the condition or well-being of another patient the nurse is visiting?

**"** *The nation that destroys its soil, destroys itself.* **"**
—*Franklin D. Roosevelt*

| Table 27-3 | Nonmarital Births by Mother's Age, 1994 | |
| --- | --- | --- |
| **Age of Unmarried Mother** | **Urban** | **Rural** |
| <20 years | 29.2% | 36.2% |
| 20–23 years | 34.4% | 36.6% |
| 24–49 years | 36.4% | 27.2% |

*Source*: Adapted from USDA, 1997, p. 68.

Rural adolescents appear to have alcohol use rates higher than the national average. Alcohol use among adolescents increases significantly as adolescents get older and is the number one substance used by eighth-, tenth-, and twelfth-grade students (NIH, 2008.). Adolescents in rural areas often participate in large outdoor drinking parties in secluded areas that are not monitored by adults. Older adolescents often initiate younger adolescents to these parties by getting them drunk. Many older adolescents reportedly purchase alcohol for younger adolescents (Wagenaar, Finnegan, Wolfson, Anstine, Williams, & Perry, 1993; Atav & Spencer, 2002).

Although cocaine has not been found to be in common use by rural adolescents, use of other drugs, especially marijuana, by adolescents continues to be a problem (Fahs et al., 1999). In fact, by the time adolescents reach the age of 17, 68% can buy marijuana within one day, 62% have friends who use marijuana, and 58% have been solicited to buy marijuana (Atav & Spencer, 2002). Anabolic steroids appear to be used equally in both rural and urban areas (Whitehead, Chillag, & Elliot, 1992).

### Sexual Activity

The birth rate has been declining over the past several years. However, even with this decline, every year more than 1 million adolescents give birth. Of these births, approximately 200,000 occur to teens in rural areas (Yawn & Yawn, 1993) (Table 27-3). In the rural areas, more unmarried mothers are likely to be adolescents.

Births to unmarried adolescent mothers are a community problem because they require additional support from community agencies. This support takes the form of additional economic resources from welfare agencies or from families who do not have monies to finance a new family unit, and from schools who must teach not only academic subjects to the young mother but parenting skills. Many rural schools have found that the best way to keep adolescent mothers in school is to provide home tutoring for them during the later stages of the pregnancy and child care later at the school. Although both require additional funds from the community, they are cost-effective because these services often make the difference between young mothers finishing or not finishing high school. Many rural schools have found that having the school nurse participate in teaching child care as part of the curriculum for adolescents returning to school with their babies enhances parenting and assists in preventing additional teen pregnancies.

Community health nurses are often the healthcare professional most consistently seen by the rural adolescents during their pregnancies. This requires community health nurses to serve in the following roles:

- An educator to prepare the adolescent and her family about the changes that will occur throughout the pregnancy
- A counselor regarding family concerns and disagreement regarding the pregnancy
- An advocate for services for the adolescent and her newborn

Research conducted on sexually transmitted diseases in both rural and urban adolescent populations found no differences. A study of rural and urban high school students by Svenson, Varnhagen, Godin, and Salmon (1992) found no differences in knowledge, attitudes, and behaviors regarding sexually transmitted diseases. Engaging in risky behaviors such as unprotected intercourse was also not found to be different between the two groups. However, the 1997 study by Spencer, Atav, and Collins found that sexual activity was

---

## ❝ *a conversation with . . .* ❞

**Faith Hill, on growing up in a rural community**

I'm so glad I am out there telling the world I'm from Mississippi right now. It's something I've always been proud of, but with all the devastation and damage from Hurricane Katrina, yes, there's a lot of concern and I'm feeling a lot of connection. All these years there's never even been a traffic light in Star, but now they just added one . . . everyone knows everyone. I grew up singing in the First Baptist Church of Star. There's not a person in this state who wouldn't give you the shirt off his back.

—From "Mississippi Rising" benefit for Hurricane Katrina Victims, Oxford, Mississippi, September 2005

---

## ◉ MEDIA MOMENT

### *Cold Comfort Farm* (1995)

When Flora Poste (Kate Beckinsale), a young society woman in 1930s London, becomes suddenly orphaned, she's forced to take up residence with a group of her unsophisticated, oddball relatives at their farm. Despite protests from the bedridden, iron-willed matriarch of the farm, the aspiring lass tries to achieve some semblance of order and class in the house—and in her own life. The cast also includes Eileen Atkins, Ian McKellen, and Joanna Lumley. Both urban and country learn from each other in this offbeat satire about life under difficult conditions.

## Research Alert

Survey data were collected from a random sample of teens working on farms in North Carolina. The teens ranged in age from 14 to 17. The researchers analyzed the data for farm-based hazard exposure and injury. The sample consisted of 141 teens (72% male) whose mean age was 16.6 years. The data indicated that these North Carolina teens were exposed to significant safety hazards throughout their farming experience. The teens in the sample were exposed to tractors, large animals, all-terrain vehicles, farm trucks, and rotary mowers. More than one-third of the sample was exposed to pesticides and tobacco harvesting equipment. Commonly reported injuries ranged from insect stings to cuts, burns, and falls.

*Source:* Schulman, M. D., Evensen, C. T., Runyan, C. W., Cohen, L. R., & Dunn, K. A. (1997). Farm work is dangerous for teens: Agricultural hazards and injuries among North Carolina teens. *Journal of Rural Health, 13*(4), 295–305.

significantly different between urban and rural adolescents. Rural adolescents reported sexual activity beginning at a younger age (9.6% of rural adolescents reporting 11 years or younger as age at first intercourse compared with 7.4% of urban adolescents). Participation in sexual activity was also significantly different between rural and urban adolescents, with 49% of rural adolescents stating they participated in sexual activity, compared with 35% of urban adolescents. Many rural school districts do not address the issue of sexually transmitted diseases or teen pregnancy because of the more conservative nature of the school boards, whose members are representatives of these districts. Community health nurses and school nurses must be advocates in rural communities for health education on these topics to be introduced in the school and at community-sponsored activities such as church groups, scouts, or 4-H clubs (Atav & Spencer, 2002; Connor, Rainer, Simax, & Thomisee, 2007).

### Agricultural Hazards

Adolescent workers on farms are at particular risk of injury as a result of the hazardous nature of agriculture and the lack of safety regulations (see Research Alert). Estimates indicate that approximately 20% of all fatalities in the U.S. each year occur on U.S. farms. Because the Occupational Safety and Health Administration (OSHA) regulates only businesses employing 11 or more people and the majority of family farms have a small labor force, children/adolescents working on farms are not subject to regulatory protections. Older adolescents and males have higher injury and death rates than do younger adolescents and females. The traditional division of labor by gender on the farm also is an important social influence on work hazards and injury rates. With increasing age, adolescents are channeled into gender-specific tasks, such as males using machines and females doing household tasks (Bartlett, 1993; Wilek, 1992; USDA, 2004).

## NOTE THIS!

Seventy percent of federally designated medically underserved areas in the United States are rural.

Urban populations have higher rates of alcohol and most illegal drug use than rural areas, with the exception of use of methamphetamine. Missouri law enforcement officers found more than 2,700 "meth labs" in 2004—more than any other state. Rural areas are becoming havens for small-time "cooks" of meth for several reasons:

- Rural areas provide cover for the pungent chemical odors from meth labs.

- Rural areas are populated with many abandoned buildings, such as farmhouses and barns on remote roads. Some of these buildings house methamphetamine labs, which can often operate undetected.

- Anhydrous ammonia is one of the key ingredients in producing meth. It is readily available in rural areas because farmers use this chemical as fertilizer.

Methamphetamine use in rural areas is being affected in the following ways:

- Rural areas are dealing with the clean-up of toxic methamphetamine lab sites, which have a severe impact on the environment. Each pound of methamphetamine produced releases poisonous gas into the atmosphere and creates five to seven pounds of toxic waste. In addition, many meth lab operators dump the toxic waste down household drains, in fields and yards, or on rural roads.

- Children are being endangered. Children who are around areas of meth labs are exposed to toxic chemicals that present significant health and environmental risks. According to research by the federal government, in 2003, 60% of children removed from lab sites had methamphetamine in their systems.

"Meth orphans" include children who are in foster care due to one or both parents being in either jail or dead due to methamphetamine use or children being born to mothers addicted to the drug. Their number is growing at an alarming rate. The number of grandparents raising their grandchildren because of this problem is also growing. According to law enforcement officials, the rise in arrests of methamphetamine users in rural America created 3,000 meth orphans in 2003.

Injury to EMS personnel can occur when first responders arrive at a meth site and deal with hazardous substances as well as people under the influence of meth who may be violent, agitated, and unpredictable. The same is true of police and other officials who are involved with responding to illegal meth labs; they are also vulnerable to toxic exposure.

Rural health resources are seldom adequate to accommodate these new health threats, which are becoming a serious public health problem for the entire United States.

*Source:* Substance Abuse and Mental Health Services Administration, U.S. Department of Health and Human Services. *The DASIS report: Trends in methamphetamine/amphetamine admissions to treatment, 1993–2003.* http://oas.samhsa.gov/2k6/methTx/methTX.cfm.

Tractor accidents are a leading cause of injuries in rural areas.

Community health nurses need to find ways to target rural adolescents for health promotion. One way is to work with school nurses in junior and senior high schools to advocate for current information to be included in school health curricula. Many rural schools are linked with the Internet, which can be a way to engage many adolescents in innovative health programming. Clubs, church youth groups, scouts, and 4-H are other arenas where young adolescents in rural areas gather, and many of these groups are often in need of programs for these teens. Community health nurses often are members of the rural community and are asked to present programs on health; they should take full advantage of these opportunities.

## ■ Isolation: Rural Elders

Isolation is fundamental to rural life. Isolation encompasses the ideas of sparse population, limited contact with others, greater distances between people, and limited transportation. Sometimes, people choose the isolation of rural life because they feel it gives them independence and opportunity for self-sufficiency. Isolation is neither a positive nor negative feature, but a reality that community health nurses need to take into account when planning and implementing health care.

Elderly people in rural areas present challenges to community health nurses that arise from both the isolation of rural life and the isolation of elderly life. Multiple losses, both physical and psychosocial, add to the isolation elderly people can experience. Physical changes of normal aging can contribute to isolation. Sensory losses such as diminished

hearing and vision result in distancing from the normal experience of life. Decreased mobility resulting from skeletal changes and disease may cause elderly people to stay at home. Fear of falling and other safety issues limit social interaction. Loss of friends because of relocation and death limit opportunities for human connections. Disease processes further isolate elders. For example, diabetes that requires a special diet and frequent blood glucose testing and insulin injections may prohibit participation in some social events.

Other problems that rural people experience can be more complex if they are older. On average, rural elders have approximately 22% lower incomes than metropolitan elderly because of lower social security payments, smaller savings, fewer opportunities for part-time work, and infrequent enrollment in Supplemental Security Income (SSI) (Krout, 1994; National Center for Farmworker Health, 2003; Rogers, 2002). Most (80%) rural elders own their homes, but these homes are likely to have been built before 1940. These homes may lack modern heating, plumbing, and insulation and may be in need of other repairs. Rural elders often need to relocate, but there are limited alternative housing opportunities in rural areas. Their houses may resell at a low price, creating another financial loss for the rural elder.

Elderly people residing anywhere may find themselves unable to drive their own cars. Lack of alternative transportation in rural areas is a problem that has wide-reaching effects on rural people. Elders have difficulty obtaining supplies, accessing health care, and meeting psychosocial needs.

Many research studies have been conducted that examine the unique characteristics and needs of this at-risk population. Community health nurses are challenged to design interventions that recognize the independence of older rural people but maintain their safety and health. Community-based services for rural elders must meet the criteria of availability, accessibility, awareness, acceptability, affordability, appropriateness, and adequacy. Parish nurse programs have had great success in rural areas because they meet these criteria. Nurses serve church members by "organizing health fairs, writing health articles for church newsletters, making presentations, providing blood pressure screening, referring to community health and social service resources, making home visits, and coordinating support groups" (Mockenhaupt & Muchow, 1994, p. 195). Healthcare providers must find a way to reduce the isolation experienced by rural elders by providing transportation, enhancing communication systems, and creating additional opportunities to bring elders together (Cosby et al., 2008; Ziller, Coburn, Anderson, & Loux, 2008).

☞ THINK ABOUT THIS ························

Ironically, rural America has become viewed by a growing number of Americans as having a higher quality of life not because of what it has, but rather because of what it does not have!

—Don A. Dillman

### Got an Alternative?

The use of herbs for health and medicinal use is common among rural and migrant populations. These natural remedies are seldom discussed with medical and nursing professionals, according to research. What is the role of the community health nurse in the use of complementary and medicinal herbal use among rural residents in the promotion of health? ◐

## ■ Culture: Migrant Farm Workers

**Migrant farm workers** represent a unique culture arising from ethnic background and a distinctive lifestyle. The migrant farm worker population is estimated to be approximately 5 million (DHHS, 1990; Lambert, 1995; Sandhaus, 1998; USDA, 2004). There are three primary streams in which they travel. The West Coast and midcontinent (or central) streams consist mostly of people of Mexican heritage. The East Coast stream is the most ethnically diverse, consisting of African Americans, Haitians, Puerto Ricans, whites, and some Mexican Americans (Lambert, 1995; Smith & Gentry, 1987).

Migrant farm workers "follow the crops." That is, they move north with the spring, living in temporary housing for days or weeks. The housing is often substandard and crowded, from shacks to mobile homes, rarely with furnishings. Sanitation and drinking water provision are also variable and often not available in the fields where the migrants work. Entire families make the season-long trip, with those who are unfit for fieldwork (elders and preteens) caring for the young children. Some areas make an effort to provide schooling for the young children, even though it is summer. Farm work provides the income that the family lives on for the entire year. Pay is hourly, at or below minimum wage, and for only the duration of the farming season.

Often, local communities react with hostility to migrant farm workers who are commonly seen as markedly different and potential carriers of disease. Thus living apart from the local communities, this population becomes more vulnerable to isolation and neglect. Fear of deportation, poverty, and limited education only serves to intensify feelings of distrust. As a result, migrant workers form cohesive communities of their own based on language, food, music, religion, social interactions, and beneficial folk practices. It is critical that community health nurses acknowledge their cultural differences and include family and social support networks when planning care for this population (Sandhaus, 1998).

In addition to understanding the culture of migrant farm workers, healthcare providers are confronted with their difficult healthcare needs. The major healthcare problems include women's health issues, high infant mortality, delayed immunization, poor dental health, mental health problems, substance abuse, family violence, malnutrition, diabetes, hypertension, respiratory illness (especially tuberculosis), anemia, and parasites. The infant mortality rate for migrant workers is 25 times higher than the U.S. national average. Parasitic infections occur 11 to 59 times more often in mi-

**MEDIA MOMENT**

***Who Says You Can't Go Home?***
I spent 20 years trying to get out of this place
I was lookin' for something I couldn't replace
It's been a long long road
Feels like I've never left, that's how the story goes
It doesn't matter where you are, doesn't matter where you go
If it's a million miles aways or just a mile up the road
Take it in, take it with you when you go, who says you can't go home

—Bon Jovi and Sugarland, 2006

grant workers than in the general population. Deaths from tuberculosis, influenza, and pneumonia are 25% higher. The life expectancy for migrant workers is 49 years, compared with a national average of 75 years (Sandhaus, 1998; NCFH, 2003).

Occupation-specific health problems are also worse for migrant workers than for other farm workers. These problems include risk of motor vehicle accident caused by high annual mileage, pesticide exposure, poor sanitation, farm accidents, skin diseases, and frequent and severe heat and cold exposures (Rust, 1990; Sandhaus, 1998). The fact that the population does not stay in one place for very long interferes with diagnosis, follow-up, and referral for any health problem (Harvey, 2008; Ziller et al., 2008).

Community health nurses have led the way in designing healthcare delivery models that respond to cultural differences, mobility, and the fundamental healthcare needs of migrant farm workers. Recognizing that migrant farm workers cannot rely on the consistency of one healthcare provider to oversee care, nursing models that emphasize education, self-care, empowerment, and responsibility for one's own health have found success with this population (Poss & Meeks, 1994; Stein, 1993; Watkins, Larson, Harlan, & Young, 1990). Successful programs often include mobile clinics with hours appropriate to migrant work schedules, sensitivity to cultural preferences, bilingual workers, and use of lay workers and peers.

The health care of migrant farm workers must be supported at the local, state, and national levels. With the identified health concerns of migrants ranging from infant mortality to communicable disease, funds must be found to support the following:

- The provision of adequate and accessible health care
- Adequate living wages
- Migrant education programs

## ■ Housing: Homeless People

Poverty in rural areas is most reflected in available housing. Rural homes are in worse condition than those in urban

---

☝ THINK ABOUT THIS ·······

The churches and people of rural North Louisiana have stepped in and done a better job than the government could have ever done.
— Scott Henderson after Hurricane Katrina, August 2004

Housing in rural areas is often substandard.

areas. Some have incomplete plumbing facilities, and others have structural problems such as inadequate heating, faulty electric, leaking roofs, and holes in the walls. Home ownership, however, is higher in rural areas than in urban areas. These two facts combined lead to rural homelessness. People have difficulty finding adequate housing to rent.

Homelessness in urban populations has been extensively examined (see Chapter 26), but little attention has been given to the problem of homelessness in rural populations. Research studies at both the state and national levels have noted that rural homelessness appears to be growing (First, Rife, & Tooney, 1990; Fitchen, 1991; Lindsey, 1995). The Housing Assistance Council, a Washington advocacy group, estimates up to 12.5% of homeless persons in the United States live in rural areas (USDA, 2004; National Advisory Committee on Rural Health and Human Services, 2004). The National Rural Health Association (NRHA) (1996) defines a family as homeless if they have no fixed place of residence. This includes living temporarily in shelters, with friends or relatives, in informal church-sponsored arrangements, in automobiles, in abandoned buildings, on the street, and in campgrounds, and, in the case of farm families, facing eminent eviction (NRHA, 1996, p. 1).

Homeless families are the largest growing subgroup of the homeless (Bassak, 1991; Helvie, 1999; Lindsey, 1995). Homeless families are often single-parent families with the woman as head of household. Approximately 3.5% of poor workers in rural areas have at least three barriers to earning a livable wage: low educational level, female head

## GLOBAL CONNECTION

Half of the world's population lives in rural areas.

of household, and a child younger than 6 at home (USDA, 1997). These workers are at grave risk of becoming homeless. Wagner, Menke, and Ciccone conducted a study in 1995 to examine the health of rural homeless families. Their study found the following similarities to previous urban studies:

- Most families were female headed.
- The ethnic distribution of homeless families mirrored the percentage of poor people in the area under study.
- Poverty was more extensive in rural than in urban areas as a greater percentage of the population was below the poverty line, and thus poverty was more difficult to escape.

Wagner, Menke, and Ciccone (1995) also found the following differences between rural and urban homeless families:

- The average number of rural homeless children was lower than reported in urban studies.
- Rural families were more likely to have been homeless for 4 to 12 months, which is longer than found for urban homeless families.
- Rural families were more likely to have doubled up with another family, which has been found to mask the degree of homelessness present in rural areas.
- Fewer rural families were found to stay in shelters, which may be attributed to the fact that fewer shelters were available.

Community health nurses who practice in rural areas are likely to encounter homeless families daily. These nurses must have an understanding of the needs of rural homeless families and be prepared to provide accessible, adequate, and appropriate care. This is not a simple task as homeless rural families are not easily identifiable, and each family will have different needs based on the length of time that they have been homeless. Case management has been found to be a particularly helpful tool in assisting homeless families or those who are near homeless find solutions. Rural community health nurses acting as case managers, are challenged to identify which services (health care or social services) are available in the community, to creatively piece together other types of services available to fill in the gaps that exist, and to make these services acceptable to the families.

Multidisciplinary teams are often created to meet the needs of homeless families identified in the rural area. These teams may be composed of healthcare professionals, clergy, local politicians, community organizations, and other social support groups available in the rural community. The community health nurse is in a perfect position to develop and lead these teams as a member of the community who is knowledgeable about community support systems and able to broker a coalition of various community members.

The need for housing for homeless families in rural areas is at crisis proportion. With the number of poor single-parent families that are now found to be homeless, affordable housing must be a prime concern for rural policy.

## Application to Practice

As a community health nurse, you are running the once-a-week well-child clinic in a rural town. As you call in the first young mother, Mrs. Boone, you recognize the strong odor of dirty clothing, soiled diapers, and unwashed children. Mrs. Boone sits down and places her youngest child, a small, pale girl, on her lap. The other two children, boys who appear to be preschool age, sit quietly on the floor at the end of the room. Mrs. Boone and the three children all are wearing grimy clothes. Mrs. Boone looks at the floor and says, "We come over from the emergency room they sent us over here because we don't have health insurance and the baby is sick. The nurse in the emergency room said you would see us even if we don't have no money."

You ask, "Tell me what's been going on," as you take a seat opposite Mrs. Boone.

"We just come here last week from Little County with my boyfriend. We're staying with his brother but we've got to find another place to live because there isn't enough room. A couple of days ago Melanie—that's the baby's name—started being real fussy and she feels hot. She didn't sleep at all last night and kept us all awake. My boyfriend got real mad and told me to do something about her. Kids drive him crazy. Anyway, it seemed like she was pulling on her ear. She had the same thing about a month ago, and we got some medicine from the nurse where we lived before and it got better. Can you give me some medicine?"

You ask, "What was wrong with Melanie when the nurse saw her, and what kind of medicine did she get?"

"The nurse said her ear was infected and gave her some kind of medicine for the infection and for the fever. I gave her the medicine until she felt better. I lost the rest of the bottle when we were getting ready to move or I could have given her the rest of it now. I've really got to do something to make her be quiet—she is driving my boyfriend crazy."

The older of the two boys on the floor begins to whine "I'm hungry." Mrs. Boone quickly turns to him and yells, "I told you to be quiet. Shut up before I smack you."

You take a deep breath and begin to get a health history on Mrs. Boone and the children. Mrs. Boone tells you that Melanie, the youngest, is 18 months old. The other two children, Travis and Jack, are 3 and 5, respectively. Mrs. Boone is 19. She did not finish high school but got married at 14, when she found that she was pregnant with Jack. She has been at home with the children, and her husband had been supporting the family with his earnings from two part-time jobs. About 2 months ago, her husband abandoned her and the children; she did not know where he was. Mr. Boone did not believe in welfare and had not let Mrs. Boone apply for any government assistance. After Mr. Boone left, Mrs. Boone managed to get some emergency food from a church food pantry and was thinking about applying for emergency assistance from welfare. Instead, she met her current boyfriend, Ashford, about 4 weeks ago, and they decided to come to Big County to see if they could find work. Mrs. Boone states that both the boys are quite healthy but that Melanie has been sick on and off since birth.

After you examine Melanie, you find that she has an ear infection and anemia. There is no money for medication for Melanie's ear infection.

1. What should you do?
2. Would you consider this family homeless?
3. What community supports should be sought to help them? ◉

---

## ■ Confidentiality: Persons with HIV/AIDS

Although most HIV/AIDS cases are still found in major metropolitan areas of the United States, the incidence of HIV/AIDS in rural areas is increasing at a greater rate than in metropolitan centers. Data from the Centers for Disease Control and Prevention (CDC) reveal that among the more than 40,000 new AIDS cases reported in 2001, 7.6% were from rural areas. New cases show a troubling pattern in rural regions, with the southern states having more than half of all the rural HIV/AIDS cases. In 2001, 70% of rural AIDS cases were in the South (NRHA, 2004).

> *Those who labor in the earth are the chosen people of God, if ever he had a chosen people.*
>
> —Thomas Jefferson

The migration of AIDS-infected people increases the rural numbers as a result of the shift in the numbers of cases from urban to rural. Unfortunately, funding to support HIV and AIDS programs is usually provided to the county of diagnosis rather than to the county of current residence; thus rural counties often do not benefit from state programs (Buehler, Frey, & Chu, 1995). In addition, transient migrant workers who harvest crops include both documented and undocumented individuals, and access to care for this population may only be through community and migrant health centers. Because of the mobility of this population, traditional methods of surveillance and prevention may be challenging (NHRA, 2004).

The spread of HIV and AIDS to rural communities has been described as the "second wave" of the epidemic (Berry, 1993). The demographic characteristics of the rural HIV and AIDS population also differ from those of the urban population. They are more likely to be young, nonwhite, and female and to have acquired their infection through risky heterosexual behaviors. In addition, rural women with AIDS have less access to health services and face greater stigma than their urban counterparts (Foster & Frazier, 2008; Johnson et al., 2008; Heckman, Somlai, Otto-Salaj, & Davontes, 1998; McCoy et al., 1999; Ziller et al., 2008).

In a 2000 report, state AIDS directors identified many issues that are often cited regarding the difficulties of prevention and care activities in rural populations. They include the following:

- Long travel distances to access services
- Inadequate supply of healthcare providers with HIV/AIDS expertise
- Lack of available medical facilities
- Limited social services and patient support
- Concern over confidentiality and stigma, which may prevent people from getting tested for HIV or seeking care if infected
- Scant substance abuse treatment services, which makes untreated addiction a barrier to dealing with one's HIV disease (NRHA, 2004, p. 2)

Rural community nurses are critical to the management of persons living with AIDS (PLWAs) because they are the

## MEDIA MOMENT

### *Mississippi Girl*

Well it's a long way from Star, Mississippi
To the big stage I'm singing on tonight
And sometimes the butterflies still get me
When I'm in the spotlight

And some people seem to think that I've changed
That I'm different than I was back then
But in my soul I know that I'm the same way
That I really always been

'Cause a Mississippi girl don't change her ways
Just cause everybody knows her name.

—Sung by Faith Hill, a native of Star, Mississippi
(population 1,500); written for her
by John Rich and Adam Shoenfeld, 2005

**Application to Practice**

Nina is a 30-year-old HIV-infected woman. When she was 17 years old, she lived with a man in New York City. Once into the relationship, she found that he was using intravenous drugs and selling drugs to supply his habit. After trying without success to get him to go for treatment, she left the relationship of 3 years. At age 22, she met and married James. They now have three children. James Jr. is 7 years old, Sheldon is 5, and Latisha is 3.

Once they started their family, they decided to move to rural Vermont, where James's mother, sister, and brother-in-law lived. When Sheldon was 3 months old, he began to have one infection after another. After almost 2 years of continuing antibiotics, the family practitioner suggested that they take Sheldon to a pediatrician. The pediatrician was located in an urban center about 45 miles from their home. The pediatrician, after reviewing the records and taking an in-depth history, requested that Sheldon be tested for HIV infection. When Sheldon tested positive for HIV, the pediatrician asked that all members of the family be tested. James, James Jr., and Latisha tested negative for HIV, and Nina tested positive. The pediatrician sat down with both James and Nina to discuss treatment and follow-up care for the family. Nina was adamant that all care should come from healthcare providers in the urban area because she did not want anyone in her community to know of the HIV diagnoses. The pediatrician suggested a referral to an infectious disease specialist from the urban center. After meeting with the infectious disease specialist, a referral was made to her local public health department, where you will be the case manager for the family.

1. Did the infectious disease specialist ignore Nina's request for services from the urban area by referring her to the local public health department?
2. What plans will you make for Nina and for Sheldon?
3. What will you advise regarding notification of the elementary school that James and Sheldon attend?
4. How will you support the family?

largest group of healthcare professionals in nonmetropolitan parts of the country. Furthermore, they are the healthcare professionals who provide the most regular, prolonged, and intimate care for rural HIV/AIDS patients. Because of geographic distances, lack of public transportation systems, a shortage of social and support services, fewer healthcare providers, and limited technological resources, care of the AIDS patient in rural America has become increasingly difficult. In addition, the poverty found in rural areas and the lack of health insurance are also barriers to care (Cosby et al., 2008; Foster & Frazier, 2008; Graham, Forrester, Wysong, Rosenthal, & James, 1995; Mayer, 2008).

Confidentiality is a concern for anyone; however, it is especially important to the rural population infected with HIV/AIDS. Rural community health nurses caring for HIV-infected patients will probably be known to both the patients and their families as neighbors, friends, or friends of friends. This informality contributes to a fear regarding lack of privacy. This fear often results in HIV-infected persons driving long distances for treatment rather than risk disclosure of their HIV status (Levi, 2000; Brumm, 2001). It also results in lack of education for both the HIV-infected person and the family members about the disease. "Fear of personal safety, loss of employment, and stigmatizing family members are strong motivators for persons who delay treatment" (Sowell & Christensen, 1996, p. 112). The concern over confidentiality is almost as great as the fear of HIV itself.

## Access to Health Care: Agricultural Workers

Agricultural workers are exposed to distinct health risks. The annual occupation-related death rate for all workers is

Agriculture is the main industry in many rural areas.

### Research Alert

This study sought to examine the relationships among stress, caregiver burden, and the health status of rural caregivers and to assess whether caregiver burden and stress predict the physical health status of caregivers in the rural setting. The study's descriptive-correlational design utilized a convenience sample of 63 rural caregivers. The subjects self-reported their perceptions of stress, burden, and health status using the Zarit Caregiver Burden Interview Scale, Lifestyle Appraisal Questionnaire, and the health status question from the National Health Interview Survey.

The relationships among stress, burden, and health status in rural caregivers were significantly related ($p < .05$), and caregivers were found to have higher rates of obesity, hypertension, and cardiovascular disease and to rate their health as poorer than the general population. Caregivers complained of experiencing uncomfortable physical symptoms and sleep disturbances. Significant variance in health status ($p < .05$) was accounted for by the model variables of stress and caregiver burden. Significant variance ($p < .05$) in caregiver burden was accounted for by the model variables of caregiver age and employment status. Caregivers who provided care for individuals with low levels of functioning experienced greater levels of caregiver burden and reported a poor health status. These findings should be considered when planning care for the chronically ill and their caregivers.

*Source:* Sanford, J. (2004). Unpublished doctoral dissertation, University of South Alabama, Mobile, AL.

9 per 100,000 workers, but the death rate for farmers is 42 per 100,000 (Gerberich, 1995). Compared with blue-collar and white-collar workers, farmers have a higher rate of amputations, arthritis, cardiovascular disease, ischemic heart disease, hypertension, skin cancer, chronic respiratory diseases, asthma, and back pain (Schenker, 1996). Farmers are exposed to excessive noise from machinery. They sometimes resist wearing the protective equipment required because it is bulky and hot and prevents them from hearing mechanical problems and warning cries (Marvel, Pratt, Marvel, Regan, & May, 1991). Entanglements in machinery, falls, and electrocution are common injuries (Ehlers, Connon, Themann, Myers, & Ballard, 1993). Chemical hazards for the farmer include pesticides, fertilizers, fumes, solvents, and sanitizing solutions. They can also experience allergic reactions to substances. Respiratory diseases arising from dusts, gases, and chemicals are prevalent in farm workers. Exposure to these hazards can occur during almost all the phases of farm work. Work with animals creates risk for communicable diseases as well as injury.

Mental health is a serious problem for farmers. They report high stress levels caused by the responsibilities placed on

## HEALTHY PEOPLE 2010

### Objectives Related to Rural Life

#### Cancer

3.9    Increase the proportion of persons who use at least one of the following protective measures that may reduce the risk of skin cancer: avoid the sun between 10 AM and 4 PM, wear sun-protective clothing when exposed to sunlight, use sunscreen with a sun protective factor (SPF) of 15 or higher, and avoid artificial sources of ultraviolet light.

#### Environmental Health

##### Toxics and Waste

8.13    Reduce pesticide exposures that result in visits to a healthcare facility.

#### Infrastructure and Surveillance

8.25    Reduce exposure of the population to pesticides, heavy metals, and other toxic chemicals, as measured by blood and urine concentrations of the substances or their metabolites.

#### Injury and Violence Protection

##### Unintentional Injury Prevention

15.23    Increase use of helmets by bicyclists.

15.24    Increase the number of states and the District of Columbia with laws requiring bicycle helmets for bicycle riders.

*Source*: DHHS, 2000.

---

one person, the risks in farm work, the necessity to maintain a great store of current knowledge, and the unpredictability of factors such as the weather, market prices, and land value. Suicide rates for farmers are nearly twice that of the general population (Ehlers et al., 1993; Fraser et al., 2005).

Farm families also experience special risks. Farm wives often help on the farm as well as having jobs out of the home. Children are at very high risk of injury on the farm. Approximately 300 children die every year on U.S. farms, and thousands more are injured (National Committee for Childhood Agricultural Injury and Prevention, 1996). Farm family members demonstrate higher than expected rates of some cancers, respiratory illnesses, and adverse reproduction outcomes (Ehlers et al., 1993). Finally, migrant farm workers are exposed to all of the same risks, but potentially without the knowledge, skills, and safety equipment that are recommended.

Many farmers face an issue of access to health care. Distance from metropolitan areas and services is definitive of rurality. Travel may be over poor roads and involve geographic barriers. When one bridge is out, the travel necessary to get to the next bridge may be prohibitive.

Farmers define *health* as "the ability to work" (Lee cited in Weinert & Long, 1994). Because farmers may be indis-

 **THINK ABOUT THIS**

Farming looks mighty easy when your plow is a pencil and you're a thousand miles from the corn field.

—Dwight D. Eisenhower

pensable to their work, they push themselves to work when they are ill or injured. They will seek health care only when they are unable to ignore the health problem. Under these circumstances, farmers often seek health care in almost an emergency state. Sometimes, they need a higher level of care because they wait until the health problem demands action. Because they are self-employed, farmers may forgo buying health insurance for themselves and their families. Furthermore, there is no law that requires farmers as employers to insure their workers. Lack of insurance also may inhibit farm workers from seeking health care.

Emergency rescue of farmers presents several barriers. Farmers work independently and their absence may not be noticed for several hours. Notification systems to call for emergency help are sporadic through rural America. The terrain and distance may delay rescue vehicles. Rescue equipment such as "the jaws of life" may be unsuited for farm machinery (Staff, 1995).

Healthcare delivery to farmers and other rural residents requires innovation that recognizes their special needs. Mobile clinics, flexible hours, prevention and screening programs, and networks for peer education and assistance are possibilities. Throughout the country, there are agricultural health and safety centers that provide grant funding, report research findings, and support community health workers' efforts to protect farm workers.

## MEDIA MOMENT

### Thank God I'm a Country Boy

Life on the farm is kinda laid back
Ain't much an old country boy like me can't hack
It's early to rise, early in the sack
Thank God I'm a country boy

—Sung by John Denver, 1975;
written by John Martin Sommers

## ❝❝ *a conversation with . . .* ❞❞

### Lynne Cameron

There is a somewhat bipolar aspect of being a small town clinic in winter and a very busy primary care/emergency room/triage center in summer. That particular aspect requires an elasticity and ability to reprioritize and change gears that takes one to the edge. My friend and I have also found that the severity of climatic change here also puts a lot of challenge into life; however, it seems that the most energy is found in the edges of greatest challenge. I find a relationship with this land to be essential to my practice and to my humanity in sharing healing with others. In short, I love my life!

—**Lynne Cameron, ANP**
Skagway Medical Center,
Skagway, Alaska, June 21, 1999

 ### Research Alert

Rural residents may have higher death rates than urban residents. This study revealed an emerging non-metropolitan mortality penalty by contrasting 37 years of age-adjusted mortality rates for metropolitan versus nonmetropolitan U.S. counties. During the 1980s, annual metropolitan—nonmetropolitan differences averaged 6.2 excess deaths per 100,000 nonmetropolitan population, or approximately 3600 excess deaths; however, by 2000 to 2004, the difference had increased more than 10 times to average 71.7 excess deaths, or approximately 35,000 excess deaths. The researchers recommended that research be undertaken to evaluate and utilize these preliminary findings of an emerging U.S. nonmetropolitan mortality penalty.

*Source:* Cosby, A., Neaves, T., Cossman, R., Cossman, J., James, W., Feierabend, N., et al. (2008). Preliminary evidence for an emerging nonmetropolitan mortality penalty in the United States. *American Journal of Public Health, 98*(8), 1470–1472.

## Conclusion

Rural life is often idealized as one of peacefulness and health. Although there are rewards associated with rural living, research is just beginning to reveal the realities of healthcare needs in this population. Healthcare planners and providers must develop innovative acceptable programs and educate healthcare providers to give accessible, acceptable, appropriate, and better than adequate care.

Community health nurses lead the way in understanding diverse rural populations and communities by recognizing the effects of lifestyle, isolation, culture, poverty/housing, confidentiality, specific health needs, and access to health care. The community nurse is capable of reaching these unique populations because often the nurse is part of the rural culture and is accepted as an insider by the people for whom he or she cares.

### Country Lanes

One more time we walk down a country lane
Not the same as when the children were small

They would dance ahead just within view
Threatening to fall or run into poison ivy

This time we walk—much slower—talk
Much less of children's clothes and scratched knees

Amber leaves rick—deep among our feet
Smoke from the dying fire of fall
Soft and blue above our heads
Our voices low—whispering the years away.

—*Ann Thedford Lanier, PhD*

 Explore Community Health Nursing on the Web! To learn more about the topics in this chapter, use the passcode provided to access your exclusive website: **http://nursing.jbpub.com/ communityhealth.** If you do not have a passcode, you can obtain one at this site.

## ■ CRITICAL THINKING ACTIVITIES

1. Richford, New York, is a rural community with a population of approximately 1,150. Most of the residents work elsewhere, and those who do not are mostly self-employed in farming. There is no local industry, grocery store, hotel, bank, library, school, or police department. There is one outreach clinic operated by a hospital system about 30 miles away, and a volunteer fire/EMS department. There is a closer community hospital (22 miles), but the residents prefer traveling the 30 miles to the metropolitan area for health services. There is very limited public transportation (twice daily stops) and no taxi services. According to the rural–urban continuum, in which type of county is Richford located? How does this understanding affect your health planning?

2. A rural community health nurse has been asked to participate on a community task force to develop a plan to stop underage drinking in the community. The task force receives $10,000 from its state senator to be used in the development and implementation of the plan. If you were the community health nurse, what would your role be as community health educator and consultant for this group?

# ■ REFERENCES

Atav, A. S., & Spencer, G. A. (2002). Health risk behaviors among rural suburban, and urban adolescents: A comparative study. *Journal of Family and Community Health, 23*(2), 1–18.

Bartlett, P. F. (1993). *American dreams, rural realities: Family farms in crisis.* Chapel Hill, NC: University of North Carolina Press.

Bassak, E. L. (1991). Homeless families. *Science America, 265*(6), 66–74.

Berry, D. E. (1993). The emerging epidemiology of rural AIDS. *Journal of Rural Health, 9,* 293.

Brent, D. A., Perper, J. A., Moritz, G., Baugher, M., Schweers, J., & Roth, C. (1993). Firearms and adolescent suicide. A community case control. *American Journal of Diseases in Children, 147*(10), 1066–1071.

Brumm, M. (2001). Duke study finds rural HIV patients wary about confidentiality. *The Chronicle.*

Buehler, J. W., Frey, R. L., & Chu, S. Y. (1995). The migration of persons with AIDS: Data from 12 states, 1985 to 1992. *American Journal of Public Health, 85*(11), 1552–1555.

Connor, A., Rainer, L. P., Simcox, J. B., & Thomisee, K. (2007). Increasing the delivery of health care services to migrant farm worker families through a community partnership model. *Public Health Nursing, 24*(4), 355–360.

Cook, P. J., & Mizer, K. L. (1994, December). *The revised ERS county typology: An overview.* Rural Development Research Report Number 89. Economic Research Service, U.S. Department of Agriculture.

Cosby, A., Neaves, T., Cossman, R., Cossman, J., James, W., Feierabend, N., et al. (2008). Preliminary evidence for an emerging nonmetropolitan mortality penalty in the United States. *American Journal of Public Health, 98*(8), 1470–1472.

Department of Health and Human Services (DHHS). (1990). *Atlas of state profiles.* Washington, DC: Author.

Department of Health and Human Services (DHHS). (1991). *Healthy people 2000.* Washington, DC: Author.

Department of Health and Human Services (DHHS). (2000a). *Healthy people 2010: Conference edition.* Washington, DC: U.S. Government Printing Office.

Department of Health and Human Services (DHHS). (2008). 2008 HHS poverty guidelines. *Federal Register, 73*(15), 3971–3972.

Eberhardt, M. S., & Pamuk, E. R. (2004). The importance of place of residence: Examining health in rural and non rural areas. *American Journal of Public Health, 94,* 1682–1686.

Ehlers, J. K., Connon, C., Themann, C. L., Myers, J. R., & Ballard, T. (1993). Health and safety hazards associated with farming. *American Association of Occupational Health Nursing Journal, 41*(9), 414–421.

Fahs, P. S. S., Smith, B. E., Atav, A. S., Britten, M. X., Collins, M. S., Morgan, L. L., & Spencer, G. A. (1999). Integrative research review of risk behaviors among adolescents in rural, suburban, and urban areas. *Journal of Adolescent Health, 24*(4), 230–243.

First, R. J., Rife, J. C., & Tooney, B. G. (1994). Homelessness in rural areas: Causes, patterns, and trends. *Social Work, 39*(1), 97–108.

Fitchen, J. M. (1991). Homelessness in rural places: Perspectives from upstate New York. *Urban Anthropology and Studies of Cultural Systems, 20*(2), 177.

Foster, P., & Frazier, E. (2008). Rural health issues in HIV/AIDS: views from two different windows. *Journal of Health Care for the Poor & Underserved, 19*(1), 10–15.

Fraser, C., Smith, K., Judd, F., Humphreys, J., Fragar, L., & Henderson, A. (2005). Farming and mental health problems and mental illness. *International Journal of Social Psychiatry, 51*(4), 340–349.

Gerberich, S. G. (1995). Prevention of death and disability in farming. In H. H. McDuffie, J. A. Dosman, K. M. Semchuk, S. A. Olenchock, & A. Senthilselvan (Eds.), *Agricultural health and safety.* Boca Raton, FL: Lewis.

Graham, R. P., Forrester, M. L., Wysong, J. A., Rosenthal, T. C., & James, P. A. (1995). HIV/AIDS in the rural United States: Epidemiology and health services delivery. *Medical Care Research and Review, 52*(4), 435–452.

Grossman, D. C. (2000). The history of injury control and the epidemiology of child and adolescent injuries. *Future Child, 10*(1), 23–52.

Hartley, D. (2004). Rural health disparities, population health, and racial culture. *American Journal of Public Health, 94*(10), 1675–1677.

Harvey P. (2008). Community work injuries: Country style. *Australian Journal of Rural Health, 16*(5), 321–321.

Heckman, T. G., Somlai, A. M., Otto-Salaj, L., & Davontes, B. R. (1998). Psychosocial differences between urban and rural people living with HIV and AIDS. *Journal of Rural Health, 14,* 138–145.

Helvie, C. O. (1999, Spring). Nursing the homeless—A vulnerable population. *American Public Health Association Public Health Nursing Newsletter,* pp. 8–9.

Johnson, A., Mink, M., Harun, N., Moore, C., Martin, A., & Bennett, K. (2008). Violence and drug use in rural teens: National prevalence estimates from the 2003 Youth Risk Behavior Survey. *Journal of School Health, 78*(10), 554–561.

Kidd, P. S., & Holton, C. (1993). Driving practices, risk-taking motivations, and alcohol use among adolescent drivers: A pilot study. *Journal of Emergency Nursing, 19*(4), 292–296.

Klein, S. J., Karchner, W. D., & O'Connell, D. A. (2002). Interventions to prevent HIV-related stigma and discrimination: Findings and recommendations for public health practice. *Journal of Public Health Management & Practice, 8*(6), 44–53.

Krout, J. A. (1994). An overview of older rural populations and community-based services. In J. A. Krout (Ed.), *Providing community-based services to the rural elderly* (pp. 3–18). Thousand Oaks, CA: Sage.

Lambert, M. I. (1995). Migrant and seasonal farm worker women. *Journal of Obstetric, Gynecologic, and Neonatal Nursing, 24*(3), 265–268.

Levi, J. (2000). The public health challenges of the HIV epidemic. *American Journal of Public Health, 90*(7), 1023–1024.

Lindsey, A. M. (1995). Physical health of homeless adults. *Annual Review of Nursing Research, 13,* 31–61.

Marvel, M. E., Pratt, D. S., Marvel, L. H., Regan, M., & May, J. J. (1991). Occupational hearing loss in New York dairy farmers. *American Journal of Industrial Medicine, 20,* 517–531.

Mayer, M. (2008). Disparities in geographic access to pediatric subspecialty care. *Maternal & Child Health Journal, 12*(5), 624–632.

Mockenhaupt, R. E., & Muchow, J. A. (1994). Disease and disability prevention and health promotion for rural elders. In J. A. Krout (Ed.), *Providing community-based services to the rural elderly* (pp. 183–201). Thousand Oaks, CA: Sage.

Muellman, R. L., Walker, R. A., & Edney, J. A. (1993). Motor vehicle deaths: A rural epidemic. *Journal of Trauma, 35*(5), 717–719.

National Center for Farmworker Health (NCFH). (2003). *Overview of America's farmworkers.* Retrieved May 30, 2007, from http://www.ncfh.org/aaf_01.php

National Committee for Childhood Agriculture Injury and Prevention. (1996). *Children and agriculture: Opportunities for safety and health.* Marshfield, WI: Marshfield Clinic.

National Institutes of Health (NIH). (2008). *Monitoring the future survey*. Retrieved November 13, 2008, from http://www.drugabuse.gov/DrugPages/MTF.html

National Rural Health Association (NRHA). (1994, Fall). *Rural Clinician Quarterly*.

National Rural Health Association (NRHA). (1996). *The rural homeless: America's lost population*. Kansas City, MO.

National Rural Health Association (NRHA). (2004). *HIV/AIDS in rural America: Disproportionate impact on minority and multicultural populations* (issue paper).

North Carolina Rural Health Research and Policy Analysis Center. (1998). *Mapping rural health: The geography of health care and health resources in rural America*. Chapel Hill, NC: Author.

Poss, J. E., & Meeks, B. H. (1994). Meeting the health care needs of migrant farmworkers: The experience of the Niagara County Migrant Clinic. *Journal of Community Health Nursing, 11*(4), 219–228.

Rausch, T. K., Sanddal, N. D., Sanddal, T. L., & Esposito, T. J. (1998). Changing epidemiology of injury-related pediatric mortality in a rural state: Implications for injury control. *Pediatric Emergency Care, 14*(6), 388–392.

Ricketts, T. C., & Johnson-Webb, K. D. (1997). *What is "rural" and how to measure "rurality": A focus on health care delivery and health policy*. Chapel Hill, NC: Federal Office of Rural Health Policy, North Carolina Rural Health Research and Policy Analysis Center, Cecil G. Sheps Center for Health Services Research.

Rogers, C. C. (2002). Rural health issues for the older population. *Rural America, 17*(2), 30–35.

Rust, G. S. (1990). Health status of migrant farmworkers: A literature review and commentary. *American Journal of Public Health, 80*(10), 1213–1217.

Sandhaus, S. (1998). Migrant health: A harvest of poverty. *American Journal of Nursing, 98*(9), 52–54.

Schenker, M. B. (1996). Preventive medicine and health promotion are overdue in the agricultural workplace. *Journal of Public Health Policy, 17*(3), 275–305.

Schulman, M. D., Evensen, C. T., Runyan, C. W., Cohen, L. R., & Dunn, K. A. (1997). Farm work is dangerous for teens: Agricultural hazards and injuries among North Carolina teens. *Journal of Rural Health, 13*(4), 295–305.

Smith, L. S., & Gentry, D. (1987). Migrant farm workers' perceptions of support persons in a descriptive community survey. *Public Health Nursing, 4*(1), 21–28.

Sowell, R. L., & Christensen, P. (1996). HIV infection in rural communities. *Nursing Clinics of North America, 31*(1), 107–123.

Spencer, G. A., Atav, A. S., & Collins, M. S. (1997). *A comparison of health risk behaviors of rural, suburban and urban adolescents*. Unpublished manuscript. Binghamton, NY.

Spencer, G. A., & Bryant, S. A. (2000). Dating violence: A comparison of rural, suburban, and urban teens. *Journal of Adolescent Health, 27*(4).

Spencer, G., & Bryant, S. (2000). Dating violence: a comparison of rural, suburban, and urban teens. *Journal of Adolescent Health, 27*(5), 302–305.

Staff. (1995). *Topics in Emergency Medicine, 17*(3).

Stein, L. M. L. (1993). Health care delivery to farmworkers in the southwest: An innovative nursing clinic. *Journal of the American Academy of Nurse Practitioners, 5*(3), 119–124.

Svenson, L. W., Varnhagen, C. K., Godin, A. M., & Salmon, T. L. (1992). Rural high school students' knowledge, attitudes, and behaviors related to sexually transmitted diseases. *Canadian Journal of Public Health, 83*(4), 260–263.

Symons, P. Y., Groer, M. W., Kepler-Youngblood, P., & Slater, V. (1993). Prevalence and predictors of adolescent dating violence. *Journal of Child and Psychiatric Nursing, 7,* 14–23.

U.S. Department of Agriculture, Economic Research Service (USDA). (1997). *Rural Conditions and Trends, 8*(2).

U.S. Department of Agriculture, Economic Research Service (USDA). (1999). *Rural Conditions and Trends, 9*(2).

U.S. Department of Agriculture, Economic Research Service (USDA). (2003). *Measuring rurality: New definitions in 2003*. Retrieved September 18, 2008, from http://ers.usda.gov/briefing/Rurality/NewDefinitions/

U.S. Department of Agriculture, Economic Research Service. (2004). *Rural development research report: Rural poverty at a glance* (Publication No. 100). Retrieved August 15, 2008, from http://ers.usda.gov/publications/rdrr100/rdrr100.pdf

U.S. Department of Agriculture, Economic Research Service (USDA). (2005a). *Measuring rurality: 2004 county typology codes*. Retrieved September 18, 2008, from http://ers.usda.gov/Briefing/Rurality/Typology/

U.S. Department of Agriculture, Economic Research Service (USDA). (2005b). *Rural population and migration*. Retrieved November 10, 2008, from http://www.ers.usda.gov/Briefing/Population/

United States Department of Agriculture (USDA). (2008). *What is rural?* Retrieved November 13, 2008, from http://www.nal.usda.gov/ric/ricpubs/what_is_rural.shtml

U.S. Department of Labor, Department of Labor Statistics. (2008). *Occupational outlook handbook, 2008–2009 edition: Agricultural workers*. Retrieved July 7, 2008, from http://www.bls.gov/oco/ocos285.htm

Ventura, S. J., Martin, J. A., Mathews, M. S., & Clarke, S. C. (1996). Advance report of final natality statistics, 1994. *Monthly Vital Statistics Report, 44*(11).

Wagenaar, A. C., Finnegan, J. R., Wolfson, M., Anstine, P. S., Williams, C. L., & Perry, C. L. (1993). Where and how adolescents obtain alcohol beverages. *Public Health Reports, 108*(4), 459–464.

Wagner, J. D., Menke, E. M., & Ciccone, J. K. (1995). What is known about the health of rural homeless families? *Public Health Nursing, 12*(6), 400–408.

Watkins, E. L., Larson, K., Harlan, C., & Young, S. (1990). A model program for providing health services for migrant farmworker mothers and children. *Public Health Reports, 105*(6), 567–575.

Weinert, C., & Long, K. (1994). Rural health and health seeking behaviors. *Annual Review of Nursing Research, 12,* 65–92.

Whitehead, R., Chillag, S., & Elliot, D. (1992). Anabolic steroid use among adolescents in a rural state. *Journal of Family Practice, 35*(4), 401–405.

Wilk, V. A. (1992). Injuries to farmers and farm families in a dairy state. *Journal of Occupational Medicine, 34*(3), 283–290.

Yawn, B. P., & Yawn, R. A. (1993). Adolescent pregnancies in rural America: A review of the literature and strategies for primary prevention. *Community Health, 16*(1), 36–45.

Ziller, E., Coburn, A., Anderson, N., & Loux, S. (2008). Uninsured rural families. *The Journal of Rural Health: Official Journal of the American Rural Health Association And the National Rural Health Care Association, 24*(1), 1–11.

# CHAPTER 28
# Adolescent Pregnancy

Loretta Sweet Jemmott, Michelle Cousins Mott,
Susan Oliver Dodds, Karen Saucier Lundy,
and Lynn Reynolds Stabler

Visit **http://nursing.jbpub.com/communityhealth** for interactive exercises, review questions, Web links, and more.

Parenting classes help teen mothers bond with their babies.

Ours is not the task of fixing the entire world all at once but of stretching out to mend the part of the world that is within our reach. Any small, calm thing that one soul can do to help another soul, to assist some portion of this poor suffering world, will help immensely. It is not given to us to know which acts, or by whom, will cause the critical mass to tip toward an enduring good.

—*Clarissa Pinkola Estes*

Adolescent pregnancy is a modern public health issue. Prior to the twentieth century, females were married and bearing children in their early teens as a societal norm. In many parts of the world, this is still an accepted cultural pattern. Think about your own beliefs and feelings about teenage pregnancy. How do they affect your nursing care of this vulnerable population?

## CHAPTER FOCUS

**Sexual Behavior and Pregnancy Rates**
- Teen Birth Rates: How Does the United States Compare?
- Teen Sexual Activity in the United States

**Factors Contributing to Adolescent Pregnancy**
- Developmental Stage
- Social and Environmental Factors

**Impact of Adolescent Pregnancy**
- Psychosocial and Health Outcomes of the Mother
- Impact on the Family

- Impact on the Adolescent Father
- Psychosocial and Health Outcomes of the Newborn

**Role of the Nurse**
- Primary Prevention
- Adolescent Pregnancy Prevention Community-Based Programs
- Program Evaluation
- Secondary and Tertiary Prevention

## QUESTIONS TO CONSIDER

After reading this chapter, you will know the answers to the following questions:

1. Which factors contribute to adolescent pregnancy?
2. What are the health outcomes for adolescent mothers?
3. What is the effect of adolescent pregnancy on the family?
4. How are adolescent fathers affected by their partner's pregnancy?
5. What are the health outcomes for babies born to adolescent mothers?
6. What kinds of community-based prevention programs are available?

7. What are effective interventions to promote the role and involvement of the teen father?
8. What is the role of the community health nurse in primary, secondary, and tertiary prevention efforts for adolescent pregnancy?
9. What are policy implications of research findings for teen pregnancy prevention?
10. How can the community nurse who works with teens use research data in the prevention of teen pregnancy?

## KEY TERMS

Abortion
Abstinence
Acculturation
Adolescent fathers
Adoption

Childhood victimization
Condoms
Contraception
Family dynamics

Gynecological age
Health outcomes
Low birth weight (LBW)
Prenatal care

Primary prevention
Repeat pregnancy
Secondary prevention
Tertiary prevention

ADOLESCENT PREGNANCY AFFECTS individuals across all ethnic groups, socioeconomic classes, and geographic boundaries in the United States. Despite our investment of significant amounts of attention, time, research, and money on prevention efforts, the results remain discouraging, as adolescent pregnancy rates in the United States remain higher than those in all industrialized countries.

Community health nurses can play a significant role in reducing the incidence of adolescent pregnancy and improving the quality of **health outcomes** of adolescent mothers, their children, and communities overburdened by this problem. By implementing creative interventions that address adolescents, families, and the community, community health nurses can play critical roles at all levels of prevention—primary, secondary, and tertiary alike.

In this chapter, adolescent pregnancy will be examined by reviewing the contributing factors and key variables and considering the impact of pregnancy on the adolescent, family, schools, community, and society. The role of community health nurses at all levels of prevention will be presented.

## Sexual Behavior and Pregnancy Rates

More than 46% of high school students in the United States are sexually active. The incidence of unplanned pregnancy and STDs statistically correlates to the early onset of sexual activity (Collins et al., 2004). Although there has been a decline in the teenage pregnancy rate since the 1990s, the United States continues to have the highest teen pregnancy rate in the industrialized world (Hoffman, 2006). One of every three teenage girls will become pregnant. More than 400,000 babies are born to teen mothers in the United States annually, and 80% of these teen mothers are unmarried (Hoffman, 2006).

There were 750,000 teen pregnancies in the United States in 2002, which resulted in 425,000 births, 215,000 abortions, and 117,000 fetal losses. These figures represent a 35% reduction in the teen pregnancy rate since 1990 (Ventura, Abma, Mosher, & Henshaw, 2006).

The Youth Risk Behavior Survey (CDC, 2006) revealed that adolescent sexual activity was more prevalent among black adolescents (67%) than among white (43%) or Hispanic (51%) adolescents. The survey also revealed that 6.2% of high school students had their first sexual intercourse prior to age 13 and 14.3% had had sexual intercourse with more than four partners.

## ■ Teen Birth Rates: How Does the United States Compare?

Despite a one-third decline since the early 1990s, the United States still has the highest rates of teen pregnancy and birth among comparable countries. In 2004, the U.S. teen birth rate was 41.1 births per 1,000 teens aged 15–19. By way of comparison, the U.S. teen birth rate is *one and a half times* higher than the teen birth rate in the United Kingdom (26.8 per 1,000), which has the highest teen birth rate in Europe; more than *twice as high* as the teen birth rate in Canada (14.5 per 1,000); and *seven* times higher than the teen birth rate in Japan (5.6 per 1,000), Denmark (5.7 per 1,000), and Sweden (5.9 per 1,000).

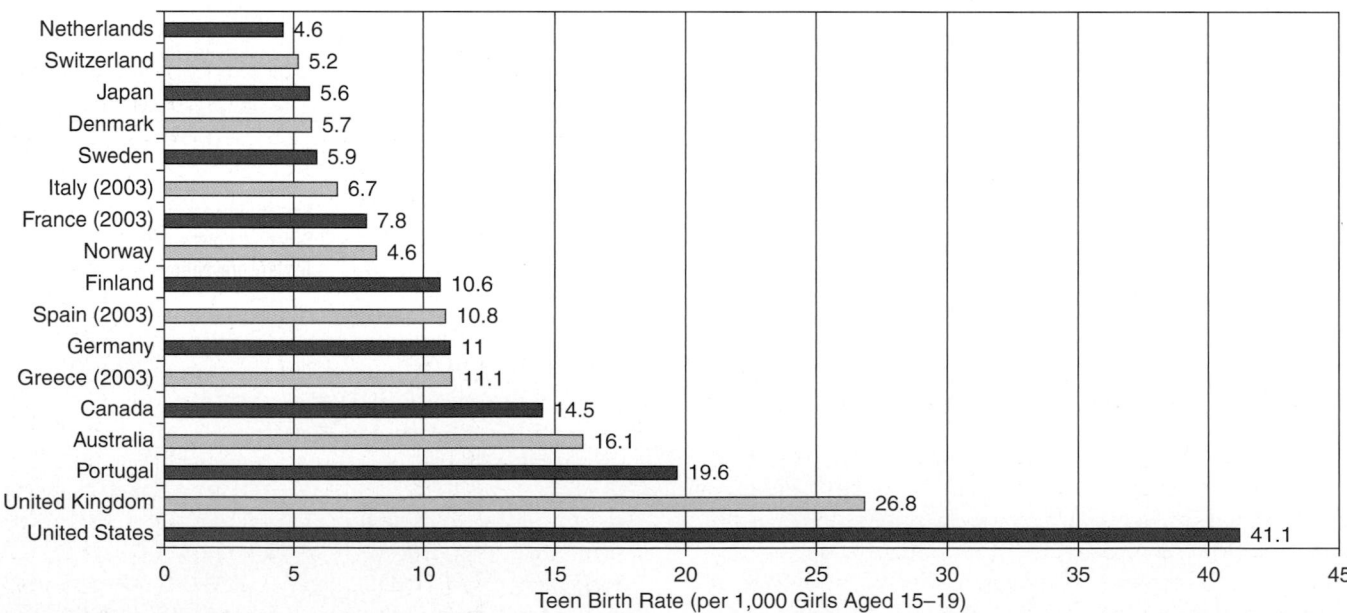

Teen birth rates, 2004

*Note:* All birth rates are for 2004 unless otherwise noted.

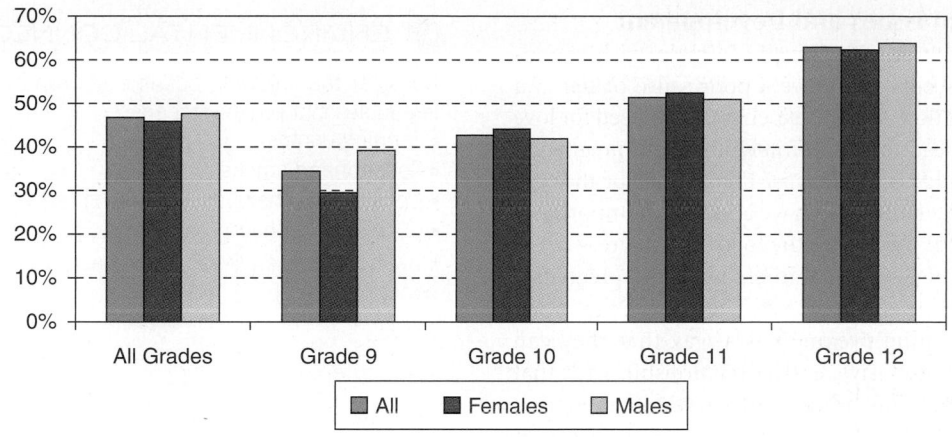

Proportion of high school students who have had sex at least once, 2005 (Grades 9–12, YRBS)

*Source*: CDC, 2006.

## Teen Sexual Activity in the United States

The Youth Risk Behavior Survey (YRBS) was developed by the Centers for Disease Control and Prevention (CDC) in 1990 to monitor teen sexual behavior, tobacco and alcohol use, and other behaviors. The survey is conducted every two years and provides data on ninth- through twelfth-grade students in public and private schools in the United States. The figure reflects the most recent data available (2005). Currently 46.8% of all high school students report they have had sexual intercourse. The percentage of high school students who have had sex decreased by 13.3% between 1991 and 2005 (54% to 46.8%).

 NOTE THIS! ●————————————

- Three of four teens used a method of contraception during their first intercourse.

- Nine percent of teen females report that their first sexual intercourse was involuntary.

- Teenage females' sexual partners are most often one to three years older than they are.

- Hispanic females are most likely (35%) to have a teen birth and non-Hispanic whites (12%) are least likely.

*Source*: Abma, 2001.

## Factors Contributing to Adolescent Pregnancy

Many factors have been associated with adolescent pregnancy. Factors including earlier age of onset of puberty, earlier age of initiation of intercourse, nonuse or inconsistent use of contraceptives, lack of knowledge about sex and conception, developmental age, early risk-taking behaviors such as smoking and alcohol/drug use (Kandel, 1990; Kaiser Family Foundation, 1998; Whitbeck, Conger, & Simons, 1993; Ventura et al., 2006; CDC, 2006), and social/environmental status all contribute to an increased risk for

teenage pregnancy. For the community health nurse to develop appropriate interventions to prevent adolescent pregnancy, it is essential to understand the contributing factors.

## Developmental Stage

Adolescence is a time of uncertainty and experimentation, as young people strive to develop their identity in preparation for adulthood. For many young people, it is a time of sexual experimentation. This experimentation is in response to the adolescents' physical, hormonal, cognitive, and psychosocial development. Unfortunately, the consequences of such experimentation far too often include increased risk of pregnancy.

### Psychosocial Development

Adolescent psychosocial development progresses through three stages: early, middle, and late adolescence. Early adolescence (ages 11 to 13) is characterized by turmoil stemming from physical changes and emotional fluctuation influenced by changing hormone levels (Drake, 1996). In this stage, adolescents are often seeking control, may show defiance to authority figures, and may use sex as an outlet for the expression of their perceived control (Drake, 1996; Flavell, Miller, & Miller, 1993). Middle adolescence (ages 14 to 16) is characterized by development of self-identity and sexual identity. In search of their identity, adolescents may imitate the behaviors they see around them from media, older peers, parents, and other adults (Foster, 1997; Males, 1993). Late adolescence (ages 17 to 20) is characterized by the adaptation of self-identity and development of coping strategies that will be used in adulthood (Drake, 1996). Adolescents who do not have a strong self-identity and sexual identity may not be able to assert themselves and apply coping strategies such as the sexual negotiation skills that are used with a sexual partner (Flavell, Miller, & Miller, 1993). As a result, adolescents may give in to sexual pressure from their peers and sexual partners.

## Intrapersonal Issues and Development

The development of self-concept is a major task of adolescence. For adolescents who have a poor sense of self and have a history of unsuccessful life experience, the need for love and attention may lead to sexual intercourse and pregnancy. As a mother, the adolescent may sense that she will be the center of attention in the family and have a feeling of importance and belonging (Fisher, 1984). See the following figure.

Adolescents may view sexual intercourse and pregnancy as a bond or link to a sexual partner. They may believe that having sex or becoming pregnant is a way that they can ensure a continued, exclusive, caring relationship with that partner. As a result, some adolescents may feel pressured into sexual relations because they fear losing their partner if they do not comply (Davis, 1980; Toledo-Dreves, Zabin, & Emerson, 1995). This is a particularly important factor for adolescents who do not feel needed or cared for within the family unit.

A 2006 report by the U.S. Department of Health and Human Services revealed that teens placed more emphasis on condom use when having sex with a casual partner. Males engaged in casual sexual relationships much more often than females. Those teens, both male and female, who had sex with casual partners were more likely to also have substance problems. Negative attitudes of teens' partners toward the use of condoms greatly affected the teens' decisions regarding condom use (U.S. Department of Health and Human Services, 2005).

In general, pregnancy as a strategy to compensate for unmet needs, to have self-esteem, or to assert independence

### ENVIRONMENTAL CONNECTION

Consider the following possible environmental threats affecting adolescent pregnant teens:
- Tanning booths
- Secondhand smoke
- Occupational hazards, such as in fast food restaurants
- Cosmetic and hair products

How do these environmental hazards pose threats to this population?

is not particularly beneficial or successful. Parenting provides ample opportunity for failures, which are not helpful to adolescents already faced with repeated failures in their lives. An infant cannot meet all the nurturing expectations of the adolescent and has significant nurturing and attention needs of its own.

## ■ Social and Environmental Factors

Environment significantly influences adolescent ideas about sexual intercourse and pregnancy and their consequences. Each society has implied messages about sexuality, social behavior, and pregnancy. The clarity of the messages the community provides influences the sexual behaviors and expectations of its members (Foster, 1997). Several social and environmental factors have been identified as contributing to the high rates of adolescent pregnancy in the United States. Influences from family, culture, socioeconomic status,

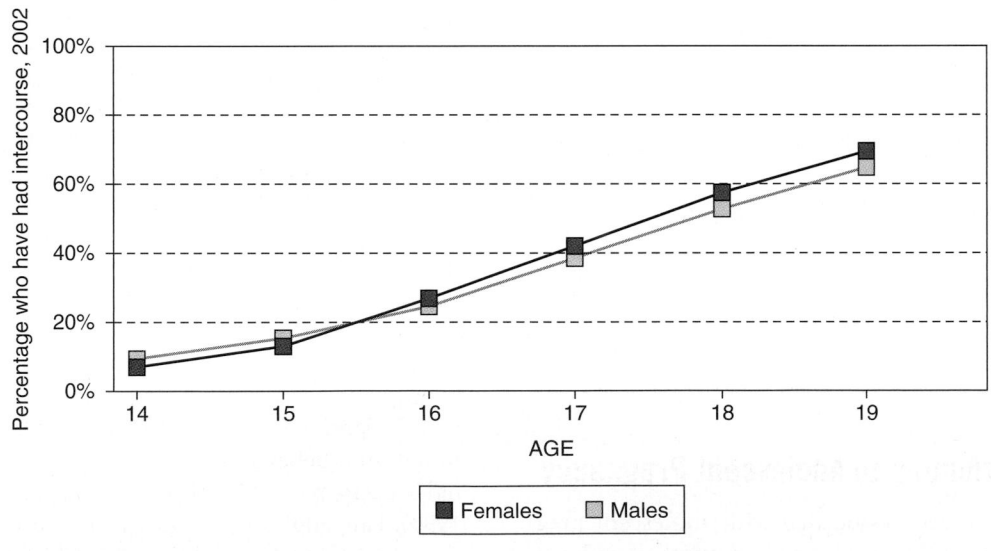

**Sexual Activity**
- Sex is rare among very young teens, but becomes more common in the later teenage years.
- Ten percent of young women aged 18–24 who had sex before age 20 reported that their first sex was involuntary. The younger they were at first intercourse, the higher the proportion.
- Twelve percent of teen males and 10% of teen females have had heterosexual oral sex but not vaginal intercourse.
- The proportion of teens who had ever had sex declined from 49% to 46% among females and from 55% to 46% among males between 1995 and 2002.

*Source*: Alan Guttmacher Institute. (2006). *Facts on American teens' sexual and reproductive health*. Washington, DC: Author. Available online: http://www.guttmacher.org/pubs/fb_ATSRH.html

peers, sexual partners, conflicting values presented in the media, feminist influences, decreasing stigma, relationships of younger girls with older boys, drugs/alcohol use, previous sexual abuse, and STDs have all been identified (Kenney, Reinholtz, & Angelini, 1997; Plouffe & White, 1996; Robinson & Frank, 1994; Toledo-Dreves, Zabin, & Emerson, 1995; Widom & Kuhns, 1996; Zoccolillo, Meyers, & Assiter, 1997; Ventura et al., 2006).

### The Family of the Adolescent

An understanding of **family dynamics** is essential for the community nurse to work effectively with the pregnant adolescent and her family. Every family is governed by its own rules and expectations, which determine expected behavior for its members (Bowen, 1971). Miller (2002) found that close parent–child relationships have a direct impact on pregnancy risk. Parental supervision is an important factor in reducing teen pregnancy. However, teens of parents who are extremely controlling tend to have higher pregnancy rates than those teens whose parents allow them a sense of freedom and privacy (Miller, 2002). Miller (2002) stresses the importance of supportive parental relationships and appropriate monitoring of teens' activities.

Problems occur when there is poor communication and conflicting messages about sex and pregnancy (DiIorio, Hockenbeery-Eaton, Maibach, Rivero, & Miller, 1996). Adolescents may hear mixed messages from the family, which often come from the family's own discomfort and embarrassment about sex and pregnancy. As a result, adolescents may perceive affirming attitudes about adolescent sexuality.

### The Ethnicity/Culture of the Adolescent

Differences in culture may affect the family and peer reactions to adolescent pregnancy, which in turn influences an adolescent's perception of pregnancy. Many factors contribute to cultural identity, and it is not suggested that all members of a particular cultural group will behave in an identical fashion; however, the community nurse must be aware of and sensitive to cultural influences on adolescent pregnancy.

Mainstream American culture has a negative view toward adolescent pregnancy, yet the rates of adolescent pregnancy remain higher in the United States than in other industrialized nations (Desmond, 1994; Trad, 1999). Hoff-

man (2006) and Jemmott and Jemmott (2007) gave the same information (U.S. pregnancy rates are highest among the world's industrialized nations). The existence of many subcultures and various culturally based beliefs may contribute to the higher rates of adolescent pregnancy. For example, in traditional, patriarchal Latino culture, females are expected to respond to male demands, and marriage and motherhood/fatherhood are viewed as catalysts to adulthood (Orshan, 1996). As a result, Latino adolescents may have a positive attitude toward pregnancy. However, the extent to which these common culturally based beliefs affect attitudes toward pregnancy may depend on the adolescent's level of acculturation. **Acculturation** is a dynamic, multidimensional phenomenon in which the ideals and beliefs of one culture are incorporated into that of another (Orshan, 1996; Reynoso, Felice, & Shragg, 1993). Acculturated American Latino adolescents from traditional Latino families may receive contradictory sexual messages from mainstream American society and the more traditional messages of their Latino culture.

### Research Alert

This research study of African American and Latina girls, among whom there is an especially high rate of sexually transmitted diseases (STDs), showed that role playing and practice applying condoms had a striking effect: The girls who received these interventions contracted fewer STDs within 12 months than did peers who had no such practice. The sample was composed of 700 sexually active African American and Latina girls ages 12 to 19 who were randomized into three groups: One group received information on STDs and condom use, one group received information on STDs but no condom use practice, and a control group received general health information unrelated to sexual activity. Each subject participated in a 250-minute group session led by a trained facilitator. At the 12-month followup, girls in the practice and role-playing group reported fewer incidents of unprotected intercourse and intoxications. Only 10.5% of girls in the practice and role-playing group had infection with STDs while 18.2% in the control group did. Although a limitation of the study was its reliance on self-report, other findings show that teaching such skills and helping girls become more self-reliant are viable prevention strategies with this at-risk group.

*Source*: Jemmott, J. B., Jemmott, L. S., Braverman, P. K., & Fong, G.T. (2005). HIV/STD risk reduction interventions for African American and Latino adolescent girls at an adolescent medicine clinic: A randomized controlled trial. *Archives of Pediatrics and Adolescent Medicine, 159*(5), 440–449.

> *Just saying 'no' prevents teenage pregnancy the way 'Have a nice day' cures chronic depression.*
> —Faye Wattleton, past president of Planned Parenthood

To the adolescent who is developing an identity, these conflicting views may lead to inconsistent feelings about sexual activity and contraceptive use and subsequent risk-taking sexual behavior.

Similarly, African American adolescents who grow up in single-parent families may receive mixed messages about adolescent pregnancy. These adolescents may see a pattern of intergenerational out-of-wedlock teen pregnancies but hear disapproving messages about adolescent pregnancy from parents, media, and school (Desmond, 1994; Youth Risk Behavior Survey, 2005; Jermott, Jermott, & O'Leary, 2007). Compounding the issue, there may be poor communication between the adolescent and parent about sexual issues.

Cultural influences are not limited to adolescents in minority cultures. Caucasian adolescents may also be influenced by cultural issues. In some European American cultures, discussion about sex and pregnancy is taboo. Adolescents who live in these environments may look to their peers and the media for rules of acceptable sexual conduct. Uneducated peers may provide misinformation. The media often depict sex as being disconnected from sexual responsibility, such as contraception and STD protection, with romanticized and idealized images of sexual behavior (Ventura et al., 2006).

### Socioeconomic Factors

Teens whose parents talked openly with them about sex were more likely to delay becoming sexually active. When these teenagers did become sexually active, they were more likely to practice protected sex. Several components of the parent–child relationship appeared to affect teen sexual behavior: family closeness, parental monitoring and supervision, and parent–child communication (Blake, Simkin, Ledsky, Perkins, & Calabresa, 2001). Family levels of education, income, and social standing in the community also appear to influence teen

 THINK ABOUT THIS

Social costs related to teen pregnancy are far-reaching:
- Teen mothers are more likely to drop out of school.
- Teen mothers are more likely to remain unmarried and live in poverty.
- Babies born to teen mothers are more likely to have a low birth weight.
- Babies born to teen mothers are more likely to experience abuse and neglect.
- Babies born to teen mothers are more likely to enter the welfare system.
- Daughters of teen mothers are more likely to become teen mothers.

*Source:* Hoffman, 2006.

sexual behavior (Kirby, 2001). Miller (2002) proposed that single and divorced parents' more permissive sexual conduct increased the adolescents' probability of becoming sexual active at a younger age. Miller (2002) also cited an earlier onset of sexual activity and unprotected sex in neighborhoods with higher crime rates. Girls who have lived in foster care are more likely to become teen mothers. Children of mothers who had first intercourse at an early age are more likely to also be sexually active at an early age (Miller, 2002).

### The Adolescent's Peers

One of the single most influential factors in adolescent sexual activity and pregnancy is the influence of peers (Coyle et al., 1996). Formation of peer groups and an increased need for peer acceptance are normal developmental milestones of adolescence. However, this increased need for acceptance may cause adolescents to give in to the requests of their peers or imitate the actions of their peers, which may include sexual experimentation and risky sexual behavior. Moreover, sexual information is often exchanged by adolescent peers and may lead to misconceptions and result in unintended pregnancy.

The attitudes, or perceived attitudes, of teens' peers regarding sexual activity greatly influence the teens' own concepts. This tendency to follow a pattern of behavior similar to that of peers relates to the decision to become sexually active and also to the use of condoms among those teens who choose to become sexually active (Kirby, 2001).

### The Adolescent's Sexual Partner

It is important to understand the male partner of female adolescents because female adolescent sexual activity often is submissive to male sexual desire (Blythe & Diaz, 2007; Heavey, Moysich, Hyland, & Druschel, 2008; Jemmott & Jemmott, 1990). In addition, the typical contraceptive methods on which adolescents rely before seeking prescription contraceptives are male methods, such as condoms, oral sex, status, and coitus interruptus (Blythe & Diaz, 2007; Morrison, 1985).

Male attitudes toward contraceptive use, especially **condoms,** have been described as negative (Jemmott & Jemmott, 1990, 1992; Jemmott, Jemmott, & Fong, 1998; Morrison, 1985; Sorensen, 1973). For instance, many males view condom use unfavorably because they believe it reduces the pleasure or spontaneity of sexual activities. Adolescent males commonly believe that **contraception** is a female's responsibility (Blythe & Diaz, 2007; Jemmott & Jemmott, 1990).

Little attention has been paid to the age of sexual partners of adolescents. It has been reported that the majority of male sexual partners of adolescent females are approximately 5 years older (average age 20 to 24) (AGI, 2008; Jemmott, Jemmott, & O'Leary, 2007; Lemay, Cashman, Elfenbein, & Felice, 2007), with only 30% of adolescent pregnancies resulting from **adolescent fathers.** Adolescent females may view their relationships with older partners as providing an escape from poverty, a show of defiance, a display of sexuality, and a boost to self-esteem. However, adolescent females with an incomplete perception of self may not feel able to negotiate and assert sexual

## Research Alert

Almost half of high school–aged teens in the United States have had sexual intercourse. Researchers have examined the time and place that teens are more likely to first have sex.

### Where Do Teens Have Sex for the First Time?

Two-thirds (68%) of 16- to 18-year-olds reported in 2000 that they first had sexual intercourse in their family home, their partner's family home, or a friend's house. More than one in five (22%) reported that their first sexual encounter occurred in their family homes. Only 4% reported having sex for the first time in a vehicle and 3% in a hotel, park, or outdoors.

### When Do Teens Have Sex for the First Time?

More than two-thirds (70%) of teens report having their first sexual experience in the evening or night (3 P.M. to 7 A.M.). The time breaks down as follows for timing of first intercourse:

- 42% during the hours between 10 P.M. and 7 A.M.
- 28% during the hours between 6 P.M. and 10 P.M.
- 15% during the hours between 3 P.M. and 6 P.M.
- 14% before 3 P.M.

Research indicated that there is no significant difference between the time of year or month when teens have sex for the first time. Teens appear to have the first sexual encounter as often during the school year as during summer vacation.

*Source:* Cohen, D. A., Farley, T. A., Taylor, S. N., Martin, D. H., & Schuster, M.A. (2002). When and where do youths have sex? The potential role of adult supervision. *Pediatrics, 110*(6), 110–116.

boundaries, such as condom use with their older partners, and may submit to the older partner's sexual demands. Consequently, many adult adolescent relationships result in an adolescent pregnancy (Kalmus, Davidson, Cahall, Laraque, & Cassell, 2003; Toledo-Dreves, Zabin, & Emerson, 1995).

Adolescent males have similar risk factors for pregnancy as their female peers. Often, adolescent males struggle with development and may attempt to demonstrate independence, belong to peer groups, and demonstrate physical and sexual maturity by engaging in sexual activity. As adolescents, males may also lack future-oriented thinking and concrete thinking abilities. Together, these factors contribute to increased potential for participating in risky sexual behaviors that may lead to pregnancy. Adolescent males may also view pregnancy as a catalyst toward manhood and may purposely have unprotected intercourse. In the African American community, the risk for an adolescent-fathered, teenage pregnancy may be higher. The mean age for sexual initiation among African American males has been estimated to be as low as 11.1 years (Blythe & Diaz, 2007; Jemmott, 1993; Jemmott & Jemmott, 1990; Terry-Humen & Manlove, 2003).

### Substance Use Among Adolescents

Several studies have found that the use of alcohol or drugs during sexual activity is associated with risky sexual

behavior, such as intercourse with multiple partners and failure to use condoms (Jemmott & Jemmott, 2007). Alcohol and drug use may change the nature of the sexual behavior in which people engage because logic and good judgment are clouded and inhibitions are loosened when people are "high" or because intoxication provides an excuse to engage in risky behavior (Crowe & George, 1989; Fortenberry, Orr, Katz, Brizendine, & Blythe, 1997; Jemmott & Jemmott, 2007; Kokotailo, Langhough, Cox, Davidson, & Fleming, 1994). However, there is a second, simpler explanation of the relationship between alcohol and drug use and risky sexual behavior. Adolescents who use alcohol and drugs more frequently than their peers may also engage in more sexual activity than their peers; consequently, they may engage in more risky sexual activity compared with their peers. The argument is not that alcohol and drug use causes adolescents to engage in different, more risky sexual behavior, but rather that adolescents who use alcohol and drugs engage in sexual activity more frequently (Jemmott & Jemmott, 1992; Jemmott, Jemmot, & O'Leary, 2007).

### Sexual and Physical Abuse of Adolescent Females

**Childhood victimization** may be linked to promiscuity and adolescent pregnancy. Adolescent females who were physically and/or sexually abused may be more likely to initiate sexual intercourse at a younger age, use drugs and alcohol, and engage in more promiscuous relationships than nonabused adolescents (Kenney et al., 1997; CDC, 2006). Childhood abuse has been associated with low socioeconomic status, unemployment, family dysfunction, substance use, and psychological dysfunction. Because many of the risk factors for childhood abuse are interrelated and linked to adolescent pregnancy, it is difficult to separate the effect of each factor in a child's environment that may influence behavior (Fiscella, Kitzman, Cole, Sidora, & Olds, 1998).

Adolescents who have experienced physical or sexual abuse may use sex in an effort to attain loving nonabusive relationships or may view pregnancy as a way out of the abusive environment at home (Widom & Kuhns, 1996). However, the adolescent who has not fully developed emotionally may not be in the position to be assertive and use sexual negotiation skills, leaving him or her at greater risk for experiencing further sexual exploitation by present and future partners.

### Knowledge Deficit Regarding Sex, Conception, and Contraception

The increased sexual activity among adolescents has not been accompanied by increased knowledge about sexual function, procreation, or birth control. Studies indicate that many adolescents remain woefully ignorant about conception and the menstrual cycle (Blythe & Diaz, 2007; Darabi, Jones, Varga, & Hourse, 1982; Davis & Harris, 1982; Jemmott & Jemmott, 1990; Jemmott et al., 2007; Landry, Bertrand, Cherry, & Rich, 1986; Villarruel, Jemmott, Jemmott, & Eakin, 2007). In addition to lack of information on sex and conception, adolescents lack correct information on birth control methods and the correct use of contraceptives (Morrison, 1985; Pollack, 1992; Collins et al., 2004; Ventura et al., 2006).

Even though contraceptive information has become more available, many adolescents do not use birth control on a regular basis (Box 28-1). Adolescents generally engage in sexual intercourse for some time before obtaining reliable contraception. Reluctance to obtain and use contraception is associated with certain attitudes and psychological and social factors. Stevens-Simon, Kelly, Singer, and Cox (1996) reported that adolescents' attitudes include "I don't mind getting pregnant" or "I want to get pregnant." Adolescents

---

✎ NOTE THIS! ●————————————

One of every five pregnant adolescents is physically and/or sexually abused (hitting, unwanted touching, sexual advances and intercourse) by a family member or partner during her pregnancy. Nurses need to assess adolescents, their partners, and their families for signs of abuse. ▲

---

**BOX 28-1**

**Why Adolescents Don't Use Contraception**
- I didn't mind getting pregnant.
- I wanted to get pregnant.
- I didn't know how to get birth control.
- I didn't think that I could get pregnant.
- I wanted to have a baby so my boyfriend would love me.
- I was afraid my family would find out.
- I was afraid of the side effects.
- I didn't want to appear to my partner to be prepared to have sex.
- I wasn't planning to have sex.
- I thought my boyfriend was sterile.
- I didn't know how to use birth control.
- I thought my partner would be angry with me if I used birth control.
- I wanted a baby to love.
- I thought other people would find out that I was using birth control.
- It's hard to talk to my partner about birth control.
- My boyfriend wanted me to get pregnant.
- My partner didn't want to use birth control.
- Using a condom interferes with sexual pleasure.
- I was embarrassed about using birth control.
- I just did not get around to it.
- Birth control can be expensive.
- Getting birth control is inconvenient.

*Sources:* Adapted from AGI, 1981; Howard & McCabe, 1992; Jemmott & Jemmott, 1990, 1992; Jemmott, Jemmott, & Fong, 1998; Loda, Speizer, Martin, Skatrud, & Bennett, 1997; Zelnik & Kantner, 1979.

---

who feel this way may neglect to use contraception or be inconsistent users of contraception.

## Impact of Adolescent Pregnancy

Adolescent pregnancy has significant, far-reaching consequences. Pregnancy can affect the adolescent's health, development, education, socioeconomic status, and, ultimately, future. The family and community may also feel the effects because the majority of adolescents are unwed, live with their families, and depend on public assistance (Coley & Chase-Lansdale, 1998). In addition to psychosocial and economical outcomes, the adolescent mother experiences physical consequences that may affect her health.

### ■ Psychosocial and Health Outcomes of the Mother

Pregnancy is a time of increased demands on a woman's body. These demands can be harmful to a developing adolescent, especially if there is no focus on the increased needs of pregnancy such as nutrition and rest. In general, adolescents experience greater health problems with pregnancy than do women older than 20 years of age. The consequences are especially severe to the youngest adolescents, those 12 to 15 years of age (Chedraui, 2008; Hoffman, 2006; Levy, Perhats, Nash-Johnson, & Welter, 1992; Trad, 1999).

- One in eight adolescents age 15–19 years in the United States becomes pregnant each year.

- One-half of all initial adolescent premarital pregnancies occur within the first 6 months after initiation of coitus; 20% occur in the first month alone.

- Media images of adolescent pregnancy often show minority adolescent teens, but adolescent pregnancy is not only a minority issue. Caucasian teenagers consistently account for the largest percentage of adolescent pregnancies and births (AGI, 1994, 1998; Pittman & Adams, 1988).

- Approximately 1 in 7 Caucasian adolescents, 1 in 4 African American adolescents, and 1 in 4 Latino adolescents are mothers by age 19. ◢

Adolescents are at greater risk for developing pregnancy-induced hypertension and toxemia (AGI, 1981), anemia, nutritional deficiencies, and urinary tract infections (Bulcholz & Gol, 1986; Chedraui, 2008; Wilson, Alio, Kirby, & Salihu, 2008; Zeck, Walcher, Tamussino, & Lang, 2008). Adolescent girls are more likely to deliver prematurely, experience rapid or prolonged labor, develop abruptio placenta, or have fetal or maternal infections (Mott, 1990; Zeck, Bjelic-Radisic, Haas, & Greimel, 2007).

### Lack of Prenatal Care

One of the major reasons for negative health outcomes for mothers and infants is lack of **prenatal care.** More pregnant adolescents delay seeking prenatal care, access less prenatal care, or do not receive regular care as often as adult women (Cockey, 1997; Geronimus, 1986; Hoffman, 2006). The same teenagers at greatest risk for pregnancy—those from poor families—are also at greatest risk for poor prenatal care. This lack of care contributes to poorer health outcomes for both mother and infant. Most adolescents do not receive prenatal care in the first trimester, with nearly 20% accessing care in the last trimester only. In general, this group tends to be more illness-oriented than prevention-oriented in their health practices. The reasons for this delayed initiation of prenatal care are varied and include denial of the pregnancy, lack of knowledge, lack of access to health care, concern about concealing the pregnancy, developmental immaturity (Cockey, 1997; Hoffman, 2006; Zuckerman, Walker, Frank, Chase, & Hamburg, 1984), and an orientation toward concrete, present-centered reasoning (Geronimus, 1986).

### Repeated Pregnancy

Several studies have shown that many young mothers have more than one child during their teen years. Obtaining exact numbers is difficult because U.S. Census data do not report **repeat pregnancy** rates, but estimates range from 15% to 60%, depending on the study (Brown, Saunders, & Dick, 1999; Cockey, 1997; Hoffman, 2006; CDC, 2006).

Adolescent mothers who have repeat pregnancies continue to be at higher risk for poor outcomes. Although it might be reasonably assumed that adolescent mothers would be more savvy in a second pregnancy, seeking and receiving more timely prenatal care, this is often not the case. One study examined the outcomes of first and second adolescent pregnancies among Caucasian and African American teenagers. The results revealed that a poor outcome in the first pregnancy was associated with a three times greater risk of repeating that outcome in the second pregnancy. The recurrence rate of preterm delivery was especially severe for African American adolescents (Blankson, Cliver, Goldenberg, Hickey, Jin, & Dubard, 1993; SmithBattle, 2007; Tocce, Sheeder, & Teal, 2008; Wilson et al., 2008). These results are critical because they provide a specific target for the **secondary prevention** efforts of nurses working in the community.

### Psychosocial Outcomes

Although pregnancy can become a stimulus for positive growth in an adolescent, generally the results are more negative than positive. Motherhood or fatherhood in the adolescent years can cause severe disruption in the normal psychosocial development of adolescents. Pregnancy places an additional psychosocial burden on teenagers, who are already attempting to cope with the normal maturational crisis of adolescence (Bulcholz & Gol, 1986; Trad, 1999).

Adolescents typically cope with the confusion and conflict in their lives by finding safety and acceptance in their peer groups. However, adolescent parents, especially mothers, may find themselves isolated from their peer groups at a critical time in their development. The degree of isolation may vary depending on the norms accepted by different cultural peer groups.

A primary goal of adolescence is attainment of independence. Although pregnancy may enhance independence in some ways by forcing the adolescent to take charge of a difficult situation, this forced rapid ascension into adulthood certainly is not without negative consequences. After delivery, as adolescent parents cope with the demands of a new infant, their own needs and desires are no longer first priority. The increased stress of being an adolescent parent can lead to more self-doubt, uncertainty, loneliness, and helplessness. The adolescent's inability to effectively cope with

Adolescent parents typically need more structured education focusing on newborn care, parenting skills, and fostering developmentally appropriate interactions.

**MEDIA MOMENT**

**Movies about Adolescent and Unplanned Pregnancy**

*Juno (2007)*
*Knocked Up (2007)*
*Junebug (2005)*
*For Keeps (1988)*
*Saved (2004)*
*Riding in Cars with Boys (2001)*

these feelings is reflected in the increased incidence of child abuse and neglect within this cohort (Ipsa, Sable, Porter, & Csizmadia, 2007; Lieberman, 1980; Marshall, Buckner, & Powell, 1991).

### Education and Economic Disruption

Adolescents who become pregnant are less likely than their non-pregnant peers to complete their education. For example, whereas 90% of women who delay childbearing beyond adolescence complete a high school education, only 70% of adolescent mothers ultimately reach this goal. Without a complete education, many adolescent mothers find employment opportunities out of their reach and rely on low-paying jobs or public assistance programs (AGI, 1994; CDC, 2006; Grogger & Bronars, 1993; Rolleri, Wilson, Paluzzi, & Sedivy, 2008).

## ■ Impact on the Family

An unplanned adolescent pregnancy can seriously jeopardize quality of life not only for the young mother and infant but also for their extended families. Families are often called on to shoulder considerable economic and emotional burdens. The strain on the family is often intensified because adolescent mothers are more likely to live in single-parent households. The long-term impact on the family is unknown, but as families compensate to deal with adolescent pregnancy, they may normalize the experience and set the stage for future adolescent pregnancy. From generation to generation, this trend may develop into a cycle. The children of adolescent parents are at increased risk of perpetuating the cycle by becoming adolescent parents themselves and dropping out of school.

## ■ Impact on the Adolescent Father

For every adolescent conception that occurs outside marriage, there is a father as well as a pregnant mother, yet there is limited research focusing on adolescent males who become fathers. The impact of adolescent pregnancy has been largely focused on adolescent females despite the obvious involvement of males. Even though adolescent males are the fathers in only 30% of adolescent pregnancies, it is important for the community health nurse to address the problem of teenage pregnancy with this group. Adolescent fathers may be more at risk for continued educational and

## ❝ *a conversation with . . .* ❞

### A Teen Mother

This teenage mom was 17 when she had her first child. She married the father of the child, finished high school, and is pursuing a college education.

On learning I was pregnant, I was really sad. My world was coming to an end. Many changes took place. My boyfriend and I both wanted to finish high school. So we were married and moved in with my in-laws.

After the baby was born, we graduated and soon moved into a trailer. I was overwhelmed with the responsibility. I lost so much sleep I thought I would never feel rested again!

We made the choice to stay married and I chose to go on to college against all odds. Now that college graduation is only a little over a year away, and I've grown up a lot, my future has hope! It has taken us more than three years, but I can truthfully say the last four months have been happy for us as a family.

Two major factors that have helped me keep from giving up on education and my marriage were the support of my mother and the teen-mom support group leader who became a real friend to me. They gave me something to hang on to and hope for when the winds of strife seemed capable of blowing me over.

After almost four years, we are beginning to see ourselves as a family mostly because of two concepts learned in the support group. The first was that I realized decisions in life were mine to make. I was responsible for my life. The second concept was learning how to effectively communicate love to my husband and son. He and I are the two people in the world that will love our son more than anyone else. We are partners in our responsibility for his nurturance, guidance, and support. How different my life might have been if I had not involved myself with this community service.

*Source*: Contributed by Arlene McFarland, DNSc, RN, from her weekly column, "Family Matters" in the Fort Payne (Alabama) *Times Journal*, May 5, 1998. Reprinted with permission.

social problems. Fagot, Pears, Capaldi, Crosby, and Leve (1998) found that adolescent fathers had more arrests and substance use problems than did nonfathers of the same age. The adolescent father's reaction to the pregnancy, his own psychosocial developmental issues and needs, and his behavior as a young father are critical to developing positive health outcomes for the child and impacting the behaviors of these young men before adulthood.

The adolescent father's reaction to the pregnancy is a crucial factor in determining what role he will play in the pregnancy and delivery and in the child's life. Some adolescent males react positively, but others do not. Reactions to pregnancy are influenced by many factors, including family reaction, peer group reaction, and relationship with the mother

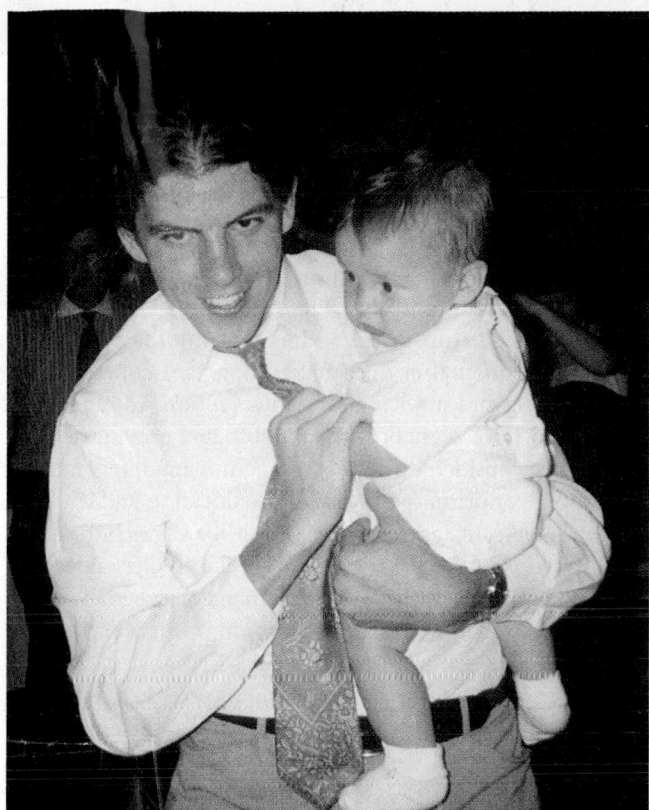

Nurses can use celebrity role models like Will Turpin, bass guitarist for Collective Soul (shown here with his son, Tristan), to demonstrate the rewards of waiting for marriage and fatherhood.

### HEALTHY PEOPLE 2010

**Selected Adolescent Pregnancy Primary Prevention Goals**

- Increase to at least 85% the proportion of people ages 10 through 18 who have discussed human sexuality, including values, with parents and/or have received information through another parentally endorsed source such as school (baseline = 66%)
- Reduce the proportion of adolescents who have engaged in intercourse to no more than 15% by age 15 and 40% by age 17 (baseline = 27% girls and 33% boys by age 15; 50% girls and 66% boys by age 17)
- Increase to at least 90% the proportion of sexually active young who use contraception (baseline = 78% at most recent intercourse; 63% at first intercourse among young women age 15 to 19)
- Reduce teenage pregnancies in all ethnic groups to no more than 50 per 1,000 girls age 17 and younger (30% decrease); African American adolescents to 120 per 1,000 (baseline = 186 per 1,000); Latino adolescents to 105 per 1,000 (baseline = 158)

*Source:* U.S. Department of Health and Human Services. (1990). *Healthy people 2000: National health objectives* (DHHS Publication No. 91-50213). Washington, DC: U.S. Government Printing Office.

of the child. Another factor that may influence the reaction is the developmental stage of the father, because many may not be able to cope effectively with a pregnancy. Problems that affect the adolescent male revolve around the acknowledgment of the child, his financial responsibility, his school commitment, and his work situation (Albert, 2004; Lowe, 2008; Males, 1993). Adolescent fathers report feeling frightened and disturbed by the responsibilities and neglected in the decision-making process, although few abandon the mother during pregnancy. Unfortunately, the young father may abandon the adolescent mother after pregnancy.

Regardless of the good intentions of most men, the fate of most adolescent fathers is similar to that of teenage mothers. Most are ill prepared to assume the role of fatherhood, and few relish the opportunity. Generally, having come from poor, relatively uneducated backgrounds, they experience serious social and economic disadvantages compared with young men who postpone fatherhood until a later age (Ispa et al., 2007; Lowe, 2008; Sonenstein et al., 1997). Most of the fathers lack the necessary skills to provide a stable home environment for their families even if they want to. In short, poverty is the tie that binds most adolescent fathers and mothers. Although some manage to cope with their situation, continue educational and vocational pursuits, and mature into self-sufficient, productive members of society, the odds are stacked against them.

## Psychosocial and Health Outcomes of the Newborn

Infants born to adolescents are at risk for various health problems as a result of complications with the adolescent mother's pregnancy and with the birth. These health problems include the increased incidence of preterm deliveries (before 38 weeks of gestation), increased incidence of **low-birth-weight (LBW)** infants (birth weight of less than 2,500 g), and increased incidence of perinatal morbidity and mortality (Abma, 2001; Blankson et al., 1993; Leppert, Namerow, & Barker, 1986; Miller, 2002; Ventura et al., 2006).

There has been considerable debate over whether young maternal age alone is an independent risk factor for complications, and the results are still unclear (DuPlessis, Bell, & Richards, 1997; Hoffman, 2006). More recent research suggests that other mediating factors (e.g., low socioeconomic status, poor prenatal care, race/ethnicity, unfavorable sociocultural circumstances) play a critical role (Hoffman, 2006; Plouffe & White, 1996; Yoder & Young, 1997).

## Role of the Nurse

It is apparent that pregnancy during the adolescent years presents some unique risks and special needs for the adolescent, her pregnancy, and her infant. Obviously, **primary prevention** of pregnancy is a crucial component of any adolescent intervention program. For effective primary prevention intervention success with teen females and males, the community health nurse must consider developmental, cultural, and socioeconomic issues as well as values in the

**Objectives Related to Family Planning**

9.2 Reduce the proportion of births occurring within 24 months of a previous birth.

9.6 Increase male involvement in pregnancy prevention and family planning efforts.

9.7 Reduce pregnancies among adolescent females.

9.8 Increase the proportion of adolescents who have never engaged in sexual intercourse before age 15 years.

9.9 Increase the proportion of adolescents who have never engaged in sexual intercourse.

9.10 Increase the proportion of sexually active, unmarried adolescents aged 15 to 17 years who use contraception that both effectively prevents pregnancy and provides barrier protection against disease.

9.11 Increase the proportion of young adults who receive formal instruction before turning age 18 years on reproductive health issues, including all of the following topics: birth control methods, safer sex to prevent HIV, prevention of sexually transmitted diseases, and abstinence.

*Source*: DHHS, 2000.

community. However, if young girls become pregnant, it is imperative that they receive secondary and tertiary preventive care, including adequate prenatal care coupled with long-term postpartum follow-up to ensure a healthy outcome for both mother and child. Community health nurses, because of their expertise in assessment, health teaching, and program development, are well suited to this task. Their accessibility to adolescent populations places them in a pivotal position to play a significant role in the delivery of care before sexual activity, during pregnancy, and during long-term follow-up with the parents and child.

*Healthy People 2010* addresses specific goals for adolescent pregnancy prevention (see the *Healthy People 2010* box for selected objectives). The community health nurse may use these national objectives to guide the development of individual, local, and regional nursing interventions.

■■ CULTURAL CONNECTION

Recent news about young teens in a conservative Mormon community in Texas marrying older men and bearing children prior to age 18 resulted in national controversy. Due to allegations of polygamy, hundreds of children were taken from these families by the state of Texas in 2008. Community health nurses should respect cultural differences in families and yet, when community norms are threatened, this can cause conflict in our roles as advocates. Read about the culture of various religions and their values about teen mothers. How can these differences be respected in the care of all families while recognizing the health risks of early pregnancy for females? ◯

> *The majority of adolescents behave as if their states were that of moratorium. That is, adolescence is a time for experimenting with how one might want to be as an adult.*
> —Rew, 1998

## ■ Primary Prevention

Because primary prevention is a critical component of effective community health nursing, there are tremendous opportunities for nurses to address the multifaceted problem of teen pregnancy and make important contributions to developing and implementing interventions to reduce the incidence of adolescent pregnancy. Table 28-1 provides a list of issues to be considered when planning nursing interventions. An example of primary prevention is education and counseling for adolescents about sexual health issues, including, but not limited to, pregnancy prevention, family life education, family planning, and the postponement of pregnancy into adulthood. A comprehensive program in primary prevention targeting adolescent pregnancy includes four goals:

1. Delaying or halting participation in sexual activity
2. Providing access to contraception and sufficient knowledge and skills to use contraception appropriately
3. Strengthening life goals and encouraging long-term planning
4. Educating teens about the relationship between all risky behaviors (i.e., substance abuse) and risk for teen pregnancy

Some prevention programs focus selectively on one goal, whereas others address all four.

One task in primary prevention is contraceptive education targeted at both males and females, encouraging adolescents to practice responsible sexual behavior. For adolescents to use contraceptives (including condoms) consistently, they need not only the correct knowledge on how to use the method, but also technical skills on how to use them correctly and on how to negotiate contraceptive use, especially condoms, with their partners (Jemmott et al., 2007). Adolescents need confidence and self-efficacy in their ability to use contraceptive methods, and the desired method must be available and accessible (Cook, Erdman, & Dickens, 2007). Finally, adolescents need positive attitudes toward contraceptive use, especially condoms (Jemmott & Jemmott, 1992, 1998). Community health nurses should carefully explore an adolescent's knowledge base and correct any misconceptions about birth control methods. This is the important first step in providing adolescents with clear, accurate directions regarding the use of birth control. Some recent trends in contraceptive use among adolescents are encouraging (Jemmott et al., 2008; Santelli, Lindberg, Finer, & Singh, 2007; Villarruel et al., 2007). For example, two-thirds of adolescents reportedly use some form of contraception at first intercourse, with a significant increase in prevalence of use at first intercourse among 15- to 19-year-old females (AGI, 1994, 2008). Kahn, Brindis, and Glei (1999) claim that

**Table 28-1** Considerations for Nursing Interventions

| Issue | Considerations |
|---|---|
| Adolescent father | ■ Acknowledge the risk factors for adolescent fatherhood and encourage involvement in the prenatal and postnatal periods. In speaking with adolescent males, it is important for the nurse to identify and assess beliefs and diagnose problems that may be specific to the adolescent male.<br>■ Personalize interventions to adolescent males, both in terms of preventing adolescent pregnancy through responsible sex and in terms of coping with the consequences of being a young father. Interventions that positively affect adolescent fathers may indirectly benefit their partners by enhancing partner support (Roye & Balk, 1996).<br>■ Talking in a nonthreatening, engaging manner with the male adolescent will facilitate effective communication that will address risk factors and beliefs and promote healthy outcomes for the father, mother, their families, and their child (Roye & Balk, 1996; Sonenstein, Stewart, Lindberg, Pernas, & Williams, 1997).<br>■ Stress male responsibility in birth control.<br>■ Increase his role in pregnancy and child care.<br>■ Improve his parenting skills and support his lifestyle changes (completing school, job training, and working). |
| Developmental stage | ■ Nurses who are knowledgeable about factors in adolescent development can better design developmentally appropriate primary interventions to prevent pregnancy, STDs, and HIV in their community.<br>■ Recognize the developmental tasks and stages of adolescence so as to understand the influence that those developmental factors have on adolescent sexual behavior. Consider the biophysical, cognitive, and psychosocial theories of development.<br>■ Answer questions and educate the adolescent about physical development and sexual issues. |
| Culture/ethnicity | ■ Assess and diagnose each adolescent patient and family to develop culturally sensitive interventions that are tailored to address cultural factors that affect sexual behavior, contraception, and potential pregnancy. |
| Peer | ■ Take advantage of the powerfully influential peer group to reach adolescents, as trained peer educators may be utilized to deliver safer sex and abstinence messages. |
| Intrapersonal | ■ Be aware that the adolescent is in a stage where he or she is developing self-identity and self-esteem, and that the adolescent may utilize sexual activity and pregnancy to bolster his or her identity. |
| Attitudes | ■ Explore nonjudgmentally the adolescent's attitudes about pregnancy. |
| Socioeconomic | ■ Assess the adolescent's economic situation and intervene to connect the adolescent and family with needed community resources. |
| Sexual abuse | ■ Identify adolescents in potentially abusive situations and assess both the adolescent and the adolescent's family for abuse. |
| Positive health outcomes | ■ Conduct home visits to adolescents during pregnancy and after birth to improve pregnancy outcomes and infant health status and to delay repeat pregnancies (Olds, 1992; Olds, Henderson, & Kitzman, 1994; Olds, Henderson, Tatelbaum, & Chamberlin, 1988). |

more than 1 million adolescent pregnancies were averted in 1995 because of consistent contraceptive use. These pregnancies would have led to approximately 480,000 live births, 390,000 abortions, 120,000 miscarriages, 10,000 ectopic pregnancies, and 37 maternal deaths.

The two most popular methods of contraception used by adolescents have traditionally been the birth control pill and the condom. Although it is beyond the scope of this chapter to fully discuss contraceptive options, it is particularly important for nurses working with adolescents to recognize the type of methods, side effects, and potential barriers that influence contraceptive choice.

Considering the variety of factors that contribute to an adolescent's increased risk for pregnancy, it is clear that there is not one reason why teens become pregnant. However, there are clear solutions and programs. These solutions and programs differ according to their target and the problem identified.

### HEALTHY PEOPLE 2010

**Selected Adolescent Pregnancy Secondary and Tertiary Prevention Goals**

- Reduce infant mortality to no more than 7 deaths per 1,000 births (31% reduction; blacks to 11 deaths per 1,000)
- Reduce low birth weight to no more than 5% of live births (28% decrease; blacks to no more than 9% of live births)
- Increase first-trimester prenatal care to at least 90% of live births (18% increase)
- Increase to at least 90% the proportion of women and infants who receive risk-appropriate care
- Increase to at least 90% the proportion of infants age 18 months and younger who receive recommended primary care services at appropriate intervals
- Reduce unintended pregnancies to no more than 30% of pregnancies (46% decrease; among African American women to no more than 40% (baseline = 78%)

*Source*: U.S. Department of Health and Human Services. (1990). *Heathy people 2000: National health objectives* (DHHS Publication No. 91-50213). Washington, DC: U.S. Government Printing Office.

## ■ Adolescent Pregnancy Prevention Community-Based Programs

A comprehensive review of adolescent pregnancy prevention research reveals many successes and failures. Kirby (1997) concludes that programs with positive outcomes share important characteristics (Box 28-2). There is no clear agreement on what exact combination of these elements makes up the ideal prevention program. Clearly, programs must be tailored to match the needs of the particular target population (Blythe & Diaz, 2007). Ideally, members of the target population, the family, and the community should be involved in the program development and implementation (Grobler, Botma, Jacobs, & Nel, 2007). There is a pressing need for prevention programs that are culturally sensitive and relevant, addressing the norms, attitudes, and beliefs of the target population (Cook et al., 2007). There are various types of programs with different approaches to pregnancy prevention, such as peer education, life options, working with parents, and working in schools and other community settings, including faith communities (Flynn, Budd, & Modelski, 2008; Kalmus et al., 2003).

### Lessons Learned

Important lessons have been learned in the area of adolescent pregnancy prevention. For example, although some prevention efforts focus solely on the importance of **abstinence** from sexual intercourse, the bulk of current evidence indicates that this approach is not successful in delaying the onset of intercourse. Furthermore, education alone is generally not sufficient to change risky behavior such as inconsistent contraceptive use (Flynn et al., 2008; Howard & Mitchell, 1993; Kalmus et al., 2003). Multidisciplinary programs are needed that combine elements such as sexuality education, enhanced negotiation and communication skills, and access to services and contraceptives (AGI, 1994; Flynn et al., 2008; Howard & Mitchell, 1993; Kalmus et al., 2003; Plouffe & White, 1996). Finally, although some have expressed concern that sexuality education and/or contraceptive distribution might encourage sexual activity among teens, recent research reviews have concluded that the opposite is actually true (Flynn et al., 2008; Jemmott & Jemmott, 2007; Kirby, 1997; Kirby, et al., 1993).

### Peer Education Approach

The peer education model shows great promise for use in adolescent pregnancy prevention (Minter, 1990) because the peer group is a common source for information about sex. In this model, peers are trained to lead prevention programs within their peer group. Community health nurses may serve as trainers and facilitators in these programs. Some of the advantages of peer education are that it provides positive role models, reinforces norms, empowers youth, and encourages personal responsibility (Albert, 2004; Coyle et al., 1996; Schaffer, Jost, Pederson, & Lair, 2008).

### Life Option Approach

A promising approach that is worthy of additional study is programs that shift the focus to enriching an adolescent's life options across the board by addressing concerns such as academic performance, self-esteem, substance abuse, and long-term goal realization (Albert, 2004; Schaffer et al., 2008). These programs may include one-on-one mentoring and role modeling with successful adults, community service participation, remedial education, tutoring services, counseling by both professional and peer groups, self-worth enhancement techniques, and exposure to new experiences to expand life options (e.g., concerts, museums, travel). This approach attempts to expand an adolescent's future goals and expectations by improving educational and employment prospects. Because future-oriented, goal-directed adolescents are less likely to become pregnant, the expected result is a reduction in the rate of adolescent pregnancies. Although this approach does not directly address adolescent pregnancy, it targets many of the factors that contribute to an adolescent's risk for unintended pregnancy (Abma, 2001; Hoffman, 2006; Kirby, 1997; Loda et al., 1997; Rolleri et al., 2008). Because the community health nurse is familiar with the community and its members, he or she may serve as a trusted mentor, educator, community liaison, and coordinator of such programs. In addition, for these programs to be effective, community health nurses must be aware of programs and resources that target adolescents in a broader sense, not only in terms of pregnancy prevention and contraception.

---

### BOX 28-2

**Characteristics of Effective Adolescent Pregnancy Prevention Programs**

Effective programs should do the following:

- Focus clearly on reducing one or more sexual behaviors that lead to unintended pregnancy or HIV/STD infection.
- Incorporate behavioral goals, teaching methods, and materials that are appropriate to the age, sexual experience, and culture of the students.
- Be based on theoretical approaches that have been demonstrated to be effective in influencing other health-related risky behaviors.
- Last long enough to allow participants to complete important activities.
- Provide basic, accurate information about the risks of unprotected intercourse and methods of avoiding unprotected intercourse.
- Employ a variety of teaching methods designed to involve the participants and have them personalize the information.
- Include activities that address social pressures related to sex.
- Provide models of and practice in communication, negotiation, and refusal skills.
- Select teachers or peers who believe in the program and then provide them with training, which often includes practice sessions.

*Source:* National Campaign to Prevent Teen Pregnancy. Used by permission.

## BOX 28-3

**Ten Tips for Parents to Help Their Children Avoid Teen Pregnancy**

1. Be clear about your own sexual values and attitudes.
2. Talk with your children early and often about sex, and be specific.
3. Supervise and monitor your children's behaviors, setting rules, curfews, standards, and other limitations.
4. Know your children's friends and their families.
5. Discourage early, frequent, and steady dating
6. Take a strong stand against your daughter dating a significantly older boy, don't allow your son to develop an intense relationship with a much younger girl.
7. Help your teenager to have options for the future that are more attractive than early parenthood.
8. Let your kids know that you value education highly.
9. Know that your kids are influenced by the media; pay attention to what they are watching, listening to, and reading.
10. Develop strong, close relationships with your children at an early age.

*Source:* National Campaign to Prevent Teen Pregnancy. Used by permission.

"Adolescence is a period of rapid changes. Between the ages of 12 and 17, for example, a parent ages as much as 20 years."
—Author Unknown

### Working with Parents and Adults

Community health nurses may work with parents and other adults significant to the adolescent, such as adult relatives, teachers, coaches, and neighbors. Recent research indicates that parents may be one of the most significant factors in preventing the onset of teen sexual behavior. This approach may be a promising avenue for prevention because parents and significant adults influence the behavior of adolescents, including sexual behavior, in their everyday interactions (Kirby, 2001; Miller, 2002). Although there is no single way for parents to effectively communicate with their children, the nurse may suggest that parents follow the guidelines provided by the National Campaign to Prevent Teen Pregnancy outlined in Box 28-3.

### School-Based Programs

A large number of pregnancy prevention programs target teens through school programs. Some of the programs in school may include sex education, family life education, and contraception education. Sex education is provided by some private schools and by public schools in approximately 75% to 80% of the United States; however, most family life programs are offered at the junior or senior high school level as an elective course, which means they do not reach many adolescents and cannot target those at greatest risk (Grobler et al., 2007). Also, most sex education teachers have little training in sex education, and it is not their primary focus. In school systems with school nurses, the nurse is involved in both sex and family life education (Lederman & Mian, 2003). Nurses can also provide factual sex education to teenagers as they provide other health services. Nurses are effective sex educators because they are equipped to provide sexual content in a factual, non-judgmental approach. They are also proficient at encouraging and guiding patient discussion, characteristics helpful in addressing sex education with adolescents (Jemmott, Jemmott, Hutchinson, Cederbaum, & O'Leary, 2008). These and other school-based programs receive limited funding, and access is limited for most students. However, school-based programs operate within a highly politicized environment. Decisions to include or exclude certain program elements within school-based programs may be made in an effort to minimize controversy rather than to maximize positive outcomes. As a result, community health nurses may need to broaden the focus of their prevention efforts beyond the domain of the school to the community at large.

### Working in Various Settings

Rather than limit the discussion of sexuality and pregnancy prevention to any one setting or a particular type of visit, community health nurses are uniquely positioned to seize opportunities to provide education and implement prevention in numerous settings. These settings, such as family planning clinics, primary healthcare clinics, school health clinics, community-based health clinics, churches, and teen centers are all ideal settings for adolescent pregnancy prevention, even when the adolescent does not present for contraceptive services. Interventions targeting adolescents who use the services of family planning clinics appear to be particularly promising in that they can effectively reach a high-risk group, adolescent females (and potentially their partners) who come to the clinic for a pregnancy test. These clinics are logical sites because of the population that they serve: More than 60% of adolescents younger than 17 use family planning clinics, and more than 82% of young

African American adolescents use them. In addition, they provide the opportunity to reach a population of vulnerable, high-risk adolescents at a timely moment (CDC, 2006; Delphisheh et al., 2007; Zabin & Clark, 1981; Zabin, Emerson, Ringers, & Sedivy, 1996).

### ■ Program Evaluation

Evaluation is an important part of the nursing process. Programs must be continually evaluated and modified by the community health nurse to ensure their effectiveness and appropriateness for preventing adolescent pregnancy. New prevention programs are constantly in the process of being designed; however, few programs are carefully and consistently developed and evaluated. Thus efforts may be wasted on interventions that are not effective. One measure of a sound design is the incorporation of theory in the design. Community nurses should have a knowledge base that includes an understanding of various behavioral theories such as the health belief model (Becker, 1974), social cognitive theory (Bandura, 1986), and the theory of reasoned action (Azjen & Fishbein, 1980). These theories can be used to understand the factors that encourage or discourage health promotion behaviors and can guide both program design and evaluation. The lack of meaningful program evaluation is a major defect in the primary prevention of adolescent pregnancy. Evaluation by the community health nurse is critical not only to identify ineffective programs or program elements but also to identify effective interventions and provide the impetus for replication and reevaluation in a different population. An effective prevention intervention is one that makes positive behavioral changes in measurable outcomes such as decreased incidence of early sexual intercourse or unprotected sex, or decreased number of sexual partners.

### ■ Secondary and Tertiary Prevention

Prevention efforts may not reach all adolescents because the risk of pregnancy may not be associated with extremely negative outcomes (Stevens-Simon et al., 1996). Therefore, the community health nurse must implement secondary and **tertiary prevention** techniques. In secondary and tertiary prevention, the community health nurse focuses attention on the health care, prevention needs, and long-term development of pregnant adolescents and adolescents who are already young mothers or fathers, with an emphasis on continuing their education to reduce the social and economic risks that can affect their future (Table 28-2). Secondary prevention efforts are designed to promote healthier outcomes from adolescent pregnancy. Its efforts are aimed at improving participation in prenatal care, childbirth preparation, and parenting activities. Interventions may include early detection of pregnancy, options counseling, prenatal care, childbirth education, parenting education, and safer sex education. Community health nurses may also be involved on a more global scale in secondary prevention efforts by working

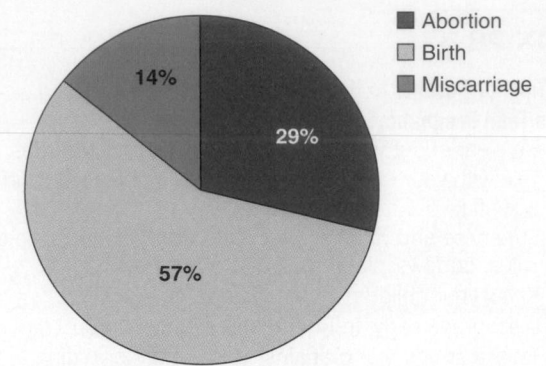

**Teen Pregnancy Outcomes**
- Nearly one-third of all teen pregnancies end in abortion.
- Black women have the highest teen pregnancy rate (134 per 1,000 women aged 15–19), followed by Hispanics (131 per 1,000) and non-Hispanic whites (48 per 1,000).
- The pregnancy rate among black teens decreased 40% between 1990 and 2000, more than the overall U.S. teen pregnancy rate declined during the same period (36%).
- Eighty-two percent of teen pregnancies are unplanned; they account for about one in five of all unintended pregnancies annually.
- Two-thirds of all teen pregnancies occur among 18- to 19-year-olds.
- Teen pregnancy rates are much higher in the United States than in many other developed countries—twice as high as in England and Wales or Canada, and eight times as high as in the Netherlands or Japan.

*Source*: Alan Guttmacher Institute. (2006). *Facts on American teens' sexual and reproductive health*. Washington DC: Author. Available online: http://www.guttmacher.org/pubs/fb_ATSRH.html

to increase access of pregnant adolescents to care. These efforts may include developing policies relevant to adolescent pregnancy in various organizations, working through coalitions and in other professional organizations.

#### Early Detection

A goal for the community health nurse is to identify pregnant adolescents early in their pregnancies, because many teens wait until they are visibly pregnant before they initiate prenatal care. Factors such as shame, denial, self-esteem issues, low value and knowledge of health, limited access to care, lack of future-oriented thinking, and lack of symptoms have all been linked to failure to receive early diagnosis and care (Baker, 1996; Lee & Grubbs, 1995; Thompson, Powell, Patterson, & Ellerbee, 1995). Community health nurses can work to identify teens early in their pregnancies by using community outreach techniques such as advertisement for prenatal services in malls, schools, public transportation, and churches.

#### Options Counseling

In counseling the pregnant adolescent, the nurse must be aware that the adolescent's decisions about her pregnancy and subsequent pregnancy prevention will affect both the adolescent mother and her entire family. Once pregnancy is confirmed, the adolescent faces an important decision about her options, which include **abortion** (Table 28-3), **adoption,** or keeping the baby. The nurse has the responsibility to provide (or refer to someone who will provide) the adolescent

**Table 28-2**   Secondary and Tertiary Prevention: Nursing Intervention

| Issue | Considerations for Nursing Interventions |
|---|---|
| Early detection | ■ Identify pregnant adolescents early in their pregnancies.<br>■ Recognize factors linked to failure to receive early diagnosis and care. |
| Pregnancy options | ■ Assess knowledge about pregnancy options.<br>■ Be sensitive to the factors that influence the mother's decision.<br>■ Assess the support the adolescent receives throughout the pregnancy.<br>■ Facilitate therapeutic relationships with the adolescent mother and father and their social support networks.<br>■ Include the father of the baby. A comprehensive assessment should include identification of his attitudes, emotional reactions, plans for education, and plans for involvement with the pregnancy, his partner, and the child.<br>■ Provide options counseling. |
| Prenatal care | ■ Encourage early and consistent prenatal care to reduce neonatal and maternal complications.<br>■ Teach the adolescent and her partner about the special needs of pregnancy.<br>■ Assess barriers to adolescent prenatal care.<br>■ Provide health screening assessments, counseling, and education for pregnant patients. |
| Adolescent father | ■ Encourage the father's participation in prenatal visits.<br>■ Invite the father to prenatal classes, encourage questions and participation in prenatal visits, and acknowledge the father's role as a partner in the pregnancy.<br>■ Encourage fathers to participate in the delivery. |
| Parenting education | ■ Assess knowledge about parenting.<br>■ Provide education about positioning and handling of infants, nutrition, hygiene, elimination, growth and development, immunization, and recognition of illnesses.<br>■ When doing health teaching, it is important to be sensitive to the ethnicity and culture of the patient and integrate those considerations into the care of the infant. |
| Postpartum care | ■ Focus on the standard postpartum areas as well on specific concerns of the adolescent, such as body image, weight loss, and fatigue.<br>■ Assess the adolescent's adjustment to her new role and the emotional support systems available to her.<br>■ Provide a health assessment of both the mother and the infant, newborn care education and supervision, prenatal education on growth and development and parenting skills, review of role adjustment and available supports and sex education and birth control information.<br>■ Encourage the adolescent to continue developing as an individual (for example, to continue education, participate in some social activities, and explore relationships with peers) and at the same time increase the adolescent's proficiency and confidence in parenting. |
| Support | ■ Assess physical and emotional available support.<br>■ Refer adolescents to other possible resources, such as parenting programs, cooperative daycare programs, or programs that pair the new mother with an older adolescent mother with a successful experience. |
| Status of the newborn | ■ Provide a newborn assessment/well-baby check.<br>■ Assess for signs of adequate maternal infant bonding.<br>■ Provide information about child care. |
| Sexual activity and contraceptive use | ■ Assess adolescents' plans for sexual activity and need for contraceptive methods.<br>■ Initiate discussion about birth control while the adolescent is pregnant so that both partners have an opportunity to identify contraceptive and safer sex methods that they will use after the pregnancy.<br>■ Provide instruction on condom use during pregnancy in your discussion of disease prevention in pregnancy.<br>■ Help adolescents explore the risks involved if they have sex without adequate protection.<br>■ Help the adolescent select the most appropriate form of contraception from several alternatives.<br>■ If the adolescent has already used birth control, it is helpful to identify the method, how it was used, and the reason for discontinuance.<br>■ Make sure that the adolescent is aware of community resources (family planning clinics) where she may be supplied with contraceptives.<br>■ Encourage clinic attendance, promote access to contraception, and provide referrals to appropriate contraceptive services. When counseling individuals or teaching sex education classes, emphasize the importance of contraceptive use by all sexually active adolescents.<br>■ Monitor compliance and encourage cooperation with adolescents. |

| Table 28-3 | Adolescents and Abortion in the United States |
|---|---|

- There were 214,750 abortions among 15–19-year-olds in 2002.
- Twenty-nine percent of pregnancies among 15–19-year-olds ended in abortion in 2002, compared with 21% among all women.
- The reasons teens give most frequently for having an abortion are concerns that how having a baby would change their lives, inability to afford a baby now, and feeling insufficiently mature to raise a child.
- Thirty-four states (as of August 2006) require that a minor seeking an abortion involve her parents in the decision.
- Six in 10 minors who have abortions do so with at least one parent's knowledge. The great majority of parents support their daughter's decision to have an abortion.

*Source:* Alan Guttmacher Institute. (2006). *Facts on American teens' sexual and reproductive health.* Washington DC: Author. Available online: http://www.guttmacher.org/pubs/fb_ATSRH.html

---

### BOX 28-4

**Adolescent Pregnancy and Nutrition Requirements**

The nutritional needs of the pregnant adolescent are often different from those of adult women. Many adolescents are experiencing rapid physical growth and maturation during their teenage years. Pregnancy increases the nutritional requirements of the adolescent.

The recommended nutritional goals of the adolescent depend on the **gynecological age** of the adolescent. Adolescents with a gynecological age less than or equal to 2 years have increased nutritional needs because of their own physical growth requirements. When the gynecological age is less than 2 years, the nutritional requirements of a pregnant teen may compete with the nutritional requirements of the fetus.

Gynecological age = number of years between the chronological age and the age of menarche

Because adolescent diets are often high in salt, sugar, and fatty foods, and low in protein, vitamins, and minerals, the nurse must be diligent about assessing and diagnosing deficits in the pregnant adolescent's diet.

---

with information about pregnancy options. Among adolescents, the most common outcome (55%) is a live birth. Only 1 in 20 pregnant adolescents chooses to place her infant for adoption, whereas 28% of adolescent pregnancies end in abortion (Ventura, Abma, Mosher, & Henshaw, 2006).

The community health nurse must recognize that many factors play a role in the decision the adolescent makes about the pregnancy. These factors may include cultural and religious upbringing, family attitude toward the pregnancy (perceived or real), partner attitude, community values and norms, and state law. Partner age plays an important role, as data have shown that adolescent females with younger partners tend to terminate their pregnancies at a higher rate than adolescent females with adult partners (Collins et al., 2004; Hoffman, 2006).

### Prenatal Care

Once an adolescent decides to continue the pregnancy, effort is directed toward ensuring a healthy outcome for the mother and infant. Early initiation and regular continuance of prenatal care significantly reduce the risk for both adolescents and their infants. The nurse should educate the adolescent and her partner about the special needs of pregnancy as they relate to adolescence, such as the following:

- Special nutritional needs (Box 28-4)
- Physical changes and demands of pregnancy
- How pregnancy affects the female adolescent's growth and development
- Emotional changes during pregnancy for both parents
- What to expect during delivery
- Preterm labor
- Signs and symptoms of pregnancy complications

Programs that address barriers to adolescent prenatal care have demonstrated positive outcomes, including reduced neonatal and maternal complications (CDC, 2006; Delpisheh et al., 2007; Rogers, Peoples-Sheps, & Suchindran, 1996; Yoder & Young, 1997).

Prenatal care services that prove successful in getting teenagers to use and comply with the overall program of care are those that provide an accepting, caring atmosphere and work to reduce obstacles to beginning or continuing care. These results have been in comprehensive community-based programs with a heavy outreach and educational emphasis, using multidisciplinary healthcare teams, especially community health nurse involvement, and home visits. The community health nurse acts as the case manager of prenatal care and sees that patients are provided with needed services. The nurse is the team member who spends the most time with the adolescent, providing most of the health screening assessments, counseling, and education for pregnant patients.

Prenatal programs should also aim to improve the quality and duration of the father–child relationship. Community health nurses can assist in these efforts by encouraging the father's participation in prenatal visits. Most fathers are curious and interested in the process of gestation and delivery but are uncomfortable asking questions and hesitant in interacting with healthcare providers. The community health nurse can invite the father to prenatal classes, encourage questions and participation in prenatal visits, and acknowledge the father's role as a partner in the pregnancy. Fathers can be encouraged, but not forced, into participation in the baby's delivery.

Three types of programs offer prenatal care to adolescents: private medical services, public health clinic programs, and school-based prenatal programs. The choice of program depends on the accessibility and the financial circumstances

### ▢ Research Alert

American Indian adolescent pregnancy rates are high, yet little is known about how Native youth view primary pregnancy prevention. This study was meant to identify pregnancy prevention strategies from the perspectives of urban Native youth to inform program development. Native Teen Voices (NTV) was a community-based participatory action research study in Minneapolis, Minnesota. Focus groups were convened with Native youth who had never been involved in a pregnancy. Participants were asked what they would do to prevent pregnancy if they were in charge of programs for Native youth. Respondents' recommendations were identified and categorized across age and sex cohorts. Participants in all cohorts emphasized the following themes: show the consequences of adolescent pregnancy; develop more pregnancy prevention programs for Native youth in schools and community-based organizations; improve access to contraceptives; discuss teen pregnancy with Native youth; and use media to reach Native youth. Native youth perceived limited access to comprehensive pregnancy prevention education, and contraceptives. They suggested a variety of mechanisms to address gaps in sexual health services and emphasized enhancing school-based resources and involving Native peers and elders in school and community-based adolescent pregnancy prevention initiatives.

Garwick, A., Rhodes, K., Peterson-Hickey, M., & Hellerstedt, W. (2008). Native teen voices: adolescent pregnancy prevention recommendations *Journal of Adolescent Health, 42*(1), 81–88.

Nurse role modeling appropriate infant care with teen mother.

of the adolescent and her family. Private medical services are provided by physicians in single or group practices or associated with health maintenance organizations. These services are available to people who have a medical insurance plan or can afford to pay. Public health clinic programs are for families without insurance or the financial resources to pay for prenatal care. School-based programs provide services in connection with other school-run clinic services or in separate schools designed for the exclusive use of pregnant adolescents (Olds, 1992). School-based prenatal services provide a comprehensive approach to care and are usually found in large school districts with high rates of adolescent pregnancy.

### Parenting Education and Contraceptive Education

Adolescent parents typically need more structured education focusing on newborn care, parenting skills, and fostering developmentally appropriate interactions. Discussion about birth control should also be initiated while the adolescent is pregnant so that both partners have an opportunity to identify contraceptive methods that they will use after the pregnancy. The community health nurse is in a unique position to provide these services at a group or individual level and promote continuity of care that focuses on the new family.

### Transition from Prenatal to Postpartum Care

After delivery of the baby, the focus is on postpartum care, which varies widely in scope and duration of services. All prenatal programs provide a postpartum check for the mother. A well-baby check is included in most services, although a private obstetrical practice may rely on the mother to make her own arrangements for all infant care. The most extensive postpartum care is delivered in community programs that rely heavily on nurses. These programs usually include the following:

- Health assessment of both the mother and infant
- Newborn care education and supervision
- Prenatal education on growth and development and parenting skills
- Review of role adjustment and available supports
- Sex education and birth control information
- Promotion of the role of continuing education to reduce future risks for the teen mother and father

One valuable component of these programs is the emphasis on regular contact with the new mothers, starting the first week after delivery. Studies show that regular nurse visits reduce anxiety and increase infant health as measured by fewer accidents and emergency department visits (Olds, 1992; Olds et al., 1994; Olds et al., 1988). Mothers experience many concerns or problems before the first scheduled clinic or physician visit. Earlier contacts allow the adolescent and nurse to address these issues and reduce anxiety. Contact need not always be in person; some care can be provided by telephone monitoring of the new mother and newer technology such as e-mail reminders.

### Health and Psychosocial Status of the Mother

At a minimum, the mother should have a 6-week postpartum examination. Some community health programs

## A Good Read

### Dear Diary, I'm Pregnant: Teenagers Talk About Their Pregnancy (1997)

*Annrenee Englander, Vancouver, BC: Annick Press.*

This book is the result of interviews with women who became pregnant during adolescence. Englander demonstrates through first-person narratives (by the women interviewed) the experiences of many teens who become pregnant. Women of differing race, ethnicity, and income levels provide a more well-rounded view of the adolescent pregnancy experience. In these different narratives, you are able to see how each teen had to make difficult decisions about the pregnancy and her life, sometimes with limited support.

### Not Our Kind of Gir: Unraveling the Myths of Black Teenage Motherhood (1997)

*Elaine Bell Kaplan, Berkeley, CA: University of California Press.*

Sociologist Elaine Bell Kaplan, based on her own experiences as an African American adolescent mother, discusses and dispels common myths and misconceptions about African American teen motherhood. She does so by looking at class, gender, and racial factors that influence black teenagers to become mothers. She examines and addresses several assumptions that are promoted in the media, such as the notion that the African American community condones teen pregnancy, single parenting, and reliance on the public health system. She provides alternatives to these misconceptions with examples from both her own experience and the experiences of others she has studied.

### Kids Having Kids: Economic Costs and Social Consequences of Teen Pregnancy (1996)

*Rebecca A. Maynard, Baltimore, MD: Urban Institute Press.*

*Kids Having Kids* is a book of essays by experts in the field of adolescent pregnancy. This book takes a look at the problem of adolescent pregnancy and estimates the economic and social effects of adolescent pregnancy on the teen, her child, her family, the community, and the U.S. economy. It provides an in-depth look at the long-term consequences of adolescent pregnancy as well.

---

start home visits at about 2 weeks postpartum. The physical assessment should focus on the standard postpartum areas as well as on specific concerns of the adolescent, such as body image, weight loss, and fatigue. In addition, the nurses should assess the adolescent's adjustment to her new role and the emotional support systems available to her. Adjusting to the role of parent during adolescence is difficult. Conflict is not unusual. Family members may expect the adolescent to instantly become an adult and mother, or the opposite, to remain a child and allow her parents to assume all the responsibilities for the infant. Ideally, the adolescent should be encouraged to continue developing as an individual (e.g., to continue her education, participate in some social activities, to explore relationships with peers). The adolescent mother needs support in increasing her proficiency and confidence in parenting and integrating her new responsibilities into her daily routine. She may be juggling school, social activities, and infant care. Fatigue and stress are common.

### Got an Alternative?

Pregnant adolescents are often fearful of gaining weight and losing their relatively new female shape. Exercise, such as yoga and aerobics, often appeal to this group and can promote a healthy pregnancy, with proper professional supervision.

The community health nurse can help the new mother look at the immediate family, other relatives, significant others, and the father of the infant and his family for support. The adolescent mother could also be referred to other possible resources, such as parenting programs, cooperative daycare programs, or programs that pair the new mother with an older adolescent mother with a successful experience. Even if support systems are adequate, the family may need some help in understanding and supporting the adolescent as a maturing individual (Zeck et al., 2007). Adequate physical and emotional support, along with health teaching and realistic expectations for their children, successfully reduces the incidence of abuse and neglect from at-risk mothers (Abma, 2001; East, Reyes, & Horn, 2007; Marshall et al., 1991; Olds, 1992; Olds et al., 1994; Olds et al., 1988).

### Sexual Activity and Contraceptive Use

Ideally, the idea of future contraception should be introduced as part of the prenatal program. The adolescent must decide whether she will continue sexual activity after delivery and must be encouraged to be honest with the nurse about her decision. Sometimes, the mother is no longer involved with the father of the infant and announces that she does not intend to be sexually active or to have another child. In this case, the adolescent mother should be helped to explore

### Application to Practice

You are a school nurse at Oak Hills High School. You have carefully followed several of your students who have become pregnant and helped them find resources for support both during and after their pregnancies. You have noticed, however, that several of your students have decided to discontinue breastfeeding. In speaking with Arlene Johnston, a 15-year-old sophomore with a 3-month-old son, Antonio, you find out that she is also reconsidering breastfeeding. She understands the benefits of breastfeeding and is able to discuss them with you. Both Arlene and her mom think that breastfeeding is good for Antonio. However, upon further questioning, you discover that her new partner, Sam, and her friends at school think that breastfeeding is "nasty." Arlene feels embarrassed that her friends know she breastfeeds and she is afraid that she will lose her friends and boyfriend.

1. Which factors in Arlene's (and the other adolescents') cognitive development support her decision to discontinue breastfeeding?
2. How can you address this to continue to promote Arlene's breastfeeding Antonio?

You decide that one means to addressing attitudes toward breastfeeding is to address the attitudes of all students at Oak Hills High.

1. Consider different ways that you, as the school (community) health nurse, can address the students at Oak Hills High.
2. Which special considerations apply for such an intervention?

---

## MEDIA MOMENT

### *Juno* (2007)

Academy Award winner Ellen Page plays a 16-year-old high school student (Juno) suddenly faced with an unexpected pregnancy after a one-time sexual encounter with her good friend. Juno faces the pregnancy with a pragmatic attitude and intent to control her and her unborn baby's future. She ultimately decides to find a suitable couple to adopt her baby, choosing a closed adoption and the prospect of never seeing her child again. An excellent film about the complexities of adolescent pregnancy and the family.

tion classes. The nurse must emphasize the importance of contraceptive use by all sexually active adolescents.

### Health Status and Care of the Newborn

In addition to the usual newborn assessment, the community health nurse should look for signs of adequate maternal–infant bonding. Evidence of attachment includes calling a child by its name, cuddling, talking to the infant, and demonstrating an interest in infant care and development. Adolescents often demonstrate difficulty in bonding simply because they have had no previous experience with infants and are afraid to do anything. Sometimes, another person has assumed the role of caregiver and the adolescent becomes an observer rather than caregiver. Bonding can be assessed in clinic settings, but home visits by the community health nurse allow for a more accurate picture of the nature and scope of the mother–infant relationship and the relationship of the adolescent father with the mother. Considering the current trend of short postpartum length of stay, the community health nurse has the opportunity to observe the interaction among the infant, teenager, father, and other caregivers for a longer time than nurses in the clinical setting.

### Tertiary Prevention

Tertiary prevention efforts may include prevention of additional adolescent pregnancies, support of positive parent–infant interaction, support groups for adolescent parents, and programs that support adolescents while they pursue educational goals. The techniques discussed previously that are used in primary prevention may be used to prevent repeat pregnancies in adolescents. The nurse may work collaboratively with organizations that provide support such as child care and allowing adolescent parents to complete and pursue further education. Other nursing interventions may include long-term child development education and parenting classes. Programs that foster maternal education, father involvement, and increased self-esteem show significant promise for better maternal and infant development (Diehl, 1997; Hoffman, 2006; Roye & Balk, 1996).

---

the risks involved if she changes her mind without adequate protection. Once an adolescent has been pregnant, she risks repeating the situation (AGI, 1981; Brown et al., 1999; Youth Risk Behavior Survey, 2005).

Access to and regular use of birth control is the goal of contraceptive services for adolescents. Family planning clinics and private physicians are one source; school-based clinics are a more recent effort. Community health nurses can encourage clinic attendance, promote access to contraception, and provide referrals to appropriate contraceptive services when counseling individuals or teaching sex educa-

## BOX 28-5

### Key Ideas

- Adolescent pregnancy is a nationwide problem, affecting more than 1 million adolescents per year in the United States—a higher rate than in other industrialized countries.
- Adolescent pregnancy transcends ethnic, racial, and cultural boundaries.
- Repeat pregnancies for adolescents are of great concern, because half of all pregnant adolescents will have a repeat pregnancy in 2 years.
- Pregnant adolescents and their children experience more complications with pregnancy and have poorer health outcomes.
- Adolescent parents may have increased psychological stress and disruption of psychosocial development. They may also have incomplete education, poor success in the job market, and higher dependence on public funds. As a result, the community and the families of adolescent parents may experience increased economic and social stress.
- Adolescent males have similar risk factors for pregnancy as their female peers. However, adolescent males (and issues particular to them) are frequently overlooked in the literature. The impact of fatherhood on adolescent boys and inclusion of fathers in the maternity and postpartum experience is an important and new phenomenon to increase father involvement.
- Pregnant adolescents and their infants are at greater risk for developing medical complications (e.g., hypertension, toxemia, anemia, low birth weight, stillbirth, and infant mortality) than are older women and their infants.
- There is no single factor that causes adolescent pregnancy, but an awareness of the personal, environmental, and social contributing factors allows the community health nurse to appropriately assess, diagnose, plan, and evaluate interventions for adolescents and their families.
- Many contraceptive options are available for the adolescent. The nurse must have an awareness of the potential barriers that the adolescent may encounter in using contraception consistently and effectively.
- The ideal manner in which to prevent the complications associated with adolescent pregnancy is to prevent pregnancy from occurring. Primary prevention efforts need to focus on the special developmental needs of adolescence, emphasize the importance of peer groups, and occur in various settings to effectively promote behavior change. Programs that include sex education, contraceptive information, and access to contraceptive services have been found to delay sexual activity and increase contraceptive use in sexually active adolescents. Successful prevention programs share important characteristics that should be considered in program development.
- The nurse should develop secondary prevention programs that include interventions that have been documented to reduce medical complications and promote healthy outcomes for the pregnant adolescent and her newborn infant, including promoting early initiation of prenatal care, childbirth education, and nutrition counseling.
- Tertiary prevention programs are largely rehabilitative—that is, they provide a variety of support services for new mothers and their infants to reduce health risks for both mother and child and to increase the chances that the mother will continue her education. Prevention programs may include activities that promote education completion, psychosocial development, and development of career goals.
- The overall goal of the community health nurse is to prevent adolescent pregnancy, promote healthy outcomes of adolescent pregnancy, prevent repeat pregnancies, and foster positive long-term development of adolescents and their children.

## Conclusion

Despite the proliferation of prevention efforts, adolescent pregnancy is a significant and enduring community health problem. It has been linked to various problems such as increased poverty, decreased educational attainment, increased psychological stress, potential isolation from peers, and increased reliance on public funds. Multiple pregnancies among adolescents are not uncommon and are particularly disturbing because the negative effect of pregnancy increases dramatically.

Many factors contribute to adolescent pregnancy, and community health nurses must be aware of potential risk factors and understand the complex interaction of these factors. Without this awareness and understanding, the nurse will not be able to adequately perform the nursing process to develop and evaluate age-appropriate, culturally sensitive, convenient, comprehensive, and affordable interventions that will meet the special needs of adolescents. It is clear that unless community health nurses and other health professionals make an effort to provide information, few adolescents will actively seek out nurses or other professionals as resources. Nurses are well suited to address the issues of adolescent pregnancy. The professional roles in schools, clinics, screening programs, health departments, and community outreach centers provide access to at-risk populations. Community health nurses have the opportunity, sensitivity, and commitment to work to achieve positive outcomes for adolescents and their children.

## BOX 28-6

### Web Sites of Interest

| Organization/Service | Web Site |
|---|---|
| ■ Advocates for Youth, Teen Pregnancy Prevention Initiative | http://www.advocatesforyouth.org/pregnanc.htm |
| ■ Alan Guttmacher Institute | http://www.agi-usa.org |
| ■ Ask NOAH (New York Online Access to Health) About Pregnancy | http://www.noah.cuny.edu/pregnancy/pregnancy.html (information in both English and Spanish) |
| ■ Campaign for Our Children | http://www.cfoc.org |
| ■ National Campaign to Prevent Teen Pregnancy | http://www.teenpregnancy.org |
| ■ Planned Parenthood Federation of America | http://www.plannedparenthood.org |

Beyond the scope of care to individuals, community health nurses are sensitive to the community in which they practice. Community health nurses are uniquely equipped to assess communities, identify needs and special risk groups, and formulate solutions (see Box 28-5, page 698). Nurses have an obligation to meet the special needs of pregnant adolescents by designing programs, organizing community support, and advocating for funding and policy changes to enhance positive health outcomes for adolescents and their infants.

Explore Community Health Nursing on the Web! To learn more about the topics in this chapter, use the passcode provided to access your exclusive website: **http://nursing.jbpub.com/communityhealth.** If you do not have a passcode, you can obtain one at this site.

## ■ CRITICAL THINKING ACTIVITIES

1. What are the social norms and cultural beliefs about adolescent pregnancy and sexuality in your community? How do you think that these beliefs affect adolescent behavior?

2. What strategies can the community health nurse implement to help the pregnant adolescent and her family cope with the changes in the family structure?

3. You are planning a pregnancy prevention intervention for adolescents in your community. Identify program characteristics that you might include in your intervention that have been shown to be effective in adolescent pregnancy prevention programs.

4. It is important for the community health nurse to be aware of community resources to appropriately refer patients. What resources are available in your community for pregnant adolescents? Adolescents with children? Adolescent fathers?

5. Does your school district provide child care for adolescents with children? Do you believe they should? Why?

## ■ REFERENCES

Abma, J. C. (2001). *Sexual activity and contraceptive practices among teenagers in the United States, 1988 and 1995.* Hyattsville, MD: U.S. Dept. of Health and Human Services, Centers for Disease Control and Prevention, National Center for Health Statistics.

Alan Guttmacher Institute (AGI). (1981). *Teenage pregnancy: The problem that hasn't gone away.* New York: Author.

Alan Guttmacher Institute (AGI). (1994). *Sex and America's teenagers.* New York: Author.

Alan Guttmacher Institute (AGI). (2008). *In brief: Facts on American Teens' Sexual and Reproductive Health.* Retrieved November 20, 2008, from http://www.guttmacher.org/pubs/fb_ATSRH.html

Albert, B. (2004). *With one voice 2004: America's adults & teens sound off about teen pregnancy.* Washington, DC: The National Campaign to Prevent Teen Pregnancy.

Azjen, I., & Fishbein, M. (1980). *Understanding attitudes and predicting social behavior.* Englewood Cliffs, NJ: Prentice Hall.

Baker, T. J. (1996). Factors related to the initiation of prenatal care in the adolescent nullipara. *Nurse Practitioner, 21*(2), 29–42.

Bandura, A. (1986). *Social learning theory*. Englewood Cliffs, NJ: Prentice Hall.

Becker, M. H. (1974). The health belief model and personal health behaviors. *Health Education Monographs, 2*, 324–508.

Blake, S., Simkin, L., Ledsky, R., Perkins, D., & Calabresa, J. (2001). Effects of a parent–child communications intervention on young adolescents' risk for early onset of sexual intercourse. *Family Planning Perspective, 33*(2), 52–62.

Blankson, M. L., Cliver, S. P., Goldenberg, R. L., Hickey, C. A., Jin, J., & Dubard, M. B. (1993). Health behavior and outcomes in sequential pregnancies of black and white adolescents. *Journal of the American Medical Association, 269*(11), 1401–1403.

Blythe, M., & Diaz, A. (2007). Contraception and adolescents. *Pediatrics, 120*(5), 1135–1148.

Bowen, M. (1971). The use of family theory in clinical practice. In J. Haley (Ed.), *Changing families*. New York: Grune & Stratton.

Brown, H. N., Saunders, R. B., & Dick, M. J. (1999). Preventing secondary pregnancy in adolescents: A model program. *Health Care for Women International, 20*(1), 5–15.

Bulcholz, E. S., & Gol, B. (1986). More than playing house: A developmental perspective on the strengths in teenage motherhood. *Theory and Review*, 347–357.

Centers for Disease Control and Prevention (CDC). (2006). *Youth risk behavior survey*. Atlanta: U.S. Department of Health and Human Services.

Chedraui, P. (2008). Pregnancy among young adolescents: trends, risk factors and maternal-perinatal outcome. *Journal of Perinatal Medicine, 36*(3), 256–259.

Cockey, C. D. (1997, June). Preventing teen pregnancy. It's time to stop kidding around. *Lifelines*, 32–40.

Coley, R. L., & Chase-Lansdale, P. L. (1998). Adolescent pregnancy and parenthood. Recent evidence and future directions. *American Psychologist, 53*(2), 152–166.

Collins, R., Elliott, M., Berry, S., et al. (2004). Watching sex on television predicts adolescent initiation of sexual behavior. *Pediatrics, 114*(3), 280–289.

Cook, R., Erdman, J., & Dickens, B. (2007). Respecting adolescents' confidentiality and reproductive and sexual choices. *International Journal of Gynecology & Obstetrics, 98*(2), 182–187

Coyle, K., Kirby, D., Parcel, G., et al. (1996). Safer choices: A multicomponent school-based HIV/STD and pregnancy prevention program for adolescents. *Journal of School Health, 66*(3), 89–94.

Crowe, L. C., & George, W. H. (1989). Alcohol and human sexuality: Review and integration. *Psychological Bulletin, 102*, 374–386.

Darabi, K. F., Jones, J., Varga, P. L., & Hourse, M. (1982). Evaluation of sex education outreach. *Adolescence, 17*(65), 57–64.

Davis, K. A. (1980). *A theory of teenage pregnancy in the U.S. adolescent. Pregnancy and childbearing*. Washington, DC: Department of Health and Human Services.

Davis, S. M., & Harris, M. B. (1982). Sexual knowledge, sexual interests, and sources of sexual information of rural and urban adolescents from three cultures. *Adolescence, 18*(66), 471–492.

Department of Health and Human Services (DHHS). (1990). *Healthy people 2000: National health objectives* (Publication No. 91-50213). Washington, DC: U.S. Government Printing Office.

Delpisheh, A., Kelly, Y., Rizwan, S., Attia, E., Drammond, S., & Brabin, B. (2007). Population attributable risk for adverse pregnancy outcomes related to smoking in adolescents and adults. *Public Health, 121*(11), 861–868.

Desmond, A. M. (1994). Adolescent pregnancy in the United States: Not a minority issue. *Health Care for Women International, 15*(4), 325–331.

Diehl, K. (1997). Adolescent mothers: What produces positive mother–infant interaction? *Maternal Child Nursing, 22*, 89–95.

DiIorio, C., Hockenbeery-Eaton, M., Maibach, E., Rivero, S., & Miller, K. (1996). The content of African American mothers' discussions with their adolescents about sex. *Journal of Family Nursing, 2*(4), 365–382.

Drake, P. (1996). Addressing the needs of pregnant adolescents. *Journal of Gynecological and Neonatal Nursing, 25*(6), 518–524.

DuPlessis, H. M., Bell, R., & Richards, T. (1997). Adolescent pregnancy: Understanding the impact of age and race on outcomes. *Journal of Adolescent Health, 20*, 187–197.

East, P., Reyes, B., & Horn, E. (2007). Association between adolescent pregnancy and a family history of teenage births. *Perspectives on Sexual & Reproductive Health, 39*(2), 108–115.

Fagot, B., Pears, K., Capaldi, D., Crosby, L., & Leve, C. (1998). Becoming an adolescent father: Precursors and parenting. *Developmental Psychology, 34*(6), 1209–1219.

Fergus, S., Zimmerman, M. A. (2005). Adolescent resilience: A framework for understanding healthy development in the face of risk. *Annual Reviews of Public Health, 26*, 399–419.

Fiscella, K., Kitzman, H. J., Cole, R. E., Sidora, K. J., & Olds, D. (1998). Does child abuse predict adolescent pregnancy? *Pediatrics, 101* (4 Pt. 1), 620–624.

Fisher, S. M. (1984). The psychodynamics of teenage pregnancy and motherhood. In M. Sugar (Ed.), *Adolescent parenthood*. Jamaica, NY: Spectrum Publications.

Flavell, J. H., Miller, P. H., & Miller, S. A. (1993). *Cognitive development* (3rd ed.). Englewood Cliffs, NJ: Prentice Hall.

Flynn, L., Budd, M., & Modelski, J. (2008). Enhancing resource utilization among pregnant adolescents. *Public Health Nursing, 25*(2), 140–148.

Fortenberry, J. D., Orr, D. P., Katz, B. P., Brizendine, E. J., & Blythe, M. J. (1997). Sex under the influence. *Sexually Transmitted Diseases, 24*(6), 313–319.

Foster, H. W. (1997). The campaign to prevent teen pregnancy. *Journal of Pediatric Nursing, 12*(2), 120–121.

Geronimus, A. (1986). The effects of race, residence and prenatal care on the relationship of maternal age to neonatal mortality. *American Journal of Public Health, 76*(12), 1412–1421.

Grobler, C., Botma, Y., Jacobs, A., & Nel, M. (2007). Beliefs of grade six learners' regarding adolescent pregnancy and sex. *Curationis, 30*(1), 32–40.

Grogger, J., & Bronars, S. (1993). The socioeconomic consequences of teenage childbearing: Finding from a natural experiment. *Family Planning Perspectives, 25*(4), 156–161, 174.

Heavey, E., Moysich, K., Hyland, A., Druschel, C., & Sill, M. (2008). Female adolescents' perceptions of male partners' pregnancy desire. *Journal of Midwifery & Women's Health, 53*(4), 338–344.

Hoffman, S. D. (2006). *By the numbers: The public costs of teen childbearing*. Washington, DC: National Campaign to Prevent Teen Pregnancy.

Howard, M., & McCabe, J. A. (1992). An information and skills approach for younger teens: Postponing sexual involvement program. In B. C. Miller, J. T. Card, R. L. Paifoff, & J. I. Peterson

(Eds.), *Preventing adolescent pregnancy.* Newbury Park, CA: Sage Publications.

Howard, M., & Mitchell, M. E. (1993). Prevention teenage pregnancy: Some questions to be answered and some answers to be questioned. *Pediatric Annals, 22*(2), 109–118.

Hutchinson, M., Jemmott, J., Jemmott, L., Braverman, P., & Fong, G. (2003). The role of mother-daughter sexual risk communication in reducing sexual risk behaviors among urban adolescent females: A prospective study. *Journal of Adolescent Health, 33*(2), 98–107.

Hutchinson, M., Jemmott, L., Wood, E., Hewitt, H., Kawha, E., Waldron, N., et al. (2007, March). Culture-specific factors contributing to HIV risk among Jamaican adolescents. *JANAC: Journal of the Association of Nurses in AIDS Care, 18*(2), 35–47.

Ispa, J., Sable, M., Porter, N., & Csizmadia, A. (2007). Pregnancy acceptance, parenting stress, and toddler attachment in low-income black families. *Journal of Marriage & Family, 69*(1), 1–13.

Jemmott, L. S. (1993). AIDS risk among black male adolescents: Implications for nursing intervention. *Journal of Pediatric Health Care, 7*, 3–11.

Jemmott, L. S., & Jemmott, J. B., III. (1990). Sexual knowledge, attitudes, and risky sexual behavior among inner-city black male adolescents. *Journal of Adolescent Research, 5*, 346–369.

Jemmott, L. S., & Jemmott, J. B., III. (1992). Increasing condom-use intentions among sexually active inner city black adolescent women: Effects of an AIDS prevention program. *Nursing Research, 41*, 273–279.

Jemmott, L. S., & Jemmott, J. B., III (2007). Applying the theory of reasoned action to HIV risk reduction behavioral interventions. In A. Icek, D. Albarracin, & R. Hornik (Eds.), *Prediction and change of health behavior: Applying the reasoned action approach* (pp. 93–100). Mahwah, NJ: Lawrence Erlbaum Associates.

Jemmott, J., Jemmott, L., & Fong, G. (1998). Abstinence and safer sex HIV risk-reduction interventions for African American adolescents: A randomized controlled trial. *Journal of the American Medical Association, 279*(19), 1529–1536.

Jemmott, L. S., Jemmott, J. B., & O'Leary, A. (2007). Effects on sexual risk behavior and STD rate of brief HIV/STD prevention interventions for African American women in primary care settings: Effects on sexual risk behavior and STD incidence. *American Journal of Public Health, 97*, 1034–1040.

Jemmott, L., Jemmott, J., Hutchinson, M., Cederbaum, J., & O'Leary, A. (2008, March). Sexually transmitted infection/HIV risk reduction interventions in clinical practice settings. *JOGNN: Journal of Obstetric, Gynecologic, & Neonatal Nursing, 37*(2), 137–145.

Kahn, J. G., Brindis, C. D., & Glei, D. A. (1999). Pregnancies averted among U.S. teenagers by the use of contraceptives. *Family Planning Perspectives, 31*(1), 29–34.

Kaiser Family Foundation. (1998). *National survey of teens: Teens talk about dating, intimacy and their sexual experiences.* Menlo Park, CA: Author.

Kalmus, D., Davidson, A., Cahall, A., Laraque, D., Cassell C. (2003). Preventing sexual risk behaviors and pregnancy among teenagers: Linking research and programs. *Perspectives on Sexual and Reproductive Health, 35*, 87–93.

Kandel, D. B. (1990). Early onset of adolescent sexual behavior and drug involvement. *Journal of Marriage and the Family, 52*, 783–798.

Kenney, J. W., Reinholtz, C., & Angelini, P. J. (1997). Ethnic differences in childhood sexual abuse and teenage pregnancy. *Journal of Adolescent Health, 21*(1), 3–10.

Kirby, D. (1997). *No easy answers: Research findings on programs to reduce teen pregnancy* (Summary). Washington, DC: The National Campaign to Prevent Teen Pregnancy.

Kirby, D. (2001). Understanding what works and what doesn't in reducing adolescent sexual risk-taking. *Family Planning Perspectives, 33*(6), 276–281.

Kirby, D., Resnick, M. D., Downes, B., et al. (1993). The effects of school-based health clinics in St. Paul on school-wide birthrates. *Family Planning Perspectives, 25*(1), 12–16.

Kokotailo, P. K., Langhough, R. E., Cox, N. S., Davidson, S. R., & Fleming, M. F. (1994). Cigarette, alcohol and other drug use among small city pregnant adolescents. *Journal of Adolescent Health, 15*, 366–373.

Landry, E., Bertrand, J., Cherry, F., & Rich, J. (1986). Teenage pregnancy in New Orleans: Factors that differentiate teens who deliver, abort, and successfully contracept. *Journal of Youth and Adolescence, 15*, 259–274.

Lederman, R., Chan, W., & Roberts-Gray, C. (2008). Parent–adolescent relationship education (PARE): Program delivery to reduce risks for adolescent pregnancy and STDs. *Behavioral Medicine, 33*(4), 137–143.

Lederman, R., & Mian T. (2003). The parent–adolescent relationship education (PARE) program: A curriculum for prevention of STDs and pregnancy in middle-school youth. *Behavioral Medicine, 3*(29), 33–41.

Lee, S. H., & Grubbs, L. M. (1995). Pregnant teenagers' reasons for seeking or delaying prenatal care. *Clinical Nursing Research, 4*(1), 38–49.

Lemay, C., Cashman, S., Elfenbein, D., & Felice, M. (2007). Adolescent mothers' attitudes toward contraceptive use before and after pregnancy. *Journal of Pediatric & Adolescent Gynecology, 20*(4), 233–240.

Leppert, P. C., Namerow, P. B., & Barker, D. (1986). Pregnancy outcomes among adolescents and older women receiving comprehensive prenatal care. *Journal of Adolescent Health Care, 7*, 112–117.

Levy, S. R., Perhats, C., Nash-Johnson, M., & Welter, J. F. (1992). Reducing the risks in pregnant teens who are very young and those with mild mental retardation. *Mental Retardation, 30*(4), 195–203.

Lieberman, E. J. (1980). *The psychological consequences of adolescent pregnancy and abortion: Adolescent pregnancy and childbearing.* Washington, DC: Department of Health and Human Services.

Loda, F. A., Speizer, I. S., Martin, K. L., Skatrud, J. D., & Bennett, T. A. (1997). Programs and services to prevent pregnancy, childbearing, and poor birth outcomes among adolescents in rural areas of the Southeastern United States. *Journal of Adolescent Health, 21*, 157–166.

Lowe, S. (2008). It's all one big circle: Welfare discourse and the everyday lives of urban adolescents. *Journal of Sociology & Social Welfare, 35*(3), 173–194.

Males, M. (1993). School-age pregnancy: Why hasn't prevention worked? *Journal of School Health, 63*(10), 429–432.

Marshall, E., Buckner, E., & Powell, K. (1991). Evaluation of a teen parent program designed to reduce child abuse and neglect and to strengthen families. *Journal of Child Adolescent Psychiatric and Mental Health Nursing, 4*(3), 96–100.

Miller, B. (2002). Family influences on adolescent sexual and contraceptive behavior. *Journal of Sex Research, 39*, 22–26.

Morrison, D. (1985). Adolescent contraceptive behavior: A review. *Psychological Bulletin, 98*, 538–568.

Mott, S. (1990). Adolescence. In S. Mott, S. James, & A. Sperhac (Eds.), *Care of children and families.* Redwood City, CA: Addison-Wesley.

Olds, D. (1992). Home visitation for pregnant women and parents of young children. *American Journal of Diseases of Children, 146*(6), 704–708.

Olds, D., Henderson, C., & Kitzman, H. (1994). Does prenatal and infancy nurse home visitation have enduring effects on qualities of parental caregiving and child health at 25 to 50 months of life? *Pediatrics, 93*(1), 89–98.

Olds, D., Henderson, C., Tatelbaum, R., & Chamberlin, R. (1988). Improving the life-course development of socially disadvantaged mothers: A randomized trial of nurse home visitation. *American Journal of Public Health, 78*(11), 1436–1445.

Orshan, S. A. (1996). Acculturation, perceived social support, and self-esteem in primigravida Puerto Rican teenagers. *Western Journal of Nursing Research, 18*(4), 460–473.

Pittman, K., & Adams, G. (1988). *Teenage pregnancy: An advocate's guide to the numbers.* Washington, DC: Children's Defense Fund.

Plouffe, L., & White, E. W. (1996). Adolescent obstetrics and gynecology: Children having children—Can it be controlled? *Current Opinion in Obstetrics and Gynecology, 8*(5), 335–338.

Pollack, A. E. (1992). Teen contraception in the 1990s. *Journal of School Health, 62*(7), 288–293.

Resnick, M. D. (2000). Protective factors, resiliency and health youth development. *Adolescent Medicine,* 157–165.

Rew, L. (1998). The adolescent. In N. C. Frisch & L. E. Frisch (Eds.), *Psychiatric mental health nursing.* Albany, NY: Delmar.

Reynoso, T. C., Felice, M. E., & Shragg, G. P. (1993). Does American acculturation affect outcome of Mexican-American teenage pregnancy? *Journal of Adolescent Health, 14*, 257–261.

Robinson, R. B., & Frank, D. L. (1994). The relation between self-esteem, sexual activity, and pregnancy. *Adolescence, 29*(113), 26–35.

Rogers, M. M., Peoples-Sheps, M. D., & Suchindran, C. (1996). Impact of a social support program on teenage prenatal care use and pregnancy outcomes. *Journal of Adolescent Health, 19*, 132–140.

Rolleri, L., Wilson, M., Paluzzi, P., & Sedivy, V. (2008). Building capacity of state adolescent pregnancy prevention coalitions to implement science-based approaches. *American Journal of Community Psychology, 41*(3/4), 225–234.

Roye, C. F., & Balk, S. J. (1996). The relationship of partner support to outcomes for teenage mothers and their children: A review. *Journal of Adolescent Health, 19*, 86–93.

Santelli, J., Lindberg, L., Finer, L., & Singh, S. (2007). Explaining recent declines in adolescent pregnancy in the United States: The contribution of abstinence and improved contraceptive use. *Contemporary Sexuality, 41*(7), 8–12.

Schaffer, M., Jost, R., Pederson, B., & Lair, M. (2008). Pregnancy-free club: A strategy to prevent repeat adolescent pregnancy. *Public Health Nursing, 25*(4), 304–311.

Silverman, J. G., Raj, A., Mucci, L. A., & Hathaway, J. E. (2001). Dating violence against adolescent girls and associated substance abuse, unhealthy weight control, sexual risk behavior, pregnancy, and suicidality. *JAMA, 286*, 572–579.

SmithBattle, L. (2007). Legacies of advantage and disadvantage: The case of teen mothers. *Public Health Nursing, 24*(5), 409–420.

Sonenstein, F., Stewart, K., Lindberg, L., Pernas, M., & Williams, S. (1997). Practical advice and program philosophy. In *Involving males in preventing teen pregnancy* (pp. 153–174). Washington, DC: Urban Institute Press.

Sorenson, D. (1973). *Adolescent sexuality in contemporary America.* New York: World Press.

Stevens-Simon, C., Kelly, L., Singer, D., & Cox, A. (1996). Why pregnant adolescents say they did not use contraceptives prior to contraception. *Journal of Adolescent Health, 19*, 48–53.

Terry-Humen, E., & Manlove, J. (2003). Just who is having sex before age 15? Dating and sexual experience among middle school youth: Analysis of the NLSY97. In B. Albert, S. Brown, & C. M. Flanigan (Eds.), *14 and younger: The sexual behavior of young adolescents (Full Report).* Washington, DC: The National Campaign to Prevent Teen Pregnancy.

Thompson, P. J., Powell, M. J., Patterson, R. J., & Ellerbee, S. M. (1995). Adolescent parenting: Outcomes and maternal perceptions. *Journal of Obstetrical, Gynecological and Neonatal Nursing, 24*(8), 713–717.

Tocce, K., Sheeder, J., & Teal, S. (2008). The road to repeat adolescent pregnancy is paved with good intentions. *Contraception, 78*(2), 176–176.

Toledo-Dreves, V., Zabin, L. S., & Emerson, M. (1995). Duration of adolescent sexual relationships before and after conception. *Journal of Adolescent Health, 17*, 163–172.

Trad, P. V. (1999). Assessing the patterns that prevent teenage pregnancy. *Adolescence, 34*(133), 221–240.

Ventura, S., Abma, J., Mosher, W., & Henshaw, S. (2006). *Recent trends in teenage pregnancy in the United States 1990–2002.* Hyattsville, MD: National Center for Health Statistics.

Villarruel, A., Jemmott, L., Jemmott, J., & Eakin, B. (2006). Recruitment and retention of Latino adolescents to a research study: Lessons learned from a randomized clinical trial. *Journal for Specialists in Pediatric Nursing, 11*(4), 244–250.

Villarruel, A., Jemmott, J., Jemmott, L., & Ronis, D. (2007). Predicting condom use among sexually experienced Latino adolescents. *Western Journal of Nursing Research, 29*(6), 724–738.

Whitbeck, L. B., Conger, R. D., & Simons, R. I. (1993). Minor deviant behaviors and adolescent sexual activity. *Youth and Society, 25*(1), 24–37.

Widom, C. S., & Kuhns, J. B. (1996). Childhood victimization and subsequent risk for promiscuity, prostitution, and teenage pregnancy: A prospective study. *American Journal of Public Health, 86*(11), 1607–1612.

Wilson, R., Alio, A., Kirby, R., & Salihu, H. (2008). Young maternal age and risk of intrapartum stillbirth. *Archives of Gynecology & Obstetrics, 278*(3), 231–236.

Wood, K., Maforah, F., & Jewkes, R. (1998). "He forced me to love him": Putting violence on adolescent sexual health agendas. *Social Science & Medicine, 47*(2), 233–42.

Yoder, B. A., & Young, M. K. (1997). Neonatal outcomes of teenage pregnancy in a military population. *Obstetrics & Gynecology, 90*(4), 500–506.

Zabin, L. S., & Clark, S. D. (1981). Why they delay: A study of teenage family planning clinic patients. *Family Planning Perspective, 13*, 205–217.

Zabin, L. S., Emerson, M. R., Ringers, P. A., & Sedivy, V. (1996). Adolescents with negative pregnancy test results: An accessible at-risk group. *Journal of the American Medical Association, 275*(2), 113–117.

Zeck, W., Bjelic-Radisic, V., Haas, J., & Greimel, E. (2007). Impact of adolescent pregnancy on the future life of young mothers in terms of social, familial, and educational changes. *Journal of Adolescent Health, 41*(4), 380–388.

Zeck, W., Walcher, W., Tamussino, K., & Lang, U. (2008). Adolescent primiparas: Changes in obstetrical risk between 1983–1987 and 1999–2005. *Journal of Obstetrics & Gynaecology Research, 34*(2), 195–198.

Zelnik, M., & Kantner, J. F. (1979). Reasons for nonuse of contraception by sexually active women age 15–19. *Family Planning Perspectives, 11*(5), 289–296.

Zoccolillo, M., Meyers, J., & Assiter, S. (1997). Conduct disorder, substance dependence, and adolescent motherhood. *American Journal of Orthopsychiatry, 67*(1), 152–157.

Zuckerman, B. S., Walker, D. K., Frank, D. A., Chase, C., & Hamburg, B. (1984). Adolescent pregnancy: Biobehavioral determinants of outcome. *Journal of Pediatrics, 105*(6), 857–863.

# CHAPTER 29
# Disabilities and Health

Valerie M. Rachal and Linda G. McDowell

Visit **http://nursing.jbpub.com/communityhealth** for interactive exercises, review questions, Web links, and more.

The move toward community services for individuals with disabilities has greatly expanded the role of the community health nurse. Although in the past this population was served primarily by nurses and physicians in institutional settings (hospitals, rehabilitation centers, nursing homes, or state residential facilities), there has been a strong movement to include people with disabilities in community life and offer a comprehensive array of individualized, community-based services.

The only disability in life is a bad attitude.

*—Scott Hamilton*

We should never walk by somebody who is in a wheelchair and be afraid of them or think of them as a stranger. It could be us—in fact, it is us.

*—Christopher Reeve, May 4, 1998*

What do you think about Scott Hamilton's and Christopher Reeve's quotes about persons with disabilities? Some have referred to people without disabilities as being "temporarily abled." How does such a description compare to the quotes? Are there disabilities that limit a person's choices in life? Have you experienced limited function either physically or mentally at any time in your life? What in your environment influenced the way that you felt?

## CHAPTER FOCUS

**Definitions**

**Incidence of Disabilities**

**Historical Context of Disability Services and Disability Legislation**

**Current Situation for People with Disabilities**
- Situation for Adults
- Situation for Children

**Legislation Protecting the Rights of People with Disabilities**

**Appropriate Language for Communicating About Persons with Disabilities**

**Community Living Needs of People Who Have Disabilities**
- Homes of Their Own
- An Accessible Community
- Meaningful Work
- Relationships
- Recreation

**Services for Individuals with Disabilities**
- Case Management
- Educational Programming
- Transition from Education to Work and Living in the Community
- Rehabilitation
- Medical Technology
- Nonmedical Assistive Technology
- Assistance Animals

**Ethical Issues Related to Disabilities**

***Healthy People 2010* Objectives Related to Disabilities**

**Roles of the Community Health Nurse**

## QUESTIONS TO CONSIDER

After reading this chapter, answer the following questions:

1. What is a disability?
2. What are the legal protections for a person with disabilities?
3. How should we communicate with a person with disabilities?
4. What are community living needs related to caring for a population with disabilities?
5. Which services are available for persons with disabilities?
6. Are there ethical issues that influence the care of persons with disabilities?
7. What are specific roles for the community health nurse in caring for a population with disabilities?

## KEY TERMS

| | | | |
|---|---|---|---|
| Assistive technology device | Early intervention | Medical assistive devices | Person-centered planning |
| Case management | Individualized education plans | Mental impairment | Physical impairment |
| Developmental disability | Individualized family service plan | People-first language | Rehabilitation |
| Disability | Informed consent | Personal care attendant | Respite care |

APPROXIMATELY 18% OF INDIVIDUALS in the United States have some kind of a disability, and 12% have a severe disability (U.S. Census Bureau, 2006). We can expect an increase in the number of people with disabilities (incidence of disability increases with age) as the baby-boomer generation ages and the life expectancy of the general population increases. Primarily through development of advanced surgical techniques and medications, medicine has made great strides in increasing the survival of infants, children, and adults with disabilities. Now, the more difficult task of improving the overall quality of life for these individuals is at hand. Society, including members with disabilities, has come to expect not only a long life, but a rich, fulfilling life as well.

Community health nursing is poised as the key profession to integrate knowledge of the healthcare needs of people with disabilities with the often more challenging needs related to full inclusion in community life. In addition to possessing the knowledge required to serve in the traditional role of caregiver, the community health nurse must be well versed in disability legislation; issues of accessibility, work, housing, transportation, and recreation; use of technology; and case management strategies required to navigate the complex and inconsistent service system presently in place.

## Definitions

Terms can be useful when people who share something in common are grouped together for easier communication about them. Terms can be harmful, however, when the focus is on the label and anticipated problems rather than on the unique capabilities of each individual. Labels usually generate predictions of what a person can or cannot do, and a person tends to act based on the expectations of others. Each person within a particular disability category has different abilities and will require varying levels of assistance and support. To offer appropriate help, the community health nurse should get to know the capabilities and needs of each person before making assumptions about their needs based on a disability label (DiLeo, 2007).

The term **disability** "is now being used to indicate that an individual has some functional limitation due to an alteration in anatomy (internal or external physical configuration, such as short stature or missing limbs) or physiology (organic processes, such as paralysis, decreased cardiac function, or ineffectiveness of the immune system)" (Hablutzel & McMahon, 1992). For the purposes of protection by the Americans with Disabilities Act (ADA), *disability* is defined as "(a) a physical or mental impairment that substantially limits one or more of the major life activities of such individual; (b) a record of such an impairment; or (c) being regarded as having such an impairment" (U.S. Department of Justice, 1992, p. 8). If an individual meets any one of these three criteria, he or she is considered an individual with a disability for the purposes covered by the ADA. When enacting the ADA in 1990, Congress adopted the same basic definition of disability first used in the Rehabilitation Act of

> ## CULTURAL CONNECTION
>
> Specific cultural groups may find it difficult to encourage independence and autonomy for a family member with a disability. They may instead value "doing for the patient" instead of promoting self-care. How can the community health nurse preserve respect for the family's cultural values while promoting the patient's autonomy?

1973 and the Fair Housing Amendments of 1988. Congress used the term *disability* rather than *handicap* in an effort to use up-to-date, currently accepted terminology. The term *handicap* is not a synonym for disability and is now rarely used other than to describe parking places and facility accessibility.

**Physical impairment** according to the ADA is "any physiological disorder or condition, cosmetic disfigurement, or anatomical loss affecting one or more of the . . . body systems," including, for example, orthopedic, visual, and hearing impairments; cerebral palsy; epilepsy; muscular dystrophy; multiple sclerosis; and human immunodeficiency virus (HIV) disease (symptomatic or asymptomatic) (U.S. Department of Justice, 1992, p. 8).

**Mental impairment** "is any mental or psychological disorder, such as mental retardation, organic brain syndrome, emotional or mental illness, and specific learning disabilities" (U.S. Department of Justice, 1992, p. 8).

As defined in the Developmental Disabilities Assistance and Bill of Rights Act Amendments of 1996, an individual is considered to have a **developmental disability** when "physical or mental impairments manifest before age 22 that continue indefinitely, resulting in substantial functional limitations in three or more life areas, and . . . reflect a need for lifelong or extended individually coordinated services."

## Incidence of Disabilities

Approximately one in five Americans has some type of disability causing difficulty in performing certain functions (e.g., seeing, hearing, walking, talking, climbing stairs, lifting, carrying); has difficulty with activities of daily living (e.g., bathing, dressing, toileting, feeding); or has difficulty with certain social roles (e.g., doing schoolwork, performing household chores, working). About one in ten Americans has a disability so severe that he or she is unable to perform certain basic activities, such as walking, dressing, or speaking; must use assistive devices such as a wheelchair or scooter for mobility; or needs personal assistance to perform basic activities. Among children ages 6 to 14, about one in eight has some type of disability. The number or percentage of adults with a disability is more difficult to determine and will not represent the same percentages as in the school-age population. Some disabilities, recognized during the school years, become difficult to detect in adult settings, even though the impact may be significant. For

**Table 29-1**    Examples of Disability, Etiology, Incidence, and Effects

| Disability | Etiology | Incidence | Effects (Selected) |
|---|---|---|---|
| ■ Amputation | Trauma, bone cancer, diabetes | Not available | Impaired mobility |
| ■ Autism | Brain damage, abnormality in brain development, genetic predisposition | 10/10,000 live births[1] | Impaired reciprocal social interaction, impaired communication and imaginative activity, markedly restricted repertoire of interests and activities |
| ■ Cerebral palsy | Perinatal anoxia, trauma, intraventricular hemorrhage, or stroke; trauma, meningitis in early childhood | 1.4–2.4/1,000 births[1] | Difficulty with balance, coordination, and movement, hypertonicity; associated with sensory impairments, seizures, mental retardation |
| ■ Down syndrome | Genetic; extra chromosome 21 | 1/700–1/1,000 live births[1] | Mental retardation, hypotonia, physical characteristics, sensory impairments, decreased immunity, frequent respiratory infections and otitis media, increased incidence of leukemia, thyroid problems, early onset Alzheimer's-type dementia |
| ■ Duchenne's muscular dystrophy (MD) | Genetic, inherited as a sex-linked trait, affects males | 1/3,500 males[1] | Increasing muscle weakness beginning with waddling gait and resulting in need for crutches or wheelchair; eventually heart and diaphragm are affected; usually causes death before adulthood |
| ■ Fetal alcohol syndrome (FAS) | Maternal alcohol ingestion resulting in prenatal exposure (leading known cause of mental retardation) | 1–2/1,000 births[1] | Mental retardation, decreased height and weight, facial characteristics, behavior problems including hyperactivity and noncompliance |
| ■ Fragile X syndrome | Genetic; inherited as a sex-linked trait | 1/1,500 males 1/500 females[1] | Mental retardation, hypotonia, physical characteristics, behavior problems such as self-stimulatory behavior, self-injurious behavior, and aggression |
| ■ Hearing impairment | Otitis media (middle ear infections), congenital malformation, genetic, exposure to maternal virus or drug, meningitis, head trauma | 1/1,000 infants born with severe to profound hearing loss[1] | Ranges from mild hearing impairment to deafness; developmental delay, language impairment, need for prenatal hearing aid, FM trainer, speech-language therapy, sign language |
| ■ Polio | Polio virus causes paralysis below part of spinal column damaged by virus | Eliminated since 1991 but 16,316 cases of paralytic polio occurred during the period 1951–1954[3] | Paralysis, complications related to immobility (decubiti, fractures), postpolio syndrome in mid to late adulthood causing increased severity of symptoms |
| ■ Spina bifida (myelomeningocele) | Multifactorial etiology; environmental causes including folic acid deficiency and genetic influences | 60/100,000 births[1] | Paralysis below level of defect, impaired ambulation requiring crutches and walker or wheelchair, lack of bowel and bladder control, hydrocephalus requiring shunt, seizures, vision problems, mental retardation, complications related to immobility |
| ■ Spinal cord injury (SCI) | Trauma from diving accidents and motor vehicle accidents | 250,000 individuals with SCI in the United States[2] | Paralysis, hypotonia and muscle wasting, incontinence, complications related to immobility and repeated catheterization; high-level injuries can also cause inability to breathe without assistance |
| ■ Traumatic brain injury (TBI) | Trauma from motor vehicle accidents, gunshots, child abuse | 71–125/100,000 (22% of those died)[2] | Motor, communication, cognitive, sensory, and behavioral deficits |
| ■ Vision impairment | Prenatal exposure to viruses or bacteria, prematurity and oxygen treatment, eye trauma, chemical burns, diabetes, glaucoma, cataracts | 1/3,000 children are blind[1]; vision impairment increases significantly in older adults | Ranges from poor sight to total blindness |

1. Batshaw, 1997.
2. Marino, 1999.
3. CDC, 1999.

| Table 29-2 | Popular Films Portraying Characters with Disabilties | | |
|---|---|---|---|
| **Film** | **Disability** | **Film** | **Disability** |
| ■ *As Good as It Gets* | Obsessive-compulsive disorder | ■ *Man Without a Face* | Craniofacial defect |
| ■ *Benny and Joon* | Schizophrenia | ■ *The Miracle Worker* | Deaf/blind |
| ■ *Best Boy* | Mental retardation | ■ *My Left Foot* | Cerebral palsy |
| ■ *Born on the Fourth of July* | Spinal cord injury | ■ *One Flew Over the Cuckoo's Nest* | Mental illness/ institutional care |
| ■ *Charley* | Mental retardation | ■ *Philadelphia* | AIDS |
| ■ *Children of a Lesser God* | Hearing impairment | ■ *Rain Man* | Autism |
| ■ *The Elephant Man* | Physical disability | ■ *Rear Window* | Spinal cord injury |
| ■ *First Do No Harm* | Epilepsy | ■ *Regarding Henry* | Traumatic brain injury |
| ■ *The Fisher King* | Schizophrenia | ■ *Scent of a Woman* | Visual impairment |
| ■ *Forrest Gump* | Mental retardation | ■ *Sling Blade* | Mental retardation |
| ■ *The Heart Is a Lonely Hunter* | Hearing impairment | ■ *There's Something About Mary* | Mental retardation |
| ■ *La Strada* | Mental retardation | ■ *What About Bob?* | Anxiety disorder |
| ■ *The Last Picture Show* | Mental retardation | ■ *What's Eating Gilbert Grape?* | Mental retardation |
| ■ *Lorenzo's Oil* | Adrenoleukodystrophy (ALD) | | |

instance, individuals with learning disabilities or mental illness may go unidentified for long periods and are often not counted in studies reporting the incidence of disabilities in adulthood. The incidence of disability increases significantly with age; about half of adults age 65 and older have a disability. As the population continues to age, we can expect the proportion of the population having disabilities to increase accordingly (Bernstein, 2006). Table 29-1 provides examples of disabling conditions, and their etiologies, incidence, and effects on the individual.

The effects of disability on the individual, family, and community vary and are related to a number of variables, including age and rapidity of onset, cause, and severity of the disability. Personal characteristics such as determination and resiliency along with available family and community support also play a role in determining the impact of a disability. Table 29-2 lists recommended popular films that portray main characters with disabilities.

## Historical Context of Disability Services and Disability Legislation

Beirne-Smith, Patton, and Kim (2006) paint a clear picture of how society's values and historical events have influenced the lives of people with disabilities. Before the 1700s, services for persons with disabilities were virtually nonexistent. In the United States, the family unit was of prime importance, so most of the responsibility for caring for a member with a disability rested on the family. The colonies also enacted laws that provided some support in the forms of poorhouses and workhouses. During the first part of the 1800s, there was an attitude of optimism, and it was believed that children with mental retardation or other disabilities could be trained, "cured," and returned to the community as productive citizens. By the late 1800s, however, society recognized that these individuals could not be "cured." People with disabilities were then pitied, resulting in decreased opportunities for systematic training and increased formation of institutions. By the end of the 1800s, the general attitude of pity shifted to fear. Citizens became concerned that "mentally defective" people were dangerous, and society responded with restricted marriages, mandatory sterilization, and institutionalization (Cegelka & Prehm, 1982). This alarmist attitude was based on a fear of the inheritability of mental defectiveness and its perceived relationship to poverty, crime, incorrigibility, and disease.

One ironically positive occurrence in the early 1900s was the return of World War I veterans with war-caused disabilities. As a result, in 1920, the Vocational Rehabilitation Act brought medical and rehabilitation services not only to veterans, but also to others who displayed a need. President Franklin D. Roosevelt's administration improved the situation somewhat with passage of the Social Security Act of 1935 and a supportive attitude toward public welfare programs. As more veterans with disabilities returned home during World War II, a concern for the rights of citizens with disabilities grew. Although government services had finally become available for individuals with disabilities in the 1920s, these services continued to be provided in ways that segregated people with disabilities from others until the 1970s (Berkowitz, 1987). During most of the twentieth century, "literally, through institutionalization, and subtly,

### ETHICAL CONNECTION

Persons with disabilities may become depressed to the point of becoming suicidal. This state is more common in persons when they become disabled because of an accident upon the realization that the disability is likely to be permanent. How would you respond to a patient whom you encounter in a home setting who asked you about assisted suicide?

**ENVIRONMENTAL CONNECTION**

Persons with a mobility and/or paralytic disability may be at greater risk for environmental toxin exposure in the home. Community health nurses should do an environmental assessment of the home at the level of the patient's interaction with the physical environment. Patient education and specific prevention measures should be implemented and evaluated to ensure patient safety and promote patient autonomy.

through negative attitudes and behaviors, people with disabilities [were] isolated from the social mainstream and denied the benefits and opportunities available to people without disabilities" (Ward, 1996, p. 4).

Fortunately, advances in medical care such as the development of antibiotics in the 1940s and 1950s and increasingly successful surgical procedures for spina bifida, hydrocephalus, and congenital heart defects since the 1970s, coupled with developmental and rehabilitation services, have enabled people with disabilities to live longer. Public outrage and court involvement in response to abusive conditions in institutions, along with research on the negative effects of institutionalization, led to the development of services in local communities in the 1960s and 1970s. With the expectation that most individuals with disabilities will live to adulthood, society and policy makers have been forced to consider strategies to protect the rights of these individuals.

## Current Situation for People with Disabilities

### ▪ Situation for Adults

In 2004, the Harris survey of Americans with disabilities reported a number of facts related to the quality of life for people with disabilities in the United States. Although a majority of Americans with disabilities believe that life improved for people with disabilities over the past 10 years, adults with disabilities still lag behind other adults in most aspects of life. Examining the areas of employment, housing/income, education, and health care highlights how the existence of a disability continues to place an individual at risk in many aspects of life. In the area of employment, three of ten adults with disabilities are working (35%), compared with eight out of ten adults without disabilities (78%); this statistic remained the same for the past 10 years. For housing/income, one in three (26%) adults with disabilities is in very-low-income housing with an annual income of less than $15,000, compared with one in eight (9%) of those without disabilities. When examining the area of education, data show that one in five adults with disabilities (21%) has not completed high school, compared with one in ten adults without disabilities (10%). Finally, in the area of health care, one in five adults with disabilities (21%) did not get needed medical care on at least one occasion during the past year, compared with one in ten adults without disabilities (11%) (National Organization on Disability, 2004).

Available statistics between 1982 and 2001 indicated a change in residential supports provided to people with cognitive and developmental disabilities. There has been a major shift from institutional services to services in relatively small community settings with three or fewer residents. Instead of state governments being the primary provider of services, state governments are now largely a purchaser of services, with 85% of people with cognitive and developmental disabilities receiving residential services supported by nonstate agencies. State financing of services has shifted to federal–state cost sharing of community service expenditures, with an increase from 18.8% to 48.0% in federal contributions to community services. There has also been a substantial growth of the total number of people with cognitive and developmental disabilities receiving services, driven in part by the aging of the U.S. population, and specifically by the aging of persons with cognitive and developmental disabilities. Additionally, the generally much more attractive residential options in 2001 as compared to 1982, with one in five residential services recipients living in their own homes in 2001, has contributed to this trend (Lakin, Prouty, Polister, & Coucouvanis, 2003).

Barriers still exist that contribute to people with disabilities continuing to live in isolated situations. The most significant barrier is related to public beliefs that people with disabilities need to be raised in seclusion because protective environments are "for their own good." Although lawmakers were supportive of the ADA, there remains a lack of federal funding to support the shift in national policy away from secluded and protective environments. The majority of federal funds to support people with disabilities continue to go directly to facility-based programs that are not designed to flow down to the individual in his or her community (West, Wehman, & Wehman, 2005; Wehman, 2003b).

The unemployment rate remains high for individuals with disabilities despite the protection afforded by laws such as the ADA, changes in the U.S. economy, advances in rehabilitation technology, some changes in public attitudes, and increases in expenditures for employment services. High unemployment affects not only the quality of life for individuals with disabilities, but also society, which is burdened with the increase in expenditures connected to benefits such as unemployment affects insurance and Social Security disability benefits—specifically Social Security Income (SSI) and Social Security Disability Income (SSDI). This increase in expenditures is due in part to the higher survival rates following injuries and the increase in younger beneficiaries who are likely to remain on benefit rolls for a more extended period of time (Yasuda, Wehman, Targett, Cifu, & West, 2002).

Although the unemployment rate for individuals with disabilities remains high, those unemployed indicate that they want to work. The challenges for work entry or re-entry include health issues, transportation, personal care needs, and Social Security disincentives (i.e., restrictions on one's ability to work without losing medical and cash benefits). A number of supports can facilitate employment for

**❝**We who live with disabilities have been silenced by those who did not want to hear what have to say. We have also been silenced by our own fear.**❞**

—Kenny Fries

individuals with limited physical abilities. Individuals with disabilities can perform the essential elements of a job when service providers focus on a person's interests and abilities during the assessment process rather than the individual's limitations, and when they provide appropriate career development, job matching, and individually tailored supports—a process known as "customized employment" (Butterworth, Gandolfo, Revell, & Inge, 2007).

Despite these areas of difficulty, many people with disabilities reported improvement over the past 10 years in access to public facilities and transportation, quality of life, public attitudes toward people with disabilities, and how the media portray people with disabilities. These improvements may in part be due to increased awareness of the Americans with Disabilities Act of 1990 or additional laws passed in recent years to protect people with disabilities.

### ■ Situation for Children

Educators are moving away from segregating students with disabilities in special classes. With recent litigation and legislation that supports inclusion, and with increasing pressure from advocates of inclusion in professional organizations, the trend toward including students with disabilities in the general education classroom will probably continue. The move toward inclusion has raised numerous questions about the roles, responsibilities, and preparedness of school personnel in providing appropriate education for and ability to address the social and academic needs of all students. Administrators and general and special educators must have a positive attitude toward inclusion and the skills for collaborative teaming and use of instructional accommodations if inclusion is to be successful (Bernie-Smith, 2000; Katz, Mirenda, & Auerbach, 2002).

## Legislation Protecting the Rights of People with Disabilities

Strongly influenced by the civil rights movements of the 1960s, the disability community began to fight for the right to integration and meaningful equality of opportunity. Although the U.S. Constitution protects the rights of all citizens, individuals with disabilities have needed additional protection under the law from exploitation, abuse, and neglect. Specific rights (affirmative rights and protection from mistreatment) of citizens with disabilities have been defined in federal and state laws and are represented in state agency policies and procedures. Affirmative rights, which are designed to meet individual needs and promote independence, include the right to effective and appropriate services as close as possible to home. Eligible individuals with disabilities and their family members have the right to participate in service

planning meetings, to be notified if and why services are terminated, and to be informed of the process for challenging the decision. Adults with disabilities have the right to manage their own affairs, including the decision of how to spend money, how to use their free time, how to manage their own possessions, where and with whom to live and work, how to worship, and whether to vote (Racino, 1999).

Both professionals and advocates have declared that individuals with mental retardation and developmental disabilities have the same basic human rights as others in society, including the right to give consent. By giving informed consent, an individual makes knowledgeable choices about programs, procedures, or activities that are potentially invasive or that could have a significant effect on that person's life. Recent discussions focus on how to reliably determine the skills an individual must possess to give consent, how to improve those skills or expand the activities he or she is able to give consent for, and which kinds of support systems are needed to promote personal autonomy. The concern continues to be balancing an individual's rights to autonomy with his or her need for protection (Lindsey, Guy, Wehmeyer, & Martin, 2001).

Guardianship is the process of a court appointing someone to have the power to make decisions for and handle the affairs of another person. There are different degrees of guardianship—namely, plenary (total or full) or partial (limited). Depending on state statutes and the extent of authority given to the guardian, a ward may lose many or all of his or her legal rights. Because of the potential loss of rights, advocates have argued that guardianship should always be considered as a last resort, and if ever imposed, should be temporary and used to encourage the development of self-determination. Efforts to promote self-determination in a young adult with disabilities may be negated if his or her abilities are challenged by another, guardianship is imposed, and his or her rights to make decisions are possibly eliminated (Millar & Renzagia, 2002).

With the requirements for the transfer of parental rights at the age of majority within Individuals with Disabilities Act (IDEA) 1997, guidance is needed by those who are a part of the lives of youth with disabilities. Education regarding the ramifications of guardianship and its alternatives should be explained on an individual basis to all who might be affected by it. Information should be provided on appropriate supports and use of effective strategies to enable youth and young adults with disabilities to assume adult roles and responsibilities without the threat of loss of their civil rights. Achieving self-determination requires that an individual with disabilities develop inner resources while taking normal life risks and that society support and respond to him or her based on an individual's worth or ability—not disability. The issuance of a court order granting authority to one individual over another curtails independence and dignity. Young adults with or without disabilities have the right to be as self-determined as possible (Millar & Renzagia, 2002).

Self-determination has been linked to positive adult outcomes and enhanced quality of life. The self-determina-

**Table 29-3** Legislative Milestones for People with Disabilities

| Title | Purpose |
| --- | --- |
| ■ PL 93-112 Sec. 504 of the Rehabilitation Act (1973) | Initiated legislation to prohibit discrimination against and to provide access to persons with disabilities in programs receiving federal funds. Amendments ensured no discrimination in education and employment. Also known as the "Bill of Rights for People with Disabilities." |
| ■ PL 94-103 (1974) | The Developmental Disabilities Assistance and Bill of Rights Act defined the term developmental disabilities and provided funding to states and university-affiliated programs. |
| ■ PL 94-142 (1975) | The Education for All Handicapped Children Act required states to provide a free appropriate education for all children with disabilities between the ages of 3 and 18. |
| ■ PL 99-457, Part H (1986) | Amended PL 94-142 to include children from birth through age 2 and their families. |
| ■ PL 101-476 (1990) | The Individuals with Disabilities Education Act (IDEA) was the reauthorization of PL 94-142 and entitles all students ages 3–21 with disabilities a free, appropriate public education in the least restricted environment. Included incentives for providing services for children from birth to 2 years old. School districts are required to identify and evaluate children with disabilities at no cost to families. The law added a further requirement for schools to provide transition services to students with disabilities. |
| ■ PL 101-336 (1991) | The Americans with Disabilities Act (ADA) reaffirmed the rights of individuals with disabilities to equal access to facilities and opportunities and expanded this right to all services offered to the public, not just those receiving federal funds. |
| ■ PL 102-569 (1992) | The 1992 Amendments to the Rehabilitation Act emphasized competitive employment outcomes, integrated settings, helping students make transitions from school to work, using profit-making organizations for on-the-job training, and the assumption that persons with disabilities can benefit from vocational rehabilitation services. |
| ■ PL 103-218 (1994) | The Technology-Related Assistance Act for Individuals with Disabilities provided grant funding for programs providing technology assistance that is responsive to consumer needs. |
| ■ PL 103-218 (1994) | The Technology Related Assistance for Individuals with Disabilities Act reactivated the 1988 "Tech Act," which was established to develop consumer-driven, statewide service delivery systems that increase access to assistive technology devices and services. |
| ■ PL 104-235 (1995) | The Child Abuse Prevention and Treatment Act (CAPTA) Amendments included a new family resource and support program that supported state efforts toward community-based, prevention-focused support programs equipped to address the additional family support needs of families with children with disabilities. |
| ■ PL 104-191 (1996) | The Health Insurance Portability and Accountability Act increased access to health care for millions of Americans by guaranteeing that private health insurance is available, portable, and renewable. |
| ■ PL 104-183 (1996) | The Developmental Disabilities Assistance and Bill of Rights Act Amendments enhanced Developmental Disabilities Councils, other programs, and Projects of National Significance. |
| ■ PL 104-104 (1996) | The Telecommunications Act ensured equal access to telecommunications for people with disabilities. |
| ■ PL 104-134 (1996) | Fiscal-year 1997. Department of Veterans Affairs and Department of Housing and Urban Development appropriations provided an initiation of veterans benefits for children with spina bifida resulting from their parents' Vietnam-era exposure to Agent Orange. The bill also prohibited insurance companies from having lower lifetime caps for treatment of mental illness versus other disabilities. |
| ■ PL 105-17 (1997) | The Individuals with Disabilities Education Act Amendments of 1997 reauthorized IDEA to strengthen and improve education programs and services for children with disabilities. |
| ■ PL 105-394 (1998) | The Assistive Technology Act provided further federal funding for state improvement of access to assistive technology devices and services for people with disabilities. |
| ■ PL 106-170 (1999) | The Ticket to Work and Work Incentives Improvement Act provided more options to people with disabilities than simply choosing between healthcare coverage and work. |
| ■ PL 106-402 (2000) | The revised Developmental Disabilities Assistance and Bill of Rights Act of 2000 included training programs for early childhood education personnel authored by Easter Seals and the American Association of University Affiliated Programs. |
| ■ PL 106-501 (2000) | The Older Americans Act Amendments of 2000 included a new National Family Caregiver Support Program, which provided funding to agencies on aging and other organizations to provide support services to family caregivers. |

tion of individuals with cognitive and developmental disabilities is limited by congregate living or work settings with fewer opportunities for choice and decision making. More typical, community-based environments and supports enhance self-determination; therefore, it is critical to consider ways to enable people with cognitive and developmental disabilities to live and work in their communities (Wehmeyer & Bolding, 2001).

Congress has passed several critical pieces of disability legislation designed to protect the rights of people with disabilities. See Table 29-3 for a summary of legislative milestones for people with disabilities in the United States. The most significant piece of legislation has been Public Law PL No. 101-336, the ADA, which reaffirmed the rights of individuals with disabilities to equal access to facilities and opportunities and expanded these rights to all services offered to the public—not just those receiving federal funds.

The ADA is the most significant disability-related legislation to date, including provisions affecting employment, state and local government services, public transportation, public accommodations, and telecommunications. Provisions stipulate that employers may not discriminate against individuals with disabilities in hiring or promotion and must provide reasonable accommodations. All government facilities, services, and communications must be accessible, as must new buses and rail cars. Places of public accommodation, including restaurants, hotels, and stores, may not discriminate against individuals with disabilities, and, in fact, must proactively make efforts to include people with disabilities in services offered. All new construction or alteration of facilities must be accessible, and telephone companies must offer telephone relay services to persons who use telecommunication devices (Jenkins, Patterson, & Szymanski, 1992).

Early books on the social psychology of disability identified the disability experience with other minority groups that have endured discrimination, and current literature continues to designate the disability community as an oppressed minority. Constructive criticism of the disability rights (DR) movement has related to its relatively homogeneous leadership and membership, compared to the wide diversity of people with disabilities. People with mobility and sensory disabilities have dominated the DR movement since the beginning, and the movement as a whole has not done a good job of recruiting people with hidden disabilities (e.g., back problems, heart conditions, brain injuries, cognitive or psychiatric conditions). Regrettably, most individuals in these groups have not identified with the DR movement and, consequently, they are served exclusively by the rehabilitation system using the medical model of disability (McCarthy, 2003).

In spite of the progress in the passing of disability rights legislation, discrimination against people with disabilities persists. Reports on the gains and failures of implementing the civil rights laws to protect people with disabilities can be found on the National Council on Disability website (www.ncd.gov). People with disabilities in prominent positions indicate that, despite their current reputations as advocates, it took time to develop a comfortable disability identity. Changes in public attitudes about the rights and responsibilities of people with disabilities to access and integration in all aspects of everyday living would be enhanced by mainstream media exposure of the DR movement activities and issues—primarily through greater exposure to the voices and visions of individuals with disabilities. However, merely increasing the interaction is no guarantee of a positive social attitude that would deem a life with a disability to be worthy of investment and protection in the same way a life without an identified disability is valued (McCarthy, 2003). Table 29-4 lists some resources on the DR movement.

---

**Table 29-4** Books on Disability Rights, 1992–2008

- Bowe (Franklin Watts, 1992), *Equal Rights for Americans with Disabilities*
- Shapiro (Three Rivers Press, 1993), *No Pity: People with Disabilities Forging a New Civil Rights Movement*
- Hockenberry (Hyperion, 1995), *Moving Violations: War Zones, Wheelchairs, and Declarations of Independence*
- Campbell & Oliver (Routledge, 1996), *Disability Politics: Understanding Our Past, Changing Our Future*
- Dybwad & Bersani (Brookline Books 1996), *New Voices: Self-Advocacy by People with Disabilities*
- Pelka (ABC-Clio, 1997), *The ABC-CLIO Companion to the Disability Rights Movement*
- Charlton (University of California Press, 1998), *Nothing About Us Without Us: Disability Oppression and Empowerment*
- Percy (Policy Studies Journal 1999), *Disability, Civil Rights, and Public Policy: The Politics of Implementation*
- Fleischer & Zames (Temple University Press, 2001), *The Disability Rights Movement: From Charity to Confrontation*
- Barton (David Falton Publishers, 2001), *Disability, Politics, and the Struggle for Change*
- Barnartt & Scotch (Gallaudet University Press, 2001), *Disability Protests: Contentious Politics in the Disability Community, 1970–1999*

- Russell (Common Courage Press, 2002), *Beyond Ramps*
- Jacqueline Vaughn Switzer (Georgetown University Press, 2003), *Disabled Rights: American Disability Policy and the Fight for Equality*
- Engel & Munger (University of Chicago Press, 2003), *Rights of Inclusion: Law and Identity in the Life Stories of Americans with Disabilities*
- Hamilton Krieger (University of Michigan Press, 2003), *Backlash Against the ADA: Reinterpreting Disability Rights*
- Blanck, Hill, Siegal, & Waterstone (West, 2005), *Disability Civil Rights Law and Policy: Cases and Materials*
- Jaeger & Bowman (Praeger, 2005), *Understanding Disability: Inclusion, Access, Diversity, and Civil Rights*
- Shakespeare (Routledge, 2006), *Disability Rights and Wrongs*
- The Ragged Edge Online Community & Johnson (The Avocado Press, 2006), *Disability Awareness—Do It Right! Your All-in-One How-To Guide*
- Owen & Griffiths (Jessica Kingsley Publishers, 2008), *Challenges to the Human Rights of People with Intellectual Disabilities*

THINK ABOUT THIS

## Personal Connections to the Disability Rights Movement

Respondents (people with polio, spinal cord injuries, spina bifida, spinal muscular atrophy, amputation, and blindness) recalled how liberating it was to have their thoughts and feelings finally validated by the worldview that early DR activists expressed with their words and their lives.

That was the turning point for me—when I met Judy Heumann and Ed Roberts. They acted and spoke like there was nothing wrong with them; that what was wrong was that the doors were too narrow, and there were no curb cuts, and there was not a way to get personal assistance if you needed it. When they articulated that the problem was not them, that they were the perfect specimen of the person they were supposed to be, and that because of the social and environmental conditions, they were somehow disenfranchised—just like black people had been—and put on the outside, that was an enormous relief to me. I wanted that so bad. So the independent living movement had an enormous effect on my personal goals and my emotional well-being. It redefined me, or helped me redefine myself.

—S. Daniels, polio

## Most Pressing Issues in the Future

Staying alive, because the resources have been spread very thin, and once you get your rights, people are not so crazy for doing stuff for you out of compassion.

—C. Vash, polio

As we have a society marching along toward genetic manipulations and wanting to contain healthcare costs, we are facing more and more desires to persuade people to die and get out of the way . . . If we can't fight that mentality, it doesn't matter what kind of ostensible civil rights victories we win in all these years, because we won't be alive. I'm not convinced you can truly fight for equal rights to employment of people that you would really prefer not be born.

—A. Asch, blindness

What the movement Not Dead Yet [www.notdeadyet.org] is currently fighting, especially about babies with genetic problems—that they should be euthanized or not allowed to live. As technology and medical advancements make it that many disabilities are curable or at least treatable, I think we are going to devalue people who are not perfect. We are going to have this attitude that we are fixable, and if you are not fixable, then your life is not worth living.

—P. Nosek, spinal muscular atrophy

It will not be some giant legislation or major technological something . . . To me, the most important thing is attitude from other people, how they accept you and how they treat you. If people with disabilities could just be in the community like everybody else, People wouldn't need to treat them with more specialness than they need; or treat them with disdain, as a lot of people do; or try to ignore them.

—T. Cook, amputation

Attitudes and communication about disability issues and real integration. That will make it easy for people to accept their disability when they first get it. The best measure of success of the disability rights movement is that an understanding of it will become so general that when people first achieve their disability, they'll be more likely to say, "Thank God I lived long enough to experience this," not, "I'd rather be dead."

—R. Hotchkiss, spinal cord injury

 ETHICAL CONNECTION

## What do you think?

"Either he didn't take his medication or he's acting." Radio host Rush Limbaugh, on October 23, 2006, accused actor Michael J. Fox, who has Parkinson's disease, of exaggerating his disease in Democratic political ads. Fox, who supported Democratic candidates nationwide in midterm elections through a series of political ads, was instrumental in moving the stem cell research debate into the public arena.

Did Limbaugh have the right to criticize Michael J. Fox for exercising his "freedom of speech"? What do you think of celebrities who advocate for scientific research simply based on their own personal experiences with the disease? What are some of the influences, in addition to celebrity involvement, that contribute to changes in policies regarding people with disabilities and their future?

## Appropriate Language for Communicating About Persons with Disabilities

The community health nurse should use language that is current and endorsed by the disability community when speaking or writing about people with disabilities. The words we choose and the way we structure sentences can create a clear, positive view of persons with disabilities or a negative, discriminatory portrayal that reinforces common stereotypes. One of the best-known guidelines is that of **people-first language,** with which the speaker puts the person first, not the disability. For example, the community health nurse should refer to "the child with mental retardation" or "a man with Down syndrome." One exception to the people-first language guideline is when speaking about deaf people. Many deaf people do not consider themselves disabled and prefer to be called a "deaf person" rather than a "person who is deaf" or a "person with a hearing impairment." Deaf people often see themselves as members of a subculture with their own language, customs, and ways of perceiving their roles in the hearing world (Craft, 1995). When in doubt, the community health nurse should ask persons with disabilities how they wish to be described.

The community health nurse must avoid using language that characterizes the person with a disability as pitiable. Do not say "afflicted with," "crippled with," or "suffers from." Rather, say "the person *has* a spinal cord injury" or speak about "the person *with* spina bifida." Words such as *crippled* or *deformed* are never acceptable. The word *handicapped*, which was once used to refer to a person with a disability, has been redefined. *Handicap* now refers to a functional limitation that varies based on the conditions in the environment of the individual. For example, although a person with a spinal cord injury has a disability, whether or not that individual has a handicap in a certain situation would depend on conditions such as lack of a ramp to a building entrance. Finally, emphasize abilities, not limitations. Healthcare providers should never say "confined to a wheelchair" or "wheelchair-bound." These negative phrases connote pity and can encourage dependency. Instead, the professional should say "uses a wheelchair" or "uses crutches" (Research and Training Center on Independent Living, 2001).

Following are some guidelines for interactions with persons with disabilities (Barking & Dagenham, Center for Independent, Integrated, Inclusive Living Consortium, 2001).

### Etiquette and Common Courtesies

- Do not make assumptions about an individual's ability to do certain things. People with disabilities develop their own methods of overcoming the everyday problems they encounter.
- Do not assume that just because a disability is not visible, it does not exist. The majority of people with disabilities do not use wheelchairs.
- Treat people with disabilities as you would treat any other person—that is, as a woman, as a man, as a parent, as a worker. If an individual needs time to do things, be patient.
- Do not be embarrassed should you use common expressions such as "see you later" or "I might run into you," then realize they may be obliquely related to a person's disability.
- Do not use behavior more appropriate for dealing with children, such as literally or figuratively patting a wheelchair user on the head.
- Do not assume that an offer of assistance will automatically be welcome. Wait until your offer is accepted. Even then, do not assume you know the best way of helping. Instead, listen to any instructions you are given by the expert (the one who receives the assistance).
- Do not insult a person with a disability by talking to him or her through a companion, "Does he or she take sugar?" syndrome.

- Relax, speak normally, and stand in front to allow eye contact to be made, in the same way you would when talking to anyone else.
- When making physical contact, whether verbal or body language, respect boundaries and personal space.

### Etiquette with People with Mobility Impairments

- When talking with wheelchair users, either get a chair or sit down or ask if they would prefer that you stand or crouch. Do not tower over them, so they get a stiff neck, but stand a little away so that you can have a conversation on an equal basis.
- When visiting your building or organization, ensure that the person with a disability has clear information about access restrictions. If it is not accessible, give the person a choice of a home visit or meeting elsewhere.
- Ask persons with disabilities if they need help rather than ignoring them or charging in.
- If trying to find suitable venues for meetings or seminars, consult with local disability organizations, which may have experience with suitable venues and their accessibility.
- If access to your building is not obvious or is difficult, meet the person at the entrance to give assistance if required.
- A wheelchair is part of the body space of the person using it. Do not lean on it unless you would usually lean on the person.
- If you wish to speak to the person who is with the wheelchair user (assuming it isn't private), take up a position so that the wheelchair user, who may be unable to turn, can also join in the conversation and does not feel left out.
- In public places or offices, ensure that items are not left lying around on the floor. Make sure there are adequate spaces for people to get around and that access is safe for everyone.

### Etiquette with People with Visual Impairments

- Identify yourself clearly, first of all, and introduce anyone else who is present and where he or she is placed in the room.
- Ask the person if he or she requires any assistance and, if so, how best this should be provided. Sometimes the offer could be accompanied by saying something like "let me offer you an arm." This will allow you to guide rather than propel the person.
- When offering a handshake, say something to indicate that you wish to shake hands.
- When meeting persons out of the home or working surroundings, ask what central point they are familiar with and arrange to meet them there. Arrive at the agreed time.
- When offering a seat, speak the person through the process (chair on right, left, back of you, and so on) and place the person's hand on the back or the arm of the chair, so that he or she becomes aware of its position.

- At the end of a conversation, do not just leave. Say when you wish to end a conversation or to move away.
- Some people have a dual sensory impairment, being both deaf and blind. Make yourself known to them by touching their sleeve gently and then wait until they have indicated the type of help they require, if any.
- If in a noisy place, speak louder and directly toward the person with a visual impairment; however, generally, you don't need to shout!
- Consider other formats for communicating, if the obvious ones are not open to you.
- Always say what you want, as gestures are useless communication tools to most people with visual impairments.
- Always talk to the person with a visual impairment and not to his or her guide dog!

### Etiquette with People with Speech Impairments

- Make eye contact and be especially attentive and patient with a person who has difficulty speaking or who uses a communicator. Wait quietly and listen while the person talks.
- Resist the temptation to speak for the person or to finish his or her sentences.
- Some people may prefer to be asked questions that require either a short answer or a nod or shake of the head.
- Be sure you understand fully what the person is meaning before making any assumptions. It may help to say what you have understood and ask the person to repeat the rest.
- Ask simpler/shorter questions rather than ones that rely on a long answer if meeting the person for the first time (if this is appropriate).
- If you don't understand what is being said, don't be afraid or embarrassed to ask the person to repeat it—maybe several times. People are usually used to repeating what they say.
- Don't make assumptions about the person's hearing or intellect just because he or she has difficult speaking.
- If noisy, take account of this and, if possible, move to a quieter area.
- Be aware that the person's first language might not be English.
- Do not rush the person. Patience and respect for what the individual has to say is very important.

### Etiquette with People with Hearing Impairments

- Do not make assumptions about a person's ability to communicate or the way in which the individual does so. Always ask the person to tell you which method he or she prefers to use.
- Remember that for many deaf people, sign language is their first language and is, therefore, the preferred method of communication.
- If an interpreter is present, remember to speak to the person you are meeting, rather than to the interpreter.

- It may seem obvious but speak in your usual voice and make eye contact when talking to a person with a hearing impairment.
- Should there be difficulties in communicating, written notes can sometimes be used (but remember, English may not be the person's first language).

### Lip Reading Etiquette

- Do not assume that everyone who has a hearing impairment can lip read. Always ask the person when you meet him or her.
- If he or she does lip read, remember the skill is never wholly reliable and requires intense concentration. It is very tiring.
- Look directly at the person and speak slowly and clearly but do not exaggerate or shout.
- Use facial expressions, gestures, and body movements with care to emphasize the words (only 3 out of 10 words are visible on the lips).
- Face the light and keep hands, cigarettes, and food away from your face when speaking.
- To attract the person's attention, do so with a light touch on the shoulder or a wave of the hand.

### MEDIA MOMENT

Think about the last time you viewed a popular television show that featured a person with a disability. Was the disability a focus of the character? Was it often mentioned as part of the plot of the show? How do such portrayals affect our views about people with disabilities?

## Community Living Needs of People Who Have Disabilities

Legislation has been passed to ensure that environments in which people with disabilities live and work follow the patterns of life and conditions that most people experience. Children and adults with disabilities have the right to live in homes and attend school or work within integrated settings with their peers without disabilities. For example, most adults live in settings of their choosing, with people of their choice, getting up and going to bed at "normal" times, eating three meals a day about 5 hours apart, going to work, and choosing their own recreational activities and friends. Social movements (e.g., "normalization" and now "inclusion") have urged the provision of opportunities and supports for individuals with disabilities to enable them to live and work in their communities (DiLeo, 2007; Wehman, 2006a).

Similar to individualized family services plans and individualized education plans, which are discussed later in this chapter as plans of service for children, individual service plans of assistance and skill enhancement can be written for adolescents and adults to identify the supports needed to transition to work, further education, or other living arrangements. These plans are written with the individual with a disability and/or family members as the most important members of the team.

**Person-centered planning** is an approach whose goals are to reduce social isolation and segregation, establish friendships, increase opportunities to engage in preferred activities, develop competencies, and promote respect. Person-centered planning brings together the most important people in the life of a person, envisions a better life for the person, and discovers ways to achieve the vision. Participation is voluntary and the group is typically diverse, not consisting solely of service providers. The views of the family members, friends, and the focus person are foremost, instead of the professional authority hierarchy of a clinical team meeting, with an orientation toward the deficiencies of the individual. The process is guided by a facilitator who keeps the group focused on creating a lifestyle based on the aspirations of the focus person. The facilitator typically partners with a recorder or maps what people say on large sheets of paper, under categories such as history, preferences, dreams, and fears; these items then become the basis for developing a vision for the future. The group continues to meet periodically to reflect on successes and setbacks and adjusts strategies to accommodate changing circumstances and sometimes changing aspirations (Holburn, 2002).

Unfortunately, service plans are still being written that segregate individuals with disabilities. Segregated situations are often established under the premise that people need to "get ready" for living and working in the community. Work and living skills, however, are best learned in real jobs, homes, and communities. Program activities with self-contained groups of people with disabilities in perpetual preparation for the real world by traveling, recreating, working, and living together do not promote the uniqueness and value of each individual with a disability, nor do they prepare individuals for life in the community (DiLeo, 2007; Wehman, 2006a).

Our society, with cultural values of productivity, skill, attractiveness, and affluence, still views people with disabilities as different in a negative way, perceived as incompetent or as children who never grew up, "funny looking," or even dangerous. The most powerful way to change negative societal attitudes is for individuals with disabilities to participate successfully in their communities, as skilled and productive workers and managers of their own homes (with the right supports). As neighbors, coworkers, and friends, people with disabilities demonstrate their adult needs for expression of personal accomplishment, responsibility, interdependence, privacy, and sexuality. The more opportunities for choice and the more competencies an individual possesses, the more self-esteem and status he or she will have in the com-

---

## MEDIA MOMENT

*My Left Foot,* 1989
Physical disability: The story of Christy Brown, who was born with cerebral palsy. He learned to paint and write with his only controllable limb, his left foot.

*A Beautiful Mind,* 2002
Mental illness: After a brilliant but asocial mathematician accepts secret work in cryptography, his life takes a turn to the nightmarish.

*Brother's Keeper,* 1992
Mental retardation: This documentary by Joe Berlinger and Bruce Sinofsky details the murder trial of Delbert Ward.

*Fight Club,* 1999
Mental illness: An office employee and a soap salesman build a global organization to help vent male aggression.

*Girl, Interrupted,* 1999
Mental illness: Based on writer Susanna Kaysen's account of her 18-month stay at a mental hospital in the 1960s.

*I Am Sam,* 2002
Mental retardation: A mentally retarded man fights for custody of his 7-year-old daughter, and in the process teaches his cold-hearted lawyer the value of love and family.

*As Good as It Gets,* 1997
Mental illness: A single mother/waitress, a misanthropic author, and a gay artist form an unlikely friendship.

*Matchstick Men,* 2003
Mental illness: A phobic con artist and his protege are on the verge of pulling off a lucrative swindle when the con artist's teenage daughter arrives unexpectedly.

*Memento,* 2000
Mental illness: A man, suffering from short-term memory loss, uses notes and tattoos to hunt for the man he thinks killed his wife.

*The Other Sister,* 1999
Mental retardation: A mentally retarded woman proves herself to be every bit as capable as her "perfect" sister when she moves into an apartment and begins going to college.

*Pumpkin,* 2002
Mental retardation: A sorority girl is drawn to a disabled man.

*Radio,* 2003
Mental retardation: The story of a high school coach and the developmentally challenged man whom he took under his wing.

*Prozac Nation,* 2001
Mental illness and treatment issues: A young woman struggles with depression during her first year at Harvard. Based on Elizabeth Wurtzel's novel.

munity. Community health nurses who provide assistance should show care in interactions, choosing moments to teach and methods of support provision that are professionally appropriate and demonstrate personal respect. For example, the community health nurse should use minimal cues, gestures, and words (the less assistance the better, to counteract dependency), watching tone and volume, to promote the dignity of the individual and not convey an attitude of pity or assume a parental role.

The movement away from a focus on an individual's deficits to a focus on self-determination and inclusion has influenced decisions on which supports are needed for individuals to participate in their communities, assume valued social roles, and experience greater satisfaction and fulfillment. Supports are defined as resources and strategies that promote the interests and welfare of individuals and result in enhanced personal independence and productivity, greater participation in an interdependent society, increased community integration, and an improved quality of life. Types of supports should be tailored to individual needs and preferences and be provided in a flexible manner. Supports are more important to some individuals than to others. Systematic assessments of support needs should consider multiple factors and guide the development and revision of individual support plans. Assessment and planning should begin with identifying an individual's desirable life experiences and goals. After determining the intensity of support needs, an individual support plan should be developed that will be monitored for progress (Thompson, et al., 2002).

## ■ Homes of Their Own

Historically, people with significant disabilities, particularly those with mental impairments, had two living options. Either the family could care for the individual at home indefinitely, with little, if any, public assistance, or the family could place the individual in a state residential facility. Current beliefs about the rights of people with disabilities support that (1) all children, including those with severe disabilities, have the right to live at home with their family; and (2) adults with disabilities have the right to the supports necessary to live in a home in the community, either alone or with another adult of their choosing.

Living options for people with disabilities are often presented on a continuum from large segregated facilities at one end to group homes or homes of their own at the other. Such a continuum reinforces the past belief that large residential institutions or large group homes can be legitimate options as places to live. Most professionals believe that "the people who were most often viewed as needing to live in larger, specialized facilities, such as institutions and group homes, were often the very people who most benefited from the opportunities a smaller place offered" (Racino & Taylor, 1993, p. 36). When these smaller group homes are managed based on the same model of services as the large facilities, however, people with disabilities are still shortchanged. The pseudo-home can be highly routinized, "run" by service providers, and "homelike" in atmosphere, but it is not truly a home.

Living arrangements can vary from a home of one's own, a semi-independent or supported apartment (with staff available to assist), a home with one's family, a foster home, or a group home (Kirk, Gallagher, Anastasiow, & Coleman, 2006; Wehman, 2006a). Regardless of the type of living arrangement a person wants, needs, and can reasonably afford, there should be opportunity for choice, ownership of personal property, and privacy. For example, the individual should choose the type of neighborhood, style of home, landscaping, furnishings, and decorations—all choices demonstrating the individual is a competent adult. Also, a person should own his or her possessions, make choices in how to spend his or her own money, and choose activities he or she wishes to participate in. If there is a roommate (by choice of the individual), arrangements should be made for privacy, such as providing personal space and securing private items.

Housing must be accessible for the individual with a disability. Contractors and builders may be unaware of modifications or regulations involving accessibility, and few accessible houses or apartments are available, particularly in rural areas. The community health nurse can educate community members and leaders regarding housing needs of adults with disabilities, which in many ways overlap the needs of older adults in the community: the need for safe, affordable, and accessible housing choices. Information related to accessibility is available through each state's Department of Rehabilitation Services or Office of Vocational Rehabilitation Services, along with ample information available on the Internet.

A person with a disability may require assistance in the home to carry out activities of daily living such as bathing, dressing, cooking, eating, and toileting (Newcomer, Kang, Kaye, & LaPlante, 2002). It is estimated that about 9 million individuals in the United States need personal assistance to carry out typical daily activities. Although most of these helpers are relatives (80%), in many cases the individual with a disability must hire a helper to come into the home (U.S. Census Bureau, 2006). A **personal care attendant** can be employed to assist with activities of daily living, transportation, pet care, and household chores and maintenance. Personal assistant services also include interpreting, mobility assistance, social support, medical assistance, reading, and recreation. Unfortunately, availability of attendants, coordinating agencies, and public funding options vary greatly from state to state.

 **GLOBAL CONNECTION**

Disabling conditions throughout the world are often the result of war and conflict. When governments in other developing countries are unable to assume responsibility for the rehabilitation of the population's veterans and war victims, how do these people recover? How does this differ from U.S. policy related to veterans?

Families who may be caring for a child or adult with a significant disability 24 hours a day need the option of **respite care** to prevent caregiver burnout. Respite care provides another caregiver to assume the round-the-clock care of the family member with a disability, allowing the caretaker a vacation, a mental health break, time to recover from illness, or merely time to oneself. Because of the significant medical problems that individuals with severe disabilities may have, the respite provider (e.g., church, civic group, the Association for the Rights of Citizens with Developmental Disabilities) often will recruit nurses in the community to serve as respite caregivers. Respite may be provided in the patient's home, at a group home, in a private home, or at an organization's facility.

## ■ An Accessible Community

Accessibility to all that a community offers is critical if persons with disabilities are to participate to the fullest extent possible in community life. Many individuals with disabilities cannot afford to own customized vehicles to drive or may be physically or mentally unable to drive. Accessible public transportation is needed by many persons who are disabled so that they may work, recreate, worship, seek medical attention, socialize, and so on, as we all do on a daily basis. Inadequate transportation was cited as a problem by 30% of adults with disabilities in a 2000 Harris poll. Many areas are lacking adequate public transportation, particularly in rural areas of the country. By the year 2002, all public buses were required to be accessible. Facility accessibility is also necessary and required by the ADA. It is accomplished by accommodations such as curb cuts, ramps, large doorways with easily opened doors, elevators, and wide hallways. The community health nurse can educate community leaders about these needs for access and may become involved in advocating for individuals with disabilities or working with legislators for policy reform. Individuals who use wheelchairs for mobility are often frustrated with the inadequate

Dr. Valerie Rachal, chapter author, consults with faculty member with disability.

involvement of people with disabilities in the development of facilities that comply with ADA accessibility requirements (Pierce, 1998). Ideally, a person who uses a wheelchair should serve on committees involved in designing buildings to ensure that they not only meet ADA requirements, but also are functional for those who use wheelchairs or who have other types of disabilities.

## ■ Meaningful Work

Work is highly valued in our society. Society often judges an individual's worth by his or her productivity; thus performing real work and paying taxes can enhance a person's dignity. The stigma associated with disability decreases when individuals are seen as productive and competent workers (Wehman, 2003c). Work, with the regular co-worker contact and shared common experience, offers opportunities for development of personal relationships, arranged social activities after work hours, and a network of social support in the community that is often lacking in the life of individuals with developmental disabilities (Green & Schleien, 1991). The wages and fringe benefits earned at work can also offer increased financial security, greater independence and mobility in the community, control over life choices, and greater personal satisfaction (Wehman, 2003c).

Vocational options for individuals with mild to severe disabilities range from day treatment programs and sheltered workshops to supportive employment and competitive employment in community businesses. Each of the options represents less and less supervision and assistance for the individual with disabilities in a work setting. For many years, the only vocational option for individuals with mental retardation or developmental disabilities was training in segregated work settings (e.g., adult activity centers, sheltered workshops, nursing homes and institutions). Maintaining an individual who can be productive on the Social Security disability rolls is not an efficient use of human resources or public funds. Individuals with developmental disabilities can and should work in competitive community employment settings (Revell, Kregel, Wehman, & Bond, 2000; Wehman, 2006b).

Competitive employment as a possibility for individuals with significant developmental disabilities has grown with the use of trained employment specialists, informed co-workers, mentors, technology supports, and legislation such as the ADA. Supported employment, with its focus on valuing the abilities of individuals with disabilities and their productivity in the workplace, has given these individuals an opportunity to be included in community business environments. The goal of supported employment is to help individuals with the most significant disabilities be successful in paid employment in the integrated work setting of their choice. Supported employment emphasizes the benefits of competitive employment for all involved. Community employment provides the individual with a disability with a real job plus the benefits and dignity that comes with contribution. The employer gets a good worker and receives specialized support to train and maintain the individual. The family is able to see its family member in a competent role in the workplace. Taxpayers spend less money than they would to support the individual in a segregated program (Wehman, Revell, & Brooke, 2003; Wehman, Targett, & Cifi, 2006).

A 1998 Harris survey cited a number of factors that facilitated beginning or continuing employment for people with disabilities. Three major factors identified as helpful were assistance from vocational rehabilitation (23%); getting equipment or a device that they needed to do their work, talk with other workers, or get around at work (21%); and getting an interpreter or personal care attendant (7%). For those individuals with disabilities who did not work full-time, reasons given included the following: employers do not recognize they are capable of doing the job (42%); they lack skills, education, or training needed to get the job (33%); they need a personal assistant to help get to work or to do the job (32%); they risk losing benefits or insurance (31%); no work is available in the line of work respondent could do (29%); and special equipment or devices are needed to do the work, talk to or hear other workers, or get around at work (28%) (National Organization on Disability, 2004).

Many businesses have made changes in how they think and act about hiring individuals with disabilities since the signing of the ADA. Supervisors are indicating they are satisfied at the same or even a higher level compared to workers without disabilities regarding the performance of workers with disabilities in the areas of timeliness of arrival and departure, punctuality, attendance, and consistency in task. The business community appears to be increasingly embracing the employment of individuals with disabilities as a sound business strategy, investing in appropriate supports to ensure these employees' success. Businesses are changing their procedures for hiring new employees to better accommodate job applicants and new hires with disabilities. Written return-to-work policies for workers with disabilities are also becoming more popular. Accommodations for workers with disabilities (and without) are including job carving, job restructuring and schedule modifications, transitional work, telework, and use of assistive technology (Wehman, 2003a).

Innovations in natural supports, co-worker training, and employer leadership within the business community have helped increase the capacity of service providers to include people with disabilities in the workforce. New methods of job development, modern marketing techniques, assistive technology, transition services from school to work, expansion of choice and self-determination, and person-centered planning have all contributed to the increase in integrated employment. Today segregated employment of activity centers and sheltered workshops are giving way to alternatives such as work crews and enclaves and now individual placements in community businesses, although these jobs are largely entry-level positions in the service industry (Mank, Cioffi & Yovanoff, 2003; Yamaki & Fujiura, 2002).

Years of research have confirmed that individuals with disabilities who need long-term employment assistance fare better in supported employment than in sheltered workshops. To assist individuals with severe disabilities to succeed in employment, professionals must identify suitable opportunities within community businesses and develop the supports that those individuals need. Inclusive employment within the community is the right of all people, including those with significant disabilities (Wehman, Brooke, Green, Hewett, & Tipton, 2008).

**Got an Alternative?**

Persons with chronic, disabling conditions often use complementary and alternative interventions. What is the role of the community health nurse as patients seek alternative treatments?

## Relationships

All people experience sexual feelings, and individuals with disabilities are no exception. Sexual activity is one of the most controversial issues pertaining to the lives of individuals with disabilities, particularly mental retardation. Sexual development for individuals with mental retardation is for the most part similar to persons without mental retardation. Many professionals argue that individuals have the right to socially appropriate sexual expression. Others disagree and are concerned about outcomes, including unwanted advances (e.g., rape, incest) and sexually transmitted diseases. Appropriate sexual expression is more difficult for individuals with mental retardation who have higher levels of supervision and support. They may not have information about sexual development and functioning and typically have fewer socialization opportunities in which to practice appropriate behaviors, roles, and expectations (Beirne-Smith et al., 2006).

Individuals with physical disabilities such as spinal cord injuries or cerebral palsy also may need education regarding sexuality. The community health nurse and other professionals assisting individuals with disabilities may have to set aside their own sexual values so as not to deny, limit, or inhibit an individual's interest in romance and sex. People with disabilities should receive sex education, sexual health-care information, and opportunities for socializing, sexual expression, and intimacy.

## Recreation

Participating in recreational activities is an important aspect of life for individuals with disabilities, just as it is for others in our society. Individuals with disabilities usually participate in sedentary leisure, commonly watching television or listening to the radio with family or possibly a few friends. This pattern of leisure does not help them maintain their health or fitness level. Without coordinated preventive health care for increasing fitness, secondary health conditions often result for individuals with disabilities, such as high blood pressure and high cholesterol levels, heart disease, diabetes, obesity, chronic skin problems, and hygiene-related issues. With inclusive community recreation programs for individuals with disabilities, not only will there be increased opportunity for improved health and fitness, but individuals also have increased opportunities for social contact—an additional critical variable for improved quality of life (Carter, 2002). Recreation may take the form of individual or team games, athletic programs in schools, college-sponsored recreational sports, employer-sponsored activities, church-sponsored activities, and family recreation. Specific activities include outdoor recreation (e.g., birding, hiking, bike riding, canoeing, softball) and indoor activities (e.g., ceramics, painting, aerobics, weight lifting, racquetball). Ideally, recreational activities in the community serve to promote physical health and conditioning, improve social skills, facilitate friendships, and develop specific skills. Although achieving a balance between work and leisure is important for everyone, it is especially critical for people with disabilities. Many individuals with disabilities who work do not have recreational outlets for evenings and weekends. Community recreation programs have been slow to accept responsibility for offering programming that includes people with disabilities. "It is not enough merely to open programs to people with disabilities; the professionals in charge of the programs must go further and actively recruit and encourage the participation of people with disabilities and provide them with successful and ongoing mechanisms of support" (Schleien, Ray, & Green, 1997, p. 19). Community recreational opportunities ranging from individual skill building to competitive international competition are becoming increasingly available to people with disabilities and are supported by recreational specialists and special equipment (e.g., modified bowling balls, walkers for ice skating, sit-skis for snow skiing). In addition to group participation in community-based opportunities for recreation, home-centered hobbies such as card games, board games, collections, and other leisure interests should be encouraged.

The camp movement for children with disabilities is on the rise. Currently there are hundreds of camps for children with diabetes, cancer, HIV/AIDS, multiple sclerosis, muscular dystrophy, cystic fibrosis, cerebral palsy, spina bifida, blindness, and hearing impairments. Camps may be sponsored on a national basis or supported by local chapters of national charitable organizations (Mayo, 2002). Children and youth with developmental disabilities usually attend separate recreation and leisure activities and need additional options to participate in community activities with other children and youth. With assistance and accommodation recommendations from knowledgeable personnel, all participants can benefit from inclusive recreation programs created by community recreation agencies, nonprofit sports organizations, schools, parks and recreation departments, universities, local governments, religious organizations, and private activity providers. Some children will need one-on-one assistance for safety or other very individualized accommodations to meet their unique learning or equipment needs and communication styles (Fennick & James, 2003).

Adults with disabilities may attend fewer social and cultural activities than adults without disabilities. Although they attend a place of worship almost as often as individuals without disabilities (54% as compared with 57%), their participation in other social events is typically less. For example, only 33% of adults with disabilities go to a restaurant at least once a week, compared with 60% of those without disabilities; 70% of people with disabilities did not go to a sporting event in the past year; only 48% went to the movies or the theater during the past year; and only 27% attended a live music performance at least once during the year (National Organization on Disability, 2004).

## Services for Individuals with Disabilities

### ■ Case Management

The vast array of services required by many individuals with disabilities requires some system of central coordination. This system is called *case management*. **Case management** has been defined as "the collaborative provision of coordinated care by professionals from multiple disciplines, in one or more settings, over a period of time, to achieve specific outcomes" (Trachtenberg & Lewis, 1996, p. 203). After its inception in the mental health field, case management was later adopted in the rehabilitation field in the 1960s and 1970s. The intent of current disability legislation, along with the special interests of third-party payers, has driven the development of case management as a way not only to coordinate services but also to allocate resources. Persons with disabilities often have complex problems requiring services from a multitude of agencies. An interdisciplinary case management team identifies problems, formulates goals, and coordinates the services needed. In the process, gaps and redundancies in the community service system may be identified and dealt with. Case management teams therefore not only serve the targeted patient, but also have the potential to improve the overall service system for persons with disabilities in the community.

The case manager may be an agency service provider, such as the community health nurse. Although the case manager may represent a particular agency, he or she must look beyond the agency's prescribed services to address the broad range of patient needs across all possible support agencies. To complicate matters further, an individual receiving services through several different agencies may have multiple case managers, assigned by health service agencies, social service agencies, or insurance companies. Communication among these case managers is essential to avoid the risk of duplication or omission of services. At this time, there are no requirements for certification of case managers. A case manager for one agency may be a master's degree–prepared social worker, and another agency may use nonprofessionals with varying educational backgrounds. Some patients, to ensure that their needs and not the needs of the agency are being met, may contract with a private case manager on a fee-for-service basis. Whether initiated to better meet the patient's needs, to better allocate scarce resources, or to ensure adherence to a treatment plan, case management has the potential to encourage communication between the parties involved to meet clearly defined goals generated by the individual with disabilities.

## ■ Educational Programming

For young children with disabilities, promoting optimal development in the gross motor, fine motor, language, cognition, adaptive/self-help, and social areas is the focus of intervention. **Early intervention** is the term used to refer to specialized services for infants and toddlers who are at risk for or are experiencing a developmental delay. Early intervention services are provided at no cost to families through each state's early intervention system, usually through the state's health department or local education agencies (public school system). An interdisciplinary team along with the parents develop an **individualized family service plan** (IFSP), which is a documented plan of care to meet the child's and family's needs. For instance, an infant born with Down syndrome could benefit from physical therapy in the first months of life to begin working on emerging gross motor skills such as head control, upper body strength, and rolling over. (Infants with Down syndrome have hypotonia and delayed gross motor skill development.) Speech language therapy would also be needed to work on sucking, spoon feeding, and making sounds in the early months. (Infants with Down syndrome have a small osseous orbit of the mouth, large protruding tongue, and poor muscle tone, causing feeding problems and delayed language development.)

Public schools are the primary agency for serving children with disabilities from 3 years of age (or younger) until 21 years of age. Schools are required by law to provide every child with a disability a free appropriate public education in the least restrictive environment. For most children with disabilities, this means integration, or education within regular education classrooms of same-age peers without disabilities. Public school districts have made varying degrees of movement toward this goal. In addition to education, public schools must provide related services needed by the child for the child to benefit from education, which may include physical therapy, occupational therapy, speech language therapy, nursing, and therapeutic recreation. Documented plans called **individualized education plans** (IEPs), developed by the parents and an interdisciplinary team provided by the school, provide direction for the child's care and a means of enforcing accountability.

The community health nurse, when serving as a school health nurse, can play a critical role in preventing disabilities and ensuring a safe and supportive school experience for children with disabilities. The school health nurse may collaborate with teachers to develop and present an injury prevention curriculum aimed at specific age groups (e.g., poisoning and preschoolers or head injuries and elementary/middle school children). Teachers will rely on the school health nurse for guidance and assistance in working with children who have physical disabilities such as spina bifida or cerebral palsy, children taking medications for behavior problems, children with compromised immune systems, and children with seizure disorders. The school nurse may also serve on an interdisciplinary team to assess children with disabilities for eligibility for special education services or conduct annual vision and hearing screening for at-risk children.

### 🖥 Research Alert

The movement toward inclusion of students with developmental disabilities in general education classrooms has been supported by research suggesting that inclusive classrooms do not hinder the academic achievement of typical students and offer many social and developmental advantages for students both with and without disabilities. Two variables commonly used to evaluate the outcomes of classroom inclusion are engaged behavior and social interaction. Classroom strategies such as small-group instruction and cooperative learning, peer tutoring, multimodality instruction, flexible response activities, curriculum-performance–based assessment, the use of technology, and community-based instruction have been found to facilitate both engaged behavior and peer social interaction. "Multiple Intelligence" practices have also been cited as potentially facilitative of inclusion without the research.

The purpose of this study was to examine the engaged behavior and social interactions of students with developmental disabilities in both the Multiple Intelligence inclusive classrooms and the more traditional inclusive classrooms. Results revealed that the experiences of the participants in both types of classroom were more alike than different. In both classroom types, participants were engaged more during whole-class, independent seatwork, and traditional classroom activities and were engaged less in small groups or multiple response activities. However, participants were engaged more frequently in multiple response activities in Multiple Intelligence classrooms. In typical classrooms, participants were engaged more frequently in noninstructional time and individual seatwork that was different from their peers. The participants spent more time interacting with their peers in the Multiple Intelligence classrooms and more time with adults in the typical classroom. These results suggest that to ensure increased engagement of students with developmental disabilities and social interaction, classrooms should use activities that allow for multiple methods of responding and small-group instruction. ▲

*Source:* Katz, J., Mirenda, P., & Auerbach, S. (2002). Instructional strategies and educational outcomes for students with developmental disabilities in inclusive "multiple intelligences" and typical inclusive classrooms. *Research and Practice for Persons with Severe Disabilities, 27*(4), 227–238.

### ■ Transition from Education to Work and Living in the Community

Students with disabilities are now placed in regular education programs as much as possible because the best preparation for living and working in an integrated environment is to be taught in an inclusive school setting. Educational programming available to students with disabilities includes four major areas: (1) general education academic content, (2) basic academic skills and social skills, (3) learning strategies, and (4) vocational and life skills. A balance of these instructional areas should also address relevant adolescent issues such as biological changes and sexuality; social values and behavioral competence; identification of personal interests, talents, and areas of need; and a desire for emotional independence (Patton, Blackbourn, & Fad, 2004; Wehman, 2006a).

Educational systems are expanding their roles in preparing students for transition to work and living in the community (Dolyniuk, Kamens, Corman, DiNardo, Totaro, & Rockoff, 2002). Employers and employees of industries and businesses should be invited to address school systems about their workforce needs. Business connections and alliances offering students opportunities for work experiences and employment before graduation are having success. Many students with disabilities are staying employed upon graduation and are not remaining dependent on their families or the social service system.

To facilitate successful transition from the school environment to more independent living and work environments, key connections should be built with community businesses, community colleges, recreation centers, and adult supports for living. Appropriate planning focusing on student/family choice is also critical. Major options for students with disabilities include (1) employment (full-time or part-time, supported or nonsupported), (2) further education (2- and 4-year colleges, technical schools, trade schools, adult education), (3) military service, (4) volunteer work, (5) "domestic engineering" (house husband/wife), or (6) absence of gainful employment or purposeful activity (Patton et al., 2004).

Transition planning is shifting the decision making to individuals with disabilities and their families. Students are now learning to make choices, be more self-determined, and be self-advocates assuming control and management responsibilities for their own lives. Professionals are shifting away from "curing" individuals with disabilities to supporting them for improved quality of life. Before students leave the school environment, they and their family members must learn how to access the supports (informal and unpaid or formal and paid) they need and want in the communities. Person-centered planning focuses on the desires of the individuals and their families and identifies the formal and informal supports the individuals will need to achieve their future dreams. A planning meeting focuses on the individual's abilities and preferences and identifies possible resources needed to provide desired assistance and support for adult living and work.

### ■ Rehabilitation

**Rehabilitation** is a term used for interventions aimed at restoring or optimizing functioning after an injury or significant medical problem. Rehabilitation nurses work to reduce the stigma associated with disabilities, restore maximum levels of independent functioning, advocate for optimal quality of life, help the individual and family adapt to an altered lifestyle, and improve the overall outcome for the individual with disabilities. Individuals having experienced spinal cord injuries or cerebrovascular accidents are examples of types of persons who would be involved in rehabilitation. Initially, after a significant injury, the individual with disabilities is involved in inpatient rehabilitation, which may use nursing, physical therapy (PT), occupational therapy (OT), speech language therapy, recreation therapy, music therapy, and counseling. Later, after discharge from the facility, the individual may receive home visits from a home health nurse and PT or OT sessions at an outpatient rehabilitation facility. Both the length of the initial hospital stay and the number of outpatient rehabilitation visits permitted after discharge have been severely curtailed in recent years by insurance providers.

### ■ Medical Technology

Many individuals with disabilities require technology assistance, nonmedical or medical, immediately after an injury, during rehabilitation, and/or throughout their lives. **Medical assistive devices** assist or replace necessary body functions and are necessary to keep the individual alive or prevent further disability. Persons using medical technologies also typically require daily skilled nursing care. Medical technology is used to assist with respiration, nutrition, excretion, and surveillance of vital functions and oxygen levels.

Individuals with chronic respiratory failure may require oxygen supplementation by nasal cannula, face mask, oxygen tent or hood, or a tracheostomy. These individuals often may require chest physiotherapy and suctioning several times a day to clear pulmonary secretions. When assistance is needed

Faculty member with disability uses service dog to function more independently.

*There are two kinds of "disabled" persons. Those who dwell on what they have lost and those who concentrate on what they have left.*

—Thomas S. Szasz

to replace or augment the individual's own breathing, mechanical ventilation and tracheostomy are used. Training nurses in rehabilitation facilities about ventilators can expedite the discharge of ventilator-dependent individuals from the hospital acute care unit to rehabilitation facilities.

Individuals with chronic serious respiratory problems may be discharged to home from an acute care setting while still using a ventilator. Home ventilator care is one of the most expensive, time-consuming, and risky types of home therapies. Equipment failure or poor judgment of the caregiver can result in immediate death of the patient (Capen & Dedlow, 1998). Young children receiving long-term mechanical ventilation are at high risk for language deficits, feeding problems, and behavior problems. A speech-language pathologist should be consulted to devise a developmentally appropriate alternative mode of communication for the individual with a tracheostomy receiving long-term oxygen supplementation or ventilation. Alternative methods of communication such as sign language, language boards, or computers can promote expressive language development and help prevent behavior problems stemming from frustration.

Neurological impairments such as cerebral palsy can cause numerous problems with feeding such as a weak suck, poor lip closure, poor tongue control, uncoordinated suck–swallow reflex, and gastroesophageal reflux. In addition, some individuals may lack the stamina to chew, swallow, and breathe without becoming totally exhausted or risking aspiration. Nasogastric tubes may be used as a short-term method to deliver food directly to the stomach but are not used for long-term feeding because of the irritation to the nose and throat and the unappealing appearance. Individuals who cannot take in enough food by mouth to be adequately nourished can benefit from a gastrostomy. A gastrostomy is an opening through the abdominal wall directly to the stomach. A gastrostomy tube or button is inserted into this opening to allow for feeding. Occasionally, the gastrointestinal tract is not able to digest or absorb nutrients, and the individual is nourished with total parenteral nutrition (TPN). TPN is infused in a central venous catheter placed in the vena cava or right atrial area to provide adequate dilution of the hypertonic solution (Krzywda, 1998; Roman, Miller, Maculuso, Dempsey, & Golden-Baker, 1998).

Medical technology or equipment may be necessary to promote excretion of wastes. Indwelling urinary catheters may be used to empty the bladder and keep the individual dry. Two main problems with long-term indwelling catheters are frequent urinary tract infections, which can cause permanent kidney damage, and the bulkiness and unsightliness of the urine collection bag. Many persons with spina bifida (accompanied by paralysis below the level of the defect) or spinal cord injuries prefer to perform clean intermittent self-catheterization throughout the day, eliminating the need for the urine collection bag and indwelling catheter. An ostomy or opening in the abdominal wall may also be used, either to empty the bladder or to allow evacuation of the bowel contents through the abdominal wall. In the past, adults with kidney failure could receive hemodialysis at home, and now children with kidney failure can receive peritoneal dialysis at home and avoid hospitalization. Peritoneal dialysis, in which fluid is passed into the abdominal cavity via an abdominal catheter and allowed to drain back out, takes several hours to complete and may be needed up to 3 to 5 days per week (Batshaw, Pellegrino, & Roizen, 2007).

Another category of medical technology commonly used at home or in rehabilitation settings includes monitoring devices such as cardiorespiratory monitors and pulse oximeters. Monitors are important for alerting caregivers to problems requiring prompt intervention, such as a kink in the oxygen tubing or an occluded airway, but the beeping and alarms of the monitors can unfortunately compete with the patient as the focus of the caregiver.

## ■ Nonmedical Assistive Technology

Nonmedical assistive technology is often a critical part of the continuum of services needed by a person with a disability. An **assistive technology device** is "any item, piece of equipment, or product system, whether acquired commercially off the shelf, modified, or customized that is used to increase, maintain, or improve functional capabilities of individuals with disabilities" (PL 100-407, the Technology Related Assistance for Individuals with Disabilities Act, 1988). Areas in which assistive technology is helpful include employment tasks, activities of daily living, environmental control, communication, mobility, transportation, and recreation. Within each of these areas, technology can be either low tech (easy to make and inexpensive) or high tech (more difficult to make, often computerized or electronic, and expensive). The physical, economic, and cultural environments in rural areas create rehabilitation facility, service, and personnel obstacles for use of assistive technology. Rehabilitation needs in rural areas may best be met by primary care professionals, community rehabilitation workers, people with disabilities, and their family members using appropriate low-tech assistive technology and adaptations in the immediate environments (Eldar, 2001).

Technology for everyday living, or those adaptations and devices that will enable the individual to perform activities of daily living, are the first needs of consumers. These needs must be met before other needs, such as transportation, can be attended to. Examples of technology to help with activities of daily living include "grabbers," adapted eating utensils, shower chairs, and Braille or large-print labels on appliances. Environmental control can be achieved through the use of switch extenders to place light switches within reach of a person in a wheelchair, adapters to convert lamps into "touch" lamps, or voice-controlled lights and heating/cooling. Personal computers are owned by 30% of people with disabilities, up from only 20% in 1994 (U.S. Census Bureau, 2006). Voice recognition software is available that enables a person with vision, motor, or coordination problems to use a computer strictly by voice commands and dictation, without ever having to touch the keyboard. The ability to communicate is a basic need of all individuals, regardless of disability or age. Communication systems (which may be based on sign language, gesturing, or Braille) may require low-tech devices such as simple communication boards at which to point or gaze, or high-tech computers that "talk" for the person such as the Liberator. TDDs (telecommunication devices for the deaf) allow individuals with severe hearing impairments to transmit and receive typed messages over the telephone. Text messaging via cellular phones and Personal Digital Assis-tants (PDAs), such as the Blackberry and the Apple iPhone, have increased communication opportunities for persons with a wide range of disabilities. Mobility devices include the traditional walkers, canes, and crutches along with scooters and wheelchairs. Scooters and wheelchairs have become costly and highly technical pieces of equipment that are custom-made to fit the size, posture, and lifestyle of the person with a disability. In addition to manual wheelchairs, power wheelchairs with joystick control and tilt and recline options are available. For persons without upper-extremity control, sip and puff or breath-controlled power chairs are available. Specialized wheelchairs have also been developed for rough outdoor terrain and for specific sports such as wheelchair basketball, track, or rugby. Technological adaptations for vehicles include wheelchair lifts for vans, mechanical or electronic hand controls, and steering devices.

Ideally, evaluations for assistive technology devices should be conducted by appropriate interdisciplinary teams that include the individual as a key member. Team members may include physical therapists, occupational therapists, nurses, speech-language pathologists, rehabilitation engineers, vocational rehabilitation counselors, teachers, and technology suppliers. Although many of the low-tech devices can be made or purchased for a moderate price, other pieces of technology such as computerized communication devices, specialized wheelchairs, and customized vans require significant financial resources (see Box 29-1).

Advances in technology are enhancing the possibilities for individuals with disabilities to communicate and move more effectively. With the knowledge of technology, service providers can provide solutions to everyday problems in school and workplace settings. However, adequate funding to make the best technology available to citizens with disabilities has still not been allocated. For example, grocery stores have laser scanners and voice synthesizers on their computers, yet people with disabilities have difficulty accessing voice synthesizers of this quality for themselves (Patton et al., 2004).

Adaptive/assistive devices have moved some individuals from dependence to independence but include sometimes costly equipment such as customized electric wheelchairs and electronic communication systems. Because of the con-

---

**BOX 29-1**

**Means of Financing Assistive Technology**

**Public Sources**
Medicaid
Medicare
CHAMPUS
Private insurance
Social Security Administration work incentive
Veterans Administration
State vocational rehabilitation agencies
State education agencies

**Private Sources**
Lions Club
Easter Seals
United Way
Sororities and fraternities
Muscular Dystrophy Association
Credit financing

---

siderable expense, school systems, insurance companies, and public assistance programs often disagree on who should pay for the devices (Kirk et al., 2006).

It has been estimated that more than 2.5 million Americans need assistive technology devices that they are unable to acquire, primarily because of the high cost of the products (Laplante, Hendershot, & Moss, 1992). Technology, both low and high tech, has made the difference for many people with disabilities between a life of dependency and limited options and an independent, productive life in which the person is included in all aspects of community life.

## ■ Assistance Animals

In addition to technological assistance, individuals with disabilities may benefit from animal assistance. Using pets to enhance health status dates back to the eighteenth and nineteenth centuries, when pets were used in Great Britain to give institutionalized people with mental retardation a sense of purpose and meaning. Caring for pets has been shown to help individuals improve mood, lower blood pressure, overcome physical limitations, and increase social skills (DeLaune & Ladner, 2006). A variety of animals can be used to provide companionship and give purpose to daily living (e.g., cats, dogs, rabbits, guinea pigs, birds) or to assist individuals in daily activities (e.g., dogs, monkeys).

The most commonly used animal to assist patients with disabilities is the dog (Eames & Eames, 2001). Assistance dogs, although commonly thought to include only guide dogs for people who are blind, actually include several types of dogs serving a variety of purposes. Guide dogs are specially trained dogs who, when working, stay at their owner's side and provide behavioral cues about the environment. Examples would be warnings of steps, streets, or other obstacles in the path of movement. Hearing dogs, also specially

Theresa Uchytil, as former Miss Iowa, was born without a left hand and adopted as her slogan for the 2000 Miss America contest: "Americans with disabilities, think ability."

trained, may be used by individuals with significant hearing impairments to cue the individual about meaningful sounds in the environment such as a doorbell, telephone, smoke detector, or an approaching person. Service dogs for persons with physical disabilities are especially useful to persons using wheelchairs. These dogs are trained to be helpful by picking up dropped objects (e.g., a pen, car keys, a wallet), carrying items in a dog backpack, and retrieving objects (e.g., a telephone) for the owner. For an individual who can walk short distances between a chair and a nearby bathroom, for instance, a large dog can help the person balance and provide stability for the short walk. A lesser known type of assistance dog is the seizure detection dog. Certain dogs seem to have an innate ability to sense an impending seizure. Dogs with this ability can be trained to warn the owner that a seizure is about to begin, enabling the owner to position himself or herself in a safe position away from sharp and hard objects and to summon help. Once the seizure begins, if no one else is present, the dog is trained to bark to get help. All of the aforementioned types of assistance dogs require specialized training for both the dog and the prospective owner, funds to purchase the dog (often available through a civic organization), and owner commitment.

The ADA (1990) protects the rights of a person with a disability who uses an assistance dog to have full access to any public facility, including hospitals and outpatient rehabilitation facilities. The community health nurse may be involved in developing or revising a healthcare agency's policies regarding service animals to ensure that the facility is in compliance with ADA guidelines (Eames & Eames, 1997). Questions about access to places of public accommodation can be directed to the U.S. Department of Justice's ADA hotline (800-514-0301).

## Ethical Issues Related to Disabilities

A number of ethical issues exist in the disability field. Newborn screening for diseases such as phenylketonuria (PKU) is one area of question. Presently, in many states, newborn screening is conducted without parental consent. This screening detects several diseases, including PKU, which respond profoundly to early treatment. It is more economical for states to detect and treat a disease such as PKU early rather than provide lifelong support for an untreated child who will develop severe mental retardation. Does this law violate parents' rights to give informed consent? Would it be ethical to expand mandatory screening of newborns for other genetic diseases such as cystic fibrosis when the disease course will not be significantly improved by newborn diagnosis?

Prenatal diagnosis is now readily available to most women in the United States and raises a number of concerns for those in the disability field. It is feared that women could be pressured to undergo abortions of fetuses with disabilities because of society's devaluing of people with disabilities and its unwillingness to pay for their care. Although the goal of prenatal diagnosis is to give information to expectant parents so that they can make an informed choice, the high rates of abortion following diagnosis of a disability suggests that service providers are biased in the information that they share. It is critical that prenatal diagnostic information be shared through a genetic counselor and that parents receive accurate information about a disabling condition before making any decisions (Warren, 2002).

Historically, another ethical debate centered on the relatively common occurrence of withholding lifesaving surgical treatment of newborns with obvious disabilities such as Down syndrome, hydrocephalus, or spina bifida. Although withholding treatment from infants with disabilities had been common, the 1982 birth of "Baby Doe" in Indiana brought this practice under public scrutiny. An infant was born with Down syndrome and tracheoesophageal fistula, a connection between the trachea and esophagus. Without corrective surgery, oral feedings would be routed into the baby's lungs via the fistula. Following the advice of their obstetrician, the parents refused to consent to the corrective surgery and the infant was not given food or water. A consulting pediatrician tried to stop the starvation of the infant, but the courts upheld the parents' decision and the infant died a number of days later. In response to the public outrage resulting from the death of this infant, the federal government enacted the "Baby Doe" ruling and notified all hospitals that such activity would be penalized. Since 1982, it has been unlawful to withhold treatment from a baby born with a disability; however, violation of this "Baby Doe" ruling carries minor penalties such as loss of federal dollars, rather than criminal or civil actions.

Professionals need to be aware of their own biases and consciously strive to prevent them from coloring the

**THINK ABOUT THIS**

Recent disasters in the United States, including the September 11, 2001 terrorist attacks and Hurricane Katrina, exposed the lack of awareness of the need for plans to accommodate those persons with disabilities in all evacuation and disaster plans. For most of the people with disabilities who were affected by these two disasters, there were virtually no plans to manage the special needs of this vulnerable population. What can be done at the local, state, and national levels to provide safe, appropriate prevention and intervention in the workplace, homes, and communities for people with disabilities? What role does the community health nurse play in promoting disaster preparation for this vulnerable population?

information shared with parents about the risks and benefits of procedures. Research has shown that nurses and physicians are often not supportive of treating infants with severe disabilities because of quality-of-life issues, cost of care, and impact on the family. Nurses and physicians have been shown to be less optimistic about achieving a positive outcome than parents, teachers, social workers, physical therapists, and occupational therapists. Because of these biases, nurses may unknowingly accentuate certain risks or underestimate the potential quality of life of an infant with a disability, thereby influencing the parents' treatment decision (Batshaw et al., 2007). Other ethical issues, including do not resuscitate orders or withdrawing life support, are based on similar issues as the withholding treatment issue discussed earlier. Personal beliefs about the value of an individual with a disability and the acceptable quality of life influence the recommendations made by medical professionals when parents face decisions about resuscitation and life support.

Another ethical issue involves the use of organs from infants born with anencephaly, a congenital absence of the brain except for a brain stem. These infants typically live only a few days, and the condition is uniformly fatal. Because of an extreme shortage of organs available for transplant in infants, newborns with anencephaly were used as organ donors (with parental consent). This practice came under scrutiny because the donor infants were not technically brain dead before the organs were harvested; allowing the infant to die first would have resulted in damage to the organs to be harvested. Since 1988, this practice has not been permitted, and there are virtually no organs available for infants in need of transplants. Ethical concerns included the fear that this practice encouraged the use of a human solely as an organ donor, that it used euthanasia by taking the organs before the donor had died, and that it could be the beginning of the harvesting of organs from the terminally ill, prisoners, institutionalized individuals, the poor, and other devalued populations.

Sexual and reproductive rights of individuals with disabilities have been another area of ethical debate. Not only have people with disabilities reported feeling violated by the personnel caring for them, but in individuals with mental retardation, the person may not learn appropriate physical boundaries. In the past, programs for individuals with mental retardation separated males and females and punished sexual behavior such as masturbation. These methods are now considered questionable because they forbid individuals to express their autonomy through activities that are pleasurable and potentially harmless to others. Of course, individuals with mental retardation need to be taught appropriate times and places to engage in sexual behaviors such as masturbation. In addition, these individuals should receive

🖉 NOTE THIS! •————————————————

President George H. W. Bush signed the Americans with Disabilities Act on July 26, 1990, the landmark law that advanced the rights of persons with disabilities.

instruction in using judgment in choosing when and with whom to engage in sexual activity, in the use of birth control, and in the prevention of sexually transmitted diseases. Sterilization is considered in some cases in which the individual is unable to learn to use birth control, would be unable to competently raise a child, or would experience a serious health risk if pregnant. Sterilization should not be done, however, strictly for the convenience of parents, schools, or institutions. If it is determined that sterilization is necessary, the individual should participate to the fullest extent possible to obtain informed consent.

**Informed consent** means that the individual understands the risks and benefits of the procedure, is presented with alternatives, and is given the opportunity to express a choice. Acquiring informed consent from an individual with mental retardation can be time-consuming, requiring simplification of information and multiple meetings. Informed consent is a sensitive issue in the United States because of the eugenics policies of the 1920s and 1930s. These policies were in some cases a model for the eugenics programs in Nazi Germany and required compulsory, involuntary sterilization of individuals who were "feeble-minded" or "mental defectives" in an effort to improve public health and the gene pool. A 1927 U.S. Supreme Court ruling defending sterilization resulted in more than 60,000 persons with mental retardation being sterilized without their consent. Before sterilization is performed, the motives of those in favor of the procedure along with documented efforts to use a less restrictive alternative must be examined (Batshaw et al., 2007).

## *Healthy People 2010* Objectives Related to Disabilities

Although people with disabilities are targeted by *Healthy People 2010* as a special population, objectives related to people with disabilities are found throughout the document. The health promotion and disease prevention needs of people with disabilities are critical. People with disabilities are at high risk for developing additional health problems, which may further decrease their level of functioning. Secondary conditions such as decubitus ulcers or urinary tract disorders are associated with the decreased mobility experienced by many individuals with physical disabilities and are often preventable. People with disabilities are also more likely to develop musculoskeletal disorders caused by lack of physical activity or respiratory problems caused by lack of physical activity or tobacco use. In addition, people with disabilities encounter many of the same risks as the rest of the population, such as drug and alcohol abuse, poor nutrition, and stress. The box on page 727 lists selected objectives related to people with disabilities found in *Healthy People 2010*.

## Roles of the Community Health Nurse

The roles of the community health nurse in working with individuals with disabilities are varied. These roles include

---

## 🏛 HEALTHY PEOPLE 2010

**Objectives Related to Disability**

### Disability and Secondary Conditions

6.1 Include in the core of all relevant *Healthy People 2010* surveillance instruments a standardized set of questions that identify "people with disabilities."

6.2 Reduce the proportion of children and adolescents with disabilities who are reported to be sad, unhappy, or depressed.

6.3 Reduce the proportion of adults with disabilities who report feelings such as sadness, unhappiness, or depression that prevent them from being active.

6.4 Increase the proportion of adults with disabilities who participate in social activities.

6.5 Increase the proportion of adults with disabilities reporting sufficient emotional support.

6.6 Increase the proportion of adults with disabilities reporting satisfaction with life.

6.7 Reduce the number of people with disabilities in congregate care facilities, consistent with permanency planning principles.

6.8 Eliminate disparities in employment rates between working-aged adults with and without disabilities.

6.9 Increase the proportion of children and youth with disabilities who spend at least 80% of their time in regular education programs.

6.10 Increase the proportion of health and wellness and treatment and facilities that provide full access for people with disabilities.

6.11 Reduce the proportion of people with disabilities who report not having the assistive devices and technology needed.

6.12 Reduce the proportion of people with disabilities reporting environmental barriers to participation in home, school, work, or community activities.

6.13 Increase the number of tribes, states, and the District of Columbia that have public health surveillance and health promotion programs for people with disabilities and caregivers.

*Source*: DHHS, 2000.

---

partner, change agent, researcher, case finder, case manager, referral agent, advocate, educator, and caregiver.

In working with individuals with disabilities, the community health nurse may assume the role of *partner*. The community health nurse can enhance partner competence by developing equal partnerships with individuals that do not place the community health nurse in the dominant role. The nurse can share professional knowledge with individuals with disabilities, but also assist them in recognizing and building on their own experiential knowledge (Paavilainen & Astedt-Kurki, 1997).

Often experiencing the flaws in the service system alongside families, the nurse may be moved to serve as a *change agent* for the service system. One nurse joined with a certified therapeutic recreation specialist (CTRS) to change a community recreation program's policy of excluding children with disabilities from its youth basketball program. After they educated the director and staff about the ADA requirements and strategies for inclusion, a child with spina bifida who used a wheelchair was placed on one of the teams and enjoyed several years of competitive basketball play with his same-age nondisabled peers. In the roles of *researchers*, the nurse and CTRS went on to examine the extent of the child's participation on the team, the extent of his contribution to team success, and the extent of his social acceptance by his teammates (Green & DeCoux, 1994).

The role of *case finder* is a more traditional role of the public health nurse. In the disability field, locating young children with or at risk for disabilities is especially important. *Childfind*, or locating, assessing, and offering services to such children, is required by federal law in all states. Both

### ✏ NOTE THIS! ●────────────

Oscar Pistorius becomes first double amputee to make a run for the Beijing Olympics in 2008.

Oscar Pistorius' lower legs were amputated at the age of 1. He has now become a world-class sprinter from South Africa and the first double-amputee to compete in trials for the 400-meter 2008 Olympics in Beijing, China. Many were so surprised at Pistorius' accomplishments; ironically, some believed that his prosthetic legs somehow gave him an advantage. The International Association of Athletics Federations (IAAF) ruled he could not compete against able-bodied athletes, once he decided to compete for the Olympics in Beijing. An IAAF-initiated study found that more energy is returned to Pistorius' upper legs from his blades than from ankles and calf muscles and that he uses less oxygen.

Pistorius, 21, is appealing, on the basis of studies with differing results. In the past, living with prosthetic legs was seen as a major barrier and yet he has turned his disability into a surprising controversy. According to Erik Weihenmayer, the only blind person to conquer Mount Everest, "He's on the cusp of a paradigm shift in which disability becomes ability, disadvantage becomes advantage. Yet we must not lose sight of what makes an athlete great. It is too easy to credit Pistorius' success to technology. Through birth or circumstance, some are given certain gifts, but it's what one does with those gifts, the hours devoted to training, the desire to be the best, that is at the true heart of a champion."

Pistorius was named in *Time Magazine's* list of The World's 100 Most Influential People of 2008.

*Source*: The Time 100 (2008). *Time Magazine, 171* (19), 64. Available online: http:/// www.time.com/time/specials/2007/0,28757,1733748,00.html

the states' early intervention system and public school system are responsible for Childfind. The community health nurse may work with a developmental screening team through the public school system or the state's early intervention system to identify children ages birth to 5 years with or at risk for disabilities. Typically, the nurse's role in developmental screening includes eliciting a family medical history and the child's medical and developmental history, conducting a physical examination, and assessing hearing and vision. The developmental component may be conducted by a specially trained nurse, early childhood special educator, developmental pediatrician, or psychologist.

*Case management*, or coordinating the individual with disability's care, is another role that may be assumed by the community health nurse. Knowledge of both community services and eligibility requirements is essential for effective case management. This knowledge is also used in the role of *referral agent*. The nurse can direct individuals with disabilities to agencies that can meet their needs by providing a contact person's name and the phone number of the agency. Some individuals, however, may need assistance with contacting agencies. The parents of a child who has recently experienced a traumatic brain injury may be emotionally and physically exhausted and in a state of denial regarding the likelihood of long-term disability, necessitating that the nurse be active in contacting potentially helpful agencies, groups, and individuals.

Serving as an *advocate*, or speaking on behalf of people with disabilities who are unable to speak for themselves, is an important role of the community health nurse. This advocacy may take place on the community level, with the community health nurse advocating for a medically fragile child to be included in a regular classroom rather than served "homebound" by a local public school system. At the policy level, the community health nurse could speak before a legislative hearing about the need for small group homes for adults with mental retardation in local communities or the need for public assistance with the cost of personal care attendants needed to allow people with disabilities to remain

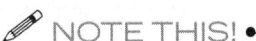

**NOTE THIS!**

Runner Marla Runyan became the first blind athlete in history to qualify for the 2000 U.S. Olympic team.

---

in their own homes. In some cases, the nurse may need to refer individuals with disabilities to the state's protection and advocacy program.

The role of the community health nurse as *educator* continues to be a cornerstone of community health nursing when working with individuals with disabilities. The nurse may educate an entire community on prevention of fetal alcohol syndrome or an individual with a spinal cord injury about preventing decubiti formation. The community health nurse can motivate adults with disabilities who have completed rehabilitation programs and returned home to resume an active productive life. Education by the nurse was credited as the key to self-care and responsibility by all persons with spinal cord injuries participating in a study looking at motivation of adults with disabilities (Brillhart & Johnson, 1997).

The role of *caregiver* is another historic role of the community health nurse. In this role, the nurse applies the nursing process by assessing, implementing, and evaluating care of a person with a disability. For individuals with significant disabilities, this care may require familiarity with medical and assistive technological devices such as ventilators and computerized communication systems (see Box 29-2).

## Conclusion

Persons with disabilities are living longer and more productive lives than ever. Community health nurses are in settings where the opportunity to promote the health of persons, families, and populations with disabilities are ample. Using knowledge gained from this chapter, community health nurses can assist these populations with preventing health problems and enhancing their ability to make informed health decisions.

Explore Community Health Nursing on the Web! To learn more about the topics in this chapter, use the passcode provided to access your exclusive website: **http://nursing.jbpub.com/ communityhealth**. If you do not have a passcode, you can obtain one at this site.

## " a conversation with . . . "

**Christopher Reeve**

Put a disabled person in the middle of a group of workers and they complain less and are more productive. Hire the disabled. They'll motivate the rest of your workforce.

(Actor Christopher Reeve was critically injured in a horse riding accident in May 1995 and sustained a spinal cord injury. He was paralyzed from the neck down. Reeve wrote his autobiography *Still Me* about his experiences with disability. He died in 2004.)

*Source*: Zaslow, J. (2000, May). The uncommon strength of Christopher Reeve. *USM Weekend*, 4–5.

## ■ CRITICAL THINKING ACTIVITIES

1. How does having a disability affect a person's self-concept?
2. Can a person with a disability ever be autonomous? Why or why not?
3. When community health nurses assist patients with disabilities in areas of health promotion, what are the most difficult challenges in regard to self-care and independence?
4. How can community health nurses promote positive self-regard for persons with disabilities in the media? Give some examples of projects that could enhance the perception of "abilities" rather than disabilities for this vulnerable population group. eLearning

## ■ REFERENCES

Barking & Dagenham, Center for Independent, Integrated, Inclusive Living Consortium. (2001). *Disability language and etiquette*. London: London Borough of Barking & Dagenham.

Batshaw, M. L., Pellegrino, M. D., & Roizen, M. D. (2007). *Children with disabilities* (6th ed.). Baltimore: Brookes Publishing Company.

Beirne-Smith, M., Patton, J. M., & Kim, S. H. (2006). *Mental retardation: An introduction to intellectual disability* (7th ed.). Upper Saddle River, NJ: Pearson Education.

Berkowitz, E. D. (1987). *Disabled policy: America's policy for the handicapped*. Cambridge, MA: Cambridge University Press.

Bernie-Smith, M. (2000). Administrators' and teachers' perceptions of the collaborative efforts of inclusion in the elementary grades. *Education, 121*(2), 331–339.

Bernstein, R. (2006). *More than 50 million Americans report some level of disability*. Retrieved December 16, 2008, from http://www.census.gov/Press-Release/www/releases/archives/aging_population/006809.html

Blackburn, J. M., Patton, J. M., Trainor, A. (2004). *Exceptional individuals in focus* (7th ed.). Princeton, NC: Merrill.

Brillhart, B., & Johnson, K. (1997). Motivation and the coping process of adults with disabilities: A qualitative study. *Rehabilitation Nursing, 22*, 249–256.

Butterworth, J., Gandolfo, C., Revell, W. G., & Inge, K. (2007). *Community rehabilitation programs and organizational change: A mentor guide to increase customized employment outcomes*. Retrieved December 16, 2008, from http://digitalcommons.ilr.cornell.edu/cgi/viewcontent.cgi?article=1361&context=gladnet collect

Capen, C. L., & Dedlow, E. R. (1998). Discharging ventilator-dependent children: A continuing challenge. *Journal of Pediatric Nursing, 13*, 175–184.

Carter, M. (2002). Inclusive fitness strategies. *Parks & Recreation, 37*(12), 54–58.

Cegelka, P. T., & Prehm, H. J. (1982). *Mental retardation: From categories to people*. Columbus, OH: Charles E. Merrill.

Centers for Disease Control and Prevention (CDC). (1999). Achievements in public health, 1900–1999; Impact of vaccines universally recommended for children, United States, 1900–1998. *Morbidity and Mortality Weekly Report, 48*(12), 243–248: www.cdc.gov/epo/mmwr/preview/mmwrhtml/00056803.htm

Craft, D. H. (1995). Visual impairments and hearing losses. In J. P. Winnick (Ed.), *Adapted physical education and sport* (2nd ed., pp. 143–166). Champaign, IL: Human Kinetics.

DeLaune, S. C., & Ladner, P. K. (2006). *Fundamentals of nursing: Standards and practice* (3rd ed.). Florence, KY: Cengage.

Department of Health and Human Services (DHHS). (2000). *Healthy People 2010.* Atlanta, GA: Author.

DiLeo, D. (2007). *Raymond's room: Ending the segregation of citizens with disabilities.* St. Augustine, FL: Training Resource Network.

Dolyniuk, C., Kamens, M. W., Corman, H., DiNardo, P. O., Totaro, R. M., & Rockoff, J. C. (2002). Students with developmental disabilities go to college: Description of a collaborative transition project on a regular college campus. *Focus on Autism & Other Developmental Disabilities, 17*(4), 236–242.

Eames, E., & Eames, T. (1997). Interpreting legal mandates: Assistance dogs in medical facilities. *Nursing Management, 28*(6), 49–51.

Eames, E., & Eames, T. (2001). Guide dog teams in the United States: Annual number trained and active, 1993–1999. *Journal of Visual Impairment & Blindness, 95*(7), 434–438.

Eldar, R. (2001). Community-based rehabilitation: Better quality of life for older rural people with disabilities. *Journal of Rural Health, 17*(4), 341–344.

Fennick, E., & James, R. (2003). Community inclusion for children and youth with developmental disabilities. *Focus on Autism & Other Developmental Disabilities, 18*(1), 20–28.

Green, F. P., & DeCoux, V. (1994). A procedure for evaluating the effectiveness of a community recreation integration program. *Therapeutic Recreation Journal, 28*(1), 41–47.

Green, F. P., & Schleien, S. J. (1991). Understanding friendship and recreation: A theoretical sampling. *Therapeutic Recreation Journal, 25(4),* 29–40.

Hablutzel, N., & McMahon, B. T. (1992). *The Americans with Disabilities Act: Access and accommodations.* Orlando: Paul M. Deutsch Press.

Holburn, S. (2002). How science can evaluate and enhance person-centered planning. *Research & Practice for Persons with Severe Disabilities, 27*(4), 250–260.

Jenkins, W. M., Patterson, J. B., & Szymanski, E. M. (1992). Philosophical, historical, and legislative aspects of the rehabilitation counseling profession In R. M. Parker & E. M. Szymanski (Eds.), *Rehabilitation counseling: Basics and beyond* (2nd ed., pp. 1–41). Austin, TX: PRO-ED.

Katz, J., Mirenda, P., & Auerbach, S. (2002). Instructional strategies and educational outcomes for students with developmental disabilities in inclusive "Multiple Intelligences" and typical inclusive classrooms. *Research & Practice for Persons with Severe Disabilities, 27*(4), 227–238.

Kirk, S. A., Gallagher, J. J., Anastasiow, N. J., & Coleman (2006). *Educating exceptional children* (11th ed.). Florence, KY: Cengage.

Krzywda, E. A. (1998). Central venous access: Catheters, technology, and physiology. *Medical–Surgical Nursing, 7,* 132–141.

Lakin, K., Prouty, R., Polister, B., & Coucouvanis, K. (2003). Change in residential placements for persons with intellectual and developmental disabilities in the USA in the last two decades. *Journal of Intellectual & Developmental Disability, 28*(2), 205–210.

Laplante, M., Hendershot, G., & Moss, A. (1992). *Assistive technology devices and home accessibility features: Prevalence, payment, need, and trends.* Washington, DC: National Center for Health Statistics.

Lindsey, P., Guy, B., Wehmeyer, M. L., & Martin, J. (2001). Age of majority and mental retardation: A position statement of the Division on Mental Retardation and Developmental Disabilities. *Education and Training in Mental Retardation and Developmental Disabilities, 36*(1), 3–15.

Mank, D., Cioffi, A., & Yovanoff, P. (2003). Supported employment outcomes across a decade: Is there evidence of improvements in the quality of implementation? *Mental Retardation, 41*(3), 188–197.

Marino, M. J. (1999, June/July). CDC report shows prevalence of brain injury. *TBI Challenge, 3*(3).

Mayo, M. (2002). Camps for children with illnesses on the rise. *Camping Magazine, 75*(6), 20–25.

McCarthy, H. (2003). The disability rights movement: Experiences and perspectives of selected leaders in the disability community. *Rehabilitation Counseling Bulletin, 46*(4), 209–223.

Millar, D. S., & Renzagia, A. (2002). Factors affecting guardianship practices for young adults with disabilities. *Exceptional Children, 68*(4), 465–484.

National Organization on Disability. (2004). *2004 N.O.D./Harris Survey documents trends impacting 54 million Americans.* Retrieved December 16, 2008, from http://www.nod.org/index.cfm?fuseaction=Feature.showFeature&FeatureID=1422

Newcomer, R., Kang, T., Kaye, H. S., & LaPlante, M. (2002). Housing changes and moves into supportive housing among adults with disabilities. *Journal of Disability Policy Studies, 12*(4), 268–279.

Paavilainen, E., & Astedt-Kurki, P. (1997). The patient–nurse relationship as experienced by public health nurses: Toward better collaboration. *Public Health Nursing, 14,* 137–150.

Patton, J. R., Blackbourn, J. M., & Fad, K. (2004). *Exceptional individuals in focus* (7th ed.). Englewood Cliffs, NJ: Prentice-Hall:

Pierce, L. L. (1998). Barriers to access: Frustrations of people who use a wheelchair for full-time mobility. *Rehabilitation Nursing, 23,* 120–125.

Racino, J. A. (1999). Statewide approaches to community integration: Moving toward technical assistance strategies that make a difference. *Journal of Vocational Rehabilitation, 13,* 31–44.

Racino, J. A., & Taylor, S. J. (1993). People first: Approaches to housing and support. In J. A. Racino, P. Walker, S. O'Connor, & S. J. Taylor (Eds.), *Housing, support, and community: Choices and strategies for adults with disabilities* (vol. 2, pp. 33–56). Baltimore: Paul H. Brookes.

Research and Training Center on Independent Living. (2001). *Guidelines for reporting and writing about people with disabilities* (6th ed.). Lawrence, KS: Research and Training Center on Independent Living, Bureau of Child Research, University of Kansas.

Revell, G., Kregel, J., Wehman, P., & Bond, G. (2000). Cost effectiveness of supported employment programs: What we need to do to improve outcomes. *Journal of Vocational Rehabilitation, 14,* 173–178.

Roman, M., Miller, L., Maculuso, S., Dempsey, R., & Golden-Baker, S. (1998). Breaking the boundaries: Collaborating to develop a model ventilator training program. *Medical-Surgical Nursing, 7,* 9–18.

Schleien, S. J., Ray, M. T., & Green, F. P. (1997). *Community recreation and people with disabilities: Strategies for inclusion* (2nd ed.). Baltimore: Paul H. Brookes.

Thompson, J., Hughes, C., Schalock, R., et al. (2002). Integrating supports in assessment and planning. *Mental Retardation, 40*(5), 390–405.

Trachtenberg, S. W., & Lewis, D. F. (1996). Case management. In L. A. Kurtz, P. W. Dowrick, S. E. Levy, & M. L. Batshaw (Eds.), *Handbook of developmental disabilities: Resources for interdisciplinary care* (pp. 203–208). Gaithersburg, MD: Aspen.

Travers, P. L. (1999). Autonomic dysreflexia: A clinical rehabilitation problem. *Rehabilitation Nursing, 24,* 19–23.

U.S. Census Bureau. (2006). *American community survey: Disability characteristics.* Retrieved December 16, 2008, from http://factfinder.census.gov/servlet/STTable?_bm=y&-geo_id=01000US&-qr_name=ACS_2006_EST_G00_S1801&-ds_name=ACS_2006_EST_G00_

U.S. Department of Justice. (1992). *Nondiscrimination on the basis of disability in state and local government services.* Retrieved December 18, 2008, from http://www.usdoj.gov/crt/ada/reg2.html

Ward, M. J. (1996). Coming of age in the age of self-determination: A historical and personal perspective. In D. J. Sands & M. L. Wehmeyer (Eds.), *Self-determination across the lifespan: Independence and choice for people with disabilities* (pp. 3–16). Baltimore, MD: Paul H. Brookes.

Warren, S. (2002). Presidential address 2002—Genes, brains, and behavior: The road ahead. *Mental Retardation, 40*(6), 471–476.

Wehman, P. (2006a). *Life beyond the classroom: Transition strategies for young people with disabilities* (4th ed.). Baltimore: Brookes Publishing Company.

Wehman, P. (2006b). Comment to Brown Shiraga and Kessler (2006) paper: Integrated employment: If not now, when? If not us, who? *Research and Practice for Persons with Severe Disabilities, 31*(2), 122–126.

Wehman, P. (2003a). Business collaboration with public sector. *Journal of Vocational Rehabilitation, 19,* 3–4.

Wehman, P. (2003b). Opening the community for persons with disabilities: How are we doing? *Journal of Vocational Rehabilitation, 19,* 121–122.

Wehman, P. (2003c). Workplace inclusion: Persons with disabilities and coworkers working together. *Journal of Vocational Rehabilitation, 18,* 131–141.

Wehman, P., Revell, W. G., & Brooke, V. (2003). Competitive employment: Has it become the "first choice" yet? *Journal of Disability Policy Studies, 14*(3), 163–173.

Wehman, P. H., Targett, P. S., & Cifi, D. X. (2006). Job coaches: A workplace support. *American Journal of Physical Medicine and Rehabilitation, 85*(8), 704.

Wehman, P., Brooke, V., Green, H., Hewett, M., & Tipton, M. (2008). Public/private partnerships and employment of people with developmental disabilities: Preliminary evidence from a pilot project. *Journal of Vocational Rehabilitation, 28*(1), 53–66.

Wehmeyer, M. L., & Bolding, N. (2001). Enhanced self-determination of adults with intellectual disability as an outcome of moving to community-based work or living environments. *Journal of Intellectual Disability Research, 45*(5), 371–383.

West, M. D., Wehman, P. B., & Wehman, P. (2005). Competitive employment outcomes for persons with intellectual and developmental disabilities: The national impact of the Best Buddies Job Program. *Journal of Vocational Rehabilitation, 23*(1), 51–63.

Yamaki, K., & Fujiura, G. (2002). Employment and income status of adults with developmental disabilities living in the community. *Mental Retardation, 40*(2), 132–141.

Yasuda, S., Wehman, P., Targett, P., Cifu, D., & West, M. (2002). Return to work after spinal cord injury: A review of recent research. *NeuroRehabilitation, 17,* 177–186.

# PART 2

# Community-Based Nursing Care

 EVIDENCE-BASED PRACTICE: A COMMUNITY APPROACH

RECENT CHANGES IN SOCIETY have had a profound impact on the health care delivery system in the United States. There has been an explosion of technology accompanied by an increase in health care costs to the consumer, with resulting changes in the *setting* and *focus* of health care delivery. Managed care and controlling health care costs are primary foci of the health care industry. The family, as the oldest and most basic of all social institutions, has undergone dramatic change in structure and function. Through the family, health care needs are identified and addressed, from birth to death. The portion of the U.S. population that is older than 65 is the fastest growing segment, as well as the group that requires the most health care dollars. Individuals with higher acuity levels, that in the past were treated in acute care institutions, are now being discharged to the community and treated in the home. The nurse of the 21st century will require a firm foundation in both acute and community-based/community-focused nursing health care to assist individuals in making the transition not only from acute care to home care but to and from other community settings, such as school and work.

Through the family, children are socialized to norms, values, and behavior. As such, the family is a powerful influence on the health beliefs and behavior of its members. The assessment of family functioning and its ability to meet the health needs of its members is a critical aspect of the community health nurse role.

Research indicates that gender influences the seeking, acquisition, and use of health services and health behavior. Women are less likely to be diagnosed with heart disease because it has long been associated as a male health problem. Men, in turn, often seek health care later than their female counterparts, which often results in less successful outcomes.

When children receive appropriate health-promotion and disease-prevention services, they are less likely to develop health problems. Nursing has a role in providing anticipatory guidance to parents and children regarding health-promotion and disease-prevention activities.

Community-based settings for mental health care have dominated for several decades. With the mental health clients, this is more cost-effective than institutionalization, and outcomes for the family are positive. Local community mental health centers provide care for all levels of mental health care needs. Lack of reimbursement and appropriate identification mechanisms for locating the mentally ill require creativity on the part of the community health nurse to meet community mental health needs.

Because Americans are living longer, myriad age-appropriate additional health care services for the aging population will be necessary. The health and care of the elder client is but one of the challenges associated with this age group. Ample research has documented that the caregiver is also at high risk from impaired health. Poor health of the caregiver is often a deciding factor in making the decision to place an elderly family member into institutionalized care. Community health nurses must develop and implement strategies that promote physical and mental health for both the elder and the caregiver.

# UNIT 6

# Care of Families

CHAPTER 30
Foundations of Family Care
*Ruth A. O'Brien*
*Karen Saucier Lundy*

CHAPTER 31
Caring for the Family in Health and Illness
*Linda Beth Tiedje*
*Karen Saucier Lundy*

# CHAPTER 30
# Foundations of Family Care

Ruth A. O'Brien and Karen Saucier Lundy

Visit **http://nursing.jbpub.com/communityhealth** for interactive exercises, review questions, Web links, and more.

If the family were a container, it would be a nest, an enduring nest, loosely woven, expansive and open.

If the family were a fruit, it would be an orange, a circle of sections, held together but separately—each segment distinct.

If the family were a boat, it would be a canoe that makes no progress unless everyone paddles.

If the family were a sport, it would be baseball: a long, slow, non-violent game that is never over until the last out.

If the family were a building, it would be an old, but solid structure that contains human history, and appeals to those who see the carved moldings under all the plaster, the wide plank floors under the linoleum, the possibilities . . .

—Letty Cottin Pogrebin

We all enter the world with fairly simple needs: to be protected, to be nurtured, to be loved unconditionally, and to belong.

—*Louise Hart*

As you reflect on the quotes on the facing page and the one above, what is your definition of family? Who do you consider your family? Does your definition include friends and non-blood-related members? How did your family of origin (the family of your childhood) affect your values about life, about health? As an adult, have your values about families changed or remained the same? As nurses, we often have "idealized" notions about family, which influences our care. Think about your own experiences as a child with your family as well as your present family as you read this chapter.

## CHAPTER FOCUS

**Definition of Family**

**Health Responsibilities of the Family**
- Development of Members' Sense of Personal Identity and Self-Worth
- Emotional Support and Guidance During Life-Cycle Transitions
- Socialization of Family Members to Value and Maintain Health
- Education About When and How to Use the Healthcare System
- Care Provision and Management for Chronically Ill, Disabled, and Aging Family Members

**Theoretical Approaches to the Family**
- Human Ecology Theory
- Family Systems Theory
- Family Development Theory

**Family-Oriented versus Family-Focused Nursing Role**

**A Conceptual Framework for Family Assessment**
- Energy
- Consciousness
- Role Structure
- Decision-Making Processes
- Communication Patterns
- Values
- Family Boundaries

**A Self-Efficacy Model of Nurse–Family Intervention**
- Identification of Family Health Concerns and Needs
- Mutual Setting of Goals
- Delineation of Alternatives
- Implementation of the Plan
- Evaluation

## QUESTIONS TO CONSIDER

After reading this chapter, you will know the answers to the following questions:

1. How is *family* defined?
2. What are the health responsibilities of the family?
3. What is the difference between family-oriented and family-focused nursing care?
4. What is an example of a conceptual framework for family assessment?
5. How is the self-efficacy model of family interventions used in promoting the health of families?

## KEY TERMS

| | | | |
|---|---|---|---|
| Affect | Environment | Interdependence | Positive feedback |
| Beliefs | Family | Meaning | Power |
| Communication | Family developmental tasks | Negative feedback | Self-regulation |
| Contracting | Function | Nonsummativity | Structure |

WHAT IS A FAMILY? Perhaps no other word in today's society would yield as many different responses from people who should know: After all, we have all been raised in some form of family. As the basic unit of society, the family has certainly undergone dramatic changes in the last 25 years. Since World War II, through the civil rights and women's rights movements of the 1960s and the economic challenges of the latter part of the twentieth century, to the national insecurity post–September 11, 2001, in this century, society has faced conflicting ideas about how and what to think about the institution we call "family." We all care about our own families, and most of us have definite ideas about how they have influenced our lives. In recent years, however, society has also moved to caring about the *idea* of family and the future of the family in the United States.

Family is not a precise or universally understood word: It has many different meanings and provokes strong reactions depending on the context in which it is used. To give us some idea of how family is used in different contexts, consider the following:

- When are you two going to settle down and raise a family? In this context, *family* means children.
- We refer to orphans as children "without a family."
- When abused children are removed from the custody of their father and mother, they are taken "from their family," so in this context, *family* means parents.

---

### 🔨 ETHICAL CONNECTION

Joyce Williams, a school nurse at Sagebrush Elementary, reflected on her recent meeting with Mrs. Carson, the first-grade teacher for Kevin Johnson. Mrs. Carson had contacted her to discuss Kevin's increasing episodes of toileting accidents and inattention in class over the past 2 months. Mrs. Carson questioned whether Kevin's behavior was indicative of problems coping with his parents' divorce; she told Joyce that the third-grade teacher who had Kevin's sister in class related that the children's father recently remarried and moved to another city about 50 miles away. According to Kevin's school file, Mrs. Johnson was a legal secretary for a large law firm downtown. Recognizing the strains that a single, working parent raising two children, 6 and 8 years old, might be experiencing, Joyce decided that she would call Mrs. Johnson to schedule a home visit to talk with her about the problems Kevin's teacher had reported. A home visit, rather than a conference at the school, would provide an opportunity for her to observe parent–child interaction and also to gain a better appreciation of how Mrs. Johnson is handling being a single parent and what other supports are available.

---

🖉 NOTE THIS! ●
What is a DINK? Dual incomes, No kids. Childless couples have doubled in number over the past 20 years.

Three of five U.S. mothers work for wages today. One in six children is in day care.

- The media often refer to the "single-parent family," but this usually means the parent is a "mother."
- When a question of care is involved (as in parenting courses, and class parents), "parent" means "mother."
- When a man is arrested for a horrible crime, neighbors often refer to their surprise at him as being a "real family man." Is a "family man" somehow distinct from other husbands? Is he less likely to commit a crime? Do you hear people refer to women as a "real family woman"?
- When a woman runs for office, she is often asked how she will manage as a "working mother." Yet, is that same question ever asked of a "working father"?

In this chapter, you will learn about how community health nurses can assist all families, whatever form they take, to live healthier lives. The family may be defined in many ways but, most importantly, *our family is who we think it is.*

🖉 NOTE THIS! ●
Denmark became the first country in the world to legalize same-sex marriage when it did so in 1989.

## Definition of Family

Dramatic changes in family structure over the past few decades are highlighted in contrasting media images portrayed in popular television sitcoms, from *Ozzie and Harriet* and *Father Knows Best* in the 1950s to the *The Simpsons, The Cosby Show, Everybody Loves Raymond,* and *Will and Grace* in more recent years. The popular image of the family as a nuclear two-parent unit raising their own children, with father as the breadwinner and mother as the homemaker, as portrayed in *Ozzie and Harriet* and *Father Knows Best,* is no longer the dominant pattern in American society. Only 1 in 5 families in the twenty-first century comes close to this stereotype.

The single-mother family has increased in number during the past decade. These families are at special risks for poverty and a lack of health insurance.

Single-parent, stepfamilies or blended families, dual-career families in which both parents work, married couples without children, cohabitating couples, and gay and lesbian families are more typical of the diverse family patterns today. Social, demographic, and economic factors have all contributed to the changing composition of the family. Close to 40% of all births in the United States are now to unmarried women (Kaiser Family Foundation, 2004). Contrary to common perceptions that teens are responsible for most of the out-of-wedlock births, rates of out-of-wedlock births are highest among single women in their 20s. Based on the trend toward a higher proportion of births to single women, coupled with the higher incidence of divorce, about half of all children today are expected to spend some part of their time in a single-parent home. Given that most people who divorce remarry, stepfamilies or blended families are fast becoming the norm in the twenty-first century. The number of dual-career families also has markedly increased, with almost three-fourths of married mothers with children reporting some paid employment. Furthermore, the continued growth of the older population will increase both the number of elderly couples and the number of frail elderly persons living alone who will require supportive services in an era when adult daughters hold jobs and are not as readily available as earlier generations to be family caregivers.

Heightened attention to demographic changes in the composition of the family over the past 40 years has generated considerable debate among social scientists on whether the family is declining in importance in our society. In reflecting on the passion that often surrounds the debate, Cowan, Field, Hansen, Skolnick, and Swanson (1992) asserted, "Families mattered in the past; they continue to matter in the present; and they will matter still, in the uncertain years of our future" (p. 481). Valuing the family, however, should not be confused with valuing a particular family form. These authors urged that, rather than viewing demographic changes in the composition of the family unit as indicative of family decline, we need to reconsider traditional definitions of family that emphasize legal and biological ties between members and conceptualize how diverse types of families fulfill different functions to address the complexity of their health needs.

How should we define the family for community health nursing assessment and intervention? Although community health nursing's primary target of service is the community, work with the family as a population is one strategy that nurses may use to improve the health of communities. Thus community health nurses need a broad conceptual perspective of the family that recognizes diverse compositions. **Family** in this chapter refers to two or more individuals who identify themselves as family and manifest some degree of interdependence in interactions with each other and their **environment** in meeting basic human needs for affection and meaning. Themes central to this definition are members' **interdependence** in meeting basic needs and members' **beliefs** that they are a family. This purposefully broad view of family encompasses the traditional two parent nuclear family, single-parent families, stepfamilies or blended families, and childless couples, as well as relationships that are not built on legal or biological ties, such as gay or lesbian families.

## Health Responsibilities of the Family

How well the family functions has a great impact on individual family members' well-being and health behaviors. Health professionals' encounters with the family are episodic, with the family assuming primary responsibility for the health care of its members. An assessment of family functioning in promoting and protecting its members' health requires a clear understanding of its responsibilities in this arena. Five major responsibilities of the family for members' health are presented.

### ■ Development of Members' Sense of Personal Identity and Self-Worth

The family plays a significant role in the development of one's mental health (Hanson & Boyd, 1996; Loveland-Cherry, 1996). Family interactions may facilitate or impede members' access to (1) **affect,** the sense of loving and being

---

**THINK ABOUT THIS** .....

What makes a happy marriage? Lauer and Lauer (1992) interviewed 351 couples who had been married for 15 years or longer. Fifty-one of these couples were unhappy with their marriages but stayed together for the children, tradition, and other reasons. The other 300 "happy" couples all had the following in common:

- Think of their spouse as their best friend
- Like their spouse as a person
- Think of marriage as a long-term commitment
- Believe that marriage is sacred
- Agree with their spouse on goals
- Believe that their spouse has grown more interesting over the years
- Strongly want the relationship to succeed
- Laugh together

*Source:* Lauer, J., & Lauer, R. (1992). Marriages made to last. In J. M. Henslin (Ed.), *Marriage and family in a changing society* (4th ed., pp. 481–486). New York: Free Press.

---

### ■■ CULTURAL CONNECTION

- Fewer than half of Hispanics and African Americans own homes, compared with 70% of whites in 2002.
- The median net worth of African American families fell 32% to $5,988 from 1999 to 2002; over the same period, the median net worth of Hispanic households dropped 24% to $7,932 and that of white households rose 3% to $88,651.

A strong and mutually respectful relationship between partners promotes healthy development in children and families.

loved; (2) **power,** the freedom to decide what one wants and the ability to obtain it; and (3) **meaning,** a sense of who and what one is. The functionally healthy family is one that maintains a balance between all members' access to affect, power, and meaning so that no member consistently and systematically is denied actualization of these basic human needs. Community health nurses often receive referrals to conduct a family assessment in situations in which parents have experienced difficulties in meeting the socioemotional needs of infants and young children, resulting in impaired attachment and inadequate weight gain associated with the syndrome referred to as *failure to thrive.* Early parent–infant attachment is critical to the development of trust and ability to form intimate relationships with others later in life. Parents who have difficulty forming appropriate attachments with their infants may have lacked appropriate role models as young children themselves. Such individuals often are suspicious of professionals, and much interpersonal skill and patience are needed to establish working relationships with them. By conveying warmth and caring, coupled with a

### ETHICAL CONNECTION

*❝The poorest people in our country today, on the whole, are working every day. But they are earning wages so low that they cannot begin to function in the mainstream of the economic life of our nation. . . . We have thousands and thousands of people working on full-time jobs, with part-time incomes.❞*
—*Martin Luther King, Jr., January 1968*

How different is today's society than it was in 1968? Are the poorest families still "outside of the mainstream"?

nonjudgmental attitude, nurses can assist parents in learning how to meet the socioemotional needs of their children.

### ■ Emotional Support and Guidance During Life-Cycle Transitions

As individuals grow and mature, they are expected to meet new performance expectations consistent with their current life stage. For example, a child is expected to learn to read when he or she goes to school. Should the child find reading difficult, school progress is slowed and the child's sense of personal worth is threatened. Support and guidance from the family are essential in helping individuals achieve their developmental tasks across the life cycle (Duvall & Miller, 1985). In fact, the family as a whole is described as having responsibilities, goals, and developmental tasks that parallel the developmental tasks of individual family members. Thus, while children are expected to learn to read and develop other cognitive skills when they go to school, the family has the corresponding developmental task of encouraging children's educational achievement and learning to relate to the educational system in an effective manner.

Community health nurses have many opportunities to provide guidance to families undergoing life-cycle transitions. Prenatal and postpartum visits for new parents can offer health teaching to ease the transition to parenthood. Changes in family structure as a result of divorce and/or remarriage also present new developmental tasks for family members, such as single parenthood and the addition of stepparent into children's lives. As noted in the introductory paragraph, Kevin's teacher in making a referral to the school nurse questioned whether his toileting accidents in school

Elder women and their family members share celebrations as opportunities to enhance family bonds.

might be symptomatic of difficulty in coping with his parents' divorce and the subsequent move and remarriage of his father.

## Socialization of Family Members to Value and Maintain Health

Family members acquire values about health and learn personal health practices relative to nutrition, exercise, smoking, alcohol consumption, and hygiene through their family of origin and later transmit these values and beliefs to children as they become parents. Recognition that lifestyle factors are the single most important determinant of most of our chronic diseases has focused attention on the importance of the family's responsibility to teach its members how to maintain and preserve health (Antonovsky, 1987).

*Healthy People 2010* (DHHS, 2000) offers a vision for preventing unnecessary death and disability, enhancing the quality of life for all Americans through the establishment of specific health promotion and disease prevention objectives. Many of the objectives focus on lifestyle risks that have their origin in health practices learned within the family context. In their interactions with families, nurses may assist members to assess health risks and to incorporate health promotion into their lifestyle (Duffy, 1988). Schools and the workplace also offer natural loci for helping children and adults to improve their health knowledge and develop attitudes that facilitate healthier behaviors.

**❝** *For good or ill, our families and the environment in which we live are the backdrop against which we play out our entire lives. Families shape our futures; our early family experiences heavily influence and to a degree determine how we forever after think and behave.* **❞**

—Hillary Rodham Clinton, It Takes a Village: And Other Lessons Children Teach Us, 1996

THINK ABOUT THIS

The 300 millionth American was born in 2006. A baby is born every 8 seconds in the United States.

## Education About When and How to Use the Healthcare System

The family also serves as the basic referent for defining illness and what should be done about it (Doherty & Campbell, 1988). The process by which the ill person seeks information and advice from family, friends, neighbors, other nonprofessionals, and Internet-media sources has been labeled the "lay referral network." Whether a family member's symptoms should be treated with home remedies

Elders today are more active. This couple climbs mountains throughout the world after retirement.

**❝** *The heart is where the home is.* **❞**

—Kenneth Keniston

and over-the-counter medications or professional help should be sought is negotiated within the family based on interpretations of the seriousness of the symptoms, the possible cause, costs versus benefits of the action, and the impact that illness may have on the member's fulfillment of role responsibilities (Doherty, 1992). While *Healthy People 2010* has shifted national attention toward primary prevention by emphasizing health promotion and health protection activities, secondary prevention, which involves early detection and treatment of illness, is recognized as another important approach for fostering healthy communities. In some families, one is defined as ill only when symptoms are severe enough to affect role performance. Teaching women the importance of breast self-examinations, Pap smears, and mammograms and teaching males the importance of regular testicular and digital rectal examinations are examples of ways nurses can encourage family members to value the early detection of disease and to use the healthcare system in a more proactive way.

With recent national disasters, there has been a greater awareness of the need for disaster preparedness for families. Additionally, families need assistance in evaluating the quality of Internet-based health information.

## ■ Care Provision and Management for Chronically Ill, Disabled, and Aging Family Members

Families assume a major share of the responsibility for intergenerational support and assistance. Among older disabled persons who live in the community, more than 90% rely in part on family for care (Kaiser Foundation, 2004). Two distinct caregiving roles that may be assumed by the family are direct care provider and indirect care manager. The direct care provider actively assists family members with those activities and tasks that they are no longer able to perform independently. The indirect care manager identifies the needed services an impaired relative requires and manages their provision by others. Problems in meeting societal expectations of families for caring for disabled and aging members are emerging because the caregiving role previously filled by women has dramatically changed as a result of the increase in dual-career families. Women still account for the largest percentage of caregivers for these family members. Recognition of this fact has led to the rapid expansion of home health services and hospice programs to facilitate care of family members within their home environment.

## Theoretical Approaches to the Family

Theory provides the practitioner with a systematic way of viewing a particular phenomenon. A variety of theoretical frameworks have been used to describe family interaction and behavior. No single theory is sufficiently broad to deal with the complex dynamics that undergird the family's competence to fulfill its health responsibilities. Thus an integrated approach that blends family systems theory with family development and human ecology theory will be used here. This ecological systems perspective is particularly relevant to the discipline of nursing because it considers interrelationships between individuals within the family as well as between the family unit and the community over time.

## ■ Human Ecology Theory

Human ecology theory emphasizes the importance of social contexts as influences on human development. Bronfenbrenner (1986) notes that the parent–child relationship is enhanced as a context for development to the extent that the family's interrelationships with social networks, neighborhoods, communities, institutions, and cultures are supportive of its efforts to care for children. A similar perspective is presented by Hillary Rodham Clinton in her 1996 book *It Takes a Village: And Other Lessons Children Teach Us*. Thus

✎ NOTE THIS! ●─────────────────────

Two-thirds of women work for pay during the same years that they are bearing and raising children.

................................................................

*Source*: International Law Office. (1999). *Maternity protection at work*. Geneva, Switzerland: International Labor Office.

the extent to which work settings provide quality day care or flexible working hours can strongly influence the success of dual-career couples in fulfilling their childrearing functions. Similarly, adolescent parents are more likely to be able to continue to meet their own developmental needs for education when school policies support pregnant teens' remaining in school throughout the pregnancy and/or provide child care for teens returning to school after the baby's birth.

Another distinctive feature of human ecology theory is its recognition that the family is both influenced by and actively influences the larger social systems with which it interacts. This perspective of human ecology theory encourages us to look at interactions between the family and its multilevel environment as reciprocal rather than unidirectional processes. For example, although governmental policies often strongly influence the healthcare services available to a family, families can also shape policy. Parents concerned about pressures from health maintenance organizations (HMOs) and insurance companies, which often forced mothers and their newborns to be discharged within 24 hours of birth, joined professional and citizen lobby groups to help pass a

❝*Nothing is more important to our shared future than the well-being of children. For children are at our core—not only as vulnerable beings in need of love and care but as a moral touchstone amidst the complexity and contentiousness of modern life. Just as it takes a village to raise a child, it takes children to raise up a village to become all it should be. The village we build with them in mind will be a better place for us all.*❞

*—Hillary Rodham Clinton, It Takes a Village: And Other Lessons Children Teach Us, 1996*

..................................................................

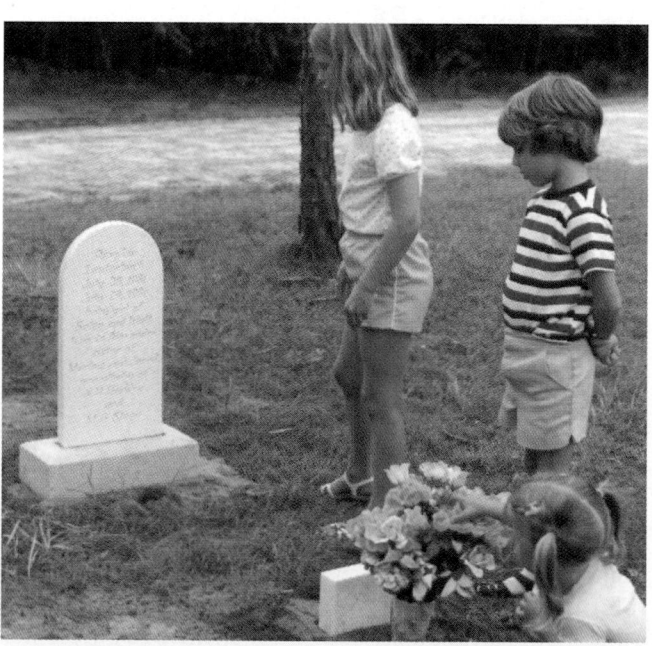

The socialization of children is one of the most important functions of the family.

1996 law titled "The Newborns' and Mothers' Health Protection Act." This bill requires insurers to cover a minimum stay of 48 hours for mothers and their newborns.

## Family Systems Theory

Although human ecology theory provides us with a conception of how interrelationships between the family and its social context influence the family's capacity to foster health, it does not address how internal processes within the family may facilitate or impede health. Family systems theory, however, does provides us with several key concepts to understand the role of internal family processes on health. First is the concept of **nonsummativity,** which states that the family as a whole is greater than the sum of its parts, such that a change in one family member affects all family members (Wright & Leahey, 1994). Because the whole is more than and different from the sum of its parts, the family's ability to fulfill its health responsibilities cannot be predicted from knowledge about an individual's behavior and health practices. Instead, the nurse must assess how family relationships and their social environments either impede or foster health (see the Research Alert).

For example, one cannot judge that an infant is developing adequate attachment without assessing the relationships between the parent and infant. Are bids of the infant to mother for attention when distressed responded to with soothing behaviors on the part of the mother? Healthfulness is reflected in the dyad's capacity to achieve patterns of interaction that are mutually rewarding (Robinson, Emde, & Korfmacher, 1997). Another example of the principle of nonsummativity is illustrated in the brief vignette presented at the beginning

### MEDIA MOMENT

**The Family in Movies**

*The Long Walk Home* (2002)
On a long walk, a man remembers the events that led to the death of his wife.

*Crimes of the Heart* (1986)
Three sisters with quite different personalities and lives reunite when the youngest of them, Babe, has just shot her husband.

*Steel Magnolias* (1989)
Revolving around Truvy's Beauty Parlor in a small parish in modern-day Louisiana, *Steel Magnolias* is the story of a close-knit circle of friends whose lives come together there.

*What's Eating Gilbert Grape?* (1993)
Gilbert has to care for his mentally disabled brother, Arnie, and his morbidly obese mother, which gets in the way when love walks into his life.

 **Research Alert**

A study of 35 mothers with multiple sclerosis and their children found that both mothers and children perceived that mothers were less physically affectionate when mothers' symptoms of illness were exacerbated. Mothers, however, significantly underestimated the changes in their physical affection compared with children's perceptions. Qualitative data further revealed that affective issues were linked with tremendous fears of the children, particularly the younger children, as reflected in the following comments: "I cry when she's sick. Sometimes I think that she is going to die."

*Source*: Deatrick, J. A., Brennan, D., & Cameron, M. E. (1998). Mothers with multiple sclerosis and their children: Effects of fatigue and exacerbations on maternal support. *Nursing Research, 47*(4), 205–210.

of this chapter. Rather than simply viewing Kevin's toileting accidents and inattention as indicators only of a potential underlying physical health problem, the school nurse and the teacher recognize the importance of considering that Kevin's symptoms may reflect problems he is having in coping with changes in family relationships. Moreover, the school nurse chooses to follow up on the problem by scheduling a home visit to gather more data on how the mother is handling the transition to being a single parent.

Two other concepts important in understanding how the family operates as a system are structure and function. **Structure** refers to the organization of relationships among family members (i.e., roles), whereas **function** defines the purposes or goals of the family, such as activities necessary to ensure health and growth of its members (Walsh, 1982). Structure and function are interrelated in that the structure of a family influences how well it is able to fulfill its purposes or goals. Roles within a family must be integrated, much like the meshing of gears in a finely tuned engine, facilitate attainment of common goals. Nurses working in the community often encounter families who are struggling with children's behavioral problems because the parents cannot agree on what are reasonable bedtimes for young children or how to consistently set limits, and consequently each defines different expectations for the child. Although adults may learn to balance multiple role expectations (e.g., spouse, parent, worker, volunteer), young children need clarity in role expectations to begin to develop a sense of identity and self-worth (one of the family's five health responsibilities).

 NOTE THIS!

Families with incomes greater than $50,000 per year have a 31% chance of divorce after 15 years as compared to families making less. If the workplace provides men and women with dignity and a semblance of economic security, that will translate within the family.

*Source*: Blumer, R. (2006). *National marriage project.* New Brunswick, NJ: Rutgers, The State University of New Jersey.

Finally, understanding the role that **self-regulation** processes play in how the family functions in meeting its health responsibilities is important for nurses working in the community. A balance between stability and change is needed for a family to effectively address the differing needs of its members over time (Klein & White, 1996). Self-regulation involves processing the internal as well as external feedback that a family receives regarding its behavior. Feedback can be positive or negative. **Positive feedback** moves the family toward change, whereas **negative feedback** tends to promote stability. In assessing a family, the nurse seeks to identify those behaviors that are detrimental to health and provides feedback in the form of health teaching. In the previous example in which parents are having difficulty in agreeing on limits for their children, teaching by the nurse about realistic expectations for the child's developmental age and the importance of consistency in parental discipline would be directed toward behavioral change. Conversely, when working with a mother who the nurse observes reads to her toddler, teaching about how parents can facilitate language development of toddlers would reinforce and expand on the mother's existing behaviors.

 THINK ABOUT THIS ················································

Bad child care is the nightmare from which no mother can escape. The professional who can run a business or save a life . . . the mother who can organize a community fundraiser while entertaining two toddlers and nursing a baby—no matter how thoroughly they've investigated a nanny, no matter how many years they've known their sitter, all walk out the door haunted by the specter that the sitter or staff member to whom they've entrusted their most precious responsibility is a Hyde masquerading as a Jekyll, or otherwise not the woman they thought her to be.

—Melinda M. Marshall

### ■ Family Development Theory

Family development theory highlights that change is an inherent aspect of family life. The family life cycle is described in terms of developmental stages characterized by major family events—in particular, the addition and exiting of members (Carter & McGoldrick, 1989). The concept of **family developmental tasks** refers to growth responsibilities that must be achieved by a family during each stage of its life cycle to successively meet the health and developmental needs of its members. For example, the birth of a child necessitates that other family members learn new role behaviors for protecting and fostering the health and development of the infant.

Variations in the family life cycle and its developmental tasks are changing with the increasing diversity of family types. Although the single-parent family experiences the same life-cycle changes as the traditional two-parent nuclear family, the absence of the second parent to carry a share

of the family tasks with respect to support, childrearing, companionship, and gender role modeling for children may result in increased stressors for single parents. Divorce and possibly remarriage, with their losses and shifts in family membership, create new developmental tasks. For example, after divorce, spouses need to work through resolution of the attachment to one another while promoting ongoing parental contact between the ex-spouse and children (Carter & McGoldrick, 1989). With step-parent or blended families, crucial developmental tasks involve the restructuring of family boundaries and roles to allow for inclusion of new family members (step-parent and possibly step-children).

Bain (1978) has advanced a theory to predict the capacity of families to cope with life-cycle transitions that helps integrate human ecology and family systems with family development theory. According to his theory, families who are likely to have the least capacity to cope with life cycle transitions, or who are at most risk, are (1) those who are experiencing a greater number of concurrent life-cycle changes involving (2) role transitions of great magnitude (e.g., blended families) and who (3) have a social support network that is small and non-supportive, and (4) live in a community that has few available services to assist them with the transitions confronting them.

*How to be a good parent:*
- *Laugh a lot.*
- *Get the family moving, be active, get away from the TV.*
- *Avoid "labels"—they stick.*
- *Read to children every night.*
- *Catch your children being 'good.'*

—Ann Pleshette Murphy

## Family-Oriented versus Family-Focused Nursing Role

Nurses working in the community generally advocate a family approach in the delivery of services. In practice, a family approach has varied meanings. Many times, nursing interventions are directed toward the health concerns of referred individuals, with other family members being considered only as a support system for helping the individual cope with his or her health concerns. This family-oriented approach is most typical of nurses working in ambulatory care centers and home health agencies. For example, in working with a person with newly diagnosed diabetes, the nurse may assess the extent to which other family members understand and support the diabetic individual's need to modify dietary patterns to manage the disease effectively and prevent further complications.

The complexity of health issues confronting families may, at times, necessitate a more sophisticated holistic approach. With a family-focused approach, as contrasted with a family-oriented approach, the family as a whole is viewed as having specific health responsibilities, and the extent to

## ⦿ MEDIA MOMENT

*Ordinary People* (1980)

Robert Redford made his Academy Award–winning directorial debut with this highly acclaimed, poignantly observant drama (based on the novel by Judith Guest) about a well-to-do family's painful adjustment to tragedy. Mary Tyler Moore and Donald Sutherland play a seemingly happy couple who lose the older of their two sons to a boating accident; Timothy Hutton plays the surviving teenage son, who blames himself for his brother's death and has attempted suicide to end his pain. The family lives in a meticulously kept home in an affluent Chicago suburb, never allowing themselves to speak openly of the grief that threatens to tear them apart. Only when the son begins to see a psychiatrist (Judd Hirsch) does the veneer of denial begin to crack. Superior performances and an Oscar-winning script by Alvin Sargent make this one of the most uncompromising dramas ever made about the psychology of dysfunctional families in grief.

*Running on Empty* (1988)

Arthur and Annie Pope, along with their two sons, Danny and Harry, have been on the run and hiding from the law for years, stemming from the parents staging a bomb attack on a napalm factory as a protest against the Vietnam War. Always keeping on the move, changing identities, and having no stability in their lives, the Popes gradually become weary of the chase and are forced to question their beliefs on family unity. Settling in New Jersey after yet another narrow escape with authorities, Annie Pope enrolls her son in a local high school, where his talent for playing the piano is quickly noticed and appreciated by his music teacher. As Danny's talent blossoms, he receives a scholarship to attend the Julliard School of Music. Arthur and Annie Pope, kept out of the loop, eventually learn of these plans plus Danny's evolving relationship with his music teacher's daughter and his fervent desire to act on the scholarship. The Pope family is forced to examine their lives, their beliefs, and their convictions regarding the impending consequences of finally breaking the family circle.

---

which family processes support these functions is the nursing focus. Assessments of the family as a group are made and interventions are directed toward helping the family grow in its abilities to meet its health responsibilities.

A typical example often encountered by nurses working in public health departments is the family with a 13-year-old pregnant adolescent. From an ecological systems perspective, the adolescent's pregnancy necessitates role changes for all family members as the new baby is incorporated into the family. Hence a family-focused approach is needed to help family members deal effectively with the life-cycle transitions triggered by the adolescent's pregnancy.

As nurses move into community settings, they need to be aware of the differences between a family-oriented and family-focused approach and select the one that is best suited to the needs of the healthcare situations they encounter. The mission of the healthcare delivery system in which the nurse works also may influence the choice of approach. For example, where the mission of the organization is disease control or rehabilitation, the family-oriented approach may be a better fit. Nurses working in organizations such as health departments, which have a population-focused perspective and emphasize health promotion and disease reduction, are likely to find more support for a family-focused approach.

## A Conceptual Framework for Family Assessment

A conceptual framework provides direction to the collection, organization, and interpretation of data about the family's health situation. The conceptual framework for family assessment presented in this chapter builds on the perspective of the family as an ecological system and is designed to assist nurses in evaluating the extent to which a family is able to fulfill its health responsibilities (Box 30-1). The conclusion reached by conducting the assessment is an evaluation that the family is functioning more or less optimally in meeting its health responsibilities, as opposed to an evaluation regarding the health status of a particular family member.

To meet its health responsibilities, a family needs to be conscious of the health needs of its members at varying stages in the life cycle and have sufficient energy to undertake the desired healthful behaviors (O'Brien, 1979; O'Brien & Robinson, 1984). At times, a family may have sufficient energy but lack the necessary awareness of members' needs

---

**BOX 30-1**

**Family Health Responsibilities**

Promote mental health of family members by providing opportunities for each to achieve a satisfactory sense of personal identity and self-worth.

Provide support and cognitive guidance for family members to achieve developmental tasks associated with life-cycle transitions.

Socialize family members to adopt health practices that foster health and reduce risks for disease.

Educate family members about when and how to use healthcare services when disruptions in health occur.

Assist ill, disabled, and aging family members to meet their basic needs either through direct care provision or through helping them access community services.

to use its energy constructively to attain desired goals. The reverse also may be true. Thus it is only when energy and consciousness interface and overlap that the family has the potential to effectively fulfill its health responsibilities (see the figure on the right).

A more detailed discussion of these two core concepts as well as those family attributes and processes that may influence the level of energy and consciousness within a family system is presented below.

### ■ Energy

To teach family members good health practices, to use the professional care system to foster health maintenance, to provide members with supportive and effective relationships necessary for positive mental health, and to actively cope with life-cycle transitions all require the investment of energy (Newman, 1994; Rogers, 1983). A critical issue in family functioning is the regulation of energy flow to attain balance as opposed to imbalance—too much or too little energy (O'Brien & Robinson, 1984). When the energy flow within families is excessive, behavior is likely to be chaotic and ineffectual, resulting in crisis-oriented problem solving when members' needs or concerns become too great to ignore. The latter is often the case in families that lack clear boundaries and where extended kin, neighbors, and friends move in and out of the household at will. In contrast, when energy is low or depleted, family members' needs are likely to be unmet, as illustrated in the following experience related by a mother suffering from postpartum depression.

In addition to assessing the energy that the family has available to invest in meeting members' health needs, it is important to identify how it replenishes its energy. The

> **"***My husband and son got back from the store. I think my 3-year-old son wanted to tell me about something that happened. It was physically so hard to listen that I really remember just trying to pull up some kind of wall so that I wouldn't be battered to death. At this point I was really sitting on the couch trying to figure out whether I could ever move again, and I started to cry. My son started hitting me with his fists, and he said, "Where are you, Mom?" It was really painful because I didn't have a clue as to where I was either. He was really trying to wake something up, but it was just too far gone. There was no way that I could retrieve the mom that he remembered and hoped he would find, let alone the mother I wanted to be for my new baby.***"***
> —*Cheryl Tatano Beck, Postpartum Depressed Mothers' Experiences Interacting with Their Children, 1996*

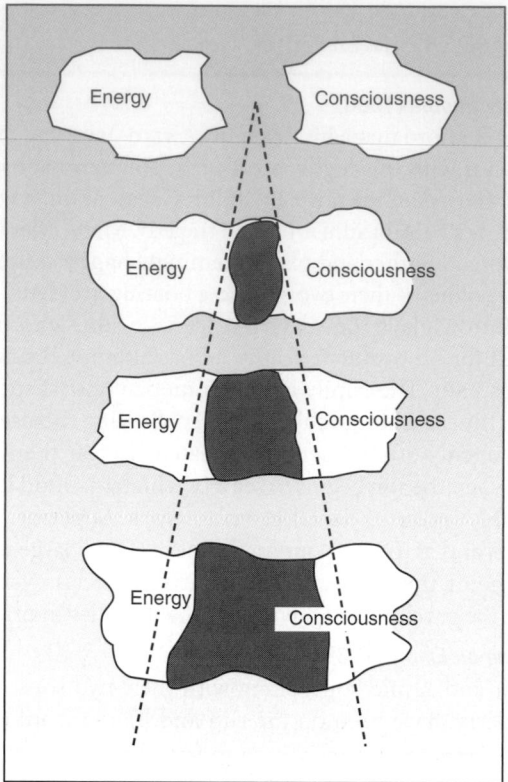

Expanding family health potential

*Source*: "Expanding Family Health Potential" by O'Brien and Robinson, from *Directions in Community Health Nursing*, edited by Judith Ann Sullivan, Blackwell Scientific Publications, 1984.

potential sources of energy vary from family to family, from individual to individual. For some, the source may be religious beliefs, cultural traditions, shared time together, school or work activities, or social relationships with friends. The nature of the sources is unimportant, provided that the family acquires sufficient energy to meet the demands placed on it. With a family that manifests a low energy level, nursing intervention may take the form of helping the family identify new ways of acquiring energy.

Pertinent questions to consider in assessing a family's energy level include the following:

- How does the family acquire energy?
- What are its sources?
- Is there sufficient energy to meet the varying needs of its members? If not, where is the family's energy directed?
- Does the expenditure of energy in meeting family demands occur repeatedly at the expense of one particular family member?

## ■ Consciousness

Consciousness is being aware of one's own feelings, needs, and actions as well as what is happening with others; in essence, it is the information that a system has available to effectively fulfill its functions (Newman, 1994). Growth and change within a family are directly linked to the family's level of consciousness, because it enables knowledge to be translated into goal-directed behavior. That is, the greater the consciousness, the more aware the family will be of its health responsibilities at any given stage of the life cycle, and the more refined repertoire of choices generated for meeting those responsibilities (Newman, 1994; O'Brien & Robinson, 1984). A thoughtful assessment of the family's level of consciousness provides the foundation for planning health promotion activities.

Another important aspect of the family's consciousness is the myths it creates about how it operates as a family (O'Brien & Robinson, 1984). For example, a family may describe relationships among members as close and intimate because all members spend a lot of time watching television together. Yet an observer might note that family members hardly ever communicate with one another during the time spent in the same room. Quite obviously, family myths may at times impede addressing family members' needs because the family is unable to recognize the need for behavioral change as a result of the belief that it is already behaving in the desired way. A useful assessment technique to begin to help family members become more aware of their own behavior is to engage them in reflective exercises. For example, in responding to a mother who complains that her son is "always misbehaving and won't listen" to her, the nurse might ask the mother to describe in detail a typical incident, including what her son was doing at the time and how she responded to his behavior. A common error that parents make in setting limits is to tell the child what not to do but offer no explanation for why the behavior is unacceptable.

Pertinent questions to consider in assessing a family's level of consciousness include the following:

- How aware and knowledgeable is the family of specific health and developmental needs of its members?
- Does it hold incorrect beliefs that are likely to lead to unsound health practices?
- Is its perception of how it functions congruent with reality?
- What are the sources that the family utilizes in acquiring knowledge?
- How do past family experiences influence its consciousness of health issues?
- Does it actively seek to expand its level of consciousness or does it respond only to crisis demands?

*"The family is changing, not disappearing. We have to broaden our understanding of it, look for the new metaphors."*

—Mary Catherine Bateson

## ■ Role Structure

Roles define the goals and actions that are expected to characterize the occupant of a specific position such as mother or father (Hardy & Conway, 1988). Identification of the varying roles of family members provides the nurse with important information about the organization of relationships among family members, such as who is expected to do what and for whom. Flexibility of role definitions enables the family to deal more effectively with developmental transitions and situational crises resulting from illness or disability of one of its members (Boss, 1988).

Difficulty in the performance of one's role is defined as role insufficiency. A basic concept in role theory is that roles are reciprocal in that they are patterned to complement that of a role partner. Thus the mothering role cannot be understood without looking at the corresponding role of the child at a particular developmental stage. Role behaviors expected of mothers of infants will differ from those expected of mothers whose children are in their adolescent years. When role insufficiency occurs, one or more family members' health and developmental needs are likely to be unmet.

In assessing family members' role performance, nurses need to be aware that role behaviors are learned according to the cultural values of the family. Collecting information about the family's customs and traditions is important for interpreting whether family members' roles are appropriate within their social context. For example, the maternal grandmother often assumes the mothering role for young children in African American single-parent families (Burton & deVries, 1995). Furthermore, it often is helpful to gather information about their early role models and to determine how these experiences have affected present role behaviors (Friedman, 1998). It is not uncommon for parents' expectations and behaviors toward children to be similar to those they experienced in their families of origin (see the Research Alert on page 744).

Role overload leading to increased stress and reduced levels of wellness has been cited as an issue for single-parent families (Burden, 1986; Popenoe, 1995). The single parent must fulfill both mother and father roles, often in addition to the work role, whereas role ambiguity and conflict are often major sources of stress in step-parent and blended families as members attempt to define whether the step-parent should assume the role of parent or nonparent and how children of the respective parents should relate as siblings. A typical example of resulting role conflict is the stepfather who disciplines his wife's child for misbehavior and is confronted by his wife for "overstepping" the boundaries of his role as a stepfather. In addition, ongoing relationships with the bio-

### GLOBAL CONNECTION

Globally, there were an estimated 33 million people living with HIV in 2007. The percentage of women worldwide among people living with HIV has remained stable at 50% for several years (UNAIDS, 2008).

Research Alert

This literature review focuses on family identity formation within a social cultural context for families, couples, and women who are in committed Black-White interracial relationships that include biracial children. This review was limited to U.S. research studies completed between 1990 and 2002. The American racial lens represented the environmental context that this article seeks to capture. Family nurses who can assess and intervene in a culturally competent manner will be essential to promoting health and eliminating health disparities for these interracial families.

Byrd, M., & Garwick, A. (2004). A feminist critique of research on interracial family identity: Implications for family health. *Journal of Family Nursing, 10*(3), 302–322.

logical parent and the addition of relationships with the kin of the step-parent further compound the clear definition of family roles (Carter & McGoldrick, 1989).

It is important for the nurse to carefully assess role strain and conflict occurring within the family because tension and conflict may negatively impact members' emotional well-being. Clarity of role expectations is crucial to helping family members develop a sense of personal identity and self-worth. Moreover, role strain and conflict, if left unresolved, may deplete the usable energy available for meeting the family's other health responsibilities, such as teaching members basic health practices to maintain health and ways to use healthcare services appropriately (Pratt, 1976, 1982).

Pertinent questions to consider in assessing a family's role structure include the following:
- Which roles do each of the family members fulfill? How competently do members perform their roles?
- How do past family experiences influence members' role performance?
- If role strain or conflict exists, what are the contributing factors?
- Is there flexibility in roles when needed?

## Decision-Making Processes

Decision making is central to the fulfillment of family responsibilities in meeting members' health and developmental needs. It is a process that involves (1) recognizing the need for a decision, (2) identifying and weighing alternatives, and (3) selecting an alternative and facilitating its implementation. Central to effective decision making is the processing of information; the decision maker must be able to discriminate between what is important and what is not, between what is relevant and what is irrelevant, between actions that will achieve goals and those that will not.

The family's use of healthcare services often provides insight into their decision-making processes. As noted, families often seek the advice of extended kin and friends about how to interpret untoward symptoms and whether they are sufficiently serious to warrant professional care. In some

❝ *The relationship of a family to its patriarch creates a paradigm for every other power hierarchy in Western culture: The team coach controls the captain, the starting lineup, and down to the last guy on the bench. The generals head the chain of command in the military. American corporations and the country itself have their own pyramids of authority, each topped by a president. Dominance depends on hierarchy and hierarchy begins at home with Big Daddy. Sophocles put these sentiments in the mouth of King Creon centuries ago:*

*. . . Nothing should come before your loyalty to your father.*
*If I allow*
*My own relations to get out of control,*
*That gives the cue to everybody else.*
*People who are loyal members of their families*
*Will be good citizens too...*
*Once a man has authority, he must be obeyed—*
*In big things and in small, in every act,*
*Whether just or not so just.* ❞

*—Letty Cottin Pogrebin, Family Politics:*
*Love and Power on an Intimate Frontier, 1983*

 A Good Read

## Love in the Driest Season: A Family Memoir (2004)

*By Neely Tucker, New York: Crown.*

This memoir was written by Neely Tucker, a writer for the *Washington Post* and a white Mississippi native, married to a black woman, Vita, whom he met in Detroit. The book focuses on their journey to Zimbabwe with their intent to adopt a Chipo, a baby black girl abandoned in a field of dry grass, one of thousands of children left orphaned by AIDS, civil war, and the Rwandan genocides. Tucker is an engag-

ing writer who combines a lively style with the emotionally moving story of the couple driven to achieve what seems to be the impossible: adopt a Zimbabwe child in a country where foreign adoptions are prohibited. They encounter impossible odds from President Robert Mugabe's policies, which eventually even endanger their own lives. Their courage and commitment to adopt Chipo makes for a creative and engaging story about love and family, all set against the backdrop of the tense situation in Africa. Overall, the story is a well-written tale of a journey between two worlds that offers many lessons about the power of love that truly can conquer all odds.

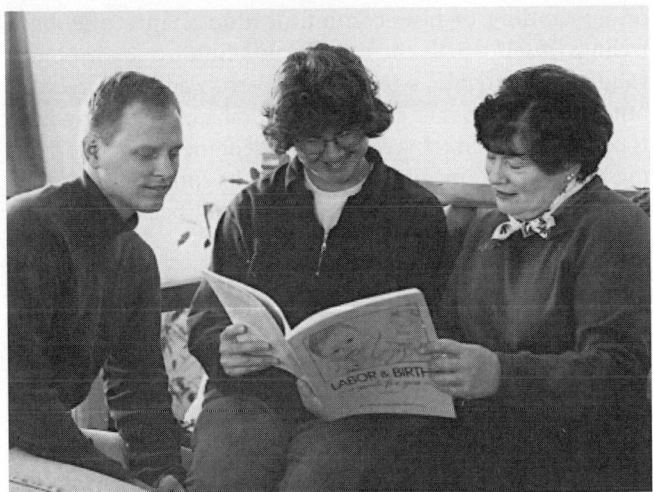

Chapter author Dr. Ruth O'Brien (right) counsels a prenatal family about their birth options.

**Research Alert**

The ability of a nurse home visitation program for first-time mothers and their infants to effect changes in the quality of the caregiving environment was found to vary with household structure. Mothers who lived alone and those who lived with their husbands or boyfriends were able to create a safer and more stimulating child-rearing environments than mothers who lived with grandmothers or with other adults. The investigators interpreted these findings as suggesting that where the mother is able to plan and take a course of action on her own, or in concert with someone over whom she is likely to exert some decision-making influence such as a husband or boyfriend, she is more able to implement changes in the home suggested by nurse home visitors.

*Source*: Cole, R., Kitzman, H., Olds, D., & Sidora, K. (1998). Family context as a moderator of program effects in prenatal and early childhood home visitation. *Journal of Community Psychology*, *26*(1), 37–48.

families, illness may be equated with inability to perform one's expected roles, resulting in a delay in seeking health care until symptoms are advanced. Studies have shown that poor health-related decision-making skills often reflect difficulty in decision making in other areas of family life. Conversely, parents who make general lifestyle decisions that are growth-oriented and motivated toward change are more likely to practice and encourage health promotion behaviors for themselves and their children (Duffy, 1988).

Nursing assessment of the family's decision-making processes focuses on identifying strengths or limitations in the information-processing function as well as the generation of alternative solutions. Immediate closure through the selection of a single option without explicit ranking or elimination of alternatives is characteristic of dysfunctional families, whereas healthy, functioning families explore numerous options, and if one alternative does not work, the family backs off and tries another, instead of trying to just make one option work (O'Brien & Robinson, 1984; Walsh, 1982).

Of equal importance to note are those situations in which families arrive at no decision. Discussions finish inconclusively and are then decided by events, as with a couple who argues about which form of birth control to use until the wife discovers she is pregnant. Such an event is called *de facto decision making* in that things are allowed to happen without planning. De facto decision making is characteristic of multiproblem families, many of whose members feel powerless and/or lack the energy to actively manage their lives. It also may occur in healthy families dealing with highly stressful situations when members' abilities to process information are reduced (Friedman, 1998).

Observations about family decision-making processes also help clarify its power structure. Families tend to reach decisions either by consensus or by accommodation (Friedman, 1998). With consensus, a particular course of action is mutually agreed on by all concerned. With accommodation, some members assent to allow a decision to be reached. Ac-

commodation occurs by use of compromising, bargaining, and coercion. Thus, by recognizing situations involving accommodation and who was identified with the decision reached, the nurse can identify the "power" brokers in the family. Identification of who has the power in family decision making is crucial for nurses working with families because interventions must be designed to include these family members (see the preceding Research Alert).

Pertinent questions to consider in assessing family decision making include the following:

- Who makes which decisions?
- Are there particular health needs or issues that are not recognized or addressed?
- Is the family able to discriminate between information that is relevant and information that is irrelevant to the decision?
- Are alternative solutions generated and weighed? Is the selected alternative implemented?
- Who holds the power in family decision making? To what extent do family decisions involve consensus or coercion?

## ■ Communication Patterns

Observation of a family's communication patterns yields valuable information about the meaning accorded to various family members as well as the clarity of interpersonal boundaries (Sieburg, 1985). **Communication** is a transactional process between two or more individuals in which feelings, needs, information, and opinions are shared. One of the most basic assessments regarding the family's communication patterns is the identification of who communicates what with whom. Individuals within the family may selectively disclose feelings, needs, and information to other members. Thus communication patterns are linked to the family's level of consciousness. When individuals share their ideas and feelings freely and completely, they have a broad base of cues and provisional solutions on which to base their final actions. Problem solving is more effective in such families because members contribute to the solution of concern and are more likely to be committed to the decisions reached.

Still another important assessment is the identification of covert rules governing communication among family members. Satir (1983) defines rules as the "shoulds" and "should nots" of family life. For example, a family rule may be that only positive feelings should be expressed or that sex is not an appropriate topic of discussion. An illustration of the importance that family rules play in understanding communication exchanges among family members may be found in a spousal argument over the wife's allowing the couple's 10-year-old son to attend a movie with a group of friends. After much heated discussion, the husband acknowledges that he did not object to his son's having gone to the movies with his friends, but he felt his wife should have consulted him before giving the son permission. In reality, the argument between husband and wife stems from the husband's perception that his wife violated a family rule—namely, that decisions about the son's peer activities are joint parental decisions.

One fundamental principle of communication theory is that every exchange not only conveys information or content, but a definitional meaning of how one views self and others (Sieburg, 1985). In fact, the recognition accorded to the other is more crucial than the content. By attending to the recognition accorded to others, the nurse can gain an understanding of how communication shapes member's feelings of self-worth and self-efficacy. Confirming messages validate the intrinsic worth of the person and endorses the other's self-experience as unique and valuable. Confirmation is conveyed by direct verbal acknowledgment of the other's message, expanding or elaborating on its content, requesting clarification of what another has said—all behaviors reflective of active listening.

Child: "Mom, look—I tied my own sneakers."

Mother: "Let me see. Yes, you did do a fine job of tying your laces. You have worked very hard at learning to do that. I'm proud of you."

In contrast, disconfirming messages question the other's perception or validity of self-experience through such behaviors as looking away from the other when speaking, interrupting the other, turning to speak to a third person while the other is still talking, interjecting comments that are irrelevant, engaging in other activities while talking, exiting while another is talking, or remaining silent when a response is required or expected (Sieburg, 1985). Obviously, such behaviors leave the recipient with a feeling of powerlessness and, over time, result in lowered self-esteem.

Child: "Mom, look—I tied my own sneakers."

Mother: "Don't bother me now. Can't you see that I'm reading the newspaper?"

Another important principle of communication relates to the congruence between the verbal and nonverbal aspects of the exchange. Verbal language conveys the substance of the message, whereas nonverbal language transmits the more subtle nature of the intent of the message. The degree of congruence and balance between the verbal and nonverbal portions of an exchange define the degree of clarity of the message for the recipient. Given that much verbal conflict among family members often stems from faulty interpretation of nonverbal aspects of communication, it is particularly important to assess the extent to which family members are able to elicit feedback and validate messages to minimize misinterpretation of cues and faulty mind reading (Sieburg, 1985).

 THINK ABOUT THIS ........................

**Words of Wisdom from Anne Morrow Lindbergh**

*A Good Relationship Has a Pattern Like a Dance*

A good relationship has a pattern like a dance and is built on some of the same rules. The partners do not need to hold on tightly, because they move confidently in the same pattern, intricate but gay and swift and free, like a country dance of Mozart's. To touch heavily would be to arrest the pattern and freeze the movement, to check the endlessly changing beauty of its unfolding. There is no place here for the possessive clutch, the clinging arm, the heavy hand; only the barest touch in passing. Now arm in arm, now face to face, now back to back—it does not matter which. Because they know they are partners moving to the same rhythm, creating a pattern together, and being invisibly nourished by it.

Marriage is tough, because it is woven of all these various elements, the weak and the strong. "In love-ness" is fragile, for it is woven only with the gossamer threads of beauty. It seems to me absurd to talk about "happy" and "unhappy" marriages.

When the wedding march sounds the resolute approach, the clock no longer ticks, it tolls the hour. The figures in the aisle are no longer individuals, they symbolize the human race.

 Research Alert

This qualitative study explored the experience of delayed parenthood for women who had children for the first time after the age of 30. Unstructured, conjoint interviews with both parents were conducted with couples. The findings suggested that older parents experience parenthood differently than younger parents concerning negotiation of childcare roles and career roles, greater interest and participation of the father in childbirth and childrearing, a general concern over career involvement among the mothers, and greater selectivity in terms of healthcare professionals. When women choose to become parents at a later age, their maturity, career status, and values about sharing of parenting responsibilities are significantly different from those of younger first-time mothers. As women age, especially for those who are childless, they tend to become more independent in their marriage roles and are more career oriented. Having a baby past the age of 30 presents somewhat different challenges to women whose lives are "already in progress." Mothers in the study consistently mentioned that the baby was "joining" a family, rather than the family adapting to the baby. This is a significant difference relative to younger women whose lives have not been well defined by work and other adult roles. The traditional norm for beginning parenthood has been slowly changing over the past 20 years. This change is clearly evidenced by the increasing number of adults who are delaying parenthood until age 30 or older. This situation appears to represent a significant change in the attitudes of some women and men toward traditional parenting roles. For example, while birth rates for younger women have decreased, the age at first birth for U.S. women aged 30 to 39 has increased steadily over the past few years.

First-time parenthood has long been recognized as one of the most important events in adult development and in the formation of the family. Changing demographic patterns of fertility have been the result of and catalyst for changes in parenting roles and statuses for men and women. With advanced reproductive technologies, women and men are facing new options regarding the decision to have children, including issues of timing, number of children, and even the method of conception. Although delayed childbearing has occurred in the past, the current trend should be of particular interest, not only because of the numbers involved, but also because the reasons for the delay may reflect general structural changes in society that may cause more and more people to delay parenthood. These reasons include changing attitudes toward marriage and family, changing parenting and gender role patterns, increasing levels of education for both men and women, greater employment opportunities for women in particular, and technological advances. These findings have implications for nurses and other caregivers who work with childbearing families, especially those involved in parent education, labor and delivery, prenatal health care, and newborn nurseries. ◯

*Source*: Saucier, K. A. (1997). *The experience of having children late: A qualitative study about delayed parenthood.* Unpublished dissertation, University of Colorado, Boulder, CO.

---

Communication patterns also are the most observable indicators of the clarity of interpersonal boundaries among family members. The use of "I" statements as opposed to "we" statements and the extent of mind reading and censorship (e.g., "You shouldn't say that," "You have no reason to feel angry") present in members' communications with one another provide important clues to the clarity of interpersonal boundaries and members' sense of separateness and personal autonomy (Sieburg, 1985). Clear and functional communication among family members is considered a cor-

nerstone of the healthy family (Goldenberg & Goldenberg, 1996; Janosik & Green, 1992; Satir, 1983). It is foundational in enabling the family to fulfill its health responsibility in assisting members to develop a sense of personal identity and self-worth. Moreover, clarity and openness of communication among family members facilitates effective decision making when disruptions to health arise. Families whose members lack good communications skills also often have difficulty accessing community services to help with their needs.

Pertinent questions to consider in assessing a family's communication patterns include the following:

- Who talks to whom?
- Which feelings or issues are closed to discussion?
- Are members able to clearly state their needs and feelings?
- Is there congruence between verbal and nonverbal aspects of communication?
- How well do members listen when others are communicating?
- Do members elicit feedback and validation in communicating with one another?
- What are the predominant patterns of acknowledgment accorded various members?
- Is communication among members age appropriate?

## ■ Values

Knowledge of the value orientations of the family provides direction to understanding the why of family dynamics. A family's configuration of values ascribes meaning to certain health events and suggests ways to respond to them (Friedman, 1998). The identification of family values, however, is often compounded by the family's own lack of awareness of how it ascribes worth to people, events, and things. It is important to distinguish both the overt and covert values operative in family behavior.

A particularly important value orientation to assess is how the family views itself in relation to the environment. The family that feels it has little control over what happens does not take the initiative to seek out new ideas, information, or resources and apply them to the solution of family problems or to minimize health risks (Boss, 1988). Similarly, the time orientation of the family influences the extent to which it actively addresses life-cycle transitions and change. Families who emphasize past traditions may experience life-cycle transitions as more stressful (Carter & McGoldrick, 1989). Likewise, a predominant focus on the present is likely to minimize anticipatory planning and emphasize de facto decision making (Duffy, 1988). As noted in the discussion of family decision making, families who rely on de facto decision making are less likely to engage in health promotion activities or use preventive health services.

Furthermore, there is a hierarchical nature to family values that influences the family's perceptions of risks and benefits of taking certain actions. The relative ranking of health in the family's hierarchy of values is important in determining the extent to which forces within the family tend to sustain or undermine healthcare behaviors. For example, the family who places a high value on home ownership may choose to forgo preventive health care if economic resources are limited. An accurate assessment of a family's value system should help tailor interventions to goals that are important to the family.

A family's values are a reflection of its subculture as well as of the community in which it resides. Obviously, the greater the degree of congruence between a family's subcultural values and the community's values, the more the community supports the family's identity. Incompatibility in values between the family and the community generates conflict that increases stress within the family as a whole or between varying members of the family who have assimilated the community's values in differing degrees. Such stress may deplete the energy available to meet health responsibilities and negatively affect members' self-esteem (Friedman, 1998; Pratt, 1982).

It is equally important to recognize that nurses often have their own personal and professional values that define how the "ideal family" should behave. Unless nurses are aware of their own values, interactions with families may become conflictual as they pursue interventions directed toward expectations they hold for the family that are incongruent with its own values and beliefs. Generally, nursing's code of ethics encourages respect for the family's autonomy to make its own choices involving health matters unless such choices are likely to result in serious harm for others, such as spread of communicable disease and physical or sexual abuse of children.

Given that values cannot be seen directly, Friedman (1998) advocates the use of a "compare and contrast" method to assist the nurse in identifying specific family values. The compare and contrast method involves using a list of central values of the dominant culture or the family's subcultural reference group to engage the family in a discussion of their own values. Through discussion with the family, the nurse seeks not only to identify values held by the family and their overall relative importance to one another, but also to identify value differences and clashes between family members.

Pertinent questions to consider in assessing a family's values include the following:

- What are the important values held by the family?
- To what extent do family values foster active coping and mastery of concerns?
- What is the family's orientation to the past, present, and future?
- What is the relative ranking of health in the family's hierarchy of values?
- Are there value conflicts evident within the family, between the family and the subculture/community, or between the family and the nurse?

## ■ Family Boundaries

Family boundaries serve to distinguish the family from the social contexts or environments with which it interacts. In essence, family boundaries serve as a conceptual filter controlling the degree of exchange that family members have with their environment (Klein & White, 1996). Having selectively permeable boundaries allows for family growth and change, because the use of resources outside the family is enhanced (see the Research Alert). The latter can contribute to family functioning by developing awareness of alternative courses of action (e.g., greater consciousness) and by increasing understanding of personal health practices and the value of self-directed action for promoting health (Pratt, 1982). Conversely, the amount of information a family can handle adequately is limited, and loose boundaries that result in an excess of information or conflicting information from the environment may amplify and create family disorganization (Walsh, 1982).

---

### MEDIA MOMENT

**Prince of Tides (1991)**
A troubled man from a dysfunctional family talks to his suicidal sister's psychiatrist about their family history and falls in love with her in the process.

**The Squid and the Whale (2006)**
Based on the true childhood experiences of Noah Baumbach and his brother, *The Squid and the Whale* tells the touching story of two young boys dealing with their parents' divorce in Brooklyn in the 1980s.

**Orange County (2002)**
A guidance counselor mistakenly sends out the wrong transcripts to Stanford University under the name of an overachieving high schooler. The student wants desperately to leave his dysfunctional family.

**Garden State (2004)**
A quietly troubled young man returns home for his mother's funeral after being estranged from his family for a decade.

---

### ⌨ Research Alert

This article presents guidelines for spiritual assessment and interventions explicitly for families, while considering each family member's unique spirituality. The category of spiritual interpretation to represent diagnosis is introduced. Case studies exemplify how to integrate the guideline, and illustrate elements that may favor specific interpretations which would guide the interventions. As nurses continually strive to assist families with their health needs, they must also attend to their spiritual needs.

Tanyi, R. (2006). Spirituality and family nursing: Spiritual assessment and interventions for families. *Journal of Advanced Nursing, 53*(3), 287–294.

## Application to Practice

### Family Life-Cycle Transition: Teenage Pregnancy

Nancy, a 16-year-old unmarried Caucasian teen, lives in a housing project with her mother, her mother's current boyfriend, and two brothers—Jerome, 17 years old, and Derrick, 3 years old. She is 25 weeks pregnant. The pregnancy was unplanned; she was not using any form of contraception. Ronald, her 26-year-old boyfriend, is the father of the expectant child. Ronald has two previous children (ages 2 and 4 years) by another woman whom he rarely sees.

Nancy did not seek prenatal care until the beginning of her second trimester of pregnancy. To date, she has gained 13 pounds. Her health practices include the use of home remedies and self-comfort measures that she learned from her grandmother. She began smoking at age 13 and now smokes 1 to 2 packs of cigarettes per day. A frequent problem is urinary tract infections. Nancy told the clinic nurse who made the referral, "I can hardly get up in the morning to face the day now that I am pregnant. Sometimes life just doesn't seem worth it."

The two-bedroom apartment is too small for the five-person family; Nancy sleeps on a pull-out couch in the living room. She complains that she never has any privacy. The home is cluttered and in need of cleaning. Much cigarette smoke permeates the environment. Nancy says she feels unsafe in her neighborhood, where groups of males congregate outside the project complex; thus she stays indoors most of the day.

Nancy dropped out of school in the ninth grade to stay home and care for Derrick while her mother works. She states that she knows that she will not be able to get a very good job in the future without finishing high school and wishes she could find a way to continue her education. Her mother works long hours as a certified care assistant in a nursing home trying to support herself and her children. The mother's current boyfriend is looking for employment because he had to quit his job in construction as a result of a back injury from an automobile accident.

Nancy is ambivalent about her pregnancy. She reports that Ronald has become more distant as her pregnancy has progressed; she is concerned that he may not assume financial responsibility for the baby and that this will be a further strain on her mother. She expresses confidence about being able to take care of a baby because she has had significant responsibility for her younger brother. The nurse observes that Nancy displays much warmth and patience in interactions with Derrick during the visit.

Nancy receives Medicaid and help from the Women, Infants and Children (WIC) Program. Although she could not be specific as to how Ronald makes a living, she states, "He always seems to have plenty of money." He has given her some money to buy baby equipment and clothes.

1. Which initial family diagnosis would you make?
2. Which other information would you need to know to assist Nancy in promoting a healthy pregnancy?
3. Which community resources could you use to promote family health in this family?

---

Markedly restricted interchange with the environment creates a greater reliance on inner family resources. Relatively closed families may exhibit more energy, in the form of tension, than they can discharge in constructive ways. Studies repeatedly have noted that child abuse clusters in families that are isolated from other families, neighbors, and society. In healthier isolated families, the members tend to believe that all or most of the needs of the members can be met within the family or the family's reference group (Sedgwick, 1981). Yet such exclusive reliance on internal resources may occur to the detriment of one or more family members in situations involving long-term chronic illness or disability, as evidenced by caregiver burden (Kramer & Kipnis, 1995; Smith, Tobin, & Fullmer, 1995).

Pertinent questions to consider in assessing family boundaries include the following:

- Are family boundaries overly rigid or overly loose?
- What ongoing relationships does the family maintain with extended kin, friends, or other social groups?
- Do interactions with its support network foster or impede the family's ability to cope with its health responsibilities?
- Is the family satisfied with its support network?
- Is the family willing and able to access community services?

Although the framework for family assessment presented in this chapter emphasizes critical areas of family functioning that have been found to contribute to the family's effectiveness in meeting its health responsibilities, one usually begins by obtaining basic identifying data about the family and its immediate environment: names and ages of family members, health history of each family member, racial/ethnic background, education, employment, income, health insurance, housing, characteristics of the immediate neighborhood, and availability of health and other basic services in the neighborhood (e.g., grocery stores, schools, churches, transportation). The purpose or reason for the nurse's contact with the family guides the initial information collected about pertinent areas of family functioning. For example, in making a home visit to the Johnson family to follow up on Kevin's toileting accidents and inattention in school, the nurse might begin by asking Mrs. Johnson what she thinks may be contributing to the changes in Kevin's behavior. Initial information shared by the family will help guide the nurse in determining what other data to collect. The data are synthesized to identify family strengths in meeting its health responsibilities and areas where the family could use help to cope more effectively. The latter serves as a guide for negotiating the nurse's continuing role and activities with the family.

## A Self-Efficacy Model for Nurse–Family Intervention

Because the family's ability to effectively fulfill its health responsibilities requires self-direction and self-governance, the nurse–family intervention should facilitate the family's active participation in dealing with the health concerns or issues that it is experiencing. Indeed, the family's active participation in nurse–family interactions may be a significant variable in determining the effectiveness of nursing intervention (Kemp et al., 2006; O'Brien & Robinson, 1984).

The **contracting** process provides a means for enhancing family participation in its own health maintenance. Contracting is based on the belief that families have the potential for self-growth and the right to self-determination. It calls for an active participative as well as a collaborative role for both family and nurse because the goal is to build family self-efficacy in addressing its needs. The contracting process may be subdivided into five interlinking, sequenced phases (Sloan & Schommer, 1982). As with any relationship, the phases denote an ebb and flow of movement rather than discrete points at which something begins or ends. In the description that follows, each phase is discussed separately, although in reality they may overlap.

### ■ Identification of Family Health Concerns and Needs

This phase begins with the initial contact between the family and the nurse. Data, both subjective and objective, are gained about each other through observation and exchange of information. The use of a conceptual framework for assessing family functioning facilitates a clear identification

of how the family is meeting its health responsibilities and any accompanying concerns (see Appendix A). The preferable outcome of this first phase is an agreement between the nurse and the family on the definition of the problems, needs, and concerns to be addressed in subsequent interactions. Two other outcomes are also possible: (1) referral to a more appropriate service or (2) termination because congruence between nurse and family does not exist and effective problem solving is not feasible (Williamson, 1981).

### ■ Mutual Setting of Goals

What does the family hope to accomplish? This is a crucial question, and one that is not asked often enough by nurses. By asking what the family hopes to gain from the intervention, the nurse assists the family to focus on its own goals and priorities. The nurse also can gain a sense of congruency between individual member and family goals, which are often a source of potential conflict (Lynch & Tiedje, 1991). In essence, this phase involves collaborative negotiations and democratic compromise rather than the nurse deciding what the goals will be. The nurse, however, expands the family's consciousness by sharing observations and knowledge that can facilitate the family's identification of goals.

The communication style used by the nurse can foster or hinder the family's acceptance of a suggested goal. For instance, "Perhaps we need to work on ways to reduce the distress your son's behavior is causing" is likely to be met with a more favorable response than "You need to work on improving your relationships with one another." The second approach will invariably raise the family's defenses, whereas the first fosters its willingness to allow the nurse to help them work toward a solution to their concern. Helping the family to set realistic, attainable goals is one of the nurse's key functions. Goals should be stated in a precise manner capable of being monitored and a time frame for accomplishment specified. For example, "Mother will spend half an hour each evening in some planned activity with children" is a more measurable goal than "Mother will improve attention given to children." Even when specific goals are set, there may be lack of progress. The family's prioritizing of goals may conflict with the nurse's. The nurse may need to support the family's priorities to free its energy for other goal attainment. If the nurse cannot offer such support because of possible injury to a particular family member, the family needs to be informed of what action will be taken.

### ■ Delineation of Alternatives

Once the goals are established, the nurse and the family need to discuss how those goals can be attained. This process involves (1) the exploration and determination of the family's strengths and available resources, (2) the steps or actions needed to attain the goals, (3) the negotiation and division of responsibilities of the family and nurse for goal attainment, and (4) the establishment of a reasonable time limit for implementing the plan.

Emphasizing the existing family strengths reinforces the family's belief in its own ability to solve problems and meet goals. In working with a mother having difficulty with limit setting and discipline with a toddler, the nurse might begin by acknowledging the attempts the mother has made to solve the problem and emphasize how well she is managing other areas of child care. Such an approach fosters esteem and confidence in the mother and facilitates her acceptance of the nurse as a helping person. A temptation to be avoided is the offering of numerous suggestions about how to do something better or differently before recognizing and drawing out the family's estimation of its own resources and potential solutions. The nurse can then supplement the family's developing knowledge base by introducing family and/or community resources not identified for its consideration.

Equally important in the planning process are decisions on the sequence of activities and the time frame needed to achieve the goal. The nurse generally plays a supportive role in this process, encouraging the family to make specific and detailed plans that are likely to maximize goal attainment. Agreement on the nurse's role and ways to monitor progress are crucial outcomes of this phase.

## ■ Implementation of the Plan

The plan and division of responsibilities mutually agreed on are tried. The nurse plays particularly vital roles during this phase. First is the anticipation of problems or setbacks that may arise, followed by helping the family recognize and deal with them in as positive a way as possible. A series of minor setbacks can discourage and demoralize family members to the extent that the carefully negotiated plan may be prematurely abandoned. Frequent contacts for guidance and support during the implementation phase can help individual family members accomplish their tasks. Second, the nurse has an important role-modeling function in that nursing responsibilities are carried out as agreed, within the given time limit. If problems are encountered in fulfilling the agreed-on nursing activities, the nurse should communicate them openly to the family and seek help in making alternative plans.

## ■ Evaluation

Evaluation is an ongoing process throughout all phases of the nurse–family transaction as well as an end phase. Results may range from successful goal attainment to discovering that the selected solution is not acceptable to the family. The latter may happen when the family and nurse fail to identify the "real" problem, they select unrealistic solutions, or unforeseen outcomes occur. As in other phases, the family should be encouraged to participate equally by sharing feelings and concerns about its course as well as about the nurse's role in accomplishing outlined responsibilities. Emphasis on positive strides, although they may be small, can bolster the family's sense of self-efficacy.

**The Long Walk**

We have walked a long way—the old woman said.
I no longer know the way—
The trees are so tall—they all look the same.
Are we near to the end?
We are close—
You see—right there—the cleared meadow on the top of the next hill—we have just one more hill to climb.
We are very close to the end my dear—the old man said.
I am growing tired—is it much farther—she asked.
See my dear we are close. Just beyond the next hill
See how the trees part—just one more hill to climb.
Are you sure this is the way? We have walked for such a long time and climbed so many hills.
We are close now my dear—you can almost see the stream.
Listen we are very close—just behind that hill—see how the valley opens.
It's growing late—have we reached the end?
My legs are tired and I would like to rest.
See the top of the hill—see how the trees are black picture cuts—you can almost see it now.
Look where the sun is setting—home is just beyond that bend—we can hear the stream if we listen—my dear.
The shadows are growing long and I would like to rest.
Are we near home?
Just one more hill to climb—then we can rest.
It is growing so dark and my eyes are not so good—do you see the end of our journey?
This is our last hill to climb. We will soon rest—my dear.

—*Ann Thedford Lanier*

Crucial questions to consider in end-phase evaluation include the following:
- Was the goal(s) achieved?
- Was the selected solution(s) appropriate?
- Which factors facilitated or impeded goal attainment?
- Should the nurse–family relationship be terminated or should other goals and plans be developed?

The manner in which the nurse–family relationship is concluded is as vital as the way in which it is begun. The establishment of a plan for continuity of care, if needed, is crucial. Often, after a period of intensive nursing supervision, a plan for periodic reassessment of the situation is warranted. This is particularly applicable to families dealing with long-term chronic illness or disability. The family should know how to contact the nurse should unanticipated changes occur before the scheduled interval for reappraisal.

## Application to Practice

### *Application of Nurse–Family Intervention Model: Johnson Family*

Mrs. Williams, the school nurse at Sagebrush Elementary, called Mrs. Johnson and scheduled a home visit for 5:30 P.M. She began the visit by clarifying for Mrs. Johnson the changes in Kevin's behavior that his teacher had noted in recent months and asked her if she had observed similar problems at home. Mrs. Johnson reported that Kevin had begun to have episodes of nighttime bedwetting and she felt he was more moody and, at times, quite argumentative with her when she would not let him "have his way." She stated that she had spoken with Kevin's pediatrician about the bedwetting, and he felt that Kevin was probably having trouble with the changes with his father. Kevin had no history of bedwetting or toileting accidents since about 3 years of age. The pediatrician encouraged her not to scold Kevin for his accidents and to try to give him a little more attention to help him deal with his separation from his father.

When asked what she thought of the pediatrician's advice, Mrs. Johnson acknowledged that she knew the divorce had been hard for the children. Their father's former job had made it possible for him to be home with them after school, and he had spent a lot of time with Kevin, helping him with schoolwork, games, and other activities. Since her ex-husband's remarriage, he had spent less time visiting with the children. She knew that Kevin missed his father's attention, but planning time to do all the things his dad had done was difficult for her along with working and managing the home. Moreover, she knew Kevin resented going to the "after-school program" because of her work hours. In fact, she sometimes had to ask her mother-in-law to pick up the children from the childcare center because she had to work late. Mrs. Johnson indicated that she didn't want to refuse her boss's request to work late because she was hoping to qualify for a promotion. One of the women she worked with was retiring in another 6 months, and her position as office manager would need to be filled. Although her mother-in-law was always willing to be helpful with caring for the children, she didn't like to ask too often. She felt that her in-laws might have some feelings that she contributed to the divorce because of her interest in "getting ahead in her career." Her own parents did not live close nearby.

During the visit, Mrs. Williams observed that Mrs. Johnson often seemed impatient with Kevin, responding rather sharply to him when he came into the room where they were meeting to ask questions. She often redirected him to go to his sister for help. At one point, Mrs. Johnson even remarked to the nurse that she had difficulty coping with Kevin's many requests of her and that it hurt her when he made comments to her about how things were different "when Daddy lived here." When she set limits with him, he often remarked, "I want to go live with my Daddy."

Using Mrs. Johnson's descriptions of the problems she was facing in dealing with Kevin at the time of the divorce (Kevin's bedwetting and increased demands for her attention, his remark that "things were different when Daddy lived here") and her own observations about parent–child interactions, and Mrs. Johnson's hesitation to turn down requests for overtime work and to ask for too much help from in-laws, the nurse felt it appeared that the family was experiencing difficulty with new family developmental tasks resulting from the divorce and remarriage of the father, such as learning to be a single parent and promoting ongoing parental contact between the ex-spouse and children. In discussing with Mrs. Johnson ways that she thought the nurse might be helpful, they identified the goal as helping Mrs. Johnson to assist her children with the divorce and developed the following immediate plan:

- The nurse would set up a conference with the school psychologist for Mrs. Johnson to have some counseling about how to deal with Kevin's reaction to the divorce and his behavior.
- Mrs. Johnson would take children to neighborhood library on the weekend and borrow some children's books that deal with parental divorce. Together she and children would read the books.
- Mrs. Johnson would try to spend half an hour each evening with children in some planned activity that the children helped choose.
- The nurse would revisit in 2 weeks to follow up on Mrs. Johnson's meeting with the school psychologist and to assess how children had responded to books on parental divorce and the mother's efforts to plan some activity with them each evening. ◯

**I Planned It This Way**

I planned it this way you know.

I planned it to happen at the very height of Spring.

I loved the Spring.

The time of rebirth, remember, this is a new beginning for me.

Bert loved the Spring too you know.

Remember our big garden?

Oh how I enjoyed our big garden, snapping the beans while sitting in the swing, Bert cooking pork chops on the grill, watermelon, ice cream . . .

Oh how I love my home and Bert, and my children, my family, my church, my community, all of you.

I liked to keep my house in order you know.

So I decided it was a good time for me to go home, back with Bert again,

At the very height of Spring.

*—Dr. Judith A. Barton, written about her*
*mother-in-law after her death*

## Conclusion

Understanding the family as a focal unit for nursing care will become more important in the future as healthcare delivery increasingly takes place in community settings. A family is two or more individuals who manifest some degree of interdependence in their interaction with each other and their environment in meeting basic needs for affection and meaning. The family life cycle is described in terms of developmental stages corresponding to major family events—in particular, the addition and exiting of members.

Families who are likely to have the most difficulty coping with life-cycle transitions are those who experience a large number of concurrent life-cycle changes involving transitions of great magnitude; who have a small, nonsupportive social network; and who live in a community with few resources to assist them.

Health responsibilities of the family include the (1) provision of opportunities for members to achieve a sense of personal identity and work, (2) emotional support and cognitive guidance for members experiencing life-cycle transitions, (3) education of members about how to maintain health and when and how to use professional services, (4) the socialization of members to value health and to accept personal responsibility for its maintenance, and (5) care provision for chronically ill, disabled, or aging family members. To fulfill its health responsibilities, the family needs sufficient energy and knowledge to invest in goal-directed behavior.

Nurses' work with families is facilitated through the use of a conceptual framework for collecting, organizing, and interpreting data about how the family is fulfilling its health responsibilities and issues and concerns they are experiencing. The self-efficacy model for nurse–family intervention involves a contracting process in which the nurse and family pursue mutually established goals.

Explore Community Health Nursing on the Web! To learn more about the topics in this chapter, use the passcode provided to access your exclusive website: **http://nursing.jbpub.com/ communityhealth.** If you do not have a passcode, you can obtain one at this site.

## ■ CRITICAL THINKING ACTIVITIES

1. Reflect on your own experience in growing up in a family. Identify how your family met each of the five health responsibilities. How are your beliefs about health and ways to maintain your health similar to or different from those practiced in your family?

2. Using the Application to Practice on "Family Life-Cycle Transition: Teenage Pregnancy," address the following questions.

   • What are some factors that may have led Nancy to become pregnant? As you answer this question, think about her life history.

   • What are the potential health threats to Nancy and her unborn baby, given her current health habits and living situation?

   • Using the framework for assessment presented in this chapter, how would you assess the family's current capacity to deal with this life-cycle transition given the information provided?

   • Which additional information would you want to gather?

   • Which ethical principles should guide your interactions with Nancy and her family?

# ■ REFERENCES

Antonovsky, A. (1987). *Unraveling the mystery of health: How people manage stress and stay well.* San Francisco: Jossey-Bass.

Bain, A. (1978). The capacity of families to cope with transition: A theoretical essay. *Human Relations, 8,* 675.

Beck, C. T. (1996). Postpartum depressed mothers' experiences interacting with their children. *Nursing Research, 45*(2), 98.

Boss, P. (1988). *Family stress management.* Newbury Park, CA: Sage.

Bronfenbrenner, U. (1986). Ecology of the family as a context for human development. Research perspectives. *Developmental Psychology, 22*(6), 723–742.

Burden, D. S. (1986). Single parents and the work setting: The impact of multiple job and homelife responsibilities. *Family Relations, 35*(1), 37–43.

Burton, L., & deVries, C. (1995). Challenges and rewards: African-American grandparents as surrogate parents. In L. M. Burton (Ed.), *Families and aging* (pp. 175–190). Amityville, NY: Baywood.

Carter, E. A., & McGoldrick, M. (Eds.). (1989). *The changing family life cycle: A framework for family therapists* (2nd ed.) New York: Gardner Press.

Clinton, H. R. (1996). *It takes a village: And other lessons children teach us.* New York: Simon & Schuster.

Cole, R., Kitzman, H., Olds, D., & Korfmacher, J. (1998). Family context as a moderator of program effects in prenatal and early childhood home visitation. *Journal of Community Psychology, 26*(1), 37–48.

Cowan, P. A., Field, D., Hansen, D. A., Skolnick, A., & Swanson, G. E. (Eds.). (1992). *Family, self, and society: Toward a new agenda for family research.* Hillsdale, NJ: Lawrence Erlbaum.

Deatrick, J. A., Brennan, D., & Cameron, M. E. (1998). Mothers with multiple sclerosis and their children: Effects of fatigue and exacerbations on maternal support. *Nursing Research, 47*(4), 205–210.

Department of Health and Human Services (DHHS). (2000). *Healthy people 2010: Conference edition.* Washington, DC: U.S. Government Printing Office.

Doherty, W. J. (1992). Linkages between family theories and primary health care. In R. Sawa (Ed.), *Family health care* (pp. 30–39). Newbury Park, CA: Sage.

Doherty, W. J., & Campbell, T. L. (1988). *Families and health.* Newbury Park, CA: Sage.

Duffy, M. E. (1988). Health promotion in the family: Current findings and directives for nursing research. *Journal of Advanced Nursing, 13,* 142–148.

Duvall, E. M., & Miller, B. L. (1985). *Marriage and family development* (6th ed.). New York: Harper & Row.

Friedman, M. M. (1998). *Family nursing: Research, theory and practice* (4th ed.). Stamford, CT: Appleton & Lange.

Goldenberg, I., & Goldenberg, H. (1996). *Family therapy: An overview* (4th ed.). Monterey, CA: Brooks/Cole.

Hall, L. A., Sachs, B., & Rayens, M. K. (1998). Mothers' potential for child abuse: The roles of childhood abuse and social resources. *Nursing Research, 47,* 87–95.

Hanson, S. M. H., & Boyd, S. T. (Eds.). (1996). *Family health nursing: Theory, practice and research.* Philadelphia: Davis.

Hardy, M. E., & Conway, M. (1988). *Role theory: Perspectives for health professionals.* New York: Appleton-Century-Crofts.

Janosik, E. H., & Green, E. (1992). *Family life.* Boston: Jones and Bartlett.

Jepson, C., McCorkle, R., Adler, D., Nuamah, I., & Lusk, E. (1999). Effects of home care on caregivers' psychosocial status. *Image: The Journal of Nursing Scholarship, 31*(2), 115–120.

Kaiser Family Foundation. (2004). *Parents, media and public policy.* Menlo Park, CA: Author.

Kemp, L., Eisbacher, L., McIntyre, L., O'Sullivan, K., Taylor, J., Clark, T., et al. (2006). Working in partnership in the antenatal period: What do child and family health nurses do? *Contemporary Nurse: A Journal for the Australian Nursing Profession, 23*(2), 312–320.

Klein, D. M., & White, J. M. (1996). *Family theories: An introduction.* Thousand Oaks, CA: Sage.

Kramer, B. J., & Kipnis, S. (1995). Eldercare and work-role conflict: Toward an understanding of gender differences in caregiving burden. *The Gerontologist, 35*(3), 273–278.

Loveland-Cherry, C. (1996). Family health promotion and health protection. In P. J. Bomar (Ed.), *Nurses and family health promotion* (2nd ed., pp. 22–35). Philadelphia: W. B. Saunders.

Lynch, I., & Tiedje, L. B. (1991). Working with multiproblem families: An intervention model for community health nurses. *Public Health Nursing, 8*(3), 147–153.

Newman, M. A. (1994). *Health as expanding consciousness* (2nd ed.). New York: National League for Nursing Press.

O'Brien, R. A. (1979). *A conceptualization of family health. Clinical and scientific sessions.* Kansas City: ANA.

O'Brien, R. A., & Robinson, A. G. (1984). Family as client. In J. A. Sullivan (Ed.), *Directions in community health nursing* (pp. 138–152). Boston: Blackwell Scientific.

Popenoe, D. (1995). The American family crisis. *National Forum, 75*(3), 15–19.

Pratt, L. (1976). *Family structure and effective health behavior: The energized family.* Boston: Houghton Mifflin.

Pratt, L. (1982). Family structure and health work: Coping in the context of social change. In H. I. McCubbin, A. E. Cauble, & J. M. Patterson (Eds.), *Family stress, coping, and social support* (pp. 73–89). Springfield, IL: Charles C. Thomas.

Robinson, J. L., Emde, R. N., & Korfmacher, J. (1997). Integrating an emotional regulation perspective in a program of prenatal and early childhood home visitation. *Journal of Community Psychology, 25*(1), 59–75.

Rogers, M. E. (1983). Analysis and application of Rogers' theory of nursing. In J. W. Clements & F. B. Roberts (Eds.), *Family health: A theoretical approach to nursing care* (pp. 219–228). New York: Wiley.

Satir, V. (1983). *Conjoint family therapy* (3rd ed.). Palo Alto, CA: Science and Behavior Books.

Sedgwick, R. (1981). *Family mental health: Theory and practice.* St. Louis: Mosby.

Sieburg, E. (1985). *Family communication: An integrated systems approach.* New York: Gardner Press.

Sloan, M. R., & Schommer, B. T. (1982). The process of contracting in community health nursing. In B. W. Spradley (Ed.), *Readings in community health nursing* (2nd ed., pp. 197–204). New York: Little, Brown.

Smith, G. C., Tobin, S. S., & Fullmer, E. M. (1995). Elderly mothers caring at home for offspring with mental retardation: A model of permanency planning. *American Journal on Mental Retardation, 99*(5), 487–499.

UNAIDS, Joint United Nations Programme on HIV/AIDS. (2008). *UNAIDS 2008 report on the global AIDS epidemic.* Geneva, Switzerland: World Health Organization.

Walsh, F. (Ed.). (1982). *Normal family processes.* New York: Guilford Press.

Williamson, J. A. (1981). Mutual interaction: A model of nursing practice. *Nursing Outlook, 29,* 104.

World Health Organization (WHO). (2005). *The world health report 2005—make every mother and child count.* Retrieved November 20, 2008, from http://www.who.int/whr/2005/en/

Wright, L. M., & Leahey, M. (1994). *Nurses and families: A guide to family assessment and intervention* (2nd ed.). Philadelphia: Davis.

## APPENDIX
# Family Assessment Guide

1. **Family Composition and Identifying Data**
   - *Names, ages of family members*
   - *Address*
   - *Racial/ethnic background*
   - *Education/school attendance*
   - *Employment*
   - *Income*
   - *Health insurance*

2. **Environmental Data**
   - *Is housing adequate to meet the family's needs?*
   - *What are the characteristics of the immediate neighborhood and community?*
   - *What health and other basic services are available in the neighborhood? In the community?*
   - *What is the availability of public transportation?*

3. **Energy**
   - *What are the sources of energy for the family?*
   - *Is there sufficient energy to meet the varying health needs of its members? If not, where is the family's energy directed?*
   - *Does the expenditure of energy in meeting family demands occur repeatedly at the expense of one particular family member?*

4. **Consciousness**
   - *How aware and knowledgeable is the family of specific health and developmental needs of its members?*
   - *Does it hold incorrect beliefs that are likely to lead to unsound healthcare practices?*
   - *Is its perception of how it functions congruent with reality?*
   - *What are the sources that the family utilizes in acquiring knowledge?*
   - *Does the family actively seek to expand its level of consciousness or does it respond only to crisis demands?*
   - *How do past family experiences influence its consciousness about health issues?*

5. **Role Structure**
   - *Which roles do each of the family members fulfill?*
   - *How competently do members perform their roles?*
   - *How do past family experiences influence members' role performance?*
   - *If role strain or conflict exists, what are the contributing factors?*
   - *How are role conflicts resolved?*
   - *Is there flexibility in roles when needed?*

6. **Decision-Making Processes**
   - *Who makes which decisions?*
   - *Are there particular needs or issues that are not recognized or addressed?*
   - *Is the family able to discriminate between information that is relevant and information that is irrelevant to the decision?*
   - *Are alternative solutions generated and weighed?*
   - *Is the selected alternative implemented?*
   - *To what extent does family decision making involve consensus or coercion?*
   - *Does the mode of decision making affect its implementation?*
   - *Is the family satisfied with the results of their choices?*

7. **Communication Patterns**
   - *Who talks to whom?*
   - *Which feelings or issues are closed to discussion?*
   - *Are members able to clearly state their needs and feelings?*
   - *Is there congruence between verbal and nonverbal aspects of communication?*
   - *How well do members listen when others are communicating?*
   - *Do members elicit feedback and validation in communicating with one another?*
   - *What are the predominant patterns of acknowledgment accorded varying members?*
   - *Is communication among members age appropriate?*

8. **Values**
   - *What are the important values held by the family?*
   - *To what extent do family values foster active coping and mastery of concerns?*
   - *What is the family's orientation to the past, present, and future?*
   - *What is the relative ranking of health in the family's hierarchy of values?*
   - *Are there value conflicts evident within the family, between the family and the subculture/community, or between the family and the nurse?*

9. **System Boundaries**
   - *Are family boundaries overly rigid or overly loose?*
   - *Which ongoing relationships does the family maintain with extended kin, friends, or other social groups?*
   - *To what degree do interactions with its support network foster or impede the family's abilities to cope with its health responsibilities?*
   - *Is the family satisfied with its support network?*
   - *To what extent is the family willing and able to access community services?*

# CHAPTER 31
# Caring for the Family in Health and Illness

Linda Beth Tiedje and Karen Saucier Lundy

Visit **http://nursing.jbpub.com/communityhealth** for interactive exercises, review questions, Web links, and more.

Caring for families in health and illness is not new to nurses. Lillian Wald, Margaret Sanger, and Mary Breckenridge are a few of the nurses who helped established a tradition of family care. Indeed, some count public health nurses as one of the unique contributions the United States has made to the cause of public health. Much has changed in the social and economic system since the days of Wald, Sanger, and Breckenridge. Each generation of nurses must reclaim this tradition of family care: keeping relevant wisdom of the past and learning new ways to help families in the ever-changing world in which we live.

Call it a clan, call it a network, call it a tribe, call it a family: Whatever you call it, whoever you are, you need one.

*—Jane Howard*

In an ideal society, mothers and fathers would produce potty-trained, civilized, responsible new citizens while government and corporate leaders would provide a safe, healthy, economically just community.

*—Mary Kay Blakely*

Community health nurses most often come in contact with families who are experiencing illnesses or family dysfunctions. Think about how your own family has reacted to health and illness. Do your values about family health influence how you evaluate a family's health status? How does U.S. society assist or hinder families who are experiencing health risks?

## CHAPTER FOCUS

**Thinking Differently About Family Health**
- Thinking Upstream
- Thinking of a Bottom-Down Health System
- The Human Ecology Model: Thinking in Layers

**Community-Based Services for Promoting Family Health**
- Preventive Support Services for All Families
- Targeted Programs for More Vulnerable Families
- Families in Crisis

**Characteristics of Successful Interventions: Creating Healthy Families and Communities**
- Relationship-Focused Care
- Intensity and Timing of Interventions
- Nursing Skills and Strategies

**Issues in Family Nursing Today**

**Values: A Challenge for the Future**

## QUESTIONS TO CONSIDER

After reading this chapter, you will know the answers to the following questions:

1. What is thinking upstream and relevance to caring for families?
2. What are community-based services in the promotion of health for families?
3. What are characteristics of successful family interventions?
4. What is the nurse's role in relationship-focused care?
5. What are necessary nursing skills and strategies in promoting positive family interventions?
6. What are current issues in family nursing?
7. What are current nursing values?

## KEY TERMS

Ad Hoc Committee to Defend Health Care
Bottom-down health system
Caring
Comprehensive community initiatives (CCIs)

Courage
Human ecology model
Inclusion
Intensity
Intensive services

Least possible contribution theory
Nursing skills and strategies
Preventive support services
Reflective thinking
Relationship-focused care

Social responsibility
Strength-based approach
Targeted programs
Think upstream
Timing

WHAT IS FAMILY HEALTH, and what does it mean to care for the family in health and illness? Family health is a whole series of activities that are designed to promote health, to prevent disease and injury, to prevent premature death, and to create conditions in which we can all be safe and healthy (Levy, 1998). There are many examples of activities nurses do every day to promote family health:

- Supporting a family with a chronically ill child to find community resources and respite care
- Working with a family with a schizophrenic young adult to establish consistent drug therapy and vocational training
- Discussing eating patterns learned in families of origin when providing support and information for weight reduction
- Reflecting on family learned values as we attempt to understand others for whom health is not a priority
- Assessing whether other women in the family have breastfed in the process of helping a new mother initiate breastfeeding
- Working for the enforcement of laws that prohibit sales of tobacco to minors
- Being part of school curriculum committees to ensure a focus on social skills so that students learn skills such as sharing, listening to others, and working cooperatively in groups
- Teaching parenting competency skills in parent education classes
- Participating in community-based sex education committees
- Promoting awareness of the need for disaster preparedness, including terrorism
- Educating families about Internet use and abuse, and the importance of parental involvement

A more specific example of family nursing to prevent disease, injury, and premature death occurred in Hawaii. A group of emergency department (ED) nurses there noted the numbers of individual children who were coming to the ED as a result of drownings and near-drownings. Some of the children were resuscitated; others died. Over time the nurses collected data from families and found that none of the pools in which the children drowned had fences. Working with families, the fire department, and other community groups, they raised funds to help families fence their private pools, and the accidental drownings among children decreased. This is an example of a family-focused, community-targeted intervention that served to prevent disease and injury and premature death. Nurses in EDs each day save children in tertiary care settings; they can also move beyond this "downstream" approach, to thinking about how to work with families in *preventing* such accidents from occurring in the first place.

## Thinking Differently About Family Health

As novice healthcare providers, we may view provision of health care to families as an "extra," a nonessential part of individually focused, technically oriented care. As we be-come more confident of our physical assessment, communication, and psychomotor skills, we learn that health care is more than the provision of individual-level physical care. Indeed, we begin to appreciate that factors at the level of the family, group, and society affect the health of individuals within them. Overall family health challenges us to think in new ways about influences on the family. Specifically, this new way of thinking challenges us to (1) **think upstream,** always asking, "What would have prevented this in the first place?" (Butterfield, 1991, 2002; McKinlay, 1979); (2) think of working with families in a **bottom-down health system** (Hancock, 1993) where homes and neighborhood meeting places are the basis of healthcare delivery, not hospitals; and (3) use the **human ecology model** (Bronfenbrenner, 1986) in thinking beyond what happens within individual families to factors outside families that influence family health.

---

**Getting Old**

Sun browned
Lined skin.
Traced by
Tiny fingers.
"Are you old daddy?"
"Soon to die baby, soon to die."

*—Ann Thedford Lanier, Ph.D.*

---

## ■ Thinking Upstream

If we think of illness as people drowning in swiftly flowing water, thinking upstream means we have to think beyond rescuing people from the water and look upstream to see what is "pushing" the people into the dangerous water in the first place (McKinlay, 1979). Rescuing people is a "downstream endeavor." In health care, downstream endeavors are short-term, individually focused interventions such as lung transplants for two-pack-a-day smokers or treating myocardial infarctions instead of the sedentary, stressful lifestyles that lead to them. Upstream interventions focus on the social and physical environments in which families live. Upstream interventions focus on changing the behavioral, social, political, and environmental factors that lead to poor health, not waiting "downstream" for poor health to occur (Butterfield, 1991, 2002).

In the late 1990s and into the twenty-first century, school violence erupted throughout the United States: Springfield, Oregon; Littleton, Colorado; Pearl, Mississippi; Paducah, Kentucky; Fayetteville, Tennessee; Jonesboro, Arkansas; and the 2006 Amish school tragedy in Lancaster, Pennsylvania. School violence was a rare and unpredictable phenomenon that fueled a search for "answers." The answers and the causes, of course, are multifaceted. A steady diet of violent media, the availability of guns, increasing feelings of alienation and unchecked rage, racism, and a lack of communication within families are all implicated as causes. School violence is a complicated phenomenon with no easy answers. In the real world, downstream thinking (dealing with consequences of school violence) and upstream think-

**CULTURAL CONNECTION**

For in the final analysis, our most basic common link is that we all inhabit this small planet, we all breathe the same air, we all cherish our children's futures. And we are all mortal.
—John F. Kennedy

 **ENVIRONMENTAL CONNECTION**

Family members with allergies can reduce allergens significantly by avoiding household products with added perfume, such as dryer sheets, carpet cleaner, and bathroom products.

ing (dealing with its prevention) are both required. To focus only on downstream thinking is a mistake. The other mistake often made is to focus blame on singular causes.

President Bill Clinton, in a radio address to the nation (May 1, 1999), urged all citizens to focus on responsibility instead of blame. What responsibility could be taken by each citizen to help prevent such violence in the future? Thinking responsibly means thinking upstream about what would prevent such school violence in the first place. Consider these comments taken from a *USA Today* story the week of the Littleton, Colorado, shootings. Recall that in Littleton the student gunmen targeted people of color and athletes:

"I think one of our jobs as students is to include everybody; I would want to do that." Mario Francisco Penaiver, 18-year-old student from Puyallup, Washington.

"These kids were not genetically programmed to be racist. They have been taught by the people around them." Stanley Wilson, 39, Montgomery, Alabama.

"We, as a society, have to ask, 'What is the impact of a steady diet of violent media content on a growing child?'" Kathryn Montgomery, the Center for Media Education.

Urging parents to take any guns in their homes to the police, Rosie O'Donnell, talk show host, said, "If you have a gun in the house, you are 43 times more likely to be a victim of gun violence."

The National Association of Attorneys General and the National School Boards Association have also published a manual with tips on preventing violence in schools, focusing on parents as a key in prevention. Some of the upstream

thinking includes encouraging parents to participate and volunteer at school and encouraging students and teachers to talk about problems. The National School Safety Center also encourages parents to talk with their children about fears and feelings and to be part of their children's lives. Community health nurses, in the spirit of such upstream thinking, could start school-based parent groups. If parental involvement is one of the keys to prevention, parents need to know *how* to communicate, offer support, and open the dialogue. Community health nurse–led parent groups would be a preventive start. See the box for selected *Healthy People 2010* objectives focusing on families.

■ Thinking of a Bottom-Down Health System

Hancock (1993) suggests that instead of thinking of a healthcare delivery system based in tertiary or hospital-/specialty-based care, we should focus on how to keep people healthy (see the following figure). Such a system would be a health system, as opposed to the current illness-focused system. Most resources would then be prevention focused at the neighborhood and community level. In a bottom-down health system, the services link people and families with others in support groups, neighborhood activities, parent training groups, early childhood education, and after-school recreation programs. Such services can be provided by primary care teams in the home and primary health centers based in schools and neighborhoods.

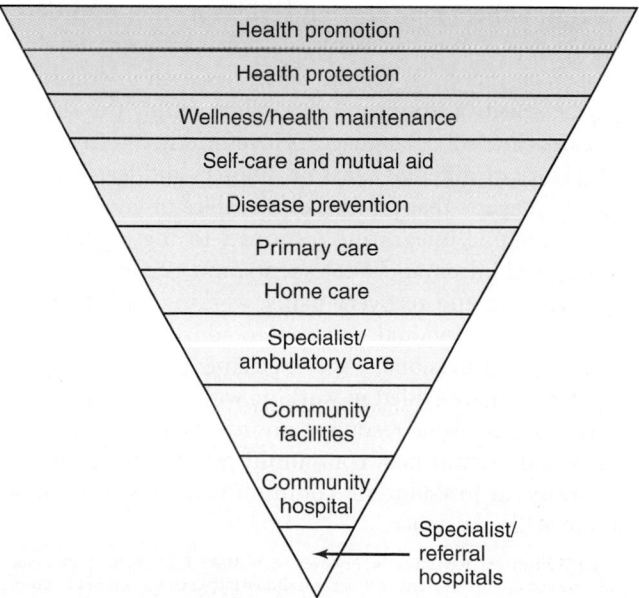

Bottom-down health system

A bottom-down health system is based on the concept of social capital (Kawachi, Kennedy, Lochner, & Prothrow-Stith, 1997; Lomas, 1998) and the importance of increasing social cohesion in communities. Features of social capital in communities include "social organization such as networks, norms and trust that facilitate coordination and cooperation for mutual benefit" (Putnam, 1995, p. 66). This can be done by creating meeting places, sports leagues, clubs, and associations. Creating spaces in communities for people to come together allows for idea exchange and fosters trust. Building a community structure is the focus for health, not the individual (Minkler, 1998). Some experts now think that social capital is the most important determinant of our health (Lomas, 1998).

An example of building social cohesion in a community occurs in Grand Ledge, Michigan, each spring. On a spring weekend, several activities are planned to bring people of all ages together. Children gather to make May baskets to deliver to friends, and a May Pole dance is held at a city park. Other activities include a teddy bear tea, a quilt show, and a pie contest. Such community building is "for health" because it increases social contact. A vast group of studies has already linked social support networks to health outcomes (House, Landis, & Umberson, 1988). But more than that, a new body of research is emerging that supports the additional health benefits of cohesive, caring communities (Lomas, 1998).

### 🖥 Research Alert

This meta review focuses on recent research to identify implications for designing sustainable programs of psychosocial care for children and young people who are affected by disasters and terrorism. Recent research confirms previous knowledge that most children and young people are resilient, but also very vulnerable to the psychosocial effects of disasters. Most children are distressed in the immediate aftermath when they recover sense of safety from adults, predictable routines, and consistent support systems. Others may develop serious mental disorders, though post-traumatic mental disorders may not develop until weeks, months, or years later. Research instruments may be sensitive to cultural variability; simply translating measures into other languages is insufficient. International experience of different types of disasters and terrorist incidents suggests that the broad principles of good service design include integrating responses to the psychsocial needs of children and adolescents into general disaster preparedness and recovery plans; working with families rather than individual children to address their needs; identifying professionals who specialize in responding to disasters and are skilled in working with children prior to events; and focusing resources on increasing the capabilities of staff members of community facilities to recognize and respond to children's common reactions to trauma and provide assistance.

*Source*: Williams, R., Alexander, D., Bolsover, D., & Bakke, F. (2008, July). Children, resilience and disasters: Recent evidence that should influence a model of psychosocial care. *Current Opinion in Psychiatry, 21*(4), 338–344.

### ■ The Human Ecology Model: Thinking in Layers

In Chapter 30, the family was presented as an ecological system using general systems and human ecology theories. These theories focus on the external influences that affect families and their ability to function. These forces outside the family have a powerful influence on what goes on inside the family. Some of these systems outside the family are neighborhoods, institutions, the media, and government. The human ecology model (see the following figure) shows how individual and family health are nested within and influenced by these macro-level forces, like Russian dolls stacked neatly one inside the other (Bronfenbrenner, 1986).

In this human ecology model, many factors inside and outside the family influence family health. Are community factors more important than family factors? Are individual factors more important than family factors? Are community factors more important than individual factors? Each of the three broad categories of factors—community, family, and individual—contributes about the same amount to making people within families—especially children—resilient and resistant to stress.

❝ *The family is the most intimate expression of self beyond the primal 'I.'* ❞

—*Letty Cottin Pogrebin, Family and Politics, 1983*

❝ *The essence of family is*
- *Who it is,*
- *How it feels, and*
- *What it does.* ❞

The human ecology model

Most traditional interventions focus mainly on individuals, occasionally on families, and less often on institutions and communities. For example, when a community health nurse makes a home visit to an adolescent mother, her baby, and her extended family, traditionally, the primary focus has been on individuals within that family, such as how much the baby weighs and health follow-up for mother and baby. Bronenfenbrenner (1986) would encourage us also to look at the family and community: Does the workplace or school have a designated place for women to privately breastfeed or pump milk? Do friends support the adolescent mother by providing child care from time to time? What encouragement is the mother receiving to return to school? Does the mother have a list of friends she can keep by the phone to call when she needs to talk? What messages do the media (e.g., television, the Internet, magazines) provide to adolescent women? Do local churches provide quality drop-in child care? What are school policies regarding child care for adolescent parents? What are government programs for employment or educational support for teen parents? Does this adolescent mother have access to contraceptive services?

The human ecology model emphasizes that "the way we organize our society, the extent to which we encourage interaction among the citizenry, and the degree to which we trust and associate with each other in caring communities is probably the most important determinant of our health" (Lomas, 1998, p. 1181).

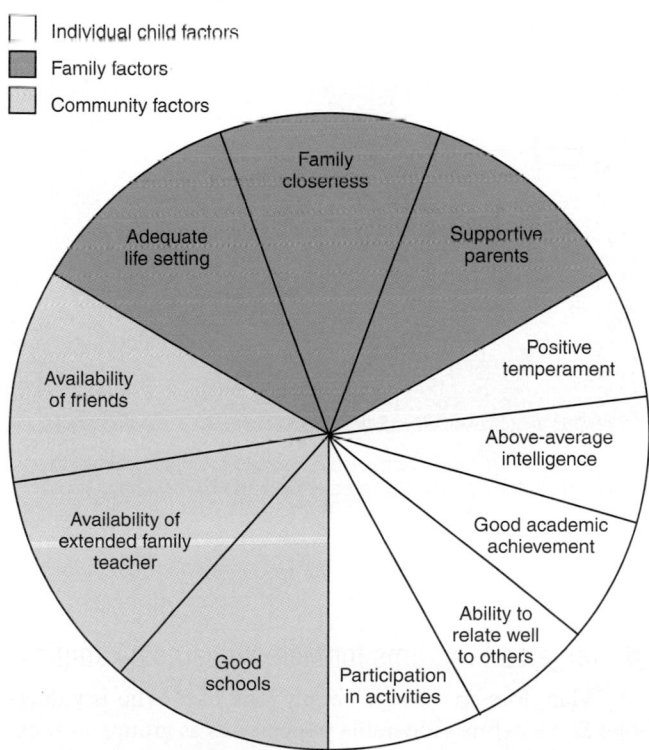

Factors that contribute to invulnerability or resistance of stress in children

## Community-Based Services for Promoting Family Health

Recall that in the introduction to this chapter one aspect of family health was to create conditions in which we can all be safe and healthy. "Every community must have a range of family-based programs, starting with **preventive support services** for all families, continuing through **targeted programs** for more vulnerable families, and ending with highly **intensive services** for families in crisis" (Children's Defense Fund, 1994, p. 4, emphasis added).

### ■ Preventive Support Services for All Families

In contrast to the United States, where programs are most commonly developed for "at-risk" groups with problems, in other parts of the world community-based social support for all families is part of a comprehensive program of health care. *All* families receive postpartum home visits after they leave the hospital, and health visitors continue to see *all* families of preschool children on a regular basis (Crockenberg, 1985; Heaman, Chalmers, Woodgate, & Brown, 2007; Kempt et al., 2006).

Another example of preventive support services for all families is a preterm birth prevention program begun in France, based on a communitywide public health approach. In contrast to approaches in the United States, which have unsuccessfully attempted to identify women at risk for preterm birth, in France all families, regardless of income, were targeted by a national media campaign. The purpose of the campaign was to make everyone more aware of symptoms of preterm labor. In addition, the effects of employment, such as long-term standing, were widely publicized as affecting preterm labor. This universal preterm birth prevention approach has become a successful national policy in France and has markedly reduced infant mortality there. France has been recognized as an international model in its efforts to focus on prevention of preterm births (Papiernik, Bouyer, Yaffe, Winisdorffer, Collin, & Dreyfus, 1986; World Health Organization, 2005).

Another example of preventive support services for all families is a widely disseminated program created by the Search Institute in Minneapolis. This program uses a **strength-based approach** and focuses on building assets broadly in all

**❝** *This is me, this is my family.* **❞**

—*Lettie Cottin Pogrebin*

### ☞ ETHICAL CONNECTION

Parents often seek advice from community health nurses about the need for circumcision of infant boys. Are there ethical considerations for the nurse in assisting parents with such decisions? ◢

Think of an individual patient you have taken care of in the past. List family, neighborhood, community, media, and government factors that influence his or her health or illness. Then identify one prevention-targeted intervention that would help prevent disease and injury or promote health. For example, research has established connections between asthma and the exposure to environmental chemicals and passive smoke. In addition to treating asthma (tertiary care), a more prevention-oriented approach would examine family, neighborhood, community, media, and government factors that influence asthma and then develop interventions targeted at prevention of these factors. For instance:

- *Government*: E-mail legislators about air quality standards.
- *Media*: Use principles of marketing, public relations, and advertising to design a public service campaign working with the state health department, such as public service announcements or a website to increase awareness of asthma and who is affected. Use experts such as William DeJong and Jay Winsten, who have written *The Media and the Message: Lessons Learned from Past Public Service Campaigns*. (This book provides guidelines and is available from the National Campaign to Prevent Teen Pregnancy, 2100 M Street NW, Suite 300, Washington, DC, 20037.)
- *Community*: Petition local restaurants to provide no-smoking sections.
- *Neighborhood*: Plan test cigarette buys using teens to see which businesses are not enforcing bans on cigarette sales to minors.
- *Family*: Role-play with patients ways to persuade those they live with not to expose them to passive smoke.
- *Individual*: Encourage those with asthma to write about their stressful experiences. One study documented the positive effects of such a writing intervention for people with asthma (Smyth, Stone, Hurewitz, & Kaell, 1999).

Chapter author Dr. Linda Beth Tiedje works to promote health with teen mothers through hands-on education and by including family members in interventions.

individuals, families, and communities (Hill, 2008; Laursen, 2000; Roehlkepartain, 1995). The assumptions include that all people and environments possess strengths that can be used toward improving their quality of life and that all environments, even the most bleak, contain resources.

## Targeted Programs for More Vulnerable Families

What does an "at-risk" family look like? Who is vulnerable? Some define vulnerable populations as groups who experience limited resources and have a consequent high risk for morbidity and premature mortality (Flaskerud & Winslow,

### Application to Practice

#### Strength-Based Approaches

At a prenatal clinic, a nurse approached a teenage mother and her boyfriend with their new baby who seemed thin for her age of 6 weeks. The father was holding the baby and burping her, vigorously pounding on her back. Overcoming her urge to negatively comment on the father's burping technique, the nurse asked how things were going. The family related that the baby had already had surgery for pyloric stenosis and had several repeat visits at child health clinic to check on her small head circumference. Later in a discussion with other families in the clinic waiting room, the father strongly voiced his opinion that babies needed lots of holding and "couldn't be spoiled." Reflecting back on this encounter, if the nurse had acted on her initial impulse to judge this teen couple and their childcare techniques, she would have missed the opportunity to see their real strengths: attentiveness at keeping healthcare appointments, shared care of the child, and knowing that the child needed holding and touch. This strength-based approach is in keeping with Search Institute programs.

1. How could the nurse be most effective in working with this young family?
2. What might be a priority intervention for these parents?

1998), such as families with a chronically ill child who do not have respite care. Families who are least likely to cope with life-cycle transitions are those defined to be most at risk, such as families with a history of abuse who are moving to a new city with a new baby. Vulnerable families might also have a small and nonsupportive social network or live in communities with few available services. All of these factors may make families at risk from time to time.

For example, during the 2005 Hurricane Katrina disaster, the most vulnerable families in New Orleans suffered the most, and not just from the storm itself. These families were unable to leave their homes because they lacked adequate transportation. When they did escape to expected safety in the New Orleans Convention Center and the Superdome, they found chaotic conditions there. Many died, and even more continue to face extreme health problems as a result of their ordeal.

Economic factors also help define risk in families, poverty being an especially potent factor. One-third of all children in the United States will live in poverty at some time before reach-

### Research Alert

This article reviews family and conceptual research on the concept of family resilience. Family resilience is the successful coping of family members under adversity that enables them to flourish with warmth, support, and cohesion. An increasingly important realm of family nursing is to identify, enhance, and promote family resiliency. Prominent factors of resilient families include positive outlook, spirituality, family member accord, flexibility, family communication, financial management, family time, shared recreation, routines and rituals, and support networks. A family resilience orientation, based on the conviction that all families have inherent strengths and the potential for growth, provides the family nurse with an opportunity to facilitate family protective and recovery factors and to secure extrafamilial resources to help foster resilience.

*Source*: Black, K., & Lobo, M. (2008). A conceptual review of family resilience factors. *Journal of Family Nursing, 14*(1), 33–55.

ing adulthood. Surprisingly, fewer than 20% of poor families live in inner-city urban areas (Federman et al., 1996; Tandon, 2007). Individuals in these poor families are indeed vulnerable, facing multiple problems such as joblessness, substance use, crime, violence, and poor schools. These multiproblem families vary in size, composition, location, and the nature of problems they present (Lynch & Tiedje, 1991).

Although not all poor families are multiproblem families, certain family qualities help define families as multiproblem. Women in multiproblem families often feel exploited and powerless in relationships with males. Men in these families, if present, often do not see themselves as responsible for taking care of children either physically or emotionally. Children in multiproblem families depend on proximal control and lack home orientation to school norms (Lynch & Tiedje, 1991; Tandon, 2007). These defining qualities are not intended as value judgments or descriptors for *each* family in this category. Multiproblem families have problems both within the family and between the family and the wider community. They often feel insecure and fearful in the wider community. Multiproblem families span both vulnerable and crisis family categories and are known for both the chronic problems that make them vulnerable and the crises they frequently experience.

### ✎ NOTE THIS!

**Refugee Families**

In 1999 in Kosovo, thousands of families were displaced, causing crisis and chaos. Once refugee camps were established to provide for basic needs, schools were set up to provide education and a unifying social support for the families. Finally, the United Nations trained preventive mental health workers to work with groups of children. Healthcare workers assisted the children in playing games, telling stories, and expressing their grief, because many of them were separated from parents. The components of these interventions are common to interventions for all families in crisis. ●

Comprehensive, community-based services targeting family economics, social support, and education are more successful with multiproblem families than services that focus narrowly on one type of problem at a time.

### ■ Families in Crisis

A family may be in crisis for several reasons. Families may run out of food. Home fires may leave a family without shelter. Families in which physical and emotional abuse occur are certainly families in crisis. Families displaced by war, terrorism, and natural disasters are also families in crisis. Regardless of the cause, interventions to help families in crisis share common components. First, their basic needs of food, clothing, and shelter must be provided for and their safety ensured. Next, both social and community support networks must be initiated or maintained. Finally, longer-term mental health prevention programs must be referred to or established.

## Characteristics of Successful Interventions: Creating Healthy Families and Communities

Launching and sustaining work with families are difficult. Successful nursing interventions with families contain several similar components: (1) **relationship-focused care**, (2) attention to **intensity** and **timing** of the interventions, and (3) particular **nursing skills and strategies.**

### ■ Relationship-Focused Care

The ability of sensitive nurses to develop ongoing, meaningful relationships with families makes a difference in the ultimate effectiveness of an intervention. Nursing is more than a series of tasks to be performed "on" families or information delivered to educate them. Through interactions with families nurses weave a "tapestry of care" (Gordon, 1997). Interpersonal connections become the foundation for effectively influencing health behaviors and helping people

The family provides the framework for learning from parents and siblings about health risks and health behavior.

*Women find ways to give sense and meaning to daily life—ways to be useful in the community, to keep mind active and soul growing even while they change diapers and cook vegetables.*

—Lillian Breslow Rubin

take charge of their health and healing (Heaman et al. 2007; Kemp et al. 2006; Remen, 1996; Tanner, 1995; Zerwekh, 1997).

### ■ Intensity and Timing of Interventions

Programs with successful results offer opportunities for multiple contacts with families over a short time. Programs during the childbearing years are particularly useful because they furnish potential continuity over time and multiple contacts. Multiple contacts in and of themselves do not ensure success, however. Other factors, such as provider credibility, are also important for successful results.

School-based clubs and groups offer opportunities for multiple contacts over time. One such group, begun by a school nurse, targeted preadolescent girls, who during the second decade of life appear to be substantially more vulnerable than boys to environmental and psychological stressors (Pipher, 1994). A school nurse started a girls club with girls from the fourth grade. The girls met weekly over the noon hour at school, at first to talk. A softball team, field trips to sporting and cultural events, and a presentation on grooming and hygiene were soon club activities. Such a club, building assets such as self-esteem and communication skills, is health promoting and helps prevent adolescent pregnancy. Positive, asset-building activities with preadolescent girls are prime examples of intensive interventions.

### 🖥 Research Alert

Several North American studies have found a connection between domestic violence and animal abuse. This article reports on the first Australian research to examine this connection. A group of 102 women recruited through 24 domestic violence services in the state of Victoria and a non–domestic violence comparison group (102 women) recruited from the community took part in the study. Significantly higher rates of partner pet abuse, partner threats of pet abuse, and pet abuse by other family members were found in the violent families compared with the non–domestic violence group. As hypothesized, children from the violent families were reported by their mothers to have witnessed and committed significantly more animal abuse than children from the nonviolent families. Logistic regression analyses revealed, for the group as a whole, that a woman whose partner had threatened the pets was five times more likely to belong to the intimate partner violence group.

*Source*: Volant, A., Johnson, J., Gullone, E., & Coleman, G. (2008). The relationship between domestic violence and animal abuse: An Australian study. *Journal of Interpersonal Violence, 23*(9), 1277–1295.

## Application to Practice

### Establishing Trust for Relationship-Focused Care

At the request of a children's clinic, a nurse made a home visit because clinic personnel were concerned that a 6-month-old child had not been brought in for cast changes. The cast was the result of treatment for congenital foot deformities. At the first home visit, the mother was guarded and uncommunicative and admitted the nurse to her home with obvious reluctance. The dominant feature in the dark, cluttered room was a slate pool table. The nurse, sensing that so costly an item in all probability was highly prized, shared that observation with the mother. The nurse then admired the pool table, noting its many features. The mother responded immediately. She explained at length about how much it meant to the family to have it, how friends and neighbors gathered to use it, and its contribution to her life. She then angrily described the previous nurse who had scolded her for spending money foolishly instead of using her resources to better meet the needs of her children. She was grateful to the current nurse for being a more understanding person and immediately switched the conversation to questions she had about her children. She then proceeded to plan with the nurse how she could arrange for necessary clinic follow-up for the 6-month-old, thanked the nurse for all her help, and asked when she would return.

*Source:* Lynch & Tiedje, 1991.

> **"** Most people learn how to avoid emotional hijackings from the time they are infants. If they have supportive and caring adults around them, they pick up the social cues that enable them to develop self-discipline and empathy. **"**
>
> —Hillary Rodham Clinton, 1996

In addition to intensity, most family interventions require time and living through difficulties. Unlike quiz shows, family interventions do not provide immediate answers. It takes time for families to experiment with new ideas and strategies. It takes time for families to come to their own solutions.

For example, there is a growing number of community-based programs for couples who present for domestic violence counseling and want to be treated jointly (Dawe & Harnett, 2007; Johannson & Tutty, 1998; LaTaillade, Epstein, & Werlinich, 2006). Although controversial, in cases of domestic abuse, the conjoint treatment of couples is increasing because unless both men and women are treated, the cycle of abuse repeats even when a relationship with a particular abusive partner ends. Conjoint treatment requires patience and

time. Most conjoint groups last 12 weeks and are preceded by gender-specific (all-men or all-women groups) 24-week treatment groups. The conjoint groups are often held in community centers, schools, or YWCAs and emphasize alternatives to domestic violence. Cessation of physical violence between the partners is a condition for group membership.

### ■ Nursing Skills and Strategies

Nurses delivering interventions to families must have skills specific to the intervention delivered. Five skills are particularly important: communicating, problem solving, listening, connecting, and evaluating.

#### Communicating

In addition to the skills nurses need to communicate, communication is a core issue in families and communities. Community health nurses can facilitate communication and also teach particular communication skills to people in families and groups. The following program example is one way nurses may provide parents with practical advice about ways of communicating with their children. The content area is human sexuality.

In New York, Jo Leonard and Marcia Siegel (1998) implemented a workshop for mothers and daughters called "Mother–Daughter Workshop: Getting Your Period." Offering the class to girls ages 9 to 13, no class is bigger than eight mother–daughter pairs. The class is based on the premise that parents are the first and most important sexuality educators and that family support and guidance have a significant effect on sexual activity. The class provides opportunities for parents and children to practice communicating about sexuality. It also provides opportunities to ask questions about sexuality in a neutral atmosphere. The class is a prime example of a strategy nurses may use to enhance family communication.

### A Good Read

## Bradshaw on: The Family: A New Way of Creating Solid Self-Esteem (1996)

*By John Bradshaw, Deerfield Beach, Florida: Health Communications, Inc.*

John Bradshaw is a well-recognized speaker and author on the family and addiction, recovery, and spirituality. This book is based on his 1984 television series. Bradshaw contends that the patriarchal model of childrearing is outdated and calls for a more democratic model of family relations. The book provides insights into the evolution of parenting and family relations and suggests how to create healthier families.

## MEDIA MOMENT

### Life as a House (2001)
Faced with a diagnosis of terminal cancer, George (Kevin Kline) decides to construct a beautiful new house on his land overlooking the Pacific Ocean, while at the same time trying to connect with his estranged son (Hayden Christensen). Kristin Scott Thomas and Mary Steenburgen co-star in a drama that speaks eloquent volumes about the fragility—and resilience—of the human condition.

### One True Thing (1998)
When tough New Yorker Ellen Gulden (Renee Zellweger) discovers that her mother (Meryl Streep) has cancer, she quits her job, breaks up with her boyfriend, and moves back in with her parents to help out. Wanting nothing more than to ease her mother's suffering, Kate inadvertently uncovers several family secrets, including one about her philandering professor father (William Hurt).

## GLOBAL CONNECTION

Families in many parts of the world are given paid leave after a child's birth. In many Scandinavian countries, women or men can take as much as 6 months paid leave to stay with their newborn baby.

### Problem Solving

Problem solving is a skill that must be done with—and not for—families and communities. Nurses may have "rescue fantasies" as helpers, wanting to take on the problem and tell others what to do. Coming to terms with who owns the problem leads to mutual goal setting and gives patients the power of solving their own problems.

For example, a nurse in a prenatal clinic was discussing the importance of finishing high school with a pregnant mother who had dropped out of school. The pregnant woman was accompanied by her mother, who also was a high school dropout. As the nurse talked with both women, it was obvious that the grandmother was proud of her long-standing job as a hotel maid. She also believed high school had been unnecessary for her achievement. For the nurse to assume an authoritarian, directive role in this situation and insist on high school completion would have been unproductive. Instead, talking with the mother and daughter about education, jobs, and life success over the course of the pregnancy helped the nurse better understand the mother–daughter perspective. The mutual problem solving that evolved enabled the daughter to "own the problem" of high school completion and take the necessary steps for it to happen.

### Listening

Nurses have vast amounts of health information to share with families and communities in an effort to improve health outcomes. Often, our first impulse is to give advice and information. Sometimes, especially in response to particular patient questions, advice is appropriate. However, we

> **❝**At work, you think of the children you've left at home. At home, you think of the work you've left unfinished. Such a struggle is unleashed within yourself; your heart is rent.**❞**
> —Golda Meir, Former Prime Minister of Israel

have entered an era in which health information is no longer a commodity exclusively owned by health systems. Many individuals, families, and communities can access health information from many sources. Self-care and wellness reflect a growing awareness that maintaining and enhancing health is a shared enterprise between providers and consumers. In such a shared enterprise, listening becomes a more vital skill. What does the patient already know? Which experiences has the patient already had? Listening through storytelling has recently been reclaimed as a powerful educational and therapeutic tool (Banks-Wallace, 1998). When a nurse truly listens to patients' or families' stories, he or she can more fully understand where they are coming from. Storytelling can reveal the way patients and families think about health issues, as well as gaps in their understanding. The use of storytelling as an educational tool also has been expanded to include groups of patients within prenatal and other clinical settings (Banks-Wallace, 1999; Carter, 2008; Nelson, McClintock, Perez-Ferguson, Shawver, & Thompson, 2008).

### Connecting

Caring for families in health and illness requires the ability to connect with other agencies and programs, to coordinate and reinforce interventions. Being assertive, phoning other providers, planning family meetings—all these actions require skill and a definite lack of shyness! Nurses often know the many other agencies involved with a family and initiate care conferences to coordinate services. Long before case managers were popular, community health nurses were coordinating services for individuals and families. It is nurses who often are the best patient advocates, articulating family needs for and with families.

During the late 1980s and the early 1990s, an approach emerged to facilitate connecting: **comprehensive community initiatives (CCIs).** Instead of focusing on one type of problem at a time, CCIs focus on creating systems of comprehensive services (e.g., health care, social services, education, housing) through a variety of programs and community building to better the lives of urban poor families (Stagner & Duran, 1997). The overall purpose is to provide neighborhood conditions in which families can succeed. CCIs share certain attributes such as emphasizing participation and providing a variety of services with their predecessors: settlement houses (early 1900s), neighborhood programs (1930s), war on poverty programs (1960s), and community action agencies (1970s).

### Evaluating

Outcomes of what community health nurses do are important. To measure outcomes, evidence-based practice guidelines are especially critical. In addition to evaluating interventions with individuals and families, nurses are often asked to serve on evaluation teams to review the impact of community planning or intervention efforts. Traditional evaluation methods include pretesting and post-testing, interviews, surveys, record review, and focus groups (Minkler, 1998). A new approach that expands on some of these traditional methods is called *empowerment evaluation*. It is used as a tool for both evaluation and community building (Fetterman, Kaftarian, & Wandersman, 1996).

Empowerment evaluation was used in the evaluation of a human immunodeficiency virus (HIV) prevention community planning effort funded by the Centers for Disease Control and Prevention and consists of four steps. The first step in the empowerment evaluation process is taking stock. This involves a review of documents (e.g., budgets, reports, organizational charts) and interviews and focus groups with community participants to uncover background experiences. The purpose of this step is to reveal a common history and broad shared experience. In the second step, setting goals, the evaluator helps community group members identify where they want to go and the kind of evaluation they want to create. Note that the evaluation process is not a preconceived idea of the evaluator.

The third step, that of developing strategies, is often difficult. Uneasy group dynamics and underfunding often create hassles and obstacles as communities struggle to decide on particular strategies to meet high expectations. In the example of the HIV prevention planning, one team encountered many difficulties when generating strategies. In an effort to overcome these difficulties, participants were asked to name the biggest hassle of community planning and to identify what they particularly appreciated in each of the other participants. The written responses were then organized into hassles, uplifts, and ways of changing course. These responses were circulated and then discussed at a community meeting. This helped the participants move beyond the difficulties to the work they needed to do: developing strategies.

The fourth and final step of empowering evaluation is documenting the process—that is, keeping a written record of what occurred and why, in a way accessible to all participants. The usefulness of this step was apparent in the HIV prevention planning process when the planning group, after nearly a year, faced some difficult decisions. Planning group members were on a 3-day retreat and faced a vote about how to proceed. Behind-the-scenes maneuvering, miscommunication, and longstanding alliances left the planners angry and divided. The empowering evaluation team found some data collected after an ice breaker exercise early in the planning process when participants had been asked to share their personal mottoes and messages for the world. One of the

messages was from a group member who had died of acquired immune deficiency syndrome (AIDS) just a few months before. Stunned, the group was reminded of their collective vision, and they were then able to vote in a more unified spirit. This use of data is a prime example of how documenting the process can be used to empower communities in evaluation efforts (Roe, Berenstein, Goette, & Roe, 1996).

The five nursing skills and strategies of communicating, problem solving, listening, connecting, and evaluating are a necessary foundation for community health nurses as they seek to provide services to individuals, families, and communities. These skills are necessary but not sufficient in a healthcare system where changes are massive, swift, and without precedent. Therefore, in the next section, issues in family nursing resulting from large-scale integrated healthcare enterprises, managed care plans, intense market competition, and a pervasive concern for operational efficiency and cost reduction are discussed.

## Issues in Family Nursing Today

The healthcare climate in which we practice may constrain what we want to do with families and communities. For example, many states have community programs in which nursing visits are reimbursed in a fragmented way for childbearing families: maternal support services for mothers; infant support services for children; Women, Infants and Children (WIC) for nutrition; and family planning services for contraception. The "family" sees many healthcare providers, with little concern for coordination of services. As nurses in that situation, we may find ourselves in situations we have not created and without much power. It is difficult to provide family-centered care in an environment that reimburses for individual services and that is not designed for time with families. Difficult, but not impossible. The nation's estimated 2.9 million nurses make up the clinical backbone of the care delivery system (USDHHS, 2004). Nurses are uniquely suited in this emerging healthcare system. We have the exact skills the healthcare delivery system needs: communicating, problem solving, listening, connecting, and evaluating.

Nursing reinvented itself in the past when social changes demanded it. Before the Depression, most nurses worked in private duty. As the Depression grew worse, nurses moved into hospitals and were employed at a salary. We can reinvent ourselves again, as we have done before (Salmon, 1999). How do we accomplish this reinvention?

One strategy is based on the **least possible contribution theory** (Weisman, 1981). A little can go a long way, and the least possible contribution is the one with the best chance of making a difference, however small. Making one small, insignificant contribution furnishes a foundation on which one can continue to add other contributions until something surprising but substantial results. Of course, least possible contribution does not mean doing as little as possible. Least possible contribution means doing something that the nurse is really good at and something that is only a little bit beyond the ordinary (Weisman, 1981).

***Got an Alternative?***
Gentle massage for infants has been linked to improvements with sleep and food intolerance.

⌨ Research Alert

A caring inquiry grounded in the hermeneutic–phenomenologic philosophical perspectives was conducted to uncover the family experience of living with childhood chronic illness. The purpose of this study was to describe and interpret the family's experience and to sensitize healthcare professionals about this experience. The presence of a child with chronic illness in a family is a unique, yet not uncommon experience. Chronic illness is both a personal misfortune and a sign of progress. No longer solely terminal, but still not thoroughly curable, these illnesses become illnesses to live with.

Data were generated from audiotaped interviews, photographs taken by the families, the artwork of the children, and the researcher's journaling. Eight family interviews and 32 individual interviews were the source of text for analysis. Data analysis was guided by a caring inquiry combining the hermeneutic–phenomenologic approaches of van Manen and Ray and other philosophers.

The analysis included several levels of reflection. The first level of reflection revealed the descriptions and themes of the families. The families' metaphor of "traveling a different road" also emerged. In the second level of reflection, literature and poetry were used to illuminate the experiences of these families and the themes were linguistically transformed into the seven meta-themes of the experience: "embodiment of illness: being in tune"; "temporal changes: living with uncertainty"; "relationships: creating a caring community"; "interacting with our environment: being aware"; "endowing the illness with meaning: understanding the illness"; "confronting death, affirming life: living with dying"; and "a spiritual transcendence: faith, hope, and love." Through deeper reflection, the unity of meaning, "a way of life: a new beginning each day," was revealed as metaphor. A theory of coming to understand the meaning of chronic illness, "a way of life: a new beginning each day" integrates the themes, meta-themes, and family metaphor. This research makes a strong plea for transforming healthcare delivery for children with chronic illnesses from a medically based, categorical, illness structure to an experiential, holistic, family-centered process. Implications for healthcare professionals in practice, education, healthcare policy development, and research are described. ◉

*Source:* Hagedorn, M. I. E. (1993). *A way of life: A new beginning each day: The family's lived experience of childhood chronic illness.* Doctoral dissertation, University of Colorado Health Sciences Center.

An example of the least possible contribution theory in action occurred in 1997 when a group of Massachusetts healthcare providers created the **Ad Hoc Committee to Defend Health Care.** Together these physicians and nurses worked to reestablish caregiving from those who were trying to make health care a business driven by the bottom line. This committee has become a national movement against "a corporate-driven health care system" (Shindul-Rothschild,

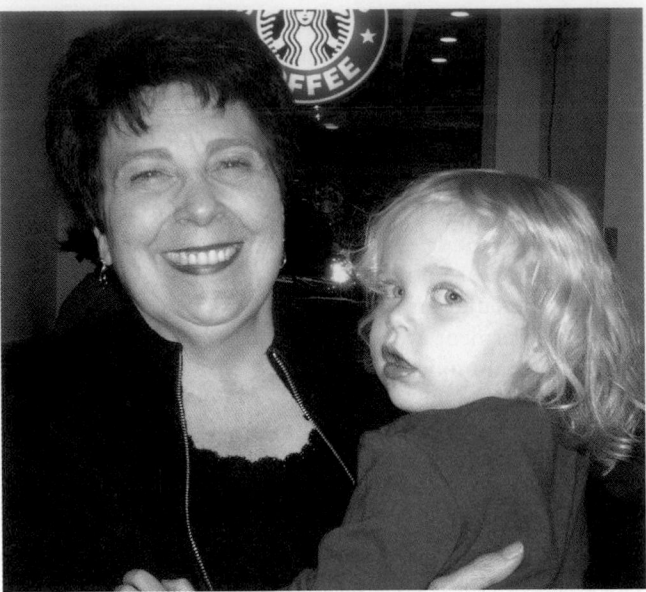

Children form a healthy self-identity through positive and caring relationships in the family.

1998). The committee's agenda is based on the following legislative initiatives: (1) Give the public information so that they can make informed choices; (2) assure patients that they will be cared for by registered nurses; and (3) extend whistle-blower protection to all healthcare workers so that they are not put in the position of choosing between a job and advocacy for patients. Only through such group efforts can the healthcare delivery scale be tilted back toward care instead of profits. Human and capital resources can then be put back into direct patient care instead of where the true inefficiencies lie in the delivery system—in the huge administrative overhead.

## Values: A Challenge for the Future

The value of inclusion rather than exclusion and the embracing of diversity as a means of enriching the social fabric remain two of our greatest challenges in community health. Perhaps the Hurricane Katrina national disaster and our perceived vulnerability to acts of terrorism have

❝*Power is also being redefined. Women often explain with care that we mean power to control our lives but not to dominate others.*❞

—Gloria Steinem

❝*Future shock: is the shattering stress and disorientation that we induce in individuals by subjecting them to too much change in too short a time.*❞

—Alvin Toffler, Future Shock, 1970

❝*A simple enough pleasure, surely, to have breakfast alone with one's husband, but how seldom married people in the midst of life achieve it.*❞

—Anne Morrow Lindbergh

made these challenges to the U.S. public more essential to our well-being as a nation. To deliver relationship-focused care to families, nurses must get emotionally free to focus on the family without judgment or bias. As nurses we may perceive people's situations differently because of our own value systems, which are created by our own experiences. We live in a heterogeneous society, a society with many different kinds of people and families. There are recent immigrant families from all over the world, as well as families whose ancestors came from Northern Europe, England, Eastern and Southern Europe, and Scandinavia. We must not simply assess minorities for cultural norms, customs, and rituals; the majority culture also has cultural norms, customs, and rituals that must be owned. To ignore cultural assessment of everyone is to imply that the majority culture is the "norm" and is beyond assessing.

The structure of families is also increasingly diverse: single parent, two parent, gay or lesbian parent, and so on. Therefore, healthcare providers often find themselves relating to families that are different from the ones they grew up in either in culture or in structure. It is common when confronting such differences to feel strange or uncomfortable. Sometimes, healthcare providers react by thinking of ways all people and families are alike, such as that we all have similar needs (e.g., food, clothing, shelter) and we all need love and affection. As healthcare providers, we also need to preserve the differences in people and families. That is more difficult. At times, we may just want everyone to be like us.

To better meet the values challenges of a diverse culture, three activities are outlined in this section. The first is a self-assessment quiz in Box 31-1 to increase value and community awareness. The second is a critical thinking exercise in Box 31-2 about providing support for families when there are scarce resources. Decisions about such family support ultimately involve values. The third activity is to recall how core nursing values may help us meet the challenges of a diverse society.

In the area of values, looking where we have come from may help us in where we are going. Nursing may provide guidance to meeting the values challenges in providing care to families and communities in a diverse culture. Salmon (1999) reminds us that there are five core values in nursing: **caring, courage, inclusion, reflective thinking,** and **social responsibility.** The value of caring is what has allowed us to move from the "doing for" approach to the current focus on enabling and empowering. The second value of courage needs to be shared and taught with exemplars and living models. We need to share and call attention to the daily courageous acts of nurses, particularly as they care for diverse groups. The third nursing value of inclusion seems most appropriate for the values challenge of working with diverse groups. But have we as nurses, so long marginalized and excluded, learned our lessons so well that we in turn oppress others? Listen to Salmon on this point: "I wonder what

---

## BOX 31-1

### Self-Assessment Quiz for Providers Working with Families and Communities

In the spirit of thinking of similarities and differences in people, this self-assessment is intended as a means for you as a provider to become more aware at your values. In addition, questions 4 to 9 are intended to assess your awareness of your community, because community cohesion and the degree to which you associate with others in creating caring communities will be important to your success as a community health nurse.

1. Do you respect others' beliefs?
2. Do you believe that life is good and positive?
3. What is your ethnic/cultural heritage? List some norms/customs/rituals.
4. When was the last time you took public transportation?
5. Have you given blood recently?
6. Have you ever served on a jury?
7. How many of your neighbors do you know by name?
8. When was the last time you went to a free public event or amusement like a museum or the zoo?
9. When was the last time you checked a book out of the local library?
10. Do you do volunteer work in your community?

*Source:* Questions 1 to 3 are based on Benson, 1996; questions 4 to 10 are based on a community quotient quiz adapted by the *Utne Reader* (Cordes & Walljasper, 1997).

---

## BOX 31-2

### Value Checkpoint: Critical Thinking

The issue of who is responsible for children affects not only how we as healthcare providers care for families, but also how resources get allocated in our society. People from widely different points of view can agree that valuing families is important in our society. What is harder is agreeing on how much the family needs to be supported by social institutions, including churches, schools, community agencies, and government (Schorr, 1989).

The conservative view is that families should be self-reliant and self-sufficient, not relying on community and government support. The liberal view is that "parents are and should be the most important people in their children's lives. But that doesn't mean they can or should raise their children without any help" (Children's Defense Fund, 1994). Liberals maintain that many forms of assistance are needed to maintain strong families, including sufficient family income and access to health care, child care, and adequate housing.

Think for a moment about your attitudes and beliefs regarding family support. How much family support is needed? What kind of support is needed? Should government ensure basic health care for all families, including children and parents? How does increasing the supply of affordable housing promote health in families? What is the best environment for families if we want to create families who are self-reliant, self-sufficient, and responsible? At what point does the conservative model threaten the overall health of the community? At what point does the liberal model threaten self-reliance in families?

## MEDIA MOMENT

### Kramer vs. Kramer (1979)

Winner of five Academy Awards, including Best Picture, Actor, and Screenplay, *Kramer vs. Kramer* remains one of the most powerful dramas ever made about divorce and child custody issues. Adapted from the novel by Avery Corman, the film chronicles the failure of a marriage and the tumultuous shift of parental roles within the family. Joanna Kramer (Meryl Streep) suddenly informs her husband Ted (Dustin Hoffman) that she is leaving him, just as his advertising career is advancing and demanding most of his waking hours. Ted's self-centeredness and Joanna's search for her own identity interplay with the 7-year-old son's future (Justin Henry). The son now finds himself living with a workaholic father he barely knows. Balancing his domestic challenge with professional deadlines, Ted is further pressured when his wife files for custody of their son. The drama of the legal battle for the child's custody explores complex issues related to gender, parenting, and legal accountability.

### Terms of Endearment (1983)

*Terms of Endearment* was adapted from Larry McMurty's novel and won five Academy Awards, including the Best Adapted Screenplay, Best Picture, Best Actress (Shirley MacLaine), Best Director (James Brooks), and Best Supporting Actor (Jack Nicholson). The cast includes Debra Winger, John Lithgow, Jeff Daniels, and Danny DeVito. The story focuses on a mother, Aurora Greenway (Shirley MacLaine), and her daughter, Emma (Debra Winger), and explores how their relationship develops over the years, from the day that their husband/father dies. Aurora disapproves of Emma's marriage to Flap Horton (Jeff Daniels), a college professor. Emma has three children with Flap, even as his infidelity continues throughout their marriage. Aurora keeps her male admirers at a distance, until she falls hard for the former astronaut next door, Garrett Breedlove (Jack Nicholson). Garrett and Aurora have an on again/off again relationship, owing to Garrett's commitment issues and Aurora's emotional distance.

The event that ties everyone together is Emma's cancer diagnosis. One of cinema's most dramatic scenes occurs when Aurora confronts the nurses at the nurses' station, demanding that her daughter's pain medication be given early. The nurses appear more concerned with protocol and schedules than with relieving her daughter's pain; Aurora's shouting match is perhaps the most memorable in the movie. After Emma's death, it becomes apparent that Flap is not the one who should be raising the children; Aurora takes the two boys and Emma's best friend raises the girl. The ending reveals the complexities of how families function in good times and in bad times. Many critics consider the film one of the best of the last century, with outstanding performances and a touching and dramatic analysis of today's family.

---

we teach our students about inclusion. Do they understand that our health care system serves only some people, and that more than 40 million others have no real access to care? . . . Does our science teach students to care only for those who are part of the system? . . . Or do we convey the value that nursing's job is not complete until all receive the care they need?" (p. 23).

The fourth nursing core value is that of reflective thinking, not easy to come by in our fast-paced lives. However, as community health nurses, we must become more than just technicians. "We must also educate people who are equipped intellectually to deal with the meaning of what they do and who they are in the context of humanity" (Salmon, 1999, p. 24). It is reflection that is needed as we deal with the issues of value conflicts in a complex and diverse society.

Finally, the last core value, the linchpin for all the others, is social responsibility. Florence Nightingale's vision of nursing's responsibility to the common good was based on social responsibility. She saw a society like ours in which certain groups were marginalized and in poor health because

 THINK ABOUT THIS

Parents who are stressed or disturbed will have more difficulty in meeting their children's needs. Parents who have little support—from friends, relatives, neighbors, or the community—are more likely to be overburdened by the demands of their babies and to be unable to respond to them adequately. Parents who experience severe poverty or economic insecurity, who cannot satisfy their own basic needs, are likely to have difficulty in responding to their children's needs.

—Sheila B. Kamerman

of unjust systems. "Her response was to engage nursing in addressing these injustices" (Salmon, 1999, p. 25). Nursing is only as good as what it does for all the people. Do we, like Lillian Wald, have a firm grasp of the way in which society functions to impact the health of individuals? Our sense of social responsibility will help us meet the challenges of values conflicts in a diverse culture.

| Highly intensive services | Targeted services | Preventive support |
| Families in crisis | Vulnerable families | All families |
| Safe houses; foster care | Multiproblem families | Parental/support |

Continuum of services

## A Good Read

## Merry Christmas 1953: A Story About Family

*Ann Thedford Lanier*

It is amazing how quickly the years go by. I can still feel the sun on my face that day, smell the turkey cooking in the kitchen, hear the sounds of the children playing, and sense the joy of being home.

I also remember that within a few minutes of this photo a neighbor child shot out our picture window with his new 22 rifle as a Christmas gift and mortally wounded our dog "Mutt." Daddy, in anger and frustration, slapped Lynda so hard that her Christmas watch flew off her arm and was broken. I ran away to hide in the playhouse next door. In my rush to get away, I fell down with my new skates and ripped the knee of my only pair of jeans. My two brothers, Howard and David, got into a fistfight—blackened each other's eyes and bloodied each other's noses. Mother screamed at all of us for being such heathens on "this Day of Our Lord's Birth." She then locked herself in her bedroom and cried. The only member of the family that got away unharmed was "Felix" the cat. Well, so much for happy childhood memories.

What are you thinking as you read this account of one family's holiday? What are ways that the community health nurse could assist this family in making positive changes in family functioning and managing conflict in a healthier way?

## Conclusion

Community health nurses must not only care for individuals and families, but also create caring and cohesive communities. Key concepts highlighted in this chapter, which serve as a foundation for a community-based family nursing, include the following:

- Family health is a series of activities designed to promote health, to prevent disease and injury, to prevent premature death, and to create conditions in which we all can be safe and healthy.
- Family health challenges us to think in new, broader ways. Thinking differently about family health means (1) thinking upstream about prevention, (2) thinking of a bottom-down health system focused on increasing cohesion in communities and providing services at the neighborhood level, and (3) thinking in layers in terms of the human ecology model about the many external influences on family health.
- There are three general strategies for promoting family health: preventive services for all families, targeted programs for more-vulnerable families, and intensive services for families in crisis.
- There are three characteristics of all successful interventions with families embedded in neighborhoods and larger social systems. Successful interventions involve (1) relationship-focused care, (2) attention to intensity and timing of interventions, and (3) the use of the nursing skills and strategies of communicating, problem solving, listening, connecting, and evaluating.
- The issues in family nursing today are varied and complex. Most important are the constraints of the healthcare delivery system.
- There are many challenges facing community health nurses as they build and organize communities for health. A special challenge is the value conflicts that result when we work with diverse families and communities.
- Salmon's five core values of nursing are proposed as ways to meet the value conflicts of diversity. The five core values are caring, courage, inclusion. reflective thinking, and social responsibility.

Explore Community Health Nursing on the Web! To learn more about the topics in this chapter, use the passcode provided to access your exclusive website: **http://nursing.jbpub.com/ communityhealth.** If you do not have a passcode, you can obtain one at this site.

## ■ CRITICAL THINKING ACTIVITIES

1. As a community health nurse you have been assigned to a community action committee to design a parent support group for parents of teens in your local high school. The purpose of the group is to teach communication, conflict resolution, and problem-solving skills and to provide a forum for social support for parents. A major emphasis will be on practicing skills. Explore the following questions and give rationales to your decisions.
   - Would you have a group for parents only, for parents and teens, or separate groups for parents and teens?
   - Which resources would you use to teach communication, conflict resolution, and problem-solving skills? Remember that a major emphasis of the groups is to practice these skills.
   - The teaching of social skills to children is important, especially children who feel alienated and left out. In a recent book, *Why Doesn't Anybody Like Me?*, Hara Estroff Marano gives several suggestions to parents. How would you incorporate some of these suggestions into your parent group? Which activities would you use to make the suggestions come alive?
   - How many weeks will the group meet, when (e.g., evening, weekend), and for how long (e.g., 1 hour, 2 hours)?
   - Who would you have lead the groups? Which experts in your community would you utilize to help you if you were chosen to lead the groups?

2. Explore the factors contributing to the gap in mortality between the rich and the poor. Especially look at factors other than health behaviors. Explain how some of the other factors suggested by the research might contribute to increased mortality in the poor. How might these factors affect physical health? What are interventions that would address these other factors?

   *Other factors:*                    *Intervention:*

   - Lack of social relationships and social supports
   - Personality factors such as a lost sense of mastery, optimism, sense of control, and self-esteem
   - Factors such as heightened level of anger and hostility
   - Chronic and acute stress in jobs and at home as a result of lack of resources
   - The stress of racism and classicism and other stress related to the unequal distribution of power and resources

- Differences in exposure to occupational and environmental health hazards (poor people tend to have more exposure to these hazards, such as lead)
- Differences in access to health care

3. Think of a family you are currently working with. Name one skill that each family member possesses that is a strength. Does the documentation system used in your nursing agency, hospital, or community clinic have a place for listing strengths of individuals and families?

4. Most conjoint domestic abuse after-treatment groups are co-led by a man and a woman. Leaders should have experience in counseling, group work, and family violence. Assume you are co-leading a conjoint after-treatment group.
   - Which safety considerations would you have for the formerly abused women in the group?

- Which skills would be particularly important for couples to practice in the groups?
- Which built-in strategies would you use to monitor current physical abuse in these relationships?
- Which kind of system would you have in place for crisis intervention if abuse developed between sessions?

5. Explain why someone in a family or community would respond differently to a problem than you do. Discuss the following questions with the family/community to enhance their problem solving (adapted from Schorr, 1997).
   - What do you think is the problem?
   - What do you think you should do?
   - What would help?
   - What have you done in the past when this happened? Did it work?
   - What are your options?
   - Who might help you?

## Toys

Color washed from years,
At awkward angles,
Tension springs still wound
Grandchildren—children no longer

Waiting to be touched—once again
To dance—march—beat the drum—play the music

Alone in the lower drawer
They wait

Company kept with
Orange green photographs of—
What summer day—what winter night?

—*Ann Thedford Lanier, PhD*

## ■ REFERENCES

Banks-Wallace, J. (1998). Emancipatory potential of storytelling in a group. *Image: The Journal of Nursing Scholarship, 30*(1), 17–21.

Banks-Wallace, J. (1999). Storytelling as a tool for providing holistic care to women. *American Journal of Maternal Child Nursing, 24*(1), 20–24.

Benson, H. (1996). *Timeless healing. The power and biology of belief.* New York: Simon & Schuster.

Bronfenbrenner, U. (1986). Ecology of the family as a context for human development. Research perspectives. *Developmental Psychology, 22*(6), 723–742.

Butterfield, P. G. (1991). Thinking upstream: Nurturing a conceptual understanding of the societal context of health behavior. In K. A. Saucier (Ed.), *Perspectives in family and community health* (pp. 66–71). St. Louis: Mosby.

Butterfield, P. G. (2002). Upstream reflections on environmental health: An abbreviated history and framework for action. *Advances in Nursing Science, 25*(1), 32–50.

Byrd, M. E. (1999). Questioning the quality of maternal caregiving during home visiting. *Image: The Journal of Nursing Scholarship, 31*(1), 27–32.

Carter, B. (2008). "Good" and "bad" stories: Decisive moments, "Shock and awe," and being moral. *Journal of Clinical Nursing, 17*(8), 1063–1070.

Children's Defense Fund. (1994). *Helping children by strengthening families: A look at family support programs.* Washington, DC: Author.

Clinton, H. R. (1996). *It takes a village: And other lessons children teach us* (p. 65). New York: Touchstone.

Cordes, H., & Walljasper, J. (Eds.). (1997). *Goodlife: Mastering the art of everyday living.* Minneapolis: Utne Reader.

Crockenberg, S. B. (1985). Professional support and care of infants by adolescent mothers in England and the United States. *Journal of Pediatric Psychology, 10,* 413–428.

Dawe, S., & Harnett, P. (2007). Reducing potential for child abuse among methadone-maintained parents: Results from a randomized controlled trial. *Journal of Substance Abuse Treatment, 32*(4), 381–390.

Federman, M., Garner, T. I., Short, K., et al. (1996). What does it mean to be poor in America? *Monthly Labor Review, 119*(5), 3–17.

Fetterman, D. M., Kaftarian, S. J., & Wandersman, A. (Eds.). (1996). *Empowerment evaluation: Knowledge and tools for self-assessment and accountability.* Thousand Oaks, CA: Sage.

Flaskerud, J. H., & Winslow, B. J. (1998). Conceptualizing vulnerable populations: Health-related research. *Nursing Research, 47*(2), 69–78.

Gordon, S. (1997). *Life support: Three nurses on the front lines.* Boston: Little, Brown.

Hancock, T. (1993). Re-designing healthcare from the bottom down. In *Healthier communities action kit* (vol. 2). San Francisco: Healthcare Forum.

Heaman, M., Chalmers, K., Woodgate, R., & Brown, J. (2007). Relationship work in an early childhood home visiting program. *Journal of Pediatric Nursing, 22*(4), 319–330.

Heinicke, C. M. (1993). Factors affecting the efficacy of early family intervention. In N. J. Anastasiow & S. Harel (Eds.), *At-risk infants: Interventions, families and research* (pp. 91–100), Baltimore, MD: Paul H. Brookes.

Hill, K. (2008). A strengths-based framework for social policy: Barriers and possibilities. *Journal of Policy Practice, 7*(2/3), 106–121.

House, J. S., Landis, K. R., & Umberson, D. (1988). Social relationships and health. *Science, 241*(4865), 540–545.

Johannson, M. A., & Tutty, L. M. (1998). An evaluation of after-treatment couples' groups for wife abuse. *Family Relations, 47*(1), 27–35.

Kawachi, I., Kennedy, B. P., Lochner, K., & Prothrow-Stith, D. (1997). Social capital, income inequality, and mortality. *American Journal of Public Health, 87*(9), 1491–1498.

Kemp, L., Eisbacher, L., McIntyre, L., O'Sullivan, K., Taylor, J., Clark, T., et al. (2006). Working in partnership in the antenatal period: What do child and family health nurses do? *Contemporary Nurse: A Journal for the Australian Nursing Profession, 23*(2), 312–320.

LaTaillade, J., Epstein, N., & Werlinich, C. (2006). Conjoint treatment of intimate partner violence: A cognitive behavioral approach. *Journal of Cognitive Psychotherapy, 20*(4), 393–410.

Lantz, P. M., House, J. S., Lepkowski, J. M., Williams, D. R., Mero, R. P., & Chen, J. (1998). Socioeconomic factors, health behaviors, and mortality: Results from a nationally representative prospective study of US adults. *Journal of the American Medical Association, 279*(21), 1703–1708.

Laursen, E. (2000). Strength-based practice with children in trouble. *Reclaiming Chidren and Youth, 9*(2), 70–75.

Leonard, J., & Siegel, M. (1998). Mother and daughter workshops. *Childbirth Instructor Magazine,* March/April, 34–35.

Levy, B. S. (1998). Creating the future of public health: Values, vision, and leadership. *American Journal of Public Health, 88*(2), 188–192.

Lomas, J. (1998). Social capital and health: Implications for public health and epidemiology. *Social Science and Medicine, 47*(9), 1181–1188.

Lynch, I., & Tiedje, L. B. (1991). Working with multiproblem families: An intervention model for community health nurses. *Public Health Nursing, 8*(3), 147–153.

McKinlay, J. B. (1979). A case for refocusing upstream: The political economy of illness. In E. G. Jaco (Ed.), *Patients, physicians, and illness* (3rd ed., pp. 9–25). New York: Free Press.

Minkler, M. (Ed.). (1998). *Community organizing & community building for health.* New Brunswick, NJ: Rutgers University Press.

Nelson, A., McClintock, C., Perez-Ferguson, A., Shawver, M., & Thompson, G. (2008). Storytelling narratives: Social bonding as key for youth at risk. *Child & Youth Care Forum, 37*(3), 127–137.

Papiernik, E., Bouyer, J., Yaffe, K., Winisdorffer, G., Collin, D., & Dreyfus, J. (1986). Women's acceptance of a preterm birth prevention program. *American Journal of Obstetrics and Gynecology, 155,* 939–946.

Pipher, M. (1994). *Reviving Ophelia: Saving the selves of adolescent girls.* New York: Ballantine.

Putnam, R. D. (1995). Bowling alone. American's declining social capital. *Journal of Democracy, 6,* 65–78.

Remen, R. N. (1996). *Kitchen table wisdom.* New York: Riverhead Books.

Roe, K. M., Berenstein, C., Goette, C., & Roe, K. (1996). Community building through empowering evaluation. In Meredith Winkler (Ed.), *Community organizing & community building for health* (pp. 308–322). New Brunswick, NJ: Rutgers University Press.

Roehlkepartain, J. L. (1995). *Building assets together.* Minneapolis: Search Institute.

Salmon, M. E. (1999). Thoughts on nursing: Where it has been and where it is going. *Nursing and Health Care Perspectives, 20*(1), 20–25.

Schorr, L. B. (1997). *Common purpose: Strengthening families and neighborhoods to rebuild America.* New York: Anchor Books.

Shindul-Rothschild, J. (1998). Nurses week tribute: A nursing call to action. *American Journal of Nursing, 98*(5), 36.

Smyth, J., Stone, A. A., Hurewitz, A., & Kaell, A. (1999). Effects of writing about stressful experiences on symptom reduction in patients with asthma or rheumatoid arthritis. *Journal of the American Medical Association, 281*(14), 1304–1309.

Stagner, M. W., & Duran, M. A. (1997). Comprehensive community initiatives: Principles, practice, and lessons learned. In R. E. Behrman (Ed.), *The future of children: Children and poverty* (vol. 7[2] pp. 44–68.). Los Altos, CA: Center for the Future of Children.

Tandon, D. (2007). Promotion of service integration among home visiting programs and community coalitions working with low-income, pregnant, and parenting women. *Health Promotion Practice, 8*(1), 79–87.

Tanner, C. A. (1995). Living in the midst of a paradigm shift. *Journal of Nursing Education, 34*(2), 51–52.

U.S. Department of Health and Human Services. (2000). *Healthy people 2010: Understanding and improving health* (2nd ed.). Washington, DC: Author.

U.S. Department of Health and Human Services. (2004). *The 2004 national sample survey of registered nurses.* Washington, DC: Author.

Weisman, A. D. (1981). Understanding the cancer patient: The syndrome of caregiver's plight. *Psychiatry, 44,* 161–168.

World Health Organization (WHO). *The World health report 2005—Make every mother and child count.* Retrieved November 20, 2008, from http://www.who.int/2005/en/

Zerwekh, J. V. (1997). Making the connection during home visits: Narratives of expert nurses. *International Journal for Human Caring, I*(1), 25–29.

# UNIT 7

# Care of Individuals

CHAPTER 32
Women's Health
*Karen Saucier Lundy*
*Norma G. Cuellar*
*Venus Callahan*

CHAPTER 33
Men's Health
*Sharyn Janes*
*A. Serdar Atav*
*Joseph F. Farmer*
*Karen Saucier Lundy*

CHAPTER 34
Children's Health
*Carole Hanks*
*Harriet Kitzman*
*Lorrie Yoos*

CHAPTER 35
Elder Health
*Virgina Lee Cora*

CHAPTER 36
Mental Health in the Community
*Sarah Steen Lauterbach*
*Janna Lesser*

Karen Saucier Lundy, Norma G. Cuellar,
and Venus Callahan

Visit **http://nursing.jbpub.com/communityhealth**
for interactive exercises, review questions,
Web links, and more.

"A woman's health is her capital."
—Harriet Beecher Stowe

Women do two-thirds of the world's work. Yet they earn only one-tenth of the world's income and own less than 1% of the world's property. They are among the poorest of the world's poor.

—*Barber B. Conable*

I will be post-feminist in the post-patriarchy.

—*Meg Sullivan*

Women never have a half-hour in all their lives (excepting before or after anybody is up in the house) that they can call their own, without fear of offending or of hurting someone. Why do people sit up so late, or, more rarely, get up so early? Not because the day is not long enough, but because they have "no time in the day to themselves."

—*Florence Nightingale, 1852*

If it is a woman's nature to nurture, she must first nourish herself.

—*Anne Morrow Lindbergh*

The sadness of the women's movement is that they don't allow the necessity of love. See, I don't personally trust any revolution where love is not allowed.

—*Maya Angelou*

When you reflect on these women's quotes, how are women different from men in their caring for themselves as well as caring for others? What are the health risks that women have as compared to men? Has the feminist movement affected changes in the way society values women? Is the feminist movement still relevant today, especially for young women?

## CHAPTER FOCUS

**Profile of Women's Health**
- Education
- Employment
- Poverty
- Marital Status/Family Configuration
- Reproductive Health and Risks
- Patterns of Health and Illness

**Health Issues, Health Promotion, and Health Prevention Across the Life Span**
- Adolescence (12 to 18 Years Old)
- Young Adulthood (19 to 35 Years Old)
- Perimenopausal/Menopausal (36 to 55 Years Old)
- Mature (55 and Older)

**Specific Disease Conditions of Women Throughout the Life Span**
- Cancer
- Osteoporosis

**Diversity and Women's Health**
- Cultural Influences
- Sexual Orientation

- Women and Aging
- Global Issues and Women's Health

**Special Issues Affecting Women's Health**
- Violence
- Homelessness
- Incarceration
- Poverty
- Workplace Health

**Toward the Future**
- Women's Ways of Knowing
- Feminism
- Empowerment
- Health Care Policy

*Healthy People 2010:* Objectives Related to Women's Health

QUESTIONS TO CONSIDER

After reading this chapter, answer the following questions:

1. How are demographic variables related to women's health status?
2. As women age, which specific health concerns and issues are most prevalent?
3. What are special health concerns of lesbians, women of color, and elder women?
4. What are the special ethical issues related to health that concern women?
5. Which populations of women are more vulnerable to health risks?
6. How can nurses provide preventive-based care to the diverse population of women in the promotion of health?
7. What are sources of empowerment for women related to improved health?
8. Which future issues will likely influence the health of women?

KEY TERMS

Caregivers
Commission on the Status of Women
Constructed knowledge
Empowerment

Feminism
Feminization of poverty
Heterosexism
Homophobia

Hormone replacement therapy (HRT)
Mammography
Perimenopausal period
Procedural knowledge

United Nations Platform for Action for Women
Urinary incontinence

WOMEN NOW LIVE an average of 30 years longer than they did 100 years ago. A woman born in 1900 was expected to live 49 years; today's baby girls can expect a life span of 80 years. Significant changes and increased opportunities in the lives of American women have broadened the focus of women's health to include physiological, emotional, social, cultural, and economic well-being. Women, as the primary caregivers of families, are key to achieving the goal of healthy communities. However, women face significant barriers in gaining access to health care and in caring for themselves, even as they care for others. Often, inadequate education, gender bias in the health care system, and low socioeconomic status prevent women from assuming the responsibilities for their own health and well-being. As consumers of health services, women must be involved in the development of health policy to achieve parity in availability and access to health care resources for women. Community health nurses play key roles in collaborating with women to achieve the national goal of health care for all. This chapter provides information about the context of women's health and describes how community health nurses can assist women of all ages to meet health needs.

For much of the twentieth century, women's health focused almost exclusively on reproductive functions such as menstruation, childbearing, and menopause. In 1990, a landmark report by the General Accounting Office (GAO) revealed shocking gaps in research on women's health issues. During the twentieth century, women had been left out of most research on cancer, heart disease, and interventions, such as the development of new technology and medications. Such inequities resulted in women's health lagging considerably behind in advances known to benefit men.

In the 1990s, the federal government mobilized the greatest effort ever to improve women's health through research and services. We now have better and safer **mammography** and breast cancer treatment, have more effective ways to prevent and treat osteoporosis, and know more about alternatives for women during the **perimenopausal period.** As the lives of women have been extended, chronic diseases and disability have taken the place of acute illness and childbirth as leading causes of death. Women are living longer lives, challenging community health nurses to help women improve the quality of these added years.

## Profile of Women's Health

The U.S. Census Bureau (2003) reports a ratio at birth of 105 males to 100 females; the mean age for females in the United States is currently 37 years. In most countries, women typically have longer life spans than men and consequently make up 52% of the world's population. In the United States, the average life span for a woman is 79.9 years, compared with 74.4 years for men. Because males are more likely to die at any given age, the proportion of females to males increases over the life span (National Vita Statistics Report, 2004). The difference in the life expectancy of men and women in the

 CULTURAL CONNECTION

Research has consistently found that mothers who create a "culture of weight fixation" are more likely to have daughters with eating disorders than are less self-conscious moms. The media influence daughters, but daughters more often tend to model their mothers' behaviors, such as noticing what they eat, how they talk about their bodies, how often they weigh themselves, and especially whether they have "self-loathing" attitudes. Self-contempt passes from generation to generation as a cultural trait; for daughters to accept their bodies, mothers need to accept their own as only a part of their self-worth. With self-awareness, the culture can become more balanced and healthy for both mothers and daughters throughout their lives.

*Got an Alternative?*

Medicinal herbs often used by women include the following:

- Black cohosh—used for treating hot flashes as symptoms of menopause
- Chaste tree berry (*Vitex agnus castus*)—for premenstrual syndrome (PMS)
- Cranberry (*Vaccinium macrocarpon*)—for prevention of urinary tract infections
- Dong quai (*Angelica sinensis*)—for general female wellness, irregular periods, fatigue
- Flaxseed (*Linum usitatissimum*)—for cardiovascular health and fiber supplement
- Feverfew (*Tancetum parthenium*)—for treatment of symptoms of migraine headache
- Turmeric (*Curcuma longa*)—as an anti-inflammatory and antioxidant
- Green tea (*Camellia sinensis*)—for cancer prevention
- Ginger (*Zingiber officinale*)—for nausea and vomiting, especially during pregnancy

Before advising patients about the use of any herbs, nurses should conduct a thorough literature review of current research on specific herbs, contraindications, and recommendations for specific use. The National Center for Complementary and Alternative Medicine (NCCAM), a division of the U.S. National Institutes of Health (NIH), is the best resource for clinical trial data on herbs and other complementary therapies. NCCAM can be accessed online at http://nccam.nih.gov/.

*Source:* Parch, L. (2006). The nine best herbs for women. *Natural Health, 36*(8), 74–79.

United States has narrowed over the years, and the difference of 5.2 years in 2004 was the smallest difference ever recorded. Among persons 65 years and older, women make up 58% of this age group. By the age of 85, women outnumber men about 2.5 to 1. For community health nurses, many gerontological health issues in the future will be those involving elder women. With a decline in mortality in certain diseases for men (e.g., cardiovascular disease) and an increase in the number of women who have assumed many lifestyle behaviors and health habits previously characteristic of men (e.g., cigarette smoking, alcohol use, stress associated with full-time work in the labor force, and added challenges of maintaining traditional gender roles, such as housekeeping and family care as well as head of household responsibilities), the differences in life spans for women and men are expected to converge even more in the future.

*We grow neither better nor worse as we get old, but more like ourselves.*

—Mary Lamberton Becker

*Since every woman's problem occurs in part because of the nature of being female in this culture, which programs us to put the needs of others ahead of our own, we need to make radical changes in our minds and in our lives to get and stay healthy.*

—Christine Northrup

## Education

Education is positively correlated with health status for both men and women. While women in the United States have high literacy rates (equal to those of men), almost 1 billion adults around the world cannot read, and two-thirds of those are women (U.S. Department of Education, 2007). In the past, the predominant roles professional women chose were in education, nursing, library science, and social work. However, in the last two decades, more women have entered professions traditionally dominated by men, such as engineering, theology, medicine, law, and dentistry. A continuing concern is that ethnic minority women have been slow to enter these major areas of study. An emerging trend, according to the U.S. Census Bureau (2003), is an overall significant increase in college enrollment among African Americans and Hispanics since 1970. Such a trend holds promise for increasing the number of all women and women of color pursing advanced specialty degrees as these cohorts move through the educational ranks.

## Employment

More women are in the U.S. workforce than ever before, and they are entering the workforce at increasingly earlier ages. As compared to 1960, when one of every three workers in the United States was female, half of all workers today are women. However, increased opportunities in the workforce are creating more challenges and risks for their families, such as child and elder caregiving issues. The job market remains male dominated, with average annual salaries differing by gender. Recent data indicate that women earn 60% of the average man's salary in the United States (*Statistical Abstract of the United States,* 2000). This ratio varies considerably throughout the world, according to educational levels and chosen professions. A contributing factor to the significant gender differences in salary relates to women choosing lower-paying jobs by career preparation: Half of the pay difference in salaries for women is attributed to this factor alone. Other factors include caring for family and children during peak earning years.

Traditional female occupations generally pay less than comparable men's jobs and have fewer health care and retirement benefits. Sixty-five percent of women are in the workforce as librarians, teachers, social workers, and nurses

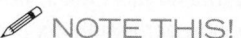 NOTE THIS!

In the United States, women live on average 7 years longer than men.

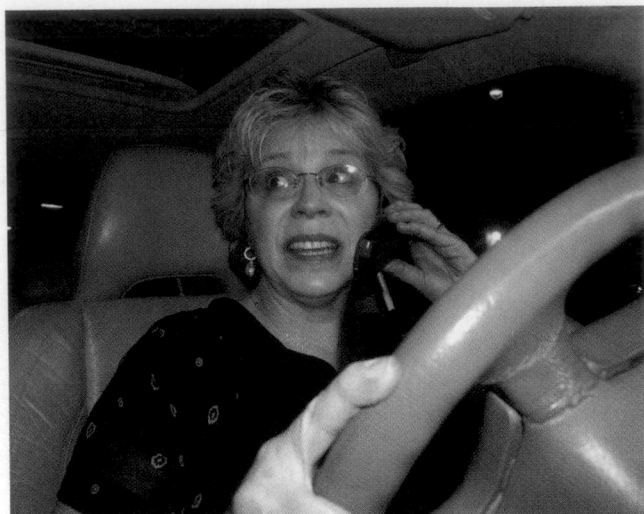

Technology has improved our lives dramatically, especially "anywhere" instant communication and availability. The use of cellular phones in automobiles, as result, has also added stress and risk for many women as they have extended their multitasking to travel time.

with lower mean salaries than members of other professions. Working women continue to assume responsibility for child care, housework, and elder care. More than 50% of women with an infant are in the workforce, up 35.3% since 1978. The percentage of new mothers who work tends to increase with both age and education. Men are more likely to be employed in higher-level management positions, with jobs that offer health benefits, medical leave, and insurance. Women continue to face the "glass ceiling" in regard to career advancement to managerial positions. The "glass ceiling" refers to the barriers that keep women from reaching the executive suite in their chosen professions. Women tend to be outside the "pipeline to success, choosing limited upward mobility options, such as public relations and human resource positions. Men tend to be in more upwardly mobile marketing and sales positions. Women often do not have mentors in

❝*Ours is not the task of fixing the entire world all at once, but of stretching out to mend the part of the world that is within our reach. Any small, calm thing that one soul can do to help another soul, to assist some portion of this poor suffering world, will help immensely. It is not given to us to know which acts, or by whom, will cause the critical mass to tip toward an enduring good. What is needed for dramatic change is an accumulation of acts, adding, adding to, adding more, continuing. We know that it does not take "everyone on Earth" to bring justice and peace, but only a small, determined group who will not give up during the first, second, or hundredth gale.*❞*

—Clarissa Pinkola Estes, Urgent Message from Mother, 2004*

❝*There was that law of life, so cruel and so just, which demanded that one must grow or else pay more for remaining the same.*❞

—Norman Mailer*

higher positions and are often stuck in the 'mommy track', limiting their overnight travel and night/weekend work" (Clarke, 2000). This translates to a major difference in total life earnings between women and men.

Universally, greater prestige is given to male work activities, regardless of what they are. For example, when most infants were delivered by midwives in the nineteenth and early twentieth centuries, the job had low prestige and an associated small salary. When men took over the job of "birthing babies" as medicine specialized in obstetrics and gynecology, the prestige of the role rose along with the salary. This is but one example of how the value of the "nature" of work changes according to the gender of the worker and societal values. Thus it is not about the work itself that promotes privilege and salary, but rather the gender of the worker.

Women with limited health benefits and lower salaries tend to have limited health care options. As a consequence, they may not seek out health care when needed and are less likely to practice preventive health care.

## ■ Poverty

Women earn less than men and, as a result, account for two-thirds of all poor adults (U.S. Census Bureau, 2003). This statistic is greatly influenced by culture and race, with the largest increases in poverty occurring among African American and Hispanic women. Women in poverty are usually 18 to 24 years old, live in the South, and reside outside central cities. Women and children make up a majority of the homeless population in the United States. Many factors contribute to poverty, including the gender wage gap, single mothers as heads of households, teenage birth rates, lack of adequate child care, and lack of enforcement of child support payments. Of all the countries in the industrialized world, the United States is the only country without a system that provides subsidized child care for working parents.

Dual-earner families are least likely to live in poverty (U.S. Census Bureau, 2003). All of these risk factors of poverty as related to women have been referred to as the **feminization of poverty** (Albelda & Tilly, 1997; Dujan & Withorn, 1996).

## ■ Marital Status/Family Configuration

Women's roles in marriage and the family are in a state of transition and have been since the 1960s. The traditional role of the unemployed mother working in the home has become a small minority. Only 6% of households have a male working full-time supporting a full-time homemaker with children in the home—and yet the image of the traditional family (stay-at-home mom, working dad) persists as the norm. We see evidence of this in the media, such as in commercials where housekeeping advertisements target women and business advertisements target men. The necessary goal of any family, however defined, is to maintain the safety, well-being, and health of the family. More than half of adult women in the United States are single, with their number having increased 50% since 1970.

Racial differences in lifestyles can affect attitudes and beliefs about health. African Americans, as compared with Caucasians, are more often single or married with no spouse present or living with extended families. More Caucasians are divorced or widowed, and they tend to have fewer children than do African Americans and Hispanics. Families maintained by women with no husband present are more likely to be poor. Among those men who are present in their families; African American and Hispanic men tend to spend more time with their family tasks than do Caucasian men.

Women, on top of their everyday family obligations, continue to care for older family members: More than 1 in 10 women cares for a sick or aging relative. Meeting these multiple obligations is demanding and leaves many women concerned about the challenge of meeting all their family and work commitments as well as managing their own health. An overwhelming majority of women are responsible for the vast majority of routine health care decisions and responsibilities for their families. For example:

- Eight in 10 women are responsible for choosing their children's health care provider.
- Thirty-four percent take their children to health care appointments and follow-up care.
- Fifty-seven percent of mothers are primarily responsible for decisions about their children's health insurance.
- One in 10 women cares for a sick or aging relative, including doing housework, providing transportation, making various financial decisions, and managing health care, medication administration, and basic care such as assisting with bathing and dressing.
- Four in ten women who are caring for others have a chronic health condition of their own. Twenty-nine percent of those caring for a sick relative provide more than 40 hours per week as a caregiver. This is even more common among low-income caregivers, 44% of whom assist their relative for more than 40 hours per week (*Kaiser Women's Health Survey*, 2005).

### ⌨ Research Alert

"That's What Makes Me Care": Empowering Women as Community Health Workers to Promote Personal and Public Health

Susan Mayfield-Johnson, PhD, MPH, CHES
Director, Education and Training
Center for Sustainable Health Outreach
University of Southern Mississippi
Hattiesburg, Mississippi

Because the cost of health care is continuing to rise and resources are not, innovative solutions must be employed to mobilize our largely untapped but most valuable resource, the people in our community and neighborhoods. The lack of coordination between various health service delivery agencies and programs has often led to duplication of efforts and widening gaps in meeting community needs. Community Health Advisors (CHAs) have emerged as a viable solution to bridge the gap between health service delivery systems and the community. As trusted community members, community health advisors are able to integrate health information about prevention of disease and the health system into the community's culture, language, and value systems, and as a result, they reduce cultural, linguistic, social, and financial barriers to health care. They can

### ⚖ ETHICAL CONNECTION

Dana Reeve lost her battle with lung cancer at age 44 on March 6, 2006, just 17 months after the death of her husband Christopher Reeve. Dana, a nonsmoker, often said, "I learned a long time ago life just isn't fair . . . you just forge ahead."

Lung cancer accounts for the most cancer deaths among women and yet often goes unrecognized as the "top killer" that it is. Smokers used to account for 95% of all lung cancer cases. Today, however, as many as 15% of lung cancer patients are nonsmokers; of those, about 60% are women. Breast cancer kills about 35,000 women each year in the United States, while lung cancer kills about twice that many—70,000 women per year. Research is unclear about the exact reasons for this trend but some factors have emerged as possible epidemiological factors: genetics, estrogen, and the increase in environmental toxins (e.g., radon gas, secondhand smoke, pollution). To further emphasize the political significance of public perception of cancer risks, in 2005 the National Cancer Institute spent $23,000 on research per breast cancer death but only $1,800 per lung cancer death.

Part of the problem is the perception that lung cancer is a "self-inflicted" disease of smokers. What are the ethical implications of this view?

For more information, go to www.lungusa.org.

increase access to care and facilitate appropriate use of health resources by providing outreach and cultural linkages between communities and health systems. Community health advisors are often described as natural helpers or individuals to whom people naturally turn to for advice, emotional support, and tangible aid.

Because community health advisors are members of the communities they serve, they are agents of change within these communities. However, little research exists that described how these women as change agents experience growth themselves in the empowerment process. The purpose of this phenomenological study was to examine and describe the empowerment change processes of community health advisors utilizing photovoice, an innovative method that incorporates documentary photography within a group setting, and separately through reflective in-depth interviews. Using photos and narratives as primary research methods, the women who served as community health advisors in this study gave voice to an often-overlooked resource in the improvement of vulnerable populations in the promotion of the public's health.

Photovoice is an innovative participatory tool based on health promotion principles and the theoretical literature on education for critical consciousness, feminist theory, and a community-based approach to documentary photography (Wang, 2003). Photovoice was chosen because it provided a means for participants to narrate their perceptions and experiences through an emic perspective. Instead of placing cameras into the hands of professional photographers or researchers who are often in control of photo data generation, the photovoice method puts cameras into the hands of the individuals whose lives are daily affected and the focus of the study. The goal of photovoice is to use people's photographic documentation of their everyday lives as an educational tool to record and reflect their needs, promote dialogue, encourage action, and inform policy. Photovoice has three main goals: (1) enable people to record and reflect their community's strengths and concerns through taking photographs; (2) promote critical dialogue and knowledge about important personal and community issues through discussion of their photographs; and (3) to reach policymakers (Wang, 1999; Wang & Burris, 1994). It is a participatory process that integrates empowerment education, feminist theory, and documentary photography. After the photovoice sessions, semi-structured in-depth reflective interviews were also chosen to complement the study design.

In this study, thirty-one female African American community health advisors in a cancer control and prevention program in Mississippi and Alabama participated in four photovoice focus groups, and fifteen additional women participated in reflective interviews. Analysis of the data in the sample revealed the following:

1. The experiences of a CHA profoundly affect her desire to help her community. The typical CHA came from a large family with little to low income and expressed a desire to make a difference in the community.

2. Most community health advisors are either the eldest child, eldest female child, or had a position of authority and/or caregiving in the family structure.

3. Most community health advisors are older women who have experienced significant hardship and struggle in their lives. They have lived through major social and political movements in history, and the significant struggle to obtain equality has left a lasting impression in their philosophy and activities.

4. community health advisors expressed dismay at the apathy and destructiveness of African Americans related to other African Americans. CHAs in the research study believed that they have a duty to their families, communities, and the African American race to change the health disparities and oppression that exist in predominantly African American communities.

5. History, culture, and family are intertwined layers that define who they are and where they come from. These layers cannot be severed in describing their experience. While the remnants of slavery still exist, progress is evident.

6. Spirituality and faith are essential components for service in the community. Their role was often described as "a calling."

7. Participation in a community health worker program served two purposes: individual change in knowledge, attitudes, and beliefs and application of efficacy in practice.

8. Community health advisors feel that they have made a difference in their communities. They see the changes in their communities.

9. Community health advisors described their role in the community as a leader, educator, caregiver, mentor, and servant. They credit these roles to the leadership development and skill building characteristics of the program.

10. Community health advisors draw on other women for support. The social networking function of a CHA group was expressed by the participants as essential to professional growth and development.

One community health advisor in Alabama described her perception of race and class in the African American community in this way:

**❝** *So we had a class system, just because you're Black doesn't mean class doesn't exist. You can have class system between light color Blacks and dark color Blacks, you have it between poor Blacks and better-off Blacks, you know, so you had the class system. And in that point, considering my dad's job status, we were the poorer Blacks and the darker color Blacks.* **❞**

*54 year-old, mother of three, who lost her daughter to cancer.*

Another community health advisor in Mississippi describes her personal growth and empowerment in the following narrative account:

> *I had a pair of black pumps and I had had them for I don't know, three or four years but anyway they were all ran over and the heel was crooked on them. You know, my mama told me that when I got ready to graduate she said, "Why don't you go and get you a new pair of shoes?" I said, "No." So every event that I had to attend when I went to school, I wore those shoes . . . I'm gonna wear these shoes and even after I graduate, I kept those shoes until they really dry rotted. And the reason why I kept those shoes, is because I didn't want to forget where I came from so everyday I looked in that closet and I saw those shoes and I remembered the struggle that I had to be where I came from. But now I look back and I see that I had to go through that to get to where I am now. And I thank God and He let me go through that. Because the people that I work with now, the abused women, the low self-esteem women, I can related to those women because I been through that. And I think that's what makes me care.*
>
> *51 year old, mother of three,*
> *sister to a lung and liver cancer survivor.*

### Implications of the Study

Describing what it means to be a community health advisor gives important recognition and value to the role of change agents in the community. Discovering how the empowerment change process takes place in community health advisors is crucial for public health professionals in their efforts to promote community health. Community health education research can be designed to enhance individual and population focused learning by understanding the needs of the people within the framework and culture of the community. Allowing the emergence of a theoretical framework shaped by the perspectives of community health advisors will enable members of the community to collaborate with researchers and practitioners in designing effective interventions in their communities. Involving community health advisors in developing and implementing interventions that are socially and culturally appropriate to their learning needs has the potential to result in changes in the paradigm of public health promotion, specifically related to health education. These implications for change go beyond how programs are developed and administered by examining empowerment, social action, and community capacity. Inclusive and consistent program design and methodology can then form the basis for true community participatory research. ◯

*Sources:* Mayfield-Johnson, S. (2007). Herstory through photovoice and reflective interviews: Describing changes in empowerment among Community Health Advisors as Research Partners in Mississippi and Alabama. *Dissertation Abstracts International: The Humanities and Social Sciences, 68*(06), UMI No. 3268458; Wang, C. (1999). Photovoice: A participatory action research strategy applied to women's health. *Journal of Women's Health, 8,* 185–192; Wang, C. C. (2003). Using photovoice as a participatory assessment and issue selection tool: A case study with the homeless in Ann Arbor. In M. Minkler & N. Wallerstein (Eds.), *Community-based participator research for health* (pp. 179–186). San Francisco: Jossey-Bass; Wang, C., & Burris, M. A. (1994). Empowerment through photo novella: Portraits of participation. *Health Education Quarterly, 21,* 171–186.

## ■ Reproductive Health and Risks

Women are uniquely at risk during pregnancy and childbirth, including the risks of induced and spontaneous abortions. Even in the twenty-first century, women continue to die during childbirth, with pulmonary embolism being the leading cause of death in pregnant women. However, thanks to partnerships between community health nurses and the health care system, maternal mortality has been dramatically reduced through prenatal care, education related to maternal risk factors, blood transfusions, anesthesia, and antibiotics. Racial discrepancies persist in the number of maternal deaths, with women of color having a threefold greater incidence of death during pregnancy than Caucasian women (*Kaiser Women's Health Survey,* 2005). Contributing factors include late or no prenatal care, poor nutrition, and substandard living conditions. Concurrent infant death rates are also disproportionate among races, with twice the number of infants of color dying as Caucasian infants during the first year of life.

Trends in U.S. birth rates have major implications for the growth of the population and the evolution of health care. Fertility rates continue to drop, with an overall decline in birth rates in the United States (U.S. Census Bureau, 2003). The number of births is expected to decline further as the baby-boomers age and pass their childbearing years. More women are delaying childbearing or choosing to remain childless. Birth rates vary by age and ethnicity, with the number of births for unmarried women declining in all age groups.

Women are beginning prenatal care earlier and seeking it out in greater numbers, although this tendency varies, with women of color and those in poverty seeking prenatal care later or not at all. Twice as many African American women deliver low-birth-weight babies compared with Caucasian women. Of women of childbearing age, 25% are not covered by insurance and 25% are insured but without maternity insurance coverage. Parenting classes, health care for children,

---

**Madam Chairperson**

Must I wear my skirts longer than most
So I can put my feet upon my desk
And smoke
And learn to drink
Jack Daniels?

"Just because you were born deformed
    doesn't mean you can't
    stand up just as straight
    and be heard just as far
    as those born with a
    talie-wacker!"

I believe gentlemen, I will
Smoke that cigar
And a brandy sounds
Quite nice
I think I'll stay
—*Ann Thedford Lanier*

### Research Alert

Rap music videos as a media genre have long concerned the public owing to their graphic depiction of violence and sexual exploitation of women. Little research has examined the effect of rap music videos on adolescent behavior. This study sought to determine whether exposure to rap music videos at baseline could predict the occurrence of health-risk behaviors and STDs among African American adolescent females over a 12-month follow-up period.

The study followed 522 single African American females ages 14 and 18 who had been sexually active in the previous 6 months. Level of exposure to rap music videos—the predictor variable—was determined by asking the subjects to estimate the number of hours they viewed rap music videos during an average day. This was multiplied by the number of days in the week that rap music videos were viewed. Music video viewing characteristics assessed included which primary type of rap music videos was viewed (gangsta, bass, or hip-hop), with whom they viewed rap music videos, and where the videos were viewed. Covariates included age, employment status, involvement in extracurricular activities and religious events, family composition, public assistance, parental monitoring, and group assignment to HIV intervention. Health-risk behaviors assessed included teacher violence, fighting in school, arrest, alcohol or drug use, multiple sex partners, condom use, and STD infection over the 12-month period.

Greater exposure to rap music videos was associated with unemployment and less parental monitoring. Greater exposure was also independently associated with a broad spectrum of health outcomes. Compared with adolescents who had less exposure to rap music videos, adolescents who had greater exposure to such videos were 3 times more likely to have hit a teacher, more than 2.4 times as likely to have been arrested, 2 times as likely to have had multiple sexual partners, and more than 1.5 times as likely to have acquired a new STD, used drugs, and used alcohol over the 12-month follow-up. Although this was one of the first studies to empirically show that greater exposure to rap music videos at baseline was prospectively associated with the occurrence of health-risk behaviors and having lab-confirmed new STDs 1 year later, the authors were careful to note that it is difficult to determine whether the relationship between exposure to rap music videos and adolescent health status was causal.

Social cognitive theory was used to explain the findings. Modeling occurs more readily when the modeled behavior is salient, simple, and prevalent and when it has functional value. Thus exposure to rap music videos—and specifically gangsta rap, which is explicit about sex and violence and rarely shows the potential long-term adverse effects of risky behaviors—may influence adolescents modeling these unhealthy practices. Moreover, African

American females desiring greater independence may rebel against parental medical restrictions and engage in risky behaviors. Implications for community health nurses are that education efforts should focus on these high-risk groups in determining risky behaviors and mediating factors.

*Source*: Wingood, G., DiClemente, R. J., Bernhardt, J. M., et al. (2003). A prospective study of exposure to rap music videos and African American female adolescents' health. *American Journal of Public Health, 93*(3), 437–440.

quality daycare facilities, and flexible employment opportunities for working mothers are not consistently available to women in the United States; the health and well-being of working families has not been a national funding priority. By contrast, many countries throughout the world have established policies that ensure protection and support of mothers, infants, and families and can serve as role models for such positive family investments.

### ■ Patterns of Health and Illness

Women are generally healthier and live longer than men, yet women miss more sick days from work, visit physicians more often than men, and are more likely to take on what sociologists refer to as the "sick role." Differences are often explained in terms of the way men and women are socialized to health and illness. Men are more likely to view illness as a sign of weakness, reflecting a macho association with being well (Klonoff & Landrine, 2000). Nearly 4 in 10 women (38%) have a chronic condition that requires ongoing medical attention, compared to 30% of men. Not surprisingly, the incidence of chronic conditions increases with age. Nearly 6 in 10 women in their senior years are dealing with hypertension (58%) and arthritis (61%), and almost half have high cholesterol (45%). The prevalence of certain chronic conditions has been increasing earlier in women's lives, too. Between 2001 and 2004, significant changes included the rise in diabetes from 5% to 8% of non-elderly women; anxiety and depression rose from 21% to 24%; and obesity rates increased from 11% to 13%. These gender differences in the incidence of chronic illnesses are still not fully understood. The three major chronic conditions women experience are heart conditions, arthritis, and hypertension, all of which increase with age (*Kaiser Women's Health Survey*, 2005).

The leading causes of death in women are heart disease, cancer, and stroke, with differences in mortality observed by age and across racial groups. The leading causes of death in women older than age 65 are heart disease, cancer, cerebrovascular accident (CVA), pneumonia, and influenza. These diseases can be attributed to lifestyle, environmental, and

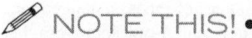

✎ NOTE THIS! ●─────────────────

For all persons who live to be 100 years of age, there will be five women for every two men.

Most women have contact with the health care system during their reproductive years. Venus Callahan, chapter author, examines an expectant mother

Elizabeth Edwards, wife of Democratic vice presidential nominee John Edwards, was diagnosed with breast cancer the week her husband and John Kerry failed in their presidential bid in November 2004. At the time, Elizabeth was 55 years old and the mother of a 6-year-old daughter, a 4-year-old son, and a teenaged daughter. She and her husband lost their 16-year-old son to a car accident in 1996. Elizabeth underwent fertility treatments that resulted in the births of her two youngest children when she was in her late forties.

Says Edwards, "This diagnosis is a reminder that this is the life you've got, and you're not getting another one. Whatever has happened, you have to take this life and treasure and protect it. In a sense, having cancer takes you by the shoulder and shakes you."

social factors and are often preventable. Alcohol and drug use and abuse, unprotected sex, cigarette smoking, lack of exercise, obesity, and environmental threats are all associated with the leading causes of death in women.

Women's health needs are reflected in their provider choices as they age. Virtually all elderly women (95%) age 65 and older have regular health providers, compared to three-fourths of women ages 18 to 44 and 90% of women ages 45 to 64. Predictably, as women age, they are also less likely to visit a women's health care specialist on a regular basis. Only 26% of senior women report a gynecological visit in the past year, and only 12% consider these women's health care specialists among their regular providers, compared to 47% of women in their reproductive years. Of concern to health professionals, there have been declines in mammogram and Pap smear rates in both younger and middle-age women. While the changes are modest, these findings cause concern, as they reverse gains in previous years as women became more aware of the value of these early detection screening tests in improving the outcomes of breast and reproductive cancer. Mammography rates reported by women ages 40 to 64 dropped from 73% to 69%; Pap testing rates for women ages 18 to 64 fell from 81% to 70%. Possible reasons for these declining rates include media attention about the accuracy of mammography in detecting early-stage breast cancer. Further, the guidance on mammography for women ages 40 to 49 can be ambiguous, with major breast cancer organizations and researchers in disagreement over the recommendations for this age group. There have also been changes in recommendations for timing of Pap smears, which are now based on risk and presence of other health conditions, rather than uniform guidelines based on age. While these changes were intended to improve the targeting of screening programs and reduce the costs of unnecessary testing, they could be creat-

ing some confusion among women and their health care providers (*Kaiser Women's Health Survey,* 2005).

Women may delay seeking care when sick because of family and work obligations, may not take symptoms of pain seriously, and may not pursue health care for themselves while focusing on the care of others. In addition, physicians may minimize women's complaints and delay necessary diagnostic tests, which results in a greater chance for a poor health outcome. One study examined the differences in women's survival rates from open-heart coronary bypass surgery as compared to men. The researchers found a significant survival rate difference between men and women. Women were almost twice as likely to die (at 4.6%) as men (2.6%) following the exact same open-heart surgical procedure. Factors identified by the researchers as explaining the difference are related to women's cardiac symptoms being different from those experienced by men, with health care providers taking women's complaints less seriously than men's. Physicians were 10 times more likely to order stress tests and scans with the first symptom for men, but they waited longer until women had clear-cut symptoms before ordering these diagnostics and doing surgery. By operating on a patient with more-severe and late-manifested cardiac damage, the mortality goes up (Bell, Grill, Garrett, Berger, Gersh, & Holmes, 1995). All of these factors may contribute to women entering the health care system at a high acuity level with a greater chance of either dying or requiring more expensive and advanced medical and health interventions.

"*Aging is very much a woman's issue. That's because women are most valued for their childbearing capacities. Once we've used up those capacities and our supposed sexual attractiveness, our social worth is gone.*"

—Gloria Steinem, 1999

Mental health is an often-overlooked but critical aspect of women's health care. One out of every four women (23%) reports that she has been diagnosed with depression or anxiety, more than twice the rate for men (11%). Even among senior women, who have lower rates of depression than young women do, these mental health issues affect 16% (*Kaiser Women's Health Survey,* 2005).

Health coverage, public or private, continues to be a major concern for women and is highly correlated with health and illness patterns in women throughout the life span. Nearly 1 in 6 women younger than age 65 is uninsured (17%). Women who are Latina, low income, single, and young are particularly at risk for being uninsured. Uninsured women are least likely to have visited a health care provider even once a year (67%), compared to women with either private insurance (90%) or public insurance—Medicaid (88%) and Medicare (93%) (*Kaiser Women's Health Survey,* 2005). Clearly, when women cannot afford insurance, pay for drugs, or qualify for public insurance, their health suffers. Compared to women with insurance, uninsured women consistently report lower rates of preventive screening tests for many conditions, including breast cancer, cervical cancer, hypertension, high cholesterol, and osteoporosis. Even insured women face barriers when seeking and accessing health care: One in 6 women with private coverage and one-third of women with Medicaid report that they postponed or went without needed health services in the past year because they could not afford it. Women are more likely (56%) than men (42%) to use prescription medicine on a regular basis and are more likely to report difficulties affording their medications. One in 5 women (20%) reports not filling at least one prescription, compared to 14% of men. Approximately 41% of uninsured women fail to fill prescriptions because of the drugs' costs. Related to these cost barriers, 1 in 7 women reports that skipping or taking lower doses of prescribed medication to make them last longer (*Kaiser Women's Health Survey,* 2005).

African American women are at elevated risk for certain health problems, and these risks increase with age. For example, African American women have arthritis and diabetes at significantly higher rates than do white women.

## Research Alert

salons. Campaigns and policy enactments are needed, much as occurred with successful antismoking campaigns, pushing laws to limit access, and raise taxes on tanning salons. Mass-media campaigns featuring celebrities who discourage tanning salons for teens would be wise as well.

Community health nurses should teach individuals about UV risk and tanning salons and promote the use of sunscreen on a daily basis, not just when tanning. Early detection of skin cancer, such as irregularly shaped moles and changes in existing skin lesions (e.g., oozing moles), should be emphasized in all contact with teenagers. Schools can be an excellent forum to warn teens about indoor tanning and encourage the use of sunless lotions. ◯

*Sources:* WHO, 2004; 2002

**❝** *Be who you are and say what you feel, because those who mind don't matter and those who matter don't mind.* **❞**

—*Dr. Suess*

**❝** *Anything you think is wrong with your body at 35, you will be nostalgic for at 45.* **❞**

—*Nora Ephron*

# Health Issues, Health Promotion, and Health Prevention Across the Life Span

Community health nurses, because of their unique relationship with clients and their awareness of community problems and resources, occupy a pivotal role in influencing women's beliefs and practices for health promotion and illness prevention. Community health nurse, as educators of women about health issues, incorporate the health promotion and disease prevention aims of *Healthy People 2010* to accomplish the primary goal of identifying and implementing behavioral and social interventions that are effective in motivating women to use preventive health services across the life span.

## ■ Adolescence (12 to 18 Years Old)

Today's teenage females in the United States face many health and social issues that their mothers and grandmoth-

ers could never have imagined. The present generation of teens is more likely to be "plugged in" to all types of media, including iPods, videocasts, instant messaging on cell phones, and the Internet. Opportunities are unlimited in the use of these media in influencing healthy behaviors, as these forms of communication are often more effective in reaching teens than in traditional clinic settings. Teens are more likely than adults to seek health information on the Internet, for example, due to the anonymity of the World Wide Web (WWW). Community health nurses can play an important role in promoting the health of adolescent females through teaching, counseling, and role modeling, and can gainfully employ these various new technologies for sharing health information.

Community health nurses need to establish trusting relationships with adolescents, thereby gaining their confidence. This is a most challenging task, as parents of teens can relate to. As nurses, we must be able to ask the tough questions that might reveal alcohol and other drug abuse, high-risk sexual activity, or emotional distress. Community health nurses working with adolescents face challenges in communication, peer influences, and the stigma of teens being seen in local health clinics or settings that offer reproductive health resources. Effective programs that have a positive impact on the health of adolescents are often specifically targeted to teens in schools, night clinics, and malls, as well as through celebrity and teen role model spokespersons.

Young women in adolescence have many issues to deal with, including puberty, menarche, body image, eating disorders, and sexual issues, including sexual identity, contraception decisions, and sexually transmitted diseases (STDs). Attitudes about these issues are influenced by the media, peers, society, and family relationships. *Healthy People 2010* objectives should guide the direction of educational efforts targeting this age group. School-based health programs for health promotion, exercise and fitness, sex education, and prevention of drug use should address social concerns related to teenage girls. Because the greatest number of new smokers are adolescent females, primary lung cancer prevention must start at the elementary school level, with aggressive counseling programs to decrease the number of new smokers among young girls. Successful programs with teen girls and the prevention of smoking initiation have focused on assertiveness training and decision-making models of accountability.

**Table 32-1** Births and Percentage of Births of Women by Age and Race, 2004

| Age Group | Total Births | Non-Hispanic White | Non-Hispanic Black | American Indian | Asian or Pacific Islander | Hispanic |
|---|---|---|---|---|---|---|
| 10–14 | 6,789 | 22% | 40% | 2% | 1% | 35% |
| 15–19 | 415,408 | 41% | 23% | 2% | 2% | 32% |
| 20–24 | 1,034,834 | 50% | 18% | 1% | 3% | 27% |
| 25–34 | 2,072,305 | 60% | 11% | 1% | 7% | 21% |
| 35–44 | 580,040 | 64% | 10% | <1% | 8% | 17% |
| 45–54 | 6,214 | 66% | 10% | <1% | 8% | 13% |

*Source:* CDC, 2004.

## HEALTHY PEOPLE 2010

### Objectives Related to Women's Health

**Arthritis, Osteoporosis, and Chronic Back Conditions: Osteoporosis**

2.9    Reduce the overall number of cases of osteoporosis.

2.10    Reduce the proportion of adults who are hospitalized for vertebral fractures associated with osteoporosis.

**Cancer**

3.3    Reduce the breast cancer death rate.

3.4    Reduce the death rate from cancer of the uterine cervix.

3.11    Increase the proportion of women who receive a Pap test.

3.13    Increase the proportion of women aged 40 years and older who have received a mammogram within the preceding 2 years.

**Family Planning**

9.4    Reduce the proportion of females experiencing pregnancy despite use of a reversible contraceptive method.

9.11    Increase the proportion of young adults who have received formal instruction before turning age 18 years on reproductive issues, including all of the following topics: birth control methods, safer sex to prevent HIV, prevention of sexually transmitted diseases, and abstinence.

9.12    Reduce the proportion of married couples whose ability to conceive or maintain a pregnancy is impaired.

9.13    Increase the proportion of health insurance policies that cover contraceptive supplies and services.

**HIV**

13.3    Reduce the number of AIDS cases among females and males who inject drugs.

**Injury and Violence Prevention: Violence and Abuse Prevention**

15.34    Reduce the rate of physical assault by current or former intimate partners.

15.35    Reduce the annual rate of rape or attempted rape.

**Maternal, Infant, and Child Health**

*Maternal Death and Illness*

16.4    Reduce maternal deaths.

16.5    Reduce maternal illness and complications due to pregnancy.

*Prenatal Care*

16.6    Increase the proportion of pregnant women who receive early and adequate prenatal care.

**Nutrition and Overweight: Iron Deficiency Anemia**

19.12    Reduce iron deficiency among young children and females of childbearing age.

19.14    Reduce iron deficiency among pregnant females.

**Sexually Transmitted Diseases: STD Complications Affecting Females**

25.6    Reduce the proportion of females who have never required treatment for pelvic inflammatory disease (PID).

25.7    Reduce the proportion of childless females with fertility problems who have had a sexually transmitted disease or who have required treatment for pelvic inflammatory disease.

25.8    Reduce HIV infections in adolescent and young adult females aged 13 to 24 years that are associated with heterosexual contact.

*Source*: DHHS, 2000.

---

Parents should be included in these targeted interventions, as one media campaign advises: "Parents: The Anti Drug." Research supports this advice, with studies linking consistent attention by parents to drug prevention in their everyday conversations and decreased risks of their children engaging in drug experimentation (including smoking) and use.

While illegal drug use has decreased in past years, over-the-counter (OTC) and prescription drug abuse have continued to increase at alarming rates. Parents should remain constantly vigilant about the availability or misuse potential of their own prescribed drugs, especially those with high risk for abuse, such as narcotics, antihistamines, antidepression drugs, and cough and cold preparations. They should also monitor online purchases via credit card on a monthly basis, checking out any suspicious charges. Drugs sold over the Internet are often charged on credit cards as innocent miscellaneous product or service sales. Nurses should be also vigilant about including this information when both counseling teens, their parents, and educators who are in frequent contact with members of this age group.

The Youth Risk Behavior Surveillance System, which exists under the auspices of the Centers for Disease Control and Prevention, monitors health-risk behaviors among youth and young adults on an annual basis. These health-risk behaviors contribute to unintentional and intentional injuries, tobacco use, alcohol and other illegal and prescription drug use, sexual behaviors, dietary behaviors, and physical activity, and should guide the community health nurse in planning interventions directed toward the female adolescent. Nurses should check the CDC website (www.cdc.gov) on a regular basis for current research and trends related to this age group, as well as review suggestions for applying the information in community settings. Schools, churches, and recreational groups all provide the community health nurse with opportunities to influence health decisions through education and media campaigns (CDC, 2008).

Adolescents' misconception that they are "immortal" sometimes leads to risk-taking behaviors that make them more susceptible to injury and death. During the past few years, females have been gaining on males as greater num-

Women who are involved in their communities, such as this community lay advisor group, are very effective in promoting health among specific populations, such as elder African American women.

hers engage in risk taking traditionally associated with males Increases in automobile accidents, often in conjunction with cell phone use, and aggressive acts toward both males and other females have increased significantly. These trends are most likely to continue as gender roles move toward less rigid stereotypical expressions and the boundaries of appropriate behavior as distinguished by gender continue to blur. Female adolescents face potential threats to health such as substance abuse, pregnancy, acne, menstrual disorders, eating disorders, and STDs. Every year, nearly one-fourth of all new HIV infections, one-fourth new STD infections, and 1 million pregnancies occur among U.S. teenagers.

The community health nurse can be a pivotal force in promoting the health of adolescents through health assessment, risk analysis, screening, anticipatory guidance, health teaching, and counseling with both adolescents and parents. The most common health care request of adolescent females is related to pregnancy, sexual choices, and pregnancy prevention. As part of any visit with a teen female, the nurse should conduct a health screening assessment, including last missed menstrual period; contraception, if any, being used; living arrangements; financial status; and significant

## MEDIA MOMENT

**Songs About Women and Women's Issues**
*Independence Day,* Martina McBride
*I Am Woman,* Helen Reddy
*Goodbye Earl,* The Dixie Chicks
*Eleanor Rigby,* The Beatles
*Hey Hey Cinderella,* Suzy Boggus
*Stand by Your Man,* Tammy Wynette
*It Wasn't God Who Made Honky Tonk Angels,* Kitty Wells
*The Pill,* Loretta Lynn

sex partners. This provides the nurse with opportunities to determine the teen's concerns about the initiation of a sexual relationship, the risks involved with such initiation, and concerns arising from the teen's own moral and ethical feelings about sex and attachment.

Young females are having sex at younger ages and approaching the percentage of teen boys who begin having sex as early as 15. Teen girls are at risk for acquaintance rape during high school, and this problem only escalates in the college years. The frequent use of the "date rape" drug Rohypnol ("roofies") placed in drinks exposes girls who overuse alcohol in social settings to an even greater risk of sexual assault and rape. Because of the effects of Rohypnol, girls have little to no memory of the sexual assault or the person involved, which lessens the likelihood of the rape being reported. The nurse should offer suggestions about how to avoid this ever-increasing problem, as teen girls' alcohol use has increased significantly in the past 5 years, leaving them even more vulnerable to date rape.

One recent study found that if an adolescent is pregnant, anticipatory guidance is needed. This includes referral to a local prenatal health clinic or health department, encouragement of open communication regarding the pregnancy with family members or the significant other, and referral to the local department of human services for Medicaid enrollment if necessary. Health teaching must include the effects of alcohol and drugs on the fetus, the potential side effects of x-rays on the fetus, nutrition, and Women, Infant and Children (WIC) nutrition program enrollment. The counseling services of the nurse should include a meeting with the adolescent and parent to inform them of the pregnancy.

For sexually active adolescents who are not pregnant, the nurse should encourage enrollment in a family planning clinic for contraceptives and STD education, and take the time to discuss sexual values and concerns that are often difficult for the teen to talk about with friends or family. Instead

**Table 32-2**   Recommended Health Care Calendar

| Test or Procedure | Who Needs It? | How Often? |
|---|---|---|
| ■ General physical exam (including blood pressure and lifestyle counseling | Everyone | Every year |
| ■ Pelvic examination | Everyone | Every year |
| ■ Dental examination | Everyone | Every year |
| ■ Eye examination | Everyone | Every year |
| ■ Breast examination | Everyone | Every year |
| ■ Breast self-examination (BSE) | Everyone | Every month |
| ■ Skin cancer check | Everyone | Every 3 years |
| ■ Rectal examination | Everyone | Every year |
| ■ Pap smear | Everyone | Every year |
| ■ Blood cholesterol | Everyone | Every 3 years (if first test was normal); as recommended by health professional if level is elevated |
| ■ Mammogram | Everyone | Every 1 to 2 years between ages 40 and once a year after age 50 |
| ■ Tests for sexually transmitted diseases | Anyone who is sexually active | Every 6–12 months if multiple partners, otherwise as recommended by health professional |
| ■ Electrocardiogram | Anyone with two or more of the following risk factors for heart disease: family history, smoking, high cholesterol, diabetes, high blood pressure | Every 3 to 5 years |
| ■ Sigmoidoscopy | Anyone over 50 | Every 3 years |
| ■ Fecal occult–blood test | Everyone | Every year |
| ■ Tuberculin skin test | Anyone who is at increased risk | Every year or as recommended by health professional |
| ■ Tetanus booster | Everyone | Every 10 years |
| ■ Diphtheria booster | Everyone | Every 10 years |
| ■ Human Papillomavirus vaccination | Girls, ages 11–26 | Once |

*Sources*: CDC, 2006.

of asking, "Do you have any other concerns?", the nurse can often open up the discussion with "Many young women your age have concerns and questions about intimacy and decisions about sex. I know that it is very hard to talk about these things with our friends and family. Do you have any questions or concerns that we might need to talk about?"

■ **Young Adulthood (19 to 35 Years Old)**

Two main concerns of women in this age group include making career choices and establishing relationships that may lead to marriage and pregnancy. Over the past two decades, women in increasing numbers are delaying marriage and children, which has led to an increase in infertility rates for women in their thirties and forties. Community health nurses can address health promotion interventions in the context of these two life tasks. Nurses need to be knowledgeable about the various resources that are available in the community to assist women in this age range with such decisions. The nurse can be an effective model/mentor for young women in this developmental stage and should be able to address such concerns as fertility counseling, parenting skills, contraception options, domestic violence, and occupational health issues. Women in young adulthood face concerns such as STDs, contraceptive choices, safety, intentional and unintentional injury, stress management, alcohol and drug

---

**BOX 32-1**

**Health-Promotion Activities for the Mature Woman**
Health screenings
Blood pressure, early cancer detection, hearing and vision screenings
Health Education
Stress reduction, nutrition, general health, smoking cessation, classes about seasonal health issues such as hypothermia, heart related illness, colds/flu
Immunizations
Influenza shots
Safety
Safe driving courses, self-protection measures
Exercise
Walking, aerobics, water aerobics, weight lifting, weight-bearing exercise

---

abuse, unhealthy dietary behaviors and relationships, physical activity, and role stress and strain. As women marry and establish families, they face issues such as learning to balance work and children, sexual harassment in the workplace, and establishing habits of self-care. The community health nurse must be cognizant of the problems of this age group and skillful in locating and accessing the resources available to intervene with this age group in setting lifelong healthy patterns.

Violent deaths, homicide, suicide, and accidents (particularly motor vehicle accidents) are responsible for the majority of deaths in this age group. For young adults and college students, as for adolescents, violent death or injury, alcohol and substance abuse, unwanted pregnancies, and STDs are major health threats. Females in this age group may find themselves more vulnerable to "date rape," especially in college, where the use of alcohol and binge drinking have increased. Most health problems in this stage are related to lifestyle behaviors and can alter individuals' chances for a healthy life in the future. Weight concerns and eating problems are often reported as concerns for young women. Media images and social influences may pressure young women desiring to be thin into abusive habits, such as purging, vomiting, laxative and diuretic abuse, and poor nutrition. Young women should be aware of interventions to delay onset of osteoporosis, including increasing calcium intake and weight-bearing exercises to promote bone density and decreasing cola intake, which decreases reabsorption of calcium. Ingesting excessive soft drinks is associated in research studies with decreasing bone mass, and many members of this age group consume soft drinks on a daily basis as a habit started during the teen years. Diet sodas have been found to be associated with a greater risk for obesity, despite the traditional belief their use reduces calorie intake. The use of diet sodas apparently keeps the need for and consequent consumption of foods and drinks that are high in sugar higher than in those who do not drink excessive diet sodas.

The community health nurse can play a vital role in educating this group regarding behaviors that will positively affect their lifestyles. The proper use of condoms to help prevent STDs and the availability and variety of contraceptive choices to prevent unwanted pregnancy must be discussed

*I am not the usual celebrity size. And I think that people who like to see images of themselves reflected back feel strongly connected to me.*

—Rosie O'Donnell

### MEDIA MOMENT

**Born into Brothels, 2004**
This Academy Award–winning documentary is a portrait of several memorable and vulnerable children who live in Calcutta's red-light district, where their mothers work as prostitutes. Zana Briski, a photographer documenting life in the brothels, finds these children fascinated with her camera and decides to teach them photography. As they begin to look at and record their world through new eyes, the kids awaken to their own talents and sense of worth. A disturbing and yet hopeful movie about children and prostitution.

**BOX 32-2**

**Acquaintance Rape: A New Name for an Old Crime?**
Acquaintance rape occurs when a friend or former acquaintance sexually molests a woman. While this act of violence was more likely to have occurred in the past, studies of young women—especially those in college—have indicated a wider incidence than previously thought. In one study, 24% of women reported that they had sex at least once when they "did not want to" (Felton, Gumm, & Pittenger, 2001). A majority of women in the study reported unwanted sexual advances, particularly when drugs and alcohol were involved. Because this crime occurs with acquaintances and can occur under the influence of "date rape" drugs, few report the incidents. A woman is often reluctant to report the incident because she knows the person and was with him voluntarily, at least to some degree. Women often define rape erroneously as occurring only with strangers. Many times, women have no memory of the incident or the identity of the man or men involved.

Young women must be educated while still in middle and high school about the additional risk of sexual assault while under the influence of alcohol and drugs and told to avoid drinking any liquid from an opened bottle or cup at any time during social gatherings. Having a "buddy system," similar to the one used in scuba diving and other risky sports, can also reduce the risk of unwanted sexual assault during college and young adulthood.

with the young adult. Many young adults continue to erroneously believe that the use of oral contraceptives eliminates the need for condom use. Nurses must be vigilant about reminding young women of the continued STD risks even with the use of alternative birth control methods; using a condom every time is a good practice for all young women who have multiple sex partners. Addressing these concerns and seeking mutual solutions together can accomplish the ultimate goal of improved health and risk reduction with young women in this age group.

### ■ Perimenopausal/Menopausal (36 to 55 Years Old)

A comprehensive assessment of women in this age group should include the changes of life that a woman goes through, including physiological, psychological, and emotional changes. The community health nurse must assess the woman's knowledge regarding the changes in her body, including her beliefs about menopause and the implications for her health. The nurse must be aware of complementary therapies women may choose for their health care and should remain open-minded about what is acceptable for their clients. Cardiovascular disease, cancer, and osteoporosis are the three major diseases that occur during the perimenopausal/

### A Good Read

*Maya Angelou: Remarks at the funeral service for Coretta Scott King, who died in February 2006. Mrs. King was the widow of Martin Luther King, Jr.*

"I open my mouth to the Lord and I won't turn back, no. I will go, I shall go. I'll see what the end is gonna be."

In the midst of national tumult, in the medium of international violent uproar, Coretta Scott King's face remained a study in serenity. In times of interior violent storms she sat, her hands resting in her lap calmly, like good children sleeping.

Her passion was never spent in public display. She offered her industry and her energies to action, toward righting ancient and current wrongs in this world.

She believed religiously in nonviolent protest.

She believed it could heal a nation mired in a history of slavery and all its excesses.

She believed nonviolent protest religiously could lift up a nation rife with racial prejudices and racial bias.

She was a quintessential African American woman, born in the small-town repressive South, born of flesh and destined to become iron, born a cornflower and destined to become a steel magnolia.

She loved her church fervently. She loved and adored her husband and her children. She cherished her race. She cherished women. She cared for the conditions of human beings, of Native Americans and Latinos and Asian Americans. She cared for gay and straight people. She was concerned for the struggles in Ireland, and she prayed nightly for Palestine and equally for Israel.

I speak as a sister of a sister. Dr. Martin Luther King was assassinated on my birthday. And for over 30 years, Coretta Scott King and I have telephoned, or sent cards to each other, or flowers to each other, or met each other somewhere in the world.

We called ourselves "chosen sisters," and when we traveled to South Africa or to the Caribbean or when she came to visit me in North Carolina or in New York, we sat into the late evening hours, calling each other "girl." It's a black woman thing, you know. And even as we reached well into our seventieth decade, we still said "girl."

I stand here today for her family—which is my family—and for my family and all the other families in the world who would want to be here, but could not be here. I have beside me up here millions of people who are living and standing straight and erect, and knowing something about dignity without being cold and aloof, knowing something about being contained without being unapproachable—people who have learned something from Coretta Scott King.

I stand here for Eleanor Traylor and for Harry Belafonte, and I stand here for Winnie Mandela. I stand here for women and men who loved her—"Dinky" Romilly. On those late nights when Coretta and I would talk, I would make her laugh. And she said that Martin King used to tell her, "You don't laugh enough." And there's a recent book out about sisters in which she spoke about her blood sister. But at the end of her essay, she said, "I do have a chosen sister, Maya Angelou, who makes me laugh even when I don't want to." And it's true. I told her some jokes only for no-mixed company.

Many times on those late evenings she would say to me, "Sister, it shouldn't be an 'either-or', should it? Peace and justice should belong to all people, everywhere, all the time. Isn't that right?" And I said then and I say now, "Coretta Scott King, you're absolutely right. I do believe that peace and justice should belong to every person, everywhere, all the time."

And those of us who gather here, principalities, presidents, senators, those of us who run great companies, who know something about being parents, who know something about being preachers and teachers—those of us, we owe something from this minute on, so that this gathering is not just another footnote on the pages of history. We owe something.

I pledge to you, my sister, I will never cease.

I mean to say I want to see a better world.

I mean to say I want to see some peace somewhere.

I mean to say I want to see some honesty, some fair play.

I want to see kindness and justice. This is what I want to see and I want to see it through my eyes and through your eyes, Coretta Scott King.

menopausal period of a woman's life. The community health nurse must address health priorities with this age group of women:

- Benefits and risks of **hormone replacement therapy (HRT)**
- Early signs and symptoms of cardiovascular disease
- Benefits of monitoring and controlling cholesterol and blood pressure levels
- Maintaining bone strength and density
- Maintaining healthy weight
- Exercising regularly
- Benefits of regular mammograms and Pap smears
- Maintaining meaningful sexual relations with the partner

- Maintaining healthy eating habits and adjusting to the nutritional needs as they age

As women delay childbearing and then resort to advanced reproductive technology, more women may be having their first child during this late reproductive stage. Women may also be caring for their own parents during this time while building careers, putting even greater time and energy demands on themselves.

During this period of a woman's life, the ovaries begin to slow down and eventually cease production of estrogen. Because of this decrease in estrogen, women may experience symptoms such as hot flashes, vaginal dryness, or night sweats. All perimenopausal women should be counseled about the benefits and risks of HRT. HRT has been associated with greater risks for certain groups of women, and research continues to help nurses better inform all women about their choices during menopause. With declining estrogen levels, bones density decreases dramatically during and after menopause, resulting in greater risks for fractures and other complications. As estrogen levels drop, a decrease in high-density lipoprotein (HDL) cholesterol and an increase in low-density lipoprotein (LDL) cholesterol increase the risk of cardiovascular problems, such as myocardial infarction and CVA. Women may react differently to these menopausal physiological changes in the body, and nurses should consider individual risk factors, tolerance of symptoms, and comfort as women face a myriad of choices and options available to them during this period of change.

## ■■ CULTURAL CONNECTION

We black women must forgive black men for not protecting us against slavery, racism, white men, our confusion, their doubts. And black men must forgive black women for our own sometimes dubious choices, divided loyalties, and lack of belief in their possibilities. Only when our sons and our daughters know that forgiveness is real, existent, and that those who love them practice it, can they form bonds as men and women that really can save and change our community.

—Marita Golden

 Research Alert

Artificial insemination by donor (AID) is an option being selected by increasing numbers of single women who desire parenthood. Although AID has been reported to have positive outcomes for couples, there is a paucity of research about the experience of single women who choose this alternative, perhaps, because of cultural and social prohibitions. Thus, nurses who provide health care with this "emerging family" have little knowledge available related to the unique needs of these patients.

This case study can be utilized by nurses as more women choose alternative ways of becoming mothers. In this case, a 38 year old single female, well established in her career, delivered her first child, a son, from insemination. The baby is now 3 months old. The nursing theory of Man-Living-Health provided the framework to elicit, organize and analyze nursing care. Research questions were derived from the principles of this theory and focused on three areas: the processes of structuring and giving meaning in situations, developing and changing relationships and transcending or actualizing one's dreams and future goals. A fourth question focused specifically on the subject's perceptions of her health care and health needs. The researcher conducted an unstructured tape-recorded interview to collect data.

Themes emerging from date analysis suggested that valuing independence, making choices related to directing health decisions and assuming self-responsibility for outcomes of decisions were associated with the decision to have insemination. A period of relationship flux appeared to occur as the woman took on the maternal role. While there were some dramatic positive effects on the new mother's perspectives about her quality of like experience, themes of vulnerability and aloneness were also predominant.

Implications to promote optimal health and effective maternal role transition were identified, especially directed towards fostering the woman's sense of security and community. The need for the nurse to initiate immediate and anticipatory guidance was viewed as critical because the mother's intense feelings of self-responsibility could conflict with the desire to ask for support and guidance. Because the new mother was acutely aware of potential censure from others, a critical element of effective nursing care was the nurse's examination of his or her own moral/ethical values about insemination. Because of the growing numbers of women who are choosing to have children through AID, there is a significant need for further research to validate health needs in this population.

*Source*: Frank, D. (1987). *The health experience of a single woman having a child through artificial insemination by donar (AID)*. Presented at the 8th Annual Research Symposium, Gamma Zeta Chapter, Sigma Theta Tau, University of North Carolina, Greensboro.

During this time, a woman may reexamine her life, which may result in a new self-identity. Women must explore what aging means to them and go through an acceptance of what their life has been and what it may still become. Sexuality of women also changes during this time. Our society, with its focus on youth and sexuality, rarely acknowledges the sexuality of women as they age. Health professionals more often than not exclude sexuality in their assessment of women in the postmenopause years. Most women continue to have healthy sex drives and, when this consideration is included as an integral part of health assessment and care, maintain their interest in sexuality as they age. Research indicates that for many women, the post-reproductive years become better sexually once children and family obligations are less demanding. Many women view this time as the best years of their lives: Children are grown, careers are more stable, career changes are possible, and acceptance of self-identity is well established. For women who have devoted their younger years to childrearing, they may be returning to school, reentering the career market, or making career changes.

## ■ Mature (55 and Older)

As more women are reaching the mature stage of the life cycle, the community health nurse must realize that a shift of health emphasis from infectious and acute diseases to chronic diseases occurs in this age group. Because of the chronic nature of diseases in this age group, the historical definition of health (absence of disease) is less applicable. Rather, the emphasis should be placed on functional health, independence, and autonomy. Health promotion should be aimed at preserving the mature woman's ability to function at the highest spectrum of wellness. Health-promoting activities to enhance wellness are listed in Box 32-1. Career choices and lifestyle changes, such as dating after divorce or death of a spouse, bring both challenges and opportunities as women move into this new phase of their lives. Most women find the freedom of this period in their lives very exciting, as it is often filled with choices and opportunities not possible or considered when younger.

### ✎ NOTE THIS! ●──────────

- Nearly 500,000 women die of cardiovascular disease every year in the United States.

- Of the 435,000 who have heart attacks each year, 83,000 are younger than 65, with 9,000 younger than age 45.

- The typical warning signs of heart attack in women are not the same as those in men. Chest pain is number one in men; the most common warning signs in women include unusual fatigue, sleep disturbances, and shortness of breath.

- Chest pain is present in only 53% of women before a coronary event.

*Source*: McSweeney, J. C., Cody, M., O'Sullivan, P., Elberson, K., Moser, D. K., Garvin, B. J. (2003). Women's early warning symptoms of acute myocardial infarction. *Circulation*, *108*(21), 2619–2623.

Mature women deal with many health care issues as they age. Many of the issues and health conditions discussed in the previous section on menopausal women apply here as well. However, as women live longer, their chronic conditions may increase in severity. Depression, dementia, and **urinary incontinence** are some of the illnesses that occur later in life. Arthritis, osteoporosis, hypertension, and cardiovascular disease continue to be health concerns for women in this age group (Fogel & Woods, 1995).

Community health nurses often must deal with depression in mature women. Many may have outlived their spouses and are dealing with the loss daily. This depression often goes untreated. Many medications may also contribute to the depression. If dementia is present, safety considerations in the surrounding environment become essential. Urinary incontinence is seen twice as often in women than in men (Fogel & Woods, 1995). Nurses must also be aware of medications that may cause urinary retention or urinary incontinence, possibly leading to urinary tract infections.

**❝***Middle age is when a guy keeps turning off lights for economical rather than romantic reasons.* **❞**
—*Lillian Carter, RN, mother of former U.S. President Jimmy Carter*

---

###  GLOBAL CONNECTION

The idea of female circumcision is so horrifying that women cannot comprehend how widespread the practice is globally. It is common in Muslim Africa, Malaysia, and Indonesia. Some 100 to 200 million young girls have been circumcised in Egypt alone, where 97% of women are circumcised in the country (Boyle, Songora, & Foss, 2001). The most common victim of this practice is 4 to 8 years of age, and the procedure is done without anesthesia. Complications include shock, excessive bleeding, and chronic urinary tract infections.

In female circumcision, the clitoris (and often the labia) is removed, with only a small opening left for urination. The cut is opened wider when the woman is married (often by her husband) and for childbirth. After birth, the opening is once again sutured shut.

Why is this practice done? Factors associated with female circumcision include ensuring the woman is a virgin from birth to marriage, removing pleasure from sex to ensure faithfulness in the marriage, and enhancing "cleanliness." A common myth is that this act enhances the fertility of the woman. Mothers often support the practice because it makes a girl "more marriageable" (Boyle et al., 2001).

There is hope on the horizon, as the horror of female circumcision has become more widely known outside of these countries. Women across the globe have condemned the practice and led political action to stop it. Charges to eliminate the practice have come from the First Ladies of Burkina Faso, Guinea, Mali, and Nigeria, all of whom have publicly condemned the cultural practice of female mutilation (Boyle & Lacy, 2003; Marhra, 1981).

Do you think that the United States should intervene in other countries' cultural practices? Are there legitimate reasons to do so? ◉

**"** *When we were young, you made me blush, go hot and cold and turn to mush. I still feel all those things, 'tis true . . . but is it menopause or you?* **"**

—*Susan D. Anderson*

## Specific Disease Conditions of Women Throughout the Life Span

Cardiovascular disease is the largest single cause of mortality among women, accounting for 38% of all deaths among females in the United States. The most effective strategies for CVD disease reduction target the primary prevention level. In reality, almost all women are at risk for cardiovascular disease; consequently, women and their healthcare providers should consider the use of guidelines as part of routine visits and preventive health education. The public health impact of CVD in women is not solely related to mortality, as advances in science and medicine now allow many women to survive heart disease. For example, in the United States, 42.1 million (36.6%) women live with CVD, and the population at risk is even larger. Modifiable risk factors for such disease include cigarette smoking, hypertension, hypercholesterolemia, and physical inactivity, with less direct but still important risk factors being obesity, diabetes, stress, and menopause. The American Heart Association publishes *Guidelines for Preventing Cardiovascular Disease in Women,* which is updated annually based on current research about risk factors and CVD in women. The *Guidelines* provide research-based health information that should be used by women and their healthcare providers to reduce CVD risks throughout a woman's lifetime.

Community health nurses need to first become aware of the modifiable risk factors and then develop a cardiovascular health plan with an emphasis on prevention. When a woman seeks health care, either for herself or for a family member, the community health nurse should seize the opportunity to emphasize heart health. The relationship between estrogen and cardiovascular disease, along with cardiac risk factors, must be discussed and assessed. The use of medications in the home should be reinforced by client teaching, including when to take prescribed nitroglycerin and when to seek medical attention for chest pains. By empowering women with knowledge, nurses can help women employ appropriate prevention strategies in their lives, as well as seek health care early, should CVD become a health problem. By following preventive measures regarding heart health, women can improve their chances for living longer and enjoying a better quality of life.

### ■ Cancer

Cancer is the second leading cause of death in women in the United States. Lung cancer has surpassed breast cancer as the leading cause of cancer deaths in women. The most common types of cancer in women are lung, breast, colorectal, ovarian, and pancreatic. Tobacco is the single most toxic carcinogenic substance responsible for the occurrence of

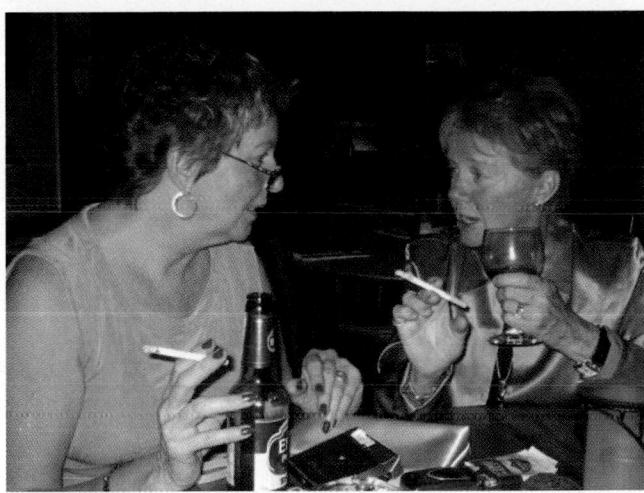

Women in high stress careers may be at greater risk for substance abuse although educated and better informed than previous years as to the problems associated with alcohol and smoking behaviors.

**"** *Cancer got me over unimportant fears, like growing old.* **"**
—*Olivia Newton John, 1998—actress, singer, and breast cancer survivor, who had a modified radical mastectomy to remove a cancerous tumor in July 1992*

lung cancer and has been linked to cancers of the mouth, pharynx, larynx, esophagus, pancreas, uterine cervix, kidney, and bladder. For this reason, smoking cessation programs for women who smoke need to be readily accessible.

Breast cancer is the second leading cause of cancer death in women overall and is the leading cause of cancer deaths in women aged 50 to 54. It is imperative that community health nurses educate women about breast self-examination (BSE), the signs and symptoms of breast cancer, and the need for age-appropriate mammography (American Cancer Society, 2008). If symptoms are detected, women must be educated that seeking health care is critical in the reduction of morbidity and mortality risks associated with breast cancer. When breast cancer is detected in the early stages (localized), the 5-year survival rate for women is more than 94%.

When a woman is receiving chemotherapy for cancer, the nurse should be aware of the side effects of this treatment and know what can be done in the home to decrease or alleviate symptoms of discomfort (e.g., nausea, vomiting, pain). Nurses must also be aware of local resources to ensure that women have prompt access to care as soon as a definite cancer diagnosis has been obtained, along with support groups and referral agencies for cancer victims. Reach to Recovery is the American Cancer Association's peer support program, which provides women with both individual and group support in the promotion of recovery from breast cancer.

### ■ Osteoporosis

Bone mass peaks at the end of the growth period, usually around age 17. Some small gains in bone mass occur up

## " a conversation with . . . "

**Deanna Favre, wife of Brett Favre, formerly quarterback of the NFL's Green Bay Packers; breast cancer survivor and activist**

Deanna Farve was diagnosed with breast cancer in 2004. She has become an activist in the fight against breast cancer and in raising the awareness about early detection.

"Brett was so supportive. He was a big shoulder for me to cry on. I'm not a crier; I never do that. And he would come in in the evening and I would be bawling and he didn't quite know what to do. But he was very sensitive and he listened and he just talked me through it," says Deanna.

"Chemo," she says, "was something I thought I would be ready for. I was going to work out, eat right, and be fine, get through it. I've always been strong. I don't depend on Brett emotionally. I've always done things myself and taken care of things myself. However, that first chemo really knocked me on my butt, and I realized there are something you can't prepare for. I was floored when I actually got my first statement from the chemo. This one little shot—Neulasta—to keep your white blood cells up—was $3500. Incredible. I was thinking about single moms because I was there. I had to work really hard for a long time, waiting tables to get through school. And I thought, 'What if I were not so fortunate? What if I were not so blessed?'"

Brett and Deanna helped established the Deanna Favre Hope Foundation to aid uninsured or underinsured women in need of breast cancer treatment. Deanna funds the Foundation, in part, through her speaking engagements and other fundraising activities.

As for Brett, he said, "All I know is that when you hear cancer, it sounds like a death sentence. It's treatable, but I still didn't want my wife to have it. I was worried sick for her safety. And for our girls [Brittany, 16, and Breleigh, 6], who could lose their mom and would run the risk of having it. Nothing positive went through my mind for a while."

What then could Brett do to show Deanna his support as she began her chemo and lost her hair? He had his head shaved by his Packers teammates!

For information about Deanna Favre's Hope Foundation, go to http://www.favrefoundationgear.com/.

*Source: Hattiesburg American, October 21, 2006.*

 **Research Alert**

This descriptive research study examined the effectiveness of exercise as an aid for smoking cessation in women. The sample was composed of 281 healthy but sedentary female smokers between the ages of 18 and 65 who had smoked routinely for at least 1 year. The subjects were followed in a 12-week smoking cessation program. Of the 134 women who exercised three times per week, 19.4% gave up smoking for at least 2 months after their program ended, compared with 10.2% of the 147 nonexercisers. Three months later, 16.4% of the exercisers were still not smoking, compared with 8.2% of the nonexercisers. One year after the study, the difference was 11.9% and 5.4%, respectively. The study provides evidence that vigorous exercise leads to improved rates of continuous abstinence from smoking in women.

*Source: Marcus, B., & Albrecht, A. (1999). The efficacy of exercise as an aid for smoking cessation in women. Archives of Internal Medicine, 159(11), 1229–1235.*

anterior rib pain, negatively changed body image, difficulty in fitting clothes, a protuberant abdomen, and abdominal discomfort (as a result of reduced lumbar vertebral height). Hip fractures occur twice as often in women older than 75 than in men and are associated with excess mortality of 5% to 20% as a result of preoperative and postoperative complications, such as deep vein thrombosis, pulmonary embolism, and pneumonia.

The community nurse must be aware of lifestyle changes that can help prevent osteoporosis, including calcium intake, weight control, and weight-bearing exercise, as well as hormone replacement therapy used to treat osteoporosis. Nurses can apply the osteoporosis profile (Table 32-3) to identify risk factors for women.

| **Table 32-3** Osteoporosis Risk-Factor Profile for Women |
| --- |
| ▪ 65 years or older |
| ▪ Family history of osteoporosis |
| ▪ Caucasian or Asian |
| ▪ Postmenopausal, especially premature |
| ▪ History of a traumatic fracture |
| ▪ Loss of 1 inch or more in height |
| ▪ Slender build |
| ▪ Estrogen deficiency |
| ▪ Sedentary lifestyle |
| ▪ Low calcium intake |
| ▪ Failure to achieve peak bone mass |
| ▪ Cigarette smoking |
| ▪ High alcohol consumption |
| ▪ Weight below normal |
| ▪ Steroid use |

to age 30; this is then followed by a progressive loss of bone mass. Osteoporosis is largely a disease affecting women, with 80% of females suffering from this preventable disorder. Osteoporosis is a major public health problem in the United States. Vertebral fractures generally occur in women 55 years and older, and result in back pain, height loss and kyphosis,

## BOX 32-3

**Cancer Support Groups**

American Cancer Society
1599 Clifton Rd. NE
Atlanta, GA 30329
800-ACS-2345

Candlelighters Childhood Cancer Foundation
1312 18th St. NW, 2nd Floor
Washington, DC 20036-1808
800-366-2223

National Alliance of Breast Cancer Organizations
1180 Avenue of the Americas, 2nd Floor
New York, NY 10036
212-719-0154

National Coalition for Cancer Survivorship
323 8th St. SW
Albuquerque, NM 87102
505-764-9956

SHARE: Self-Help for Women With Breast Cancer
19 W. 44th St.
New York, NY 10036
212-719-0364
hotline 212-382-2111

Y-ME National Organization for
Breast Cancer Information and Support
18220 Harwood Ave.
Homewood, IL 60430
800-221-2141
24-hour hotline 708-799-8228

### Research Alert

The American Heart Association's 2007 *Guidelines for Preventing Cardiovascular Disease in Women* emphasize the following points:

- Make lifestyle changes to help manage blood pressure, include weight control, increased physical activity, alcohol moderation, sodium restriction, and an emphasis on eating fresh fruits, vegetables, and low-fat dairy products.
- Cease of all tobacco use through counseling, nicotine replacement, or other forms of smoking cessation therapy.
- Physical activity recommendations for women who need to lose weight or who want to sustain weight loss include a minimum of 60 to 90 minutes of moderate-intensity activity (e.g., brisk walking) on most, and preferably all, days of the week.

- Reduce saturated fats intake to less than 7% of calories, if possible.
- Consume oily fish at least twice weekly, for omega-3 fatty acid intake; use a capsule supplement of 850 to 1,000 mg of EPA (eicosapentaenoic acid) and DHA (docosahexaenoic acid) in women with heart disease, and 2 to 4g for women with high triglycerides.
- Hormone replacement therapy and selective estrogen-receptor modulators (SERMs) are not recommended to prevent heart disease in women.
- Antioxidant supplements (such as vitamin E, vitamin C, and beta-carotene) should not be used for primary or secondary prevention of cardiovascular disease (CVD).
- Folic acid should not be used to prevent CVD.
- Routine low-dose aspirin therapy may be considered in women age 65 or older regardless of CVD risk status if benefits are likely to outweigh other risks.
- The upper dosage of aspirin for high-risk women is up to 325 mg per day.
- Reduce LDL cholesterol to less than 70 mg/dL in very high-risk women with heart disease, which may require a combination of cholesterol-lowering drugs.

*The 2007 Guidelines for Preventing Cardiovascular Disease in Women* are published by the American Heart Association and written by an expert panel of cardiovascular specialists and researchers. The *Guidelines* are updated based on new research findings and designed for use by women to reduce their cardiovascular risks. Emphasis in the latest version of the *Guidelines* is on the *lifetime* risk of women for CVD, and as such includes a new paradigm for risk assessment based on risk factors and family history. Women and health professionals focusing on the prevention of CVD should use the *Guidelines* over the life span.

The new *Guidelines* include expanded recommendations on lifestyle factors, such as physical activity, nutrition, and smoking cessation, as well as more in-depth recommendations on drug treatments for blood pressure and cholesterol control.

*Source*: Evidence-based guidelines for cardiovascular disease prevention in women: 2007 update. (February 20, 2007). *Circulation: The Official Journal of the American Heart Association*, 115, 7.

## Diversity and Women's Health

### Cultural Influences

Gender roles are greatly influenced by culture and affect where, when, and how women seek health information and advice. The impact of culture on women is imperative for the community health nurse to understand. An awareness of family dominance patterns is essential when teaching clients and communicating with family members about the specific health issues affecting women. Although many cultures are still largely patriarchal, matriarchal influences are also important. Acceptable ways of communicating and touching should be assessed by community health nurses and included in any interventions for the client. In some cultures, women may not speak unless they are given permission to do so by a spouse or father. In other cultures, the elder female in the household may speak for the entire family. Men and women interact with each other according to their cultural values. Community health nurses should always remain sensitive to a woman's cultural influences in the promotion of healthy interventions (Lipson, Dibble, & Minarik, 1996; Purnell & Paulanka, 1998). Guidelines for a cultural communication assessment appear in Box 32-4.

## ■ Sexual Orientation

As lesbianism has become more widely accepted, its effects on families and health care should be acknowledged by the community health nurse. Family structures are no longer made up only of the typical married couple with children. Gay and lesbian couples are more open in today's society and may live with other persons, including communal communities where responsibilities are shared, based on their common beliefs. Many lesbian women choose to adopt children or conceive a child through artificial insemination or heterosexual intercourse. Women whose sexual orientation is lesbian or bisexual still face discrimination and insensitivity in the health care system, where heterosexuality is still considered the norm. Health care providers may continue to employ narrow definitions of families and partners and often exhibit prejudice by ignoring the specific health care considerations of this population.

Lesbian women are more likely to neglect their own health care needs and avoid examinations by health care providers because of the stigma and humiliation that often accompany the disclosure of being a lesbian. They are more likely to reveal their identity to nurses and other healthcare providers who are open and nonjudgmental (Stevens, Tatum, & White, 1996). Lesbians are at low risk for vaginal infections, STDs, and HIV. In contrast, they are at higher risk for breast and uterine cancer than their heterosexual cohorts (Brandenburg, Matthews, Johnson, & Hughes, 2007; Dibble, Eliason, DeJoseph, & Chinn, 2008; Rosser, 1994). They also are more likely to experience stress and depression because of social isolation. Substance abuse has been reported in 30% of lesbian women, compared with 7% of the general female population (Roberts, 2006). **Heterosexism** and **homophobia** contribute to prejudice, fear, and continued discrimination against lesbians, which in turn places these women at higher risks for health problems.

The community health nurse should learn to communicate without bias with women of all sexual orientations. Lesbians are often insulted when health care workers assume they are heterosexual and ask gender-specific questions, such as "What form of birth control do you use?" Alternative questions should be phrased in the form of open-ended, nongender statements such as "Tell me about your sexual activity." The nurse should encourage lesbian women to have regular pelvic examinations and to avoid unprotected oral sex by using latex barriers (Zeidenstin, 1990). Mental health counseling and support networks are also options for dealing with troublesome psychosocial issues, such an addiction and depression.

## ■ Women and Aging

The elderly population will more than double by the year 2050, with the oldest old—those older than 85—the most rapidly growing segment in the United States (U.S. Census Bureau, 2003). These women are much more likely to be widowed, live alone, and live in poverty. Women belonging to racial and ethnic groups are in "quadruple jeopardy" because they are elderly, minority, female, and poor. Elderly women are also at greater risk than their younger counterparts for depression related to loneliness and isolating health conditions.

As women age, friendships become more important in promoting a sense of well-being.

**Old Ladies**

Hurrying, late again,
I rounded the corner too fast.
They were caught, frozen on one
frame of my mind's camera.
Two old ladies sitting on the porch swing
so near the narrow winding road
I could have touched them.
Both were white-haired and
comfortably padded,
both wearing red dresses,
turned to almost face each other,
both laughing, faces lined but serene.
Old ladies are sometimes poor,
sometimes stuck with raising children's
children. I know. But still
I think of those two old ladies
wearing red dresses, swinging and laughing.
A measure of wisdom and grace
and peace seem theirs.
Oh sure, they must peer into the dark tunnel
and see the train growing larger. And maybe
they lie alone in silent dark room. And maybe
wisdom and grace and peace
sometimes elude them.
But still
I hope I live to be an old lady
and wear red dresses
and sit in a porch swing
and laugh.

—Jeanne Ezell, 1993

Differences have been identified regarding why women are living longer, including differences related to gender, exposure to environmental hazards, health habits, personality styles, and reactions to illness. Men have traditionally held jobs that expose them to more hazardous environmental factors, such as asbestos and carcinogens. Women have traditionally smoked less and managed stress better. These differences are expected to narrow in the future as a result of changes in our society, equal rights for women, and greater participation of women in the workforce.

 **MEDIA MOMENT**

**The Turning Point, 1977**
This movie is about the friendship between two professional ballerinas who chose different paths. One becomes a world-renowned ballerina, while the other chooses homemaking and raising children. Their often-conflicted relationship surfaces when the daughter of the stay-at-home mom wins a role as a prima ballerina in the friend's dance company.

**Circle of Friends, 1995**
Set in Ireland in the 1950s, high school girls come of age in a small village.

**Soul Food, 1997**
Lives and family are the focus of this outstanding movie about the African American family.

**Woman Thou Art Loosed, 2004**
Based on the best-selling book, this movie follows the life of a woman in jail who meets weekly with a kind and forgiving minister.

**Thelma and Louise, 1991**
The classic women's freedom, take-to-the-highway movie. Thelma and Louise take off on a vacation road trip to escape their unsatisfactory relationships with their spouses and end up facing rape, committing murder, and engaging in crime. Ultimately, they are cornered by police. The ending alone is worth watching this movie.

**Extremities, 1986**
Farah Fawcett plays one of several roommates who face a rapist in their home. After an attempted rape, the women tie him up and torture him, which sets off a soul-wrenching ethical conflict among the women. This is the first movie of its kind—where the woman is not the victim, the man becomes the trapped and vulnerable rapist.

**Like Water for Chocolate, 1992**
A Mexican-produced movie, which combines food and passion effectively in a mystical setting where one daughter has exceptional powers regarding male and female interactions. This is a must-see film about the value of love and family.

**Places in the Heart, 1984**
This award-winning movie stars Sally Field as a struggling widow in a rural area, with her farm in danger of repossession. She enlists the help of two strangers to help her learn about farming and saving her home.

**Beaches, 1988**
Story about a long-time friendship and dealing with terminal cancer.

**Steel Magnolias, 1989**
The story follows older Southern women in a small town in Lousiana, where the daughter of one of the women has developed diabetes but decides to have a baby even with the risks. A story about the power of women's friendships.

**Crimes of the Heart, 1986**
Based on the Pulitzer Prize–winning play by Beth Henley, the movie is set in Mississippi and chronicles three sisters as they face the impending death of their father and the accusation of one sister of shooting her abusive husband. Racial issues and gender issues in the family are featured.

> *Freedom is what you do with what's been done to you.*
> —Jean-Paul Sartre

Because women generally outlive men, more women live alone or live in long-term care facilities. Women currently outnumber elderly men by 6 to 5 from age 65 to 69, and by 5 to 2 at ages older than 85 (U.S. Census Bureau, 2003). More families are opting to care for their elderly parents at home; however, women (especially Caucasian women) continue to make up a larger percentage in nursing homes, with 50% childless or having outlived their own children. The financial consequences for elderly women are of major concern. Elderly women often have saved little, because many grew up in a male-dominated era in which women did not manage their finances. The few resources that these women have must last for a longer period. Additionally, older women may have limited Social Security benefits owing to their lack of participation in the workforce. With rising healthcare costs, many elderly women rely on Medicare and Medicaid resources with fewer Social Security benefits of their own, due to limited contributions during their lifetime.

Elderly women often report they are disappointed with health care and their treatment by health care personnel. As the women age, they report that physicians often dismiss their complaints as compared with their male cohorts. An example of this phenomenon is often seen in women with cardiac conditions. Until recently, women have been largely ignored in cardiovascular research and have not had the benefits of the same interventions as men, such as early intervention and cardiac rehabilitation. Many elderly women report feeling disrespected and mistreated by their health care providers. Discrimination based on race and sexual orientation is also a concern. Elderly lesbian women are often discounted in healthcare practices, with their significant other being eliminated from major healthcare decisions. Elderly women may not have been socialized to deal with finances, and this lack of knowledge may place them at significant risk. Rural elderly women may also be disadvantaged because of the greater risks associated with their often low educational and socioeconomic status.

Community health nurses must acknowledge the diverse needs of elderly women. Health promotion should be encouraged, including sleeping, exercising, weight control, and diet. Nurses in the community should work with elderly women, listening to their needs and problems, and promoting autonomy as they age. The cultural prejudices against the elderly in the United States influence how women perceive themselves as they age, how they care for themselves, how they relate to health care providers, and ultimately how healthy they remain in their later years of life.

## ■ Global Issues and Women's Health

The **Commission on the Status of Women** was one of the first bodies established by the United Nations Economic and Social Council to monitor the situation of women and promote their rights in all societies around the world. The United Nations Fourth **World Conference on Women** was held in Beijing, China, in 1995. Ethical issues related to women were explored, and universal standards regarding equality between women and men were set. Women's concerns should be brought to the forefront with issues related

---

### Three of Us

Three of us
Talk among the simmering pots
And bubbling ham

Of gifts and debts
And years behind—ahead
Of pimples and diaper rash
And falling out of love

Of bombs and war
And Mary Kay

The posts boil over and we rush about
Finding ways to save the family dinner.
—*Ann Thedford Lanier*

---

### The Death of a Soft Snowflake

My friend Babs always reminded me of a soft snowflake, From her outward appearance to her inner core.

Her outward appearance was a soft one—her perpetual sweet smile, her blond hair, her radiant light complexioned skin, her preference for pastels.

Her inner core a caring one—for family, friends, and strangers; Never an unkind thought or word towards anyone.

It is hard to say what will be missed the most about my friend Babs, She was a wonderful loving daughter, wife, and mother; She was a true friend;

She was a tireless community worker.

The qualities that I will probably miss the most about my friend Babs will be her smiling face, and her authenticity.

It was almost unnerving to be in the company of someone as authentic as Babs—could she be real?

But it was genuine—the softness, the caring, the tenderness.

My heart is broken over the loss of my friend Babs. My heart is also broken for her family;

I know she had to be a sparkling light in their lives—a sparkling soft snowflake.

Our prayer for this family is for strength to go on without her, for thankfulness for having had Babs in their lives.

Please dear Lord, take care of Babs—our sparkling soft snowflake.
—*Judith A. Barton, PhD, RN*

GLOBAL CONNECTION

In 2004, a woman's life expectancy in the United States was 80 years, as compared to 85 years in Japan, 73 years in Saudi Arabia, 63 years in India, 53 years in Haiti, and 47 years in Ethiopia.

*Source*: Population Reference Bureau, 2004 world population data sheet.

to human rights. Mutilation of female body parts, prostitution for survival, and female child slavery are all considered culturally acceptable in some countries. Women must participate in the political arena and in decision making related to legislation to fully address these ethical concerns. Women should also have a role in the development of their countries, including in the realms of policy, employment, education, the economy, and the environment.

**I Planned It This Way**

I planned it this way, you know.
    I planned it to happen at the very height of Spring.
I loved the Spring.
    The time of rebirth, remember, this is a new beginning for me.

Bert loved the Spring too, you know.
    Remember our big garden?
Oh how I enjoyed our big garden, snapping the beans while
    sitting in the swing, Bert cooking pork chops on the
    grill, watermelon, ice cream . . .
Oh how I love my home and Bert, and my children, my family, my church, my community, all of you.

I liked to keep my house in order, you know.
    So I decided it was a good time for me to go home, back
    with Bert again,
    At the very height of Spring.

—*Judith Barton*

This poem is about an elderly woman's death. How do you interpret this poem's meaning concerning gender roles and culture?

## Special Issues Affecting Women's Health

### ■ Violence

Violence against women takes many forms, including physical and verbal assault, sexual assault, and homicide. Age has been identified as the most significant trait that puts women at risk for a violent attack: Younger women are more likely to be victims of abuse. The health consequences of vio-

lence against women are vast, including physical, psychological, and social effects. Societal consequences are more subtle, but are nonetheless damaging to women's sense of security and safety. More than 1.3 million physical or sexual assaults are committed by current or former partners each year in the United Sates. One in 4 women reports having been harmed by an intimate partner during her lifetime (Wiebe, 2003). On a personal level, violence touches 1 in 4 families and is responsible for more than 1 in 3 female murder victims (Tjaden & Thoennes, 2000). To put this in perspective, acts of violence in the United States kill as many women every 5 years as the total number of U.S. citizens killed in the Vietnam War. Violence is the single largest cause of injury to women in the United States—it is more common than automobile accidents and muggings combined. While evidence from research in the past 10 years reveals that 1 in 4 women will experience violence at some point in her life, health care providers rarely assess women as potential victims of violence, even when symptoms of abuse present as the primary complaint (Scholle, Buranosky, Hanusa, Ranieri, Dowd, & Valappil, 2003).

While abuse in a marriage or relationship is commonly assumed to involve men abusing women, sociologists for many years have found that men and women are about equally likely to attack each other. An important distinction that should be of concern to nurses, however, is that 85% of the injured parties are women (Goetting, 2001; *Statistical Abstract*, 2004). A primary reason for this discrepancy is that men are generally larger and stronger than women, putting women at a physical disadvantage in the relationship. Men are much more likely to use not only their strength, but also firearms, which leaves women more vulnerable to severe and often life-threatening injuries (Strauss, 1992).

Violence directed toward women is related to the sexist structure of our society. Because men are socialized with norms that encourage aggressive behavior and the use of violence, men who abuse often feel it is their right to control women. When the inevitable frustrations of life occur within a relationship—and sometimes as a result of events outside the couple's lives—male abusers may turn violent toward their partners. Equality between the sexes in the United States has certainly become more valued than in previous generations, yet we have made less progress in socializing males to handle frustration and disagreements without resorting to aggressive and violent behavior (Strauss, 1992).

**NOTE THIS!**
The National Resource Center on Homelessness and Mental Illness provides technical assistance and information about services and housing for the homeless and mentally ill population. It is sponsored by the Center for Mental Health Services, Substance Abuse and Mental Health Services Administration, and can be found at http://www.samhsa.gov

### Got an Alternative?

Naomi Judd, country music singer and registered nurse, contracted hepatitis when she was a nurse in an ICU. She has approached this chronic illness with a combination of traditional treatments and complementary interventions by seeking out consultation with Dr. Deepak Chopra, a leading researcher in mind–body healing.

Most of what they teach us in nursing school is like a mental enema. Let's separate the wheat from the chaff and start emphasizing nutrition, music, humor altruism, support system, faith, and an open belief system. We need to be freed of the useless, time-consuming, soul-draining stuff. When you combine psychology and spirituality, healing takes place. This is the mind–body connection. The mind controls the body and our bodies want to heal us. My motto these days is "Slow down, simplify, and be kind."

Your belief becomes your biology. For instance, if you're having a bad day and all of a sudden you realize that you're holding the winning lottery ticket, everything just completely changes. Unfortunately, data shows that 3 months later, you return to your prior emotional state. So the mind is the body's control tower, and it tells the body what hormones, neuropeptides and neurochemicals to secrete. The brain is like a drug store.

Naomi is the author of the book *Naomi's Breakthrough Guide: 20 Choices to Transform Your Life* (Simon and Schuster, 2004).

*Sources*: Siegler, B. (2004). Love built a bridge. *Better Nutrition*, 66, 10. Lee, M. (1994). Naomi Judd: One of country music's brightest stars is also a nurse living with a chronic illness. *American Journal of Nursing*, March, 40–45.

### NOTE THIS!

Emergency contraception (EC) is often confused by the public and health professionals alike. EC, which is commonly referred to as the "morning after" pill, is a form of backup birth control that can be taken up to a few days after intercourse and still prevent pregnancy. Approved by the FDA in 1999 for distribution by prescription, EC supporters believe that this contraceptive has enormous potential to reduce the rate of unintended pregnancies.

EC consists of a series of pills containing progestin, the same hormone found in daily oral contraceptives. It is not intended for use as a regular contraceptive method, but rather as a backup in the event of unprotected sex or contraceptive failure. EC does not affect an established pregnancy, nor is it a medical abortion drug like mifepristone or RU-486. Plan B, the most widely used form of EC, is a two-dose regimen that must be taken within days of unprotected sex to be effective.

EC prevents pregnancy by inhibiting or delaying ovulation or by preventing implantation of a fertilized egg in the uterus. It reduces the likelihood of pregnancy by 81% to 90% when taken within 72 hours of intercourse. There are no known serous side effects of EC, through approximately 23% of women report nausea and vomiting. Researchers estimate that widespread use of EC could potentially prevent as many as half of the approximately 3 million unintended pregnancies that occur annually in the United States and as many as 700,000 pregnancies that now result in abortion. In 2003, only 6% of women aged 18 to 49 reported ever using EC. A major factor in the lack of use of EC is confusion about the difference between EC and medical abortion medication, such as RU-486.

*Source*: *Women's health policy facts*. (2005). Henry J. Kaiser Family Foundation.

A common question asked about women in abusive relationships is "Why do women stay in abusive relationships?" Researchers have studied such issues for many years and have found some common characteristics of women who stay and those who leave a violent relationship. Goetting (2001) studied women who had left their abusive partners and provides insights into why other women stay. She found the following common characteristics among the women who had made ?? an abusive relationship: The women: had a positive self-concept and believed that they could "do better"; broke with traditional values about staying in a relationship "for better or worse"; found adequate finances; and had supportive friends and family who provided a social network that helped them "rescue" themselves. Conversely, women who tolerate abuse don't have good self-worth, believe in the duty of staying with a relationship at any cost, do not believe they can make it financially, and may lack a supportive network.

These findings are not all equally important in explaining why women stay or leave a destructive relationship, and they do not apply to all women. However, community health nurses should be aware of the possible barriers and solutions to assisting women who are victims of abuse. This includes assisting these women in improving their abilities to care for themselves, financially and emotionally, and affirming their right to living in a safe and healthy relationship. Safe houses for women and families can provide job and financial counseling, as well as a supportive network for helping them envision a new life outside of the abusive relationship. Although fewer studies have addressed lesbian relationships, abuse can and does occur in these partnerships as well (Gershick, 2002). Nurses should not consider the sexual orientation of the woman as either greater or lesser risk for abuse.

Community health nurses should be aware of "red flag" identifiers associated with domestic violence, such as women who (1) often have bruises on the limbs, torso, and face; (2) come to the clinic with vague symptoms of illness, such as pain in lower abdomen, chronic diarrhea, or pain of undetermined origin; (3) have trouble making eye contact; (4) have controlling partners; and (5) consistently wear sunglasses indoors. Because of the significant number of women at risk for abuse, community health nurses should assess every woman's relationship as part of their routine health assessments, regardless of the individual's sexual orientation. The stigma and fear associated with relationship abuse keep most women from expressing or admitting any information about this very serious "invisible" health problem in our society.

Community health nurses should be aware of local resources that can be accessed to assist women who find themselves in an abusive situation. National crisis lines such as the Domestic Violence Crisis Line and the Sexual Assault Crisis Line are accessible nationwide and safe houses are available in most cities throughout the United States.

 ## ETHICAL CONNECTION

### Stand by Your Man—But Keep a Gun Just in Case

As women have become more unwilling to tolerate abusive relationships and risky social situations, one of the more controversial outcomes has been the increase in the number of women who buy and use firearms. Current or former partners commit more than 1.5 million physical or sexual assaults against women each year in the United States. An intimate partner has harmed an estimated one in four women during their lifetime (Tjaden & Thoennes, 2000). Most of these women fail to press charges against the accused or even to report repeated attacks and harassment to proper authorities. Emergency room health care professionals are often faced with obvious physical and sexual abuse of women presenting for treatment, only to have the woman refuse to report her abuser's name or contact authorities. For women who do report such abuse, the legal system often puts her "on trial" and convictions, especially of present or former partners, are difficult to obtain.

In a study by Sorenson and Wiebe (2004), the researchers found that the common weapons used against and by women during a violent incident with a partner were words, hands/feet, household objects (e.g., telephones, pots, pans, dishes, ashtrays), kitchen knives, hammers, screwdrivers, and belts. A majority of the women had had a door slammed against their bodies or limbs and had been slammed against a door or wall.

Approximately one-third of the women interviewed had a firearm in the home. Previous research has linked firearm ownership with a greater potential for abuse in the family. The proportion of homes with a firearm in which abuse occurs is about 20% higher than in the general population (Lund, 2002; Smith & Martos, 2002). In two-thirds of these households, the partner eventually used the gun against the woman, usually threatening to shoot or kill her. The women in the Sorenson and Wiebe (2004) study expressed the need for partner/spousal notification regarding gun purchases by partners and stated that a personal firearm in the home creates greater risk for harm to them.

Implications for nurses include the assessment of household presence of firearms and experiences of women at risk for abuse concerning other forms of violence. The presence of firearms in the home poses an especially dangerous threat to women, given the lethality of guns. Firearms can also be used to intimidate or threaten a woman into doing something or allowing something to be done to her. Although physical harm may not result, emotional abuse occurs just the same. Further research in this area should go beyond gunshot wounds to the role of firearms in the home used to harass abuse and intimidate women.

### "Goodbye Earl"

In 2001, the Dixie Chicks released a song about a subject rarely broached in country music: spousal abuse. *Goodbye Earl* asked an age-old question about violent relationships: What does an abused wife (Mary Ann) do with a mean, unrepentant, and drunk partner (Earl) after all legal options have failed? The song, which was banned by many radio stations as being too controversial, presented an equally violent solution: Earl had to die, and the wife's best friend became her enthusiastic partner. In the song, Earl physically abused Mary Ann from the beginning of their marriage. When she reported his attacks, nothing changed: "He walked right through that restraining order and put her in intensive care." The two friends plotted the only permanent solution to Mary Ann's plight—they poisoned Earl's black-eyed peas, put him in the back of the car trunk, dumped his body, and reported him as a "missing person, that no one missed at all." The two get away with the murder and live happily ever after selling home-grown fruit on a roadside stand.

A similar country song that won numerous awards, *Independence Day* by Martina McBride, is about a young girl's account of her mother burning down their house after abuse from her alcoholic father. Both her mother and father are killed in the blaze. The song reflects an association with "freedom" and eliminating the problem through her mother's death. Again, lyrics reflect the community "looking the other way" even though the abuse was a widely known occurrence.

Women make up the fastest-growing demographic group in the United States who buy handguns. This fact has caught the attention of both pro- and anti-gun advocacy groups, because women have traditionally avoided the purchase or use of firearms. For a man to die at the hand of a woman (or women) has rarely been the subject of songs in any musical genre, whereas men killing their "cheating" women is common in songs. One such example is Jimi Hendrix's song *Hey Joe*, about a woman who is shot because of her philandering ways, and the immortal *Pretty Polly*, who also does not make it to the end of the song alive.

1. What are the ethical implications of a popular song, such as *Goodbye Earl*, when violence is presented as a solution to spousal abuse?

2. Can songs change the way we think about social problems, such as abuse?

3. Do you think such a song should be banned from the public, why or why not?

## ■ Homelessness

Homelessness is a growing problem in all urban and rural regions of the United States. Women and children continue to make up the fastest-growing segment of the homeless and, as such, are among the most vulnerable in this already hazardous environment. For women, many factors can lead to homelessness, including divorce, poverty, eroding work opportunities, decline in public assistance, domestic violence, substance abuse, and mental illness. Substance abuse often accompanies homelessness and increases the risk of homeless women engaging in prostitution and experiencing other health-related conditions such as HIV, STDs, tuberculosis, and malnutrition.

The community health nurse can assist homeless women and families through primary, secondary, and tertiary prevention interventions at individual, community, and national levels. The community health nurse may be a first-line defense for the homeless woman and her family. Maintaining a long-term relationship with this vulnerable group is perhaps the most challenging among all populations. Establishing trust is difficult because of sporadic and infrequent contact with these families, so the nurse must be creative and take immediate steps to provide safe and acceptable care at the time of contact. Knowledge about community resources

### 🖥 Research Alert

This research study of African American and Latina girls, among whom there is an especially high rate of sexually transmitted diseases (STDs), showed that role playing and practice applying condoms had a striking effect: The girls who received these interventions contracted fewer STDS within 12 months than did peers who had no such practice. The sample was composed of 700 sexually active African American and Latina girls ages 12 to 19 who were randomized into three groups: One group received information on STD and condom use, one group received information on STDs but no condom use practice, and a control group received general health information unrelated to sexual activity. Each subject participated in a 250-minute group session led by a trained facilitator. At the 12-month follow-up, girls in the practice and role-playing group reported fewer incidents of unprotected intercourse and intoxications. Only 1.0.5% of girls in the practice and role-playing group had infection with STDs, whereas 18.2% in the control group did. Although a limitation of the study was its reliance on self-reported data, other findings show that teaching such skills and helping girls become more self-reliant is a viable prevention strategy with this at-risk group.

*Source*: Jemmott, J. B., Jemmott, L. S., Braverman, P. K., & Fong, G. T. (2005). HIV/STD risk reduction interventions for African American and Latino adolescent girls at an adolescent medicine clinic: A randomized controlled trial. *Archives of Pediatrics & Adolescent Medicine, 159*(5), 440–449.

### 🖥 Research Alert

Women's increasing alcohol consumption has come under intense scrutiny from the British press. The coverage overall presents women who drink as problematic. Although feminist researchers have examined media constructions of gender, and although men's drinking has been the subject of critical analyses, there appears to be little feminist work on women's drinking per se. This is a significant omission, because gender representations related to eating, drinking, or sex tend to draw on conventional ideals of femininity and, as such, invite feminist deconstruction. It is also necessary for feminists working in this area to examine critically scientific thinking on women's drinking, as media constructions and everyday understandings will inevitably be distilled from mainstream psychological knowledge. ◢

*Source*: Day, K., Gough, B., & McFadden, M. (2004). Warning! Alcohol can seriously damage your feminine health. *Feminist Media Studies, 4*(2), 165–183.

is vital; the nurse can act as an advocate to assist the client through the "red tape" of the bureaucratic process.

Working with the community to prevent homelessness through policy changes should also be a priority for nurses who work with this vulnerable and often forgotten population. Nurses must work in the community by challenging government officials to examine the homeless problem and soliciting concerned citizens to develop shelters and programs for homeless individuals and families.

## ■ Incarceration

In the last 10 years, due to the decline in economic conditions and the crackdown on drugs and crime, the number of women in U.S. prisons has increased dramatically. The typical conviction of an incarcerated women is for property crimes—for example, check forgery and illegal credit card use. The increase in the female population in jails and prisons over the last 5 years is attributed to drug possession and abuse, often as a result of partner involvement. Women are increasingly more likely to be arrested for drug crimes, even though they may have been simply residing with a drug user or distributor. Single mothers account for 90% of women inmates. Poverty, age, race, and lack of education are primary risk factors for women in prison.

The majority of incarcerated women have a dependency on drugs and/or alcohol and have incomes at or below the poverty level. Given these lifestyle patterns, health care has often been neglected before incarceration. Many of these women have a host of chronic medical problems, such as tuberculosis, HIV, and other STDs. Historically, prison systems have not had enough resources to provide sufficient or appropriate health care for women.

Community health nurses need to be politically active and act as advocates for this hidden population of vulnerable women. The community health nurse should assume the role of client advocate in regard to child care and visitation while incarcerated. Parenting and childcare classes should be made available to the inmates. Programs that provide occupational training and that promote self-esteem and assertiveness have been linked with better outcomes for women who are released from prison.

### The Unplanned Gift

I hold my breath
My head up high
Now I breathe deep and smooth,
Straighten my shoulders

I hear your voice
    "Don't let them see you blink."

God I wish I could remember
What happened?
When I heard your voice
The first time?

Were you really there
Standing beside me?
Or was I so frightened
I conjured your spirit?

And your voice comes to me now
    "Do what you have to do
        and don't look back."

A wealth of wisdom in such simple phrases.

A wealth of strength when I have needed it.

There are times when such down-home guidance
Comes in handy,

There are times when I must stand and be a man.

What thing for a mother to teach
A Southern daughter!
—*Ann Thedford Lanier*

## Poverty

Poverty dramatically affects women's health. Women who are poor, sick, uninsured, or members of a racial minority are at particularly high risk for experiencing barriers in affording and accessing appropriate preventive care. Poor women have limited access to health care and preventive health care services, which results in delay of diagnosis of disease and injury, and consequently leads to shorter life

spans. For women in poverty, healthcare problems often exacerbate other existing challenges in their lives. Half of poor women and 38% of near-poor women (100–199% of poverty) report that they have delayed or did not get needed health care because of the cost.

Medicaid serves the poorest and sickest populations of women in the United States. Almost 1 in 4 women on Medicaid (23%) reports being turned away by a physician or health care provider who was not taking new patients or did not accept Medicaid (*Kaiser Women's Health Survey*, 2005).

Factors unique to women in regard to poverty include the following:

- Women are usually responsible for children, and many are single parents with no extended support.
- Women are not traditionally socialized to assume the breadwinner role and usually accept lower-paying jobs, often leading to a choice between public assistance and inadequate child care while they work.
- Health care is an expendable luxury when placed alongside child care, food, and lodging.
- Jobs women take may not have healthcare benefits comparable to the benefits associated with men's jobs.

Community health nurses need to be knowledgeable about local resources if they are to assist women who are poor to gain access to appropriate health care. Church-based programs and other community resources can provide community health nurses with excellent opportunities to both identify this vulnerable population and provide much-needed health interventions. Some local resources that are available in most areas include religious groups, county and state health departments, federal health clinics, United Way support, Medicaid, and the Social Security Administration.

## Workplace Health

Women represent half of the current workforce in the United States. Many factors have contributed to the increasing number of women in the workforce, including economic necessity, fewer children, changes in women's attitudes toward work, and changes in society. Women face a variety of concerns in the workplace, including reproductive risks, job stress, role conflict, sexual harassment, discrimination, and salary inequality.

Women account for the largest percentage of healthcare workers in the United States. Major occupational hazards for health care workers include biological, chemical, environmental, physical, and psychosocial hazards. All of these factors may influence a woman's physical and emotional/mental health at work, in the family, and in her community. The community health nurse in the occupational setting should address sensitive issues for women, including effects of cancer, reproductive problems (e.g., menstrual disorders,

*If I have to, I can do anything. I am strong, I am invincible. I am Woman.*

—Helen Reddy, 1972

### Research Alert

Eighty-nine percent of female veterans who served in the Vietnam War were nurses. Agent Orange, a toxin used in Vietnam to clear out dense vegetation and crops, is well known for its serious adverse health affects and role in cancer and Hodgkin's disease in men. Virtually no research had been conducted on the women who were exposed to Agent Orange. Dr. Linda Schwartz has studied this "forgotten population" and found that they are at great risk for increased cancer rates and miscarriages. Agent Orange was used to keep down weeds around the camps, and the empty containers often used to store supplies and as barbecue grills. Nurses handled the containers and were exposed to the toxin as well. The outcome of this study has been to influence policy in the Veterans Administration to compensate women for these damages.

*Source:* Trossman, S. (1999, May/June). RN explores Agent Orange's lasting effects on women vets. *American Nurse*, 24.

Women who remain active after retirement are generally healthier than more sedentary counterparts. This woman at 65 is on a five day dog sledding excursion in Alaska.

reduced fertility, genetic damage, spontaneous abortion, stillbirths), back problems, carpal tunnel syndrome, and sexual harassment issues (Fogel & Woods, 1995).

Occupations known to place women at a greater risk for health problems should be considered by nurses in the community when assessing personal health. Even though many factors affect health in the workplace, very little research has been conducted with regard to women and work. Instead, most research has been conducted with male workers, resulting in gender-biased findings. This bias has led to designs and practices in the work environment that may compromise the working woman's health and safety. Community health nurses must act as advocates for women in the workplace by promoting research specific to female workers and educating women about gender-specific risks associated with work.

## Toward the Future

### ■ Women's Ways of Knowing

Women must play a major role in their acquisition of knowledge to make informed health decisions. Historically, most women have not been as well educated as men in basic or health sciences. The way in which women have been educated directly influences their health knowledge. Poorly educated women may participate in the health care system in silence—afraid to ask questions, feeling inadequate, with minimal knowledge of their own health care. They may accept answers without question. They may not be able to understand the complex healthcare system or understand why they are expected to change from old patterns. Some distrust anyone of authority and reject science and medicine, relying on tradition or family influence.

As women become better educated through college, life and work experiences they learn **procedural knowledge,** including critical thinking and logical reasoning skills. Some women acquire **constructed knowledge** and are able to synthesize knowledge from many areas. The logic of women's ways of knowing is related to a degree to the lack of formal education for many women programs (Rosser, 1995). Education can play a key role in eliminating the subservient way women react to the healthcare industry. Community health nurses play a critical role in the education of women throughout the life span.

*When you don't like a thing, change it. If you can't change it, change the way you think about it and stop complaining and whining. Whining is not only graceless, it is hazardous—it can alert a bully a victim is in the neighborhood.*

—Maya Angelou

*For us who nurse, our nursing is a thing, which unless we are making progress every year, every month, every week, take my word for it, we are going back.*

—Florence Nightingale, Graduation address, St. Thomas School of Nursing, 1872

## ■ Feminism

The politics of women's health care issues have long been priorities of the feminist movement. Traditionally, few women have been invited to attend or participate in legislative forums related to women's health. Women have often been absent in the establishment of research priorities related to their health until recently. **Feminism** and the promotion of women's rights in society today are closely associated with the promotion of a national women's health agenda.

Feminist theory deals with gender by race and class, along with individuals, groups, and communities. There are many feminist theories, including liberal feminism, Marxist feminism, socialist feminism, African American feminism, lesbian separatist feminism, conservative feminism, existential feminism, psychoanalytic feminism, and radical femi-

> ❝ *Feminism's agenda is basic . . . that women be free to define themselves instead of having their identity defined for them by their culture and their men.* ❞
>
> —Susan Faludi

### ❝ *a conversation with . . .* ❞

> *I get accused a lot of talking too much, but if you don't tell people the problem, how can you expect them to solve it?*
>
> —Margie E. Richard

Retired schoolteacher Margie E. Richard became a local hero when she took on Shell petrochemical plants in her small community of Norco, Louisiana, upriver from New Orleans. Shell was the main employer in the community, which surrounded the African American community, and was illegally venting toxic chemicals from its plant. Richard convinced the petroleum giant to clean up its act and pay each homeowner in a four-block area surrounding the plant a minimum of $80,000 to buy a house elsewhere—an offer all homeowners accepted. She set up a Webcam to show the venting of chemicals, installed her own atmospheric monitors, and even traveled to Shell headquarters in the Netherlands to invite company executives to "take a whiff" of Norco's air for themselves. The end result—Shell agreed to invest more than $20 million in emission reduction and relocation, which was a historic victory for the "fence-line communities" living with energy industries.

Richard became the first African American to win the Goldman Environmental Prize in 2004.

*Source: AARP Magazine,* January/February 2006. "Margie Richards: Pollution Fighter."

### A Good Read

Gail Sheehy wrote the landmark book *Passages* in 1974 about the stages of continuing development of adulthood. More than 30 years later, as she reflected on the changes in women's lives:

> The incredible shrinking traditional family with a stay-at-home mom and breadwinner dad is down to only one-tenth of all American households. More and more contemporary women are choosing to remain single or to raise a child on their own. This dramatic demographic shift is driven only in part by women's desire for independent; their male contemporaries also have more choices, including prolonged bachelorhood or dual-income, childfree cohabitation.

*Source:* Sheehy, G. (2004). Passages redux. *More*, July/August, 62–65.

nism. Women's issues focus on economics, health care, and violence toward women. The correlation between the feminist movement and the political arena and the impact on women's health is obvious. Women must continue in their quest for a voice in health care policy and the implementation of policies that affect women (Rosser, 1995). Community health nurses can promote the feminist agenda through public policy activism and service on boards where women's health issues are concerned.

> ❝ *I myself have never been able to find out precisely what feminism is: I only know that people call me a feminist whenever I express sentiments that differentiate me from a door mat.* ❞
>
> —Rebecca West, 1913

### ■ Empowerment

**Empowerment** is based on the assumption that all people are created equal. Each person has the opportunity to recognize one's assets and develop from them on a professional, physical, spiritual, and emotional level. Recognizing and respecting the fact that all people have assets supports humility and dismisses the threat that others are better or more deserving. People feel powerful in themselves when they feel secure and safe. Community health nurses can be the "mirror" that reflects the woman's steps toward recognizing her own special assets. By affirming and reinforcing a woman's ability to recognize these assets, women can gain confidence to move forward in the search for security, well-being, and improved self-esteem.

One of the most empowering events for women was the formation of the **United Nations Platforms for Action for Women** with the purpose of challenging governments

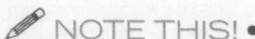 NOTE THIS!

Some medical historians say that the development of a foolproof contraceptive for women in 1960 influenced the role of women more than any single factor in the history of humankind. In 1950, the Planned Parenthood Federation provided funds to conduct research on the development of a safe, reliable oral contraceptive to a biologist, Gregory Pincus. Ten years later, the oral contraceptive, marketed under the name Enovid-10, was approved by the U.S. Food and Drug Administration. Within 2 years, 1.2 million women were taking it to control the size of their families. In 1999, 10 million women used an oral contraceptive. The "pill" was, indeed, revolutionary in changing lives, attitudes, values, and society for both women and men.

to raise the status of women. Global conferences are held on a regular basis and focus on the identification of commonly held beliefs about women's rights to health care, global health care needs of women and children, and proposed solutions for these identified problems. Some recent strategic objectives for women's health are listed in Box 32-5. A specific action plan was developed for achievement of each of the four objectives.

## ■ Health Care Policy

Policy makers in health care have historically ignored women's issues when developing health care policy. However, many policies were established in the last decade of the twentieth century that influence the health promotion and well-being of women.

The Women's Health Equity Act of 1990 identified the inequality of research into women's health issues and required that women and underrepresented racial and ethnic groups be included in research. At the same time, the National Institutes of Health established the Office of Research in Women's Health, based on the concept that women's research must expand from its traditional focus on women's reproductive systems to include all body systems and behavioral factors that influence women's health care. Recommendations for priority research for the next two

decades for women include health promotion and wellness, elimination of barriers to health care services, prevention of illness, health education, and recognition of differences among women. Box 32-6 identifies areas of research needed for women across the life span.

The Family Medical Leave Act of 1993 allows for 12 weeks of unpaid leave time from work for family or medical reasons. Employees are guaranteed the same job, pay, and benefits when they return to work after a leave. Because women are the primary family **caregivers** in the United States, this legislation is considered a major victory for working women with families.

Although women are the dominant caregivers in our society, policy development at the national level has been slow to formally recognize the "second shift" so many women work when caring for sick family members. Caring for family members has long been an expectation of women. In addition to working outside the home, women are required to care for children, spouses, and aging parents. Women often must give up their employment to care for family members, with loss of wages, employee benefits—health and retirement—and social support. Many women who lack health insurance, may not have adequate resources for health care. Owing to the extra stresses of caregiving, women may end

---

### BOX 32-5

**Strategic Objectives of the World Conference on Women**
- Increase women's access throughout the life span to appropriate, affordable, and quality health care, information, and related services
- Strengthen preventive programs that promote women's health
- Undertake gender-sensitive initiatives that address sexually transmitted diseases, HIV/AIDS, and sexual and reproductive health issues
- Increase resources and monitor follow-up for women's health

---

### BOX 32-6

**Research Areas for Women Across the Life Span**
- Adolescence:
  Prevention of accidents, suicide prevention, HIV, sexuality, alcohol, tobacco, diet and exercise
- Young adult/college:
  Low-birth-weight babies, pregnancies dangerously complicated by hypertension, ectopic pregnancies resulting in death, infertility, sexually transmitted diseases, cancer prevention (breast), safety (alcohol/drugs), health education, contraception, eating disorders, discomforts of pregnancy, obesity, HIV, family planning
- Midlife:
  Disease prevention (cancer, hypertension, stroke, heart disease), health promotion, health education, strengths of single-parent head of households, multiple role adaptation, obesity, influence of diet on osteoporosis, domestic violence, early detection of cancer, arthritis, pain
- Perimenopausal:
  Heart disease, health promotion, health education, impact of diet on osteoporosis, domestic violence, urinary incontinence, hormone replacement therapy, dietary influence on breast cancer, calcium and vitamin D supplements
- Mature:
  Coping with chronic illnesses and disability, urinary incontinence, depression, institutionalization, respite care, social and economic contributions to health status, older women and health policy, racial/cultural influences on health care, caregivers, cost-effectiveness of health care to elder women

## ❝*a conversation with . . .*❞

While the education of girls and women is obviously desirable for its own sake, it is especially crucial to lowering birthrates because of the different possible futures it opens up. . . . By opening the doors of education and social participation for the world's women and children, we can not only help our human family to a better life, but reduce our pressure on the planet as well.

—Carl Pope, Executive Director of the Sierra Club

*Source:* Pope, C. (1999). Solving the population problem: The key is to improve the lives of women. *Sierra Magazine, 84*(5), 14–15.

up divorced, with the additional loss of security from the employee benefits of their spouses (e.g., health insurance).

Health care policy for female caregivers should be promoted as a critical social need that benefits not only women but also society as a whole. Examples of policy issues related to unpaid caregiver responsibilities of women in their families include reimbursement and respite services. Changes in health care policy that relate to the challenges of female caregivers will serve to improve the quality of women's lives and the lives of their families and communities. These critical policy issues are not just about women, but affect the health of the entire nation.

Health behaviors of women are affected by the availability of health care resources and influenced by both education and income. Women get health insurance either through employment or marriage. Well-educated women are more likely to practice positive health-promotion activities such as healthy eating, exercising, not smoking, and drinking less alcohol (Fogel & Woods, 1995). Poverty and lack of education have a negative influence on health, however, often leading to stress, depression, and poor health-promotion habits. Usually, poor women wait until an acute episode to seek health care. Many may rely on home remedies or alternative interventions for health care. Inadequate health care access for women, especially the most vulnerable, results in needless personal suffering and economic losses for society.

Despite the reality that women are the major caregivers for families in the United States, they play a small role in public decision making regarding health care issues. Women have traditionally remained outside the circle of influence in the national political arena. This trend is changing, however, as more women become better educated and assume roles with greater power in their professional lives. More women are being elected to public office, as evidenced by the outcome of the 2006 elections. In that year, Representative Nancy Pelosi of California became the first woman in history to serve as Speaker of the House of Representatives. Women in the United States are entitled to equal health care, and community health nurses are in a position to lead the way toward a healthier future for all women.

 Research Alert

This research examined mental health and birth outcomes among women exposed to Hurricane Katrina. Data were collected prospectively from a cohort of 301 women from New Orleans, Louisiana. Pregnant women were interviewed about their experiences during the hurricane, and whether they had experienced symptoms of post-traumatic stress disorder (PTSD) or depression. High hurricane exposure was defined as having 3 or more of the 8 severe hurricane experiences, such as feeling that one's life was in danger, walking through floodwaters, or having a loved one die. Study results found that the frequency of low birth weight was higher in women with high hurricane exposure (14.0%) than women without high hurricane exposure (4.7%), with an adjusted odds ratio (aOR): 3.3; 95% confidence interval (CI): 1.13–9.89; $P < 0.01$. The frequency of preterm birth was higher in women with high hurricane exposure (14.0%) than women without high hurricane exposure (6.3%), with aOR: 2.3; 95% CI: 0.82–6.38; $P > 0.05$. Rather than a general exposure to disaster, exposure to specific severe disaster events and the intensity of the disaster experience may be better predictors of poor pregnancy outcomes. To prevent poor pregnancy outcomes during and after disasters, future disaster preparedness may need to include the planning of earlier evacuation of pregnant women to minimize their exposure to severe disaster events. ◐

Xiong, X., Harville, E., Mattison, D., Elkind-Hirsch, K., Pridjian, G., & Buekens, P. (2008). Exposure to Hurricane Katrina, post-traumatic stress disorder and birth outcomes. *The American Journal of the Medical Sciences, 336*(2), 111–115.

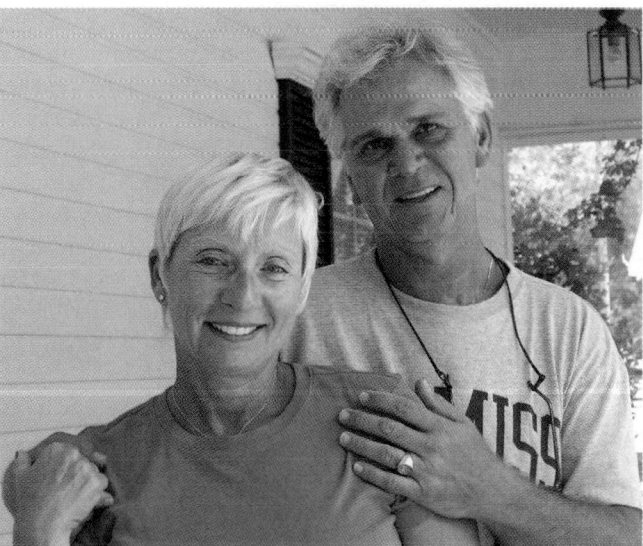

Healthy relationships are characterized by open communication, a sense of humor, and truly liking one's mate.

### Application to Practice

Frances Benton is a 68-year-old widow who has recently been referred to your community health clinic by Rachel Jackson, a concerned neighbor. According to Ms. Jackson, Mrs. Benton's husband died about 8 months ago. Mr. Benton had been Mrs. Benton's caretaker. The couple did not have children, and there are no close relatives. Mrs. Benton had fallen and sustained a hip fracture approximately 1 year ago, and she recently cracked a vertebra. She has begun to have lapses of memory and has lost her way home from the grocery store. Two days ago, Mrs. Benton was out in the yard with only her slip on, which is definitely out of character according to Ms. Jackson. The landlord stopped by several times to collect the rent but could not get Mrs. Benton to understand that she had not paid it in 3 months. He had spoken with Ms. Jackson and was planning to evict Mrs. Benton.

1. What are your nursing diagnoses in this situation?
2. Which secondary and tertiary preventive measures might be appropriate in working with Mrs. Benton?
3. Which community resources could you collaborate with to address the health risks for Mrs. Benton?

## Conclusion

Community health nurses are invaluable in assisting women with health care needs in the community. They should be knowledgeable regarding the various health concerns that women face, such as violence, homelessness, incarceration, poverty, and health conditions such as osteoporosis and cancer, and they must be able to define these women's needs. Community health nurses should be aware of the local resources that are available and be skilled in linking these resources with clients and their communities. Finally, they should be able to evaluate the process, fill in the gaps, and provide continuity of care for the individual client and the community as a whole.

Explore Community Health Nursing on the Web! To learn more about the topics in this chapter, use the passcode provided to access your exclusive website: **http://nursing.jbpub.com/communityhealth.** If you do not have a passcode, you can obtain one at this site.

## ■ CRITICAL THINKING ACTIVITIES

1. You are a rural community health nurse working on a mobile van visiting a large migrant community at a local farm. Selena King, a 16-year-old Hispanic female, comes into the van to have her blood pressure checked because she has been feeling tired and nauseated lately and is having difficulty working in the fields. She is also complaining of a coin-shaped rash on her arms, palms, and trunk. In completing your history, you find that she has not had any medical care since she was 8, when she had her appendix removed in Florida. Her blood pressure is 100/68 mm Hg. Selena cannot remember when her last menstrual period was, but she thinks it was 2 months ago. She is sexually active and uses condoms occasionally. She lives with her mother, four sisters, two brothers, and her father (who has forbidden her to see her boyfriend, Juan) in a travel trailer that they pull from town to town.
   - What are your nursing diagnoses in this situation?
   - How would you address the two dimensions of secondary prevention (diagnosis and treatment) of pregnancy and secondary syphilis?
   - Which secondary and tertiary preventive measures might be appropriate in working with Selena?
   - Which resources could you as a community nurse tap to assist Selena?

2. Mrs. Wise, a 67-year-old woman, is being discharged from the hospital after having surgery to repair a broken hip and bilateral wrist fractures. She will have bilateral casts for 8 weeks. Mrs. Wise is a widow and has two sons who live within 2 miles of her. She lives alone. Her daughters-in-law will be the main caretakers. Both daughters-in-law work outside the home, neither has had any medical training, and both are afraid of assuming the health care of their mother-in-law. Mrs. Wise is reluctant to move in with her sons and would rather return to her small townhouse. The discharge diagnosis includes hip and wrist repair as a result of osteoporosis, diabetes, hypertension, and obesity.
   - What are your nursing diagnoses in this situation?
   - How would you address considerations of competence, time management, and supervision in planning the care of Mrs. Wise?

- Which resources could you as a community nurse use to assist this family in caring for Mrs. Wise and at the same time address Mrs. Wise's concerns regarding her independence?
3. Empowerment of women may well be seen in a depiction of the Hindu goddess Sarasvati (sa-RAS-vah-tee). The goddess of knowledge, she is credited with the creation of the fruits of civilization, arts, and music. Her color and brightness represent the powerful, pure light of education, which destroys the darkness of ignorance. Sarasvati is depicted with four arms, showing that her power extends in all directions. In one of her hands, she holds a book (representing learning) and in another a strand of beads (representing spiritual knowledge). In the other hands, she holds and plays the vina, an Indian lute, representing the art of music (Waldherr, 1996).

- How does this depiction reflect our society's view of women in the United States today?
- Is education encouraged in women?
- What is spirituality, and how is it seen in our society? How is it seen in Sarasvati?
- What does music represent to Sarasvati or to the women of many other cultures and diversities?
- What is the darkness of ignorance?

## ■ REFERENCES

Agency for Healthcare Research and Quality. (2005). *Selected findings on child and adolescent health care: From the 2004 national healthcare quality disparities reports.* Retrieved September 3, 2008, from http://www.ahrq.gov/qual/nhqrchild/nhqrchild.htm

Albelda, R., & Tilly, C. (1997). *Glass ceilings and bottomless pits: Women's work, women's poverty.* Cambridge, MA: South End Press.

American Cancer Society. (2008). *All about breast cancer.* Retrieved November 11, 2008, from http://www.cancer.org/docroot/CRI/CRI_2x.asp?sitearea=&dt=5

Bell, M. R., Grill, G. E., Garrett, K. N., Berger, P., Gersh, B. J., & Holmes D. R. Jr. (1995). Long-term outcome of women compared with men after successful coronary angioplasty. *Circulation, 91,* 2876–2881.

Boyle, E. H., Songora, F., & Foss, G. (2001). International discourse and local politics: Anti-female-genital-cutting laws in Egypt, Tanzania and the United States. *Social Problems, 48*(4), 524–544.

Brandenburg, D., Matthews, A., Johnson, T., & Hughes, T. (2007). Breast cancer risk and screening: A comparison of lesbian and heterosexual women. *Women & Health, 45*(4), 109–130.

Centers for Disease Control and Prevention (CDC). (2004). *Total births and percentage of births with selected demographic characteristics.* Retrieved November 5, 2008, from http://www.cdc.gov/nchs/data/hestat/prelimbirth04_tables.pdf

Centers for Disease Control and Prevention (CDC). (2006). *HPV Vaccine recommendations.* Retrieved November 5, 2008, from http://www.cdc.gov/STD/hpv/STDFact-HPV-vaccine-hcp.htm#vaccrec

Centers for Disease Control and Prevention (CDC). (2008). Youth risk behavior surveillance—United States, 2007. *MMWR: Morbidity and Mortality Weekly Report, 57*(SS-4), 1–136.

Clarke, R. D. (2000). Has the glass ceiling really been shattered? *Black Enterprise, 30*(7), 145–158.

Dibble, S., Eliason, M., DeJoseph, J., & Chinn, P. (2008). Sexual issues in special populations: Lesbian and gay individuals. *Seminars in Oncology Nursing, 24*(2), 127–130.

Dujan, D., & Withorn, A. (1996). *For crying out loud: Women's poverty in the United States.* Cambridge, MA: Southend Press.

Felton, L. A., Gumm, A. & Pittenger, D. J. (2001). The recipients of unwanted sexual encounters among college students. *College Student Journal, 35*(1), 135–143.

Fogel, C., & Woods, N. (1995). *Women's health care: A comprehensive handbook.* Thousand Oaks, CA: Sage Ps.

Goetting, A. (2001). *Getting out: Life stories of women who left abusive men.* New York: Columbia University Press.

*Kaiser women's health survey.* (2005). Henry J. Kaiser Family Foundation.

Lipson, J., Dibble, S., & Minarik, P. (1996). *Culture and nursing care: A pocket guide.* San Francisco: UCSF Nursing Press.

Lund, L. E. (2002). *Incidence of non-fatal intimate partner violence against women in California, 1998–1999.* Sacramento, CA: California Department of Health Services, Epidemiology for Prevention and Injury Control Branch, Report No. 4.

Marhran, N. (1981). Medical dangers of female circumcision. *International Planned Parenthood Association Medical Bulletin, 2,* 1–2.

Purnell, L., & Paulanka, B. (1998). *Transcultural health care: A culturally competent approach.* Philadelphia: F. A. Davis.

Roberts, S. (2006). Healthcare recommendations for lesbian women. *JOGNN: Journal of Obstetric, Gynecologic, & Neonatal Nursing, 35*(5), 583–591.

Rosser, S. (1995). *Women's health—missing from U.S. medicine.* Bloomington, IN: Indiana University Press.

Scholle, S. H., Buranosky, R., Hanusa, B. H., Ranieri, L., Dowd, K., & Valappil, B. (2003). Routine screening for intimate partner violence in an obstetrics and gynecology clinic. *American Journal of Public Health, 93*(7), 1070–1073.

Smith, R. W., & Martos, L. (1999). *Attitudes towards and experience with guns: A state level perspective.* Chicago, IL: National Opinion Research Center.

Sorenson, S. B., & Wiebe, D. J. (2004). Weapons in the lives of battered women. *American Journal of Public Health, 94*(8), 1412–1417.

*Statistical abstract of the United States: The national data book.* (2000, 2003, 2004). Washington, DC: U.S. Government Printing Office. Published annually.

Stevens, P., Tatum, N., & White, J. (1996). Optimal care for lesbian patients. *Patient Care, 30*(5), 121–134.

Strauss, M. A. (1992). Explaining family violence. In J. M. Henslin (Ed.), *Marriage and family in a changing society* (4th ed., pp. 344–356). New York: Free Press.

Tjaden, P., & Thoennes, N. (2000). *Full report of the prevalence, incidence and consequences of violence against women.* Washington, DC: U.S. Department of Justice, Office of Justice Program, National Institute of Justice. Publication NCJ 183781.

U.S. Census Bureau. (2003). *National Center for Health Statistics: National vital statistics reports.* Washington, DC: U.S. Government Printing Office.

U.S. Department of Education. (2007). *Secretary Spelling's Remarks at UNESCO General Conference Plenary Debate in Paris, France.* Retrieved November 11, 2008, from http://www.ed.gov/news/speeches/2007/10/10182007.html

Waldherr, K. (1996). *The book of goddesses.* Hillsboro, OR: Beyond Words.

Wiebe, J. (2003). Firearms in the home as a risk factor for homicide and suicide: A national case-control study. *Annals of Emergency Medicine, 4,* 771–782.

World Health Organization. (2002). *Ultraviolet radiation: Global solar UV index.* Retrieved September 3, 2008, from http://www.who.int/mediacentre/factsheets/fs271/en/

Zeidenstein, L. (1990). Gynecological and childbearing needs of lesbians. *Journal of Nurse Midwifery, 35,* 10–18.

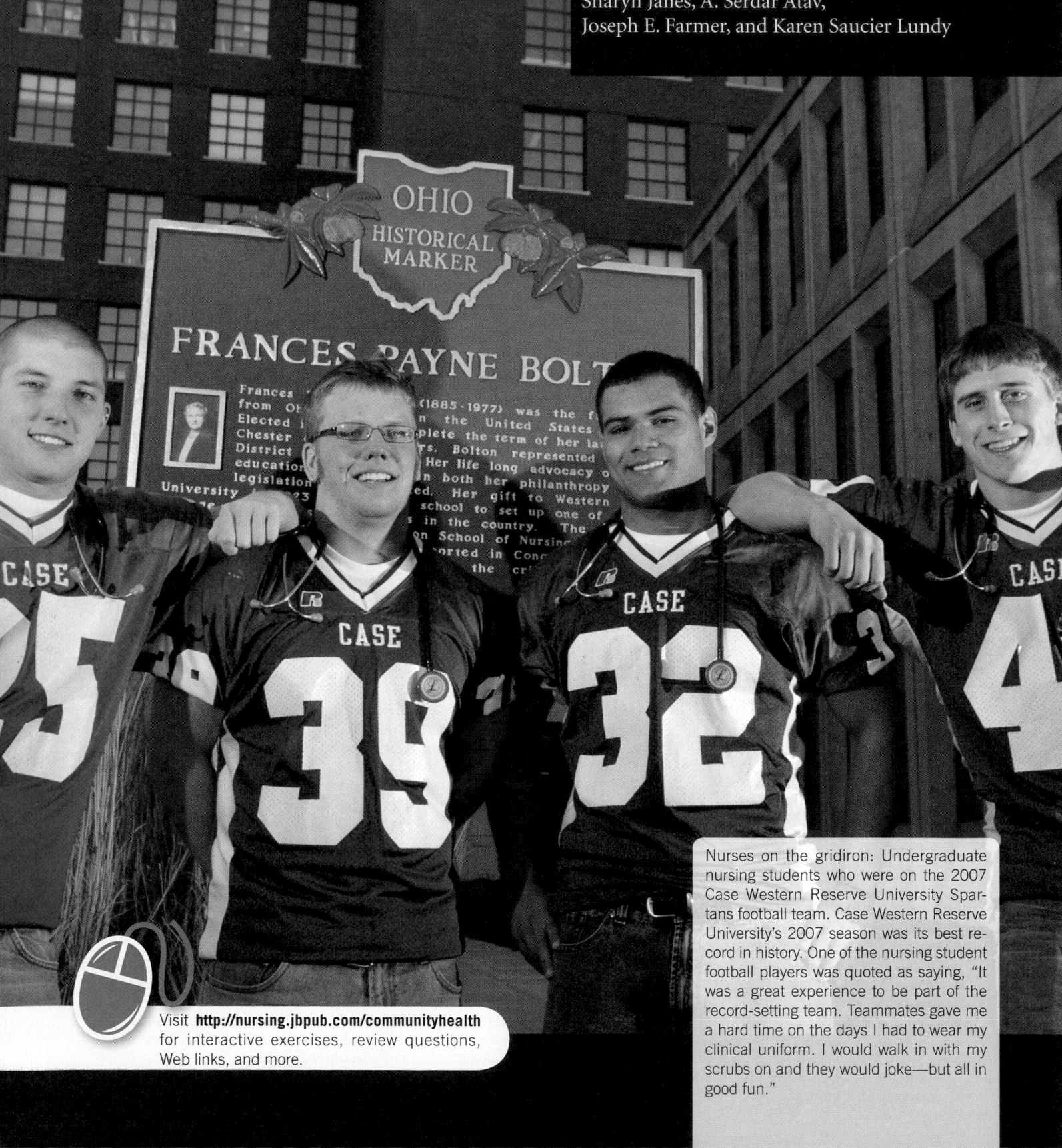

Sharyn Janes, A. Serdar Atav,
Joseph E. Farmer, and Karen Saucier Lundy

OHIO
HISTORICAL
MARKER

FRANCES PAYNE BOLT

Frances ... (1885-1977) was the f...
from Oh... ... n the United States
Elected ... plete the term of her la...
Chester ... rs. Bolton represented ...
District ... Her life long advocacy o...
education ... n both her philanthropy ...
legislation ... ed. Her gift to Western ...
University ... 23 school to set up one of ...
... s in the country. The ...
... n School of Nursin...
... orted in Conc...
... the cri...

Visit **http://nursing.jbpub.com/communityhealth** for interactive exercises, review questions, Web links, and more.

Nurses on the gridiron: Undergraduate nursing students who were on the 2007 Case Western Reserve University Spartans football team. Case Western Reserve University's 2007 season was its best record in history. One of the nursing student football players was quoted as saying, "It was a great experience to be part of the record-setting team. Teammates gave me a hard time on the days I had to wear my clinical uniform. I would walk in with my scrubs on and they would joke—but all in good fun."

Historically, most research studies have been based on male subjects. In many Western cultures, years of a predominantly male workforce have resulted in health care systems and policies being established by men. Despite this dominance of men in health care systems, women still have longer life expectancies than men.

It has been said that the most dangerous substance on earth is testosterone. What do you think? How do biology, gender, and culture affect the health of men?

Gender matters. Men and women have different death rates from the same diseases. Most men have shorter life spans than women, particularly among minorities. What are your stereotypes of men and how they differ from women? How do these images affect nursing care? This chapter will explore the specific threats to men's health based on physiological, social, and cultural differences.

## CHAPTER FOCUS

**Men's Health**
- Genetic Factors
- Sociocultural and Ethnic Factors
- Environmental Factors
- Behavioral Factors
- *Healthy People 2010*

**Health Care System Utilization**
- Ambulatory Care
- Hospital Care
- Preventive Care

**Specific Male Health Issues**
- Prostate Cancer
- Testicular Cancer

- Erectile Dysfunction (Impotence)
- Cardiovascular Disease

**Selected At-Risk Populations**
- Men with HIV/AIDS
- Homosexual Men and Families

**Community Health Nursing Roles**
- Patient Advocate
- Educator
- Facilitator

**Men's Health Research Issues**

***Healthy People 2010:* Objectives Related to Men's Health**

## QUESTIONS TO CONSIDER

After reading this chapter, you will know the answers to the following questions:

1. What are some of the major factors affecting men's health?
2. How are risk factors for illness or injury different for men compared with women?
3. How does the threat of testicular and prostate cancer affect the lives of young and middle-aged men?
4. What is the nurse's role in the treatment of erectile dysfunction?
5. What are some roles for the community health nurse in the promotion of men's health?

## KEY TERMS

| | | | |
|---|---|---|---|
| Erectile dysfunction | Health status | Socialization process | Viagra |
| Fertility | Homosexuality | Stress | Violence |
| Gender differences | | | |

As a nursing student, you have most likely had a course in women's health. What you most likely have *not* had is a specific course on men's health. The male gender has been neglected as the "other half" of the human population. Especially today, men are most likely to be in need of health care. When you hold clinics in community-based settings, it is unlikely that you will have seen many men in waiting rooms where primary health and prevention health services were provided. Whether through media campaigns or in focused efforts by health professionals, few health efforts have been directed toward men. Poor men and men of color are even more at risk in a society that rewards wealth and career success, particularly for men. Men typically die earlier than women, have fewer contacts with the health care system as compared to women, and have the highest risks for most diseases such as heart disease and cancer, and for accidents, including those associated with violent behavior. More than women, many men focus more intensely on work and providing for their families on a daily basis, and do not see health as a priority.

This chapter focuses on men's health, the risks that men face, and the role of the community health nurse in making the well-being of men a priority.

## Men's Health

Women live longer than men. Men are many times more likely to die of lung cancer, motor vehicle accidents, cirrhosis of the liver, heart disease, and acquired immune deficiency syndrome (AIDS) than women. Suicide rates are three times higher for men. **Gender differences** in health are genetic, sociocultural, environmental, and behavioral factors (Harrisson, Chin, & Ficarotto, 1992).

### ■ Genetic Factors

Genetic factors related to gender influence a man's physiological and psychological well-being. According to the genetic approach, some gender differences are natural in origin. They are driven by instinctual, hormonal, structural, or neurological characteristics of the male gender (Blekham et al., 2008; Galdas, Cheater, & Marshall, 2005; Sabo & Gordon, 1995). For example, gender differences in ischemic heart disease mortality may be a result of the protective effects of female sex hormones and men's tendency to accumulate fat in the upper abdomen (Courtenay, 2000b; Fackelmann, 1998; Waldron, 1995). Higher levels of testosterone contribute to men's predisposition to **violence.** Some of the other physiological differences between men and women include the following (Tanne, 1997):

- Men's brain cells die faster than women's as they age.
- There are structural differences between men and women in the mitral valve, which separates the left atrium of the heart from the left ventricle.
- Women's hearts beat more rapidly than men's hearts.
- Men have weaker immune systems than women.
- Men and women often react differently to medications, therapies, and diagnostics.

 **Research Alert**

A study used a qualitative research design to assess 70 stay-at-home fathers in Canada. The research explored the ways that work and family interact for fathers who "trade cash for care." While fathers are at home, they also remain connected to traditionally masculine sources of identity such as paid work and take on unpaid masculine self-provisioning work at home and community work that builds on traditional male interests. In this way, they carve out complex sets of relationships between home, paid and unpaid work, community work, and their own sense of masculinity. Narratives from stay-at-home fathers speak volumes about the ways in which the long shadow of hegemonic masculinity hangs over them, while also hinting at resistance and change as fathers begin to critique concepts of "male time" and market capitalism approaches to work and care. The research study offers theoretical contributions to research on fatherhood and masculinity in society.

*Source:* Doucet, A. (2004) "It's almost like I have a job, but I don't get paid": Fathers at home reconfiguring work, care, and masculinity. *Fathering: A Journal of Theory, Research, & Practice about Men as Fathers,* 2(3), 277–304.

### ■ Sociocultural and Ethnic Factors

In many cultures, particularly Western cultures, the male **socialization process** has emphasized traits such as the following (Torres, 1998):

- Assertiveness
- Preoccupation with achievement and success (individualism, status, aggression, toughness, and winning)
- Restricted emotionality and affectionate behavior
- Concerns about power and control
- Fear and bias related to **homosexuality**

As a result, most males tend to conform to these stereotyped gender expectations and behaviors, leading to definite health consequences. Some men may experience and endure more trauma because of their belief that taking physical risks is a sign of masculinity. Boys are socialized into competitive games at an early age and learn to endure physical punishment as part of having fun or as a prerequisite to becoming a man (Charles & Walters, 2008; Courtenay, 2000b; Stillion, 1995; Williams, 2008). From Little League on, a boy is told to "act like a man." Hence, to admit to having pain or some other health problem may be seen as a reflection of weakness. This male denial factor is pervasive and not related to occupation, age, race, or socioeconomic status. High death rates from coronary heart disease for men in the United States may be due in part to these stereotyped gender expectations, which increase the risk of the disease (Charles & Walters, 2008; Glassner, 1992; Harrisson et al., 1992; Men's Health Network, 2008; Pease, 1997).

THINK ABOUT THIS

**President Bill Clinton and Heart Surgery: Did He Ignore the Early Warnings of a Pending Heart Attack?**

Former president Bill Clinton was hospitalized in 2004 and had successful coronary bypass surgery immediately. He had complained of shortness of breath and chest pain, and drove himself to the hospital.

Physicians were alarmed enough to insist that Clinton, 58, undergo bypass surgery with minimal delay at Manhattan's New York–Presbyterian Hospital.

In a call from the hospital to CNN's *Larry King Live*, Clinton said: "I guess I'm a little scared, but not much. I'm looking forward to it. I want to get back; I want to see what it's like to run five miles again.

"My blockage is so substantial, I think if I don't do this, there's virtually a 100% chance that I'll have a heart attack," he said.

Clinton's health scare took most of the nation by surprise for a man who had been declared in good health after years of intensive annual physicals in his White House years and afterwards

The former president, though he has labored against a tendency toward chubbiness, has been particularly fit over the years after the presidency. He has lifted weights and uses an elliptical trainer and has lost weight using a modified version of the South Beach Diet. However, he told CNN last night that he had regained 10 pounds during a tour promoting his memoir, *My Life*.

Clinton has a family history of heart disease and a history of eating fast-food meals. "Some of this is genetic, and I may have done some damage in those years when I was too careless about what I ate," the former president said.

Clinton has described himself as a child as "fat, uncool, and hardly popular with the girls." His grandmother was 5 feet tall and 180 pounds, and one of her main goals in life was to get people to eat. "When I was little, it was generally believed that a fat baby was a healthy baby."

Heart bypass surgeries are performed when one or more of the arteries feeding the heart are blocked or choked off by buildups of fatty plaque—high cholesterol levels are the leading culprit. The chest pains that brought Clinton into the hospital appear to have developed abruptly, but the root causes of the problem are likely to be several years old: During his last physical before he left the White House, Clinton had a total cholesterol count of 233 and a "bad" cholesterol count of 177. Clinton acknowledged he needed "to keep my cholesterol down, keep my blood pressure down." The American Heart Association recommends that total cholesterol should be below 200.

Men often ignore the early signs of heart failure. President Clinton admitted that he had experienced a few symptoms in the past, but he thought it was reflux. This is a common misconception about heart disease because of the overlap of the symptoms. The two conditions are very different, even with similar symptoms. Men who experience symptoms of reflux should have a complete workup to rule out heart disease.

*Sources:* Harris, J. F., & Vedantam, S. (September 4, 2004). *Washington Post*, p. A01; A look at heart disease. (September 11, 2004), *CNN House Call with Dr. Sanjay Gupta.*

The lack of healthy emotional channels for men contributes to higher risks among men for suicide, heart disease, accidents, and violence. The traditional male socialization process has historically emphasized restricted emotionality and affectionate behavior. This traditional male gender role is inconsistent with the provision and receipt of social support, particularly emotional support that includes expressiveness and disclosure. Such characteristics may have adverse health consequences (Galdas, Cheater, & Marshall, 2005). The lack of expressiveness becomes especially significant in the way men deal with **stress** and depression. Most men tend not to cry and try to keep emotions hidden (Williams, 2008). They are far less likely to seek psychological counseling than are women. Along with other cultural messages that men need to be strong, powerful, and independent, men are taught not to react to physical, psychological, or spiritual pain. Some men are unwilling to seek health care simply because they fear the risk of appearing "unmanly" or the exposure of their sense of vulnerability (Charles & Walters, 2008; Harrisson et al., 1992; Will, 1998).

**"***I think we have a national crisis of boys in America. For some boys who are not allowed tears, they will cry with their fists or they will cry with bullets.***"**

—Dr. William Pollack, psychologist, Harvard Medical School

### ENVIRONMENTAL CONNECTION

Men are more vulnerable to accidents due to their risk-taking behavior. How does the environment in which we live affect the choices we make about health? For example, in rural areas, four-wheeler accidents occur almost exclusively among men. Compared to their female counterparts, teenage boys in the United States remain at higher risk for death from automobile accidents and acts of violence, most notably in urban environments. How does the environment affect these outcomes?

The sociocultural differences between men and women must be considered when planning and developing intervention and prevention programs. Strategies that target the general population may not consider the diversity of expectations and behaviors of men. Although some publicly funded programs may attempt to target as many people as possible, programs with more specifically focused segments or populations may be more effective with men. The nurse must consider the vast number of socialization possibilities that exist within male societies (Isenhart & Silvermith, 1994). This gender difference in regard to socialization also extends to nursing. The media image of a nurse as female has often been cited in research as a deterrent in the recruitment of males in nursing. Health interventions directed toward men may be more effective when men are separated from women, divided into age-specific groups, or grouped into a larger audience. For example, instead of a smoking cessation program for all people, with an emphasis on the long-term effects of smoking, a program targeting men ages 15 to 25, with an emphasis on the sex appeal of nonsmokers, may be more effective.

■ Environmental Factors

Physical and occupational environments affect the **health status** of men. More men are employed than women, and male-dominated occupations such as mining, construction, and farming are often more hazardous. Accidents on the job are a major contributor to higher death rates among men. In addition, men in these types of occupations are more likely to be exposed to carcinogens and other toxins that are associated with higher rates of pneumoconiosis (black lung), asbestosis, leukemia, and cancer of the bladder. Men's greater exposure to occupational hazards account for about 5% to 10% of the gender difference in mortality (Hudak & Hagan, 2002; Parker, 2002; Roman & Carroll, 2003; Miniclier, 2002; Waldron, 1995).

The high number of men in high-risk employment settings may be advantageous to community health nurses, who can use these environments to introduce men to health care. Prevention and screening programs in the workplace can be effective interventions for men who would not seek health care in traditional settings. Recent West Virginia coal mining accidents have exposed the public to the often invisible, yet hazardous work of men. Fire fighters, especially those involved in the September 11, 2001, terrorist attacks, have suffered extraordinary health consequences (Delsohn, 1996; Hauser & Sokol, 2008; Poppius, Virkkunen, Hakama, & Tenkanen, 2008).

■ Behavioral Factors

Unlike genetic factors, behaviors such as diet, tobacco use, alcohol consumption, illicit drug use, lack of physical exercise, physical and sexual risk taking, and suicide and violence are controllable and subject to human influence and intervention. Individuals can make wiser choices such as wearing seatbelts; exercising and eating right; not using tobacco, drugs, or alcohol, or at least not driving while under the influence of alcohol or drugs; not bungee jumping; or not committing acts of violence against themselves or others (Courtenay, 2000c; Harrisson et al., 1992; Steenbergh, Whelan, Meyers, Klesges, & DeBon, 2008). Partly as a result of the cultural expectations of society and the gender socialization process, men's behavior is consistently less healthy than that of women. As a result, behavior is the cause of the largest differences in mortality between men and women (Courtenay, 2000a; Galdas et al., 2005; Stillion, 1995; Stoltenberg, Batien, & Birgenheir, 2008).

Data in the United States indicate that men's diets have had higher ratios of saturated to polyunsaturated fat, which contribute to higher ischemic heart disease mortality among men (Power & Schulkin, 2008). More males than females smoke cigarettes and drink heavily. Men's smoking habits account for as much as 90% of gender differences in cancer mortality and roughly one-third of gender differences in ischemic heart disease mortality. Similarly, men's drinking contributes to higher mortality in liver disease, accidents, suicide, and homicide (Courtenay, 2000a; Galdas et al., 2005; Stoltenberg et al., 2008; Waldron, 1995).

**Diet**

Obesity and consumption of fatty foods increase the risk of cardiovascular disease, which is a major killer for men. Men consume a large amount of fatty foods and are

---

■■ CULTURAL CONNECTION

Antonio Villaraigosa is the first Hispanic mayor of Los Angeles since 1872. He was elected to the office on May 17, 2005.

Born Antonio Villar in the Boyle Heights neighborhood of Los Angeles' east side of Mexican American parentage, Villaraigosa had a troubled childhood. He added his wife's surname, Raigosa, after he married Corina Raigosa and, combining their names, changed his name from Villar to Villaraigosa.

Although he dropped out of high school, Villaraigosa received an honorary degree from Theodore Roosevelt High School. He was a gang member but eventually shook off that lifestyle and went on to attend East Los Angeles College and the University of California at Los Angeles (UCLA). While at UCLA, he was active in MEChA, a student-based civil rights organization. He obtained his degree in history, and then attended the People's College of Law, an unaccredited law school. After failing the bar four times, he moved on to labor.

As early as fifteen years old, Villaraigosa had been volunteering with the farm workers movement. He has been active in labor, the American Civil Liberties Union, and the American Federation of Government Employees. He has also campaigned for smaller school districts, sought more funding for the homeless, and is an advocate for the environment.

Los Angeles is the second largest city in the United States, with a population 3.7 million. The city is plagued by school violence, racial and ethnic tensions, and poverty. Approximately 40% of people in Los Angeles are foreign born, according to the U.S. Census. Nearly half of the population is Hispanic, 11% is black, and 11% is Asian.

The Academy Award–winning *Crash,* which was released in 2005, is about the brutal ethnic and racial tensions in Los Angeles.

I was born here. I raised my family here. I've always said to my children that we're all going to make mistakes in our lives. We'll be defined not by our mistakes but what we did to overcome them.

—Antonio Villaraigosa, May 2005

Young males are likely to be involved in risk-taking behavior. However, as role model Leonardo DiCaprio and friends demonstrate, risk can be decreased through the use of protective gear.

less likely than women to change their eating habits, even though more than 33% of men meet the definition of obesity (a body mass index [BMI] of 27.8 kg/m²). Researchers suggest that low-fat diet programs for men should target work site and peer-group organizations and include meal modifications with all family members (Coakley, Rimm, Colditz, Kawachi, & Willett, 1998; Nguyen, Otis, & Potvin, 1996; Power & Schulkin, 2008).

### Tobacco

Gender differences in smoking prevalence have been decreasing for decades, but still more males than females smoke cigarettes. Smoking is positively correlated with men's higher mortality from bronchitis, emphysema, and asthma.

Men, especially rural men, are more likely to use smokeless (chewing) tobacco. Despite the general declining trends in the use of cigarettes, there has not been a concomitant decline in the use of smokeless tobacco. Smokeless tobacco use is associated with higher risks of cardiovascular disease and cancers of the oral cavity, as well as gum recession and nicotine addiction. Heavy marketing efforts by tobacco companies toward rural men might explain the slight increase in the use of smokeless tobacco (Dutta & Boyd, 2007; Hede, 2007; Nelson, Tomar, Mowery, & Siegel, 1996).

### Alcohol and Drug Use

Alcohol abuse is well known for its devastating effects on physical and emotional health. More men drink than women, and men are five times more likely to drink heavily. Higher numbers of male drinkers contribute to males' higher mortality, related to chronic liver disease, cirrhosis of the liver, accidents, and homicide. In addition, male drivers have substantially higher risk of fatal motor vehicle accidents because they are more likely to have high blood alcohol levels when driving and are also more likely to exhibit riskier driving behaviors (Gough & Gareth, 1998; Gefou-Madianou, 1992; Poppius et al., 2008; Stoltenberg et al., 2008; Thornton, 2004; Waldron, 1995).

Alcohol use must be taken into consideration in developing strategies to prevent the transmission of sexually transmitted diseases (STDs), including human immunodeficiency virus (HIV), because alcohol consumption is related to risky sexual behavior. A number of studies have suggested that people who drink more heavily are more likely to have multiple partners, and among young men, consistent use of condoms decreases at higher levels of alcohol use (Graves, 1995; Isenhart & Silversmith, 1994). It is estimated that two-thirds of all alcoholics are men; more than 80% of those who have serious drug addictions are men; more than 80% of those who die of drug abuse are men; and 90% of those arrested for alcohol or drug abuse are men (Thornton, 2004).

### Suicide and Violence

Deaths by suicide and violence are a predominantly male phenomenon. Approximately four of five deaths by suicide are men. Between the ages of 20 and 24 men are six times more likely to commit suicide than women; and over the age of 85, men are more than 11 times more likely to kill themselves than women (Men's Health Network, 2008). Suicide rates for specific groups of men, such as veterans, divorced men, and homosexual teenagers, are even higher. Researchers argue that men's higher suicide rates are due to men's greater frequency of substance abuse, subjection to more stress, lack of emotional channels, and use of more violent, lethal means of taking their lives in comparison with women (Femquist, 2001; Williams, 2008).

The world of men is much more violent than that of women. White men are three times more likely to die in a homicide than white women; and African American men are

### Research Alert

In this study, risk factors for college male sexual aggression that were both theoretically and empirically based were tested using multivariate regression analyses. These risk factors included substance abuse patterns, pornography consumption, negative gender-based attitudes, and child sexual abuse experiences. Regression analyses indicated that some gender attitudes, pornography use, and alcohol abuse were significant predictors of perpetration of sexual violence. Although a number of men were sexually abused as children, this risk factor did not predict sexual aggression as an adult. Many men reported alcohol-related sexual coercion and held many rape-supportive attitudes and beliefs. These practices by college men contribute to the pro-rape cultures found on many campuses. Strategies are needed to identify and intervene with high-risk men to prevent sexual victimization of women in college.

*Source*: Carr, J., & VanDeusen, K. M. (2004) Risk factors for male sexual aggression on college campuses. *Journal of Family Violence,* 19(5), 279–90.

## HEALTHY PEOPLE 2010

### Objectives Related to Men's Health

**Cancer**

3.2   Reduce the lung cancer death rate.

3.7   Reduce the prostate cancer death rate.

3.10  Increase the proportion of physicians and dentists who counsel their at-risk patients about tobacco use cessation, physical activity, and cancer screening.

**Family Planning**

9.6   Increase male involvement in pregnancy prevention and family planning efforts.

**Heart Disease and Stroke**

*Heart Disease*

12.1  Reduce coronary heart disease deaths.

*Stroke*

12.7  Reduce stroke deaths.

*Blood Pressure*

12.8  Reduce the proportion of adults with high blood pressure.

**HIV/AIDS**

13.2  Reduce the number of new AIDS cases among adolescents and adult men who have sex with men.

13.3  Reduce the number of new AIDS cases among females and males who inject drugs.

13.4  Reduce the number of new AIDS cases among adolescent and adult men who have sex with men and inject drugs.

**Injury and Violence Prevention**

*Unintentional Injury Prevention*

15.15  Reduce deaths caused by motor vehicle crashes.

15.21  Increase the proportion of motorcyclists using helmets.

15.22  Increase use of helmets by bicyclists.

*Violence and Abuse Prevention*

15.32  Reduce homicides.

15.33  Reduce physical fighting among adolescents.

15.34  Reduce weapon carrying by adolescents on school property.

**Mental Health and Mental Disorders**

*Mental Health Status Improvement*

18.1  Reduce the suicide rate.

**Occupational Safety and Health**

20.1  Reduce deaths from work-related injuries.

**Substance Abuse**

*Adverse Consequences of Substance Use and Abuse*

26.1  Reduce deaths and injuries caused by alcohol- and drug-related motor vehicle crashes.

26.2  Reduce drug-induced deaths.

*Substance Use and Abuse*

26.12  Reduce average annual alcohol consumption.

26.13  Reduce steroid use among adolescents.

**Tobacco Use**

*Tobacco Use in Population Groups*

27.1  Reduce tobacco use by adults.

27.2  Reduce tobacco use by adolescents.

*Source*: DHHS, 2000.

---

five times more likely to die in a homicide than black women (Black & Breiding, 2008; Stillion, 1995). The persons at greatest risk for violence victimization, as well as becoming the perpetrators of violence, are young males who are members of underrepresented ethnic groups and live in poor urban communities. These young men risk injury to themselves, disrupted personal lives, damaging criminal records, extended imprisonment, and in some cases, capital punishment.

Much of the violent actions of men are directed at women. In the United States female murder victims are most often killed by their husbands, boyfriends, other male family members, or close male friends (Carr & Van Deusen, 2004; Gerlock, 1997; Glassner, 1992; National Center for Health Statistics, 2002). Violence against women will not cease until greater emphasis is put on prevention, treatment, and rehabilitation programs for the men who perform the violent acts. The nursing literature that addresses the issue of working with men who batter women and children is almost nonexistent, yet nurses who work in hospitals and community settings deal with the results of domestic violence every

day. Because nurses are on the front line, they are in the best position to intervene in ways that are sensitive to both the perpetrators and the victims of family violence. Nurses working in settings such as schools, churches, and work sites can conduct education programs to promote awareness of the potential for and prevention of family violence (Carr & Van Deusen, 2004; Goldstein, Chesir-Teran, & McFaul, 2008; Greenwood et al., 2002; Rynerson & Fishel, 1998).

### ■ *Healthy People 2010*

The purpose of *Healthy People 2010* is to improve the health of Americans with specific objectives in many health-related areas. Although men are not specifically listed as a

 THINK ABOUT THIS

Men are more likely to speed, drive aggressively, fail to wear seat belts, and drive drunk (Thornton, 2004).

Research Alert

**Osteoporosis: Not Just a Woman's Disease—2 Million American Men Have Osteoporosis, and Another 12 Million Are at Risk**

Osteoporosis . . . isn't that a woman's disease? While it is true that more women than men have been diagnosed with osteoporosis, men have no "immunity" to osteoporosis. Some of the factors that contribute to the gender differences in bone density are:

1. Men usually have larger bones than women do.
2. The life expectancy for men in the United States is shorter than that of women. One of the factors in the development of osteoporosis is age-related loss of bone density. Women live long enough to be diagnosed with osteoporosis.
3. Bone density is affected by estrogen and testosterone. Decreases in estrogen usually occur in the late forth or early fifth decade of life for women, while testosterone decreases in the fifth or sixth decade. Another variable that affects women is surgical menopause; many women in the United States have lost the bone-protective effects of estrogen earlier than age 50. There are very few medical indications for male castration, so men do not suffer from surgical andropause!

**The bad news for men is:**

Even though there are fewer cases of osteoporosis in men, and fewer osteoporotic fractures in men, the chance of dying from an osteoporotic fracture are higher for a man than for a woman! Men, such as the Pope and former President Ronald Reagan, suffered from osteoporosis-related complications, which contributed to their deaths.

**The good news for men is:**

1. Even at the same bone mineral density level, men generally do not fracture at the same rate as women.
2. Effective treatments are available.

**Risk factors for men include:**

1. Alcohol use of more than two drinks per day
2. Use of corticosteroids for diseases such as asthma, Addison's disease, and Crohn's Disease
3. Advanced age (70 years or more)
4. Use of anticonvulsants (such as Dilantin)
5. Use of thyroid supplements (such as Synthroid)

Recommendations for slowing progress in osteoporosis, according to the National Osteoporosis Foundation (2008), include:

- 1200 mg of calcium per day for adults 50 and older
- 800–1,000 I.U. of vitamin $D_3$ per day for adults 50 and older
- Fortified dairy products are among the best food sources of calcium and vitamin D.
- For those concerned with fat and cholesterol counts, reducing fat content does not adversely affect calcium and vitamin D content of dairy products.
- Exposure of the forearms to sunlight for 15 minutes three of four times a week is recommended to stimulate the production of vitamin D.
- In addition to calcium and vitamin D intake, weight-bearing exercise is known to be protective for bones. Walking for 20 minutes three to four times a week will help maintain bone mass.

—Dr. Cynthia Luther, ANP
Assistant Professor
The University of Southern Mississippi
School of Nursing

Source: National Osteoporosis Foundation. (2008). *Clinician's guide to prevention and treatment of osteoporosis*. Washington, DC: Author.

targeted group, several objectives do focus on either racial or ethnic groups of men. Selected objectives are listed in the *Healthy People 2010* box.

## Healthcare System Utilization

Patterns of health care utilization by men are cited as an important contributor to the inferior health status of men. One-third of American men do not have a checkup every year. Men visit doctors 25% less often than women. At the same time, men account for the majority of the patients admitted to emergency rooms (Courtenay, 2000a, 2000b). Men tend to have fewer contacts with the healthcare system, perhaps as a result of psychological and sociological factors such as a reluctance to admit that they need assistance. This situation is exacerbated by the fact that the U.S. health care system tends to focus on health from an illness perspective, with relatively little attention paid to prevention. As a result, unlike women who have annual gynecological examinations that include screening for other conditions, men are less likely to enter the healthcare system for a physical examination on a routine basis. Moreover, although men come in contact with many health care professionals in a wide variety of settings, they have no specialist to whom they can go for their specific care needs. Men have to be to attended by generalists, such as family practitioners, or by other specialists such as urologists who also see women. There is a growing national movement to create men's health as a medical and nursing specialty, a long overlooked but necessary change in improving the health of men (Treadwell & Ro, 2003).

Strategies to improve men's utilization of preventive health care must target all ages. Men must establish a committed relationship with preventive health care as early as possible. For men to use preventive health care, programs

**A Good Read**

## It's Hard to Be a Man These Days

*Doris Lessing*

At the beginning of the twenty-first century, it is difficult to avoid the conclusion that men are in serious trouble. Throughout the world, developed and developing, antisocial behavior is essentially male. Violence, sexual abuse of children, illicit drug use, alcohol misuse, gambling—all are overwhelmingly male activities. The courts and prisons bulge with men. When it comes to aggression, delinquent behavior, risk taking, and social mayhem, men win gold.

With a big dollop of generalization, male angst can be reduced to three grievances. Men have been emasculated by the loss of traditional functions, women have not; women have choices, men do not; men are emotionally illiterate, women are not.

Men, goes the first complaint, have been robbed of their traditional roles as providers, protectors, and even procreators. The heavy muscular jobs—building ships, digging coal, banging metal—from which men derived an assertive, productive masculinity have disappeared. They have been replaced by jobs that favor nimble fingers, flexible minds, and ready smiles: answering telephones, assembling computers, scanning bar codes. Not only have women snapped up these jobs, but also such occupations seem unmanly. For this predicament, blame whatever best fits your prejudices. Have newly assertive women, freed by contraception to postpone childbearing for careers, and liberated from material dependence on men, undermined contemporary manhood? Alternatively, has the shift from a blue-collar to a white-collar economy placed demands on all workers for "feminine" qualities such as flexibility, an ability to cope with uncertainty, and no expectation of power?

Men, it seems, cannot win. They are the new guilty and the new victims. Worse, increasingly beset by self-doubt, men are confronted with the breezy self-confidence of independent young women as depicted in popular culture. Take *Sex and the City*, a TV series about the sexual conquests of single New York women. On the other hand, Renault's "Size matters," a commercial for a motor car narrated by a mocking woman wielding a tape measure. Or *The Simpsons*, a cartoon family of feckless men and savvy women.

Worse, an accompanying cult of physical perfection—pectoral body-sculpting, plastic surgery, penile implants, Viagra—has taken root, too, celebrated in men's fitness magazines. "No wonder men are in such agony," writes Ms. Faludi. "Not only are they losing the society they were once essential to, they are 'gaining' the very world women so recently shucked off as demeaning and dehumanizing."

Unsurprisingly, male health, too, is under stress. According to a recent British government report, men are more likely than women to commit suicide, suffer from coronary heart disease, have a serious accident or drink too much alcohol. Male sperm counts, too, are declining. Dr. Clare, [a] British psychiatrist, says that his patients used to be middle-aged women whose children had left home. Today, they are "middle-aged men, who gave their lives loyally to this company or that corporation, who sacrificed everything for it, now ruthlessly put out to grass, compulsorily retired, downsized, rendered redundant."

Doris Lessing is a noted feminist. After reading Lessing's essay, do you think men are becoming the discriminated-against gender?

*Source*: Lessing, D. (2001). Sometimes it's hard to be a man, *Economist*, *361*(8523), 32–35.

that present health prevention as masculine and strengthening must be developed and implemented. The required school physical before participation in extracurricular activities may be used in the resocialization of men for the active and lifelong usage of preventive health care.

### ■ Ambulatory Care

Men have significantly lower rates of visits to ambulatory care settings, such as physician offices and outpatient services, than women, but the visit rates to hospital emergency departments do not differ by gender. By age 75, men have approximately half of the contacts with health care providers compared to women. This discrepancy persists even when the contribution of pregnancy and birth

control–related issues is not counted in women's contacts. The patterns in provider contacts indicate that, for all ages, the difference between men and women has been increasing. Although the total number of health care provider contacts is lower for men, men are seen more frequently than women for chronic diseases, such as heart and lung disease, which are more prevalent among men (Galdas et al., 2005; Harrisson et al., 1992; Pattison, 1998).

### ■ Hospital Care

Hospitalization rates and length of stays in hospitals vary by gender. Hospital discharge rates, the numbers used to determine usage, from short-stay hospitals are higher for women than for men (Galdas et al., 2005; Harrisson et

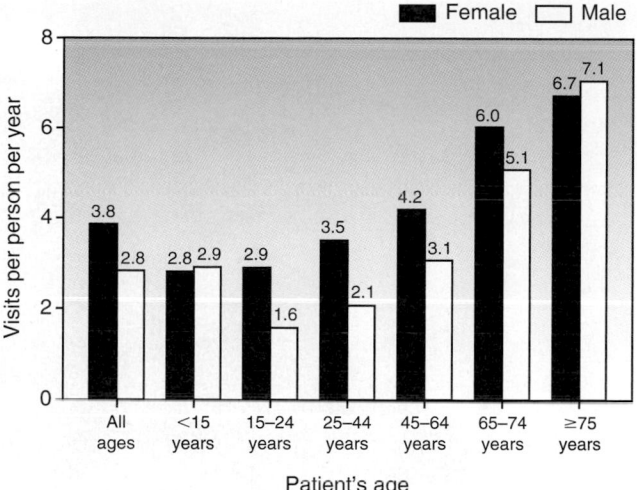

Annual rate of ambulatory care visits by patient's age and gender

*Source*: Adapted from Schappert, 1997.

al., 1992; Pattison, 1998). When gynecological disorders in women and reproductive disorders in men are excluded, rates of hospitalization for men are about the same as for women. The lower rate of discharge and longer hospital stays may be due to the fact that when men are hospitalized their conditions are more severe.

> **"** *Hope for the best.*
> *Expect the worst.*
> *Life is a play.*
> *We're unrehearsed.* **"**
>
> —Mel Brooks

### ■ Preventive Care

Men and women differ in their ability to seek preventive care for the early diagnosis of health care problems. Unlike women, who seek routine reproductive health screening, most men do not have routine checkups that would detect health problems at an early stage. Men are more likely to have examinations at the insistence of their employers, and they do not perceive that they need a regular source of care. More often than women, men perceive their health as very good or excellent and therefore may not think that they need to be involved in health promotion activities (Clark, 1999; Galdas et al., 2005; Harrisson et al., 1992). Women are more likely than men to exhibit stronger health promotion behaviors in terms of blood pressure checks, dental flossing, diet, smoking, drinking, physical activity, weight, and hours of sleep. Men tend to view exercise as sufficient to compensate for unhealthy behaviors such as fatty diets. As a result, men are at greater risk for several of the top killers such as heart disease, cancer, suicide, accidents, and violence. Because most of these killers are preventable, changes in eating habits, workplace environments, and educational strategies are needed to improve preventive care for men (Pattison, 1998).

 NOTE THIS! •

Several high-profile men came forward in the 1990s to talk about their experiences with prostate cancer in an effort to remove the embarrassment surrounding the disease. As a result of the openness of men like former U.S. Senator and presidential candidate Bob Dole, professional golfer Arnold Palmer, and retired General H. Norman Schwarzkopf, many books and journal articles appeared and support groups surfaced all over the country.

## Specific Male Health Issues

### ■ Prostate Cancer

The American Cancer Society lists prostate cancer as the second leading cause of cancer death in American men after lung cancer. Prostate cancer is most common in men older than 40, and the risk increases with each decade thereafter. Most often, prostate cancer is asymptomatic until the disease has progressed. Symptoms that may indicate prostate disease include the following (O'Rourke, 2007; Turner, 2007):

- Difficulty or pain with urination
- Painful ejaculation
- Blood in urine or semen

Although prostate cancer is the second leading cause of cancer deaths in American men, how many prostate cancer prevention and awareness campaigns have you seen? Can the same be said for breast cancer? Consider the financial appropriations and expenditures for cancer in the United States detailed in Table 33-1.

Information about the necessity of digital rectal examinations beginning at age 40 for all men, with possible earlier intervention for those with signs and symptoms of problems or a positive family history, must be included and incorporated into health fairs and promotions. Information related to prostate-specific antigen (PSA) blood testing that is used in conjunction with the digital rectal examination should also be provided. In 1986, the U.S. Food and Drug Administration approved the PSA test for prostate cancer screening. Many physicians believe that the subsequent fall in prostate cancer mortality rates can be attributed to early diagnosis with PSA testing (Courtenay, 2001, Feuer & Merrill, 1999).

**Table 33-1** Breast Versus Prostate Cancer Expenditures

|  | Breast | Prostate |
|---|---|---|
| ■ National Cancer Institute research | $1.8 billion | $376 million |
| ■ Department of Defense research | $455 million | $20 million |
| ■ U.S. government: | | |
| Per person diagnosed | $3,000 | $250 |
| Per death | $12,000 | $2,000 |

*Source*: Jaffe, 1997.

## " *a conversation with . . .* "

### Lance Armstrong, Tour de France winner and testicular cancer survivor

Lance Armstrong, diagnosed with testicular cancer in October of 1996, went on to make history winning the tour de France bicycle race from 1999–2006. Lance stated "I always had the size difference there [testicle size], but I didn't know. I would have still been waiting, if it hadn't started hurting. It got so painful that I couldn't sit on my bike any more. Lance was diagnosed by ultrasound with testicular cancer, began chemotherapy, and with further scans, cancer was also found in his lungs, abdomen, and brain. The cancer was so advanced he eventually needed four cycles of chemotherapy. Lance was diagnosed with an aggressive form of testicular cancer, containing 60% choriocarcinoma, 40% embryonal, and less than 1% teratoma. Lance underwent two surgeries, one to remove his cancerous testicle and another to remove two cancerous lesions on his brain. Lance took an active role in educating himself about the disease and treatment, as well as maintaining his high level of fitness. He declared himself "not a cancer victim but a cancer survivor." Lance underwent aggressive treatment and is now in remission. "It's like breast cancer. Women don't really want to talk about it, men don't really want to talk about it, at first I didn't understand; it's like, man what's the big deal." Lance created his LiveStrong Foundation to increase awareness about testicular cancer. He has worked tirelessly to promote education and research in the most common cancer in men aged 15–35. If detected early, its cure rate is a promising 90%.

*Source*: http://www.livestrong.org

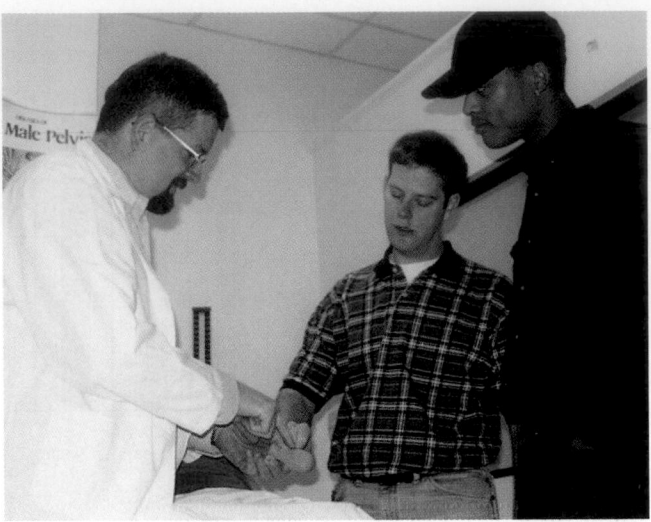

Chapter author Joseph Farmer uses a model to teach young men how to do a testicular self-examination.

34 (Anderson, 2002). It is the second most common cancer for men between the ages of 35 and 39 and the third most common for men between the ages of 15 and 19. This type of cancer is 4.5 times more common among Caucasian men than African American men, with rates for Hispanics/Latinos, Native Americans, and Asians falling somewhere in between.

Epidemiological data show an increase in the incidence of testicular cancer over the past 20 years (Clore, 1993; Koshti-Richman, 1996). As recent as the early 1980s, testicular cancer was fatal for 8 of 10 patients (Brock et al., 1993; Walbrecker, 1995). Today, because of advances in chemotherapy and improved surgical techniques, testicular cancer is one of the most curable forms of cancer (Rosella, 1994). Testicular cancer has a nearly 100% cure rate with early detection and treatment (Brakey, 1994; Clore, 1993; Peate, 1997; Rosella, 1994; Walbrecker, 1995). This optimistic prognosis with early intervention makes testicular self-examination (TSE) a critical component of health teaching for young men, especially because most cases of testicular cancer are found by the patients themselves. Boys should begin TSE around age 13 and make it a lifelong practice because, although testicular cancer is most likely to occur before the age of 40, it can occur at any age. In fact, the incidence rises again after the age of 70.

The characteristics that put men at higher risk for testicular cancer include Caucasian race, young age, high socioeconomic status, or family history, as well as having a

The importance of the procedure and information regarding signs, symptoms, and the screening process should be emphasized in promotions. Nurses should also include written information for distribution because some men are ill at ease discussing the procedure and testing in public (Turner, 2007).

The community health nurse can also organize targeted prostate-specific screenings, during which the men have the digital rectal examination and PSA blood tests on site. In a study that explored the relationship between attitudes toward digital rectal examinations and prostate screening among African American men, the results revealed that fear of the procedure did not prevent men from participating in the screening (Gelfand, Parzuchowski, Cort, & Powell, 1995; Gleason, 2006; Treadwell & Ro, 2003).

### ■ Testicular Cancer

Testicular cancer accounts for only 1% of all cancers in men. However, testicular cancer is the most common form of cancer in men between the ages of 20 and

" *I'm prouder of being a cancer survivor than I am of winning the Tour de France. If I never had cancer, I never would have won the Tour de France. I'm convinced of that. I wouldn't want to do it all over again, but I wouldn't change a thing.* "
—*Lance Armstrong, winner of the Tour de France (21-day, 2287-mile bicycle race) and testicular cancer survivor (Montville, 1999)*

**Testicular Self-Examination**

- Self-examination should be done once a month after a warm bath or shower because heat relaxes the scrotum and loosens the skin, making the testes easier to examine.
- Visually inspect the scrotum for any swelling or changes in color.
- Examine each testicle with both hands by placing the index and middle fingers under the testicle with the thumbs placed on top. Roll the testicle gently between the fingers and thumbs, feeling for any changes such as lumps, swelling, or painful spots.
- The first sign of testicular cancer is usually a hard, painless lump about the size of a pea. However, if there are any kinds of changes or abnormalities, immediately notify your health care provider, because only he or she can make a positive diagnosis.

*Sources*: Adapted from Henkel, 1996; "Testicular Cancer," 1999; Walbrecker, 1995.

Young men are less likely than young women to practice preventive health care.

mother who took estrogen during her pregnancy (Bertuccio et al., 2007; Brakey, 1994; Cheung et al., 2007; Feldman, Bosl, Sheinfeld, & Motzer, 2008; Kinkade, 1999; Wigle, Turner, Gomes, & Parent, 2008). Males with undescended testicles or late descending testicles (after age 6) have a 3 to 17 times higher than average risk for developing testicular cancer. Despite this information, the health education literature suggests that most of the men who are most susceptible to testicular cancer are unaware of the signs and symptoms of the disease and how to detect them (Rosella, 1994). Research has indicated that although information has been readily available to young women regarding breast self-examination (BSE) and the importance of regular Pap smears, the information related to TSE has not been as widely communicated.

Nurses are in the best position to provide young men with the information to learn the self-examination techniques needed for early detection and cure (Peate, 1997; Walbrecker, 1995). TSE education and screening programs can be set up in high schools and presented simultaneously with BSE and screening programs. Models can be used for practicing self-examination with lifelike lumps and abnormalities to teach young men what they should be looking for. Testicular examination and TSE education should be part of every routine physical examination for adolescent and young adult males. Instructions for self-examination of the testicles are given in Box 33-1.

The only way a positive diagnosis of testicular cancer can be made is through surgical removal (orchiectomy) of the affected testicle for direct examination. Because testicular cancer occurs most often in men of reproductive age, **fertility** is a major concern. Although sperm count may be lowered, a unilateral orchiectomy usually does not affect sexual function or fertility (Brakey, 1994; Henkel, 1996; Walbrecker, 1995). However, abnormalities in the remaining testicle or the effects of radiation and chemotherapy may have adverse effects on sexual function and fertility (Brakey, 1994), although studies have shown that many men recover fertility within 2 to 3 years after chemotherapy (Bertuccio et al., 2007; Blekhman et al., 2008; Feldman et al., 2008; Henkel, 1996; Paduch, 2006; Petterson, Richiardi, Nordenskjold, Kaijser, & Akre, 2007).

### ■ Erectile Dysfunction (Impotence)

Many sexual topics are now discussed openly, but **erectile dysfunction** (ED) is still a subject that causes fear and anxiety for many men and women. Although a significant amount of scientific data are available about erectile dysfunction (also called *impotence*), large segments of the public, including health care professionals, are still uninformed, or even worse, misinformed. A lack of accurate information,

**"**At my age, 'getting a little action' means I don't have to take a laxative. **"**

—Bruce Lansky

## ETHICAL CONNECTION

Should health care providers address men differently than women in their assessments of behaviors, such as the number of sex partners, risky behavior, and rate of seeking primary health care? Women go to health care providers much more frequently than men do; they also take more prescription medications over a lifetime than men do. How would this information affect your care of men as patients?

 THINK ABOUT THIS

The Peyton family is football royalty. Archie Manning, the father, was a legendary quarterback at the University of Mississippi and with the New Orleans Saints. His middle son Peyton, an All Pro with the Indianapolis Colts, is one of the most popular and respected players in the game. Youngest son Eli led the New York Giants to victory in the 2008 Super Bowl.

Cooper Manning was the first son born to Archie and Olivia Manning in 1974. In the beginning, he was the most gifted athlete among Archie's sons—smart, witty, and fearless. His problems began in his sophomore year at Ole Miss, when he began dropping balls and experiencing numbness on his right side. He was eventually diagnosed at Baylor Medical center as having spinal stenosis, a congenital disorder. In 1993, Cooper underwent surgery on his spine and had to learn to walk again. He is now a stock trader for an energy investment company, but cannot do any kind of risky sports. He is married and has a daughter.

*Source:* Bradley, J. E. (November 10, 2003). The other brother. *Sports Illustrated*, 79–86.

as well as reluctance on the part of many health care providers to deal openly with sexual issues, has left many patients without a source of help for their sexual concerns. Improving both public and professional knowledge and attaining a comfort level in talking about erectile dysfunction will provide both men and their sexual partners with an avenue for obtaining needed information and effective treatment.

### What Is Erectile Dysfunction?

Erectile dysfunction is the inability to achieve or maintain a penile erection sufficient for sexual intercourse. Approximately 15 million American men suffer from erectile dysfunction, and the incidence increases with age. Approximately 5% of men experience erectile dysfunction by the age of 40, increasing to between 15% and 25% by the age of 65 (National Kidney and Urologic Disease Information Clearinghouse, 2008). Erectile dysfunction is often assumed erroneously to be a normal part of the aging process (NIH, 2006). Sex researchers Masters and Johnson discovered that although sexual activity slows down with advancing age, it does not end. Most men and women between the ages of 50 and 60 are still interested in remaining sexually active.

## "a conversation with . . ."

I love my job. I absolutely love what I do. Cancer controls your life, and I didn't want cancer to take me off the ice.

Shock and fear are the first two things that you feel. Then you feel a feeling of anxious desperation. And then when the diagnosis was complete, and I heard there was a treatment, it was nonstop humor. My goal is to find a way to laugh every day.

For people with testicular cancer that are going through their treatments and challenges, feel fortunate that there is a treatment. Understand that it will be a hard episode in your life. Understand that the treatment will try to defeat you and damage your spirit. But you can fight back and win.

—Scott Hamilton,
Olympic figure skating champion
and testicular cancer survivor

*Source:* A chat with Scott Hamilton (excerpts from a chat on ABC News: http://vix.com/menmag/tcschotth.htm).

### Causes

Most cases of erectile dysfunction have a physical cause such as disease, injury, or drug side effects. Diabetes mellitus, kidney disease, multiple sclerosis, atherosclerosis, chronic alcoholism, hypertension, and vascular disease account for approximately 70% of all cases of erectile dysfunction. Of men with diabetes mellitus, 35% to 50% experience erectile dysfunction (Herbert et al., 2008; National Kidney and Urologic Diseases Information Clearinghouse, 2008). Various kinds of surgeries are also associated with increased incidence of erectile dysfunction. The most common are surgeries that can cause injury to nerves and arteries near the penis. These include surgeries for prostate, colon, rectal, and bladder cancers. Any type of vascular surgery can increase a man's risk for ED. Many common medications list erectile dysfunction as a side effect, including drugs used to treat hypertension, antihistamines, antidepressants, sedatives, tranquilizers, appetite suppressants, and pain medications. Smoking has also been shown to have an adverse effect on erectile function by increasing the effects of other risk factors such as vascular disease or hypertension. Vasectomy, however, has not been associated with increased risk for erectile dysfunction (Herbert et al., 2008).

In 10% to 20% of cases of erectile dysfunction, the cause is deemed to be psychological. Factors such as stress, anxiety, guilt, depression, low self-esteem, and fear of sexual failure can cause erectile dysfunction without the presence of any physical problems or can be secondary reactions to underlying physical causes (Herbert et al., 2008). Important facts that should be emphasized when counseling a man and his sexual partner about erectile dysfunction include the following:

- Most men experience erectile dysfunction related to stress or alcohol at some time in their lives.
- Past sexual practices, including masturbation, do not cause erectile dysfunction.

### Research Alert

We have neglected a significant part of the population most in need of health care. We have been blind to the fact that when we visited clinics and worked with communities to address their health needs, there were few men in the waiting rooms of the clinics where primary health and prevention services were being provided. Virtually no health efforts were directed toward men. Poor men had become invisible and their health needs neglected. Poor men and men of color live with tremendous emotional and physical pain, are demeaned and devalued in a system that rewards wealth and values some people over others, and die early. Poor men are less likely to have health insurance, less likely to seek needed health service, and less likely to receive adequate care when they do. Even among the poor, some men are less than equal.

Those men of African descent demonstrate the great peril that poor men have to face (Treadwell & Ro, 2003). Life expectancy for African American men is 7.1 years shorter than that for men overall. Forty percent of African American men die prematurely from cardiovascular disease, compared with 21% of white men (Burnett, et al., 2001). Death rates for HIV/AIDS are nearly 5 times higher for African American men that for white men (Anderson, 2002).

Society has no system in place to support the health and health-seeking behaviors of men who work at lower wage levels or who are unable to work because of poor education, absence of jobs, mismatch in skills, or other reasons. Men are so concerned about their daily survival—that is, caring for their families and having a good job—that they do not make health a priority. Working conditions of low-income men are frequently hazardous, and policies designed to protect these workers are often grossly inadequate. Most often, low-paid and low-skilled workers are not offered health insurance coverage through work. Low-income men who are childless are excluded from publicly funded insurance programs (Hudak & Hagan, 2002; Miniclier, 2002; Parker, 2002; Roman & Carroll, 2003; Barstow & Bergman, 2003).

Sadly, the penal system is the only place where men have the right to health care, under the U.S. Constitution's protection against "cruel and unusual punishment." There are currently more than 1.4 million inmates in federal and state prisons and more than 600,000 are released during each year. Some 93% of U.S. inmates are male and 44% are people of color (Harrison, & Beck, 2002).

- Physical disorders can directly affect sexual functioning.
- An occasional problem with erectile dysfunction does not mean a chronic problem will develop.
- A man can sabotage his ability to have an erection by worrying about it.

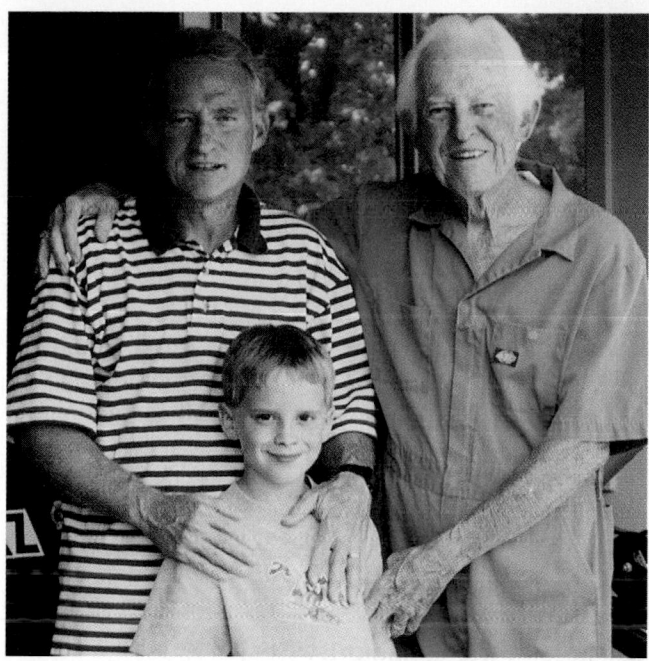

Men with at least two close relatives with prostate cancer have a very high risk of developing the disease before the age of 70. Men with a family history of prostate cancer should have PSA screening and prostate examinations between the ages of 50 and 70.

❝I do have one big regret. I left Harvard with no real awareness of the awful inequities in the world . . . the appalling disparities of health and wealth and opportunity that condemn millions to lives of despair.❞

❝I have been waiting 30 years to say this: 'Dad, I always told you I'd come back and get my degree.'❞

—Bill Gates, upon receiving an honorary degree from Harvard in 2007, 30 years after dropping out

The Bill and Melinda Gates Foundation was founded to address health and education issues and has an endowment of more than $33 billion, making it by far the largest charitable foundation in the world.

### Treatment

Treatment varies according to the severity and cause of the dysfunction. Health care providers start with the least invasive treatment and progress to more invasive treatments until erectile dysfunction is corrected. Reducing the dosage or eliminating drugs that may be causing erectile dysfunction is the first step. Psychotherapy and behavior modifications are next. Vacuum devices, oral drugs, drugs injected into the urethra, and finally surgically implanted penile devices or vascular surgery are offered as treatment if the problem persists (National Kidney and Urologic Disease Information Clearinghouse, 2008; NIH, 2006).

In 1998, a new "wonder drug" called *sildenafil citrate* (commonly known as **Viagra**) was approved by the U.S. Food and Drug Administration. Viagra is taken 1 hour before sexual intercourse and works by boosting the effects of nitric oxide, a chemical produced by the body to relax smooth

THINK ABOUT THIS

Men experience notable midlife physical changes. After age 40, testosterone decreases; muscle mass loss, cognition problems, and osteoporosis risk increase. Lower testosterone levels are known to increase a man's prostate cancer risk.

muscle in the penis and allow increased blood flow during sexual stimulation. This drug does not trigger automatic erection as other drugs used to treat erectile dysfunction do, but rather just allows the man to respond to sexual stimulation (National Kidney and Urologic Disease Information Clearinghouse, 2008). The drug is very successful in treating many forms of erectile dysfunction, although some fear the drug may be overused by middle-aged and older men who may not actually suffer from erectile dysfunction but just want to "boost" their sex lives.

### Role of the Community Health Nurse

The most important things the community health nurse can do for men with erectile dysfunction are to provide accurate and easily understandable information and to encourage the man and his sex partner to talk openly and comfortably about the problem. Including the man's sex partner in the discussion acknowledges his or her importance in the relationship. The partner may also have questions, doubts, and insecurities that need to be addressed. Many persons whose partners are impotent blame themselves for the problem. The partner may also feel hurt and angry because the male has withdrawn physically and emotionally. Understanding that he or she is not to blame can go a long way in enabling the partner to support the diagnosis and treatment. It is important for the nurse to be sensitive to the needs of patients whose values or sexual orientation may be different from the nurse. Whatever the relationship of the partners, all couples should be treated with dignity and respect.

## ■ Cardiovascular Disease

Cardiovascular disease is the single greatest cause of death in men. Approximately 1 in 3 male deaths is related to cardiovascular disease. Similarly, more than one-third of men dying between the ages of 45 and 65 die of a heart attack. Cardiovascular disease is caused by the accumulation of fatty deposits within the artery wall that causes stiffness and reduced blood flow. When the brain interprets reduced blood flow as low blood pressure, it sends a signal to the heart to compensate. The heart works faster with less rest and increases the pressure on each contraction. Although there are many explanations for higher cardiovascular disease rates among men than women, research points to two major factors:

1. Men's diets have higher ratios of saturated to polyunsaturated fat, which contributes to cardiovascular disease (Power & Schulkin, 2008).
2. Men's sociocultural environments lead to higher levels of stress, which contributes to cardiovascular disease (Hall, 2007; Williams, 2008).

 Research Alert

Socialization of men into the masculine role influences their health-related beliefs, attitudes, perceptions, and risk-taking behavior. Yet traditionally men's health has been primarily defined in terms suggesting that biological factors, such as hormones, are the main determinants of morbidity and mortality. Men's health must be viewed within the broader context of family health. Across the population, the main differences in mortality and morbidity are related to variations in exposure to risk factors. Men stress the importance of being fit, strong, energetic, physically active, and in control, whereas women stress not being ill and not needing to see a doctor. Men see their body as a machine and view exercise as more important than nutrition and rest, whereas women place more emphasis on nutrition, rest, and relaxation and less emphasis on exercise.

Men are not encouraged to express their feelings, such as pain and other symptoms of illness. Instead, men often mask their feelings by engaging in aggressive and risk-taking behaviors, which can expose them to illness, injury, or death.

STD incidence is higher in men, especially among the 25- to 34-year-old age group, because men in this age cohort tend to have more sexual partners than women of the corresponding age do.

Male infertility appears to be on the increase, possibly due to environmental factors and chemicals that increase risk of testicular disease and affect sperm production.

What can nurses do to correct this imbalance? Here are some practical steps:

- Establish men's health-awareness-raising groups, and involve women in seeking a solution to the problem.
- Educate nurses and others on risk-reduction strategies, and help men ventilate their feelings in a healthy way.
- Teach men testicular self-examination.
- Organize campaigns to increase men's contact with health services.
- Identify and focus interventions on high-risk groups such as young men, poor men, men of color, single divorced and widowed men with chronic disease, and men who abuse substances.
- Promote safer sex practices.
- Promote regular screening for rectal, prostate, and other cancers.

*Source*: Lloyd, R. (1996). Men's health review. Men's Health Forum, London Royal College of Nursing.

 *Got an Alternative?*

Men are less reluctant to use alternative and complementary health measures than are women. How can you explain this difference according to gender?

Cardiovascular disease and hypertension can often be prevented by changes in behavior, including stopping smoking, increasing activity, and improving diet. Community health nurses can design educational programs that target men to promote behavior changes that reduce the risk of cardiovascular disease (Burnett et al., 2001; Gregory, Blanck, Gillespie, Maynard, & Serdula, 2008; Noloshin, Schwartz, & Welsh, 2008). These recommendations may include the following:

- Losing weight
- Reducing salt intake
- Smoking cessation
- Eating foods rich in natural sources of fiber and antioxidant vitamins
- Exercising
- Relaxing

In addition, consumption of moderate amounts of alcohol and sexual activity are associated with reduced risks of cardiovascular disease.

## Selected At-Risk Populations

### ■ Men with HIV/AIDS

According to the Centers for Disease Control and Prevention, by 1994 HIV/AIDS had become a leading cause of death in the United States for men between the ages of 25 and 44. With the introduction of new medications in recent years, HIV/AIDS-related death rates have steadily declined, but the incidence of new HIV/AIDS cases continues to rise. HIV/

 Research Alert

This research study explored young men's perceptions of and participation in hip hop culture—urban social and artistic expressions, such as clothing style, breakdancing, graffiti, and rap music—and how contextual factors of the hip hop scene may be associated with their condom use, condom-use self-efficacy, and sense of community. A cross-sectional survey design was conducted of 95 African American and Latino men aged 15 to 25 years as part of a 4-year ethnographic study in New York City. Results indicated that differences in young men's perceptions of and levels of affiliation with hip hop culture were not statistically associated with differences in their sense of community or condom-use self-efficacy. Frequency of participation in the hip hop nightclub scene was the strongest factor negatively associated with condom use. The researchers concluded that popular discourses on young men's health risks often blame youths' cultures such as the hip hop culture for increased risk practices but do not critically examine how risk emerges in urban young men's lives and what aspects of youths' culture can be protective. Further research needs to focus on contextual factors of risk such as the role of hip hop nightlife on increased HIV risk.

*Source*: Muñoz-Laboy, M., Castellanos, D., Haliburton, C., Del Aguila, E., Weinstein, H., & Parker, R. (2008). Condom use and hip hop culture: The case of urban young men in New York City. *American Journal of Public Health, 98*(6), 1081–1085.

"The young always have the same problem—how to rebel and conform at the same time. They have now solved this by defying their parents and copying one another." —Quentin Crisp

AIDS has historically been viewed in the United States as a disease targeting a specific population—homosexual men. Although the initial cases in the United States, Canada, Australia, and Western Europe were found among this population, this was not the case for the rest of the world. After three decades of the pandemic, many still view HIV/AIDS as something that will not affect them (Stoltenberg et al., 2008). As a result of this apathy, the safer sexual practices adopted in the homosexual communities have not been applied as readily in heterosexual communities. High-risk behaviors, such as alcohol and drug use and unprotected sex with numerous partners, continue to put heterosexual men at risk (Williams, 2008). Heterosexual transmission rates continue to escalate, especially in the African American and Hispanic communities (Anderson, 2002).

The introduction of new medications has reduced the number of HIV/AIDS-related deaths, which means persons with HIV/AIDS are living longer. HIV/AIDS, when appropriately treated, is now considered more of a chronic illness. What does this mean to younger men? An entire generation of sexually active men has never known of a world without HIV or AIDS. To some, this may be interpreted as, "Why bother to protect myself, because I can always take the medications." Some are applying safer sexual practices haphazardly, thus allowing the introduction of drug-resistant strains of HIV into their bodies. To others, especially an alarming number of young homosexual men, the principle of "I'd rather die young and beautiful" applies. Intervention and prevention programs must address these issues and concerns. The community health nurse's best

### ■■ CULTURAL CONNECTION

Gender matters. For example, men and women have different death rates from the same diseases. Most men have shorter life spans than women, particularly among minorities.

What are your stereotypes of men and how do they differ from women? How do these images affect nursing care? This chapter explores the specific threats to men's health, based on physiological, social, and cultural differences.

## Application to Practice

You are a nurse working in a community clinic. One of your patients is Rick Fernandez, a 34-year-old married man who complains about fever and swollen glands. Fearing the possibility of HIV/AIDS, you ask Rick the typical textbook questions to assess his HIV/AIDS risk behaviors: You ask if he uses intravenous drugs, if he has had any blood transfusions, if he has sex with men, and if he is homosexual. He responds with a no to all questions. Based on his replies, you do not pursue HIV/AIDS testing. When he comes back a few months later with complaints of recurrent skin lesions, you again ask about his HIV/AIDS risk behaviors and receive the same answers as before. Rick insists that he is a happily married man in a monogamous relationship and does not use any sort of drugs. Rick seems offended by your questions. You approach the physician and ask if he has considered testing Rick for HIV/AIDS. The physician has assessed the risk behaviors and concluded that Rick does not have any of the risk factors associated with HIV/AIDS. When Rick returns to the clinic for a third visit, you are more assertive and convince Rick to have an HIV test. The test comes back positive. Rick reveals to the HIV/AIDS counselor that he had been imprisoned a while back and that his only potential exposure to HIV/AIDS might have been through another inmate who raped him.

1. What is your reaction to Rick's situation?
2. Do you feel that your personal beliefs and values influenced your reaction?
3. Why do you think Rick did not disclose the key information earlier?
4. What could you have done to obtain the accurate information?
5. What specific questions could you have asked Rick to obtain this information?

*The reasons for unhealthy behaviors are not that the public does not fully understand healthy ones: It is something more deeply rooted in the ills of our society. Unhealthy behaviors start in part as a response to a social environment that fosters no alternatives. To change that environment is the challenge. Where do we start? We start at the beginning.*

Geoges C. Benjamin, Executive Director of the American Public Health Association, 2003

### ✏ NOTE THIS!

Men account for 66% of all deaths caused by extreme heat, according to the CDC.

Eighty percent of drowning victims are men.

option would include the education of young men who would act as role models for their peers.

What does the increase in HIV/AIDS cases within the African American and Hispanic communities mean to the community health nurse? Intervention and prevention programs need to specifically target these communities. The church is an institution generally accepted as having a powerful influence within both of these communities. By securing the commitment from religious leaders and their congregations, the community health nurse can create positive change from within the system. Developing role models and implementing prevention programs that include members of the community results in much more effective outcomes.

For example, the community health nurse working within a community often develops a relationship with community members. Once a trusting relationship has been established, the nurse can approach some of the unofficial leaders within the community to enlist their support and discuss strategies and objectives to decrease the epidemic of infection affecting the population. This needs to be done in a nonjudgmental manner, in which the nurse details the problems and possible solutions without passing blame or creating fear. By enlisting the members' support in the initial stages, the nurse can formulate plans and develop goals that are perceived as important to the community, thus securing support for the intervention.

### ■ Homosexual Men and Families

The special needs of homosexual men include more than just HIV/AIDS education. Homosexual men and their families exist in virtually every community, regardless of how restrictive or liberal the community proclaims to be. However, societal stigmatization of homosexuality forces many

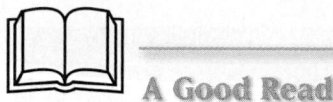

## A Good Read

# Age Proofing—My Way

*David Cartwright*

*What does a man do when the "medical system" takes over his life? Go on a bicycle trip across the country!*

Why would a man over the age of 60 ride a bicycle half way across the country? I have no idea; I had never done anything like this before. Maybe we ride because we're mad—we want to do the wild thing. For men of a certain age, it is called the *Ulysses Factor.*

How else can one explain chafing your backside, battling heat and thirst, living with numbness in your feet and hands—and being literally scared to death at the mercy of those on four wheels who claim to "share" the road with you. There is certainly no money in it for most of us, in this boot camp approach to well-being. In this complex world, I can barely manage myself. The simple life of an adventure cyclist is a wonderful tonic. It's a fine thing, to do—a kind of age proofing. I get outdoors. It keeps me in good physical shape. For me, it helps me keep a good mental attitude and have the time to reflect on that meaning of life.

I am no romantic cycling bum but I talked myself into this last long trip. I kept it a secret. Why? Because there is always somebody who will find something wrong with what you are doing or about to do.

The germ of the idea began when I saw myself as a growing victim of the medical system, mentally, physically and emotionally—undergoing surgeries, popping pills, and receiving reassurance with recommendations for more treatments—in short I was rapidly becoming a crock. Somehow I had to break the chains and regain control. I did it by hopping on a bicycle, laden with tent and sleeping bag, waving goodbye to my loved ones—for a test of my survival skills. For a nonthinker, I even did some planning—such as how far, best routes, what to take, when to go, and whom to avoid. And I just did it.

1,700 miles later, I am back to my old life, back to work. But I am ready to do it again. The best thing about my trip was the hospitality I found on my trip and the people I met. I'm a new man now with an extraordinary sense of freedom and energy, looking forward to the weekends for those short rides and forever planning the next really long one. You know the one that keeps me age-proofed.

---

to remain "in the closet." Homosexual myths and stereotypes abound, particularly in cultures that value male dominance or masculinity. Homosexual men and their sexual practices run the entire spectrum, just as in the heterosexual community. Also, homosexual men may be married or have children, live alone or with a partner. Individuals define who makes up their family group, not nurses or official definitions.

Although there is little research on violence between male homosexuals, early reports indicate that abusive behavior in these relationships is significant (Harrison & Beck, 2002; El Bassel, 2007).

The community health nurse's role in interactions with any group of men is inclusion instead of exclusion. Nurses should ask questions in such a manner that the man does not feel obligated to give an answer he believes the nurse expects. When using such items as risk assessments, questions should be phrased in a general manner. For example, the nurse should ask about "the number of sexual partners" instead of "the number of female sex partners." Nurses should maintain a nonjudgmental tone and manner throughout all interactions. Just as in any interaction, including the entire family whenever possible is recommended. By developing a trusting and honest relationship, the nurse can be instrumental in generating assistance and implementing change of unsafe or risky behaviors (Kaufman & Gregory, 2007).

## Research Alert

Rooted in a qualitative research project with 70 stay-at-home fathers in Canada, this paper explores the ways that work and family interact for fathers who "trade cash for care." While fathers are at home, they also remain connected to traditionally masculine sources of identity such as paid work and they take on unpaid masculine self-provisioning work at home and community work that builds on traditional male interests. They thus carve out complex sets of relations between home, paid and unpaid work, community work, and their own sense of masculinity. Narratives from stay-at-home fathers speak volumes about the ways in which the long shadow of hegemonic masculinity hangs over them while also pointing to hints of resistance and change as fathers begin to critique concepts of "male time" and market capitalism approaches to work and care. The researchers concludes by pointing to several theoretical contributions to research on fatherhood and masculinities as well as to policy implications that arise from this study on the social valuing of unpaid work.

*Source:* Doucet, A. (2004) "It's almost like I have a job, but I don't get paid": Fathers at home reconfiguring work, care, and masculinity. *Fathering: A Journal of Theory, Research & Practice about Men as Fathers*, 2(3), 277–302.

**Table 33-2**

| Life Expectancy at Birth | 2003* | 1970** | 1950** | 1920** |
|---|---|---|---|---|
| Classification | | Life Expectancy | | |
| ▪ Population | 77.6 | 70.8 | 68.2 | 54.1 |
| ▪ All females | 80.1 | 74.7 | 71.1 | 54.6 |
| ▪ All males | 74.8 | 67.1 | 65.6 | 53.6 |
| ▪ White females | 80.5 | 75.6 | 72.2 | 55.6 |
| ▪ Black females | 76.1 | 68.3 | 62.9*** | 45.2*** |
| ▪ White males | 75.4 | 68.0 | 66.5 | 54.4 |
| ▪ Black males | 69.2 | 60.0 | 59.1*** | 45.5*** |

*Hoyert, D. L., Kung, H.-C., & Smith, B. L. (2005). Deaths: Preliminary data for 2003. *National Vital Statistics Reports, 53*(15), 1–48.
**Anderson, R. N. (2001). United States life tables, 1998. *National Vital Statistics Reports, 48*(18), 33–34.
***Prior to 1970, data for the black population are not available; data shown prior to 1970 are for the nonwhite population.

*Source*: Men's Health Network, 2008.

Most American children suffer too much mother and too little father.
—Gloria Steinem, *New York Times*, 26 August 1971

### MEDIA MOMENT

**My Life**
Bob and Gail Jones are expecting their first child, but Bob has been diagnosed with kidney cancer, which may take his life before his child is born. Heartbroken at the prospect of not ever getting to know his child, he decides to make a video about himself and his life so that his child will know him.

# Community Health Nursing Roles

The community health nurse assumes a wide range of duties and responsibilities while providing health care to men. A typical week could include hundreds of miles traveled, diverse teaching methods and strategies, and numerous new encounters. Community health nursing roles may include patient advocate, educator, and facilitator.

## ▪ Patient Advocate

As a patient advocate, the role of the community health nurse includes interfacing with healthcare providers and healthcare agencies to support the best care for the patient. For instance, a nurse realizes that a recently diagnosed HIV-positive man has been prescribed AZT alone, rather than the more effective cocktail combination medications and latest research-based interventions. A proper assessment must be made to determine whether alternative medications should be prescribed. With the permission of the patient, the nurse can contact the appropriate healthcare provider and discuss the patient's options with a nonthreatening and nonjudgmental stance to allow for future interactions. Any new information must be shared with the patient.

## ▪ Educator

The role of a health educator for men can often be challenging. Education can occur in any setting from the stockyards to the corporate boardroom. Safety issues, violence, diet, sexual relationships, stress, and physical exercise are examples of topics that may be addressed. The community health nurse must customize education efforts to the specific needs of the patient population. The first step involves a correct assessment of the educational needs of the individuals. The nurse determines the level of the learners to ensure that the level of the educational program is neither too low nor too high for the specific group. Providing educational programs for men in their own environments requires versatility, flexibility, and consideration of cultural issues.

Research Alert

Risk factors for college male sexual aggression that were both theoretically and empirically based were tested using multivariate regression analyses. These included substance abuse patterns, pornography consumption, negative gender-based attitudes, and child sexual abuse experiences. Regression analyses indicated that some gender attitudes, pornography use, and alcohol abuse were significant predictors of perpetration of sexual violence. Although a number of men were sexually abused as children, this risk factor did not predict sexual aggression as an adult. Many men reported alcohol-related sexual coercion and held many rape-supportive attitudes and beliefs. These practices by college men contribute to the prorape cultures found on many campuses. Strategies are needed to identify and intervene with high-risk men to prevent sexual victimization of women in college.

*Source*: Carr, J., & VanDeusen, K. M. (2004). Risk factors for male sexual aggression on college campuses. *Journal of Family Violence, 19*(5), 279–90.

### ■ Facilitator

The community health nurse as facilitator brings various people and groups together to talk about issues and needs. The most significant facilitator role involves helping people and groups with different views to reach a compromise so that they can find a common ground to solve problems and bring about positive changes to alleviate a specific community health issue. For instance, a community health nurse, as the facilitator, may initiate positive change through programs with specific targeted groups such as adolescent boys. This can be accomplished by teaching safer sexual practices to prevent STDs and teenage pregnancies by bringing together parents, school administrators, politicians, health care providers, and teens.

## Men's Health Research Issues

Despite the advances in medical technology and research, men continue to live an average of 7 years less than women. Although most medical research was historically based on men, men's health issues no longer dominate the research agenda because of recent federal mandates. Research on men's health must focus on the areas where prevention, early detection, and treatment efforts will significantly improve the quality of life of men across the life span. Men's health should be considered a specialty, including clinics and programs especially designed for men.

In addition, research studies must be more inclusive and utilize subjects that represent the diversity within the male population. Studies need to report findings based not only on middle-aged, middle class, Caucasian males, but also on other males representing various ethnic and socioeconomic groups.

✎ NOTE THIS! ●──────────────
Men who smoke a pack of cigarettes or more per day are nearly 40% more likely to have erectile dysfunction compared to nonsmokers.

Historically, most research studies have been based on male subjects. In many Western cultures, years of a predominantly male workforce have resulted in healthcare systems and policies being established by men. Despite this dominance of men in healthcare systems, women still have longer life expectancies than men.

## Conclusion

Men's health care is not easily defined as a single issue with a limited focus or target population. Although men constitute half the population, their needs and health system utilization vary greatly from those of women. Men's health has failed to be recognized as a specialty, and the declining health of men in the United States may be a result of this lack of specialization. Issues faced by men must be addressed to improve their overall health and decrease the variance in life expectancy between men and women.

The community health nurse can be instrumental in securing access to and promoting the utilization of health care by men. Health promotion and screening programs can be implemented with specifically targeted groups of men. The community health nurse also assumes the roles of patient advocate, educator, and facilitator to secure the most advantageous outcomes for the improvement of men's health.

Explore Community Health Nursing on the Web! To learn more about the topics in this chapter, use the passcode provided to access your exclusive website: **http://nursing.jbpub.com/ communityhealth.** If you do not have a passcode, you can obtain one at this site.

## ■ CRITICAL THINKING ACTIVITIES

1. Smoking is a behavior issue that plays an important role in the reduction of the length and quality of life of men. As a community health nurse, which programs would you develop to improve this situation? Which groups would you specifically target? How would you most effectively implement your plans?

2. Based on the information provided regarding men's utilization of preventive health care, what would be the most effective intervention(s) to ensure participation? Where should the intervention(s) be implemented? How would the intervention(s) be modified to address differences in age, religion, education, or socioeconomic status?

## ■ REFERENCES

Anderson, R. N. (2002). Deaths: Leading causes for 2000. *National Vital Statistics Report 2002, 50*(16), 1–85.

Barstow, D., & Bergman, L. (2003). At a tax foundry, an indifference to life. *New York Times,* January 8, p. A1.

Bertuccio, P., Malvezzi, M., Chatenoud, L., Bosetti, C., Negri, E., Levi, F., et al. (2007). Testicular cancer mortality in the Americas, 1980–2003. *Cancer (0008543X), 109*(4), 776–779.

Black, M., & Breiding, M. (2008). Adverse health conditions and health risk behaviors associated with intimate partner violence—United States, 2005. *JAMA: Journal of the American Medical Association, 300*(6), 646–649.

Blekhman, R., Man, O., Herrmann, L., Boyko, A., Indap, A., Kosiol, C., et al. (2008). Natural selection on genes that underlie human disease susceptibility. *Current Biology, 18*(12), 883–889.

Brakey, M. R. (1994, September). Myths and facts . . . About testicular cancer. *Nursing, 24.*

Brock, D., Fox, S., Gosling, G., et al., (1993). Testicular cancer. *Seminars in Oncology Nursing, 9*(4), 224–236.

Burnett, R., Casper, M. L., Halverson, J. A., et al. (June 2001). *Men and heart disease: An atlas of racial and ethnic disparities in mortality.* Morgantown, WV: West Virginia University, Office for Social Environment and Health Research.

Carr, J., & VanDeusen, K. M. (2004) Risk factors for male sexual aggression on college campuses. *Journal of Family Violence, 19*(5), 279–90.

Charles, N., & Walters, V. (2008). "Men are leavers alone and women are worriers": Gender differences in discourses of health. *Health, Risk & Society, 10*(2), 117–132.

Cheung, W., Demers, A., Hossain, D., Owen, T., Ahmed, S., & Czaykowski, P. (2007). Appropriateness of testicular cancer management: a population-based cohort study. *The Canadian Journal of Urology, 14*(3), 3542–3550.

Clark, M. J. (1999). *Nursing in the community* (3rd ed.). Stamford, CT: Appleton & Lange.

Clore, E. R. (1993). A guide for the testicular self-examination. *Journal of Pediatric Health Care, 7*(6), 264–268.

Coakley, E. H., Rimm, E. B., Colditz, G., Kawachi, I., & Willet, W. (1998). Predictors of weight change in men: Results from the Health Professionals Follow-Up Study. *International Journal of Obesity, 22,* 89–96.

Courtenay, W. H. (2000a). Behavioral factors associated with disease, injury, and death among men: Evidence and implications for prevention. *Journal of Men's Studies, 9*(1), 81–142.

Courtenay, W. H. (2000b). Constructions of masculinity and their influence on men's well-being: A theory of gender and health. *Social Sciences Medicine, 50*(10), 1385–1401.

Courtenay, W. H. (2000c). Engendering health: A social constructionist examination of men's health beliefs and behaviors. *Psychology of Men & Masculinity, 1*(1).

Courtenay, W. H. (2001). Men's health: Ethnicity matters. *Social Work Today, 1*(8), 20–22.

Delsohn, S. (1996). *The fire inside: Firefighters talk about their lives.* New York: HarperCollins.

Dutta, M., & Boyd, J. (2007). Turning smoking man images around: Portrayals of smoking in men's magazines as a blueprint for smoking cessation campaigns. *Health Communication, 22*(3), 253–263.

Fackelmann, K. (1998). An enzymatic sex difference. *Science News, 153*(13), 204.

Feldman, D., Bosl, G., Sheinfeld, J., & Motzer, R. (2008). Medical treatment of advanced testicular cancer. *JAMA: Journal of the American Medical Association, 299*(6), 672–684.

Femquist, R. M.(2001). Education, race/ethnicity, age, sex, and suicide: Individual-level data in the United States. *Current Research in Social Psychology, 3,* 277–290.

Feuer, E. J., & Merrill, R. M. (1999). Cancer surveillance series: Interpreting trends in prostate cancer—Part II: Cause of death misclassification and the recent rise and fall in prostate cancer mortality. *Journal of the National Cancer Institute, 91*(12), 1025–1032.

Galdas, P. M., Cheater, F., & Marshall, P. (2005). Men and health help-seeking behaviour: Literature review. *Journal of Advanced Nursing, 49*(6), 616–623.

Gefou-Madianou, D. (Ed.). (1992). *Alcohol, gender, and culture.* London & New York: Routledge.

Gelfand, D. E., Parzuchowski, J., Cort, M., & Powell, I. (1995). Digital rectal examinations and prostate cancer screening: Attitudes of African American men. *Oncology Nursing Forum, 22,* 1253–1255.

Gerlock, A. A. (1997). New directions in the treatment of men who batter women. *Health Care for Women International, 18,* 481–493.

Glassner, B. (1992). Men and muscles. In M. Kimmel & M. Messner, (Eds.), *Men's lives* (2nd ed.). New York/Toronto: Macmillan/Maxwell.

Goldstein, S., Chesir-Teran, D., & McFaul, A. (2008). Profiles and correlates of relational aggression in young adults' romantic relationships. *Journal of Youth & Adolescence, 37*(3), 251–265.

Gough, B., & Edwards, G. (1998). The beer talking: Four lads, a carry out and the reproduction of masculinities. *Sociological Review, 46*(3). 409–435.

Graves, K. L. (1995). Risky sexual behavior and alcohol use among young adults: Results from a national survey. *American Journal of Health Promotion, 10*(1), 27–36.

Gregory, C., Blanck, H., Gillespie, C., Maynard, L., & Serdula, M. (2008). Perceived health risk of excess body weight among overweight and obese men and women: Differences by sex. *Preventive Medicine, 47*(1), 46–52.

Hall, R. (2007). Racism as health risk for African-American males: Correlations between hypertension and skin color. *Journal of African American Studies, 11*(3/4), 204–213.

Harrison, P. M., & Beck. A. J. (2002). *Prisoners in 2001.* Washington, DC: U.S. Department of Justice, Bureau of Justice Statistics.

Harrisson, J., Chin, J., & Ficarotto, T. (1992). Warning: Masculinity may be dangerous to your health. In M. Kimmel & M. Messner (Eds.), *Men's lives* (2nd ed.). New York/Toronto: Macmillan/Maxwell.

Hauser, R., & Sokol, R. (2008). Science linking environmental contaminant exposures with fertility and reproductive health impacts in the adult male. *Fertility & Sterility, 89*(2), e59–e65.

Hede, K. (2007). Lung cancer may be different for men and women, but researchers ponder what to do. *Journal of the National Cancer Institute, 99*(24), 1830–1832.

Henkel, J. (1996, January/February). Testicular cancer: Survival high with early treatment. *FDA Consumer*. Retrieved November 13, 2008, from http://www.menweb.org/fdatesti.htm

Herbert, K., Lopez, B., Castellano, J., Palacio, A., Tamari, L., & Arcemen, L. (2008). The prevalence of erectile dysfunction in heart failure patients by race and ethnicity. *International Journal Of Impotence Research, 20*(5), 507–511.

Hudak, S., & Hagan, J. F. (2002). Asbestos: The lethal legacy, families of workers blame deaths on plants' use of asbestos. *Plain Dealer* (Cleveland, OH), November 4, p. A1.

Isenhart, C. E., & Silversmith, D. J. (1994). The influence of the traditional male role on alcohol abuse and the therapeutic process. *Journal of Men's Studies, 3*(2), 127–135.

Jaffe, H. (1997, September). Dying for dollars. *Men's Health*, p. 134.

Johnson, J. V., Stewart, W., Hall, E. H., Fredlund, P., & Theorell, T. (1996). Long-term psychological work environment and cardiovascular mortality among Swedish men. *American Journal of Public Health, 86*(3), 324–331.

Kaufman, K., & Gregory, W. (2007). Discriminators of complementary and alternative medicine provider use among men with HIV/AIDS. *American Journal of Health Behavior, 31*(6), 591–601.

Keane, H. (2005). Diagnosing the male steroid user: Drug use, body image and disordered masculinity. *Health, 9*(2), 189–208.

Kinkade, S. (1999, May 1). Testicular cancer. *American Family Physician, 59*(9), 2539–2544.

Koshti-Richman, A. (1996). The role of nurses in promoting testicular self-examination. *Nursing Times, 92*(33), 40–41.

Men's Health Network. (2008). *Men's health network*. Retrieved November 13, 2008, from www.menshealthnetwork.org

Miniclier, K. (2002). Coal miners dig for pay, perks: Workers at Rangeley site brush aside issue of danger. *Denver Post*, August 25, p. B01.

Montville, L. (1999, August 9). Tour de Amerique. *Sports Illustrated, 91*(5), 68–72.

National Center for Health Statistics. (2002). *Health, United States, 2002, with chartbook on trends in the health of Americans*. Hyattsville, MD: Department of Health and Human Services.

National Kidney and Urologic Disease Information Clearinghouse. (2008). *Impotence*. Retrieved November 13, 2008, from http://kidney.niddk.nih.gov.

Nelson, D. E., Tomar, S. L., Mowery, P., & Siegel, P. Z. (1996). Trends in smokeless tobacco use among men in four states, 1988 through 1993. *American Journal of Public Health, 86*(9), 1300–1303.

Nguyen, M. N., Otis, J., & Potvin, L. (1996). Determinants of intention to adopt a low-fat diet in men 30 to 60 years old: Implications for heart health promotion. *American Journal of Health Promotion, 10*(3), 201–207.

Paduch, D. (2006). Testicular cancer and male infertility. *Current Opinion in Urology, 16*(6), 419–427.

Parker, D. (2002). Hazardous job workers learn to live with fear. *Corpus Christi Caller-Times*, August 11, p. H1.

Pattison, A. (1998). *The M factor: Men and their health*. East Roseville, NSW: Simon & Schuster.

Pease, B. (1997). Masculinity and health: The emotional and physical costs of dominance. In B. Pease (Ed.), *Men and sexual politics: Towards a profeminist practice*. Adelaide: Dulwich Centre Publications.

Peate, I. (1997). Clinical. Testicular cancer. The importance of effective health education. *British Journal of Nursing, 6*(6), 311–316.

Pettersson, A., Richiardi, L., Nordenskjold, A., Kaijser, M., & Akre, O. (2007). Age at surgery for undescended testis and risk of testicular cancer. *New England Journal of Medicine, 356*(18), 1835–1841.

Poppius, E., Virkkunen, H., Hakama, M., & Tenkanen, L. (2008). The sense of coherence and risk of injuries: Role of alcohol consumption and occupation. *Journal of Epidemiology & Community Health, 62*(1), 35–41.

Power, M., & Schulkin, J. (2008). Sex differences in fat storage, fat metabolism, and the health risks from obesity: Possible evolutionary origins. *The British Journal of Nutrition, 99*(5), 931–940.

Roman, S., & Carroll, S. (2003). Migrant farmworkers live their lives in shadows. *Sarasota Herald-Tribune*, January 16, p. A1.

Rosella, J. D. (1994). Testicular cancer health education: An integrative review. *Journal of Advanced Nursing, 20*(4), 666–671.

Rynerson, B. C., & Fishel, A. H. (1998). Expressions of men who batter: Implications for nursing. *Journal of the American Psychiatric Nurses Association, 4*(2), 41–47.

Sabo, D., & Gordon, D. F. (1995). Rethinking men's health and illness. In D. Sabo & D. F. Gordon (Eds.), *Men's health and illness: Gender, power, and the body* (p. 21). London: Sage.

Schappert, S. M. (1997). Ambulatory care visits to physician offices, hospital outpatient departments, and emergency departments: United States 1995. *Vital Health Statistics, 13*(129).

Steenbergh, T., Whelan, J., Meyers, A., Klesges, R., & DeBon, M. (2008). Gambling and health risk-taking behavior in a military sample. *Military Medicine, 173*(5), 452–459.

Stillion, J. (1995). Premature death among males. In D. Sabo & D. F. Gordon (Eds.), *Men's health and illness: Gender, power, and the body* (pp. 47–67). London: Sage.

Stoltenberg, S., Batien, B., & Birgenheir, D. (2008). Does gender moderate associations among impulsivity and health-risk behaviors? *Addictive Behaviors, 33*(2), 252–265.

Tanne, J. H. (1997). Medicine's new motto: One sex does not fit all. *American Health For Women, 16*(5), 54–58.

Testicular cancer—What to look for. (1999, May 1). *American Family Physician, 59*(9), 2549–2550.

Thornton, J. (2004). Driving while male. *Men's Health, 19*(7), 96–99.

Torres, J. B. (1998). Masculinity and gender roles among Puerto Rican men: Machismo on the US mainland. *American Journal of Orthopsychiatry, 68*(1), 16–26.

Treadwell, H. M., & Ro, M. (2003). Poverty, race, and the invisible men. *American Journal of Public Health, 93*(5), 705–707.

Walbrecker, J. (1995, January). Start talking about testicular cancer. *RN*, pp. 34–35.

Waldron, I. (1995). Contributions of changing gender differences in behavior and social roles to changing gender differences in mortality. In D. Sabo & D. F. Gordon (Eds.), *Men's health and illness: Gender, power, and the body* (pp. 22–35). London: Sage.

Wigle, D., Turner, M., Gomes, J., & Parent, M. (2008). Role of hormonal and other factors in human prostate cancer. *Journal of Toxicology & Environmental Health: Part B, 11*(3/4), 242–259.

Will, H. (1998). Better to die than cry? A longitudinal and constructionist study of masculinity and the health risk behavior of young American men. Doctoral dissertation, University of California at Berkeley. *Dissertation Abstracts International, 59*(08A), (publication number AAT 9902042).

Williams, D. (2008). The health of men: Structured inequalities and opportunities. *American Journal of Public Health, 98*, S150–S157.

Woloshin, S., Schwartz, L., & Welch, H. (2008). The risk of death by age, sex, and smoking status in the United States: Putting health risks in context. *Journal of the National Cancer Institute, 100*(12), 845–853.

# CHAPTER 34
# Children's Health

Carole Hanks, Harriet Kitzman, and Lorrie Yoos

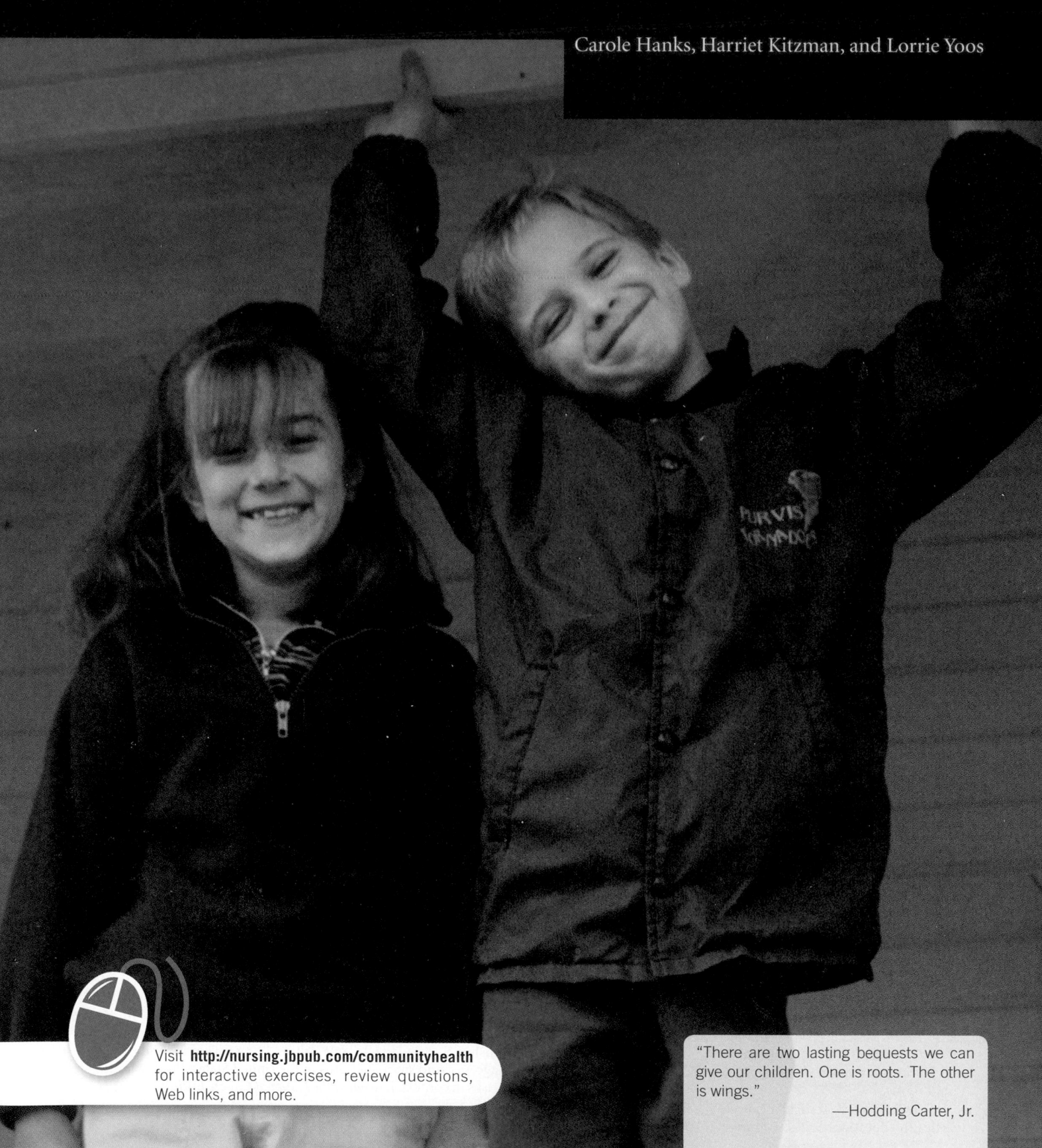

Visit **http://nursing.jbpub.com/communityhealth** for interactive exercises, review questions, Web links, and more.

"There are two lasting bequests we can give our children. One is roots. The other is wings."

—Hodding Carter, Jr.

Ring-a-round o'roses
A pocket full of posies,
A-tishoo! A-tishoo!
We all fall down.

Old English children's rhyme that dates back to the Great Plagues refers to the "rosy rash"; "posies" of herbs were kept in pockets as protection from the disease, and sneezing was often a final, fatal symptom with resulting death and "falling down."

—*The Oxford Dictionary of Nursery Rhymes*

You have most likely heard this children's rhyme throughout your childhood. Until the last century, children were at greatest risk of dying from infectious diseases. How have the changes in antibiotics and vaccines affected children's health care in the twentieth and twenty-first centuries? What are the vulnerabilities of children today as compared to those in "Ring Around the Rosies"? Are there some that are still the same?

## CHAPTER FOCUS

**Improving Children's Health: Working with Families**
- Preventing Mother and Infant Deaths
- Immunizing Children
- Preventing Childhood Injuries
- Promoting Children's Mental Health

**Selected Nursing Interventions**
- Transition from Hospital to Home
- Weaving Spirituality into Nursing Interventions
- School-Based Programs
- Home-Based Programs

**Improving Children's Health: Systems of Care**

**Ecology of Children's Health: Contexts for Growth and Development**
- Poverty
- Neighborhood Contexts
- Parents' Work Context
- Childcare Context
- Public Policy Context

## QUESTIONS TO CONSIDER

After reading this chapter, you will know the answers to the following questions:

1. What is the significance of the infant mortality rate in the assessment of a community's health?
2. What are three common health problems of children?
3. How is chronic disease manifested in children?
4. How are risk-taking behaviors of adolescents related to health?

5. What are common behavioral problems that have health consequences during adolescence?
6. What is the scope of maltreatment of children in the United States?
7. What is the ecology of child health?
8. What are delivery of care issues related to child health?
9. How does the role of the community health nurse in child health differ from the acute care setting?

## KEY TERMS

Children's Defense Fund
Externalizing behaviors
Individuals with Disabilities Education Act (IDEA)

Mild mental retardation
Multi-systemic therapy model
The Nurse–Family Partnership

Recidivism
System of care

Temporary Assistance to Needy Families (TANF)

COMMUNITY HEALTH NURSES have traditionally had a strong focus on children's health. In the early twentieth century, nurses from settlement houses taught immigrant families how to care for their children. In the twenty-first century, community nurses are involved in many programs addressing children's health, from giving immunizations, to helping communities identify unmet needs, to finding ways to improve the health of mothers and infants as members of local child fatality review (CFR) teams.

It makes sense for a society to be child centered. In European nations, where the "aging" of the population is even more marked than in the United States, it is national policy to provide extra resources to families with newborns and young children. For example, the French government provides paid pregnancy and infancy leaves for mothers, stipends for each additional child, and free preschools. As a result, France has some of the best health outcomes in the world, including a longer life expectancy and a lower infant mortality rate than the United States and most post-industrialized nations.

To some degree, focusing on children's health is self-serving for adults: Children are the wage-earners of the future. But children's health is more important to a thriving nation than just having new young workers to pay taxes. If children are not healthy in the broadest sense—physically healthy, but also well-educated, mentally healthy, competent citizens—then a nation lacks future leaders, scientists, and parents capable of continuously renewing human capital.

Community nurses use all of the themes presented in this text, but especially upstream programming, family, environmental health, and systems of care, to plan and carry out effective child health programs. In many states, public health nursing is changing from providing direct services, such as well-child clinics, to assessing community needs and resources, developing policies to improve population health, and assuring the quality and accessibility of health services. This change in roles from direct care to population-based care offers nurses an opportunity to lead the community in providing comprehensive, excellent services addressing children's physical, mental, spiritual, and social health.

The chapter has three sections. The first section addresses progress in improving children's health at the individual and family levels. The *Healthy People 2010* goals

Father's involvement with babies is a critical part of healthy development.

for children and family health focus on salient, preventable children's diseases and causes of death, especially those that unfairly affect children of certain social classes, races, or ethnicities. Stories of successful nursing interventions—many of them related to the 2010 goals for children—confirm the promise of upstream or preventive measures. These stories bring to life how nursing research and practice in the community or in the transition from hospital to home address common childhood illnesses.

The second section of this chapter addresses systems of care for children—not only the health care system, but also systems of justice, welfare, education, and public housing. Surprisingly, in addition to the large number of children whose parents are involved with the justice system, 7% to 9% of U.S. children aged 10 to 17—nearly one out of 10—are arrested every year (Office of Justice Programs, 2006). Knowledge of systems of care helps community health nurses find resources and coordinate care.

Finally, the third section considers the contexts or settings other than the family that make a difference in children's health. The home and the family context are most important to children, but nurses must attend to the health consequences of other contexts. The air children breathe, their parents' workplaces, neighborhoods, and public policy all affect children's health and development.

## Improving Childrens' Health: Working with Families

Community health nurses must always see the child both as an individual and as a member of a family. Our society tries to balance the right of the family to make decisions for children against older children's rights for self-determination and against society's responsibility to keep children safe. Ideally, families will understand and meet their children's needs on their own. Unfortunately, at least 23 of every 1,000 children, or 2% of children, experience maltreatment, including neglect and physical, emotional, and sexual abuse (DHHS Healthy People 2010). Economic stress on families, such as occurs in single-parent and low-income families, increases the risk of abuse or neglect of children.

🏛 **HEALTHY PEOPLE 2010**
**Objectives Related to Children**

**Maternal, Infant, and Child Death**
16.1  Reduce the rate of child death.

**Immunizations and Infectious Disease:**
**Vaccination Coverage and Strategies**
12.44  Achieve and maintain effective vaccination coverage levels for universally recommended vaccines among young children.

**Mental Health and Mental Disorder:**
**Treatment Expansion**
18.7  Increase the proportion of children with mental health problems who receive treatment.

**Overweight and Obesity**
19.3c  Reduce the proportion of children and adolescents who are overweight or obese.

When families need support in meeting a child's health and development needs, the nurse's approach to the family is important. Nurses should spend the time needed to create a partnership with the family using a warm, nonjudgmental approach. When families feel threatened and defensive, use your nursing knowledge and experience of adult health to open doors. Remember that by showing interest and concern for parents, nurses can "get in the door" to address the child's needs.

As a result of our sometimes contradictory values—family privacy and children's safety, for example—the United States has more violence against children than any developed country. Two of the nursing interventions discussed later in the chapter—nurse home visits and nurse-run parenting clinics—show promise in helping parents decrease harsh parenting and foster their children's safety, growth, and development.

Discrepancies in health outcomes between racial or ethnic groups within the United States, and between the United States and other countries, led to a government task force setting the 2010 goals for health. The *Healthy People 2010* box lists some of these goals for infants and pregnant women. The bar charts show differences between race/ethnicities in infants' and pregnant women's mortality. For example, black infants are twice as likely to die as white infants. Few women die during childbirth, but black women are more than three times as likely to die as white women.

### ■ Preventing Mother and Infant Deaths

While there has been progress in meeting the *Healthy People 2010* goals to decrease mother and baby deaths, there is still work to do, particularly in decreasing health disparities among children of different ethnic and socioeconomic groups. Some health researchers believe that disparities such as the difference in infant mortality between blacks and other groups suggest a need for more social justice in access

Mothers and babies during the first half of the twentieth century were at a greater risk for dying from acute infection.

■■ **CULTURAL CONNECTION**

Youths who identify themselves with the "Goth" culture may be more at risk for suicide attempts and self-mutilation than those in the general population of adolescents. Research is not clear on whether participation in the Goth culture leads to self-destructive behavior or whether adolescents with more tendencies gravitate toward the Goth culture. Goth culture is defined as "a dark and sinister aesthetic, with aficionados conspicuous by the range of distinctive clothing and makeup and tastes in music." A recent British study found that self-identification with a Goth subculture was associated with a 14-fold increase in the risk for self-harming behavior and a 16-fold increase in the risk for suicide attempts as compared with non-Goth youth. These findings held true even after adjusting for other known predictive factors, such as being female, having divorced or separated parents, smoking, drug use, and depression. Goth identification remained the single strongest predictor of self-harm and suicide attempt. ◯

*Source*: Young, R. (April 13, 2006). Prevalence of deliberate self-harm and attempted suicide within contemporary Goth youth subculture: A longitudinal cohort study. *British Medical Journal*, 10. 1136/bmj.38790.495544.7C.

to basic resources—better access for minorities to good jobs and education, not just more health care.

Nurses have traditionally been strong advocates of social justice. You can learn more about these issues by doing community participatory research about local causes of disparities in child health outcomes. For more background information on racial and ethnic health disparities, start at the Maternal and Child Health Library (www.mchlibrary. info), which has several "knowledge paths" including one on racial and ethnic disparities in health.

### ■ Immunizing Children

Another *Healthy People 2010* goal focuses on childhood immunizations. Vaccines are the true "miracle drugs." Before the polio vaccine became available in 1955, summers were a time of terror for parents. A child's neck ache could turn into paralyzing polio overnight. As well as preventing suffering, childhood immunizations save billions of dollars in health-related and other expenditures.

The *Haemophilus influenzae* B (HIB) vaccine is one of the newest vaccines. Today, more than 90% of U.S. infants receive three doses by 2 years of age. Prior to wide use of this vaccine, hundreds of infants were hospitalized with severe *Haemophilus* infections, such as meningitis, epiglottitis, pneumonia, and cellulitis. The HIB vaccine alone saves about $3.50 in medical and nonmedical costs for every $1 spent on manufacturing and giving the vaccine to children (Zhou, Bisgard, Hussain, Deuson, Bath, & Murphy, 2002).

The 2010 goals for vaccine coverage have been met for four out of seven recommended vaccinations of children aged 19 to 35 months: HIB, hepatitis B, measles–mumps–rubella (MMR), and polio (U.S. Department of Health and Human Services, 2007). Despite these vaccine success stories, we cannot let our guard down. For example, more than 11,000 cases of whooping cough (pertussis) were reported in 2003.

Tips for increasing immunization levels and other vaccine information can be found at the website of the Immunization Action Coalition (http://www.immunize.org). The Centers for Disease Control and Prevention site (http://www.cdc.gov) also has up-to-date information on vaccines and immunization schedules.

### ■ Preventing Childhood Injuries

A *Healthy People 2010* goal is to reduce the number of older children dying. After age 1, the most common cause of child death is injury. While rates of childhood injuries have

**ENVIRONMENTAL CONNECTION**

We must protect the forests for our children, grandchildren, and children yet to be born. We must protect the forests for those who can't speak for themselves such as the birds, animals, fish, and trees.

—Qwatsinas (Hereditary Chief Edward Moody),
Nuxalk Nation

**ETHICAL CONNECTION**

Parents who practice certain religions may choose not to immunize their children and instead homeschool them to avoid the school-mandated schedule of required immunizations. How do you feel about this practice? How does it affect public health in the community?

dropped over the last decade, injury is still a leading cause of death from infancy to adolescence. Dying due to a motor vehicle accident is the number one cause of all such injury deaths. Safety restraints appropriate to the age and size of the child can save lives, but the family must make their use a habit at all times.

The racial and gender disparities in child deaths send a compelling message that we must act to prevent violent deaths. Black adolescents and young men are nearly twice as likely to die as their peers of other races. As we will discuss later in this chapter, school and neighborhood violence pose a mental and physical health threat to all children.

### ■ Promoting Children's Mental Health

The 2010 goal for improved mental health for children is as important as the goals for improving children's physical health. Surveys estimate that 20% of children have mental health problems, but fewer than half of those children receive treatment for the problem. Mental health problems that are not treated in childhood do not just go away; many tend to linger or even flare up and become more serious in adulthood. Mental health problems such as depression are among the most costly health problem for adults, due to loss of wages as well as the cost of care.

Clearly, there is a lot of work to be done to protect and improve children's physical and mental health. In this work it is important to see the child in an ecological framework. Children's physical and mental health is affected by factors at many levels: biological, family, neighborhood, and national

The health of an infant is greatly influenced by the ability of the mother to meet the infant's security needs.

health policy. The book *From Neurons to Neighborhoods*, published by the Institute of Medicine in 2000, has this ecological view of child development. This book told parents and professionals that young children need early emotional responsiveness and spoken language from their parents as well as protection from neighborhood violence. The third section of this chapter more specifically addresses the ecological factors that affect children's health and development.

## Selected Nursing Interventions

The excitement of being a community health nurse is best communicated by learning about real nurses who have created and carried out programs addressing common child health problems at various ages and in various community settings. Two examples of interventions specifically focused on mental health and child development are presented here. However, nurses also address mental health and development when intervening with children with any physical illness, such as asthma or cancer.

### ■ Transition from Hospital to Home

The transition from hospital to home is an opportunity for community health nurses to improve children's health. Children are rarely hospitalized, but when they are, the nurse must prevent long-term physical or mental health effects from the trauma of illness and being in strange surroundings. Two nurses have had important impacts on this transition. Dorothy Brooten and colleagues (1986) asked why healthy, but low-birth-weight infants were being kept

#### ✎ NOTE THIS! •──────

Melanoma—the most serious and potentially deadly form of skin cancer—was until recently almost unheard of in children. The incidence of pediatric melanoma, while still rare, has risen from 3 per million in 1982 to 7 per million in 2002, according to the National Cancer Institute. Recent studies have also reported increases in England, Sweden, and Australia. Although the reasons for the increase are uncertain, many researchers speculate that depletion of the ozone layer might be allowing children to be exposed to more of the sun's damaging ultraviolet radiation. Other factors may be excessive sun exposure and blistering sunburns in early childhood and use of tanning beds. The rate of melanoma has more than doubled among adults as well.

Melanoma is often missed in children, not only because of its rarity but also because of its very different appearance than in adults. Melanoma in children comprises lighter-colored lesions that have well-defined borders. Also, unlike adults, most children presenting with melanoma have no family history of the disease. ◣

in the hospital so long. She and her colleagues then designed a research study that answered this question and changed the protocols for keeping low-birth-weight children in the hospital. In their work, these researchers found that, as long as the infant had no serious complications, parents with support and instruction from advanced practice nurses could provide care at home at less cost and less distress for the infant and the parents.

Another nurse, Bernadette Melynk, identified the need to support, educate, and involve parents of sick children in their children's care. In her evaluation of Creating Opportunities for Parent Empowerment (COPE), Melynk and her colleagues (2004) found that when parents of low-birth-weight infants or children needing intensive hospital care for other reasons received preventive educational–behavioral support from specially trained nurses, fewer child adjustment problems (such as post-traumatic stress disorder) occurred when children went home.

Nursing interventions for chronically, as well as acutely, ill children also address the transition from hospital to home. Cancer is a serious chronic illness that kills more children than any cause other than injuries. Pamela Hinds and her colleagues (2001) at St. Jude Children's Research Hospital in Memphis value improving the quality of life for children, even when they have incurable cancer. As well as inquiring into ways to support nurses who work with very sick and dying children, these nurses developed guidelines to involve adolescents and their parents in making decisions about their care. These nurses concluded that adolescent patients want to know about their treatment and are able and willing to help make decisions. The research team published guidelines to help nurses in the hospital or the community give the best quality of care from diagnosis to end-of-life decision making (Hinds et al., 2001).

### ■ Weaving Spirituality into Nursing Interventions

Nursing interventions are an excellent place to address children and spirituality. Hinds and her colleagues found that both parents and children identified "religious beliefs" as "belief in a god and the certainty of life after death" as

#### ◉ MEDIA MOMENT

Each day, most 8- to 18-year-olds spend an average of 4 hours watching television, videos, and DVDs; more than 1 hour on the computer; and about 50 minutes playing video games. ◣

### Got an Alternative?

Yoga and tai chi can be effectively used as stress-relieving exercises as well as flexibility-enhancing interventions for children.

important factors in making an end-of-life decision. The 31 factors considered by physicians in making end-of-life decisions addressed staff recommendations, family preferences, therapeutic options, and the family and child's comfort and preferences, but not spiritual issues. This indicates that caregivers may often not help children and their parents explore and integrate their spiritual beliefs into the care plan.

Children, like adults, see themselves as part of a narrative or a story with meaning. While considering the child's developmental stage and respecting religious and cultural beliefs, the nurse can help the child tell his or her own story and find meaning not just in the stress of illness or violence, but also in the joy of living. By asking a few questions appropriate for the child's developmental age, the nurse can explore the child's preconceived ideas about illness or death, fears, fantasies, and concerns about separation, isolation, or death. Simple questions that might work with children or adults are "What is most important to you?", "What do you think is happening to you?", "What brings you joy?", and "What scares you?"

### ■ School-Based Programs

Community health nurses are in contact with children and can see important trends in children's health even before they become newsworthy. For example, nurses in schools and community clinics knew that children's asthma and obesity were serious problems long before official statistics confirmed the fact.

In the United States, asthma is a major cause of morbidity in children. This chronic condition affects 5.8% of children and is responsible for 25% of missed school days. The prevalence and severity of asthma have both increased in the past 20 years. From 1980 to 1996, the rates for children ages 5 to 14 years nearly doubled. Since 1996, these rates have decreased, but are still higher than those in 1980 (CDC, 2002). Although medications and therapeutic regimens to control the disease have improved, asthma continues to have devastating effects on the lives of large numbers of children and their families. The prevalence and severity of the disease are greater in African American children living in poverty and in crowded conditions (Yoos & McMullen, 1997).

Viral respiratory infections as well as exposure to specific allergens, such as cigarette and other smoke, dust mites, molds, cockroaches, and pet dander, often provoke this disease. Nurses and nurse researchers working in schools have developed and implemented asthma education programs in schools that increase adherence to prescribed medical regimens and reduce exposure to allergens (Yoos et al., 1997).

### MEDIA MOMENT

**Born into Brothels (2004)**

This Academy Award–winning documentary is a study of several unforgettable children who live in Calcutta's red-light district, where their mothers work as prostitutes. Zana Briski, a photographer documenting life in the brothels, decides to teach these children photography. They are fascinated with the camera. As they begin to record their world, the children come to a recognition of their own worth and talents.

These programs have had varying degrees of success in helping families change their lifestyles. One of the explanations for limited adherence to asthma-prevention regimens is that the disease produces intermittent symptoms. It is often difficult for families to maintain regular day-to-day prevention practices during times when the child is well.

Prevention of childhood obesity is one of the *Healthy People 2010* goals. In the 1990s, the percentage of overweight children aged 6 to 11 in the United States more than doubled and the percentage of overweight adolescents more than tripled. Nearly 15% of all school-aged children are overweight. There are also racial and ethnic disparities in these percentages, with black and Hispanic children twice as likely to be overweight as white children (Salinsky & Scott, 2003).

A nurse researcher, Margaret Grey, and her colleagues have studied the connection between childhood obesity and diabetes for many years. These nurses believe that community health nurses have a key role in identifying and addressing the lifestyle changes needed to prevent and treat childhood obesity and diabetes. These nurses understood that obesity has spiritual, physical, cultural, and psychosocial causes.

### GLOBAL CONNECTION

Teenagers in the United States weigh more than their counterparts in most other industrialized countries, and fast food availability and consumption is most likely the leading cause. According to a study of 15-year-olds in 15 developed nations, 15% of U.S. girls and nearly 14% of U.S. boys are classified as obese. The next highest numbers (5.5% of girls and almost 11% of boys) come from Greece. By comparison, only 4% of French girls and not quite 3% of French boys were obese. (Lissau, Overpeck, Ruan, Due, Holstein, & Hediger, 2004). In another study, one-third of U.S. children aged 4 to 19 were found to eat at least one fast-food meal daily and take in 187 calories more a day than those who don't, for an average of about 6 extra pounds per year (Bowman, Gortmaker, Ebbeling, Pereira, & Ludwig, 2004).

*Sources*: Lissau, I., Overpeck, M. D., Ruan, W. J., Due, P., Holstein, B. E., & Hediger, M. L. (2004). Body mass index and overweight in adolescents in 13 European countries, Israel and the United States. *Archives of Pediatric and Adolescent Medicine, 158*(1), 27–33. Bowman, S. A., Gortmaker, S. L., Ebbeling, C. B., Pereira, M. A., & Ludwig, D. S. (2004). Effects of fast-food consumption on energy intake and diet quality among children in a national household survey. *Pediatrics, 113*(1), 112–118.

| Table 34-1 | APHA Action Plan: Childhood Obesity |
|---|---|

- **Goal 1:** Increase daily physical activity among children and adolescents.
- **Goal 2:** Reduce the amount of time kids spend watching television, video games, and the Internet.
- **Goal 3:** Decrease the consumption of energy-dense, high-sugar/high-fat foods such as soda, ice cream, junk food, and fast food.
- **Goal 4:** Increase the consumption of nutritious foods such as fruits, vegetables, whole grains, and skim milk.
- **Goal 5:** Create social, monetary, and policy-driven incentives that reinforce long-term environmental and behavioral change.

*Source*: http://www2.apha.org/ppp/obesity_toolkit/005_action_plan.htm

Children are one third of our population and all of our future.

Preliminary testing of a school health program designed by Grey to address these various causes of obesity found that minority youth could increase their dietary knowledge and improve food choices resulting in lower blood sugar. Parents of the children enrolled in the program also benefited from working with the school nurses. These parents themselves made healthier nutrition choices, took more responsibility for their health, used stress management skills, and increased their physical activity (Grey, Berry, Davidson, Galasso, Gustafson, & Melkus, 2004).

The American Public Health Association (APHA) has developed an action plan to address the goal of preventing childhood obesity. Table 34-1 outlines its recommendations.

A mental health program designed by a creative community health nurse, Carolyn Webb-Stratton, focuses on elementary-school-age children with behavior problems that could escalate into antisocial behavior or crime if not addressed. This work is very important because as many as 1 out of 4 high-risk children may already exhibit aggressive, disruptive behavior in preschool. Furthermore, if these children are not helped to learn more positive behaviors, they are at high risk of adopting criminally delinquent behavior and/or dropping out of school. (Le Blanc, Swisher, Vitaro, & Tremblay, 2007).

Her work with children, teachers, and parents earned Webster-Stratton a prestigious Research Scientist Award from the National Institute of Mental Health. In a nurse-run parenting clinic, and in the schools, nurses help parents and teachers understand how to change from negative to positive teaching and parenting strategies (Webster-Stratton & Reid, 2008). It is counterintuitive to most adults, but praising children when you "catch" them behaving well works better than focusing on punishing misbehavior. Children are also taught to recognize and express their emotions, to solve problems without fighting, and to apologize and pay compliments to other children. Learning new positive social skills helps suppress children's misbehavior.

**BOX 34-2**

### Challenging Question for Students

Compare the action plan and explanation of the causes of obesity in children cited by the APHA with the areas addressed by nurse researcher Margaret Grey. Why would Grey include measures of spirituality in her school health program to decrease obesity in minority youth? What does it mean to be holistic in addressing obesity in children? How is a child's spirituality different at different ages, and how would that affect your treatment plan for an obese child?

Here are more resources on children's spirituality:

Catlin, E. A., Guillemin, J. H., Thiel, M. M., Hammond, S., Wang, M. L., & O'Donnell, J. (2001). Spiritual and religious components of patient care in the neonatal intensive care unit: Sacred themes in a secular setting. *Journal of Perinatology, 21,* 426–430

Coles, R. (1990). *The spiritual life of children.* London: Harper Collins

Smith, J. & McSherry, W. (2004). Spirituality and child development: A concept analysis. *Journal of Advanced Nursing, 45*(3), 307–315

❝*I think, at a child's birth, if a mother could ask a fairy godmother to endow it with the most useful gift, that gift would be curiosity.*❞

—Eleanor Roosevelt

### ■ Home-Based Programs

**The Nurse–Family Partnership** links low-income families with nurses who visit in the home from pregnancy until the baby is 2 years of age. These visits focus on the mother's health and life choices as well as her knowledge of child development and other needs. They not only prevent child abuse and neglect, but also improve the child's health and development. More importantly, even after the visits stop,

Video games, on television and portable devices and via computers, should be carefully monitored by parents for violent and inappropriate content as well as setting time limits on their use.

both mothers and children make wiser, healthier choices that save money in welfare and other costs. You can learn more about this program at the website of the Nurse Family Partnership (http://www.nccfc.org/nurseFamilyPartnership.cfm) or from special reports on the program on the website of the Robert Wood Johnson Foundation (http://www.rwjf.org/news/special/nurseFamily_1a.jhtml).

These kinds of programs involving community health nurses, ranging from helping tiny newborn babies move safely from the hospital to the home and visiting new mothers at home, highlight the importance of systems of care. As well as forming partnerships with families, nurses in these programs must collaborate with many other community agencies to provide holistic care. Children and their families also need resources from the justice, welfare, housing, and political systems. The next section of the chapter addresses these systems of care and explores how they affect children and offer opportunities for nursing leadership.

## Improving Children's Health: Systems of Care

Community health nurses must often intervene at the system level to assure that children receive needed and effective education, housing, economic assistance, and spiritual guidance as well as health care. The term "system of care" was coined to describe comprehensive mental health care for disabled children. We will first address the system of mental health

 NOTE THIS!

Children's illnesses—the top four causes of missed school:

1. Colds

2. Gastroenteritis ("stomach flu")

3. Conjunctivitis ("pink eye")

4. Strep throat

*Source*: The Mayo Foundation for Medical Education and Research, August 8, 2005.

care for children. We will use the term "system of care" generically to address health care, justice, education, welfare, spiritual/religious, and public housing systems.

The mental health system of care aims to bring together many agencies and service providers into a coordinated network to meet the "multiple and changing needs of children and adolescents [and their families] with severe emotional disturbances" (Stroul & Friedman, 1986, p. xx). The visionary system of care has core values that are also important to community health nurses. The values shared by systems of care and community nurses are

- Being child centered and family focused
- Being community based so that children could live at home
- Being culturally competent about racial, ethnic, and cultural differences among families
- Providing individualized services that build on the strengths of families
- Providing integrated, coordinated, effective, and efficient services
- Identifying and treating problems early (Cook & Kilmer, 2004)

These values are important but hard to achieve.

One of the oldest mental health systems is the system of services for children with disabilities funded by the **Individuals with Disabilities Education Act (IDEA)**. The Early Intervention program is part of IDEA. Early Intervention grants to each state are used for comprehensive statewide programs to work with children (and their families) from birth to age 2 with disabilities or slowed development. The expectation is that, by providing early intervention measures such as physical therapy and developmental child care, children will be less likely to have permanent disabilities with the attendant extra human and financial costs. This system of screening, diagnosis, and treatment for infants and young children is run by different agencies in different states. You can find out which government agencies have grants at the website of the National Early Childhood Technical Assistance Center (www.NECTAC.org).

IDEA is more than just early intervention. Public law No. 94-142 (Education for All Handicapped Children, now known as Individuals with Disabilities Act [IDEA]) was first passed in 1975 and was most recently reauthorized by Congress in 2004. IDEA covers children with disabilities ranging from Down syndrome to attention-deficit/hyperactivity disorder (ADHD) from birth to age 18. The public school system is responsible for providing educational and assistive services to children from age 3 to age 18. Parents, sometimes the child, and school representatives meet to set goals for the child and to agree on which special resources the school

**"***Common sense is the collection of prejudices acquired by age eighteen.***"**

—*Albert Einstein*

**❝***Naked or clothed, you walk with a dignity and grace that only comes from having been cherished.***❞**

—Anne Rice

must provide to ensure that the child has the best chance of meeting his or her educational and developmental goals.

In most states, mental health systems of care focus on children already diagnosed with serious mental health problems such as emotional disturbance. Except for early identification of children with developmental delays, the concept of "upstream programming" is rare in the mental health system. There are two main reasons that mental health care is usually remediation-based, rather than preventive, care: Mental health care is stigmatized and poorly funded.

For many persons, there is a negative stigma connected with seeking mental health care. Depression, obsessive thoughts, and oppositional behavior are often considered personal weaknesses rather than illnesses that can be treated with medications or counseling. Consequently, parents may not want to get care for their mental health problems even when those problems also harm family relationships. Perhaps because of this stigma, policy makers do not believe that mental health care should be funded on an equal basis with physical health care.

The Commonwealth Fund (Leatherman & McCarthy, 2004) reports that, in any given year, 20% of U.S. children aged 6 to 17 years need mental health care for serious problems. Fewer than half of the children needing care actually receive it, however. This problem is equally shared by children of all races and ethnicities. In fact, children on Medicaid public insurance are *more* likely than privately insured children to receive developmental and mental health screening (Kataoka et al., 2002).

Evaluations of the impact of creating a formal interagency system of care for severely emotionally disturbed children have yielded mixed results. The children served by these systems have significant functional impairment at home and school. They have diagnoses of one or more of the following: ADHD, oppositional defiant disorder, conduct disorder, and/or depression (often bipolar). The families of these children often have economic, social, mental, and legal problems. Many agencies, as well as informal helpers such as churches and neighbors, must work together to help these families and children. While there was variation across community sites where systems of care were funded and put in place, overall the outcomes were no better for children provided with services from a formal system of care (Cook & Kilmer, 2004) compared to children with usual community care.

**❝***My heart is singing for joy this morning! A miracle has happened! The light shone upon my little pupil's mind, and behold, all things are changed!***❞**

—Anne Sullivan, teacher of Helen Keller

**⬤ NOTE THIS! ⬤**

The Child Health Insurance Program (CHIP) was approved in 1997 by the U.S. government to cover uninsured children whose families earn too much to qualify for Medicaid. More than a dozen states have expanded the program, which also insures about 693,000 adults.

The explanation for the lack of improved outcomes in these funded interagency systems of care for severely emotionally disturbed children and their families is unclear. Traditionally, community agencies have had their own unique cultures and are accustomed to working alone. It takes skilled leadership to create long-term collaboration among agencies.

There may be more hope in single agencies using multiple therapists to address all the problems of these children and families. In the **multi-systemic therapy model** (Henggeler, 2003), one agency works intensively with families and connects them with other community resources. This model has improved children's school performance, kept more children living at home, decreased substance abuse, and improved families functioning.

There may be a take-home lesson from these efforts for community health nurses trying to create coordinated, integrated systems of care for children. Groups of agencies and informal helpers can learn to work together by solving specific, immediate problems of a real family in crisis. Trying to reform a system by convening meetings to address abstract needs of generic families may not lead to efficient collaboration among agencies. In other words, community systems seem to learn to work together using inductive, bottom-up processes rather than top-down, deductive processes.

It is an easy transition from talking about children in the mental health system for children to talking about other systems of care and children. Mental health is an important factor in the justice, school, health care, welfare, and public housing systems:

- Most of the children in the justice system have mental health problems.
- School systems are the largest providers of mental health services for children.
- Mental health problems increase the cost of care for physical health problems.

**❝***We cannot fashion our children after our desires; we must have them and love them as God has given them to us.***❞**

—Johann Wolfgang von Goethe

**❝***Your children are not your children. They are the sons and daughters of Life's longing for itself. They came through you, but not from you, and though they are with you, yet they belong not to you.***❞**

—Kahlil Gibran

- Medicaid public insurance for poor children covers more mental health services than most private insurance.
- Public housing systems provide housing specifically for homeless mentally ill persons because it is nearly impossible for them to get well without safe housing.

When systems of care work well for children, they are efficient, comprehensive, and just. Unfortunately, systems, like individuals, can get "stuck" and fail to adopt the best practices or to meet new and growing needs of those who depend on them. For example, starting in 1970 the justice system began punishing juvenile offenders with rough, scare tactics and "adult punishment for adult crimes." More juvenile offenders who are sent to boot camps or to adult jails end up being chronic criminals than those who receive more developmentally appropriate support and guidance (Peters, Thomas, & Zamberlan, 1997).

It is hard to know the exact number of children arrested or the percentage of crimes attributed to juveniles. The juvenile justice system in the United States is actually 51 separate systems in each state and the District of Columbia. One report estimates that more than 100,000 youths are incarcerated on any given day. Juvenile arrests have been declining since the 1980s, whereas adult arrests have continued to increase. However, four times as many youths are stopped,

"You are worried about seeing him spending his early years in doing nothing. What! Is it nothing to be happy? Nothing to skip, play, and run around all day long? Never in his life will he be so busy again."
—Jean Jacques Rousseau, 1762

 *If women ruled the world, there would be greater attention to issues involving women and children.*
—Former U.S. Attorney General Janet Reno

✐ NOTE THIS! •—————————————

Children raised with pets are less allergic. In one study, children who were raised in households with two or more dogs or cats in infancy were about half as likely to develop common allergies as children who had no pets in the home. Research found that the group exposed to animals had fewer positive skin tests to both indoor allergens (e.g., pet dander, dust mites) and outdoor allergens (e.g., ragweed, grass). The children exposed to cats and dogs were almost half as likely to have hyperresponsive and easily irritated airways—a risk factor for asthma. Researchers propose that the difference may lie in endotoxins, the breakdown products of bacteria found in the animals' mouth. These endotoxins are thought to force the body's immune system into developing a response pattern that is less likely to lead to allergic reactions. ◢

*Source*: Ownby, D. R., Johnson, C. C., & Peterson, E. L. (2002). Exposure to dogs and cats in the first year of life and risk of allergic sensitization at 6 to 7 years of age. *Journal of the American Medical Association, 288*(8), 963–972.

interrogated, and searched than are actually arrested. Minority youth, and particularly black males, are stopped and arrested at higher rates than other youth. More than half of all incarcerated youth have a severe mental disorder such as conduct disorder, depression, ADHD, learning disability, post-traumatic stress disorder, or developmental disability. Such disorders contribute to risky or violent behaviors leading to arrest. There is little or no treatment for mental disorders in the juvenile system; indeed, the harsh conditions found there often exacerbate these disorders.

Intensive treatment of mental disorders and problem behaviors aimed at the child and the family can divert the child from incarceration and prevent further criminal behaviors. Harsh, punitive treatment, which occurs when a child is forced to move to the adult justice system for serious crimes, usually increases **recidivism** or chances of rearrest and more jail time.

Community health nurses may feel helpless to change this situation or even to continue contact with youthful patients who happen to be arrested and incarcerated. The National Mental Health Association provides descriptions of programs aimed at children involved with the juvenile justice system (http://www.nmha.org/children/justjuv/index.cfm). It also provides descriptions of programs that do not work. Sharing knowledge of best practices in juvenile justice with parents and politicians is a first step to changing the juvenile justice system where you practice.

School systems usually have their own health component. Even without designated health programs, schools are so central to children's healthy growth and development that the community health nurse must collaborate with this system. The "health" program at a school can vary from a

**Antique Doll**

Hair set with sugar
Face painted
Brittle she waits

Patient in the dark room
Petals are lost
From the wedding bouquet

Children are grown
More children are on the way
The house fills with sound

For a brief span
Time will pass more rapidly.

—*Ann Thedford Lanier*

secretary handing out Band-Aids to a comprehensive program with the following standards set by the CDC:

- Community based
- Integrated within and supportive of the educational system
- Managed by a qualified nursing leader who is integrated into the school administrative structure as part of the management team
- Advised by a school and community group, including parents and students
- Based on accepted standards, regulations, and statutes
- Supported by a health service management information system
- Offering a range of prevention and treatment services, including tobacco control
- Implemented by sufficient numbers of qualified school nurses and support personnel during the entire school day
- Culturally competent and linguistically relevant
- Coordinated with the eight components of a comprehensive school health program, as defined by the CDC: health education, health services, social and physical environment, physical education, guidance and support services, food service, school and worksite health promotion, and integrated school and community health promotion
- Linked with community primary care, mental health and dental health providers, local youth and family serving agencies, local and state public health and emergency providers, and public insurance outreach programs
- Making maximum use of available public and nonpublic funds (e.g., Municipal Medicaid, grants, insurance reimbursement, business partnerships, Foundation Budget, Community Benefits Program)
- Evaluated regularly to determine its effectiveness and efficiency

 **THINK ABOUT THIS**

Children exposed to high levels of secondhand smoke score 7 points lower on standardized tests than those exposed to little or no smoke (www.cdc.gov).

School clinics are becoming more common. Those clinics were first implemented in high schools, but can now be found in middle and elementary schools. While children must have their parents' permission to receive care from a school clinic, these clinics increase access to health care and improve school attendance and school performance. Evaluations of school clinics show that they can decrease emergency room use (Key, Washington, & Hulsey, 2002), improve immunization coverage, promote responsive sexuality, and identify serious untreated health problems ranging from asthma to heart disease.

Unfortunately, community health nurses seldom work in or with the school systems unless they are school employees. Providing a continuing nursing education program or collaborating on a school health fair is a great way to break the ice and start working together. If you can collaborate with the school system, you will have access to all but the youngest children in your community. There are wonderful opportunities for health promotion and health education with school children.

Health care systems are addressed in Chapter 2. The community nurse focusing on child health should remember that almost all divisions of the health care system are potential partners in promoting health and preventing disease in children. Home health agencies have child patients with

### Research Alert

This study looked at the protective effectiveness of speed bumps in reducing child pedestrian injuries in residential neighborhoods. A matched case-control study design was conducted over a 5-year period among children seen in a pediatric emergency department after being struck by an automobile. A multivariate conditional logistic regression analysis showed that speed bumps were associated with lower odds of children being injured within their neighborhood and being struck in front of their home. Children living within a block of a speed bump had significantly lower odds of being struck. Living within a block of a speed bump was associated with a roughly two-fold reduction in the odds of injury within one's neighborhood. This protective effect was even more pronounced among the subset of children who were injured on the block immediately in front of their house.

*Source*: Tester, J. M., Rutherford, G. W., Wald, Z., & Rutherford, M. W. (2004). A matched case-control study evaluating the effectiveness of speed humps in reducing child pedestrian injuries. *American Journal of Public Health, 94*(4), 646–649.

diagnoses ranging from cancer to cerebral palsy. Occasionally children must be placed in nursing homes when their families can no longer care for them at home. To care for children in the transition from hospital to home, the community nurse must have contacts with local hospitals to receive referrals when children are discharged.

The last two systems of care addressed here are essential resources for low-income children and their families. There resources are not thought of as health resources, but a child cannot be healthy and develop well if the family has no money for food and other essentials or if the family does not have a safe place to live. The human services or welfare department has traditionally provided financial assistance to poor families. The Housing and Urban Development (HUD) agency oversees most of the publicly owned housing in the United States as well as a program that discounts the amount of rent paid in private housing.

In 1996, drastic changes were made in a cash-payment program formerly called Aid to Families with Dependent Children (AFDC). In addition to changing its name to Temporary Assistance to Needy Families (TANF), the program was redesigned to provide only short-term cash assistance while adults in the family were getting education and/or job placement help so that they would support themselves. There are many requirements for families receiving cash assistance. Adults must be looking for work, in school, or in some other worthy endeavor such as job training or volunteering to keep getting assistance. Furthermore, adults must immediately report changes of address and income or risk losing their cash grant or even being prosecuted.

At the same time that AFDC was abolished, Medicaid health insurance was separated from the cash grant system. While the federal government provides part of the money to pay for Medicaid insurance, each state must also fund a portion of this publicly funded insurance. Two-thirds of the Medicaid-insured population are poor children and their families; the other third are low-income elderly or disabled adults. Medicaid is one of the largest expenses of state governments and is frequently seen as a place to cut benefits.

☞ THINK ABOUT THIS ········································

Leaving children alone in vehicles can result in death from overheating and injuries from power windows. A 2002 report by the Centers for Disease Control and Prevention found that at least 9,000 children younger than age 14 were injured in vehicle-related incidents between July 2000 and July 2001 (www.cdc.gov). Additionally, Kids and Cars (www.kidsandcars.org) reported 213 child fatalities from nontraffic incidents in 2005, which is a 29% increase over the previous year. The American Nurses Association, along with its member state constituents, is supporting the Ad Council's national campaign to make people aware of the dangers through a national campaign, similar to the ones on preventing forest fire and promoting designated drivers. ▲

As a community health nurse interested in children, you should know that the one-third of patients who are elderly or disabled adults account for two-thirds of the costs incurred by Medicaid programs. One of the largest costs of Medicaid is elderly people who use this insurance to pay for care in nursing homes. Compared to the cost of nursing home care, children's health care is inexpensive.

Safe housing is very important to a child's health and development. HUD agencies provide safe public housing and other services in almost every city in the country. Just as for people receiving cash assistance, there are also many rules for families living in public housing. Families must keep the apartment clean and agree to regular inspections. Families can be evicted if they allow anyone who has been convicted of dealing illegal drugs to live with them in public housing. While these rules may seem harsh, the resources are so important to family survival that adults can usually understand and follow the rules. Furthermore, there was a time when public housing projects were considered the most unsafe place to life; these harsh rules help make the needed housing option safer. The community health nurse should learn about agencies providing cash grants and housing and understand their regulations to help in providing referrals to families who need these services.

**Captured**

I saw you this morning
  holding your oldest son

Love can be captured—only the color will change

Locked inside the plastic case
  of paper and chemicals

Miniature hands grasping

He smiles up at you—mouth open for your breast.

—*Ann Thedford Lanier*

## Ecology of Children's Health: Contexts for Growth and Development

In the first section of this chapter, we addressed the family context and the need for community nurses to work as partners with families to improve children's health and development. Other, larger contexts also affect children's growth and development. The neighborhood, work, and public policy contexts form the child's ecology (see Bronfenbrenner, 1979, for a discussion of the theory of human ecology) and are of particular interest for children.

### ■ Poverty

Living in the context of poverty places children at risk for poor health and developmental outcomes (Wagmiller et al., 2006). Kids Count, a project of the Annie E. Casey Foun-

Creating a healthy environment is critical to raising a healthy child. This toilet has a safety latch to prevent accidents

dation, estimates that 18% of children in the United States live in families whose income is below the federal poverty line. Nearly half of these children live in extreme poverty, which means the family of four has an annual income of less than $10,000 per year. The risks of being poor increase with single parenthood, low educational attainment, part-time employment, or low wages. The educational level of parents is a strong predictor of family income.

### Effects of Poverty on Children's Physical Health

There is evidence that family poverty and neighborhood physical and socioeconomic conditions affect a child's health status.

Low birth weight and prematurity are highly correlated with poor health status in the infancy period. Sequelae of both these conditions (neurologic damage or poor respiratory function, for example) or their treatment (retinopathy of prematurity from high concentrations of administered oxygen) may be long-lasting. There are two mechanisms of low birth weight—fetal growth retardation and preterm delivery; both are more common in low-income families and neighborhoods (Pless, 1994). Predisposing factors for fetal growth retardation include pregnancy in an adolescent or unsupported mother; intrauterine exposure to drugs, nicotine, or alcohol; intrauterine infection; maternal ill health; maternal short stature or underweight; multiple births; and fetal anomalies. Preterm deliveries are related to vaginal infections, which are in turn related to the number of sexual partners.

The chances of a child's thriving if born preterm or with low birth weight are strongly related to the socioeconomic status of the family. Factors that appear to explain why children are born at low birth weight and are more likely to die in infancy

in poverty neighborhoods include public and substandard market housing, high crime rates, single-parent and female-headed families, and high male unemployment (Anthony, Vu, & Austin, 2008; Pless, 1994). These neighborhood conditions have direct effects on the child, but also indirectly affect the child's chance of thriving by shaping the home environment (Cohen & Reutter, 2007; Klebanov, Brooks-Gunn, Chase-Lansdale, & Gordon, 1997).

Respiratory illnesses are the most common illnesses for which children seek medical care and are hospitalized. They are still important causes of death. The number of respiratory illnesses appears to be constant at 6 to 8 episodes per child per year throughout the world (Durani et al., 2008). Children living in poverty are more likely to have severe viral or bacterial infections that progress to the lower respiratory tract and cause pneumonia, bronchitis, bronchiolitis, or croup. The following factors are related to the severity of respiratory infections:

- Air pollution, both outdoor and indoor (Bateson et al., 2008)
- Crowding, particularly with many young children in a home (Collins, Kasap, & Holland, 1971)
- Malnutrition (Harsten, Prellner, & Heldrup, 1990)
- Daycare attendance (Harsten et al., 1990)

Maternal stress, perhaps by increasing the child's stress and causing related declines in immunity, increases the risk of a child's having respiratory infections (Graham, Ryan, & Douglas, 1990).

Gastroenteritis is yet another common physical illness that is more prevalent and more serious when children live in poverty and when sanitation is poor. In the United States, 10% of preventable postneonatal infant deaths are attributable to diarrhea and occur primarily in the most disadvantaged groups (Pless, 1994).

It would be expected from discussions of the increased severity of illness that the likelihood of sequelae of low birth weight and prematurity for children in poverty would have lower average reported health status. Children have have better access to health care since implementation of Medicaid in 1965, but when health status is controlled, poor children still make far fewer visits to physicians and are less likely to have a personal physician than nonpoor children (Coir & Bloom, 1994).

### Cognitive Skills in the Context of Poverty

Family and neighborhood conditions also have important influences on children's ability to take in and process information. The effects can be subtle or devastating. The presence of both biological risks and poor environmental conditions can be disastrous. Physical illness, which is more common in poor families and neighborhoods, causes a child to miss school or perform poorly when present. The combination of physical illness, stress, and living in communities where most adults are poorly educated and lack the energy, vision, and skills to spend time helping children learn can place the young child at higher risk of school failure.

As children grow, they need a stimulating environment for optimal development.

**A Good Read**

## The Secret Life of Bees
*By Sue Monk Kidd (2003)*

*Penguin Publishers, New York*

In Sue Monk Kidd's *The Secret Life of Bees*, 14-year-old Lily Owen, neglected by her father and isolated on their Georgia peach farm, spends hours imagining a blissful infancy when she was loved and nurtured by her mother, Deborah, whom she barely remembers. This coming of age story set in the turmoil of the early 1960s takes the reader on a journey with Lily and her beloved nanny, Rosaleen, to the colorful world of the Black Madonna. The search for a mother, and the need to mother oneself, are themes of this critically acclaimed bestseller. The women who take Lily and Rosaleen into their homes and hearts teach her about love, life, and beekeeping, all metaphors for healing and growing up.

We have long known that children raised in poverty are at a disadvantage at school entry (Zigler, 1967). While some claim this inequality is a result of poor genetic endowment, others fault the lack of cognitive and sensory stimulation. **Mild mental retardation** (MR) is defined as an IQ between 51 and 69. It is more prevalent in populations with lower socioeconomic status. Mild MR has no apparent biological basis and its prevalence varies widely across populations; from 5 to 12 children per 1,000 are affected. Mild MR accounts for at least one-third of school failure.

Social deprivation is related to both mild and severe mental retardation. However, unlike the wide variation in mild MR, the prevalence of severe MR has stayed in the range of 3 to 5 children per 1,000 since it was first measured by Lewis in 1929. Furthermore, there are often clear biological causes (genetic factors such as chromosomal abnormalities; infections and intoxications; conditions related to low birth weight or prematurity; and endocrine disorders) of severe MR (Pless, 1994).

In view of a lack of biological cause and variation across populations, many consider mild MR to be preventable (Pless, 1994). Early intervention programs have temporarily increased IQ by as much as 10 points in special populations of premature children and institutional populations (Head Start programs) (Olds & Kitzman, 1993). However, continuing services into the elementary school grades does appear to prolong the effects (Berlin, Brooks-Gunn, McCaron, & McCormick, 1990). Excellent preschool programs, such as the High Scope Program, can also have effects that persist into adulthood (Congressional Quarterly, 1993).

Poverty and poor neighborhoods are also the major risk factors for childhood injuries. Poor children are more than twice as likely to die from trauma as nonpoor children, and they are five times more likely to die from fires and burns (Nersesian, Petit, & Shaper, 1985; Rodgers & Payne, 2007). Poor housing, violence, high traffic volume, and lack of smoke detectors in poor neighborhoods put children at very high risk of injury.

While children are able to report their own emotional disorders, they are less able to report **externalizing behavior** such as disrupting others (Pless, 1994). Externalizing behaviors have an early onset, and without treatment or a change in environment can lead to patterns of escalating hostility between the child and adults. Children who have externalizing behaviors often have poor self-esteem as well as problems with personal and work relationships (Pless, 1994).

Interactions with adults are essential for infants and children to develop emotional and social intelligence. Risk factors for poor adult–child interactions include age and education of the mother, family dysfunction, birth order of the child, and physical illness, such as being preterm or suffering from respiratory illness. A wide variety of interventions, from mothers viewing and analyzing videotapes of themselves feeding their infant, to general social support counseling, can improve scores on social interaction. Improvement occurs most often when the professional first develops a therapeutic alliance with the parent, and when the intensity of the intervention is appropriate to the family's risk status. Middle-class, educated parents may benefit from a short, one-time

☞ THINK ABOUT THIS ················

**Children and Terrorism**

Parents, teachers, and caregivers were challenged with how to communicate with children and adolescents about the cataclysmic events surrounding the terrorist attacks on September 11, 2001. As nurses, it is important that we take a leadership role in raising awareness of how children may understand, interpret, and respond to related and persistent fears and concerns of these events. Although being honest with our children and reassuring them about their safety is important, it is critical to provide information that is developmentally appropriate. By providing information that is appropriate to the age and circumstances of the child, stress and fear can be reduced and children can better understand the chaotic events facing our nation in terms of terrorism and war. This interaction can also lay the foundation for future communication should additional terrorist attacks or acts of war occur. ◯

*Source:* Adapted from DeRanieri, J. T., Clements, P. T., Clark, K., Kuhn, D. W., & Manno, M. S. (2004). War, terrorism and children. *Journal of School Nursing, 20*(2), 69–72.

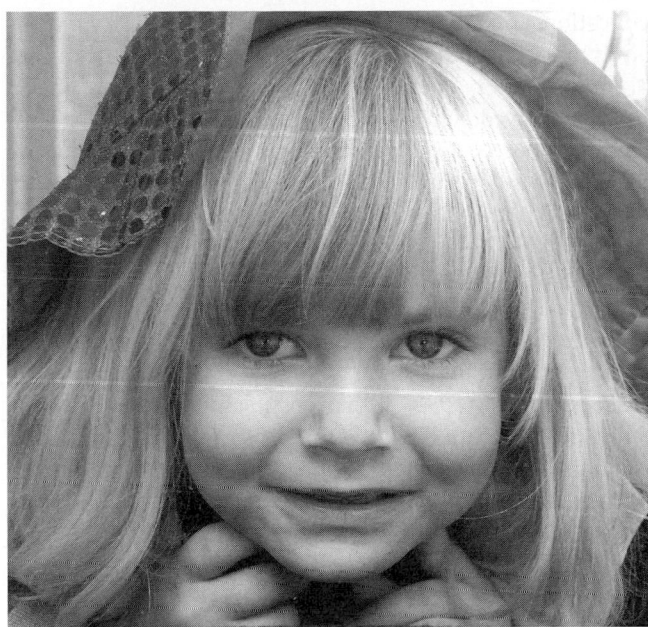

Female children learn early healthy habits which can promote their well-being as adults.

intervention, whereas parents of low socioeconomic status need more intensive and longer interventions.

This review provides evidence that family poverty and various correlates of being poor, such as young maternal age, crowding, low birth weight, malnutrition, parental stress, and dysfunctional adult relationships, are important predictors of poor outcomes in physical health, cognitive performance, and emotional or behavioral problems (Holzer, Schanzenbach, Duncan, & Ludwig, 2008). The family environment is very important to a child's health and development. There is also evidence that neighborhoods have direct and indirect effects on health and development (Guthrie, 2007; Prentice, 2007).

### Environmental Hazards in the Poverty Context

Pollutants such as tobacco smoke or nitrous oxide in the air we breathe inside and outside the home increase the risk for impaired lung growth, middle ear infection, respiratory infections, asthma attacks, and even cancer. Community health nurses can provide information to parents about the risks of secondhand smoke to children and can support parents as they try to stop smoking.

In addition to the toxins in the air, toxic chemicals such as lead, diazinon, and mercury are found in common household objects and substances. Young children are most at risk for harm from exposure to toxins. Children who eat large amounts of flaking old paint containing lead can get sick, and even be left mentally retarded. Children crawling in grass that has been sprayed with insecticides may absorb the insecticide through their skin.

### ■ Neighborhood Contexts

Protective factors in families and neighborhoods are more important than risk factors for important outcomes such as developmental test scores. That is, low-risk family status and neighborhoods with affluent families have positive effects with respect to average family risk and average income neighborhoods. High-risk scores for a family and few affluent families in the neighborhood do not further decrease child developmental test scores. Family protective or risk status has been measured by proxies for human capital (e.g., maternal education, maternal verbal comprehension, maternal age, employment of head of household) and proxies for social capital measures (e.g., child-to-adult ratio, low social support network score). Neighborhood protective status is based on the percentage of affluent families; risk status is based on the percentage of families below the poverty line.

When neighborhood risk factors rise above a threshold level, they become important. Neighborhoods with extreme impoverishment and a high childcare burden (high child-to-adult ratio, high population turnover, and many female-headed households) tend to have high rates of child abuse and neglect (Anthony et al., 2008; Korbin & Coulton, 1994; Rodgers & Payne, 2007). Furthermore, residents in these neighborhoods perceive that neighborhoods with crime, drugs, and violence are poor places to raise children. High levels of criminal behavior and physical evidence of poverty and neglect, such as broken windows, abandoned cars, and weeds, may either elicit or be markers for fear and hopelessness.

Research suggests that neighborhood effects on child development start after family effects, but exist as early as age 3. For a population of low-birth-weight infants, Klebanov et al. (1998) concluded that there are significant nonlinear effects of family risk factors, such as maternal education, employment of head of household, and child-to-adult ratio, on child developmental test scores as early as age 1. Family poverty became significant at age 2. Neighborhood income showed significant nonlinear effects at age 3. Thus living in poverty during early childhood appears to be more harmful than the same duration of living in poverty in later childhood (Anthony et al., 2008; Rodgers & Payne, 2007).

Neighborhood poverty, family risk status, and family poverty effects have been shown to be mediated by the quality of the home environment—primarily by learning opportunities within the home, such as appropriate toys, books, pets, and interaction with male and female caregivers (Klebanov et al., 1998). Other possible mediators of the effect of neighborhood poverty and its sequelae (e.g., violence, isolation, and lack of basic services) are the mother's depression or lack of self-efficacy. These mediators have not been extensively studied, but will be considered in this research.

Perhaps the clearest statement from research is the vulnerability of black children, particularly black males. Black children are more concentrated in poor neighborhoods than white or Hispanic children (Massey & Kanaiaupuni, 1993). Male joblessness is significantly related to black children's, but not white children's, internalizing and externalizing problems (Chase-Lansdale, 1997).

The detrimental effects of long-term exposure to neighborhood risks are clear in African American male adolescents. Spencer and co-authors (1977) concluded from their research on African American adolescents living in high- and low-risk neighborhoods in Atlanta that African American "boys require more protection from adverse circumstances in the most extreme neighborhood conditions" (p. 217).

■ Parents' Work Context

The family friendliness of the workplace affects children's health and development indirectly. If parents cannot take leave to care for a sick child without the fear of losing their job, the child suffers.

■ Childcare Context

A dramatic increase in the number of women with children who work occurred in the last part of the twentieth century. Nearly three out of four U.S. mothers work. Even among mothers with very young children, nearly two out of three are employed outside the home. Unmarried mothers are more likely than married mothers to work (Bureau of Labor Statistics, www.bls.org). While most children of working mothers are still cared for by other family members, more children than ever are now in site-based child care.

It is difficult for parents to balance work, time with children, caring for the home, and adult social life. The stress and resultant anxiety of feeling that, as a parent, you are not spending enough time with your child can contribute to depression and fatigue. Parents can feel better about their work if they are sure that their child is in a safe, developmentally rich childcare setting. Unfortunately, there are not enough or

government-funded childcare programs such as Head Start and Early Head Start. Furthermore, government subsidies to working parents needing child care are limited. Parents often must take whatever child care they can afford. While childcare providers want to provide good care, that is expensive, and childcare care workers are typically paid little more than minimum wage.

■ Public Policy Context

One of the challenges for community health nurses focusing on children's health and development is the lack of a public policy system focused on children's rights and needs. Why should children have their own policy system? Because it works. For example, elderly persons in the United States have a network of public agencies called Area Agencies on Aging in every medium-size or larger city to advocate for their rights.

Nothing like this exists for children. The state of California and certain cities have attempted to establish and fund formal agencies to plan and implement a well-thought-out set of programs to assure that children grow and develop into productive and happy citizens. One of the most powerful policy advocates for U.S. children is the **Children's Defense Fund**, a nonprofit agency. See its website for news on children's policy issues (http://www.childrensdefense.org/).

Another public policy dilemma for children is that children don't vote and low-income parents struggling to work and care for their children often don't vote either. These parents are the last to know when Medicaid insurance or child care for the working poor is cut to balance the budget.

As a community health nurse, you can find out which agencies in your town advocate for children and their families. Encourage families you work with as a nurse to tell their political representatives how public programs help their children. Encourage people to vote.

## Conclusion

Nurses working in the community have a unique opportunity to provide individualized services to families in their homes and community. Nurses observe parents struggling to do the best for their children, often in the face of tremendous adversity. Nurses then have unique perspectives and information from their work with children and families. Consequently, community nurses are critical members of community efforts to plan services for children and families.

Explore Community Health Nursing on the Web! To learn more about the topics in this chapter, use the passcode provided to access your exclusive website: **http://nursing.jbpub.com/ communityhealth.** If you do not have a passcode, you can obtain one at this site.

## Application to Practice

Ben is a 16-year-old, Hispanic male with severe asthma. Originally diagnosed at 6 months of age, Ben's asthma has escalated in severity over the past 3 years. He has experienced multiple emergency department visits and hospitalizations, often requiring intensive care.

Ben's parents are divorced. He lives with his father but often spends time at his mother's home or at his maternal grandmother's residence. Ben has experienced many school absences throughout this academic year as a result of the persistent nature of his symptoms and frequent need for hospitalization. He thinks his grades are suffering because of his absences. Ben's usual asthma triggers include dust, cigarette smoke, upper respiratory infection, and weather change.

Ben is currently being discharged after a 3-day hospitalization for an asthma exacerbation. One week before admission, Ben began to experience nasal congestion and cough On the day of admission, he developed labored breathing and wheezing despite increased use of his albuterol inhaler. In the emergency department, Ben did not respond to continuous albuterol nebulizer treatments and was transferred to the pediatric intensive care unit. His condition gradually improved with supportive medical therapy. Because of Ben's anxiety associated with his asthma attacks, the psychiatry service was consulted and relaxation therapy was initiated.

At the time of discharge Ben was feeling well, with peak-flow readings of 560 before and after albuterol treatments.

Chest examination at discharge revealed an occasional expiratory wheeze but was otherwise clear to auscultation. His discharge medications included the following: prednisone 30 mg/day orally; fluticasone (Flovent) twice daily; nedocromil (Tilade) MDI 2 puffs twice daily; albuterol MDI 2 puffs every 6 hours, increasing to 2 puffs every 4 hours for cough or wheeze. A community health nursing referral was initiated.

1. Which lifestyle changes might you recommend to Ben and his family for avoiding his asthma triggers? Be sensitive to his family situation and needs and consider cultural influences.

2. Education about asthma and its management is an essential part of your care. Develop a teaching plan for Ben and his family including learning objectives, content, and appropriate teaching strategies.

3. His father is very concerned about Ben's absences from school and the work that he has missed. Which options might you consider for approaching this problem? How might you work with school personnel to help Ben remain in school?

4. Community-based, comprehensive service programs are needed to provide the full continuum of required services to asthmatic children and their families. Describe the role of the community health nurse in advocating for and developing such services. Which resources are available in your community? ▲

## ■ CRITICAL THINKING ACTIVITIES

1. Is it necessary for prospective parents to be prepared for pregnancy and parenthood?

2. The United Nations Convention on the Rights of the Child suggests that a woman planning on becoming pregnant should be in a state of optimal health. She should schedule a pre-conception health examination (including a review of nutritional status); have a plan for regular prenatal care with early detection and treatment of complication and have a plan for managing day-to-day demands during pregnancy; be free from infections and chemical agents that may affect the sperm, ovum, and fetus; be emotionally, psychologically, and economically committed to being a parent and be socially connected with a supportive network and living in a community that values the rights of children.

- Are these suggested conditions feasible?
- What are the social implications of these recommendations?
- Do these recommendations conflict with the rights of individuals as they have been operationalized?
- What is the role of the community health nurse in education and advocacy regarding the bases for these recommended conditions?
- What role should nurses play when working with families who do not meet these conditions?

# ■ REFERENCES

Aber, L. J., Bennett, N. G., Conley, D., & Li, J. (1997). The effects of poverty on child health and development. *Annual Review of Public Health, 18,* 463–485.

Anthony, E., Vu, C., & Austin, M. (2008). TANF child-only cases: Identifying the characteristics and needs of children living in low-income families. *Journal of Children & Poverty, 14*(1), 1–20.

Bateson, T. E., & Schwartz, J. (2008). Children's Response to Air Pollutants. Journal of Toxicology and Environmental Health, *71*(3), 238–243.

Berlin, L. J., Brooks-Gunn, J., McCaron, C., & McCormick, M. (1990). The effectiveness of early intervention: Examining risk factors and pathways to enhanced development. *Preventive Medicine, 27*(2), 243–245.

Bronfenbrenner, U. (1979). *The ecology of human development: Experiments by nature and design.* Cambridge, MA: Harvard University Press.

Brooten, D., Kumar, S., Brown, L. P., et al. (1986). A randomized clinical trial of early hospital discharge and home follow-up of very-low-birthweight infants. *New England Journal of Medicine, 315*(15), 934–939.

Centers for Disease Control and Prevention (CDC). (1997). Atlanta GA.

Centers for Disease Control and Prevention (CDC). (2002). Surveillance for asthma—United States, 1980–1999. *Morbidity and Mortality Weekly, 51*(SS01), 1–13.

Chase-Lansdale, P. L. (1997). Neighborhood and family influences on the intellectual and behavioral competence of preschool and early school-age children. In G. J. Duncan, J. Brooks-Gunn & J. L. Aber (Eds.), *Neighborhood poverty* (vol. 1). New York: Russell Sage Foundation.

Cohen, B., & Reutter, L. (2007). Development of the role of public health nurses in addressing child and family poverty: A framework for action. *Journal of Advanced Nursing, 60*(1), 96–107.

Coiro, M. J., Zill, N., & Bloom, B. (1994). Health of our nation's children. *Vital Health Statistics, 10,* 191.

Colley, J. R. T., & Reid, D. D. (1970). Urban and social origins of childhood bronchitis in England and Wales. *British Medical Journal, 2,* 213–217.

Collins, J. J., Kasap, H. S., & Holland, W. W. (1971). Environmental factors in child mortality in England and Wales. *American Journal of Epidemiology, 93,* 10–22.

Congressional Quarterly. (1993). The Perry Preschool success story. *CQ Researcher, 3*(13), 294.

Cook, J. R., & Kilmer, R. P. (2004). Evaluating systems of care: Missing links in children's mental health research. *Journal of Community Psychology, 32*(6), 655–674.

Durani, Y.; Friedman, M. J.; Attia, M. W. (2008). Clinical predictors of respiratory syncytial virus infection in children. *Pediatrics International, 50*(3), 352–356.

Graham, N. M. J., Ryan, P., & Douglas, R. M. (1990). Acute respiratory illness in Adelaide children. II: The relationship of maternal stress, social supports and family functioning. *International Journal of Epidemiology, 19*(4), 937–940.

Grey, M., Berry, D., Davidson, M., Galasso, P., Gustafson, E., & Melkus, G. (2004). Preliminary testing of a program to prevent type 2 diabetes among high-risk youth. *Journal of School Health, 74*(81), 10–15.

Guthrie, B. (2007). An inconvenient truth. *Journal for Specialists in Pediatric Nursing,* 213–214.

Harsten, G., Prellner, K., & Heldrup, J. (1990). Acute respiratory tract infections in children: A three year follow-up from birth. *Acta Paediatrica Scandinavia, 79,* 402–409.

Henggeler, S. (2003). Advantages and disadvantages of multisystemic therapy and other evidence-based practices for treating juvenile offenders. *Journal of Forensic Psychology Practice, 3*(4), 53–59.

Hinds, P. S., Oakes, L., Furman, W., et al. (2001). End-of-life decision making by adolescents, parents, and healthcare providers in pediatric oncology: Research to evidence-based practice guidelines. *Cancer Nursing, 24*(2), 122–134.

Holzer, H., Schanzenbach, D., Duncan, G., & Ludwig, J. (2008). The economic costs of childhood poverty in the United States. *Journal of Children & Poverty, 14*(1), 41–61.

Kataoka, S. H., Stein, B. D., Jaycox, L. H., et al. (2002). A school-based mental health program for traumatized Latino immigrant children. *Journal of the American Academy of Child and Adolescent Psychiatry, 42*(3), 311–319.

Key, J. D., Washington, E. C., & Hulsey, T. C. (2002). Reduced emergency department utilization associated with school-based clinic enrollment. *Journal of Adolescent Health, 30*(4), 273–278.

Klevbanov, P. K., Brooks-Gunn, J., Chase-Lansdale, P. L., & Gordon, R. A. (1997). Are neighborhood effects on young children mediated by features of the home environment? In J. Brooks-Gunn, G. J. Duncan, & J. L. Aber (Eds.), *Neighborhood poverty: Context and consequences for children* (vol. I, pp. 119–145). New York: Russel Sage.

Klebanov, P. K., Brooks-Gunn, J., McCarton, C., & McCormick, M. C. (1998). The contribution of neighborhood and family income to developmental test scores over the first three years of life. *Child Development, 69*(5), 1420–1436.

Korbin, J. E., & Coulton, C. J. (1994). *Neighborhood impact on child abuse and neglect* (Final Report Gov. Doc. 90CA-1494). Cleveland, OH: Case Western Reserve University.

Leatherman, S., & McCarthy, D. (2004). *Quality of health care for children and adolescents: A chartbook.* New York: Commonwealth Fund.

Le Blanc, L., Swisher, R., Vitaro, F., Tremblay, R. E. (2007). School Social Climate and Teachers' Perceptions of Classroom Behavior Problems: A ten-year longitudinal and multilevel study. *Social Psychology of Education, 10*(4), 429–442.

Massey, D. S., & Kanaiaupuni, S. M. (1993). Public housing and the concentration of poverty. *Social Science Quarterly, 74*(1), 109–122.

Melnyk, B. M., Alert-Gillis, L., Feinstein, N. F., et al. (2004). Creating opportunities for parent empowerment: Program effects on the mental health/coping outcomes of critically ill young children and their mothers. *Pediatrics, 113*(6), 597–607.

Nersesian, W. S., Petit, M. R., & Shaper, R. (1985). Childhood death and poverty: A study of all childhood deaths in Maine, 1976 to 1980. *Pediatrics, 75,* 41–50.

Office of Justice Programs. (2006). *Juvenile offenders and victims: 2006 national report.* Washington, DC: U.S. Department of Justice.

Olds, D. L., & Kitzman, H. (1993). Review of research on home visiting for pregnant women and parents of young children. *Future of Children, 3*(Winter), 53–92.

Peters, M., Thomas, D., & Zamberlan, C. (1997). *Boot camps for juvenile offenders program summary.* Washington, DC: Office of Juvenile Justice and Delinquency Prevention, U.S. Department of Justice.

Pless, I. B. (Ed.) (1994). *The epidemiology of childhood disorders.* New York: Oxford University Press.

Prentice, S. (2007). Less access, worse quality. *Journal of Children & Poverty, 13*(1), 57–73.

Rodgers, Jr., H., & Payne, L. (2007). Child poverty in the American states: The impact of welfare reform economics, and demographics. *Policy Studies Journal, 35*(1), 1–21.

Salinksy, E., & Scott, W. (2003). Obesity in America: A growing threat. National Health Policy Forum Background paper. Retrieved November 13, 2008, from http://www.nhpf.org/pdfs_bp/BP%5FObesity%5F7%2D03%2Epdf.

Shonkoff, J. P., & Phillips, J. A. (Eds.). (2000). *From Neurons to Neighborhoods: The science of early childhood development.* Available from The National Academic Press: http://search.nap.edu

Spencer, M. E. (1977). History and Sociology: An Analysis & Weber's The City. *Sociology, 11*(3), 507–525.

Stroul, B. A., & Friedman, R. M. (1986). *A system of care for children and youth with severe emotional disturbances.* (revised ed.). Washington, DC: Georgetown University Child Development Center, CASSP Technical Assistance Center.

U.S. Department of Health and Human Services. (2007). Progress Review: Immunization and Infectious Diseases. Retrieved November 13, 2008, from http://www.healthypeople.gov/data/2010prog/focus14/

Wagmiller, R. L., Kuang, L.; Aber, J. L.; Lennon, M. C.; Alberti, P. M. (2006). The dynamics of economic disadvantage and children's life chances. *American Sociological Review 71*(5), 847–866.

Webster-Stratton, C., Jamila, R. M., & Stoolmiller, M. (2004). Preventing conduct problems and improving school readiness: Evaluation of the Incredible Years teacher and child training programs in high-risk schools. *Journal of Child Psychology and Psychiatry and Applied Health Disciplines 59*(5), 471–488.

Yoos, H. L., McMullen, A., Bezek, S., et al. (1997). An asthma management program for urban minority children. *Journal of Pediatric Health Care, 11*, 66–74.

Zigler, E. (1967). Mental Retardation, *Science 157*(788), 578–579.

Zhou, F., Bisgard, K. M., Hussain, R. Y., Deuson, R. R., Bath, S. K. & Murphy, T. V. (2002). Impact of universal *Haemophilus influenzae* type b vaccination starting at 2 months of age in the United States: An economic analysis. *Pediatrics, 110*(4), 653–661.

# Elder Health

Virginia Lee Cora

Visit **http://nursing.jbpub.com/communityhealth** for interactive exercises, review questions, Web links, and more.

As community health nurses stand at the dawn of a new century, more than one-third of our nation's citizens are elderly. How can we prepare for the future of a generation of more than 76 million whose numbers, demands, expectations, and diversity have no precedent?

Just remember, once you're over the hill, you pick up speed.

*—Charles Schultz*

Grow old with me, for the best is yet to be!

*—Rabbi Ben Ezra*

You can't help getting older.
But you don't have to get old.

*—George Burns*

When we are younger, it is almost impossible to imagine what it is like to grow old, lose some of our physical strength, and face sensory limitations and mortality. What is your idea of growing old? Are you comfortable with the elderly? What is your experience living or working with people older than yourself? The answers to these questions will help you learn that aging is not to be feared, but rather celebrated as another stage in life.

## CHAPTER FOCUS

**Aging**
- Aging Terminology
- Gerontological Nursing
- Aging and Health

**Nursing of Elders**
- Elders in the Community
- Elders in the Family
- Elders as Individuals

**Preventive Health Care**
- Sensory Integrity
- Nutrition and Sleep
- Elimination

- Mobility and Communication
- Cognition and Affect
- Employment and Retirement
- Thermal Regulation and Skin Integrity
- Comfort and Spirituality

**Special Elder Health Issues**
- Immunizations
- Medications
- Chemical Addictions
- Ethical Dilemmas

***Healthy People 2010:* Objectives Related to Older Adults**

## QUESTIONS TO CONSIDER

After reading this chapter, answer the following questions:

1. What are the various meanings of *aging*?
2. What is gerontological nursing?
3. What are the major health concerns of the aging population?
4. How are ideas and misconceptions about aging related to the care of elders?

5. What are the major preventive health issues of the elderly?
6. What are specific intervention strategies for the community health nurse in promoting the health of elders?
7. What are special health considerations that the community health nurse should be aware of in caring for the elder?
8. Which ethical issues are involved when working with the elderly?

## KEY TERMS

Activity of daily living (ADL)
Age
Ageism
Aging
Advance directives
Alzheimer's disease
Cohort
Confusion
Delirium

Dementia
Depression
Elder abuse (maltreatment)
Elder neglect
Elders geriatrics
Gerontology
Instrumental activity of daily
    living (IADL)

Life expectancy
Life review
Life span
Longevity
Mild cognitive impairment
Osteoporosis
PLISSIT model

Polypharmacy
Presbycusis
Presbyopia
Primary aging
Respite care
Secondary aging
Senescence

IN CARING FOR ELDERLY ADULTS, nurses cannot look to the past for direction, for never have so many people lived to such old ages and in such relatively good health. Traditionally, all persons who survived childhood and adolescence were grouped together as "adults." Only in the last generation have health care providers begun to realize that older adults represent a unique population with aging and health care needs requiring specialized knowledge and skills. The old ways of thinking about aging and models of caring for elderly populations are outdated and do not provide much guidance for today's elders and their families. As nurses work with ever-increasing numbers of older adults in a variety of settings, we must develop more progressive attitudes about aging and health and improved ways of promoting independence, dignity, and self-care among these elderly patients.

In the past, most of society's investments in health care have focused on child and adult healthcare issues. Health care for older adults has been poorly organized, with greater emphasis on institution-based secondary and tertiary prevention strategies, and little attention paid to preventive, holistic "aging-in-place" centered care. Yet, home- and community-based alternatives are slowly but surely becoming the norm for healthcare of elders, and nurses provide the leadership to promote maximum levels of independence and the highest possible quality of life for elders and their families. Addressing these evolving views of aging and health from the perspective of community health nursing is the focus of this chapter on elders and their families.

## Aging

Elders differ from young and middle-aged adults in many ways. Persons 80 years old obviously are not the same as persons 20 or 50 years old. **Aging** is the sum of all the changes that normally occur in a person with the passage of time; it begins at conception and ends at death. Aging is a natural, lifelong, and total process that varies among individuals and within various domains and organ systems of each individual. Aging is *universal*—it occurs at different rates and degrees; *progressive*—it interferes with lifestyle; *decremental*—it has a general gradual decline; and *intrinsic*—it is unmodifiable, as opposed to *extrinsic* (modifiable by lifestyle changes) (Busse & Blazer, 1996).

**Primary aging** is "a biologic process whose first cause apparently is rooted in heredity" (Busse & Blazer, 1996, p. 4). **Secondary aging** refers to "defects and disability whose first cause comes from hostile factors in the environment, particularly trauma and disease" (Busse & Blazer, 1996, p. 4). Increasingly, health care providers are influencing primary aging, but they have the most impact on secondary aging by

> ❝*I'm not afraid of growing old, because I am. That's just a fact of life. I'm not out to "arrest" life, the way some people do. I'm living with it. That's a part of your journey, that's part of who you are. You carry it with you.*❞
>
> —*Robert Redford, actor, at age 60*

**One Last Song**
Above the flag-draped coffin
The manboy stands.

Silent seconds hang.

Cool old church
Creaks in pain.

The voice comes slow, gentle, high, clear.
    Eyes move heavenward
    He sings

One last time for grandpa.

—*Ann Thedford Lanier*

identifying genetic predispositions in family health histories, using data from screening tests, and teaching appropriate changes to alter risk factors associated with lifestyle, safety, and the like (e.g., healthy diet, regular exercise, weight management, pollution reduction). For example, in an elder with heart disease in both parents and a sibling, total cholesterol levels greater than 200, and low-density lipoprotein (LDL) levels greater than 100, the nurse can encourage a low-fat diet and exercise; the primary care provider may prescribe hypolipidemic agents.

## ■ Aging Terminology

In working with elderly populations, community health nurses must differentiate among several age-related terms: age, life span, life expectancy, longevity, senescence, and cohort. **Age,** of course, is the length of time a person has existed. **Life span** is the maximum potential for survival of a particular species. The maximum duration of existence for a human being currently is believed to be 115 to 120 years.

**Life expectancy** ("expected life") is the average observed years of life of a species from birth to death or at any stated age. For example, the life expectancy of a child born today is 77.2 years; the life expectancy of an 85-year-old person is 6.3 more years (NCHS, 2003, Table 27). Living most of the

### ■□ CULTURAL CONNECTION

In *An Hour Before Daylight* (Simon & Schuster, 2001), former U.S. President Jimmy Carter remembers the type of nursing his mother practiced:

> Since we lived several miles from town among neighbors who were very poor and whose best transportation, if any, was a mule and wagon, my mother cared for many of them almost as a doctor, often providing both diagnosis and treatment. There may have been other nurses who did this, but I never heard of it. Mama was a special person, who refused to acknowledge most racial distinctions and spent many hours with our black neighbors. She never charged them anything for her help, but they would usually bring her what they could afford—a shoat, some chickens, a few dozen eggs, or perhaps blackberries or chestnuts.

potential human life span is a relatively contemporary phenomenon. The life expectancy during the Stone Age was 15 years; in the time of Hippocrates (460–377 B.C.), it was about 18 years; in the time of George Washington (1732–1799), it was 30 years; in the time of Florence Nightingale (1820–1910), it was 50 years. Thus the "graying of America" refers to the longer life expectancy of the U.S. population.

**Longevity** ("long life") usually is the expected length of an individual's life, based on the lives of their immediate family members. **Senescence** ("grown old") is the last stage of a lifelong process of aging. This period culminates in changes in behavior with decreased power of survival and adjustment (Comfort, 1990). In the United States, old age, or senescence, was designated by the 1935 Social Security Act as being over age 67.

**Cohort,** a term derived from the Roman military unit, is a group of people who share a particular age, historical moment, or geographical area (i.e., born between 1900 and 1920, in the Depression era, or in an urban ghetto). Cohorts of people who share experiences of a certain place or period tend to develop similar attitudes and values (e.g., the frugality seen in many elders who survived the Great Depression).

Language used to designate elderly persons is more poorly differentiated than it is for children. It is inexact to lump together all individuals aged 65 to 120 years simply as "old." **Elders** usually are persons age 65 years or older. They often are referred to as pre-old, ages 55 to 64 years; young-old or "almost-old," ages 65 to 74 years; middle-old or "already-old," ages 75 to 84 years; old-old or "very-old," ages 85 and over; and "elite-old," the centenarians 100 years and older (Ebersole, Hess, Touhy, & Jett, 2005).

**Geriatrics** (*geras*, "old age"; *iatros*, "physician") is the branch of health science concerned with the diseases and problems of old age. **Gerontology** (*geron*, "old man"; *logos*, "word") is the study of old age and aging. It is a multidisciplinary, applied science that can be examined from several perspectives: myths and folk wisdom, efforts to prolong life, demographics, and scientific inquiry (Ebersole et al., 2005). Gerontology has no core, unifying theory of aging. Instead, there are biologic theories at the molecular, cellular, and system levels; psychologic theories of the life span; and sociologic theories of elders as social beings (see Appendix A).

> ❝ *To learn from the old, we must love them, not just in the abstract, but in the flesh, beside us in our homes, businesses, churches, and schools. We must work together as a people to build the kinds of rituals, communities, institutions, and language that allow us to love and care for one another.* ❞
>
> —Mary Pipher

## Gerontological Nursing

Although elderly populations in almshouses and rural settings were the focus of nurses from the turn of the century (Burnside, 1988), the evolution of a nursing specialty concerned with older people is a recent phenomenon (see Box 35-1). Gerontological nursing—the nursing of older adults—began evolving as an arena of practice in the early

---

**BOX 35-1**

**Evolution of Gerontological Nursing**

| | |
|---|---|
| 1966 | American Nurses Association (ANA) established a Division of Geriatric Nursing Practice |
| 1968 | ANA developed the first standards of geriatric nursing practice |
| 1973 | ANA established certification in geriatric nursing as generalists (1974), nurse practitioners (1976), and clinical nurse specialists (1989) |
| 1979 | National League for Nursing (NLN) began integrating gerontological content in nursing education |
| 1981 | ANA developed the first statement of the scope of gerontological nursing practice |
| 1983 | Creation of the National Conference of Gerontological Nurse Practitioners (NCGNP) |
| 1984 | Creation of the National Gerontological Nursing Association (NGNA) |
| 1985 | Creation of the Canadian Gerontological Nursing Association (CGNA) |
| 1986 | Creation of the National Association of Directors of Nursing Administration in Long-Term Care (NADONA/LTC) |
| 2000 | American Association of Colleges of Nursing (AACN) publishes *Older Adults: Recommended Baccalaureate Competencies and Curricular Guidelines for Geriatric Nursing Care* |
| 2005 | The John A. Hartford Foundation awards the AACN a $2.6 million grant to support a new initiative: Enhancing Gerontology Content in Baccalaureate Programs |

---

1960s. The standards and scope of gerontological nursing practice are well defined by the American Nurses Association. *Gerontic nursing* also is a nursing term coined by Gunter and Estes (1979) to define "a health service for the aged." The American Association of Colleges of Nursing, in collaboration with the John A. Hartford Foundation Institute for Geriatric Nursing, published competencies for the care of older adults by baccalaureate and advanced practice nurses (AACN, 2000; see Appendix G). Because most elders live in the community, especially in rural settings, as opposed to being in institutions, the needs of elders have been a focus of community health nurses throughout their history.

## Aging and Health

With this country's many advantages, most Americans are able to live long enough to grow old. As community health nurses, we must examine our own attitudes and values about aging and elderly people to gain holistic, realistic views and provide age-appropriate care for this elderly population.

*Aging does not equal health.* The changes associated with normal aging are differentiated from the changes associated with health problems. For example, a 65-year-old may be confined to bed with end-stage rheumatoid arthritis, while an 85-year-old may run a 26-mile marathon.

*Aging changes are both relative and absolute.* For example, the individual who has poor eye–hand coordination as a young adult will have poorer eye–hand coordination as an elder than his or her peers, a *relative* change. A person with 10% reduction in vital capacity of the lungs has an *absolute* change. The *principle of individual variation* is that the best predictor of a person's current performance is that person's previous performance. Elders should not be judged by the average age-related decline seen in cross-sectional studies (Kane, Ouslander, & Abrass, 2003).

*Aging is a comprehensive process.* It is not only an accumulation of biological changes, but also a complex series of psychosocial, socioeconomic, and spiritual changes that influence and are influenced by the elders, their families, communities, and society. Any changes that affect one domain simultaneously affect all other domains.

*Old age is a time of continued growth, development, and fulfillment* (i.e., achieving self-actualization or ego integrity). This culmination of the life cycle is a balance of both gains and losses in the processes of change. As with other transitional periods of life, old age is a time of holding on and letting go. Some performance may be enhanced by age. For example, with greater wisdom, perspective, and problem-solving skills, an elder's cognitive function may improve.

*The elderly population is heterogeneous and diverse.* Human beings tend to be more homogeneous (similar) at birth and become quite heterogeneous (different) in old age. As with other age or ethnic groups, the nurse must avoid simplistic generalizations and neither romanticize elders nor stereotype and stigmatize them. Rather, we must balance their positive aspects with their negatives to accept them as they are with specific health problems countered by many real strengths.

*Elders are tough.* Very few elders are frail; a great majority are hardy, vigorous, and active through the very end of their lives. They are not *victims* of aging processes, but rather *survivors* of life's experiences as part of family systems within their environment. They usually appreciate direct, factual information rather than ambiguous indirect statements.

**❝***You don't get old from calendar years. You get old from inactivity.***❞**

—Jack LaLanne

## Nursing of Elders

The "age wave" of baby-boomers is arriving throughout the first decade of the twenty-first century. Society needs well-educated and experienced nurses to meet the challenge of providing care to this ever-increasing, complex segment of the population. In providing holistic care, community health nurses consider these elders with the context of their community, their family, and their individual selves. Recent disasters in the United States, such as Hurricane Katrina, demonstrate the need of society to recognize the specific needs of elders as compared to the younger population. In New Orleans, Hurricane Katrina caused unprecedented damage to property and demands for mass evacuation of an entire city. Disaster plans had not included the special issues related to the elder population, such as mobility, driving ability, awareness of disaster risk, and specific health needs. As a result, many elders remained in their homes, had limited ability to evacuate to safe shelters, and made up a large percentage of those who died. This is but one example of society's failure to address the complexities and unique risks of this vulnerable population.

### ■ Elders in the Community

The status and roles of elderly people in the community are influenced by the values placed on aging by society. In some cultures, elders and their collective wisdom are held in very high esteem; in other cultures, old age exemplifies loss of productivity with subsequent loss of status and stigmatization. **Ageism** is the systematic stereotyping of and discrimination against people because they are old (Butler, 2003). Learned at an early age, these prejudices may surface in younger people's negative beliefs about older people as well as in the elders' beliefs about themselves. These views can influence the outcomes of health care. For example, elders may be viewed as too old for surgical procedures, even-though most tolerate surgery well. Demented elders may be seen as not needing analgesics or comfort measures when in pain. Nurses need to listen for ageism in themselves and others, and confront it as they would racism or sexism through the education of adults and children about the realities of old age, both positive and negative.

#### Demography of Elders

The aging population is growing by both absolute and relative numbers (U.S. Bureau of the Census, 2001). In 1990, persons aged 65 years and older numbered 3 million, or 3% of the U.S. population. With a 12% increase since 1990, they currently number 35 million, 12.4% of the total population, and 1 of every 8 persons—thus the "graying of America." In 2010–2030, as the baby-boomers turn 65, an "age wave" will hit all of American society, including health care. In 2050, older adults will account for 20% of the U.S. population and number 80 million, representing 1 in 5 Americans. Elders make up 6% of the world population. The old-old (age 85 and older) are the fastest-growing segment of the population, projected to increase from 50,000 in 2000 to 1 million in 2050.

Elderly women outnumber men by a ratio of 100 women to 70 men. This gender ratio increases by age: the ratio for the 65–74 age group is 82:1, the ratio for the 75–84 age group is 65:1, and the ratio for the 85+ group is 41:1. Most older men (75%) are married, and most older women (41%) are not (National Center for Health Statistics, Center for Disease Control & Prevention, 2003).

The elderly population in the United States also is becoming more racially, ethnically, and culturally diverse: 87% are Caucasian, 7.7% are African American, 3.4% are His-

**Walk with Me**

Long ago I was a young man
I had children and friends
Remember?

Moments I recall slip away.

Brown and gray
    Orange and green still life

Between paper and plastic

Memories
    child, wife, mother
Fade

Remember for me.

—*Ann Thedford Lanier*

panic, 1.4% are Asian/Pacific Islanders, and 0.4% are Native American (U.S. Bureau of the Census, 2001). By 2050, African American elders will increase to 12% of the U.S. population, the Hispanics population will grow eightfold, and Asian and Native American groups will increase significantly. Cultural and ethnic differences in aging and health are reflected in the life expectancy of men and women. For example, the life expectancy of white men and women is 73 and 80 years, respectively; the life expectancy of black men and women is 65 and 74 years, respectively. Elders of various cultural groups may have different responses to health problems, modifiable risk factors, and health promotion activities such as education. Community health nurses need to determine the distributions and values of elderly populations within their area and figure out how these cultural differences affect health care. For example, elderly family members may be immigrants to the United States. They may not understand or speak English; they may not be literate in any language. These individuals may delay seeking health care because of fear of the system.

The distribution of the elderly population is biased 4:1 rural over urban settings. Rural elders are the oldest old, are poorer, and have more chronic illnesses, compounded by greater problems with access, transportation, and inadequate health care facilities. In 1990, nine states had more than 1 million elders: California, Florida, New York, Pennsylvania, Texas, Illinois, Ohio, Michigan, and New Jersey. The largest percentage of the oldest old are clustered in five farm states: Iowa, South Dakota, Nebraska, North Dakota, and Kansas.

Economically, the median annual income of elderly men and women is $15,000 and $8,500, respectively. Only 11% are below the poverty line, but 27% are near poor. Women account for 74% of poor elders; blacks account for 24% of these poor. The major source of income for elders is the federal Social Security program; more than half have pensions and 19% have private pensions. Eight percent are on public assistance, 6% receive food stamps, and 12% have Medicaid.

The education of elders is improving from a median level of 9 years in 1970 to 12 years in 1990, but only 55% have a high school education and 13% have completed college. As many as 50% to 80% of elders have inadequate *functional health literacy*—that is, they are unable to read prescription bottle labels, comprehend health literature and appointment slips, complete health insurance forms, follow diagnostic test instructions, and perform other reading comprehension tasks (Williams et al., 1995).

Of U.S. households, 21 million are headed by elders; 78% are owners and 22% are renters. Approximately 15% of elderly men and 79% of elderly women live alone. Because of their economic status, disabilities, or social needs, many elders resort to a wide variety of living arrangements, including senior housing units, home sharing, home equity conversion, group homes, "granny flats," and others. Although only 4.5% of U.S. elders age 65 live in nursing homes, at age 85 years 18.2% live in these facilities, with more women and Caucasians than men or other ethnic groups being part of this population (U.S. Bureau of the Census, 2001). A growing variety of alternative housing arrangements and number of facilities for frail and/or demented elders are emerging. These newer services include adult daycare centers, personal care homes, assisted-living facilities, and dementia care units.

With regard to health care access, the elderly population accounts for 36% of U.S. health care expenditures—$72 billion from Medicare, $20 billion from Medicaid, and $10 billion from other sources. Health care consumes as much as 20% of the income of elders, who average $1,500 in out-of-pocket expenses per year. Although only 12% of the total U.S. population, older adults account for approximately 50% of patients in hospitals, 85% of home health patients, and 90% of nursing home residents. Most of these health care expenditures are made in the last six months of life. Individual, family, cultural, and health provider beliefs and values all may influence choices for health care during this period. For example, family members may refuse to "give up" on an elder and want everything to be done for a terminal illness, while the elder may believe the "only cure for old age is death" and resist further interventions, even pain management.

### Healthy People 2010 for Older Adults

For the elderly population, *Healthy People 2010* goals are to maintain their health and functional independence and compress morbidity and dependence into the shortest possible time. The 10 leading health indicators (i.e., physical activity, overweight and obesity, tobacco use, substance abuse, responsible sexual behavior, mental health, injury and violence, environmental quality, immunization, and access to health care) all have implications for older adults. Community health nurses can help address the need for more health education and programs for older adults. For example, only 30% of elders participate in moderate physical activity (e.g., walking, gardening) and less than 10% in vigorous physical

## HEALTHY PEOPLE 2010
### Objectives Related to Older Adults

**Physical Activity**

22.2 Increase the proportion of adults who engage regularly, preferably daily, in moderate physical activity for at least 30 minutes per day. (By age 75, one in three men and one in two women engage in *no* regular physical activity.)

**Obesity and Overweight**

19.2 Reduce the proportion of adults who are obese. (More than half of adults in the United States are estimated to be overweight or obese, especially women with lower incomes.)

**Tobacco Use**

27.1a Reduce cigarette smoking by adults. (Following years of steady decline, rates of smoking among adults leveled off at 24% in the 1990s.)

**Mental Health**

18.9b Increase the proportion of adults with recognized depression who receive treatment. (Depression rates are higher among older adults with coexisting medical

conditions. For example, 12% of older persons hospitalized for problems such as hip fracture or heart disease are diagnosed with depression. Rates of depression for older persons in nursing homes range from 15% to 25%.)

**Injury and Violence**

15.15a Reduce deaths caused by motor vehicle crashes. (People aged 75 years and older have the second highest rate of motor vehicle-related deaths in the United States.)

**Immunizations**

14.29a,b. Increase the proportion of noninstitutionalized adults who are vaccinated annually against influenza and ever vaccinated against pneumococcal disease. (In 1998, influenza immunization rates were 64 percent in adults aged 65 years and older—almost double the 1989 immunization rate of 33 percent. In 1998, only 46 percent of persons aged 65 years and older ever had received a pneumococcal vaccine.)

---

activity; only 10% have received the pneumococcal vaccine; less than 20% get an annual influenza vaccination; and elders have seen the largest increase in sexually transmitted diseases (STDs). Selected objectives for older adults are summarized in the *Healthy People 2010* box. Some programs and organizations concerned with improving the living situations and health of elders are identified in Box 35-2.

### ■ Elders in the Family

As the basic social unit mediating between the individual person and the whole of society, the family is the focus of intervention for elders in the community. A family is "a social system of multiple, interdependent generations of persons who identify each other as being related by birth, marriage, adoption, or mutual consent, as being committed to one another over time, and as having common properties, rights, and responsibilities" (Cora, 1985). By helping families maintain positive attitudes toward aging, nurses can assist elders to enjoy their longevity and life experiences. Elders then give their families one final gift: a positive model of old age.

#### Aging Families

Aging families are assessed according to their structure, functions, or development, or as systems that encompass all of these attributes. No matter the setting, elders should be approached as members of multigenerational families.

The structural approach to aging families is demonstrated by the family *genogram*, including at least three generations. Even when elders live alone, their families influence their needs, behaviors, and health care. When assessing elders' families, nurses may need to develop brief genograms

of immediate, distant, or extended family members to understand their beliefs and values and explain their behaviors. Nurses may need to help contact these family members to establish support systems for frail or demented elders or to create surrogate families to assist with health care.

The functional approach is described by activities to meet the sexual, economic, reproductive, and educational needs of aging family members (see Duvall in Box 35-3). However, in modern societies the state has assumed many responsibilities for family functions that were previously within the family purview. Care of elders may be added to the list of services performed by the state in the form of elder care centers, residential centers, and nursing homes. Examining the functional tasks of aging families is helpful in assessing their patterns of control and levels of involvement with their elders. For example, when helping adult children adjust to familial roles and responsibilities as caregivers, knowledge of family tasks may assist nurses to support family members and prevent burnout from overtaxing the system.

The developmental approach emphasizes the synchronization of several dimensions of time: individual time, family time, and historical time (Erikson, 1963). Individual time is the chronological movement of a person over a lifetime. Family time is the timing of epoch events in the family—for example, birth, death, and transitions of persons from one role to another. Historical time is the chronology of a society over an extended period of time, such as decades or centuries. Elders nearing the end of their individual time are experiencing role changes that involve the transition of power from themselves to younger family members. These changes become important events in the evolving of family time, but

## BOX 35-2

### Legislation, Programs, and Organizations Concerned with Older Adults

#### Federal Programs

- Social Security Act of 1935: Social Security Administration (SSA); Old Age, Survivors, and Disability Insurance (OASDI); Social Security (SS); Supplemental Security Income (SSI).
- Older Americans Act (OAA) of 1965: Is administered by the Department of Health and Human Services' (DHHS) Administration on Aging (AoA). Provides state and area agencies on aging with multipurpose senior centers (social, recreational, educational, and nutritional services for senior citizens), senior employment and volunteer programs (ACTION: Foster Grandparents, RSVP, Senior Companions), senior nutrition programs, health education and prevention activities, senior transportation services, and in-home health care. National Aging Information Center (202-619-1116). Eldercare Locator (800-677-1116).
- Research on Aging Act of 1974: Created the National Institute on Aging (NIA) within the National Institutes of Health. Publishes a resource guide for older Americans (*Age Pages*).
- Centers for Medicare and Medicaid Services (CMS): Renamed in 2001 (formally the Health Care Financing Administration [HCFA]); administers Medicare and Medicaid insurance programs.
- Department of Agriculture: Offers food and nutrition programs, including food stamps.
- Department of Veterans Affairs: Provides services and benefits to veterans.
- Department of Housing and Urban Development: Provides low-cost public housing for elders.
- Department of Treasury, Internal Revenue Service (IRS): Offers assistance with income tax problems and filing.
- Department of Interior: Provides access to federal park system; Gold Age Passports (free), Golden Eagle Passports (low-cost).

#### National Private and Voluntary Nonprofit Organizations

- National Council on Aging (NCOA): Established in 1950 as a national resource for information, consultation; sponsors publications, special programs, advocacy activities, research, training, Health Promotion Institute.
- American Association of Retired Persons (AARP): Founded in 1958 by Dr. Ethel Percy Andrus (also founder of the National Retired Teachers Association); 36 million members; more than 4,000 local chapters; largest nonprofit, nonpartisan membership organization in the world; purpose is to enhance quality of life for older persons; promote independence, dignity, and purpose for older persons; provide leadership in determining the role of older persons in society; and improve the image of aging. Members 50+. *Modern Maturity* magazine, AARP news *Bulletin*. Driver safety program, tax assistance, health insurance, mail order drugs, information.
- National Eldercare Institute on Health Promotion.
- Andrus Foundation on gerontological research.
- American Society on Aging (ASA): Enhances knowledge and skills of those working with older adults and their families.
- Gerontological Society of America (GSA): A multidisciplinary professional and scientific organization for those working in the field of gerontology.
- Gray Panthers: Founded by Maggie Kuhn (1905–1995) as an intergenerational activist group dedicated to social change. "Speak your mind. Even if your voice shakes, well-aimed slingshots can topple giants. . . . The best age to be is the age you are."

---

must also be interpreted in the context of the historical moment of the society of which they are a part (Erikson, 1963). (See Carter and McGoldrick in Box 35-3.)

### Family Caregivers

As part of the intergenerational family life process, family members accept familial responsibility in times of crisis. More than 23% of U.S. households include at least one caregiver, of whom more than 76% are caring for a relative or friend who is at least 50 years old (AARP, 2004). The average age of caregivers is 46 years. These individuals often represent the "sandwich generation"—adults who may be both raising children and caring for elders, often while working outside the home. However, elders aged 65 years and older are 12% of caregivers. More than 2.4 million grandparents also are raising grandchildren (AARP, 2004).

More than 73% of the caregivers are female; two-thirds are working. The average American woman will spend

More women than men survive, and the very old are often cared for by their older children.

## BOX 35-3

**Checklists of Aging Family Tasks and Processes**

### Duvall's (1977) Family Developmental Tasks for Elderly Family Members

- Do the elders have satisfactory living arrangements for their current situation?
- Have the elders established comfortable routines for their old age?
- Are the elders adjusting to retirement income?
- Is the family helping to safeguard the elders' physical and mental health?
- Are the elderly couple maintaining love, sex, and marital relations?
- Are the elders remaining in touch with other family members?
- Are the elders keeping active and involved with family and community?
- Are the elders and family finding meaning in the elders' life?
- Are the elders and family finding meaning in the elders' death?

### Carter and McGoldrick's (1980) Family Life Cycle of Aging Families

Primary emotional transition:
- Are the elders and family members accepting their shifting generational roles?

Second-order changes in family status required to proceed developmentally:
- Are the elders maintaining their own and/or the couple's functioning and interests in face of physiological decline? Are they exploring new familial and social role options?
- Are the elders providing support for a more central role for middle generation?
- Is the family making room in the system for the wisdom and experience of the elderly, supporting the older generation without over-functioning for them?
- Are the elders dealing with loss of spouse, siblings, and other peers and preparation for own death? Is there life review of the elders and integration of the family?

---

**Lost Things**

What's his name?
    Don't know.
He's a nice man.
Hope he come back.
    Sure reminds me
    of someone I knew
    long time ago.

Charlie's his name
Rode a big gray mule

    I'm going home
        Can't stay here
    They'll be looking for me
        At supper time.

You know that woman,

Won't let me drive,
    keeps my money

Good lady
    means well,

Took my keys
    to the old blue truck.

—*Ann Thedford Lanier*

---

16 years caring for children and 17 years caring for elderly relatives. A majority of the care recipients are female relatives.

Twenty-one percent of caregivers live in the same household as the care recipient, and 94% live within two hours' commuting distance. The average time of care provided per week is 18 hours, but 57% of caregivers provide 40 or more hours of care per week. While the average outlay for caregiv-

ing expenditures is $171 per month, the average for high-intensity caregivers is $357 per month.

Most caregivers provide assistance with at least one **instrumental activity of daily living (IADL),** about one-half assist with one **activity of daily living (ADL),** and one-third help with at least three ADLs. Most view caregiving as having some impact on family life, leisure time, work life, and personal finances. They also see caregiving as an overall positive experience (AARP, 2004).

Community health nurses need to assess caregivers for their *competence* (i.e., caregiving knowledge, skills, confidence, and objectivity), *burden* (number of hours of caregiving per day/week, nature of tasks to be completed), and *burnout* (psychological stress related to nature of illness and necessary care and support system). Because many caregivers are elderly themselves, their own health issues needs to be addressed, especially if they are too frail to give care. When problems are identified, caregivers may need to expand their support systems through family, friends, or community agencies (e.g., home health social services, area agencies on aging, religious groups). Caregivers may need assistance to manage financial and legal concerns, or they may benefit from participation in caregiver groups for their educational and social support. They usually need to increase their access to resources and may need respite services for relief of stress.

A respite ("look back") is an interval of rest; **respite care** provides family members with temporary relief of caregiving responsibilities for elders. The availability of these services varies widely in rural and urban areas and across different regions of the country. Respite may be offered in the home by other family members, religious organizations, or federal or state programs; alternatively, this service may be offered in institutional settings by adult daycare centers, assisted-living facilities, or nursing homes. Social workers may be helpful in locating respite services in various communities, or the community health nurse may need to help create opportunities for respite for overburdened caregivers.

### Elder Abuse, Exploitation, and Neglect

With most caregiving for elders occurring in homes, community health nurses must be aware of the potential for abusive, dysfunctional family relationships. More than 1 million elderly women are victims of abuse each year. They often fail to report maltreatment because of shame, fear of retaliation, or previous unsatisfactory experiences with police, district attorneys, or social workers who may have lacked sensitivity to the concerns and needs of older people. As a form of domestic violence, **elder abuse** or **maltreatment** is defined as the willful infliction of physical pain, injury, debilitating mental anguish, unreasonable confinement, or willful deprivation by a caregiver of services which are necessary to maintain physical and mental health (O'Malley, 1987). **Elder neglect** refers to elderly persons who are either living alone and not able to provide for themselves the services that are necessary to maintain physical and mental health or are not receiving necessary services from responsible caretakers (O'Malley, 1987). Types of elder maltreatment are described in Table 35-1.

Maltreatment occurs with 5% to 10% of elders, typically by family members. The most frequently abused, exploited, and neglected elders are those who are frail, confused, and dependent with functional disabilities; are older than 70 years of age, female, and of minority status; and have poor social networks. The abuse often is invisible—it is repeated, not reported. Adult protective service laws require mandatory or voluntary reporting of suspected abuse or neglect in all states. Also, elders can be abusive to their family members and caregivers. Sensitivity to these dysfunctional family relationships is essential for community health nurses.

Nurses who encounter elders in the community have opportunities to assist with both primary and secondary prevention of elder maltreatment. The goals of primary prevention are to support caregivers and reduce the potential for abuse. The goals of secondary prevention are early case finding of abusive situations and crisis intervention, referrals, and follow-up with elders and family caregivers. Techniques for interventions in the maltreatment of elders are summarized in Box 35-4.

## ■ Elders as Individuals

The goals of health care for individual elders are to maximize independence and to minimize dependence. For nurses working directly with elders in the community, the focus of intervention is on health promotion and primary prevention to maintain autonomy of the elders as members of family systems with their environment. Emphasis is on the elders' abilities (i.e., what can be built upon) rather than disabilities (i.e., what's been lost). Functional ability depends on individual characteristics and the setting/environment. The health care provider's role is to enhance coping ability by careful clinical assessment and management of remediable problems and by facilitating changes in the environment to

---

**Table 35-1  Types of Elder Maltreatment**

| Types | Behaviors of Abusers and/or Elders |
|---|---|
| **Abuse** | |
| ▪ Physical or sexual | Slapping, pushing, restraining, molesting |
| ▪ Psychological | Threats, intimidation |
| ▪ Exploitation | Misappropriation of funds or property |
| ▪ Medical | Withholding necessary medications, treatments, or assistive devices |
| **Neglect** | |
| ▪ Passive | Unintentional lack of caregiving because of lack of knowledge and/or skills |
| ▪ Active | Abandonment or intentional failure to provide caregiving |
| ▪ Self-neglect | Intentional or unintentional lack of attention to self-care |

---

**BOX 35-4**

**Techniques for Intervention in the Maltreatment of Elders**

**Primary Prevention**
- Be aware of the risk factors for potentially abusive situations—in both elders and caregivers (e.g., frailty, confusion, dependence, functional disabilities, age 70+ years, female, minority status, poor social networks).
- Provide anticipatory guidance to help families plan for future needs of frail and/or demented elders.
- Broaden support systems for families with dependent elders by involving other family and friends in caregiving activities.
- Teach families stress management techniques and provide information about caregiving and local resources (e.g., caregiver classes, support groups, respite and day care, financial aid, counseling).

**Secondary Prevention**
- Observe for physical injuries (e.g., bruises, lacerations, burns, fractures, pressure sores, malnutrition, poor hygiene, dehydration, recurring injuries) and/or psychological damage (e.g., unusual fears, caregiver not letting elder be alone with providers).
- Ask direct questions while alone with the elder: "Has anyone tried to hurt you or make you do things you didn't want to do?"
- Do a complete physical examination, including the skin, head, neck, breasts, abdomen, genitals, and rectum.
- Document findings with the elder's own words, detailed descriptions, and, if possible, photographs of injuries.
- Assess the severity and frequency of the abuse and the safety of the elder. Report findings to adult protective services. If potentially lethal, make immediate referrals (call the police).
- Provide follow-up with the elder and family, as many abusive situations are repetitive.

## NOTE THIS!

### Elders Have Their Own Dreams

John Glenn, Osceola McCarty, and Lillian Carter are well-known public figures who pursued their dreams throughout their lives. Each took different paths toward realizing their dreams as they grew older.

John Glenn took his first ride in space in 1962, becoming the first man to orbit the earth. Thirty-six years later, he became the oldest person in space when at the age of 77, he returned as part of the crew of the *Discovery*. When Glenn went into space in 1962 as a young man, the thought of sending a 77-year-old into orbit seemed unthinkable; today it is not only possible but expected. Glenn states, "Just because we grow older, doesn't mean we give up our dreams."

Ms. Osceola McCarty never set out to get attention. McCarty, a tiny 87-year-old woman, washed clothes all her life. She lived a simple life, never married and never had children, yet amazingly she was able to amass a small fortune of $250,000. When she donated $150,000 to the University of Southern Mississippi to fund scholarships for African-American students, she was surprised at the reaction. Her generosity so touched people the world over that she became a cultural heroine. She shared the spotlight with Oprah Winfrey and Jesse Jackson and received the Presidential Citizen's Medal from President Bill Clinton. She simply said, "If you can help somebody, help them." She dreamed of a future in nursing but was forced to drop out of school in the sixth grade. The USM College of Nursing made her an honorary graduate of its nursing program in 1996. Because of Miss McCartney's generosity, Ted Turner was inspired to give $1 billion to the United Nations.

Ms. Osceola McCarty with her "honorary nurse" certificate from the Mississippi Nurses Association.

Mrs. Lillian Carter greets her son, President Jimmy Carter, in 1977, upon her return from India, where she spent 2 years working as a nurse in the Peace Corps.

Lillian Carter, mother of President Jimmy Carter, was a retired RN at the age of 68 when she joined the Peace Corps and served as a nurse in Bombay, India, for 2 years.

### Miss Lillian Sees Leprosy for the First Time

When I nursed in a clinic near Bombay,
A small girl, shielding all her leprous sores,
Crept inside the door. I move away,
But then the doctor called, "You take this case!"
First I found a mask, and put it on,
Quickly gave the child a shot and then,
Not well, I slipped away to be alone
and scrubbed my entire body red and raw.
I faced her treatment every week with dread
and loathing—of the chore, not the child.
As time passed, I was less afraid,
and managed not to turn my face away.
Her spirit bloomed as sores began to fade.
She'd raise her anxious, searching eyes to mine
To show she trusted me. We'd smile and say
a few Marathi words, then reach and hold
Each other's hands, and then love grew between
Us so that, later, when I kissed her lips
I didn't feel unclean.

—Jimmy Carter
*Source*: Carter, 1995. Used with permission.

maximize function in the face of those problems that remain (Kane et al., 2003).

Elders usually exhibit multiple health problems with complex interactions. As a consequence, health care interventions often require multidisciplinary approaches. Nurses work in collaboration with primary care providers (e.g., physicians, nurses practitioners, physician assistants), therapists (e.g., physical, occupational, speech therapists), pharmacists, dietitians, social workers, psychologists, and many others. Health care for these elders must consider the issues of access, quality, and cost.

In the community, providers of health care become integral to the elder's environment. Nurses may be viewed as friendly visitors or surrogate family members rather than as health care providers. Nurses must be aware of factors that foster dependency, including their own attitudes and behaviors. The aversion to risk of health care providers, families, and the elders themselves can bias thinking toward conservative interventions without a full consideration of quality-of-life issues (Kane et al., 2003). For example, fear of falling in an elder may lead to a suggestion of using a wheelchair, which promotes further deconditioning, rather than emphasizing walking to strengthen muscles and improve balance and gait. Nurses can help keep elders as active and healthy as possible, encourage their independence, and support their health decisions.

### Chronic Illness

The cost of surviving the acute illnesses and injuries of young and middle age is the chronic illnesses of old age. Approximately 85% of elders have at least one chronic disease, and 30% of the aged have three or more chronic conditions (Cobb, Duthie, & Murphy, 2002). There is also an increase in functional disabilities with age, with 20% of elders being dependent in at least one ADL. The causes of morbidity and mortality in elders are summarized in Table 35-2.

With the focus of nursing for health promotion being on self-care, a universal prescription for patients of every age, including elders, is reduction of health risks. In the United States, ample evidence shows that at the start of the twenty-first century, we are living better as well as longer. The disability rate, although high for elders, has been falling steadily since the early 1980s. Fewer (percentage-wise) elders older than 65 have hypertension, arteriosclerosis, and dementia. All of this improvement is most likely the result of the improved treatment of disease and the accelerated study of aging. A growing body of knowledge confirms that chronic illness and disability are not inevitable consequences of aging, as previously believed. Those individuals who suffer the most and the longest

**NOTE THIS!**

President George W. Bush, the most powerful man in the world, turned 60 in 2006. He was in good company among the baby-boomer generation that, many have said, changed the world. Among those who turned 60 in 2006: Bill Clinton, Cher, Dolly Parton, Donald Trump, Reggie Jackson, and Jimmy Buffett. Bush is among the first wave of the 78 million strong baby-boomers to enter their senior years. Upon turning 60, Bush remarked that, while he considered 60 practically "ancient" when he was younger, he has been inspired by changing circumstances and has adjusted his perspective: "It's all in your mind. It's not that old, it really isn't."

from disabilities are often the victims of their own unhealthy lifestyle choices, such as smoking, obesity, sedentary lifestyle, or poor adaptation to stress. The way we age is often more dependent on how we live than who our parents are.

### Assessment of Elders

Nurses in community health emphasize wellness with the goal of maintaining optimal function—physically, mentally, socially, and spiritually—so as to be as independent as possible for as long as possible. The four primary domains of geriatric assessment are functional ability, physical health, mental health, and socioenvironmental factors.

#### Functional Assessment

As a measure of physical and mental abilities to manage ADLs and IADLs, functional assessment is an important parameter for determining an elder's potential for self-care at home (see Appendix B). In addition to self-reports by the elder and family member, the ability to perform the ADLs needs to be observed by the nurse by having the elder perform as many

---

**Table 35-2** Causes of Morbidity and Mortality in Elders

**Morbidity: Incidence of chronic diseases of persons aged 65+ years**

| | | | |
|---|---|---|---|
| Arthritis | 50% | Orthopedic impairments | 16% |
| Hypertension | 36% | Sinusitis | 15% |
| Heart disease | 32% | Diabetes | 10% |
| Hearing impairments | 29% | Visual impairments | 10% |

**Mortality: Causes of death in persons aged 65 years or older**

| Cause | Risk Factors | Risk Reduction |
|---|---|---|
| Heart disease | Smoking, hypertension, hypercholesterolemia | Take aspirin, estrogen, low-fat diet, exercise |
| Cancer | Tobacco use, radiation | Screen breast, colon, skin, prostate, uterus, mouth |
| Stroke | Hypertension, tobacco | Aspirin, smoking cessation |
| Lung disease (COPD pneumonia/influenza) | Tobacco use, allergens | Immunization, smoking cessation |
| Accidents/falls | Weakness; imbalance; polypharmacy; environmental, home, and community safety hazards | Exercise, drug review |
| Diabetes | | Screen, diet, exercise |
| Kidney disease | Hypertension, diabetes | Treat infections |
| Liver disease | | Avoid toxic substances, ETOH; immunization |

| Table 35-3 | Preventive Studies for Older Adults |
|---|---|

| Health Problems | Diagnostic Studies | Frequency |
|---|---|---|
| **Primary Prevention** | | |
| ■ Osteoporosis | Bone densitometry | Women: at least once after 65 |
| | | Men: at least once after 75 |
| ■ Hyperlipidemia | Lipid profile | Every 5 years; more often in CAD, diabetes mellitus, peripheral arterial disease, and prior stroke |
| ■ Hypertension | Blood pressures | Yearly |
| ■ Influenza | Immunization | Yearly after age 65 |
| ■ Pneumonia | Vaccination | Once at age 65 |
| ■ Obesity/cachexia | Height and weight | Yearly |
| ■ Lung cancer/COPD | Smoking cessation | At every office visit |
| **Secondary Prevention** | | |
| ■ Alcohol abuse | Screening | Unspecified but should be done periodically |
| ■ Depression | Screening | Unspecified but should be done periodically |
| ■ Hypothyroidism | TSH | Every 1–2 years after age 65 |
| ■ Colorectal cancer | FOBT and/or sigmoidoscopy | Yearly/every 3–5 years/every 10 years |
| | or colonoscopy | Yearly |
| ■ Hearing impairment | Screening | Every 1–2 years |
| ■ Breast cancer | Mammography, clinical breast examination | At least every 3 years |
| ■ Skin cancers | Skin examination | Yearly |
| ■ Visual impairment | Screening | Yearly |

*Source*: Adapted from American Geriatric Society. (2004). *Geriatrics at your fingertips* (4th Edition). Available online at www.geriatricsatyourfingertips.org.

of these activities as possible (e.g., put on a button-front shirt, get on the toilet, pick up a penny). Individuals' risk for falls is assessed by checking balance and gait (see Appendix C.)

### Physical Assessment

In the physical assessment of elders, emphasis is placed on those areas that most directly affect functional ability (i.e., vision, hearing, strength). The health history for older adults must include frequent inquiries about exercise, nutrition, medications, substance use (tobacco, alcohol, caffeine), incontinence, memory and depression, social activities, and isolation. In addition to the usual height, weight, and vital signs, blood pressures need to be checked sitting, lying, and standing for orthostasic hypotension (a frequent problem in elders). Along with the usual adult physical examination, vision and hearing, mouth, skin, breasts (women), prostate (men), and feet need to be checked regularly. Diagnostic screening tests performed by primary care providers for asymptomatic, low-risk older adults usually include primary and secondary prevention studies (see Table 35-3). Complete blood count, urinalysis, and PSAs are done periodically depending on the situation. Pap smears usually are not indicated after age 70 or after a hysterectomy.

Nurses should be aware that the normal values for diagnostic laboratory tests and other physical findings may differ between younger and older adults. For example, uric acid and alkaline phosphatase increase slightly with age; erythrocyte sedimentation rate (ESR) and C-reactive protein increase significantly with age.

### Mental Assessment

The assessment of mental health in elders focuses primarily on memory and mood. The Folstein, Folstein, and McHugh (1975) Mini-Mental State Examination is an 11-item instrument designed to screen five areas of cognitive functioning: orientation, registration, attention and calculation, recall, and language and praxis. Scores may be adjusted for educational and visual deficits, but generally a score of 24 to 30 indicates no cognitive impairment, 18 to 23 is mild impairment, and 0 to 17 is severe impairment (see Appendix D). The Clock Drawing Test, a performance test of freehand clock drawing, measures constructional skills and visual–spatial abilities, usually with scoring on a 10-point system.

The 30-item Yesavage and Brink (1983) Geriatric Depression Scale is used to screen for depression in elders with intact cognition or only mild cognitive impairment (see Appendix E). The 15-item short form is used for initial screening and, if depression is indicated by missing 5 or more items, the remaining 15 items are administered. Depression is suspected if the elder misses 11 or more items on the full instrument (sensitivity = 84%, specificity = 95%). Elders

### MEDIA MOMENT

#### *Driving Miss Daisy* (1989)

This four-time Academy Award–winning story about a strong-willed Southern matron, Daisy Wethan (Jessica Tandy), and her elderly chauffeur, Hoke (Morgan Freeman), is based on Alfred Uhry's Pulitzer Prize–winning play. It is a contest of wills as the pair learn that for two people so different, they have much in common. The bumpy road they travel ultimately leads to the friendship of a lifetime.

NOTE THIS!

## Clinical Pearls for the Community Health Nurse

- *Ten pennies make one dime.* Loss of independence in elders may be the result of many subtle changes accumulated over time rather than sudden, dramatic events. Look for multiple simple interventions (the pennies) to support existing strengths and maximize function (the dime). For example, correcting poor vision, losing a few pounds of excess weight, and strengthening deconditioned extremities through a walking program may enable elders threatened with impending relocation to become more mobile and remain in their own homes living independently.

- *Never ask an elder's age.* Rather than ask elders their ages, ask when they were born to identify their cohort. This fact provides rich information about the physical, psychological, and social factors that have influenced elders' lives. For example, to know a man is 91 identifies him as old-old; to know he was born in 1917 places him at the end of the Great Depression and prior to World War II during his early adulthood while trying to establish work and family roles.

- *Listen to be heard.* Community health nurses usually are younger than their elderly patients. There is a tendency for nurses to "preach" about health care and for elders to "turn off" these young "know-it-alls." After all, elders are the survivors of many hardships in their life experience (not victims). If you are talking more than 50% of the time, you are not listening. To avoid this common pitfall, each nurse needs to center the self, ask clarifying questions and then listen the elder's answers; reinforce the positive and support the elder's control, and then listen to the elder's concerns; verify understandings and then listen to the elder's responses; reinforce outcomes and enable maximum autonomy, and, yes, *listen* to the elder!

- *To hydrate elders, encourage them to drink fluids in small, frequent amounts.* Offer a 4- to 6-ounce juice glass every 1 to 2 hours; or provide a 1-pint, covered plastic mug sipped frequently between breakfast and lunch, refilled, and consumed again between lunch and supper; or a half-gallon plastic carton of water kept in the refrigerator and drunk throughout the day. Avoid fluids after the evening meal to reduce nocturia.

- *Be realistic about weight management goals for elders.* Rather than using ideal body weight (IBW), ask about the usual body weight (UBW) at about age 30 to 50 to establish more individualized goals for gaining or losing weight.

- *For health teaching with elders, remember the four S's:* Start Small and Stay Simple. Take more time, break content into smaller units, present one idea at a time, be concrete (not abstract), increase repetitions (three to seven times), and use more than one modality (visual, verbal, and written).

- *Be aware of bowel function.* Any time an elder presents with anorexia, nausea and vomiting, constipation, abdominal pain, loose stool, fecal incontinence, urinary retention or incontinence, confusion, delirium, fever, dysrhythmia, or tachypnea, inquire about the last bowel movement and check for a fecal impaction.

- *Teach elders to use it or lose it.* "The right amount of exercise in old age is 'more than yesterday.' If you don't do it today, you can't do it tomorrow." ◢

with significant mental/emotional impairments are referred to their primary care provider for further evaluation and treatment.

### Socioenvironmental Assessment

Socioenvironmental factors are assessed to identify family and living situations, social support systems, financial status, and environmental hazards. A home and community safety checklist may be administered on the initial visit and periodically thereafter to monitor for the hazards contributing to accidents, falls, and injuries (see Appendix G). A community assessment can be completed as described elsewhere in this textbook.

### Interpreting Assessment Data

In analyzing the findings of geriatric assessments, nurses must remember that the effects of normal aging are continuously being redefined. The presentation of signs and symptoms of illnesses in older adults may be atypical. They may under-report or over-report symptoms of illnesses or have multiple, nonspecific complaints that require explication. Older adults may have a lessened tolerance for stress, yet have difficulty communicating their health needs. The remainder of this chapter covers ways to maintain abilities for a vigorous old age through health promotion and environmental management and prevent disabilities through disease prevention in elders.

## Preventive Health Care

In providing preventive health care for elders in the community, nurses can use 16 verbs that represent basic functions. These eight verb sets are easily understood by elders and their families and provide a framework for a functional approach to this section on preventive health care:

How well does the elder
- See and hear?
- Eat and sleep?
- Eliminate bladder and bowel?
- Walk and talk?
- Think and feel?
- Work and play?
- Heat/cool and touch/feel?
- Hurt and believe?

### ■ Sensory Integrity

The elderly person depends on accurate perception of environmental information from all the senses to maintain independence. Interventions to maximize perception are essential for success in living alone or with families. In addition to regular assessment of seeing and hearing, the community health nurse needs to be aware of the potential for sensory overload or sensory isolation in elders.

#### Vision

Normal aging is associated with increasing impairment of vision, most commonly a progressive farsightedness called **presbyopia.** In addition, four major ocular diseases

---

**BOX 35-5**

**Techniques for Visually Impaired Elders**

- Increase background color contrast between surfaces; use warm tones.
- Increase light intensity, but avoid or reduce glare by using blinds, unwaxed floors, and other measures.
- Check corrective glasses daily for cleanliness and fit; use magnifying lenses.
- Simplify and unclutter the environment; check for safety hazards (i.e., throw rugs).
- Caution about altered perception when using uneven surfaces (e.g., stairs, escalators, ramps).
- Avoid night driving; assess driving ability every year.
- Increase print size; use large-print books.
- Consult the local library for the Library of Congress directory of publishers of large-type books, talking books, and catalogues of visual aids, appliances, and computer training.
- Check radio reading services that offer the weather, news, sports, and readings of interest.
- Have annual visual acuity screening; refer the patient to an ophthalmologist as indicated.

---

**BOX 35-6**

**Techniques for Hearing-Impaired Elders**

- Minimize background noise (i.e., turn off or down the television or radio).
- Stand within 2–3 feet of the person when talking.
- Speak face-to-face, on the same level, and toward the best ear.
- Speak at a normal level or slightly louder volume—do *not* shout (it distorts sound).
- Speak a little more slowly in a clear, slightly lower-pitched voice.
- Get the person's attention; call his or her name first.
- Use short, simple sentences; pause at the end of each sentence (e.g., "Ms. Smith, here is a glass of water.").
- Repeat by paraphrasing the message in a different way (e.g., "I brought your water glass.").
- Provide extra time for responses and give visual clues or transitional sentences to preface a message (e.g., pointing to the door, "It's time for lunch."); avoid appearing frustrated.
- Write down key words if the person can read.
- Have the person repeat the information to be certain the message was understood.
- Be sure hearing aids are worn, functioning (check batteries), clean, and fit properly.
- Inspect ears at least every 3 months for impacted cerumen.

---

frequently are seen in elders older than age 75: cataracts (46%), macular degeneration (28%), glaucoma (7%), and diabetic retinopathy (7%) (Kane et al., 2003). Approximately 92% of adults older than age 65 wear eyeglasses; however, the vision of only 65% of those older than 85 is corrected well enough to be able to recognize a friend across the street or read newsprint. Yellowing of the lens reduces color clarity so that reds, oranges, and yellows are seen more clearly than greens, blues, and purples. Decreased lens elasticity and pupil size (miosis) decrease accommodation and contribute to central ("tunnel") vision and night blindness. Diminished lacrimation may cause xerophthalmia ("dry eyes"). Loss of skin elasticity may result in entropion (inversion) or ectropion (eversion) of the eyelids, both of which are associated with conjunctivitis and blindness.

Visual acuity should be assessed annually. Individuals with scores greater than 20/40 should then be referred to an ophthalmologist. Correction typically involves magnification with bifocal glasses. Other interventions to improve function in visually impaired elders are summarized in Box 35-5.

### Hearing

Because of its implications for social interactions and safety, hearing is an essential component of sensory integrity. Hearing impairment is the most common sensory problem experienced by elders: It occurs in 25–30% of people older than 60, especially males. It is the most poorly recognized and under corrected sensory deficit. Only 25% of those who might benefit from a hearing aid actually use one (Cobb et al., 2002). The most common impairment of aging is **presbycusis,** a gradual, progressive bilateral sensorineural hearing loss of predominately higher frequencies and impairment of speech discrimination (especially the consonants *f, s, th, h,* and *sh*). Hearing sensitivity may be assessed with the simple

whisper test: whisper random numbers about 12 inches from each ear while covering the opposite ear. Elders with hearing deficits require referral to an audiologist for amplification with a hearing aid or an assistive listening device such as the "pocket talker." Techniques to improve communication with hearing-impaired elders are summarized in Box 35-6.

Healthy elders often find assisted living facilities provide them with privacy, modified and accessible compact living quarters, and supervision of health issues by registered nurses on site.

Because of the increased viscosity of cerumen and coarseness of hairs lining the auditory canal, another common problem found in elders is cerumen impaction. A simple intervention is to soften the ear wax daily for 3 or 4 days with a cerumenolytic agent (e.g., Cerumenex or Debrox), then irrigate with warm water until the wax is removed (see the package instructions). Refer the elder to a primary care provider if the impaction is not resolved.

## ■ Nutrition and Sleep

In every culture, meals have great social significance as well as nutritional value. Changes in appetite and weight may be the first indicators of altered health status. A balance of activity and rest are important for feelings of well-being. Therefore, "eat and sleep" are functions to be assessed thoroughly and often in elderly individuals.

### Nutrition

Of community-dwelling elders, 15% to 50% are believed to have poor nutrition or be malnourished. Because of this major health problem, the Nutrition Screening Initiative (1992), a coalition of the American Academy of Family Physicians, the American Dietetic Association, and the National Council on Aging, was developed to identify nutritional problems, improve nutrition, and improve delivery of nutrition programs. Three interdisciplinary nutrition risk-screening tools were developed to assess older adults, including the brief DETERMINE checklist. The Mini-Nutritional Assessment (MNA; Nestle Clinical Nutrition, 1999) was developed to evaluate the risk of malnutrition among frail elders and identify those who may benefit from early intervention. Factors often associated with malnutrition in community-dwelling elders include physical illness, medications, lack of hydration, social isolation, oral health problems, limited mobility, lack of transportation, poor vision, poverty, dementia, depression, and alcoholism.

The nutritional needs of elders change significantly with advanced age. For example, calorie requirements progressively decrease, about one-third from a lowered metabolic rate and two-thirds from reduced physical activity. There is a decrease in the acuity and differentiation of taste (dysgeusia) and smell (anosmia), which contributes to anorexia and malnutrition. With loss of salty and sweet tastes, foods taste more bitter and sour. Less volume and acidity of salivation contributes to xerostomia (dry mouth), dysphagia (difficult swallowing), and difficulty digesting starches. Loss of gingiva and wearing down of teeth contributes to gingivitis, loss of teeth, edentulism, ill-fitting dentures, and potentially mouth ulcers. Thinning of the esophageal wall and relaxation of the cardiac sphincter contributes to early satiety (feeling of fullness) and dyspepsia (acid indigestion/heartburn), as does less mucin, decreased gastric juices (HCl, enzymes) and slower peristalsis in the stomach. Thinning of the intestinal wall and slower peristalsis in the colon contributes to increased flatulence, polyps, and diverticula. As with other age groups, the nutritional requirements for elders differ in some

| Table 35-4 | Nutritional Requirements of Elders |
|---|---|
| **Macronutrients** | |
| ■ Protein | 1.0–1.25 g/kg/day |
| ■ Calories | 1,800–2,100 kcal/day |
| ■ Water | 2 L/day; 30 mL/kg/day |
| ■ Sodium | Minimum: 0.5 g/day; maximum: 2.4 g/day |
| ■ Sodium chloride | Minimum: 1.3 g/day; maximum: 6.0 g/day |
| ■ Dietary fiber | Typical: 8–17 g/day; ideal: 20–35 g/day |
| **Micronutrients** | |
| **Vitamins** | |
| ■ Water-soluble (B and C) | Become deficient over weeks to months |
| ■ Fat-soluble (A, D, E, and K) | Become deficient over many months to years |
| **Minerals** | |
| ■ Calcium | 1,200–1,500 mg/day |
| ■ Zinc | 12–15 mg/day |

*Source:* Adapted from Cobb, Duthie, & Murphy, 2002.

categories (Table 35-4). The health problems and associated nutritional deficits of elders are summarized in Table 35-5.

Changes in weight may be early indicators of health problems in older adults (e.g., depression, dementia, congestive heart failure, diabetes). Height and weight need to be measured and the body mass index (BMI; 24 to 29 is ideal in elders) calculated with the initial assessment of the elder's nutritional status. Then, on *every visit*, the weight is rechecked and the percentage of change is calculated. The elder is referred to the primary care provider if the percentage of change is significant or severe. The formulas for calculating the caloric needs and BMI and the standards for

**A Good Read**

## What's Happening to Grandpa? (2004)

*by Maria Shriver, New York: Little, Brown*

This book for children facing the challenge of having a grandparent with Alzheimer's disease helps children understand not only the disease, but also ways they can communicate and keep a relationship with their grandparents. Shriver does an excellent job of presenting the relationship between a young girl and her grandfather, questions she has about the changes produced by Alzheimer's disease, and ways, such as photos and scrapbooks, to stay connected through the progression of the disease. Resources for families facing this situation are included as well.

**Table 35-5    Health Problems and Nutritional Deficits of Elders**

| Health Problem | Nutritional Deficiency |
|---|---|
| ■ Resistance to infection | Protein, calories |
| ■ Poor wound healing and skin friability | Vitamins A, B$_6$, C, D, E; selenium, zinc, copper, iron, protein, zinc |
| ■ Osteopenia and risk of fractures | Calcium, vitamins D, K; estrogen |
| ■ Anemia | Iron, folate, vitamin B$_{12}$ |
| ■ Cardiovascular disease | Folate, vitamins E, B$_{12}$; excess fat |
| ■ Cataracts, age-associated macular degeneration | Zinc, selenium, vitamins A, C, E |
| ■ Constipation | Water, dietary fiber |

*Source*: Adapted from Cobb, Duthie, & Murphy, 2002.

estimating the significance of weight change over time are shown in Box 35-7.

The community health nurse can begin the nutritional assessment with a 3-day diet recall and calorie count. Consider *financial* (fixed income, buying habits), *physical* (transportation, limited mobility, poor vision), and *personal barriers* (food preparation, preferences, eating problems, medications). Oral assessment includes checking for ill-fitting dentures, lost teeth, periodontal disease, and the last dental visit.

## BOX 35-7

**Formulas for Calculating the Nutritional Status of Elders**

**World Health Organization calorie estimates for adults older than age 60 years:**

$$\text{Women} = (35.5) \times (\text{weight in kg}) + 596$$
$$\text{Men} = (13.5) \times (\text{weight in kg}) + 487$$

**Harris–Benedict equations for estimating resting calorie requirements:**

$$\text{Women} = 655 + (9.6)(\text{weight in kg}) + (1.7)(\text{height in cm}) - (4.7)(\text{age in years})$$
$$\text{Men} = 66 + (1333.7)(\text{weight in kg}) + (5.0)(\text{height in cm}) - (6.8)(\text{age in years})$$

**Body mass index** $= \dfrac{\text{weight in kg}}{(\text{height in m})^2}$ **or** $\dfrac{\text{weight in lb}}{(\text{height in in})^2 \times 703.1}$

where    kg = weight in pounds × 0.45
         m = height in inches × 0.025

**Percentage of change** $= \dfrac{\text{usual weight} - \text{actual weight}}{\text{usual weight}} \times 100$

**Importance of weight change:**

| Time Interval | Significant | Severe |
|---|---|---|
| 1 week | 1%–2% | >2% |
| 1 month | 5% | >5% |
| 3 months | 7.5% | >7.5% |
| 6 months | 10% | >10% |

### As We Grow Old

We will pick the wildflowers along the road
And sit upon the ground when we grow tired
And laugh between us at our conservative children
And walk in the summer rain because it is warm and fresh,
And fall asleep upon the new grass,
And hold each other as we sleep
And dream of when we were young
And made love
And were afraid of growing old.

—*Ann Thedford Lanier*

The goals for nutrition are to assist elders to plan and provide a well-balanced diet with a variety of foods from each food group and to maintain a desirable weight. They need to be encouraged to eat low-fat, high-fiber foods and to avoid fried, fatty, concentrated sweet and salty foods.

Nutritional services may start with shopping assistance, which can be provided by family, friends, religious groups, senior centers, and local homemaker services. Grocery stores may offer senior parking and electric shopping carts. Community services include aggregate meal sites in senior centers, Meals on Wheels, area agencies on aging, and county extension services.

For elders with limited income, stretching money to purchase both food and medications can be a challenge. They may buy easy-to-prepare "empty-calorie" foods (concentrated sweets or salty snacks) rather than foods for a balanced diet. The nurse can suggest a variety of foods that will not break the budget: dried legumes, beans, whole cereal grains, poultry, fish, dried fortified milk, less expensive cuts of meat, low-fat cheeses, yogurt, and dried instant breakfast mixes.

The goal of weight management is help elders approach an ideal body weight (IBW) for their age, sex, and body frame. As individuals age, they may involuntarily gain or lose weight and may need to stabilize their weight; or they may have a long history of being seriously overweight or

 THINK ABOUT THIS

More baby-boomers and Middle Americans are getting motorcycles as the baby-boomer generation continues to defy previous trends of "aging gracefully." Unfortunately, aging adults often buy more machine than their aging and out-of-practice bodies can handle. The annual number of motorcycle fatalities among age 40-plus riders in the United States tripled over the past decade to 1,674 deaths in 2003, even as deaths among riders younger than age 30 dropped slightly, according to the National Highway Traffic Safety Administration. The average age of motorcyclists killed in accidents rose from 32 in 1994 to 38 in 2003.

*Source*: National Highway Traffic Safety Administration, 2003.

Elders are living longer than in generations past and are healthier than their predecessors.

for weight loss are difficult to accomplish and maintain at any age, and no less so with elders. In addition to reducing amounts or eliminating certain types of foods, elders must incorporate exercise into daily routines to achieve their goals. They are especially prone to fads and gimmicks rather than adjustment of lifelong eating and exercise patterns. Appetite suppressants are to be avoided because they generally are ineffective and may have serious side effects in elders.

To assist with weight loss, many nutritionally sound, holistic commercial weight-loss programs (e.g., Weight Watchers) are available. Public television may offer low-impact exercise programs, such as chair aerobics. Community and religious groups also may offer weight-loss and exercise programs, or the nurse can facilitate the formation of a neighborhood weight-loss group. Whatever the approach, overweight elders often need weight-loss programs that are relatively inexpensive, easily accessible, and socially supportive. Obese persons on weight-loss diets also need to be weighed weekly.

### Hydration

Often overlooked as part of nutrition, adequate hydration is a key factor to prevent dehydration, soften stools, increase salivation and expectoration, maintain skin and renal function, and aid in absorption of medications and high-fiber foods. Elders usually require at least 1.5 quarts (1,500 mL) of fluids per day, especially water. For diabetic or overweight elders or those who dislike the taste of water, sugar-free liquids (e.g., Crystal Light, Sugar-Free Kool-Aid) can be encouraged.

Like infants, elders are particularly vulnerable to variations in fluid volume (overhydration or underhydration) because of their decreased cardiovascular and renal reserves. Signs of dehydration include weight loss; concentrated urine and decreased output; elevated temperature; sunken eyeballs; dry, parched coated tongue; poor skin turgor; and dry mucous membranes. Depending on thirst for the intake of fluids is unreliable in elders. A weight loss of 2% to 4% is considered mild dehydration, 5% to 9% is moderate dehydration, and 10% or more is severe dehydration with danger

underweight and now are experiencing health problems. Techniques for improving the nutritional status of elders are suggested in Box 35-8.

### Underweight

For elders who are malnourished or underweight (BMI less than 20 or more than 10% *below* IBW), the goal is to increase the calorie intake, including taking a daily multivitamin with mineral supplementation. Loss of smell affects taste and enjoyment; loss of appetite may be from loneliness and depression. The nurse calculates the caloric needs based on the desired weight for these elders. For example, if an 83-year-old frail man's current weight is 130 pounds; his height is 5 feet, 11 inches; and his usual body weight is 160 pounds, his caloric needs are between 1,460 calories (World Health Organization [WHO] formula) and 2,160 calories (estimated formula) per day.

### Overweight

For elders who are obese or overweight (BMI greater than 29 or more than 20% *above* IBW), the weight management goals are to decrease calories and increase activity levels. Diets to promote weight loss generally limit intake to 1,500 to 1,800 calories per day (including a daily multivitamin with mineral supplementation) with adjustments for age, sex, and body frame. The lifestyle adjustments required

### Got an Alternative?

Many elders, especially those with chronic health conditions, take herbal and alternative medications, as mobility/pain issues persist despite the availability of better treatment options. While science has made significant progress in the treatment and management of chronic conditions, elders' expectations of health care providers and these advancements often meet with disappointment in this vulnerable population. Community health nurses should ask elders about *all* that they do in the management of their own health, not just prescription and over-the-counter drug use, as part of their assessments.

of circulatory collapse and death. These individuals require immediate referral to their primary care provider for careful rehydration.

### Sleep

Adequate periods of sleep and rest are essential for the restoration of energy in all living beings. Elderly persons commonly experience changes in both sleep pattern and sleep structure. These changes can result in initial insomnia (disturbances and difficulty falling asleep), interim insomnia (frequent awakenings), and terminal insomnia (earlier morning awakenings), or hypersomnolence (excessive sleep).

Community health nurses can prevent or intervene in many of these problems by thorough assessments of patterns of activity and rest. Consider the nature of the sleep problem by determining its onset and duration (i.e., acute, transient, chronic [more than 3 weeks]). A sleep history can be obtained by having the elder keep a "sleep log" for several days and nights. The log is analyzed for patterns of wakefulness and sleep: total sleep time, total time in bed, nap times, night problems and day problems that interfere with sleep. The nurse inquires about changes in behavior or performance and evaluates use of caffeine (e.g., coffee, tea, cola), xanthine (e.g., chocolate), nicotine, alcohol, and medications that interfere with sleep (prescription and over-the-counter [OTC] drugs). Health problems that may interfere with sleep are considered (e.g., arthritis, heart failure, chronic obstructive pulmonary disease [COPD], gastroesophageal reflux disease [GERD], diabetes, anxiety, depression, dementia, nocturnal myoclonus, sleep apnea). Finally, the nurse teaches the elder and family good sleep hygiene (see Box 35-9).

### ■ Elimination

Problems with elimination can have devastating consequences for elders. Fear of "accidents" may contribute to social withdrawal and isolation. Inability to control the bladder and bowels are major precipitants to institutionalization. Therefore, nurses must take every opportunity to maintain elimination patterns in older adults.

---

## BOX 35-9

### Techniques for Sleep Hygiene

- Standardize bedtime and rising time: Go to bed at the same time each night and get out of bed at the same time each morning, regardless of sleep during the night. Avoid drastic shifts in the sleep–wake cycle.
- Minimize daytime napping to 30 to 60 minutes in early afternoon.
- Encourage daily exercise and both daytime and evening activities with adequate exposure to bright light during the day.
- Avoid large meals and fluids within 4 hours of bedtime. Eliminate or limit caffeine, xanthines, nicotine, and alcohol, especially within 4 hours of bedtime. Avoid diuretics within 8 hours of bedtime.
- Engage in bedtime rituals (e.g., personal hygiene, toileting, relaxation activities, prayer, meditation).
- If in pain, provide comfort measures (e.g., acetaminophen 500 or 650 mg one to two tablets HS, if indicated [maximum 4,000 mg daily]).
- If hungry, have a light bedtime snack with milk (contains tryptophan).
- Wear comfortable sleep clothes and keep the bedroom cool, clean, and quiet with only a night light, if desired. Use the bedroom only for sleep and sex (not for watching reading, television, eating, or working).
- If unable to sleep within 30 minutes, go to another room and engage in restful activities (reading, soft music, hobbies); avoid active television. Return to bed only when sleepy.
- Avoid over-the-counter drugs for sleep (especially diphenhydramine [Benadryl], which interrupts the sleep cycle, can be cumulative, and may cause delirium in elders). Avoid regular use of hypnotics (they cause interruption of the sleep cycle, tolerance, and habituation); limit their use to three times per week.
- Consult with the primary care provider concerning health problems and medications that interfere with sleep.

---

### Urinary Elimination

Although aging alone does not cause urinary incontinence, several age-related changes can contribute to its development (e.g., childbirth, menopause, prostate surgery, stroke). Urinary incontinence is the involuntary loss of urine severe enough to have social or hygienic consequences. Its prevalence is 15% to 30% of community-dwelling men and women, respectively (Cobb et al., 2002). Stress, urge, and overflow incontinence are caused by failure to store urine or empty the bladder. Functional incontinence is caused by an inability to toilet efficiently. Neurogenic incontinence is usually associated with urinary retention; it often requires an indwelling catheter or intermittent catheterizations and is managed on an individual basis. As much as 80% of incontinence can be eliminated with bladder rehabilitation programs (AHCPR, 1996b).

To assess the nature of urinary incontinence, the nurse determines previous patterns of urination and daily activities. The elder or family member is asked to record fluid intake and voiding patterns for at least 3 days to establish the current schedule of urination. In collaboration with the primary care provider, the nurse determines the cause, duration, and degree of incontinence.

Factors commonly associated with this problem include medications, caffeine, and fecal impactions. With frail or confused elders, it is especially helpful to observe toileting activities (e.g., walking, dressing, transfers, hygiene). When establishing realistic goals for urinary incontinence, the nurse considers the level of cooperation anticipated from the elder and family for bladder rehabilitation activities (e.g., total continence, daytime continence with night-time padding).

Treatments for urinary incontinence include pelvic muscle rehabilitation (Kegel exercises, biofeedback, vaginal weight training, pelvic floor electrical stimulation), behavioral therapies (bladder training, toileting assistance), medi-cations (e.g., oxybutynin [Ditropan], tolterodine [Detrol], desmopressin [DDAVP]), estrogen creams), and surgery (Cobb et al., 2002). Techniques for bladder rehabilitation in elders are summarized in Box 35-10. By working with these elders, their caregivers, and primary care providers, community health nurses often can prevent or minimize this condition with significant impact on overall functioning and quality of life.

### Fecal Elimination

Bowel elimination has significant implications for elders' comfort and quality of life. Bowel regularity and fecal continence take on near-spiritual significance for some elders. Common problems include diarrhea, constipation, and fecal incontinence.

#### Diarrhea

For diarrhea in elders, the criterion is the volume of stool per day, rather than the number or consistency of stools, which may be altered with changes in food or fluid intake but still be within normal limits. Diarrhea can be infectious or non-infectious and is a significant cause of morbidity and mortality among those elders who are frail and more susceptible to fluid and electrolyte imbalances. This condition is prevented by scrupulous food preparation and storage, frequent hand washing, and avoidance of

## BOX 35-10

### Techniques for Bladder Rehabilitation in Elders with Urinary Incontinence

- Explain the nature of urinary incontinence and establish mutual goals to encourage participation and cooperation in bladder rehabilitation activities.
- Provide adequate fluid intake— at least 1,500 mL per day—to dilute urine and minimize bladder and skin irritation and odor.
- Check for medications that precipitate incontinence (e.g., diuretics) and give them early in the day. Check caffeine use (e.g., coffee, tea, or colas) and reduce or eliminate them (switch to decaffeinated beverages).
- When usual voiding times have been established, prompt the elder to toilet one-half hour prior to these times, usually hourly at first, then every 2 hours, and finally every 3 hours, if tolerated. Encourage the elder to void before meals, after naps, before bed, and before any special activities, such as walks or outings. Advance times only when the elder is successful during shorter periods of continence for several days.
- Encourage the elder to empty the bladder completely at each voiding by leaning forward and gently pushing down with abdominal muscles (Crede maneuver).
- Observe the amounts of urine voided (i.e., bladder capacity). If the quantity is very large, schedule more frequent visits to the toilet; if it is very small, schedule less frequent voiding.
- For women with stress incontinence, teach Kegel exercises to help recondition the pelvic muscles and improve sphincter control. With the woman on the toilet, instruct her to stop the flow of urine for a few seconds; repeat several times. When she has learned to interrupt her flow of urine, have

her execute the same contractions while sitting in a chair, starting with 5 repetitions and advancing to 10 repetitions held for 5 seconds with each set done four or more times per day. An alternate activity is to contract and relax successively the urethral, vaginal, and rectal sphincter muscles in the same manner described above.
- For urge incontinence, once on the commode, teach elders to hold back the urine as long as possible by tightening the pelvic musculature.
- If elders are confused, demented, or demonstrate anxious behavior, check them frequently for the need to void. During activities, place these elders nearest the bathroom and remove barriers in their path.
- Encourage the elder and family to use incontinent pads (*not* diapers!), such as Attends or Depends, to promote dryness until continence is reestablished. These products are not much more bulky than regular underwear and can be worn with confidence under everyday clothing. If skin breakdown is a problem, coat the perineum with a thin layer of petroleum or zinc oxide ointment (e.g., Vaseline, A&D Ointment, or Desitin).
- Monitor rehabilitation activities daily and evaluate them at least weekly until a voiding pattern is established. Check for dryness and odor, use of toilet for voiding, skin integrity, and self concept. Encourage the elder frequently, praise successes, reinforce teaching frequently, and do not permit discouragement when accidents occur. Reconditioning of the bladder may require several weeks, but with patience and persistence, it usually is successful.

## " a conversation with . . . "

General Colin Powell, former Secretary of State for President George W. Bush, says that he prefers to look through the front windshield rather than the rearview mirror: "There is nothing I can do about what's in the rearview mirror," he explains, "and if I go fast, that which is behind me will disappear more rapidly." Powell, who turned 60 in 2006, is a two-time winner of the Presidential Medal of Freedom, a knight commander of the British Empire, and one of the most decorated and respected leaders of our time. Since leaving office, he has headed up the Revolution Health Group, a company led by former AOL chair Steve Case that focuses on using information technology to give older citizens greater choice in how they spend their health care dollars.

"People are able not only to live longer but to live active lives longer. I am working with a company involved in consumer-driven health care, to put choice more in the hands of the consumer. But the more we got into it, the more we realized it's not just health care, meaning giving you care when you need it. It's also health—making choices about how you live to *avoid* needing health care that is about preventive health care."

*Source*: Staying power: The former Secretary of State talks. (July–August 2006). *AARP Magazine*, pp. 41–46.

---

### BOX 35-11

**Techniques for Common Diarrhea in Elders**

- Place the bowel at rest for 36 to 72 hours. Give clear liquids for first 12 to 24 hours, full liquids or soft diet for next 24 to 48 hours, then a regular diet as tolerated. Maintain adequate hydration (1,500 to 2,000 mL per day).
- Give an OTC antidiarrheal agent, if needed:
  - Absorbent agents (Kaopectate) 15 to 30 mL every 4 to 6 hours PRN loose stool for 24 hours, **or**
  - Bismuth subsalicylate (Pepto-Bismol) 15 to 30 mL every 4 to 6 hours PRN loose stool for 24 hours, **or**
  - Opioid (Immodium AD) 2 mg one to two tablets initially, then one tablet PRN loose stool for 24 hours (maximum, 16 mg/day).
- Teach the elder to avoid irritating foods until clear of diarrhea for at least 24 hours.
- If not improved in 24 hours, refer to the primary care provider for prompt evaluation.
- Check sanitation and hygiene, especially if diarrhea recurs.

---

fecal contamination and polypharmacy. Initial assessments include onset, volume, number, consistency of stools; duration (acute versus chronic); the presence of bright red blood (hematochezia) or black, tarry stool (melena); the presence of other symptoms (e.g., abdominal cramping or distention, lassitude, thirst, nausea, vomiting, fever, malaise); diet; and medications. The nurse evaluates the elder's general appearance, vital signs, and weight and performs an abdominal exam for pain or tenderness.

Although common diarrhea often is treated in the home (Box 35-11), any condition lasting more than 24 hours in elders should be referred to the primary care provider for evaluation and possible rehydration. The protocol for chronic diarrhea, which is often a part of irritable bowel syndrome, is developed in collaboration with the primary care provider and usually includes a high-fiber diet, possibly with a bulking agent (e.g., methylcellulose or psyllium hydrophilic mucilloid [Citrucel or Metamucil]) or loperamide (Immodium AD).

### Constipation

For elders, the most common bowel problem is constipation, a difficulty in passing stools or incomplete or infrequent passage of stools (usually less than three per week). The usual causes of small, hard, or infrequent stools are poor bowel habits, including a lack of dietary fiber, poor fluid intake, inadequate exercise, psychological factors, and medications, often with inappropriate use of laxatives. Common complications are fecal impaction and fecal incontinence.

To assess the nature of constipation, the nurse must determine previous patterns of bowel habits and daily activities. The elder is asked to record food and fluid intake (noting dietary fiber and free water) and bowel movements (frequency, timing, difficulty) for at least 3 days. The elder's general physical and mental condition is evaluated and, if frail or confused, the level of function for toileting activities (e.g., walking, dressing, transfers, hygiene) is observed. The nurse considers possible associated factors (e.g., medications, fecal impactions, illnesses) and makes a referral to the primary care provider, if indicated. When setting goals for bowel elimination, the nurse considers the level of cooperation anticipated for the elder and family with bowel rehabilitation activities. By working with these elders, their caregivers, and primary care providers, community health nurses often can prevent and intervene with a bowel rehabilitation including a high-fiber diet, adequate fluids, daily exercise, and elimination of laxatives (Box 35-12).

Monitor rehabilitation activities daily and evaluate them at least weekly until a bowel pattern is established. Check for constipation, use of the toilet for defecation, fecal impaction, skin integrity, and self concept. If relapses occur, restart the program with suppositories for 3 days. Encourage the elder frequently, praise successes, reinforce teaching frequently, and do not permit discouragement when accidents occur. Reconditioning of the bowel may require several weeks to overcome years of poor bowel habits, but with patience and persistence, it usually is successful.

## ■ Mobility and Communication

The ability to move about the environment is crucial for independent living. The ability to communicate thoughts and feelings to others is also essential for well-being. There-

## BOX 35-12

### Techniques for Bowel Rehabilitation in Elders with Constipation

- Explain the nature of constipation and establish mutual goals to encourage participation and cooperation in bowel rehabilitation activities.
- Encourage a high-fiber diet that adds bulk to stool. This diet usually starts with high-fiber cereals (i.e., more than 10 g of dietary fiber per serving, such as All Bran, Bran Buds, 100% Bran, or Fiber One) and/or supplemental wheat bran (miller's bran) 1 to 4 tablespoons per day added to moist foods (e.g., cereals, grits, oatmeal, cream of wheat, applesauce, soup, cottage cheese, ice cream). Vegetables and fruits also add bulk to stools (at least five servings per day of whole-wheat breads, green leafy vegetables, raw fruits, and vegetables).
- Provide adequate fluids to make the stool softer and easier to pass. Include at least 1.5 to 2 quarts (1,500 to 2,000 mL) of fluids per day, unless contraindicated (see Hydration, page 871).
- Encourage exercise daily to promote circulation to the bowel and stimulate evacuation. For example, walk at least 1 mile per day, ride a stationary bicycle, or swim for at least 30 minutes per day, unless contraindicated (see Exercise, page 886).
- Establish a regular evacuation time to correspond with daily activities or family lifestyle patterns. Defecation is a learned, conditioned response that generally occurs at the same time each day. Most elders prefer an early-morning time for bowel evacuation, but, if scheduling of family activities in the morning precludes sufficient time for bowel hygiene, an evening bowel program is recommended (i.e., after supper and before bathing).

- Start the bowel program with a clean bowel (i.e., give a laxative or enema the day before if necessary). For 3 consecutive days, insert a bisacodyl (Dulcolax) suppository into the rectum approximately 30 minutes before the established evacuation time. Wait 30 minutes, and then assist the elder to toilet with a book or magazine to promote relaxation. Another approach is to use 1 to 3 tablespoons of an osmotic agent (lactulose or sorbitol) daily for 3 to 5 days to get a bowel pattern established. Stool softeners (e.g., docusate [Colace, Dialose]) make the stool more difficult to evacuate and generally are ineffective for constipation in elders.
- Absolutely avoid laxatives, especially the long term use of stimulant laxatives with phenolphthalein (e.g., Correctol, Ex-Lax, & Feen-A-Ment) because of their blunting of natural evacuation and purging of the bowel. A daily bowel movement is not necessary, but avoid going for more than 3 days without defecation. If no BM occurs in 2 days, use a bisacodyl (Dulcolax) suppository. If no BM occurs in 3 days, use a phosphate enema (e.g., Fleets). If the enema is not successful, use 1 ounce (30 ml) of Milk of Magnesia to get the bowels restarted. Daily osmotic agents may be needed; consult the primary care provider.
- Observe the consistency of stools (i.e., normal, soft, hard, or watery). If stools are hard or painful, increase the water intake. If stools are small or scant, increase the bulk with dietary fiber. Recommend a stool softener, such as docusate sodium (e.g., Colase, Dialose) only if needed because of hemorrhoids or other rectal problems.

fore, nurses must take an active role in maintenance of an elder's ability to "walk and talk" while striving to remain in the community.

### Mobility

Adequate mobility is critical for elders to maintain their functional independence. Even brief periods of immobility can lead to rapid deconditioning and loss of flexibility and strength in elders, increasing the risk of falls and injury. Conversely, daily exercise helps the elder to prevent diseases (e.g., osteoporosis, arterial/venous insufficiency, gastrointestinal stasis, musculoskeletal stiffness, coronary heart disease, obesity, stroke, depression, anxiety, dementia); improve sleep, mobility, strength, flexibility, and mood; increase life expectancy; and improve quality of life. Community health nurses can encourage elders to exercise individually, with families, or in groups.

**❝***To age gracefully means to let nature take its course while doing everything in our power to deal with the onset of age-related disease. Or in other words . . . to live as long and as well as possible, then have a rapid decline at the end of life.***❞**
—*Andrew Weil*

Impaired mobility usually involves multiple factors, including an initial physical deficit (i.e., a fractured hip or degenerative joint disease), compounded by a sedentary lifestyle, deconditioning, inadequate daily exercise patterns, sensory impairment (i.e., vision and hearing), confusion, inappropriate medications, improper assistive devices, and/or environmental hazards. To assess mobility in elders, the nurse determines the elder's previous types and levels of exercise and daily activity patterns, any history of activity-related injuries and falls, and possible associated factors influencing mobility (e.g., medications, confusion, illnesses). The nurse evaluates the elder's general physical and mental condition, food and fluid intake, environmental safety, and availability of assistive devices, and observes the individual's level of function for physical activities (e.g., posture, gait, balance, strength, endurance). When establishing a program for exercise or physical rehabilitation, the nurse considers the level of cooperation anticipated from the elder and family for physical activities and addresses both the physical deficits and any contributing factors (Box 35-13).

### Falls

Accidents are the fifth leading cause of death among elders, and falls account for two-thirds of these deaths. Seventy percent of fall injuries occur in persons older than 75 years

## BOX 35-13

### Techniques for Exercise and Mobility in Elders

- Explain to the elder and family the benefits of an exercise program and set mutual, realistic goals to encourage participation and cooperation in physical rehabilitation activities. It is important to emphasize functional independence rather than an arbitrary physical goal (e.g., ability to walk to the bathroom unassisted rather than ability to walk 100 feet).
- Maximize visual and hearing functions by referral to an ophthalmologist and/or otologist and wearing corrective glasses and/or hearing aids (see Sensory Integrity, page 867).
- In collaboration with the primary care provider, evaluate the medication regimen for drugs that alter cardiovascular function, impair central nervous system function, interact, and polypharmacy. Simplify the drug regimen by eliminating all nonessential drugs.
- Check footwear for proper fit and condition. Athletic shoes with shock-absorbent soles and good support are ideal for an exercise program; shoes with Velcro closures are more easily managed by elders with hand problems. Check clothing for comfort and fit. Athletic apparel (e.g., cotton fleece or wind breakers) is designed for maximum movement, comfort, and convenience, and should be worn if acceptable to the elder.
- In collaboration with the primary care provider, refer the elder to a physical therapist or rehabilitation facility for correction of major physical decrements (e.g., stroke, arthritis).
- Provide for gait retraining through a program of physical exercise—basically walking outside or at a covered mall for at least 30 to 60 minutes per day for at least 5 to 6 days per week. *Start low, go slow* with regular, low-impact, unstressed, but progressive exercise. Begin with a distance the elder can manage (e.g., 100 feet or 1/4 mile), increase the distance at 1- to 2-week intervals until the elder is walking 1 to 2 miles, then gradually increase the speed until a comfortable cadence is achieved (i.e., mild perspiration, increased breathing and heart rate). Alternatively, use stationary exercise machines, bicycling, swimming, or low-impact aerobic, strengthening, flexibility programs (tai chi, YMCA/YWCA, fitness centers, community parks, senior programs, televised chair aerobics, Senior Olympics). Exercise is better maintained if done with a partner (spouse, friend) at the same time every day.
- Use assistive devices (e.g., straight cane, four-prong cane, or walker) for balance and support, and/or support stockings for venous return. Check these devices for proper fit and safety, including non-skid tips on canes and walkers.
- Use mild analgesics for relief of soreness, aches, and pains. Acetaminophen 500 or 650 mg one to two tablets a few times daily (maximum, 4,000 mg/day) is recommend over aspirin or ibuprofen which have increased side effects in elders. Taking analgesics 30 minutes before exercise may minimize discomfort from deconditioning.
- Encourage the use of adaptive behaviors (e.g., rising slowly, using rails or furniture for balance) to minimize the risk of falls and, when appropriate, teach techniques for falling and getting up after a fall to minimize complications.
- Avoid physical restraints that actually increase, rather than decrease, fall injuries and compound immobility.
- Monitor the exercise program daily and evaluate at least weekly for improvement in muscle strength, flexibility, and gait stability. Check for orthostatic hypotension, falls, pain, motivation, and self concept. Encourage elders frequently, praise successes, reinforce teaching frequently, and do not permit discouragement when problems occur. Reconditioning of muscles may require several weeks or months, but with patience and persistence, some progress will be made.

---

**❝** *Wrinkles should merely indicate where smiles have been.* **❞**

—*Mark Twain*

of age; 50% of those hospitalized for such an injury do not survive for 1 year. Fear of falling further inhibits many elders from performing activities that would prevent falls and contributes to functional decline, depression, helplessness, and social isolation. Falls may be caused by environmental hazards, deconditioning, sensory deficits, and impaired central processing. The best prevention for falls is a combination of rehabilitative, environmental, and behavioral strategies. For example, correcting vision, using assistive devices, installing bathroom grab bars, and implementing a progressive exercise program that emphasizes conditioning of the lower extremities all help reduce the occurrence of falls.

### Osteoporosis

A multifactorial disease of increased skeletal fragility, **osteoporosis** places elders at risk of fractures during activities of daily living. Postmenopausal women usually are affected initially, but men are also subject to this type of bone loss. Given that they have a bone mineral density more than 2.5 standard deviations below normal values of young adults, the vertebral bodies, proximal femur, and distal radius are common fracture sites in elders. In collaboration with primary care providers, community health nurses can assist with preventive strategies for osteoporosis (Box 35-14).

### Communication

Other than development of slower speech, verbal communication usually is unaffected by aging. The most common causes of language disorders in elders are strokes and dementia resulting in some form of aphasia. Strategies for improving communication are summarized in Box 35-15.

### ■ Cognition and Affect

Because people are sentient beings, attention, memory, and emotion are integrally interwined with personal identity, environmental adaptation, and quality of life. Changes in thinking cognitive abilities may be stereotyped as "senility" and either minimized or maximized by elders and family members. Altered mood and emotional responses may further confound the situation. Impaired cognition and affect may exhaust family resources and precipitate relocation from the home to a long-term care facility. Therefore, nurses can assist elders to remain independent in their own environments by being sensitive to changes in how they "think and feel."

### Cognition

Cognitive functioning changes very little with normal aging. Intelligence is unchanged and, with the wisdom gathered from life experience, problem solving often is improved. Memory involves pattern recognition and is both declarative (factual, "what") and procedural (process, "how"). With diminished attention and immediate recall, elders may have some declarative memory loss (forgetfulness), but their procedural memory usually is not affected by the aging process. Learning, which depends on memory, also is undisturbed, although it proceeds more slowly. Performance may be slower, but it is more precise. **Confusion** is a common problem in elders and may result from alterations in sensory or central processing. The most common causes of confusion are delirium, dementia, and depression.

### Delirium

Acute confusional state (**delirium**) is a physiological state that usually is reversible and is characterized as an altered level of consciousness and disorganized thinking (incoherent speech, repetitive speech and behavior), with a rapid onset and fluctuating course, often worse at night. Delirium has an underlying medical cause (e.g., pneumonia, urinary tract infection, fecal impaction, septicemia). Prevention involves adequate oxygenation, hydration, nutrition, elimination, sensory stimulation, exercise, and avoidance of certain medications.

### Dementia

**Mild cognitive impairment** (MCI; previously called age-associated memory impairment or benign senescent

> **"**The old believe everything.
> The middle-aged suspect everything.
> The young know everything. **"**
>
> —Oscar Wilde

forgetfulness) is the mild, gradual deterioration in memory performance, speed of cognitive processing, and executive functions that may accompany normal aging but does not interfere with activities or relationships. Elders with MCI may have *subjective* memory complaints and *objective* memory impairments, yet may be within the normal or range in early dementia (i.e., about 15% per year of persons with MCI progress to Alzheimer's disease) (Cobb et al., 2002).

**Dementia** is a syndrome of progressive decline that relentlessly erodes intellectual abilities, causing cognitive function deterioration and leading to impairment in social and occupational functioning (AHCPR, 1996a, p. 1). Dementia occurs in 5% of persons aged 65; the rate doubles every 5 years after age 65, until dementia affects almost 50% of persons age 85 or older. This cognitive impairment is irreversible, has an insidious onset, and is relatively stable over time, though it leads to progressive amnesia (loss of memory), aphasia (loss of language), agnosia (loss of object recognition), apraxia (loss of motor function), and loss of executive function (abstract thinking and complex behavior). **Alzheimer's disease** is a cortical degeneration that accounts for 80% of dementia.

Most elders with mild or moderate dementia live at home and are cared for by family members. Community health nurses can assist with early case finding and referral to a primary care provider or specialist (geriatrician, neuropsychologist, or psychiatrist). Assessment includes elimination of reversible causes (e.g., drugs, depression, delirium, thyroid dysfunction, vitamin $B_{12}$ deficiency). Cognitive functioning is screened in community settings with mental status exams, which test orientation, memory, attention, language, and praxis.

The basic principles for working with elders who have cognitive deficits are to *simplify the environment, provide a*

## BOX 35-16

### Strategies for Management of Dementia in Elders

- *Structure time and place.* Use daily and weekly schedules that provide consistency, predictability, and repetition. Structure and simplify activities of daily living, family activities, specific tasks, and the environment to maximize ability in conjunction with less clutter, complexity, and hurry. For example, activities may be done in the same order and at the same times and places each day (e.g., arise at 7:00, breakfast at 7:30); certain activities take place on certain days of the week every week (e.g., bathe on Tuesday and Saturday, laundry on Monday).

- *Anticipate change.* Known events, such as holidays and family gatherings, may be anticipated several weeks in advance by mentioning every day the names of people who will be involved and using photos, stories, or other aids to familiarize the elder with the anticipated situation. Persons with cognitive deficits can learn, but the key is repetition—as many as 7 × 7 times!

- *Modify the environment.* Reorganize the elder's living situation to compensate for sensory and functional impairments. Use memory aids (e.g., clocks, calendars, simple written cues) for orientation and identification of items and places. Keep the environment as simple and uncluttered as possible. Avoid situations that stress intellectual capabilities. For those with early dementia, newspapers, television, telephone calls, and email may be helpful. For those with severe dementia, security devices and electronic monitoring may be indicated. Recommend identification jewelry, photo ID, and current photos; suggest Medialert or the Alzheimer's Association Safe Return Program (800-272-3900).

- *Manage problem behavior.* Analyze each behavioral problem in three parts:
  - **A:** Antecedents (which happens before to trigger or cause the behavior)
  - **B:** Behavior (which specific actions can be seen and described)
  - **C:** Consequences (what happens after or because of the behavior)

  Develop a plan to either avoid or prevent problem behaviors by changing either the antecedents or the consequences of the behavior. Avoid catastrophic reactions by minimizing the common antecedents (too much too fast, fatigue).

- *Support the caregiver.* Since persons with dementia may not be able to change as a result of their illness, the caregivers have to be the ones to change. Altering problem behaviors is not easy and not every attempt will be successful. If the plan isn't working, look at the situation again and try another approach. Be flexible and willing to try new approaches as the elder changes over time. Reward successes, no matter how small. Remember to laugh.

- *Provide information and referral:* Encourage family members to contact the Alzheimer's Association (800-272-3900), Alzheimer's Disease Education and Referral (ADEAR), area agency on aging, community mental health centers, and/or Internet groups.

- *Community-based care:* adult day centers, home health agencies.

- *Caregiver burden:* caregivers support groups, respite care.

- *Long-term care:* personal care/assisted living homes, skilled care nursing homes.

---

**❝** *It has begun to occur to me that life is a stage I'm going through.* **❞**

—Ellen Goodman

---

*structure* for daily activities, *minimize changes* in that structure, and, when changes are necessary, *prepare for changes* well in advance. The goals of cognitive behavioral programs are to help elders maintain their highest level of function, enable them to continue living at home, and offer support to caregivers. These programs are based on strengths, areas of deficit, and realistic goals for their living situations. Strategies for the management of dementia are summarized in Box 35-16.

### Affect

Self-concept evolves from what persons think and feel about themselves, what they think and feel about others, and what they think and feel others think and feel about them (Satir, 1964). Assurance of personal worth is based on feeling valued, useful, and competent. Old age is accompanied by many epoch events—retirement, altered health, relocation of home, deaths of family and friends, and finally one's own transition from life to death. With the frequent, multiple losses associated with old age, elders may experience feelings of powerlessness, hopelessness, and spiritual distress. These feelings may result in the anxiety, fear, and anger of depression.

### Depression

The most common disturbance of mood experienced by elders is **depression**. Its prevalence varies by setting: 5% to 20% in community-dwelling elders, 25% in hospitalized elders, and 40% in nursing home residents (Cobb et al., 2002). Its presentation may differ from younger populations, with somatic complaints being more likely than emotional statements about guilt, anger, or depressed mood in elders. The etiology may be exogenous (situational)—resulting from finances, disability, bereavement, loneliness, or social isolation—or endogenous (biochemical)—resulting from physical illnesses, pain, or medications—or both. Among community-dwelling elders, depression can be clinical (1%) or subsyndromal (15%) (Cobb et al., 2002).

The assessment of depression in elders requires information from the elder and family members. New physical complaints or exacerbations of previous pain, gastrointestinal symptoms, cardiovascular symptoms, preoccupation with poor health or physical limitations, diminished interest in pleasurable activities (anadonia), sleep disturbances, fatigue, poor concentration, patchy memory loss, and expressions of negativism should be noted. The Geriatric Depression Scale is administered to screen for depression, and the elder is referred to the primary care provider as indicated by assessments. In collaboration with the primary care provider, the nurse checks for physical problems and medications that cause depression. Interventions for depression in community-dwelling elders are summarized in Box 35-17.

### Suicide among Elders

Given the high prevalence of depression among elders, it is not surprising that they have the highest suicide rate among any demographic group. Suicides among elders are characterized more by physical illnesses and functional losses than by the problems with employment, finances, and family relations that are more frequently encountered among younger adults who attempt suicide. Suicides are more often completed by men (60%); suicides are more often attempted by women (75%). The methods include guns, hanging, drug overdose, and cutting or slashing. Threats are real, and first attempts usually are successful. One half to two-thirds of individuals see primary care providers within the month prior to the suicide, 10% to 40% have seen providers within the week of their death (Cobb et al., 2002). These visits represent a cry for help and provide a window of opportunity during which to intervene. More insidious suicide activities among elders include refusal to eat, take medications, or follow simple safety procedures and overuse of alcohol and drugs.

Nurses should consider the potential for suicide in any elders who are depressed or exhibit negativism and hopelessness. Elders fear loneliness, abandonment, loss of control, and pain, but not always death. Incidence of suicide is higher among elders who are white, male, Protestant, or widowed; they often live alone, have financial problems, have a history of alcoholism, and have poor health, especially a recent diagnosis of terminal illness. The nurse must not hesitate to inquire about suicidal fantasies and ideation. If these thoughts are present, the elder is asked directly about plans, method, and means. Behavioral clues such as putting personal affairs in order, giving away possessions, making wills and funeral arrangements, self-neglect, erratic behavior, suspiciousness,

---

### BOX 35-17

**Strategies for Management of Depression in Elders**

- Offer unconditional positive regard for the changes of aging and altered function.
- Emphasize with the elder and family that depression is very manageable and reversible; offer hope.
- Encourage the elder to maintain control over self and the situation by offering choices for simple decision making.
- Assist the elder to identify the positives of the situation and opportunities for gains as well as losses.
- In collaboration with the primary care provider, encourage the use of medications, psychotherapy, and exercise to treat the depression.

---

### BOX 35-18

**Strategies for Prevention of Suicide in Elders at Risk**

- Reduce immediate danger by removing hazardous articles.
- Refer any potentially suicidal elder promptly to his or her primary care provider (same day). Provide a constant companion (family, friend) en route.
- Extract a promise from the elder not to attempt suicide before the agreed intervention (e.g., clinic visit, your next visit).
- Mobilize resources by restoring a sense of control in the elder's life, reconnecting the elder with significant others, and developing life lines of support systems and community resources.
- Follow up with regular calls on the elder and maintenance of support systems.

---

hoarding pills, and personality changes must be addressed. Community health nurses have unique opportunities for suicide prevention through early case finding and enrichment of resources and support systems (Box 35-18).

## ■ Employment and Retirement

Approximately 12% of older adults are employed or actively seeking employment (18% of elder men and 10% of elder women), up from 1990 and with an increasing trend toward women working in their later years. Of these working elders, more than 50% work part-time (often without benefits) and 24% are self-employed (U.S. Bureau of Census, 2001). With a life expectancy of 20 or more years at age 65, transition from work into retirement which is a twentieth-century phenomenon—is the major normative event of the second half of life. Issues to be considered in retirement planning include financial security; role restructuring; location; new or part-time careers; educational, recreational, and leisure activities; and relationships with family and friends. With the loss of a formal work role and more leisure time, many elders enjoy volunteering with community agencies or through programs such as the Retired Senior Volunteer Program (RSVP) through the local area agency on aging. Others pursue lifelong learning by way of community education programs through schools (including high school equivalency programs), colleges, and universities, and elderhostel programs throughout the world. Travel about the country or abroad may be an option.

By being aware of the meanings of "work and play" for elders, community health nurses can be alert for the problems that may arise during these transition periods. For those who are able to redefine themselves with meaningful activities, the latter stages of life can be times for achieving ego integrity (Erikson, 1963) and self-actualization (Maslow, 1968) through lifelong learning and creativity. For those who are unable to make these transitions, old age may become a time of loneliness, hopelessness, and boredom. Quality of life rather than quantity of life becomes the issue. Mastery of the past is the basis for adaptation to the present and hope for the future. Family, friends, and faith are integral to self-concept and spirituality.

Nurses can help alert elders to the characteristics and normality of aging and the **life review** process to find purpose in life (Ebersole et al., 2005). Interventions to facilitate these transitions are summarized in Box 35-19. For frail and/or demented elders, special programs (e.g., the Eden Alternative) are needed to combat the plagues of loneliness, boredom, and helplessness in nursing homes by using

Although as a culture we often associate romance, dating, and marriage with youth, elders can continue to have healthy, loving, and passionate relationships throughout the life span. This couple dated for two years and married at the age of ninety, after being widowed for several years.

companionship, variety, and helpfulness. The integration of resident animals, abundant plants, children, and community activities into this environment makes it a more human habitat. For example, a nursing home may adopt suitable dogs and cats from animal shelters, sponsor a scout troup, offer its meeting rooms for local gardener groups, and provide summer day camps for children.

### Sexuality

Aging is no deterrent to the need for love and belongingness. The desire for intimacy usually is with one's own generation (spouse, partner, friend), rather than with previous generations (parents) or subsequent generations (children). Elders in any community setting need social interactions with their peers. Their sexual expressions may take a variety of forms, including touching, holding, kissing, fondling, petting, and intercourse, and may be heterosexual or homosexual. For older adults living with children or in institutions, nurses may need to facilitate their needs for privacy and intimacy. For those with no spouse or partner, masturbation or fantasy may be alternatives. As with any age group, sexually active elders are at risk for sexually transmit-

## THINK ABOUT THIS

The endlessly youthful baby-boomer generation turns 60 in 2005 and they are *not* in their rocking chairs!

The baby-boomer generation that "couldn't get no satisfaction" are now senior citizens. Kathleen Casey has the distinction of being the first baby born in the baby-boomer generation at 12:01 A.M. on January 1, 1946. She was the first of 76 million Americans brought into the world between 1946 and 1964 when, in a sharp reversal of a steady century of decline, the national birth rate skyrocketed, creating a massive demographic upheaval. This generation is showing no signs of slowing down or changing the lifestyles that changed the world more than 40 years ago. For example, 40 years after the Rolling Stones hit the top of the charts with *I Can't Get No Satisfaction*, the Stones launched their 2005 world tour at Boston's Fenway Park. The band continues to be among the top five grossing concert groups in the United States. This generation gained unprecedented affluence—no matter how much they have, they can't ever seem to get enough or do enough. Here are just a few well-known Americans who are in their fifties and sixties.

Dolly Parton (1946)
Former President Bill Clinton (1946)
President George W. Bush (1946)
Katie Couric (1957)
Condoleezza Rice (1954)
Oprah Winfrey (1954)
Bill Gates (1955)
Bruce Springsteen (1949)
Cher (1946)
Donald Trump (1946)
Jimmy Buffett (1946)
Reggie Jackson (1946)

## BOX 35-19

### Strategies for Late-Life Transitions

- Encourage spontaneous reminiscence and life review that provide opportunities for elders and their families to recapitulate events in their lives, for elders to create material and/or symbolic legacies, and for families to develop their family and cultural heritage.
- Facilitate connections between past hopes, present events, and future expectations. Support the elder's spiritual belief system. Confront conflicts and anxiety regarding death, guilt, and dependency; instill a sense of hope.
- Use an eclectic approach with counseling, coaching, and listening based on individual situations. Be a dependable confidante, and be aware that life review may be carried out sporadically over several months or years.
- Recommend motivation and remotivation, purpose in life, or validation therapies for frail and/or demented elders.
- Avoid stereotyping and premature closures by elders, families, and caregivers, including nurses.
- Suggest age-appropriate social, recreational, and diversional activities with family and peers to establish support systems and prevent social isolation (e.g., volunteerism, educational programs, 50 Plus, RSVP, civic and religious groups, senior citizens centers).

## BOX 35-20

### Safety Precautions for Elders

- Check to see that stairs are well lighted, are free of clutter, and have nonskid surface and hand rails.
- Check bathrooms for hand rails, nonslip adhesive surfaces in tubs/showers, and nonslip flooring.
- Provide rooms with adequate, nonglare lighting; eliminate clutter and throw rugs, casters on chairs, dangling cords, and waxed floors. Avoid sedation with narcotics and sedatives. Use carbon monoxide and smoke detectors.
- Encourage defensive driving; suggest the local AARP mature/defensive driving program.
- Provide for easy access to the local emergency system, including telephone numbers. If the individual is frail and/or homebound, suggest "Friendly Caller" or lifeline services.
- Recommend identification jewelry (i.e., bracelet or necklace) and have current photo identification readily available.
- When accidents occur, investigate as to specific information on location, time, and environmental factors, and intervene to prevent their recurrence.

ted diseases (STDs), including human immunodeficiency virus (HIV) infection and acquired immune deficiency syndrome (AIDS).

The **PLISSIT model** (Permission, Limited Information, Specific Suggestions, Intensive Therapy) is helpful to assess and intervene in sexual problems with elders (Annon, 1976). For example, nurses can support the sexuality of elders indirectly by saying gently that romance does not end at a certain age and wonder if the person has any questions or concerns in this area (e.g., getting permission to discuss sexuality). If men indicate a problem, the nurse can ask more directly, but tactfully, if they are having problems with erections or intercourse; if women indicate a problem, the nurse can ask about lubrication; both can be asked about satisfaction and what they want to do about their intimacy needs. The nurse can provide limited information and make specific suggestions for simple problems (e.g., mild analgesia and alternative positions for painful joints), and then make referrals to a primary care provider for intensive therapy as indicated.

### Safety and Security

As an aspect of work and play, safety for elders is concerned with accidental injuries in the home and community, especially from falls, fires, and motor vehicle accidents. Older adults with generalized weakness, slow reaction time, unstable gait, visual changes, hearing loss, and on multiple medications are at greater risk for accidents and crime. Unfortunately, their vulnerability makes them frequent targets of purse snatchings, pickpocketing, fraud (e.g., fraudulent claims, confidence games, medical quackery), theft, vandalism, and harassment. Community health nurses need to assess home safety to eliminate hazards (see Appendix F), teach elders and caregivers basic safety measures, and advocate for greater safety in the community. Safety precautions for elders are summarized in Box 35-20.

## ■ Thermal Regulation and Skin Integrity

With less efficient thermal regulation, elders are at higher risk for health problems during temperature extremes. As the largest organ of the body, the skin of elderly people undergoes many age-related changes, and it is subject to serious complications. Nurses are at the forefront of preventive health care for the functions of both "heat/cool" and "touch/feel."

### Thermal Regulation

Internal body temperature is a balance of cellular metabolism, muscle activity, and heat loss by radiation, convection, and evaporation through the skin (Ebersole et al., 2005). The ability to feel heat and cold is impaired in elders, and their return to core body temperature in response to heating or cooling takes twice as long as in their youth. Drugs such as sedative-hypnotics, phenothiazines, and alcohol may further impair thermoregulatory mechanisms (Cobb et al., 2002). Fear of costly utility bills may inhibit their use of air conditioning or heating systems during extreme temperatures. These factors place community-dwelling elders at high risk for hypothermia and hyperthermia during very hot and cold weather.

Community health nurses can help prevent life-threatening emergencies and death by encouraging elders and families to check homes for insulation and caulking to maintain heat and cool. Assistance with fuel costs, which is available in most states, also may be needed. Nurses can help establish "buddy" systems among family, friends, and neighbors to make daily checks on elders during weather extremes. A low threshold of suspicion should be used for referrals of at-risk elders to primary care providers or emergency care centers for thermal regulatory problems.

### Hypothermia

Elders produce less heat per kilogram of body weight. They usually have decreased muscle mass and subcutaneous fat, reduced muscle activity, and less efficient shivering. The vasoconstriction response of their skin arterioles to cooling is diminished, so heat within the body is not conserved. Elders are also less able to discriminate temperature differences and may have delayed perception of being cold. These age-related changes contribute to an increased risk of hypothermia in elders when indoor temperatures are below 65°F. Symptoms of hypothermia include a body temperature of 95°F (96°F rectal) or less, cold to touch, absent shivering and piloerection, slow capillary refill, pallor or cyanosis, bradypnea, arrhythmia and bradycardia, hypotension, slurred speech, and lethargy. Treatment requires slow warming and may require hospitalization for metabolic imbalances if cooling is prolonged or extreme. See Box 35-21 for techniques to prevent hypothermia.

### Hyperthermia

The vasodilatation response of the arterioles to heating is diminished in elders, such that heat is not delivered to the skin for dissipation. As a consequence, a greater threshold temperature is needed to initiate perspiration, and less sweat is produced in response to heating. Elders also are less sensitive to thirst. Individuals with cardiovascular and peripheral vascular diseases, diabetes, and infections, well as those taking certain medications (e.g., anticholinergics, antihistamines, diuetics, beta blockers, antidepressants, antiparkinsonian drugs), are at risk for hyperthermia.

The three types of hyperthermic emergencies are heat syncope, heat exhaustion, and heat stroke. Symptoms include increased body temperature (especially 105°F and higher), flushed skin, tachypnea, headache, weakness, and seizures. Suggested techniques to prevent hyperthermia in elders are listed in Box 35-21.

### Skin Integrity

Owing to increased elasticity, decreased surface acidity, dryness of the epidermis (xerosis), thinning of the dermis, and loss of subcutaneous fat, skin integrity is an ever-present potential problem in elders. Skin also has strong symbolic significance and influence on self-esteem. Some elders feel "untouchable" as they experience the wrinkling associated with aging. Gentle touch on the hand, arm, or shoulder helps establish contact with many elders. Nurses need to inspect the skin during any clinical encounter or procedure to check for the many skin disorders of elders (e.g., pruritis [itching], urticaria, intertrigo, seborrheic dermatitis and keratosis, rosacea, psoriasis). Several skin cancers are common in elders (e.g., actinic keratoses [precancerous], basal-cell and squamous-cell carcinomas, and melanomas). The nurse should check skin lesions for the ABCDs of cancers: Asymmetry, irregular Borders, multiple Colors, and Diameter greater than 1 cm. Suspicious findings should be reported promptly to the primary care provider. Lacerations (especially skin tears), abrasions, and pressure ulcers also are common in elders.

---

**BOX 35-21**

**Techniques to Improve Thermal Regulation in Elders**

**Prevention of Hypothermia**
- Drink adequate warm fluids and eat hot, calorie-rich foods.
- Warm hands and feet; cover them with warm blankets. Warm the room to 68 to 70 °F when elders are inactive, and use electric blankets at night.
- During the day, wear head coverings; warm, layered clothing; and socks and shoes. Use leg warmers on arms and legs. At night, wear a bed cap and leg and foot warmers.
- Encourage indoor physical activity.
- Avoid alcohol and drugs that lower regulatory mechanisms.

**Prevention of Hyperthermia**
- During heat extremes, drink 2,000 to 3,000 mL of cool fluids per day, if tolerated.
- Avoid exertion, especially during the heat of the day, between 10 A.M. and 4 P.M.
- Alternate periods of heat exposure with cooling; stay in air conditioning or use fans when possible.
- Avoid alcohol and drugs that inhibit thermal regulation.

---

Maintenance of skin integrity can be accomplished by limiting bathing (i.e., two to three times per week in warm weather, once or twice per week in cold weather), liberally using emollients (e.g., Eucerine lotion, Vaseline ointment), and avoiding prolonged direct sun exposure (i.e., wearing protective clothing or sunscreens). Bath oils are to be avoided because they may exacerbate skin problems and increase the risk of falls; water softeners and perineal wipes often are too harsh for the thin skin of elders and are to be avoided.

### Pressure Ulcers

Maintenance of skin integrity and prevention of pressure ulcers require an ever-present vigilance of elders, family caregivers, and nurses in the community. As with other age groups, skin problems are prevented with adequate nutrition and avoidance of pressure, friction, shear, and moisture

---

**A Good Read**

## Tuesdays with Morrie: An Old Man, a Young Man, and Life's Greatest Lessons (1997)

*by Mitch Albom, New York: Doubleday*

This book details the relationship between a former student and his professor, Morrie, as the professor battles Lou Gehrig's disease (amyotrophic lateral sclerosis). A nonfiction best-seller, this book is an outstanding story about life, death, and the meaning of it all.

## BOX 35-22

### Techniques to Prevent Pressure Ulcers in Elders

- Teach elders and family members to inspect the skin daily, especially the sacrum, hips, and heels. Use a hand mirror for pressure sites not easily seen. Nurses should directly observe the skin of vulnerable elders on *every* visit.
- Improve skin tolerance to pressure by cleansing vulnerable areas with mild soap; avoid hot water, excessive friction, and prolonged soaking. Treat dry skin with moisturizers or emollients. Avoid massage over bony prominences.
- Minimize exposure to moisture. Check persons with incontinence at least every 2 hours, clean the skin, and change clothing or pads immediately. Use topical moisture barriers if necessary.
- While in bed, absolutely reposition the elderly every 2 hours (post a schedule); use positioning devices (i.e., pillows, foam wedges) at no more than 30 degrees lateral inclined position; avoid positioning on the trochanters. Use pressure-reducing devices (30 degrees maximum) and limit time of head elevation. Keep both heels off the bed—no doughnuts.
- Use lifting devices (i.e., trapeze, lifts, bed linens) to avoid friction and shear.

(AHCPR, 1992). Individuals most at risk are immobile, incontinent, malnourished, frail, or confused. With elders who are confined to bed or wheelchairs, the most common sites of pressure ulcers are the ischium (24%), sacrum (23%), trochanters (15%), and malleolus (7%). Community health nurses can help prevent these painful, costly, and life-threatening complications by being systematic, comprehensive, and routine about skin care. Two instruments often used for assessment of risk factors are the Braden Scale, for predicting pressure sore risk, and the Norton Risk Assessment Scale. Techniques to prevent pressure ulcers in elders are listed in Box 35-22.

## ■ Comfort and Spirituality

Elders may not complain of discomfort or pain; health care providers may treat it inadequately; and poorly managed pain may aggravate other health problems. Given the many age-related health and lifestyle changes experienced by elders, an intact spiritual belief system is essential. "Hurt" and "believe" conclude this functional approach to preventive health care.

### Comfort

Altered proprioception is more common in elders, who typically have increased light touch and pain thresholds. Maintaining comfort and managing pain—both acute and chronic—are essential to keep elders mobile and fully involved in their daily activities. Community health nurses need to assess comfort levels frequently using standard pain scales for persistent problems. Gentle massage, warm (*not* hot) baths, and fragrances are just a few of the techniques that may be helpful for common discomforts. In collabora-

tion with the primary care provider, *regular* use of analgesics may be helpful to lower the pain threshold and improve comfort and mobility (e.g., acetaminophen 500 or 650 mg one or two tablets three or four times daily as needed for discomfort [maximum 4,000 mg/day]). Nurses must be vigilant for overuse of OTC nonsteroidal anti-inflammatory drugs (NSAIDs; e.g., aspirin, ibuprofen, naproxen), which can lead to gastrointestinal bleeding in elders. They must also be cautious with narcotic and sedative drugs, which can contribute to delirium and falls in this age group.

### Spirituality

With the experiences of aging and changes in health status, many elders and families are faced with the need to discover a continuing purpose in the elder's life, find new meanings in their existence, and prepare for their transcendence from life to death. As they approach the end of their lives, elders may contemplate their movement from the concrete reality of their physical existence toward more abstract, metaphorical conceptualizations of their oneness with God, a divine being, or a higher power. Spirituality—the essence of the soul—may be integral to elders' beliefs, hope, energy, creativity, acceptance of life and death, and transcendence (Ebersole et al., 2005).

As with other age groups, nurses assess the spiritual health of elders by inquiring discretely about their spiritual perspectives and religious commitments. Observations include their ability to discover continuing meaning and purpose in life, give and receive love, have hope, be creative, and share humor. The goals of spiritual care are to preserve the elders' unique beliefs and values and support their religious practices. Nurses may need to help elders make contact with religious advisors (e.g., minister, priest, rabbi, shaman) and use religious articles (e.g., Bible, Koran, crucifix, medals, prayer shawls, incense). They may need to have privacy for prayer and meditation or may want to sing hymns, read or write poetry, or offer other forms of self-expression. Elders may ask the nurse to share in these practices, as is appropriate for the situation. Other spiritual issues, life review, and advance directives are discussed elsewhere in this chapter. However the elders express their spirituality, it is important that nurses recognize these needs and assist with their being met.

### ◉ MEDIA MOMENT

Don't miss these movies about aging:
*On Golden Pond*
*Driving Miss Daisy*
*The Notebook*
Songs about aging include these:
*Old Man*, Neil Young
*100 Years*, Five for Fighting
*Living Years*, Mike and the Mechanics
*When I'm 64*, The Beatles
*Eleanor Rigby*, The Beatles

## Special Elder Health Issues

Community health nurses must consider special aspects of health care in elderly populations. Comprehensive health care for elders includes immunizations, medication review, chemical abuse, and ethical dilemmas.

### ■ Immunizations

Taken together, pneumonia and influenza are a leading cause of death in the United States. Elders with chronic illnesses are at the highest risk for these respiratory illnesses (e.g., individuals with heart disease, lung disease, diabetes, immunocompromised status, and other chronic conditions). In the elderly population, immunizations usually are limited to four vaccines: influenza, pneumococcal, tetanus/diphtheria and Zostavax for shingles (Herpes zoster) (CDC, 2008). For elders who travel to foreign countries, other immunizations may be indicated. Elders should be referred to their local health department immunization clinic for information about the requirements for specific countries.

### ■ Medications

Elderly individuals purchase 40% of all prescription drugs (most commonly cardiovascular, anti-infective, antipsychotic, antidepressant, and diuretic agents) and 40% of OTC medicines (mostly analgesics, laxatives, and antacids). An average of five prescription drugs and three OTC drugs are taken by 90% of elders (USFDA, 2003). Because aging changes affect the absorption, distribution, metabolism, and elimination of pharmacological agents, elders are more prone to drug interactions, adverse reactions, and toxicities.

**Polypharmacy** (use of many drugs simultaneously) is a multifactorial problem that results from a "pill-oriented" society, elders' beliefs about health care and their various acute and chronic health problems, the prescribing practices of primary care providers, and the use of multiple primary and specialty providers. Problems of adherence to drug regimens occur with 25% to 50% of medications, including underuse, overuse, and misuse; many of these errors contribute to unnecessary hospitalizations (Ebersole et al., 2005). In 2005, Medicare began to provide limited funding for some prescription drugs; in most states, Medicaid limits recipients to five prescriptions per month. Some insurance plans also offer assistance with drugs (www.med.care.gov/pdp_basic_information.asp. Because of the expense of these drugs, elders may not fill prescriptions or may discontinue medications or decrease dosages and/or frequencies to stretch their medicines.

Community health nurses must be attentive for errors of omission (e.g., unfilled prescriptions, skipped doses, discontinuing medicines) and errors of commission (e.g., self-medication by increasing or decreasing dosages, changing times, using another person's drugs, taking OTC drugs). Nursing interventions for drug therapies are summarized in Box 35-23.

---

### BOX 35-23

**Strategies to Improve Medication Use by Elders**

- Obtain a medication history and consider the ability of elders to manage their medications, including financial status (purchase), environmental situation (storage), educational level (literacy), cognitive status (memory), visual acuity (reading labels), functional status (opening containers), and drug allergies.
- Remind elders to bring their medicines to each clinic visit; do a drug review ("brown-bag check") for correct medications, dosages, instructions, refills, and drug knowledge.
- Check medications frequently during home visits, including storage arrangements and the disposition of old medications.
- In collaboration with primary care providers, simplify drug regimens and eliminate all unnecessary drugs, both prescribed and OTC. Use once- or twice-daily dosing whenever possible.
- Teach elders and family members about all their medications and prepare a written schedule, including each drug name and strength, size/color, purpose, frequency with specific times or days (e.g., 8 A.M. and 4 P.M. instead of "twice daily"; Monday, Wednesday, Friday instead of "every other day"), and important side effects.
- Encourage elders and family members to purchase all medications through the same pharmacy to check for drug allergies and interactions.

- Encourage elders to take medications at the same time and place every day with 4 to 6 ounces of water. Use memory aids to assist with adherence to drug regimens (e.g., written lists, medication calendars, pill boxes).
- Store all medicines together in a safe dry place, in their original containers, and out of the reach of small children. Some medications require refrigeration.
- Remind elders to take a sufficient supply of all medicines when traveling away from home.
- If elders have memory problems, functional impairments, or complicated drug regimens, suggest the use of medication boxes prefilled by the elder or caregiver either daily or weekly.
- If elders have arthritic problems, suggest easy-opening containers; if they have visual problems, use large print for labels; if they have swallowing problems, use liquid forms. Caution against crushing tablets or emptying capsules into food or fluid before checking with a pharmacist.
- Monitor elders continually for efficacy and side effects of medications. Use the Abnormal Involuntary Movement Scale (AIMS) to monitor drugs (especially antipsychotics) with extrapyramidal side effects such as tremors, akinesia, akathesia, and rigidity (tardive dyskinesia).

## ■ Chemical Addictions

Among elders, chemical addictions include all of the psychoactive chemicals used by younger populations, with alcohol being the substance that is most frequently abused. Alcoholism is estimated to affect 10% to 15% of community-dwelling elders. Given their decreased tolerance to alcohol, combined with normal aging changes and use of multiple prescription and OTC drugs, elders are at higher risk for falls, accidents, and burns. Nurses in the community can help identify these individuals by noting changes in behavior (e.g., anxiety, memory loss, depression, blackouts, confusion), health status (e.g., weight loss), hygiene, falls, and injuries. Elders can be screened with the TWEACK test (Cobb et al., 2002).

| | |
|---|---|
| Tolerance | How many drinks before you feel the effects of alcohol? |
| Worry | Have you ever felt worried by criticism of your drinking? |
| Eye opener | Have you ever taken a morning "eye opener"? |
| Amnesia | Are there times after drinking when you can't remember what you did? |
| Cut down | Have you ever felt the need to cut down on drinking? |
| Drinking | How many drinks before you fall asleep or pass out? |

Those persons and families found to have alcohol problems may be referred to their primary care providers, community mental health centers, Alcoholics Anonymous, or other local agencies for chemical abuse. Because denial of alcohol abuse is so prevalent and the necessary lifestyle changes are so difficult to maintain, recovery often is a long, irregular process. Nurses need to persist in their support, referral, and follow-up for these individuals and their families.

Other substances abused by elders include nicotine, food, caffeine, prescription and OTC drugs, illicit street drugs, and food. Assessments and interventions for these chemicals are similar to those for younger populations.

## ■ Ethical Dilemmas

Because community health nurses become so involved with elderly people in their own environment, they often encounter ethical dilemmas and end-of-life issues. All too often, there is no simple, easy, "right" answer to these complex situations—if there was, the dilemma would not exist. Usually the choice is between two or more "bad" options. Beware of simple solutions, which usually ignore the complex nature of dilemmas. For example, when a frail, demented elder is anorexic, losing weight, and at risk for complications, one option is to insert an enteral feeding tube. That measure may improve nutrition, but it may also prolong the person's suffering and dying and may be against his or her wishes for end-of-life care.

In American society, critical values in most ethical dilemmas are concerned with autonomy (freedom of choice), nonmaleficence or beneficence (do no harm/do good), and distributive justice (use of resources). Because elders consume large amounts of healthcare resources, ethical conflicts occur around the issues of old versus young, and quantity of life (adding years to life) versus quality of life (adding life to years). For many elders, the finality of death must be weighed against dependence, pain, abandonment, and loneliness. Clarification of beliefs and values of the elder, the family, and the healthcare providers may offer insights into these differing perspectives and facilitate satisfactory resolution of these conflicts.

**Advance directives** can help clarify elders' desire for health care interventions in the event of life-threatening situations. Nurses can encourage families to discuss end-of-life issues (e.g., cardiopulmonary resuscitation, hospitalization, antibiotics, intravenous and enteral feedings) while elders are relatively young, healthy, and competent to express their wishes. The elder can complete a durable power of attorney for health care in accordance with state statutes to assist family members and healthcare providers in implementing these wishes. In elders, intellectual competence for informed consent can be determined with the FMMSE (see Appendix E).

For elders who have no advance directives and are very frail or demented, the occurrence of end-of-life issues frequently can be anticipated. Nurses can take the initiative to approach families with these decisions *early*, encourage them to talk with extended family members as appropriate, and consider what the elders would prefer if they were able to express their wishes. Criteria for decision making are to be considered (e.g., reversibility or irreversibility of the condition), communicated with the primary care provider, and decisions documented appropriately. If elders are able to participate in these decisions, the nurse should encourage them to do so. Supporting the spiritual integrity of all concerned helps sort out the issues and maintain positive attitudes and behaviors.

---

### ⚖ ETHICAL CONNECTION

The number of older female drivers will increase dramatically as baby-boomers continue to work past 65 years of age. Currently, 75% of women older than 55 have a driver's license, but 90% of women younger than 55 drive. As the percentage of the population older than age 65 rises sharply after 2010, a key question will be how many continue to work and, therefore, commute in their cars.

Retired people have traditionally been very careful about staying off interstate highways, taking back roads, and not driving after dark. If you are still working, you may not have that choice. That leads to a safety question that remains to be answered.

What are the ethical implications for nursing, the healthcare system, and society? ◯

*Source*: Pisarski, A. (October 16, 2006). *Commuting in America III*. Transportation Research Board, National Research Council.

## Application to Practice

Ten years ago, I had the opportunity to work as a beginning nurse practitioner and clinic manager for a new outpatient clinic offering services exclusively to men and women aged 65 years and older. In addition to offering traditional clinic health services such as visits for health problems and illnesses, lab work, and diagnostic procedures, one of the goals of the clinic was to focus on health promotion for older adults. In designing the clinic facility, we dedicated space for a classroom for community events, such as education classes and health screenings.

Recognizing that most exercise programs in the community involved joining a fitness club and fees, we developed a senior exercise class, to be held in the community classroom. The senior exercise class was offered without charge to senior adults in the community. The only requirement was that the senior's primary care provider complete a brief health history and permission for participation in exercise. We provided age-appropriate videotapes to the seniors, and a group of "faithful" exercisers began to form. Within a year, this community of "exercisers" outgrew their classroom, necessitating offering additional sessions. As the program expanded, our facility had to move the sessions to a larger room to accommodate their demands for walking around the room's perimeter. Our senior exercisers continued to make additional requests over the years, such as equipment for weight-bearing exercise, which we gladly provided.

Ten years later, the group is now at least 50 members strong who participate in the program on each of the 3 days that the facility is open for exercise. In addition to the obvious health benefits of exercise, the participants enjoy this fellowship of friends, old and new. If there is an illness, surgery, or death, group members send cards and visit their exercise "community."

One of the most remarkable outcomes of this self-governed group is that the group members have assumed total responsibility for leading the exercises, choosing whether to use videotapes, selecting music, and generally running the program with little to no assistance from the clinic's staff. The group has sustained itself for over a decade, demonstrating "if you build it, they will come"—as long as we create *with* our patients, not *for* them!

**—Cynthia Luther, ANP, PhD**

Thoughts from the Seniors:

Our program starts at the top of the head and progresses downward until every part receives a share of the exercise. This is followed with a session of aerobics. As "icing on the cake," each class is accompanied by appropriate music as a method of putting the participants "in the mood" and removing any drudgery that may accompany a session. At the beginning of the aerobics, participants are invited to dance, using steps of their choice, to music selected by the group. This serves to add a bit of pleasure to a session . . . Another advantage of a class session is the development of friendships by providing for meeting of people they may otherwise never know. Then there is the possibility and innate pleasure of engaging in activities that enlarge their lives at a time when such may be badly needed.

"The Music Man"

Walking around the carpeted indoor track for about 15 minutes before exercise class increases my heartbeat. This may not be for everyone, but I like it. When class begins, we are seated in armed chairs for the first 50 exercise movements. We move our heads, shoulders, arms, fingers, hands, legs, feet, and toes. If I experience any discomfort, I don't move beyond that point. I try to keep up with the background music. The last part of the exercise program is spent standing behind our chairs, which includes aerobics.

By attending the "early bird" class, I still have time for other things during the day. When class ends, I feel better than when I left home. Class members are friendly; the fellowship is very good!

Monday, Wednesday, and Friday we rise early, so as to get to the senior early-bird exercise class. We both have arthritis and know this helps keeps those joints moving. Our leader is in her 80s but can still bend to touch her toes! We have our "Music Man" who provides great tapes to exercise by, and that breaks the monotony. However, we do laugh a lot at the various joints popping! We are a unique group of approximately 30 seniors who really enjoy each other's company—so much that we get together in one of the member's homes for spring brunch and Christmas luncheon. ◉

Source: Photos courtesy of Cynthia Luther, PhD, ANP.

## An Old Woman Lives in My Mother's House

An old woman lives in my mother's house;
she sits alone and watches TV.
An old woman lives where my mother once did,
in the house Daddy built in '53.

An old woman wears my mother's clothes
though they don't fit; they hang on her back.
The old woman shuffles in Mother's shoes
when we go for a walk at the walking track.

An old woman cries in my mother's bed,
cries for the things she thinks someone took.
The old woman stops and scratches her head
And looks for her keys or her puzzle book.

The old woman says no one ever comes
to visit, though we go every day.
My mother would not complain like that
but the old woman took my mother away.

The old woman wants my mother's checks,
screams that she has no money at all.
My sister patiently pays the bills,
takes the old woman to shop at the mall.

They buy more yarn for my mother to knit,
to make afghans for little ones' toes.
The old woman bundles the skeins in bags
and hides it away where only she knows.

The old woman screams when I clean her house;
I shut the door and change the bed.
Sometimes I cry when she throws me out,
though I know it's not Mother's anger I dread.

My brothers help out whenever they can.
The old woman swears they never come.
We write in a book, keep a daily log,
for Mother to read, should she ever come home.

—*Brenda Finnegan*

This poem was written by the author about her experiences with her mother, who has Alzheimer's disease.

Research Alert

This article presents information on a new Great Britain National Health Service (NHS) report titled "Prescriptions Dispensed in the Community 1997–2007," which has revealed that polypharmacy is on the rise in older people in England. It also says that people over age 60 are prescribed twice as many drugs as they were 10 years ago. The report further says that older people receive more prescription items per head than any other group, 42.4 items on average compared with 9.5 items for those aged 16–59.

*Source*: Birmingham, K. (2008). Older people take twice as many drugs. *Nursing Older People, 20*(7), 4–4.

## Conclusion

With the "graying of America," elders have became an integral concern for the delivery of community health care. These older adults were socialized in a reactive health care system that focused on illness. Until recently, they have not been especially proactive or focused on wellness or preven-tion. Community health nurses in the twenty-first century can help elders by promoting the three A's: awareness, assessment, and advocacy. Nurses can help elders practice health promotion and primary disease prevention through good nutrition, regular exercise, family and community involvement, stress management, anticipatory guidance, and safety checks. Secondary prevention requires self-monitoring activities (e.g., breast or testicular self-examinations), periodic screening, regular physical and oral health exams, and adherence to therapeutic regimens. By working collaboratively with primary care providers, nurses can improve the health and quality of life of older adults—and help them celebrate the joy of aging.

 Explore Community Health Nursing on the Web! To learn more about the topics in this chapter, use the passcode provided to access your exclusive website: **http://nursing.jbpub.com/ communityhealth.** If you do not have a passcode, you can obtain one at this site.

## ■ CRITICAL THINKING ACTIVITIES

1. After reading the following, what are some ways that community health nurses can help "reconnect" elders with other patients in the health care delivery system? Identify settings where health promotion interventions might be created to meet this need.

   On the need to reconnect with elders . . .

   A great deal of America's social sickness comes from age segregation. . . . We segregate the old for many reasons: prejudice, ignorance and a lack of good alternatives. . . . If we aren't around dying people, we don't have to think about dying . . . and, the more involved we are with the old, the more pain we feel at their suffering. . . . The old often save the young. And the young save the old. . . . If 10 people ages 2 to 80 are grouped together, they will fall into a natural hierarchy that nurtures and teaches them all . . . the incredible calculus of old age—that as more is taken, there is more love for what remains.

   Mary Pipher (1999, March 19–21). The new generation gap: For the nations health, we need to reconnect young and old. *USA Weekend*, p. 12.

2. Using photographs, assist an elderly patient with visualizing independence in his or her life today. How can photographs throughout our lives assist in maximizing our ability to care for ourselves and promote our autonomy? Think of times in your own life when you were dependent and had limitations. What kinds of images helped improve your confidence in becoming self-sufficient again?

# ■ REFERENCES

Agency for Health Care Policy and Research (AHCPR). (1992). *Pressure ulcers in adults: Prediction and prevention.* Rockville, MD: U.S. Government Printing Office.

Agency for Health Care Policy and Research (AHCPR). (1996a). *Recognition and treatment of Alzheimer's disease and related dementias.* Rockville, MD: U.S. Government Printing Office.

Agency for Health Care Policy and Research (AHCPR). (1996b). *Managing acute and chronic urinary incontinence.* Rockville, MD: U.S. Government Printing Office.

American Association of Colleges of Nursing (AACN). (2000). *Older adults: Recommended baccalaureate competencies and curricular guidelines to geriatric nursing care.* Washington, DC: Author.

American Association of Retired Persons (AARP). (2004). *Care and family.* Washington DC: Author.

Annon, J. (January 1976). The PLISSIT model: A proposed conceptual scheme for behavioral treatment of sexual problems. *Journal of Sex Education and Therapy*, pp. 18–20.

Burnside, I. (1988). *Nursing and the aged: A self-care approach* (2nd ed.). New York: McGraw-Hill.

Busse, E., & Blazer, D. (1999). *Textbook of geriatric psychiatry* (2nd ed.). Washington, DC: American Psychiatric Press.

Butler, R. (2003). *Why survive? Being old in America.* Johns Hopkins University Press. Baltimore, MD.

Carter, E., & McGoldrick, M. (1980). *The family life cycle: A framework for family therapy* (pp. 3–20). New York: Gardner.

Carter, J. (1995). *Always a reckoning.* New York: Random House.

Centers for Disease Control and Prevention (CDC). (2008). *National immunization project: Adult immunization schedule.* Washington, DC: Centers for Disease Control and Prevention. Atlanta, GA. Retrieved November 13, 2008, from http://www.cdc.gov/vaccines/recs/schedules/adultschedule.htm

Cobb, E., Duthie, E., & Murphy, J. (Eds.). (2002). *Geriatrics review syllabus: A core curriculum in geriatric medicine* (5th ed.). Malden, MA: Blackwell Publishing for the American Geriatrics Society.

Comfort, A. (1990). *Say yes to old age: Developing a positive attitude toward aging.* New York: Crown.

Cora, V. L. (1985). *Family life process of intergenerational families with functionally dependent elders.* Dissertation. University of Alabama at Birmingham.

Duvall, E. M. (1977). *Marriage and family development.* Philadelphia: Lippincott.

Ebersole, P., Hess, P., Touhy, T., & Jett, K. (2005). *Gerontological nursing and healthy aging.* St. Louis, MO: Mosby.

Erikson, E. (1963). *Childhood and society.* New York: Norton.

Folstein, M., Folstein, S., & McHugh, P. (1975). Mini-mental state: A practical method for grading the cognitive state of patients for the clinician. *Journal of Psychiatric Research, 12,* 189–198.

Gunter, L., & Estes, C. (1979). *Education for geronic nursing.* New York: Springer.

Kane, R., Ouslander, J., & Abrass, I. (2003). *Essentials of clinical geriatrics* (5th ed.). New York: McGraw-Hill.

Katz, S., Ford, A., Moskowitz, R., et al. (1963). Studies of illness in the aged: The index of ADL. *Journal of the American Medical Association, 185,* 914.

Lawton, M., & Brody, E. (1969). Assessment of older people: Self maintaining and instrumental activities of daily living. *Gerontologist, 9,* 179–186.

Maslow, A. (1968). *Toward a psychology of being* (2nd ed.). Princeton, NJ: Van Nostrand.

National Center for Health Statistics (NCHS), Centers for Disease Control and Prevention. (2003). *Health, United States,* Table 27. U.S. Public Health Service, DHHS Publication No. 94-1232. Washington, DC: U.S. Government Printing Office.

Nestle Clinical Nutrition. (1999). *A guide to completing the Mini Nutritional Assessment (MNA).* Nestle Healthcare Nutrition, Minnetonka, MN.

Nutrition Screening Initiative. (1992). *Consensus conference.* Washington, DC: Author.

O'Malley, R. (1987). *Inadequate care of the elderly: A health care perspective on abuse and neglect.* New York: Springer.

Satir, V. (1964). *Conjunct family therapy: A guide to theory and technique.* Palo Alto, CA: Science & Behavioral Books.

U.S. Bureau of the Census. (2001). *Statistical abstract of the United States: 2000.* Washington, DC: U.S. Government Printing Office.

U.S. Food and Drug Administration (USFDA). (2003). Medications and Older People. FDA Consumer. Retrieved November 13, 2008, from http://www.fda.gov/fdac/features/1997/697_old.html

Williams, M., Parker, R., Baker, D., et al. (1995). Inadequate functional health literacy among patients at two public hospitals. *Journal of the American Medical Association, 274,* 1677–1720.

Yesavage, J., & Brink, T. (1983). Development and validation of a geriatric depression screening scale: A preliminary report. *Journal of Psychiatric Research, 17,* 37–49.

## APPENDIX A
# Selected Theories of Aging

## Biological Theories

### ■ Molecular Theories

Gene: selected genes become active in later life, causing the organism to fail to survive
Error, error catastrophe
    Somatic mutation
    Transcription
Programmed, programmed senescence
    Run-out-of-program

### ■ System-Level Theories

Neuroendocrine control (pacemakers)
Immunologic/autoimmune

### ■ Cellular Theories

Free radicals, antioxidants
Cross-link/connective tissue
Clinker
Wear-and-tear

## Sociological Theories

Disengagement (Cummings & Henry, 1961)
Activity (Lemon, 1972)
Continuity (Havighurst, 1963)

Age stratification
Person–environment fit
Sociological aging: life course, life transitions, status and role changes, social supports

## Psychological Theories

Maslow's hierarchy of human needs
Jung's individualism
Course of human life
Erikson's (1963) eight stages of life: Sense of ego integrity versus sense of despair
Peck (1968): ego differentiation versus work-role preoccupation; body transcendence versus body preoccupation; ego transcendence versus ego preoccupation
Feil (1982): resolution of the past versus vegetation
Butler's (1963) life review
Levinson's (1977) seasons of life
Lowenthal's (1973) life transitions
Havighurst's (1974) developmental tasks: establishing satisfactory living arrangements, adjusting to retirement and reduced income, adjusting to decreasing physical strength and health, establishing an explicit affiliation with one's age group

## APPENDIX B
# Activities of Daily Living and Instrumental Activities of Daily Living

|  | Independent | Assisted | Dependent |
|---|---|---|---|
| ■ Bathing | 0 | 1 | 2 |
| ■ Dressing | 0 | 1 | 2 |
| ■ Toileting | 0 | 1 | 2 |
| ■ Transfer | 0 | 1 | 2 |
| ■ Continence | 0 | 1 | 2 |
| ■ Feeding | 0 | 1 | 2 |
| ■ Telephoning | 0 | 1 | 2 |
| ■ Shopping | 0 | 1 | 2 |
| ■ Transporting | 0 | 1 | 2 |
| ■ Medicating | 0 | 1 | 2 |
| ■ Handling money | 0 | 1 | 2 |
| ■ Preparing food | 0 | 1 | 2 |
| ■ Housekeeping | 0 | 1 | 2 |
| ■ Laundry | 0 | 1 | 2 |

| ADL Score (0–12) ____ | | IADL Score (0–16)____ | | Total Score (0–28)____ | |
|---|---|---|---|---|---|
| 0 | Independent | 0 | Independent | 0 | Independent |
| 1–6 | Assisted | 1–8 | Assisted | 1–14 | Assisted |
| 7–12 | Dependent | 7–16 | Dependent | 15–28 | Dependent |

*Source*: Adapted from Katz et al., 1963, and Lawton & Brody, 1969 (alternate scoring).

# APPENDIX C
## Tinetti Fall Assessment Scale

| Balance | (Seated in Hard, Armless Chair) | Scoring |
|---|---|---|
| ■Sitting balance | Leans or slides in chair | = 0 |
| | Steady, safe | = 1 ____ |
| ■Arises | Unable without help | = 0 |
| | Able, uses arms to help | = 1 |
| | Able without using arms | = 2 ____ |
| ■Attempts to rise | Unable without help | = 0 |
| | Able, requires 1 attempt | = 1 |
| | Able to rise, 1 attempt | = 2 ____ |
| ■Immediate standing | Balance (first 5 seconds) | |
| | Unsteady (staggers, moves feet, trunk sway) | = 0 |
| | Steady but uses walker or other support | = 1 |
| | Narrow stance without other support | = 2 ____ |
| ■Standing balance | Unsteady | = 0 |
| | Steady but wide stance and uses other support | = 1 |
| | Narrow stance without support | = 2 ____ |
| ■Nudged | Begins to fall | = 0 |
| | Staggers, grabs, catches self | = 1 |
| | Steady | = 2 ____ |
| ■Eyes closed | Unsteady | = 0 |
| | Steady | = 1 ____ |
| ■Turning 360° | Discontinuous steps | = 0 |
| | Continuous steps | = 1 |
| | Unsteady (grabs, staggers) | = 0 |
| | Steady | = 1 ____ |
| ■Sitting down | Unsafe (misjudged distance, falls into chair) | = 0 |
| | Uses arms or not a smooth motion | = 1 |
| | Safe, smooth motion | = 2 ____ |
| ■Balance Score: | | ____/16 |

| Gait: | (Stands, walks about 10 feet at usual pace, then back at rapid, but safe pace with aids) | Scoring |
|---|---|---|
| ■Initiation of gate | Any hesitancy or multiple attempts to start | = 0 |
| | No hesitancy | = 1 ____ |
| ■Step length and height | | |
| Right swing foot | Does not pass left stance foot with step | = 0 |
| | Passes left stance foot | = 1 |
| | Right foot does not clear floor completely | = 0 |
| | Right foot completely clears floor | = 1 |
| Left swing foot | Does not pass right stance foot with step | = 0 |
| | Passes right stance foot | = 1 |
| | Left foot doesn't clear floor completely | = 0 |
| | Left foot completely clears floor | = 1 |
| ■Step symmetry | Right and left step length not equal (estimate) | = 0 |
| | Right and left step appear equal | = 1 ____ |
| ■Step continuity | Stopping or discontinuity between steps | = 0 |
| | Steps appear continuous | = 1 ____ |
| ■Path | Marked deviation | = 0 |
| | Mild/moderate deviation or uses walking aid | = 1 |
| | Straight without walking aid | = 2 ____ |
| ■Trunk | Marked sway or uses walking aid | = 0 |
| | No sway but flexion of knees or back or spread arms out while walking | = 1 |
| | No sway, no flexion, no use of arms, and no use of walking aid | = 2 ____ |
| ■Walking time | Heels apart | = 0 |
| | Heels almost touching while walking | = 1 ____ |
| ■Gait Score: | | ____/12 |
| ■Balance 1 Gait Score: | | Score ____/28 |

| Key to Risk for Falls: | Score |
|---|---|
| Low | 25–28 |
| Moderate | 19–24 |
| High | 0–18 |

## APPENDIX D
# Mini-Mental State Exam

### FOLSTEIN MINI-MENTAL STATE EXAM

Highest school grade completed _____

| Maximum | Score | |
|---|---|---|
| | | **Orientation** |
| 5 | _____ | What is the (year), (season), (date), (day), (month)? |
| 5 | _____ | Where are we: (state, (city), (county), (facility), (floor)? |
| | | **Attention and Calculation** |
| 5 | _____ | Serial 7s. One point for each correct. Stop after five answers. 93 86 79 72 65. |
| | | alternatively, spell "world" backward: D L R O W |
| | | **Recall** |
| 3 | _____ | Ask for three objects repeated above. Give 1 point for each correct answer. |
| | | **Language and Praxis** |
| 2 | _____ | Name a pencil and a watch. |
| 1 | _____ | Repeat the following phrase: "No ifs, ands, or buts." |
| | | **Registration** |
| 3 | _____ | Name three objects: 1 second to say each; ask person all three objects after they are said. Give 1 point for each correct answer. Then repeat objects until all three are learned. Count trials and record: _____ |
| 3 | _____ | Follow a three-stage command: "Take this paper in your right hand, fold it in half, and put it on the table." |
| 1 | _____ | Read and obey the following command: |
| | | **CLOSE YOUR EYES** |
| 1 | _____ | Write a sentence: |
| 1 | _____ | Copy this design: |
| ___ | | |
| 30 | | |

**Key to FMMSE Scores:**

| | |
|---|---|
| No cognitive impairment | 24–30 |
| Mild cognitive impairment | 18–23 |
| Severe cognitive impairment | 0–17 |

*Source*: Folstein, Folstein, & McHugh, 1975.

# ▥ APPENDIX E
# Geriatric Depression Scale

| Mood Scale | | |
|---|---|---|
| 1. ARE YOU BASICALLY SATISFIED WITH YOUR LIFE? | yes | NO |
| 2. HAVE YOU DROPPED MANY OF YOUR ACTIVITIES AND INTERESTS? | YES | no |
| 3. DO YOU FEEL THAT YOUR LIFE IS EMPTY? | YES | no |
| 4. DO YOU OFTEN GET BORED? | YES | no |
| 5. Are you hopeful about the future? | yes | NO |
| 6. Are you bothered by thoughts that you just can't get out of your head? | YES | no |
| 7. ARE YOU IN GOOD SPIRITS MOST OF THE TIME? | yes | NO |
| 8. ARE YOU AFRAID THAT SOMETHING BAD IS GOING TO HAPPEN TO YOU? | YES | no |
| 9. DO YOU FEEL HAPPY MOST OF THE TIME? | yes | NO |
| 10. DO YOU OFTEN FEEL HELPLESS? | YES | no |
| 11. Do you often get restless and fidgety? | YES | no |
| 12. Do you prefer to stay home at night rather than go out and do new things? | YES | no |
| 13. Do you frequently worry about the future? | YES | no |
| 14. DO YOU FEEL THAT YOU HAVE MORE PROBLEMS WITH MEMORY THAN MOST? | YES | no |
| 15. DO YOU THINK IT IS WONDERFUL TO BE ALIVE NOW? | yes | NO |
| 16. Do you often feel downhearted and blue? | YES | no |
| 17. DO YOU FEEL PRETTY WORTHLESS THE WAY YOU ARE NOW? | YES | no |
| 18. Do you worry a lot about the past? | YES | no |
| 19. Do you find life very exciting? | yes | NO |
| 20. Is it hard for you to get started on new projects? | YES | no |
| 21. DO YOU FEEL FULL OF ENERGY? | yes | NO |
| 22. DO YOU FEEL THAT YOUR SITUATION IS HOPELESS? | YES | no |
| 23. DO YOU THINK THAT MOST PERSONS YOUR AGE ARE BETTER OFF THAN YOU ARE? | YES | no |
| 24. Do you frequently get upset over little things? | YES | no |
| 25. Do you frequently feel like crying? | YES | no |
| 26. Do you have trouble concentrating? | YES | no |
| 27. Do you enjoy getting up in the morning? | yes | NO |
| 28. Do you prefer to avoid social gatherings? | YES | no |
| 29. Is it easy for you to make decisions? | yes | NO |
| 30. Is your mind as clear as it used to be? | yes | NO |

**Score**     Circled capitalized answers        _____
          Crossed-out lowercase answers     _____
          Total                              15 or 30

| Key to Scoring | GDS |
|---|---|
| No depression | 0–4 capitalized on 15-item screen |
| Mild depression | 5–10 capitalized on 30-item scale |
| Severe depression | 11–30 capitalized on 30-item scale |

**Directions for Scoring:** This scale is intended to be administered orally to the elderly person in a quiet, private setting. Circle the capitalized *answer* if the elder answers the question with the capitalized response. Draw a line through the lowercase *answer* if the elder answers with the lowercase response.
   Score 1 point for each circled capitalized answer.
   Score 0 for each lowercase answer.
For screening purposes, use the 15 short-form *questions,* which are capitalized. If the elder scores more than 5 points, administer the full 30-item scale.

**Interpretation:** A score of 5 or more capitalized responses on the 15-item screen is suggestive of depression and indicates the need to administer the full scale. A score of 0–10 is normal range; a score of 11 or more capitalized responses on the 30-item scale is positive for depression.
   According to Yersavage and Brink (1983), a cut-off score of 11 has a sensitivity of 84% and a specificity of 95%. A cut-off score of 14 has a sensitivity of 80% and a specificity of 100%.

*Source*: Yesavage & Brink, 1983.

## APPENDIX F
# Home Safety Checklist

## Home Interior

Floors: clean, clutter-free, rugs anchored and in good repair (no scatter rugs), surface smooth and nonskid wax

Electrical appliances: cords in good repair and out of traffic lanes

Lighting: adequate not-glare lighting; stairs illuminated; night lights where needed

Temperature: range 70–75 °F; adequate heating, cooling, and ventilation; insulation; fireplace/heaters with protective screens

Furniture: sturdy, good repair

Stairs: sturdy railings; nonskid steps; uncluttered

Organization: uncluttered, navigable traffic lanes

## Communication

Lock/unlock door; reach light switches

Emergency telephone numbers posted, legible (fire, ambulance, doctor, family)

If no telephone, life line, neighbor, "buddy," or other means to summon help

Smoke alarms available with working batteries

## Kitchen

Food: adequate supply, fresh

Stove: free of grease and flammables, baking soda or fire extinguisher

Refrigerator: cooling effectively, food available and fresh

Sink: draining properly, hot (check temperature) and cold water; dishes washed

Cleaning supplies: stored separately and clearly marked

Garbage: taken out; regular pick-up

Ladder or step stool: sturdy with handle

## Bathroom

Hand rails for tub and toilet

Skid-proof mats for tub and/or shower

Nonskid rug on floor

Electrical outlets safe distance from tub

## Medications

Stored safely; current; disposal of old medicines

Current list with times, dosage, description, purpose

## Outside

Walks, driveways, and stairs: smooth surfaces in good repair (no raised or uneven places); edges painted or clearly visible; hand rails secure

Doors and windows: panes and screens in good repair

Fire escape or alternate exit from house

*Source*: Adapted from Burnside, 1988.

## APPENDIX G
# Baccalaureate Competencies for Geriatric Nursing Care

The following competencies are necessary for nurses to provide high-quality care to older adults and their families:

1. Recognize one's own and others' attitudes, values, and expectations about aging and their impact on care of older adults and their families.
2. Adopt the concept of individualized care as the standard of practice with older adults.
3. Communicate effectively, respectfully, and compassionately with older adults and their families.
4. Recognize that sensation and perception in older adults are mediated by functional, physical, cognitive, psychological, and social changes common in old age.
5. Incorporate into daily practice valid and reliable tools to assess the functional, physical, cognitive, psychological, social, and spiritual status of older adults.
6. Assess older adults' living environment with special awareness of the functional, physical, cognitive, psychological, and social changes common in old age.
7. Analyze the effectiveness of community resources in assisting older adults and their families to retain personal goals, maximize function, maintain independence, and live in the least restrictive environment.
8. Assess family knowledge of skills necessary to deliver care to older adults.

9. Adapt technical skills to meet the functional, physical, cognitive, psychological, social, and endurance capacities of older adults.

10. Individualize care and prevent the morbidity and mortality associated with the use of physical and chemical restraints in older adults.

11. Prevent or reduce common risk factors that contribute to functional decline, impaired quality of life, and excess disability in older adults.

12. Establish and follow standards of care to recognize and report elder mistreatment.

13. Apply evidence-based standards to screen, immunize, and promote healthy activities in older adults.

14. Recognize and manage geriatric syndromes common to older adults.

15. Recognize the complex interaction of acute and chronic comorbid conditions common to older adults.

16. Use technology to enhance older adults' function, independence, and safety.

17. Facilitate communication as older adults transition across and between home, hospital, and nursing home, with a particular focus on the use of technology.

18. Assist older adults, families, and caregivers to understand and balance "everyday" autonomy and safety decisions.

19. Apply ethical and legal principles to the complex issues that arise in the care of older adults.

20. Appreciate the influence of attitudes, roles, language, culture, race, religion, gender, and lifestyle on how families and assistive personnel provide long-term care to older adults.

21. Evaluate differing international models of geriatric care.

22. Analyze the impact of an aging society on the health care system.

23. Evaluate the influence of payer systems on access, availability, and affordability of health care for older adults.

24. Contrast the opportunities and constraints of supportive living arrangements on the function and independence of older adults and on their families.

25. Recognize the benefits of interdisciplinary team participation in care of older adults.

26. Evaluate the utility of complementary and integrative health care practices on health promotion and symptom management for older adults.

27. Facilitate older adults' active participation in all aspects of their own health care.

28. Involve, educate, and, when appropriate, supervise family, friends, and assistive personnel in implementing best practices for older adults.

29. Ensure that quality of care is commensurate with older adults' vulnerability and frequency and intensity of care needs.

30. Promote the desirability of quality end-of-life care for older adults, including pain and symptom management, as essential and desirable, and integral components of nursing practice.

*Source*: American Association of Colleges of Nursing. (2000). *Older adults: Recommended baccalaureate competencies and curricular guidelines for geriatric nursing care.* Washington, DC: Author.

# CHAPTER 36

# Psychiatric Care and Mental Health in the Community

Sarah Steen Lauterbach and Janna Lesser

Visit **http://nursing.jbpub.com/communityhealth** for interactive exercises, review questions, Web links, and more.

Given today's stresses, it is imperative that nurses in psychiatric–mental health take self-care and caring for one another seriously. Nurses must develop self-care strategies that ensure they enjoy balanced, healthy, meaningful lives.

Much madness is divinist sense
To a discerning eye;
Much sense the starkest madness.
'Tis the majority
In this, as all, prevails.
Assent, and you are sane;
Demur,—you're straightway dangerous,
And handled with a chain.

—*Emily Dickinson*

Mental health is a neglected area of public health. Community health nurses work within a holistic framework and address the entire spectrum of a community's health. After reading Emily Dickinson's poem, reflect on your own ideas about what contributes to mental well being.

## CHAPTER FOCUS

**The Unique Role and Perspective of Psychiatric–Mental Health Nursing in Caring for the Public's Health**

**Definitions of Mental Health**

**History of Mental Health in the Community**
- Early Humanitarian Reform in Mental Health
- Community Mental Health Reform in the 1960s

**Historical Context for Professional Nursing**

**History and Spirit of Psychiatric–Mental Health Nursing in the Community**
- State of the Science of Psychiatric–Mental Health Nursing
- Levels of Psychiatric–Mental Health Nursing Practice

**Individuals and Population Groups Needing Psychiatric–Mental Health Services**

**Current Assessment of the Public's Mental Health Status**
- Ethics of Psychiatric–Mental Health Services

**Psychiatric–Mental Health Nursing's Roles and Phenomena of Concern**
- Guiding Philosophical and Theoretical Frameworks for Mental Health Nursing

**Models for Psychiatric–Mental Health Nursing Practice**
- Public Health Model
- Primary Care Model
- Primary Mental Health Care Model
- Using Reflection in Nursing Education and Practice
- Using a Phenomenological Perspective: Understanding the Public's Mental Health Lived Experience, One Person at a Time

**The Future of Psychiatric–Mental Health Nursing**

## QUESTIONS TO CONSIDER

After reading this chapter, you will know the answers to the following questions:

1. What is the definition of *mental health in the community*?
2. What is the history of community mental health nursing?
3. What is the current mental health status of Americans?
4. What are some of the conceptual and theoretical frameworks for psychiatric–mental health nursing?
5. What are some of the models for psychiatric–mental health nursing practice?
6. What will psychiatric–mental health nursing practice be like in the future?

## KEY TERMS

Advocacy
Community mental health centers (CMHCs)

Mental health
Phenomena of concern
Phenomenology

Presence
Prevention
Psychiatric–mental health nursing

Seriously mentally ill
Universal human experiences

THE IDEA OF MENTAL HEALTH in this chapter is embedded within cultural, social, political, and economic contexts of the time, and within a historical—as well as contemporary—perspective. The chapter presents psychiatric–mental health (P-MH) conditions and treatment as being contextually bound, and ultimately responding to the state of knowledge and science surrounding mental health. Additionally, the influence of nursing history and professional **psychiatric–mental health nursing** practice are considered as relevant to the idea of mental health. Mental health and illness are viewed as playing a key role in determining the state of the public's health. This chapter examines the American public's mental health and illness continuum, using current information (i.e., demographic, population, and epidemiological data).

Although population and numerical data are tremendously useful, it is also important to use qualitative, humanistic perspectives and lenses in assessing and understanding mental health. Conceptual frameworks, interdisciplinary theory, nursing theory, philosophical perspectives, and models for reflective practice are particularly useful in understanding current care and practice.

The central context used for defining the scope of P-MH nursing is the state of knowledge and research and nursing's historic role in social reform and activism. Receiving particular emphasis in the chapter is the unique contribution made by P-MH nursing to professional nursing. Specifically, this contribution lies in articulating for professional nursing a primary role in facilitating and developing therapeutic relationships with persons, families, groups, and populations at risk. It is rooted in Hildegard Peplau's (1952) nursing work and text, *Interpersonal Relations in Nursing*. This classic work established therapeutic relationships as a primary focus, a focus underpinning the entire nursing discipline.

The multiple theoretical perspectives nursing uses contributes to its unique role, which will be discussed in detail here. The focus on facilitating and developing relationships underpins nursing in every care context and role, and is proposed to serve as a primary task for all nurses. It underlies nursing's potential role in promoting health and wellness, preventing disability and dysfunction, and treating and restoring the mental health of the public.

Public health policy and care provision needs to be inclusive of mental health, and P-MH services and treatments need to be mainstreamed into the primary health care system. Currently, the private/public split in P-MH care establishes and promotes disparities in the public's mental health. Public programs carry the burden of serving the **seriously mentally ill** (SMI) with inadequate resources. Where privatization has become lucrative for private P-MH programs, it has resulted in the creation of a second-class citizenship status for the SMI population. The inequity and disparities relate to access, quality, and

cost of care, and they have direct effects on mental health, especially for vulnerable groups. The dual nature of P-MH care system serves to further impoverish especially vulnerable and at-risk populations, such as the homeless, incarcerated SMI, and people with both physical and mental disabilities. It is time for the *Healthy People 2010* goal of reducing these disparities to be taken seriously. Responsible, ethical, social and health policy reform is drastically needed.

The chapter includes textual contributions from creative writers, artists, and public figures as reflective of classic struggles that many humans face. Many of the most accomplished people who have made tremendous contributions to science, literature, and art have lived with serious mental health conditions. Their contributions and wisdom have been very helpful in articulating what it is like to be human. These sources are especially informative for health care professionals and the public in understanding what it is like to live with mental health and/or illness. Additionally, the comments of students are included as they reflect on their growing awareness and understanding of mental health and illness and learn what it is like to provide therapeutic healing care and relationships.

Universal human phenomena are discussed as still in need of research and public policy attention. Many common human conditions and experiences need to be explored by using reflection to explicate the meanings in experiences. These conditions are often involved in the etiology of P-MH problems and dysfunction. Conditions and experiences particularly needing exploration include dealing with loss, death, change, anxiety, stress, crisis, inadequate coping, depression, and disappointment. Reflection offers an opportunity to enhance understanding through reflecting on meanings in experiences. As understanding grows, enhanced care and treatment potentially become better informed and facilitated.

---

**Quiver of Fear**

Quiver of fear down the spine
    Black towers of
      Never ending hallways

Florescent lit
White coated men

Come Daddy.
    Why?

There is no merciful prayer,
    No merciful answer
    Not for me
    Not for you.

—*Ann Thedford Lanier*

## The Unique Role and Perspective of Psychiatric–Mental Health Nursing in Caring for the Public's Health

The unique and special contribution of psychiatric nursing in caring for the public's mental health comes from the specialty's history, commitment, and expertise in therapeutic communication and relationship development. The Psychiatric–Mental Health (P-MH) nurse engages in *therapeutic use of self*, a concept that involves the nurse becoming and being an *instrument of care*. Through using self in communication therapeutically, and through using expert relationship building knowledge, "We can literally, become the healing environment" (Quinn, 1992).

Becoming the healing environment in caring for the public's mental health often involves providing both very vulnerable people and functional people with basic human needs for trust, support, and security, as well as specialty treatment and care. Many P-MH nurses see the specialty as underpinning all of nursing, with professional nursing literally, becoming the healing environment, and being the instrument of care in each nursing encounter regardless of specialty or practice arena.

Nursing's professional commitment to holistic care, providing the public with a holistic, caring presence, is actualized in the P-MH concept of relationship. The focus on providing comfort care, caring for persons in the present as well as in the future, provides a temporal relationship in caring for the public that is unique to nursing. Nursing caring involves *doing for, being with, helping and healing through relationships* when the person is incapable of self-care. The nursing focus is on understanding a person's history using strengths and resources to address areas of needed change.

**Presence** is another concept used to describe nursing work. *Being fully present for another*, with an intention to facilitate and promote healing and comfort, and *being with* people are nursing intentions and goals. It is critical that the nurse understands the experience from the perspective of the person in need of care. In being fully present, often the nurse must look at and explicate past personal experience, biases, and attitudes.

Self-reflection is a critical activity and process in P-MH nursing. Reflective education and practice activities are provided throughout this chapter. Through reflection, the nurse is able to become more aware of, and use bracketing to put aside, personal material consciously, so that the nursing presence is focused on those in need. Reflection and bracketing become critical in understanding the person. Reflection and bracketing pre-understandings and biases, values, and attitudes make it possible for the nurse to become fully present in caring for the mental health needs of the other.

In P-MH nursing, the nurse is involved with implementing treatment programs, and with facilitating, developing, and using groups and the therapeutic milieu. The context of

**Application to Practice**

**Reflective Education and Practice Exercise 1**

*Caring for Self*

The idea of caring for self was a hard concept for me to undertake. I've always been a person who enjoyed helping others, and often would get so caught up in others that self could be considered a foreign thing at times. It is sometimes easier to avoid looking at myself and my own problems by making other people the focus of my attention.

However, when this assignment began, I wanted to make a legitimate effort to look at my needs, and the areas where I needed improvement.... There were several areas that needed to be addressed, including the need for appropriate amounts of sleep, leisure, and relaxation. I found these to be very important, especially when going through the mental health clinical experiences. I was feeling drained and would go home and just sleep for hours and hours, sometimes not waking until the next morning. I recognized that this was an ineffective coping method for the stress I felt. To combat those feelings, I started doing meditation and prayer on the mornings of the clinical or when I knew I would have a challenging day. Doing these activities completely changed my attitude and the experiences that I had. During the rest of my clinicals, I was much more mentally and emotionally prepared to learn what the experience had to teach me, and I slept soundly at night, not during the day.

—Nursing student, spring 2003

As we all know, nursing school is no walk in the park. It has to be one of the most difficult, time-consuming things I've ever had to go through in my life. I've never had to work as much or as hard as I have for these classes. I realize, however, that during these trying times, I need to take care of myself as well as working for the grades I am attempting to achieve.... In my life after college, I hope to live as much of a holistic life as possible: I want to go to work, exercise regularly, and eat well. I think that when working in health care, it is important to be healthy yourself—otherwise, you might be contradictory. If you tell your patient to do something like exercise a few times a week, and you yourself don't do it, then it makes you look bad. Of course, I want to exercise for my life . . . I want to live a long, happy life so I need to take care of the body I have because it's the only one I'll get.

—Nursing student, spring 2003

caring for persons 24/7 puts P-MH nurses in a similar role as nurses in other nursing specialties. Nurses assist people in their activities of daily living. P-MH patients often have difficulty in navigating through self-care routines. Similarly, in chronic care, self-care deficits are often the norm.

The nurse is often the point person in case management of mental health patients. The P-MH nurse has a history of accepting responsibility for and demonstrating a long-term commitment for care. P-MH nursing has an ethic of responsibility for caring for persons, especially vulnerable groups and populations over the life span. Follow-up care, communication, and partnering with other disciplines and agencies is critical in providing comprehensive, holistic care.

Finally, nursing work is often very private, especially when considering the stigma attached to, and attitudes of many people toward people suffering from, mental health problems. Just as cancer was once a dreaded, stigmatized condition, so mental health problems are often associated with stigma. Education and research, along with improvements in treatment, should eventually eliminate this phenomenon that surrounds mental health care. Further, knowledge and understanding must be consciously implemented and planned.

Nursing often involves body work, up close and personal. In P-MH, the personal aspects of the disease often involve lack of ability to function, or problematic behaviors and symptoms. Mental health symptoms are often complex and difficult to manage or control. This unique vantage point taken by the caregiver provides the P-MH nurse with an opportunity to know the person intimately and, therefore, makes the nursing role potentially sensitive and complicated. Nurses are involved with people who experience alterations in health and, in many cases, intolerable suffering.

As stated earlier, in P-MH nursing the therapeutic relationship is the primary instrument of care. It is through the development and maintenance of relationships with people over time that nursing P-MH work is accomplished.

Nurses learn from the beginning of the nursing educational experience that therapeutic use of self and communication are critical in intervention and healing. Through the proximity of nursing involved in intimately engaging in patients' lives, the nurse can become a role model for relationships and communication. Just as Dewey stated of education, the P-MH nurse mentors, guides, coaches, and assists persons in becoming more fully functional.

To become a fully functioning P-MH nurse requires that opportunities provided by nursing education and nursing practice for self-reflection are fully embraced. Reflection is a process that enhances one's awareness of values, perceptions, and meanings in life experience. Through reflection, there is an enhanced understanding of self and others, a heightened awareness of meanings in experiences, and potential for taking action.

### 🖥️ Research Alert

Nurse researcher and scholar, Patricia L. Munhall, ARNP, EdD, FAAN, PsyA, was an invited keynote speaker for the Nursing Research Conference in Biloxi, Mississippi, sponsored by Gamma Lambda Chapter Sigma Theta Tau International of The University of Southern Mississippi, November 12–13, 1998. Her address, titled "Out of the Box," challenged nurses and researchers to question assumptions and preunderstandings in nursing and education that inhibit thinking, behaving, and creative nursing action. She states in an editorial in *Image, the Journal of Nursing Scholarship*, that "Boxes are useful for storage and keepsakes. Out of the box is going off the block. Staying in the box is standing still, stripped of awe" (Munhall, 1998, p. 203).

❝*No temper could be more cheerful than hers, or possess, to a greater degree, that sanguine expectation of happiness which is happiness itself.*❞

—Jane Austen, 1775–1817

To care for others fully, the nurse must first care for self (Lauterbach & Becker, 1996; Lauterbach & Becker Hentz, 1998, 2005). This issue is especially important considering the nursing shortage. Many see nursing as an oppressed profession, with nurses' burnout further threatening the public's health. Given today's stresses, it is imperative that nurses in P-MH take self-care and caring for one another seriously. Nurses—and P-MH nurses in particular—must develop self-care strategies that ensure they enjoy balanced, healthy, meaningful lives. Self-care is no longer just a choice or a nice thing to do, but rather a necessity. Otherwise, nurses' and the public's care and safety will suffer, stress and anxiety will be exacerbated, and personal feelings of security will be unattainable for nurses. The reader is referred to the boxes throughout this chapter, which focus on reflection, journaling, and caring for self.

In summary, through interaction and development of relationships, P-MH nursing is committed to caring and facilitating healing for persons, families, groups, communities, populations, nations, and the planet/environment. It is through the context of helping relationships that nurses respond to and care for self and others, interacting with patient systems, other professions, and community partners in a diversity of health and human life contexts.

## Definitions of Mental Health

Definitions of mental health in literature range from a focus on the absence of disease to the attainment of one's potential.

**❝** *Everything has been figured out, except how to live.* **❞**
—Jean Paul Sartre, 1905–1980

.................................................................

The definition provided by *Healthy People 2010* "refers to an individual's ability to negotiate the daily challenges and social interactions of life, without experiencing undue emotional or behavioral incapacity" (U.S. Department of Health and Human Services, 1990). Missing in this definition is the human expectation and experience of living happily, as well as functionally, mentally healthy.

Concepts of mental health and illness have changed drastically over the last few centuries. In the fifteenth century the mentally ill were thought to be witches "possessed" by demons. Some cultures historically regard persons with psychiatric conditions as worthy of great respect, as having uncanny abilities and visionaries. At one time, mental illness was thought to be caused by a lesion or physical injury to the brain. If no objective injury or lesion was found, mental illness was thought to be a defect in morality and character.

Since the early 1900s, identifying the mentally ill has been the focus of psychiatry. Great efforts were made toward the diagnosis and treatment of specific mental disorders and conditions. The development of the *Diagnostic and Statistical Manuals (DSM)* by the American Psychiatric Association (APA) since the 1950s (APA, 1980, 1987, 1992) has contributed to differentiation and research. Designated as "the decade of the brain," the focus of research in the 1990s has contributed to a fuller understanding of biological determinants of behavior (Hedaya, 1996). The major psychiatric milestones of the twentieth century included the development of the diagnostic manual and assessment procedures; psychotherapy, including psychoanalysis; developmental theories; behavioral, cognitive, and psychological foci for psychotherapy, including crisis intervention, short-term, group, family, and long-term therapy; psychopharmacology; and knowledge concerning the biological determinants of behavior.

The definition of *mental health* is still in need of our attention and continued thinking in nursing. Many believe that the focus on biology has obscured, once again, the understanding of mental illness or mental health. The view of mental health in this chapter encompasses the notion that **mental health** involves connection of body, mind, and spirit, in mental and physical wholesomeness. The concept of "balance" is common in holistic literature. Mental health is further viewed as involving a process through which a (w)holistic balance between mind, body, and spirit (of individuals, families, groups, and the public) is pursued through meaningful life activities. The mentally healthy person seeks experiences that promote well-being, productivity, and happiness as fully as possible given the particular situational contexts and limitations.

This notion of health is consistent with the aim of phenomenological inquiry. The ultimate aim of phenomenology is to assist persons, through understanding, to "become fully human." Nursing has historically embraced a role with caring that has focused on maximizing human potential. A focus on maintaining harmony and balance is needed in many areas of human endeavor and experience: in meaningful work, occupation or pursuit; in relationships with loved ones, significant others, and in social relationships, friendships, and work relationships; in meaningful relaxation, leisure, balanced nutrition, and fitness activities; and in having a respect and responsibility for the planet and world.

Mental illness or dysfunction, although it exists more in vulnerable population groups, is not wholly a respecter of vulnerability. There have been and currently are many gifted as well as ordinary people who have periodic mental health issues and conditions. The arts and sciences are filled with examples of brilliant and revolutionary contributions from people who had mental health problems. For example, the symbolist artist Edvard Munch, born in 1863, was an alcoholic and experienced depression throughout his life. His work focuses on themes of life and death and his experience with mental illness. The lithograph *The Scream* is one of his most important and popularized pieces. Of particular interest are three other works, *Anxiety*, *The Sick Child*, and *Death in the Sick Room*. As a young child, Munch experienced the death of his mother, and when he was 14, his sister died. *Death in the Sickroom* depicts the family scene years earlier. The following quote by Munch illustrates this anguish:

> I was born dying . . . Sickness, insanity, and death were the malevolent angels that guarded my cradle and have followed me through my life ever since.
>
> I must retain my physical weaknesses; they are an integral part of me. I don't want to get rid of illness, however unsympathetically I may depict it in my art.

## History of Mental Health in the Community

In the United States today, the public community mental health program has been the primary model of care for people with serious mental illness. Beginning in 1963, President John Kennedy raised awareness of and attention to mental health with the Community Mental Health Centers Act. Federal funds were committed for the construction and staffing of **community mental health centers (CMHCs),** using the catchment area concept, which distributed mental health services throughout states all over the country. Today these programs provide access to a range of services that before this legislation were nonexistent.

Community mental health development was closely associated with legislation. Box 36-1 describes the major mental health legislative efforts and its influence on the development of mental health services. Understanding that

## BOX 36-1

**Mental Health Legislation And Its Influence on Mental Health Services**

1935    Social Security Act
Shifted care for ill people from state to federal government.

1943    National Institute for Mental Health
Established as one of the Institutes of Health, where funds for research and development were committed to mental health.

1955    Mental Health Study
Established Joint Commission on Mental Illness and Health.
Led to the transformation of state hospitals to establishment of CMHCs.

1963    Community Mental Health Centers Act
Marked beginning of CMHCs and deinstitutionalization of large psychiatric hospitals.

1960s   Funds were committed from federal government for grants for education for mental health disciplines, including nursing; stipends were made available for traineeships for undergraduate and graduate nursing students; gradually these were less frequent and finally were no longer available.

1975    Developmental Disabilities Act
Addressed rights of developmental disabilities and provided for similar actions for individuals with mental disorders.

1977    President's Commission on Mental Health
Reinforced importance of community based services, protection of human rights, and national health insurance for mentally ill persons.

1978    Omnibus Reconciliation Act
Rescinded much of the 1977 commission's provisions and shifted funds for all health programs from federal to state governments in the form of block grants.

1986    Protection and Advocacy for Mentally Ill Individuals Act
Legislated advocacy programs for mentally ill persons.

1990    Americans with Disabilities Act
Prohibited discrimination and promoted employment opportunities for people with disabilities, including mental disorders.

*Source*: Adapted from Stanhope & Lancaster, 2008.

---

**ʕʕ** *Mental illness is the last great stigma of the twentieth century. Most people treat someone with a mental illness as if it's their fault or as if they can just snap out of it.* **ʔʔ**

—*Tipper Gore*

community mental health as a humanitarian reform is seen when considering the early reform history of mental health. It is still in need of reform today.

### ■ Early Humanitarian Reform in Mental Health

Early treatment for people with mental illness was both cruel and inhumane. In 1843, Dorothea Dix, a school teacher, started the reform movement for the treatment of criminals, the mentally ill, and later, victims of the Civil War. Her work led to the establishment of asylums dedicated to humane treatment for the mentally ill. States built institutions for housing and treating persons with severe mental disorders. Intended as a humane movement, the large numbers of patients, combined with little knowledge and information about either cause or cure of mental illness, the establishment of asylums was, in retrospect, anything but humane. Within a few years, these large state institutions provided the only mental health treatment and grew to be overcrowded. Patients were not discharged to families in communities that had no treatment services. Psychiatric treatment was limited to somatic therapies and did very little to handle difficult symptoms. The asylum

population continued to grow as new people were admitted and the long-term residential population grew. It was not uncommon for "back ward" patients to have stays of 20 to 40 years. The asylum became the home.

### ■ Community Mental Health Reform in the 1960s

The community mental health centers movement, a century after Dorothea Dix's reform efforts, was another mental health reform movement. Some progress had been made in mental health science and treatment. The development of psychopharmacology was a milestone in treatment reform. Previously untreatable conditions were opened to the possibility of treatment. Since the early 1900s, psychotherapy had also been the focus of scholarship from several disciplines, including psychiatry, psychology, social work, and nursing. Psychotherapies that developed included long- and short-term and crisis intervention with individuals, groups, and families.

The community mental health centers movement was short-lived as the ideal solution to mental health care. Currently, large numbers of patients discharged from the state institutions and those who would have required institutional care in years past are residing in communities. A large number of the homeless population in urban centers are chronically mentally ill. They continue to have exacerbating mental conditions and experience environmental stresses, including the stress of meeting basic needs. This group of homeless, chronically mentally ill is especially vulnerable.

### Application to Practice

### Reflective Education and Practice Exercise 2

*Therapeutic Use of Self in Nursing Relationships*

I could not believe how unsure and anxious I was about my first therapeutic conversation in the mental health nursing course. Never before had I even considered what to say in relationships. And then, all of a sudden I was very uncomfortable. I realized that most of my interactions with patients in the first course were all about me . . . not focused on the patient at all. I talked about my family, being a student, and whatever came into my mind.

Until mental health, I hadn't really thought about the differences in helping or therapeutic relationships. The course came at a good time for all of us, since we are just beginning the really hard nursing clinicals. All of us had made similar mistakes, continually chatted with patients, and unaware of their real needs. The realization that it really matters what you say to mental health patients really hit home. It really made me think. All of a sudden, it seemed important to know and understand something about the condition a mental patient has in order to respond in a helpful therapeutic way. After the class, when we discussed the differences in therapeutic and social relationships, I felt completely like a fish out of water. I realized that therapeutic communication involved more than just having a nice conversation. It demands a thoughtful, careful approach to be used along with very careful listening. I realized that this would be harder than I had expected.

After the first couple of weeks in postconferences, where much of the discussion was focused on therapeutic interactions, I finally began to be more comfortable. By using active, careful listening and taking time to respond, I realized that if I made mistakes, I could always correct a response. I am confident that my communication with all patients, regardless of where I work, will be much improved by the experience of analyzing interactions with patients in mental health.

—Nursing student, spring 2002

As individuals were discharged from state mental institutions, private fee-for-service psychiatric services sprang up quickly in communities all over the country. Although care and a full range of treatment services are now more easily accessible within the community, there is inequity in access as a result of economic issues. Often, the families of the seriously mentally ill are unable to do what is necessary to ensure continuity of care or to get any care.

The inequity in access and economics of mental health care and physical care continues to dominate the environment of mental health care. Within most communities, supportive services have been developed, primarily by the consumer movement, to meet particular support needs of the general population. Box 36-2 identifies vulnerable populations who are in need of preventive, health promotion, and specialized treatment. Box 36-3 provides a listing of support services and groups available in many communities.

Beginning with the consumer movement of the 1970s, the groups focusing on support and psychoeducational issues with particular conditions have grown. These groups are available to the public, are listed in the telephone directories, and are advertised in varying community bulletin boards.

Mental health programs offer many services to the seriously mentally ill. Box 36-4 provides a listing of examples

---

### BOX 36-2

**Vulnerable Populations**
- Young and old
- Experiencing developmental transitions— adolescents, with young families
- Experiencing work and vocational problems and transitions
- Unemployed
- Part of the growing aggregate of the very old, older than 85, elderly
- Living in poverty
- Single parents of young children
- Adolescent parents
- Grandparents in parenting roles because adult children are suffering with dysfunction
- Uneducated
- Isolated and marginalized
- Dealing with learning and attention deficits, have disabilities
- Living as minority populations
- Depressed
- Angry
- Acutely or chronically ill
- Have histories of incarceration
- Have been victims of human and environmental abuse
- Victims of oppressive political systems
- Seeking asylum
- Experiencing stress, crisis, and change

## BOX 36-3

### Support Groups

- Compassionate Friends: focus on death, bereavement and loss (spouses, sudden infant death syndrome, perinatal, sibling)
- Cancer Support: focuses on variety of phenomena, including breast cancer and ostomy
- Caregivers Support Group: for caregivers of elderly, cancer, mentally ill
- Infertility Support: for couples experiencing infertility
- Parents without Partners
- Suicide Survivors
- Addictions Anonymous: for alcohol, gambling, exercise, shopping, food
- Smoking Cessation: including smokeless tobacco
- Families of Murdered Victims
- Families of Seriously Mentally Ill
- Medication follow-up and education: for patients and families
- Parenting Groups: for parents of adolescents, learning disabilities, autism, incarcerated
- Grandparenting
- Homeless Mothers
- Diabetes Education
- Alzheimer's Family Support: including Parkinson's
- Fibromyalgia Support
- Cardiac: Mended Hearts
- Organ Donor Group Support: families of donors and recipients of organs
- Physical Disabilities Support
- Homeless Mothers and Families Support

## BOX 36-4

### Community Mental Health Services

**Services**
- Seriously mentally ill day treatment
- Acute partial hospitalization for seriously mentally ill
- Children's services
- Adult day care
- Day Treatment Club House: for those with chronic conditions who live in the community
- Alcohol and chemical addictions programs
- Outpatient follow-up
- Group living

**Possible Treatment Modalities Available in These Programs**
- Resocialization, remotivation, and life skills assistance
- Social services
- Psychological services, including testing
- Medical services management and referral
- Psychopharmacological management
- Occupational therapy
- Recreational therapy
- Group, family therapy, and individual therapy
- Outreach and home visiting
- 12-step program
- Vocational rehabilitation
- Psychotherapy, long and short term

### A Good Read

## A Beautiful Mind

*S. Nasser*

This book about the brilliant mathematician and Nobel Laureate John Nash, who lapses into schizophrenia psychosis at the height of his career and remains there for 30 years, gives the reader an impression about what the experience of living with a serious mental illness is like. It also describes the extraordinary effort that returning to his theoretical work requires. At times, Nash thinks he can escape the ravages of time, picking up where he left off. And there are days when he cannot work; other days when he is full of remorse. The film that is based on the text is also informative, and gives one a virtual experience of auditory and visual hallucinations. Chronicity and long-term disability often accompany schizophrenia. The book also addresses the effects of illness on Nash's family, his community of scholars, and his life's work.

of mental health services available in a community mental health center in Mississippi.

Increasingly, community programs are being called to provide consultation to schools and communities in dealing with sensitive issues needing professional mental health attention. The *Healthy People 2010* priority areas are listed on p. 905. Even though mental health and mental disorders are listed separately, it is clear that mental health underpins many other priority areas, such as those listed in preventive services and health promotion.

Inpatient services for the seriously mentally ill are still provided by the state hospital system. Patients experiencing acute problems or acute exacerbations of chronic conditions are usually housed within jails in holding facilities, which usually have consultative psychiatric services. Despite attempts to build in continuity and access to care, there are needed reforms in all systems that use holding rather than inpatient treatment facilities. Inpatient services for the private system exist within relative geographic access in most communities. However, as cost-containment measures have been instituted, inpatient care is often too brief. Insurance

**HEALTHY PEOPLE 2010**

**Leading Health Indicators**

These 10 health indicators reflect the major health issues of the twenty-first century. They were selected based on their ability to motivate change, availability of data to monitor progress, and their importance as public health issues.

| | |
|---|---|
| Physical activity | Mental health |
| Overweight and obesity | Injury and violence |
| Tobacco use | Environmental quality |
| Substance abuse | Immunizations |
| Responsible sexual behavior | Access to health care |

*Source*: U.S. Department of Health and Human Services, 2000.

and economics are currently the greatest barriers to access to comprehensive, appropriate, and timely care in both the private and public systems.

## Historical Context for Professional Nursing

Nursing as a profession was part of a social reform movement, with professional roots in "women's suffrage, abolition, missionary work, and social reform" (Lynaugh & Brush, 1999, p. xi). Professional nursing represents the emergence of women from a private role to a public, humanitarian role, caring for the public's suffering and illness just as they had traditionally cared for their own families. In 1987, in a classic study of American nursing during the period 1850–1945, Reverby (1987) stated that "nursing's contemporary difficulties are shaped by the factors that created its historical obligations to care in a society that refuses to value caring" (p. i).

Nightingale defined nursing as the finest of the fine arts, stating that the role of nursing is to "put the patient in the best possible condition for nature to work upon him [sic]" (1859). Close to 100 years later, Virginia Henderson declared,

> As a nurse, I try to do for [patients] what they would do for themselves if they had the strength, the will, and the knowledge that a nurse has. And I try to do it in such a way that I don't make them dependent on me, any more than is necessary. (Baer, 1990, interview with Virginia Henderson)

Nursing is defined by the authors of this chapter as an open, caring art, spirit, human science, holistic practice, and discipline that uses a commitment to research, knowledge, humanity, education, the creative arts, and peace to facilitate, transform, actualize human potential, and promote wellness and healing for all people and the planet in the present, future, and beyond. Nursing work, according to Wolf (1988), is work that is both "sacred and profane." It is personal, involves up-close and personal work, is private, and often involves body work. In many cases, it is surrounded by an atmosphere of phenomenological silence (Lauterbach, 2003). Nursing work is very hard work and is often challenging,

> **"**I come to present the strong claims of suffering humanity. I come to place before the Legislature of Massachusetts the condition of the miserable, the desolate, the outcast. I come as the advocate of helpless, forgotten, insane men and women; of beings sunk to a condition from which the unconcerned world would start with real horror.**"**
>
> —Dorothea Dix, memorial to the Legislature of Massachusetts, 1843

especially in P-MH. It often involves caring for the most vulnerable, without resources, or using methods that have not been researched, or using untested, reliable treatments. Nursing often involves dealing with tremendous human suffering, as well as hope and opportunity for improving the human condition. In mental health, nursing involves *knowing*, *caring for*, *and being with* persons whose lives have often been dominated and altered forever by acute exacerbations in mental functioning, change, dysfunction, and serious mental illness.

## History and Spirit of Psychiatric–Mental Health Nursing in the Community

As influenced by the social, political, and economic forces and the tenor of the times, the dilemma faced by modern nursing is highlighted by P-MH nursing. P-MH nurses care for persons and populations suffering from mental conditions that do not resolve readily. They care for those who experience the devastating effects of tormenting, chronic mental conditions, often over the course of a lifetime. The asylum movement actually began and continued as a social reform movement. P-MH nurses care for people who represent a growing "Third World" community residing within America's borders. Mentally ill citizens include many of the United States' vulnerable, oppressed, disenfranchised, ethnic, and often hopeless people.

Box 36-5 identifies important events in the history of P-MH nursing. Hildegard Peplau is considered the founder

## BOX 36-5

**Important Events in Psychiatric Nursing History, 1773–1955**

| | |
|---|---|
| 1773 | First mental hospital in the United States established in Williamsburg, Virginia |
| 1846 | First use of the term psychiatry by physicians attempting to upgrade the status of their work with the mentally ill |
| 1882 | First school for psychiatric nurses (or mental nurses) established at the McLean Asylum in Somerville, Massachusetts |
| 1913 | Johns Hopkins Hospital included psychiatric nursing in the course of study for general nurses |
| 1920 | Publication of the first psychiatric nursing textbook, *Nursing Mental Diseases*, by Harriet Bailey |
| 1946 | Passage of the National Mental Health Act, which established the National Institutes of Mental Health (NIMH) |
| 1948 | Publication of the Brown Report, which recommended that psychiatric nursing be included in general nursing education |
| 1952 | Publication of *Interpersonal Relations in Nursing* by nurse theorist Hildegard Peplau |
| 1955 | National League for Nursing made psychiatric nursing a requirement for accreditation of basic nursing programs |

*Source*: Adapted from Frisch & Frisch, 1998.

of P-MH nursing; she is referred to fondly as "the mother of psychiatric nursing." Interestingly, she was one of the first nursing theorists, and her book *Interpersonal Relations in Nursing* has been translated into more than 50 languages. The text was ready for publication in 1949, but Peplau was unable to find a publisher who would publish it with a female nurse as the sole author. She refused to seek out a first author who was a physician, and finally was able to publish the book under her own name in 1952. At the time, Peplau had a very collegial relationship with the famous interpersonal theorist and psychiatrist, Harry Stack Sullivan. At the International Council of Nursing Biennial Convention in 1999, nurses from all over the world honored her at a specially convened memorial service, speaking about Peplau as a "formidable" international nursing leader and woman.

Orlando's 1961 text, *The Dynamic Nurse–Patient Relationship*, is another classic work that has been used in nursing education—not only in P-MH nursing, but in foundations and skills courses. Travelbee's *Intervention in Psychiatric Nursing* (1971) continued the work on relationships; her major contribution was in her conceptualization of the *therapeutic use of self*. Other work related to the thesis that the nurse is the primary instrument of nursing and therapeutic care includes Quinn's (1992) conceptualization of the healing environment.

The authors of this chapter and many other nursing faculty have used the classic works of Peplau, Orlando, and Travelbee in developing guidelines for reflection on developing therapeutic relationships in undergraduate and graduate students in nursing. Such therapeutic relationships underpin all of nursing, regardless of specialty or practice level.

The experience of P-MH nurses today is reflective of the struggles of the profession as a whole and of the struggles of women around the world. The nursing profession needs to bring a heightened awareness and consciousness of the phenomenon of misogyny, the hatred of women. This phenomenon demands attention, awareness, and global critical action. Other oppressed marginal people are also worthy of attention. The Research Alerts in the chapter highlight work investigating the experiences of women, oppressed people, and vulnerable groups within society who need attention and mental health intervention.

Though short-lived, the community mental health centers established in the mid-1960s through the late 1970s provided P-MH nurses with opportunities to develop significant roles for themselves in **advocacy,** community liaison building, consultation, crisis stabilization, case management, medication management, research, and education, as well as to develop the role of therapist in working with individuals, families, and groups.

Unfortunately, the P-MH nurses and professionals involved with the CMHC reform movement experienced lost hopes and dreams as the needed mental health care revolution and reform failed to materialize. Many nurse researchers were originally involved in the CMHC movement but took other paths as the movement all but disappeared. Through the application of partisan politics in the early 1980s, the U.S. federal government established block grants for states to administer mental health services. With that act, the federal oversight role, along with the CMHC movement, was abolished.

Deinstitutionalization of the large public asylums and state hospitals began with the development of CMHCs and was finally completed by the late 1970s, just in time for the state block grants to take over the public mental health program. In response to this trend, a new group of private psychiatric hospitals sprang up. Mental health care for the private hospitals became a lucrative business, which further motivated privatization of mental health treatment. The state-funded public programs, in turn, began shouldering the primary burden of caring for the seriously mentally ill.

The public–private split in mental health care exists today, and P-MH care remains desperately in need of revolution and reform. For a nation so advanced in technology and advanced physical care, the gap in research into and knowledge of mental health care in the United States is a national embarrassment. Further, for a large number of state and federal professionals and residential care providers, caring for the nation's most seriously ill and incarcerated population is often considered an undesirable assignment.

**Application to Practice**

**Reflective Education and Practice Exercise 3**

*Constructing a Multigenerational Genogram*

Sometimes the things you think you know the most about are the things that can teach you so much. When the family assessment was assigned, I was sure that I already knew everything there was to know about my family. Yet, as I began to talk to my parents, grandparents, aunts, and uncles, I realized that there are many stories, traits, and patterns that run throughout. I learned new things about people I thought I knew everything about. . . . But, most importantly, researching my family allowed me to learn new things that I may have never had the opportunity to learn. I am lucky to have grandparents who know about family medical history and even better who know about the traditions that our family is based on. . . . The things I have learned are not only valuable to me personally, but will also be priceless in my career as a nurse. This was an opportunity to see family in a whole new light, to analyze relationships and see patterns among members. I learned the effect that one conflict in a relationship can have on an entire family. I also learned the value of having family close by. This assignment has allowed me to see the big picture . . . to see how much family can impact a person, especially in hard times. This will be precious in helping to treat patients.

—Nursing student, spring 2003

The first and most obvious pattern in my family is for men and women on my mother's side to be alcoholics or to marry alcoholics. . . . I mention this because they have impacted me in way that I myself do not even understand. . . . So, I unwittingly followed the pattern set by my mother and grandmother. I married a recovering alcoholic . . . I love my family. The strength of character, although it may not be obvious from what I have reported, is a predominant theme. Despite their faults, [my family members] have overcome many trials of faith and I have learned from the stories they tell.

—Nursing student, spring 2003

Conducting the analysis was pretty simple. It is easy to see the trends that flow through our family. . . . It brought my attention to many of the health issues in my family. Any nurse should be aware of family histories. Creating a genogram can be a good way to give tips on preventing certain diseases that run in a patient's family. ◐

—Nursing student, spring 2003

As a consequence, the most seriously ill are cared by the least educated, least supported healthcare providers.

## ■ State of the Science of Psychiatric–Mental Health Nursing

The 1990s were considered the decade of the brain, during which great strides were made in understanding the biological component of mental disorders and functioning and developing drugs to treat these conditions. Atypical antipsychotic medications have continued to be developed and, although they are not without adverse consequences, have provided some hope for relief of symptoms. Long-term studies of these drugs are still needed. The weight gain associated with use of many antidepressants and antipsychotics has been associated with the development of type 2 diabetes. Clearly, there is a continuing need for research. Complementary and alternative modalities are in great need of research as well.

There is a growing need for public education focused on anxiety, stress and coping with stress, depression, integration of complementary and alternative therapies with traditional approaches, and assisting in people developing balanced lives. Large-scale community violence and terror experiences in the United States in the mid- to late 1990s have continued to be of national concern. The Oklahoma City bombings; school violence in Pearl, Mississippi, and Columbine, Colorado; and continuing community experiences related to sniper and perpetrator violence have produced significant anxiety in the general population. In the aftermath of the threats to national security following the terrorist attacks on September 11, 2001, large scale community education and intervention programs are needed. The aftermath of the war on terrorism, the Iraq war, and the continuing concern about terrorism and violence has caused great stress for those serving in the U.S. military, their families, the rest of the country, and the world. Further, widespread corporate scandals and unethical practices exposed around the same time as the 2001 terrorist attacks have further threatened personal as well as national security for many U.S. residents. The notion of safety in the United States and all over the world, as terrorists' takeover of a Russian elementary school demonstrates, has been altered forever.

There is also a need for further exploration of human and basic sciences and research in the areas of treatment, prevention, and health promotion. Nursing research and the social sciences disciplines have begun to make significant contributions to our understanding of the person and experience of mental illness. A growing body of literature is devoted to evidence-based practice and outcome-focused research. Nevertheless, there is an unmet need for research that identifies qualitative outcomes and qualitative evidence for practice. The growing wealth of research literature delves into both quantitative and qualitative research and studies new methodologies. Both foci add to the knowledge and understanding of the human condition and human experience.

**Application to Practice**

**Reflective Education and Practice Exercise 4**

*Student Reflection: Journaling*

The first time I approached journaling was 12 weeks ago. At that point I was still trying to grasp an understanding of what it was I was trying to accomplish through the journaling process. Now, 12 weeks later, I have a greater appreciation of what journaling can do. It has helped me grasp some of the thoughts that fly rapidly through my head, and turn them into something legible that I can view. The whole process has helped me understand my thought processes and turn the abstract into a somewhat tangible reality.

—Nursing student, spring 2002

Journaling has also helped me to express my thoughts and feelings, which is something I have persistently had a problem with. Even to this day, I struggle in sharing with others when I am having trouble either in my personal life or in my life as a student. I tend to keep issues bottled up inside, but those around me can clearly see that something is bothering me. This lack of communication has affected some of my relationships in the past and present, but journaling has provided me with a means of expression.

—Nursing student, fall 2002

 Research Alert

Using street ethnography while interviewing homeless men in San Francisco and St. Louis, researchers examined the nexus and interaction between homelessness and incarceration. Among the men in the study, crimes of desperation, aggressive policing, and close proximity of homeless men and many ex-cons created a strong likelihood of incarceration and reincarceration. For incarcerated men, time inside eroded employability, family ties, and other defenses against homelessness. For several men, homelessness had occurred for the first time following release from prison or jail. The following phrase is worthy of close scrutiny: "[the] homelessness/incarceration cycle, more powerful than the sum of its parts, a racialized exclusion/punishment nexus which germinates, isolates, and perpetuates lower-class male marginality" (p. 500).

Where the plight of homeless women is different from that of homeless men, the homeless/incarceration cycle for women is different in that "historically, poor women have been positioned differently vis-á-vis the law" (p. 502).

For the homeless untreated mentally ill, this phenomenon is in need of continued scrutiny.

*Source*: Gowan, T. (2002). The nexus: Homelessness and incarceration in two American cities. *Ethnography*, *3*(4), 500–534. This special issue of the journal *Ethnography* is entitled "In and Out of the Belly of the Beast: Dissecting the Prison."

process underlying human experience. Narratives and stories, in "their own words" accounts, and naturalistic settings further inform and serve to fully describe human experience. Quantitative studies, using large random population samples, have the potential for generalizing findings to the population at large. Each methodology scrutinizes a slice of human experience and, when combined with other perspectives, plus triangulation of methods and data collection strategies, presents a fuller understanding of human experience.

Many P-MH phenomena have been investigated by advanced practice nurses to date, including the work of the following authors: Douglas, (2004); Frank (1987); Hutchinson (1986); Becker (1991); Becker Hentz (1994); Lauterbach (1992, 1995, 2003); Lesser, Oakes, & Koniak-Griffin (2003); Lesser, Tello, Koniak-Griffin, Kappos, & Rhys (2001); Lesser, Koniak-Griffin, & Anderson (1999); Munhall & Boyd (1983); Swanson-Kaufmann (1993); and Munhall (2007). All of these authors are advanced practice P-MH nurses involved with qualitative inquiry.

Loss, change, and bereavement, along with stress and anxiety, are universal human phenomena that involve human suffering. These conditions often underlie mental health conditions. As examples of **universal human experiences,** they occur throughout the life span, and require specific and general resources for coping and resolution. Research into these and other universal human experiences is of particular interest to P-MH nursing. Lauterbach's (1992, 1995, 2008) doctoral and follow-up research, for example,

Additionally, there is a growing need for development of and research into integrative complementary alternatives in mental health treatment. Many people suffering with depression, anxiety, or stress use complementary and alternative therapies, often exclusively. In addition, professional groups that face undue stress because of the nature of their work or the state of the profession, such as nursing, need to research the stress related to the practice discipline. Further, research findings related to human phenomena need to be shared directly with the public, as it often has direct practice application, particularly research emerging from qualitative methodologies.

Research carried out using qualitative perspectives offers new understanding of the human experience. Phenomenological research uncovers and discovers meanings in human lived experience and leads to better understanding of the human experience. Ethnography offers an understanding of the culture and mores that surround human experience and phenomena. Grounded theory seeks to explicate the basic human

## BOX 36-6

**Psychiatric–Mental Health Nursing: Areas of Practice**

**Basic-Level Functions**
- Health promotion and health maintenance
- Intake screening and evaluation
- Case management
- Preventive management of a therapeutic environment
- Self-care activities
- Psychobiological interventions
- Health teaching, including psychoeducation
- Crisis intervention
- Counseling
- Community action
- Advocacy

**Advanced-Level Functions**
- Psychotherapy
- Psychobiological interventions
- Medication management and prescriptive authority (in some states)
- Clinical supervision/consultation
- Consultation/liaison building

*Source*: Adapted from Nurses for a Healthier Tomorrow, 2008.

focused on perinatal loss—specifically, on uncovering meanings surrounding mothers' experience with having a wished-for baby die.

## ■ Levels of Psychiatric–Mental Health Nursing Practice

Psychiatric–mental health nursing practice includes practice at both basic levels and advanced levels. The basic levels included in Box 36-6 are registered nurses (RNs) who have associate or baccalaureate degrees. There are still a small number of RNs in practice who were trained in diploma programs. Currently, assistive-level personnel in public institutions provide most of the day-to-day supportive care and assistance for patients. These personnel are called mental health technicians (techs), patient care assistants, or a similar designation. Private programs and institutions often have technicians who have college degrees. Medication supervision is provided by an RN with an associate or baccalaureate degree, or by a licensed practical nurse (LPN).

Nurses at the advanced practice level have master's degrees in nursing and may also have doctoral degrees. Specialization in the clinical area of P-MH is available at the master's level, with board certification available as a clinical specialist (CS) since the late 1970s and 1980s and for the nurse practitioner (NP) since the early 2000s. The nurse practice act of the state determines whether prescriptive privileges and independent practice are available for the advanced-practice-level nurse.

**Application to Practice**

**Reflective Education and Practice Exercise 5**

*Attending a Support Group*

I have tried my best to apply some of the steps that I acquired from attending the AA meeting to my eating habits. I have been on Weight Watchers off and on throughout the semester. I find myself feeling so much lighter and healthier when I stay on it. It is hard to eat healthy today when every restaurant is pushing "biggie size." With technological advances, energy expenditures are not promoted. It is much easier to say yes to the food that tempts me than to the food that is good for me. All of my life I have had to watch my weight, but all I seem to watch is it go up! I have found, though, that journaling about it helps me express my feelings instead of eating them away. Hopefully, I will continue to stay motivated and will not allow myself to become a statistic.

—Nursing student, spring 2002

Sitting in on a CA and AA meeting was a quick way to learn about their general purposes, the audience, and group procedures and process. The content of the discussion presented a picture of life as a drug user. Although each person's story was unique, several themes surfaced. The prevailing themes were the bondage to the drug, feelings of total defeat, and enslavement to the drug. Drug use had had a marked impact on their work performance, which usually led to their unemployment. They exploited family and friends to maintain their addiction. Many spoke about how their drug-using friends abandoned them when they faced trouble or prison.

The group process impressed me the most. The meetings seemed to be desperately needed by the members. In both meetings, people were eager to participate and share their lives and situation. Those who were clean offered their experiences and encouragement. Mutual respect for each other was high. When one man picked up his chip, there was applause and encouragement and celebration. . . .

This experience was highly beneficial to me. As a nurse, I can confidently recommend such support group to drug-abusing patients. As a nursing student, I have a better grasp of mental health concepts. As a FSU [Florida State University] student, the sad stories I heard warn of the horrors of drug and alcohol abuse. As a friend, I have a better understanding of the life and struggles that drug users experience.

—Nursing student, spring 2003

**Objectives Related to Mental Health and Mental Disorders**

**Mental Health Status Improvement**

18.1    Reduce the suicide rate.

18.2    Reduce the rate of suicide attempts by adolescents.

18.3    Reduce the proportion of homeless adults who have serious mental illness.

18.4    Increase the proportion of persons with serious mental illnesses who are employed.

18.5    Reduce the relapse rates for persons with eating disorders, including anorexia nervosa and bulimia nervosa.

**Treatment Expansion**

18.6    Increase the number of persons seen in primary health care who receive mental health screening and assessment.

18.7    Increase the proportion of children with mental health problems who receive treatment.

18.8    Increase the proportion of juvenile justice facilities that screen new admissions for mental health problems.

18.9    Increase the proportion of adults with mental disorders who receive treatment.

18.10    Increase the proportion of persons with co-occurring substance abuse and mental disorders who receive treatment for both disorders.

18.11    Increase the proportion of local governments with community-based jail diversion programs for adults with serious mental illnesses.

**State Activities**

18.12    Increase the number of states and the District of Columbia that track consumers' satisfaction with the mental health services they receive.

18.13    Increase the number of states, territories, and the District of Columbia with an operational mental health plan that addresses cultural competence.

18.14    Increase the number of states, territories, and the District of Columbia with an operational mental health plan that addresses mental health crisis interventions, ongoing screening, and treatment services for elderly persons.

*Source*: DHHS, 2000.

An example of a relatively new specialty role, which has emerged from the P-MH specialty, is that of forensic nursing. This specialty area integrates nursing and forensic science in bridging the gap between the health care and criminal justice systems. As a response to the increasing epidemic of violence, this specialty attempts to meet care needs of both victims and perpetrators. Although it is quite different in scope and purpose from the P-MH clinical specialty and nurse practitioner role, this specialty is of growing interest to nursing. Board certification is becoming available for advanced practice nurses in forensic roles.

Increasingly, there is a need for primary mental health care within primary care organizations. Many P-MH NPs work in primary care practice settings, such as college health care programs. **Prevention** and early intervention are key to reducing the ultimate societal and human costs in treating mental disorders. Over time, many disorders escalate out of control because they are overlooked and/or undertreated. Providing timely, appropriate, and supportive care for

people who experience common human problems such as trauma, loss, or anxiety, or for those who experience intolerable suffering seems to be critical in preventing patterns of dysfunctional and inadequate coping.

Public education remains an area of great unmet need. This need has been partially addressed by the National Alliance for the Mentally Ill (NAMI) and state mental health

---

🖳 Research Alert

Research has provided us with a better understanding of the experience of obsessive–compulsive disorder (OCD). Using a phenomenological perspective, the author of one study investigated the lived experience of the phenomenon of OCD, a personality disorder according to the *DSM-IV-R*. In its severe form, OCD is similar to the psychoses, in that it completely dominates the conscious experience with obsessive thoughts and compulsions that are directed to lessening the anxiety, and it renders the person unable to function in activities of daily living or work.

This work and the text of which it is a part represent a collection of writings aimed at explicating and understanding the human experience. The researcher author uses subjects' descriptions "in their own words." The beauty of this qualitative method and research is that *knowing about* and *understanding* the condition have direct practice applications. ◬

*Source*: Haase, M. (2002). Living with "obsessive compulsive disorder." In M. van Manen, *Writing in the dark: Phenomenological studies in interpretive inquiry*. London: Althouse Press.

❝*Nursing is an art; and if it is to be made an art,*
*Requires as exclusive a devotion, as hard a preparation;*
*As any pointer's or sculptor's work;*
*For what is the having to do with dead canvas or cold marble,*
*Compared with having to do with the living body—*
*The temple of god's spirit?*
*It is one of the fine arts;*
*I had almost said, the fines of the Fine Arts.*❞
—*Florence Nightingale*

## HEALTHY PEOPLE 2010

**Highlights of *Healthy People 2010* Progress Review**

Nearly half of all Americans will meet the criteria for a mental disorder at some time in their lives, with first onset usually in childhood or early adolescence.

More than 25% of adult Americans have at least one mental disorder and approximately 5% have three or more.

The four most widespread disorders are anxiety disorders, mood disorders, impulse disorders, and substance disorders.

Mental disorders are a leading cause of disability, absenteeism, and lost productivity in the workplace.

Emerging factors contributing to the prevalence of mental illness in the US include an aging population and the large proportion of veterans returning from Iraq and Afghanistan with post-traumatic stress disorder, depression, and anxiety.

To help address the increased risk of male veteran's dying by suicide, a national suicide hotline is being made available to veterans. Options for providing telephone crisis counseling and referrals to active duty military personnel and their families are also being explored.

Advances in research have shown that depression and certain cognitive losses are not an inevitable part of aging. This should lead to improved diagnostic precision and enhance the provision of age-appropriate treatment.

Too few primary care providers are trained to recognize depression and the variety of disabilities associated with it.

Five states have legislated parity in insurance benefits for treatment of mental disorders and physical illnesses.

The provision of mental health services in schools provides an opportunity for early intervention. For example, the city of Baltimore through collaboration with local universities is able to offer the services of full-time mental health professionals in more than 60 of its public schools.

*Source:* Adapted from DHHS, 1999.

---

**❝**We are more alike, my friends,
than we are unalike.
We are more alike, my friends,
than we are unalike.**❞**

—Maya Angelou

associations, but much remains to be accomplished. Reducing the resistance to treatment and societal stigma attached to mental health problems through education, research, and knowledge-based treatment should be a *Healthy People* public health goal.

## Individuals and Population Groups Needing Psychiatric–Mental Health Services

Mental health and mental disorders are included in *Healthy People 2010* as part of health promotion, and the *Healthy People 2010* boxes identify mental health problems and populations in need. The *Healthy People 2000* 1996 review report refers to an increasing problem of drug and alcohol use among teens, but it seems to be more serious than even the statistics show. Parents with young teens are aware of

 Research Alert

This article examines the health-related issues of the spouses of deployed military personnel who are living in community settings. It focuses on increasing the knowledge of healthcare providers regarding the stressors these spouses may experience and providing resources in case they may require extra support and assistance. Suggestions of possible community health nursing interventions in dealing with these spouses and the role of nurse practitioners in their coping strategies are discussed.

*Source:* Tollefson, T. (2008). Supporting spouses during a military deployment. *Family & Community Health,* 31(4), 281–286.

---

**BOX 36-7**

**Common Human Experiences**
- Loss, death, separation
- Crisis
- Relationships with significant others—family, friends, work, society
- Anxiety
- Sadness, depression, and mood conditions
- Developmental eras and transitions—individual, family, group, societal
- Illness—acute and chronic
- Stress and coping
- Coping with change

---

this growing population of youth who are encountering very serious substance use, including cigarettes, smokeless tobacco, an incredible variety of inhalants, abuse of prescription "pills," and daily and large quantities of marijuana use, coupled with alcohol. In addition, the epidemics of rape, violence, legal entanglements, and pregnancy among junior and senior high school students are, from the perspective of the youth, much greater than statistics demonstrate. The pattern of misuse and abuse that is reflected in the aforementioned behaviors, along with a recognition of problems with anxiety, depression, and attention to school and learning, warrant careful investigation, research, and concurrent social action. Many of the behaviors are seen by professionals as attempts to self-medicate. However, research is needed to identify factors that are associated with and contribute to "using" behaviors. We need to understand more about these human phenomena.

There are a growing number of individuals and populations at risk in need of primary mental health nursing as well as specialized P-MH. This reflects the growing consumer and public recognition that specialized support is needed to cope with particular human phenomena and experiences. Box 36-7 lists universal human experiences that are often in need of special support and crisis or continuing care. The potential direction and roles for P-MH nursing will focus on

## Application to Practice

### Reflective Education and Practice Exercise 6

#### *The Shelter Experience*

. . . as you looked around, you could see some people with very definite mental illnesses, and there were some whom you couldn't really decide if they had an illness or not. . . . It was interesting because when I looked around at the people there, I didn't see just the people; I saw individual stories . . . stories that I wanted to learn about, but did not want to intrude. . . . Maybe if I volunteered more of my time, they would become able to trust me and then possibly confide in me. One will never know unless the time is dedicated. . . .

—BSN Nursing student, Florida State University School of Nursing

Each experience in life presents us with a unique situation to observe and learn from. The Shelter is no exception. Approaching the experience was intimidating, much like the first experience at Florida State Hospital. But, by simply participating, sitting back and watching the people who call this their home offered many insights into a side of life I have never considered before.

As I arrived at The Shelter, I surveyed what was around me: hand-me-down blankets, well-worn clothes, used towels and sheets. I smelled the smells of people who had not bathed in days. I smelled tobacco, so strong that it made my eyes water. I wondered, How anyone could live there?

Soon the people who lived there taught me an important lesson. This life was better than sleeping in a cardboard box on the streets, and better than freezing out in cold weather. When they began to file into The Shelter, I realized as they signed in that they were real people. There were women released from jail to find their homes repossessed, women who had nowhere else to go. There were men with families, men who had been kicked out of their homes, men who fought for their country and came home to nothing. I realized that they were thankful to have a place to sleep, to be safe, where they didn't have to worry about someone taking the few things they carried in their bag.

It became obvious that the life they had lived had taken a toll on them. Physically they seemed drained. Their hands showed scars and years of work with no care. Many were sick, coughing, and were grateful for a glass of water. Mentally, many were plagued with illness. One man hid in a corner. Many were alcoholic. Each person who came through the door had a story.

This experience changed my attitude toward the homeless. Many are employed, working long hours and not getting paid enough to get back on their feet. They have hopes and dreams and goals like the rest of us. Perhaps the biggest eye opener for me was the way they interacted with each other. They were careful to see that the older men had extra blankets, or were able to have their special mat, or that everyone got a blanket. They joked and laughed and told stories about their families and experiences. This experience was perhaps one of the most meaningful experiences in my life. Two nights with these people drastically changed my ideas. It made me realize that many are trying their hardest to survive and to make it on their own. In the meantime, they are grateful and appreciative of the care received. I will take away a compassion for those who have been humble enough to admit that they need help and have graciously accepted it.

—BSN Nursing student, Florida State University School of Nursing

To be homeless and not to have any place to go is an overwhelming reality to many people in our society. That notion is difficult for me to comprehend. How could someone not have family or friends who would love him or her unconditionally and give [the person] simple shelter? Where can such people go? The Shelter is one place. It is an unconditional place that will accept anyone and only ask the residents to obey limited rules for their own safety and the safety of others. The Shelter provides the basic needs of residents. . . . In this place they can be treated with respect. Some of the new residents were unsure at first, but they quickly felt comfortable. The residents were thankful for everything and they expressed it openly. . . .

My experience at The Shelter was humbling. It made me appreciate my family in many different ways. I also felt like helping at The Shelter made a small difference in the lives of homeless people. Leaving The Shelter, I felt like I needed to do much more, and I plan to volunteer again in the future. They say that most of us are only a couple of paychecks away from living on the streets. What a scary thought!

—BSN Nursing student, Florida State University School of Nursing assisting persons and groups in handling living through difficult human experience.

As a focal phenomenon, changes in the American family warrant particular attention. A growing number of children grow up in single-parent homes, usually with the father absent. There are changes in the structure and function of families. Single parents and working women are growing aggregates. This combined with poverty serves to compound vulnerability.

The growing elderly population with cognitive impairments, institutionalized elders, and those with Alzheimer's disease and their families further reflect the concept of compounding vulnerability. More work, more research, and more preventive efforts are needed for serious mental health conditions and diagnoses, such as schizophrenia, which involve exacerbations of acute symptoms of distress and disturbance. This population represents a large number of persons and families who experience periods of acute exacerbation of chronic illness. Other chronic illnesses, such as diabetes, have patterns involving crisis and management and need psychiatric-mental health nursing attention.

## Current Assessment of the Public's Mental Health Status

In 1978, the President's Commission on Mental Health established by U.S. President Jimmy Carter estimated that nearly 15% of the population needed some type of mental health services at any given time. This estimate was found to be very conservative. Data from the *Diagnostic Statistical Manual* (DSM) correlated with data from the World Health Organization's (WHO) International Classification of Dis-

### Research Alert

The article cited below reviews literature and data supporting the links between substance abuse and men's violence toward women partners. It also examines critical issues in treatment for men who batter and discusses particular treatment issues for black men who abuse substances and batter women partners.

Common explanations of substance abuse and violence discussed are disinhibition owing to lower brain functioning caused by substance use, cognitive distortion, learned disinhibition, disavowal of responsibility ("It was the alcohol"), and power and control.

Effective treatment needs to involve an integration of services and agencies, and a coordinated effort by all involved, including the community. The following elements were identified as critical in helping black men change their behavior:

- Confront and take ownership of the problem and associated negative behavior
- Challenge the current method of addressing problems in their lives
- Identify other models for life and problem solving
- Develop alternative life codes of conduct
- Build the capacity to problem-solve in challenging situations

Further, it is important to view black men's partner violence not only as a personal problem, but also as a larger social community problem. Women's abuse occurs within the context of the larger society and cultural group. A lower tolerance for partner violence in the community is needed.

When considering a population-focused approach to the problem of substance abuse and violence, this theoretical exploration has implications for other human phenomena. Substance abuse is often related to criminal behavior, and it is a critical component in other relationship problems, health-related conditions, morbidity, and mortality data.

*Source*: Bennett, L., & Williams, Oliver, J. (2003). Substance abuse and men who batter. *Violence Against Women*, 9(5), 558–575.

eases (ICD) has been used in the *DSM-III* epidemiological study. This program estimated that 32% of adults in the United States report symptoms meeting criteria for one or more psychiatric disorders during their lifetime (Tsuang, Tohen, & Zahner, 1995).

Mental disorders occur across the life span and affect people from all racial, ethnic, and geographic areas. They affect both genders and cut across all socioeconomic groups. However, these conditions are distributed differently between population groups and genders: 36% of men and 30% of women meet the criteria for a diagnosis of disorder, and 20% of men and women have symptoms of active disorder within the last year. These population figures show few

### Research Alert

The purpose of this study was to systematically review qualitative research that addresses how people live with suicidality or recover a desire to live. Suicide is a pressing social and public health problem. Much emphasis in suicide research has been on the epidemiology of suicide and the identification of risk and protective factors. Relatively little emphasis has been given to the subjective experiences of suicidal people, but this is necessary to inform the care and help provided to individuals. A systematic review of the literature and thematic content analysis of findings was conducted. The findings were extracted from selected papers and synthesized by way of content analysis in narrative and tabular form. Twelve studies were identified. Analysis revealed a number of interconnected themes: the experience of suffering, struggle, connection, turning points, and coping. Living with or overcoming suicidality involves various struggles, often existential in nature. Suicide may be seen as both a failure and a means of coping. People may turn away from suicide quite abruptly through experiencing, gaining, or regaining the right kind of connection with others. Nurses working with suicidal individuals should aspire to be identified as people who can turn people's lives around.

*Source*: Lakeman, R., & FitzGerald, M. (2008). How people live with or get over being suicidal: A review of qualitative studies. *Journal of Advanced Nursing, 64*(2), 114–126.

Dr. Sarah Steen Lauterbach, chapter author, in an encounter with an elder patient.

differences from the results of Leighton, Harding, Macklin, MacMillan, and Leighton's 1963 study, which found that SMI typically affects the impoverished (low-socioeconomic) population.

In the United States, approximately 40 million people aged 18–64, or 22% of the population, had a diagnosis of mental disorder alone in the previous year. One in five children and adolescents between age 9 and 17 years has a diagnosable mental disorder in a given year. Serious emotional disturbances in this population often lead to school failure, alcohol or illicit drug use, violence, or suicide. An estimated 5% of children and adolescents are extremely impaired by mental, behavioral, and emotional disorders. An estimated 25% of older people (age 65 and older) experience depression, anxiety, substance abuse, or dementia that is not part of aging. Approximately 8–15% of this population group experience Alzheimer's disease, and the size of this group doubles for every 5 years of age after 60. Alzheimer's disease is thought to be responsible for 60–70% of dementia, which is a leading cause of nursing home placement (Healthy People 2010, 2004).

Serious mental illnesses (SMIs) such as schizophrenia, mood disorders (major depression and bipolar disorder), and severe anxiety disorders (obsessive–compulsive disorder and panic disorder) can be, and often are, enormously dis-

abling. Schizophrenia affects 2 million people each year, or approximately 1.5% of the population. Affective (mood) disorders affect roughly 9.8% of the population, including both women (6.5%) and men (3.3%). Bipolar disorder affects approximately 1% of the population, with men and women being equally affected. A high rate of suicide is associated with mood disorders. Anxiety disorders (panic disorder, obsessive–compulsive disorder, post-traumatic stress disorder, and phobia) are more common than other disorders and affect as many as 19 million people in the United States annually (*Healthy People 2010*, 2004).

Rates of the most severe forms of SMI have been estimated to be between 2.6% and 2.8% of adults aged 18 and older during any given year. Only 25% of these individuals obtain help for their condition through the health care system. In contrast, 60–80% of all persons with heart disease seek and receive care. More importantly, 40% of people with SMI do not receive help from either general or specialty mental health providers, and most do not receive any help. Of those aged 9–17 years who have a mental disorder, 27% receive help from the health sector, but 20% of children and adolescents with mental disorders use only mental health services in their schools. Comorbidity (more than one mental disorder existing at the same time) is a growing problem and requires specialized treatment and understanding, such as is needed for concomitant depression and substance abuse.

Substance abuse and related problems are among society's most pervasive health and social concerns. Each year, 100,000 deaths in the United States are related to alcohol consumption. Illicit drug use accounts for another 12,000 deaths. Further, a substantial proportion of the population uses alcohol. Alcohol and alcohol-related problems are common among adolescents. The age of onset of use is associated with dependence, with approximately 40% of those who drink at 14 years or younger developing dependence at some point in their lives.

## ⌨ Research Alert

Pregnant adolescents and young mothers living in Los Angeles County are vulnerable to acquiring HIV/AIDS through sexual transmission because they lack the resources, social status, and power to protect themselves. This article describes adolescent mothers' ($n = 76$) responses to an HIV prevention program. The design of the study was based in ethnography, the anthropological tradition of qualitative research. Many of the pregnant teens and young mothers described how the experience of becoming a mother helped empower them to improve their lives. Yet efforts to decrease risky sexual behavior were overshadowed by more immediate concerns and by relationship issue of gender and power and of trust.

*Source*: Lesser, J., Oakes, R., & Koniak, O. (2003). Vulnerable adolescent mothers' perceptions of maternal role and HIV risk. *Health Care Women International*, 24(6), 513–528.

Alcohol has been linked to injuries, accidents, and violent acts and deaths. People who drink only a relatively small amount can nevertheless create tremendous consequences if they drink and drive. Alcohol consumption is associated with close to 40% of all fatalities in automobile crashes. These fatalities due to alcohol use continue to fall—likely due to more strigent laws, enforcement, and education.

Alcohol is often a factor in homicides, suicide, family violence, and child abuse. The SMI population is especially vulnerable to substance abuse. Many are polysubstance users and commit the crimes for which they are incarcerated during intoxication. The forensic SMI population experiences compounded vulnerability, and members of this group are at risk of becoming permanently incarcerated owing to being incompetent to proceed (ITP) or not guilty by reason of insanity (NGI).

There are great disparities in the occurrence of mental disorders in the population and treatment opportunities. Disparities in P-MH treatment merely serve to increase and compound disparities in the occurrence of mental disorders within a population. Since the early 1980s, with the changes in allocation of funds in block grants and oversight of the federal government to states, private P-MH hospitals have served the insured; state programs have served the SMI population. Additionally, within health care systems, there are marked differences in how disorders present themselves, and how they are prevented, diagnosed, and treated by gender, racial, ethnic groups, and age. Depression affects twice as many women as men, but women who are poor, have little formal education, are unemployed or on welfare, and live in rural areas are more likely to experience depression than women in the general population. Many of these women have no access to health care or are underserved. This gender gap in care and disorder is seen from adolescence on.

Suicide is one of the leading causes of death in the population aged 15–24 years. Recently, attention has focused on the increasing suicide rate for returning Iraq war veterans. Research has consistently shown that approximately 90% of all people who kill themselves have a mental disorder, a substance abuse problem, or combination of these disorders. Suicide is sometimes associated with a copy-cat phenomenon. This phenomenon is also seen in violent acts involving the taking of hostages, situations of school violence, and terrorism acts. Examples of this phenomenon are school shootings that followed the 2007 Virginia Tech massacre. Although much is known about suicide prevention, it is increasingly evident that violence needs particular research support.

Marginal, oppressed individuals and groups, for example, are at risk of perpetrating violent acts on society. Fundamentalism in politics, religion, and social programs, where only one solution is considered the "right" solution, seems to breed violence. Multicultural and reflective perspectives offer strategies to understand experiences from the perspective of the other. This phenomenon needs particular attention, as terrorism has been an increasingly global problem since the dawning of the twenty-first century.

Following violent acts, such as the September 11 terrorist attacks, or other large-scale crises, such as the Hurricane Katrina disaster, experiences of severe anxiety and depression increase. Post-traumatic stress disorder (PTSD) is an acute anxiety disorder that develops as a response to overwhelming anxiety. Following the Vietnam War, PTSD proved debilitating for many returning veterans and their families. In military personnel returning from the Iraq war, approximately 16% have PTSD, though this disorder is probably grossly under-reported.

Following the September 11 attacks, there was an increase in anxiety and depression in the general population, and a much higher incidence of anxiety and depressive symptoms in survivors, individuals who were relatively close in geographic proximity to the events, and individuals who had family members and friends who lost their lives. For recovery workers, the direct and protracted nature of the rescue and recovery made them especially vulnerable. Data from the Mount Sinai School of Medicine's evaluation of September 11 rescue and recovery workers and volunteers, many of whom worked 4 months of 8-hour workdays, indicated that 51% met threshold criteria for a clinical mental health evaluation. The top three emotionally related disabilities were in the area of problems with social life, work, and home life. Seven years after these events, the nation continues to deal with bereavement and coping with change and loss. The feeling of safety, security and freedom in everyday life seems gone forever (*MMWR*, 2004).

**❝***Never doubt that a small group of thoughtful, committed citizens can change the world; Indeed, it is the only thing that ever has.* **❞**

—*Margaret Mead*

## Research Alert

Although there is a growing body of research in the area of adolescent pregnancy and parenting, little is known about the more personal experiences of these teens. Ethnographic research methods were used in one with the goal of narrowing existing gaps in knowledge about the affective component of adolescent mothers' maternal role attainment. The sample consisted of 15 voluntary informants who reported depressive symptoms during pregnancy or postpartum. The findings suggest that for some adolescent mothers the experience of motherhood may help them improve their previously self-destructive lives. Many adolescent mothers have engaged in impulsive high-risk activities prior to their pregnancies. Through the establishment of a strong sense of maternal identity and simultaneous development of a strong sense of maternal protectiveness, these young women begin making realistic, future-oriented decisions that motivate them to leave gang life, finish high school, go to college, and get vocational training. However, a subset of adolescent mothers who experience chronic depressive mood along with social isolation in the postpartum period may be at increased risk for development of problematic maternal behaviors.

**❝**I used to be part of a gang but I got out of it when I was pregnant with him. When you are a gang member, you do drugs or do anything. And when I got pregnant, I thought I should look out for my kid now, I should not gang bang, drink, do drugs with my friends . . . I was going crazy in the gang. So I told my friends, you know what, I'm pregnant. I'll see you guys later. And they just let me go. Since my baby was born, I left everything; I left all my gang member friends. **❞**

—Ophelia, teen mother (fictitious name)

Source: Lesser, J., Koniak-Griffin, D., & Anderson, N. L. R. (1999). Depressed adolescent mothers' perceptions of their own maternal role. *Issues in Mental Health Nursing, 20*, 131–149.

Another population group needing special attention and understanding is the homeless population. Approximately 25% of the homeless in the United States have a SMI. Although new approaches and attention have been focused on this group, the population remains especially vulnerable. Treatment is not enough for this population: A complex array of human services, health care, and affordable housing solutions is needed to address their problems. Further, homeless shelters are often very restrictive in who they will serve and how long housing is provided, and they are top heavy with rules about who can gain admission and use services. For example, many refuse to give shelter to a person under the influence of alcohol. For a person in a small city in northern Florida living on minimum wages, it would require 96 hours of work per week to afford a one-bedroom apartment. About one-fourth of shelter residents have jobs

## MEDIA MOMENT

*Mental health parity* was the topic of *Justice Talking* on a National Public Radio broadcast on September 22, 2004. Margot Adler said the following: "A federal law 8 years ago started to address the inadequate pay for mental health care. Now there are attempts to limit it further. If you want to have limits on mental health care, the limits should be no different than care for any other illness." The entire broadcast can be downloaded from www.justicetalking.org.

In his address "Inequality Matters" on June 3, 2004 at New York University, Bill Moyers described many things to get mad about. He ended with the following, "What we need is a mass government of people like you. Get mad, yes—there's plenty to be mad about. Then get organized and get busy. This is the fight of our lives." Visit www.inequalitymatters.org for more information.

and return to the shelter for housing and meals. They see the shelter as a primary group, similar to that of a family. In fact, many refer to the shelter as "home" and as being "family."

Violence in the United States has reached epidemic levels. More than 100,000 youths are placed in U.S. juvenile justice facilities annually. There is an increasing trend in childhood violent deaths, with infant homicides considered to be fatal child abuse. Males are more often perpetrators, and African Americans are more than five times as likely as whites to be murdered. Factors such as low income, racism and discrimination, lack of education and employment opportunities are associated with greater rates of violence. In addition, substance use and abuse, including use of illicit drugs and alcohol, are often associated with violence.

There is a growing concern about the increase in personality disorders in the general larger population. Of special concern is the growing number of individuals with antisocial personality disorders and their lack of response to psychosocial therapies and treatment. There is a need for research in all disorders, but particularly in the Axis II disorders. The person with antisocial personality does not experience anxiety, which is often used as part of therapy and is associated with learning. Such an individual does not experience distress or assume responsibility for his or her acts and behavior. This general lack of anxiety or distress, coupled with feeling no responsibility, is common among forensic residents in prisons and mental health units. These individuals do not experience discomfort or guilt from behaviors that harm or take away the rights and privileges of another. In fact, the pleasure taken in another's suffering is a common feature of their disorders.

Statistics and rates of mental disorders, although impressive on their own, need to be personalized. Numerical data need personalized interpretations. Such figures do not

## MEDIA MOMENT

**Portrayal of Mental Illness and Psychiatric Conditions in Media**

Embedded within the mental health nursing course were opportunities for planned, structured reflective exercises. The following films and tapes are examples of audiovisual materials that have been used for in-class or outside-class viewing. These films, combined with reflective journaling, dialogue, and class discussion, help develop the skills needed in reflective nursing practice. The following list is only a few of the wonderful films available to the public that support the development of reflective practice:

*Wit* (2001)
*Ordinary People* (1980)
*Whose Life Is It, Anyway?* (1981)
*The Days of Wine and Roses* (1962)
*When a Man Loves a Woman* (1994)
*A Beautiful Mind* (2001)
*Fight Club* (1999)
*Reign over Me* (2007)
*The Bucket List* (2007)

*Three Faces of Eve* (1957)
*Tuesdays with Morrie* (1999)
*Asylum* (1972)
*Chattahoochee*
*Fried Green Tomatoes* (1991)
*Girl, Interrupted* (1999)

**Student reflection focused on The Three Faces of Eve**

I have always been fascinated with split personalities. This movie helped me see that behind the turmoil of all these personalities vying for control was a suffering young lady in need of help. It is easy in situations where someone is disturbed to want to probe and inspect the mind, forgetting that there is a person who is affected by that mind. The movie gave me a greater understanding of the disorder and the suffering of another human being.

—BSN Nursing student, spring 2002,
Florida State University School of Nursing

---

inform alone, nor do they tell the human story behind the condition. Each statistic represents a person, an individual—someone's child, or spouse, or father or mother, or sibling, or friend. Each person represented suffers often unbearable pain and anxiety, along with failed hopes and dreams, as do all of the people connected to that person, such as the family, community, work, or social group.

### Ethics of Psychiatric–Mental Health Services

Inequity that exists around mental health care impoverishes a group of people who are already at risk. Furthermore, the cost of services is a factor in access and serves to compound risk in an already vulnerable population. This is in direct conflict with prevention concepts and health promotion, which require delicate timing and appropriate intervention within the least restrictive environment. The right to fair and equal mental health treatment is a human rights issue. Interestingly, the community mental health movement was concurrent with the civil rights movement in the United States and was just about as successful. Where civil rights and care are much improved today, there is great need for equity and mainstreaming of mental health services into the health care system of services.

Mental health problems, in contrast to physical health problems, are often very complex, involving an interaction of many factors, including heredity, cultural, social class, living conditions, lifestyle, family relationships, occupation, and economic and political factors. There are often unrecognized mental health issues surrounding and involved with physical health and illness conditions that, if treated along with the physical illness, would promote a healthier adjustment.

> **"** *There is nothing more dangerous than to build a society, with a large segment of people in that society who feel that they have no stake in it; who feel that they have nothing to lose. People who have a stake in their society, protect that society, but when they don't have it, they unconsciously want to destroy it.* **"**
>
> —Martin Luther King, Jr.

The separation of mental health services from other health services creates problems of access to treatment. Problems occur both for those with major or chronic and debilitating mental health conditions and for those who have symptoms that, if treated appropriately at the time, would contribute to the recovery, health, and well-being of the person.

## Psychiatric–Mental Health Nursing's Roles and Phenomena of Concern

The preceding discussion is particularly important in understanding the complexities of the art and science of P-MH nursing care. The American Nurses Association (ANA, 1994) identified a list of actual or potential mental health problems presented in Box 36-8 that comprise **phenomena of concern** for P-MH nursing. These include phenomena presented earlier as universal human experiences in need of attention, care, and research. Basic-level functions of P-MH nursing presented previously are inclusive of both prevention and promotion activities as well as treatment and intervention activities. Advanced-level functions further delineate the specialty and therapist role of the advanced practice P-MH nurse.

**Psychiatric–Mental Health Nursing's Phenomena Of Concern**

Actual or potential mental health problems of patients pertaining to the following:

- The maintenance of optimal health and well-being and the prevention of psychobiological illness
- Self-care limitations or impaired functioning related to mental and emotional distress
- Deficits in the functioning of significant biological, emotional, and cognitive systems
- Emotional stress or crisis components of illness, pain, and disability
- Self-concept changes, developmental issues, and life process changes
- Problems related to emotions such as anxiety, anger, sadness, loneliness, and grief
- Physical symptoms that occur along with altered psychological functioning
- Alterations in thinking, perceiving, symbolizing, communicating, and decision making
- Difficulties in relating to others
- Behaviors and mental states that indicate the patient is a danger to self or others or has a severe disability
- Interpersonal, systemic, sociocultural, spiritual, or environmental circumstances or events that affect the mental and emotional well-being of the individual, family, or community
- Symptom management, side effects/toxicities associated with psychopharmacological intervention and other aspects of the treatment regimen

*Source*: © 2007 ANA, APNA, and IPNA. *Psychiatric Mental Health Nursing: Scope and Standards of Practice*. Silver Spring, MN: Nursesbooks.org. Reprinted by permission.

The P-MH nursing role includes health promotion, health maintenance, health teaching, community action, and advocacy; however, this area encompasses one of the greatest needs in community mental health program development. Currently, nurses in practice within community programs function primarily as managers of care, overseeing care, administering medication, and maintaining records. Community action and advocacy activities are often limited. Some nurses are involved in developing and maintaining the therapeutic milieu, but staffing issues are prevalent throughout the private and public programs.

Missing from the list of functions is the nurse's key role in providing continuity of care. The nurse's unique role and position with persons and groups over time provide opportunities for support and intervention that others on the treatment team simply do not have. In addition, the commitment to using strengths of people and active involvement of those cared for place nursing in a key position.

Since the beginning of modern nursing, the concept of *prevention as intervention* has been a key concept of public health care. The unique vantage provided by the nursing perspective, nursing presence, and the temporality of this role is often under-used in therapeutic relationships with individuals, groups, and communities. This is an area in need of attention in both public and private programs.

The P-MH nurse of the twenty-first century has assumed more coordinating, collaborative, and case management activities than ever before. At the same time, the role encompasses direct service and therapeutic interventions with individual and groups within services and programs that are located at a variety of locations, within community agencies, and the home. The role of nursing in the public's mental health needs continued assessment and evaluation.

In primary mental health care environments, basic-level P-MH nurses are key professionals who are ideally positioned to assume a variety of roles in multiple settings ranging from acute inpatient to community settings. They are often the only member of the health care team who has knowledge to monitor general health as well as mental health needs and care (see Box 39-9 for leading health indicators). They are prepared in early identification of problems, including preventive intervention, primary prevention, and health promotion. They possess skills in assessment, social intervention, and psychoeducational processes connected with understanding illness and experience of mental illness, and also have knowledge of symptom management, pharmacology, and rehabilitation. The advanced practice P-MH nurse is prepared to manage the care of persons, including monitoring medications.

**❝***The time is always right to do what is right.***❞**

—*Martin Luther King, Jr.*

## ■ Guiding Philosophical and Theoretical Frameworks for Mental Health Nursing

The purposes of theory are description, explanation, prediction, and control of human phenomena. In addition, nursing theory serves the purpose of providing understanding of human experience and phenomena. Nursing, as a practice discipline, until the last 40 years, operated based on theories related to a biological model of health. It also used interdisciplinary theory. In addition, the use of practice experience as described in the discussion of "tacit understanding" provided a basis for nursing intervention. Nurses have always borrowed and "cut and pasted" theory, sometimes without enough concern for the relevance or "fit." Increasingly, with the development of qualitative research that focuses on developing theory and quantitative research, which requires a theoretical structure, clarity, and operationalization of concepts, mid-level nursing theory is being developed. The 1960s and 1970s were the decades for development of nursing grand conceptual models (Table 36-1). In addition, the development of doctoral programs in nursing has provided the impetus for theory analysis, theory derivation, and theory construction. Advanced-level P-MH nurses involved with theory development can be seen in dissertations and writings of several qualitative nurse researchers, including Becker (1991), Hutchinson (1986), Lauterbach (1992, 1995), Swanson-Kaufmann (1983), and Swanson (1993). Aguilera's (1994) classic nursing text is in its seventh edition and is almost universally used in nursing education curriculums that teach crisis intervention. Aguilera's model of crisis intervention assesses the presence of balancing factors.

More recently, writings from psychiatric-mental health nurses such as Boyd (1988), Lauterbach and Becker (1996), Lauterbach and Becker Hentz (1998, 2004), Munhall (1994, 2007), Munhall and Boyd (1993), and others also embrace the philosophy of phenomenology. Jean Watson's writings

and contributions identify caring as the central focus of nursing. There is need for continuing theory development in P-MH nursing. Researchers and scholars such as Janice Morse and her colleagues' (1997) symposium on the Comfort Project and other qualitative nurse researchers show potential for theory development.

**❝** *Millions of nurses throughout the world hold the key to an acceptance and expansion of primary health care because they work closely with people . . .* **❞**
—*Dr. Halfdan Mahler, Director-General of World Health Organization, at the time of the Alma Ata Declaration*

## Models for Psychiatric–Mental Health Nursing Practice

The writings of educator John Dewey in the early 1900s, who was a friend and colleague of Isabel Stewart, then Chair of the Department of Nursing at Teachers College, Columbia University, are informative. The 1938 writings of Horace Mann (Cremin, 1957) are appropriate considering his views on the value of universal education as the "great equalizer" of human conditions, the "balance wheel of the social machinery," and the creator of wealth undreamed of. He believed that poverty would disappear as an educated public discovered new "treasures of natural and material wealth." Mann also stated that "a nation cannot remain ignorant and free." Education is the key to an informed public and underpins P-MH nursing practice at all levels.

**Table 36-1    Chronology of Conceptual Models in Nursing, 1950–1986**

| Year | Author | Key Emphasis, Publication, and/or Model |
|------|--------|------------------------------------------|
| ▪ 1952 | Hildegard E. Peplau | Interpersonal Relations in Nursing |
| ▪ 1960 | Faye Abdellah | Client's problem is focus of nursing care |
| ▪ 1961 | Ida Jean Orlando | The Dynamic Nurse–Patient Relationship |
| ▪ 1964 | Ernestine Weidenbach | Clinical Nursing: A Helping Art |
| ▪ 1966 | Virginia Henderson | The Nature of Nursing |
| ▪ 1966 | Lydia Hall | Nursing Care—Use of Self |
| ▪ 1967 | Myra E. Levine | Four Conservation Principles of Nursing |
| ▪ 1970 | Martha Rogers | Science of Unitary Human Being |
| ▪ 1971 | Imogene King | General Systems Framework |
| ▪ 1971 | Dorothea Orem | Self-care framework for model |
| ▪ 1971 | Joyce Travelbee | Therapeutic Use of Self |
| ▪ 1974 | Betty Neuman | Systems Model |
| ▪ 1976 | Sr. Callista Roy | Adaptation Model |
| ▪ 1976 | Josephine G. Patterson & Loretta T. Zderad | Existential philosophical foundation of nursing |
| ▪ 1978 | Madeleine M. Leininger | Caring and transcultural perspectives |
| ▪ 1980 | Dorothy E. Johnson | Behavioral System Model |
| ▪ 1981 | Rosemarie Rizzo Parse | Man-Living–Health |
| ▪ 1985 | Jean Watson | Nursing: Human Science and Human Care |
| ▪ 1986 | Margaret Newman | Health as Expanding Consciousness |
| ▪ 1989 | Patricia Benner and Judith Wrubal | Caring is central to the essence of nursing |

## ■ Public Health Model

The traditional public health model includes all levels of prevention: primary, secondary, and tertiary. It has been a viable model for P-MH nursing practice. Central to this model is the critical role of public education. This model uses concepts of mental health and illness, epidemiology, and population-focused statistics in assessing mental health needs as well as risks. Population statistics, when combined with knowledge of mental health issues, are useful in identifying populations vulnerable to experiencing dysfunction.

Currently, the major thrust of U.S. mental health care is toward secondary prevention efforts, providing treatment and minimizing disability. There is a need for research and funding in all areas of prevention, but particularly within primary prevention. The following primary prevention activities are in need of public policy inquiry and research: mental health promotion and dysfunction prevention; holistic, meaningful, mind–body wellness activities; personal and community education; acquisition of effective coping skills; wholesome early attachments and healthy lifelong relationships; facilitating environments conducive to meaningful work and mental and physical health; and finally, self-empowerment. There is need for a large-scale community studies of stress and crisis conditions.

Secondary prevention activities are the major thrust of care and include early diagnosis and intervention, accessible services, and timely, appropriate treatment. One of the most important contributions of the community mental health movement of the 1960s and since has been the development of crisis intervention services. This, combined with the consumer movement of the 1970s, has made a significant contribution to support services for individuals and communities. Still, major primary prevention work is needed to address the conditions and environments that create and perpetuate interpersonal crises. Situational crises, which are superimposed on predicted developmental crises, further create risk, but with proper attention, they can be addressed. Consumer involvement has been helpful in the development of suicide prevention programs, services for rape crisis and victim recovery, and other phenomena needing support and therapeutic intervention. However, more research into crisis prevention, intervention, and impact of crises on life is needed. The phenomenon of human abuse and violence needs to be researched and better understood. Where treatment usually is focused on the victim, more work is needed in addressing the treatment and rehabilitation of the perpetrator, facilitating a violence-free environment. Phenomena need to be reconceptualized and investigated as a community and social phenomenon as well as an individual phenomenon.

Tertiary care has been the focus of community mental health programs and currently provides most of the care for the seriously mentally ill public, including state hospitalization. The community mental health care system includes a range of community-based services addressing a full range of needs and particular groups needing care. These programs address ongoing and acute exacerbations of conditions and chronic care. Activities aimed at rehabilitation and reducing the discomfort and suffering associated with particular mental health problems need research.

Community studies of health have provided information that is potentially useful in articulating nursing's future role in community mental health. Early studies such as Hollingshead and Redlich's (1958) work associated social class

## CULTURAL CONNECTION

Domestic violence is of concern throughout the world, and is present in all economic, racial, and ethnic groups. The status of women and the oppression of women in economic, social, and political roles are underlying causes of such violence. Intimate-partner violence is a major public health issue for all women and for people who are oppressed. There is a great need for health care providers to be culturally aware and competent to provide services and intervention. The dual discrimination that black women face predisposes them to black male aggression. Further, the cultural and spiritual conditions trap battered black "women into silence, submission, and continued victimization" (p. 535).

There are also structural, cultural, and situational issues surrounding the violence. The structural context is defined as the macro-level structural arrangements and social conditions that have a direct effect on access to opportunity and the quality of life. Intergenerational exposure to racial and gender oppression is a major feature of many black men's experience. Chronic unemployment and underemployment have profound effects on black women and children.

The cultural-community context provides the socialization that black men have, which instills in them views similar to the white male views about their superiority over women. Subordinated masculinity for black men and other lower-class men has prompted many of them to redefine masculinity in a manner consistent with the context of their subordinated status. For all these reasons, black women wives and girlfriends are at increased risk for becoming victims of black men committing violent crimes against their partners.

The situational context is that most intimate-partner violence occurs close to home, between 6:00 P.M. and midnight. It typically occurs within the normal context of everyday life.

Although no single program can eliminate this violence, successful efforts might include early intervention in the form of school retention programs, high school–based programs providing job readiness, low-interest loans for education, and placement centers for employment in inner cities. When black men are employed, they are less available on the street—organizing their daily activities, rather than hanging out and getting in trouble with their wives or girlfriends, which in turn increases the likelihood of conflict.

*Source*: Hampton, R., Oliver, W., & Magarian, L. (2003). Domestic violence in African American community: An analysis of social and structural factors. *Violence Against Women, 9*(5), 533–557.

and mental health. Studies that also show the promise of stress and education include Folkman and Lazarus's analysis of coping in a middle-aged community (1980). Antonovsky's (1979, 1987) work on health focuses on "salutogenesis," the origins of health, and "what healthy people have in common." This mid-level theory, along with Selye's (1956, 1974) classic work on the biological model of stress and the work of Benson (1975, 1984), have contributed much to the field. The value of theories such as these comes from the combination of the idea of the connection between mental and physical health and a sociological model for conceptualizing stress.

## ■ Primary Care Model

Since the beginning of modern nursing, nursing has offered two different perspectives for the focus of care: caring for the individual and caring for the needs of populations. There is often tension between these two different perspectives. This is especially true for P-MH nursing, where the individual often is seen as the identified patient but in reality

### GLOBAL CONNECTION

The publication of *Nurses of All Nations* marks the one-hundredth anniversary of the International Council of Nurses (ICN). This text is the culmination of more than a decade of scholarly inquiry, research, and planning. The first chapter, entitled "Above All Other Things—Unity," begins by identifying the roots of the ICN in "women's suffrage, abolition, missionary work, and social reform" (p. xi). The text is organized around five perspectives that trace ICN's 100-year history: self-image; race, class, and gender; meaning(s) attached to professional nursing; nursing diplomacy; and friendship. In 1997, the new president of ICN, Kristen Stallknect (from Denmark), urged nurses to continue to stress "humanity," regardless of whether governments or others do, urging nurses to demonstrate their values (p. 198). In addition to urging nurses to demonstrate concern for public health, ICN has since its inception been concerned about the "special" needs of women around the globe. The history of the ICN and professional nursing worldwide reflects the history of women in society.

Unity, as a theme for nursing, is of particular interest for the chapter author. Nursing's history is also a history of friendships. Unity is a critical phenomenon in past, current, and future nursing work. We acknowledge that often nurses fail to provide individual and collective support to one another, even as care is provided the public. Nursing work is often anxiety provoking, sensitive, and private; involves human suffering; and is often surrounded by a phenomenological silence. It is imperative that nurses value and provide care for themselves and for one another to provide the care the public needs and deserves.

*Source*: Bush, B. L., Lynaugh, J. E., Boschma, G., Rafferty, A. M., Stuart, M., & Tomes, N. J. (1999). *Nurses of all nations: A history of the International Council of Nurses 1899–1999*. Philadelphia: Lippincott.

reflects dysfunction within a family, community, or larger social system. Taking the example of the state of the mental health care system within the nation, there is dichotomization, stigma, and economic differences within systems providing physical care and mental health care. Privatization of mental health care, reimbursement differences between physical and mental care, and the current contrast with public mental health care's focus on tertiary care are reflective of sentiment and thinking in a society that values economics and physical care over mental health.

Nursing has traditionally been able to provide care to both individuals and groups, using both paradigms for providing care: the public health model and person-focused or family-centered model. Nurses have seen the need for the current "illness care" system to be transformed into a "health care" system.

Primary health care is increasingly being viewed as synonymous with provision of health care (Haber & Billings, 1995). If this concept is to be fully actualized, then primary care will necessarily have to include mental health care. Whether this concept will be fully realized is doubtful. Rather than be a reactive profession, nursing needs to take a position for advocating planned change, advocating for the right for each citizen to have responsive, quality mental health care alongside responsive quality health care. Access to the health care system needs to include both.

## ■ Primary Mental Health Care Model

Increasingly, the discussion of a primary mental health care model is being proposed as a model for delivering community-based, comprehensive P-MH nursing (Haber & Billings, 1995). It has the potential to integrate the two traditional models of care and posits nursing in a key role meeting needs of both individuals and communities. There is need for continued dialog between psychiatric nurses themselves, represented by the Coalition of Psychiatric Nursing Organizations (COPNO), including the ANA Council on

**Primary Mental Health Care: A Model for Psychiatric—Mental Health Nursing**

Haber and Billings (1995) stated that primary care is increasingly becoming synonymous with the provision of health care. In addition to discussing roles of basic- and advanced-level nursing practice in primary mental health care, these authors state that anxiety disorders, depression, and substance abuse are among the most commonly misdiagnosed categories in primary health care practice. In addition, they propose that the boundaries of mental health care delivery must be redefined and expanded from a specialty focus to a primary mental health care model. Furthermore, they state that nurses are beginning to find their niche in nontraditional settings. ◉

**❝**We do not see things as they are, we see them as we are.**❞**

—Talmud

It involves carefully attending to and focusing on the other and the experience itself. It includes the unfolding interaction, focusing on the *content* of communication, the possible meanings, and the unfolding communication *process*. By using a reflective and thoughtful, attentive posture, it becomes possible to "see" much more fully the meanings in the experience of another. This practice increases awareness and leads to greater understanding of the other. As a result of this enhanced understanding, the nursing process can be more fully, appropriately, and timely implemented and evaluated.

Many examples of reflective activities have been provided that have been particularly useful in nursing education and in P-MH nursing practice. Reflection on personal attitudes, feelings, and values, as well as reflection on life and educational experience, is a critical process in nursing education; it is a critical process in becoming a nurse.

Using publications and teaching experiences (Lauterbach & Becker, 1996; Lauterbach & Becker Hentz, 1998, 2005), the use of reflection is introduced and used in nursing courses and elective university courses in several nursing programs. Since the early 1990s, reflective practice has been

Psychiatric Mental Health Nursing, the American Psychiatric Nursing Association (APNA), and the International Society of Psychiatric–Mental Health Nurses (ISPN), which includes the following divisions:

- Association of Child and Adolescent Psychiatric Nurses (ACAPN)
- International Society of Psychiatric Consultation Liaison Nurses (ISPCLN)
- Society of Education and Research in Psychiatric–Mental Health Nursing (SERPN)
- Adult and Geropsychiatric–Mental Health Nurses (AGPN)

Primary care roles need to be conceptualized to include providing P-MH care within front-line health care and should include more than case management of the large population of psychiatric patients receiving tertiary and chronic P-MH care.

### ■ Using Reflection in Nursing Education and Practice

Throughout this chapter, we have made many references to P-MH nursing's use of reflection as a critical activity in nursing education and practice Becoming a reflective practitioner is specially critical in P-MH nursing. It is imperative that self-reflection be developed early in the educational experience and continued in nursing practice.

Reflective practice involves a bending back of attention to self and others and to the therapeutic encounter. Reflection takes place throughout the nursing encounter.

---

**⚑ ETHICAL CONNECTION**

Costello and Dunaway have focused on "threatened egotism" as a major condition of violent behavior. Where the social sciences in the last several years have attempted to test the hypothesis that low self-esteem is associated with violent behavior, this research addresses the association between inflated self-esteem and violent behavior. The researchers conducted a preliminary test with participants from a small junior and senior high school in a Southern city. Their results showed that egotism is positively associated with violent and nonviolent delinquency and that the relationship holds when a number of important predictors of violent behavior are controlled, including self-control and social control.

Substance use is often associated with a person developing an overly self-focus, inflated self-esteem, or narcissism. This may be a contributing factor in the development of egotism, where inflated esteem and overly self-focus prevent the person from developing appropriate, reality-based self-esteem.

Are there ethical implications of this research linking inflated self-esteem and delinquency? As nurses we tend to focus on promoting self-esteem in patients. How would you plan nursing intervention in a school setting using these findings? ◯

*Source*: Costello, B. J., & Dunaway, R. G. (2003). Egotism and delinquent behavior. *Journal of Interpersonal Violence, 18*(5), 572–590.

integrated into human sciences disciplines and practice. In nursing education, reflective practice and activities have become critical strategies to enhance learning. The following are examples of the types of reflective education and practice activities used for this purpose. Student reflections are included in boxes throughout the chapter.

### Journaling to Learn: A Strategy to Develop the Art, Science, and Practice of Reflection in Nursing

Journaling has been used as an educational strategy in P-MH nursing and other nursing and elective courses. Reflective activities have been developed that are geared to increasing awareness of meanings in self and in others. Through journaling, students become aware of their own attitudes, values, and biases regarding mental illness. Journaling has been used as a critical activity in developing a habit of reflection, using informal yet disciplined writing. It has helped to create a greater depth of awareness and more expansive breadth of understanding. This activity has been especially helpful in developing therapeutic communication and relationships in P-MH nursing courses where students are placed in a variety of settings, including community programs and civil and forensic units in a state mental hospital.

Self reflection activities have been and continue to be developed in the following areas: understanding the family as it moves through time, with an emphasis on changing family structures, functionality, family process, patterns of health and illness, and patterns of stress and coping; caring for persons who are residents in The Shelter in a small Southern city, including the homeless SMI residents; and serving as observer-participants in support groups. In addition, class material, films, and other mental health materials were used as focal topics for guided reflection. Students kept a weekly clinical journal and wrote a short reflection and critique of the course experiences at three times during the semester. The written reflective critique was found to be especially helpful in students' continued reflection and processing experiences.

### Reflecting on Experiences with the Homeless

Students participated in a service learning clinical experience with The Shelter, a residential care facility for homeless persons in a small Southern city. They helped check residents in for the evening, provided supplies for bath and personal care, and assisted with the evening meal. They had brief interactions focused on these activities. Students found this experience to be especially transformative.

### Reflecting on Support Group Experiences

Students in the following nursing courses attended and wrote reflective papers on their support group experience: the core P-MH clinical course; an RN/BSN concepts course; and elective university-wide substance abuse course; and a university-wide required communication course. Examples of groups attended were Alcoholics Anonymous (AA), AlAnon, Narcotics Anonymous (NA), Alzheimer's Support,

Caring for the Caregiver, Hospice and Palliative Care, Cancer Support, Victims of Violent Crimes, Breast Cancer Survivors, and MADD.

### Reflecting on Family Experiences: Constructing a Multigenerational Family Genogram

The concept of family has been explored in nursing courses in several nursing programs, including P-MH nursing courses, an RN/BSN concepts course, a communication course, and a substance abuse course. The students were required to construct a multigenerational genogram of their own family going back three generations. They identified issues related to health and illness, stress and coping patterns, family structure, and family process using a family systems theory framework. Through focusing on issues and family process in their own family, students became more self-aware and understanding of the issues in their own lives that needed attention. They also developed an understanding of family processes that was applicable to their nursing practice. Students became more aware of the complexity of issues in working with patients and their families. In working with SMI patients and forensic SMI residents, they understood the care and needs of this population group, who cry out for a revolution in care. They saw the profound impact of SMI on the family.

### Self-as-Patient Clinical Reflection: Caring for Self

Self-as-patient clinical activities have been included in several courses in a variety of nursing programs. This activity was used in a professional development course, in the first theory course in the nursing curriculum, in P-MH nursing courses, and in a variety of holistic nursing courses. Students used a personal journal for reflection, and conducted an assessment of and identified priorities for care in the following areas: personal health issues and status; patterns of stress and coping; nutrition; rest and leisure; relaxation; fitness; and family relationships. A plan of care focused on areas of need, priority, and interest. At the end of the semester, students shared their work in several formats, including posters and portfolio, oral presentations, and a written paper about the experience. Examples of these experiences are captured in photographs of students' posters throughout the chapter.

### Therapeutic Use of Self Clinical Reflection

Using guidelines developed for a focus on therapeutic use of self (TUS), students in several courses in several nursing curricula have been introduced to the concept of using the self therapeutically. The thesis underlying this approach is that the nurse is an instrument of healing and care. TUS activities have been used in P-MH nursing, communication, and substance abuse courses, for example. Reflecting on interactions with patients has been especially informative to students. Immediately following these interactions, students recalled the verbatim conversation and wrote process recordings. Interactions were processed and analyzed in post-conferences using the readings and theories underlying human development, therapeutic communication, and relationship development. The reflection on conversations with patients helped students identify possible interpretations of the conversation and possible meanings as they reflected on their use of therapeutic communication strategies. Such guided reflective activities help students learn to critically process, evaluate, and identify appropriate, effective communication strategies.

### Using a Phenomenological Perspective: Understanding the Public's Mental Health Lived Experience, One Person at a Time

**Phenomenology** as a philosophical human science and research perspective has been embraced by P-MH nurses as a perspective for understanding human experience. Max van Manen (1990), stated that phenomenology is the "study of the lifeworld—the world as experienced rather than as conceptualized categorized or reflected upon" (p. 9). It is the observation and experience of lived experience as it happens, as presented to our consciousness. It involves seeking for meaning in everyday, commonplace experiences. The writings of nurse researcher Munhall (1994) and others have further developed phenomenology as a perspective that provides a vantage point for "knowing" others as well as a research methodology. In P-MH nursing, this perspective is especially illuminating.

Understanding underpins the nursing process from the beginning assessment, planning, and therapeutic intervention and evaluation. Sartre (1984, orig 1967) asserted that the goal of literature, or the written word, is, "to reveal the world and particularly to reveal man [sic] to other men [sic] so that the latter may assume full responsibility before the object which has been thus laid bare" (p. 18). Further, he stated, "If you name the behavior of an individual, you reveal it to him [sic]; he [sic] sees himself [sic]. And since you are at the same time naming it to all others, he [sic] knows that he [sic] is seen at the moment he [sic] sees himself [sic]" (p. 16). Insight and understanding in therapeutic encounters are enhanced for both nurse and patient.

Phenomenology as a perspective in P-MH practice offers strategies for uncovering meanings in lived experiences. It reveals meanings and insight to the patient and the nurse about what it is like to be a person with the particular experience. Understanding is the ultimate goal of using a phenomenological perspective. The nurse who uses a phenomenological perspective has a goal of facilitating the patient's personal understanding of behavior, of understanding more fully the patient's experience, and of helping others to understand through better communication and more coordinated and integrated care.

### CULTURAL CONNECTION

I could have been dead by now, you know, I was gang related, on drugs, really big time. Like now, I'm not gang related. I have, next month, one year clean with drugs. You just change (as a father) automatically. And when you see your son crying or you see your son smiling at you it's like, oh, I want to be at home with him . . . all the time I have to spend, I spend with my family now.

—Robert, age 19 (fictitious name)

Young Latino fathers' feelings about their fathering role and perceptions of risk for HIV were the focus of this cultural study. Many teen parents have engaged in activities that place them at risk for exposure to HIV. Compared with young mothers, little is known about teen fathers. Young Latino fathers ($N = 45$) living in the inner-city participated in focus groups interviews; 10 also completed individual interviews. Participants provided an account of the influence of lifelong poverty and social oppression on their worldviews and life choices, describing experiences with community violence, substance abuse, and risky sexual activity. Findings illustrate the profound changes that some young men make after becoming fathers, including developing an understanding of the importance of relationships based on equality. Because of these youths' ability to make difficult behavioral changes for the sake of their children, young Latino fathers are excellent candidates for intervention programs, such as HIV prevention.

*Source*: Lesser, J., Tello, J., Koniak-Griffin, D., Kappos, B., & Rhys, M. (2001). Young Latino fathers' perceptions of paternal role and risk for HIV/AIDS. *Hispanic Journal of Behavioral Sciences, 23*(3), 327–343.

A phenomenological stance in nurse caring and relating involves listening carefully, imagining what it is like to be the other person with the experience, and being open to multiple meanings attributed to experience. It requires listening carefully for themes that emerge in the descriptions and paying attention to their emergence in therapeutic conversations. From a phenomenological perspective, we learn about the meaningful, relevant experiences from the perspective of the person in focus.

To understand the person requires that we listen actively to the patient's experiences and elicit rich descriptions of life experience. Often, the novice nurse fails to fully glean an understanding of the patient because of not taking the time, or hastily jumping to conclusions, or simply not being comfortable with the meanings underlying the descriptions and stories.

This perspective also helps in discovering themes in universal human experiences as well as discovering unique and differences in people and experiences. Further, living through a difficult experience is common to many mental health patients and their families. In developing phenomenologically focused therapeutic relationships, the nurse develops a deeper, broader understanding of persons and differences among and between people. This broadened understanding contributes to the development of consciousness. There is a need for a public consciousness regarding the status of mental health care and the growing disparities in needs and care for particular population groups. For nursing, this recognition could potentially facilitate planning, developing, and participating in social and human advocacy with renewed and fuller understanding.

A quote by the poet T. S. Eliot (1936) describes the temporal nature of human experience: "Time present and time past are contained in time future . . . And time future contained in time past" (p. 175). The understanding and insight gleaned from every therapeutic relationship and encounter are intimately connected to past and future experiences for each nurse and patient. Through the process of caring for and of understanding one person, the nurse affects the experience of all those connected to the person and the encounter leads to a potentially transformative relationship for many.

## The Future of Psychiatric–Mental Health Nursing Practice

Current P-MH nursing practice operates within the managed care, cost-containment drive behind health care. A growing number of persons, groups, and communities are not receiving care, do not have basic needs met, and are being lost between services and programs. Preventive care, although identified in *Healthy People 2000* as being targeted (Table 36-2), is still in need of development. P-MH nurses need to be integrated into primary health care environments and community-based programs, such as in schools, daycare programs, parenting programs, and self-help and support programs. Most importantly, there is need for P-MH advocacy in the area of health policy and healthcare planning.

Increasingly, communities are experiencing acts of violence. Since the September 11 terrorist attacks, there has been national security anxiety and depression. Following the invasion of Iraq, there has been heightened anxiety, depression, and post-traumatic disorders among the population. Grandparents are parenting their dysfunctional adult children's children. The future looks bleak as the future grandparents are today's dysfunctional adults. Within this day of information and technology, the growing Third World vulnerable populations, within the larger affluent American society, are cause for concern. Unless we support and care for all our population's needs, health and human rights, including

### 🖥 Research Alert

An ethnographic approach was selected to generate an explanatory model for minority young offenders in the juvenile justice system receiving mental health services. Thirty (10 female, 20 male) youths between the ages of 13 and 17 years participated. Five themes were identified in the group: a desire for caring and stable families; lack of personal control; a love–hate relationship with school; feeling depressed and hopeless; and "it's better to be tough than sick." These youths felt they had no control over their lives. Reliance on peers (gangs) was commonly used as a means of protecting themselves when they had no reliable family. Expressions of sadness and anxiety were common, and the youths were regressed, appearing very childlike as they expressed themselves. They were secretive about their mental health problems and expressed distrust of counselors even though they needed to talk to someone and indicated that they might use mental health services if they could be assured of confidentiality. This study concluded that further research is needed about this phenomenon.

*Source*: Shelton, D. (2004). Experiences of detained youth offenders in need of mental health care. *Journal of Nursing Scholarship, 36*(2), 129–133

| Table 36-2 | Problems and Populations Targeted in National Health Objectives for Mental Health |
|---|---|
| **Problem** | **Target Population** |
| ■ Persistent mental disorders | Children |
| | Adolescents |
| | Adults |
| ■ Adverse health effects from stress | Adults |
| ■ Injurious suicide attempts | Adolescents |
| ■ Suicide | Adolescents |
| | Adult and elderly men |
| | Native Americans and Alaska natives in reservation states |
| ■ Maltreatment | Children and youth age 18 and younger |
| ■ Assault injuries | Children aged 12 and older |
| | Adults |
| ■ Physical abuse | Women |
| ■ Rape and attempted rape | Women and adolescents age 12 and older |
| ■ Homicide | Children age 3 and younger |
| | Spouses |
| | African American men and women |
| | Hispanic American men |
| | Native Americans and Alaska natives in reservation states |

*Source*: Adapted from U.S. Department of Health and Human Services, 1990.

**MEDIA MOMENT**

"Never doubt that a small group of thoughtful, committed citizens can change the world: Indeed, it is the only thing that ever has."

—Margaret Mead

"There is nothing more dangerous than to build a society, with a large segment of people in that society, who feel that they have no stake in it; who feel that they have nothing to lose. People who have a stake in their society, protect that society, but when they don't have it, they unconsciously want to destroy it."

—Dr. Martin Luther King, Jr.

"The time is always right to do what is right."

—Dr. Martin Luther King, Jr.

**On Mental Health Parity**

Mental health parity was the topic of *Justice Talking* with Margot Adler on a National Public Radio (NPR) broadcast on September 22, 2004. The following is an excerpt:

"A federal law 8 years ago started to address the inadequate pay for mental health care. Now there are

attempts to limit it further. If you want to have limits on mental health care, the limits should be no different than care for any other illness."

The entire broadcast can be downloaded at www .justicetalking.org

**On Civic Responsibility**

In his address during *Inequality Matters* on June 3, 2004, at New York University, Bill Moyers ended his broadcast with the following:

"What we need is a mass movement of people like you. Get mad, yes—there's plenty to be mad about. Then get organized and get busy. This is the fight of our lives."

See www.inequalitymatters.org

*On October 28, 2008, the Mental Health Parity bill passed with bipartisan support. This ensures that more than one-third of all Americans will be able to receive equal coverage for mental and physical illnesses. The law goes into effect January 1, 2010. This represents a major accomplishment for mental health coverage for Americans. See www.nami.org*

shelter, nutrition, and meaningful life, the health and happiness of the public is threatened. Caring comprehensively for a multicultural population and world is key.

## Conclusion

"There, but by the grace of God, go I." This phrase is often used when referring to those suffering from mental illness. Often very little separates those with a P-MH condition and those without such a disorder. Accidents of birth, geography, culture, and the tenor of the times are all factors contributing to the distinction between *those who have* and *those who have not*. Mental health epidemiology demonstrates that *those who have not* are also those who have a greater risk of having a mental disorder. Equal opportunity lies in the accident of birth.

Today, as in the past, mental illness, disorder, and dysfunction are surrounded by a pervasive atmosphere of misunderstanding and social stigma. The stigma is fueled by a lack of knowledge, scientific advances, and reliable treatment and cure. Further, little value is assigned to mental health and treatment of P-MH disorders, and an impoverished and universal lack of public understanding is all too common.

Stigma has been attached to many serious illnesses, such as cancer, in the not too distant past. Over time, however, research and scientific advances in physical health have greatly expanded our knowledge base and treatment options, resulting in positive outcomes and ultimately diminishing stigma.

Even though the 1990s was called the decade of the brain, and many advances were certainly made in treatment modalities, there is still a lack of reliable, tried-and-true

treatments for mental health disorders. We know more about the biological basis of many mental conditions, and we have developed many new psychopharmacological agents that target specific symptoms and produce fewer negative side effects. Nevertheless, we have a long way to go in translating the research into effective treatment. We have not invested the time, energy, and intellectual and economic resources needed to do so.

It was not until the 1950s, with the first advent of psychiatric medications, that many troublesome mental health symptoms were treated. Until then, the reliance on somatic therapies, such as hydrotherapy, insulin shock, and physical restraints, produced even more fear and stigma in association with these disorders.

Mental health problems are often very complex and have roots in social, economic, and political injustices, as well as in problematic behavior patterns. We have made progress in greatly enhancing the treatment of serious episodes and acute exacerbations of chronic mental conditions. With knowledge and treatment success has come a greater openness and acceptance of mental illness. However, our work has just begun. We must take on the *lack of parity* for mental health care and physical health care, for research and treatment. It is only by achieving equity in the research and science underpinning mental disorders that treatment success and understanding will occur.

As members of a specialty, P-MH nurses continue to lead the way in developing reflective practice strategies for nursing and other disciplines. We continue to support the public in experiencing better mental health and self-actualization through developing timely, targeted, and critical interventions. We continue to advocate for the development of therapeutic, facilitative environments and relationships for treatment to thrive. We continue our efforts to revolutionize mental health care and advocate for its status to be equal to physical health care in terms of research support, with affordable, quality, accessible treatment for all people. We hope to ensure the improvement of the public's mental health by caring for people, one person at a time, including self, in families and groups, populations, and nations.

Explore Community Health Nursing on the Web! To learn more about the topics in this chapter, use the passcode provided to access your exclusive website: **http://nursing.jbpub.com/communityhealth.** If you do not have a passcode, you can obtain one at this site.

## ■ CRITICAL THINKING ACTIVITIES

1. Consider what is it like to experience the following:
   - Serious mental illness, such as schizophrenia, mania, or depression
   - Paranoid feelings, to the degree that you know that if you do not take medication, you will get sicker and sicker
   - Feeling that the medication dulls your attention, which helps you stay vigilant; feeling that something bad will happen if you let down your guard

2. What is it like to experience the following?
   - Having no one who you feel understands you and likes you just the way you are
   - Having no friends
   - Experiencing your little brother's death after he was sick so long with leukemia
   - Watching your dad begin to drink heavily in the evenings
   - Feeling fat, even though you ate only lettuce today, weigh 105 and are 5 feet, 7 inches tall
   - Wanting and feeling very independent but still being told by your parents what time you must come in

3. What is it like to experience the following?
   - Wanting your parents to stop fighting
   - Wanting your parents to get back together even though you remember how awful it was before they separated
   - Being devastated when your dad moved out
   - Living with your mom, who works too hard and still does not have enough money even though she gets some child support
   - Visiting your dad, who has forgotten what it is like to have anyone, much less a child, around

4. What is it like to experience the following?
   - Being so depressed that you simply are too tired to get out of bed
   - Feeling that you have nothing to live for
   - Feeling that the world and your family would be better off if you just died
   - Being 17 and suddenly discovering that you had lost all your dreams and goals

## ■ REFERENCES

Aguilera, D. (1994). *Crisis intervention: Theory and methodology.* St. Louis: Mosby.

American Nurses Association (ANA). (1994). *A statement on psychiatric–mental health clinical nursing practice and standards of psychiatric–mental health clinical nursing practice.* Washington, DC: American Nurses Publishing.

American Psychiatric Association (APA). (1980). *Diagnostic and statistical manual of mental disorders* (3rd ed.). Washington, DC: Author.

American Psychiatric Association (APA). (1987). *Diagnostic and statistical manual of mental disorders* (3rd ed., rev.) Washington, DC: Author.

American Psychiatric Association (APA). (1992). *Diagnostic and statistical manual of mental disorders* (4th ed.) Washington, DC: Author.

Antonovsky, A. (1979). *Health, stress, and coping.* San Francisco: Jossey-Bass.

Antonovsky, A. (1987). *Unraveling the mystery of health: How people manage stress and stay well.* San Francisco: Jossey-Bass.

Baer, E. (1990). *Editor's notes. Nursing in America: A history of social reform, a video documentary.* New York: National League for Nursing Press.

Becker, P. (1991). *Perspectives of ethical care: A grounded theory approach.* Ann Arbor, MI: University Microfilms International Dissertation Service.

Becker Hentz, P. (1994). Out of silence. In P. Munhall, *In Women's Experience* (pp. 27–46). New York: National League for Nursing Press.

Becker Hentz, P., Lauterbach, S. S. (2005). Becoming self-reflective: Caring for self and others. *International Journal of Human Caring, 9*(1), 24–28.

Bennett, L., & Williams, O. J. (2003). Substance abuse and men who batter. *Violence Against Women, 9*(5), 558–575.

Benson, H. (1975). *The relaxation response.* New York: Avon Books.

Benson, H. (1984). *Beyond the Relaxation Response.* New York: Times Books.

Boyd, C. (1988). Phenomenology: A foundation for nursing curriculum. In *Curriculum revolution: Mandate for change.* New York: National League for Nursing Press.

Bush, B. L., Lynaugh, J. E., Boschma, G., Rafferty, A. M., Stuart, M., & Tomes, N. J. (1999). *Nurses of all nations: A history of the International Council of Nurses 1899–1999.* Philadelphia: Lippincott.

Costello, B. J., & Dunaway, R. G., (2003). Egotism and delinquent behavior. *Journal of Interpersonal Violence, 18*(5), 572–590.

Cremin, L. (1957). *The republic and the school: Horace Mann on the education of free man.* New York: Teachers College University Press.

Department of Health and Human Services (DHHS). (1999). *Healthy People 2000: Mental health and mental disorders progress review.* Retrieved November 13, 2008, from http://www.cdc .gov/nchs/about/otheract/hp2000/mentalhlth.htm

Department of Health and Human Services (DHHS). (2000). *Healthy People 2010: Conference edition.* Washington, DC: U.S. Government Printing Office.

Douglas, D. (2004). The Lived Experience of Loss: A Phenomenological Study. *Journal of the Psychiatric Nurse's Association, 10*(1), 9–15.

Eliot, T.S. (1936). *Collected Poems 1909–1962.* New York: Harcourt, Brace and World.

Folkman, S., & Lazarus, R. (1980). An analysis of coping in a middle-aged community sample. *Journal of Health and Social Behavior, 21*(3), 219–239.

Frank, D. (1987). The health experience of a single woman having a child through AID. Presented at the 8th Annual Research Symposium, Gamma Zeta Chapter, Sigma Theta Tau International, UNC, Greensboro & Northwest AHCC, April 2, 1987.

Frisch, H., & Frisch, L. (1998). *Psychiatric mental health nursing.* Albany, NY: Delmar.

Gowan, T. (2002). The nexus: Homelessness and incarceration in two American cities. *Ethnography, 3*(4), 500–534.

Haase, M. (2002). Living with "obsessive compulsive disorder." In M. van Manen, *Writing in the dark: Phenomenological studies in interpretive inquiry.* London: Althouse Press.

Haber, J., & Billings, C. (1995). Primary mental health care: a model for psychiatric–mental health nursing. *Journal of the American Psychiatric Nurses Association, 1*(5), 154–163.

Hampton, R., Oliver, W., & Mararian, L. (2003). Domestic violence in the African American community: An analysis of social and structural factors. *Violence Against Women, 9*(5), 533–557.

Healthy People 2010. (2004). *Leading Health Indicators.* Retrieved November 13, 2008, from http://www.healthypeople.gov/Document/html/uih/uih_4.htm

Hedaya, R. (1996). *Understanding biological psychiatry.* New York: W. W. Norton & Company.

Hollingshead, A., & Redlich, F. (1958). *Social class and mental disorder.* New York: Wiley.

Hutchinson, S. (1986). Grounded theory: The method. In P. Munhall & C. Oiler (Eds.), *Nursing research: A qualitative perspective.* New York: National League for Nursing Press.

Lauterbach, S. (1992). *In another world: A phenomenological perspective and discovery of meaning in mothers' experience of death of a wished-for baby.* Ann Arbor, MI, University Microfilms International Dissertation Service.

Lauterbach, S. (1995). (Issue Ed.) The experience of loss. *Holistic Nursing Practice, 9*(3).

Lauterbach, S., & Becker, P. (1996). Caring for self: Becoming a self-reflective nurse. *Holistic Nursing Practice, 10*(2), 57–68.

Lauterbach, S. S. (2003). Phenomenological silence underlying sensitive human phenomena. *International Journal for Human Caring, 7*(2).

Lauterbach, S. S., & Becker Hentz, P. (1998). Becoming a reflective nurse: Caring for self (pp. 97–107). In Guzetta, *Essential readings in holistic nursing.* New York: Aspen.

Lauterbach, S. S., & Becker Hentz, P. (2005). Journaling to learn: A nursing educational strategy for developing the art and practice of reflection. *International Journal of Human Caring.*

Leighton, D., Harding, J., Macklin, D., MacMillan, A., & Leighton, A. (1963). *The character of danger: Psychiatric symptoms in selected communities.* New York: Basic Books.

Lesser, J., Koniak-Griffin, D., & Anderson, L. R. (1999). Depressed adolescent mothers' perceptions of their own maternal role. *Issues in Mental Health Nursing, 20*, 131–149.

Lesser, J., Oakes, R., & Koniak-Griffin, D. (2003). Vulnerable adolescent mothers' perceptions of maternal role and HIV risk. *Health Care Women International, 24*(6), 513–528.

Lesser, J., Tello, J., Koniak-Griffin, D., Kappos, B., & Rhys, M. (2001). Young Latino fathers' perceptions of paternal role and risk for HIV/AIDS. *Hispanic Journal of Behavioral Sciences, 23*(3), 327–343.

Lynaugh, J. E., & Brush, B. L. (1999). *Nurses of all nations: A history of the International Council of Nurses, 1899–1999.* Philadelphia: Lippincott.

Morbidity and Mortality Weekly Report (MMWR). (2004). Physical health status of world trade center rescue and recovery workers and volunteers—New York City, July 2002–August 2004. Retrieved November 13, 2008, from http://www.cdc.gov/mmwr/preview/mmwrhtml/mm5335a1.htm

Morse, J. (1997, December 1–6). *The comfort project.* Presentation at 75th Anniversary Sigma Theta Tau Conference, Indianapolis.

Munhall, P. (1994). *Revisioning Phenomenology: Nursing and Health Science Research.* New York: National League for Nursing Press.

Munhall, P. (1998). Editorial—Out of the box. *Image: The Journal of Nursing Scholarship, 29*(3), 203.

Munhall, P. (2007). *Nursing research: A qualitative perspective* (4th ed.). Sudbury, MA: Jones & Bartlett.

Munhall, P., & Boyd, C. (1993). *Nursing research: A qualitative perspective.* New York: National League for Nursing Press.

Nasser, S. (1998). *A beautiful mind.* New York: Simon & Shuster.

Nightingale, F. (1859). *Notes on nursing: What it is and what it is not.* New York: Dover.

Nurses for a Healthier Tomorrow. (2008). *Psychiatric-mental health nursing.* Retrieved December 4, 2008, from http://www.nursesource.org/psychiatric.html

Orlando, I. J. (1961). *The dynamic nurse–patient relationship: Function, process, and principles.* New York: Putnam.

Peplau, H. (1952). *Interpersonal relations in nursing.* New York: G. P. Putnam's Sons.

President's Commission on Mental Health. (1978). *Report to the President from the President's Commission on Mental Health.* Stock # 040-000-00390, Vol. 1. Washington, DC: US Government Printing Office.

Quinn, J. F. (1992). Holding sacred space: The nurse as healing environment. *Holistic Nursing Practice, 6*(4), 26–36.

Reverby, S. (1987). *Ordered to care: The dilemma of American nursing 1850–1945.* New York Cambridge Univ. Press.

Sartre, J. (1984, orig. 1967). *Existentialism and Human Emotions.* Sacramento, CA: Citadel Press.

Selye, H. (1956). *The stress of life.* New York: McGraw-Hill.

Selye, H. (1974). *Stress without distress.* New York: Signet.

Shelton, D. (2004). Experiences of detained young offenders in need of mental health care. *Journal of Nursing Scholarship, 36*(2), 129–133.

Stanhope, M., & Lancaster, J. (2008). *Public health nursing: Population-centered health care in the community* (7th ed.). St. Louis: Mosby.

Swanson, K. (1993). Nursing as informed caring for the wellbeing of others. *Image: The Journal of Nursing Scholarship, 45*(4), 352–357.

Swanson-Kaufmann, K. (1983). *The unborn one: A profile of the human experience of miscarriage.* Ann Arbor, MI: University Microfilms International Dissertation Service.

Travelbee, J. (1971). *Interpersonal aspects of nursing.* (2nd ed.). Philadelphia: F. A. Davis.

Tsuang, M., Tohen, M., & Zahner, G. (1995). *Textbook in psychiatric epidemiology.* New York: John Wiley and Sons.

U.S. Department of Health and Human Services. (1990). Healthy People 2000. Hyattsville, MD: Author.

van Manen, M. (1990). *Research on lived experience: Human Science for action-sensitive pedagogy.* New York: SUNY Press.

Walker, L., & Avant, K. (1988). *Strategies for theory construction in nursing* (2nd ed.). Norwalk, CT: Appleton & Lange.

Wolf, Z, (1988). *Nurses' work: The sacred and the profane.* Philadelphia: University of Pennsylvania Press.

# Diversity in Community Health Nursing Roles

 EVIDENCE-BASED PRACTICE: A COMMUNITY APPROACH

COMMUNITY HEALTH NURSING may offer nurses more diversity than most any other specialty because of the focus on population groups rather than on individual clients. Community health nursing roles are unique in their diversity because of the nature of their implementation, not simply because of the setting where the care occurs. Community health nursing has always embraced a variety of roles due to the diversity and complexity of public health problems. Because the focus of the care is on the group or population, community health nurses are involved in the identification of populations at risk for illness or disability. Community health nurses assist communities, groups, and populations, such as schools and churches, in the prevention of health problems through self-care and accountability. For example, a public health nurse may administer immunizations to preschool children in a day care to prevent and control communicable diseases in the community at large. Although the focus of these roles remains health promotion and protection, specializations such as occupational health nursing, school nursing, public health nursing, advanced practice, home health, and the care of faith communities through health ministries have emerged as challenging career opportunities for community health nurses.

# UNIT 8

# Community Health Nurse Roles

CHAPTER 37
Public Health Nursing: Pioneers of Health Care
Reform
*Kaye W. Bender*
*Marla E. Salmon*

CHAPTER 38
The Home Visit
*Karen Saucier Lundy*

CHAPTER 39
Home Health and Hospice Nursing
*Karen Saucier Lundy*
*Karen B. Utterback*
*Debra K. Lance*
*Ilene Purvis Bloxsom*

CHAPTER 40
School Health Nursing
*Frances Martin*

CHAPTER 41
Occupational Health Nursing
*Bonnie Rogers*

CHAPTER 42
Advanced Nursing Practice in the Community
*Mary H. Huch*
*Karen Saucier Lundy*

CHAPTER 43
Health Ministries: Health and Faith Communities
*Emily Chandler*
*Ruth Berry*

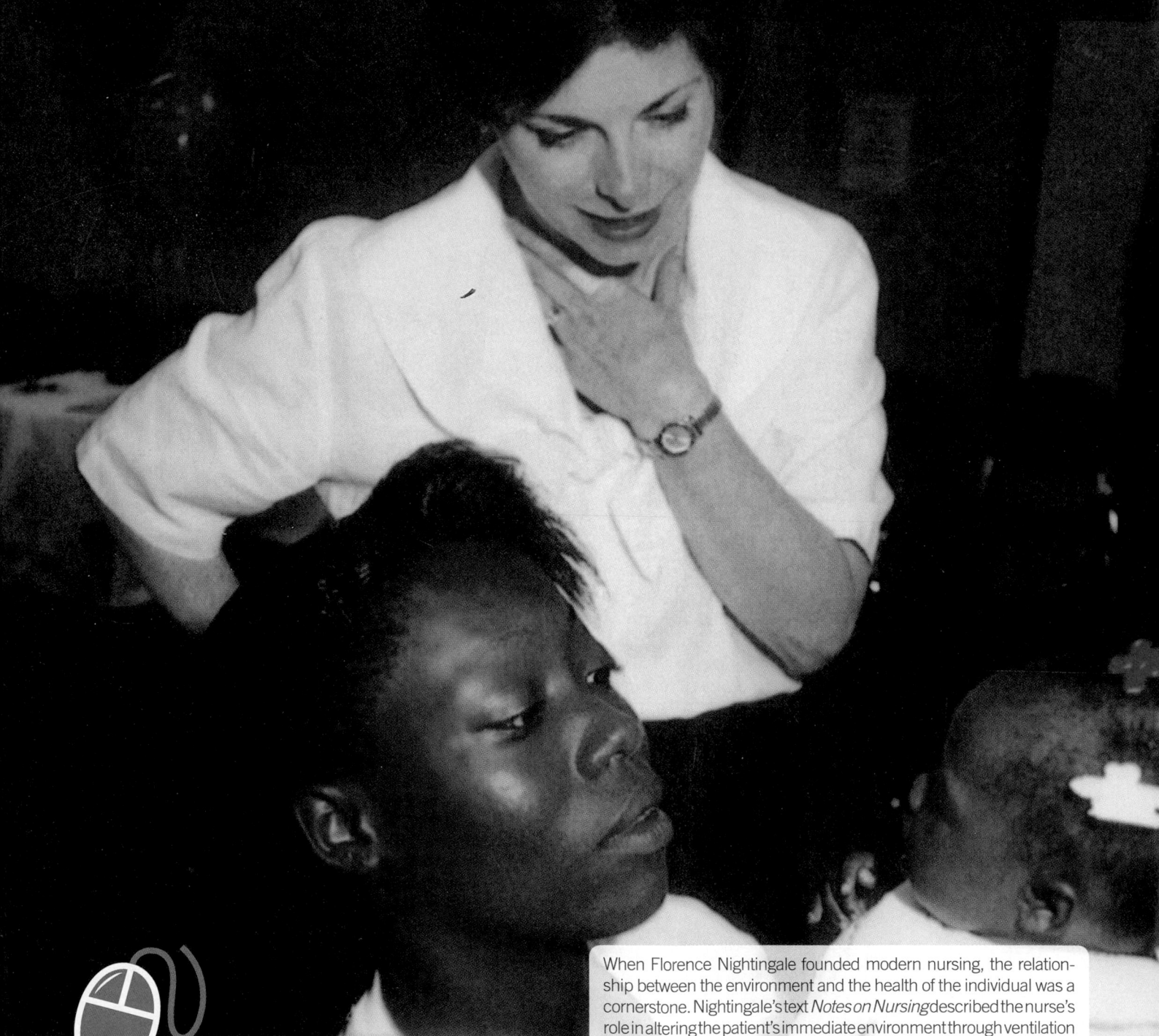

# CHAPTER 37

# Public Health Nursing: Pioneers of Health Care Reform

Kaye W. Bender and Marla E. Salmon

Visit **http://nursing.jbpub.com/communityhealth** for interactive exercises, review questions, Web links, and more.

When Florence Nightingale founded modern nursing, the relationship between the environment and the health of the individual was a cornerstone. Nightingale's text *Notes on Nursing* described the nurse's role in altering the patient's immediate environment through ventilation and heating, cleanliness of housing, modification of noise, provision of light, and proper preparation and availability of food. These factors were found by Nightingale to be of importance to the health and well-being of individuals and, therefore, relevant to nursing intervention. The public health nurse role emerged from these early links between health and the environmental conditions under which we live.

Home Health bringing requires different, but not lower, qualifications and more varied. They require tact and judgment unlimited to prevent the work being regarded as interference and becoming unpopular. They require initiative and real belief in Sanitation and that Life and Death may lie in a grain of dust or drop of water or other such minutiae which are not minutiae but Goliaths and the Health Missioner must be Davids and slay them.

*—Florence Nightingale, 1891*

Over broken asphalt, over dirty mattresses and hcaps of refuse we went . . . there were two rooms and a family of seven not only lived here but shared their quarters with boarders . . . I felt ashamed of being a part of society that permitted such conditions to exist. . . . What I had seen had shown me where my path lay.

*—Lillian Wald, 1893; Wald coined the phrase "public health nursing" and organized the first public health agency, the Henry Street Settlement in New York City*

As you reflect on these quotes, what comes to mind when you think of "public health"? The term "public health" in the past century has been associated with government programs, such as immunizations and blood tests for marriage licenses. What do you think of when you hear "public health nurse"?

## CHAPTER FOCUS

**History of Public Health Nursing**
- Early Health Care Reform
- The Later Years

**Public Health Nursing Philosophy**
- Institute of Medicine Study
- Conceptual Basis for Public Health Nursing Practice
- Definition and Development of Public Health Nursing
- Essential Public Health Services
- Activities for Essential Services

**Challenges and Issues for Public Health Nursing in the New Millennium**
- Impact of the Nursing Shortage on Public Health Nursing
- Further Development of Public Health Nursing Models and Competencies
- National Public Health Performance Standards
- Other Challenges for Public Health Nursing

## QUESTIONS TO CONSIDER

After reading this chapter, you will know the answers to the following questions:

1. What were the early public health reform efforts?
2. Who were the early public health nursing leaders?
3. What were the primary contributions of public health nurses during the early part of the twentieth century?
4. What are characteristics of nursing from the 1960s through the 1980s?
5. What is the role and focus of public health nursing practice?

6. What is the significance of the institute of Medicine's report of 1988?
7. How are conceptual models used in public health nursing?
8. What is the Construct for Public Health Nursing, and what is its usefulness in present public health nursing practice?
9. What is meant by *essential public health services*?
10. What is the future of public health nursing in the twenty-first century?

## KEY TERMS

Commonwealth Fund
Conceptual model
Construct for Public Health Nursing:
  A Framework for the Future
Essential public health services
Hospital and Reconstruction Act
  of 1946
Institute of Medicine
Medicare
Milbank Report
Mary D. Osborne
Salk vaccine
Social Security Act of 1935
Lillian Wald

# History of Public Health Nursing

There have been public health problems in the United States since colonization, but it was not until after the Civil War that concerted efforts were made to improve morbidity and mortality and to control infectious diseases. Poverty, unsanitary living conditions, rampant spread of communicable diseases, natural disasters such as floods, malnutrition, and lack of health care were contributing factors to morbidity and mortality. Public health nursing pioneers emerged as public health efforts began, the most notable being **Lillian Wald,** who is recognized as the leader of public health nursing in the United States. Wald was the first to use the term *public health nurse* to describe visiting nurses who provided direct care to the sick in their homes. These nurses also taught basic hygiene, sanitation, care of children, and proper care and preparation of food. Public health nurses proved versatile: Their skills seemed endless, with a mission to prevent disease, promote health, and to provide care. Their communities truly became their workplace as they became involved in health concerns associated with access to health care, labor movements, maternal and child health, reproductive health, mental health, prison reform, and school health.

## ■ Early Health Care Reform

Organized public health efforts were initiated across the United States in the late 1800s and early 1900s. This early health care reform movement was aimed at improving the health status of all citizens. Leading causes of death were tuberculosis, pneumonia and influenza, diarrhea, malaria, heart and cerebrovascular diseases, and infectious diseases in early infancy; complicating factors were the deplorable living conditions and malnutrition of many citizens. Most notable among the early public health nursing activities were services to river travelers in the South and seaports along the nation's coasts and preventive health services to immigrants in large Eastern Seaboard cities.

Many of the early efforts to establish public health nursing occurred as a result of collaborative agreements between municipalities and the American Red Cross. It was not uncommon for public health nurses to be assigned to posts in geographical areas other than the ones in which they lived at the time of their employment. One such early pioneer was **Mary D. Osborne,** who came to a rural Southern state to work toward the improvement of infant mortality. Her philosophy of public health nursing is reflected in her writings, in which she described qualities she deemed essential for public health nurses of the time: "nurses chosen for public health needed vision, a great desire to do community work,

## CULTURAL CONNECTION

Motorcyclists often believe that they alone should decide if they will wear a helmet. In states where helmets are mandatory for all ages, how do you address the concerns of autonomy for the motorcyclist and the protection of the public's health?

## ENVIRONMENTAL CONNECTION

**How Can Climate Change Harm the Public's Health?**
The climate is changing and these changes impact the nation's health. The ebb and flow of disease is linked to climate. For example, warmer temperatures are often associated with increases in diseases such as West Nile virus. Scientists estimate that the changes in our climate are associated with increasing rather than decreasing risks of disease. Climate change may cause extreme weather events and changes in environmental conditions, leading to increases in disease and death. Populations already at increased risk from death and disease, such as communities of color, the elderly, young children, and the poor, will bear the burden of disease and death from climate change. The existing conditions that already cause worse health among these populations—lack of clean air and water and unhealthy living conditions—will be exacerbated by the adverse effects of climate change. These communities are not only at increased risk for disease, they are also the least able to prepare, respond, and recover from effects of climate change.

*Source*: American Public Health Association. (2008). *Climate change is a public health issue.* Washington, DC: Author.

the ability to work up resources at hand, the adaptability to meet situations as they arose, and most of all infinite patience with people they serve" (Mississippi Department of Archives, 1920–1980); these qualities are as essential today for public health nurses as they were in Osborne's time. Osborne received national and international recognition in 1929 for her work in forging a strong network of public health nurses and for their accomplishments in lowering maternal and infant mortality through improved midwifery practice.

The Great Depression is remembered today as one of the most dramatic times in U.S. history, and most states felt the difficult economic effects of the early 1930s. Public health and public health nursing struggled through this era; however, federal initiatives through Roosevelt's New Deal programs and private entities such as the **Commonwealth Fund** provided funding to expand public health nursing services. The hope was to place one public health nurse in each county in many of the states. Immunization efforts against smallpox, diphtheria, and typhoid were one of the special initiatives with the expanded public health nursing workforce. New initiatives were integrated with previously established activities centered around communicable diseases, perinatal and infant care and midwifery supervision, and tuberculosis control. Their place of service delivery was literally all places in their community, as public health nurses made home visits, initiated school visits, and often set up clinic sites in rural churches or under shade trees.

The public health nurse was equipped with a large brown leather bag to carry essential items such as needles, syringes, a Sterno stove, and matches to set up clinic sites. A black nursing bag was added to provide a mechanism for carrying needed items for home visits. To get where they needed to be, the nurses might travel down muddy paths by riding a mule, borrowing a horse and buggy, or walking lengthy distances. Sometimes a boat might be the mode of transportation. An automobile was a luxury item and a prized possession when available.

### Early Health Outcomes

The dramatic results of this health care movement are noted in mortality and morbidity statistics from 1926 to 1936, with reductions in typhoid fever, diphtheria, pulmonary tuberculosis, pellagra, puerperal septicemia, and eclampsia. One state health official gave much credit to public health nursing by noting that the public health nursing service had come to be recognized as a vital part of an efficient public health administration.

Syphilis had been recognized for several years as a major source of morbidity and mortality. Several boards of health participated with the United States Public Health Service (USPHS) in major studies in the 1930s and 1940s to develop means to conquer the disease. Public health nurses were recognized by the USPHS project director as the chief means to find cases, access medical care for treatment, provide education, find contacts, and follow up on lapsed cases.

Despite interferences of World War II, public health nurses continued to receive education in prevention and treatment of disease processes, including tuberculosis, vaccine-preventable diseases, maternal and child health, and syphilis. Remarkable advances in medical prevention and diagnostic and treatment measures such as the introduction of penicillin were changing public health service delivery and opening new challenges for public health nurses. After World War II, social and economic changes in the states (e.g., improved housing and transportation, movement from farms to towns, expansion of industry) also brought challenges for public health nursing. A public health nurse was employed to institute industrial nursing, which would focus on disease prevention, improvements of hazardous work conditions, promotion of personal health (including nutrition), and first aid.

The country had experienced cyclic polio epidemics since 1934, but disaster struck with the most virulent and widespread epidemic in 1951–1952. Public health nurses made home visits to assist in rehabilitative measures for persons affected with this crippling disease. Regional orthopedic clinics were manned by public health nurses to support access to medical care and set up patient treatment plans. With the availability of the injectable **Salk vaccine** in 1955, public health nurses set up mass immunization sites, while using needles and syringes that required sterilization between each use. These efforts prevented the occurrence of any further polio epidemics.

Health care reform was again under way as federal funds were made available through the **Hospital and Reconstruction Act of 1946.** The increased availability of local hospitals resulted in more physician-attended births, another significant contribution to lower maternal and infant mortality rates. A dilemma resulted, however, as newly constructed hospitals, expanding industry, and public health were competing for the short supply of nurses in the country. Concerns

Dr. Kaye W. Bender, chapter author, on a well child home visit for the public health department.

such as the turnover of nursing personnel, the below-average ratio of public health nurse to population, inadequate salaries, and increased responsibilities caused by a shortage of medical directors in county health departments were prevalent. During this era, public health nursing services shifted significantly from the community to the clinic, rendering the large brown bag used to set up outlying clinics extinct. A shift from family health to more technical, disease-oriented services occurred as a result of limited medical coverage and increased demands for nursing services.

The individual states, along with the rest of the nation, were flourishing economically as the 1960s began. Tuberculosis and several other infectious diseases were no longer the leading causes of death. Typhoid fever, diphtheria, malaria, smallpox, and pellagra had been leading causes of death in 1930–1931; by 1959–1960, only a few deaths were reported from these diseases. Heart disease, circulatory diseases, cancer, accidents, and diabetes were reported as the leading causes of death.

Changes in morbidity and mortality required evaluation by public health and, consequently, new strategies and public health programs were needed to continue the public health mission. Public health nursing established chronic illness objectives to identify cases and treat diabetic and hypertensive patients. Nursing interventions included referrals to local physicians to initiate treatment plans, nutrition and general health education, administration of medication, and teaching administration of insulin. In addition, new vaccines to prevent measles and rubella were integrated into routine immunization standards.

Tuberculosis, although no longer a leading cause of death, remained a public morbidity threat. Medications and treatment modalities had greatly advanced, however. Recognizing the value of early detection of persons susceptible to tuberculosis and providing prophylactic treatment, public health nurses accepted the challenge of a major initiative by boards of health to eradicate tuberculosis. Public health nurses identified contacts to active cases and others determined to be infected, coordinated medical evaluations, initiated plans of care for further diagnostic measures, and administered INH medication.

Landmark federal legislation in 1965 transformed health care with an amendment to the **Social Security Act of 1935,** establishing **Medicare,** a health insurance plan for people 65 years and older and for those with long-term disabilities. Many boards of health supported expanded efforts to meet the federal conditions of participation and, over a 4- to 5-year period, implemented certified home health services. Educational opportunities provided public health nurses with knowledge and skills to provide skilled rehabilitative nursing care to persons who were essentially confined to their homes. Public health nurses had been providing home nursing services on a limited basis since the 1920s, but this would be the first reimbursement established for direct nursing services.

Another new federal initiative for public health nursing by the mid-1960s was family planning. The objective was aimed at lowering maternal and infant mortality rates and improving the general health of women and children, primary interests of public health nurses since the 1920s. With the development of oral contraceptives and the sexual revolution of the 1960s, public health nurses promoted family planning, taught contraception methods, and were key in identifying women at higher risk for such services.

The quantity and variance of public health nursing activities continued to increase. The number of public health nursing visits increased in the areas of communicable disease, maternal and child health, school health, tuberculosis control, sexually transmitted disease, home health, mental health, accident prevention, and chronic disease. Particularly in the Southern states, the work of public health nurses in all health programs was perhaps the greatest force in delivering health services to all citizens.

### ■ The Later Years

Social and political unrest begun in the 1960s continued into the 1970s, and simultaneously the nation was faced with inflation. Travel budgets were cut; public health nursing activities were again evaluated and were relocated from the field to the clinic setting. Continued vigilance in protecting the public's health was in order, and public health nursing rose to the occasion. Increased teen pregnancy rates, a higher incidence of premature births in poorer women, and frequent pregnancies were the focus for public health nursing interventions. More intense family planning initiatives and high-risk tracking systems were implemented to reduce unintended pregnancies and ensure quality, continuous care. In addition, public health nurses supported program implementations to improve nutrition to mothers and children and newborn screening with follow-up for select genetic diseases.

Public health was confronted in the 1970s with increasing demands for services and a limited availability of physicians. Federal funds were made available to provide education to expand the scope of nursing in primary care. Many nurse practice acts were revised by legislation to allow for the expanded role of public health nurses. Boards of health, recognizing the value of this level of practitioner in public health, selected public health nurses to return to school with primary areas of study in maternal and child health. This proved to be an added advantage as nurses returned to more patient- and family-centered care, which had been the traditional philosophy of public health nursing.

Public health nurses of the 1980s and 1990s have continued to provide an array of public health services to the general public, to medically underserved populations, and to culturally diverse populations. Their workplace remains the

At the groundbreaking for the Nell Hodgson Woodruff School of Nursing of Emory University's new building, James Curran, MD, MPH, dean of the Rollins School of Public Health, and Marla Salmon, ScD, RN, FAAN, dean of the School of Nursing and chapter author, broke ground together. Drs. Curran and Salmon hold joint faculty appointments in each other's schools, concrete evidence of a collaboration and partnership between the two schools.

same, as they provide services in individual homes, schools, industry, jails and prisons, and the county health departments; and their mission, to prevent disease and to promote health, remains constant. With today's national and state focus on healthcare reform, public health nurses are positioned to assist both communities and individuals within to bridge the transitions of health care. Their versatile skills include assessing the health status of communities, translating and interpreting among health care disciplines, promoting and teaching health, delivering primary community-based health care, and sustaining measures to control communicable disease (Cohen & Reutter, 2007; Gebbie & Turnock, 2006).

History reveals that health care reform is a continuous process, not a new phenomenon. The elements currently influencing healthcare reform are both old and new—tremendous technology advances, explosive and diverse population growth, political changes, an array of extreme social problems, escalating healthcare costs, access to care, financing for acute care rather than preventive health, and the need to encourage individual responsibility for health (Abrams, 2007; Kulbok & Reed, 2006; Polivka et al., 2008).

## Public Health Nursing Philosophy

Fundamental to the philosophy of public health nursing are holistic beliefs about humanity, health, and nursing. Public health nursing has been defined as "the practice of promoting and protecting the health of populations using knowledge from nursing, social, and public health sciences."

Public health nursing practice is a systematic process that accomplishes the following:

1. The health and health care needs of a population are assessed to identify subpopulations, families, and individuals who would benefit from health promotion or who are at increased risk of illness, injury, disability, or premature death.

2. A plan for intervention is developed with the community to meet identified needs that take into account available resources and the range of activities that contribute to health and the prevention of illness, disability, and premature death.

3. A plan is implemented effectively, efficiently, and equitably.

4. Evaluations are conducted to determine the extent to which the interventions have an effect on the health status of individuals and the population.

5. The results of the process are used to influence and direct the current delivery of care, deployment of health resources, and the development of local, regional, state, and national health policy and research to promote health and prevent disease.

This systematic process is based on and is consistent with (1) community strengths, needs, and expectations; (2) current scientific knowledge; (3) available resources; (4) accepted criteria and standards of nursing practice; (5) agency purpose, philosophy, and objectives; and (6) the participation, cooperation, and understanding of the population. Other services and organizations in the community are considered, and planning is coordinated to maximize the effective use of resources and enhance outcomes. The philosophy of public health nursing is based on the belief that patients (individuals, families, groups, or communities) have the right to quality health care that is available, accessible, and acceptable and that will include them in the planning of their health care (APHA, 1996; Easley & Allen, 2008; Gebbie & Turnock, 2006).

## ■ Institute of Medicine Study

Recognizing that organized public health efforts had been vital to ensuring the health of the nation, the **Institute of Medicine** (IOM) completed a 2-year study of the future of public health in 1988. During that 2-year period, the committee members interviewed an array of public health workers, policy makers, members of the general public, and public health academicians. The study's final recommendations have become a cornerstone for guiding public health's organizational development. Those recommendations included a description of the mission of public health.

**THINK ABOUT THIS** · · · · · · · · · · · · · · · · · · · · ·

Can this really be true? Public health efforts are the reason we are living longer!

Public health's prevention efforts are responsible for 25 years of the nearly 30-year improvement in life expectancy at birth in the United States since 1900. Only 3.7 years can be attributed to medical treatment, and clinical preventive services (such as immunizations and screening test) account for 1.5 years. The remaining 25 years have resulted primarily from prevention efforts in the form of social policies, community actions, and personal decisions. Examples that have added years to our life spans are infectious disease control, improved nutrition to targeted populations (women and children), clean drinking water, environmental risk reduction, prenatal care, contraception use, and self-risk reduction and education (Turnock, 1997). And yet today, less than 5% of the federal budget is allotted to preventive health services.

What do you think? Are we putting our money on the right horse?

*Source*: Turnock, B. J. (1997). *Public health: What it is and how it works*. Gaithersburg, MD: Aspen.

The resulting mission statement said succinctly what public health nurses had been practicing for many years. With the goal of improving the health of the public as a whole, public health nurses systematically provide nursing interventions at both individual and community levels. These interventions vary with the changing health status of the citizens of the country. In the early years when living conditions and crowded housing created opportunities for diseases to spread, public health nurses provided assessment, treatment, and education on tuberculosis, sexually transmitted diseases, and general personal hygiene. In later years, as lifestyles and personal health habit choices became more significant to the causes of morbidity and mortality, public health nurses added education about the prevention of tobacco use, exercise benefits, and domestic violence to their menu of interventions (Cohen & Reutter, 2007; Gebbie & Turnock, 2006).

The role of ensuring that the public remains as healthy as possible is shared between government and the private sector. The Institute of Medicine described government's role in ensuring the public's health as follows:

- *Assessment*: Public health agencies systematically collect, analyze, and publish information on the health status of the community.
- *Policy development*: Public health agencies promote the use of scientific knowledge as the basis for formulating public policy about health.
- *Assurance*: Public health agencies assure that services that are needed to ensure the health of the public are in place and are of high quality.

Several levels of responsibility were attached to these roles. Local, state, and federal governments were all challenged with their respective responsibilities in ensuring the health of the public. Special linkages to environmental health, mental health, and the care of the indigent were also described in the study.

Public health nurses have the potential to develop roles in all of the areas described in the IOM report. Although the most commonly defined role of the public health nurse has been that of providing services to control communicable diseases, there are numerous other roles for public health nurses. At the beginning of the twenty-first century, public health nurses are working in epidemiology, policy development, administration, specialized research areas, and nurse-managed projects aimed at improving the health of special populations.

 GLOBAL CONNECTION

Public health nurses in many countries are responsible for geographical areas, such as city blocks or rural areas defined by miles. They care for all families in their "district" and are considered generalists.

 *Got an Alternative?*

Public health nurses, perhaps more than other specialties, are confronted with "folk remedies" used by their patients. Because of the bond that exists between nurse and patient influenced by long-term contact, the public health nurse is often aware of what the patient and her family uses outside of traditional medical interventions. These items may include folk remedies such as medicinal herbal preparations, beliefs about childbearing and menstruation, and use of meditation and prayer. How can the public health nurse promote the health of patients, as well as prevent potential risks, considering his or her unique position with families?

## ■ Conceptual Basis for Public Health Nursing Practice

The new millennium has brought forth countless predictions about the nature of tomorrow's health care delivery system. These scenarios range from visions of health care being delivered through primarily technological means as part of the many services provided by one of a few large health-related corporations to more humanistic portrayals of high-touch, community-based programs that reflect the unique nature of where people live and work. What is common to almost all scenarios is that they seem to ignore two very important factors: the changing social context worldwide and the ongoing role of government in the protection and assurance of the health of the public.

Clearly, it is difficult to predict what the world will be like over the next two to three decades; however, there are some crucial themes that will undoubtedly play major roles in shaping the health of all people. The first of these is globalization and the resulting interconnectedness of all people. Through increasingly interlaced economies, markets, and the media, it is now virtually impossible to remain unaffected by what is happening in other countries and cultures. In addition, travel, migration, and the forced movement of masses of people by political and natural disasters have mixed peoples together in ways never before seen. Communities based on shared culture and history are disappearing rapidly. The global disruption of people and communities, coupled with the rise in religious fundamentalism and nationalism worldwide, promises a highly unstable and challenging future for the health of all people.

Global changes of the magnitude described here place heavy burdens on individuals, communities, and governments. The United States is not immune to these changes and is already struggling to address these at all levels. Rising violence of all types and growing gang membership; increasing diversity in language, culture, and race; and growing separation between the rich and the poor are challenging every social institution and community. In the face of these enormous challenges, it is difficult to imagine any health care system without considering how governments at all levels will work to ensure that the health of the public is protected.

It is in the context of ensuring the health of the public that the future of public health nursing will emerge. We will now look at those key themes that are critical to the creation of the future roles of public health nurses and propose the application of a fundamental **conceptual model** in the development of future public health nursing interventions.

When one examines most every health systems scenario for the twenty-first century, there is an implicit assumption that the system of health care will be deeply embedded in the marketplace and governed by the principles of competition and a market economy. Often accompanying this assumption is the belief that the market has the ability in and of itself to deal with the problems of access and quality that plague our system. There is a view that the more troubling issues of equity and social justice—who receives care and in what ways—will be solved by letting the market do its work. As noted financier George Soros has observed, there are inherent dangers in this optimistic view of relying heavily on the marketplace to address these crucial issues (Soros, 1997). Our economy has as its fundamental purposes the creation of goods, services, and profit, based on willingness and ability to pay. Unfortunately, when health services become a commodity, not everyone can afford them or pay for them.

The reality that large sectors of the U.S. population are denied access to reasonable health care is not in the interest of these individuals, nor does it work to the benefit of the overall public. The failure or inability of the marketplace to address public health needs—whether in provision of health care, protection of the environment, or containing and preventing disease and injury—is where much of public health's future lies (O'Fallon, 2006). It is comforting to know that this mandate of acting in the overall interest of the public has been in existence for well over a century. The historic **Milbank Report** on Higher Education for Public Health offered a timeless definition of public health:

> Public health is the effort organized by society to protect, promote and restore the people's health. The programs, services, and institutions involved emphasize the prevention of disease and the health needs of the population as a whole. Public health activities change with changing technology and social values, but the goals remain the same: to reduce the amount of disease, premature death and the disease-produced discomfort and disability. (Milbank Memorial Fund Commission, 1976, p. 3)

The history of public health nursing clearly illustrates both the changing nature and timelessness of ensuring the health of the people. For more than 100 years, public health nurses have filed multiple roles and created an endless variety of strategies, interventions, and programs to fulfill their

Clara Barton founded the American Red Cross by convincing Congress to ratify the Treaty of Geneva, and was the driving force behind the creation of the Army Nurse Corps.

mission. It is in both the constancy of the mission and the flexibility of its means that public health nursing will find its future (Chaudry, 2008; Salmon, 1993).

What this means in practical terms is that public health nursing needs to clearly understand the effects of the changing society on health and the forces that are at work either enhancing or eroding the health of the people. To do so, public health nurses need an overall operating framework that encompasses public health values, health determinants, practice priorities, types of interventions, and an understanding of the interplay of these at all levels. The model presented in this chapter is **Construct for Public Health Nursing: A Framework for the Future** (White, 1982).

In 1982, the Construct for Public Health Nursing first appeared in *Nursing Outlook*. The purpose of the construct or model was to provide a systematic model through which public health nursing could be both understood and practiced. Since that time, the model has been incorporated into both education and practice through its adoption in curricula, incorporation in a variety of texts and articles, and extensive use in the creation of public health nursing programs at a variety of levels.

 THINK ABOUT THIS

Florence Nightingale referred to public health nurses as District Nurses, because they were responsible for districts or geographical areas in their responsibilities of caregiving in the community. She held fast that District Nurses must have one year of experience in hospital nursing (which is still a widely held belief today for community health nurses) and additional formal training as a District Nurse. The additional training included patient teaching, the care of houses, preventive care, and hygiene education. Nightingale (December 16, 1896) believed that District Nurses would be "a great civilizer of the poor, training as well as nursing them out of ill health into good health, out of drink into self control, but all without preaching, without patronizing—as friends, in sympathy."

*The scope of practice is an open-ended continuum extending from individuals through
such aggregates as groups, communities, entire populations to include the entire globe.

Construct for Public Health Nursing Model

*Source*: From *Nursing Outlook, Nov-Dec 1982*, "Construct for Public Health Nursing Model" by Maria Salmon White,
pages 30 & 527. Copyright Elsevier, 1982. Used by permission.

This model is particularly useful as public health nursing grapples with understanding and shaping the health of the public in the twenty-first century. The model itself is built on the premise that the fundamental difference between public health nursing and all other nursing rests in its commitment to the health of the public. This notion of the public good is understood to be both the ethical base for public health nursing practice and the consequences of fundamentally social and political processes. As a result, the model depicts a practice that is based on explicit valuing of the public good and a "form follows function" approach to actual interventions. The values of public health nursing are interlaced in the circular depiction of the public health nursing process: assessing, diagnosing, planning, implementing, and evaluating. In other words, each of those actions is based on the primacy of the public's health and good.

This notion of valuing the public's good does not sit easy with most health professionals, whose ethics are grounded in advocacy for individual patients. It is for this reason that the explicit delineation of public health values is critical to the successful future practice of public health nursing. Most of our health care system has been built on the notion of serving individuals—very little consideration has been given to the impact on the well-being of the public.

In the model, the health of the public is seen as being impacted by four determinants of health: social, human/biological, environmental, and medical/technological/organizational. The first three are fairly well understood—it is the fourth that continues to be less a part of most practitioner's concept of health determinants. Another way of describing these determinants is that they are *made up* of the technology, organization, and policies relating to healthcare delivery. It is the content and organization of health care itself. This determinant has shown itself to be an extremely important point of consideration during this last decade of "health care reform," which has focused entirely on this factor.

In understanding the determinants of health and their dynamics, public health nursing has the knowledge on which to target interventions. In other words, public health nursing practice is fundamentally focused on influencing determinants of health as the primary mechanism for enhancing and protecting the health of people.

The practice of public health nursing that is described in the model has three priorities: prevention, protection, and health promotion. Understood as somewhat overlapping concepts, each is given its own prominence because of the importance of considering all three in actual practice. These priorities serve to focus the ways in which public health nurses interface with health determinants. The message in all three of these priorities is that early intervention is always most desirable, with prevention being the primary goal.

When one considers the mandate of ensuring the health of the public, the nature of health determinants, and the utilitarian notion that the form of public health nursing is sharpened to fulfill its function, it becomes apparent that public health nursing practice can occur in a variety of contexts at many levels. The magnitude of public health nursing practice possibilities is depicted through a scope of practice that extends from the individual at one end to the world at another. Along this continuum sit families, groups, communities, populations, and geopolitical entities, such as towns, counties, states, and countries. This enormous scope of practice provides tremendous latitude and opportunity; it also presents great challenges to the field. The successful practice of public health nursing requires practitioners with a variety of knowledge and skills. The foundations of these skills are found in the core content of both nursing and public health.

The Construct for Public Health Nursing describes three categories of interventions: education, engineering, and enforcement. These general classifications are consistent with the notion that their content is shaped by the priorities for practice, the determinants of health to be targeted, and their "location" on the scope of practice. An educational intervention that is aimed at prevention of lead poisoning, for example, is quite different at an individual level than one aimed at a family, group, community, or group of legislators. So also would be engineering strategies, which would be designed to alter the environment in a manner that protects people. Some of these strategies might focus on retrofitting plumbing at a community level or working on a house-to-house basis to reduce the presence of lead-based paint. Engineering strategies also include those of a societal nature—changing the social environment to prevent exposures. Consider, for example, preventing crime through changing social factors in a community—increasing employment, developing neighborhood watch strategies, encouraging community policing, and so on. Last, enforcement strategies are aimed at putting into place mechanisms for "compelling" behavior that results in better health. Laws that require motorcycle helmets are one such example. Enforcement strategies can also be used on an individual level, such as individually observed therapy for high-risk patients with drug-resistant tuberculosis.

The underlying theme throughout this model is that actions are guided by commitment, context, clear priorities, public health values, flexibility, and the melding of nursing and public health knowledge and skills. This means that public health nursing is really a practice that is shaped by intent, not by convention. The intent, of course, is serving the public's health.

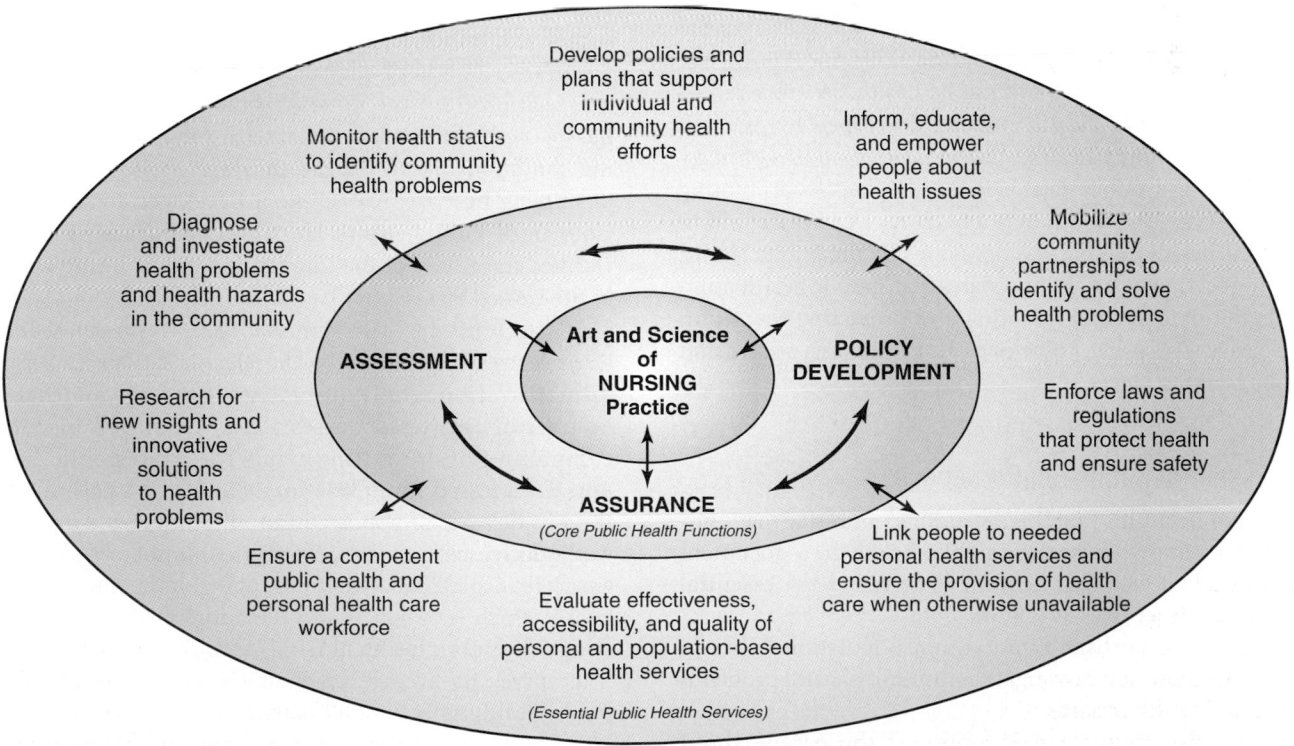

ASTDN Public Health Nursing Practice Model: Essential Public Health Services and Public Health Nursing, 1999

## ■ Definition and Development of Public Health Nursing

There are four organizations that work together to develop policy and practice-related guidelines for public health nursing. Those organizations, collectively called the *QUAD Council*, include the American Nurses Association's Council on Community, Primary, and Long-Term Care (ANA); the American Public Health Association's Public Health Nursing Section (APHA, PHN); the Association of State and Territorial Directors of Nursing (ASTDN); and the Association of Community Health Nurse Educators (ACHNE). In the 1990s, these four organizations came together to develop descriptions of the scope of practice for public health nursing that are reflective of the diversity of the roles across the country. One key element in the work of these groups is the fundamental understanding that what it takes to maintain the health of the public differs across life spans, across cultures, and across state and territorial boundaries. The process of public health nursing, however, combines the knowledge base of both public health and nursing to guide the intervention (see Appendix A and Chapter 1).

Many attempts have been made to clarify the definition between public health nursing and community health nursing. The most recently developed attempt is a white paper resulting from a national discussion on the differences between population-focused care (care aimed at improving health of the whole population), community-oriented care (care aimed at improving the health of a particular segment of the population), and community-centered care (care provided in a community setting). A 1986 definition of community health nursing developed by the ANA states that "Community health nursing practice promotes and preserves the health of populations by integrating skills and knowledge relevant to both nursing and public health." A 1995 definition of community health nursing developed by ACHNE stated: "Community health nursing is the synthesis of nursing theory and public health theory applied to promoting and preserving the health of populations." A 1996 definition of public health nursing was developed by the Public Health Nursing section of APHA and states that "public health nursing is the practice of promoting and protecting the health of populations using knowledge from nursing, social, and public health sciences."

## ■ Essential Public Health Services

A public health functions steering committee made additional attempts to describe public health in a document published in 1994. This document describes the **essential public health services** as follows:

- Monitor the health status of the population.
- Diagnose and investigate community health problems and health hazards.
- Inform, educate, and empower the people about health issues.
- Mobilize community partnerships to identify and solve health problems.
- Develop policies and plans that support individual and community health efforts.
- Enforce laws and regulations that protect health and ensure safety.
- Link people to needed personal health services.
- Ensure a competent public health and personal health care workforce.
- Evaluate effectiveness, accessibility, and quality of personal and population-based health services.
- Research for new insights and innovative solutions to health problems.

## ■ Activities for Essential Services

In an attempt to provide practice guidance to public health nurses in official governmental agencies, the directors of public health nursing throughout the country developed examples of nursing activities for each essential service (Table 37-1).

# Challenges and Issues for Public Health Nursing in the New Millennium

## ■ Impact of the Nursing Shortage on Public Health Nursing

Numerous nursing organizations and health care agencies have documented the existing nursing shortage throughout the United States. This shortage is predicted to continue and become more acute by the year 2010, when the nursing supply will no longer be able to meet the demand, regardless of distribution or educational preparation. Much of the information from the nursing profession on this shortage has focused on the institutional setting and associated working conditions. However, the shortage is affecting all areas of nursing practice. A document developed by the QUAD Council of Public Health Nursing Organizations in 2002, clarified the effects of the shortage on public health nursing in the United States.

Data from the 2000 National Sample Survey of Registered Nurses (conducted by the Health Resources Services Administration, Division of Nursing) indicate that the number of registered nurses (RNs) employed in public/community health settings with the title "public health nurse" decreased from 39% in 1980 to just 17.6% in 2000. Even in the overall public/community nursing group, there was a decrease of almost 16% in the number of nurses between 1996 and 2000. Finally, the aging of the nursing population, which is of concern to the entire profession, is more critical for public health nursing. According to data from the 2000 survey, the average age of all RNs is 45.2 years, while for public health nurses it is 49 years.

The impact of a shortage on public health nursing differs in a number of respects from that in other settings. For

**Table 37-1    ASTDN Public Health Nursing Practice Model:**
**Essential Public Health Services and Public Health Nursing, 1999**

| Essential Service | Public Health Nursing Activities | Example |
|---|---|---|
| ▪ Monitor health status | Community assessment | A public health nurse asked a civic group and local health providers to participate in a study of major risk factors for disability in their community. As a result, the community developed a walking trail and wrote a federal grant for a health center. |
| ▪ Diagnose health hazards | Disease case identification | Public health nurses provided tuberculosis skin testing to a plant's workers. As a result, two cases of tuberculosis were identified early and contacts were placed on preventive therapy. |
| ▪ Inform and educate public | Community education | Public health nurses provided classes to a local community group on prevention of disease transmission in daycare centers. |
| ▪ Mobilize community partnerships | Community organization | A public health nurse called a community meeting to discuss accident prevention. As a result of several meetings, the community raised funds for streetlights. |
| ▪ Develop policies | Advocate for funding | Public health nurses organized efforts to secure funding for a school nurse in a community with high teen pregnancy rates, high school dropout rates, and increased drug use among the teen population. |
| ▪ Enforce health regulations | Implementation of health regulations | After hearing a complaint from a member of the public about finding needles and syringes in a public garbage area behind a medical clinic, the public health nurse assessed the complainant for potential blood and body fluid exposure testing and contacted the appropriate authorities to work with the local clinic to develop proper disposal policies. |
| ▪ Link people to services | Provision of health services | In an undeserved area, public health nurses provide prenatal care to women and then refer them to a nearby physician for delivery. |
| ▪ Ensure competency | Participation in organized educational sessions | Public health nurses attend a workshop on a new treatment for HIV-infected individuals. |
| ▪ Evaluate effectiveness | Participation in research | Public health nurses collaborate with a local university on a study to determine the effectiveness of a new home visiting program for pre-term babies. |
| ▪ Research for new ideas | Implementation of new strategies | Public health nurses test a new health education model for reducing youth tobacco use. |

example, job vacancy rates are not an adequate indicator of the shortage in public health nursing because vacant positions are generally eliminated to cover local or state budget deficits or RN positions are converted to other types of positions. According to the Association of State and Territorial Directors of Nursing, 22 of the 36 member states have experienced these conversions. While other professionals in public health perform excellent jobs of connecting these individuals with community resources, they are not able to integrate the clinical status of the patient with their social needs—namely, the skill set of nurses. A better indicator of the shortage in public health nursing is the decreasing number of qualified applicants for vacant positions (resulting in agencies hiring people who are not qualified to do the job and trying to provide on-the-job training, or leaving positions open longer and, therefore, increasing the risk for elimination or transition to a position that does not require an RN). If the essential contributions that nursing can make to the health of a community are to continue, it is critical to have a public health nursing workforce that is educationally

prepared at the baccalaureate or higher degree level with a strong knowledge base and skills in public health nursing.

During 2003 and 2004, major professional organizations such as the American Nurses Association, the American Public Health Association, and the National Association of City and County Health Officials have passed policy statements reflecting their concern about a potential national shortage of public health nurses.

■ Further Development of Public Health Nursing Models and Competencies

The Council on Linkages between Academia and Public Health Practice (COL) developed a set of core competencies for public health professionals based on the Ten Essential Public Health Services framework in 2004. Recognizing the need for this work to become relevant for the specific specialty of public health nursing, the QUAD Council for Public Health Nursing Organizations initiated a national dialogue to explore nursing-specific application of the public health core competencies (QUAD Council of Public Health Nursing Organizations, 2004). The four national nursing organizations that addressed public health nursing issues included the Association of Community Health Nurse Educators (ACHNE), the American Nurses Association's Congress on Nursing Practice and Economics (ANA), the American Public Health Association–PHN Section (APHA), and the Association of State and Territorial Directors of Nursing (ASTDN).

In 2000, the QUAD Council began work on developing a set of national PHN competencies, culminating with the release of the ground-breaking document entitled "QUAD Council Public Health Nursing Competencies," published in the September–October 2004 issue of *Public Health Nursing*. These competencies complement the 1996 APHA definition of PHN practice and the 1999 Scope and Standards of Public Health Nursing Practice. Through this collaborative effort, the generalist level in public health nursing would reflect preparation at the baccalaureate level, public health practice would be population focused, and one of the unique contributions of public health nurses would be the ability to apply these principles at individual and family levels within the context of population-focused practice. See Appendix B for these public health core competencies.

By placing public health nursing in this context, many of the competency statements indicate a level of awareness, knowledge, and proficiency at the individual and family levels. QUAD Council Public Health Nursing Competencies includes the following domains:

Domain 1: Analytic Skills
Domain 2: Policy Development/Program Planning Skills
Domain 3: Communication Skills
Domain 4: Cultural Competency Skills and Cultural Dimensions of Practice Skills
Domain 5: Community Dimensions of Practice Skills
Domain 6: Basic Public Health Sciences Skills
Domain 7: Financial Planning and Management Skills
Domain 8: Leadership and Systems Thinking Skills

The Minnesota Department of Health, Center for Public Health Nursing, has developed a Public Health Interventions wheel to guide public health nursing practice based on the Ten Essential Public Health Services and related competencies. The Minnesota Model builds on a novice-to-expert population-focused nursing framework. A strong partnership between governmental public health and nursing education has encouraged incorporation of the model into public health nursing education as well.

## ■ National Public Health Performance Standards

A consortium of national public health organizations, under the leadership of the Centers for Disease Control and Prevention (CDC, 1998) recognized the need for a national set of performance standards for public health systems. Utilizing the Ten Essential Public Health Services as a framework, the National Public Health Performance Standards (NPHPS) provide guidance to state and local health Departments on self-assessment of system performance.

In many public health jurisdictions, public health nurses working on public health system quality improvement initiatives have embraced NPSHS standards. The most significant difference in the application of the standards and a more familiar model of health facility regulatory standards lies in the definition of the public health system. The NPHPS employ a broad definition of public health system partners (Bender, 2007).

## ■ Other Challenges for Public Health Nursing

During the first years of the new millennium, public health nurses were confronted with new technology, the re-emergence of "old" infectious diseases, bioterrorist threats to the public's health, and a larger population of people at risk. As a nation, we are faced with the growing problem of a "too little, too late" attitude about protecting the public's health through preventive measures. The health care system continues to focus on personal health care and expensive disease interventions, while public health resources for preventive health services declines. The value of prevention has long been recognized in economic as well as humanistic terms. Yet in the United States, less than 5% of the GNP is spent on preventive health services (Chattopadhyay & Carande-Kulis, 2004). Access to care continues to challenge our patient populations, requiring even more skills on the part of the public health nurse in the maze of managed care.

Public health nursing is destined to play a vital part in the evolution of the health care system as we continue in this new century. There are three major areas that will affect these changes: personal responsibility in health promotion and disease prevention, international health, and biological and chemical terrorism (Jakeway, LaRosa, Cary, & Schoenfisch, 2008). If the nation and the states are to adequately address the escalating costs of health care, the individual must be a key factor in the design of a new system of care. To this end, public health nurses are the best equipped to deal with these changes.

### 🖥 Research Alert

Collaboration with community partners and developing linkages with key stakeholders is included in the QUAD Council's Public Health Nursing Competencies and is an important aspect of the development of community health. Maltby's article describes a community–campus partnership between a school of nursing and the community that also included social work, physical therapy, and medical students. A shared learning experience was structured through the presentation of health fairs in collaboration with community agencies. An evaluation of the process, relationships, and outcomes of the health fairs demonstrated that the students attained beginning competencies in all public health nursing competency domains of the QUAD Council's Public Health Nursing Competencies.

*Source:* Maltby, H. (2006). Use of health fairs to develop public health nursing competencies. *Public Health Nursing, 23*(2), 183–189.

Adequate attention to the health and related socioeconomic problems in this country will require community level interest and intervention. The public health nurse will be called on to once again mobilize communities to meet the needs of their citizens for the improvement of society as a whole. In empowering the community to act, the public health nurse will be challenged to develop a greater understanding of the significant effect that culture has on the individual's response to health promotion, intervention, and education. The explosive population growth and the resultant migration of families will result in a variety of cultures to be served, even in rural communities.

The greatest number of elderly ever seen in this country will emerge as the typical patient as the baby-boomers reach retirement age. This phenomenon will occur as the workforce is getting smaller and more diversified, thereby creating a need to evaluate the role of the public health nurse. Health promotion and disease prevention activities will be primary among the services offered by the public health nurse. The created health care system will place greater emphasis on what public health nurses have known all along—that prevention is more cost-effective than technological intervention.

This millennium should be an exciting one for public health nurses. The challenges will be great, but the opportunity to practice traditional public health nursing will also be more available than it has been since its inception.

As public health nurses consider the future for their practice, there are a number of questions that surface over and over again. The framework provided by the Construct for Public Health Nursing is useful in helping public health nurses address these, given both the rapidity and magnitude of changes that we are encountering. *As clinical services seem to be moving out of health departments, what will public health nurses' role be in the future?* Clinical services should be understood as a strategy for providing needed services when they are otherwise not available. These services need to be seen as a way of ensuring health, not an end unto themselves. Public health nurses offer a tremendous breadth and depth of skills that are important to almost *any* public health intervention. When public health and public health nursing are understood through the frazmeworks of core functions and models like the Construct for Public Health Nursing, future roles are envisioned based on their utility, not their history.

*Is it possible to be a public health nurse in a managed care setting?* There is no question that the skills that public health nurses bring to managed care are extremely useful and needed, but the important distinction is the purposes for which these skills are used. The organizational values of public health and the mandate of ensuring the health of the public reside in the public sector; it is that sector alone that has this responsibility. Public health nurses can and do practice in a variety of settings, some of which focus on the health of populations. Their practice may be one of community health, but it lacks the essential public nature of public health.

*Should public health nurses practice in the private sector?* Having public health nurses practicing in the private sector benefits everyone. The skills certainly benefit patients, and

### Application to Practice

***Case Presentation:*** **Staphylococcus** *Food Poisoning in a University Cafeteria*

Stephanie is a 19-year-old white female who is a sophomore at a local university. She lives on campus in one of the dormitories. After dinner one evening, she became ill with nausea, vomiting, diarrhea, and abdominal cramps. Five other women who live in Stephanie's building became ill that same evening with similar symptoms. When others in the dorm became aware of the symptoms, most of the women thought that there was a gastrointestinal virus that was making the women ill. None of these six women became ill enough to seek medical attention.

That same evening Mary, a 20-year-old African American female who lives on campus in another dormitory, also became ill with nausea, vomiting, and severe abdominal cramps. Mary was not able to get the vomiting under control, so her roommate brought her to the local hospital emergency department. Mary was hospitalized and placed on replacement intravenous fluids and medication for nausea and diarrhea.

The hospital, which serves the university town, is relatively small, and the staff soon became aware that nine individuals—all students from the university—had been admitted with the same symptoms within a period of approximately 6 hours that evening. The hospital staff notified the campus clinic physician. He verified that he had treated eight students that same evening for nausea, vomiting, and abdominal cramps. He notified the local county health department that he suspected a food-borne illness outbreak. The public health nurses organized the follow-up of the problem utilizing the core functions of public health and the definition of public health nursing.

1. Discuss the activities that the public health nurse might conduct in this follow-up.
2. Identify the core functions and essential services that are described in this case.

## MEDIA MOMENT

*And the Band Played On* (1993)

Film, starring Matthew Modine as a doctor with the Centers for Disease Control and Prevention at the time when the first reports of a disease plaguing the gay community were heard. Modine and his colleagues embark on an investigation that resembles a compelling detective story as they try to track the source of the disease and discover a cure. Their efforts are thwarted by an ambivalent government and a turf war between French physicians and a celebrated American researcher (Alan Alda) who seems to place his own glory above the dead and the dying. The cast includes Richard Gere, Glenne Headly, Anjelica Huston, Steve Martin, Ian McKellen, Saul Rubinek, and Lily Tomlin.

*And the Band Played On* (1987)

Acclaimed book by Randy Shilts: As the first major book on AIDS, *San Francisco Chronicle* reporter Randy Shilts chronicled the making of one of the most devastating epidemics of the twentieth century. Shilts researched and reported the book exhaustively, chronicling almost day-by-day the first 5 years of AIDS. His work is critical of the medical and scientific communities' initial response, as well as the indifference of the mass media and country at large. The movie effectively captures Shilts book on film and marks the early struggles in this monumental epic, and the politics that all too effectively wiped out these victims of this devastating epidemic.

the overall values and commitments help pave the way for networking and partnerships between the public and private sectors. It is important for these individual nurses to understand that there are some critical differences between the public and private sectors in their values, priorities, and "bottom lines."

*What are the biggest challenges that public health nursing faces in the new decade?* Perhaps the most significant challenge facing public health nursing and public health in general is finding ways to address the broader issues of equity and social justice that are currently so much a part of the health "equation." As long as there are such huge inequities—disparities between the "haves" and "have nots"—the major health problems that we see today will only continue.

Public health nurses must now consider the public health threat of terrorism and how to best prepare communities for human-generated disasters, such as the World Trade Center attack; bioterrorism, such as anthrax and smallpox; and devastating natural disasters, such as Hurricane Katrina. As a society, we have learned that a healthy and well-prepared society can strengthen the entire country, in contrast to the unprecedented public health breakdown that occurred during Hurricane Katrina. Public health nurses must view their practice in global terms, going beyond the narrow boundaries of personal health services, if they are to truly enhance the health for all people.

## Conclusion

Shakespeare's *The Tempest* contains a sage observation: "The past is prologue. The future is yours and mine to dispatch." So it is with public health nursing. Our history is our prologue, our foundation. Our future is what we create within the framework of what we value, what we understand, what we know, and what we can do. When one considers the work of Lillian Wald, which included her own "hands-on" reaching out to destitute individuals and families and helping create the League of Nations and the United States Children's Bureau, it is clear that our foundation can provide us with the inspiration and wisdom that we need to move forward. There are no promises for public health nursing in the twenty-first century. There is only the ironic assurance that within the significant challenges that will confront societies around the world will be opportunities for public health nurses. The ways in which we define ourselves and our practice will either limit or enable our abilities to take hold of these opportunities. In the final analysis, public health nursing in the future will be what we make it.

Explore Community Health Nursing on the Web! To learn more about the topics in this chapter, use the passcode provided to access your exclusive website: **http://nursing.jbpub.com/ communityhealth.** If you do not have a passcode, you can obtain one at this site.

## ■ CRITICAL THINKING ACTIVITIES

1. What are the advantages of public health nurses working in the private health sector?
2. Compare the role of the public health nurse of today with that of public health nurses at the turn of the twentieth century. What are the challenges common to both roles?
3. Using the three priorities of prevention, protection, and health promotion identified by Dr. Salmon in her model Construct for Public Health Nursing, give examples from your own practice in community health nursing that illustrate these three priorities.

## ■ REFERENCES

Abrams, S. (2007). For the good of a common discipline. *Public Health Nursing, 24*(3), 293–297.

American Public Health Association (APHA). (1996, March). *The definition and role of public health nursing. A statement of the Public Health Nursing Section.* Washington, DC: Author.

Bender, K. (2007). Recommendations from the exploring accreditation for state and local health departments: Do we have the political will? *Public Health Nursing, 24*(5), 465–471.

Centers for Disease Control and Prevention (CDC). (1998). *National public health performance standards.* Atlanta, GA: Author. www.cdc.gov.

Chattopadhyay, S. K., & Carande-Kulis, V. G. (2004). Economics of prevention: The public health research agenda. *Journal of Public Health Management, 10*(5), 467–471.

Chaudry, R. (2008). The precautionary principle, public health, and public health nursing. *Public Health Nursing, 25*(3), 261–268.

Cohen, B., & Reutter, L. (2007, October). Development of the role of public health nurses in addressing child and family poverty: A framework for action. *Journal of Advanced Nursing, 60*(1), 96–107

Council on Linkages between Academia and Public Health Practice (COL). (2001). *Core competencies for public health practice.* Washington, DC: Author. www.trainingfinder.org.

Easley, C., & Allen, C. (2008). A critical intersection: Human rights, public health nursing, and nursing ethics. *Advances in Nursing Science, 30*(4), 367–382

Gebbie, K. M., & Turnock, B. J. (2006). The public health workforce, 2006: New challenges. *Health Affairs, 25*(4), 923–933.

Institute of Medicine (IOM). (1988). *The future of public health.* Washington, DC: National Academy Press.

Jakeway, C., LaRosa, G., Cary, A., & Schoenfisch, S. (2008). The role of public health nurses in emergency preparedness and response: A position paper of the Association of State and Territorial Directors of Nursing. *Public Health Nursing, 25*(4), 353–361.

Kulbok, P., & Reed, J. (2006, March). PHN Competencies. *Public Health Nursing, 23*(2), 97, 98.

Milbank Memorial Fund Commission. (1976). *Higher education for public health: A report.* New York: Prodist.

Mississippi Department of Archives. (1920–1980). *Correspondence, memoranda, and reports.* Mississippi Department of Health, Record Group 51, Public Health Nursing Division, Vol. 36. Jackson, MS: Author.

O'Fallon, L. (2006). Fostering the relationship between environmental health and nursing. *Public Health Nursing, 23*(5), 377, 380.

Polivka, B., Stanley, S., Gordon, D., Taulbee, K., Kieffer, G., & McCorkle, S. (2008). Public health nursing competencies for public health surge events. *Public Health Nursing, 25*(2), 159–165.

QUAD Council of Public Health Nursing Organizations. (2004). *Public health nursing competencies. Public Health Nursing, 21*(5), 443–452.

Salmon, M. F. (1993). Public health nursing: The opportunity of a lifetime. *American Journal of Public Health, 83*(1), 674–675.

Soros, G. (1997). The capitalist threat. *The Atlantic Monthly, 279*(2), 45–58.

White, M. S. (1982, November–December). Construct for public health nursing. *Nursing Outlook, 30,* 527.

## Ⅲ APPENDIX

# QUAD Council's PHN Competencies (April 3, 2003)

http://www.astdn.org/downloadablefiles/PHN%20competencies%20final%20comb.pdf

http://www.astdn.org/publications.htm

The QUAD Council of Public Health Nursing Organizations is an alliance of the four national nursing organizations that address public health nursing issues: the Association of Community Health Nurse Educators (ACHNE), the American Nurses Association's Congress on Nursing Practice and Economics (ANA), the American Public Health Association–Public Health Nursing Section (APHA), and the Association of State and Territorial Directors of Nursing (ASTDN; http//www.astdn.org/publications.htm). In 2000, prompted in part by work on educating the public health workforce being done under the leadership of the Centers for Disease Control (CDC), the QUAD Council began work on drafting a set of national public health nursing competencies.

The approach utilized by the QUAD Council was to start with the Council on Linkages between Academia and Public Health Practice's (COL's) "Core Competencies for Public Health Professionals" and to determine their application to two levels of public health nursing practice: the staff nurse/generalist role and the manager/specialist/consultant role. It was the QUAD Council's intent to examine these COL competencies for their fit with public health nursing and to continue to identify and refine unique competencies for public health nursing. By selecting the COL competencies as the framework, the QUAD Council felt that the competencies could provide a guide for agencies that employ public health nurses and academic settings to facilitate education, orientation, training, and lifelong learning using an interdisciplinary model where appropriate.

The COL list of core competencies "represents ten years of work on this subject" by the 15 member organizations whose missions include improving public health education and practice. More than 1,000 public health professionals reviewed the list during a public comment period. "The Council utilized several mechanisms to receive feedback from reviewers, including e-mail, focus groups, sessions at various conferences, and the competencies website. The comments from public health professionals in a broad array of disciplines and practice settings led to this consensus set of core competencies for guiding public health workforce development efforts. . . The core competencies represent a set of skills, knowledge, and attitudes necessary for the broad practice of public health. They transcend the boundaries of the specific disciplines within public health and help to unify the profession" (www.trainingfinder.org/competencies). The actual competency statements are the "property" of the COL and could not be modified by public health nursing or the QUAD Council during the process of looking at applicability to public health nursing practice. The QUAD Council's focus was on how public health nurses apply those competencies and the expected level of performance for each competency statement.

Nursing-specific application of the competencies is necessary for specialized roles within public health nursing, and the COL's competencies have been used as the framework to develop them. However, because the COL's list captures only the cross-cutting competencies for all public health professionals, it does not contain competencies that are specific to public health *nursing*. Given that the COL's competencies are for all public health professionals, even this public health nursing-specific draft does not include nursing competencies that are broader than public health (i.e., that apply to many or all nurses).

The "QUAD Council's PHN Competencies" document is designed for use with other documents. It complements the "Definition of Public Health Nursing" adopted by the APHA's Public Health Nursing Section in 1996 and *Scope and Standards of Public Health Nursing* (QUAD Council, 1999). Differentiating PHN competencies at the generalist and specialist levels will help to clarify the PHN specialty for both the discipline of nursing and the profession of public health. In addition, the ability to identify PHN competencies should facilitate collaboration among public health nurses and other public health professionals in education, practice, and research so as to improve the public's health.

In developing the competencies, the QUAD Council members concurred that the generalist level would reflect preparation at the baccalaureate level. While recognizing that in many states much of the public health nursing workforce is not baccalaureate-prepared, the QUAD Council believes that those nurses may require job descriptions that reflect a different level of practice and/or may require extensive orientation and education to achieve the competencies identified herein. Further, the specialist-level competencies described in this document reflect preparation at the master's level in community/public health nursing and/or public health. Again, while recognizing that there may be other public health nurses who are promoted or appointed to managerial or consultant positions that require specialist competencies, master's-level education prepares public health nurses for the specialist-level competencies identified in this document. At both levels, it is expected that a major focus of on-the-job training and continuing education for nurses hired for these positions who have less than a baccalaureate or master's degree (as appropriate to the level) will be on ensuring that these competencies are attained.

The QUAD Council determined that, although the COL competencies were developed with the understanding that both public health practice and public health nursing are population focused, one of the unique contributions of public health nurses is the ability to apply these principles at individual and family levels *within the context of population-focused practice*. Therefore, many of the competency statements indicate a level of awareness, knowledge, or proficiency at the individual/family level. Because of their population or system-focused language, however, it was decided that several specific competency statements and three entire domains would not include application at the individual/family level: "Domain 5—community dimensions of practice skills," "Domain 7—financial planning and management skills," and "Domain 8—leadership and systems thinking skills." Finally, it was recognized that "groups" are entities that can be addressed at the individual/family level and at the population/system level. Therefore, when PHNs use the group format primarily to convey information targeted to individual or family approaches to health issues (e.g., a group format is used to teach newly diagnosed diabetics about the importance of diet and exercise, but the information targets individuals), this represents an application at the individual/family level.

Finally, the QUAD Council based this document on the following additional assumptions:

- Public health nurses must first possess the competencies common to all baccalaureate-prepared nurses (not addressed in this competency list) and then demonstrate these additional competencies specific to their roles in public health.
- The progression from awareness to knowledge to proficiency is a continuum, and there are no discrete boundaries between those levels of competence (definitions of each of these three levels appear at the bottom of each page of the competencies list).
- Both levels reflect competencies for a reasonably prudent PHN who has experience in the role (i.e., not a "novice" and not in a specialized or limited focus role).
- These competencies are intended to reflect the standard for public health nursing practice, not necessarily what is occurring in practice today.
- In any practice setting, the job descriptions may reflect components from each level, depending on the agency's structure, size, leadership, and services.

In preparing this document, the QUAD Council sought feedback on a draft of these competencies from nurses across the country who are members of one or more of its member organizations; more than 220 nurses, most of whom are directly involved in public health practice, provided specific comments on the draft. The QUAD Council is grateful to all those public health nurses who took the time to review the draft and provide thoughtful comments. Their feedback was carefully considered in developing this final document.

## Public Health Nursing Competencies (April 2003)

| | Generalist/Staff PHN | | Manager/CNS/Consultant/ Program Specialist/Executive | |
|---|---|---|---|---|
| | Individuals and Families | Populations/ Systems | Individuals and Families | Populations/ Systems |
| **Domain 1: Analytic Assessment Skills** | | | | |
| 1. Defines a problem | Proficiency | Knowledge | Proficiency | Proficiency |
| 2. Determines appropriate uses and limitations of both quantitative and qualitative data | Knowledge | Awareness | Proficiency | Proficiency |
| 3. Selects and defines variables relevant to defined public health problems | Knowledge | Knowledge | Proficiency | Proficiency |
| 4. Identifies relevant and appropriate data and information sources | Proficiency | Knowledge | Proficiency | Proficiency |
| 5. Evaluates the integrity and comparability of data and identifies gaps in data sources | Knowledge | Awareness | Proficiency | Proficiency |
| 6. Applies ethical principles to the collection, maintenance, use, and dissemination of data and information | Proficiency | Knowledge | Proficiency | Proficiency |
| 7. Partners with communities to attach meaning to collected quantitative and qualitative data | N/A* | Knowledge | N/A* | Proficiency |
| 8. Makes relevant inferences from quantitative and qualitative data | Knowledge | Awareness | Proficiency | Proficiency |
| 9. Obtains and interprets information regarding risks and benefits to the community | Knowledge | Knowledge | Proficiency | Proficiency |
| 10. Applies data collection processes, information technology applications, and computer systems storage/retrieval strategies | Knowledge | Awareness | Proficiency | Proficiency |
| 11. Recognizes how the data illuminates ethical, political, scientific, economic, and overall public health issues | Knowledge | Awareness | Proficiency | Proficiency |
| **Domain 2: Policy Development/Program Planning Skills** | | | | |
| 1. Collects, summarizes, and interprets information relevant to an issue | Knowledge | Awareness | Proficiency | Proficiency |
| 2. States policy options and writes clear and concise policy statements | Awareness | Awareness | Proficiency | Proficiency |
| 3. Identifies, interprets, and implements public health laws, regulations, and policies related to specific programs | Knowledge | Knowledge | Proficiency | Proficiency |
| 4. Articulates the health, fiscal, administrative, legal, social, and political implications of each policy option | Awareness | Awareness | Proficiency | Proficiency |
| 5. States the feasibility and expected outcomes of each policy option | Awareness | Awareness | Proficiency | Proficiency |
| 6. Utilizes current techniques in decision analysis and health planning | Knowledge | Awareness | Proficiency | Proficiency |
| 7. Decides on the appropriate course of action | Knowledge | Awareness | Proficiency | Proficiency |
| 8. Develops a plan to implement policy, including goals, outcome and process objectives, and implementation steps | Knowledge | Awareness | Proficiency | Proficiency |
| 9. Translates policy into organizational plans, structures, and programs | N/A* | Awareness | N/A* | Proficiency |
| 10. Prepares and implements emergency response plans | Knowledge | Knowledge | Proficiency | Proficiency |
| 11. Develops mechanisms to monitor and evaluate programs for their effectiveness and quality | Knowledge | Knowledge | Proficiency | Proficiency |
| **Domain 3: Communication Skills** | | | | |
| 1. Communicates effectively both in writing and orally, or in other ways | Proficiency | Knowledge | Proficiency | Proficiency |
| 2. Solicits input from individuals and organizations | Proficiency | Knowledge | Proficiency | Proficiency |
| 3. Advocates for public health programs and resources | Proficiency | Knowledge | Proficiency | Proficiency |
| 4. Leads and participates in groups to address specific issues | Proficiency | Knowledge | Proficiency | Proficiency |
| 5. Uses the media, advanced technologies, and community networks to communicate information | Knowledge | Awareness | Knowledge† | Knowledge† |
| 6. Effectively presents accurate demographic, statistical, programmatic, and scientific information for professional and lay audiences | Knowledge | Knowledge | Proficiency | Proficiency |
| 7. Attitudes: Listens to others in an unbiased manner, respects points of view of others, and promotes the expression of diverse opinions and perspectives | Proficiency | Proficiency | Proficiency | Proficiency |

*(continues)*

Public Health Nursing Competencies (April 2003)—Continued

| | Generalist/Staff PHN | | Manager/CNS/Consultant/Program Specialist/Executive | |
| --- | --- | --- | --- | --- |
| | Individuals and Families | Populations/Systems | Individuals and Families | Populations/Systems |
| **Domain 4: Cultural Competency Skills** | | | | |
| 1. Utilizes appropriate methods for interacting sensitively, effectively, and professionally with persons from diverse cultural, socioeconomic, educational, racial, ethnic and professional backgrounds, and persons of all ages and lifestyle preferences | Proficiency | Proficiency | Proficiency | Proficiency |
| 2. Identifies the role of cultural, social, and behavioral factors in determining the delivery of public health services | Knowledge | Knowledge | Proficiency | Proficiency |
| 3. Develops and adapts approaches to problems that take into account cultural differences | Proficiency | Knowledge | Proficiency | Proficiency |
| 4. Attitudes: Understands the dynamic forces contributing to cultural diversity | N/A* | Knowledge | N/A* | Proficiency |
| 5. Attitudes: Understands the importance of a diverse public health workforce | N/A* | Knowledge | N/A* | Proficiency |
| **Domain 5: Community Dimensions of Practice Skills** | | | | |
| 1. Establishes and maintains linkages with key stakeholders | | Knowledge | | Proficiency |
| 2. Utilizes leadership, team building, negotiation, and conflict resolution skills to build community partnerships | | Knowledge | | Proficiency |
| 3. Collaborates with community partners to promote the health of the population | | Knowledge | | Proficiency |
| 4. Identifies how public and private organizations operate within a community | | Knowledge | | Proficiency |
| 5. Accomplishes effective community engagements | | Knowledge | | Proficiency |
| 6. Identifies community assets and available resources | | Knowledge | | Proficiency |
| 7. Develops, implements, and evaluates a community public health assessment | | Knowledge | | Proficiency |
| 8. Describes the role of government in the delivery of community health services | | Knowledge | | Proficiency |
| **Domain 6: Basic Public Health Sciences Skills** | | | | |
| 1. Identifies the individual's and organization's responsibilities within the context of the essential public health services and core functions | Knowledge | Knowledge | Proficiency | Proficiency |
| 2. Defines, assesses, and understands the health status of populations, determinants of health and illness, factors contributing to health promotion and disease prevention, and factors influencing the use of health services | Knowledge | Knowledge | Proficiency | Proficiency |
| 3. Understands the historical development, structure, and interaction of public health and health | Knowledge | Knowledge | Proficiency | Proficiency |
| 4. Identifies and applies basic research methods used in public health | Awareness | Awareness | Knowledge | Knowledge |
| 5. Applies the basic public health sciences, including behavioral and social sciences, biostatistics, epidemiology, environmental public health, and prevention of chronic and infectious diseases and injuries | Awareness | Awareness | Knowledge | Knowledge |
| 6. Identifies and retrieves current relevant scientific evidence | Knowledge | Knowledge | Proficiency | Proficiency |
| 7. Identifies the limitations of research and the importance of observations and interrelationships | Awareness | Awareness | Knowledge | Knowledge |
| 8. Attitudes: Develops a lifelong commitment to rigorous critical thinking | Proficiency | Proficiency | Proficiency | Proficiency |

## Public Health Nursing Competencies (April 2003)—Continued

| | Generalist/Staff PHN | | Manager/CNS/Consultant/Program Specialist/Executive | |
|---|---|---|---|---|
| | Individuals and Families | Populations/ Systems | Individuals and Families | Populations/ Systems |
| **Domain 7: Financial Planning and Management Skills** | | | | |
| 1.  Develops and presents a budget | | Awareness | | Proficiency |
| 2.  Manages programs within budget constraints | | Knowledge | | Proficiency |
| 3.  Applies budget processes | | Awareness | | Proficiency |
| 4.  Develops strategies for determining budget priorities | | Awareness | | Proficiency |
| 5.  Monitors program performance | | Knowledge | | Proficiency |
| 6.  Prepares proposals for funding from external sources | | Awareness | | Proficiency |
| 7.  Applies basic human relations skills to the management of organizations, motivation of personnel, and resolution of conflicts | | Knowledge | | Proficiency |
| 8.  Manages information systems for collection, retrieval, and use of data for decision making | | Awareness | | Proficiency |
| 9.  Negotiates and develops contracts and other documents for the provision of population-based services | | Awareness | | Proficiency |
| 10.  Conducts cost-effectiveness, cost–benefit, and cost utility analyses | | Awareness | | Proficiency |
| **Domain 8: Leadership and Systems Thinking Skills** | | | | |
| 1.  Creates a culture of ethical standards within organizations and communities | | Knowledge | | Proficiency |
| 2.  Helps create key values and shared vision and uses these principles to guide action | | Knowledge | | Proficiency |
| 3.  Identifies internal and external issues that may affect delivery of essential public health services (i.e., strategic planning) | | Knowledge | | Proficiency |
| 4.  Facilitates collaboration with internal and external groups to ensure participation of key stakeholders | | Knowledge | | Proficiency |
| 5.  Promotes team and organizational learning | | Knowledge | | Proficiency |
| 6.  Contributes to development, implementation, and monitoring of organizational performance standards | | Knowledge | | Proficiency |
| 7.  Uses the legal and political system to effect change | | Knowledge | | Proficiency |
| 8.  Applies theory of organizational structures to professional practice | | Awareness | | Proficiency |

**Definitions:**
Awareness: Basic level of mastery of the competency. Individuals may be able to identify the concept or skill but have limited ability to perform the skill.
Knowledge: Intermediate level of mastery of the competency. Individuals are able to apply and describe the skill.
Proficiency: Advanced level of mastery of the competency. Individuals are able to synthesize, critique or teach the skill.
* These competencies, because of their population- or system-focused language, do not apply at the individual/family level, but are applicable to the broader context of population-focused public health services and systems.
† Reflects ability to determine need for and to utilize experts in these areas.

Source of competencies: Core Competencies for Public Health Professionals, a project of the Council on Linkages Between Academia and Public Health Practice funded by the Health Resources and Services Administration.

# CHAPTER 38
# The Home Visit

Karen Saucier Lundy

Visit **http://nursing.jbpub.com/communityhealth** for interactive exercises, review questions, Web links, and more.

Home health nurses can assess the patient's living environment and set realistic health goals with the patient.

And though home is a name, a word, it is a strong one; stronger than magician ever spoke, or spirit answered to, in strongest conjuration. . . . When I speak of home, I speak of the place where—in default of a better—those I love are gathered together; and if that place were a gypsy's tent, or a barn, I should call it by the same good name notwithstanding.

—*Charles Dickens*

No matter how dreary and gray our homes are, we people of flesh and blood would rather live there than in any other county, be it ever so beautiful. There is no place like home.

—*L. Frank Baum, The Wizard of Oz*

Where thou art, that is home.

—*Emily Dickinson*

Home is where the heart is.

—*Pliny the Elder*

The heart is where the home is.

—*Kenneth Keniston*

Hospitals are an intermediate stage of civilization. While devoting my life to hospital work I have come to the conclusion that hospitals are not the best place for the poor sick except for surgical cases.

—*Florence Nightingale, 1860*

The home was the earliest setting for nursing care. In today's society, most of us expect to go away from home to receive health care. What is your idea of home? Have you ever been on a home visit for providing health care? Think about how you might feel as a patient receiving a home visit from a nurse.

## CHAPTER FOCUS

The Home Visiting Process

Advantages of Home Visits

Effectiveness of Home Visits

Challenges of Home Visits

Distractions in the Home Environment

## QUESTIONS TO CONSIDER

After reading this chapter, you will know the answers to the following questions:

1. What is a home health visit?
2. How is a home visit conducted?

3. What are the stages of a home visit?
4. What are the advantages and challenges of a home visit?
5. How effective are home visits in improving health for populations?

## KEY TERMS

Behavioral distractions    Environmental distractions    Nurse-initiated distractions    Visiting nurse

The acceleration of home health nursing came during the 1960s, when Medicare approved home health visits for reimbursement.

SINCE THE BEGINNING OF TIME, humans have cared for their own at home, both in sickness and in health. Historically, homes were the earliest practice settings for nurses who worked in the community. Patients were seldom in hospitals, but rather recovered from illness at home and learned about disease prevention and treatment at home; as always, nurses reached out to them through the home visit. During the latter part of the nineteenth century and throughout the twentieth century, community health nurses always had the home as a common setting for practice. As hospitals became more accessible and technology advanced, roles for nurses in the community became more specialized. One specialized role that emerged was that of the visiting nurse, organized by visiting nurse associations that were funded by philanthropic donations (Howse, 2007).

The evolution of home care in the United States resulted from social, economic, technological, demographic, and political forces that continue to shape our health care delivery system (NAHC, 2006). By the end of World War II, the physician shortage and the continued explosion of medical technology in the hospital moved many physicians into hospitals, and physician home visiting became a thing of the past (Hafkenschiel, 1990). By the early 1960s, home care was primarily provided by public health and visiting nurses, who assessed patients, provided the necessary services, and managed the therapeutic plan of care. Public health nurses focused on prevention and education; visiting nurses provided sick care in the home. By 1963, according to the National Association for Home Care (NAHC, 2006), the number of home health agencies, primarily private philanthropic organizations, had grown to 1,100. The services they provided involved a variety of professional disciplines, including skilled nursing.

Nurses who make home visits today are employed by a variety of agencies, and their roles can encompass elements of both the **visiting nurse** (sickness care) and the public health nurse (health promotion, case finding, disease prevention,

and education). However, in the current reimbursement-driven health care system, most nurses who visit patients at home tend to specialize in home health services, with an emphasis on illness care and posthospital follow-up, or public health services, which deliver care in the home and health education. With the increase in outpatient surgeries, prevention, chemotherapy, and other services previously done on an inpatient basis, follow-up care at home will continue to be even more critical in a managed care environment. The role of the home care nurse is increasingly more important as a specialty within community-based health care.

Home health nurses may be employed by home health agencies, hospices, hospitals, public health departments, or clinics. Public health nurses may see patients at home through the auspices of the state health department, a local hospital, or a rural clinic. In this chapter, the home visit as a practice environment is described in the context of the emerging community-based health care system. Home health nursing and hospice as specialties in community-based care will follow in Chapter 39.

## The Home Visiting Process

One simply has to look around any local hospital to see that it would seem to be much more efficient for patients to come to the nurse and other health care providers, where resources are plentiful. Certainly, one of the primary reasons that hospitals were first developed in the Middle Ages was so that caregivers could see more patients and observe them throughout the day and night. Yet there are very good reasons for seeing patients in their own homes. Box 38-1 lists common purposes of home visiting; Box 38-2 details the stages of the home visit, with information about the sequential steps in the home visiting process; and Box 38-3 provides information about differences between the home setting and the acute care setting. Box 38-4 provides hints on communicating effectively in the home setting.

❝*Example isn't another way to teach. It is the only way to teach.*❞

—Albert Einstein

## MEDIA MOMENT

### *Magnolia* (1999)

This movie follows the lives of several people, both family and caregivers, in one day. Through a series of interlocking comedic and poignant episodes, human relationships and their complexities play out on a one random day in Los Angeles. The lives of these people are linked by blood, coincidence, and the way in which their lives seem parallel. Themes emerge—the death of a father, resentment and unresolved conflicts of the children, the failure of expectations, and the way all plans and ambitions can be undermined by sudden events. Phillip Seymour Hoffman plays a major character in the movie as the compassionate, skilled, and devoted nurse for the dying father.

Jessica Winter, film critic of the *Village Voice*, provides a poignant description of the nurse in *Magnolia* played by Hoffman:

> Hoffman delivered one of his most indelible performances, as the empathic nurse who eases the passing of

Jason Robards's agonized patriarch as would a guardian angel. "That's the guy's life and that's his job, and my point was, that doesn't make it any easier," Hoffman says. "He has a strong understanding of the importance of helping someone die, even though he knows that every time he goes through it, it's going to be painful."

Film critic Richard Propes writes 5 years after seeing *Magnolia*:

> There is no film . . . EVER . . . that has made me think and made me feel and made me question like *Magnolia*. It made me laugh and cry and squirm and giggle with nervous laughter. Yet, I can't deny that five years later my life is changed because I've seen *Magnolia*. I sit here at my computer getting goosebumps at the tenderness of Phillip Seymour Hoffman. . . .

---

### BOX 38-1

**Purposes of Home Visits**

**Casefinding**
- Public health and protection
- Abuse, neglect cases
- Communicable disease
- School-related health conditions

**Illness Prevention and Health Promotion**
- Prenatal and well-baby care
- Child development
- Elder care

**Care of the Sick and Terminally Ill**
- Home health
- Hospice

## Advantages of Home Visits

Community health nursing is holistic. Seeing patients in the artificial and controlled environment of a hospital reveals little to the nurse about the family's health influences and ability to carry out the plan of care (Persily, 2003). In the home, the nurse gets the complete picture, including environmental factors that affect health, social and psychological influences, relationships between and among family members, and the interaction of the patient with family and social networks. In a hospital, patients are separated from the context of their everyday lives: Health care providers control their every movement (including self-regulated body func-

Home health visits take an average of 45 to 60 minutes to complete.

tions), they wear institutional clothes, and care is organized around physician and nurse schedules. Such separation of patients from the context of their lives makes it easier for nurses in the hospital to focus only on the biomedical aspects of disease (Liaschenko, 1994; Williams, 2004).

This is not the case in the home, where illness is but one aspect of the totality of the patient's living experience (Coffman, 1997; Williams, 2004). Hazards and resources are

## BOX 38-2

### From Beginning to End . . . Selecting a Successful Home Visit

#### Previsit / Planning Stage

- Determine which patients need to be seen.
- Prioritize the scheduled visits based on patient need, distance between visits, laboratory work, and coordination with other professionals and physician.
- Review the chart, orders, patient diagnosis, goals of care, and reasons for the home visit.
- Telephone the patient for validation of scheduled visit; ask patient about specific needs, such as supplies, and any special hazards, such as pets or environmental concerns; caregiver schedule.
- Secure directions to the home.
- Conduct inventory of bag, needed equipment and supplies for patients, and educational materials.
- Review safety considerations, such as timing of visit, environmental assessment.

#### Implementing the Visit

- Initiate the visit: introduction and identification of nurse to patient, brief social phase to establish rapport.
- Practice appropriate hygienic practices before patient assessment.
- Review plans for visit with patient.
- Determine expectations of patient regarding home visits.
- Conduct assessment: environment, patient, medication, nutrition, functional abilities and limitations, psychosocial issues, and evaluation of previous visit intervention effectiveness.
- Modify the plan of care based on patient need and situational dictates.
- Perform nursing interventions.
- Deal with distractions: environmental, behavioral, and nurse initiated.

#### Evaluating the Visit

- Evaluate effectiveness of interventions based on established short-term (response during visit) and long-term outcome criteria (effects of intervention at subsequent visits or other patient contact).
- Evaluate as to primary, secondary, tertiary interventions.
- Evaluate conduct of visit: availability of appropriate supplies, preparation of nurse for visit.

#### Documentation

- Document based on established outcome criteria and agency requirements.
- Validate diagnoses and additional health needs based on visit.
- Evaluate goals and objectives.
- Review actions taken, response of patient, and outcome of interventions (short and long term).
- Record both objective (nurse-based) and subjective (patient-based) data.
- As appropriate, use federal agency reimbursement guidelines, such as Medicare, for progress documentation and certification/recertification requirements.

#### Termination

- Termination begins with the first visit as nurse prepares the patient for time-limited nature of home visiting.
- Review goal attainment with patient/family and make recommendations and referrals as necessary for continued health care issues.
- Develop strategies for appropriate closure with patients who die, refuse visits, or are terminated because of nonreimburseable services.

## BOX 38-3

### Challenges in Home Settings

*Control belongs to the patient* because care is being provided in his/her home.

*A feeling of isolation and lack of support* often results from the nature of the home setting. There are no nurses or other team members in the next room to confirm an assessment or to distinguish an abnormal finding.

*The home environment and family support system* are unpredictable and not always conducive to optimal care.

*Dealing with multiproblem families* is difficult emotionally for the nurse, especially in the home setting where family dynamics and interactions are more intense and visible.

*Difficulty in communicating with the various team members* can be a stressor.

*The volume of documentation* required can be difficult as a result of the variety and demands of various funding sources and standards.

*Frustrations with the system* are a common concern. There is often difficulty explaining Medicare or Medicaid's ever-changing requirements to patients and families, as well as to other providers.

*Complex case loads* that encompass all age groups with diverse problems are common in home care. The skills and knowledge required are broad, requiring the nurse to become a strong generalist.

*Concern for personal safety* is an issue, because violence has increased in all delivery settings.

**BOX 38-4**

**Secrets of Professional Conversation: The Home Visit**

1. *Break the ice with a warm topic.* Try opening with a cliché such as the weather, pets, sports, children, yard flowers, garden, or any subject that interests *most* people. This often establishes a conversational bond that helps make the transition to other more sensitive topics easier. Example: "How has all this rain lately affected your garden?" or while pointing to pictures in home, ask "Are these your children?"

2. *If you are extremely uncomfortable or have a sense of un-identified anxiety, explore possible source with the patient.* Often, nurses can sense nonverbal conflict in the home, with the patient, or with the family. By acknowledging that this is valuable information can be elicited from the patient. Example: "Things seem a little unsettled today. Do you want to talk about anything before we get started with your assessment?"

3. *Pick up the pace by asking open-ended questions.* This forces discussion because questions can't be answered with a simple yes or no. Answers will be longer so you will be able to notice other things that are being said to keep the conversation going. Example: "Why do you like living out in the country? What do you think about the new road going through town? What if . . .?"

4. *Show sincere interest.* Listening is a skill that must be practiced daily. This means make good eye contact. When the patient is speaking, our tendency is to spend that time planning what we will say next. This is not only discourteous and nontherapeutic, but also causes us to miss important information. Flatter your patient/family with sincere comments: All people crave appreciation. Make sure you *individualize* compliments with details, such as commenting on how much more energetic your patient is or noting that a young mother is attending to her new baby's cries very well. Listening is an excellent way to demonstrate your respect for your patient! Example: Instead of rehearsing your next line, focus on your *genuine* response to what he/she is saying. Challenge yourself to come up with questions about the points the person has raised.

5. *Develop a broad outlook.* Avoid using the word *I* too often. Watch the great conversationalists— Oprah Winfrey, Jane Pauley, Barbara Walters, Katie Couric, or Larry King—they seldom mention themselves, know a little bit about a lot of subjects, and demonstrate a curiosity about a broad range of topics. Example: Read the local newspaper daily and try to listen to at least one news show every other day. This ensures that you will expand your consciousness about community and national issues that concern your patients. Read a variety of opinions about a wide range of issues. Challenge yourself to think about things in new ways.

6. *Avoid judging others in advance (i.e., "prejudice").* Try to suspend judgment about your patient. Coming to conclusions about people before you have even entered their homes, based on what you have read in their chart or know about their income, shuts down your curiosity and prevents you from learning what you need to know about their health status. Example: In a home visit with a new mother who consistently misses clinic appointments, keep an open mind and ask her about other aspects of her life. Listen to her accounts of how her life has changed since giving birth.

7. *Quote your patient when possible.* A very flattering and confirming strategy to promote your patient's self-confidence is to use actual quotes from previous conversations (either from the same visit or previous visits, which means you have to really listen!) to illustrate health information. Example: "Since you mentioned last visit that you felt a 'bit better when I am able to cook my own breakfast,' I think that taking care of yourself as much as possible really makes a difference."

8. *End a conversation gracefully.* Breaking away from a conversation in the home can often be more difficult than starting one. After we "connect" with someone, most of us are hesitant to interrupt when you need to move on to other topics or to end the visit. The reality is that there will eventually come a point in any conversation when you will have to end it. Prepare when you enter the home to end the conversation. Example: Prepare an exit early on in a polite and friendly way. "I have so enjoyed our visit, but I must get going in order to see my other patients," or, "I see from the clock that it is near lunch and I know you must be hungry."

*Source*: Adapted from King, L. (1994). *How to talk to anyone, anytime, anywhere: The secrets of good conversation*. New York: Crown.

quickly evident and allow a more realistic plan of care to be established, which promotes the achievement of mutually set health strategies and goals. In addition, on a home visit, the nurse can see firsthand how well the patient can perform self-care and can make a more accurate evaluation of medical and nursing interventions. Such information can provide the nurse with valuable indicators in the evaluation of the effects of therapeutic interventions, as compared with the limited time and artificial constraints of the clinic or hospital environment (Liepert, 1996).

There are distinct advantages to the patient when care is provided in the home. For example, rather than having to obtain transportation to a health care facility, a home visit may

> **"** *Besides nursing the patient, she shows them in their own homes how they can call in official sanitary help to make their own poor room healthy, how they can improve appliances, how their homes may not be broken up.* **"**
>
> *—Florence Nightingale, 1890*

be a more appropriate way to reach a patient. Transportation can be an obstacle for many patients, including those who do not have access to a private car or mass transit, are unable to drive, or are confined to their homes, especially those who live in rural areas. Another advantage is that patients are able to exercise more autonomy on their own turf, which allows

**Home Call: Mother and Child**
There's so little here: one table,
not laden, one blind
shut. One bulb
hung straight down. One woman,
not well (that look
of someone who won't talk
because they've been beaten
so the bruises don't show), and one
boy, dancing over, no
diaper, eager for the coin
of candy you lay in his
hand. He leans into your
yellow dress, reaching up,
a tendril attaching, lifting
out of the dark, unfurling
his last leaf. She watches him
watch you,
you with a house
she imagines half glass, where light
pours in, and everything
is already paid for: your
dress, the shine of health you wear
as though you own it, the look
of wealth, and (this too is
visible) the knowhow
to make the right phone calls,
calls to those, who, when you call,
will do what you say, pay
what you tell them, when
and to whom. You, she imagines,
who have at least two
of everything, you lift her son
to your yellow breast, that
well lighted place, where the air's
clean, and you don't
hate yourself, waiting in line
to pay for a sack of potatoes
you can't afford, She watches him
cling to you, she waits to see
what you will do; you who
have things, you who can
do things, you who can do
what you choose to, you
who can do something for them,
if you choose to, a little something
or nothing.

—*Marilyn Krysl*

*Source*: Krysl, M. (1989). *Midwife and other poems on caring*. New York: National League for Nursing, pp. 11–12.

 **GLOBAL CONNECTION**

Home visiting in other countries may take the form of mandatory visits for mothers and babies, such as in Cuba. For remote villages, such as in the mountains of Nepal, how could home visiting be used as an efficient way of improving the health of community residents?

 **MEDIA MOMENT**

***Marvin's Room* (1996)**
Bessie, played by Diane Keaton, is a straight-laced, devoted daughter providing total care for her ill father (Hume Cronyn) who faces her own health crisis and must ask her estranged, bohemian sister, Lee (Meryl Streep), for help after Bessie suffers a health catastrophe. Bessie lives with her father and eccentric older aunt and has devoted her life to their care. Lee left the family years before and expresses little interest in the welfare of either her sister or her ailing father. She eventually makes the trip home to Florida with her two sons in tow. Leonardo Di Caprio effectively portrays the older, disturbed son who finds comfort with his newly found family. Old wounds are opened, and the movie provides an outstanding examination of life-choice consequences and the rewards of caring for others. Bessie has put her life on hold for years to care for her father, who "has been dying for 20 years—slowly, so that I won't miss anything." She doesn't see the years as wasted but rather says, "I've been so lucky to have been able to love someone so much."

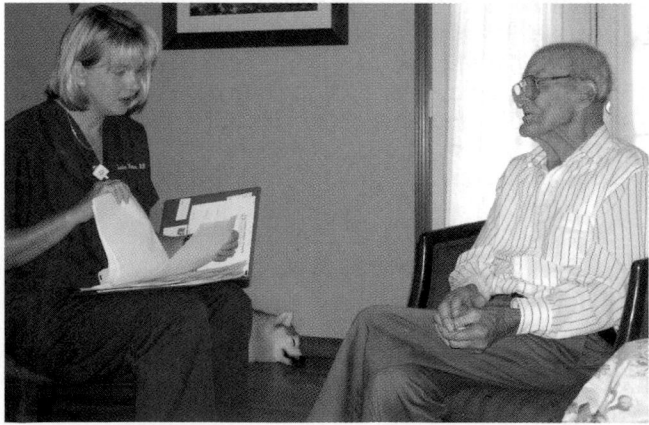

Home health nurses can assist elders to recover more quickly from acute episodes of age related conditions.

### Knowing in Nursing

I stepped outside of myself so that I could know
So that I could know the meaning of the earth
Its green springs and quiet winter nights.
So that I could know the depths
of the great, blue ocean
A place from which we all came.
I stepped outside of myself so that I could know
that there was more than the moon,
and the sun, and the stars . . .
And that when I looked upon the earth
so that I could know the meaning of life and
appreciate its continuance in death.
I stepped outside of myself so that I could know
how to raise my arms in loving, caring ways
And say to those who would listen
Let me share myself with you and all that I know . . .

*—Robyn Rice, RN, MSN, Ph.D.*

**❝** *Doing more things faster is no substitute for doing the right things.* **❞**

—Stephen R. Covey

the nurse to promote a sense of empowerment in the patient and family (Ruetter & Ford, 1996). The patient becomes part of the interdisciplinary team, rather than a dependent, passive recipient of care. As such, effective community health nurses can use the visit as a way to increase the patient's ability for self-care and enhance the sense of accomplishment in meeting health goals for self and family.

Home visits often take place over long periods, which affords the nurse ample opportunities for developing the authentic trust relationship necessary for a true collaborative partnership to develop between nurse and patient. A result is that patients are often more willing to share sensitive and more intimate issues in the home setting, which allows the nurse to gain insight into complex interpersonal influences (Stulginsky, 1993a, 1993b, Williams 2004).

## Effectiveness of Home Visits

Research from a variety of studies indicates that successful home visiting programs have resulted in improved health outcomes. But how effective are home visits—such as those that are preventive in nature—in the long run?

 Research Alert

### The Home Visit and the Nurse–Family Partnership: Evidence-Based Practice Research

The Nurse–Family Partnership (NFP), created by Dr. David Olds as an applied evidence-based practice home visiting model, is considered to be the most rigorously tested home visiting model in the United States. This Research Alert provides details of the actual research that supports the validity and successful outcomes of the NFP.

The cornerstone of the NFP model is the extensive research on the model conducted over the last three decades. Randomized trials were conducted with three diverse populations beginning in Elmira, New York, in 1977; in Memphis, Tennessee, in 1987; and Denver, Colorado, in 1994. All three trials targeted first-time, low-income mothers. Follow-up research continues today, studying the long-term outcomes for mothers and children in the three trials.

The program effects that have the strongest evidentiary foundations are those that have been found in at least two of the three trials.

#### Consistent Program Effects[1]
- Improved prenatal health
- Fewer childhood injuries
- Fewer subsequent pregnancies
- Increased intervals between births
- Increased maternal employment
- Improved school readiness

Employing new and improved statistical analysis methods, Olds and his research team at the Prevention Research Center have been involved in an extensive reanalysis of certain outcomes from the 15-year follow-up of the Elmira trial of NFP. An updated summary of the positive program effects found in the first trial in a child at age 15 is given here:

#### Benefits to Mothers
- 61% fewer arrests
- 72% fewer convictions
- 98% fewer days in jail[2]

#### Benefits to Children at Child Age 15
- 48% reduction in child abuse and neglect
- 59% reduction in arrests
- 90% reduction in adjudications as PINS (person in need of supervision) for incorrigible behavior[3]

Whereas the original analysis indicated that program effects were limited to the higher-risk portions of the sample (where the mother was unmarried and from a low-income family at registration), the reanalysis indicates that the benefits of the program on the outcomes listed previously are present for the entire nurse-visited sample, irrespective of risk. Many of the program-control differences remain larger for the higher-risk families, but the significance of the program effects now holds for the entire sample.

Earlier reported impacts of the Elmira program on "maternal behavioral problems due to substance abuse" and number of times the teens ran away were no longer statistically significant in the new analysis. Program effects on "conviction rates among 15-year-old children" and "number of sex partners among 15-year-old children" are more accurately characterized as trends.

Olds and his research team are committed to continually subjecting their work and earlier findings to the highest scientific standards and state-of-the-art statistical analysis.

### About the Research Design

A randomized trial is the most rigorous research method for measuring the effectiveness of an intervention. It is the type of study that the FDA requires of new drugs or medical devices to determine their effectiveness and safety before they are made available to the public. Because of their cost and complexity, these kinds of trials are not often used to evaluate complex health and human services.

In addition, important data are continuously collected from NFP replication sites through the web-based Clinical Information System (CIS). These data are analyzed and returned to local NFP-implementing agencies to provide them with evidence of their progress toward NFP's three goals. For more details on the research, visit: http://www.nursefamilypartnership.org.

---

1. Effects observed in at least two of three trials (Elmira, Memphis, and Denver).
2. Impact on days in jail is highly significant, but the number of cases that involve jail time is small, so the magnitude of program effect is difficult to estimate with precision.
3. Based on family-court records of 116 children who remained in the study community for a 13-year period following the end of the program.

---

*Sources*: Eckenrode, J., Ganzel, B., Henderson, C. R., et al. (2000). Preventing child abuse and neglect with a program of nurse home visitation: The limiting effects of domestic violence. *Journal of the American Medical Association, 284* (11), 1385–1391; Izzo, C., Eckenrode, J., Smith, E., et al. (2005). Reducing the impact of uncontrollable stressful life events through a program of nurse home visitation for new parents. *Prevention Science, 6*(4), 269–274; Kitzman, H., Olds, D. L., Sidora, K., et al. (2000). Enduring effects of nurse home visitation on maternal life course: A 3-year follow-up of a randomized trial. *Journal of the American Medical Association, 283*(15), 1983–1989; Olds, D. (2003). Reducing program attrition in home visiting: What do we need to know? *Child Abuse & Neglect, 27*(4), 359–361; Olds, D., Luckey, D., & Henderson, C. (2004). Can the results be believed? *Pediatrics, 115*(4), 1113–1114.

---

In a landmark research study, prenatal and early childhood home visits by nurses reduced subsequent antisocial behavior and experimentation with drugs in adolescents born into high-risk families. The study, which evaluated the effects of home visits by nurses over the course of 15 years to low-income, unmarried women, found long-term benefits that included fewer episodes of children running away from home, arrests and convictions, and drug abuse when compared with similar groups of women who received prenatal and well-child care in a clinic. The adolescent children of

---

## MEDIA MOMENT

### One True Thing (1998)

In this adaptation of Anna Quindlen's novel, when tough New Yorker Ellen Gulden (Renee Zellweger) discovers that her mother (Meryl Streep) has cancer, she quits her job, breaks up with her boyfriend, and moves back in with her parents to help out. Wanting nothing more than to ease her mother's suffering, she inadvertently uncovers several family secrets, including one about her philandering professor father (William Hurt). The movie's lesson is that we go through life telling ourselves a story about our childhood and our parents, but we are the authors of that story, and it is less fact than fiction.

---

these mothers also improved in terms of having fewer sexual partners, and they smoked and drank less than their peers who were not part of the home visiting programs (Olds & Kitzman, 1993; Kitzman et al., 2000; Izzo et al., 2005).

Zeanah, Larrieu, and Boris (2006) used the Nurse–Family Partnership (NFP) program in Louisiana, focusing on the use of mental health professionals paired with visiting nurses, to successfully improve maternal and child health, especially in relation to social and developmental issues. In this and other settings where the NFP model has been used, the long-term preventive mental health impact has been impressive. Brown, McLaine, Dixon, and Simon (2006) found that focused home visits to children with elevated blood lead levels resulted in improved parent–child interaction and family housekeeping practices at the end of one year of visits, as well as a 47% decrease in blood lead levels in the children.

Other research has revealed that successful home visiting programs should be broad in focus (e.g., "improved pregnancy outcome" versus "hypertension management during pregnancy"), so as to contribute to the most lasting effects in health status. Also, home visits that occur over time and in greater frequency accomplish more in terms of improved health status for the patients than single visits (Barkauskas, 1983; Persily, 2003). Home visiting to targeted high-risk groups who have complex and multiple needs have been linked with more significant changes health status than those at medium or low risk (Byrd, 1998; Deal, 1994; Olds & Kitzman, 1993; Brown et al., 2006; Persily, 2003; Zotti & Zahner, 1995; Roberts, Kramer, & Suissa, 1996, Izzo et al., 2005). Numerous studies have demonstrated that home visiting by nurses to pregnant and postpartum women and their infants reduces risk factors that result in preterm births, abuse and neglect, and maternal health problems. In addition, home visits improve healthy behaviors and are cost-effective (Gomby, Larson, Lewit, & Behrman, 1993; Olds, 1992; Olds, Henderson, Phelps, Kitzman, & Hanks, 1993; Izzo et al., 2005).

Home health visits have been linked with fewer hospital readmissions, fewer emergency department visits, and cost

## ◼◼ CULTURAL CONNECTION

The Nurse–Family Partnership (NFP) model has been utilized successfully in the remote swamps of southern Louisiana. This program was in place before Hurricane Katrina hit the area in August 2005.

Southern Louisiana is perhaps one of the most challenging locales for implementing the highly successful NFP project. Professional nurses, also referred to as "professional nurturers," visit poor and isolated mothers in the Cajun communities of Terrebonne and Lafourche parishes as part of the NFP program in Louisiana. Nurses visit mothers and babies up to the age of two to role-model good parenting practices and teach young families how to raise healthy children. This program is particularly challenging owing to the Cajun culture's resistance to government intervention programs and outsider intrusion. The area targeted by the NFP program was one of the poorest in the South before Hurricane Katrina struck, and it was hard hit by the hurricane. Yet due to the historically harsh living conditions of the swamps, few residents seemed to be concerned about the hurricane, according to one of the nurses in the program.

The Louisiana program focuses on an area an hour's drive southwest of New Orleans, along foggy, cypress-tree-lined winding roads to the Gulf of Mexico. The Mississippi River sediment shaped this marshy delta, to which French Acadians migrated in the eighteenth century after being expelled by the British from Nova Scotia. Cajuns now live in one of the harshest environments in the United States and have built their lives for two centuries on one of the fastest-sinking lands on earth.

Louisiana has some of the lowest literacy and child poverty rates in the United States. Thirty percent of Louisiana's children grow up in poverty. Childrearing practices often reflect Cajun cultural beliefs, such as the notion that giving a baby a haircut before his first birthday will stunt his growth and damage his brain.

The NFP visiting nurse program has resulted in improved statistics, although the gains are modest when considered against most standards in public health. After four years, the Louisiana legislature doubled funding for the program, mainly through Medicaid. With more than 1,000 mothers and children who have finished the two-year program, results are encouraging. By the time these children turned two years of age, almost 60% of the mothers who had started the program without a high school diploma or GED had one. Thirty percent of toddlers had scored in the top quartile of a national test for language development.

1. Why are the Cajuns of southern Louisiana seldom considered an ethnic group in the United States?
2. What are the political implications and possible blocks to implementing this type of program on a national basis?
3. Would these programs be in opposition to widely held American values of the sanctity of the family—for example, the idea that such programs intrude into a family's private life?
4. Does a program such as the NFP undermine other community efforts to fund public quality daycare centers, such as Head Start? Why or why not? What are possible compromises in funding these programs to promote better family outcomes and improve the community's overall health? ◉

*Sources*: Boo, K. (February 6, 2006). Swamp nurse. *New Yorker*, p. 55; Izzo, C., Eckenrode, J., et al. 2005. Reducing the impact of uncontrollable stressful life events through a program of nurse home visitation for new parents. *Prevention Science*, 6(4), 269–274.

---

❝*They may forget what you said, but they will never forget how you made them feel.*❞

—*Carl N. Buechner*

---

savings when compared with acute care. A study of patients with congestive heart failure who were visited by home health nurses linked fewer hospital admissions, from 3.2 admissions per year to 1.2 admissions per year, with home health visits. The length of stay decreased from 26 days per year to 6 days per year (Kornowski, Zeeli, Averbuch, & Finkelstein, 1995).

Schoen and Anderson (1998), in their extensive review of the effectiveness of home visiting programs, found that the most successful programs have the following elements:

- A focus on families in greater need of services rather than universal programs
- Interventions that begin in pregnancy and continue through the second to fifth years of life
- Flexibility and family specificity regarding the duration and frequency of visits, according to the family's need and risk level
- Active promotion of positive health-related behaviors
- Use of a broad, multiproblem focus to address the full complement of family needs
- Assistance to the family with reduction of stress by improving the social and physical environment
- Use of nurses and professionals specifically prepared in home visiting

## Challenges of Home Visits

Paradoxically, many of the aspects of home visiting that make it more advantageous for the nurse and patient than the hospital environment also contribute to the challenges of home visiting. Because the nurse is more independent and less tied to the physical constraints of the agency, professional isolation can be a problem, especially for a novice nurse. In the clinic or hospital, help or consultation with other professionals is only a few steps away. For the home visiting nurse, finding that help becomes more difficult and can be a source of considerable anxiety. With advanced technology, such as laptop computers, pagers, and cellular phones, and remote

## Research Alert

Recent advances in telecommunication technologies have enabled the direct provision of services to patients in the home using tools such as videophones and data transmission over phone lines. The present study compared nurse–patient interaction using two different video platforms designed for telehome care. One platform uses existing telephone lines (POTS video), and the other uses the Internet (IP video). The specific aims of this study were (1) to assess the degree of acceptance by nurses and patients of home video visits for nurse–patient interaction and (2) to compare preferences for delivery of home care between the two platforms, between video and live interaction, and between video and less frequent or no interaction.

The study used a quasi-experimental cross-over design. Nurse–patient pairs were assigned to conditions using a predetermined assignment procedure, alternating each new pair to start with one of the two platforms. Following that session, each participant pair then tested the second platform. Three simulated health problem scenarios, which focused on depression, anticoagulation therapy, and diabetes, were created for the study. A convenience sample of 26 practicing nurses and 18 volunteers serving as simulated patients participated in the study. Nurse case managers at the Iowa City Veterans Affairs Medical Center (VAMC) served as the nurse sample. Volunteer participants were recruited from the volunteer department at the same facility. Most of the volunteers (72%) were age 70 or older; 61% of the nurses were younger than 50 years old.

Most participants regularly wore corrective lenses (81% of nurses and 94% of volunteers); 11% of volunteers wore a hearing aid; and 17% reported having other hearing problems, while none of the nurses reported hearing problems. Forty percent of the volunteer patients reported that they were very or somewhat comfortable using a personal computer; 27% ($n = 4$) reported having a personal computer (PC) at home; and 20% ($n = 3$) had Internet access at home. All of the nurses regularly used computers at work, whereas most of the volunteers did not use the computer on a regular basis while at the medical center.

### Description of POTS Video and IP Video Systems

The system selected for the plain old telephone service (POTS) video portion of the study was composed of a television monitor and a camera kit that combined a telephone, microphone, and video camera. To establish contact, the nurse activates the system using the remote control to enter the patient's telephone number. The patient at home responds by pushing the start button on the remote control device. During the visit, the nurse and the patient see and talk to each other, with all functions controlled by the nurse. At the end of the interaction, the patient presses the end-call button on the remote. The remote control device has one large green button to start

the system and one large red end-call button to turn it off. This facilitates ease of use by older patients who may have limited dexterity or vision. In this study, the calls were placed on commercial telephone lines.

The Internet Protocol (IP)-based teleconferencing system consists of a small video camera with an integrated microphone that mounts on top of a PC monitor and connects to the PC via a USB port. To communicate using this platform, both the nurse and the patient need a PC, the video camera and software, and an Internet connection. To establish contact, the nurse activates the communication software, enters the patient's IP address, and clicks the dial button. When the patient has also activated the software on his or her PC and has established an Internet connection, the patient's software will recognize the incoming call and will emit an audible ring, much like a telephone call. The patient can then click a button to answer the call, and within a few seconds, the nurse and patient will be able to see and hear each other. To end the call, the nurse or patient clicks on the end-call button.

Each healthy adult volunteer played the role of a patient and was paired with a nurse. Seated in separate rooms, each patient–nurse pair conducted two simulated home visits on one of the video units being tested using a script prepared by the investigators. Scripts included typical patient problems addressed during a home care visit. Using the script, the nurse conducted a standard set of tasks or assessments that mimicked a home care visit. The nurse and patient each completed a short evaluation rating. The patient–nurse pair then conducted the same two simulated home visits using the same scripts on the second video unit, after which the nurse and patient again completed the same short evaluation rating. Following completion of the two simulated visits, the study coordinator conducted a brief open-ended interview with participants to discuss perceptions of the two platforms. These qualitative responses were recorded in notes taken by the study staff.

The three interaction scenarios simulated a nurse interacting with a patient with depression, a patient on anticoagulant therapy, and a patient with newly diagnosed diabetes. The scenarios were designed to maximize the features of the video component. The depression scenario required the nurse to observe the patient's facial expressions and body language. The anticoagulant scenario required the nurse to read the patient's medication bottle and to observe the patient's arms for signs of bruising. The diabetes scenario required the nurse to demonstrate the use of an insulin syringe to the patient. Each scenario was designed to be completed within 10 to 15 minutes.

### Outcome Measures

An investigator-developed instrument was used that addressed patient–nurse communication using the video platforms. All items were scored using a six-point Likert-type scale (1 = strongly disagree to 6 = strongly agree).

The first aim of the study was to assess the degree of acceptance of home video visits for nurse–patient interaction. For the first analysis, nurse and patient ratings were combined to compare POTS video to IP video. The IP video system was rated significantly higher ($p \leq 0.05$) in the following acceptance categories: trust that privacy is maintained; video visits as a replacement for nurse home visits; preference for the video visit compared to a nurse home visit; willingness to recommend the platform to others who need home care; willingness to use the platform if home care was needed; and recommending the platform to friends/patients. There were no significant differences between the POTS and IP system ratings for ease of use, visit taking too much time, and perceived expense of visit.

A separate analysis was conducted to compare patient and nurse ratings for each system. Patients rated the POTS video system significantly more favorably than did nurses, on the following criteria: acceptance of video visits as a replacement for nurse home visits, between the two platforms, and between video and live interaction.

Patients and nurses both preferred the IP video over the POTS system, citing superior visualization. Overall, patients ranked both platforms more favorably than did the nurses on acceptance of home video visits and preferences for more frequent visits relative to less frequent face-to-face visits.

Although the IP platform had higher overall ratings, a critical difference between the two platforms was ease of use. For example, some patients had a difficult time answering the call on the IP video system because they were not familiar or comfortable using a computer. Although the study was initially designed to have both nurses and patients log on to the IP system, technical and end-user difficulties were so common in the first few sessions that the connection was instead established for the participants. Thus ease of use is a critical consideration when selecting a home technology system.

Although participants preferred more frequent video visits compared to less frequent face-to-face visits, nurses emphasized the value of home visits. In the follow-up interviews, nurses often mentioned the importance of seeing a patient's surroundings and living conditions when conducting a home visit—a task that would be hampered by the narrow field of vision afforded by a video camera. Nurses expressed the need for personal contact with patients. However, they also acknowledged that video visits could be a good way to supplement face-to-face visits.

Home telehealth monitoring devices are quickly being adopted in practice settings. This study, by examining patient and nurse preferences for use, concluded that ease of use, clinical appropriateness, training, and support will affect the future growth of home telehealth. ◯

*Source*: Wakefield, B. J., Holman, J. E., Ray, A., Morse, J., & Kienzle, M. G. (2004). Nurse and patient preferences for telehealth home care. *Geriatric Times, 5*(2), 27–30.

❝*What you do speaks so loud that I cannot hear what you say.*❞

—*Ralph Waldo Emerson*

...............................................................

monitoring devices, the nurse must use different strategies for connecting with other professionals.

The intimacy of the home visit can create boundary issues for both the nurse and the patient. For example, the boundary between professional distance and social intimacy because of the informality of the home is a constant challenge for the community health nurse. Certainly, there is a certain amount of socialization that occurs in all home visits as the nurse maintains therapeutic rapport and extends courtesy to her patient hosts. Nurses are always guests in the patient's home, and courtesies normally not extended in the hospital become critical in the home. Nurses also may find themselves disclosing more about themselves than they would in a hospital setting. Such self-disclosure must be monitored carefully so that the patient–nurse relationship remains therapeutic. For example, a nurse's concern about her own child's illness might be mentioned in casual comments and then become a significant source of anxiety for the elder patient who becomes overly worried about the child's well-being.

The nurse must also deal with the challenge that providing care may actually increase a person's feelings of vulnerability, simply by being seen at home by a nurse. The patient may perceive that by accepting the nurse's help, his or her own ability to give self-care is inadequate. In their ethnographic study, Magilvy, Brown, and Dydyn (1988) found that home health patients often expressed concerns about relying on a home health nurse as a sign of vulnerability. They expressed a need to maintain their independence and mobility and saw the nurse as a reminder of their dependency or reliance on outside help. Therefore, the nurse must constantly promote the collaborative nature of the patient–nurse relationship and frequently praise the patient for efforts to improve health, no matter how small or insignificant the changes might be. Nurses accustomed to using "take charge" skills such as are rewarded in the hospital often find that they may lead to failure in the home setting (Coffman, 1997; Liaschenko, 1994; Millard, Hillett, & Luke, 2006; Moser, Houtepen, & Widdershoven, 2007).

In the home setting, the patient has the right to self-determination and can reject or accept the therapeutic interventions offered by the nurse. This important aspect of

■■
■■ CULTURAL CONNECTION

People who live in the United States value home ownership as a sign of a successful life. For other cultures, a home is defined and valued very differently. For the homeless, home may be under a bridge, in an abandoned car, or in an alley. How does the definition of home affect nurses who visit patients "at home"?

### ENVIRONMENTAL CONNECTION

A home visit provides the community health nurse with exceptional opportunities of assessing environmental risks, practicalities of implementing a plan of care, and the limits of patients' ability to care for themselves and for others. The hospital is an artificial environment, created for the convenience of health care providers. As nurses, we know very little about how patients live on a daily basis without visiting where they call "home." When the natural environment of home is experienced by the community health nurse during home visits, more realistic and acceptable plans of care *with* the patient can be executed with greater chance of success.

autonomy cannot be overemphasized when in the patient's home. The nurse must remember that true collaboration means that the nurse and the patient set goals, develop strategies, and evaluate outcomes of care together, no matter how difficult that sharing of power may be for the nurse who has been taught that "the nurse always knows best" (Millard et al., 2006; Zerwekh, 1997).

In a study by Jack, DiCenso, and Lohfeld (2002), researchers determined that factors which influenced relationship development with patients in the home-related "family–nurse engagement occurred through 'finding common ground' and 'building trust'." For example, a prenatal patient may refuse to stop smoking during pregnancy, explaining to the nurse that she is too nervous to do so because her mother-in-law has moved in with the family. The nurse may be able to provide the patient with assistance in reducing the number of cigarettes smoked per day, especially if the nurse is a former smoker. Successive approximations in the attainment of patient goals means that progress is measured in small increments, rather than in the dramatic turnaround of the acute care setting (Stulginsky, 1993a). For

### THINK ABOUT THIS

Oh, I have my material longings—ever so often I will throw a pity party for the house I'll never have. But quite a few of us nurses are working, you could say, in the context of our own memories.

—Luwana Marts, RN, BSN

Marts is a visiting nurse with the Nurse–Family Partnership. Here she describes her reasons for working as a nurse in the swamps and bayous of southern Louisiana for half the salary she could make in a hospital. Marts became a BSN RN after nearly 14 years of childrearing and working as a nurse's aide.

*Source:* Boo, K. (February 6, 2006). Swamp nurse. *New Yorker*, p. 55.

many nurses, this is perhaps the most difficult challenge of all, especially for nurses who have primary experience in the hospital specialty units, such as the emergency department or intensive care unit. The community health nurse cannot solve all of the patient's problems during home visiting, nor should such attempts be made. Only those health problems that are amenable to therapeutic nursing interventions and that are mutually agreed on by the patient and nurse should be the focus during home visits. For example, the patient with diabetes may not be able to eliminate sugar from her coffee and tea but over time has discontinued using sugar with her cereal.

Another challenge that often emerges is when the nurse faces the immediate pressing demands of the family and a different, preset agenda determined by the agency, typically as a result of the funding source's policy (Cowley, 1995). Usually, the funding source states a specified number of visits or a specified time frame for the care (e.g., 60 days). The dilemma occurs for the community nurse when the patient needs additional care but not specifically at the skilled level. For example, a patient may express the need for more assistance in learning to exercise with an artificial hip appliance. The nurse could refer the patient to local support groups and community senior centers that offer specialized exercise classes. Community health nurses may be some of the most creative nurses working today as they struggle to find myriad ways of meeting patient needs when conventional reimbursement sources end. Consulting with other team members and using support groups may provide resources and support in

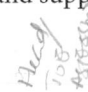

### MEDIA MOMENT

#### *Passion Fish* (1992)

May-Alice Culhane (Mary McDonnell) is a soap opera star who's left paralyzed after a car accident and, with few other options, returns to her Louisiana home. Her heavy drinking and bad attitude drive away all of her caregivers, until Chantelle (Alfre Woodard) comes to work for her. The two women form an unlikely friendship in this John Sayles film, which earned McDonnell an Oscar nomination for best actress.

At the heart of the movie is the uneasy relationship between May-Alice and Chantelle. May-Alice is used to being willful and spoiled; Chantelle does not find her behavior acceptable. But May-Alice has the money and Chantelle needs the job, for more urgent reasons than we first realize, and so it seems that Chantelle may have to put up with May-Alice's behavior. Yet in a deeper sense—one that reveals itself only gradually to May-Alice—what she needs most of all from Chantelle is the other woman's ability to stand up to her.

these complex and frustrating situations, which are becoming all too common in the managed care arena.

## Distractions in the Home Environment

Conducting a visit in the home, as compared with the nurse-controlled environment of the hospital, is unique in that the nurse must compete with many distractions. Although the distractions that nurses encounter on home visits may seem on the surface negative and interfere with the plan of care, Pruitt, Keller, and Hale (1987) contend that distractions can also provide valuable information about the patient's world. Distractions can generally be classified as environmental, behavioral, or nurse initiated.

**Environmental distractions** take the form of excessive stimuli, such as television and radio, children playing and making noise, phone calls, traffic, or construction noise. Other environmental sources of distraction may come from crowded or cluttered living conditions; the nurse almost always faces less than ideal living conditions on home visits. Nurses have their own picture of what an ideal living environment should look like, and such values influence the way distractions affect assessment and interventions. For example, the nurse may find a cluttered home a sign of a patient's depression or disinterest in a healthy environment. By remaining open to other explanations, the nurse may discover that the patient feels comforted by the various objects, furniture, and photos. How we "clutter" our homes has much to do with what is important to us—and to our patients–and thus can be a valuable way for us to learn about the patient's values. How we "use" our space, no matter how large or how small, reflects our values and lifestyles (Pruitt et al., 1987). Noticing how the furniture is arranged, the number and kinds of photographs around the home, and the kinds of objects displayed can help nurses understand a patient's family circle and ties as well as those things that bring the patient joy. The "doggie smell" and dog hair throughout the house may be what makes an elderly woman's house a home. Elders often have cluttered homes because they have accumulated the memories and possessions of a lifetime; they also may place furniture close together to make it easier to hear conversations.

The nurse can learn to minimize environmental distractions—for example, by asking to turn down or "mute" the television or avoiding visiting when the patient is most likely to be watching favorite television programs. Experienced home health nurses who visit patients over a long period of time are well aware of how important it is to avoid

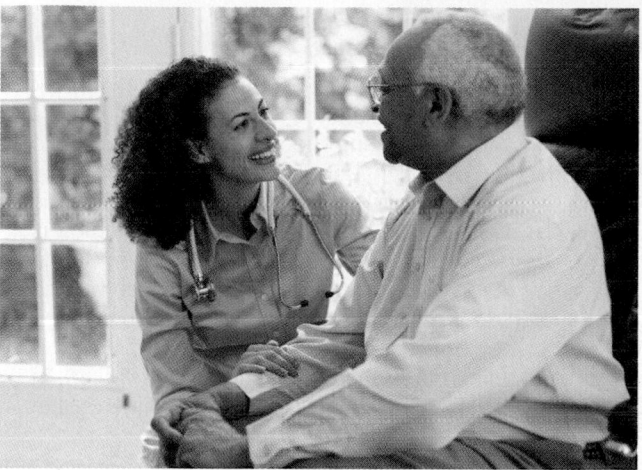

A nurse on a home visit.

certain times of the day, such as when the patient's favorite soap operas are on! If interruptions become a problem, observing how the patient reacts can provide the nurse with clues to how much of a threat the distraction is to the patient's health (Pruitt et al., 1987). One solution in visiting a pregnant woman with a 3-year-old child who may be distracting her is to have the child draw a picture for the nurse. Such a strategy can provide the nurse with ample time to perform assessment tasks with the mother. In a multiperson household where privacy is at a premium, retreating to a back room or even outside to a porch is often all that is necessary to obtain a few moments of distraction-free assessment time. Balancing courtesy with objectives for the visit becomes a skill that requires tact, humor, and creativity.

Another type of distraction is **behavioral distractions.** That is, the patient may exhibit behaviors that distract the nurse from the plan of care and goals of the home visit. Patients may avoid talking about health problems for a variety of reasons and may instead engage in social communication. Patients may have very real concerns that are not consistent with what the nurse sees as priority problems (Pruitt et al., 1987). By examining such avoidance, the nurse may find that these concerns should be addressed first. For example, a nurse who is seeing an older woman with diabetes may find that the patient refuses to discuss her daily blood sugars, but instead wants to talk about an auto accident that occurred the night before near the patient's home. Upon closer examination, the nurse finds that the accident has claimed the life of an elderly woman only casually known to the patient, and the patient then remarks, "It isn't too much longer that I will be able to drive, and then what will I do?" The patient was exposing her feelings of vulnerability about losing her mobility and independence. Other behaviors that may hinder the goals of the home visit include blocking or silence in response to inquiries related to health status. The nurse must use appropriate therapeutic communication techniques, such as refocusing, as well as exhibiting patience to provide optimal comfort for the patient in the home environment.

### *Got an Alternative?*

On a home visit, nurses often find out about folk remedies used by families for common health problems. In determining the appropriate response to these nontraditional or alternative health practices, the nurse should assess whether the practice is harmful, neutral, or beneficial. If the practice is neutral (such as keeping a good-luck charm in the baby's room), should the nurse take action with the family concerning the practice? How should the nurse intervene appropriately when the practice is determined to be harmful (such as pica eating), in contrast to being beneficial to the family's health (such as meditation and chanting)?

**Nurse-initiated distractions** can evolve from prejudices, fears, preoccupation with the tasks of home visiting, and reactions to lifestyles and living conditions different from the nurse's own. Homes of patients may be cluttered or appear unkempt, and these distractions can result in the nurse making judgments about the patient, even on an unconscious level. This "baggage" that all nurses carry with them on home visits should be carefully acknowledged and examined to prevent negative effects on nurse–patient interactions. Nurses may fear home visiting because of safety concerns, concerns over being alone without colleagues for support and consultation, and fears of being rejected by the patient. Practicing nursing in the uncontrolled environment of a patient's home can threaten even the most secure nurse in terms of autonomy and control. Other distractions that are common are talking on the phone with the home office or other health care professionals or making arrangements for other patients while in the patient's home. The nurse must be aware of how such distractions influence the nurse–patient relationship. While in the home, the patient should remain the focus as much as possible. By being preoccupied with staying on schedule, tasks, and documentation of the visit, the effectiveness of home visiting can be seriously threatened.

The nurse may also become frustrated with patients who are labeled as noncompliant or who seem to have contributed in some way to their health problems, such as emphysema in a smoker or liver cancer in an alcoholic. Understanding that these feelings are shared at one time or another by most nurses can be the first step to prevent them from affecting the care delivered. Talking with colleagues and having an open dialogue with other professionals in similar settings can help nurses understand not only the source of these distractions but also helpful ways that others have used to minimize their effects on patient care (Pruitt et al., 1987).

## Conclusion

The origins of home visiting began with organized health care. Visiting families and patients in the home can provide the community health nurse with more realistic expectations of the family's needs and more appropriate interventions. Advantages and disadvantages of home visiting should be considered when choosing this setting for community-based nursing care.

Explore Community Health Nursing on the Web! To learn more about the topics in this chapter, use the passcode provided to access your exclusive website: **http://nursing.jbpub.com/ communityhealth.** If you do not have a passcode, you can obtain one at this site.

**Application to Practice**

A community health nurse is following a child with high blood lead levels. During a follow-up visit to the clinic, the mother was distracted and kept looking at her watch while the nurse explained how important it was to keep the child from coming in contact with leaded paint. The child failed to keep an appointment with a university clinic for a chelation treatment. The community health nurse could not reach the mother because the phone had been disconnected.

On a home visit, the nurse found out that the father had been injured while working at his car repair service shop, located on the same lot as the family's mobile home. He had taken a temporary job while he recovered from the back injury, on an "as-needed" basis for a local garage, and used his own tow truck for jobs. He was on call 24 hours a day. Because of his business, many old cars were scattered all over the yard, explaining a potential source for the lead poisoning in the child. Also, the father's injury had kept him from repairing the family car, so the only transportation was the tow truck.

1. Identify three of the most serious health threats in this family.
2. Identify two nursing goals for this family.
3. What is the first action you would take on the first home visit?
4. What further information would be important to know about these family members?
5. Identify two strengths of his family.

# ■ CRITICAL THINKING ACTIVITIES

1. Read the poem *Home Call: Mother and Child* by Marilyn Krysl on page 960.
   - How does the mother perceive the nurse in terms of power?
   - Do the status differences in the nurse and the mother affect the outcome of this home visit as intervention?
   - How could the nurse be culturally sensitive in this situation while educating the mother about appropriate child care?
   - How is power represented in this poem?
   - Identify one appropriate nursing intervention in the described home visit.

2. The following questions are common ones that student nurses ask about home visiting. As you read this chapter, reflect on your own responses to the questions.
   - What do patients in the home think of student nurses caring for them, especially if an instructor is not present?
   - What if the patient or family member asks me a question to which I don't know the answer?
   - What will I be expected to do as far as skills in the home setting?
   - What about safety issues?
   - What do I do if a patient "codes" while I am there?
   - Are there specific legal implications that I should be aware of in the home setting?

# ■ REFERENCES

Barkauskas, V. H. (1983). Effectiveness of public health nurse home visits to primarous mothers and their infants. *American Journal of Public Health 73*(5), 573–580.

Brown, M. J., McLaine, P., Dixon, S., & Simon, P. (2006). A randomized, community-based trial of home visiting to reduce lead levels in children. *Pediatrics, 117*(1), 147–153.

Byrd, M. E. (1998). Long-term maternal-child home visiting. *Public Health Nursing, 15*(4), 235–242.

Coffman, S. (1997). Home-care nurses as strangers in the family. *Western Journal of Nursing Research, 19*(1), 82–96.

Cowley, S. (1995). In health visiting: A routine visit is one that has passed. *Journal of Advanced Nursing, 22,* 276–284.

Deal, L. W. (1994). The effectiveness of community health nursing interventions: A literature review. *Public Health Nursing, 11,* 315–323.

Gomby, D. S., Larson, J. D., Lewit, J., & Behrman, R. (1993). Home visiting analysis and recommendations. *The Future of Children, 3,* 6–22.

Hafkenschiel, J. (1997). Minding our business. Home health reimbursement and the 1997 Budget Act. *Home Care Provider, 2*(6), 279–281.

Howse, C. (2007). "The ultimate destination of all nursing": The development of district nursing in England, 1880–1925. *Nursing History Review, 15,* 65–94.

Izzo, C., Eckenrode, J., Smith, E., et al. (2005). Reducing the impact of uncontrollable stressful life events through a program of nurse home visitation for new parents. *Prevention Science, 6*(4), 269–274.

Jack, S., DiCenso, A., & Lohfeld, L. (2002). Opening doors: Factors influencing the establishment of a working relationship between paraprofessional home visits and at-risk families. *Canadian Journal of Nursing Research, 34*(4), 59–69.

Kitzman, H., Olds, D. L., Sidora, K., et al. (2000). Enduring effects of nurse home visitation on maternal life course: A 3-year follow-up of a randomized trial. *Journal of the American Medical Association, 283*(15), 1983–1989.

Kornowski, R., Zeeli, D., Averbuch, M., & Finkelstein, A. (1995). Intensive home care surveillance prevents hospitalization and improved morbidity rates among elderly patients with congestive heart failure. *American Heart Journal, 4,* 762–766.

Liaschenko, J. (1994). The moral geography of home care. *Advances in Nursing Science, 17,* 16–26.

Liepert, B. D. (1996). The value of community health nursing: A phenomenological study of the perceptions of the community health nurses. *Public Health Nursing, 13,* 50–57.

Magilvy, J. K., Brown, N. J., & Dydyn, J. (1988). The experience of home health care: Perceptions of older adults. *Public Health Nursing, 5*(3), 140–145.

Millard, L., Hillett, C., & Luker, R. (2006). Nurse-patient interaction and decision-making in care. *Journal of Advanced Nursing, 55*(2), 142–150.

Moser, A., Houtepen, R., & Widdershoven, G. (2007). Patient autonomy in nurse-led shared care. *Journal of Advanced Nursing, 57*(4), 357–365.

National Association of Home Care (NAHC) (2006). *Basic statistics about home care.* Washington, DC: Author.

Olds, D. L. (1992). Home visitation program for pregnant women and parents of young children. *American Journal of Diseases of Children, 146,* 704–708.

Olds, D. L., Henderson, C. R., Phelps, C., Kitzman, H., & Hanks, C. (1993). Effect of prenatal and infancy nurse home visitation on government spending. *Medical Care, 31,* 155–174.

Olds, D. L., & Kitzman, H. (1993). Review of research on home visiting for pregnant women and parents of young children. *The Future of Children, 3*(3), 53–92.

Persily, C. (2003). Lay home visiting may improve pregnancy outcomes. *Holistic Nursing Practice, 17*(5), 231–238.

Pruitt, R. H., Keller, L. S., & Hale, S. L. (1987). Mastering the distractions that mar home visits. *Nursing and Health Care, 8,* 344–347.

Roberts, I., Kramer, M. S., & Suissa, S. (1996). Does home visiting prevent childhood injury: A systematic review of randomized controlled trials. *British Medical Journal, 3122*(7022), 22–23.

Ruetter, L. I., & Ford, J. S. (1996). Perceptions of public health nursing: Views from the field. *Journal of Advanced Nursing, 24,* 7–15.

Schoen, S., & Anderson, S. (1998). The role of home visitation programs in improving health outcomes for children and families. *Pediatrics, 101*(3), 486–490.

Stulginsky, M. M. (1993a). Nurses' home health experience. Part 1: The practice setting. *Nursing and Health Care, 14,* 402–407.

Stulginsky, M. M. (1993b). Nurses' home health experience. Part 2: The unique demands of home visits. *Nursing and Health Care, 14,* 476–485.

Williams, A. M. (2004). Shaping the practice of home care: Critical case studies of the significance of the meaning of home. *International Journal of Palliative Nursing, 10*(7), 333–342.

Zeanah, P. D., Larrieu, J. A., & Boris, N. W. (2006). Nurse home visiting: Perspectives from nurses. *Infant Mental Health Journal, 27*(1), 41–54.

Zerwekh, J. V. (1997). Making the connection during home visits: Narratives of expert nurses. *International Journal of Human Caring, 1*(1), 325–333.

Zotti, M. E., & Zahner, S. J. (1995). Evaluation of PHN home visits to pregnant women on WIC. *Public Health Nursing, 12*(5), 294–304.

Karen Saucier Lundy, Karen B. Utterback,
Debra K. Lance, and Ilene Purvis Bloxsom

Visit **http://nursing.jbpub.com/communityhealth**
for interactive exercises, review questions,
Web links, and more.

"No matter how dreary and gray our
homes are, we people of flesh and blood
would rather live there than in any other
country, be it ever so beautiful. There is
no place like home."

*The Wizard of Oz*
—L. Frank Baum

"My view you know is that the ultimate destination is the nursing of the sick in their own home. I look to the abolition of all hospitals . . . but no use to talk about the year 2000."

*—Florence Nightingale, 1867*

The home was the earliest setting for nursing care. Why do you think Florence Nightingale believed that care should ideally return to the home? How does home health differ now from Nightingale's era? It is often said that almost anything that can be done in the hospital, can be done in the home today. How do you feel about being a nurse in someone's home? How is this different from the secure environment of the hospital?

## CHAPTER FOCUS

**Home Health Nursing**
- Standards of Home Health Nursing

**The Medicare Era**

**Types of Home Health Agencies**
- Home Health Documentation

**Financing and Payment Systems for Home Health Services**
- Medicare
- Medicaid
- Private Insurance
- Payment by Individual

**Quality Assurance and Public Accountability**
- Regulation and Licensure
- Accreditation

**Managed Care and Home Health**

**Interdisciplinary Team Approach in Home Health**

**Role of Family Caregivers in Home Health**

**Legal and Ethical Issues in Home Health**
- Home Care Bill of Rights
- Advance Medical Directives

**Information and Technology in Home Health**
- Communication and Data Management
- Delivery of Care

**Hospice Care in the Home**
- Hospice Care for Children
- Holistic Care

**The Future of Home Health Care**

## QUESTIONS TO CONSIDER

After reading this chapter, you will know the answers to the following questions:

1. Which factors have contributed to the increased growth in home health care in the past 30 years?
2. What is a typical home health patient like in terms of diagnosis and age?
3. What are common reimbursement sources for home health services?
4. How does home health nursing differ from nursing that takes place in other health care settings?
5. How are technologies being used in home care?
6. What is hospice, and how does it differ from home health?
7. What is the future of home care nursing?

## KEY TERMS

Capitated rate
Conditions of participation (CoP)
Disease state management (DSM)

Fee-for-service rate
Home health care
Home health care nurses

Home health care nursing
Hospice
Informal caregivers

Palliative care
Plan of care (POC)
Skilled nursing visits (SNVs)

HOME HEALTH CARE was established in the latter part of the nineteenth century, as nursing schools began graduating more and better-trained professional nurses. Influencing this movement to home care was the explosion of scientific knowledge about microorganism transmission and communicable disease and the accompanying advancement in technology.

## Home Health Nursing

**Home health care** refers to the delivery of health services in the home setting for purposes of restoring or maintaining the health of individuals and families. The purpose of home health care is to provide the support, treatment, and information that caregivers and patients need to successfully manage their healthcare needs at home. The home health nurse's role is that of facilitator of home independence through patient education, patient advocacy, and case management. Managed care and technological advances and research have all contributed to the movement from the hospital to the home as a diverse and dynamic service delivery setting for care (NAHCH, 2008; Rice, 2005). Providing home care services to some 7.6 million individuals who require health care, **home health care nursing** is the choice for many community health nurses who are attracted by the autonomy, flexibility, and challenge of caring for persons in their own home. Home health care nursing, involves the same primary preventive focus with home health patients and the secondary and tertiary prevention foci on the care of individuals in collaboration with the family and caregivers. **Home health care nurses** provide care to a broad spectrum of ages and clinical diagnoses (Rice, 2005; Duke, 2003).

Home based health care has been one of the most rapidly growing areas in the healthcare sector in the United States and other Western countries for the past two decades.

**❝**I've told my children that when I die, to release balloons in the sky to celebrate that I graduated. For me, death is a graduation. **❞**

—Elisabeth Kübler-Ross

### ■■ CULTURAL CONNECTION

As a home health nurse, you will experience many different cultural practices from your own. When entering the home of a person of the Muslim faith, it is customary to remove one's shoes at the door. Compare this to the hospital setting and our attempts to be sensitive to our patients' cultural values. Would you be likely to remove your shoes in the hospital when entering the room of a patient with similar values as above? Why or why not? ◓

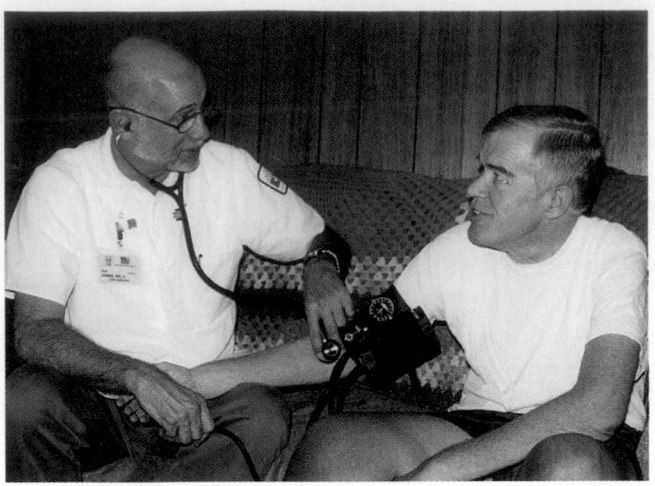

Home health nurse Jim Jones, RN, conducts a physical assessment.

Market forces and the development of government policies to control cost increases in the health sector have driven health care to move to the home. Trends which have influenced the move to home health care include economic pressure to reduce the escalating cost of healthcare systems, the movement of healthcare delivery away from acute care into the community, the rapid growth of managed care systems, and the increasing percentage of older people in populations. Home health care nursing presents a challenge to nurses who must incorporate new technology, increasing patient acuity, and complex patient and family needs into their practice. Home care serves a number of functions for acute, continuing, preventive, and palliative care; each of these functions necessitates a different care provider mix, level of care, and need for health management in the home (Congdon & Magilvy, 1998). Some examples of the type of activities of home health nurses include:

- Acute care: facilitates early discharge, reduces admission or readmission to hospitals and other more costly facilities, such as long-term care.
- Continuing care or long-term care: allows individuals to remain in their current home environment in the community as long as possible.
- Preventive care: prevents occurrence of injuries, illnesses, chronic conditions, and their resulting disabilities.
- Palliative care: offers total care to a person and supports caregiver(s) to improve the person's quality of life for life-threatening and terminal conditions.

Home health care is holistic and focused on the individual patient, integrating family, caregivers, and environmental and community resources to promote optimal health for the patient confined to the home. Boxes 39-1 and 39-2 describe the typical home health nurse's day and patient load.

In the United States, annual expenditures for home health care were projected to be $57.6 billion for 2007. Almost any care that can now be provided in the hospital can also take place in the home, which has created numerous practice opportunities for home health nurses. Home care services are provided to persons with acute care needs, long-term health conditions, permanent disabilities, or terminal illnesses and makes up 3% of total personal care expenditures in the U.S. (NAHCH, 2008).

Home health care is that component of the continuum of comprehensive health care whereby health services are provided to individuals and families in their places of residence for the purpose of promoting, maintaining, or restoring health, or of maximizing the level of independence while minimizing the effects of disability and illness, including terminal illness. The appropriate services to meet the needs of the individual patient and family are planned, coordinated, and made available by providers organized for the delivery

> ### ENVIRONMENTAL CONNECTION
>
> A home visit provides the community health nurse with ample opportunities of assessing environmental risks. When you enter a patient's home for the first time, what kinds of things do you notice first? How does this differ from a visit to a friend's house?

of home care through the use of employed staff, contractual arrangements, or a combination of the two patterns. (Rice, 2005; Shick & Balinsky, 2006)

Changes in the health care system and advances in technology and information are challenging nurses to redefine the terms "home" and "care" (Franz, 1997). Clarke and Cody (1994) have challenged nurses to rethink the central concepts of nursing: person, environment, health,

---

## BOX 39-1

### Summary Description of Patients in Sample Home Health Daily Nursing Schedule

On each skilled nursing visit:

1. Wash hands.
2. Set up equipment, including laptop computer.
3. Obtain complete assessment with review of systems. DOCUMENT.
4. Contact physician with assessment results, if indicated. DOCUMENT.
5. Ask the patient or caregiver to recall previous instruction, making corrections if needed. DOCUMENT.
6. Wash hands. Perform procedures; wash hands. Note response to care. DOCUMENT.
7. Instruct patient/caregiver from plan of care. Note response to instruction. Review as needed. DOCUMENT.
8. Schedule next visit with the patient/caregiver.
9. Clean equipment; wash hands.

Ms. Lottie AAA. Hx: 74 y/o with a longstanding history of osteoarthritis, using a walker for mobility in her small rural home. She has a recent diagnosis of type 2 DM. The physician has requested daily SNVs to instruct her in blood glucose monitoring, diabetic diet, and medication regimen after the initiation of an oral hypoglycemic agent. She lives alone but receives assistance from her many children and grandchildren in the community.

Mr. Ali BBB. Hx: 81 y/o with CHF for several years and is particularly forgetful since the death of his wife last year. His physician has requested SNVs because he has had two recent hospitalizations with exacerbations of his disease. Although he lives alone, his daughter drops by each morning at 09:00 to offer help. The nursing visit is set so that instruction can be given to both.

Mr. Carlo CCC. Hx: 26 y/o with paraplegia and development of a stage II sacral ulcer. He has a roommate who helps with shopping and some activities of daily living. He previously spent most of his day in the wheelchair but has begun to take rest periods midmorning, midafternoon, and early evening. He is pleased with the air cushion for his wheelchair and the gel overlay for his bed.

Ms. Helaria DDD. Hx: 78 y/o with recent onset of idiopathic HTN. She lives with her elderly husband and a very active dog, Maggie. Her children have hired a caregiver for ADLs and housekeeping. The physician has ordered BP assessments 2–3 times per week for 3 weeks to assess the effects of her new medication, quinapril HCl. Systolic pressure at 160 or greater and diastolic pressure at 94 or greater are to be reported. One dosage adjustment has been made, and she has been normotensive on the last two visits. Visit times are varied to give the physician an across-the-day view.

Mr. Paul EEE. Hx: 34 y/o with congenital lower-extremity malformation, type 1 DM, and open wounds on both lower limbs. He helps his elderly father with financial matters and record keeping. The patient meticulously records his wound progress and e-mails any concerns to the nurse and physician. He provides wound care to the areas he can reach, and the nurse performs care to the area outside his reach. He is well educated about his health conditions. He depends on home health aides for most of his personal care. A supervised home health aide visit is planned.

Key for abbreviations: ADLs, activities of daily living; BP, blood pressure; CHF, congestive heart failure; DM, diabetes mellitus; HTN, hypertension; Hx, history; SNVs, skilled nursing visits; y/o, years old.

*Source*: Contributed by Jim Jones, RN, BEd, Case Manager Home Health Nurse, South Mississippi Home Health, Hattiesburg, Mississippi.

## BOX 39-2

**Sample Home Health Daily Nursing Schedule***

- 7:00 Get ready for the day:
- Check laptop and ensure that the nightly transfer of schedule and patient information completed successfully.

[The laptop stores the vital scheduling information and the patients' electronic medical record and crucial teaching tools to assist the clinician in carrying out the specific plan of care or care path for the patient.] If so, unplug and pack up the laptop for the day. If the transfer did not complete successfully, this message will be present on the laptop and the process must be attempted again. If problems continue, contact the helpdesk at the office for assistance.

- Call office, check overnight voice mail for any last-minute messages.

[Night on-call nurses may have taken calls that require a schedule change, such as notification that a patient has entered the hospital for care.]

- Organize patient visits by priority.

[Some patients require a timed visit due to needed lab studies or the presence of a caregiver to receive instruction.]

- Check nursing bag and automobile to see that all needed supplies are available for assessment and procedures.
- 07:30 Turn on pager and cell phone, grab the lunch cooler. You need to travel about 30 minutes to the outlying community to see your first two patients.
- 08:00 Arrive at Ms. Lottie AAA. Ms. AAA is now testing her blood glucose with minimal prompting. She is praised for her performance and correct entry of the WNL results. Her meal plans for the day are reviewed, and suggestions are made. Instruction on signs and symptoms of hyperglycemia/hypoglycemia is given with handouts of this in pictorial and text form. She is reminded to fast for tomorrow's visit. The visit has lasted an hour and you will travel back toward town to see your next patient.
- 09:15 Arrive at Mr. Ali BBB. His daughter greets you at the door with his daily wt. record and the information that he has gained 3 pounds overnight. He is SOB, resp. 34, pulse is 100, BP is 150/92 mm Hg, temp. 98.3 °F. His 14:00 dose of furosemide is in the mediplanner for the past 2 days. Ausc. of his lung fields, posterior, indicate fine crackles in the lower lobes bilaterally, and the mid lobe on the right. Physician contact is made, and furosemide is given IV as ordered. The patient admits to forgetting medications that don't come at mealtimes. Instruction is given to move the 14:00 dose to noon, and his daughter will call after lunch as a reminder on medications. Signs and symptoms that require contact with the nurse/physician are reiterated. Now vital signs indicate resp. at 26, pulse 92, and BP 132/84. He has voided twice. Arrangements are made to return later in the afternoon for reassessment. A call is placed to the office to move an afternoon visit to tomorrow and the other patient is notified. You have spent an hour and 15 minutes here, and now you travel back into town for your remaining patients.

- 10:50 Arrive at Mr. Carlo CCC. You arrive at his home 15 minutes after the scheduled time with sincere apologies. The old dressing is removed, and the wound is gently cleaned with normal saline. The 0.5-cm measurement reveals that healing is rapidly occurring. Skin preps are applied to the intact skin, a hydrocolloid dressing is placed, and the edges are secured with tape. You continue discharge planning because the wound is nearly healed. A review of pressure relief measures and self-inspection using a mirror are discussed. The patient is eager to return to a more regular routine, and you encourage his plans. His roommate offers coffee, which you graciously decline. Your 40-minute visit is ended with traveling a short distance to the next patient.
- 11:40 Arrive at Ms. Helaria DDD. Maggie, an energetic poodle, has loudly announced your arrival, and she meets you at the door before the bell is rung. You are led to the bedroom for her positional BP checks, but extracting Maggie from the patient's lap is a problem. This accomplished, you find her sitting BP is 138/82, standing BP is 128/80, and supine BP is 144/88. She denies headache, dizziness, back pain, fatigue, dry mouth, or GI upset. She is still unclear about taking the medication because she feels "just fine." You repeat the silent threat of HTN, and the need to take her medication as ordered. She agrees and promises to call if any side effects are noted. At 12:10 you are ready to travel toward the next patient, with a pull-over for lunch.
- 12:15 After your fruit and cheese, you check your voice mail for any messages that may affect your afternoon travel.
- 12:50 Arrive at Mr. Paul EEE. The door is open when you arrive, and he calls out to "come on back." The aide has arrived just before you and is performing his routine care. You check the aide worksheet and note that the POC isn't being followed. You provide the needed supervision and document your findings. Before care can begin, a trip back to the car is needed to bring in sterile syringes. His wound self-care is observed and the wound characteristics noted. The distal wound is irrigated with ½ $H_2O_2$/½ normal saline using an 18-gauge blunt needle. The wound is rinsed with normal saline, packed with NS-moistened gauze packing, covered with gauze sponges, and wrapped with roll gauze. Tape is applied to secure the dressing. Your pager goes off and requires a brief call to one of the patients with medication instruction. Your visit, with interruptions, has lasted an hour and 10 minutes.
- 14:15 Arrive at Mr. Ali BBB. He reports voiding several times since you left. You note that there is no apparent SOB, resp. is 22, pulse is 80, BP is 132/82, and temp. is 98.8 °F. His lungs have only faint scattered crackles in the bases. Instruction is given again regarding which high-potassium foods to include in his diet. He has several bananas on hand and eats one while you talk. His daughter is called at home and reminded to call the agency if signs and symptoms

| BOX 39-2 (CONT.) |
|---|

indicate a fluid increase. This visit is over after 30 minutes, and you leave to return to the office.

- 15:05 Arrive at the office. Attend scheduled in-service training and competency testing at office. Submit notes, verbal order, and check voice mail for tomorrow's assignments and schedule. Load supplies, and return any calls. Make a note in your daily planner about the in-service on laptop use in the home for next Wednesday. Check the on-call schedule and leave a report for the night nurse should Mr. BBB call with continuing problems.
- 15:30 GO HOME. (Your own!) Plug laptop into phone jack and electrical outlet to recharge and be available for the automated data transfer set to occur during the night.

Key for abbreviations: Ausc., auscultation; BP, blood pressure; GI, gastrointestinal; $H_2O_2$, hydrogen peroxide; HTN, hypertension; IV, intravenous; NS, normal saline; POC, plan of care; resp., respirations; SOB, shortness of breath; temp., temperature; WNL, within normal limits; wt., weight.

* Refer to Box 39-1 for a summary description of each patient.

*Source:* Contributed by Jim Jones, RN, BEd, Case Manager Home Health Nurse, South Mississippi Home Health, Hattiesburg, Mississippi.

---

✎ NOTE THIS! •————————————

**What is ADL (Activities of Daily Living)?**
Activities of daily living (ADL) refer to six activities (bathing, dressing, transferring, using the toilet room, eating, and walking) that reflect the patient's capacity for self-care.

---

🔨 ETHICAL CONNECTION

During a home visit to an elderly patient, you notice several empty liquor bottles in the trash and on the kitchen table. The patient's husband is a recovering alcoholic and their 22 year old grandson is living with them while attending college. Would you respond to this observation? What ethical issues exist in the home setting, using this example, as compared to the hospital environment?

---

and nursing. In the home, boundaries between nurse and family as caregivers become blurred, with each party providing essential care to the patient. The home has long been considered the private domain of the family—but it is increasingly becoming the "employment setting" for the home health nurse, where nurse and patient needs intersect. In the hospital, there are often dramatic changes from illness to health; in the community home setting, the changes are often subtle as a chronic disease state emerges as the dominant mode of health and illness. The physician remains the central authority in the hospital; in the home, the autonomy of the family and patient is vital, and maintaining it requires a collaborative effort between caregivers and health providers.

■ Standards of Home Health Nursing

The ANA has endorsed the Standards of Home Health Nursing as the basis for home health nursing practice; these standards are found in Box 39-3. These standards, similar to other nursing practice standards, use the nursing process and identify two levels of nursing practice—the generalist and the specialist—to detail the role and function of the home health nurse. Generalist roles include direct care provider, educator,

resource manager, collaborator, and supervisor of ancillary personnel. The nurse as specialist has a master's degree and serves as consultant, administrator, researcher, and clinical specialist. The nurse in the specialist role may develop and evaluate agency policy, perform staff development, and be responsible for organizing and managing interdisciplinary staffing services.

The nurse in home health nursing must have excellent critical thinking and decision-making skills. In the home health setting, the nurse practices autonomously and without the support of a traditional peer group. In addition, giving care in the home of the patient necessitates a sensitivity for the patient's environment and culture to a much greater degree than does delivering care in other practice settings (Ward-Griffin & McKeever, 2000). Current advances in technology and pharmacology have also resulted in the need for the home care nurse to be increasingly more competent in infusion therapies, complex wound therapies, and advanced computer technologies.

## BOX 39-3

### ANA Standards of Home Health Nursing Practice

**Standard I: Organization of Home Health Services**
All home health services are planned, organized, and directed by a master's-prepared professional nurse with experience in community health and administration.

**Standard II: Theory**
The nurse applies theoretical concepts as a basis for decisions in practice.

**Standard III: Data Collection**
The nurse continuously collects and records data that are comprehensive, accurate, and systematic.

**Standard IV: Diagnosis**
The nurse uses health assessment data to determine nursing diagnoses.

**Standard V: Planning**
The nurse develops care plans that establish goals. The care plan is based on nursing diagnoses and incorporates therapeutic, preventive, and rehabilitative nursing actions.

**Standard VI: Intervention**
The nurse, guided by the care plan, intervenes to provide comfort; to restore, improve, and promote health; to prevent complications and sequelae of illness; and to effect rehabilitation.

**Standard VII: Evaluation**
The nurse continually evaluates the patient's and family's responses to interventions to determine progress toward goal attainment and to revise the database, nursing diagnoses, and plan of care.

**Standard VIII: Continuity of Care**
The nurse is responsible for the patient's appropriate and uninterrupted care along the health care continuum and, therefore, uses discharge planning, case management, and coordination of community resources.

**Standard IX: Interdisciplinary Collaboration**
The nurse initiates and maintains a liaison relationship with all appropriate health care providers to assure that all efforts effectively complement one another.

**Standard X: Professional Development**
The nurse assumes responsibility for professional development and contributes to the professional growth of others.

**Standard XI: Research**
The nurse participates in research activities that contribute to the profession's continuing development of knowledge of home health care.

**Standard XII: Ethics**
The nurse uses the code for nurses established by the American Nurses Association as a guide for ethical decision making in practice.

*Source*: © 2008 American Nurses Association. *Home Health Nursing: Scope and Standards of Practice.* Silver Spring, MD: Nursesbooks.org. Reprinted by permission.

## The Medicare Era

Following the establishment of the Medicare program in 1965, significant growth and change throughout the U.S. health care system created a broad spectrum of health services for the elderly population (Davitt and Choi, 2008). Medicare made home care services, primarily **skilled nursing visits (SNVs)** and curative or restorative therapy, available for all persons older than 65. These services were extended to the disabled population in 1973, and hospice services were added in 1983. **Hospice** services provide **palliative care** and supportive social, emotional, and spiritual services to the terminally ill and their families (NAHCH, 2008).

There were 9,284 Medicare-certified agencies in the United States in 2007 that provided home health services (NAHCH, 2008). The total national expenditure for all health care in the United States was approximately $1.8 billion in 2006. Approximately 62% of total personal care, which is a subset of health care as goods and services used by individuals, went to hospitals and physicians, whereas only 3% was spent on home care (Heffler et al.,

 Research Alert

Hospice nurses know that all their patients will die. There are several potential benefits of including rituals and healing practices into the hospice care setting for staff. Evidence suggests that not only does it provide an outlet for hospice workers to express their grief and reflect on their work in an accepting environment; it provides closure for their patient's passing and has also been shown to decrease the risk of burnout and compassion fatigue. This article discusses the important aspects of grief rituals and provides an illustrative example of one such ritual. ◯

*Source*: Running, A., Tolle, L, & Girard, D. (2008). Ritual: The final expression of care. *International Journal of Nursing Practice, 14*(4), 303–307.

2007; NAHCH, 2008). Medicare is the largest single payer of health care services in the home.

Certainly, one of the primary benefits of health care in the home is that it is significantly less expensive than

BOX 39-4

**Top Five Most Common Diagnosis-Related Groups Referred to Home Health Care**
1. Diabetes
2. Essential Hypertension
3. Heart Failure
4. Chronic Ulcer of the Skin
5. Osteoarthritis

*Source*: Department of Health and Human Services, Office of the Inspector General. (2001). Medicare home health care community beneficiaries 2001 OEI-02-01-00070. Washington, DC: U.S. Government Printing Office.

**MEDIA MOMENT**

***Magnolia* (1999)**
This movie follows the lives of a family and nurse caregiver over the course of one day. Phillip Seymour Hoffman plays the compassionate, skilled, and devoted nurse for the dying father in the home.

in the hospital. Home health care can reduce per-patient expenditures, as well as reduce the number, length, and frequency of hospitalization episodes. For example, an average Medicare charge on a per-day basis for hospital care in 2005 was $5000.00 compared with $504.00 for a skilled nursing facility and only $121.00 for a home health charge per visit (NAHCH, 2008).

More than half the patients who receive home health care are older than 65, and the amount of home health they use tends to increase with age. Approximately 40% of these patients have one or more functional limitations. The most common single diagnostic category for home health services is for diabetes. Diseases and conditions associated with the circulatory system are next, including hypertension and heart failure. These diagnoses are followed in frequency by chronic ulcers of the skin and osteoarthritis. The services provided by home health care nurses focus on assisting the patient to reach or maintain an optimal state of health, independence, and comfort in their home setting. Box 39-4 lists the most common diseases and disorders seen in the home health patient.

The persons who most need home health care require assistance in activities of daily living (National Institute on Disability and Rehabilitation Research, 1996; NAHCH, 2008). **Informal caregivers,** such as family members, friends, and others who provide services on an unpaid basis, provide the bulk of home care with guidance and support from home health professionals.

The provision of care in the patient's place of residence contributes to the unique nature of this part of the health care delivery system. Home care represents a cost-effective and satisfying means of meeting the patient's health care needs (Rice, 2005; Shamansky, 1988). Many factors have contributed significantly to the growth of the home care industry in recent years, including the aging of the U.S. population, advances in technology, shorter inpatient hospital stays, and the increasing availability of outpatient services (Curtin, 2008; Davitt & Choi, 2008). According to Maraldo

(1989, p. 303), "Home care is most suited to become the centerpiece of a new health care delivery system, because survey after survey demonstrates that consumers prefer home care to other types of care."

Many complex therapies previously administered only in hospital intensive care units are now safe and available in the home setting. For example, intravenous (IV) therapy has now become common in the home setting, infusing antibiotics, chemotherapy, analgesics, total parenteral nutrition (TPN), and blood products (Sheldon & Bender, 1994). Pediatric hospitalizations have dropped by 46% significantly in the past 25 years as more procedures and treatments have been done on an outpatient basis and in the home. Pediatric postoperative recovery often occurs in the home (Dougherty, 1998; Curtin, 2008). The ability to provide sophisticated pain control and other comfort measures to the terminally ill, along with an increased understanding and recognition of the importance of preserving dignity in the dying process, have contributed to the growth of hospice services. Often, with the provision of an intermittent skilled service along with the assistance of the home health aide for personal care and exercise therapy, the patient is able to remain in the comforts of his or her own home rather than requiring institutional care (Milone-Nuzzo, 1998; Davitt & Choi, 2008). (See Box 39-5.)

**Research Alert**

This qualitative study of 38 hospice patients examines how people answered questions about what mattered the most to them or was of ultimate concern in their lives at the time of the interviews. Responses participants gave when asked what they found most troubling and of ultimate concern at the time of the interviews are reported here. While this sample of hospice recipients reported that dependence, religious or spiritual matters, incapacitation, and money were matters of concern, the largest response category by far was concern for others.

*Source*: Pevey, C. (2008). Death, god, flesh, and other: Hospice recipients reflect on what matters: *Illness, Crisis & Loss, 16*(3), 203–226.

---

**BOX 39-5**

**Sample Role Description of a Staff Home Health Nurse**

- Establish effective relationships with the patient, family, and other health professionals.
- Collaborate with other health professionals and providers in evaluating the patient's response to the plan of care.
- Develop a discharge plan with the patient and the caregivers as well as the other health professionals.
- Use principles of teaching and learning to educate patients and caregivers in the knowledge and skills that promote self-care and prevention or control of disease progression or disability.
- Participate with patients, their caregivers, and other health professionals in decision making that reflects knowledge of care that is ethical, legal, and informed.
- Identify and discuss ethical conflicts and act as advocate for the patient regarding confidentiality and informed consent.

*Source*: South Mississippi Home Health Agency. (1999). *Hattiesburg, Mississippi, staff registered nurse job description*. Hattiesburg, MS: Author.

---

**BOX 39-6**

**Home Health Agency Classifications**

**Public/governmental agency:** A public or governmental agency is an agency operated by a state or local government. Examples are state-operated health departments and county hospitals.

**Nonprofit agency:** A private, nongovernmental agency exempt from federal income tax. These agencies are often supported, in part, by private contributions or other philanthropic sources, such as foundations. Examples include Visiting Nurse Associations and Easter Seal Societies, as well as nonprofit hospitals.

**Proprietary agency:** A private, profit-making agency or profit-making hospital.

**Institution-based agency:** An institution-based agency can be propriety, nonprofit, official, or voluntary and operates within the organizational structure of a hospital or HMO. The nature of the home health agency will be dictated by the type of hospital structure.

*Source*: Home Health Agency (HHA). (1998). *Med-Manual 2180. Citations and description, state operations manual* (CMS Publication No. 7). Washington, DC: U.S. Government Printing Office.

---

## Types of Home Health Agencies

Home health agency structures vary depending on the type of organization and their corporate structure (Shick & Balinsky, 2006). These differences affect the entity's obligations to local, state, and federal law and regulations. The structure also determines the agency's tax obligation. Agencies are classified as official, nonprofit, proprietary, and institution-based. Box 39-6 describes the various classifications of agencies.

Official agencies are publicly funded units in state or local health departments that are supported by taxes. These agencies provide home health services through legislative statutes. Home health services when offered through official agencies may be provided by community health nurses who also function in various other roles, such as in health promotion and communicable disease prevention. Medicare, Medicaid, and private insurance companies all reimburse for home health services, though the reimbursement formulas used are often complex. Because of the proliferation of private agencies as well as a reevaluation of the priorities for public health for disease prevention, most public health services that provide home health are located in underserved and isolated areas.

Nonprofit home health agencies are made up of voluntary agencies, as well as private, nonprofit agencies. Voluntary agencies are supported by charities such as United Way or private endowments. The earliest Visiting Nurse Associations are examples of voluntary agencies. This type of agency is privately owned and exempt from federal income tax. Such agencies do not receive any state or local tax revenues. Certain nonprofit hospitals may also have home health agencies as part of their community services. These types of agencies are usually governed by boards of directors composed of representatives from the community from which they serve. With the increase in the number of for-profit private agencies in the United States, the number of these agencies has declined in recent years. With voluntary agencies, service is provided based on the patient's need for home health rather than on his or her ability to pay.

Proprietary agencies include private, profit-making agencies and profit-making hospitals. These agencies receive the largest percentage of their revenue through third-party payers. Because of a trend toward a highly competitive, managed care market, many proprietary agencies are now part of national health care organizational chains managed through corporate headquarters. Another trend is the development of alliances among home health care agencies and other agencies that become contracting partners in networks. Proprietary agencies make up approximately 40% of all Medicare-certified agencies.

Institution-based agencies emerged in the 1970s as hospitals began putting a greater emphasis on continuity of care. As the high cost of hospitalization and movement toward diagnosis-related groups (DRGs) led to earlier discharges, hospitals developed their own home health agencies, with their inpatient population serving as the major source of referrals to home health. Under such a structure, patients have the advantage of staying within the same system and enjoy greater ease of movement between and among services. These agencies are second only to proprietary agencies in total number of Medicare-certified agencies in the United States, accounting for approximately 30% of these agencies.

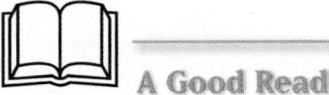

# The House on Henry Street (1915)

*By Lillian Wald, New York: Holt, Rinehart and Winston*

Lillian Wald, who coined the term *public health nursing* and founded the historic Henry Street Settlement in New York City in 1893 for home visiting, is truly a larger than life figure in the field of home health. One of the most influential and respected social reformers of the 20th century, Henry Street Settlement founder Lillian Wald was a tireless and accomplished humanitarian. Born into a life of privilege, Wald came to Manhattan to attend the New York Hospital School of Nursing at age 22. In 1893, Wald founded the Henry Street Settlement and began teaching health and hygiene to immigrant women on the impoverished Lower East Side.

This book, written by Wald, is a fascinating look at her background, passion for delivering quality professional nursing care in the home, and the art and science of providing nursing care in the home. In 1915, at the peak of her career, Wald published the history of Henry Street and her work in *The House on Henry Street*. Dedicated to "the comrades who have built the house," the book became a classic for generations of nursing, sociology, and social welfare students. The settlement's services continued to grow; in 1915 alone 100 nurses cared for more than 26,575 patients and made more than 227,000 home visits.

One day, while teaching, a little girl approached Wald and asked her to attend to her sick mother. The child led her through the tenements, "over broken roadways . . . between tall, reeking houses . . . across a court where open and unscreened closets were promiscuously used by men and women, up into a rear tenement, by slimy steps . . . and finally into the sickroom" where Wald attended to the child's mother. Her encounter with the young girl's family prompted Wald to dedicate her life's work to the tenement community. Wald wrote, "That morning's experience was a baptism of fire. Deserted were the laboratory and academic work of college. I never returned to them . . . I rejoiced that I had training in the care of the sick that in itself would give me an organic relationship to the neighborhood in which this awakening had come." With funding from philanthropists and friends, Wald and Mary Brewster, her friend and colleague, established the Visiting Nurses Service in 1893. By January 1894, the two had visited over 125 families and offered advice to many more. Wald wrote of one of her home visits in a poor, immigrant neighborhood. "Over broken asphalt, over dirty mattresses and heaps of refuse we went . . . There were two rooms and a family of seven not only lived here but shared their quarters with boarders . . . [I felt] ashamed of being a part of society that permitted such conditions to exist . . . What I had seen had shown me where my path lay."

Wald provided leadership to the Settlement until 1930. During that time, she established herself as a national leader of social reform, and as an international crusader for human rights. Wald pioneered public health nursing by placing nurses in public schools and with corporations, and by helping found the National Organization for Public Health Nursing and Columbia University's School of Nursing.

For more information on the Henry Street Settlement that still serves patients in New York City today go to: http://www.henrystreet.org

## ■ Home Health Care Documentation

Before the advent of Medicare and federal reimbursement of home health services, home health care was paid for by patients, primarily through donations and philanthropic organizations. Today, Medicare and Medicaid make up the principal funding sources for home health. Part A (hospital insurance) and Part B (supplemental medical insurance) of Medicare include coverage for home health services. Because Medicare and Medicaid together finance more than 75% of home health services in the United States, the discussion of financing and documentation of care presented here is directed primarily toward meeting Medicare requirements. Medicaid, as a state-administered program, provides a range of home care benefits that vary widely from state to state. Private, third-party health insurance also provides some reimbursement for home health services (Davitt & Choi, 2008).

Because of the reimbursement policies of the Medicare program, accurate and appropriate documentation by the home health nurse is critical to ensure current and future reimbursement of the agency and maintenance of certification of the agency. Documentation activities affect home health to a much greater degree than care delivered in perhaps any other setting (Rice, 2005). Documentation requirements are defined in the Medicare **conditions of participation (CoP).** These documentation requirements have a direct impact on reimbursement for the home health agency. Put simply, the documentation requirements for home health care are among the most stringent seen in any health care settings. Each professional note of documentation must demonstrate a skilled level of care and must be inclusive of all care rendered. The professional nurse is responsible for documenting the supervision of the licensed practice nurse (LPN) as well as the home health aide. As Lovejoy (1997) states, "Because visits and supplies translate to costs, nurses enter the front-line of margin producing responsibility when moving from hospital or other settings to home care" (p. 12).

Disease state management (DSM) is an emerging approach to population disease managed care that considers all elements of home health care in an integrated fashion, rather than each one factor separately as in traditional outcome management (Davitt & Choi, 2008). Clinical pathways are outcome driven, with specific time frames outlined for expected courses of recovery. The home health nurse participates in controlling the timing and coordination of the practice patterns to achieve the desired outcome set for the patient. Because multiple providers and team members from different practice settings are involved, they all share in the responsibility and accountability of outcomes.

DSM identifies a standardized approach to patients within a population defined by a particular disease they all have in common (Davitt & Choi, 2008; Schneider et al., 2008). Disease management improves the health of certain patient populations while cutting the costs to the health care delivery system. Although DSM is not strictly equivalent to managed care, it is associated with managed care as an effective way to reduce total costs of care. DSM has been most effective when applied to management of chronic diseases. Many managed plans are implementing DSM, which standardizes care in all settings, including the home.

Martin, Scheet, and Stegman (1993) provide this example of how DSM works. Consider the population of people with diabetes and the role played by the examination of feet. Diabetes is an expensive disease, and amputations are common, costly outcomes of poorly managed diabetes. The following question might be asked by managers of a health care facility: "Do we have more diabetic amputations in our home health agency than the national average?" (A benchmark, such as a state or national statistic, is always used as the basis for DSM.) If the answer is yes, an examination begins with a review of all patients with diabetes in that agency. Data from the electronic clinical records, which are housed within the agency's database, are analyzed to determine how patients with diabetes are cared for, from the physician to the home health nurse to the family caregiver to the patient himself or herself. Through such an analysis, it might be discovered that observation of the feet, while widely known to be a part of the assessment of a person with diabetes, has not been consistently executed by all caregivers. Research directs this intervention, based on the knowledge that routine observation of the feet not only provides the opportunity to detect early signs of poor circulation, but also gives the patient a chance to learn what to look for in a self-examination. If the caregivers conduct these assessments, along with the home health patient, fewer amputations should occur. A new policy is implemented: "At every patient encounter, examine the feet of diabetic patients and at that time, teach them to do the exam themselves." This policy is shared with everyone who has any contact with the patient.

A year later, amputation rates are again examined. A predicable change should have occurred: There should be a decline in the amputation rate. As this example suggests, populations with other chronic conditions, such as asthma, hypertension, and sinusitis, can also benefit from the application of DSM (Hickey, 1998).

The challenges of DSM are related to the expense of implementing such an approach. When DSM is applied to a population, there will be additional time and visits on the front end, patient education programs will be necessary, and additional staff may need to be hired to manage the information system. Patients are managed by protocol and are given the information they (and their caregivers) need in a standardized format at every encounter. Support is provided so that patients can manage their chronic disease. All members of the health care team must be involved, from the pharmacist to the social worker. There is a heavy emphasis on teaching patients why, when, and how to take medications and how to manage the plan of care. Community organizations, such as the American Lung Association, are used for support and educational resources.

Clinical practice guidelines are now available for the most commonly seen chronic diseases in the population (Schwartz, 1997). Disease management programs will continue to expand in the future as outcomes research and database integration provide a continuum of care from hospital to home (Remington, 1997; Schneider et al., 2008). Box 39-7 describes DSM concepts and guidelines. Box 39-8 provides proper documentation language.

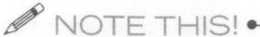

**NOTE THIS!**

**How is home health paid for?**
- Medicare
- Medicaid
- Private insurance
- Payment by individual or "out of pocket"

---

## BOX 39-7

**Disease State Management Concepts**

**Coordination of Primary and Specialty Care**
1. Referrals are coordinated from one provider to another.
2. Patients are treated by the most appropriate caregiver in the most appropriate setting.

**Practice Guidelines**
1. The optimal approach to patient care is established.
2. Providers are educated to follow the established practice guidelines given the patients' individual needs.
3. Patient care and cost-effective treatment are enhanced.
4. Patients achieve optimal outcomes.

**Patient Education and Empowerment**
1. Patients are educated in appropriate self-care.
2. Health awareness is increased, and complications are decreased.

**Preventive Care and Wellness**
1. Individuals at risk for a given disease are targeted.
2. Individuals are taught wellness and prevention strategies.
3. Future complications and costs are minimized.

# Financing and Payment Systems for Home Health Services

## ■ Medicare

The U.S. federal government, through the Centers for Medicare and Medicaid Services (CMS), contracts with regional insurance companies or fiscal intermediaries to provide reimbursement for home care services. To qualify for Medicare benefits for their patient population, home health agencies must follow the federal regulatory requirements called conditions of participation (CoP). The CoP for home health agencies and hospice services define the requirements that an agency must meet to participate in the Medicare program. They are detailed and prescriptive. Requirements related to organizational structure, patients' rights, and the covered disciplines, which include skilled nursing, physical therapy, speech therapy, occupational therapy, home health aides, and medical social services, are all specified in the CoP. The CoP also address the specific skilled services that each of these disciplines can provide, training requirements for aides, and other requirements that the agency must abide by to become an approved provider of Medicare home care or hospice services. The standards set forth in the CoP not only stipulate what agencies must do to qualify for Medicare, but also form the basis for evaluation of the quality of the services provided. Each agency must incorporate these requirements in its policies and procedures. The home health agency must follow these policies and procedures with absolute compliance to the regulations to ensure Medicare reimbursement of visits.

### Medicare Payment for an Episode of Care

Under the current Medicare program, home health services are paid for either on a fee-for-service basis, or on an episode-of-care basis. The Medicare Program defines an episode of care as being 60 days in length. Payment for the 60-day episode of care is determined by the results of the Outcomes and Assessment Information Set (OASIS)—an assessment data set that groups patients into payment episodes for reimbursement purposes. This data set, which is used to determine patient outcomes of care, is completed at specific time points throughout the patient's course of home health care. A number of circumstances might result in the payment rate for the episode being prorated for the agency—for example, if the patient required four or fewer visits in a 60-day episode (Schneider et al., 2008).

As previously discussed, documentation requirements and record-keeping standards must be adhered to strictly and are primary responsibilities of the home health care nurse. The completion of these tasks is required to ensure coverage for the care rendered. The visit and progress notes completed by the direct care staff are essential to justifying the need for the services rendered. Each visit made by the agency must be considered "reasonable and necessary" to the plan of treatment established by the physician for Medicare to consider the service to be covered. The fiscal intermediaries for Medicare are responsible for reviewing a portion of the agency's clinical documentation on an ongoing basis. This scrutiny is intended to ascertain that the services provided by the agency were appropriately ordered by the physician, were reasonable and necessary, and met the qualifying and coverage criteria for payment.

Agencies are responsible for filing detailed cost reports. These cost reports identify expenditures made by the agency in providing direct care to the patient, including the number of complete and prorated episodes of care, the number of visits made per discipline, the number of Medicare patients, and indirect care such as administration and other overhead expenses. This cost report is used to determine the future rate setting and payment levels for the Medicare Home Health Program.

The CoPs require that the patient meet several qualifying criteria to receive covered services by the Medicare program. These qualifying criteria for home health services are that the patient (1) be under the care of a physician, (2) be essentially confined to the home, and (3) require skilled services of a registered nurse, physical therapist, or speech pathologist on an intermittent basis. Box 39-9 lists

### Got an Alternative?

On a home health visit, a nurse discovers that his patient is using numerous over-the-counter vitamins and herbal supplements not previously identified by the home health agency admission nurse on a previous visit. The patient states, "I told the first nurse who came here that I was taking these but did not want my doctor to know so to please not write them down in my record." How should the nurse respond to the patient and to the other agency nurse about these unidentified vitamins and supplements?

some general questions that can guide the nurse in the documentation of homebound status.

The physician must certify that the patient is essentially homebound and establish an individual **plan of care (POC)** for the patient. The POC is established by the physician in collaboration with the home health team and must be updated as changes occur in the patient's condition, or at least every 60 days. The nurse plays a key role in establishing the POC for both home care and hospice, in collaboration with the physician and with other health team members. The POC is based on the patient's health history and a current comprehensive assessment of the patient's physical, psychological, social, and spiritual needs inclusive of the OASIS data set. The nurse's knowledge of the resources available in the community is very important to establish the plan that will optimally meet the patient's needs (Cho, 2005). Box 39-10 summarizes the concepts of Medicare criteria for home health patients.

### ■ Medicaid

Medicaid is authorized by Title XIX of the Social Security Act and provides health services to low-income persons. As a source of reimbursement for home health services, Medicaid is federally aided but state operated and state administered. Each state determines program eligibility, benefits covered, and the rates of payment for providers in that state.

Clinical guidelines for Medicaid reimbursement basically follow those of the Medicare program. Medicaid covers home health services, including skilled and unskilled services. If a

---

#### BOX 39-9

**General Questions to Guide the Nurse in Documentation of Homebound Status**

- How often does the patient leave home for social reasons?
- How long does he or she stay gone?
- How taxing or difficult is it for the patient to leave home?
- What kind of assistive devices are used when the patient leaves home?

*Source:* Courtesy of North Mississippi Medical Center Home Health and Hospice.

---

patient qualifies for both Medicare and Medicaid, Medicare is generally the primary reimbursement source. A comparison of Medicare and Medicaid benefits appears in Table 39-1.

### ■ Private Insurance

For a growing number of home health patients, private insurance offered by a third-party payer in the private sector provides reimbursement for home health care services. Three

---

### GLOBAL CONNECTION

Home health in the United States is often very different from home visiting programs in other countries. Do an Internet search on home health services in France or Canada and identify the differences in purpose, funding, and utilization of home health services as compared to the United States.

---

### Research Alert

Patients with heart failure represent a common patient population in home health care, yet little is known about their outcomes. Patients with heart failure, regardless of site of care, experience substantial numbers of rehospitalizations in the United States. Home health care is a common post-acute care service for patients with heart failure. The study used a retrospective design and employed a large administrative data base from 2003—the Outcomes and Assessment Information Set, which is required for all U.S. Medicare and Medicaid patients receiving home health care. There were 145,191 patients with a primary diagnosis of heart failure represented in the data set. The outcomes of interest were the trajectory of care (point of entry and discharge from home health care), hospitalization, length of stay, and change in functional status. Almost three-quarters (73.9%) of patients entered home health care following a hospital stay. Nearly two-thirds (64%) remained at home at discharge from home health care. Approximately 15% of patients are hospitalized during the home health care episode, most often for symptoms consistent with exacerbation of the heart failure, if a reason could be identified. The average length of stay in home health care was 44 days. There was only a small improvement in functional status: 0.50 points for activities of daily living and 0.57 points for instrumental activities of daily living. Similar small improvement occurred in depressive symptoms, 0.68. There may be room for improvement in these outcomes with more recent evidence that suggests strategies for reducing hospitalization and improving patient functional status abilities. Yet, the chronic progressive nature of heart failure may also provide a limiting factor in the outcomes that can be attained.

*Source:* Madigan, E. A. (2008). People with heart failure and home health care resource use and outcomes. Journal of Clinical Nursing, 17(7B), 253–259.

## BOX 39-10

### Summary of Medicare Criteria for Home Health Patients

**Qualifying Criteria for a Medicare Beneficiary to Receive Home Health Services**
- Essentially confined to the home
- Under a plan of care established by a physician
- In need of intermittent skilled nursing, physical, or speech therapy

**Covered Services for Home Health**
- Skilled nursing
- Physical therapy
- Speech therapy
- Occupational therapy
- Home health aide
- Medical social services

**Qualifying Criteria for a Medicare Beneficiary to Receive Hospice Services**
- A life expectancy of 6 months or less
- Seeking palliative treatment only

**Hospice Interdisciplinary Team**
- Registered nurse
- Physician
- Pastor/counselor
- Medical social services

major types of organizations provide this type of reimbursement: indemnity insurance companies that pay a percentage of billed charges, nonprofit Blue Cross and Blue Shield, and health maintenance organizations (HMOs). As more managed care networks emerge as reimbursement mechanisms, HMOs are growing in number and scope in comprehensive health care services. The services provided in the private sector vary by payer, but most often the documentation and clinical guidelines follow Medicare standards for reimbursement (Cochran & Brennan, 1998; Shick & Balinsky, 2006).

### ■ Payment by Individual

Individuals who do not have health insurance, those who do not meet their insurance coverage requirements, or those who do not qualify for federal assistance may pay the established charges by the agency or be allowed to pay on a sliding scale based on income. Patients who no longer qualify for Medicare or Medicaid may also desire home health care services and continue to pay after certification has expired. Each agency has its own policies concerning both payments by individual and medically indigent care, which may be provided at no charge.

## Quality Assurance and Public Accountability

### ■ Regulation and Licensure

In addition to Medicare requirements, most states require that home health and hospice agencies be licensed to operate within their state. Agencies operating in states that require licensure must abide by the state's minimum standards for licensure, in addition to the regulations included in the CoPs. The CMS, under the direction of the Department of Health and Human Services, contracts with state licensing and certification authorities to provide survey and audit services for the purposes of certifying home care agencies to participate in the Medicare program. Surveys are performed at regular intervals, and at least every 3 years to ensure compliance with state licensure requirements and continued certification to participate in the Medicare and Medicaid programs. These surveys may be conducted more often for new providers or providers that had deficiencies on their previous evaluations. These surveys involve record reviews, staff and patient interviews, and home visits. The purpose of the survey process is to ascertain that all regulations are being met in providing home care services to the Medicare and Medicaid beneficiaries. State authorities are responsible for responding to and investigating any complaints lodged against the agency and initiating any action indicated through the appropriate regulatory body.

### ■ Quality Assurance in Home Health

In 2000, as part of a broad quality improvement initiative, the federal government began requiring that every Medicare-certified home health agency complete and submit health assessment information for their patients. The instrument/data collection tool used to collect and report performance data by home health agencies is called the Outcome and

**Table 39-1**  A Comparison of Medicare and Medicaid in Home Health Reimbursement

| Medicare (Title XVIII) | Medicaid (Title XIX) |
|---|---|
| ■ Age 65 and older or disabled | ■ Income-based eligibility |
| ■ Homebound status | ■ Homebound status not always required |
| ■ Intermittent service | ■ Intermittent service |
| ■ Skilled service | ■ Skilled service not always required |
| ■ Restorative services | ■ Custodial and maintenance services |
| ■ Physician certification required | ■ Physician certification required |
| ■ Medical, therapy, or social service | ■ State option: medical, therapist, or social service |
| ■ Provides rental and purchase payments | ■ Provides purchase payments |
| ■ Reimbursement: "reasonable cost" | ■ Reimbursement: maximum allowed, determined by state |

Assessment Information Set (OASIS). Since fall 2003, CMS has posted on www.medicare.gov a subset of OASIS–based quality performance information showing how well home health agencies assist their patients in regaining or maintaining their ability to function. Measures of how well people can get along in their homes performing activities of daily living (ADLs) form a core of the measures, but these are supplemented with questions about physical status and use-of-service measures (hospitalization and emergent care).

In 2004 and 2005, a private nonprofit organization, the National Quality Forum (NQF), convened technical experts representing varying perspectives to review quality measures for home health care. Following a long review and consensus development process, the group endorsed measures for use in public reporting. The 2005 measures (all collected via the OASIS data set) are:

- Improvement in ambulation/locomotion
- Improvement in bathing
- Improvement in transferring
- Improvement in management of oral medication
- Improvement in pain interring with activity
- Acute care hospitalization
- Emergent care
- Discharge to community
- Improvement in dyspnea (shortness of breath)
- Improvement in urinary incontinence

NQF had previously endorsed additional measures and two of those related to wounds were added to Home Health Compare in December of 2007. Several more previously endorsed measures may be added in 2009 (CMS, 2008).

Another part of the HHS/CMS quality initiative includes Quality Improvement Organizations (QIOs). QIOs exist in each state and are private organizations that contract with CMS to help improve the quality of care provided to Medicare patients. In addition to assisting beneficiaries with complaints about the quality of care they receive, physicians and other healthcare experts work with home health agencies to encourage the adoption, use, and monitoring of best practices and quality measures. These best practice measures will assist agencies in adapting to process measures in testing for future OASIS revisions.

While the current home health assessment and reporting tool, OASIS, will remain in use in the foreseeable future, several new priorities have emerged and are expected to be part of planning for the future, including Pay for Performance which ties a portion of reimbursement to delivery of care. The generalist nurse will always be involved in the quality improvement process, whether data collecting, planning, implementing, evaluating or being the performance improvement project quality manager. Quality improvement is a continuous process tool used to assist in the goal of delivering excellent patient care (Schneider, Barkauskas, & Keenan, 2008; CMS, 2008).

Monitoring systems have been established which require agencies to report certain quality indicator data to CMS for the Home Health Quality Initiative. These quality indicator data are linked to payment, thus being a critical influence in the home health nurse's documentation and reporting of care. Agency submission of quality data was mandated beginning in 2007, with financial penalties for failure to submit (CMS, 2007; Davitt & Choi, 2008). The focus is on providing consumers with information on the practice effectiveness of home health agencies. In addition, some analysts have recommended incorporating Medicare–agency risk sharing in relation to profit–loss margins and/or tying agency payment to outcome indicators.

The Home Health Compare Web site is one of the central features of the Home Health Quality Initiative (http://www.medicare.gov/HHCompare/Home.asp). The goal of Home Health Compare is to provide quality of care information to consumers to help them make more informed decisions about home health care service providers (Home Health Compare, 2008). The Home Health Quality Initiative is part of an ongoing Department of Health and Human Services effort that also focuses on improving the quality of care in nursing homes and hospitals. Public reporting is also intended to stimulate and support providers and clinicians to improve the quality of care provided. Home Health Compare is one of a number of search tools and other valuable information available at the public Medicare Web site, http://www.medicare.gov/. Consumers can search for Medicare certified home health agencies by selecting a state and entering a county or zip code. The result is a list of agencies with addresses and phone numbers as well as the Medicare-covered services the agencies offer, the initial date of Medicare certification, and type of ownership. The search function is based on the zip code entered for OASIS item M0060,

---

### 🖥️ Research Alert

Applying Roy's Adaptation Model, the purposes of this study were to explore hospice support of family caregivers in their decision to provide care at home and the relationships between hospice support, coping, and spiritual well-being. Data were collected in home visits of 21 recently bereaved family caregivers of hospice patients. Instruments included a demographic questionnaire, a Hospice Social Support questionnaire, the Jalowiec Coping Scale, the Spiritual Well-Being Scale, and a postbereavement interview. Hospice workers were frequently identified as providing significant emotional support making the caregiver feel highly cared for, respected, and supported. Subjects scored moderately high on the SWB Scale and reported low use of coping strategies. A significant negative correlation was found between reported use of coping strategies and hospice support. Hospice family caregivers rated this support highly as a major factor in making and sustaining the home care decision. ◯

*Source*: Hunt Raleigh, E., Robinson, J., Marold, K., & Jamison, M. (2006). Family caregiver perception of hospice support. *Journal of Hospice & Palliative Nursing,* 8(1), 25–33.

## Application to Practice

Mrs. Mae Thompson is a 68-year-old woman. Her referral diagnosis is congestive heart failure. Mrs. Thompson was discharged from Baxterville General Hospital after a 5-day stay. She lives with her 75-year-old sister in a two-bedroom house in a small rural community.

Upon arrival at the home, the health nurse finds Mrs. Thompson lying in bed. Her sister is watching television in the living room. During the visit, Mrs. Thompson relates the history of her illness. About a month ago, she noticed swelling in her feet and legs and extreme shortness of breath while picking tomatoes from her garden. She had to rest after picking only a small bucket of tomatoes. She also noticed that she had to stop midway between the house and the mailbox to catch her breath. Mrs. Thompson recalled that she had to use two or more pillows to breathe easy enough to sleep. She began awakening during the night with shortness of breath and had to sit up in the bedside chair to "get her breath back again" before going back to sleep. She also reported getting up several times a night to urinate, which was a change in her usual habits. She grew increasingly more concerned about herself when she became so fatigued that she neglected her garden crops.

The nurse, when conducting a medication review, found that Mrs. Thompson had been taking digoxin following a myocardial infarction 9 months earlier. Immediately before the present symptoms began, Mrs. Thompson has discontinued taking the digoxin because "I felt fine and didn't think I needed it anymore."

Mrs. Thompson's present medications are as follows: digoxin 0.25 mg/day, furosemide (Lasix) 40 mg/day, and KCl 20% tsp per day in juice. She reports that she is taking the "heart pill" but has stopped the "fluid pill" because it makes her have to urinate frequently and getting up makes her dizzy. She took the "other liquid" for about 2 days but has since quit taking it "because it makes the juice taste funny." Since her discharge from the hospital, Mrs. Thompson has required assistance with self-care and is using a wheelchair for most ambulation. She spends much of her day in bed, because "I feel so weak, I can't stand for very long." Her physician told her to "cut down on her salt," and she was given a diet sheet in the hospital, which she misplaced before reading it. She has a return appointment to see her physician in 2 weeks.

Mrs. Thompson's breakfast today consisted of two fried eggs, two pork sausage patties, two slices of toast with butter and jelly, and two cups of regular coffee. She is complaining of shortness of breath and is expressing frustration that "I will never be able to grow my own vegetables again." Her legs are extremely swollen with 3+ pitting edema; they are cool to the touch. Mrs. Thompson does not have socks on. She reports that she is concerned about her sister's "back problems" and that she fears relying on her too much for care such as bathing and ambulating. Her vital signs are as follows: blood pressure, 140/90 mm Hg; pulse, 54 beats/min; and respiratory rate, 24 breaths/min.

1. Based on the preceding information, is Mrs. Thompson homebound?
2. Identify two nursing goals for Mrs. Thompson.
3. What action would you take regarding Mrs. Thompson's physical findings?
4. Identify one nursing goal related to Mrs. Thompson's caregiver.
5. What further information would you need about Mrs. Thompson?

and finds any agency that provided service in the area specified within the last year.

Once agencies are located in the search, consumers can view data on 11 quality measures that provide information about how well the home health agency provides care for some of their patients. This information should assist the healthcare consumer to make an informed decision when choosing a home health agency.

## ■ Accreditation

Accreditation of agencies is another aspect of quality assurance. Unlike state licensure, however, it is not required for Medicare or Medicaid participation. Accreditation is a demonstration of a commitment to providing a high standard of excellence in the delivery of care. Some third-party payers, such as managed care networks or insurance companies, may require accreditation. To meet the stringent standards of accreditation, an agency must demonstrate a team effort from all involved in the delivery of care (Lovejoy, 1997).

Three nationally recognized organizations provide voluntary accreditation for home health agencies: the Joint Commission's Home Care Accreditation Program (JCHCA); the Community Health Accreditation Program (CHAP), a subsidiary of the National League for Nursing (NLN); and the National Home Caring Council.

Home health nurses work with the family caregiver to implement the plan of care.

## Managed Care and Home Health

Managed care has become the dominant pattern of organizational reimbursement in the United States. As a result, most persons in the United States with private health insurance are in some type of managed care arrangement or network. A majority of states are in some form of Medicaid managed care program. Managed care will influence nursing practice as agencies respond to strong incentives to lower costs. As has been discussed, nursing interventions and their effectiveness will be measured against patient outcomes and patient satisfaction of care (Lin et al., 2006). Home health nurses will continue to focus on the family as caregiver, with a greater emphasis on teaching the family/caregiver more effective ways of caring for the patient. With increasing responsibilities resting with the caregiver, more efficient use of the nurse's time can occur resulting in shorter illness episodes. All home health nurses must be effective case managers to ensure that the highest quality care is delivered in the shortest time possible (Peters & Eigsti, 1991; Duke & Street, 2003).

The Balanced Budget Act of 1997 mandated that the CMS implement a prospective payment system (PPS) for home health by federal fiscal year 2000. The prospective payment system for home health is similar to the methodology used for hospitals since 1981 and for skilled nursing facilities beginning in 1998. In 1981, hospital reimbursement by the Medicare program changed from a cost-based reimbursement system to a prospective payment system using DRGs as the basis for reimbursement (Jester & Hicks, 2003). Skilled nursing facility reimbursement is a prospective rate varied by a "case-mix adjuster." This case-mix adjuster is determined from information collected in a standardized data collection tool designed to measure patients' need for additional care and services. Case-mix adjustment in the home health setting is accomplished in a similar manner using the OASIS data set. Managed health care plans, such as HMOs,

preferred provider organizations (PPOs), and networks, are providing home care services as part of their health plans at an increasing rate (Schneider et al., 2008; Kim et al., 2006).

Managed care plans generally reimburse home health agencies based on a fee-for-service or capitated rate methodology. A **fee-for-service rate** is generally based on a per-visit or hourly rate for each discipline. A **capitated rate** is generally awarded based on a population or group of "lives" for which the agency is paid a "per member per month" rate. Reimbursement of this nature requires that the agency make an estimation of the anticipated needs of the population to determine if the arrangement is financially feasible (Spector et al., 2004; McKnight, 2006).

As the focus in managed care shifts to outcomes of care, research linking outcomes to care delivery has resulted in Medicare's OASIS: Standardized Outcome and Assessment Information Set for Home Health Care. Shaughnessy (1996) developed the OASIS instrument as a data set with the following categories of items: demographics and patient history, living arrangements, supportive assistance, body systems, activities of daily living/independent activities of daily living (ADL/IADL), medications, equipment management, and emergent care. Data are collected for a patient upon admission to the home health agency, at a specified time during care, and upon discharge of home health services. OASIS is used to measure outcomes of care based on the home health interventions provided. The instrument is mandated by Medicare and is the condition of participation for certified home health agencies. These data are being used by the CMS to provide information about the population of Medicare and Medicaid patients receiving home health care and their clinical outcomes.

### 🖳 Research Alert

Although disease management is often considered oriented toward treatment, the emerging paradigm for prevention of osteoporotic fractures in postmenopausal women is changing. Conventional wisdom backed by previous research has considered menopausal women to have little opportunity for building bone resulting from calcium loss of aging. With new diagnostic procedures, such as bone densitometry, and recently developed drugs, such as biphosphonates and deselective estrogen-receptor modulators, there is increasing optimism that bone mass can be regained. Even when treatment is begun in women in their sixties and seventies, fractures can be prevented through increased bone-building interventions. Implications for home health nurses are to educate older women about the use of such pharmacological agents, weight-bearing exercises, calcium intake, and the need for bone density screening tests. ◯

*Source*: Ettinger, B. (1998). Disease management: Maintaining skeletal health among postmenopausal women. *American Journal of Managed Care*, 4(3), 387–396.

## *a conversation with . . .*

You have to be prepared for anything in home health. Home health nurses use the nursing process just like other nurses; one difference is that they begin the assessment when they pull into the driveway or yard. The nurse may see a 2-month-old for an evaluation for failure to thrive at 8:00 A.M., a 10-year-old for post-appendectomy nonhealing surgical wound care at 9:30 A.M., and a 101-year-old for catheter care at 10:45 A.M. I believe that more than any other nursing care, the art and science of nursing must hold hands in home health. You must know how to administer a high-powered antibiotic IV, know the science and possess the skill it calls for to do it properly. And at the same time, the home health nurse must use the art of caring when a patient hammers a nail into his wall for you to hang that IV on when the medical equipment company fails to deliver the IV pole on time. The true art is to use the patient's nail and tell him how important he is in the delivery of his care.

—Ilene Purvis Bloxsom, RN, BSN, MSHA
home health nurse

Home health nurses see a variety of patients with diverse health care needs.

## Interdisciplinary Team Approach in Home Health

Collaboration is mandatory in home health nursing. In fact, Medicare requires an interdisciplinary team approach for agencies to be Medicare certified. A collaborative approach is clearly evident in the definitions and standards of home health nursing. Collaboration is necessary to ensure the continuity of care as the patient moves from hospital to home. *Discharge* has traditionally referred to the patient's exit from the hospital to the home; in today's fluid health care system, patients are transitioned in and out of different realms of agency service, necessitating complex professional referrals. To be in legal compliance with federal regulatory statutes, the physician must certify the plan of treatment for the patient. In most instances, it becomes the responsibility of other team members to evaluate the patient's status and response to treatment and then, with the physician, modify the plan of treatment accordingly.

The nurse serves as manager or coordinator of care for this interdisciplinary team effort. To function in this role, the nurse must have a clear understanding of the roles of the other team members as well as a working knowledge of community resources. Traditionally, the roles and functions of the home care nurse have been that of direct care provider, educator, and case manager or coordinator of care. Direct care activities or skills include assessments, performing procedures and treatments, and patient and family teaching. Indirect care includes ancillary personnel supervision, refer-

rals, consultation, and team conferences. The nurse assesses and identifies the problems and needs. Referrals to other disciplines and community agencies may be needed, and this care is coordinated by the nurse under the direction of the physician. For example, if a nurse identifies a home health patient who is having financial difficulty owing to out-of-pocket deductibles for necessary equipment, a referral to a social worker would be appropriate (Boxer & Meadows, 2008).

Within an interdisciplinary model, the unit of care should be the family, and nursing care is designed and provided within the context of the community in which the patient lives. The home care nurse cares for patients across the life span with multiple medical diagnoses and responses to illness. Health promotion and disease prevention are the focus of care. The nurse develops a POC under the direction of a physician with the assistance of a multidisciplinary team, which becomes the home health care team and may include social workers, therapists, chaplains, nutritionists, and others as appropriate. The patient also participates in developing his or her plan of care, and evaluating, along with the team, the outcomes of care. The nurse and team members plan their visit schedule around patient preferences, other

## BOX 39-11

### Members of the Home Health Care Interdisciplinary Team

- *Home health nurse* is the traditional provider of care in the home. Home health nurses provide skilled nursing services and coordinate care within the interdisciplinary team.
- *Physician* refers patients for home care services and approves the plan of care.
- *Home health aides* provide personal care that includes activities such as bathing, shaving, and skin and nail care. The home health aide also performs basic tasks that include things such as emptying urinary drainage bags, taking vital signs, assisting with ambulation and performing exercises assigned, and light homemaking activities such as preparing a meal, changing linens, cleaning room, and laundry.
- *Physical therapists* provide evaluation of the patient's rehabilitation needs and potential, which may include areas such as range of motion, strength, balance and coordination, gait analysis, muscle tone, pain, endurance, equipment needs, and home safety. The physical therapist then develops and implements the treatment plan that includes teaching the patient and family the home therapy regime and establishing a maintenance therapy program.
- *Speech therapists* provide services related to the evaluation of rehabilitation needs and potential in patients with speech and language disorders and swallowing disorders. The speech therapist develops and implements a restorative treatment program involving the patient and family.
- *Occupational therapists* focus on evaluation and treatment of the patient's upper extremities by assisting to restore muscle strength and mobility for functional skills. The program established is designed to restore physical function and sensory-integrative function or develop compensatory techniques. Vocational and prevocational assessment and training, as well as design and fitting of orthotic and self-help devices, are also provided by the occupational therapist.
- *Medical social workers* provide assessment of the social and emotional factors related to the patient's illness and plan of treatment. This includes assessment of the relationship of the patient's medical/nursing requirements to the home situation, financial resources, and community resources. The Medical social worker may provide counseling for the patient related to areas such as depression, addictions, reaction/adjustment to illness, and strengthening family support systems. Counseling for the patient's family may be necessary to treat the patient's illness/injury in resolving family problems that are obstructing or preventing the patient's treatment.

discipline visits, physician appointments, and geographic areas (Milton 2005).

Appropriate planning by all disciplines before the visit is essential. This includes laboratory work or any supplies needed, along with the activities of the visit that center on the goals set for the patient in the previously established POC. Some agencies have care maps or critical paths that define the day-to-day activities and outcomes to be met during each visit; others use goals established on admission and modify them as appropriate. Detailed descriptions of mem-

ber roles of the home health care interdisciplinary team can be found in Box 39-11.

## Role of Family Caregivers in Home Health

As community health nurses have long been aware, home health nurses contribute less to the well-being of a home health patient than the more significant influence of family caregivers. Informal caregiving provided by family caregivers is an integral part of our health care system (Milton, 2005; Bradley, 2003). Among people 45 and older, approximately 2 in 5 report some experience with long-term care in their families. As the population ages, the demand for informal, family caregivers will escalate over the next 30 years. Home health patients would be unable to stay in their homes even to be the recipient of home health nursing care were it not for the family members and other caregivers who dedicate themselves to their care.

Community health nurses have traditionally been family oriented when conducting home visits. One need only look at our legacy of Lillian Wald and the Henry Street nurses to see the foundation of family-oriented care. (See A Good Read on p. 977.) Only when the family becomes recognized as the unit of service within the context of the larger community can significant, long-lasting change occur.

With the ever-present influence of Medicare and other funding sources, however, today's nurses often focus their care efforts on providing only those services that are reimbursable in the home setting. The individual ill patient has steadily become the focus in home care, with the family and other caregivers fading to a contextual backdrop (Bradley, 2003; Davitt & Choi, 2008; Kenyon, Smith, Hefty, Bell, McNeil, & Maraus, 1990).

Recent research has revealed that the family caregivers of home health patients often have unmet health needs and

 NOTE THIS!

### Who Are the Caregivers?

The 2004 caregiving in the United States survey, sponsored by the National Alliance for Caregiving and AARP, documented the prevalence of caregiving in the United States. The study found that more than one in five U.S. households (an estimated 44.4 million caregivers over age 18) are informal caregivers for a person older than age 18. This report also showed that 62% of caregivers are married and/or living with a partner, and nearly two-thirds (61%) are women. The typical caregiver is a 46-year-old woman with at least some college experience who provides more than 20 hours of care each week to her mother.

*Source:* National Alliance for Caregiving and AARP. *Caregiving in the U.S.* (2004). Retrieved September 7, 2008, from http:www.caregiving.org/data04finalreport.pdf

**"** *What you do speaks so loud that I cannot hear what you say.* **"**

—*Ralph Waldo Emerson*

### Research Alert

The aim of this research study was to explore and interpret the diverse subject of positions, or roles that nurses construct when caring for patients in their own home. Ten interviews were analyzed and interpreted using discourse analysis. The findings show that these nurses working in home care constructed two positions: "guest" and "professional." They had to make a choice between these positions because it was impossible to be both at the same time. An ethics of care and an ethics of justice were present in these positions, both of which create diverse ethical appeals, that is, implicit demands to perform according to a guest or to a professional norm. ◯

*Source*: Öresland, S., Määttä, S., Norberg, A., Winther Jörgensen, M., & Lützén, K. (2008). Nurses as guests or professionals in home health care. *Nursing Ethics, 15*(3), 371–383.

that the role of caregiver is associated with high stress and increased illness when compared with similar populations. This role, which is often unpaid, is associated with isolation and selfless dedication to the health of the home health patient (Levine, 1999). Quite often, the caregiver is the only other adult in the home and, as such, has little choice about being the one responsible for the household and ill patient. Many studies report that family caregivers tend to be female and themselves in late adulthood (see Bradley, 2003; Bull, 1990; Pruchno & Potashnik, 1989; Kiecolt-Glaser, Glaser, Shuttleworth, Dyer, Ogrocki, & Speicher, 1987).

The community health nurse must strive to consider these caregivers in the assessment of the environment and resources, because if the family caregiver has unmet health needs, eventually his or her caretaking abilities will be affected. Zelwesky and Deitrick (1987, p. 77) go so far as to state, "Accurate needs assessment of the patient and his or her family may prevent family burn-out, extend care-giving abilities, conserve family resources, and delay or prevent institutionalization." In her 1996 study, Bradley contends that, although prevention activities are not covered by Medicare in home health, "We depend on the family caregiver to provide needed care to many of our patients. If the caregivers become ill, their caregiving ability decreases. The likelihood of our losing the original home health patient to nursing home care or hospitalization increases when we do not promote the family caregiver's health" (p. 287). Thus, although a financial gain might be apparent in the short term, there may be significant long-term financial benefits in caring for the ones who care for our patients day in and day out.

The home health nurse must assess the role of the family caregiver in the context of how well the patient functions in the home environment (Bradley, 2003). Supporting the caregiver may mean little more than listening carefully to his or her needs regarding personal health status and providing suggestions for health promotion and time management apart from the patient. Support groups for caregivers can also provide valuable resources that ultimately strengthen the care provided to the patient. The home health nurse has many opportunities to praise the caregiver and remind him or her of the need to pay attention to self for the sake of the patient. Daycare programs and respite care can provide needed breaks for the family caregiver and should be encouraged by the home health nurse. As the need for informal caregiving increases in the future, home health nurses will need to become more involved in the promotion of local, state, and national health care policy development related to the support of family caregivers as a health care resource.

## Legal and Ethical Issues in Home Health

Home health nurses are confronted with legal and ethical issues related to nursing practice daily. Complex family situations create daily dilemmas for the home health nurse, such as questions regarding caretaking abilities of the family caregivers, financial constraints, and respect for autonomous decision making with the vulnerable patient. In the home, nurses are often caring for patients over a long period, as compared with the acute care setting; as a result, they face boundary issues related to professionals and self-responsibility for care (Gremmen, 1999; Liaschenko, 1997).

One source of ethical dilemma in health care is in providing necessary nursing care for identified patient needs when financial coverage is no longer available. Agency policy may include options for temporary services or the nurse may assist the patient and family in making alternative plans for care. Patient's noncompliance with treatment plans is an ongoing challenge, and ethical issues related to use of resources can be sources of significant ethical conflict. Reporting abusive, neglectful, and unsafe conditions, care, or practices may often be necessary as a legal and ethical mandatory practice.

Knowing a patient's rights and responsibilities, as well as the rights and limitations of the home health care nurse, is a critical component of home health care nursing practice (Gremmen, 1999). Referral to social work, support groups, and appropriate agencies is often the appropriate response.

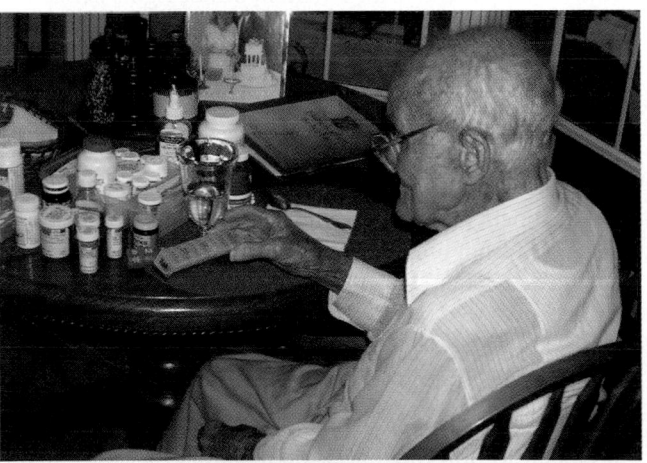

The home health visit provides nurses with opportunities to assist elders with learning how to properly take medications, as well as to support the entire therapeutic plan of care.

Lovejoy (1997) recommends the creation of agency support groups for home health care nurses and other professionals. A support group can provide needed discussion and conflict resolution in the environment of shared experiences with others. Lovejoy (1997) makes the following recommendations in the creation of an efficient support group in home health:

- A clinical nurse specialist should facilitate and coordinate the support group. This clinical nurse specialist should have experience in leading support groups and ideally should have experience in the field as a home health staff nurse.
- Support group meetings should not be mandatory. Nurses should be encouraged to attend meetings but never required to attend.
- Support groups should include a mix of new and experienced nurses. All other health professionals should be encouraged to be a part of the group as well.

The support group should be sponsored by the agency, be a part of the formal organizational structure, and have rules and bylaws as appropriate. If the group is informal, minimal rules should relate to frequency of meetings, commitment of members, confidentiality issues, and termination of membership.

An effective support group should help make members feel better about themselves and their abilities and more at ease in the complex home environment. One unexpected benefit of the support group in home health agencies is that members often are able to see co-workers in a new light and learn to trust them as resources. Home care is often a lonely profession, because nurses do not have the benefit of working closely with colleagues on a daily basis. The support group, along with modern telecommunication strategies, can bridge the isolation of "nursing on the road" (Lovejoy, 1997).

## ■ Home Care Bill of Rights

Medicare-certified agencies are required to provide home health patients with a written bill of rights before the initiation of service. Each home health patient is required to be informed of his or her right for health care treatment, and this education must be documented in the patient's permanent record. To assist home health provider agencies with this requirement, the National Association of Home Care and Hospice has developed a Home Care Bill of Rights. This document provides the patient with details of what can be expected from home care agencies in the delivery of their care. Agencies often use a modified form of the NAHCH Bill of Rights.

## ■ Advance Medical Directives

Home health nurses must also be involved in the requirements for informed decision making as specified in the Home Care Bill of Rights related to treatment options and

**Application to Practice**

With the recent public health concerns related to increased rates of Community Acquired MRSAs, infection control in the home setting is even more critical than before. Home visits should be made in sequence based on vulnerability of the patient and risk to other patients. The home health nurse should prioritize his or her visit schedule to go from the least infectious patient to the one with greatest risk for infection or existing infection. Using these guidelines, the following visits would be conducted in this order: blood pressure check for patient on new hypertensive medication, diabetic instruction for newly diagnosed patient, pediatric wound care post appendectomy patient, and HIV patient with MRSA wound.

refusal when the patient is unable to make decisions and communicate those decisions to the health care provider. An advance medical directive is a document that describes patient intent and wishes regarding various types of medical treatment in selected situations (Pevey, 2008). Medical directives were developed in the early part of the 1990s in response to increased technology in the treatment of acute and chronic illnesses and the increased awareness by the consumer population of the need to make informed decisions regarding treatment options and the refusal of medical interventions.

Two types of advance medical directives are distinguished: living wills and health care proxies. Either type of directive specifically addresses the patient's desire for health care or refusal in the event of becoming incapacitated and unable to make decisions. The living will documents a patient's decision to decline life-prolonging interventions if that patient becomes terminally ill. A health care proxy, also known as durable power of attorney, specifies the name of a person who will make health care decisions if the patient becomes incapacitated and cannot make them.

The patient maintains the right to change any of these documents at any time. Each state differs in terms of its laws and regulations related to the implementation of advance directives, and the home health nurse must remain informed about such statutes.

## Home Health Bill of Rights

### South Mississippi Home Health, Inc.
### Bill of Rights & Responsibilities

Each patient referred to South Mississippi Home Health, Inc. (henceforth referred to as SMHH), has the right to be informed in writing of his or her rights and responsibilities prior to care being rendered. The patient's family or guardian may exercise the patient's rights when the patient has been judged incompetent. SMHH has an obligation to protect and promote the rights of their patients.

### Quality of Care

Patients have the right:

- To have a relationship with SMHH that is based on honesty, ethical standards of conduct, and compliance with state and federal laws;
- To be assured of service without regard to age, race, religious preference, sex, marital status, national origin, handicapping condition, or whether or not he or she has executed an advance directive;
- To expect kindness, consideration, and respect;
- To discuss problems regarding services by calling locally _____;
- To voice a formal complaint with SMHH by calling corporate headquarters at _____, and requesting the Patient Rights Coordinator;
  - To know about the disposition of such complaints;
  - To voice their grievances without fear of discrimination or reprisal; and
- To know the state's home health hotline; the purpose of the hotline is to receive complaints or questions about home health agencies.

### Decision Making

Patients have the right:

- To be notified in writing of the care that is to be furnished and the proposed frequency of the visits;
- To participate in the planning of the care and in any changes;
- To accept or refuse services or request a change in home health care provider without fear of reprisal or discrimination;
- To make advance directives concerning his or her care; and
- To refuse to participate in experimental research.

### Privacy

Patients have the right:

- To expect confidentiality; and
- To expect SMHH to release information only as required by law or authorized by the patient.

### Financial Information

Patients have the right:

- To be informed of the extent to which payment may be expected from Medicare, Medicaid, or any other payer known to SMHH;
- To be informed of the charges that will not be covered by Medicare;
- To be informed of the charges for which the patient may be liable;
- To be notified of any changes in the above, orally and in writing, within thirty working days.

### South Mississippi Home Health Policy

South Mississippi Home Health, Inc., nurses, aides, and therapists are CPR certified. It is the policy of this company that, in the event of a cardiac arrest and in the absence of a Do Not Resuscitate order from your physician, CPR efforts will be initiated.

SMHH will comply with a patient's advance directives in providing care, to the extent allowed by state law. However, SMHH respects the right of our employees not to implement your advance directive due to personal convictions. In this case, SMHH will make every effort to comply with your advance directive or transfer you to another provider. SMHH may discharge or refer the patient to another source of care if the patient's inability or refusal to comply with the plan of care compromises SMHH's commitment to quality care.

Patients have the right:

- To know SMHH policies that apply to his/her conduct.

A patient and/or his family shall be responsible for:
  a. Cooperation with SMHH staff in the plan of care
  b. Providing SMHH personnel with accurate information as to the symptoms and condition as well as compliance with the prescribed plan of care

- To be given notice of the reason for transfer or discharge from SMHH, which may be any of the following:
  a. Goals have been met
  b. Requires a different level of care
  c. Refuses the continuation of care
  d. Ill will on the part of the patient and/or family toward SMHH
  e. Danger to SMHH staff
  f. Noncompliance with Bill of Rights and Responsibilities
  g. Noncompliance with Patient Account Policies
  h. Unsigned physician's Plan of Care

# Information and Technology in Home Health

## ■ Communication and Data Management

Home health care nurses depend on the use of information technology in clinical practice. There is continued demand for and improvement in the information systems available for use in the home. Chapter 8 provides a detailed look at how technology is changing the way patient care is being delivered in all settings. As health care becomes more mobile, remote points of access within a safe and secure infrastructure will become the norm (Seibert et al., 2008; Lind et al., 2007). Computerized records and care planning tools, such as critical pathways, are helping the home care nurses achieve greater time and patient management. Many home health nurses now practice almost exclusively from home and use laptop computers to document visits. Although working from home does not allow for the camaraderie of team communication that occurs in other settings, it does provide many nurses with more work flexibility (Neal, 1997). Along with tools to manage this information, many health care organizations have decision-support systems that would benefit the management of patient care in the home by issuing reminders, offering a menu of options, or linking the nurse to important educational tools and information needed (Pare et al., 2006).

As improvements in health networks continue, the nurse will be able to access test results from the laboratory, and information from other providers involved in the coordination of care in the home. Electronic commerce may replace traditional home health methods of communicating with partners in health care, especially as disease management programs continue to grow (Doolittle et al., 2005).

Security programs within the organization should protect the confidentiality of individually identifiable health care information. This includes training, security audits, and policies regarding access to different types of information (Pare et al., 2006; Lind, et al., 2007).

Health care information systems of the twenty-first century should guide quality improvement efforts, improve the coordination of care, advance evidence-based health care practice, and support continued research (Monsen et al., 2006). Because the health care industry is so fragmented, it will be important to work toward data sharing as is common now in so many nonhealth industries (Waters, 2007; Doolittle, et al., 2005). Although all health care organizations collect information, it is uncommon for this information to be brought together in a way that can shed light on how variations in the process of care affect outcomes. Information on the experiences and perspectives of patients and the health care team can now be collected with available computer systems. The home health nurse also works with patients as they research their health online, assisting them in evaluating the vast amount of information as to quality and application. Information on health care outcomes is becoming standard practice in most home care settings (President's Advisory Commission on Consumer Protection and Quality in the Health Care Industry, 1998; Waters, 2007).

## ■ Delivery of Care

Home care nursing must redefine the assessment parameters that are critical to be performed in person and those that can be done through technology such as telenursing. Nurses must also redefine "touch." Do we touch a patient physically, as in palpation, or do we also use the term generically, in that we can touch a patient with a few therapeutic words over the phone, television, or computer (Franz, 1997; Waters, 2007)? The home care nurse can now deliver care and information through a lens, a screen, or a telephone into the home. Home telenursing can never fully replace in-person home health care, of course. Nevertheless, the appropriate mix of in-person and electronic visitation, along with the appropriate level of providers to accomplish both, will provide better and more holistic care for the home patient and family. Telenursing technology can assist the home care nurse in managing the plan of care remotely to capture vital signs and in teaching patients and their families self-care management.

Laptop-based medical management systems have been used in the home setting for monitoring wound care and linking the home health nurses to physician consultation. This allows the physician consultants to view patient wounds from a live video image. The traditional method in the home requires the nurse to take Polaroid photographs of wounds and forward them to the physician for review. Using the telemedicine system, visiting nurses dial the physician and forward the image in real time; decisions regarding treatment protocols are then exchanged between the providers and the patient (Kincade, 1997; Waters, 2007; Seibert et al., 2008).

As home telemedicine and telenursing systems mature, they will evolve so that physical therapy can be administered, nutrition counseling conducted, and occupational therapy supervised. As computer ownership and use in the home become as common as television use, e-mail can be used to communicate with patients and patients can report directly to health care providers. Successful programs have used e-mail to remind patients about medication dosing and educational information for postsurgery patients on a daily basis (Jerant, 1999). Patient access to the Internet is becoming more common. Such systems allow nurse's aides to conduct physical home visits and be supervised by nurses at an agency or at home. The home care industry now uses these technologies to track patient outcomes, reduce service redundancy, and supplement care provided by visiting nurses and other disciplines.

**❝***Healing a person does not always mean curing a disease.***❞**

—*Dr. Dame Cicely Saunders, founder of St. Christopher Hospice in London*

## Research Alert

The Center for Total Access at the Department of Defense Southeast Telemedicine Testbed at Fort Gordon, Augusta, Georgia, in clinical partnership with Eisenhower Army Medical Center and its regional hospitals, has ongoing research trials of telenursing applications. Telenursing is the use of telemedicine technology to deliver nursing care. The word "telemedicine" comes from the Latin word *tele*, meaning "distance," and *mederi*, meaning "healing." Telenurses "visit" patients at home using telemedicine technology developed by the Eisenhower Army Medical Center, the Georgia Institute of Technology, and the Medical College of Georgia. A real-time connection over the local cable network allows audio and video contact and measurement of physiological parameters in the patient's home. The system, called the Electronic Housecall, includes blood pressure cuff, oxygen saturation monitor, temperature probe, three-lead electrocardiogram monitor, and stethoscope. Patients with common chronic conditions, such as diabetes, heart disease, asthma, and chronic obstructive pulmonary disease, are the target population for study. Findings are that these frequent electronic home visits result in fewer expensive emergency department encounters and inpatient admissions. Home telenursing enables closer monitoring so that problems are identified and acted on before they escalate into crises.

*Source*: Jerant, A. F., Schlachta, L., Epperly, T. D., & Barnes-Camp, J. (1998). Back to the future: The telemedicine house call. *Family Practice Management, 5*, 18–22, 25–26, 28.

**Beyond the Grave**

Rattling tin piano
Voices crying softly,
Through sun flecked
Tabernacle roof.

We stand,
Singing of life beyond
That open grave.

Beyond early summer jam,
Beyond racing through her
Fall dry cornfield,
Beyond rocking to sleep,
Feet drag softly,
Beyond the smell of lilac talc,
Starch, snuff, Ponds Soap,
Beyond the Christmas lights,
Story of magic
Beyond
Just beyond
The better life.

—*Ann Thedford Lanier*

## Hospice Care in the Home

Hospice services for the terminally ill became covered expenses under Medicare in 1983. Hospice nursing provides palliative nursing care for terminally ill patients and their families, with an emphasis on physical, psychosocial, emotional, and spiritual needs. Palliative care is comfort-oriented care and refers to interventions that alleviate or lessen the severity of disease or illness without curing it. The goal of the hospice program for home care is to improve the quality of life for people who are no longer able to benefit from curative interventions, with an emphasis on treating the symptoms of the disease to promote comfort. The word "hospice" comes from Latin *hospitium*, meaning "guesthouse." Hospice is holistic in nature and views dying as a normal part of living. Through hospice care in the home, the patient can live in dignity and comfort in the context of home and family. Hospice care is primarily provided at home, although facilities also exist that provide these services in an inpatient setting while still offering support for families in a homelike environment. Patients in long-term care facilities can also receive hospice services, with the facility being considered by Medicare as the place of residence of the patient (Brooks, 1997; Acorn, 2008). Medicare may pay for bereavement counseling for as long as a year after the loved one's death. Patients who most often benefit from hospice care and are most commonly seen in hospice care are individuals with cancer, acquired immune deficiency syndrome (AIDS), end-stage lung or heart disease, and those with chronic diseases.

Many HMOs and insurance companies also cover hospice services for their patients and the majority of states in the U.S. now offer hospice coverage under their Medicaid programs. Although each hospice service has individual policies concerning payment for care, a common principle of hospice care is to offer services based on a need rather than the ability to pay. For this reason, hospice services may often rely more than other home health services on grants and voluntary donations (Forcina Hill, 2008).

### Quality Assurance and Hospice

Quality Assurance (QA)/Performance Improvement (PI)/Outcome Based Quality Improvement (OBQI) and Quality Improvement (QI) have all been associated as a priority focus in the home health care arena for many years. Hospice care was thought to have an anticipated outcome of inevitability and hospice agencies were not required to develop the types of lengthy quality performance improvement plans and programs mandatory for the home health agency.

**❝***Do not go gentle into that good night, Old age should burn and rave at close of day; Rage, rage against the dying of the life.***❞**

—*Dylan Thomas*

Research Alert

Three out of every four hospice patients (74.1%) died in a private residence, nursing home, or other residential facility versus acute-care hospital settings in 2006. This exceeds the rate seen in the general population, in which about 50% die in acute hospitals.

While the majority of patient care is provided in the place the patient calls home, 19.6% of hospices also operate a dedicated inpatient unit or facility. Most of these facilities (87.1%) are either freestanding or located within a hospital and provide a mix of acute and residential care. These facilities are typically found in larger agencies with an average daily census greater than 200 patients. Only 8.8% of hospice patients died in a hospital setting that was not managed by the hospice organization.

*Source*: Brown University Center for Gerontology and Health Care Research. (2004). *Facts on dying: Policy relevant data on care at the end of lie*. Retrieved September 7, 2008, from http://www.chcr.brown.edu/dying

However, in 2005, CMS published proposed Conditions of Participation for hospices that included a new requirement that hospices develop, implement, and maintain an effective, datadriven quality assessment and performance improvement (QAPI) program. These QA plans may look at such activities as patient place of death, patient pain medication status, and bowel status to determine how the agency may improve the care of the patient. See Medicare's Quality Improvement Community Web site (www.medqic.org) for updated information on the latest requirements for hospice quality assurance.

With the emphasis on quality of care in the proposed Conditions of Participation, the National Association for Home Care & Hospice (NAHCH) and its Hospice Advisory Board identified a priority to develop resources to assist its hospice members to measure quality of care. The purpose of this set of quality measures is to facilitate quality assessment and improvement of hospice care, fulfill some of the QAPI CoP requirements for quality measures, and provide standardization to allow for comparisons (within a hospice or with other hospices; CMS, 2008b).

For hospice services, the physician must certify that the patient has a life expectancy that would normally be expected to be 6 months or less and is seeking palliative treatment only. Hospice patients must be recertified every 60 days.

Patients and family are encouraged to be involved in all decisions about caregiving and medical interventions. Admission to a hospice should not be viewed as a failure of other therapies. Rather, a more holistic approach would

✏ NOTE THIS!

In 2006, hospices served 964,614 Medicare patients throughout the United States.

*Source*: Hospice Association of America (2008). *Hospice facts and statistics*. Retrieved November 11, 2008, from http://www.nahc.org/HospiceStats08.pdf

suggest that previous treatments had become inappropriate and referral to a hospice as movement into another model of more appropriate therapy for terminal care (Hospice Foundation of America, 2008).

The nurse has traditionally cared for the dying and the bereaved, whether on the battlefield or in the trauma unit or in the home—so how is hospice different? Hospice emerged as an organized movement in England with the founding of the first hospice at St. Christopher in London in 1950 by Dr. Dame Cicely Saunders. Saunders defined hospice care as follows: "Hospice is not a place to go to die, but rather a concept of care based on the promise that when medical science can no longer add days to life, more life will be added to each day." She inspired the hospice movement in the United States, where the first home care hospice services was founded by Florence Wald in 1974 in Connecticut (Box 39-12).

The hospice movement was strongly influenced by the research of Dr. Elisabeth Kübler-Ross, who conceptualized death as the final stage of growth as contrasted with the prevailing fear of death and the dying process as failure on the part of the medical system (Kübler-Ross, 1969, 1975). Over the past 30 years, with the prolongation of life, advanced technology, and a growing recognition that dying and terminally ill patients require a special kind of care, hospice as a community health nursing specialty has grown. Thousands of persons with life-limiting diseases have relied on hospice services for comfort, dignity, and compassion at the end of life.

Medicare hospice care for the terminally ill in the home generally costs significantly less than care for patients in the standard Medicare program. Reasons for this difference include less technology used in the care of the patient and family and friends who provide most of the daily care at home. Although hospice care does not provide 24-hour-a-day care in the home, hospice staff members are usually on call 24 hours a day. Volunteers make up an integral part

❝ *Hospice does not speed up or slow down the dying process. It does not prolong life and it does not hasten death.* ❞

—*National Hospice Foundation*

**BOX 39-12**

**Florence Wald, RN, Founder of U.S. Hospice Home Care**
Florence Wald introduced America to the hospice tradition by founding the first home care hospice program in the United States in New Haven, Connecticut, in 1974. Wald, at age 81, was inducted into the National Women's Hall of Fame in July 1998 in recognition of her work to bring care for the terminally ill through palliative and psychological care. Wald believed that although medical science has given doctors new ways to understand and control disease, "their focus on the patient as a human being was being eroded."

*Source*: Florence Wald, RN, Founder of U.S. Hospice Home Care. Associated Press, (1998, July 14). Reprinted by permission of YGS Group-A/R.

*I look up in the night sky. Is anything more certain that in all those vast times and spaces, if I were allowed to search them, I should nowhere find her face, her voice, her touch? She died. She is dead. Is the word so difficult to learn?*

—C. S. Lewis

of hospice care and are required to be a part of Medicare-certified hospice service. Inpatient respite care is available for the family, which provides family caregivers with periodic relief. A written POC is also required.

Medicare mandates that four core services be provided directly by the hospice: nursing, medical, social work, and counseling (Wilson, 1993). Services provided by hospice are as follows:

- Nursing service on an intermittent basis
- Physician services
- Drugs for pain relief
- Physical, occupational, and speech therapy
- Home health aides
- Medical supplies
- Spiritual and pastoral services
- Continuous care during a crisis
- Bereavement services for the family, up to a year following death

Hospice provides coordinated services for the family of the patient with a terminal illness. Hospice, as a specialized kind of home health care, is designed to provide comfort and support to patients and families in the final stages of terminal illness. Goals center on providing care in which patients can spend their last days with dignity, at home or in a homelike setting, surrounded by family members and loved ones. Comfort involves physical and spiritual comfort and emotional support of the patient, family, and caregivers (Reese & Brown, 1997; Acorn, 2008). See Box 39-13 for a sample agency hospice philosophy.

## ■ Hospice Care for Children

Although hospice services have traditionally been associated with adults, recognition has grown among health

### BOX 39-13

**Hospice Philosophy: One Agency's Commitment**

Hospice affirms life. Hospice exists to provide support and care for persons in the last phases of incurable disease so that they might live as fully and comfortably as possible. Hospice recognizes dying as a normal process, whether or not resulting from a disease. Hospice exists in the hope and belief that, through appropriate care and the promotion of a caring community sensitive to their needs, patients and families may be free to attain a degree of mental and spiritual preparation for death that is satisfactory to them.

*Source:* Courtesy of North Mississippi Medical Center Home Health and Hospice.

### ✎ NOTE THIS! ●

**Home Health Care During and After a Disaster**
On August 30, 2005, displaced residents of New Orleans first learned that the levees of their city had been overtopped and then breached by the storm surge from Hurricane Katrina. New Orleans would soon be 80% flooded. Within a month, Hurricane Rita arrived in New Orleans, making cleanup and recovery an even more difficult process. This article discusses the preparation and follow-up still going on in 2007 and the role of healthcare providers, particularly home care providers, in the aftermath of Hurricanes Katrina and Rita.

*Source:* Weeber, S. (2007). Home health care after Hurricanes Katrina and Rita: A report from the field. *Home Health Care Management & Practice, 19*(2), 104–111.

care professionals that children with terminal illnesses can also benefit from hospice care. The epidemic of children with AIDS has prompted the development of pediatric hospice services for children with life-limiting illnesses (Oleske & Czarniecki, 1999). The first hospice home for children, The Helen House, was established in 1982 in the United Kingdom.

Palliative care for children with terminal diseases, such as AIDS and cancer, can ensure the child's comfort through the course of his or her illness. Oleske and Czarniecki (1999) advocate that children with life-limiting illnesses, regardless of diagnosis, socioeconomic status, or geographic location, should receive a continuum of palliative care and have access to hospice services that enhance life and ease the burden of dying. They contend that "children should know, in an age appropriate way, that death is near but that it will not be painful, not faced alone, but rather in the company of those they love" (Oleske & Czarniecki, 1999, p. 1291). Opportunities for hospice nursing with children will most likely increase in the future.

## ■ Holistic Care

Nurses who work in hospice care have specialized training in grief and bereavement management. Although spiritual care has been a major component of nursing practice since its inception, nurses are often uncomfortable with spiritual components related to death (Brant, 1998). Hospice nurses must be especially comfortable in their skills related to the spiritual needs of their patients. Holistic nursing care for the hospice patient means assessing for suffering in the spiritual realm, because the total person is incomplete without such consideration (Running et al., 2008). Providing spiritual care does not mean that hospice nurses must hold the same beliefs of those for whom they care. Hospice nurses who provide palliative care approach patients with a nonjudgmental, listening ear. Nurses provide spiritual care by assisting patients in their final days in their search for meaning of past, present, and future events. Patients attempt to make sense of their life experiences, and nurses, in the holistic tradition, must be involved in this healing aspect of this last stage of life (Reese & Brown, 1997; Acorn, 2008).

Hospice provides patients with the comfort and support of their families in the home as they face terminal illness.

Nurses as team members in hospice care are often the ones with the prolonged, close contact with patients and family members and, as such, can provide comprehensive information about the well-being of the family and caregivers to the physician and other members of the hospice team (Goldstein, et al., 2004).

Ethical issues have special considerations for hospice workers. Working with families during a family member's imminent death brings challenges related to professional boundaries, family responsibilities, and complex decisions about care (Hunt, 1991). The threat of legalized suicide is of concern to all nurses but is an especially significant issue in the field of hospice nursing. Legalized suicide and euthanasia practices threaten the natural cycle of dying and the final stage of growth. Providing appropriate, holistic, and comforting end-of-life care, as larger numbers of the baby-boomer generation age, will continue to emerge as critical professional issues for home health nurses who specialize in hospice care (Tilden et al., 2004; Ekman Ladd et al., 2008).

Other future issues for hospice nursing care include the expansion of community-based residential hospice care facilities, which include respite care, home care, acute inpatient care, and expanded bereavement counseling for

### Research Alert

When the U.S. hospice community was established in the 1970s, cancer patients made up the largest percentage of hospice admissions, but today cancer diagnoses account for fewer than half of all hospice admissions (44.1%). In fact, less than 25% of U.S. deaths are now caused by cancer, with the majority of deaths due to chronic conditions. In 2006, the top five chronic conditions served by hospice included heart disease (12.2% of admissions), debility unspecified (11.8%), dementia (10.0%), and lung disease (7.7%).

Source: Miniño, A. M., Heron, M. P., Murphy, S. L., Kochanek, K. D. (2007). Deaths: Final data for 2004. National Vital Statistics Reports, 55(19). Hyattsville, MD: National Center for Health Statistics.

families (Pevey, 2008). With the growing number of elders, adults with AIDS, and children with prolonged terminal illnesses, hospice services will be challenged to provide myriad home- and community-based services for families caring for the terminally ill. Humane care for the dying strains families who are already overburdened with dual career demands and child care. Such facilities can provide nurse-managed, holistic care for the terminally ill in a noninstitutional, natural environment more conducive to the promotion of health in the final stage of life (Brannstrom et al., 2005; Doolittle et al., 2005; Wilson, 1993).

**"**We need to continue to educate nurses in the art of palliative care, emphasizing holistic care that encompasses the mind, body, and spirit. Total suffering encompasses all three of these components, and end-of-life care must include the same. We can instill hope that goes beyond the grave.**"**
    —Jeannine M. Brant, RN, MS, AOCN, oncology clinical nurse specialist, Saint Vincent Hospital and Health Center, Billings, Montana

### Life Goes On

I felt like a rainbow covered with dirt in this room.
I couldn't bear seeing
my uncle and aunt washed
with sad feelings.
My grandpa's hand had no life to it.
Though life went on and the
trees kept swaying.
I wondered what would life
be like without his hand to
cross my hair.
My rainbow just did not shine that day.
The wind took over everything.
I love the wind.
It changed everything in that room.
It made me feel like a hundred
butterflies had flown from his
chest.
His stuck together lips and
hard breathing harmed me.
I couldn't stand there.
Water was pulled from my eyes.
Our hands parted and I
kissed him and walked into
reality.

—Alexandra Zacharias, age 10, on the occasion of the death of her grandfather

Source: The Educational Forum, 55(3), Spring 1991.

## The Future of Health Care in the Home

As the home health industry continues to evolve, the home care nurse will require advanced clinical skills in community health nursing as well as an understanding of data management and information technology systems. Knowledge of

### Research Alert

This study reported that hospice care may prolong the lives of some terminally ill patients. Among the patient populations studied, the mean survival was 29 days longer for hospice patients than for nonhospice patients. In other words, patients who chose hospice care lived an average of 1 month longer than similar patients who did not choose hospice care. Researchers selected 4,493 terminally ill patients with either congestive heart failure (CHF) or cancer of the breast, colon, lung, pancreas, or prostate. They then analyzed the difference in survival periods between those who received hospice care and those who did not. Longer lengths of survival were found in four of the six disease categories studied. The largest difference in survival between the hospice and nonhospice cohorts was observed in CHF patients where the mean survival period jumped from 321 days to 402 days. The mean survival period was also significantly longer for the hospice patients with lung cancer (39 days) and pancreatic cancer (21 days), while marginally significant for colon cancer (33 days).

*Source*: Connor, S. R., Pyenson, B., Fitch, K., Spence, C., & Iwasaki, K. (2007). Comparing hospice and nonhospice patient survival among patients who die within a three-year window. *Journal of Pain Symptom Management, 33*(3), 238–246.

case management concepts to reach positive clinical and financial outcomes by using resources more effectively will be required. Case managers within home care will have clinical nursing expertise and a sense of measuring nursing impact on specific patient populations, such as individuals with heart disease or cancer. These case managers will be increasingly required in home health nursing practice to possess problem-solving and decision-making skills that require negotiation and a strong sense of patient collaboration. Principles of managed care and practicing in coalitions are important skills for all healthcare workers, but especially for those who work in the home health field.

The opportunity for professional growth in home care nursing is endless. The quest to provide patients and their caregivers with the best of home care continues to be a challenge given the myriad changes in health care today. Growth in information systems and advances in decision-making technology are offering business solutions to home health care. These advances enhance the practice of home care nursing by offering additional resources to manage patient care to achieve quantifiable positive health outcomes (Hartung, 2005).

Advanced practice nurses and nurse specialists will become required roles on the interdisciplinary team that offer direction, education, and support (Hartung, 2005; Rice, 2005). As advanced practice nurses assume service privileges in acute care facilities, it is expected that they will eventually demand the ability to discharge patients to home health. Home health nurses not only will be increasingly accountable for patient outcomes but will also be called on to use business skills, such as cost–benefit analysis, to objectively support the total cost of care. The planning for care based on expected outcomes and participating in policy-making decisions that involve nursing practice will be an expectation of all staff home health nurses (Blaha, 1997; Boxer & Meadows, 2008; Duke & Street, 2003).

> ❝One's suffering disappears when one lets oneself go, when one yields—even to sadness.❞
>
> —Antoine de Saint-Exupery

> ❝Who looks outside, dreams. Who looks inside, awakens.❞
>
> —Carl Jung

## Conclusion

In a managed care environment where the most efficient and effective delivery setting is chosen, nurses will find the home setting a likely practice environment. Community health nursing will continue to include the home as a viable and attractive setting for practice in sickness and in health. See Box 39-14 for some nurses' thoughts about being home health nurses.

### BOX 39-14

**Thoughts on Being a Home Health Nurse—from the Field**

"Probably the best part of the job is being on your own and being able to spend quality time with patients who really believe you can help them."

"There have been so many good memories and experiences—all of my patients are very special, they are like family. I really get to know them, their families, their fears, and their dreams. Home health is very rewarding."

"After working for many years in intensive care, I had grown weary of less and less time getting to know my patients as I was getting better and better at managing the machines that really cared for them. In home health, each day I am doing exactly what I went into nursing for—helping people feel better, using the skills I have worked so hard to develop."

"One of the more memorable home visits was the time the patient's pigs got out of the pen and the physical therapist and I had to chase the pigs before we could attend to the patient's needs."

Explore Community Health Nursing on the Web! To learn more about the topics in this chapter, use the passcode provided to access your exclusive website: **http://nursing.jbpub.com/communityhealth.** If you do not have a passcode, you can obtain one at this site.

## ■ CRITICAL THINKING ACTIVITIES

1. Home health care is one of the fastest-growing nursing roles in health care today. Managed care has created incentives for hospitals to limit acute care episodes and patient admissions. Patients continue to be discharged earlier than ever after surgery, childbirth, and acute episodes of chronic diseases. More and more "high-tech" health care can be replicated in the home, such as chemotherapy, IV therapy, and assisted ventilation. Given that this trend is likely to continue as all health agencies struggle to contain costs, consider the following opinions about home health nursing. Respond to each statement and document your agreement or disagreement with the opinion.

- Home health nursing is more accurately described as "hospital care at home."
- Home health nursing is a new emerging specialty in preventive acute care and is not really a community health role or a hospital role.
- Home health nurses are generalists who can provide health promotion services to well patients, such as newly discharged mothers and babies, as well as newly discharged post–heart transplant patients with complex intravenous immunosuppressive drug therapy.

## ■ REFERENCES

Acorn, M. (2008). In-home palliative care increased patient satisfaction and reduced use and costs of medical services. *Evidence-Based Nursing, 11*(1), 22.

American Nurses Association. (2007). *Home health nursing scope and standards of practice.* Silver Spring, MD: Author.

American Nurses Association (ANA). (1995). *Position statement: Informal caregiving.* Washington, DC: Author.

American Nurses Association (ANA). (2007). *Standards of home health nursing practice.* Washington, DC: Author.

Anderson, M., Pena, R., & Helms, L. (1998). Home care utilization by congestive heart failure patients: A pilot study. *Public Health Nursing, 15*(2), 146–162.

Blaha, A. (1997). The current and future national voice for home healthcare nursing. *Home Healthcare Nurse, 15*(12), 873.

Boxer, M., & Meadows, B. (2008). Improving care transition from hospital to home health care through collaboration: The referral process between hospital and home health agency. *Remington Report, 16*(2), 32–34.

Bradley, P. J. (1996). Home healthcare nurses should regain their family focus. *Home Healthcare Nurse, 14*(4), 281–288.

Bradley, P. (2003). Family caregiver assessment: essential for effective home health care. *Journal of Gerontological Nursing, 29*(2), 29–36.

Brant, J. (1998). The art of palliative care: Living with hope, dying with dignity. *Oncology Nursing Forum, 25*(6), 995–1004.

Brännström, M., Brulin, C., Norberg, A., Boman, K., & Strandberg, G. (2005). Being a palliative nurse for persons with severe congestive heart failure in advanced home care. *European Journal of Cardiovascular Nursing, 4*, 314–323.

Brooks, S. (1997). Of hope and hospice. *Contemporary Longterm Care, 20*(7), 56–61.

Bull, M. J. (1990). Factors influencing family caregiver burden and health. *Western Journal of Nursing Research, 12*, 758–776.

Center for Medicare and Medicaid Services (CMS). (2007). Home health prospective payment system refinement and rate update for calendar year 2008: Final rule. *Federal Register, 72*(167), 49762–49810.

Center for Medicare and Medicaid Services (CMS) (2008). *OASIS, Health and Human Services, Center for Medicare and Medicaid Services.* Retrieved September 7, 2008, from http://www.cms.hhs.gov/oasis

Center for Medicare and Medicaid Services (CMS). (2008b). *Medicare announces new proposed rule to improve hospice care.* Baltimore, MD: Health and Human Services, Center for Medicare and Medicaid Services.

Children's Defense Fund. (1998). *The state of America's children yearbook 1998.* Washington, DC: Author.

Cho, S. (2005). Older people's willingness to use home care nursing services. *Journal of Advanced Nursing, 51*(2), 166–173.

Clarke, P., & Cody, W. (1994). Nursing theory-based practice in the home and community: The crux of professional nursing education. *Advances in Nursing Science, 17*, 41–53.

Cochran, M., & Brennan, S. (1998). Home healthcare nursing in the managed care environment: Part I. *Home Healthcare Nurse, 16*(4), 214–219.

Congdon, J., & Magilvy, J. (1998). Home health care: Supporting vitality for rural elders. *Journal of Long Term Home Health Care, 17*(4), 9–17.

Curtin, M. (2008). News from CCMC. Home health care: An integral part of the continuum. *Care Management, 14*(1), 6.

Davitt, J., & Choi, S. (2008). Tracing the history of Medicare home health care: The impact of policy on benefit use. *Journal of Sociology & Social Welfare, 35*(1), 247–276.

Davitt, J.K. (2003). *Access to Medicare home health care in the wake of the Balanced Budget Act.* Bryn Mawr, PA: Bryn Mawr College.

Doolittle, G., Whitten, P., Mccartney, M., Cook, D., & Nazir, N. (2005). An empirical chart analysis of the suitability of telemedicine for hospice visits. *Telemedicine Journal & E-Health, 11*(1), 90–97.

Dougherty, G. (1998). When should a child be in the hospital? A. Frederick North, Jr, M.D. Revisited. *Pediatrics, 101*(1), 19–25.

Duke, M., & Street, A. (2003). Hospital in the home: Constructions of the nursing role—A literature review. *Journal of Clinical Nursing, 12,* 852–859.

Ekman Ladd, R., Pasquerella, I., & Smith, S. (2000). What to do when the end is near: Ethical issues in home health care nursing. *Public Health Nursing, 17,* 103–110.

Fitzgerald, J. D., Mangione, C. M., Boscardin, J., Kominski, G., Hahn, B., & Ettner, S. L. (2006). Impact of changes in Medicare home health care reimbursement on month-to-month home health utilization between 1996 and 2001 for a national sample of patients undergoing orthopedic procedures. *Medical Care, 44,* 870–878.

Forcina Hill, J. (2008). Factors associated with hospice use after referral. *Journal of Hospice & Palliative Nursing, 10*(4), 240–252.

Franz, A. (1997). Prognosis: Home care nursing. *Home Healthcare Nurse, 15*(12), 876–877.

Goldstein, N., Concator, J., Fried, T., Kasl, S., Johnson-Hurzeler, R., & Bradley, F. (2004). Factors associated with caregiver burden among caregivers of terminally ill patients with cancer. *Palliative Care, 20*(1), 38–43.

Gremmen, I. (1999). Visiting nurses' situated ethics: Beyond "care versus justice" *Nursing Ethics, 6,* 515–527.

Hartung, S. (2005). Choosing home health as a specialty and successfully transitioning into practice. *Home Health Care Management and Practice, 17*(5), 370–387.

Health and Human Services, Centers for Medicare and Medicaid Services (CMS). (2008). *Home Health Care.* Retrieved September 7, 2008, from http://www.medicare.gov/HHCompare/Home.asp

Hickey, M. (July 1998). Disease management improves patient care, cuts costs. *Physicians Management,* p. 214.

Hoak, V. (2008). Making the case for home health care. *Caring, 27*(3), 20–22.

Hospice Foundation of America. (2008). What is hospice? Retrieved November 13, 2008, from http://hospicefoundation.org

Hunt, M. (1991). Being friendly and informal: Reflected in nurses' terminally ill patients' and relatives' conversations at home. *Journal of Advanced Nursing, 16,* 929–938.

Jerant, A. (1999). Home telemedicine: Merging the old and new ways. *American Family Physician, 60*(4), 1096–1098.

Jerant, A. F., Schlachta, L., Epperly, T. D., & Barnes-Camp, J. (1998). Back to the future: The telemedicine house call. *Family Practice Management, 5,* 18–22, 25–26, 28.

Jester, R., & Hicks, C. (2003). Using cost-effectiveness analysis to compare hospital at home and in-patient interventions. *Journal of Clinical Nursing, 12*(1), 20–27.

Kaye, L. W., & Davitt, J. K. (1999). *Current practices in high-tech home care.* New York: Springer.

Keehan, S., Sisako, A., Truffer, C., Smith, S., Sisko, A., Cowan, C. et al. (2008). "Health spending projections through 2017: The Baby Boom generation is coming to Medicare." *Health Affairs, 27*(2), W145–W155.

Kenyon, V., Smith, E., Hefty, L. V., Bell, M. L., McNeil, J., & Maraus, T. (1990). Clinical competencies for public health nursing. *Public Health Nursing, 7,* 33–39.

Kiecolt-Glaser, J. K., Glaser, R., Shuttleworth, E. C., Dyer, C. S., Ogrocki, B. S., & Speicher, C. E. (1987). Chronic stress and immunity in family care givers of Alzheimer's disease victims. *Psychosomatic Medicine, 49,* 523–535.

Kim, E., Cho, E, & June, K. (2006). Factors influencing use of home care and nursing homes. *Journal of Advanced Nursing, 54*(4), 511–517.

Kincade, K. (1997). Growing home-care business benefits from telemedicine TLC. *Telemedicine,* p. 4.

Kübler-Ross, E. (1969). *On death and dying: What the dying have to teach doctors, nurses, clergy and their own families.* New York: Macmillan.

Kübler-Ross, E. (1975). *Death: The final stage of growth.* New York: Simon and Schuster.

Levine, C. (1999). Home sweet hospital: The nature and limits of private responsibilities for home health care. *Journal of Aging and Health Care, 11*(2), 341–360.

Liaschenko, J. (1997). Ethics and the geography of the nurse-patient relationship: Spatial vulnerabilities and gendered space. *Scholarly Inquiry Nursing Practice, 11,* 45–49.

Lin, W., Kane, R. L., Mehr, D. R., Madsen, R. W., & Petroski, G. F. (2006). Changes in the use of postacute care during the initial Medicare payment reforms. *Health Services Research, 41*(4), 1338–1356.

Lind, L., Karlsson, D., & Fridlund, B. (2007). Digital pens and pain diaries in palliative home health care: Professional caregivers' experiences. *Medical Informatics & the Internet in Medicine, 32*(4), 287–296.

Lovejoy, D. (1997). *Making the transition to home health nursing.* New York: Springer.

MacLaren, E. (1994). Basics of managed care. *NurseWeek,* pp. 10–11.

Maraldo, P. (1989). Home care should be the heart of a nursing sponsored national health plan. *Nursing and Health Care, 10*(6), 301–306.

Martin, K., Scheet, N., & Stegman, M. (1993). Home health patients: Characteristics, outcomes of care, and nursing interventions. *American Journal of Public Health, 83*(12), 1730–1734.

Martinson, I. M. (1993). Hospice care for children: Past, present and future. *Journal of Pediatric Oncology Nursing, 10,* 93–98.

McCall, N., Petersons, A., Moore, S., & Korb, J. (2003). Utilization of home health services before and after the Balanced Budget Act of 1997: What were the initial effects? *Health Services Research, 38*(1), 85–106.

McKnight, R. (2006). Home care reimbursement, long-term utilization, and health outcomes. *Journal of Public Economics, 90*(1), 293–323.

Medicare Payment Advisory Commission (MedPAC). (2007). *Report to the Congress: Medicare payment policy: Home health services* (Ch. 3B). Washington, DC: Author.

Milone-Nuzzo, P. (1998). Beyond venipuncture as the qualifying service for Medicare: Seeing the forest for the trees. *Home Healthcare Nurse, 16*(3), 177–183.

Milton, C. L. (2005). The metaphor of nurse as guest with ethical implications for nursing and healthcare. *Nursing Science Quarterly, 18,* 301–303.

Monsen, K., Fitzsimmons, L., Lescenski, B., Lytton, A., Schwichtenberg, L., & Martin, K. (2006). A public health nursing informatics date-and-practice quality project. *CIN: Computers, Informatics, Nursing, 24*(3), 152–158.

Murtaugh, C. M., McCall, N., Moore, S., & Meadow, A. (2003). Trends in Medicare home health care use: 1997–2007. *Health Affairs, 22*(5), 146–156.

National Association of Home Care (NAHC). (2000, 2001). *Basic statistics about home care.* Washington, DC: Author.

The National Association for Home Care & Hospice (NAHCH, 2008). Basic statistics about home care. Washington, DC Author.

National Hospice & Palliative Care Organization (NHPCO), (2007). *Facts and figures: hospice care in America.* Alexandria, VA: Author.

National Institute on Disability and Rehabilitation Research and Training Center. (November 1996). U.S. Department of Education disability statistics abstract (Number 17). University of California, San Francisco.

Neal, L. (1997). Current clinical practice of home care nursing. *Home Healthcare Nurse, 15*(12), 881–882.

Nugent, D. (1999). Providing solutions for the growing trend toward home health care. *Health Management Technology, 20*(8), 28–31.

Oleske, J., & Czarniecki, L. (1999). Continuum of palliative care: Lessons from caring for children infected with HIV-1. *Lancet, 354*(9186), 1287–1891.

Pare, G., Sicotte, C., St. Jules, D. & Gauthier, R. (2006). Cost minimization analysis of a telehome care program for patients with chronic obstructive pulmonary disease. *Telemedicine Journal and e-health, 12*(2), 114–121.

Peters, D., & Eigsti, D. (1991). Utilizing outcomes in home care. *Caring, 10,* 44–51.

Pevey, C. (2008). Death, God, flesh, and other: Hospice recipients reflect on what matters. *Illness, Crisis & Loss, 16*(3), 203–226.

The President's Advisory Commission on Consumer Protection and Quality in the Health Care Industry. (1998). *Quality first: better health care for all Americans.* Washington, DC: U.S. Government Printing Office.

Pruchno, R. A., & Potashnik, S. L. (1989). Caregiving spouses: Physical and mental health in perspective. *Journal of the American Geriatric Society, 37,* 697–705.

Reese. D., & Brown, D. (1997). Psychosocial and spiritual care in hospice: Differences between nursing, social work, and clergy. *Hospice Journal, 12*(1), 29.

Remington, L. (1997). Disease management programs. *The Remington Report, 5*(4), 1.

Rice, R. (1996). *Home health nursing: Concepts and application* (2nd ed.). St. Louis: Mosby.

Rice, R. (2005). Home Care Nursing Practice: Concepts and Application. Mosby Publishers: St Louis, MO.

Running, A., Tolle, L., & Girard, D. (2008). Ritual: The final expression of care. *International Journal of Nursing Practice, 14*(4), 303–307.

Schaffer, C., & Behrendt, D. (1997). Disease state management across the continuum: Bettering lives, providing value. *The Remington Report, 5*(4), 20–23.

Schneider, J., Barkauskas, V., & Keenan, G. (2008). Evaluating home health care nursing outcomes with OASIS and NOC. *Journal of Nursing Scholarship, 40*(1), 76–82.

Schwartz, R. (1977). News from Washington. *The Remington Report, 5*(4), 12–13.

Seibert, P., Whitmore, T., Patterson, C., Parker, P., Otto, C., Basom, J., et al. (2008). Telemedicine facilities CHF home health care for those with systolic dysfunction. *International Journal of Telemedicine and Applications, Article ID 235031,* 7 pages.

Sezer, K. (2008). Turkish nurses' concerns about home health care in Turkey. *Australian Journal of Advanced Nursing, 25*(4), 97–106.

Shamansky, S. (June, 1988). Providing home care services in a for-profit environment. *Nursing Clinics of North America, 23*(2), 387–398.

Shaughnessy, P. W. (June 14, 1996). Using outcomes to build a continuous quality improvement program for home care. 11th National Nursing Symposium on Home Health Care, University of Michigan School of Nursing, Ann Arbor, MI.

Sheldon, P., & Bender, M. (1994). High-technology in home care. *Nursing Clinics of North America, 29*(3), 508–519.

*South Mississippi Home Health orientation manual for registered nurses.* (1996). Hattiesburg, MS: Author.

Shick, R., & Balinsky, W. (2006). Home health care services: Management and effectiveness in changing times. *Journal of Health and Human Services Administration, 28*(3), 423–462.

Spector, W. D., Cohen, J. W., & Pesis-Katz, I. (2004). Home care before and after the Balanced Budget Act of 1997: Shifts in financing and services. *The Gerontologist, 44*(4), 39–47.

Tilden, V., Tolle, S., Dracb, L., & Perrin, N. (2004). Out-of-hospital death: Advance care planning, decedent symptoms, and caregiver burden. *American Geriatric Society, 52,* 532–559.

U.S. Senate. (1979). Medicare and Medicaid Home Health Benefits. Hearings before the Subcommittee on Health, Committee on Finance (May 2 and 22, 1979). 96th Cong., Session.

Vanderboom, C., & Madigan, E. (2008). Relationships of rurality, home health care use, and outcomes. *Western Journal of Nursing Research, 30*(3), 365–378.

Ward-Griffin, C., & McKeever, P. (2000). Relationships between nurses and family caregivers: Partners in care? *ANS Advances in Nursing Science, 22*(3), 89–103.

Warhola, C. (1980). *Planning for home health services: A resource handbook.* DHSS Pub. No. (NRA) 80-14017. Washington, DC: Public Health Service, Department of Health and Human Services.

Waters, R. (2007). Technology. Measuring quality: an important tool in ensuring top notch home health care. *Caring, 26*(8), 54.

Weeber, S. (2007). Home health care after Hurricanes Katrina and Rita: A report from the field. *Home Health Care Management & Practice, 19*(2), 104–111.

Wilson, S. (1993). Hospice and Medicare benefits: Overview, issues, and implications. *Journal of Holistic Nursing, 11*(4), 356–368.

Zelwesky, M. G., & Deitrick, E. P. (1987). Rx for caregivers: Respite care. *Journal of Community Health Nursing, 4,* 77–84.

Frances Martin

School nurses provide invaluable assistance in improving students' educational outcomes.

Common sense is the collection of prejudices acquired by age eighteen.

*—Albert Einstein*

Wisdom is not a product of schooling, but of the lifelong attempt to acquire it.

*—Albert Einstein*

The illiterate of the twenty-first century will not be those who cannot read and write, but those who cannot learn, unlearn, and relearn.

*—Alvin Toffler*

All of us have experienced an educational system of some type, even home schooling. How was your school experience? Was elementary school different than high school? Did you experience unhealthy conditions in your school that threatened your safety or health? Did you develop health habits during your high school years that still influence you as a nursing student? Do you see college health as a school health setting? Why or why not?

## CHAPTER FOCUS

**History of School Health Nursing**
- Origins
- Evolution of School Nursing
- Federal Mandates in School Health

**The Education System and the School Nurse**

**Education and Credentials of the School Nurse**
- Continuing Professional Education of the School Nurse

**Role Definition of the School Nurse**
- Provider of Health Care
- Communicator
- Planner and Coordinator of Student Health Care
- Teacher
- Investigator
- Role within the Profession

**Healthy People 2010**
- At-Risk Populations
- Nurse as Team Member

**School Health Nursing Practice**
- Health Related Services
- Case Finding
- Practice Issues in School Health

**Legal Issues in School Nursing**
- Documentation
- Delegation
- Supervision and Accountability
- Funding Issues in School Health
- Violence and Terrorism in U.S. Schools

**Community Issues in School Health**
- School–Health Linkages
- Collaboration
- Resources

**Innovations**
- School-Based Clinics and Primary Health Care
- Increased Role of the Media in School Health
- Technology

## QUESTIONS TO CONSIDER

After reading this chapter, you will know the answers to the following questions:

1. What is school nursing?
2. Which services are typically offered as school health services?
3. Who was the first school nurse in the United States?
4. What role did Lillian Wald play in the development of school nursing?
5. What is a school nurse practitioner?
6. What are the major federal programs that relate to school health?
7. What is the relationship between educational goals and school nurse goals?
8. What are educational requirements of the school nurse?
9. Which kinds of health issues do school nurses deal with?
10. Which kinds of roles do school nurses play?
11. What are current practice issues in school nursing?
12. What are community issues related to school health?
13. What is a school-based clinic?

## KEY TERMS

Delegation
Health-related services
Inclusion ("mainstreaming")
Individualized educational plan (IEP)
Individualized family service plan (IFSP)
Individualized health plan (IHP)
Medically fragile children
School-based clinic
School-based services
School health services
School nursing
Unlicensed assistive personnel

EFFECTIVE SCHOOL NURSES are "bilingual"; they speak "education" as well as "health" (Costante, 1996).

> School nursing [emphasis added] is a specialized practice of professional nursing that advances the well-being, academic success, and lifelong achievement of students. To that end, school nurses facilitate positive student responses to normal development; promote health and safety; intervene with actual and potential health problems; provide case management services; and actively collaborate with others to build student and family capacity for adaptation, self management, self advocacy, and learning. (National Association of School Nurses, 1999)

Since 1975, Congress has required that students with disabilities receive an education in the "least restrictive environment." Data since 1988 suggest that U.S. schools have found regular education classrooms to be the "least restrictive environment" for increasing numbers of students with disabilities. In the 1998–1999 school year, 47% of students with disabilities spent 80% or more of their day in a regular education classroom (NCES, 2004). This number had risen from 31% just ten years previously. The largest increase occurred among students with specific learning disabilities (from 20% to 45%) (NCES, 2004).

> Schools by themselves cannot, and should not be expected to, address the nation's most serious health and social problems. Families, health care workers, the media, religious organizations, community organizations that serve youth, and young people themselves also must be systematically involved. (Schwartz & Laughlin, 2008)

There is a natural relationship between schools and child health care (Chauvin & Davis, 1994; Concepcion et al., 2008). Since 1992, the Centers for Disease Control and

## NOTE THIS!

A survey of 1,546 school districts with an identifiable school health program showed that in only 60% of these was "nursing" listed as the major field of the person in charge of school nursing.

Prevention (CDC) has provided funding for Coordinated School Health Programs (CSHP), as a means for reducing chronic disease risk factors. The CDC supported CSHPs in 20 states in 2003 (www.cdc.gov/HealthyYouth/CSHP).

Today's children are different in many ways from those of the last generation. There are children today who may have been exposed in utero to cocaine and opiates; studies are under way to evaluate these effects (Messinger et al., 2004). Almost all children entering school will have had experience with a computer; a study of participants in a Head Start program in the United States during 2001–2002 with 122 preschool children enrolled in a rural county showed that 53% had a computer at home. Of those families who did not have a home computer, 49% reported that their children had access to a computer somewhere outside the home. There was no gender difference in computer frequency use among the participating children. Children who had access to a computer performed better on measures of school readiness and cognitive development, controlling for children's developmental stage and family socioeconomic status (Li & Atkins, 2004).

Terrorism and war worries have become a part of our society (Laraque et al., 2004). Television coverage of news from war zones, for example, has created a climate of anxiety new to this country (van der Molen, 2004).

How can school nurses make a difference for children growing up with these problems today? There is both a short-term answer and a long-term answer. In the short

## Application to Practice

### *A Day in the Life of a School Nurse*

Pleasantville Elementary School, early September: The school nurse, Ms. Davis, RN, plans to do the first-grade vision screening today, but first she will see the children who are waiting outside her clinic office door. First in line is Jason. Jason's mother wants him to be "checked out for chicken pox." Jason's cousin, Tommy, a second-grader, now has chicken pox.

The school secretary knocks on the door. She has Mrs. Perez, who is visibly upset, and her three children with her. "We have a problem," says the secretary. "These children, ages 8, 6, and 5 years old, have not had any shots since their birth in Mexico. School policy will not allow me to register them. I told the mother that you could help them."

In the hallway sits 8-year-old Shelly Strong. Mr. Bullen, her teacher, is concerned because Shelly says she has asthma and needs a "breathing treatment." This is Mr. Bullen's first year to teach school. He is not sure what Shelly is talking about and says that he never has seen a breathing machine like the one Shelly brought to school in her backpack today.

Out in the hall, 9-year-old Steven (who is taking Ritalin for ADHD) and Hiram (who has a physical disability and uses crutches) are yelling and shoving each other. Both 9-year-olds have a history of poor anger control. Mr. Bullen assists Ms. Davis in breaking up the fist fight. Their teacher, Mrs. Adams, has become very frustrated with their behavior.

Ms. Davis seems to be in control of the situation. She has learned to be flexible with her schedule and to prioritize her nursing duties. Ms. Davis assesses Shelly's respiratory condition. Shelly has the signed papers from her mother and the physician giving permission for the inhalation treatment. The school nurse documents her condition and begins Shelly's treatment. She also records the time of treatment and the amount of albuterol as prescribed by her physician. She calls Mrs. Strong, Shelly's mother, at work and sets up an appointment for that afternoon to discuss Shelly's emergency care plan for future asthma attacks. Ms. Davis informs Mr. Bullen of the meeting and requests his presence. She makes a note to schedule a staff in-service on asthma: its signs, symptoms, medications, and treatments.

Ms. Davis assesses Jason for chicken pox and finds him presently free of eruptions. She sends him back to class with an excuse, then records the office visit in a nurse's note for the day. She schedules herself to check Jason in 1 week, because he has been exposed to herpes zoster and has not had chicken pox.

Ms. Davis has not forgotten about the Perez family. She discusses the immunization schedule with the mother. She teaches her about the diseases covered by the immunizations, reviews their medical records and a brief medical history for each child, and then prepares the correct immunizations for each one. Ms. Davis administers the immunizations and discusses possible side effects with the mother. Ms. Davis gives the mother and the school secretary the proper paperwork for the children to be registered in school that day.

Mrs. Perez speaks mostly Spanish. Ms. Davis has been taking Spanish night classes at a local college to communicate with the growing Spanish population in her area. Mrs. Perez requests information on applying for Medicaid. Ms. Davis sets up an appointment with the Medicaid office for Mrs. Perez to discuss this and draws a map for the mother. Ms. Davis asks if she can visit with her and the children at home to assess for other needs. The mother agrees.

Shelly's treatment has been completed. Ms. Davis assesses her respiratory condition and allows her to return to Mr. Bullen's class. Ms. Davis then schedules an appointment with Mrs. Adams (Steven's and Hiram's teacher). She wants to share some resource materials on behavior management that are now available. Also, she wants to discuss Steven's medication dosage and classroom behavior. Ms. Davis then makes a referral to the school psychologist regarding the repeat incident between the two boys. She schedules time on her calendar for classroom education regarding children with disabilities in grades K–6. By 10 A.M. she is ready to begin calling on her first class for vision screening. ◉

term, school nurses will need to grasp the impact that values and certain relevant societal problems have on education's goals. The school nurse shows evidence of understanding these issues by promoting physical, mental, and environmental health in the school. In this way, children may obtain and maintain appropriate learning experiences.

In the long term, there is a need to emphasize prevention of chronic diseases while the child is still in childhood. Among adults older than 25 years, 62.9% of all deaths result from two causes: cardiovascular disease and cancer (CDC, 2008). The majority of risk behaviors associated with these two causes of death are initiated during adolescence.

---

**▪▪ ▪** CULTURAL CONNECTION

The Columbine High School shootings apparently resulted from a complex series of events where the two shooters had experienced perceived harassment (according to their online journals). How can school nurses mediate and introduce positive primary health intervention strategies to reduce harassment in an increasingly more diverse school population? ⬤

---

Research has shown that chronic disease is often the outcome of modifiable lifestyle choices.

In the United States, more than 6 million adults work in school-related activities. The school setting is the workplace for more than 20% of the U.S. population (children and adults). Fifty-three million young people attend 129,000 public and private schools for about 6 hours of classroom time each day, for as many as 13 years of the most formative years of their lives (Snyder & Hoffman, 2002). More than 95% of youth ages 5 to 17 years are enrolled in school. Many of these children come to school with learning disabilities. The high school completion rate has remained relatively steady, reaching 72.5% in 2001 (NCES, 2003), with 77.1% being the highest rate ever attained (in 1968–1969).

High-risk behaviors can lead to substantial morbidity and social problems among young people in the ninth to twelfth grades. During the past 20 years, the percentage of children and adolescents who are overweight has doubled. The increase in type 2 diabetes may be one of the first consequences of this epidemic of obesity among young people. Statistics and trends show that "a choice is at hand: invest now in children's physical and emotional health to create tomorrow's healthy citizens, or pay ten-fold down the road" (NCSBN, 1990).

There have been encouraging statistics showing improvement in certain health indicators. The percentage of children immunized before the age of 3 was up from 67% in 1999 to 77% in 2006 (Federal Interagency Forum on Child and Family Statistics, 2008).

Data from 2001 showed that the average percentage of children younger than age 18 years who were below poverty in urban areas was 15.8%, down from 21% in 1994. The percentage range differed by geographic area (The Annie E. Casey Foundation, 2008).

Mental health needs continue to require more attention than there are resources to meet them. The school nurse may become involved when a teacher suspects child abuse or neglect. For calendar year 2002, an estimated 1.8 million referrals alleging child abuse or neglect were accepted by state and local child protective services (CPS) agencies for investigation or assessment. The referrals included more than 3 million children; of those children, approximately 896,000 were victims of child abuse or neglect, with neglect being present in 60% of the cases reported. In 2002, there were 1,400 fatalities (Child Welfare Information Gateway, 2008).

Abuse and other mental health challenges will involve more than just the child; they involve families, too. Home visits are the best strategy for assessing the child's living conditions more accurately.

The National Longitudinal Study of Healthy Adolescents (NLSHA—a congressionally mandated study of 90,000 teenagers across the United States) highlighted the importance of a child feeling "connected" to the school for greater success (Resnick et al., 1997). Continued data collection by Blum (2004) has contradicted the widely held assumptions of the predictive value of race, income, and family structure on an adolescent's choice of participating in unhealthy behaviors. "Failure in school, too much unstructured time, and poor family relationships were shown to be three to eight times more likely to predict the kinds of risk behaviors studied" (Resnick et al., 1997).

Immigration numbers have increased in the United States. Unlike previous immigrants, who often came from countries where education was valued, immigrant children today tend to come from countries where survival has taken precedence over education. The language barriers they experience have implications for health access, learning, and socialization. The percentage of children who are linguistically isolated ranged from 23.1% in Texas to 7% in Colorado (The Annie E. Casey Foundation, 2008). Members of this group are also at risk for poor physical and mental health, as well as challenges to their learning ability.

Many children currently in schools do not constitute an at-risk population but still can be healthier with school nurse interventions. Rates of "lifestyle-related" diseases such as diabetes, hypertension, obesity, cardiovascular disease, and cancer have risen dramatically, even among children. School nurses are in a strategic position to help address these issues. Currently, however, only limited school resources have been devoted to prioritized areas, such as meeting the needs of medically fragile students with severe asthma, diabetes, behavioral problems requiring medications, seizures, and HIV/AIDS, as well as students dependent on medical devices for life and health (Schwartz & Laughlin 2008).

• Nurses provide a variety of health services at schools. These services include assessing, promoting, and maintaining the health of staff as well as students. One school nurse, for example, arranged for her three schools to have a contest among staff and teachers at each school. Each school worked from January to May, striving to have the lowest cholesterol

---

✦ ENVIRONMENTAL CONNECTION

How do the cultural and physical environments of a school affect both health and learning? Compare an urban high school to a rural high school.

levels, the most normal blood pressures, the greatest numbers of average body mass index (BMI), and the most normal glucose levels. Health problems identified through this contest required referral to primary healthcare providers in the community. Health promotion in school staff has improved productivity, decreased absenteeism, and reduced health insurance costs (Schwartz & Laughlin 2008).

Prevention and control of communicable diseases, management of chronic medical conditions, and emergency care for illness or injury can be well managed by school nurses. School health services that include mental, emotional, and social components contribute not only to the well-being of the individual student, but also to the school environment. School nurses are in a key position to foster better health, thereby handling concerns about promoting safe and sanitary school environments. The health curriculum also provides educational opportunities. Counseling needs are many and varied, and at times may require family involvement. If a school-based clinic is available, follow-up may be expedited.

Initially, school health services had limited meaning for many educational administrators; they viewed the scope of school health as compliance with regulatory laws regarding immunizations, and monitoring health screening results. Boyer (1991), and many others since, have supported the findings that a direct link exists between health and academic performance.

The U.S. Secretaries of the Department of Education (DOE) and the Department of Health and Human Services (DHHS) formally recognized the importance of school health to a community's health in a joint statement supporting comprehensive school health programs (see Box 40-1). School nurses, therefore, work under two entities: education and health; school nurses provide services in these two worlds. The joint document issued by these agencies supported school-based centers as a means of facilitating access to health care.

**School health services** may consist of basic health, expanded health, or comprehensive health services. School nurses provide episodic or emergency care, monitor health status through screenings, identify health problems that ad-

versely affect students' progress, administer medications, and assist students with medical devices such as tracheostomies, urinary catheters, and orthopedic devices (Passarelli, 1996). They supervise medical care that has been delegated to non-professionals, develop programs and evaluate outcomes, and monitor family outreach as part of their expected practice. In addition, school nurses often participate in health education to staff and students. In 1998, Congress encouraged the CDC to promote comprehensive school health programs (CSHP).

At the local school district level, the principal may choose which health service model to implement. Funding often dictates the extent of services chosen for implementation. According to the Secretary of Education, "Some schools have been run as centralized, bureaucratic, monopolies with little accountability and few standards of measurement. . . . When budgets are tight, and funds needed elsewhere, many of these schools are fiscally plundered by their state or local politicians. . . . As a result, millions of students have suffered from bureaucratic imprisonment and poorly delivered services" ("Paige," 2004).

## History of School Health Nursing

### ■ Origins

School nursing grew out of a need identified by a school official in England around 1891. Without immunizations or antibiotics, children were losing school time to "minor ailments and infectious troubles" (Oda, 1981). A lack of parental support for education was pervasive; poorer families often used children as breadwinners or as baby-sitters for younger siblings. A school official and a nurse were concerned that some children's education was being hampered by absenteeism due to poor health, so the school official asked the nurse to visit the children at home. This was the beginning of school health nursing.

Around the same time (1902) in the United States, Lillian Wald became concerned about the education and general welfare of tenement children in New York. In particular, the health and education status of tenement children excluded from school due to illness or disabilities distressed Wald. At Wald's suggestion, Lina Rogers Struthers, the first school nurse in America, was hired by the Board of Education. Her task was to treat children in the school, if possible, or visit homes to monitor environmental conditions in need of attention (Pollitt, 1994).

Wald worked out of her home, known as the Henry Street Settlement. Wald's lifetime efforts brought nurses into the New York schools. Even though she was a nurse, she addressed social problems such as child labor. She established the first neighborhood playgrounds, centers, youth clubs, vocational classes, and foster homes. With remarkable foresight, Wald was the forerunner of comprehensive school health services: special education classes began with her development of the first ungraded classrooms for "defectives," or children with disabilities.

---

**BOX 40-1**

**Selected Federal Mandates Related to School Health**

| | |
|---|---|
| 1973 | Section 504, Rehabilitation Act |
| 1975 | Education for all Handicapped Children Act (PL 94-142) |
| 1978 | Health Education Act (PL 95-561) |
| 1979 | Office of Comprehensive School Health |
| 1988 | Office of School Health (Health, Education, and Welfare) |
| 1990 | Birth to Twenty-One legislation (PL 99-457) |
| 1991 | IDEA (Individuals with Disabilities Education Act) |
| 2001 | No Child Left Behind federal mandates |
| 2004 | CDC Healthy Schools Initiative |

# JOINT STATEMENT ON SCHOOL HEALTH

by

## The Secretaries of Education and Health and Human Services

Health and education are joined in fundamental ways with each other and with the destinies of the Nation's children. Because of our national leadership responsibilities for education and health, we have initiated unprecedented cooperative efforts between our Departments. In support of comprehensive school health programs, we affirm the following:

- ***America's children face many compelling educational and health and developmental challenges that affect their lives and their futures.***

  These challenges include poor levels of achievement; unacceptably high drop-out rates; low literacy; violence; drug abuse; preventable injuries; physical and mental illness; developmental disabilities; and sexual activity resulting in sexually transmitted diseases, including HIV, and unintended pregnancy. These facts demand a reassessment of the contributions of education and health programs in safeguarding our children's present lives and preparing them for productive, responsible, and fulfilling futures.

- ***To help children meet these challenges, education and health must be linked in partnership.***

  Schools are the only public institutions that touch nearly every young person in this country. Schools have a unique opportunity to affect the lives of children and their families, but they cannot address all of our children's needs alone. Health, education, and human service programs must be integrated, and schools must have the support of public and private health care providers, communities, and families.

- ***School health programs support the education process, integrate services for disadvantaged and disabled children, and improve children's health prospects.***

  Through school health programs, children and their families can develop the knowledge, attitudes, beliefs, and behaviors necessary to remain healthy and perform well in school. These learning environments enhance safety, nutrition, and disease prevention; encourage exercise and fitness; support healthy physical, mental, and emotional development; promote abstinence and prevent sexual behaviors that result in HIV infection, other sexually transmitted diseases, and unintended teenage pregnancy; discourage use of illegal drugs, alcohol, and tobacco; and help young people develop problem-solving and decision-making skills.

- ***Reforms in health care and in education offer opportunities to forge the partnerships needed for our children in the 1990s.***

  The benefits of integrated health and education services can be achieved by working together to create a "seamless" network of services, both through the school setting and through linkages with other community resources.

- ***GOALS 2000 and HEALTHY PEOPLE 2000 provide complementary visions that, together, can support our joint efforts in pursuit of a healthier, better educated Nation for the next century.***

  GOALS 2000 challenges us to ensure that all children arrive at school ready to learn; to increase the high school graduation rate; to achieve basic subject matter competencies; to achieve universal adult literacy; and to ensure that school environments are safe, disciplined, and drug free. HEALTHY PEOPLE 2000 challenges us to increase the span of healthy life for the American people, to reduce and finally to eliminate health disparities among population groups, and to ensure access to services for all Americans.

In support of GOALS 2000 and HEALTHY PEOPLE 2000, we have established the Interagency Committee on School Health co-chaired by the Assistant Secretary for Elementary and Secondary Education and the Assistant Secretary for Health, and we have convened the National Coordinating Committee on School Health to bring together representatives of major national education and health organizations to work with us.

We call upon professionals in the fields of education and health and concerned citizens across the Nation to join with us in a renewed effort and a reaffirmation of our mutual responsibility to our Nation's children.

Richard W. Riley
*Secretary of Education*

Donna E. Shalala
*Secretary of Health and Human Services*

Joint Statement on School Health

Early school nurses screened for hearing, vision, and orthopedic problems.

## Evolution of School Nursing

During the first half of the twentieth century, school nurses were seen as the people at school who made sure immunizations were up-to-date, who identified communicable diseases, who did vision and hearing screening, and who helped students in wheelchairs. Lina Rogers Struthers is considered the first school nurse in the United States, serving with Lillian Wald at the Henry Street Settlement in New York City during the early part of the twentieth century. Miss Wald placed Lina Rogers Struthers in four NYC schools October 1, 1902. New York City became the first city in the world to publicly fund school nursing services (Wold, 2001). Often, parents or support staff viewed their role at school as "Band-Aid" nurses, taking care of minor emergencies occurring at school. When mainstreaming began, the school nurse trained the teachers if a child needed medical attention (children with asthma, hearing impairments, or domestic abuse situations).

Drs. Loretta Ford and Henry Silver proposed the vision for the nurse practitioner movement in the early 1960s, in collaboration with nursing and medicine programs at the University of Colorado. A new role, school nurse practitioner, evolved along with the rest of the nurse practitioner movement. An impetus for the school nurse practitioner movement was the obvious need to improve children's access to health care, and to prepare practitioners who could focus on the needs of children and adolescents.

In 1969, the School Nurse Practitioner (SNP) program was first implemented. Under this model, the school nurse practitioner provided primary care in schools. This practice was funded through partnerships with managed care models and third-party reimbursements to school-based clinics. There was also the possibility of patient-generated revenue at such clinics (Urbinati, Steele, Harter, & Harrell, 1996).

In the 1970s, changes in funding and in public expectations of the government's role in health care reduced school health services to episodic and uncoordinated situational care. Parents and educators disagreed about how to teach sensitive and value-laden materials. To some parents, school health services became synonymous with sex education—a controversial position, to say the least. Schools began to decline as centers for providing primary care to children and the community. As increasing numbers of disabled and technology-dependent children were integrated into regular classrooms, the focus of school nursing changed to one of increased responsibility for training teachers and staff in how to meet the needs of these children. The school nurse provided in-service and one-on-one education for school personnel as needed.

Landmark research conducted during the 1980s by Judith Igoe and colleagues in Colorado (Igoe, 1990, 2002; Igoe & Giordano, 1992) highlighted the great potential for impacting the health and academic experiences of school children when adequately prepared nurses are present in the schools. Their federally funded research addressed issues such as shifting student health needs, volatile societal expectations, unpredictable legislation, and the need for reliable sources of funding. These authors even suggested a new paradigm for delivering services: the **school-based clinic.** Patient outcomes in school nursing were measured in educational terms such as school attendance and test scores, rather than as changes in morbidity. This work gave a broader context for school health nursing, which was now seen as relevant both within and outside the school setting (Gustafson, 2005).

## Federal Mandates in School Health

In 1973, Section 504 of the Rehabilitation Act required that schools provide "free and appropriate education" for children with disabilities. Included in Section 504 were mandates for specially designed classroom instruction, and additional services such as specialized transportation. The school nurse became a necessary part of "special education" at schools attended by **medically fragile children** with chronic disorders such as cerebral palsy, seizure disorders, mental retardation, and emotional or behavioral problems.

In 1975, Public Law (PL) 94-142 (the Education for All Handicapped Children Act) broadened the definition of "free and appropriate education" by bringing children with various disabilities into regular classrooms. Called **inclusion** (or **mainstreaming**), this legislation-mandated movement focused on appropriate in-class support to students with various educational risks or disabilities, for the maximum time possible during each school day. The nurse's role was to train staff and teachers in the care of children with spina bifida, asthma, attention-deficit/hyperactivity disorder (ADHD), and other medical conditions on an individual basis.

Congress passed the Health Education Act (PL 95-561) in 1978. This act proposed that comprehensive school health services be delivered in the least restrictive environments for handicapped children, in settings outside the home. Subsequent state court cases gave legal weight to allowing severely disabled students to enter public schools in record numbers.

The Department of Health, Education, and Welfare established the Office of Comprehensive School Health

(OCSH) in 1979 in which school health services were extended to include preschool children (Head Start) and expanded to cover school nutrition. Two years later, the OCSH was abolished. In 1983, school health services were placed with the U.S. Public Health Service, Department of Maternal–Child Health. Funding was not sufficient to meet the increased demands brought about by funding of school health nursing on that department's budget, so funding for school health services was divided between multiple agencies.

In 1988, Congress authorized the establishment of the Office of School Health in the Department of Education. School health services were now no longer funded from health-related departments. Since 1988, as many as 300 federal agencies related to child health, school health, mental health, and environmental health have taken an interest in school children and adolescents. These agencies include the CDC, the Health Resources Services Administration (HRSA) in the Department of Health and Human Services, the Department of Agriculture, and agencies that focus on physical fitness and environmental issues.

The initial legislation passed in 1975 (PL 94-142) was modified through the passage of the Individuals with Disabilities Act (IDEA) in 1991. This legislation (PL 99-457) mandated school health services for specific conditions, starting from birth and continuing to age 21 years. Thirteen conditions included in the 1991 IDEA legislation were amended to 12, as follows: autism, deaf-blindness, emotional disturbance, hearing impairments, mental retardation, multiple disabilities, orthopedic impairments, other health impairments (chronic diseases such as asthma, epilepsy, or diabetes), specific learning disabilities, speech or language impairments, traumatic brain injury, and visual impairments (NCES, 2004a). However, IDEA is still funded at 17% of full funding (NASN, 2004).

In 1965, the Elementary and Secondary Education Act (EASA) was enacted to provide guidance and funds to K–12 schools. Since then, Title 1 of EASA has provided trillions of dollars in financial assistance to schools educating low-income students. Half of all public schools in the United States currently receive funds under Title 1.

Funding and coordination of services are major issues for school nurses and other health professionals providing care to school children. The CDC's Healthy Schools Initiative forms the basis for coordination of agencies serving schools. An increasing number of states are availing themselves of CDC funding for these programs (CDC, DASH, 2004).

The most sweeping federal education legislative changes in decades were enacted into law in 2001. The No Child Left Behind (NCLB) legislation is the most recent reauthorization of EASA; it addresses all areas of K–12 education. NCLB seeks to address educational equity on the basis of educational *opportunity,* rather than on equalized *funding* for schools. In 2004, the General Accounting Office released a study showing that the NCLB initiative is not an "unfunded mandate." Other economists agreed ("Paige," 2004). Federal funding for education increased 36% from 2002 to 2004.

## MEDIA MOMENT

### *Mean Girls* (2004)

With parents as world-trekking zoologists, Cady Heron has never known what "high school" truly meant. She lived her first 15 years in the African jungle, home-schooled, living life with only her parents and the animals of the wilderness, knowing all of the rules of survival. However, when she moves out of Africa, she has to learn the rules of high school, a jungle in itself. She instantly makes friends with two sweet teenagers, Damian and Janis, who, in the terms of the high school, are in the "out crowd." Soon she meets the Plastics, three crude, beautiful, popular girls: Regina, the unofficial leader; Gretchen, Regina's full-time follower; and Karen, "one of the dumbest people you will ever meet." They immediately let her into their group, but Cady, wanting to keep her first friends, is unsure. The two convince Cady to keep her relationship with the Plastics, only so that they can know their dark secrets.

However, events take a turn for the worse when Cady falls for Regina's ex-boyfriend, Aaron. When Regina finds out, she seeks revenge on Cady by taking Aaron back. When Cady finds out, what began as a game to discover secrets turns into a plan to destroy Regina. Now, Cady, Janis, and Damian plot together to bring Regina's status down. However, as Cady spends more time with the Plastics, she, too, begins to become one.

Under NCLB, schools must make "annual yearly progress" (AYP) reports as a basis for funding. Without documented progress, distribution of federal monies is adversely affected, or parents are entitled to change their child's school.

This legislation has implications for schools that serve students with disabilities. There is a group of children, referred to as "gap kids" in the past, to whom the term "significant cognitive impairment" is applied. These children might have language barriers; be homeless; have parents in the military and have moved frequently; or have significant disabilities. Despite their unique challenges, the federal mandate of "no child left behind" still applies to this population. Initially, the definition of "significant cognitive impairment" could affect the AYP data on which school funding was based. Today, waivers are available to schools that provided adequate documentation. The National Center on Educational Outcomes (NCEO) has even developed a PowerPoint presentation that addresses the implications for IDEA legislation of the passage of NCLB.

## The Education System and the School Nurse

Educators and school administrators measure school success, in large part, by first whether a student successfully completes each school year, and then whether each completes the

K–12 curriculum. Costante (1996) has said, "Health-related activities that affect daily class attendance are perhaps the hallmark of school nursing services" (p. 5). Teachers find that students who are not distracted by unmet health needs in themselves or their classmates are more motivated and attentive in class. Decreased vision or hearing, emotional

### ETHICAL CONNECTION

Colleges and universities in the United States are increasingly taking a more cautious approach to students who demonstrate suicidal tendencies and severe depressive symptoms. Faced with the threat of liability suits from parents when students kill themselves on campus, schools are taking more of an aggressive approach with students they believe are a risk to themselves and to the morale and mental health of those around them. With suicide ranking as the number two cause of death for college students (claiming 1,100 lives each year), college mental health officials defend their concerns about how to address the problem.

As the number of students with mental health issues who enter college each year grows, who should bear the responsibility for their safety? Will this trend toward identifying at-risk students affect their likelihood of seeking treatment for depression in student health services if this may eventually lead to their dismissal? How can nurses in school health settings both serve as advocates for students and comply with university policies?

distress, or adolescent pregnancy, by contrast, can affect the educational experience.

Having qualified nurses in schools has been shown to decrease student absenteeism (Allen, 2003). Absenteeism affects funding; it is, therefore, an important indicator for school administrators. Absenteeism is often an indication of family problems, neglect or abuse, or lack of resources and medical access. These issues might not be addressed without the assistance of a school nurse.

For many years, principals of each school district considered the school nurse as their employee (Zimmerman, Wagoner, & Kelly, 1996). Meeting health service needs in the educational setting poses a dilemma—not because the needs are questioned or the benefits disputed, but rather because the responsibilities and priorities for service are poorly funded.

School administrators have many constituents. They often operate in a more politicized arena than most nurses do, and they know that health issues can be surrounded by conflicting values. Administrators face societal mores that vary greatly within each individual school, in terms of cultural, religious, and even language differences. As one principal stated, "If I make even one parent unhappy, it may cost me my job."

Since "mainstreaming" came to schools in 1975, school resources have been stretched to cover the special health needs of disabled or chronically ill students. Services to just

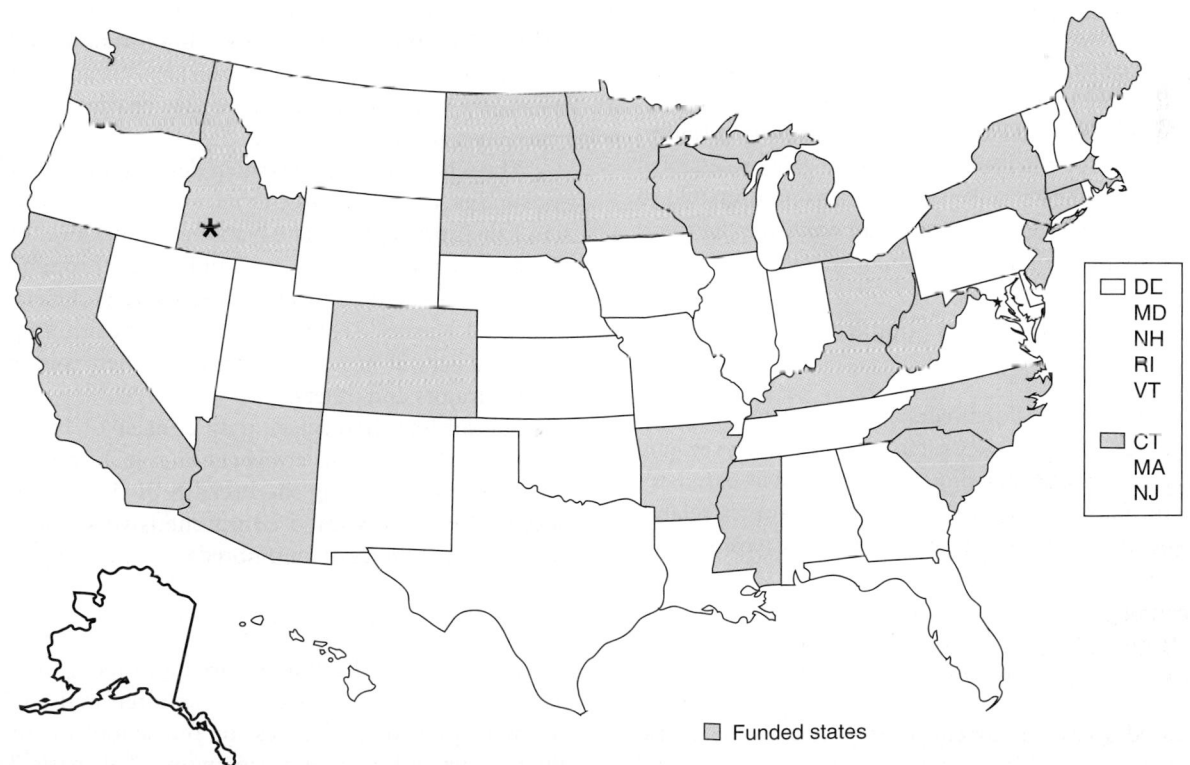

* Nez Perce reservation

CDC Funding for Coordinated School Health Programs, Fiscal Year 2008

Centers for Disease Control and Prevention (2002). Division of Adolescent School Health. *Healthy Youth*. Atlanta, GA: CDC. http://www.cdc.gov/HealthyYouth/about/healthyyouth.htm#map

one child with disabilities in Alabama ran as high as $30,000 per year in 1999, compared with $15,000 budgeted per year to educate a nondisabled child. Efforts to cut their budgets have often forced schools to cut nursing positions and replace them with health aides.

A coordinated school health program (CSHP) has eight components. The CSHP is meant to provide a way for schools to become facilities where many agencies can cooperate and address the health needs of school children and staff. The CDC supported CSHPs in 20 states in 2003.

## Education and Credentials of the School Nurse

The broad scope of knowledge expected of school nurses requires a minimum of a baccalaureate degree in nursing. Passarelli (1994) proposed that academic institutions design graduate-level and practitioner programs that correspond to the broad scope of school nursing. A National Association of School Nurses (NASN) strategic goal for 1994–1997 was "to pursue and advocate for greater access to undergraduate, graduate, and practitioner programs by influencing higher education to provide appropriate professional content to a larger school nursing enrollment" (NASN, 2004, p. 9).

In recent years, the family nurse practitioner (FNP) specialty has thrived, while the school nurse practitioner focus has become too restrictive, particularly in light of higher-education funding issues. Family nurse practitioner programs include content related to child and adolescent health, which makes FNPs educationally prepared to provide appropriate care in the school setting, particularly in school-based clinics.

The NASN and the National School Health/Education Coalition (1991) have helped school nurses gain professional status. However, the school nurse remains accountable to education. Budgetary constraints could continue the trend toward cutting nursing from the school system.

### ■ Continuing Professional Education of the School Nurse

Continuing professional education is crucial, particularly given that school nurses often practice alone. Updates on clinical skills, pharmacology, and evidence-based research help maintain clinical competence. Topics related to management, supervision, and **delegation** have specific relevance to administrative expectations of the school nurse. The networking and collegiality of continuing professional education meetings may also help prevent the burnout that characterizes the careers of many otherwise motivated nurses.

Increased access to current information via the World Wide Web has provided greater opportunities for school nurses to research a current need or to continue professional education. Nurses may negotiate for the use of staff development days to continue their own professional development. In addition, NASN offers an annual update program for school nurses. Journals addressing child health and illness, mental health, family health, and educational theory have increased in number.

Many school districts continue to require their school nurses to hold a valid school nurse certificate if they are to remain on the teacher's salary schedule. Every state requires that school nurses have an active nursing license to practice. State Departments of Education generally require school nurse certification as Education Specialists 1. School nurse specialists are educationally prepared to evaluate and care for children at risk and for medically fragile children. School nurses also support the educational goals of health promotion to students, staff, and (sometimes) families.

An increasing number of institutions of higher education are offering courses that meet these requirements for continuing professional education. Generally, school nurse certification requires 12 semester hours of coursework. Course offerings include courses on management of school nurse practice, educational psychology, physical assessment of the school-aged child, and nursing care of the child with developmental disabilities.

## Role Definition of the School Nurse

"School nursing is at once the best and least understood form of practice on the part of the lay public and nursing professionals," wrote Oda in 1979. This is still largely true. The dual-focused role is ripe for role ambiguity.

Igoe (1990) coined the term "boundary-dwellers" to describe school nurses. Frequently school nurses must decide between two competing priorities: health and education. What may be prudent healthwise may be disruptive of education, because screening takes class time.

The school nurse role is often defined for nurses by others, such as school administrators, who do not clearly understand the nursing role. The National Association of School Nurses has addressed this role ambiguity through its 2002 position statement "Education, Licensure and Certification of School Nurses" (NASN, 2002). The position statement can assist school nurses in translating their role to school administrators and others.

School health services may consist of basic health, expanded health, or comprehensive health services (Table 40-1). Reflecting the breadth of these services, the NASN (1993) illustrated comprehensive school nursing practice in the figure of an umbrella.

### ■ Provider of Health Care

Assessment of healthy children and recognition of the potential for health problems in children and adolescents are main preventive focuses for the school nurse. Minor emergencies and illnesses come up on a daily basis. Technology-dependent or chronically ill children also require competent nursing care. Nursing interventions may range from education and screening, to providing direct care to students with disabilities.

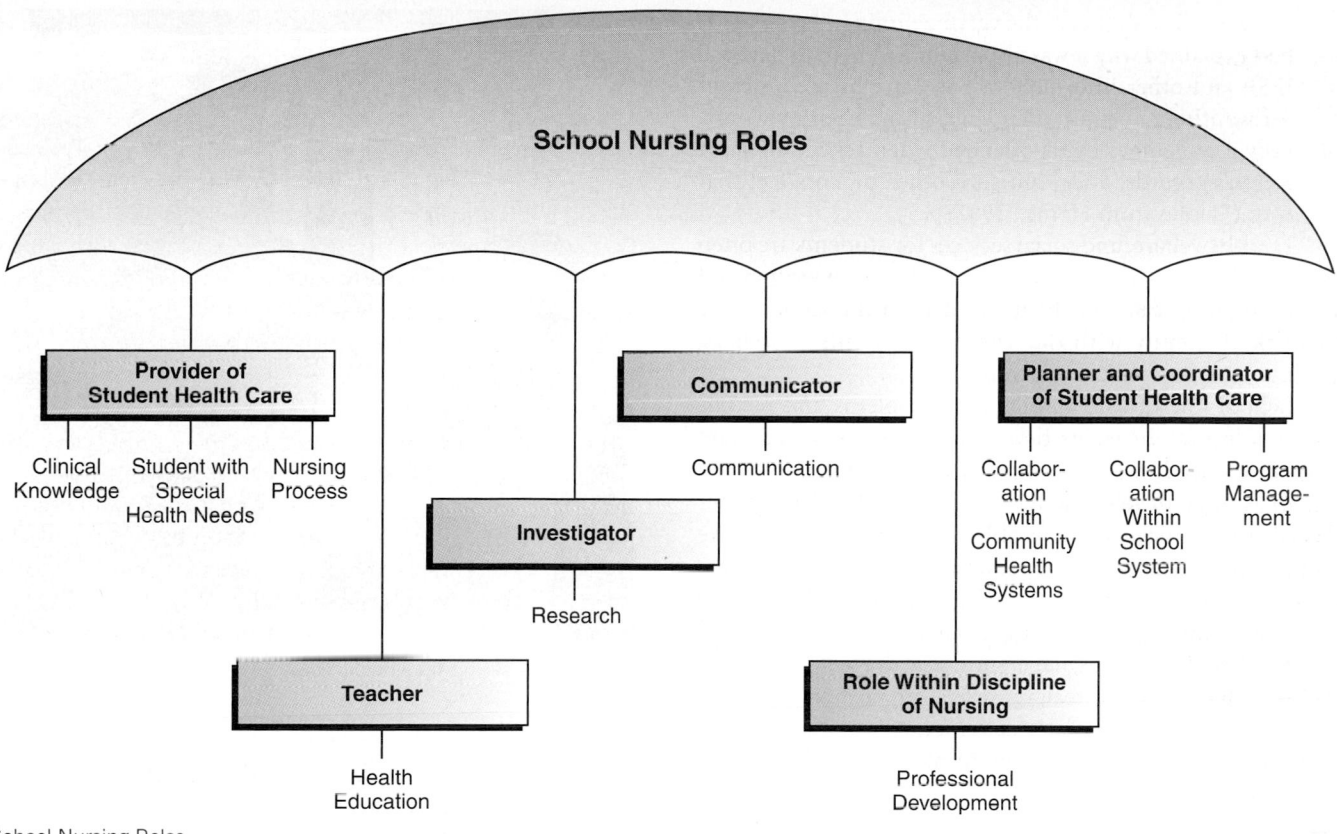

School Nursing Roles

Adapted from NASN, 1993.

**Table 40-1**  Examples of Selected Health Services Provided in Schools

**Type of Service**
- Administration of first aid
- Administration of medication
- Screens (height/weight, sensory)
- Abuse evaluation/follow-up
- Emotional/behaviors
- Monitoring of vital signs
- Cleaning/changing of dressings
- Health component of IEP
- Case management
- Nutritional counseling
- Mental health counseling
- Cardiovascular screenings
- Complex nursing to at-risk students
- Employee wellness
- Fitness screenings
- Urinary catheterizations
- Health risk appraisals

Nurses can provide health services for school staff. Educational personnel often have chronic, stable medical conditions. School nurses are concerned for the health of the bus driver and the cafeteria worker as well as the health of teachers and students.

Familiarity with theory can guide decision making by the school nurse. Besides nursing theory, such theories include change theory, developmental theory, management theory, role theory, and systems theory. School nurses, like all other nurses, use the nursing process as the framework for all assessment, diagnosis, planning, intervention, and evaluation activities.

## ■ Communicator

The following parent's story illustrates the importance of communication with parents:

I was adamant that our daughter would have at least one setting where she was treated as a "typical" kid. Because she has spina bifida, we see a lot of specialists. I wanted her child care program to be a place where we could escape the disability focus. So when the program director asked me to sign an information request form so she could get a copy of Karen's records, I refused. I wanted the child care staff to treat Karen just like all the other children.

A few months later, Karen's teacher again asked if I would be willing to share information from the IFSP (Individualized Family Service Plan). She explained that it would help her develop better lesson plans if she knew more about what Karen could do, and the skills we were working on. It was the first time I realized that Karen's special needs could be incorporated into the games and activities that happened in her school day. A little reluctant, I gave my permission.

Now, I wish that at the very beginning, the Director had explained why it was important for them to have the IFSP and other information. You can't blame a parent for wanting to protect their child's (and their own) privacy. I remember being offended when asked to release Karen's records, and I am sure other parents feel that way. ("Notes from Home," 1997, p. 7)

Health, welfare, and social services for students are often complex, fragmented, or even unavailable. Good written and verbal communication skills are needed for the school nurse to work efficiently with the learners (students), teachers, parents, and the medical community.

School nurses who can identify problems and recommend solutions in terms that evoke policy responses are desperately needed. To date, this fourth component of school health (policy development) is lagging behind the other three. Communicating the problems as well as the positive contributions that school nurses make to the school's mission is an important part of nursing activities, often directly affecting funding for school nurse positions.

Student health has been shown to have "peace dividends" (intangible, but real, rewards), but cost containment is a byword of current policy activities. A long-term investment in health makes sense—but immediate needs with potential for quick success may receive greater attention from policy makers. Unless the school nurse's voice is heard loud and clear, policies may not reflect school health as a priority.

Many school nurses provide health education inside and outside the classroom, with individuals, with groups, and with families. Good communication skills help get important messages across to the children, school staff, and the community.

## Planner and Coordinator of Student Health Care

Case management is a demanding component of school health services. Children with complex health problems may require home visits and referrals to medical services or resource agencies such as the Health Department. One individual responsible to coordinate this activity is the school nurse.

The school nurse must be self-motivated, organized, and flexible, while performing multiple activities. Many times, the school nurse is assessing rapidly changing situations, planning with teachers for addressing behavioral and emotional problems, evaluating the student and sometimes the family, or coordinating care with a physician. School nurses must also be ready to deal with unforeseen events (e.g., emergencies) in the midst of everything else.

Monitoring school health through record keeping and tracking is a part of coordinating services. The area of sexual health is often an area of discomfort in terms of documentation.

## Teacher

School nurses serve as teachers to students as well as to school staff, to parents as well as to community agencies.

School nurse seeing student in office.

Staff consultation regarding individual students is a major component of the school nurse activity (Anderson, 1994). Teachers and staff are open to assistance with behavioral problems, conflict resolution, and student performance in general. School nurses may also be asked to provide training on how to render first aid or handle emergency situations (e.g., injuries, fighting).

Students with disabilities and their parents may need individualized education provided by the school nurse. However, it is not only the chronically ill or at-risk students who need the teaching role of the nurse; all students benefit by receiving specific health-related information about nutrition, maintaining a safe environment, and proper rest and exercise.

## Investigator

Currently, there are very few meaningful data on school health nursing services. In the past, outcome parameters have included (1) number of teen pregnancies, (2) degree of substance abuse, (3) school attendance, and (4) dropout rates.

School nurses collect data from health records, home visits, and teacher conferences. These data have been used to demonstrate improved school performance in a child receiving glasses following a vision screening, for example.

School nurses may note an increased number of obese children during a weight screening. The school nurse may recommend, and then implement, a weight-management intervention for such an aggregate group, often in conjunction with nutrition and physical fitness school personnel.

School health records maintained by school nurses were used by Swanson and Leonard (1994) to provide (with 85% accuracy) an estimate of actual dropout rates. Students who dropped out of school used school health services less than those who did not drop out and who received follow-up on identified health problems. Capturing the cost–benefit data of health services validates the benefits of having qualified nurses to provide such services. Studies that demonstrate the need for programs, or the impact of school nurses on absenteeism, for example, speak to educational leaders.

Utilization of the school as a research site is on the rise (Puskar, Weaver, & DeBlassio, 1994). A national survey to identify nursing interventions used in school settings (Cavendish, Lunney, Luise, & Richardson, 1999) found that there were 60 core interventions with school children. These interventions covered a wide range of nursing diagnoses. Their research supports the need for consistent language to document school nurse activities.

### ■ Role within the Profession

The school nurse is a member of a profession now seriously committed to looking at school health. The American Nurses Association has established a Nursing Center for School Health, in collaboration with the National Nursing Coalition for School Health. In 1990, more than 50 organizations participated to form the National Health and Education Consortium (NHEC), which was formed to bridge the health and education fields (Passarelli, 1994). NHEC conducts research and develops policy to promote the education of children.

Even in systems employing more than one nurse, school nurses often work alone. Remaining an active member of the profession is important for the professional development of school nurses. "Obsolescence and isolation are therefore everpresent dangers, thus the necessity of involvement in professional school nurse organizations and for continuing education becomes most important" (NASN Standards 10, p. 55).

## Healthy People 2010

Although no single plan of action can be applied to all schools, a body of problems common to school-aged and adolescent youth has been identified in *Healthy People 2010*. Indicators include physical activity, overweight and obesity, tobacco use, substance abuse, responsible sexual behavior, mental health, injury and violence, environmental quality, immunization, and access to health care (DHHS, 2004). Health risk behaviors have been measured by the CDC's Youth Risk Behavior Survey (YRBS) since 1991, and the survey's results provide data related to the national goals. See Table 40-2.

Of deaths in persons aged 10–24 in the United States, 70.8% result from only four causes: motor vehicle crashes, other unintentional injuries, homicide, and suicide. Encouraging data trends from 1991 to 2003 from the YRBS show significant decreases in the percentage of students who never or rarely wore their seatbelts, a decreased percentage of students who rode with a driver who had been drinking alcohol, and fewer students driving after drinking alcohol.

**Table 40-2** Indicators from the Youth Risk Behavior Survey for Students in Grades 9–12, 1991–2003

| Indicator | 1991 (%) | 1997 (%) | 2003 (%) |
|---|---|---|---|
| ■ Never or rarely wore seatbelts | 25.9 | | 18.2 |
| ■ Rode with driver who had been drinking alcohol | 39.9 | | 30.2 |
| ■ Drove after drinking alcohol | 16.7 | | 12.1 |
| ■ Carried a weapon | 26.1 | 18.3 | 17.1 |
| ■ Plan to attempt suicide | 18.6 | | 16.5 |
| ■ Cigarette smoking | 70.1 | 70.4 | 58.4 |
| ■ Smokeless tobacco | | 11.4 | 6.7 |
| ■ Ever used alcohol | 81.6 | | 74.9 |
| ■ Ever used marijuana | 31.3 | 47.1 | 40.2 |
| ■ Ever used cocaine | 5.9 | 9.5 | 8.7 |
| ■ Sexual activity with more than four partners | 54.1 | | 46.7 |
| ■ Used condoms | 46.2 | | 63 |
| ■ Drank or used drugs before sex | 21.6 | | 25.4 |
| ■ Insufficient physical activity | | | 33.4 |
| ■ Not eaten fruits or vegetables (ate less than five per day) | | | 13–28 |

🏛 HEALTHY PEOPLE 2010

**Objectives Related to School Health**

**Disability and Secondary Conditions**

6.9 Increase the proportion of children and youth with disabilities who spend at least 80% of their time in regular education programs.

**Educational and Community-Based Programs**

*School Setting*

7.1 Increase high school completion.

7.2 Increase the proportion of middle, junior high, and senior high schools that provide comprehensive school health education to prevent health problems in the following areas: violence; suicide; tobacco use and addiction, alcohol and other drug use; unintended pregnancy; HIV/AIDS and STD infection; unhealthy dietary patterns; inadequate physical activity; and environmental health.

7.3 Increase the proportion of college and university students who receive information from their institution on each of the six priority health-risk behavior areas.

7.4 Increase the proportion of the nation's elementary, middle, junior high, and senior high schools that have a nurse-to-student ratio of at least 1:750.

**Injury and Violence Prevention**

*Unintentional Injury Prevention*

15.31 Increase the proportion of public and private schools that require use of appropriate head, face, eye, and mouth protection for students participating in school-sponsored physical activities.

**Violence and Abuse Prevention**

15.39 Reduce weapon carrying by adolescents on school property.

**Physical Activity and Fitness**

*Physical Activity in Children and Adolescents*

22.8 Increase the proportion of the nation's public and private schools that require daily physical education for all students.

22.9 Increase the proportion of adolescents who participate in daily school physical education.

**Tobacco Use**

*Exposure to Secondhand Smoke*

27.11 Increase smoke-free and tobacco-free environments in schools, including all school facilities, property, vehicles, and school events.

*Source*: DHHS, 2000.

The percentage of students who carried a weapon also decreased significantly from 1991 to 1997. However, the rate then remained constant from 1997 to 2003. Fewer youths also reported a plan to attempt suicide in 2003 than in 1991.

There was little change reported by students in their use of tobacco from 1991 to 1997, but from 1997 to 2003 a significant decrease occurred both in the use of cigarettes, and in use of smokeless tobacco by ninth- to twelfth-graders. The percentage of students who reported ever using alcohol also significantly decreased from 1991 to 2003.

Health education is one strategy for meeting the *Healthy People 2010* goals. However, coordinated health education is not the norm. Some risk behaviors have worsened, despite educational efforts. The percentage of students who reported ever using cocaine increased significantly from 1991 to 1999, then leveled off through to 2003. Those reporting current marijuana use increased significantly from 1991 to 1997.

Trends from 1991 to 2003 show a decrease in the percentage of students who reported having sexual activity with four or more partners. There was also an increase in the number reporting use of a condom during sexual intercourse.

Despite the fact that since 1991 selected risk behaviors monitored by the YRBS have shown some decreases among high school students nationwide, the risk for chronic health problems might actually have increased: 13.5% of students are overweight. Thirty-three percent reported that they had not participated in sufficient physical activity. The prevalence was higher among females, and higher among ninth-graders versus twelfth-graders. Only a median of 18.4% had eaten five or more servings of fruits or vegetables each day. (Prevalence ranged from 13.2% to 28.4% across state surveys.) Paxton, Valois, and Drane (2004) found little correlation between BMI, weight goals, and weight management in a large group of adolescents they studied. Students attending alternative schools have their own views on healthy behavior (Kubik, Lytle, & Fulkerson, 2004).

Yet despite improvements in certain behaviors over time, far too many high school students continue to engage in health risk behaviors, according to the YRBS. For example, in the 30 days prior to the 2003 survey:

- 2.6 million high school students rarely or never wore seatbelts.
- 2.3 million carried a weapon.
- 3.1 million students smoked cigarettes.
- 6.4 million drank alcohol.
- 3.23 million used marijuana.

## At-Risk Populations

Students at risk, such as technologically dependent children, may experience stigma from other children in the classroom because of their disability. Helping the child with socialization and addressing mental health needs are relevant school nurse roles.

Poverty may influence a child's ability to learn because parents lack the resources or the education to teach the child. When their problems are compounded with a chronic illness, these children constitute an at-risk population. Because of advancing medical technologies that have allowed tiny premature infants or children born with fetal alcohol syndrome and chromosomal abnormalities to survive, increasing numbers of medically fragile children now attend public schools across the country.

Blum (2004) found that "how young people do in school and what they do with their free time are the most important determinants for every risky behavior studied—regardless of whether they were rich or poor; white, black or Hispanic; or come from one- or two-parent families," Blum makes the following recommendations on the basis of findings from the most recent NLSHA study on healthy adolescents: "Policies must move away from the notion that youngsters' behavior choices are predetermined by their race, economic status, or family background—factors they cannot change. Efforts need to focus instead on the strong influences in children's lives that cut across demographic frameworks—the quality of involvement with friends, family, and school."

Peer pressure has significant impact on youth behaviors. The data show that when teenagers band together on prevention issues such as not drinking and driving, lifestyles are modified much more successfully than with a course on driving sober (Blum, 2004).

## Nurse as Team Member

A model of nursing services proposed by the School Nurse Organization of Minnesota (SNOM) captures the complexity of school nursing. Nursing services to children from birth to 21 years include case management, health assessment, disease-prevention activities, nursing care, policy development, and health promotion. In addition to this load, many school nurses collaborate with managed care organizations or private providers and with public health agencies.

Roles are fluid. Collaboration is the key to building an effective team. Schools operate under three levels of rules and regulations, as well as under parental and business community expectations (*Bridging the Gap,* 1992). Educators often feel they are "under siege" just to educate.

The entire school community is the school nurse's patient. School nurses work with families, with access health services, and with the environment in which learning activities occur. The health of the greater community is important to school nurses. Issues of concern to school nurses are similar to those of public health nurses. Bachman (1995) says that "as the school nurse role expands to accommodate the multiple needs

### Research Alert

Teenage pregnancy outcomes remain an increasing concern in the United States. Education and support of pregnant teens are critical factors that may determine good or poor pregnancy outcomes. Poor outcomes may include low birth weight, developmental delays, and poor academic performance. Although the number of teenagers experiencing pregnancy and parenting has declined in the United States, school-based health clinics can be used to provide support and guidance designed to avoid the negative outcomes associated with teenage pregnancy and parenting. By having school-based health clinics, nurse practitioners and school nurses can provide much-needed services to pregnant and parenting teens: These services should include educational support, counseling, and community resources. This inquiry provides a metasynthesis of the literature and reviewed, examined, and summarized the literature relating to the effect of school-based clinics on teenage pregnancy and parenting outcomes.

*Source*: Strunk, J. A. (2008). The effect of school-based health clinics on teenage pregnancy and parenting outcomes: An integrated literature review. *Journal of School Nursing, 24*(1), 13–20.

of a diverse patient population, a wide variety of collaborative practitioners is essential to the school setting" (p. 22).

## School Health Nursing Practice

Health problems exist in every school, but the nature of these health problems varies. The National Longitudinal Study of Healthy Adolescents (NLSHA) elucidated geographic, economic, and gender differences among the 20,000 teens and families surveyed (Blum & Rinehart, 1997).

The scope of clinical knowledge required ranges from wellness, to developmental delays, to other special needs of children and families. Screening for communicable diseases (e.g., lice, fever) and for developmental disorders (e.g., impairments in vision, hearing, emotional health, and scoliosis) is a large component of school nursing practice. Immunization surveillance is another important duty. Great strides have been made regarding immunization in the United States; however, healthcare providers should maintain a high index of suspicion regarding communicable diseases, especially in those persons who have traveled abroad recently.

The cost of providing one-on-one care is more than the hourly cost of the care provider. In addition to actually caring for patients, school nurses spend many hours coordinating care; developing, implementing, and monitoring individual health plans; determining the qualifications of care providers; delegating procedures and training designated personnel. Being able to provide one-on-one care also takes time from other staff time for training on how to be prepared to provide services in the absence of the care provider, or to help the care provider in an emergency. Each of these elements is an essential part of continuous nursing care and must be considered in planning. Districts will need added resources to provide such comprehensive school health services.

It is, therefore, difficult to proscribe one specific set of health promotion guidelines for all school districts in the United States. Exercise, fitness activities, and good nutrition clearly affect physical and mental health in children and adolescents.

### ■ Health-Related Services

**Health-related services** is a term used to describe services that meet the distinct needs of medically fragile students: The child with tracheostomy equipment needs extra physical space, as will a child in a wheelchair. Other children may require medication administration for asthma, seizures, diabetes mellitus, ADHD, hemophilia, or other chronic illnesses such as HIV. Children using inhalers and oxygen may be common in regular classrooms.

At times, children in schools may need technology (e.g., catheters, respirators, gastrostomies) for survival. School personnel may be asked to perform tasks such as suctioning children with tracheostomies, providing parenteral nutrition in gastrostomies, and performing catheterization. Medication administration and emergency measures are often required as well.

An **individualized educational plan (IEP)** is written for at-risk students in regular classrooms. The IEP is an educational plan tailored to each child's unique needs to assist each child in meeting educational needs. IEPs may be written for exceptionally bright, as well as at-risk, children.

**Individualized health plans (IHPs)** are plans of care used in the educational setting to identify, communicate, and document an individual student's healthcare needs. IHPs are the health-related component of the IEP. IHPs are based on the nursing process and are required by law to be written by a health team (Grabeel, 1996). Each child's IHP contains medical data, as well as plans for medication administration and emergency care (e.g., bee stings or anaphylaxis). Emergency care plans for IHPs must be written by a nurse. Emergency care plans anticipate injuries on the school grounds, exacerbation of chronic disease, and needed resources for health care.

The IHP is equivalent to the nursing care plan but is often implemented by non-nurses. The IHP is used along with the IEP to plan educational goals and activities.

For the medically fragile child, a multidisciplinary team writes an IHP. The school nurse is part of this team, which may consist of administrator, teachers, a local physician, social worker, speech pathologist, nutritionist, or occupational/physical therapists, and parents.

The composition of the team is determined by district administration. An educational coordinator is responsible for the child's assessment, training, and monitoring. Input from parents or guardians is critical for optimal educational placement.

### ■ Case Finding

Early intervention programs to identify children from birth to 3 years of age who have disabilities may utilize schools to conduct screening. Input from primary physicians becomes part of the **individualized family service plan (IFSP).** The IFSP is designed to assist in fostering the optimal development of children with disabilities from birth to 3 years of age.

All school personnel assist with identification of children and youth at risk for physical, emotional, or educational problems. The school nurse has a health perspective that can supplement the observations of teachers and staff, but teachers play a crucial role in assessing student health needs. Observation of children in the hallway, in the lunchroom, or on the playground provides teachers and school nurses with tips on physical, nutritional, or emotional needs.

Planned screening by the school nurse for developmental progress or vision, hearing, and dental screening are also important components in case finding. Review of attendance records is another form of case finding. Students who miss more than 10 days of school may need a home visit and/or family assessment, because high-risk families sometimes are unable to manage the tasks of getting their students off to school.

When a physician identifies a special need, referral to the school system may be less efficient. Hospital discharge planning may not include consideration of school needs. It may take months between the time a need is identified, the school is notified, and the child is actually enrolled in the school. This is particularly true for children experiencing the life changes that occur from a motor vehicle accident or other major trauma events. A school nurse is a key contact for healthcare providers in the community.

Collaboration with the community healthcare providers requires case management, which begins with identifying the child's healthcare needs. The school nurse has all parents complete an emergency information card that includes the name of child's healthcare provider (if any), as well as where the parent can usually be found during the day. If a student needs referral to a healthcare provider, parental permission is required to discuss the case with the provider.

Chapter author Dr. Frances Martin conducts a scoliosis screening for a girls basketball team at a local middle school.

Good documentation of the reason for referral, and requests for feedback, improve coordination of care with key contacts in the medical community. Some school nurses produce a newsletter with the goal of keeping community resource persons informed about school health.

All school personnel should assist with the identification of children and youth at risk for physical, emotional, and educational problems. Community issues such as war fears, violence and suffering in television news and other media, implications of terrorism, and sexual orientation issues may all affect the mental health of many school children. Teachers play a crucial role in identifying student health needs, but the school nurse has a health perspective that can supplement the observations of teachers and staff.

Many schools have delegated routine mandated school screenings (such as vision and hearing) to interdisciplinary teams for case finding and follow-up. As mentioned earlier, review of attendance records is another form of case finding.

## ■ Practice Issues in School Health

Funding of school health care is a major practice issue. Many physical morbidities (such as childhood diseases and malnutrition) have steadily decreased as a result of immunizations and other screening programs [such as Early Periodic Screening and Developmental Testing (EPSDT)]. However, many uninsured children with chronic diseases such as dia-

betes, asthma, recurrent otitis media, and poor vision (which are significant enough to affect functioning at school) are less likely to receive appropriate medical attention. Eye exams and eyeglasses, for example, may not be a priority for a low-income family.

The State Children's Health Insurance Program (SCHIP) offers health insurance to children 18 years and younger. This insurance covers children who are not eligible for Medicaid funding. Despite concerns that having insurance would lead families to abuse the healthcare system, the contrary has been found to be true (Lave, 1998). The school nurse is in a unique position of helping families enroll their children in this program. Each state has specific coverage.

In 1997, Congress passed legislation that allows states to provide health insurance to more children of working families. These programs build on the Medicaid program that started covering children and adults in the mid-1960s. For little or no cost, this insurance pays for physician and nurse practitioner visits, prescription medicines, hospitalizations, and much more. Most states also cover the cost of dental care, eye care, and medical equipment. Each state has a website that provides specific coverage and enrollment information, which can be accessed at http://www.insurekidsnow.gov/about.asp.

The changing structure of school health services is another practice issue. Other morbidities have taken center stage, as very tiny infants now survive into childhood, and the severely injured child may attend school despite the

School Nursing Services in the Greater School Community

*Source*: From "School Nursing Services in a Reformed Health Care System," SNOM Ad Hoc Committee on Health Care Reform, 1995. Used by permission of School Nurse Organization of Minnesota.

disabilities. In utero exposure to cocaine, marijuana, and alcohol is on the rise (Messinger et al., 2004). Health-risk behaviors of youth in alternative schools, those in the legal system, and those with no permanent home challenge the school health system (Kubik et al., 2004). Sexual orientation has emerged as a health issue as well (Frankowski, 2004).

There is a need to train leaders for school health programs. Expanding technology, changing disease trajectories, and increased accountability for patient outcomes contribute to the need for visionary innovations in school health services. School nurses work with a highly diverse population of well children and staff, as well as chronically ill children.

There are insufficient numbers of school nurses to cover all these needs. The nursing shortage has implications here, too. In fact, a membership survey of school nurses by NASN (Johnson, 2002) found that almost half of respondents were older than age 50. In 2000, the average elementary school teacher earned $13,600 more than the average registered nurse. The number of school children younger than age 18 in the United States is expected to grow from 72.6 million to 77.2 million between 2000 and 2020. School nurses are clearly necessary in the educational system, as they have a central role in implementation of school health services.

Funding needs depend on a multitude of variables and cannot be assumed to be equal across regions. Common variables are socioeconomic status of the region, numbers of special needs students, the complexity of families and diversity of cultures, the number of sites being served by each nurse, and the distance between schools. However, nurse funding may not be based on student or program needs. A critical need in school health is to find sustainable funding.

Typical sources of funding for school-based health programs serving indigent children (IDEA Book, 1996) are federal grants (usually Public Health Service Act section 329, 330, or 340); state block grants, especially for maternal–child health; local government funds; grants from national or local foundations or local hospitals; and Medicaid reimbursement (primarily EPSDT).

According to the Secretary of Education, the United States spent more than half a trillion dollars on K–12 education in 2003 ("Paige," 2004). The No Child Left Behind Act has added new requirements for testing, which are expensive. Services that are not mandated by law, as is the case with

---

 **GLOBAL CONNECTION**

Select a country outside the United States and examine the differences in the school environment that influence the health of students. Why is the United States virtually the only school system where violent outbreaks, including mass shootings, occur?

---

some nursing services, may be cut disproportionately, regardless of their benefit to students.

Our awareness of the complex environmental impact on human health has grown exponentially in recent decades. Exposures to lead and to secondhand smoking are more damaging to growing children than they are to adults. Exposure may occur in the school setting (to cockroach parts, mold, ultraviolet light, and dust mites) or at home. The school nurse is also concerned about exposures that occur outside of the school setting. One asthmatic student was riding the bus home when another student sprayed a perfume to which the asthmatic child was very allergic. The bus turned around and returned to the school to call for emergency assistance. Fortunately for the child, a clinic was located right across the street. Emergency inhalation treatment and parenteral medication assisted the needy student. It took the ambulance more than 45 minutes to reach this rural school. School policies are needed to address such emergencies (Reilly, 2002).

New infectious diseases, such as West Nile virus infection and SARS, will require school nurses to maintain vigilance and monitor the CDC's recommendations via the publication *Morbidity and Mortality Weekly Report*. Increased global travel raises the possibility of diseases in the United States for which no immunizations are available (such as malaria and HIV).

A number of students may see alcohol and drug use as a rite of passage. In fact, alcohol use may be combined with other adolescent behaviors such as sexual intercourse and reckless driving. These students put their academic achievement at risk and can be a profound challenge to the schools that serve them (NASN, 2004). Substance use may also reflect problems experienced in living with alcohol or drugs at home, or as coping methods for dealing with depression and anxiety.

The use of psychotropic medications to control behavioral problems in children has captured the attention of both lawmakers and the public. Following the Columbine High School shootings, lawmakers in Colorado explored the relationship between prescription drugs and school violence after hearing that one of the Columbine shooters was on a psychotropic medication (Delaney, 2000). A Colorado Board of Education resolution states, "Psychiatric prescription drugs have been utilized for what are essentially problems with discipline." The rate of prescribing psychotropic medications for preschool children has risen significantly frm 1990 through the first decade of the 21st century. One of the reasons cited for the rise was the larger role of school health personnel in identifying medical needs.

---

**MEDIA MOMENT**

**Heathers (1989)**
Veronica mingles with Heathers I, II, and III so that she can be as popular as them, even though she hates them. Veronica hates them enough to wish they were dead, though she would never want to be their cause of death. When she starts dating Jason Dean, however, she finds herself involved in the murders of most of her enemies, whose deaths are covered up as suicides.

**Application to Practice**
**Blog Entry**
Age: 18
Location: Colorado
Gender: Female
Date: 07 May 2008
Time: 13:01:43

I first got prescribed Paxil when I was seventeen. At that point in my life I was going through major depression and really bad anxiety attacks. I missed the first week of my senior year in high school because of my anxiety. When my mom decided to take me to the doctor, I had asked the doctor about Paxil since I had seen the advertisements on TV. He went ahead and wrote me the prescription, and I was put on therapy. I wasn't sure what to expect, but all I wanted was to feel like a normal person again.

I continued taking Paxil for a couple of months but when my insurance was up, I had no choice but to get off completely. I had no side effects at that point but my mom insisted that I get back on Paxil just to help me while I was still in school. I've been on it now for the past year and a half.

I've tried getting off Paxil, but it is so hard to do. I began experiencing extreme dizziness, shaking, nausea—any other bad feeling you can think of, I had. I'm not really all that sure what to do anymore. I still continue taking Paxil, but every other day. Even though it is every other day, I know I am addicted to this drug. As I try to shorten my dosage, it gets more and more difficult to go through each day at work and my first year at college.

My boyfriend tries so hard to help me but he's not sure how. I tell him how maybe I should see a doctor, but since he sees the side effects, he thinks they'll just try to give me another so-called wonder drug. So I guess I'm left to handle this alone and on my own. I can't believe my own doctor couldn't tell me the side effects of this drug that has now ruined my life and future.

How would you as a school nurse respond to this anonymous blog? Think of ways technology can expand the role of the school nurse beyond the physical school building.

## Legal Issues in School Nursing

All nurses practice under their state's nurse practice act. Many legal and ethical considerations arise daily. Nurses are taught the importance of documentation, but in the school setting the perspective differs. Because of the lack of sufficient numbers of nurses to cover certain school health needs, delegation of tasks such as medication administration, and documentation of that care, may fall to unlicensed personnel (such as the school secretary). State nurse practice acts have clear guidelines related to delegation. Accountability in one's practice can place a tremendous burden on many school nurses. Although many school districts carry liability insurance on school nurses, school nurses should carry their own liability insurance as well.

Parental consent is required to provide health services to children. These services include health screening for psychological or learning disabilities, medication administration, immunization, medical treatment such as catheterization, and education on human sexuality. School districts must establish health policies that follow state and federal guidelines, especially for dealing with medical emergencies when a parent is not available or consent is urgently needed.

Legal issues sometimes clash with ethical issues, as when a child's guardian has "do not resuscitate" (DNR) orders on file. In one case, when CPR was administered to such a child, responsible personnel were charged with assault.

In schools, medico-legal aspects of care, such as confidentiality, may receive different emphasis than in the traditional nursing arena. Student confidentiality and parental consent are viewed differently; the school acts *in loco parentis* (that is, in the place of the parent). Sexuality, related sexually transmitted infections (STIs), mental health, and substance abuse are recurring confidentiality issues among school children in traditional care settings.

Because of these differences, medico-legal aspects of medication administration, child abuse and neglect, documentation, and relevant licensure for care providers often challenge the school nurse. Many times these instances are managed by delegation, but the school nurse may ultimately be held responsible for the outcome. An example is medication administration to a child with ADHD. When no nurse is present at the school, but the time for the dose has come, a school staff member may be called on to "produce" the medication from a safe place, while the student is responsible for actually picking up the pill or pouring the liquid and swallowing it.

*Got an Alternative?*

Teens are often a targeted population for "quick fix," alternative diet products, including herbal products and bodybuilding enhancements. How can the school nurse educate students to make healthy, informed choices about these marketing campaigns?

The federal Health Insurance Portability and Accountability Act (HIPAA) regulations cover personally identifiable health information. Initially (2000), it was applied only to healthcare providers, health plans, and health clearinghouses. Schools were exempted from HIPAA rules, because schools were covered under the Family Education Rights and Privacy Act (FERPA) of 1974. Later, however, the federal government mandated confidentiality for health information held by schools.

The American Academy of Pediatrics (APA) has proposed the following recommendations for consideration by school officials and school health personnel:

The personally identifiable health information of students in schools should be protected in the same manner as such information elsewhere: Many schools are involved in providing health care on a day-to-day basis; however, their management of health records is a significant problem. Confidential student health information can be found in various locations throughout the schools (e.g., academic files, teachers' records). This information may be kept or accessed by a range of individuals with little or no training related to confidentiality requirements. A consistent, fair, and reasonable system must be designed to protect a student's health information in health care and educational settings.

School health providers and community health providers should be able to communicate directly concerning treatment issues, including immunization records. There is a lack of clarity concerning the intersection of FERPA and HIPAA that results in barriers to effective communication for the treatment of students in the school setting. The current environment is one of confusion that results in school health providers, who are often the people immediately responsible for a child's welfare during the day, being unable to communicate with community healthcare providers.

More stringent health privacy standards need to be put in place within the school setting in order to provide adequate privacy to a student's health information. Schools are not uniformly careful with a student's personally identifiable health information. Simply liberalizing the HIPAA privacy rule to allow school nurses to be included for purposes of receiving/sharing health treatment information is not an adequate resolution to ensuring that health information remains private.

NASN (2004a) is tracking changes in the law as they apply to schools. Confidentiality of information may be breached all too easily, as in a lunchroom conversation between teachers. Nevertheless, confidentiality of medical records is critical to parents as well as to administrators. FERPA gives parents the right to review and appeal records about their child, and it prohibits the release of student records without authorization.

Advance directives such as DNR orders raise serious ethical concerns for parents or guardians of a medically fragile child, as well as for teachers and other school personnel (Grant, Cureton, & Yahiro, 1998). Although any group of school nurses could list many other ethical concerns in school nursing, discussion of these issues is just beginning to take place on a broader scale (Proctor, 1998). Examples of ethical dilemmas include the following:

- The right of the school to exclude a child with chronic head lice, versus the need of the child to return to class for social and educational reasons
- The right of a school district to cut staff, including caregivers for severely disabled students, versus the child's right to safe, adequate, and competent care
- The refusal of a school district to implement DNR orders for a medically fragile child, versus the right of parents as guardians to forgo extraordinary procedures to prolong life (www.schoolnurse.com)

## ■ Documentation

Documentation is the only way to prove in a court of law that the nursing care was actually administered and that the standard of care was met. Malpractice suits against school nurses are rare; however, the increasing complexity of care and greater public expectations of healthcare accountability may increase the nurse's legal exposure if adequate documentation is lacking.

School health records also provide a way for the school nurse to communicate with families, students, multidisciplinary teams, emergency personnel, and other healthcare providers. Data can be used to identify student health problems, evaluate programs, provide quality assurance, and allow for continuity of care should the student move to another school district.

Student health records include documents such as immunization records, screening records, progress notes,

---

### 🖥 Research Alert

Researchers examined how schools in the U.S. Gulf Coast region perceived the mental health needs of students after Hurricanes Katrina and Rita and how schools responded. According to the report, despite strong initial efforts to support the mental health needs of students displaced by Hurricanes Katrina and Rita, many schools have not been able to fulfill students' mental health needs over the long term. Cited barriers include: (1) Problems communicating with parents; (2) Administrative pressure to "get back to normal" and focus on academics; (3) Inadequate resources and insufficient staff training; (4) Burnout among staff in charge of implementing and running the programs; and (5) Difficulties balancing the needs of displaced students with the continuing needs of preexisting students. Further research is needed to examine how future disaster planning can include school mental health needs and prevention.

*Source*: Jaycox, L. H., Tanielian, T. L., Sharma, P., Morse, L., Clum, G., & Stein, B. D. (2007). Schools' mental health responses after Hurricanes Katrina and Rita. *Psychiatric Services, 58*(10), 1339–1343.

☞ THINK ABOUT THIS ·····················

About one in five ninth-graders reports having had oral sex. The teenagers (average age 14 ½), say oral sex is less risky, more common, and more acceptable for their age group than intercourse. To study this issue, researchers surveyed 580 ethnically diverse ninth-graders in two California public high schools. Gender was not a factor, as girls and boys reported similar opinions and experiences. The study's lead author, Bonnie Halpern-Felsher, associate professor of pediatrics at University of California–San Francisco, said, "I think the stereotypes don't exist as much anymore," she said. "Girls and boys both see oral sex as not being a big deal." Teens often view oral sex as less risky, especially in regard to STDs and pregnancy.

While we know less about the risks of oral sex among heterosexuals, parents and school nurses should still inform teens about the potential risks for contracting STDs with oral sex. Further, there is the potential damage to the teen's relationships and self-esteem, which should also be discussed by healthcare providers and parents. While adults are focusing on avoiding sexual intercourse, teens are finding other ways to practice what they perceive as "safe sex" and parents are often "clueless" about these common and accepted practices among their children. ⬭

*Source:* Halpern-Felsher, B. L., Cornell, J. L., Kropp, R. Y., & Tschann, J. M. (2005). Adolescents and oral sex: Perceptions, attitudes, and behavior. *Journal of Adolescent Health, 36*(2), 443–456.

physician orders, physical examination records, medication and treatment logs, individualized healthcare plans, emergency healthcare plans, third-party medical records, consent forms, Medicaid and other insurance billing forms, and flow charts (NASN, 2004b). These may be in paper format. If so, these paper records should be kept in locked files. Records may also be stored via a number of electronic technologies, such as telephone databases, fax, e-mail, and personal digital assistants (PDAs).

Ensuring security and privacy of data is critical. Computers have streamlined record keeping, but may also convey information inadvertently if a file is left open. Information transmitted electronically is particularly subject to confidentiality regulations (HIPPA-FERPA).

Traditional health agencies view school nursing as being largely unregulated, whereas primary care sites are typically heavily regulated. The totally different types of documentation further highlight differences from primary care.

### ■ Delegation

Delegation is a legal issue. The American Nurses Association defines delegation as the transfer of responsibility for the performance of an activity from one individual to another, while retaining accountability for the outcome.

NASN recommends that the school nurse-to-pupil ratio be 1:750. Many school district administrators, not having this ratio of school nurses to students, may assign or delegate health-related activities to teachers, teachers' assistants, sec-

retaries, or others. Such staff members are called **unlicensed assistive personnel** ("working with, or in the absence of, the school nurse"). A principal is not legally licensed to delegate such activities as medical treatments or use of assistive devices. A key duty of the school nurse, therefore, is to train persons to whom activities such as notification of a parent when the child is ill or injured may be delegated. Before agreeing to accept responsibility for these staff members' actions, the school nurse will be familiar with state and federal regulations regarding delegation.

A curriculum for basic training of school paraprofessionals is available from the School Health Resources Service's Project ASSIST. Other training aids related to appropriate medication administration or specific medical procedures are available from NASN and from state nurses' associations. Training also makes sure the paraprofessional is aware of school policies related to issues such as student self-administration of medication (e.g., an albuterol inhaler).

### ■ Supervision and Accountability

Who is the school nurse's supervisor? Questions related to appropriate supervision of school nurse activities may arise almost daily. Some school nurses practice alone in their school settings and are accountable to school administration. Others work out of school health units in public health departments. The nurse must be clear on which decisions regarding health care rest with the school administration and which rest with her state's nurse practice laws.

Accountability involves meeting deadlines and following through with commitments, as well as providing competent nursing care. Being accountable involves risk. School nurses should request and welcome performance evaluations from peers.

An unlicensed assistive person (sometimes called a paraprofessional or a health aide) is an individual who is trained to function as an assistant to the licensed registered nurse in the provision of patient care activities as delegated by the RN (NCSBN, 1990). These individuals have had specific training by the nurse related to tasks delegated to them—tasks such as catheterization, suctioning, or gastrostomy feedings.

### ■ Funding Issues in School Health

Parents become strong advocates for increased school health programs when they appreciate the valuable services provided by their school nurse (Brandt, 2002). There must be adequate pay to keep nurses and other providers in the workplace where they are needed. Funds from grants and contracts

✎ NOTE THIS!

More than 52 million children attend schools in the United States. It is estimated that 10% to 20% have chronic, social, emotional, and/or health problems.

*Source:* National center at ANF addresses school nurse issues. (1998, May/June). *American Nurse,* p. 7.

**Application to Practice**

*Teachers Challenge Ruling on Medical Procedure*

Teachers at the Burkett Center for the Multihandi-capped in Birmingham, Alabama, appealed a state ruling that forces them to perform medical proce-dures on their students. They argued that because they must handle complicated medical procedures for students in their classrooms, they were violating state nursing codes. They were also concerned that their li-ability insurance would not cover them if something went wrong. Among the procedures the teachers were required to perform were catheterization, tube feed-ing, suctioning, and certain blood tests.

The circuit court judge ruled that while they were in college they should have known they would have to perform medical procedures at work. He also said that the state nursing code exempts the "gratu-itous nursing for the sick by friends or members of the family" and that due to the close nature of teacher and student work, the teachers are friends. The presi-dent of the county Federation of Teachers points out that if teachers are "friends" of the students, why do they have to get written permission to do such things as take them on field trips? If teachers are "friends," why are they paid employees? "Our teachers want to educate rather than medicate."

*Source*: Teachers Challenge Ruling on Medical Procedure, 1993.

often do not suffice to meet financial realities, and they are not reliably renewed or increased over time (Igoe, 2002).

Creative fee structures have been used to fund school health care, including managed care (Igoe & Giordano, 1992), and business and school partnerships (Lever, Stephan, Axelrod, & Weist, 2004). SNOM (1995) has assisted local school districts to access federal funds for immunizations, Mantoux testing, and for EPSDT. Some states have des-ignated money from tobacco settlements to fund school nurses. School nurses now have an increased number of partners and agencies to which they can appeal for support and innovation in school health nursing.

Business involvement in school health services has been used to fund coordinated school health programs. A hospital on the Mississippi Gulf Coast helped set up six school-based, nurse-run clinics to provide health services (Clemen, 1997). The "Cities in Schools" model is an example of a program developed by city governments to connect appropriate human services with youth at risk for dropping out of school.

One example from business is the support provided by the American Cancer Society. About 10 years ago, the American Cancer Society realized that eliminating cancer in the United States required more than delivery of cancer-prevention materials (Seffrin, 2004). Representatives went to the schools and listened to their needs. They heard about the need for community involvement, for collaboration with materials and curricula that addressed "their" area (cancer). They accepted the agenda for comprehensive school health education, viewing the full educational and school health picture. The American Cancer Society then moved from delivery of cancer-prevention materials to facilitating the ex-pertise inherent in every community. Their mission became to create the strongest health environment for all school children.

Other community-based voluntary agencies are now beginning to creatively advocate for funding of school health care, as they strive to improve the health of children, and the adults these children will become.

### Violence and Terrorism in U.S. Schools

Schools must be safe places if students are to fulfill their potential in school. Recent violence in our schools over the past few years has captured the nation's attention. Between 1992 and 2000, youths ages 5–19 were at least 70 times more likely to be murdered away from school than in school. Comparable data from crimes outside of school show that a much larger number of serious violent victimizations (e.g., rape, sexual assault, robbery) take place away from school rather than in schools. Crime in the nation's schools contin-ued to fall between 1992 and 2002, reflecting the decline in the national crime rate, according to the Department of Jus-tice's Bureau of Justice Statistics (BJS) and the Department of Education's National Center for Education Statistics (NCES) (Bureau of Justice Statistics, 2004). During these years, school crime dropped from 48 violent victimizations per 1,000 students to 24 per 1,000. Between 1995 and 2003, the percentage of students who reported being a victim of a crime of violence or theft at school also declined—from 10% to 5%. In 2002, as in previous years, students from 12–18 years of age were more likely to be victims of nonfa-tal serious violent crime away from school than at school. In 2003, about 7% of public and private school students ages 12–18 reported that they had been bullied at school within the past 6 months. Students age 12–18 were vic-tims of about 309,000 serious violent crimes away from school, compared with about 88,000 at school. Between 1993 and 2003, the percentage of students in grades 9–12 who reported being in a fight anywhere declined from 42% to 33%. In 2003, 5% of students ages 12–18 reported being victims of nonfatal crimes, 4% reported being victims of theft, and 1% reported being victims of violent incidents. Media coverage of school shootings may lead to parents and students with a sense of vulnerability in the school setting. The school nurse should be involved in efforts to provide accurate information while continuing to address student, family, and school staff concerns about the threat of violence within the school setting.

The NCES (2003) has developed indicators for school crime and safety, which cover such topics as victimization, fights, bullying, disorder, teacher injury, weapons, and student perception of school safety, among others. In 2001, students ages 12–18 were victims of nearly 2 million nonfatal crimes of violence or theft at school. The majority (62%) of all school victimizations were theft. Bullying behaviors are on the rise, however (Janssen, Craig, Boyce, & Pickett, 2004). In 2001, 80% of students reported that they had been bullied in the last 6 months at school, up from 5% in 1999.

Children as well as adults have recently endured catastrophic events, which have resulted in death and injury to children and loved ones. The Oklahoma City bombing; the terrorist attacks on September 11, 2001; the Washington, D.C., sniper incidents where random persons were targeted for death; and the wars in Afghanistan and Iraq have created a need to remain "on alert," which contributes to great anxiety (Webb, 2004). Children respond differently from adults, who are at the same time processing their own reactions. Since the September 11 attacks, researchers have identified more children with post-traumatic stress disorder (PTSD) symptoms than at any time in history (Hoven, Mandrell, & Duarte, 2003). There has been far less scientific research about children's exposure to the news than there has been to exposure to other entertainment media.

Disaster preparedness is an important part of the school health program. Disasters can occur within the school walls or beyond. Both types of disasters can impact the schools. In recent years, our country has experienced unprecedented disasters, from Hurricane Katrina to 9/11 and bioterrorism. Nurses in schools have special responsibilities and skills to act as first responders in mass casualty emergencies. They are in ideal positions to prepare school populations in disaster planning and preparedness. Schools are often utilized as shelters in disasters. The National Association of School Nurses contend in their position paper *School Nurse Role in Bioterrorism Emergency Preparedness and Response* that well-prepared nurses within the school environment have significant potential for minimizing the effects of disasters in school settings and, subsequently, in the community at large (NASN, 2005).

## Community Issues in School Health

### School–Health Linkages

**School-based services** are services delivered on the school grounds. School-linked services, by comparison, may be delivered across the street or across town, but are initiated by school personnel. The definition of which services are "eligible" as school-linked services varies greatly from state to state.

Parental involvement and community linkages are crucial for success in each local school–health linkage. Unless the community is involved in planning and supporting the services, one single component of the program, such as

pregnancy prevention education, can derail an entire health education program. President George W. Bush's recent emphasis on increased federal funding for faith-based organizations may provide incentive necessary to seek the support of dissenters (Button & Rienzo, 2002).

An example of a school–health linkage is the school-based clinic. This type of clinic offers primary care to students, their families and siblings, and school personnel. School-based clinics have been shown to be effective primary care providers of services to school children and youth, families, and their communities (Igoe & Giordano, 1992).

### Collaboration

The trend toward delivery of health care in a community setting amounts to a paradigm shift for providers and consumers alike. Service through collaboration will become the norm, not the exception. The 1993 State Adolescent Health Coordinators Conference underlined the need for collaboration as a strategy for fostering healthy children. Parents, teachers, healthcare providers, mental health services, social workers, and physical fitness and nutrition agencies all have vested interest in the health of children.

*Interdisciplinary practice* is a term used in academia, but seldom do students practice with other disciplines before graduation. Thus, after graduation, interdisciplinary practice is seldom implemented. It will increasingly be required. Education majors, particularly those going into educational administration, may welcome interdisciplinary practice with

## " a conversation with . . . "

### From School Nurse to a Career in Politics
*Marge Whaley, BSN, RN, MEd*

My career in school nursing started at Howe High School in Indianapolis in 1963. I was all of 22 years old and newly married. There were 2,500 students enrolled and for the first 2 years, I taught health classes two periods a day. I think that is when I learned to love being in the classroom.

I had the opportunity to start a school nurse program in Pasco County, Florida, in 1977. We first hired five nurses for our 25 schools. Therefore, everyone was stretched pretty thin. We did have the advantage of having a health assistant at each school, so someone else took care of the daily "boo boos."

From the beginning, Pasco nurses were in the classroom. At first, it was simple lessons on cleanliness and nutrition. We soon advanced to STDs and birth control. Every year, when I interviewed for new positions, as we grew in numbers, I would ask each applicant to bring a lesson plan for a class they might offer. This usually surprised the applicants—this was not part of their perceived school nurse role. In addition, the new nurses mainly wanted to start an IV or dress a wound the first few months until they grew more comfortable in the education setting.

Each new nurse also had to learn how to make a good presentation in front of students. Other nurses were their mentors after they had attended my orientation class. I demanded they be as effective as any other teacher in the school was, so our classes on health would be requested.

As we grew, the needs of our students grew. The number of children on ADHD meds had tripled in the last 15 years. The number of profoundly mentally retarded children and those with severe developmental disabilities continued to grow as well. Our first student with acute health issues had a brain stem tumor, was 8 years old, fed through a stomach tube, and was blind and deaf. I was privileged to witness the dramatic improvement in conditions for a 7-year-old with a rare syndrome, who was at home with no services, incontinent, and fed mostly baby food. At the end of 1 year, he was in a standing box, toilet trained, and feeding himself. It was almost a miracle for his family and for us as well.

Today our nurses are still in the classroom, counseling girls about birth control and helping them manage pregnancies, referring kids with ruptured eardrums and creeping eruption, and dealing with the ever-present head lice in the student population, However, there are also children with catheters, heart monitors, nebulizers, communication boards, and more. Parents expect many of these children to be mainstreamed into the student population, so it takes a great deal of support from nurses to help their nervous teachers cope with these challenges in their classrooms. However, our school nurses continue to take time for classroom presentations as well.

I believe we have one of the best models for school nurses anywhere in Pasco County because our nurses do not use their professional skills taking care of tummy aches and

Marge Whaley is serving her 14th year as a board member of the Pasco County School Board and is retired as school nurse coordinator of the Pasco County, Florida, school system.

putting on Band-Aids. A trained school paraprofessional— a health assistant—should do that, always under the guidance of the school nurse. This frees the school nurses to do population-focused care, such as screenings, referrals, and follow up for acutely ill students, helping teachers with mainstreamed students, counseling, and health education. I have *always* thought the nurse who must see every child who walks through the door with a minor health complaint is an inappropriate use of school nurses.

After several years of coordinating school health service, I decided to run for the county school board. I ran my first campaign in 1992 and have been a member for 14 years, serving as chair of the board three different times. Campaigning was terrible and foreign for me as a nurse—I hated asking people for money. What I learned after my first three elections where I had opposition is that most people pay almost no attention to the school board elections. We rank right above mosquito control in voters' concerns. Of course, when their child has a problem in the school system, they suddenly become much more interested.

I had a huge learning curve in my first term as a school board member; I thought, since I had been in the district for 17 years as a school nurse, I would be well prepared about school management and politics. Wow, was I ever surprised when I was the one at the orientation workshops asking the most questions. For instance, when I found out that giving the bus drivers a 50-cent raise would cost over $800,000 dollars, I was stunned. Because I know our health program is so good, I found my priorities focused on reading competency of our students in the district. Every child must learn to read or else nothing else matters. However, once a nurse, always a nurse, so I continue to keep my eye on the health of our student population.

As a school board member, I visit schools every month, staying the entire day. One of the joys of doing that is being asked to do a brief lesson in someone's classroom, often about health. So when asked if nurses should be involved in politics, I answer, "Haven't we always been?"

schools of nursing preparing school nurses. Partnerships are no longer a wonderful idea, but an idea whose time has definitely come.

### ■ Resources

The School Health Resource Services (SHRS), from the Office of School Health, University of Colorado Health Sciences Center, provides a school health reference collection. Timely updates, linkages with programs already in operation in schools and communities across the United States, "starter kits" for specific topics in school health, information links with other projects, and bibliographic services for drawing together educational and health databases are available.

## Innovations

Expanding technology, changing disease trajectories, and increased accountability for patient outcomes provide impetus for visionary innovations for school health services. The school-based clinic (SBC) movement began in the late 1960s in West Dallas. Staffed with nurse practitioners, part-time physicians, and social workers, the SBC in this town provided primary care. Funding was separate from the education budget and came from both private and public funds (Urbinati et al., 1996). The SBC movement has since grown and gained widespread acceptance as a means to address access to care.

Policy makers report that system-related factors may exacerbate poor health utilization. Examples of these factors include inaccessible hours of operation, inadequate number of health providers, and lack of continuity of care. School-based clinics have helped overcome these obstacles. Nevertheless, young people needing medical care may find lack of transportation, lack of information, and lack of money to be formidable barriers to care.

### ■ School-Based Clinics and Primary Health Care

School-based clinics have grown sevenfold in number, from 200 in the United States in 1990 to 1,400 in 2000 (Button & Rienzo, 2002). One teacher explained the benefit to children and their families of the school-based clinic:

> A lot of our kids are here without shots, without the appropriate care that they need because their parents can't reach the services—they don't have transportation or the motivation of getting up and going across town. Whereas at the school, the teachers can make sure the kids get the services. If health care providers can't get the kids to the health centers, then bring the health centers to the kids. (IDEA Book, 1996, p. 4)

A study of teenagers who used health clinics based in elementary and secondary schools found that they were nearly twice as likely to graduate from high school as those who didn't (Button & Rienzo, 2002). Thus school-based clinics are getting credit for keeping children in school, as well as decreasing parental absenteeism from work caused by the need to take a child to a doctor.

State funding for SBCs has increased dramatically, from $17 million in 1992 to $61.9 million in 2000. With the downturn of the economy and greater numbers of uninsured persons in the United States, these clinics are more important now than ever, in that they offer everything from physical examinations and mental health services to immunizations and reproductive counseling.

Some people have voiced concern over the scope of services offered in school-based clinics, particularly the contraceptive and STI programs. However, Button and Rienzo (2002) found that there is currently less opposition from religious and other groups than there was in the early 1990s.

At present, there are insufficient numbers of educationally prepared BSN nurses, much less nurse practitioners, to meet the demands for staffing in SBCs. If these clinics were set up to provide care for only 5% of the 129,000 public schools, for example, it would create an immediate demand for 6,000 more nurse practitioners.

Some school nurses have expressed concerns that SBC staff will take on all of the school nurse's responsibilities, leading to confusion among students and staff about who does what. At one site, such concerns led to a grievance (IDEA Book, 1996, p. 49).

School-based clinic nurses are covered by the health center's liability insurance and, therefore, are legally permitted to provide more services than school nurses can. Many school nurses are worried about their own liability, as discussed earlier.

Nurse practitioners who are knowledgeable about chronic illness in children as well as educational requirements for children have a valuable role at SBCs. School nurse practitioners do not replace school nurses, however.

SBCs are portable in some geographic locations. For some communities, mobile clinics, like the bookmobiles of old, provide accessible health care. In rural states, physicians and nurse practitioners may schedule travel to provide predictable in-school opportunities for check-ups and immunizations.

### ■ Increased Role of the Media in School Health

Print media represent an untapped source for developing school health linkages and for advertising for school nurses. The media are always looking for news to disseminate: Nurses should step up and speak out! Coverage of successful programs like the CDC's "Closer Look," updates on regional meetings, family training activities, and information from newsletters can be disseminated to the print media.

Television can also be very effective in portraying health providers at work (as in the show *ER*). Updates on regional meetings and family training activities could make for very exciting programming on local newscasts.

School nurses must keep in touch with events occurring in their community as well as in the world. These events are publicized through the news media. Events associated with war, violence against strangers, kidnappings (especially those involving children), natural disasters, and sexual assaults or well-touted murders show up all too frequently in news media outlets. The school nurse can take positive action by volunteering to participate in community efforts, educating both adults and children on coping strategies, or making referrals to mental health services. Experts at New York University's Child Study Center have also encouraged journalists to consider the way in which they cover tragic or traumatic events and how that perspective might affect children.

## ◾ Technology

Information technology has become critical to group work, data management, and research. E-mail is often the quickest way to cover thousands of miles. Smith, Cureton, Hooper, and Deamer (1998) found that school nurses consistently express a need for more access to computers as a means for record keeping, information updating, and communication. Examples of computerized resources include Healthmaster and SNAP Health Center. Healthmaster has two products that can handle the networking needs of large districts. HealthOffice 2000 Network is written for MSDE and is designed for districts with fewer than 20 schools or 20,000 students.

Telemedicine is another innovative networking concept. Many rural health centers have gained access to large medical centers through this technology. Network-based linkages with students at the school may give an attending provider a diagnosis, a plan of care, and educational opportunities for the patient and family.

Increased telecommunication facilities are an innovation for education as well as for practice. PDAs, cell phones, and paging equipment expedite the sharing and retrieving of information; they may even make the process much more satisfying. School nurses can be valuable resources to both students and teachers in using and evaluating web-based health information.

## Conclusion

This chapter has highlighted the unique niche of school nursing found within the greater nursing profession. School districts face overwhelming constraints and competing demands. They need the invaluable assistance of school nurses to meet their agendas of improving student educational outcomes.

Significant factors that influence public and private schools as well as school nursing include the following:

- Societal and cultural contexts of school nursing
- Federal mandates
- Educational preparation of school nurses and FNPs
- At-risk children in school
- Legal–ethical considerations
- Violence and terrorism
- School-based health centers for primary care
- Increased role of the media
- Technology

A paradigm shift is required for both providers and the public if school nursing is to continue to provide basic nursing care. Nursing is not just part of the acute care setting; it is a critical element for the community. Formative use of media and far-reaching technologies may be better utilized to catch the attention of the government and the public. All nurses can contribute to enhancing the image of school nursing.

Explore Community Health Nursing on the Web! To learn more about the topics in this chapter, use the passcode provided to access your exclusive website: **http://nursing.jbpub.com/ communityhealth.** If you do not have a passcode, you can obtain one at this site.

## ◾ CRITICAL THINKING ACTIVITIES

1. Juan, a 10-year-old boy, has spina bifida and hydrocephalus. As a result, he has limited bowel function, wears a brace for severe curvature of the spine, and uses a wheelchair for mobility. In addition, Juan has only one kidney and wears a urine collection bag under his clothing. This appliance requires frequent emptying during the school day. He takes several medications to prevent infection and promote waste elimination. Juan lives in a single-parent family with his mother and two brothers. His extended family of aunts, uncles, and cousins is 200 miles away in another state. As a community health nurse, discuss four health outcomes that you and his family would plan for Juan's care. Give the rationale for each one.

2. Danielle, a 15-year-old student, recently learned that she is 3 months pregnant. When she informed her mother, Danielle was "thrown out" of the house and is now staying with her 28-year-old boyfriend. Danielle has been absent from school four times in the last 2 weeks. Select nursing interventions at the primary, secondary, and tertiary levels for Danielle. Include holistic interventions.

# ■ REFERENCES

Allen, G. (2003). The impact of elementary school nurses on student attendance. *Journal of School Nursing, 19*(4), 225–231.

Anderson, J. (1994). The changing role of school nurses: One state's experience. *Journal of School Nursing, 10*(3), 22–26.

The Annie E. Casey Foundation. (2008). *Create a report.* Retrieved December 3, 2008, from http://www.kidscount.org/datacenter

Bachman, B. (1995). A university's response to a need for school nurse education. *Journal of School Nursing, 11*(3), 20–23.

Bonaiuto, M. M. (2007). School nurse case management: Achieving health and educational outcomes. *Journal of School Nursing, 23*(4), 202–209.

Blum, R. (2004). Success in school, healthy relationships can offset risky teen behavior. *NASP Communique, 30*(3), 12–14.

Blum, R., & Rinehart, P. (1997). *Reducing the risk: Connections that make a difference in the lives of youth.* Minneapolis: Division of General Pediatrics and Adolescent Health, University of Minnesota.

Boyer, E. (1991). *Ready to learn: A mandate for the nation.* Carnegie Foundation, Princeton, NJ: Princeton University Press.

Brandt, C. (2002). Enhancing school nurse visibility. *Journal of School Nursing, 18*(1), 5–10.

*Bridging the gap: Education primer for health professionals.* (1992). National Health/Education Consortium.

Bureau of Justice Statistics. (2004). Indicators of School Crime and Safety, 2004. U.S. Department of Justice Office of Justice Programs, Washington, DC. Retrieved October 6, 2008, from http://www.ojp.usdoj.gov/bjs/abstract/iscs04.htm

Button, J., & Rienzo, B. (2002). *The politics of youth, sex, and health care in American schools.* Philadelphia: Haworth Press.

Cavendish, R., Lunney, M., Luise, B., & Richardson, K. (1999). National survey to identify the nursing interventions used in school settings. *Journal of School Nursing, 15*(2), 14–21.

Centers for Disease Control and Prevention (CDC), Division of Adolescent School Health (HealthyYouth). (2004). *About us.* Retrieved November 10, 2008, from www.cdc.gov/HealthyYouth/about/healthyyouth.htm

Centers for Disease Control and Prevention (CDC). (2008). *School health guidelines and strategies.* Retrieved November 11, 2008, from http://www.cdc.gov/HealthyYouth/Publications/guidelines.htm

Chetney, R. (2008). Using telehealth to avoid urgent care and hospitalization. *Home Health Care Management & Practice, 20*(2), 154–160.

Child Welfare Information Gateway. (2008). *National clearinghouse on child abuse and neglect information.* Available from http://www.childwelfare.gov

Clemen, P. (1997). Status of school health services in Mississippi: Executive summary. *HPER Journal, 14*(2), 19–21.

Concepcion, M., Murphy, S., & Canham, D. (2007). School nurses' perceptions of family-centered services: Commitment and challenges. *Journal of School Nursing, 24*(1), 315–321.

Costante, C. (1996). Supporting student success: School nurses make a difference. *Journal of School Nursing, 12*(3), 4–6.

Delaney, T. (2000). Psychotropic medication and children. *National Conference of State Legislatures, 8*(40), 56–67.

Department of Health and Human Services (DHHS). (2000). *Healthy people 2010: Conference edition.* Washington, DC: U.S. Government Printing Office.

Federal Interagency Forum on Child and Family Statistics. (2008). *America's children in brief: Key national indicators of well-being, 2008.* Retrieved September 7, 2008, from http://www.childstats.gov/americaschildren/glance.asp

Frankowski, B. (2004). Sexual orientation and adolescents. *Pediatrics, 113*(6), 1827–1832.

Grabeel, J. (1996). Nursing practice management: IHPs revisited. *Journal of School Nursing, 12*(4), 28–29.

Grant, L., Cureton, V., & Yahiro, M. (1998). Advance directives and do not resuscitate orders: Nurses' knowledge and the level of practice in school settings. *Journal of School Nursing, 14*(2), 4–13.

Gustafson, E. M. (2005). History and overview of school-based centers in the U.S. *Nursing Clinics of North America, 40*(4), 595–606.

Halpern-Felsher, B. L., Cornell, J. L., Kropp, R. Y., & Tschann, J. M. (2005). Adolescents and oral sex: Perceptions, attitudes, and behavior. *Journal of Adolescent Health, 36*(2), 443–456.

Howard, K. R. (2007). Childhood overweight: Parental perceptions and readiness for change. *Journal of School Nursing, 23*(2), 73–79.

Hoven, C., Mandrell, D., & Duarte, C. (2003). Mental health of New York City public school children after 9/11: An epidemiologic investigation. In S. Coates, J. Rosenthal, & D. Schecter (Eds.), *September 11: Trauma and Human Bonds.* Hillsdale, NJ: Analytic Press, pp. 46–54.

Idea Book. (1996). *Linking community health centers with school serving low-income children.* Washington, DC: Health Resources and Services Administration.

Igoe, J. (1990). School nursing and school health. In J. Natapoff & R. Wicczoirek (Eds.), *Maternal–child policy: A nursing perspective* (pp. 153–188). New York: Springer.

Igoe, J. (2002). School nursing today: A search for new cheese. *Journal of School Nursing, 16*(5), 9–15.

Igoe, J., & Giordano, B. (1992). *Expanding school health services to serve families in the 21st century.* Washington, DC: American Nurses Publishing.

Janssen, I., Craig, W., Boyce, W., & Pickett, W. (2004). Associations between overweight and obesity with bullying behaviors in school-aged children. *Pediatrics, 113*(5), 1187–1194.

Jaycox, L. H., Tanielian, T. L., Sharma, P., Morse, L., Clum, G., & Stein, B. D. (2007). School's mental health responses after Hurricanes Katrina and Rita. *Psychiatric Services, 58*(10), 1339–1343.

Johnson, M. (2002). Choosing where we're going by knowing where we are: Results of the 2002 membership survey. *NASN Newsletter, 17*(6), 18–19.

Kubik, M., Lytle, L., & Fulkerson, J. (2004). Physical activity, dietary practices, and other health behaviors of at-risk youth attending alternative high schools. *Journal of School Health, 74*(4), 119–124.

Laraque, D., Boscarino, J., Fleischman, A., et al. (2004). Reactions and needs of tristate area pediatricians after the events of September 11th: Implication for children's mental health services. *Pediatrics, 113*(5), 1357–1366.

Lave, J. (1998). Impact of a children's health insurance program on newly enrolled children. *Journal of the American Medical Association, 279*(22), 1820–1825.

Lever, N., Stephan, S., Axelrod, J., & Weist, M. (2004). Fee-for-service revenue for school mental health through a partnership with outpatient mental health centers. *Journal of School Health, 74*(3), 91.

Li, X., & Atkins, M. (2004). Early childhood computer experience and cognitive and motor development. *Pediatrics, 113*(6), 1715–1722.

Messinger, D., Bauer, C., Das, A., et al. (2004). The Maternal Lifestyle Study: Cognitive, motor and behavioral outcomes in cocaine-exposed and opiate-exposed infants through three years of age. *Pediatrics, 113*(6), 1677–1685.

National Assembly on School-Based Health Care. (2000). *Medicaid reimbursement in school-based health centers: State association and provider perspectives.* Washington, DC: Author.

National Association of School Nurses (NASN). (1999). *Definition of school nursing.* North Branch, MN: Sunrise River Press.

National Association of School Nurses (NASN). (2002). *Position statement: Education, licensure, and certification of school nurses.* Scarborough, ME, & Castle Rock, CO: Author.

National Association of School Nurses (NASN). (2003). *Position statement: Medication administration in the school setting.* Scarborough, ME, & Castle Rock, CO: Author.

National Association of School Nurses (NASN). (2004a). *Issue Brief: School health records.* North Branch, MN: Sunrise River Press.

National Association of School Nurses (NASN). (2004b). *Issue brief: State children's insurance program.* North Branch, MN: Sunrise River Press.

National Association of School Nurses (NASN). (2004c). *Privacy standards for school health records: Issue brief.* http://www.nasn.org

National Association of School Nurses (NASN). (2004d). *Substance use and abuse: Issue brief.* Retrieved November 10, 2008, from http://www.nasn.org/Default.aspx?tabid=282

National Association of School Nurses (NASN). (2005). *School nurse role in bioterrorism emergency preparedness and response position paper.* Retrieved December 1, 2008, from http://www.nasn.org/Default.aspx?tabid=205

National Center for Education Statistics (NCES). (2003). *Indicators of school crime and safety.* Available from http://nces.ed.gov/programs/crimeindicators/crimeindicators.2004/

National Center for Education Statistics (NCES). (2004). *Contexts of elementary and secondary education.* Available from http://nces.ed.gov/annuals

National Center for Education Statistics (NCES). (2007). *Indicators of school crime and safety: 2007.* Retrieved September 7, 2008, from http://nces.ed.gov/programs/crimeindicators/crimeindicators2007

National Council of State Boards of Nursing (NCSBN). (1990). *Delegation: Concepts and decision-making process.* Chicago: Author.

Notes from home: Parents want to know why. (1997). *Child Care Plus, 7*(2).

Oda, D. (1979). School nursing: Current observations and future projections. *Journal of School Health, 49,* 437–439.

Oda, D. (1981). A viewpoint on school nursing. *American Journal of Nursing, 9,* 674–678.

Paige links business and education. (2004, June 28). http://www.ed.gov/news/speeches/2004/06/06282004.htm

Passarelli, C. (1994). School nursing: Trends for the future. *Journal of School Nursing, 10*(2), 10–21.

Passarelli, C. (1996). School nursing services: Exploring national issues and priorities. *Journal of School Nursing, 12*(3), 24–36.

Paxton, R., Valois, R., & Drane, W. (2004). Correlates of body mass index, weight goals, and weight management practices among adolescents. *Journal of School Health, 74*(4), 136–143.

Pollitt, P. (1994). Lina Rogers Struthers: The first school nurse. *Journal of School Nursing, 10*(1), 34–36.

Proctor, S. (1998). School nurses and ethical dilemmas: Are schools short on ethics? *Journal of School Nursing, 14*(2), 3.

Puskar, K., Weaver, P., & DeBlassio, K. (1994). Nursing research in a school setting. *Journal of School Nursing, 10*(4), 8–14.

Reilly, D. (2002). *Managing asthma triggers keeping students healthy: Air quality issues.* Castle Rock, CO: National Association of School Nurses.

Resnick, M., Bearman, P., et al. (1997). Protecting adolescents from harm: Findings from the National Longitudinal Study on Adolescent Health. *Journal of the American Medical Association, 278*(10), 823–832.

School Nurse Organization of Minnesota (SNOM). (1995). *Role for school nursing: A vision statement.* Ad Hoc Taskforce on Health Care Reform.

Schwartz, M., & Laughlin, A. (2008). Partnering with schools: A win-win experience. *Journal of Nursing Education, 47*(6), 279–282.

Seffrin, J. (2004). A changing view of schools. *Journal of School Health, 74*(3), 75.

Shalala, D. (1999). *Report to the president: Interagency Task Force on Children's Health Insurance Outreach.* Available from: http://www.hrsa.gov

Smith, C., Cureton, V., Hooper, C., & Deamer, P. (1998). A survey of computer technology utilization on school nursing. *Journal of School Nursing, 14*(2), 27–34.

Snyder, T., & Hoffman, C. (Eds.). (2002). *Digest of education statistics, 2001.* National Center for Education Statistics (Pub. # 2002130), Table 2.

Swanson, N., & Leonard, B. (1994). Identifying potential dropouts through school health records. *Journal of School Nursing, 10*(2), 22–26, 46.

Urbinati, D., Steele, P., Harter, B., & Harrell, D. (1996). The evolution of the school nurse practitioner: Past, present and future. *Journal of School Nursing, 12*(2), 609.

van der Molen, J. (June 2004). Violence and suffering in television news: Toward a broader conception of harmful television content for children. *Pediatrics, 113*(6), 1771–1775.

Wales, S., & Crisp, J. (2007). The views of nurses on adherence in school-aged children with a chronic illness. *Journal of Neonatal, Paediatric & Child Health Nursing, 10*(2), 5–8, 10.

Webb, N. (2004). *Mass trauma and violence: Helping families and children cope.* New York: Guilford Press.

Wold, S. J. (2001). School health services: History and trends. In N. Schwab & M. Gelfman (Eds.), *Legal issues in school health services* (pp. 8–9). North Branch, MN: Sunrise River Press.

Zimmerman, B., Wagner, E., & Kelly, L. (1996). A study of role ambiguity and role strain among school nurses. *Journal of School Nursing, 12*(4), 12–18.

## ■ WEBSITES

www.firstgov.gov Useful for searching the many websites linked with health and education from the federal level.

www.ashaweb.org The American School Health Association site.

www.cdc.gov/shpps Fact sheets; addresses issues such as staffing, HIV/AIDS policies, school-based health centers, and screening requirements.

www.cdc.gov/HealthyYouth *Morbidity and Mortality Weekly Report* facts from the Youth Risk Behavior Survey.

www.cdc.gov/nccdphp/ Facts and figures related to chronic diseases.

www.ed.gov Federal legislative initiatives in education.

www.aecf.org Website for the Annie E. Casey Foundation. "Kids Count." Statistical information is available at this website.

www.foodsafeschools.org Information related to food allergies; pharmacologic information when concerns over foods exist; and nutrition and strength training games.

www.schoolnurse.com/med_info/ Updated briefs on many topics and concerns in school nursing.

www.peds.umn.edu/peds-adol/ National Association of School Psychologists website, where you can find information about the National Longitudinal Study on Adolescent Health.

www.nasn.org National School Nurse Association resource.

www.childstats.gov Updated statistics compiled by U.S. government on comprehensive health issues of children.

www.peds.umn.edu/peds-adol/ Information on the National Longitudinal Study of Healthy Adolescents.

Bonnie Rogers

Visit **http://nursing.jbpub.com/communityhealth** for interactive exercises, review questions, Web links, and more.

"It is not wealth, nor splendor, but tranquility and occupation which gives happiness."

—Thomas Jefferson

Three Rules of Work: Out of clutter find simplicity; From discord find harmony; In the middle of difficulty lies opportunity.

—*Albert Einstein*

It is for us to pray not for tasks equal to our powers, but for powers equal to our tasks, to go forward with a great desire forever beating at the door of our hearts as we travel toward our distant goal.

—*Helen Keller*

Work gives meaning to our lives, yet also involves health risks according to what we do, how we react to our work, and under what conditions we work. What does "doing work" mean to you? Are you ever able to stop being a nursing student when you are "not at work"? How does this affect your health on a daily basis?

## CHAPTER FOCUS

**History of Occupational Health Nursing**
- Definition

**Work and Workplace Hazards**
- Allergic and Irritant Dermatitis
- Asthma and Chronic Obstructive Pulmonary Disease
- Fertility and Pregnancy Abnormalities
- Hearing Loss
- Infectious Diseases
- Low Back Disorders
- Musculoskeletal Disorders of the Upper Extremities
- Traumatic Injuries

**Work/Workplace Change**

**Occupational Health Nursing Practice**
- Scope of Practice
- Occupational Health Nursing Roles

**Governmental Influence**

**Professionalism in Occupational Health Nursing**
- Education and Certification
- Nurse-Managed Models in Occupational Health

**Future Expansions**
- Environmental Health
- Migrant Health
- Health Promotion in the Workplace

## QUESTIONS TO CONSIDER

After reading this chapter, you will know the answers to the following questions:

1. What is occupational health nursing, and how does it relate to community health?
2. Why has the practice of occupational health nursing changed so dramatically over time?
3. What are the work and workplace hazards that result in illness, injury, and loss of life to the worker?
4. How have these hazards changed over the years, and what is the role of the occupational health nurse in dealing with work-related illness and injuries?
5. What are the major laws governing occupational safety and health, and how have they affected workers and the role of the occupational health nurse?
6. What are the five models for worksite primary healthcare management in occupational health care?
7. How can the goal to provide quality, accessible, and cost-effective care be reached?
8. What is the critical link between occupational health nursing and environmental health?
9. Why will the occupational health nurses need additional competencies in environmental health in the coming years and what "competencies" will be needed?

## KEY TERMS

American Association of Occupational Health Nurses
Ergonomics
National Institute for Occupational Safety and Health (NIOSH)
Occupational health nurse case manager
Occupational health nurse clinician
Occupational health nurse consultant
Occupational health nurse coordinator
Occupational health nurse corporate director
Occupational health nurse educator
Occupational health nurse health-promotion specialist
Occupational health nurse manager
Occupational health nurse practitioner
Occupational health nurse researcher
Occupational health nursing
Occupational Safety and Health Act of 1970
Worker/workplace assessment and surveillance

WORK IS GENERALLY considered one of life's worthwhile and exciting experiences. Most adults spend approximately one-fourth to one-third of their time at work, which becomes an integral part of their life. Work can be viewed as a source of strength helping people build lives and communities. Americans work in a wide range of industries and jobs, which are displayed in Tables 41-1 and 41-2.

Although most workers may never face any serious adverse health effects from workplace exposures, all types of work have hazards (Box 41-1). These hazards can have short- and long-term health consequences, and every effort must be made to prevent and control work-related illness and injury. Thus, the necessity to provide occupational health and safety services to prevent and manage occupational health illness and injuries is paramount in this mission. This chapter provides an overview of the practice of occupational health nursing, with emphasis on the scope of practice. Examples of work-related illnesses and injuries and a discussion of governmental and professional influences are also provided.

**"**_Doing more things faster is no substitute for doing the right things._**"**

—Stephen R. Covey

## History of Occupational Health Nursing

**Occupational health nursing,** then called _industrial nursing,_ began in the latter half of the nineteenth century in Norwich, England, when Phillipa Fowerday was hired by the J. & J. Coleman Company in 1878. Her work in the mustard company was primarily to work in the dispensary and provide home care services to employees and their families (Godfrey, 1978). Although the company provided acute and tertiary care services for employees, the belief was that preventive care was better than cure in terms of healthy and quality liv-

ing. Nurses were soon employed by other companies to provide healthcare services for employees who became ill and injured at work as well as health education services related to sanitation and hygiene, particularly given the high rates of tuberculosis at the time (Slaney, 1984).

In the United States, industrial or occupational health nursing, as it is now called, began in the late nineteenth century. In 1888, it is reported that a group of Pennsylvania coal mining companies hired Betty Moulder, a graduate of Philadelphia Blockley Hospital School of Nursing, to provide nursing care for ill and injured workers and their families

**Table 41-1** Civilian Labor Force, United States, by Industry

| Industry | Workforce Size (in millions) |
|---|---|
| Agriculture | 3.1 |
| Mining | 0.6 |
| Construction | 9.6 |
| Manufacturing | 19.0 |
| Transportation and public utilities | 9.7 |
| Wholesale and retail trade | 27.7 |
| Finance, insurance, real estate | 8.8 |
| Services | 50.5 |
| Public administration | 6.1 |
| TOTAL | 135.1* |

*Because of rounding, the sum of the components does not add up to the total.

_Source_: Bureau of Labor Statistics, U.S. Department of Labor, 2001.

**Table 41-2** Labor Force by Job

| Occupational Category | Number of Workers (in millions) |
|---|---|
| Managerial and professional specialty | 41.9 |
| Technicians, sales, and administrative support workers | 39.0 |
| Precision production, craft, and repair workers | 14.8 |
| Operators, fabricators, and laborers | 17.7 |
| Service workers | 18.4 |
| Farming, forestry, and fishing industry workers | 3.3 |
| TOTAL | 135.1* |

* Because of rounding, the sum of the components does not add up to the total.

_Source_: Bureau of Labor Statistics, U.S. Department of Labor, 2001.

**BOX 41-1**

**Categories of Work-Related Hazards**

_Biological/infectious hazards_: infectious/biological agents, such as bacteria, viruses, fungi, or parasites, that may be transmitted via contact with infected patients or contaminated body secretions/fluids to other individuals

_Chemical hazards_: various forms of chemicals, including medications, solutions, gases, vapors, aerosols, and particulate matter, that are potentially toxic or irritating to the body system

_Enviromechanical hazards_: factors encountered in the work environment that cause or potentiate accidents, injuries, strain, or discomfort (e.g., unsafe/inadequate equipment or lifting devices, slippery floors, workstation deficiencies)

_Physical hazards_: agents within the work environment, such as radiation, electricity, extreme temperatures, and noise, that can cause tissue trauma

_Psychosocial hazards_: factors and situations encountered or associated with one's job or work environment that create or potentiate stress, emotional strain, and/or interpersonal problems

_Source_: Rogers, 2003.

(AAIN, 1976; McGrath, 1945; Wright, 1919). However, little more is known about her or the services she provided. In 1895, Ada Mayo Stewart, who is often credited as being the first industrial nurse, was hired by the Vermont Marble Company. She had previously worked as a district nurse in several cities. During her tenure, she visited sick employees in their homes, provided emergency care, taught healthy living habits, taught mothers about child care, and gave speeches on health and hygiene to school children. In this era, there was much ethnic diversity, and Ada Stewart incorporated cultural customs and methods of caring for the sick and their families into her practice. She was later joined by a second nurse, her sister Harriet, who provided health care to employees in the west and central sections of the state (Felton, 1985; Rogers, 2003).

In the early 1900s, industrial health services proliferated rapidly across the country as it became apparent that nursing care related to worksite health issues could have a positive impact on productivity, could decrease illness and injury, and could reduce absenteeism. Working conditions in many factories were harsh and unrelenting, as the industrial ethic often placed the importance of profit above human rights. This type of ethic was not supported by the public, and the advent of worker's compensation (discussed later) came to being.

In 1913, the first organized effort in U.S. industrial nursing began in New England with the establishment of the first industrial nurse registry and the formation of the New England Industrial Nurses' Association in 1918. In 1917, Boston University's College of Business Administration offered the first specialty education course for industrial nurses that focused on industrial health issues and economics. This was followed in the 1920s by several colleges and universities offering short courses in industrial hygiene in which industrial nurses participated (Godfrey, 1978). The advent of World War II in the 1940s supported industrial growth and the concomitant demand for nursing services, with a reported 4,000 nurses employed in industrial health (Brown, 1981). With a viable group of nurses in need of professional support, the American Association of Industrial Nurses (AAIN) was created in 1942, with Catherine Dempsey as the first president. The purposes of AAIN were to improve industrial nursing practice, provide education, and increase interdisciplinary work (AAIN, 1976).

In the 1960s and 1970s, occupational health and safety became a public issue, with particular concern focused on mining accidents, cave-ins, and black lung disease, as well as the need for professional education and hiring in several disciplines. As a result, several laws were enacted to protect the health and safety of workers (e.g., Federal Coal Mine Safety and Health Act, 1969; Toxic Substances Control Act, 1976). The **Occupational Safety and Health** (OSH) **Act of 1970** was the first comprehensive law promulgated to ensure safe and healthful working conditions.

As the occupational health nurse's scope of practice broadened considerably, AAIN changed its name to the **American Association of Occupational Health Nurses** in 1977, with a current membership of approximately 13,000 occupational health nurses. The 1980s brought more role expansion into health promotion, management, policy development, research, and entrepreneurism. Several standards were promulgated to protect workers from unwarranted exposures (e.g., Hazard Communication Standard, 1983), and in 1988, the Occupational Safety and Health Administration (OSHA) hired the first occupational health nurse consultant to provide technical assistance in standards development, field consultation, and occupational health nursing expertise. In 1993, the Office of Occupational Health Nursing was established within the agency.

In 1990, AAOHN published its first occupational health nursing research priorities, updated in 1999, which provide the direction for occupational health nursing research (Box 41-2) (AAOHN, 1999; Rogers, Agnew, & Pompeii, 2000).

---

## BOX 41-2

### Research Priorities in Occupational Health Nursing

1. Effectiveness of primary healthcare delivery at the worksite
2. Effectiveness of health-promotion nursing intervention strategies
3. Methods for handling complex ethical issues related to occupational health
4. Strategies that minimize work-related adverse health outcomes (e.g., respiratory disease)
5. Health effects resulting from chemical exposures in the workplace
6. Occupational hazards of healthcare workers (e.g., latex allergy, blood-borne pathogens)
7. Factors that influence worker rehabilitation and return to work
8. Effectiveness of ergonomic strategies to reduce worker injury and illness
9. Effectiveness of case management approaches in occupational illness/injury
10. Evaluation of critical pathways to effectively improve worker health and safety and to enhance maximum recovery and safe return to work
11. Effects of shift work on worker health and safety
12. Strategies for increasing compliance with or motivating workers to use personal protective equipment

---

## ■■ CULTURAL CONNECTION

Some workers, such as Orthodox Jews and Seventh Day Adventists, consider Saturday to be the Sabbath and a holy day. How would you be culturally sensitive to a patient who refuses to seek emergency treatment or use needed electricity for a health condition on the Sabbath?

The priorities will be used to target grant funding by AAOHN for occupational health nursing research. In 1996, the first National Occupational Research Agenda (NORA) was developed, spearheaded by the **National Institute for Occupational Safety and Health (NIOSH)** in partnership with more than 500 groups and individuals. NORA has identified 21 research priorities for occupational health and safety for which its funding is targeted. NORA priorities (NIOSH, 2006) are listed in Box 41-3.

## ■ Definition

In today's work environment, the delivery and management of occupational health services and programs are provided primarily by occupational and environmental health nurses. Collaboration with and referral to related occupational health and safety disciplines to resolve occupational health problems are essential to the practice. By definition, occupational and environmental health nursing is the specialty practice that focuses on the promotion, prevention, and restoration of health within the context of a safe and healthy environment. It includes the prevention of adverse health effects from occupational and environmental hazards. It provides for and delivers occupational and environmental health and safety services to workers, worker populations, and community groups. Occupational and environmental health nursing is an autonomous specialty, and nurses make independent nursing judgments in providing healthcare services (AAOHN, 2004).

## Work and Workplace Hazards

Workers are exposed to many workplace hazards that result in illness and injury. There are about 154 million workers in the United States (Bureau of Labor Statistics, 2008). Each

### BOX 41-3

**National Occupational Research Agenda**
**Priority Research Areas**

| Category | Areas |
|---|---|
| ▪ Disease and injury | Allergic and irritant dermatitis |
| | Asthma and chronic obstructive pulmonary disease |
| | Fertility and pregnancy abnormalities |
| | Hearing loss |
| | Infectious diseases |
| | Low back disorders |
| | Musculoskeletal disorders of upper extremities |
| | Traumatic injuries |
| ▪ Work environment and workforce | Indoor environment |
| | Mixed exposures |
| | Emerging technologies |
| | Organization of work |
| | Special populations at risk |
| ▪ Research tools and approaches | Cancer research methods |
| | Control technology and personal protective equipment |
| | Surveillance research methods |
| | Exposure assessment methods |
| | Risk assessment methods research |
| | Intervention effectiveness research |
| | Health services research |
| | Social and economic consequences of workplace illness and injury |

*Source*: National Institute for Occupational Safety and Health (NIOSH). (2006). *The team document: Ten years of leadership advancing the National Occupation Research Agenda.* Washington, DC: Author.

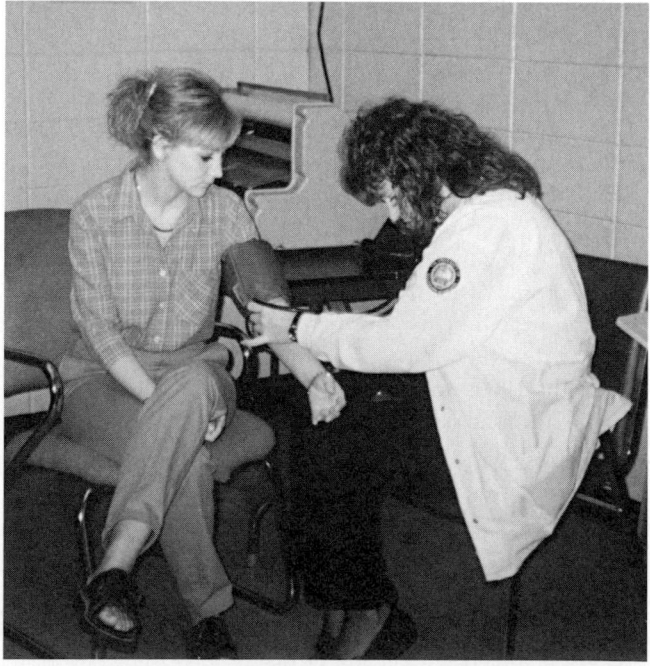

An occupational nurse conducts an assessment in the office setting.

**Table 41-3  Nonfatal Occupational Injury Incidence Rates in the United States by Industry, Private Sector**

|  | Work-Related Nonfatal Injuries (per 100 full-time workers) |
|---|---|
| ▪ Air transportation | 13.6 |
| ▪ Nursing and personal care facilities | 13.0 |
| ▪ Motor vehicles and equipment | 10.9 |
| ▪ Trucking and courier service | 8.3 |
| ▪ Hospitals | 8.2 |
| ▪ Grocery stores | 7.8 |
| ▪ Department stores | 7.7 |
| ▪ Eating/drinking places | 5.2 |

Each of these 8 industries (ranked by occupational injury rate) reported more than 100,000 injuries in 2001. Air transportation reported the highest rate in the group (13.6 per 100 workers) followed by nursing and personal care facilities (13.0 per 100 workers). Together these 8 industry sectors accounted for about 1.4 million nonfatal injuries, or 29% of the 4.9 million total.

*Source*: Bureau of Labor Statistics, U.S. Department of Labor, 2002.

day, an average of 137 individuals die from work-related diseases, and an additional 16 die from injuries on the job. Every 5 seconds, a worker is injured; every 10 seconds, a worker is temporarily or permanently disabled. NIOSH estimates that at least 10 million injuries occur on the job each year, approximately 3 million of which are severe, and every workday more than 10,000 people sustain injuries that result in lost work time. Table 41-3 shows the highest work-related injuries by specific industry. Occupational injuries alone cost billions of dollars yearly in lost wages and productivity, administrative expenses, health care, and other costs. This figure does not include the cost of occupational illnesses.

Reports of injuries among nursing home workers and other personal caregivers have increased, with back injuries accounting for more than 40% of these reports. Construction workers have the highest injury rate in private industry, while trucking and warehousing have the highest injury rates in the service sector. Mining injuries, while declining, remain high. The January 2006 mining disaster at the Sago Mine in West Virginia, in which an explosion took the lives of 12 miners, is a grim reminder of the hazards of this occupation. Nearly half of the farm injuries in the United States result in permanent, disabling conditions; back injuries account for more than 40% of these injuries.

Vision and hearing problems due to exposure to noise and chemical exposure are also on the rise. Because of the

### ✒ NOTE THIS! ●──────────────

Back injuries are the most prevalent and most costly injury in the occupation of nursing.

### ☝ THINK ABOUT THIS ··············

Many people worry so much about managing their careers, but rarely spend half that much energy managing their *lives*. I want to make my life, not just my job, the best it can be. The rest will work itself out.

> —Reese Witherspoon, Academy Award-winning actress, whose mother is a professor of nursing.

long latency period between exposure and some of the long-term effects, such as cancer and asbestosis, adequate numbers are not available to account for all industrial hazards contributing to these chronic, and often fatal, diseases. Workers in nuclear power plants have been especially concerned about this issue because of the long period of exposure resulting in diseases (Landels, 2002).

In today's climate, bioterrorism has emerged as a serious occupational threat. There is an immediate need for occupational disaster plans and strategies to cope with bioterrorism in workplaces. Dealing with bioterrorism requires occupational nurses to become familiar with the various types of organisms and chemicals used in bioterrorism and to develop a plan of action for the work environment (Salazar & Kelman, 2002).

Illnesses are much more difficult to capture because of the often long latency period between initial workplace exposure and disease occurrence and the lack of recognition on the part of the clinician that the disease manifestations are work related. Thus the relative incidence and prevalence of occupational illness may be grossly underreported. What this means is that diseases such as skin disorders, which may be more easily recognized, are more likely to be reported and treated. This may give a misleading representation of both the magnitude and severity of work-related illness. Of the 5.2 million nonfatal occupational injuries and illnesses reported in 2001, 4.9 million (93.6%) were injuries. The remainder (333,800 cases or 6.4%) were work-related illnesses. Sixty-five percent (216,400 cases) of the nonfatal occupation illnesses were disorders associated with repeated trauma (Bureau of Labor Statistics, 2002; see Table 41-4). Let's

**Table 41-4  Number of Cases of Occupational Illnesses in the United States by Category of Illness**

| Category of Illness | Number of Cases |
|---|---|
| ▪ Diseases associated with repeated trauma | 216,400 |
| ▪ Skin diseases or disorders | 38,900 |
| ▪ All other occupational illnesses | 78,500 |

*Source*: Bureau of Labor Statistics, U.S. Department of Labor, 2002.

examine the eight groups of occupational diseases/injuries as targeted in the NORA priorities (NIOSH, 2006).

## ■ Allergic and Irritant Dermatitis

In the workplace, the skin is an important route of exposure to chemicals and other contaminants. According to the U.S. Bureau of Labor Statistics, occupational skin diseases—mostly in the form of allergic and irritant (contact) dermatitis—are the second most common type of occupational disease. From 1983 to 1994, the rate of occupational skin diseases increased from 64 to 81 cases per 100,000 workers. Moreover, occupational skin diseases are believed to be severely underreported, such that the true rate of new cases may be many-fold higher than documented. In 2001, 4,714 cases of dermatitis resulted in lost work days (Bureau of Labor Statistics, 2001). Estimated total annual costs, including lost workdays and loss of productivity associated with occupational skin diseases, may reach $1 billion annually. Workers' compensation claim rates for occupational skin diseases vary by state and range from 12 to 108 per 100,000 workers per year.

Irritant contact dermatitis is the most common occupational skin disease, usually resulting from toxic reactions to chemical irritants such as solvents and cutting fluids. Allergic dermatitis is estimated to constitute approximately 20% to 24% of all contact dermatitis; it is caused by a wide variety of substances such as latex and some pesticides that trigger an allergic (delayed hypersensitivity) reaction. Contact urticaria (hives occurring soon after an allergen or irritant contacts

### ⦿ MEDIA MOMENT

**Antz (1998)**

In an anthill with millions of inhabitants, Z 4195 is a worker ant. Feeling insignificant in a conformity-based system, he accidentally meets beautiful Princess Bala, who has a similar problem on the other end of the social scale. To meet her again, Z switches sides with his soldier friend Weaver—only to become a hero in the course of events. By doing so, he unwittingly upsets the sinister plans of ambitious General Mandible (Bala's fiancé, by the way), who wants to divide the ant society a superior, strong race (soldiers) and an inferior, to-be-_____ated race (workers). Z and Bala, both unaware of the _____us situation, try to leave the oppressive system by ___for Insectopia, a place where food paves the streets.

the skin) is considered here also because it may evolve ___ contact dermatitis. A number of substances may cause bo__ irritant and allergic dermatitis as well as contact urticaria. For example, latex, which has been reported to cause skin disorders in as many as 10% of exposed healthcare workers, most commonly causes irritant dermatitis; however, it also results in allergic contact dermatitis and, least commonly, contact urticaria.

Because the prognosis of occupational irritant and allergic dermatitis is poor, prevention is imperative. Patients with occupational contact dermatitis often develop chronic skin disease. With thousands of potentially harmful chemicals being introduced into the workplace each year and with the threat of rapidly emerging skin diseases such as latex allergy, interventions need to be developed to reduce irritant and allergic contact dermatitis.

## ■ Asthma and Chronic Obstructive Pulmonary Disease

Asthma and chronic obstructive pulmonary disease (COPD—primarily chronic bronchitis and emphysema) are diseases of the lung airways. More than 20 million U.S. workers are potentially exposed to occupational agents capable of causing these diseases, including nearly 9 million workers occupationally exposed to known sensitizers such as toluene diisocyanate CTDI, a major ingredient in polyurethane manufacture, and irritants, such as ammonia, used in the manufacture of dyes, chemicals, plastics, and explosives (Levy & Wegman, 2000). Occupational asthma is now the most common occupational respiratory disease diagnosis among patients examined in occupational medicine clinics (Tarlo et al., 2008).

In 1992, asthma and COPD caused nearly 92,000 deaths in the United States, making airway diseases the fourth leading cause of death overall. Mortality from asthma and COPD is increasing annually. Estimated yearly costs for occupational asthma are approximately $400 million. NIOSH reports that asthma currently affects more than 10 million individuals in the United States and is increasing in prevalence. Recent evidence suggests that as many as 20% of adult asthma cases may be attributable to work settings (DHHS, 1999; Kallstrom, 2008). In addition to those who develop occupational asthma as a result of workplace exposure to sensitizers or irritants, many workers are unaware that pre-existing asthma may be worsened by the work environment. Each year, the number of asthma cases is increasing, and major new problem areas are emerging (Tarlo et al., 2008). For example, as a result of increased use of protective gloves, due to the introduction of universal precautions and the OSHA regulations on blood-borne pathogens, latex allergies have become a major problem for healthcare workers. A significant number of these workers (2.5% in one study) have developed latex-related asthma.

## ENVIRONMENTAL CONNECTION

Workers who are employed in highway construction may face a new health threat: silicosis from concrete destruction. Given the more than 163,000 miles of rural and urban roads, which also includes the aging interstate system, more workers are involved in this type of occupation. Silicosis is a disabling, nonreversible, and sometimes fatal lung disease caused by inhaling dust containing extremely fine particles of crystalline silica. Crystalline silica is found in materials such as concrete, masonry, and rock. Working with these materials can produce airborne respirable dust, causing lung damage. Unfortunately, silicosis is a disease with a long latency period and usually takes 20 or more years to develop. Other diseases associated with the inhalation of crystalline silica are chronic obstructive pulmonary disease (COPD), connective tissue disease, renal disease, and lung cancer.

While the dangers of silica exposure and silicosis have been well established as risks in the mining, iron, and steel manufacturing industries, the danger to construction workers is less clear. Highway workers seldom use protective face gear, so this problem will be a continuing threat for highway workers. Some states have begun surveillance of silicosis cases, but the issue is not yet a national priority at this time.

*Source*: Valiante, D. J., Schill, D. P., Rosenman, K. D., & Socie, F. (2004). Highway repair: A new silicosis threat. *American Journal of Public Health, 94*(5), 876–880.

---

Morbidity from occupational asthma is preventable. Early diagnosis holds substantial promise for effective intervention. Complete resolution of symptoms and pulmonary function abnormalities is most likely when an affected individual's exposure is terminated early in the course of the illness, so early diagnosis holds substantial promise for effective intervention and reduces employer costs (Paton, 2008).

The relationship of COPD to workplace exposures is also well documented in studies of several occupational agents (e.g., coal dust, grain dust, cotton dust). Investigations of the health consequences of particulate exposure in the general environment, where exposures are at a far lower level than in the workplace, also suggest that COPD resulting from generally dusty conditions may be an important cause of preventable disease and death. Those with lung disease from other causes are especially vulnerable to occupational respiratory hazards. Although cigarettes remain the primary cause of pulmonary diseases in the United States, many occupational and environmental exposures, both by themselves and in combination with smoking, are known to cause COPD. One estimate of the proportion of COPD attributable to occupational exposure in the general population is 15%.

## ■ Fertility and Pregnancy Abnormalities

Disorders of reproduction include birth defects, developmental disorders, spontaneous abortion, low birth weight, preterm birth, and various other disorders affecting offspring; they also include reduced fertility, impotence, and menstrual disorders. Infertility is currently estimated to affect more than 2 million American couples. One in 12 couples finds themselves unable to conceive after 1 year of unprotected intercourse. Although numerous occupational exposures have been demonstrated to impair fertility (e.g., lead, some pesticides, solvents), the overall contribution of occupational exposures to male and female infertility is unknown (Paul, 1997). Moreover, observed global trends in men's decreasing sperm counts have increased concerns about the role of chemicals encountered at work and in the environment at large (Winker & Rudiger, 2006).

Birth defects are the leading cause of infant mortality in the United States, accounting for 20% of infant deaths (more than 8,000) each year. Every year, approximately 120,000 babies are born in the United States with a major birth defect—about 3 per 100 live births. Neural tube defects, which include spina bifida and anencephaly, affect 4,000 pregnancies each year. Of all children in the United States, 18% have some type of developmental disability. The major developmental disabilities of mental retardation, cerebral palsy, hearing impairment, and vision impairment affect approximately 2% of all school-age children.

Most birth defects and developmental disabilities are of unknown cause. The overall contribution of workplace exposures to reproductive disorders and congenital abnormalities is also not known. Although some specific reproductive hazards have been identified in humans, most of the more than 1,000 workplace chemicals that have shown abnormal reproductive effects in animals have not been studied in humans. In addition, most of the 4 million other chemical mixtures in commercial use remain untested. Substances and activities that upset the normal hormonal activity of the reproductive system (e.g., shift work or pesticides that possess estrogenic activity) also need evaluation. Similarly, the effects of physical factors such as prolonged standing, reaching or lifting, or the interactive effects of workplace stressors and exposures on pregnancy and fertility have not been rigorously investigated.

Although the total number of workers potentially exposed to reproductive hazards is difficult to estimate, three-fourths of employed women and an even greater proportion of employed men are of reproductive age. More than half of U.S. children are born to working mothers. The vast number of workers of reproductive age together with the substantial number of workplace chemical, physical, and biological agents suggest that a considerable number of workers are potentially at risk for adverse reproductive outcomes.

Although the causes of reproductive disorders and adverse pregnancy outcomes are poorly defined, lost productivity and deep suffering by affected individuals and families are evident. The contribution that may be made by occupational

### *Got an Alternative?*

Musicians and other artists often develop health problems because of repetitive movements, poor technique, and poor posture due to the unique nature of their chosen professions. Damage can result from repetitive stress and overuse—that is, practicing the same movements repeatedly or increasing the workload prior to a concert or exhibit.

Dr. Kenneth Brandt founded the Performing Arts Medicine Program at Indiana University Medical Center in the early 1980s. Along with athletic trainers and occupational therapists and other specialists, he assists artists by developing exercises for them and offering pain management. Additionally, Dr. Brandt treats artists with diverse health problems, such as opera singers with throat problems, brass players with dental problems, and guitarists with rheumatism. Patients are treated with a holistic approach, including yoga, stress management, and other complementary therapies. 

*Source*: Performing Arts Medicine Program, Indiana University School of Medicine, 541 Clinical Drive, Indianapolis, IN 46223, (317) 274–4225, Director: Dr. Kenneth D. Brandt

### Research Alert

A recent study examined the effects of smoking, quitting, and time since quitting on absences from work. To do so, the researchers used data from the nationally representative Tobacco Use Supplements of the 1992–1993, 1995–1996, and 1998–1999 Current Population Surveys. The study included full-time workers aged 18–64 years, yielding a sample size of 383,778 workers. A binary indicator of absence due to sickness in the lost week was analyzed as a function of smoking status, including time since quitting for former smokers. Extensive demographic variables were included as controls in all models.

In initial comparisons between current and former smokers, smoking increased absences, but quitting did not reduce them. However, when length of time since quitting was examined, it was discovered that those who quit within the last year, and especially within the last 3 months, had a much greater probability of absences than did current smokers. As the time since quitting increased, absences returned to a rate somewhere between that of never smokers and current smokers. Interactions between health and smoking status significantly improved the fit of the model. Smokers who quit reduced their absences over time but increased their absences immediately after quitting. The benefits from smoking cessation appear to emerge over the long term rather than in the short term regarding work absenteeism.

*Source*: Sindelar, J. L., Duchovny, N., Falba, T. A., & Busch, S. H. (2005). If smoking increases absences, does quitting reduce them? *Tobacco Control, 14*(2), 99–106.

factors is largely unexplored, because the reproductive health of workers has only recently emerged as a serious focus of scientific investigation. Identifying reproductive hazards in the workplace has the potential for significantly reducing the multibillion-dollar costs and alleviating the personal suffering associated with disorders of reproduction.

### ■ Hearing Loss

Occupational hearing loss is the most common occupational disease in the United States. It is so common that it is often accepted as a normal consequence of employment. More than 30 million workers are exposed to hazardous noise, and an additional 9 million are at risk from other ototraumatic agents. Occupational hearing loss knows no boundaries with respect to industries. Any worker, young or old, male or female, risks hearing loss when exposed to ototraumatic agents. Once the loss is acquired, it is irreversible.

Although noise-induced occupational hearing loss is the most common occupational disease and is the second most commonly self-reported occupational illness or injury, it has not been possible to create a sense of urgency about this problem. Efforts to prevent occupational hearing loss have been hindered because the problem is insidious and occurs without pain or obvious physical abnormalities in affected workers.

Problems created by occupational hearing loss include (1) reduced quality of life because of social isolation and un-relenting tinnitus (ringing in the ears); (2) impaired communication with family members, the public, and co-workers; (3) diminished ability to monitor the work environment (e.g., warning signals, equipment sounds); (4) lost productivity and increased accidents resulting from impaired communication and isolation; and (5) expenses for workers' compensation and hearing aids.

### ■ Infectious Diseases

Infections acquired in the work setting are diverse, with many different modes of transmission. Of particular concern are infectious diseases transmitted by humans (e.g., from patient to worker, from worker to worker) in a variety of work settings. Blood-borne and airborne pathogens represent a significant class of exposures for the 6 million U.S. healthcare workers. Occupational transmission of blood-borne pathogens (including hepatitis B and C viruses and the human immunodeficiency virus [HIV]) occurs primarily by means of needlestick injuries but also through exposures to the eyes or mucous membranes. The risk of hepatitis B virus infection following a single needlestick injury with a contaminated

## ETHICAL CONNECTION

U.S. workers are paying more for their health insurance and getting less for their money than they did 4 years ago. The number of uninsured Americans during 2004 was more than 85 million, and 16 million lacked enough insurance to cover all their medical bills. Premiums for employer-sponsored health plans rose an average of 35.9% from 2000 to 2004, nearly three times the average growth in earnings. For family coverage, the employee's portion of the average annual premium grew to $1,947 from $1,433. This is the fourth consecutive year of double-digit growth, according to the Kaiser Family Foundation.

The United States is the richest country in the world. What are the ethical implications for workers who can no longer afford healthcare premiums and the deductibles for their care in this country?

## THINK ABOUT THIS

The kind of work we do provides important clues about our health. For example, taxi drivers have an increased prevalence of knee pain, which increases with drive time. Knee pain increases when taxi drivers have constant driving time of greater than 6 hours and can lead to work-related knee joint disorders. Which preventive measures can be taken to reduce the long-term disability risk among taxi cab drivers based on this research?

*Source*: Chen, J. C., Dennerlein, J. T., Shih, T. S., et al. (2004). Knee pain and driving duration: A secondary analysis of the Taxi Drivers' Health Study. *American Journal of Pubic Health, 94*(4), 575–578.

needle varies from 2% to more than 40%, depending on the antigen status of the source individual. Similarly, the risk of hepatitis C virus transmission depends on the status of the source and ranges from 3.3% to 10%. Before widespread use of hepatitis B virus vaccine, approximately 8,700 acute cases of hepatitis B virus infection were reported among healthcare workers each year. Although the incidence of occupational hepatitis C virus infection among these workers is unknown, antibody to hepatitis C virus (evidence of previous infection) is found in 1% of hospital-based healthcare workers.

Transmission of tuberculosis (TB) within healthcare settings, especially multidrug-resistant TB, has re-emerged as a major public health problem. Since 1989, outbreaks of this type of TB have been reported in U.S. hospitals. In addition, among workers of healthcare, social service, and corrections facilities who work with populations at increased risk of TB, hundreds have experienced tuberculin skin test conversions. Reliable data are lacking on the extent of possible work-related TB transmission among other groups of workers at risk for exposure. Some cases of influenza and other communicable respiratory infections are surely the result of exposure to infected persons at work. These are not generally considered occupational diseases, and the proportion acquired at work from co-workers, customers, patients, and the general public is unknown. The cost of lost work time and decreased productivity is likely to be substantial.

### ■ Low Back Disorders

Low back pain is one of the oldest and most common occupational health problems reported. Approximately 80% of workers will experience low back pain sometime during their active working life, and 11% of Americans report reduced functional ability. In 2001, back disorders occurred at a rate of 41 per 10,000 workers and accounted for 372,683

nonfatal occupational injuries and illnesses involving days away from work in the United States. The economic costs of low back disorders are staggering. In one study, the average cost of a workers' compensation claim for a low back disorder was $8,300, which was more than twice the average cost of $4,075 for all compensable claims combined.

As many as 30% of American workers are employed in jobs that routinely require them to perform activities that may increase their risk of developing low back disorders. For example, female nursing aides and licensed practical nurses were about 2.5 times more likely to experience a work-related low back disorder than all other female workers. Male

### A Good Read

## Nickel and Dimed: On (Not) Getting By in America (2001)

*By Barbara Ehrenreich, New York: Metropolitan Books.*

Ehrenreich left behind her middle-class life as a journalist to live as a member of the working class. In 1999 and 2000, she worked as a waitress in Key West, Florida; as a cleaning woman and a nursing home aide in Portland, Maine; and in a Wal-Mart in Minneapolis. During the application process, she endured routine drug tests and "personality tests"; once on the job, she dealt with constant surveillance and punishing scoldings about minor infractions. She learned how to survive from her co-workers, some of whom slept in their cars, and many of whom suffered from job-related back problems and arthritis. Ehrenreich's income barely covered her month's expenses, even when she worked two jobs. This book is a must-read for exposing the working world for many women in the service industry today.

## Research Alert

The Sago mining disaster on January 2, 2006, in Sago, West Virginia, claimed 12 men's lives. The mining accident occurred at the beginning of the first shift after the mine had closed for the New Year's holiday weekend. An examination conducted by a mine fireboss at 5:50 A.M. cleared the mine for use. Two carts of miners were making their way into the mine to begin work. The first group entered the mine approximately 8 to 10 minutes before the second.

The explosion occurred at approximately 6:30 A.M. and was heard and felt by many people outside the mine. The 13 trapped men were located about 2 miles inside the mine at approximately 280 feet below ground. Forty-one hours after the incident began, 12 of the miners were found dead in the early morning hours of January 4. One miner, Randal L. McCloy, Jr., was found alive, but in critical condition.

Hearings conducted during 2006 tentatively named the following as contributing causes of the explosion and fatalities:

- Sparks from restarting machinery after holiday.
- Use of "Omega blocks," a dense foam product, to seal the mine, rather than the required concrete blocks. The deputy director of the West Virginia Office of Miners' Health, Safety and Training told the state board of that group that "The seals, made with foam, could withhold pressures of five pounds per square inch."
- A lightning strike and seismic activity. Weatherbug, a Germantown, Maryland–headquartered weather tracking system reported on January 6, 2006, that "The evidence suggests that the lightning strike could have caused the explosion due to the correlation between the timing and location of the lightning strike and seismic activity."
- Carbon monoxide levels. The levels in the area where the miners were found were in the range of 300–400 ppm when the rescue team arrived. This is near the safe threshold level to support life for 15 minutes. Carbon monoxide poisoning was the likely cause of the miners' deaths.

In 2005, the federal Mine Safety and Health Administration (MSHA) had cited the Sago mine 208 times for violating regulations, up from 68 citations in 2004. Of those, 96 violations were considered significant and substantial. Additionally, West Virginia's Office of Miners' Health, Safety and Training had issued 144 citations to the mine over that year, up from 74 in the previous year.

Some of those citations were for violations that could have been factors in the accident, such as failure to control methane and coal-dust accumulation and failure to properly shore up shafts against collapse. Former MSHA official Davitt McAteer also suggested that restarting operations after a holiday weekend may have caused sparks to ignite an excess buildup of methane gas and coal dust; he also noted that the mine had deficiencies in emergency planning. At least four natural gas wells were in close proximity to the mine. One appeared to be adjacent to the sealed area where the explosion was believed to have occurred.

*Source*: Mine Safety and Health Administration. (2006, March 9). Emergency mine evacuation. *Federal Register*, pp. 12252–12271.

---

construction laborers, carpenters, and truck and tractor operators were nearly two times more likely to experience a low back disorder than all other male workers.

The diagnosis of low back pain is primarily made by history and physical examination. The possibility of work-related origin must be explored in detail. Occupational factors often associated with the occurrence of low back pain include heavy physical work, static work postures, frequent bending and twisting, lifting, pushing and pulling, repetitive work, and vibrations.

In general, individuals with low back pain recover from an acute episode in a few days to a few weeks, requiring little treatment. Modifying work activities or work restriction may be needed in the short term. However, if indicated, employees with this problem may need to be placed in new jobs, even though this is not usual.

Prevention of work-related low back pain is key and involves several measures. These measures include a work process that is ergonomically sound, optimal work levels, good work organization to reduce repetitive loading and fatigue, and training and education of workers, managers, healthcare providers, and union representatives about disease etiology and control and prevention strategies.

Despite the overwhelming statistics on the magnitude of the problem, more complete information is needed to assess how changes implemented to reduce the physical demands of jobs will affect workplace safety and productivity in the future. A tremendous opportunity exists for prevention efforts to reduce the prevalence and costs of low back disorders.

## ■ Musculoskeletal Disorders of the Upper Extremities

Musculoskeletal disorders of the neck and upper extremities from work factors affect employees in every type of workplace and include such diverse workers as food processors, automobile and electronics assemblers, carpenters, office data entry workers, grocery store cashiers, and garment workers. The highest rates of these disorders occur in the industries with a substantial amount of repetitive, forceful work. Musculoskeletal disorders affect the soft tissues of the neck, shoulder, elbow, hand, wrist, and fingers. These include the nerves (e.g., carpal tunnel syndrome), tendons (e.g., tenosynovitis, peritendinitis, epicondylitis), and muscles (e.g., tension neck syndrome). The costs associated with these disorders are high, with more than $2.1 billion in workers' compensation costs and $90 billion in indirect costs (hiring, training, overtime, and administrative costs) incurred annually for these musculoskeletal disorders. The number of musculoskeletal disorder cases declined from 784,145 cases in 1992 to 522,528 cases in 2001.

The most commonly reported musculoskeletal disorders of the upper extremities affect the hand–wrist region. In 1993, carpal tunnel syndrome, the most widely recognized condition, occurred at a rate of 3.0 per 10,000 full-time workers (Bureau of Labor Statistics, 2001). This syndrome required the longest recuperation period of all conditions resulting in lost workdays, with a median 25 days away from work.

## ■ Traumatic Injuries

### Fatal Occupational Injuries

From 1980 through 1992, more than 77,000 workers died as a result of work-related injuries. The leading causes of occupational injury fatalities over this 13-year period were motor vehicles, machines, homicides, falls, electrocutions, and falling objects. There were four industries—mining, construction, transportation, and agriculture—with occupational injury fatality rates that were notably and consistently higher than all other industries. Motor vehicle–related deaths in the transportation sector, machine-related deaths in agriculture, electrocutions and fatal falls in construction, homicide in retail trade and public administration, and deaths due to falling objects in mining and logging appear

to be important because of particularly high rates of death from injury.

### Nonfatal Occupational Injuries

In 1997, more than 5.7 million workers sustained job-related injuries that resulted in lost work time, medical treatment other than first aid, loss of consciousness, restriction of work or motion, or transfer to another job. The leading causes of nonfatal occupational injuries involving time away from work in 1997 were sprains, strains, and tears (Soll, 1999). Industries experiencing the largest number of serious nonfatal injuries include eating and drinking establishments, hospitals, and grocery stores. Industries facing higher risks of serious nonfatal injuries are concentrated in the manufacturing sector and include workers in shipbuilding, wooden building and mobile home manufacture, foundries, special products sawmills, and meat packing plants.

Clearly, work-related injuries and fatalities result from multiple causes, affect different segments of the working population, and occur in myriad occupational and industrial settings. The total cost of work-related injuries and fatalities to industry and to society at large has not been fully recognized, but it is estimated to be greater than $121 billion annually.

## Work/Workplace Change

The U.S. workplace is rapidly changing and becoming more diverse. Jobs in our economy continue to shift from manufacturing to services, with the service sector now employing 70% of all workers. Major changes are also occurring in the way work is organized. Longer hours, compressed work weeks, shift work, reduced job security, and part-time and temporary work are realities of the modern workplace. New chemicals, materials, processes, and equipment (e.g., latex gloves in health care, fermentation processes in biotechnology) are developed and marketed at an ever-accelerating pace.

The workforce is also changing. As the U.S. workforce grows (it totaled approximately 147 million in 2005), it will become older and more racially diverse. By 2005, minorities accounted for approximately 28% and women approximately 48% of the workforce. These changes are accompanied by new issues, such as potential language barriers and women's health issues.

Although much has been accomplished in controlling work-related illness and injury and reducing workplace fatalities, more needs to be done to ensure that worksites are safe and healthy for America's workforce (DHHS, 2000b). *Healthy People 2010* outlines objectives related to reducing work-related risk and injury, improving worker health, supporting research, and increasing efforts in training and education of occupational health and safety professionals (see the following box for selected *Healthy People 2010* objectives).

---

### ⦿ MEDIA MOMENT

#### *Working Girl* (1988)

This witty, romantic look at life in the corporate jungle stars Melanie Griffith as Tess McGill, an ambitious secretary with a unique approach for climbing the ladder to success. When her classy but villainous boss (Sigourney Weaver) breaks a leg while skiing, Tess simply takes over her office, her apartment, and even her wardrobe. She then creates a deal with a handsome investment banker (Harrison Ford) that will either take her straight to the top or finish her off for good.

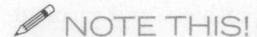

**HEALTHY PEOPLE 2010**

**Objectives Related to Occupational Safety and Health**

**Occupational Safety and Health**

20.1  Reduce deaths from work-related injuries.

20.2  Reduce work-related injuries resulting in medical treatment, lost time from work, or restricted work activity.

20.3  Reduce the rate of injury and illness cases involving days away from work due to overexertion or repetitive motion.

20.4  Reduce pneumoconiosis deaths.

20.5  Reduce deaths from work-related homicides.

20.6  Reduce work-related assault.

20.7  Reduce the number of persons who have elevated blood lead concentrations from work exposures.

20.8  Reduce occupational skin diseases or disorders among full-time workers.

20.9  Increase the proportion of worksites employing 50 or more persons that provide programs to prevent or reduce employee stress.

20.10  Reduce occupational needlestick injuries among health care workers.

20.11  Reduce new cases of work-related noise-induced hearing loss.

*Source*: DHHS, 2000a.

## Occupational Health Nursing Practice

The practice of occupational and environmental health nursing has changed dramatically over time, with increasing emphasis on autonomous decision making, independent practice, prevention and health promotion, analytical and investigative skills, management, and policy development (Rogers, 2003). This evolution is a result of the need to better deal with issues of changing workforce hazards, necessity for cost containment, and increased efforts to promote health and productivity at work.

This specialty practice has always been closely linked to public health nursing, which provides the practice underpinnings from a synthesis of the public health and nursing sciences directed at population health improvement (Rogers, 2003). Thus familiarity with the definition of public health nursing is also important. The American Public Health Association (APHA), Public Health Nursing Section (1996), has defined public health nursing as follows:

> Public health nursing is the practice of promoting and protecting the health of populations using knowledge from nursing, social, and public health sciences. Pub-

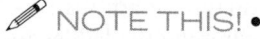

**NOTE THIS!**

With 879 fatalities, truck drivers suffered more workplace deaths in 1998 than any other profession.

*Source*: National Safety Council, 1999.

lic health nursing practice is a systematic process by which:

1. The health and health care needs of a population are assessed in order to identify sub-populations, families, and individuals who would benefit from health promotion or who are at risk of illness, injury, disability, or premature death.

2. A plan for intervention is developed with the community to meet identified needs that takes into account available resources, the range of activities that contribute to health and the prevention of illness, injury, disability, and premature death.

3. The plan is implemented effectively, efficiently, and equitably.

4. Evaluations are conducted to determine the extent to which the interventions have an impact on the health status of individuals and the population.

5. The results of the process are used to influence and direct delivery of care, deployment of health resources, and the development of local, regional, state, and national health policy and research to promote health and prevent disease.

Occupational and environmental health nursing practice is guided by the *Standards of Occupational and Environmental Health Nursing Practice* (AAOHN, 2004), which are developed and published by the American Association of Occupational Health Nurses. The professional standards provide the framework for evaluating the practice and a mechanism through which accountability with the public is maintained. Standard elements are shown in Box 41-4.

AAOHN also establishes the *Code of Ethics with Interpretive Statements* for occupational health nurses, which acts as a guide for the professional occupational heath nurse to maintain and pursue professionally ethical behavior in providing occupational health services. The *Code of Ethics* (AAOHN, 2003) is shown in Box 41-5.

**NOTE THIS!**

Women are more likely to be murdered at work than to die in a traffic accident.

## BOX 41-4

**American Association of Occupational Health Nurses**
*Standards of Occupational and Environmental Health Nursing Practice**

### STANDARD I: ASSESSMENT
The occupational and environmental health nurse systematically assesses the health status of the patient(s).

### STANDARD II: DIAGNOSIS
The occupational and environmental health nurse analyzes assessment data to formulate diagnoses.

### STANDARD III: OUTCOME IDENTIFICATION
The occupational and environmental health nurse identifies outcomes specific to the patient(s).

### STANDARD IV: PLANNING
The occupational and environmental health nurse develops a goal directed plan that is comprehensive and formulates interventions to attain expected outcomes.

### STANDARD V: IMPLEMENTATION
The occupational and environmental health nurse implements interventions to attain desired outcomes identified in the plan.

*Criteria*
### STANDARD VI: EVALUATION
The occupational and environmental health nurse systematically and continuously evaluates responses to interventions and progress toward the achievement of desired outcomes.

### STANDARD VII: RESOURCE MANAGEMENT
The occupational and environmental health nurse secures and manages the resources that support occupational health and safety programs and services.

### STANDARD VIII: PROFESSIONAL DEVELOPMENT
The occupational and environmental health nurse assumes accountability for professional development to enhance professional growth and maintain competency.

### STANDARD IX: COLLABORATION
The occupational and environmental health nurse collaborates with the patient(s) for the promotion, prevention and restoration of health within the context of a safe and healthy environment.

### STANDARD X: RESEARCH
The occupational and environmental health nurse uses research findings in practice and contributes to the scientific base in occupational and environmental health nursing to improve practice and advance the profession.

### STANDARD XI: ETHICS
The occupational and environmental health nurse uses an ethical framework for decision-making in practice.

*Note: This reflects only the category headings. Refer to the original source for the entire document.

*Source:* Copyright © 2004 by the American Association of Occupational Health Nurses, Inc. Used with permission. All rights reserved.

To apply practice skills, occupational health nursing practice requires more specific knowledge in fields nurses have some understanding of, including business and management, legal-regulatory fields, and behavioral sciences. In addition, it is essential that nurses be knowledgeable about the occupational health sciences, including industrial hygiene, toxicology, safety, and ergonomics (Rogers, 2003). A brief description of each of these occupational health science areas is provided next.

By definition, industrial hygiene includes the anticipation, recognition, evaluation, and control of occupational hazards, arising in or from the workplace, which may cause sickness, impaired health and well-being or significant discomfort, and inefficiency among workers or community citizens (AIHA, 1976). This is done through identifying and quantifying exposures, through sampling techniques, and through implementation and evaluation of control strategies to mitigate exposures.

Toxicology is the study of harmful effects of chemicals on biological systems. In the occupational setting, toxicology is primarily concerned with evaluating human health effects posed by workplace chemical exposures, including dusts, gases, fumes, mists, and vapors. This involves the recognition of routes of exposure, the relativity of these exposures to acute and latent health effects such as burns or cancer, and dose-response relationships.

Safety in the workplace is everyone's responsibility, and safety is concerned with the design and implementation of strategies to prevent and control workplace exposures that result in injury or death.

The term **ergonomics** is derived from two Greek words *ergos*, meaning "work," and *nomos*, meaning "laws"; thus the laws of work. The National Safety Council offers a simple but consistent definition: "Ergonomics is the science of designing the job and the workplace to fit the worker. The goal of ergonomics is to allow work to be done without undue stress." Within the framework of these definitions, the goal remains the same—that is, to match job demands and requirements to the abilities and capabilities of the worker (Sluchak, 1992). However, note that ergonomics is concerned with matching work and job design to fit the capabilities of most people by adapting the product to fit the user rather than vice versa.

## ■ Scope of Practice

The scope of occupational health nursing practice as depicted in the figure on this page is broad and dynamic and includes the following areas (Rogers, 2003).

**Worker/workplace assessment and surveillance** focus on identification of potential worker health problems and determination of worker health status. This is accomplished through knowledge of worker jobs and their demands, work processes and related hazards, and working conditions and exposures. Expert occupational health history taking is essential, as are appropriate assessments that help match the job to the worker. In addition to general health information, the history must include an examination of all previous jobs and exposures that may indicate potential interactions (e.g., smoking, antineoplastic agent exposure). An example of an occupational health history form is shown in Box 41-6.

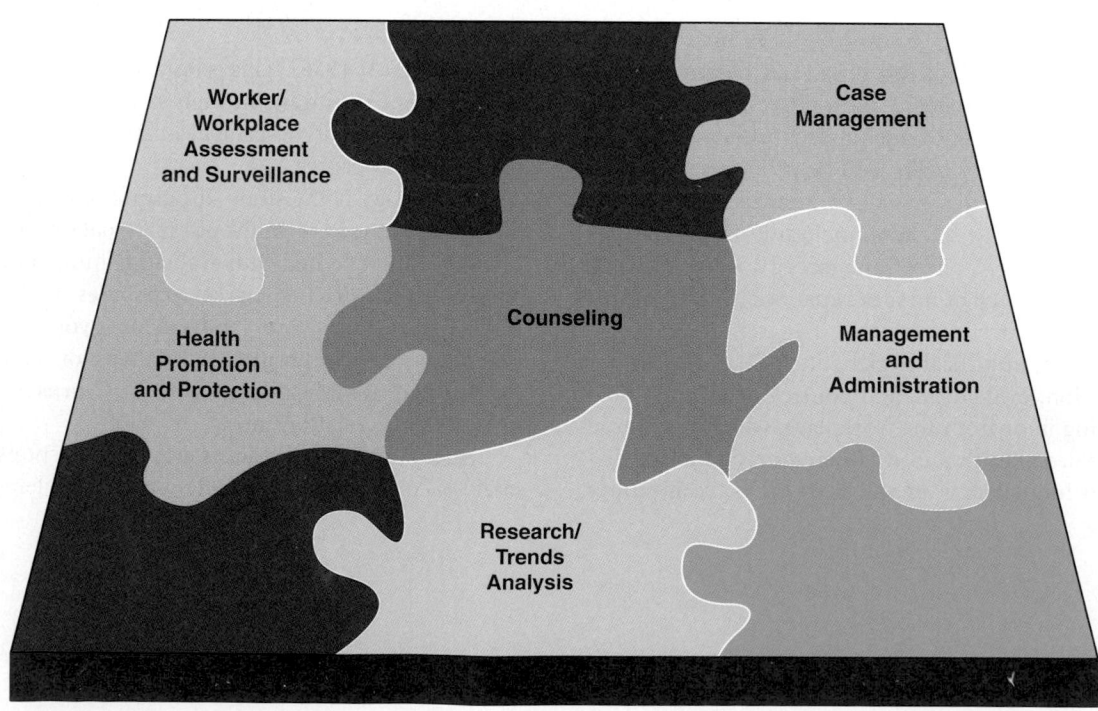

Scope of occupational health nursing practice

## BOX 41-6

**Occupational and Environmental Health History Form**

**Work History**

1. List your current and past longest-held jobs, including the military.

| Company | Dates employed | Job title | Known exposures |
|---|---|---|---|
| _____ | _____ | _____ | _____ |
| _____ | _____ | _____ | _____ |
| _____ | _____ | _____ | _____ |
| _____ | _____ | _____ | _____ |
| _____ | _____ | _____ | _____ |

2. Do you work full-time?   No ___   Yes ___   How many hours per week? ___
3. Do you work part-time?   No ___   Yes ___   How many hours per week? ___
4. Please describe any health problems or injuries that you have experienced in connection with your present or last jobs:


5. Have you ever had to change jobs due to health problems or injuries? If so, have any of your co-workers experienced similar problems?


6. In what type of business do you work currently?


7. Describe your work:


8. Have you had any current or past exposure (through breathing or touching) to any of the following?

| | | | | | |
|---|---|---|---|---|---|
| ___ acids | ___ carbon | ___ dichlorobenzene | ___ manganese | ___ pesticides | ___ toluene |
| ___ alcohols | ___ tetrachloride | ___ ethylene dibromide | ___ mercury | ___ phenol | ___ TDI or MDI |
| ___ alkalis | ___ chlorinated | ___ ethylene dichloride | ___ methylene | ___ phosgene | ___ trichloroethylene |
| ___ ammonia | naphthalenes | ___ fiberglass | ___ chloride | ___ radiation | ___ trinitrotoluene |
| ___ arsenic | ___ chloroform | ___ halothane | ___ nickel | ___ rock dust | ___ vibration |
| ___ asbestos | ___ chloropurine | ___ heat (severe) | ___ noise (loud) | ___ silica powder | ___ vinyl chloride |
| ___ benzene | ___ chromates | ___ isocyanates | ___ PBBs | ___ solvents | ___ welding fumes |
| ___ beryllium | ___ coal dust | ___ ketones | ___ PCBs | ___ stryrene | ___ x-rays |
| ___ cadmium | ___ cold (severe) | ___ lead | ___ perchloroethylene | ___ talc | |

9. Did you receive any safety training about these agents?


10. Are you involved in any work processes, such as grinding, welding, soldering, or polishing, that create dust or fumes?


11. Did you use any of the following personal protective equipment when exposed?

___ respirator   ___ gloves   ___ earplugs or muffs   ___ safety shoes
___ shield   ___ sleeves   ___ glasses or goggles   ___ boots
___ welding mask   ___ coveralls

12. Is your work environment generally clean? Describe:


13. What ventilation systems are used in your workspace?


14. Do the ventilation systems seem to work? Are you aware of any chemical odors in your environment?

**BOX 41-6**

**Occupational and Environmental Health History Form (Cont.)**

**15.** Where do you eat, smoke, and take your breaks when you are on the job?

**16.** Do you use a uniform or have clothing that you wear to work only?

**17.** How is this laundered?

**18.** How often do you wash your hands at work, and how do you wash them?

**19.** Do you shower before leaving the worksite?

**20.** Do you have any physical symptoms associated with work?

**21.** Are other workers similarly affected?

**22.** Do you have any home exposures (e.g., pesticides, household cleaners), hobbies, or community exposures (e.g., live near waste site, landfill)? Please describe:

---

*"Don't go around saying the world owes you a living. The world owes you nothing. It was here first."*

—*Mark Twain*

In addition, preplacement examinations to evaluate health status related to the work and gather baseline data, periodic examinations to determine any adverse work-related health effects, return-to-work evaluations to make certain the employee is fit for duty, screenings to detect health problems, and surveillance activities to monitor health status are needed.

The workplace also needs to be assessed and monitored to identify potential unhealthy working conditions. A collaborative walk-through assessment provides for observation of the workforce doing the work, observation of the work processes for each specific job, and observation of the working conditions and work milieu. Box 41-7 provides elements in the conduct of a worksite assessment.

The occupational health nurse should be knowledgeable about all work/work processes, the total work environment, and workforce characteristics so that hazards and potential

**BOX 41-7**

**Elements of a Worksite Assessment**
- The work, work processes, and related hazards, products, exposures
- Work environment (e.g., cleanliness, clutter, ventilation, noise, temperature, lighting, safety signs, wash disposal mechanisms)
- Worker population characteristics
- Staffing and personnel
- Corporate culture and philosophy
- Written policies/procedures for occupational health care
- Safety committee (frequency, interdisciplinary, measurements, recommendations)
- Occupational health and safety programs/services and types of occupational health visits
- Types and expenditures for medical/workers' compensation claims
- Most common illnesses/injuries
- Health-promotion/education programs
- Regulatory compliance with OSHA standards

THINK ABOUT THIS

That the birds of worry and care fly over your head, this you cannot help. But that they build nests in your hair, this you can prevent.

—Chinese Proverb

Nurses who care for seriously ill patients can experience various stressors because of personal, interpersonal, healthcare system, and professional variables. We are caregivers who often fail to "care for ourselves"! As a profession the following stressors can affect our health:

- Personal variables: perfectionism and over-involvement with patients, compassion fatigues, burnout
- Interpersonal variables: patient and family stressors, such as how the family is responding to the patient's illness; identification with the family and the nurse's own personal family situation
- Healthcare system variables: heavy workloads, scheduling conflicts, compromised time with family; physician–nurse conflicts
- Professional variables: moral and ethical dilemmas between nurse and family such as prolonging life and suffering, adverse effects of treatments, professional liability

Potential consequences of burnout and stress include the following problems:

- Eating disorders
- Gastrointestinal disturbances
- Somatic complaints: headaches, fatigue, insomnia
- Memory disturbances
- Hopelessness
- Depression
- Increased isolation
- Impaired judgment and reasoning
- Self-doubt
- Anger
- Low self-esteem
- Lack of meaning in profession
- Substance abuse
- Detachment from patients and colleagues

**Self-Care: What Can You Do Each Day to Be Healthy?**
At the end of each day (or night!) ask yourself, "Which areas in my life are unhealthy and what have I done today to keep myself balanced and well?" Keep a journal and write *something* each day in response to this question.

- Physical health: eat well, exercise, rest, use relaxation techniques, do yoga, participate in support groups.
- Emotional health: use meditation; listen to quiet music after work on the drive home; play; speak with colleagues and friends about concerns; read fiction and watch funny movies; connect with friends outside of nursing; take long, hot baths.
- Mental health: set priorities, say *no*, let go of the day and the conflict, keep your mind open to possibilities, and find new hobbies that do not involve nursing.
- Intuitional health: Meditation and relaxation can balance your sense of inner peace, harmony, and wholeness. Be still at least once a day, create your own "sacred space," and learn to "self-comfort" no matter what the setting. Take a walk every day, rain or shine. Think about one good thing that you gave of yourself at work that day.

**Contemplative Exercise**
Find your sacred place and be still. Focus on the rhythm of your breathing and then read each of the following statements:

- May I offer my care and presence unconditionally, knowing that I may be met with gratitude, indifference, anger, or anguish.
- May I offer love, knowing that I cannot control the course of life's suffering and death.
- May I remain in ease and let go of my expectations.
- May I view my own suffering with compassion as I do the suffering of others.
- May I be aware that my suffering does not limit my good heart.
- May I forgive myself for things left undone.
- May I forgive those who have hurt me.
- May those whom I have hurt forgive me.
- May all beings and I live and die in peace.

*Sources:* Halifax, J. (2000). Art of Dying III. Open Center and Tibet House, New York City. As cited on p. 54 in Sherman, D. W. (2004). Nurses' stress and burnout. *American Journal of Nursing, 104*(5), 48–56.

interventions can be adequately identified. In addition, knowledge of the corporate culture and mission related to occupational health and safety, as well as policies, staffing, and programmatic initiatives, will provide a sense about the relative importance of occupational health and safety at the worksite. The occupational health nurse will also want to know the most common illnesses and injuries at the worksite so that appropriate healthcare interventions can be made. These data will also provide information for problem solving, research, and determination of cost-effective healthcare delivery strategies.

During assessment and surveillance activities, preventive and corrective strategies such as engineering, work practice, administrative, and personal protective controls can be discussed as approaches to reduce risk and minimize health problems. Occupational health nurses critically analyze each job task to detect task situations that place employees at risk. They also note work-related risk factors, such as bending or

## Research Alert

A 1999 research study examined associations between workers' reported exposure to occupational hazards and their risk for alcohol use. The sample was drawn from the National Health Interview Survey (NHIS) and included 15,907 working adults. *Occupational hazard exposures* were defined as chemical or biological substances, physical hazards, injury risk, and mental stress. *At-risk drinking* was defined as binge drinking and driving while drinking. Of the workers in the sample, 60% reported exposure to one or more occupational hazards, 31% of the sample reported binge drinking, and 15% drove after drinking too much. In a multivariate analysis that controlled for background of the subjects, workers who reported occupational hazard exposure were 1.2 to 1.4 times more likely to engage in binge drinking than workers without exposures. Similar results were found for drinking and driving and occupational exposure. All multivariate statistical analyses were statistically significant. Findings suggest that workers who perceive themselves as being at risk for occupational hazards are at greater risk for binge drinking and driving after drinking. Occupational nurses can lead workplace initiatives to reduce occupational risk exposures and, at the same time, reduce risks for workers at risk for alcohol consumption.

*Source*: Conrad, K. M., Furner, S. E., & Qian, Y. (1999). Occupational hazard exposure and at risk drinking. *American Association of Occupational Health Nurses Journal, 47*(1), 9–16.

Woman working in a cigar factory

## MEDIA MOMENT

### Office Space (1999)

Peter Gibbons just can't seem to catch a break. His girlfriend is cheating on him, he has an obnoxious neighbor, and he's completely miserable in his job as a small cog in a soul-less company called Initech. Then he visits a hypnotherapist, who dies just after putting Peter into a state of complete bliss. Free of worrying about making a living, he no longer feels the need to keep his job, just as the company is going through a massive downsizing. His new, carefree attitude only makes him more valuable in the company's eyes, and his friends Michael and Samir are fired instead. Together, they scheme to plant a virus inside Initech's computer system that will pull money into their own account.

twisting, that may compromise the worker. The occupational health nurse is usually the first person to receive a complaint and must be prepared to recognize potential exposures and initiate exposure monitoring usually performed by an industrial hygienist.

*Occupational health and primary care* for both occupational and nonoccupational illness and injury is provided in most worksites by the occupational health nurse within the context of a collaborative multidisciplinary approach. Direct care is provided for emergency or urgent illness and injury (e.g., burns, head injuries), work-related acute illness and injury (e.g., back strain), minor health problems (e.g., headaches, lacerations), healthcare monitoring (e.g., high blood pressure), and preventive health care (e.g., immunizations, breast cancer screening). Also included here are mandatory or special programs such as hearing conservation, travel health, or drug and alcohol testing.

*Case management* is an integral component of occupational healthcare management involving conditions that may be occupational in origin (e.g., from an exposure) or nonoccupational in origin (e.g., cardiovascular disease). Coordination and management of cost-effective quality health-

care services from the onset of illness or injury to the return to work or optimal recovery are key. Early intervention and evaluation of outcomes, including cost savings, are essential components that provide for immediate problem identification and engage the worker in care planning from the beginning of the illness/injury to recovery. Early interven-

## Research Alert

Nearly three out of every four workers who participated in rescue and recovery efforts at the site of the collapsed World Trade Center towers in the wake of the September 11, 2001, terrorist attacks have experienced some health problems, a federally funded study found. The study, which was conducted by the National Institute for Occupational Safety and Health and Mount Sinai Hospital, was based on the screenings of 3,500 workers at Ground Zero and the Staten Island landfill, where tons of debris was trucked after the attacks. The preliminary results, based on 250 of the first screenings, suggest lingering health issues for a majority of the workers, and for many, a delayed diagnosis.

"Seventy-three percent of the sample had ear, nose, and throat symptoms, or abnormal ear, nose, and throat physical exam findings, or both," said Dr. Robin Herbert, co-director of the screening program. Herbert said 57% of those tested had lung problems and 20% had symptoms of post-traumatic stress disorder.

An estimated 35,000 workers—who responded from all across the country after the worst terrorist attacks on U.S. soil—were exposed to concrete dust that may have contained asbestos, lead, fiberglass, and other particles released when the twin towers collapsed after being hit by two hijacked aircraft.

*Source*: Herbert, R., Moline, J., Skloot, G., Metzger, K., Baron, S., Luft, B., et al. (2006). The World Trade Center disaster and the health of workers: Five-year assessment of a unique medical screening program. *Environmental Health Perspectives, 114*(12), 1853–1858.

tion helps prevent fragmented and delayed care by engaging appropriate healthcare providers at the beginning of care rather than later after complications may have developed. Case management requires knowledge of all factors that have an impact on worker health, including financial, spiritual, and cultural issues, and intense follow-up.

*Health promotion/health protection* activities are directed toward enhancing health and increasing the level of well-being toward optimal health. Activities are implemented at individual, group, and population levels through educational, behavioral, and environmental levels. Health protection is best described as preventive health behaviors designed to guard or defend an individual or group against specific illness or injury. Health protection is best achieved through a total range of prevention efforts incorporating primary, secondary, and tertiary prevention strategies. Primary, secondary, and tertiary prevention strategies, such as improved personal protective equipment, screening and surveillance activities, and return-to-work or cardiac rehabilitation programs, are used to reduce risks and restore health. Implementing a concept of health that is integrated into the

business structure will be key to a healthy environment. This means that health and safety must be a priority in terms of program planning and resource allocation.

*Counseling* is provided about health with regard to prevention and management of occupational illness and injury, work-related stress, productivity issues, family, conflicts, finances, personal issues, interorganizational relationships, and other areas. Knowing risk factors about employees such as recurrent absenteeism, substance abuse, social withdrawal, or changes in mood or appearance is critical for successful interventions, including referrals. The occupational health nurse is in the best position to provide counseling services to the worker because he or she is the healthcare provider most available to the employee. Some issues may interfere with the worker's ability to work or perform the job, and the employee will probably benefit from some form of intervention, such as listening, supporting, or referral.

The occupational health nurse should have specific counseling knowledge and skills such as problem recognition; building a supportive, trusting, and confidential relationship; crisis intervention approaches; and knowledge about community resources for referral to effectively assist the employee and in some cases the family.

*Management and administration*, including the development of health policy, is a major role that focuses on ensuring effective occupational health and safety programs and services. Defining a corporate culture that is supportive of a healthy work environment is necessary for an effective occupational health and safety program. Increasingly, the occupational health nurse is assuming a major role in the management and administration of the occupational health unit and in policy-making decisions to ensure effective occupational health and safety programs and services for workers. At the unit level, the occupational health nurse manager is responsible for the overall operational management of the occupational health service, including program planning, organization, staffing, budget development and management, service coordination, and evaluation. Strategic or long range planning shapes the future of the company and is key to the long-term success and growth of the occupational health program. When engaged in the strategic planning process, the occupational health nurse can use valuable expertise to set forth new ideas and positions and engage in policy development about furthering the occupational health and safety program within the context of the business mission. Understanding the business mission, the needs of the organization, and resource consumption variables is vital to a successful program. Keeping the workforce healthy and productive within the context of the cost containment is a major objective.

*Community orientation* emphasizes the development of partnerships and collaboration in the delivery of workplace health care. If used, services provided by voluntary or governmental agencies, such as parenting programs, cardi

🖊 NOTE THIS! •————————————————

Since the war in Iraq began, the number of veterans returning home with limb amputations has increased dramatically. Prosthetic science has exploded, with NASA-tested titanium and carbon fiber that is strong and light enough for artificial limb replacement being developed. Today's artificial limb for an above the knee amputee will typically weigh 5 pounds; in previous years, it was twice that heavy. This makes it easier for an amputee to move. In addition, today's prosthesis contains a microprocessor that enhances life-like movement. These microprocessors anticipate what the person is doing, thereby helping the amputee prepare to absorb the impact as he or she is about to plant the foot on the ground.

Unfortunately, such progress has always come in an era of global conflict. The injuries in World War II inspired products that meshed wood and rubber, as well as the "soft heel," which featured a more flexible toe for the amputee. In the wake of the Vietnam War, prostheses bent and bounced in such a way that energy was returned to the amputee much like a spring on a diving board.

Today's veterans—both men and women—expect to live full lives, including returning to their previous careers and sports. With recent advances in the field of prosthetics, this expectation is becoming much more of a reality.

or drug rehabilitation services, or home health care, can be cost beneficial to both the employee and employer. The occupational health nurse can help the industry create a health partnership with the community by working together on programs. Providing or sponsoring health fairs for workers, their families, and the community is another example of successful partnerships. Use of community programs and development of referral networks will aid the occupational health and safety program.

*Research and trend analysis* is necessary to improve and foster the health and well-being of the worker and workforce, to improve working conditions by eliminating or minimizing hazards, and to build a body of occupational health nursing knowledge. Research and practice go hand in hand with the mission to improve and foster the health and well-being of the worker and workforce and to improve working conditions by eliminating or minimizing potential or actual hazards. For example, understanding the effects of toxic exposures, designing strategies to prevent work-related accident/injuries or illnesses, evaluating the cost-effectiveness of health interventions, and understanding human behavior and motivation related to health promotion activities are important occupational health nursing investigations. Occupational health nursing research is essential in both preventive health management and control of workplace hazards.

*Legal-ethical monitoring* is paramount to ensure a safe and healthful work environment consistent with the OSH Act, related standards, and the Nurse Practice Acts. The occupational health nurse must be aware of occupational health

and safety statutes and recommend programs and strategies to comply with mandated requirements. The nurse also should work to influence or help develop legislation such as confidentiality of employee health records protection or legislation specific to worker/workplace health protection.

Ethical issues abound in the work environment, and the occupational health nurse is faced with many challenges in ethical decision making. Issues related to confidentiality of employee health records, hazardous exposures, truth telling, inappropriate screening of employees, discrimination, and professional incompetence or illegal practice are but a few of these ethical challenges. As mentioned, the AAOHN *Code of Ethics* will help guide practice and acts as a framework for implementation of values related to occupational health and safety. The nurse is obligated to always act in the best interest of the worker and provide effective leadership skills in ethical health care. In this role, the occupational health nurse not only brings a special expertise to occupational health dilemmas but also structures the issues so that sound and deliberate decisions are made using a reasoned approach.

## ■ Occupational Health Nursing Roles

Occupational health nursing roles have expanded enormously (Rogers & Cox, 1998) to match the increased scope of practice. The AAOHN describes the varied roles of occupational health nurses (see the figure on the next page).

The **occupational health nurse clinician** provides direct care for both occupational and nonoccupational illness and injuries using established protocols; performs health assessments, screenings, surveillance, and counseling; and conducts workplace walkthroughs/assessments and exposure follow-up.

The **occupational health nurse case manager** coordinates healthcare services for the employee from the onset of injury or illness to a safe return to work or an optimal alternative. Quality outcome-focused care is delivered in a cost-effective manner.

The **occupational health nurse coordinator** functions as the single occupational health nurse for a company responsible for the occupational and environmental health and safety services. The occupational health nurse coordinator conducts needs assessments of the patient population and worksite and develops programs designed to address these needs. Evaluation is a component of the process.

The **occupational health nurse health-promotion specialist** has primary responsibility for the overall management of the health-promotion program. This includes the development of a comprehensive program that meets the needs of the workforce population within the context of supporting organizational business objectives for a healthy workforce and work environment. These initiatives might include exercise, nutrition, or smoking-cessation programs.

The **occupational health nurse manager** is responsible for setting occupational health unit policy and directing, administering, and evaluating an occupational and environmental health and safety service. This includes the operational management of the occupational health unit, financial management consistent with organizational goals and objectives, and quality improvement of occupational health services.

The **occupational health nurse practitioner** uses independent and collaborative critical judgments in conducting health assessments, making differential diagnoses, promoting optimal health, and providing pharmacological and nonpharmacological treatments in the direct management of acute and chronic illness and injuries within the scope of state regulations. Services may range from preplacement physical examinations to comprehensive primary care for employees and their families.

The **occupational health nurse corporate director** functions as a policy maker at the corporate level and develops and directs the overall occupational and environmental health and safety programs in consultation with other health and safety specialists and corporate management. This individual also evaluates quantitative outcomes of occupational and environmental health and safety programs using cost–benefit analysis, engages in strategic planning and trend analysis in occupational and environmental health, and provides vision for the direction of the occupational health and safety program.

The **occupational health nurse consultant** provides advice for developing occupational and environmental health and safety services and for structuring the delivery of services, including managed care and case management. In addition, this individual consults about specific services such as hazard analysis, disability management review, hearing conservation, regulatory programming, and health promotion.

The **occupational health nurse educator** plans curricula appropriate to various levels of educational preparation and has responsibilities for occupational and environmental health nursing curricula and clinical experiences in college or university academic education, continuing professional education, or unit staff development programs. Evaluation is a continuous process.

The **occupational health nurse researcher** develops researchable questions, designs studies, conducts research, writes grants, and disseminates research findings to improve practice and build knowledge in the discipline.

These roles are multi-integrated, meaning that occupational health nurses often act in many capacities at the same time.

Within the knowledge context for role implementation, occupational health nurses must have a lifelong knowledge base in the public health and occupational health sciences (e.g., epidemiology, toxicology, industrial hygiene, safety/

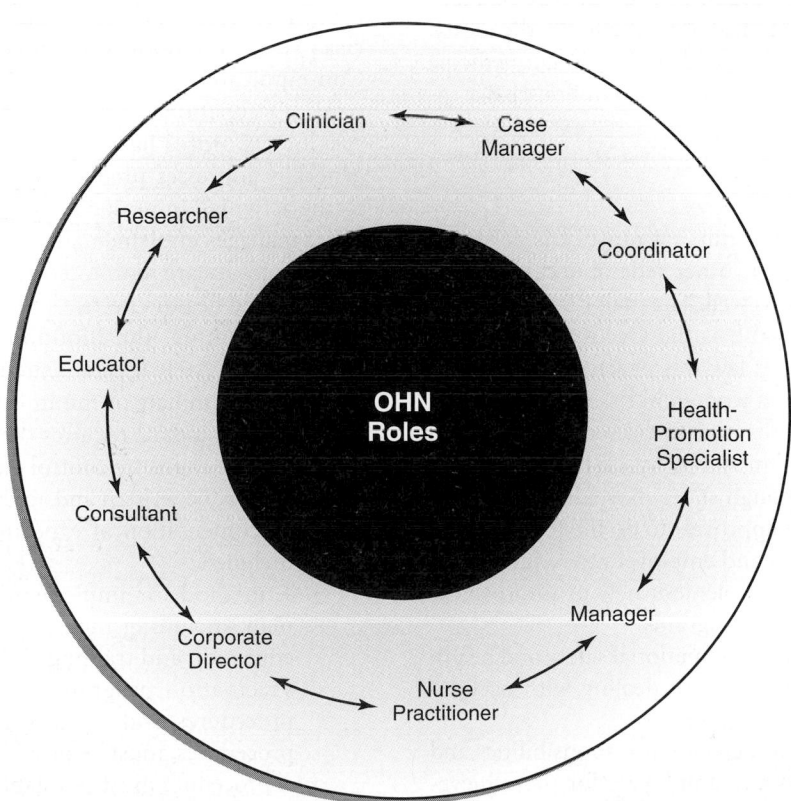

Occupational Health Nursing Roles

## BOX 41-8

**Interdisciplinary Fields of Practice Specific to Occupational Health Nursing**

**Occupational Medicine**

The assessment, maintenance, restoration, and improvement of the health of the worker through the principles of preventative medicine, and promotion of worker health and productivity

**Industrial Hygiene**

The science devoted to the anticipation, recognition, evaluation, and control of environmental factors and stresses associated with work and work operations

**Safety**

The design and implementation of strategies aimed at preventing and controlling workplace exposure that result in unnecessary injuries and death

**Ergonomics**

The study of humans at work and the evaluation of the stresses that occur in the work environment and the ability of people to cope with these stresses so that the job demands are matched with human capabilities

ergonomics), environmental health, business and economics, social and behavioral sciences, and legal and ethical parameters of practice. To implement the roles effectively, occupational health nurses must work within an interdisciplinary framework with other health disciplines, typically the industrial hygienist, safety specialist, and occupational medicine physician. These fields are briefly described in Box 41-8.

## Governmental Influence

Although occupational health nursing practice is governed by state nursing practice acts, other federal and state laws affect these nurses' practice as well. The major law governing occupational safety and health is the Occupational Safety and Health Act of 1970. This law was enacted to "assure so far as possible every man and woman in the Nation safe and healthful working conditions and to preserve our human resources." The act is administered by OSHA within the Department of Labor (although states may administer their own programs with OSHA approval) to do the following:

- Encourage employers and employees to reduce workplace hazards and to implement new or improve existing safety and health programs
- Provide for research in occupational safety and health to develop innovative ways of dealing with occupational safety and health problems
- Establish separate but dependent responsibilities and rights for employers and employees for the achievement of better safety and health conditions

- Maintain a reporting and record-keeping system to monitor job-related illnesses and injuries
- Establish training programs to increase the number and competence of occupational safety and health personnel
- Develop mandatory job safety and health standards and enforce them effectively
- Provide for the development, analysis, evaluation, and approval of state occupational safety and health programs

Within the legislation for the OSH Act, several bodies were created to help carry out the mandates of the act. OSHA is the agency responsible to set and enforce the rules and regulations of the act and standards the agency develops. NIOSH conducts research and training and makes recommendations for the prevention and control of work-related illnesses and injuries. It also funds education and research centers that provide academic, research, and continuing education training for occupational safety and health professionals.

The Occupational Safety and Health Review Commission is a quasi-judicial body charged with reviewing disputes, forwarded to it by the Department of Labor, regarding OSHA inspections.

The National Advisory Committee on Occupational Safety and Health is a consumer and professionally appointed group that makes occupational and safety recommendations to OSHA and the NIOSH. The agency also promulgates numerous standards to eliminate or reduce risks (e.g., Bloodborne Pathogens Standard, Hazardous Communication Standard, Lead Standard, Asbestos Standard). Occupational health and safety standards related to specific exposures have a health/medical component that generally addresses preplacement, surveillance, and monitoring activities. In most companies, the occupational health nurse manages implementation of these standards to ensure that employees are monitored appropriately for any adverse work-related health effects.

For example, the Bloodborne Pathogens Standard (29CFR 1910.1030), established by OSHA in 1992, was designed to eliminate or minimize blood and body fluid exposure. The standard requires the employer to develop and implement an exposure control plan as follows:

- It must be written and accessible to employees.
- Documentation of exposure determination must be included.
- A method for implementing the exposure control plan, including methods of compliance, employee education and training, description of the hepatitis B vaccination program and postexposure follow-up procedures, and record-keeping and communication procedures, must be provided.
- A procedure must be established for evaluating exposure incidents.

Hairdressers are exposed to hazardous chemicals, such as hair dye, bleach, and other skin and pulmonary irritants on a daily basis. Contact dermatitis and pulmonary problems are among the most common work-related heath conditions that require preventive health care, such as well-ventilated mixing areas and the use of disposable gloves. They are also at risk for knee and back injuries.

The occupational health nurse assists management in developing an effective program consistent with the standard's elements. Occupational health nurses also serve as consultants to assist in establishing methods of compliance, such as engineering and work practice controls.

The occupational health nurse is usually the person responsible for the development and implementation of the hepatitis B vaccination program and postexposure follow-up. The standard requires that the hepatitis B vaccine be offered, at no expense, to all exposed employees. If the employee chooses not to accept the offer of the hepatitis B vaccination, he or she must sign a mandatory declination statement. The postexposure evaluation and follow-up are critical to employee safety and health; therefore, the most important component of effective postexposure evaluation is the method for reporting exposures. Exposures must be reported and acted upon immediately. Counseling the employee about the risk of infection, importance of early

testing to determine whether transmission has occurred, and recommendations for postexposure prophylaxis and prevention of transmission of disease are essential and should occur over several sessions.

Employee education and training are also provided by the occupational health nurse. Information about the hazards of bloodborne pathogens and methods to prevent transmission to workers may be introduced at employee orientation. These programs are an ideal time to introduce the method for and importance of appropriate reporting of exposures. The occupational health nurse plays an active role in partnering with OSHA and the employer to reduce morbidity and mortality associated with exposures to blood-borne pathogens (BBP), such as hepatitis B and HIV. Occupational health nurses participate in all aspects of compliance with the BBP Standard, beginning with development of and implementing an exposure control plan and ending with maintaining the health and training records for the appropriate number of years.

Within the OSH Act, the general duty clause states that employers are required to furnish all employees "employment and a place of employment which are free from recognized hazards that are causing or likely to cause death or serious physical harm." If a specific hazard is not covered by a standard, the general duty clause can be invoked. OSHA also provides consultative services to identify and correct hazards, provide technical assistance, and provide education and training for health and safety personnel. Occupational health nurses must be fully cognizant of all occupational health and safety laws, standards, and the regulatory implications in the workplace.

In addition, the OSH Act requires most employers with 11 or more employees to prepare and maintain records of work-related illnesses and injuries. There are detailed rules and regulations regarding what constitutes a recordable event and how these events are to be recorded. In most instances in which there is an occupational health nurse, he or she is usually delegated this responsibility. Data are recorded in logs that are analyzed in aggregate form (by OSHA and the Bureau of Labor Statistics) to identify companies with high-risk illnesses and injuries that may need enforcement and consultation efforts.

In addition to the OSH Act, examples of other pertinent laws affecting health and safety at the worksite include the following:

- Americans with Disabilities Act of 1990 (ADA): This act is intended to prevent discrimination against persons with disabilities. Under Title I of the act, persons with disabilities are entitled to equal employment opportunities without regard to their disability. Health assessments can be performed only after an offer of employment has been made, and applicants can be evaluated only in terms of their ability to perform essential job functions. In some situations, reasonable accommodations must be made by the employer for the disabled person to perform the work. The occupational health nurse may be actively involved in developing and implementing the company's ADA policy. This is done through the appropriate conduct of health examinations, review of job functions to determine job suitability, and recommendations for job accommodations.

- Family Medical Leave Act: This act requires employers with 50 or more employees to provide a maximum of 12 weeks unpaid job-related leave in a 12-month period to eligible employees. The occupational health nurse has the responsibility to educate eligible employees about what constitutes an eligible leave of absence and counsel the employee regarding health issues.

- Worker's Compensation: The worker's compensation system in each state and the District of Columbia is designed to cover monetary loss as a result of work-related injuries, including salary; medical, hospital, or funeral expenses; and dependent support in case of occupational death. In turn, there is no employer negligence or fault, safeguarding the employer from legal action. Federal civilian employees are covered by federal statutes.

The occupational health nurse often manages worker compensation claims, ensuring that injured workers are medically treated and managed. In addition, the occupational health nurse monitors the employee's return to work, cautioning against reinjury, but getting the employee back to functional work in a reasonable period.

## Professionalism in Occupational Health Nursing

The professional society in occupational health nursing is the American Association of Occupational Health Nurses (AAOHN). AAOHN does the following:
- Promotes the health and safety of workers
- Defines the scope of practice and sets the standards of occupational health nursing practice
- Develops the *Code of Ethics* for occupational health nurses with interpretive statements
- Promotes and provides continuing education in the specialty
- Advances the profession through supporting research
- Responds to and influences public policy issues related to occupational health and safety

The official journal is the *AAOHN Journal.*

### ■ Education and Certification

One must be a registered nurse to gain entry into professional occupational health nursing practice. Most companies

**GLOBAL CONNECTION**

Many hospitals and other healthcare organizations recruit nurses from developing countries to work in U.S. healthcare facilities. What about the healthcare needs of these nurses' native countries? Should we be "poaching" these healthcare professionals from countries that have greater health needs than the United States simply because we are able to provide higher salaries? What do you think?

prefer to hire occupational nurses with previous experience in occupational health, public health, or emergency care. A baccalaureate in nursing is the preferred degree (AAOHN, 1996). As stated, specialty academic education in occupational health and safety is generally offered at the graduate level (master's and doctoral) through NIOSH-funded Occupational Safety and Health Education and Research Centers (Table 41-5).

These centers provide academic, research, continuing education, and outreach programs. Grants support training and education of occupational health and safety professionals, including occupational health nurses, industrial hygienists, physicians, and safety specialists. In addition, a nurse practitioner option in occupational health is offered. Doctoral-level education prepares nurses as scientists in occupational health and safety research.

Certification in occupational health nursing is conducted by the American Board for Occupational Health Nursing. Certification is met through educational qualifications, experience, continuing education, and examination.

As the occupational health nurse professionally progresses, the use of technology, in addition to print materials, may be the preferred approach to seek state-of-the-art information.

### ■ Nurse-Managed Models in Occupational Health

In 1993, an initiative of the American Nurses Association and the American Association of Occupational Health Nurses about cost-effective healthcare services resulted in the publication *Innovations at the Worksite* (Burgel, 1993), which is still in use today. This document addresses five models of worksite primary health care managed and delivered by occupational health nurses as cost-effective healthcare providers. These models apply principles of health promotion and risk reduction through continuing integration of these strategies in practice. The goal is to provide quality, accessible, and cost-effective care. Following are brief descriptions of each model.

#### Model 1: One-Nurse Unit, On-Site

This model may be the best choice for companies with limited resources, few workplace hazards, or a small workforce. The nurse acts as the in-house expert on health-related issues and develops a network of quality, community-based referrals for services not provided in-house.

| **Table 41-5** National Institute for Occupational Safety and Health Education and Research Centers | |
|---|---|
| ■ **Alabama Educational Resource Center**<br>University of Alabama at Birmingham<br>School of Public Health<br>Birmingham, AL 32594-0008<br>205-934-7032 | ■ **Michigan Educational Resource Center**<br>University of Michigan<br>School of Public Health<br>Department of Environmental and Industrial Health<br>Ann Arbor, MI 48109<br>313-936-0735 |
| ■ **California Educational Resource Center, Northern**<br>University of California, Berkeley<br>School of Public Health<br>322 Warren Berkeley, CA 94720<br>510-642-0761 | ■ **Minnesota Educational Resource Center**<br>University of Minnesota<br>School of Public Health<br>1158 Mayo Memorial Building<br>420 Delaware Street, SE<br>Minneapolis, MN 55455<br>612-626-0900 |
| ■ **California Educational Resource Center, Southern**<br>University of Southern California<br>Institute of Safety and Systems Management<br>University Park<br>Los Angeles, CA 90089-0021<br>213-740-4038 | ■ **New York/New Jersey Educational Resource Center**<br>Department of Community Medicine<br>Mt. Sinai School of Medicine<br>PO Box 1057<br>10 E 102nd Street<br>New York, NY 10029<br>212-966-5001 |
| ■ **Cincinnati Educational Resource Center**<br>University of Cincinnati<br>Department of Environmental Health<br>3223 Eden Avenue<br>Cincinnati, OH 45267-0056<br>513-558-5701 | ■ **North Carolina Educational Resource Center**<br>University of North Carolina<br>School of Public Health<br>Rosenau Hall, CB #7400<br>Chapel Hill, NC 27599-7410<br>919-966-5001 |
| ■ **Harvard Educational Resource Center**<br>Harvard School of Public Health<br>Department of Environmental Health<br>665 Huntington Avenue<br>Boston, MA 02115<br>617-432-3325 | ■ **Texas Educational Resource Center**<br>The University of Texas Health Science Center at Houston<br>School of Public Health<br>PO Box 20186<br>Houston, TX 77225<br>713-792-4638 |
| ■ **Illinois Educational Resource Center**<br>University of Illinois at Chicago<br>School of Public Health<br>PO Box 6998, M/C 922<br>Chicago, IL 60680<br>312-996-7887 | ■ **Utah Educational Resource Center**<br>University of Utah<br>Rocky Mountain Center for Occupational and Environmental Health<br>Building 512<br>Salt Lake City, UT 84112<br>801-581-8719 |
| ■ **Johns Hopkins Educational Resource Center**<br>Johns Hopkins University<br>School of Hygiene and Public Health<br>615 North Wolfe Street<br>Baltimore, MD 21205<br>301-955-3602 | ■ **Washington Educational Resource Center**<br>University of Washington<br>Department of Environmental Health, SC-34<br>Seattle, WA 98195<br>206-543-6991 |

### Model 2: Multiple Nurses, On-Site

This model is ideal for medium to large employers. Essential services are offered on-site in a nurse-managed care center. The focus is on primary care as well as work-related illnesses and injuries.

### Model 3: Consortium Model—Company Coalitions

This model is designed for groups of small employers to provide services in a centralized, nurse-managed, free-standing clinic. Essential services are provided on-site during expanded hours of service, with a local hospital providing services during off hours through a preferred provider arrangement.

### Model 4: Large Employers with Outreach to Small Employers

This model is best for a large employer with on-site services (as in model 2) that provides services to neighboring small employers through a contractual arrangement.

### Model 5: Occupational Health Nurse Consultant

This model focuses on providing services by an occupational health nurse acting as consultant to small employers in geographically scattered locations. The occupational health nurse consultant is on-site at each employer location on a periodic basis, providing some direct services and coordinating other services through a local hospital and nearby specialty providers.

In all of these models, a basic set of services is provided (e.g., direct care, health surveillance, regulatory compliance, case management, health promotion), either directly or by contracted arrangements. However, depending on the model, services may be modified to reflect the need.

## Future Expansions

### ■ Environmental Health

More than ever before, the importance of integrating environmental health into occupational and environmental health nursing practice is well recognized. Environmental health can be defined as the interaction between individual and environmental agents that may affect health states. The workplace is included because this is the place in which many of the most significant hazards occur. Environmental health has been a concept central to general nursing practice since its beginning. The nursing profession has long recognized that health is affected by many variables and has engaged a holistic approach to nursing care. Florence Nightingale viewed the environment as a fundamental aspect of nursing practice, and her interventions focused on modifying the environment as a primary means of promoting health. She cited five essential points in securing the health of individuals: pure air, pure water, efficient drainage, cleanliness, and light (Nightingale, 1869). Nightingale believed that the nurse was responsible for identifying any conditions that could affect the health of individuals and populations, such as ventilation, noise, heat, cold, and cleanliness, and for developing ways to alter the environment so that health and healing could flourish. Environmental health is a natural extension of occupational health nurses to identify environmental health hazards, explore their interaction, and work with members of the interdisciplinary team, management, workers, and communities to reduce environmental and occupational health risk (Rogers & Cox, 1998).

The Institute of Medicine issued a report describing the importance of this integration and citing the important link between occupational health nursing and environmental health, which is supported by the professional organization AAOHN. Occupational health nurses therefore need additional competencies in environmental health, including the following:

- Understanding the interaction of environmental agents, such as lead and waste products, with human systems, and related signs and symptoms of disease
- Developing prevention, protection, and control strategies for environmental health problems, such as indoor air pollution, and using environmental health resources, including information from the Agency for Toxic Substances and Disease Registry
- Discussing ethical implications of environmental health exposures such as right to know about community toxic spills

**Application to Practice**

Polluted indoor air has become increasingly recognized as a potential public health problem. As an occupational health nurse, you have been asked to assess a small company with 75 workers who manufacture plant food. The workers have complained of headache, eye and throat irritations, and fatigue. Upon assessment, you find the company housed in a 30-year-old building with inconsistent maintenance. The ventilation system is old and has had cooling problems. The workers complain of inconsistent heating and cooling and "stuffiness." You find a greater-than-expected incidence of asthma, worker sick days, and headaches requiring neurologist care.

1. What are some likely contributing factors to worker illness?
2. What should the nurse suggest that the owner do next in determining the contributing causes to the worker health problems?
3. What role could the occupational health nurse play in the prevention of future problems in this work environment?

- Influencing regulatory controls such as community residential exposures in environmental health as appropriate

### ■ Migrant Health

According to the National Center for Farmworker Health (2008), the migrant population is a diverse one, and its composition varies from region to region. However, it is estimated that 85% of all migrant workers are minorities, of whom most are Hispanic (including Mexican Americans as well as Mexicans, Puerto Ricans, Cubans, and workers from Central and South America). The migrant population also includes African Americans, Jamaicans, Haitians, Laotians, Thais, and other racial and ethnic minorities.

Migrant and seasonal farmworkers hand-pick apples or peaches, harvest asparagus or chilies, stake up tomatoes, dig potatoes or beets, or work in packing plants. Hand labor is especially vital to the production of the blemish-free fruits and vegetables that U.S. consumers demand. The fruit, vegetable, and horticultural industries, in particular, rely on the labor of migrant and seasonal farmworkers. More than

*Got an Alternative?*

As an occupational health nurse in a high-tech environment, you might assess that many workers are stressed on the assembly line due to repetitive and boring work. Which kinds of complementary and alternative health interventions could you recommend to these workers that would not affect their work but would increase their relaxation?

85% of the fruits and vegetables produced in this country are hand harvested and/or cultivated. Although many people believe that fruit and vegetable production is declining in this country, in reality, domestic production has steadily increased in recent years.

Farm labor is seasonal and intensive. Planting, thinning, and harvesting are not year-round activities. However, they are crucial to crop production, and the time frame in which they must occur is determined by the seasons and the weather. Failure to perform any of these activities at the appropriate time can result in a lost crop. The urgency to accomplish tasks according to nature's timetable compels farmworkers to work in the fields in all seasons and in all weather conditions, including extreme heat, extreme cold, rain, intense sun, and dampness.

Farmworkers' work hours accommodate the crops, not vice versa. Their work often requires stoop labor, working with the soil, climbing, carrying heavy loads, and having direct contact with plants. The plants and the soil are often treated with pesticides and chemical fertilizers. Some plants, such as tobacco and strawberries, exude chemicals that are toxic to humans or that can cause severe allergic reactions such as contact dermatitis. The Environmental Protection Agency estimates that 300,000 farmworkers experience acute pesticide poisoning each year. Anecdotal reports from clinicians indicate that many cases of pesticide poisoning are unreported because patients do not seek treatment or are misdiagnosed because the symptoms of pesticide poisoning can resemble those of viral infection.

Many of the health problems found in the general population, particularly among minorities and the poor, also affect migrant farmworkers. The hardships of life as a farmworker result in unique challenges to the health of these workers and their families.

Some health concerns are clearly attributable to the occupational hazards of farm work. Dermatitis and respiratory problems caused by natural fungi, dusts, and pesticides are common. Lack of safe drinking water contributes to dehydration and heat stroke. Other health conditions such as TB, diabetes, cancer, hypertension, depression, and HIV, which require careful monitoring and frequent treatment, pose a special problem for farmworkers who must move frequently.

Migrant and seasonal workers are a group of workers who could greatly benefit from occupational and environmental health nursing services. This can be done by providing direct care clinic services, educating workers about occupational health and safety hazards, and initiating workplace/community outreach. The occupational and environmental health nurse can have a major impact on health promotion and protection in this vulnerable population of workers.

## ■ Health Promotion in the Workplace

In 2003, the Department of Health and Human Resources launched a new initiative called Steps to a Healthier United States, aimed at promoting healthier behaviors, actions, and programs in the context of both personal and social responsibility. As part of this effort NIOSH has introduced Steps to a Healthier US Workforce, which focuses on both personal and workplace risk factors (NIOSH, 2004). The vision of this initiative is to integrate occupational safety and health protection with health promotion activities into

**❝**With employee health costs soaring to more than $1 trillion annually, the presence of an occupational health nurse (OHN) in a work environment can not only guarantee healthy, safe conditions for workers, but also can save employers the costs of illness- and injury-related absenteeism and disability claims.**❞**

—Richard Kowalski, Board President,
American Association of Occupational Health Nurses

 NOTE THIS!

**Labor Day Holiday: Why Do We Celebrate It?**
Labor Day is usually celebrated with barbecues and picnics and is associated with the beginning of school. We rarely remember that Labor Day was created as a way for us to remember the tremendous labor struggles to improve worker conditions in the United States. In the nineteenth century, workers often worked 16-hour days, 6 and 7 days a week. Children were commonly used as a labor resource. Injuries were common, thousands of workers died, "caught in the grinding machinery of our growing industries" (p. 1319).

In the labor market of today, despite improvements, workers continue to die in the workplace, while many more are injured, sometimes for life. We should remember all workers, past and present, on Labor Day. Rosner and Markowitz (1999) encourage us to remember the "historical toll in lives and limbs that workers have paid to provide us with our modern prosperity . . . the continuing toil is far too high and that workers who died and continue to die in order to produce our wealth" (p. 1320). They deserve to be remembered and honored on Labor Day.

*Source:* Rosner & Markowitz, 1999.

a coordinated system that addresses both workplace and worker health. Given that Americans spend an average of 8–12 hours per day at work, the workplace is an ideal locus for developing a healthier U.S. workforce. This initiative strongly supports the view that all illness and injury should be prevented when possible, controlled when necessary, and treated where appropriate. It emphasizes (1) preventing work-related illness, injury, and disability, and (2) promoting healthy living and lifestyles to reduce and prevent chronic disease. Health promotion programs have traditionally focused on the individual's personal and lifestyle risk factors, such as lack of physical activity, poor nutrition, and tobacco use, whereas workplace safety and health programs have focused on workplace risks such as chemicals, noise, and other unsafe working conditions. Steps to a Healthier U.S. Workforce creates an opportunity for both the occupational and safety community and the health promotion community to develop and implement workplace illness and injury programs collaboratively that prevent workplace illness and injury, promote health, and optimize the health of the U.S. workforce and workplace.

Many occupational and environmental health nurses are already engaged in developing and implementing heath promotion and health protection programs in the workplace. These efforts represent a wonderful opportunity to engage workers and employers in a significant movement to improve the health of America's workforce.

## Conclusion

Occupational health nursing is a specialty that provides nursing care to worker populations, creating and sustaining healthy and safe work environments. The specialty practice has grown enormously, encompassing expanded roles as independent practitioners, consultants, and policy makers. Expansion to focus on issues external to traditional workplace settings, including environmental health and migrant health, will be a significant and far-reaching opportunity. Prevention and health promotion are the cornerstones of care in occupational health nursing within an interdisciplinary framework. Research is critical in identifying work-related health issues and testing interventions to mitigate the risk. The specialty focus supports a healthy, productive workforce with not only a quality of work life but also a quality of life.

Explore Community Health Nursing on the Web! To learn more about the topics in this chapter, use the passcode provided to access your exclusive website: **http://nursing.jbpub.com/ communityhealth.** If you do not have a passcode, you can obtain one at this site.

## ■ CRITICAL THINKING ACTIVITIES

1. The next time you go to a fast-food restaurant, observe the potential for occupational hazards in the workers who serve your food. Are there prevention strategies that could prevent those hazards?

2. Ask one of the staff members at your nursing school about workplace hazards in the office. Ask him or her to describe what the most prevalent injury or illness associated with his or her work is. What could be done to prevent this risk?

3. Investigate your nurses association's position on workplace violence in health care. How can nurses protect themselves from this occupational hazard?

# ■ REFERENCES

American Association of Industrial Nurses (AAIN). (1976). *The nurse in industry.* New York: Author.

American Association of Occupational Health Nurses (AAOHN). (2003). *Code of ethics.* Atlanta: Author.

American Association of Occupational Health Nurses (AAOHN). (2004). *Standards of occupational health nursing practice.* Atlanta: Author.

American Association of Occupational Health Nurses (AAOHN). (2007). *Delivery of occupational and environmental health services.* Atlanta: Author.

American Public Health Association. (1996). *The definition and role of public health nursing. A statement of the public health nursing section.* Washington, DC: Author.

Brown, M. L. (1981). *Occupational health nursing.* Philadelphia: Springer.

Bureau of Labor Statistics. (2002). *Survey of occupational injuries and illnesses.* Washington, DC: U.S. Department of Labor.

Bureau of Labor Statistics. (2008). *Current Population Survey.* Washington, DC: U.S. Department of Labor.

Burgel, B. (1993). *Innovations at the worksite: delivery of nurse-managed primary care services.* Washington, DC: American Nurses Association.

Centers for Disease Control and Prevention (CDC), U.S. Department of Health and Human Services (DHHS). (1999). *National Institute for Occupational Safety and Health: National Occupational Research Agenda,* Publication Number 99-108. Atlanta: U.S. Government Printing Office.

Department of Health and Human Services (DHHS). (2000a). *Healthy people 2010: Conference edition.* Washington, DC: U.S. Government Printing Office.

Department of Health and Human Services (DHHS), Public Health Service. (1999). *NHANES III.* Washington, DC: U.S. Government Printing Office.

Felton, J. (1985). The genesis of American occupational health nursing: Part I. *Occupational Health Nursing, 33,* 615–621.

Godfrey, H. (1978, November 30). One hundred years of industrial nursing. *Nursing Times,* pp. 1966–1969.

Kallstrom, T. (2008). Focus on allergies & asthma. *AARC Times, 32*(5), 18–19.

Landels, M. (2002). Day in the life: An occupational health nurse at a nuclear power station. *Nursing Times, 98*(12), 65.

Levy, B., & Wegman, D. (2000). *Occupational health: Recognizing and preventing work-related disease.* Boston: Little, Brown.

McGrath, B. J. (1945). Fifty years of industrial nursing. *Public Health Nurse, 37,* 119–124.

National Center for Farmworker Health. (2008). Migrant and farmworker demographics factsheet. Retrieved November 10, 2008, from http://www.ncfh.org/docs/fs=Migrant%20Demographics.pdf

National Institute for Occupational Safety and Health (NIOSH). (2004). Steps to a healthier US workforce. Retrieved November 10, 2008, from http://www.cdc.gov/niosh/steps/default.html

National Institute for Occupational Safety and Health (NIOSH). (2006). *The team document: Ten years of leadership advancing the National Occupation Research Agenda.* Publication no. 2006-121. Washington, DC: U.S. Government Printing Office.

Nightingale, F. (1869). *Notes on nursing: What it is and what it is not.* New York: Dover Press.

Paul, M. (1997). Occupational reproductive hazards. *Lancet, 349*(9062), 1385–1388.

Rogers, B. (2003). *Occupational health nursing: Concepts and practice.* Philadelphia: W. B. Saunders.

Rogers, B., Agnew, J., & Pompeii, L. (2000). Occupational health nursing research priorities. *AAOHN Journal, 48*(1), 9–16.

Rogers, B., & Cox, A. (1998). Expanding horizons: Integrating environmental health in occupational health nursing. *AAOHN Journal, 46,* 9–13.

Rosner, D., & Markowitz, W. (1999). Labor Day and the war on workers. *American Journal of Public Health, 89*(9), 1319–1321.

Salazar, M., & Kelman, B. (2002). Planning for biological disasters: Occupational nurses as first responders. *AAOHN Journal, 50*(4), 174–181.

Slaney, B. (1984). *The development of occupational health nursing.* Philadelphia: W. B. Saunders.

Sluchak, T. J. (1992). Ergonomics: Origins, focus, and implementation considerations. *AAOHN Journal, 40*(3), 105–112, 147–149.

Soll. (1999). *Survey of occupational injuries and illnesses.* Washington, DC: U.S. Department of Labor, Bureau of Labor Statistics.

Staff TRAK - TB. (1999). *Surveillance for tuberculosis infection in health care workers, 1994 to 1998.* Atlanta, GA: Department of Health and Human Services, Public Health Service, and Centers for Disease Control and Prevention.

Tarlo, S., Balmes, J., Balkissoon, R., Beach, J., Beckett, W., Bernstein, D., et al. (2008). Diagnosis and management of work-related asthma. *CHEST, 134,* 1S–41S.

Winker, R., & Rüdiger, H. (2006). Reproductive toxicology in occupational settings: An update. *International Archives of Occupational & Environmental Health, 79*(1), 1–10.

Wright, F. S. (1919). *Industrial nursing.* New York: Macmillan.

## CHAPTER 42

# Advanced Nursing Practice in the Community

Karen Saucier Lundy and Mary H. Huch

Visit **http://nursing.jbpub.com/communityhealth** for interactive exercises, review questions, Web links, and more.

Life's picture is constantly changing. The spirit beholds a new world every moment.

—Rumi, Persian Sufipoet

Never forget that the most important descriptor of the role of the nurse practitioner is the word "nurse." Your professional home is the profession of nursing. It is nursing that provides you with the historical, philosophical, structure, missions and a social mandate for your practice, education, research and leadership.

Nurse practitioners have become embedded in every aspect of health care. In a great sense, nurse practitioners have transformed the profession of nursing.

—*Loretta Ford, EdD, FAAN, co-founder, Nurse Practitioner Education and Practice,*
*University of Colorado School of Nursing, July 23, 2005*

For over four decades, advanced practice nurses have delivered competent, cost-effective health care, serving their patients in settings ranging from rural areas and prisons to schools, homes, and international settings. What is your experience with advanced practice nursing? Have you personally received care from a nurse practitioner? Why or why not?

## CHAPTER FOCUS

**Advanced Practice Defined**

**Historical Development of Advanced Practice Roles**
- Certified Registered Nurse Anesthetists
- Certified Nurse Midwives
- Clinical Nurse Specialists
- Nurse Practitioners

**Education Issues and Scope of Practice**
- Certified Registered Nurse Anesthetists
- Certified Nurse Midwives
- Clinical Nurse Specialists
- Nurse Practitioners

*Healthy People 2010*

**Credentials**

**Reimbursement**
- Medicare
- Medicaid
- Private Insurance

**Role Differentiation**

**Practice Arenas**
- Acute Care Settings
- Clinics
- Long-Term Care Facilities
- Educational Institutions

**Innovations in Healthcare Delivery in the Community**
- Nursing Centers
- Case Management
- Holistic Practice

## QUESTIONS TO CONSIDER

After reading this chapter, you will know the answers to the following questions:

1. What is advanced practice nursing?
2. What are the different roles for advanced practice nurses?
3. How have advanced practice roles developed?
4. What are the practice settings for advanced practice nurses?
5. How are advanced practice nurses reimbursed for their services?
6. What are future trends in community advanced practice nursing?

## KEY TERMS

Advanced practice nurse
Certification
Certified nurse midwives

Certified registered nurse anesthetists
Clinical nurse specialists

Clinical nurse leader (CNL)
Doctorate of Nursing Practice (DNP)

Nurse practitioners
Primary care

THE SPECIFIC ROLE ACTIVITIES of advanced practice nurses are highly diverse, and role expansion is likely to continue well into the twenty-first century. New practice settings are emerging daily. These new practice arenas are continually being developed to meet health needs rather than just illness needs. Many people are looking for ways to stay healthy. People want to take control of their lives and health outcomes. The advanced practice nurse roles discussed in this chapter explore the ways these nurses contribute to the health and well-being of many individuals. The advanced practice nurses of the twenty-first century will be hindered only by their own reluctance to think in creative, innovative ways.

### ENVIRONMENTAL CONNECTION

The professional nursing environment was initially skeptical and resistant when the nurse practitioner (NP) movement began in 1965. Physicians were equally resistant to the role, which they deemed competitive and an attempt to "practice medicine" as "mini-docs."

By carefully collecting evaluation data early on, Drs. Ford and Silva, founders of the NP program at the University of Colorado, were able to demonstrate the cost-effectiveness and quality of NPs. With a strong emphasis on primary care, NPs focus on health maintenance, disease prevention, counseling, and patient education. They strive to empower patients to improve their health by providing education and counseling, focusing on prevention and self-care.

## Advanced Practice Defined

The term *advanced practice* has been in the nursing literature for many years. In simplest terms, the **advanced practice nurse** is one whose preparation includes education and experience beyond the entry level for nursing practice.

The categories of providers included under the advanced practice umbrella have changed considerably since the term was first used. Originally, nurse anesthetists and nurse midwives were the only practitioners considered advanced practice nurses. Both specialties were well accepted and commonplace within the nursing profession in the early to mid-twentieth century. It was not until the 1960s that the roles of the clinical nurse specialist and nurse practitioner were described in the nursing literature.

Advanced nursing practice is broadly defined by the American Association of Colleges of Nurses (AACN, 2004) as "any form of nursing intervention that influences health care outcomes for individuals or populations, including the direct care of individual patients, management of care for individuals and populations, administration of nursing and health care organizations, and the development and implementation of health policy."

In 2004, the AACN voted to move advanced practice nurse preparation from the master's level to the doctoral level—doctorate of nursing practice (DNP)—by 2015. This new AACN policy will make the DNP the standard for APN

education (AACN, 2004). The AACN DNP position statement calls for a transformational change in the education required for professional nurses who will practice at the most advanced level of nursing. The recommendation that nurses practicing at the highest level should receive doctoral level preparation emerged from multiple contributing factors, including the expansion of scientific knowledge required for safe nursing practice and recent concerns regarding the quality of patient care delivery and outcomes (Loomis, 2007; Lenz, 2005; Dracup et al., 2005). Nurses currently practicing in advanced practice nurse roles without the DNP may choose to enroll in post-master's DNP programs or practice within current state licensure and national certification standards according to those requirements (AACN, 2004, 2005, 2006; Loomis et al., 2007). Because of these revolutionary changes in the advanced practice nurse role, student nurses are encouraged to seek information about educational and licensure requirements about the future ANP role as they become available (Loomis, 2007; Lenz, 2005; Fitzpatrick & Marecki, 2007). An excellent resource for these changes can be found at the AACN Web site: www.aacn.nche.edu.

Presently, four categories of nurse providers are considered advanced practice nurses: **certified registered nurse anesthetists, certified nurse midwives, clinical nurse specialists,** and **nurse practitioners.** Although all four of these groups are included as advanced practice nurses, the specific practice focus for each group is quite different (AACN, 2004; O'Grady, 2004; Huch, 1995). See Box 42-1 for definitions of the four advanced practice nurse roles.

### NOTE THIS!

**Clinical Nurse Leader: An Emerging New Role in Health Care**

A new emerging role in nursing is that of the **clinical nurse leader (CNL)**. The CNL is considered an advanced generalist role, but does not meet the criteria set forth by the AACN for advanced practice nursing scope of practice. The CNL is a leader in the healthcare delivery system across all settings in which health care is delivered, including the community setting. The implementation of the CNL role, however, will vary across settings. The CNL role is not one of administration or management. The CNL functions in the healthcare system as a generalist and assumes accountability for healthcare outcomes for a specific group of patients in a setting through the assimilation and application of research-based information to design, implement, and evaluate patient plans of care. The CNL is a provider and a manager of care at the point of care to individuals and populations. The CNL designs, implements, and evaluates patient care by coordinating, delegating, and supervising the care provided by the healthcare team, including licensed nurses, technicians, and other health professionals. The CNL provides and manages care at the point of care to individuals, clinical populations, and communities.

*Source*: American Association of Colleges of Nursing. (2007). *White paper on the education and role of the clinical nurse leader*. Washington, DC: Author.

The following Application to Practice features examples of the range of activities undertaken by advanced practice nurses.

## BOX 42-1

### Definitions of Advanced Practice Nursing Roles

A *nurse anesthetist* is a registered nurse who completed a program of instruction for managing and sustaining life processes of a patient while he or she is anesthetized during surgery.

A *nurse midwife* is a registered nurse who is educated to care for women during pregnancy, delivery, and afterward for issues related to women's health care. The newborn infant is also cared for by the nurse midwife.

A *clinical nurse specialist* is a registered nurse who has advanced educational preparation with study in a specialized area of clinical nursing.

A *nurse practitioner* is a registered nurse who has advanced educational preparation in the diagnosing, treating, and prescribing of medical and health therapies for disease processes.

## BOX 42-2

### Consensus Model for APRN Regulation: Licensure, Accreditation, Certification, and Education: The Future of Advanced Practice Nurses in the United States

This document was endorsed in 2008 by the American Nurses Association and more than 20 other professional nurse organizations representing advanced practice nursing education, licensure, and practice as a landmark "future-oriented" model that streamlines and standardizes the education and regulatory processes involved in advanced practice nursing (APRN). The model further promotes the position that all advanced practice nurses nationwide should function independently. The model was developed and approved through a consensus of representatives from all major professional organizations in the United States for advanced practice. The groundbreaking, visionary document defines APRN roles, practice and populations served, regulatory, educational, and certification issues, APRN titles, and strategies for implementation. Under the consensus model, future APRNs would have to meet certain standardized educational requirements and would be educated in one of the four currently recognized roles: nurse practitioner, clinical nurse specialist, nurse-midwife, or nurse anesthetist. These APRNs would also be educated in one of the following defined population areas: family-individual across the lifespan, adult-gerontology, women's health/gender-related, neonatal, pediatrics, or psychiatric-mental health. Specialization is optional and would be completed after the core APRN curriculum, built on the role and population focused competencies. Legislative changes include a separate license for all APRNs, with licensure being the highest regulatory standard. The new model, once fully implemented, would provide APRNs flexibility in moving from state to state with standardized regulatory practice statutes and legislative policies. Current APRNs will not be required to go back and complete additional coursework, provided they meet professional state licensure and certification requirements for their current practice, retaining their present roles in the healthcare system.

*Source*: APRN Consensus Work Group & the National Council of State Boards of Nursing APRN Advisory Committee. Consensus model for APRN regulation: Licensure, accreditation, certification, and education (2008). *The American Nurse, 40*(4), 1–8.

### Application to Practice

Ms. Jones is a 51-year-old woman who comes to a primary care clinic for the first time because she has experienced "hot flashes" and "night sweats" for the past 2 weeks. As her primary care provider, the nurse practitioner elicits a detailed history of what has occurred. The symptoms are extensively explored, along with menstrual history, methods of birth control used, medications taken, and a complete health history. When comprehensive data are obtained, the nurse practitioner does a complete physical examination, including a pelvic examination. Various diagnostic tests are done, such as follicle-stimulating hormone (FSH) and luteinizing hormone (LH) levels, blood chemistries, a lipid profile, liver function studies, and a Pap smear.

Once the nurse practitioner has all of the necessary information, a return appointment with Ms. Jones is scheduled. During the next visit, the nurse practitioner explores what options are available to handle the annoying "hot flashes" and "night sweats" Ms. Jones is continuing to experience. The benefits and risks of hormone replacement therapy are thoroughly discussed with Ms. Jones to assist her in making a decision about beginning hormone replacement therapy. Other health-promotion measures such as a regular mammogram and monthly breast self-examination are also included in the discussion. Daily calcium carbonate supplementation along with regular exercise are prescribed for Ms. Jones. If Ms. Jones is a smoker, this is a good time for her to consider stopping. If Ms. Jones desires it, alternative therapies for dealing with the symptoms are also explored. If the FSH and LH levels are not indicative of the presence of menopause, counseling her on the use of birth control methods is important because pregnancy can occur if she is sexually active. A follow-up visit to the nurse practitioner in 1 to 2 months is scheduled to determine whether the planned therapies are effective in treating Ms. Jones's symptoms.

---

**BOX 42-3**

**Fast Facts About the Doctorate of Nursing Practice (DNP)**

- The practice doctorate (DNP) will be the educational requirement for advanced nursing practice preparation, including but not limited to the four current advanced practice nursing (APN) roles: clinical nurse specialist, nurse anesthetist, nurse midwife, and nurse practitioner.
- Most DNP programs of study will be 3 calendar years, or 36 months of full-time study including summers or 4 years on a traditional academic calendar.
- Post-master's programs are anticipated based on the DNP candidate's prior education, experience, and choice of specialization and may be shorter in duration.
- Preparation for specialization as an advanced practice nurse will occur at the doctoral level by 2015.
- Practice-focused doctoral programs will be accredited by a nursing accrediting agency recognized by the U.S. Secretary of Education (i.e., the Commission on Collegiate Nursing Education [CCNE] or the National League for Nursing Accrediting Commission).

*Sources:* American Association of Colleges of Nursing. (2004). AACN position statement on the practice doctorate in nursing. Retrieved July 24, 2008, from http://www.aacn.nche.edu/DNP/pdf/DNP.pdf; American Association of Colleges of Nursing. (2005). Frequently asked questions concerning the AACN position statement on the practice doctorate in nursing. Retrieved July 24, 2008, from http://www.aacn.nche.edu/DNP/AboutDNP.htm; American Association of Colleges of Nursing. (2006). *AACN essentials of doctoral education for advanced nursing practice.* Retrieved July 24, 2008, from http://www.aacn.nche.edu/DNP/pdf/Essentials5-06.pdf.

## Historical Development of Advanced Practice Roles

The roles of advanced practice nurses are always changing. Examining each group of providers from a historical perspective provides a clearer understanding of the distinct roles and leads to an exploration of the usual work settings.

### ■ Certified Registered Nurse Anesthetists

The nurse anesthetist is one who, with advanced education, is responsible for keeping a patient insensible to pain while maintaining vital functions during surgery. Nurses have long been involved in administering anesthesia in hospitals and outpatient surgery centers. As early as 1877, nurses administered anesthesia at St. Vincent's Hospital in Erie, Pennsylvania (Garde, 1996; Thatcher, 1984).

### ■ Certified Nurse Midwives

Mary Breckinridge, a British-trained nurse midwife, recognized the need for well-prepared midwives in rural Appalachia. She established the Frontier Nursing Service in 1925 and used British-trained nurse midwives because so few American nurse midwives were available. Traveling by horseback, these nurses helped with births and provided care for all women and babies in their assigned districts (Burkhardt, 1996; Frontier Nursing Service, 2008). From these humble

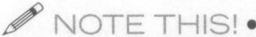 **NOTE THIS!**

**Community Clinical Nurse Specialist: A View from the Field**

Dr. Smyth is a community clinical nurse specialist with an interest in geriatrics. He contracted with a retirement center to visit twice a week to address the health issues of the residents. Some of his activities include providing instructions on various medications the residents take, giving nutritional guidance to provide for an optimal diet, developing individualized exercise programs, and counseling patients about matters of concern. Besides the individualized information provided, he assesses the community to determine whether problems currently exist or whether there is the potential for the development of problems. The community health clinical nurse specialist's mission is to promote the health of the community. A proactive stance is taken rather than waiting for problems to occur.

---

beginnings, certified nurse midwives made a significant impact on reducing infant and maternal mortality.

In 1995, the American College of Nurse-Midwives (ACNM) was formed to meet the professional needs of nurse midwives. This group began to focus on the care of normal newborns and women (Burkhardt, 1996). Many contemporary nurse midwives practice in neighborhood health centers in urban and rural areas to provide total health care for women of all ages (Avery & Howe, 2007; Dorroh & Norton, 1996).

The American Association of Colleges of Nursing published a policy statement calling for the requirement of the doctor of nursing practice for entry into practice as an advanced practice nurse by the year 2015. Certified nurse midwives, defined as those educated in both nursing and midwifery, are commonly included in the definition of advanced practice nurses (Avery & Howe, 2007).

### ■ Clinical Nurse Specialists

In the late 1960s, the nursing literature included many articles about clinical nurse specialists and nurse clinicians. About this time, nurses began to enroll in greater numbers in graduate programs of study and to focus on a particular area of practice (Georgopoulos & Christman, 1970; Reiter,

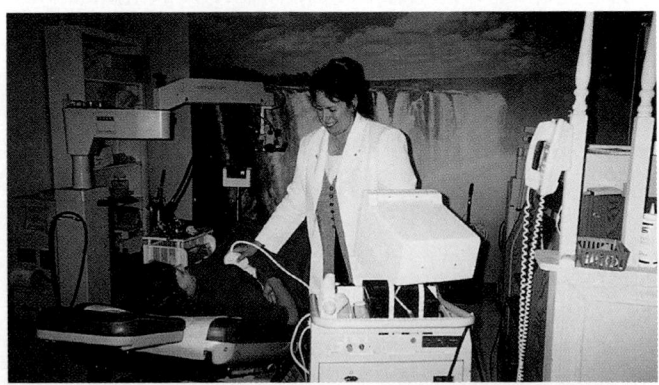

A family nurse practitioner conducting a sonogram of a prenatal patient.

1966). It was shortly thereafter that the American Nurses Association provided a definition of the clinical nurse specialist, stating that the nurse possessed a master's degree and an area of clinical concentration (ANA, 1976).

For many years, acute care settings provided the primary area for employment of most clinical specialists. An exception to this acute care focus was the psychiatric clinical nurse specialist (Boyle, 1996; England, 2008; Schroeder, 2008). Within the acute care setting, the clinical specialist had a medical–surgical nursing focus, whereas the psychiatric clinical nurse specialist functioned in both inpatient and outpatient settings. Over time, the role of clinical nurse specialists has changed, and today they can be found in a wider variety of places: acute care settings (general units and intensive care units), rehabilitation centers, home health care, schools, and community settings (AACN, 2007; Daly & Mitchell, 1996; Good, 1992; Shapiro, 2007).

The community health clinical nurse specialist has a focus on the community as a whole rather than the individuals who constitute the community. This nurse tries to ascertain which individuals are in the high-risk populations. These activities are accomplished from the perspective of the entire community. The steps of the nursing process are used in promoting, maintaining, protecting, and restoring health of the populace. In addition, efforts are directed toward disease and disability prevention (Association of Community Health Nursing Educators, 1991).

Recent changes in the advanced practice nurse role, as indicated in a previous section, will move the educational requirements for all clinical specialists to the DNP degree level (AACN, 2004, 2005, 2006). Clinical specialists in community health nursing without the DNP *may* continue to practice in this role, depending on specific professional and state requirements. Students are encouraged to seek additional current information from professional specialty nursing organizations about present and future regulatory policies and issues concerning the CNS in community and public health.

### ■ Nurse Practitioners

In the 1960s, nurse faculty member Loretta Ford, EdD, RN, from the University of Colorado School of Nursing, and Henry Silver, MD, from the University of Colorado School of Medicine, developed a post-baccalaureate pediatric nurse practitioner program at the University of Colorado. The faculty was intimately involved in evaluating nurses in this expanded role (Ford & Silver, 1967).These early nurse practitioners were taught new skills, such as using an otoscope and doing urinalysis, that today have become common activities for all nurses. A 20-month period of clinical training followed an intense 4-month period of classroom instruction. One important component of the nurse practitioner's education was the development of the ability to decide when the situation was beyond his or her scope of practice and to make the appropriate referral (see the "A Conversation With" box on page 1073).

From these origins, various other nurse practitioner programs have been instituted throughout the United States. Many early programs awarded a certificate at the completion of a course of study that varied from a few weeks to as long as 2 years. As the role of nurse practitioner gained greater acceptance, more programs were offered at the master's level. By the late 1990s, it was necessary to have a master's degree to take most nurse practitioners certification examinations.

Recent changes in the advanced practice nurse role, as indicated in a previous section, will move the educational requirements for all nurse practitioners to the DNP degree level (AACN, 2004, 2005, 2006). Nurse practitioners without the DNP *may* continue to practice in this role, depending on specific professional and state requirements. Students are encouraged to seek additional current information from professional specialty nursing organizations about present and future regulatory policies and issues concerning the nurse practitioner role and practice requirements.

 **ETHICAL CONNECTION**

A patient refers to a nurse practitioner who has an MSN as "Doctor." How should the nurse practitioner respond to the patient's salutation?

 **Research Alert**

This research explored advanced practice nurses' perceptions on wireless personal digital assistant (PDA) technologies in their role. The wireless PDA is becoming established as a hand-held computing tool for healthcare professionals. A qualitative design was used to explore advanced practice nurses' perceptions on the value of wireless PDA technologies to support their practice. The data were collected using survey questionnaires and individual and focus group interviews with nurse practitioners, clinical nurse specialists, and information technology managers based in British Columbia, Canada. An open-coding content analysis was performed using qualitative data analysis software. Researchers found that wireless PDA use supports the principles of pervasitivity and is a technology rapidly being adopted by advanced practice nurses. Some nurses indicated a reluctance to integrate wireless PDA technologies into their practices because of the cost and the short technological life cycle of these devices. Many of the barriers that precluded the use of wireless networks within facilities are being removed. Nurses demonstrated a complex understanding of wireless PDA technologies and gave good rationales for their integration into practice. Nurses identified improved patient care as the major benefit of this type and range of tools they can use to this end.

*Source*: Garrett, B., & Klein, G. (2008). Value of wireless personal digital assistants for practice: Perceptions of advanced practice nurses. *Journal of Clinical Nursing, 17*(16), 2146–2154.

## Education Issues and Scope of Practice

Although there are some similarities in educational preparation, the scope of practice for each role is different. Each of these advanced practice nurses functions in a different way when providing care for patients.

### ■ Certified Registered Nurse Anesthetists

Although this group of providers is included under the title of advanced practice nurses, they do not ordinarily practice in a community setting. Information related to education and scope of practice can be obtained from the American Association of Nurse Anesthetists.

### ■ Certified Nurse Midwives

Pathways to becoming a midwife are quite varied. Some programs are available for non-nurses who take the national examination and then become certified midwives. These individuals include physicians' assistants, family physicians, and other non-nurse learners (Burkhardt, 1996; Avery & Howe, 2007). Three types of programs are available to registered nurses who want to become certified nurse midwives. An education outcome can be a precertification, certificate (requires a bachelor's degree), or graduate program. Graduates of these nursing programs are eligible to sit for the certification examination of the ACNM, and the graduates are identified as certified nurse midwives.

The ACNM has been active in setting guidelines for directing the practice of all midwives. Midwives care for women during the antenatal, intrapartal, and postpartal periods and also care for their newborns after delivery. Midwives play a large part in family planning and gynecological care.

Whatever the educational background, certified nurse midwives are an essential force in providing better outcomes for pregnant women and their infants. Because of the focus

---

### 💻 Research Alert

This article is an excellent review for advanced practice nurses in pandemic influenza planning and response. Recent public health emergencies have brought to light the need for APNs to become educated regarding disaster emergency planning and response. Key epidemiological terms and pandemic alert designations are reviewed. Influenza surveillance activities at the local, state, and national levels are summarized. Responsibilities of the APN are discussed, and resources are provided. Current research and practice guidelines from the U.S. Department of Health and Human Services (USDHHS) Pandemic Influenza Plan, state pandemic influenza plans, U.S. Centers for Disease Control and Prevention, and the World Health Organization are included. ◯

*Source*: Hoffman, D., & Nannini, A. (2008). Planning, surveillance, and reporting for pandemic influenza: A briefing for advanced practice nurses. *Journal of the American Academy of Nurse Practitioners, 20*(1), 11–16.

---

> ❝*I look to the day when there are no nurses to the sick but only nurses to the well.*❞
>
> —*Florence Nightingale*

on preventive care, nurse-midwifery practice has resulted in lower rates of infant mortality (ACNM, 2005; Dorroh & Norton, 1996).

The American Association of Colleges of Nursing has endorsed the DNP as the requirement for entry into practice as a certified nurse midwife and advanced practice nurse (APN) by the year 2015. These changes are new, and educational programs are emerging to accommodate advanced degrees for the certified nurse midwife. Practice and licensure issues for the certified nurse midwife are specific to state and institutional requirements and students should seek information about these changes in order to remain current about this important role in maternal and infant health (Avery & Howe, 2007).

### ■ Clinical Nurse Specialists

The clinical nurse specialist evolved to meet the ever-changing demands of specialized population needs in the healthcare system. The clinical nurse specialist has traditionally been a nurse with a master's degree in an advanced clinical area. As an advanced practice nurse, clinical nurse specialists in the future will be educated at the doctoral level (AACN, 2004).

Nurse educators were responsive to this role and supported it from its inception. The strong focus on providing patient care lent credibility to the usefulness of this role. The 1964 Nurse Training Act provided financial support for nurses wishing to become clinical nurse specialists. Receiving financial support made it easier for a nurse to return to school for a master's degree. The funding also provided tuition and a monthly stipend to assist with living expenses (Hamric, 1989).

Beyond advanced study of a clinical practice area, the clinical nurse specialist curriculum focuses on specific competencies to be acquired for future practice. These competencies include being an expert practitioner, educator, consultant, and researcher. The clinical nurse specialist uses these competencies to improve the quality of life of the patient or community (Hamric, Spross, & Hanson, 1996; Robertson & Baldwin, 2007).

Clinical nurse specialists can be found in many practice arenas. As an expert practitioner, the clinical nurse specialist provides critical thinking, expert decision making, a high level of clinical judgment, and skill in determining care for selected patients or populations.

The community health clinical nurse specialist provides instruction for staff, consumers, and the community because education is at the forefront of clinical activities for this practitioner. Staff instruction can occur in planned or informal settings. When an unexpected teaching situation arises, the clinical nurse specialist acts to provide needed information

### Got an Alternative?

Advanced practice nurses are much more likely to prescribe and advise patients about complementary and alternative interventions than are physicians. Patients are also more likely to share their use of these interventions with advanced practice nurses. Why do you think this is true?

 NOTE THIS!

There are more than 240,500 RNs in the United States currently prepared to practice as advanced practice registered nurses (APRNs). The largest group of APRNs are nurse practitioners (NPs) at just over 140,000, followed by clinical nurse specialists (CNSs), nurse anesthetists (CRNAs), and nurse midwives (CNMs).

*Source:* U.S. Department of Health and Human Services, Health Resources Administration. (2006). *2004 national sample survey of registered nurses.* Washington, DC: Author.

for the staff or care recipient. The clinical nurse specialist may meet the learning needs of consumers by providing information on newly available therapies or means to improve the health of a community (Jordan, 2008; Kupina, 1995).

As a consultant, the clinical nurse specialist is called on to share expert knowledge with other professionals who are possibly from a complementary discipline. In this role, the clinical nurse specialist must not only provide information and possible recommendations for action, but should also help the other professionals develop their own problem-solving skills (Davis, 2007; Menard, 1987).

The role of the researcher involves a range of activities. Because of educational preparation, the clinical nurse specialist should have the academic preparation to apply research to practice in the public health fields (Robertson & Baldwin, 2007).

Clinical nurse specialists can be found in many practice sites. Healthcare settings employ clinical nurse specialists to provide the in-depth knowledge base needed for complex patient care. Both children and adults are the recipients of this specialized knowledge base. As with other areas in nursing practice, the clinical nurse specialist is becoming even more specialized. The clinical nurse specialist is now an integral part of many critical care units. The role of the psychiatric specialist has moved beyond the traditional inpatient and outpatient settings into the home (Broom et al., 2008; Delaney, 2008; Ward-Miller, 1996).

One of the most positive aspects of this movement is that the nurse can see patients in their own environment. Community health clinical specialists have the unique ability to merge nursing practice and public health to affect the health of the community. Another vital activity of the clinical nurse specialist in the community is functioning as a case manager (Daly & Mitchell, 1996; Good, 1992; Robertson & Baldwin, 2007).

These advanced practice nurses can be found in some private and joint practices with physicians. The community health clinical specialist has much to offer in implementing a community-based model of care. Independent practice is an area in which the community health clinical specialist can be of value. The community health clinical nurse specialist will play a vital role in the public's health as we continue in the twenty-first century.

### ■ Nurse Practitioners

As with most of the other advanced practice nurses, educational pathways have been variable for nurse practitioners. The first educational programs occurred out of the mainstream of higher educational institutions. Rogers (1972) was an outspoken critic of nurse practitioner programs, insisting they were not nursing practice, but medical practice. Other nursing leaders at the time held a similar viewpoint. Often, in these early programs, graduates received a certificate upon completion of their studies even when instruction took place within a university setting (Huch, 1992; Meleis & Dracup, 2005).

It was during the 1970s that concerted efforts were made to establish standards for the education of nurse practitioners. The National League for Nursing took the lead and stated that a nurse practitioner should have a master's degree as the outcome of the educational program. The National Organization of Nurse Practitioner Faculties (NONPF) has established accreditation criteria for nurse practitioner educational programs (NONPF, 1997). By the late 1990s, almost all education programs for nurse practitioners were in higher education settings, with a master's degree awarded upon completion of the program.

As an advanced practice nurse, the nurse practitioner of the future will be educated at the doctoral level (AACN, 2004, 2005). While most nurse practitioners in the community setting are family nurse practitioners (FNPs), specialties continue to emerge in order to meet the primary healthcare needs of the population.

As with the first practitioners, the **primary care** setting is where the greatest abundance of practitioners can be found. Primary care is any setting that accords the first entry into the healthcare system. Practice sites include pediatric, adult health, geriatric, obstetrical/gynecological, and family care clinics (Hawkins & Thibodeau, 1996).

A more recent trend is the development of acute care nurse practitioners. The number of medical residents available to provide care in the acute care setting was declining; thus, a need for another caregiver was created. To meet the need, many universities began acute care nurse practitioner programs. The goal for this practitioner, as with other nurse practitioners, is to provide high-quality, cost-effective care and to do so from a nursing perspective (Cheng & Chen, 2008; Magill, 2007; Hoffman & Nanning, 2008).

Within these various settings, nurse practitioners assist patients in managing illness through diagnosis and pharmacological and nonpharmacological means, providing health-promotion teaching, and counseling. Nurse practitioners in

GLOBAL CONNECTION

Advanced roles in nursing often have different educational and training requirements in other countries, as well as different responsibilities. Prior to accepting an international position, an advanced practice nurse should explore all legal and institutional policies regarding licensure and educational requirements for that country and institution.

all states have some measure of prescriptive authority, but the extent of that authority is quite variable (Berry & Dahl, 2007). Some states allow the nurse practitioner to legally prescribe any drug without requiring a collaborative physician. Some states limit nurse practitioners to writing prescriptions only for noncontrolled drugs, but still without requiring a collaborating physician. Yet other states require a physician's signature along with the nurse's for both noncontrolled and controlled substances.

Each state's nurse practice act regulates the specific scope of practice for this subgroup of advanced practice nurses. The rules and regulations of the state board of nursing further delineate the legal activities for the nurse. Nurse practitioners should consult the legal statutes for the states in which they plan to practice.

## Healthy People 2010

The objectives of *Healthy People 2010* provide a blueprint for the practice of community health clinical specialists and primary care nurse practitioners into the twenty-first century and beyond. The following box lists a sample of *Healthy People 2010* objectives that community health clinical nurse specialists and nurse practitioners can use.

## Credentials

Credentialing is the process of obtaining a certificate or diploma attesting to a predetermined fact. Most advanced practice nurses are required to have certification showing that a minimal competency level has been achieved. The **certification** process involves the submission of evidence of completion of a program of study, verification of a minimum number of clinical practice hours, the application for the certification examination, and documentation of a current registered nurse license (Chornick, 2008).

The American Association of Nurse Anesthetists Council on Certification of Nurse Anesthetists is the certifying body for nurse anesthetists. The Division of Accreditation that accredits educational programs of the ACNM oversees nurse-midwifery educational programs. The ACNM Certification Council administers the national certification examination. The Certification Council also administers an examination to non-nurse midwives, although they are designated as clinical midwives rather than clinical nurse midwives.

The American Nurses Credentialing Center (ANCC) administers many certification examinations to clinical specialists and nurse practitioners. For a nurse to be eligible for one of these examinations, specific clinical preparation in

---

### HEALTHY PEOPLE 2010

**Sample Objectives to Be Used by Nurse Practitioners and Community Health Clinical Nurse Specialists**

#### Access to Quality Health Services

*Primary Care*

1.4    Increase the proportion of persons who have a specific source of ongoing care.

1.5    Increase the proportion of persons with a usual primary care provider.

#### Arthritis, Osteoporosis, and Chronic Back Conditions

2.7    Increase the proportion of adults who have seen a health care provider for their chronic joint symptoms.

#### Cancer

3.11    Increase the proportion of women who receive a Pap test.

3.12    Increase the proportion of adults who receive a colorectal cancer screening examination.

#### Diabetes

5.4    Increase the proportion of adults with diabetes whose condition has been diagnosed.

5.14    Increase the proportion of adults with diabetes who have at least an annual foot examination.

#### Immunization and Infectious Diseases

*Infectious Diseases and Emerging Antimicrobial Resistance*

14.12    Increase the proportion of all tuberculosis patients who complete curative therapy within 12 months.

14.18    Reduce the number of courses of antibiotics for ear infections for young children.

#### Maternal, Infant, and Child

*Prenatal Care*

16.6    Increase the proportion of pregnant women who receive early and adequate prenatal care.

*Risk Factors*

16.10    Reduce low birth weight (LBW) and very low birth weight (VLBW).

16.11    Reduce preterm births.

#### Mental Health and Mental Disorders

*Treatment Expansion*

18.6    Increase the number of persons seen in primary care who receive mental health screening and assessment.

*Source:* DHHS, 2000.

the examination area is needed. Applicants can be certified in more than one area if they meet the educational and practice requirements of the examination. Most states require that nurse practitioners be certified before recognizing them as advanced practice nurses with prescribing privileges.

A nurse practitioner can be certified in more than one area through ANCC, but it is also possible to be certified by a different group. The American Academy of Nurse Practitioners administers a national certifying examination for adult and family nurse practitioners. Individual state boards of nursing make the determination of which certifying examination will be recognized.

The National Association of Pediatric Nurse Associates and Nurse Practitioners (NAPNAP) provides the certification mechanism for pediatric nurse practitioners. Similar requirements described for the other groups hold for this application process.

The National Certification Corporation (NCC) offers certification in women's health (OB/GYN) and neonatal nursing. This group reviews course content, clinical experiences, and learning activities to decide whether a nurse is qualified to take the examination.

## Reimbursement

### ■ Medicare

Medicare is the U.S. federally funded health insurance program for elders and persons with disabilities. Advanced practice nurses should be adequately compensated for the care they provide, but federal law regulates who can be compensated and in what amount (Lancaster & Lancaster, 1993). Safriet (1992) advanced the position that advanced practice nurses should be adequately compensated for their services, and until this is done, there will be a barrier to effective use of advanced practice nurses.

The Rural Nursing Incentive Act of 1991 provided funds for direct reimbursement of nurse practitioners and clinical nurse specialists practicing in rural areas. The Omnibus Budget Reconciliation Act (OBRA) made provision for indirect reimbursement to nurse practitioners and clinical nurse specialists. With indirect reimbursement, a physician must also have been involved in the care of the patient for payment of funds to occur. Legislative appropriation of these reimbursement funds led to an increase in the number of nurse practitioner positions.

The Balanced Budget Act of 1997 (Section 4511) brought about a major change in Medicare reimbursement practices. Nurse practitioners and clinical nurse specialists were eligible

for direct reimbursement for services without regard for the setting of the practice. The intent of the law was to provide cost-effective, quality care to all U.S. citizens.

### ■ Medicaid

Medicaid programs are joint federal and state efforts to provide for the healthcare needs of low-income persons of an individual state. The federal government provides matching funds to each state, but the state is the body that sets specific guidelines for its program. Benefits offered through Medicaid are highly variable depending on the state. Advanced practice nurses are eligible to receive reimbursement based on individual state statutes.

Likewise, certified registered nurse anesthetists and certified nurse midwives can file applications for reimbursement to the appropriate funding source. It is important that all states enact legislation to provide for nondiscrimination of healthcare providers when performing services within their scope of practice (Safriet, 1992).

### ■ Private Insurance

Guidelines for reimbursement for advanced practice nurses are highly variable due to the many private insurance plans in existence in the United States. The plans sometimes include the nurse provider in the preferred provider network, but other times, the advanced practice nurse is viewed as outside the network; generally less coverage is then afforded for the nurse's services. This places an undue burden on those with minimal resources. More and more networks are seeking to include nurse practitioners among their credentialed providers (Kremer & Faut-Callahan, 1998; O'Grady, 2004).

Of particular concern when discussing reimbursement issues is the fact that advanced practice nurses often receive less payment than a physician when the same service is provided. Advanced practice nurses have been shown to provide

---

✎ NOTE THIS! •————————————————

The nurse practitioner movement started at the University of Colorado Medical Center in 1965 as a collaborative effort between Dr. Loretta Ford and Dr. Henry Silver, primarily as a response to a shortage of primary care physicians in rural areas. ◉

---

■■ **CULTURAL CONNECTION**

**The Advanced Practice Nurse Role in Great Britain and Australia**

Davis explores the role and practice from current research about the different aspects of advanced nursing practice and nurse practitioners in Great Britain. The author further presents current role confusion of advanced nursing practice and future trends. Davis also cited the discourse analysis of the introduction of nurse practitioners in rural and remote Australia.

What are possible cultural differences in Great Britain and Australia that may affect the public and professional acceptance of the advanced practice nurse as compared to the United States?

*Source:* Davis, K. (2007). Advanced nursing practice and nurse practitioners. *Primary Health Care, 17*(7), 31.

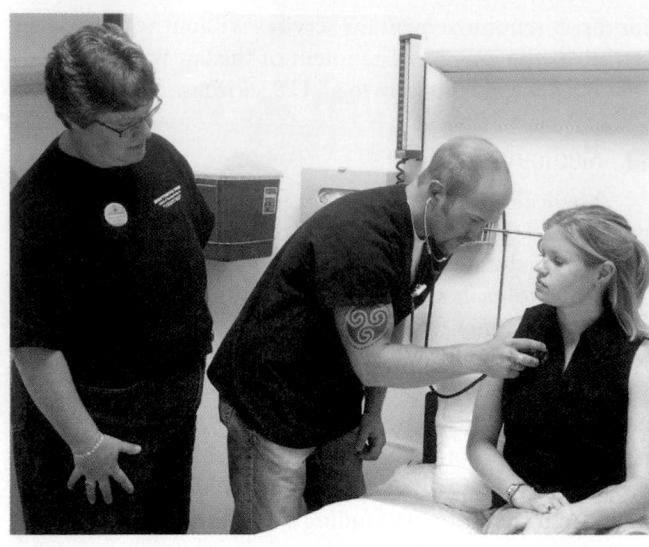

Advanced practice nurses often specialize in such areas as women's health. Women are more likely than men to share health concerns with each other.

high-quality care that is equivalent to that provided by physicians. Therefore, advanced practice nurses should be paid an equitable fee for services. Efforts of organized nursing must continue to be directed toward correcting these inequities (O'Grady, 2004; Safriet, 1992).

## Role Differentiation

The specific role functions of clinical nurse specialists and nurse practitioners are somewhat blurred, as these roles continue to evolve within the healthcare arena (Boyer, 1996). Nurse practitioners originally practiced in primary care settings in the community, and clinical nurse specialists provided services within an acute care setting. An exception to this pattern was the community health clinical specialist who had a focus on individuals, families, and groups within the community. This healthcare provider was positioned to be a leader in meeting public health needs.

Because of declining revenues within the higher education setting, administrators are examining ways of consolidating programs for greater cost-effectiveness. Although advanced practice nurses are moving into a greater variety of practice settings, research is showing that there are many similarities between the roles of nurse practitioners and clinical specialists (Elder & Bullough, 1990; Fenton & Brykczynski, 1993; Forbes, Rafson, Spross, & Kozlowski, 1990; Hunsberger et al., 1992; Schroer, 1991; Sheehy & McCarthy, 1998; AACN, 2006).

There are some marked benefits and liabilities to the merger of these roles. By merging the titles, the number of advanced practice nurses under one title would increase considerably (Schroer, 1991). The clinical nurse specialists could potentially increase their scope of practice to include prescriptive privileges and, therefore, benefit from direct re-

imbursement from third-party payers (Page & Arena, 1994). One liability of a combined role is the need to lengthen programs of study to provide enough time to truly develop the new role. Given that so many graduate students attend class part-time because of job and family commitments, it seems this would be a major burden on these students. Time will tell whether this role merging will continue or whether there will be a clearer delineation of the roles.

**❝** *Life's pictures are constantly undergoing change. The sprit beholds a new world every moment.* **❞**

—Rumi, Persian Sufi poet

## Practice Arenas

### ■ Acute Care Settings

All four types of advanced practice nurses can be found in acute care settings. In each instance, the nurse has specialized education and experience to fulfill the roles. As an expert practitioner, the clinical nurse specialist may be found on a general hospital unit such as neurology, oncology, or pediatrics. Often, the clinical nurse specialist will become even more specialized and practice only in a neonatal intensive care unit or a specialized adult critical care unit (Williamson & Le Blanc, 2008).

Nurse practitioners prepared for practice in acute care settings are working with groups of patients to manage care while the individuals are hospitalized. Some nurse practitioners have hospital admitting privileges and see patients in both the acute care and primary care settings. Often, the acute care practitioners are "on call" and respond to the unexpected events that can occur during hospitalization (Magill, 2007; Shapiro, 2007).

 **GLOBAL CONNECTION**

**Advanced Practice Nurses and World Health**
Organizations, health systems, and interested individuals globally are assessing and investigating issues related to community healthcare services, home health management, and advanced nursing practice. Scarcity of financial and human resources has motivated healthcare policy makers to rise to the challenge to explore skill mix in the healthcare workforce in the hope of improving multidisciplinary collaboration in the provision of care for the world's populations. Nurses with advanced knowledge and skills are at the forefront of providing health care in home-based and community settings. This article describes the extent of this global phenomenon as it relates to advanced nursing practice and identifies a variety of international strategies utilized to introduce advanced practice nurses into healthcare systems.

*Source*: Schober, M. (2007). The global emergence of advanced practice nurses in providing home and community health care services. *Home Health Care Management & Practice*, 20(1), 34–40.

Hospitals or groups of emergency department physicians employ nurse practitioners to see persons who come to the emergency department when the situation does not warrant emergency treatment. Free-standing emergency care centers in the community are growing in number. This setting is known as a *fast track*. These practitioners may be prepared as acute care nurse practitioners, adult nurse practitioners, emergency nurse practitioners, or family nurse practitioners. Individuals with acute problems such as sore throats, earaches, low back pain, or diarrhea are seen by these practitioners. After a thorough examination, the problem is treated and usually resolves relatively quickly. The emergency department staff physicians see those persons with urgent problems. If the nurse practitioner finds a more complex situation than originally determined, the emergency physician may be consulted or the person may be transferred to the care of the physician (Shapiro, 2007; Broom et al., 2008).

### Clinics

Primary care clinics (places of first entry into the healthcare system) have long been the sites of care of certified nurse midwives and nurse practitioners. For many people in rural or economically depressed areas, advanced practice nurses may be the only resource for health care. Any of the specialties of nurse practitioners focusing on primary care may be found in healthcare clinics. Funding for health clinics may be provided by state or federal government and at times a combination of the two. Other clinics are funded through private sources. Private sources include foundations, groups of individuals, and single owners. It is common for a nurse practitioner or group of practitioners to open a health clinic to serve the general public (Sheehy & McCarthy, 1998). These clinics often have a strong focus on health teaching in addition to providing care for individuals with acute illnesses. For persons with stable chronic illnesses, the nurse practitioner can follow and treat according to accepted protocols (AACN, 2004).

A growing trend is for nurse practitioners to be hired by physicians who have a specialty practice. Orthopedic surgeons may have a collaborating nurse practitioner who may do the initial history and physical examination, make rounds at the hospital, do patient teaching, and provide follow-up. Gastroenterologists have hired nurse practitioners to do sigmoidoscopies in addition to history and physical examinations, as well as follow-up with stable patients. These are just two examples of other areas where nurse practitioners may be found (Schroder, 2008).

An important group of clinics that must be considered is those administered by the National Health Service Corps (NHSC), which is part of the U.S. Public Health Service. The NHSC is charged with providing primary health care to underserved areas. Those communities with the greatest need are targeted to receive services. Nurse practitioners and some

Family nurse practitioners (FNPs) see patients across the life span.

other groups of healthcare providers can receive financial assistance for their education, while making a commitment to work in an underserved area.

The Indian Health Service (IHS) is another agency of the U.S. Public Health Service that provides health care to Native Americans. Various types of clinics are established as needs are identified. Nurse practitioners often serve as primary care providers for the Native American population. The nurse-managed clinic usually has a cost savings over the alternative of a physician-managed clinic or a visit to the emergency department (Berry, 1997).

### Long-Term Care Facilities

Many residents of long-term care facilities are frail elders. Changes in health status can occur quickly because so many of them have more than one chronic disease. Regular, routine medical visits are mandated by federal regulations to provide cost-effective, quality care. The regulations allow for a nurse practitioner and physician to share a nursing home practice; thus the residents receive an enhanced level of care. The knowledge base of advanced practitioners can be

✎ NOTE THIS! •————————————————————————————————————————

When nurse practitioners were surveyed in 2004, their responses to questions about their practices were sometimes surprising.

*What are the most common specialties of nurse practitioners?*

Adult (41.9%) and family (41.2%) nurse practitioners (FNPs) make up the largest number of NPs. While pediatric and women's health NPs account for only 7% and 2%, respectively, of these providers, large numbers of FNPs care for women and children.

*Where do nurse practitioners practice?*

The majority (60.1%) of NPs practice in ambulatory settings, including HMOs, school health, and private clinics or offices, including 4.7% who self-describe their practices as independent. A relatively small (17.6%) but growing number of NPs describe their practice sites as hospital inpatient settings. This is reasonable given the trend toward NPs assuming acute care roles. A surprising number of NPs (14.7%), however, select "other" as their practice settings, clearly pointing to the need to obtain more specific details about these settings in future years.

*How many patients does a nurse practitioner see in a day?*

A very small number of respondents (3.8%) see fewer than 5 patients per day. These NPs are predominantly in home care or hospice practices, where the intensity of the patient encounters and the need for travel restrict their ability to see larger numbers of patients. By com-parison, 20.8% see more than 20 patients per day. The majority of nurse practitioners see between 11 and 15 patients per day (28.8%) or 16 to 20 patients per day (24.2%). These numbers illustrate the growing demands for increasing productivity, which is inevitably accompanied by a decrease in time allowed for individual patient encounters.

*What about prescriptive authority of NPs?*

Most state laws allow NPs to write for both legend drugs and controlled substances. Every year of the survey, more NPs have reported that they have their own Drug Enforcement Administration (DEA) number; 69% of respondents in 2004 had their own DEA number, the largest percentage ever reported. This is a reflection of the increasing recognition of the role of NPs as primary care providers. It does not appear to have heralded a significant change in NP prescribing practices, as there has not been a large increase in the number of NPs reporting that they routinely prescribe controlled substances.

U.S. Nurse Practitioner Prescribing Law: A State-by-State Summary Map is available on the following website: http://www.medscape.com/viewarticle/440315. To view a summary of the NP prescribing law in any state or the District of Columbia, click on the state. ◯

*Source: Longitudinal nurse practitioner prescribing data 2004 cohort.* (2004, September 27). Ellicott City, MD: Nurse Practitioner Alternatives, Inc.

Dr. Mary Huch, chapter author (right), adult nurse practitioner, with elder patient in a long-term care facility.

a means of securing needed care before complications occur. While practicing in long-term care facilities, the advanced practice nurse also serves as a role model and teacher to the nursing home staff (Snyder & Mirr, 1995).

### ■ Educational Institutions

Advanced practice nurses bring a wealth of information to the school health setting. At one time, the nurse was the person who applied a bandage and had students lie on a cot until they felt better. Nurses are now involved in many aspects of health promotion for students. (Chapter 40 furnishes a broader discussion of the school health nurse role.) In many states, school-based clinics that provide primary health care for the students and their families have been established. Services range from providing care for minor illnesses and injuries to family planning and pregnancy counseling. Most of these school-based clinics are managed by nurse practitioners.

### *Got an Alternative?*

This article discusses the appropriate use of healing touch (HT) and therapeutic touch (TT) therapies in the *advanced practice nurse* role to patients in psychiatric settings. The uses of the therapies are described within the theoretical frameworks of Martha Roger's Science of Unitary Human Beings (SUHB) and Susan Leddy's Human Energy Model (HEM). Evidence-based research is reviewed and case studies provided that demonstrate how HT and TT can be integrated as cost-effective interventional strategies in patients with mental health needs.

*Source*: Vickers, C. (2008). Healing touch and therapeutic touch in the psychiatric setting: Implications for the advanced practice nurse. *Visions: The Journal of Rogerian Nursing Science, 15*(1), 46–52.

Nurse practitioners are also commonly found in college health centers as first-line providers of care. Within these settings, the full gamut of nurse practitioner functioning is called into play. The college health center, like any other primary care clinic, offers a range of services from physical examinations, treatment for minor illnesses, x-ray examinations, and dispensing of pharmaceuticals, to counseling for problems.

## Innovations in Healthcare Delivery in the Community

### ■ Nursing Centers

The need for an alternative way of meeting the healthcare needs of underserved citizens throughout this country prompted nursing faculty in schools of nursing to open nursing centers. Both clinical nurse specialists and nurse practitioners are critical to the operation of these centers. Nursing centers have multiple purposes that include providing direct patient care, functioning as sites for faculty clinical practice, and providing clinical experiences for both graduate and undergraduate students. Health teaching, routine physical examinations, maternal–infant care, primary care services, and counseling are some of the services provided by these centers. Funding for nursing centers is provided in many ways, including grant funds, private payment, Medicare, Medicaid, private insurance, and private donors. In some centers, there is no fee for services, but other centers do charge fees as either a flat fee or on a sliding scale. Nursing centers are often located in places that are more accessible to those who are uninsured or underinsured (AACN, 2004; Watson, 1996).

### ■ Case Management

The increased cost of care delivery and earlier discharge of patients from hospitals has opened the door for nurses to

## " *a conversation with . . .* "

Dr. Loretta Ford, who with Dr. Henry Silver started the first nurse practitioner program in 1965 at the University of Colorado Health Sciences Center, was asked to share some thoughts about advanced practice nurses.

**Have advanced nurse practitioners contributed to improved outcomes in health care?**
Advanced practice nurses have contributed positively to improved outcomes in health care by putting "health" back into a medicalized system through the advanced practice nurses' orientation, preparation, commitment, and scholarship in professional nursing principles of prevention, patient education and empowerment, and political acumen in changing the systems of care.

Advanced practice nurses have provided quality care while decreasing costs of service, and though some data have been collected on cost savings, more needs to be done. Longitudinal studies are especially needed to document behavioral changes in patients' lifestyles, use of health care services, and outcomes. Common sense would tell that the different costs of professional education, pay scales, role flexibility of advanced practice nurses as well as the growing recognition that many so-called health problems are not medical in nature and require different approaches.

**The practice arenas for advanced practice nurses increased very rapidly in recent years. Do you think this will affect the scope of practice in the future?**
The scope of nursing practice has been expanding since the early 1900s and there's no reason to suspect it will diminish. Indeed, it will expand rather wildly. The expansions in knowledge, and technology, communication, transportation, etc., will not only enlarge the scope of practice, but open many avenues of practice heretofore not imagined or even dreamed of. The challenge will be for professional nursing to envision the future in its broadest configuration and begin the preparation of those who will inherit the future. Advanced practice nurses who are creating the future will leave a legacy of knowledge, research, and philosophical thought upon which future generations can build. There's no time to lose—"carpe diem."

—**Loretta Ford, EdD, RN, FAAN**
Personal communication, March 1998

help patients through the maze known as healthcare delivery. Determining measurable, realistic outcomes takes a person with advanced knowledge. Advanced practice nurses are well positioned to serve as case managers, which may include interactions while patients are well, during hospitalization, and after discharge. Case managers strive to increase self-care abilities in the most cost-effective manner (Papenhausen,

### A Good Read

## Primary Care: The Art and Science of Advanced Practice Nursing (2nd edition, 2007)

*by Lynne M. Dunphy, Jill E. Winland-Brown, Brian O. Porter, and Debra J. Thomas, Philadelphia: F. A. Davis Company*

This book offers a holistic approach to advanced nursing practice that provides population-based care as well as individual focused care. The authors' purpose is to provide APN students with the necessary introductory information to plan and provide direct care in diverse clinical settings and to evaluate clinical outcomes. The authors use a model of advanced practice nursing, grounded in "The Circle of Caring," an epistemology structured by the nursing process, superimposed upon the medical model, grounded in the lived experience, and bound by caring. Other chapters address population- and cultural-based caring, health promotion, the art of diagnosis and treatment, and clinical outcomes. The authors contend that "this is not your mother's nurse practitioner textbook," setting forth in bold relief the expanded potential for today's ambulatory care clinical specialist or nurse practitioner.

Dr. Karen Saucier Lundy, community health nursing clinical specialist, collaborates with a community activist and elected community school board member.

include massage therapy, acupuncture, relaxation techniques, herbal therapy, meditation, and prayer. (Chapter 16 explores complementary health practices in great detail.) To use such therapies effectively, all nurses must have additional knowledge of the effects and hazards of selected approaches. Advanced education and the autonomy of independent practice make advanced practice nurses effective advocates for these therapies (Vickers, 2008).

## Conclusion

Although the advanced practice nurse role is a relatively new one, dramatic progress has been made in the evolution and implementation of the advanced practice nurse. The historical development of the role has been shaped by consumer and system demands and has faced role challenges from within the nursing profession and with other healthcare professionals. Advanced practice nurses can now function in all 50 states.

1990). Community health clinical nurse specialists are often case managers. Home health agencies are an ideal work setting in which to implement this advanced practice nursing role (AACN, 2004; Zwanziger et al., 1996).

The move to more standardized educational preparation has become a reality, with significant changes in moving educational requirements to the doctoral level (DNP). Licensure and certification issues will remain concerns and challenges for the advanced practice nurse in the community health setting. With full integration into the healthcare delivery system, the advanced practice nurse provides quality health care to diverse populations in varied settings in the promotion of health.

### ■ Holistic Practice

One of the emerging trends among nurse practitioners is to function from a holistic perspective, moving beyond traditional medical therapies. What this means is that traditional care is provided along with what are known as *complementary approaches*. The complementary approaches

### ✎ NOTE THIS! ●─────────────────

**Prescriptive Authority and Advanced Practice Nursing**
A review of state laws and regulations shows that although advanced practice nurses have some degree of prescriptive authority in all 50 states and the District of Columbia, there are restrictions on their prescribing of controlled substances. In 40 states, advanced practice nurses have differing authorities to prescribe schedule II–V controlled substances; in eight states they can prescribe only schedule III–V drugs. Three states do not allow advanced practice nurses to prescribe controlled substances.

*Source:* Berry, P., & Dahl, J. (2007). Advanced practice nurse controlled substances prescriptive authority. *Journal of Hospice & Palliative Nursing, 9*(5), 238–245.

Explore Community Health Nursing on the Web! To learn more about the topics in this chapter, use the passcode provided to access your exclusive website: **http://nursing.jbpub.com/ communityhealth.** If you do not have a passcode, you can obtain one at this site.

## ■ CRITICAL THINKING ACTIVITIES

1. Mr. Johnson is an 85-year-old, widowed nursing home resident. He has lost 20 pounds over 4 months. He is very close to his ideal body weight. He is able to eat, but he often refuses to do so, even when the staff attempts to feed him. Occasionally, he drinks a nutritional supplement that is left at his bedside. Mr. Johnson is cognitively aware of his surroundings, although he often just closes his eyes when a care provider approaches. His family wants everything possible to be done for him, including insertion of a feeding tube. Mr. Johnson does not verbally express his wishes about the feeding tube placement. As the clinical nurse specialist in the nursing home, you are called to work with Mr. Johnson and his family. What course of action would you take in this situation?

2. Explore the similarities and differences in the roles of advanced practice nurses.

3. Appraise the value of advanced practice nurses being reimbursed by third-party payers for patient care visits.

4. Research how people decide who their primary care provider will be.

## ■ REFERENCES

American Association of Colleges of Nursing. (2004). *AACN position statement on the practice doctorate in nursing.* Retrieved July 24, 2008, from http://www.aacn.nche.edu/DNP/pdf/DNP.pdf

American Association of Colleges of Nursing. (2005). *Frequently asked questions concerning the AACN position statement on the practice doctorate in nursing.* Retrieved July 24, 2008, from http://www.aacn.nche.edu/DNP/AboutDNP.htm

American Association of Colleges of Nursing. (2006). *AACN essentials of doctoral education for advanced nursing practice.* Retrieved July 24, 2008, from http://www.aacn.nche.edu/DNP/pdf/Essentials5-06.pdf

American Association of Colleges of Nursing. (2007). *AACN white paper on the education and role of the clinical nurse leader.* Washington, DC: Author.

American College of Nurse Midwives (ACNM). (2005). *About ACNM.* Retrieved December 2, 2008, from http://www.midwife.org/about.cfm

American Nurses Association (ANA), Congress on Nursing Practice. (1976). *Description of practice: Clinical nurse specialist.* Kansas City, MO: Author.

Association of Community Health Nursing Educators. (1991). *Essentials of master's level nursing education for advanced community health nursing practice.* Louisville, KY: Author.

Avery, M., & Howe, C. (2007). The DNP and entry into midwifery practice: An analysis. *Journal of Midwifery & Women's Health, 52*(1), 14–22.

Berry, P., & Dahl, J. (2007). Advanced practice nurse controlled substances prescriptive authority. *Journal of Hospice & Palliative Nursing, 9*(5), 238–245.

Berry, R. A. (1997). A nurse practitioner-managed after-hours clinic for a Native American reservation. *Journal of the American Academy of Nurse Practitioners, 9,* 165–170.

Boyer, E. (1996). Clinical practice as scholarship. *Holistic Nursing Practice, 3,* 1–6.

Boyle, D. M. (1996). The clinical nurse specialist. In A. B. Hamric, J. A. Spross, & C. M. Hanson (Eds.), *Advanced nursing practice: An integrative approach* (pp. 299–336). Philadelphia: W. B. Saunders.

Broom, C., Shirk, M., Pehrson, K., & Peterson, K. (2008). Perspectives on psychiatric consultation liaison nursing psychiatric-mental health-advanced practice nurses: Transforming nursing practice. *Perspectives in Psychiatric Care, 44*(2), 131–134.

Burkhardt, P. (1996). Nurse midwifery: Advanced practice nursing? *Nursing Clinics of North America, 31,* 439–448.

Pan, S., Geller, J. M., Gullicks, J. N., Muus, K. J., & Larson, A. C. (1997). A comparative analysis of primary care nurse practitioners and physician assistants. *Nurse Practitioner, American Journal of Primary Health Care, 22*(1), 14–17.

Cartwright, C., & Reed, C. (2005). Policy and planning perspectives for the doctorate in nursing practice: An educational perspective. *Online Journal of Issues in Nursing, 10*(3). Available from http://www.nursingworld.org

Cheng, H., & Chen, S. (2008). Medical team satisfaction with nurse practitioner clinical performance. *Journal of Nursing Research, 16*(1), 26–35.

Chornick, N. (2008). NCSBN focus. Advanced practice registered nurse educational programs and regulation: A need for increased communication. *JONA's Healthcare Law, Ethics & Regulation, 10*(1), 9–11.

Daly, C. M., & Mitchell, R. D. (1996). Case management in the community setting. *Nursing Clinics of North America, 31,* 527–534.

Delancy, K. (2008). ACAPN news addressing children's mental health needs: Educational preparation of advanced practice nurses. *Journal of Child & Adolescent Psychiatric Nursing, 21*(1), 57–59.

Dorroh, M., & Norton, S. F. (1996). The certified nurse-midwife. In A. B. Hamric, J. A. Spross, & C. M. Hanson (Eds.), *Advanced nursing practice: An integrative approach* (pp. 395–420). Philadelphia: W. B. Saunders.

Dracup, K., Cronenwett, L., Meleis, A. I., & Benner, P. E. (2005). Reflections on the doctorate of nursing practice. *Nursing Outlook, 53,* 177–182.

Elder, R. G., & Bullough, B. (1990). Nurse practitioners and clinical nurse specialists: Are the roles merging? *Clinical Nurse Specialist, 4*, 78–84.

England, M. (2008). Psychotherapy for the advanced practice psychiatric nurse—Kathleen Wheeler, PhD, APRN. *Perspectives in Psychiatric Care, 44*(3), 219–220.

Fenton, M. V., & Brykczynski, K. A. (1993). Qualitative distinctions and similarities in the practice of clinical nurse specialists and nurse practitioners. *Journal of Professional Nursing, 9*, 313–326.

Fitzpatrick, J., & Marecki, M. (2007). Is the doctor of nursing practice (DNP) the appropriate doctoral degree for nurses?... Writing for the PRO position. . . Writing for the CON position. *MCN: The American Journal of Maternal Child Nursing, 32*(3), 138–139.

Forbes, K. E., Rafson, J., Spross, J. A., & Kozlowski, D. (1990). The clinical nurse specialist and nurse practitioner: Core curriculum survey results. *Clinical Nurse Specialist, 4*, 63–66.

Ford, L. C. (1998, March). Personal communication.

Ford, L. C., & Silver, H. K. (1967). The expanded role of the nurse in child care. *Nursing Outlook, 15*(8), 43–45.

Frontier Nursing Service, Inc. (2008). *History information.* Retrieved December 2, 2008, from http://www.frontiernursing.org/history/history.shtm

Garde, J. F. (1996). The nurse anesthesia profession. A past, present, and future perspective. *Nursing Clinics of North America, 31*, 567–580.

Georgopoulos, B. S., & Christman, L. (1970). The clinical nurse specialist: A role model. *American Journal of Nursing, 70*, 1030–1039.

Good, M. E. (1992). The clinical nurse specialist in the school setting: Case management of migrant children with dental disease. *Clinical Nurse Specialist, 6*, 72–76.

Hamric, A. B. (1989). History and overview of the CNS role. In A. B. Hamric & J. A. Spross (Eds.), *The clinical nurse specialist in theory and practice* (2nd ed., pp. 3–18). Philadelphia: W. B. Saunders.

Hamric, A. B., Spross, J. A., & Hanson, C. M. (1996). *Advanced nursing practice: An integrative approach.* Philadelphia: W. B. Saunders.

Hawkins, J. W., & Thibodeau, J. A. (1996). *The advanced practice nurse* (4th ed.). New York: Tiresias Press.

Hoffman, D., & Nannini, A. (2008). Planning, surveillance, and reporting for pandemic influenza: A briefing for advanced practice nurses. *Journal of the American Academy of Nurse Practitioners, 20*(1), 11–16.

Huch, M. H. (1992). Nurse practitioners and physician assistants: Are they the same? *Nursing Science Quarterly, 5*, 52–53.

Huch, M. H. (1995). Nursing sciences as a basis for advanced practice. *Nursing Science Quarterly, 8*, 6–7.

Hunsberger, M., Mitchell, A., Blatz, S., et al. (1992). Definition of an advanced nursing practice role in the NICU: The clinical nurse specialist/neonatal practitioner. *Clinical Nurse Specialist, 6*, 91–96.

Jordan, K. (2008). Sexually transmitted infections: A major public health challenge for advanced practice nurses. *Advanced Emergency Nursing Journal, 30*(1), 63–74.

Kremer, M. J., & Faut-Callahan, M. (1998). Reimbursement for expanded professional nursing practice services. In C. M. Sheehy & M. C. McCarthy (Eds.), *Advanced practice nursing: Emphasizing common roles.* Philadelphia: F. A. Davis.

Kupina, P. S. (1995). Community health CNSs and health care in the year 2000. *Clinical Nurse Specialist, 9*, 188–190, 198.

Lancaster, J., & Lancaster, W. (1993). Nurse practitioners: Health care providers whose time has come. *Community Health, 16*(2), 1–8.

Langner, S. R., & Hutelmyer, C. (1995). Patient satisfaction with outpatient human immunodeficiency virus care as delivered by nurse practitioners and physicians. *Holistic Nursing Practice, 10*, 54–60.

Lenz, E. (2005). The practice doctorate in nursing: An idea whose time has come. *Online Journal of Issues in Nursing, 10*(3). Available from http://www.nursingworld.org

Loomis, J., Willard, B., & Cohen, J. (2007). Difficult professional choices: Deciding between the PhD and the DNP in nursing. *Online Journal of Issues in Nursing, 12*(1), 4–44.

Magill, J. (2007). The evolution of the advanced clinical nurse role in emergency nursing: CIN-er to saint: A practice development journey in one metropolitan emergency department. *Australasian Emergency Nursing Journal, 10*(4), 218–219.

Meleis, A., & Dracup, K. (2005). The case against the dnp: History, timing, substance, and marginalization. *Online Journal of Issues in Nursing, 10*(3). Available from http://www.nursingworld.org

Menard, S. W. (1987). The CNS as consultant. In S. W. Menard (Ed.), *The clinical nurse specialist* (pp. 127–143). New York: John Wiley and Sons.

National Center for Health Statistics. (1999). *Healthy people 2000 review, 1989–99.* Hyattsville, MD: Public Health Service.

National Council of State Boards of Nursing. (1992). *National Council of State Boards of Nursing position paper on the licensure of advanced nursing practice.* Chicago: Author.

National Organization of Nurse Practitioner Faculties. (1997). *Criteria for evaluation of nurse practitioner faculties.* Washington, DC: Author.

O'Grady, E. (2004). Advanced practice nursing and health policy. In J. Stanley (Ed.), *Advanced practice nursing emphasizing common roles* (2nd ed., pp. 374–394). Philadelphia: F. A. Davis.

Page, N. E., & Arena, D. M. (1994). Rethinking the merger of the clinical nurse specialist and the nurse practitioner roles. *Image: Journal of Nursing Scholarship, 26*, 315–318.

Papenhausen, J. L. (1990). Case management: A model of advanced practice? *Clinical Nurse Specialist, 4*, 169–170.

Pearson, L. J. (1999). Annual update of how each state stands on legislative issues affecting advanced nursing practice. *Nurse Practitioner, American Journal of Primary Health Care, 24*(1), 16–24.

Reiter, F. (1966). The nurse-clinician. *American Journal of Nursing, 66*, 274–280.

Robertson, J. F., & Baldwin, K. B. (2007.) Advanced practice role characteristics of the community/public health nurse specialist. *Clinical Nurse Specialist: The Journal for Advanced Nursing Practice, 21*(5), 250–254.

Robinson, D. K., Mead, M. J., & Boswell, C. R. (1995). Inside looking out: Innovations in community health nursing. *Clinical Nurse Specialist, 9*, 227–229, 235.

Rogers, M. E. (1972). Nursing: To be or not to be. *Nursing Outlook, 20*, 42–46.

Rosenfeld, A., Brown, R., Crabtree, K., Eldredge, D., Howe, C., LeCuyer, E., et al. (2007). Making a case for the DNP (doctor of nursing practice): The OHSU experience. *Communicating Nursing Research, 40*, 232.

Safriet, B. J. (1992). Health care dollars and regulatory sense: The role of advanced practice nursing. *Yale Journal on Regulation, 9*, 417–488.

Schroeder, J. (2008). Acute care nurse practitioner: An advanced practice role for RN first assistants. *AORN Journal, 87*(6), 1205–1215.

Schroer, K. (1991). Case management: Clinical nurse specialist and nurse practitioner, converging roles. *Clinical Nurse Specialist, 5,* 189–194.

Shapiro, S. (2007). Evidence-based practice for advanced practice emergency nurses. *Advanced Emergency Nursing Journal, 29*(4), 331–338.

Shapiro, S. E., & Donaldson, N. A. (2008). Evidence-based practice for advanced practice emergency nurses, part II: Critically appraising the literature. *Advanced Emergency Nursing Journal, 30*(2), 139–150.

Sheehy, C. M., & McCarthy, M. (1998). *Advanced practice nursing: Emphasizing common roles.* Philadelphia: F. A. Davis.

Snyder, M., & Mirr, M. P. (Eds.). (1995). *Advanced practice nursing: A guide to professional development.* New York: Springer.

Thatcher, V. S. (1984). *History of anesthesia with emphasis on the nurse specialist.* New York: Garland.

U.S. Department of Health and Human Services (USDHHS). (2000). *Healthy people 2010.* McLean, VA: International Medical Publishing.

Varney, H. (1987). *Nurse-midwifery* (2nd ed.). Boston: Blackwell Scientific.

Vickers, C. (2008). Healing touch and therapeutic touch in the psychiatric setting: Implications for the advanced practice nurse. *Visions: The Journal of Rogerian Nursing Science, 15*(1), 46–52.

Ward-Miller, S. (1996). The psychiatric clinical specialist in the home care setting. *Nursing Clinics of North America, 31,* 519–525.

Watson, L. J. (1996). A national profile of nursing centers. *Nurse Practitioner, American Journal of Primary Care, 21*(3), 72–81.

Williamson, L., & LeBlanc, D. (2008). A genetic services practice model: Advanced practice nurse and genetic counselor team. *Newborn & Infant Nursing Reviews, 8*(1), 30–35.

Zwanziger, P. J., Peterson, R. M., Lethlean, H. M., et al. (1996). Expanding the CNS role to the community. *Clinical Nurse Specialist, 10,* 199–202.

# CHAPTER 43
# Health Ministries: Health and Faith Communities

Emily Chandler, Ruth Berry, and Karen Saucier Lundy

Visit **http://nursing.jbpub.com/communityhealth** for interactive exercises, review questions, Web links, and more.

Wouldn't it be wonderful if faith groups adopted one small area and made sure that every single child was immunized . . . that every person had a basic medical exam . . . that every woman who became pregnant would get prenatal care? Are these possible? We believe the answer is yes.

Prayer does not use up artificial energy, doesn't burn up any fossil fuel, doesn't pollute. Neither does song, neither does love, neither does the dance.

—*Margaret Mead*

Never worry about numbers. Help one person at a time, and always start with the person nearest you.

—*Mother Teresa*

You never see a hearse pulling a U-Haul and death shrouds do not have pockets. Enjoy your wealth while alive—no need for it after that.

—*Ruth Landers*

Health is my expected heaven.

—*John Keats*

People are often unreasonable, illogical, and self-centered; forgive them anyway. If you are kind, people may accuse you of selfish, ulterior motives; be kind anyway. The good you do today, people will often forget tomorrow; do good anyway. Give the world the best you have, and it may never be enough; give the world the best you've got anyway. You see, in the final analysis, it is between you and God; it was never between you and them anyway.

—*Mother Teresa*

Blessed are those who have not seen and yet believe.

—*Jesus, John 20:29*

Every human being is the author of his own health and disease.

—*Buddha*

For what is Mysticism? Is it not the attempt to draw near to God, not by rites or ceremonies, but by inward disposition? Is it not merely a hard word for "The Kingdom of Heaven is within"? Heaven is neither a place nor a time.

—*Florence Nightingale, 1873*

I will shed the sins and struggles I have carried all these years. And I'll leave my heart wide open; I will love and have no fear.

—*Dolly Parton*

These quotes represent many different expressions of spirituality. How do you define spirituality? What are common themes in the quotes? Are religion and spirituality the same? As you read this chapter, consider the ways in which community health nurses can include the spiritual aspect of health in caring for populations.

## CHAPTER FOCUS

**Development of Health Ministries**
- History of Ministering: Hospitals, Hospitality, and Religious Communities
- Nightingale's Legacy: Relationship of Nursing to Early Models
- Philosophical Underpinnings

**Health Ministry in Action**
- The Faith Community
- Models of Health Ministry
- Structure of Health Ministries

**Relationship Between Community Health Nursing and Faith Communities**
- Parish Nursing
- Activities of Parish Nurses
- Missionary Nursing
- Roles and Practice of Missionary Nurses

## QUESTIONS TO CONSIDER

After reading this chapter, you will know the answers to the following questions:

1. What are health ministries?
2. How did health ministries begin?
3. How does spirituality relate to health?
4. How is the faith community an ideal setting for the role of the community health nurse?

5. What are examples of models of health ministries?
6. What is parish nursing?
7. How can nurses function to promote health in health ministry programs?

Assets mapping
Congregational health partnership
Extrinsic religiosity

Faith community/parish/
  congregation
Health ministry

Intrinsic religiosity
Missionary nursing

Parish nursing
Religion

## Development of Health Ministries

### ■ History of Ministering: Hospitals, Hospitality, and Religious Communities

**Health ministry,** in its broadest sense, is a concept that encompasses spirituality, spiritual well-being, and activities that may be carried out by a specific faith community either alone or in partnership with other organizations. Health ministries incorporate the spiritual foundations and practices of the faith community to promote mutual caring for the greatest potential of whole-person wellness.

The notion of ministering to the sick has ancient roots that reach back beyond Nightingale. The history of "ministering" comes from the earliest accounts of efforts to help and to care for the unfortunate, often those who were unable to afford private care in their homes. "Hospitality" was offered by religious communities who saw it as their responsibility to provide comfort and care. Hospitals originated as places where this ministering to (care of) the sick took place. Religious communities, both lay and formal, have a history of providing both advocacy and access to care. Concern for the underserved focused on the disadvantaged, the elderly, women and children, the disabled, and the chronically ill (Wall & Nelson, 2003).

Health ministries have again become a viable option in community health care because of numerous trends in society. The aging U.S. population is not only increasing in number, but also raising issues of values, quality of life, and caring for those who now are living longer. Vulnerable and frail persons continue to be underserved. Responsibility for self-care is promoted in a managed care environment. Patients are encouraged to remain out of the illness care system by staying healthy.

Individuals, families, and communities all need to know how to make healthy choices. The holistic health centers of the 1970s were instrumental in bringing individuals and families together with physicians, clergy, and nurses to determine strategies for achieving better health. This team approach emphasized preventive health practices and personal responsibility for health care. The World Council of Churches (1990), for example, entered into a dialogue regarding wholeness, health, and healing as central to faith and the Creator. The Council endorsed the caring community as a means of restoring wholeness and healing. According to this view, building community can enhance mutual concern and overcome barriers of suffering and injustice with faith communities as the focus of interventions.

The Carter Center at Emory University (Box 43-1) and the Park Ridge Center for the Study of Health, Faith, and Ethics have also addressed faith communities as an important public health resource and emphasized the advantages of churches having an active role in attaining the *Healthy People 2010* objectives. Formed in 1995, the Faith and Health Caucus of the American Public Health Association has as a major objective encouraging partnerships between faith and health institutions to promote health.

The most destructive natural disaster to ever hit the U.S. mainland, Hurricane Katrina has become a metaphor for the "perfect disaster"—not just in terms of its catastrophic devastation of the Mississippi Gulf Coast and New Orleans, but also in terms of the failure of state, federal, and voluntary organizations to respond in a timely and appropriate manner. Those who have been given credit with providing immediate and long-term aid to those in the disaster areas, often at personal risk to themselves and their fellow volunteers, include churches and their outreach disaster services. For example, members of the Seventh Day Adventist Church were in south Mississippi delivering hot meals and handing out ice, household goods, diapers, and even cat and dog food within 2 days of the disaster. By comparison, federal and American Red Cross services were not accessible for at least a week in most rural areas of Mississippi, and many of these official disaster relief services did not reach people in rural areas for as long as a month. People in the affected area were without electricity and water for as many as 6 weeks, and churches provided relief in many small towns that were isolated due to road obstructions and lack of resources available to larger towns. Church members continued their relief efforts for 2 months, providing shelter, assistance with federal and state relief funds, and, most of all, comfort for those who faced unimaginable personal losses.

 **MEDIA MOMENT**

Popular medical television programs, such as *ER, House, Scrubs,* and *Grey's Anatomy,* seldom address religious or spiritual aspects of care. Why do you think these aspects of health are avoided?

## BOX 43-1

**The Carter Center's Interfaith Health Program: Realigning Community Assets Through Collaboration of Faith Communities and Health Organizations**

### Aligning Assets of Faith and Health Communities in Building Healthier Communities

The Carter Center's interest in the role of faith communities in improving community health began in the 1980s. A national symposium, "Closing the Gap," signaled the beginning of concerted efforts to bring together the most significant health science and the most relevant knowledge and experience from theology for both the faith community and health science and health service institutions. At that time, the Carter Center identified faith communities as the most underused resource group, with potential to help in closing the gap for improving America's health.

In 1989, a conference on *Striving for Fullness of Life: The Church's Challenge in Health* was sponsored by the Carter Center and the Wheat Ridge Foundation. This conference focused on building healthy lives through public health measures such as preventing disease, disability, and premature death. This proved to be an important step forward, but it did not address the need for shifts in how congregations viewed their roles in the larger community and how health institutions and organizations perceived the assets of congregations.

The Interfaith Health Program was formed in 1992 to respond to the challenge of helping to build healthier communities by engaging leaders from the health sciences and theology along with community representatives from health services and congregations to find ways to realign faith and health assets for the good of the community.

The Five Gap Model was used to ask the right questions when searching for strategies. The gaps include the following:
- The gap between what is already known and what is applied
- The gap between what every faith group affirms as their concern for social justice and what they do

Anna Frances Wenger, PhD, RN, FAAN, the Carter Center.

- The gap between successful working models and general application in other communities
- The gap perpetuated by faith groups working in isolation from each other and health agencies
- The gap between present wants and future needs

Using the Five Gap Model, we focused on promotion of congregational health ministries, one of the key strategies of the Interfaith Health Program. The Atlanta Health Ministry Model was developed and then used in two African American communities and one multicultural community in Atlanta. This health ministry model was based on the participatory approach proposed by Paulo Freire, the Brazilian grassroots educator and author of *Pedagogy of the Oppressed*. Some of the core principles of the Atlanta Health Ministry Model (Droege & Wenger, 1997, p. 14) are as follows:
- Education is never neutral; it is either liberating or domesticating.
- People will act on issues that evoke strong feelings.
- People are creative and intelligent with the capacity for action.
- Genuine dialogue is needed if communities are to share, listen, and learn.

Several key action steps characterized the approach used in Atlanta. First, a working group of 15 religious leaders participated in a 6-month planning process to determine the most effective way to enlist faith communities to increase engagement in health-promotion activities. This process served to nurture a network of potential collaborators.

Second, in each neighborhood, local pastors (or priests, rabbi, and imam) were invited to join a network of congregations, with each network governed by a Health Ministry Council. This council was formed by the participating congregations and staffed by a network coordinator. Third, the training of Congregational Health Promoters was at the heart of the program. The training program was coordinated by the Neil Hodgson Woodruff School of Nursing at Emory University, with nursing instructors who understood the participatory teaching–learning process leading the training sessions.

The goal of this approach was to build on the capacities of the congregations and communities rather than to fix problems or to predetermine what needs to be learned.

Each participating congregation designated two natural leaders from within the congregation to join the training program, which consisted of 20 to 24 hours of 2- to 3-hour sessions. Although the emphasis was on lay health leadership, some professionals such as nurses and social workers participated in the training. As the need was expressed by the participants, local health resource persons came to discuss specific health services in the community. When the trainees recognized the need to learn more about a resource, such as nutritional information or heart health resources, the nursing instructor would make the connections for them, always emphasizing how they can assume that role in the future.

So, what has happened in these neighborhoods since the initial training period? In a largely African American community, Atlanta Health Ministries, a nonprofit organization

*(continues)*

**BOX 43-1**

**The Carter Center's Interfaith Health Program: Realigning Community Assets Through Collaboration of Faith Communities and Health Organizations—Cont'd**

with 501(c)3 status, was established. It has several active committees, with one of them being Congregational Health Promoters. In a very multiethnic community, there is a Congregational Health Ministry program as part of the Chamblee–Doraville Ministry Center. A Congregational Health Ministry Coordinator, who is a parish nurse employed by St. Joseph's Mercy Care System, conducts training sessions in Spanish and English and serves as a mentor for all of the congregational health promoters in the neighborhood, which includes Korean, Vietnamese, African American, Hispanic, and dominant-culture American congregations.

A commitment to cultural openness is inherent for all of the initiatives of the Interfaith Health Program. As boundaries are spanned among disciplines and within communities, the persons engaged in faith and health ministries need to constantly renew their commitment to learn about the meaning of faith and health within the worldviews of the people. "Cultural openness refers to a life-long stance that promotes cultural self awareness and continuing development of transcultural skills" (Wenger, 1998, p. 164). Respect for differences, although important, is not enough (Wenger, 1998). Transcultural knowledge and skills are essential components when engaging in health ministries and building partnerships.

Two other initiatives of the Interfaith Health Program are directed toward moving the faith and health movement forward. Whole Communities Collaborative is a network of faith and health leaders from five specific communities within the United States where local working groups exchange ideas and develop local activities that bring faith-based communities and health organizations together for the good of the larger community or neighborhood. The other initiative is referred to as the Faith and Health Consortium. This network focuses on academic/community partnerships. There are five sites in the United States and one in South Africa where at least a school of theology or seminary and a school of public health have formed an agreement to promote disciplinary and interdisciplinary courses, research studies, and service projects that involve the integration of faith and health concepts. Schools of nursing, medicine, social work, and allied health are included whenever possible. The Faith and Health Consortium working groups always include community partners because of the underlying premise that the education of professionals, in addition to research and service projects, needs ongoing

involvement with representatives from the community to keep the academic endeavors grounded within socio-cultural contexts. Both of these networks have developed collaborative relationships through regular monthly conference calls and periodic meetings attended by representatives from the local site working groups.

Building partnerships between health institutions and faith communities requires an appreciation of assets or strengths that are already present within the community. Most of the work of the Interfaith Health Program focuses on alignment of assets for improvement of community health. Faith-based congregations are one of the most enduring assets within a community. Gary Gunderson (1997, 1998), director of the Interfaith Health Program, has outlined eight key strengths of congregations that highlight congregations as strategic partners in building healthier communities. These strengths are as follows:

1. The power to accompany, to be physically present
2. The power to convene in small and large groups across interest lines
3. The power to connect, to form human networks across which resources flow
4. The power to frame, to story, to set events and data in a meaningful context
5. The power to give sanctuary to people, programs, ideas, and dialogue
6. The power to bless, forgive, and nurture hope amid its opposite
7. The power to pray and to mark the boundary between holy and human
8. The power to endure and to maintain the sense of time and development

The challenge for health professionals and congregational leaders is to intentionally search for ways that the assets of both health and faith structures can be aligned for the benefit of the community at large. Our aspiration is that the most relevant health science and the most mature faith will guide the alignment of assets that will build strong partnerships for healthier communities.

*Source*: Anna Frances Z. Wenger, PhD, RN, FAAN, Affiliate Faculty, Neil Hodgson Woodruff School of Nursing; Faith and Health Consortium Coordinator, Interfaith Health Program, Rollins School of Public Health, Emory University, Atlanta, Georgia.

---

## ■ Nightingale's Legacy: Relationship of Nursing to Early Models

Early models of health ministry can be traced to Florence Nightingale and her own preparation for nursing. Believing that her purpose was to care for the sick, the underserved, and the disadvantaged, Nightingale sought nursing training, but the only formal education in caring for the sick available to her was a 3-month experience at the Institution of Deaconesses at Kaiserworth, Dusseldorf, Germany. The

Institution had 100 beds, where 116 deaconesses (so-called Protestant nurses) were in training to provide care. It has been argued that her primary purpose was not necessarily religious, but spiritual (Dossey, 1998). Historically, Nightingale followed a long line of healers—shamans, witches, midwives, and deaconesses. She wanted to answer what she believed to be her vocation—her call. Her primary commitment was to actualizing her spiritual convictions in acts of social justice.

### ■■ CULTURAL CONNECTION

Organized religion has many icons and symbols that represent values related to good and evil, the sacred and profane, and the expected actions of believers. Think of your own experiences with these symbols and your reaction to them. Now consider your reaction to religious symbols unfamiliar to your own values. How difficult is it to accommodate your patients' religious beliefs and values associated with their symbols in healthcare settings?

Read the "A Conversation with" feature by Donna Dowerty and consider how one nurse dealt with this conflict. Was she accepting or did she simply tolerate her patients' religious values? Why or why not? ▲

> **"***A bodily disease, which we look upon as whole and entire within itself, may after all be but a symptom of some ailment in the spiritual part.***"**
>
> —*Nathaniel Hawthorne, The Scarlet Letter, 1850*

Nightingale was raised in a Unitarian and Anglican home. Although she came to disdain organized religion, she was an intensely spiritual person. She wrote in 1852 of her dissatisfaction with the Church of England and the Catholic Church:

> The wound is too deep for the Church of England to heal. I belong as little to the Church of England as to that of Rome—or rather my heart belongs as much to the Catholic Church as to that of England—oh, how much more. The only difference is that the former insists peremptorily upon my believing what I cannot believe, while the latter is too careless and indifferent to know whether I believe it or not. (Dossey, 1999)

While Nightingale believed in the messages of Christianity, she demonstrated an unconventional tolerance and acceptance of other world religions. She wrote, "To know God we must study Him in the Pagan and Jewish dispensations as in the Christian" (Dossey, 1999, p. 48). This thread of unity to the whole continued throughout her life's writings. Dossey noted that Nightingale studied the St. James version of the Bible with great intensity, providing written annotations on almost every page. She wrote her own ideas, meanings, and interpretations in English, French, Greek, and Italian, with a blank page between most every printed page of the Bible (Dossey, 1999).

> **"***We shall not cease from exploration***
> *And the end of all our exploring*
> *Will be to arrive where we started*
> *And know the place for the first time.***"**
>
> —*T. S. Eliot*

> **"***Something began me***
> *And it had no beginning:*
> *Something will end me*
> *And it has no end.***"**
>
> —*Carl Sandburg*

Dossey, through her extensive research of Nightingale's writings, casts her as a genuine nineteenth-century mystic: "I plotted her life as such and found it to be similar to recognized mystics, such as St. Catherine of Siena, St. Catherine of Genoa, and St. Teresa of Avila" (Dossey, as quoted in Manthey, 1999, p. 3). Nightingale heard the voice of God for the first time on February 7, 1837, at the age of 16. She wrote, "God spoke and called me to his service" (Dossey, 1999). Although many have compared Nightingale's experience to Joan of Arc's experience, for Nightingale, there were no further "instructions" from God for another 16 years. From that point on, her life was a journey of spiritual enlightenment, through her writings, research, and obsession with the creation of the professional nurse.

Recent attention to Nightingale's philosophical leanings shows how committed she was to the integration of spirituality in nursing, clearly differentiating between spirituality and **religion**, which she saw as only one possible expression of spiritual life. Nightingale distinctly articulated a concept of spirituality that was broader than religion. Spirituality was, for her, a connection between an inner self and a higher reality through creative energy. Such energy was the most powerful resource for healing (Macrae, 1995; Anderson, 1996).

Nightingale, it seems, was as ahead of her time in health ministry and spirituality in nursing as she was in epidemiology and community health nursing. Today the growing commitment to holistic care is pushing nursing and medicine, as well as other disciplines, to reexamine the place of spirit in relationship to body and mind. Differences between spirituality and religion, and **extrinsic** and **intrinsic religiosity** are poorly understood and often badly articulated (Zinnbauer et al., 1997; Dossey, 1998; Couture, 2003).

### ■ Philosophical Underpinnings

The philosophical underpinnings of faith communities remain essentially unchanged. At their best, communities of faith seek ways to continue a tradition of service, often to those who need it most.

The commitment is to health and wholeness for self and others. Participation in advocacy, health education, promotion, and illness prevention are intrinsically linked to spiritual health. Such a health ministry functions within a self-understanding of compassion and care that encompasses faith, lived out in the concept of care; hope, actualized within a context of care; and love, which becomes the blueprint for the conduct of care.

## Research Alert

A study of 1,931 older residents of Marin County, California, analyzed the association between attending religious services and all-cause mortality over a 5-year period looking at six confounding factors: demographics, health status, physical functioning, health habits, social functioning, and support and psychological state. Persons who attended religious services had lower mortality rates than those who did not, and religious attendance tended to be slightly more protective when coupled with high social support. This study lends credence to the existence of a "protective effect" of religious attendance on health; a broad implication is the potential benefit of partnerships between religious organizations and health promotion efforts.

*Source*: Oman, D., & Reed, D. (1998). Religion and mortality among the community-dwelling elderly. *American Journal of Public Health, 88*(10), 1469–1475.

## Health Ministry in Action

### ■ The Faith Community

The **faith community** gives professional nursing a unique setting to practice with a diverse population. Members of the faith community represent the entire developmental age span. Families, as members of faith communities, comprise the entire array of "family-makeup" represented in this country. Families consisting of the elderly never-married, widow, or widower living alone; the single mom; the unmarried young adult, career male or female; "blended" families; and other one-parent families are all members of faith communities or congregations. The traditional two-parent family with one or more children also participates in activities, subscribes to the religious dogma, and embraces the faith community rituals to add a spiritual dimension to their lives.

Gaining inner strength to cope with life situations; giving meaning to life's existence and its joys, concerns, and challenges; and collectively finding support from members of the group are values gained by faith community members. Congregations with predominately young families might concentrate on early childhood education efforts or activities of a more active and younger adult population. Congregations that include predominately middle-aged and older adults might find that their focus will be primarily on life transitions of that age group, caregiving concerns, faith maturation issues, and life fulfillment later in one's life journey. By comparison, congregations that encompass a broader age spectrum have the challenge and opportunity to deal with cross-generational and intergenerational issues. Members can learn from one another by participating in the various age groupings, and they can find service opportunities within their congregation.

> **"**Nothing is so firmly believed as what is least known.**"**
> —Montaigne, 1588

Another feature of the faith community is the cohesiveness inherent in the group. The term "connectedness" more aptly describes the cohesiveness and belongingness often found among members of a faith community. Connectedness with the Creator (identified as God, or a Higher Power, or the Supreme Being) of the faith community is a unique attribute of this community cohesiveness. The bond of connectedness with the Creator becomes the basis for the common bond of the faith community, which is evident in the interactions among families and various age groups (Winslow & Winslow, 2003). The strength of these relationships provides a protective effect for members of the faith community and often extends beyond the benefit of simple social support (Strawbridge, Shema, Cohen, Roberts, & Kaplan, 1998; Abrums, 2004).

Connectedness is also evidenced in marking significant life passages. Members across the entire life span experience connectedness with family, friends, preceding generations, future generations, and the faith community around major transitions such as birth, marriage, and death. Events pivotal in the life of faith communities include baptism, christening, bris, confirmation, bar mitzvah, anniversaries, and funerals. In addition to the comfort that ritual provides at nodal events, attendance at religious services has been found to have a significant beneficial effect on health and longevity (Abrums, 2004; Kark, Shemi, Friedlander, Martin, Manor, & Blondheim, 1996; Koenig, Cohen, George, Hays, Larson, & Blazer, 1997; Strawbridge, Cohen, Shema, & Kaplan, 1997).

Assisting families to make choices with their loved ones for a peaceful death and dealing with the associated grief are major responsibilities for nurses in faith communities (Chandler, 1999). The opportunity to intervene with people whose histories are known within a faith community is especially meaningful. Walking beside individuals and families in times of joy, sorrow, and celebrations of beginnings and endings fosters connectedness of members with one another, with caregivers, and with the entire faith community (Wall & Nelson, 2003).

 THINK ABOUT THIS

I have an almost complete disregard of precedent and a faith in the possibility of something better. It irritates me to be told how things always have been done. . . . I defy the tyranny of precedent. I cannot afford the luxury of a closed mind. I go for anything new that might improve the past.
—Clara Barton, *A Chosen Faith*

What do you think Clara Barton means in her last statement, "I go for anything new that might improve the past"?

Issues of health and wholeness, respect for the body, responsibility, and respect for life in its fullest and richest dimensions are important to congregations that take health ministry seriously. When individuals and congregations are themselves healthy, or whole, they are more likely to be responsive to needs in the wider community.

### ■ Models of Health Ministry

Within the local congregation (church, mosque, or temple), health ministries often interact with smaller groups on formal and informal bases, such as age-appropriate faith educational classes, women's and men's services, prayer groups, governing councils, and congregational staffs. Incorporating appropriate health concerns with these groups may occur as a consequence of identifying needs in a particular group, media or public policy concerns, or the prompting of a health professional such as the community health nurse. For example, a group of women who have a women's prayer circle may have concerns about menopause changes.

There are as many examples of health ministry activities a congregation can initiate as there are creative ideas within the congregation. The vision of a **congregational health partnership** is enhanced by the input of many different people, often bringing their personal and professional gifts to the enterprise (Abrums, 2004; Couture, 2003). Starting a health ministry can have a galvanizing effect on a community; few people are politically opposed to health, and the resultant shared goals have the serendipitous effect of forging bonds in disparate groups within the community. Knowledge of how systems, subsystems, and interfaces operate is invaluable, as is expertise in group behavior and a sense of humor. Most of all, the effort is more likely to come to fruition if goals are mutually agreed upon in advance. For example, a group of ministers within a church district may be having stress-related health concerns. The nurse could meet with the

> **❝** *Rise and go your way: your faith has made you well.* **❞**
> —Jesus, in response to a Samaritan who was healed and then threw himself at Jesus's feet and thanked him, Luke 17:19

> **❝** *I confused things with their names: that is belief.* **❞**
> —Jean-Paul Sartre

group and assist them in identifying concerns and developing networks within the larger church community as results.

Health promotion at all levels of promotion is a good place to begin planning. Which resources can be matched with which needs? Which partnerships can be explored? There is good reason that many parish nurses have come from the ranks of community health nurses. They bring savvy, experience, and the ability to coalesce groups to the effort.

Health education in the church community takes the form of classes, literature, newsletters, and Web-based information. Support groups, especially those that are age focused, such as day care for preschool children or for elderly community members, make a real contribution to a community's well-being, as do issue-focused groups that provide a forum for shared experiences such as separation or bereavement.

Community service initiatives such as care teams, providing housing with Habitat for Humanity (a housing volunteer group), and Operation Read and Stephen's Ministries (literacy programs) are all health ministries. Giving space and time to support groups such as Alzheimer's caregivers and self-help groups, such as Alcoholics Anonymous, fills a larger community health need. Programs for children might focus on terrorism and its roots. Current events in the United States, such as Hurricane Katrina and the September 11, 2001, terrorist attacks should be addressed in health ministries. Classes on disaster planning should be offered as well.

### ■ Structure of Health Ministries

Congregations respond to the mandate for care in a variety of ways. In formal or informal fellowship, they generate discussion of areas of interest or concern within the congregation. Sometimes a single incident or experience in a faith

---

☝ THINK ABOUT THIS ·····················

Our common threads: How world religions express "The Golden Rule."

Christian: Do unto others as you would have them do unto you.

Bahai: Blessed are those who prefer others to themselves.

Buddhism: Hurt not others in ways that you yourself would find hurtful.

Judaism: What is hateful to you, do not do to your neighbor. That is the entire Torah. The rest is commentary. Go and learn.

Islam: No one is a believer until you desire for another that which you desire for yourself.

Sikhism: Be not estranged from one another for God swells in every heart.

Jainism: In happiness and suffering in joy and grief, regard all creatures as you would yourself.

---

**A Good Read**

## For One More Day (2006)

*By Mitch Albom, New York: Hyperion.*

What would we do if we had just 24 more hours to spend with our deceased loved ones? Author Mitch Albom gives us a glimpse into one suicidal man's experience of 24 hours with his mother, who died 12 years before.

community is an impetus for concerted dialogue or action. At other times one individual might be instrumental in stirring interest in a group that evolves into a working committee. The faith community as an entirety and the groups that function within it are representative of Lassiter's "established groups" (1996, p. 441). These groups have the advantage of existing bonds because they are members of the faith community. Members already know how groups function within the congregation, how to work together cooperatively, and who some of the effective leaders are. These ties and a common interest in health are helpful in the formation of a committee intentionally focusing on wellness (Couture, 2003).

A wellness committee gathers together persons with a common interest who are willing to further explore health and health-related issues. Wellness committees may be called Faith and Health Cabinets, Wholeness in Health Teams, Parish Nurse Advisory Committees, or Congregational Health Councils, among other names. Whatever the term, the purpose is that a group forms around the faith and health of the congregation—physical, emotional, and spiritual.

The membership of a wellness committee includes both lay and professional members. Seven to 12 persons generally

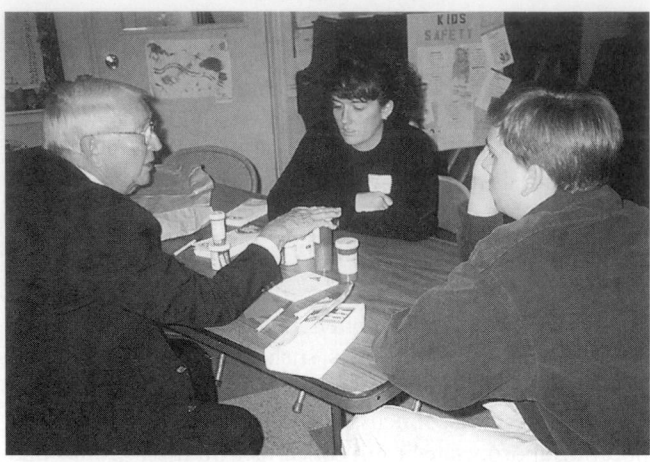

Pharmacist counseling church members at health fair about prescription drug therapy.

### Research Alert

In a recent study, researchers sought to examine the role of religious organizations in the provision of HIV/AIDS-related assistance in Africa. Data were collected from Christian religious organizations in southern Mozambique. Bivariate comparisons and logistic regression analysis of survey data were performed, and an analysis of the qualitative data complemented the quantitative data.

The analysis revealed little involvement of religious organizations in provision of assistance. Instead, most assistance was decentralized and consisted of psychological support and some personal care and household help. Material or financial help was rare. Assistance to nonmembers of congregations was reported more often than to members. Members of larger and better secularly connected congregations were more likely to report assistance than were members of smaller and less secularly engaged ones. Assistance was reported more in cities than in rural areas. Women were more likely to report assisting congregation members than men were, but the reverse was true for assistance provided to nonmembers. The cooperation of religious organizations in provision of assistance was hindered by financial constraints and institutional rivalry. The conclusion and implications for policy were to involve religious organizations in provision of HIV/AIDS-related assistance by taking into account that organization's resources, institutional goals, and social characteristics.

*Source:* Agadjianian, V., & Sen, S. (2007). Promises and challenges of faith-based AIDS care and support in Mozambique. *American Journal of Public Health, 97*(2), 362–366.

work well together. Membership should represent the life and interests of the congregation as well as various health disciplines. The charge is to uncover the many dimensions of what it means to be a healthy and caring congregation. Nurses, social workers, physicians, dentists, hospice workers, caregivers, widows, youth, childcare staff, clergy, and representatives of the church governing body are all potential volunteer professionals who can lead rich discussions for program planning.

The initial assessment of the congregation needs to include any previous surveys or assessments of the congregation and the components within it. A simple walk by the nurse with members elicits comments that are invaluable in assessing the values and priorities of individuals:

"This room is a lively place when the young moms get together, watch their little ones play, and talk about the joys and challenges of parenting."

"I recall when Alice began the first home-delivered meals for our town in this church kitchen."

"This mural of names painted by youth is so important to the Fellow and Senner families because the names of their deceased children are there."

"This is where the Women's AA group meets."

In addition to listening and recording, taking a visual survey of spiritually significant symbols and items is helpful. An environmental assessment would include indoor and outdoor signage, physical accessibility, reading materials, lighting, and emergency equipment.

Following the walk-through, an important next step is to acknowledge and catalogue the skills, gifts, talents, and possible capabilities of members and groups within the church. This approach, patterned after the **assets mapping** described by Kretzman and McKnight (1993; Ammerman & Parks, 1998), emphasizes the strengths and abilities of the congregation and will form the framework of subsequent possibilities and activities. The model emphasizes both strengths and competencies. The assets mapping model is particularly adaptable to faith communities because terms such as *gifts,*

## CULTURAL CONNECTION

### Caring for People of the Muslim Faith

Those who practice the religion of Islam are called Muslims; there are approximately 1.1 billion Muslims worldwide. Some 10–26% of Muslims are Arab; the majority of Muslims worldwide are Asian or African. Islam is one of the largest and fastest-growing religions in North America, yet nurses in the United States are often unfamiliar with the cultural needs of this faith.

Islamic beliefs include the revealed word of God to the Prophet, Muhammad, and are based on the belief in one God, Allah. *Islam* means surrender or obedience to the will of God. Its scripture is called the Quran and is considered God's revelation to the Prophet Muhammad through the Angel Gabriel, which began in about the year A.D. 610.

Muslims strive to live their lives in surrender to Allah through the five basic pillars or requirements of the faith: the affirmation that "there is no god but God, and Muhammad is the Messenger of God; the five daily ritual prayers; the giving of alms to the poor; the observance of Ramadan (fasting from dawn to sunset during the month of Ramadan); and the religious pilgrimage to Mecca. Muslims see Muhammad as the continuation of a lineage of prophets including Adam, Noah, Abraham, Moses, David, and Jesus, so they seek a sense of community with the People of the Book, including Jews and Christians. Jihad is a duty to God and is to be both individual and communal.

Health is very much a part of Muslims' everyday life, from food practices, exercise, and the seeking of outside medical treatment for illness. Modesty through dress customs is often the most unfamiliar practice to U.S. nurses when interacting with Muslim families. There is considerable diversity in dress according to individual and cultural identities. Both men and women are modest and uncomfortable with unnecessary body exposure. Women may wear a body covering called a *hijaab,* a *burka'a,* and the *khumar.* The specific wearing of these garments is cultural rather than religious. Diet restrictions include consumption of only kosher or halal-prepared meat, as well as prohibition of pork and alcohol. Muslims should be well informed and provided alternatives in the use of medications that contain alcohol.

Islamic teachings regulate relationships between men and women. It is preferred to have healthcare providers who are of the same sex as the patient and Muslim if possible.

When a patient is dying, in either the home or the hospital, the nurse can respect the Muslim faith by turning the patient on his or her right side to face Mecca and allowing visitors to recite the prayer of allegiance to Allah. When death occurs, the body must be covered at all times. Muslims prefer that only health professionals of the same gender as the patient touch the body. Preparations are extensive and include washing and perfuming the body and then wrapping it in a white sheet by family members of the same gender. Autopsies are usually not performed and the body is buried with a simple prayer. The body is buried directly into the ground without a coffin, again facing Mecca. All of this takes place within a very short period of time, often within hours after death. The bereavement period is confined to 3 days and children are not exposed to death or death rituals.

Nurses in the community should ask the patients and families of the Muslim faith which practices are comforting for them. One suggestion is to ask: "Do you have spiritual or religious beliefs that are important for your health care?" and respond in kind. ◯

*Source*: Ott, B. B., Al-Khadhuri, B., & Al-Junaibi, S. (2003). Preventing ethical dilemmas: Understanding Islamic health care practices. *Pediatric Nursing, 29*(3), 227–230.

## *a conversation with . . .*

### Elisabeth Kübler-Ross

It's only when we truly know and understand that we have a limited time on earth—and that we have no way of knowing when our time is up—we will then begin to live each day to the fullest, as if it was the only one we had.

There is no joy without hardship. If not for death, would we appreciate life? If not for hate, would we know the ultimate goal is love? . . . At these moments, you can either hold on to negativity and look for blame, or you can choose to heal and keep on loving.

The most beautiful people we have known are those who have known defeat, known suffering, known struggle, known loss, and have found their way out of the depths. These persons have an appreciation, a sensitivity, and an understanding of life that fills them with compassion.

*Elisabeth Kübler-Ross*
*is a pioneer in research of death*
*experiences in children and adults.*

*talents, interests,* and *journeys* or *experiences* are common language in congregations. Members have opportunities to share their skills in church activities and may be able to redirect the skills to achieve new goals. Focusing on the capabilities, talents, and potentials of selected populations motivates the community or, in this case, the congregation and wellness committee to view healthy potential outcomes.

Traditionally, assessments result in the generation of a number of problems or needs. Community health nurses also engage in assessments that include multiple sources of data, such as demographics, health status indicators, group beliefs, and expressed needs. A concentrated effort to build on the identified strengths of the congregation is important. These interests and abilities, which represent positive assets endorsed by Kretzmann and McKnight (1993), would also yield comprehensive involvement in health outcomes with traditional methods. Successful use of traditional community health nursing assessment processes with faith communities has been described by Miskelly (1995). This program skillfully employed the needs assessment process and incorporated *Healthy People 2000* objectives in an assessment for

### ETHICAL CONNECTION

Health ministry programs are often associated with specific religious denominations (e.g., Catholic, Protestant). How can community health nurses implement healthy lifestyles in the role of a parish or missionary nurse when the specific religious doctrine contradicts the nurse's values about health and disease intervention?

program planning within the church community. Interventions such as education, support groups, and counseling can be effectively constructed around strengths and needs identified in the assessment.

Additional assessment information may be gained from the experiences of others who have embarked on health ministry services. The denominational or national faith community body can be contacted. Surveys of websites, literature, and videos are helpful as well, and selected resources are noted at the end of this chapter. The committee could also ask a nurse to attend one of the meetings to assess the ways in which the congregation might benefit from this resource (Abrums, 2004).

Health fairs are often a valuable first activity for the wellness committee. Not only do they engage a large number of persons in providing and receiving help at one time, but they also serve to create awareness of a wide variety of issues. In addition, health fairs generate data that are helpful for further planning and evaluation. The scope of the activity can be very broad and comprehensive to involve multiple congregational members who have a personal interest in health and wholeness. The events can also include agencies represented in the community. In some cases, health fairs focus on narrower topics and thus respond to very intentional wishes and concerns that are identified.

Health fair at church provides opportunities for the nurse to discuss drug use with children.

## Relationship Between Community Health Nursing and Faith Communities

### ■ Parish Nursing

An appropriate and challenging intervention for the community health nurse is putting the theological foundations of health ministries into action. Given that the professional discipline of nursing incorporates the physical, emotional, cultural, and spiritual domains of practice, and because professional nursing partners with professionals from a variety of disciplines and community members with varying life experiences, health ministry activities are a natural arena for nurses working in community-based and population-focused practice.

**Parish nursing** is one response to the societal trends and healthcare delivery system changes of the last decades of the twentieth century. During the mid-1980s, professional nursing practice expanded into more independent practice arenas with the development of nursing centers, and parish nursing evolved out of holistic health centers. The movement's early beginnings included both the model of six congregations guided by Lutheran General Hospital of Chicago, and the collaborative efforts in rural Iowa with the Northwest Center on Aging. By the mid-1990s, more than 2,000 parish nurses were serving congregations in the United States as well as other countries; the nurses were in faith communities that included Christian, Muslim, and Jewish gatherings. Today parish nurses are often key facilitators in health ministries of faith communities (Patterson, 2006).

### MEDIA MOMENT

***What Dreams May Come*** (1998)
This movie features Robin Williams and his search for heaven after losing his own life, and the lives of his children and his wife. Cuba Gooding, Jr., is the angel who guides his journey into the afterlife and search for his family, which is his "heaven." The movie does not venture into specific religious doctrine, which allows for people of all faiths to appreciate the experience of good and evil in a beautifully filmed story.

***Oh, God!*** (1977)
This movie stars George Burns as God and John Denver as his unwilling messenger. Although it is a comedy, the movie deals with important topics such as the relevance of God and the Bible in today's society.

❝ *I've looked at life from both sides now*
*From win and lose, and still somehow*
*It's life's illusions I recall*
*I really don't know life at all.* ❞

—*Joni Mitchell, Both Sides Now, 1969*

☝ THINK ABOUT THIS ······························

Where do I start? How do health ministries really "get off the ground"?

1. **Start small.** Focus on a minimum of time, money, and people. Start with blood pressure screening; involve the congregation in the planning and involvement of the activity.

2. **Be visible at all times.** This can be done easily with a monthly bulletin board in the religious structure, which features new information about healthy lifestyles each month.

3. **Don't waste time.** Avoid meetings if possible; do not get bogged down in structure, policy, and committees, which can lead to unnecessary work and time. Most health ministries are made up of volunteers; requiring too many meetings, and creating too much structure can lead to burnout and lack of participation from church members.

4. **Ask others what you need.** Many health projects can be very inexpensive if you ask local businesses to provide services or goods in exchange for public recognition of their donation. Health fairs are excellent ways to involve the religious community.

5. **Play it safe.** Avoid hands-on care; make home visits, use referrals and consultation as primary interventions, and focus on education. Avoid any medical treatments and always make sure you are covered through the religious organization's insurance.

6. **Know your congregation.** Do assessments of members' needs often, and plan health projects *with* them, not *for* them.

7. **Document all health-related activities** associated with health ministry, no matter how small. This practice provides the nurse and the ministry with outcome data that serve as evidence of effectiveness and promote continuation of health services.

8. **Think broadly.** Include health professionals in community and congregation, as well as those who are interested in health. Keep your "arms open" for health ministry involvement.

9. **Don't give up.** Ministers and congregations come and go, priorities change, and some programs are successful and some are not. Keep your eye on the long-term goal of keeping spirituality and health as an expected part of ministries. 🔘

*Source*: Adapted from Klammer, L. M. (January 2006). Starting a church ministry. *Clergy Journal*.

·······························································

## A Good Read

# A Faith Like Mine: A Celebration of the Worlds' Religions Through the Eyes of Children (2005)

*By Laura Buller, New York: DK Publishing.*

This book provides an illuminating and comprehensive look at the world's many and diverse religions through the eyes of children. It gives parents and caregivers a theological tour of faith as seen through the perspectives of children growing up in each of the religious traditions. From Buddhism, Islam, Judaism, Christianity, and Sikhism to lesser-known religions, such a Zoroastrianism and Shintoism, hardly any religions are left out. Having a clearer view of what it means to be people of "faith" can provide nurses and others with an introduction to the world's faiths and an appreciation of how much they all have in common. Respect for life, beauty, tradition, and a reassuring faith emerge as common patterns that can promote understanding and acceptance for all faiths, even as we embrace our differences. 🔘

The document entitled *Scope and Standards of Parish Nursing*, prepared by the Health Ministries Association (HMA), was adopted by the American Nurses Association in 1998. The HMA is a professional interfaith organization that encourages faith communities to work with professionals, lay individuals, and agencies to promote health and wellness. Both nurses and others interested in health ministries make up its membership. The 1998 document describes to the profession and to the public this evolving "specialty practice

of nursing and of health ministry" (HMA/ANA, 1998, p. 3). Further, the document clearly describes the independent practice of nursing, as defined by the jurisdiction's nursing practice act, in health promotion within the context of the patient's values, beliefs, and faith practices. The patient focus of a parish nurse is the faith community, including its family and individual members and the community it serves (p. 3).

Basic preparation courses recommended for the parish nurse and endorsed by the International Parish Nurse Resource Center consist of at least 30 hours of coursework in parish nursing. Information can be obtained from this center, which advocates, develops, and promotes quality programs and current resources. The center provides consultation and is on the cutting edge of research in parish nursing. The annual Westberg Symposium provides the valued benefits of education and networking. Spiritual maturity, professional practice experience, competent communication and negotiation skills, and a commitment to assessment of personal holistic health are necessary to achieve success in parish nursing.

Parish nursing's philosophy first of all maintains that the spiritual dimension is central to the practice (Patterson, 2006; Solari-Twadell & McDermott, 1999); see Box 43-2. The intentional and compassionate caring of nursing evolves from the spiritual dimension inherent in all humankind.

Second, parish nurses affirm that their focus is the faith community and its ministry. Third, strengths of the congregation are seen as paramount. The fourth component supports congregational and community partnerships that become vital aspects of programs. The fifth component addresses the continuous, dynamic process among health, spiritual health, and healing. From the philosophy, parish nurses have a basis for appropriate educational and experience preparation, for functions of the specialty, and for wide-reaching health ministry activities.

## ■ Activities of Parish Nurses

In collaboration with the wellness committee, the parish nurse assists with and often initiates the effort for the congregational assessment. The appendix to this chapter shows an assessment form compiled by a wellness committee. The committee reviewed survey forms and guidelines and decided that it wanted a manageable questionnaire that could be administered during a 10-minute period of the worship service. It also wanted to offer options that were nonthreatening and readily acceptable by persons with a wide experience of wellness and illness. Thus nonthreatening educational literature was offered and followed by classes and support groups. Topics were intermingled; parenting, spiritual support practices, caregiving, and chronic illnesses were listed with concerns such as substance abuse, mental illness, communicable disease, violence, and disaster preparedness that are more often inadequately addressed in communities. The resulting health questionnaire can be altered to meet the unique wishes or interests of any wellness committee and its congregation. The survey should be evaluated, its results prioritized, and a report submitted with recommendations for

## ❝ *a conversation with . . .* ❞

*Donna Doherty, MSN, RN*

### Working with Patients of Different Faiths

The following home health story will challenge your approach to religious beliefs with your patients and within yourself. Nursing is more than science. It is a true healing art that touches the soul when practiced with love.

Allen M. was an 84-year-old man who was dying. He had lived a full life and had personal photos on the walls with presidents, mayors, governors, and movie stars. He was comfortable with himself and his surroundings. He always had a smile. His walls were covered with hundreds of books, books on every subject. His paintings and drawings mirrored a love of life and people that I rarely have seen.

Allen practiced a healing modality called Reiki. He would constantly send energy and prayers for other people even though he was very ill. He would say, "In healing others, I heal myself." His favorite reply to good conversation was, "That's beautiful."

Every day that I visited, as his home health nurse, was an eye-opening experience. Most days Allen would be in prayerful meditation. He would be kneeling in front of an altar on his sun porch . . . soft music playing, incense burning, a Chinese gong standing on the altar, a laughing Buddha in position, and an artificial waterfall in place. This made the area an optimal healing environment for him.

I would assess his health status, answer questions, and teach him information about his illness. In the course of evaluating issues that were of concern to him, the conversation turned to the terminal part of his illness. He openly discussed funeral plans. I had assumed that he would have a Buddhist service. I was surprised to learn that he had been a lifelong Episcopalian. His church had been planning an elaborate service. He was very pleased with this but he wanted to honor the Buddhist part of his life. He asked me to help him plan the service. It would be a memorial ceremony.

The conflicts in me arose. Would I be dishonoring my beliefs in honoring his? Was it really my place to help Allen with this task? Nurses are placed in unusual circumstances sometimes. I prayed about this and in doing so realized that the greatest gift that we have been given is free will. Right or wrong, good or bad, we can choose who we are. The freedom that Allen demonstrated in his personal worship was dear to him. He had lived a full life in service to others. He never forced his views on others.

I carry these special memories with me always. Honoring the spiritual beliefs of my patients comes naturally to me. If I had constructed a boundary between the spiritual belief, it would not have served any purpose but to create a stagnation in the healing process. I allow the spiritual interaction to flow like water, always moving, cleansing, and ending at its natural conclusion.

The memorial service was, in Allen's words, "beautiful."

CULTURAL CONNECTION

### Prayers from the World's Religions

When you arise in the morning, give thanks for the morning light, for your life and strength, give thanks for your food and the joy of living. If you see no reason for giving thanks, the fault is in yourself.

—Tecumseh, Native American

Mystery of Life, Source of All Being, we are thankful for the gifts of life and being, of love and connection. We are thankful for all the wonders of the world around us. We are thankful for each other and for all the members of our global family. As we make our Family Pledge, may we have eyes that see, hearts that love, and hands that are ready to serve in love and in kindness, with caring and with courage. Blessed Be.

—Unitarian Universalist Prayer

Even as a mother at the risk of her life watches over and protects her only child, so with a boundless mind should one cherish all living things. Let none by anger or hatred wish harm to another. May all beings be happy. May they live in safety, free from fear and distress.

—Buddhist Prayer

O Thou kind Lord! These lovely children are the handiwork of the fingers of Thy might and the wondrous signs of Thy greatness. O God, protect these children. Graciously assist them to be educated and enable them to render service to the world of humanity. O God, these children are pearls. Cause them to be nurtured within the shell of Thy loving kindness. Thou are the Bountiful, the All-Loving.

—Baha'I Prayer

All praise is due to You, our Lord, Guardian, and Cherisher of the Universe, who has sent the prophets to teach us how to live as full human beings. Make us among those who can truly say, "We hear and obey." Awaken in our hearts those attributes you love the best, and help us to be Merciful, Compassionate, Forgiving, Truthful, Just, and Patient with each other and with all those around us. Make us worthy to be counted in the community of Your Beloved, who said, "The best of you are those who are the best to their families."

—Islamic Prayer

Loving God, you sent Jesus to show us how to live in peace and love for one another. Jesus, you are our rock and our salvation. You showed us to love as you have loved us and to care for those who are less fortunate. You forgave those who hurt you. Your heart went out to people no one else cared about. Jesus, send us your Spirit to help each of us be truthful whenever we speak, loving whenever we act, and courageous whenever we find violence or injustice around us. We ask this in your holy name and that of the Father, the Son, and the Holy Ghost.

—Christian Prayer

O God, God of my brothers and sisters, relations and friends, God of my ancestors, God of all connections with all things; You, through all obstacles; You, in our emptiness and in our abundance; You, in our search for peace, You, We have given ourselves to sacred collation with You in the Repair of the world, *Tikkun*. As You make peace there, let there be peace among us, among all peoples, changing the world one person at a time, one family at a time, one community at a time, one world. Amen.

—Jewish Prayer

*This feature graciously edited by Jean Haspeslagh, DNS, RN.*

---

action. The implementations and outcomes should then be evaluated. This process would be repeated annually.

Overall, parish nurse services address health, wholeness, and healing within the context of the faith community served. With an emphasis on health promotion at all levels of prevention, the nurse considers individuals and families across the life span and partners with the congregation as community. Sometimes the parish nurse may even serve several congregations that may form a cluster or alliance.

In addition to working closely with wellness committees, usual functions of the parish nurse include personal health counseling, health education and teaching of personal lifestyle management skills, initiating and facilitating referrals to congregations and community resources, advocating and encouraging support resources, and integrating faith and health (Abrums, 2004; Berry, 1994; Solari-Twadell & McDermott, 1999). Providing pastoral care is a major priority. Nursing activities corresponding to these functions are valued by members of the faith community. Responsibilities of parish nurses include group programs; making visits

 *Got an Alternative?*

People are like stained glass windows. They sparkle and shine when the sun is out, but when the darkness sets in, their true beauty is revealed only if there is a light from within. There is no need to go to India or anywhere else to find peace. You will find that deep place of silence right in your room, your garden, or even your bathtub.

—Elizabeth Kübler-Ross

Research has associated stained glass with inducing relaxation and a sense of peaceful self-consciousness and promoting meditation. How can our knowledge of the influence of color be used in creating a therapeutic environment for our patients, either in a healthcare facility, in a church, or at home?

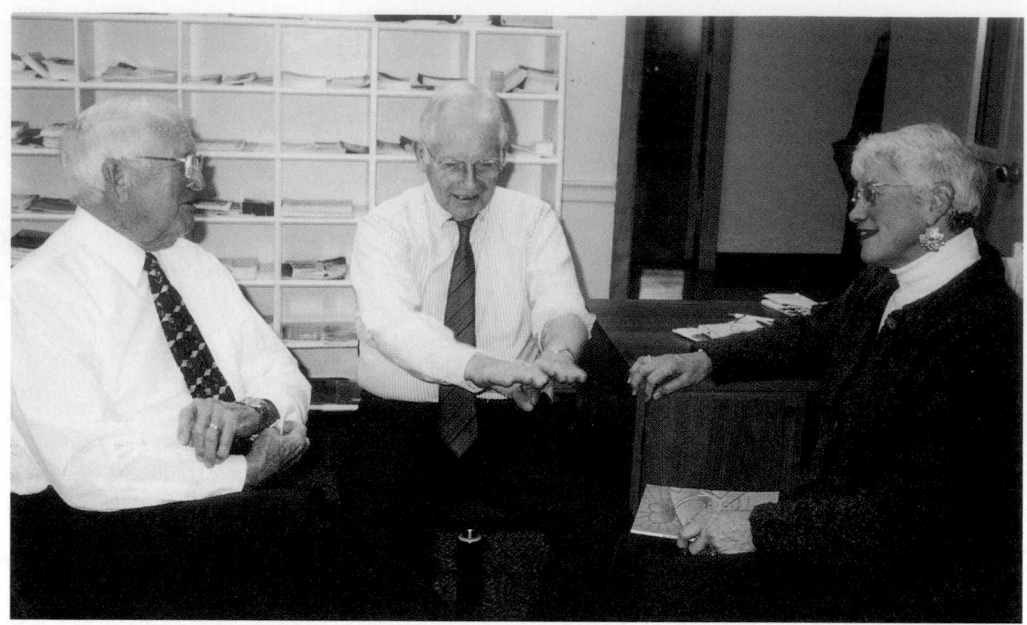

Chapter author Ruth Berry (right) counseling church members between church services.

## ENVIRONMENTAL CONNECTION

Expand your definition of environment to include the physical and symbolic aspects of a church or religious gathering place. How does the religious "environment" affect the health and well-being of the church population?

to homes, hospitals, and nursing homes; meeting regularly with the pastoral staff; and participating in worship services of the community. The implementation of both the concept of the specialty and the functions of the practice has resulted in creative, innovative, compassionate activities and nursing interventions (Berry, 1994; Culp, 1997; Klammer, 2006; Magilvy & Brown, 1997; Patterson, 2006; Solari-Twadell, Truty, & Ryan, 1994; Weis, Matheus, & Schank, 1997).

Nurses as community health nurses working in health ministries incorporate these community-based and population-focused roles in the practice with faith communities. Nurses may monitor care provided by other providers to ensure members the most seamless care possible and communicate with healthcare providers, discharge planners, family members, and others. They may also engage congregation members in posthospital supportive activities at home. To embrace the population focus as well, the skills of partnering with community members and agencies, advocating for the most appropriate framework of care, facilitating health promotion at all three levels of prevention, and evaluating results are important components of parish nurse practice.

While assisting the congregation to strive for positive physical, spiritual, and emotional health outcomes, the parish nurse experienced in community health can interpret and incorporate the goals of *Healthy People 2010* (Magilvy & Brown, 1997; Marty, 1990; Miskelly, 1995; DHHS, 1998; Weis,

**"** *Our scientific power has outrun our spiritual power. We have guided missiles and misguided men.* **"**
—Martin Luther King, Jr.

**"** *During a very busy week in November 1889, sister-nurses from the Congregation of the Sisters of Charity of the Incarnate Word at St. Joseph's Infirmary, Fort Worth, Texas, admitted 19 patients, discharged 6 patients, and cared for the 24 patients already there. Many of the patients were critically ill and the nurses were frantically trying to care for all the needs of the patients. This prompted one nurse to remark, 'Our heels are praying very hard all day.'* **"**

B. M. Wall & S. Nelson. (2003). Our heels are praying hard all day. Holistic Nursing Practice, 17(6), 320–328.

et al., 1997). The numerous objectives that target schools, workplace, and communities with health issues, which are also likely represented in the congregation, are readily addressed in faith communities for reasons mentioned in the description of the structure of health ministries. Put simply, faith communities should become aware of the leading health indicators included in *Healthy People 2010*. Congregations will continue endeavors to achieve these goals because they are consistent with overall missions of justice and mercy in faith communities. The integration of responsibility for individual and collective health and wholeness is consistent with eliminating health disparities, increasing quality and years of healthy life, improving systems for personal and public health, and promoting healthy behaviors and communities (Klammer, 2006; Patterson, 2006).

## ■ Missionary Nursing*

A discussion of health ministries and parish nursing would be incomplete without reviewing the role of missionary nurses. In the United States, the number of nurses who serve/work as missionary nurses continues to increase yearly. Exact figures are unavailable because these nurses may serve/work on a private, local, state, national, or international level. Another reason that exact numbers are unavailable is to protect the safety of missionary nurses, some of whom work in countries where their faith is at risk due to unstable political environments.

Many of the major denominations in the United States have nurses who serve/work as missionary nurses. Examples include the International Mission Board of the Southern Baptist Convention, the Presbyterian Church in America, the General Board of Global Ministries, and the United Methodist Church.

Some missionary nurses may serve/work on a short-term or part-time basis, for a period of weeks or months. Many work full time in other nursing roles and participate in focused mission projects on their vacation days or take temporary leave time to do so. These short-term or part-time missionary nurses routinely participate in mission trips to areas of the United States or to areas abroad (e.g., Mexico, Honduras, Ukraine) where underprivileged and underserved populations are in dire need of food, clothes, medicine, and health care. The missionary teams that travel to these areas to meet the specific needs of patients and communities include various combinations of nursing, medical, surgical, dental, and lay people. Each mission trip is as unique as the patients and communities to which it ministers. Interpreters are used, as needed, to overcome language and cultural barriers. Often, makeshift healthcare clinics are set up in churches, in schools, or outside under canopies. Many of these clinics are primitive; others may be equipped with some modern technology, if electricity is available. Missionary teams may not only provide health care, but also assist with the building of churches, houses, and schools.

Other missionary nurses may be career missionary nurses, working for years or even a lifetime in this capacity. Missionary nurses may work as a "home missionary" in the United States or as a "foreign missionary" in other countries. Career (i.e., full-time) missionary nurses who work abroad become totally immersed in the culture of the people whom they serve and learn to speak the native language fluently. Many of the foreign countries in which they reside are impoverished, war-torn, and desperate for physical, nursing,

The stained glass of the windows at Notre Dame Cathedral in Paris, France depicts spiritual connectedness to the Creator, light, warmth, comfort, conscience, hope, and continuity. Stained glass has long been part of organized religion.

medical, and spiritual attention. Missionary nurses who work full-time often find themselves in unsafe conditions owing to governments that are resistant to outside interventions.

## ■ Roles and Practice of Missionary Nurses

Missionary nurses focus on meeting the physical, spiritual, and emotional needs of their patients. They often report that serving in this role provides almost indescribable personal fulfillment and job satisfaction and consider missionary nursing to be a "calling." These nurses often refer to **missionary nursing** as "pure nursing," unencumbered by the demands of paperwork, documentation, and other system restraints. Nursing schools are seeing an increase in the number of students who seek to become missionary nurses or who begin mission work as nursing students during school vacations; many nursing students receive credit for clinical hours by participating in mission trips. Missionary nursing is based on the principles and philosophy of community health nursing.

The needs of patients and communities vary greatly, depending on the location, culture, economy, type of government, and access to affordable health care. Missionary nurses must be committed to serving and ministering to the differing needs of patients and communities with diverse

GLOBAL CONNECTION

Missionary nursing is a specialty within health ministries. How can nurses provide care in other cultures and faiths than their own without experiencing ethical and professional conflicts?

*This section (from pp. 1093–1096) is authored by Barbara Foster, RN, MSN, Instructor, Division of Associate Degree Nursing, Copiah–Lincoln Community College, Wesson, Mississippi, and adapted from Lundy, K. S., Sutton, V., & Foster, B. (2003). The nurse's role in ambulatory health settings. In K. S. Lundy & S. Janes (Eds.), *Essentials of community-based nursing* (pp. 259–291). Sudbury, MA: Jones and Bartlett.

## Application to Practice

### *A Health Fair: Medicines and More*

"Medicines and More" was the result of interest expressed on the part of members of the Wellness Committee of Second Presbyterian Church, Lexington, Kentucky. Comments from a retired health professional and from an older adult caregiver noted that they were concerned about numerous conversations and observations regarding confusion with medications. Quickly, the committee's discussion included stories of inquiries regarding multiple names for medicines, complex over-the-counter preparations, duplicate medicines for the same ailment, values and dangers of herbal preparations, problems eating or not eating food with medicines, medication errors indicating the need for reinforcement of emergency assistance, and others.

Members decided a fair would reach many people quickly. Although a major target was the older population, the committee believed that the information was valuable for members of all ages, for families as well as for individuals who were living alone. Because members already gathered on Sunday mornings for educational and worship services and because many elderly persons regularly participated in the monthly "Retirees Lunch," it was decided to plan the event to coincide with established habits. The committee further decided that because they wanted to provide information applicable for all ages and for the total congregation, they would schedule the fair during and following the Retirees Lunch in a room adjacent to the dining room. Families and those members not participating in the lunch were guided directly to the fair location following worship service. Retirees would be the special fair participants after lunch.

Upon agreeing on a number of objectives, the members listed tasks and eagerly offered to take responsibility for the many jobs. These jobs included marketing and publicity, obtaining resources, volunteering for hosting the various exhibits, taking blood pressure readings, greeting community presenters, and monitoring flow on the day of the fair.

The parish nurse contacted the local health department nutritionist and the university's college of pharmacy. A pharmacy brown-bag event was very popular, and the nutritionist provided helpful information regarding food–medicine interaction, supplements, and herbal preparations. Committee members contacted a local hospital's home care agency for information on Lifeline emergency calling. The senior nursing student contacted the local police department for 9-1-1 guidelines, supplied various phones for demonstration and practice, and obtained literature and posters at the State Pamphlet Library. In collaboration with the parish nurse, a County Cooperative Extension "Look-a-Likes" display was updated. Children and adults were able to view models and a brochure depicting potentially dangerous and confusing foods, medicines, and household products.

To encourage participation at all exhibits and to obtain evaluation data, members who completed surveys were eligible to win loaves of whole-wheat variety breads. The committee reviewed the evaluations within 2 weeks, reported the results and extended thanks to planners and attendees in the congregation's newsletter, and gained information for planning future programs regarding nutrition and exercise.

Effective and enjoyable health fairs can be simpler or more elaborate than the one described. The community presenters gained a new resource for their information. Both the pharmacists and the nutritionist expressed that they had never envisioned the benefits of providing health information in a faith community setting, and the county's extension agency appreciated help in renewing their display and obtaining feedback for additional outreach options. Collaborating with these professionals and their agencies created new partnerships with mutual benefits.

### A Good Read

## Lessons from the Lotus Sutra

*Karen Rich, PhD, RN*

The *Lotus Sutra*, one of the Buddha's last teachings, is sometimes referred to as the "King of Sutras" (Thich Nhat Hanh, 2003). In the *Lotus Sutra*, the Buddha introduced many bodhisattvas to his followers. A bodhisattva is an enlightened being who vows, though compassion, to help all other beings attain enlightenment. Bodhisattvas realize the teachings of the Buddha "to look and listen with the eyes of compassion" and understand that "compassionate listening brings about healing" (Thich Nhat Hanh, 1998, p. 86).

In caring for elderly patients and populations, nurses can be compared to compassionate bodhisattvas that facilitate elders' well-being. Elders suffer from many losses in their lives, both large and small. Loss of loved ones, health, mobility, beauty, and status are only a few of these losses. Although their patients' losses may go unnoticed by nurses, the events can have intense effects on elderly patients. Simmons (2000) has called "the work of learning to live richly in the face of loss . . . learning to fall" (p. xi). Letting go can be terrifying for elders. Living can be terrifying, too, because one must learn to let go to live.

The ubiquitous losses and changes that occur with old age can result in anxiety about life's unpredictability. Elderly patients must depend on and trust in the moral goodness of healthcare professionals even when they are confronted with attitudes of ageism and when their care is not given serious consideration because no cure can be achieved. When an elder reacts to these insults by developing a hardened resistance toward life's fluctuations, impermanence, and loss, the outcome may be anger and depression.

Compassion is the desire to separate others from suffering and the desire for others to experience well-being. Like the bodhisattvas described in the *Lotus Sutra*, compassionate nurses can dedicate themselves to helping patients overcome suffering and its causes. Nurses who exhibit the virtue of compassion can help elders learn to relax in the face of life's changes rather than tightening into an unhealthy resistance. All people suffer, yet all people desire well-being regardless of their age. "Compassion is not a relationship between the healer and the wounded. It is a relationship between equals" (Chodron, 2001, p. 50).

Compassion requires communicating with patients from one's heart. For many elders, the world is a lonely place with no one to listen to their feelings or understand their lives. Nurses who have a sincere desire to take action to alleviate the suffering of this vulnerable group are widening the circle of compassion in the world. Research has shown that elders have a higher response to placebo treatment than is normally expected (Soloman, 2001). This higher response has been attributed to the attention that elderly persons receive because of their participation in research studies. Elders must be very lonely indeed for this slight attention to be so important to them.

Unpredictability is inherent in the daily life of elders, and impermanence and loss have a glaring presence that is difficult for the aged to ignore. Nurses might do well to remember the teachings of the *Lotus Sutra* when caring for elderly individuals and populations—to look and listen with the eyes of compassion and that compassionate listening brings about healing.

Karen Rich, PhD, RN
Assistant Professor
The University of Southern Mississippi School of Nursing
Hattiesburg, Mississippi

---

**❝** *They must be true Nurses to be true Missionaries.* **❞**
—*Florence Nightingale, 1892*

cultures and populations. The primary purpose of missionary nursing is to meet the spiritual, physical, and emotional needs of persons in need throughout the world.

Communication skills and therapeutic communication are essential to the role of missionary nurses. Often, different languages and cultures represent barriers to communication. Missionary nurses must exhibit flexibility, patience, and a willingness to work within different health systems. Patients' values regarding health and nursing roles are often dramatically different from the values of the nurse. Missionary nurses tend to focus on basic professional values, such as compassion and nonjudgmental attitudes, rather than the

proscribed roles typical in U.S. health care, so as to provide culturally appropriate care.

Missionary nurses utilize population-based skills of the community health nurse, such as community assessment, to provide culturally relevant care as defined by the community. Specific needs are then prioritized by the community and the mission healthcare team. Collaboration among fellow members of the missionary team and community members enables missionary nurses to plan ways to meet specific needs, often in a very short time span. Goals may be set so as to meet the needs of these communities on a short-term basis and then provide direction for subsequent mission trips.

Missionary nurses may utilize and apply nursing research and outcomes management in various ways. For example, the specific needs of various populations and diverse cultures may be compared on private, local, state, national, and international levels. Data may be analyzed and used in different ways to meet the unique needs of each culture and population group. Various caring interventions and missionary nursing activities then focus on these findings to provide needed services.

Missionary nurses should learn all they can about the cultures of the populations and communities they serve, both prior to leaving their home country and after comparing this information upon arrival. Teaching is also an important component of missionary nursing. For example, in some countries cholera is a constant threat to the health of a community, so missionary nurses may teach ways to prevent cholera. Language and cultural barriers are frequently encountered and must be overcome to enable nurses to establish helping, trusting relationships.

Missionary nurses may formally or informally manage the care of patients and communities from diverse cultures. Managing care requires spiritual maturity, therapeutic communication, negotiation skills, and a personal commitment to the overall health and well-being of patients and communities. Missionary nurses pay particular attention to the spiritual needs of patients. Whenever possible, basic needs, such as food, water, clothing, and housing, are provided.

## Conclusion

New and innovative endeavors are emanating out of the convergence of faith and health in health ministries. Growth of the partnerships between health and faith came about because of the increasing need to fill the ever-widening

gaps brought about by economic and legislative constraints. Faith communities' history of caring and volunteerism were sought to be part of the solution to healthcare access, especially in health education, health promotion, and advocacy. Welfare reform legislation certainly demanded numerous community responses to care for those who could not speak for themselves.

Faith communities are also beginning to be seen as a neutral place to increase awareness of justice and social concern in relation to health care. The confusion and dilemmas brought about by the changes and complexity of the healthcare delivery system have created consumers at all economic levels who are poorly informed about how to navigate and use the system. Community health nursing has emerged as significant participant in these new developments. Nursing's traditional concern for the disadvantaged and underserved coincides with the mandate of the faith communities to care for those same populations. Creative forms of health ministries allow nurses to carve out innovative roles, thereby bringing the best of community health nursing to the task.

Explore Community Health Nursing on the Web! To learn more about the topics in this chapter, use the passcode provided to access your exclusive website: **http://nursing.jbpub.com/ communityhealth.** If you do not have a passcode, you can obtain one at this site.

## ■ CRITICAL THINKING ACTIVITIES

1. Identify a health problem in your home community that could be addressed by building a potential partnership with a local faith community.
   - In what ways could a faith community address the problem to enhance public sector efforts?
   - What kind of partnerships could be forged with the faith community to enhance their contribution?

- What are the steps that need to be taken to initiate a plan?
- How will your own faith experience influence your participation?

## ■ REFERENCES

Abrums, M. (2004). Faith and feminism: How African American women from a storefront church resist oppression in health care. *Advances in Nursing Science, 27*(3), 187–201.

Ammerman, A., & Parks, C. (1998). Preparing students for more effective community interventions: Assets assessment. *Family and Community Health, 21,* 32–45.

Anderson, A. A. (1996). Florence Nightingale: Construction of a profession. *Anglican Theology and Review, 78*(3), 404–420.

Berry, R. (1994). A parish nurse. In Office of Resourcing Committee on Preparation for Ministry, *A day in the life of. . . . A kaleidoscope of specialized ministries* (pp. 38–49). Louisville, KY: Presbyterian Church (USA); Distribution Management Service.

Chandler, E. (1997). *Spirituality and well-being in older adults.* Unpublished doctoral dissertation. Claremont, CA: Claremont School of Theology.

Chandler, E. (1999). Care of dying patients and their families. In T. Buttaro, J. Trybulski, T. Bailey, & J. Kook (Eds.), *Primary care: A collaborative approach.* St. Louis: Mosby.

Chodron, P. (2001). *The places that scare you: A guide to fearlessness in difficult times.* Boston: Shambhala Publications.

Couture, P. (2003, January 7). *When public health and faith groups encounter each other: Overcoming obstacles.* Paper for the Carter Center Interfaith Health Working Group on Congregations and Public Health. Atlanta: Carter Center.

Culp, L. (1997). Health ministries: Caring for body and soul. *Registered Nurse Journal, 9,* 8.

Department of Health and Human Services (DHHS), Public Health Service. (1998, June). *Healthy people in communities: A guide for community leaders.* Washington, DC: U.S. Government Printing Office.

Dossey, B. M. (1998). Florence Nightingale: A 19th century mystic. *Journal of Holistic Nursing, 16*(2), 111–165.

Droege, T., & Wenger, A. F. Z. (1997). *Starting point, empowering communities to improve health: A manual for training health promoters in congregational coalitions.* Atlanta: Carter Center.

Gunderson, G. R. (1997). *Deeply woven roots: Improving the quality of life in your community.* Minneapolis: Fortress Press.

Gunderson, G. R. (1998). Aligning assets for community health improvement. *Medical Journal of Allina, 7*(4), 2–5.

Health Ministries Association/American Nurses Association (1998). *Scope and standards of parish nursing practice.* Washington, DC: American Nurses Publishing.

Kark, J. D., Shemi, G., Friedlander, Y., Martin, O., Manor, O., & Blondheim, S. H. (1996). Does religious observance promote health? Mortality in secular vs religious kibbutzim in Israel. *American Journal of Public Health, 86,* 341–346.

Klammer, C. M. (2006, January). Starting a church-health ministry. *Clergy Journal,* 14–18.

Koenig, H. G., Cohen, H. J., George, L. K., Hays, J. C., Larson, D. B., & Blazer, D. G. (1997). Attendance at religious services, interleukin-6, and other biological parameters of immune function in older adults. *International Journal of Psychiatry in Medicine, 27*(3), 233–250.

Kretzmann, J. P., & McKnight, J. L. (1993). *Building communities from the inside out: A path toward finding and mobilizing a community's assets.* Chicago: ACTA Publications.

Lassiter, P. G. (1996). Group approaches in community health. In M. Stanhope & J. Lancaster (Eds.), *Community health nursing: Promoting health of aggregates, families, and individuals* (4th ed., pp. 385–410). St. Louis: Mosby.

Macrae, J. (1995). Florence Nightingale's spiritual philosophy and its significance for modern nursing. *Image: Journal of Nursing Scholarship, 27*(1), 8–10.

Magilvy, J. K., & Brown, N. J. (1997). Parish nursing: Advanced practice nursing model for healthier communities. *Advanced Practice Nursing Quarterly, 2,* 67–72.

Marty, M. (Ed.). (1990). *Healthy people 2000: A role for America's religious communities.* Chicago: Park Ridge Center.

Miskelly, S. (1995). A parish nursing model: Applying the community health nursing process in a church community. *Journal of Community Health Nursing, 12,* 1–14.

Oman, D., & Reed, D. (1998). Religion and mortality among the community-dwelling elderly. *American Journal of Public Health, 88*(10), 1469–1475.

Ott, B. B., Al-Khadhuri, B., & Al-Junaibi, S. (2003). Preventing ethical dilemmas: Understanding Islamic health care practices. *Pediatric Nursing, 29*(3), 227–230.

Patterson, D. (2006, March). The head bone's connected to the heart bone: Parish nurses as teachers. *Clergy Journal,* 21–24.

Simmons, P. (2000). *Learning to fall: The blessings of an imperfect life.* New York: Bantam Books.

Solari-Twadell, P. A., & McDermott, M. A. (Eds.). (1999). *Parish nursing: Promoting whole person health within faith communities.* Thousand Oaks, CA: Sage.

Solari-Twadell, P. A., Truty, L., & Ryan, J. A. (1994). *Congregational health services.* Park Ridge, IL: Lutheran General Hospital.

Soloman, A. (2001). *The noonday demon: An atlas of depression.* New York: Scribner.

Strawbridge, W. J., Cohen, R. D., Shema, S. J., & Kaplan, G. A. (1997). Frequent attendance at religious services and mortality over 28 years. *American Journal of Public Health, 87*(6), 957–961.

Strawbridge, W. J., Shema, S. J., Cohen, R. D., Roberts, R. E., & Kaplan, G. A. (1998). Religiosity buffers effects of some stressors on depression but exacerbates others. *Journal of Gerontology, 53B*(3), S118–S126.

Thich Nhat Hanh. (1998). *The heart of the Buddha's teaching: Transforming suffering into peace, joy, and liberation.* New York: Broadway Books.

Thich Nhat Hanh. (2003). *Opening the heart of the cosmos: Insights on the Lotus Sutra.* Berkeley, CA: Parallax Press.

Wall, B. M., & Nelson, S. (2003). Our heels are praying very hard all day. *Holistic Nursing Practice, 17*(6), 320–328.

Weis, D., Matheus, R., & Schank, M. J. (1997). Health care delivery in faith communities: The parish nurse model. *Public Health Nursing, 14,* 368–372.

Wenger, A. F. Z. (1998). Cultural openness, social justice, global awareness: Promoting transcultural nursing with unity in a diverse world. In P. Merilainen & K. Vehvilainen-Julkunen (Eds.), *The 23rd annual nursing research conference 1997, Transcultural nursing—Global unifier of care, facing diversity with unity* (pp. 162–168). Kuopio, Finland: Kuopio University Publications.

Winslow, G. R., & Winslow, B. W. (2003). Examining the effects of praying with patients. *Holistic Nursing Practice, 17*(4), 170–177.

World Council of Churches. (1990). *Healing and wholeness: The churches' role in health.* Geneva: World Council of Churches.

Zinnbauer, B., Pargament, K., Cole, B., et al. (1997). Religion and spirituality: Unfuzzying the fuzzy. *Journal for the Scientific Study of Religion, 36*(4), 546–564.

## ■ INTERNET RESOURCES

Healthy People 2010: http://web.health.gov/healthypeople

Carter Center: www.cartercenter.org

International Parish Nurse Resource Center: www.parishnurses.org

Health Ministries Association: www.hmassoc.org

Wayne E. Oates Institute, Center for Study of Spirituality, Ethics and Pastoral Care: www.oates.org

🏛 APPENDIX
## Parish Nurse Service

## Health Questionnaire

Dear Friends

To plan for the ongoing wellness program parish nurse service, it is important to know what the congregation's needs are in regard to health issues. This questionnaire was designed to gather that information primarily from adults. Another survey will address the young people more specifically. We would appreciate your assistance in answering the following questions. All information will be anonymous and will be used for planning services for this congregation.

Please return your questionnaire today if at all possible. If you have any health-related concerns that you would like to discuss with the parish nurse, or if you would like to have literature we might have, please call the church, or leave a message so that the parish nurse will be able to contact you.

Thank you for your time and help.

Wellness Committee—Second Presbyterian Church
Ruth D. Berry, Parish Nurse

1. Classes, support groups, or information packets may be developed to meet interests and needs of people at Second Presbyterian Church to enhance physical, emotional, and spiritual health. Please indicate if you would be interested in any of the following. You may mark as many as you like.

_____Living with chronic illness            _____First aid

_____Adolescent health issues               _____Weight control

_____Coping with cancer                     _____Divorce recovery

_____Caring for elderly parents             _____Exercise groups

_____Parenting                              _____Normal aging process

_____Single parenting                       _____Values clarification

_____Step-parenting                         _____Healthy eating

_____Humor                                  _____Adult children of alcoholics

_____Substance abuse                        _____Living wills/advance directives

_____Alcoholics Anonymous                   _____Loss and grief

_____Smoking cessation                      _____Marriage enrichment

_____Interpersonal relationships            _____Prayer

_____Safe babysitting                       _____Bible study

_____Spiritual direction                    _____Healthcare access

_____Women's health issues                  _____Childbirth preparation

_____Men's health issues                    _____Values clarification

_____Childbirth preparation                 _____Memory disorders

_____Pre-retirement planning                _____Alzheimer's disease

_____CPR instruction                        _____Conflict resolution

_____Human sexuality                        _____Hormone replacement therapy

_____Psalm study                            _____Attention-deficit disorders

_____Coping with AIDS                       _____Other

**2.** Which of the health promotion classes or groups do you think that Second Presbyterian Church needs most? Place a star to the right of the item.

**3.** How would you rate your health? Excellent_____ Good_____ Fair_____ Poor_____

**4.** Do you engage in regular exercise? Yes_____ No_____

If yes, how often?_____

**5.** Do you have a regular physical exam? Yes_____ No_____

If yes, how often?_____

**6.** Do you have regular dental exams? Yes_____ No_____

If yes, how often?_____

**7.** Do you regularly wear a car seatbelt? Yes_____ No_____

**8.** Check any of the following conditions that you have or have had in the past:

| | |
|---|---|
| _____Heart disease | _____Allergies |
| _____High blood pressure | _____Depression |
| _____Arthritis | _____Lung disease |
| _____Diabetes | _____Physical disability |
| _____Cancer | _____Substance abuse |
| _____Emotional problems | _____Other |

Please provide the following information about yourself:

**9.** Sex: Male _____ Female _____

**10.** Age _____

**11.** Marital status: Single_____ Married_____ Separated_____ Divorced_____ Widow(er)_____

**12.** Education:

| | |
|---|---|
| _____Elementary | _____Two years college |
| _____High school | _____Four years college |
| _____Technical school | _____Beyond college |

**13.** Number of children at home:

| | | |
|---|---|---|
| _____ Younger than 1 year | _____6–10 years | _____15–18 years |
| _____1–4 years | _____11–14 years | _____Older than 18 years |
| _____5–6 years | | |

**14.** Employment:

| | |
|---|---|
| _____Not working | _____Work full-time |
| _____Work at home | _____Plan to retire in 5 years |
| _____Work part-time | _____Retired |

**15.** Which worship service do you usually attend?

| | | |
|---|---|---|
| _____8:30 A.M. | _____11:00 A.M. | _____Neither |

**16.** On which day of the week would you be interested in attending classes or a group?

Sun_____ M_____ Tu_____ W_____ Th_____ F_____ Sat_____

**17.** Would you need child care? Yes_____ No_____

**18.** Need transportation? Yes_____ No_____

**19.** Which health concern is most important to you?

_____Chronic illness            _____Related financial issues        _____Aging

_____Catastrophic illness       _____Stress                         _____Grief

_____Substance abuse            _____Fitness                        _____Other

**20.** Are there other topics that you would like the Wellness Committee to consider?

# Index

Page numbers in italics indicate figures; page numbers followed by *t* indicate tables; page numbers followed by *b* indicate boxes.

## A

AARP (American Association of Retired Persons), 863, 883, 988
Abandonment of elders, 519*b*
Abortions, *107*, 108, 692, 694, 694*t*
Absolutism, health education and, 342–43
Abstinence, 690
Abu Ghraib prison, 531
Abuse, protection from, 712
Abuse shelters, 133
Access to care
  for agricultural workers, 671–73
  barriers to, 122, 149*b*, 164–66, 237
  challenges of, 946
  health behaviors and, 811
  health plan coverage and, 145*t*
  *Healthy People 2010* objectives, 167
  influences on, 167–68
  insurance coverage and, 166
  meaning of, 626
  Medicare and Medicaid, 96, 807
  in rural communities, 661
  STDs and, 470
  in the U. S., 11, 941
  for vulnerable populations, 625*b*, 626, 646, 711, 787, 861
  waiting periods, 559
Accessibility, community-level, 720
Accident prevention, for the elderly, 883
Accountability, of school nurses, 1021
Accreditation. *See also* certification; licensing
  CAAHEP in, 127
  of home health agencies, 985–86
  of managed care organizations, 146–48
Acculturation, 681
Acquaintance rape, 793. *See also* date rape
Acquired immune deficiency syndrome (AIDS). *See* HIV/AIDS
Active humoral immunity, 429
Activism, 628
Activities of daily living (ADLs)
  assessment of, 892–93*t*
  description, 975

facilitation of, 562, 864
fatigue and, 553
Acute care settings
  advanced practice nurses in, 1072–73
  benefits for nurses, 15
  community health nursing *versus*, 15–16
  facilities for, 128
  home health nurses and, 972
  nurse practitioners in, 1069
  nursing interventions, 15*t*
Acute illnesses, 551–52
Ad Hoc Committee to Defend Health Care, 770
Adaptations, 725
Addiction, definition of, 480
Adherence, absolutism and, 342–43
Adjusted rates, 109–10
Administration for Children and Families (ACF), 194
Administration on Aging (AoA), 194
Administrative costs, 168
Administrative Orders of Consent (AOC), 22
Adolescence
  psychosocial development, 679
  research areas related to, 810*b*
  serious mental illness in, 916
  stages of, 679–80
  teenage female health issues, 789–92
Adolescent pregnancies, 678–703
  anticipatory guidance in, 791
  birth rates, 678, *678*
  community-based prevention programs, 690–92, 690*b*
  contraception information, 693*t*, 696–97
  costs of, 682
  data collection, 1014
  early detection of, 692, 693*t*
  economic disruption by, 686
  education disruption by, 686
  factors contributing to, 679–84
  family vulnerability and, 617
  fathers, 693*t*
  health outcomes, 684–86, 695–96
  HIV/AIDS risk and, 917
  impacts of, 684–87, 686
  nursing interventions, 687–89, 689*t*, 693*t*
  nutritional requirements, 694*b*
  options counseling, 692–94

  parenting education, 693*t*, 695
  postpartum care, 693*t*, 695
  prenatal care, 693*t*, 694–95
  psychosocial outcomes, 684–86, 685–86
  repeat, 685
  risk factors, 617
  in rural areas, 664–65
  sexual activity and, 693*t*, 696–97
  status of newborns, 693*t*
  support, 693*t*
Adolescents
  alcohol use by, 481*b*
  chronic illness and, 554–55
  drug use by, 482
  environmental factors, 680–84
  families of, 681
  as fathers, 682–83, 686–87, 693*t*, 926
  feelings of immortality, 790–91
  high-risk behaviors, 1006
  homeless, 646
  intentional injuries to, 662–63
  issues in rural communities, 662–66
  as mothers, 918
  peer groups, 682
  pregnancy in, 678–703
  risk of HIV infection, 465–66
  sexual activity by, 664, 678–79, *680*
  sexual partners, 682–83
  social factors, 682–84
  substance abuse interventions, 493–94
  suicide, 917
  unintentional injuries to, 662
  use of contraception, 684*b*
  vulnerability of, 622–23
Adoption, option of, 692, 694
Adult learning theory, 344
Adult Protective Services, 519, 865
Advance directives, 887, 1022
Advance medical directives, 990–91
Advanced practice nurses (APRNs)
  case management, 1075–76
  curriculum for, 1065*b*
  education issues, 1068–70
  liability issues, 1072
  prescriptive authority, 1076
  regulation of, 1065*b*
  reimbursement issues, 1071–72
  roles of, 1065*b*
  world health and, 1072

Advanced practice nursing, 137
    community health focus in, 563–64
    definition of, 1064
    history of, 1066–68
    home health discharges and, 997
Advertising, policy making and, 220
Advocacy. *See also* patient advocates
    for community health education,
        358–59
    definition of, 342*t*
    for HIV/AIDS patients, 832
    nurses' role in, 149
    by parents, 1023–24
    for patients, 148–49, 288
    the political process and, 201–2
    in psychiatric-mental health
        nursing, 908
    for public health, 217
    tools for, 224
    for vulnerable populations, 559, 628,
        649–50, 730
Affect
    in the elderly, 878–81
    role of the family, 737–38
Affective domain, health education, 350–51
African-American nurses
    American Nurses Association
        membership, 96
    bibliography on history of, 82
    discrimination against, 83
    Lillian Wald and, 84
African-American populations
    caregiving responsibilities, 558, 562
    college enrollment statistics, 781
    elderly persons in, 860–61
    family structures, 783
    homicide rates, 918
    male life expectancy, 827
    in rural areas, 660
    STDs among adolescents, 806
Age/aging
    birth mothers' race and, 789*t*
    of families, 862–63
    family caregivers, 740
    generational roles, 864*b*
    health and, 859–60
    home health care utilization and, 977
    of men, 816
    pain management in, 555
    process of, 858
    quality of life and, 557–58
    terminology of, 858–59
    theories of, 892
    women and, 800–802
Ageism, definition, 860
Agency for Health Care Research and
        Quality (AHRQ), 193
Agency for Toxic Substances and Disease
        Registry (ATSDR), 192, 289*t*

Agents
    of bioterrorism, 446*b*
    of infectious disease, 426
Agnosia, 879
Agricultural hazards, 665–66
Agricultural workers, 671–73
Aid to Families with Dependent Children
        (AFDC), 172–73, 848
*Air, Water and Places* (Hippocrates), 65
Airplanes, drinking water, 22
Alaska, 8, 48
Alcohol consumption. *See also*
        substance use
    in the American culture, 481–82
    at-risk drinking, 1050
    by childbearing-women, *112*
    date rape and, 533, 541, 791, 793
    depression and, 1020
    erectile dysfunction and, 826
    in high school, 485
    by men, 818, 819
    by rural adolescents, 663–64
    serious mental illness and, 916–17
    traffic deaths and, 483
    by women, 806
Alcohol–drug interactions, 499*t*, 500
Alcoholism, 485–86
Aldrin, health effects of, 300*t*
All-terrain vehicle injuries, 662
Allergic dermatitis, 1038
Allergies, 549, 846
Alternative medical systems, 370
Alternative therapies, economics of,
        179, 179*b*
Alzheimer's disease, 879
Ambulatory care, visits by men, 822
Ambulatory care center nursing, 135
Ambulatory care sites, 129
Ambulatory patient groups (APGs), 172
Ambulatory surgery centers, 135–36
America, first hospital in, 71
The America Project (TAP), 636
American Academy of Ambulatory Care
        Nursing, 135
American Academy of Nurses (AAN), 531
American Academy of Pediatrics (AAP),
        600, 1022
American Academy of Physician
        Assistants, 127
American Accreditation Healthcare
        Commission (URAC), 147*b*
American Association for Ambulatory
        Health Care (AAAHC), 147*b*
American Association of Industrial Nurses
        (AAIN), 1035
American Association of Managed Care
        Nurses (AAMCN), 152
American Association of Occupational
        Health Nurses, 1035

American Association of Occupational
        Health Nurses (AAOHN),
        289*t*, 1045
American College of Nurse-Midwives,
        1066, 1068
American Heart Association (AHA), 44,
        797, 799, 817
American Holistic Nurses Association,
        367, 368*b*
*American Journal of Nursing (AJN)*, 81
*American Nurse,* 12
American Nurses Association (ANA)
    on advanced practice nursing,
        563–64
    African-American nurses in, 96
    *Code of Ethics for Nurses with
        Interpretive Statements,* 22
    Council on Community, Primary, and
        Long Term Care, 944
    Department of Labor Relations and
        Workplace Advocacy, 12
    foundation of, 81
    health policy and, 137
    Nursing Center for School Health, 1015
    Steering Committee on Databases to
        Support Nursing Practice, 329
American Psychiatric Nursing Association
        (APNA), 924
American Public Health Association
        (APHA), 309, 843*b*, 843*t*, 1044
American Red Cross (ARC)
    disaster management, 589
    disaster services, 592–93
    early health care reform and, 936
    enrollment campaign for nurses, 577
    online disaster preparedness
        resources, 588
    PTSD among volunteers for, 606
    roles during disasters, 599
    shelter management, 598–99
American Society for Addiction Medicine
        (ASAM), 485
Americans with Disabilities Act of 1990,
        191, 485, 550, 711, 713–14, 727,
        1055–56
Ammonia gas, 297*t*
Amnesia, 879
Amputations, 709*t*
Amputations, diabetes-related, 980
Analgesics, mobility and, 878
Analytic epidemiology, 114–15
Ancylostomiasis, 444
Anemia, substance abuse and, 483
Anthrax attacks, 588
Antibiotic resistance, 424, 425*b*, 444
Antibiotics, historical impact, 424, 425*b*
Anxiety
    coping with, 909
    impact on children, 1004

Aphasia, 878, 879
Appropriations, for policies, 222
Aristotle, 251, 251*b*
Armed conflict, 393–94
Army and Navy Nurse Corps, 88
Aromatherapy, 377–78
Arsenic, health effects of, 293*t*
Arsine, health effects of, 293*t*
Art therapy, 376
Arthritis, 546*t*, 549*t*, 551*t*
Artificial intelligence, 332
Ascariasis, 444
Asian and Pacific Islanders, 861
Asphyxiant gases, 298*t*
Aspirin, benefits of, 13
Assessments. *See also* Outcomes and
    Assessment Information Sets
    (OASIS)
  of activities of daily living, 892–95*t*
  at-risk populations, 37
  attitude self-assessment, 488
  of body weight, 869
  of bowel function, 869
  of caregivers, 864, 989
  of communities, 39–44, 39*t*, 56–59,
    **355, 357**
  community-focused interventions
    and, 42*b*
  complementary health and, 372–73
  of elderly populations, 867–69
  environmental assessments, 283*b*
  of families, 743–52, 757
  health education tasks, 348–50, 349*t*
  of home environments, 283*b*
  of homeless populations, 650–51
  of listening skills, 349–50, 869
  of literacy levels, 350
  locations for, 349
  of mental health, 868, 915–19
  nutritional, 57–58, 371, 483
  oral, 872
  of providers, 771*b*
  QUAD Council Public Health Nursing
    competencies, 951*t*
  questions used in, 349, 349*t*
  of reading levels, 350
  self-assessment quizzes, 771*b*
  of spirituality, 375
  of STD risk, 473
  of technology, 175–76
  timing of, 349
  of vision, 869–70
  worker/workplace, 1046–57, 1048*b*
Assets mapping, 1088–89
ASSIST project, 1023
Assistance animals, 726–27
Assisted-living facilities, 563
Assistive Technology Act, 713*t*
Assistive technology devices, 725, 726*t*

Association of Community Health Nurse
    Educators (ACHNE), 12, 36, 944
Association of Occupational and
    Environmental Clinics, 289*t*
Association of State and Territorial
    Directors of Nursing (ASTDN),
    944, 945*t*
*Assuring the Health of the Public in the 21st
    Century* (IOM), 96
Asthma
  experience of, 553
  *Healthy People 2010* objectives, 551*t*
  household items and, 549
  school-based programs for, 842
  work-related, 1038–39
At-risk drinking, 1050
Atherosclerosis, 826
Athletics, by people with disabilities, 722
Attention-deficit/hyperactivity disorder
    (ADHD), 629, 844–45, 1021
Audiologists, 870
Authoritarian leadership, 415–16, *416*
Authorization, of policies, 222
Autism, 709*t*
Automobile accidents, 629, 847
  injuries due to, 662
Autonomic dysreflexia, 730*b*
Autonomy
  conflicts with beneficence, 262*b*
  cultural factors, 708
  health education and, 342
  impact of chronic illness, 555
  of the individual, 255
Avian influenza (H5N1), 442
Ayurvedic medicine, 370

**B**
Baby-boomer generation, 95–96, 882. *See
    also* age/aging; elderly populations
"Baby Doe" issues, 727
Back pain
  chronic, 554
  *Healthy People 2010* objectives, 551*t*
  work-related, 1041, 1042
Balanced Budget Act of 1997, 171, 173,
    986, 1071
Bargaining, policy development and, 219–21
Barriers, definition, 342*t*
Barton, Clara, 86–87, 592
*Bartonella henselae*, 443
Behaving, community assessment, 43
Behavior, biological determinants of, 903
Behavior change, 355–58, 843
Behavior change theories, 344, 346, 473–75
Behavioral distractions, 967
Behavioral Risk Factor Surveillance System
    (BRFSS), 110, 309
Behavioral violence, 509, *510*, 512*b*. *See also*
    violence

Beliefs, 737. *See also* cultural factors;
    religion; spirituality; values
Belonging, community, 44
Beneficence, 257, 257*b*, 262*b*
Benefit periods, 171
Benefits, definition of, 342*t*
Benefits interpreters, 149
Benevolence, definition, 255
Benzene, health effects of, 295*t*
Beryllium, health effects of, 293*t*
Bicycles, injuries due to, 662
Bikers, risks to, 115–16
Bill and Melinda Gates Foundation, 386,
    390–91
Bill of Rights, 188
Bioelectromagnetics, 371
Bioethics, 250, 254, 255. *See also* ethical
    issues
Biofield healing practices, 371
Biologically-based therapies, 370–71
Bioterrorism, 445, 446*b*, 1025, 1037
Bipyridyls, health effects of, 300*t*
Birth control, access to, 697
Birth defects, work-related, 1039–40
Births, by age and race of mothers, 789*t*
Black Death (bubonic plague), 67–68
Bladder rehabilitation, 875*b*
Blogs, community interactions and, 57
Blood pressure, 551*t*. *See also*
    hypertension
Bloodborne Pathogens Standard
    (OSHA), 1054
Blue Cross, 123, 162
Blue Shield, 162
Body-based methods, 371
Body mass index (BMI), 871, 872*b*
Body weight, 869, 871–73, 872*b*
Bolton, Frances Payne, 88
Bone mass, in women, 797–99
Booth, William, 593
*Borrelia burgdorferi*, 440
Bottom-down health systems, 760–62
Bowel function, 869, 875–76, 877*b*
Breast cancer, 25, 556, 618, 823*t*
Breast self-examination, 797
Breckenridge, Mary, 87
Brewster, Mary, 84
British Nurses Association
    (BNA), 78
Brown, Esther Lucille, 81
Brucellosis, 81
Burnout
  after disasters, 1022
  avoiding, 32, 608
  of caregivers, 563, 862, 864
  in health ministries, 1091
  of nurses, 902, 976, 1012, 1049
Bush–Clinton Fund for Hurricane Katrina
    Recovery, 601

**C**

CAAHEP. *See* Commission on Accreditation of Allied Health Education Programs
Cadet Nurse Corps, 88, 90
Cadmium, health effects of, 293*t*
Calorie requirements, calculation of, 872*b*
*Campylobacter jejuni,* 441, 443
Campylobacteriosis, 439
Canada
    gun control, 527
    hand gun deaths, 215
    health care spending, 129
    health care system in, 175, 399–400
    Healthy Cities project, 35
    HIV in, 466, 829
    homicide rates, 529
    life expectancy, 164, 165, 170
    teen birth rates, 678
Canada Health Act (CHA), 399
Cancer. *See also specific* cancers
    costs of, 546*t*, 549*t*
    death in women and, 786
    fatigue associated with, 561
    *Healthy People 2010* objectives, 551*t*
    morbidity, 546*t*
    mortality from, 546*t*
    patients in hospice, 996
    STDs and, 457
    support groups, 799*b*
    surveillance of, 566
    vulnerable populations, 549–55
    in women, 797
    world health issues, 392
Capitation, 132, 143, 145, 986. *See also* insurance coverage; managed care; reimbursement
Carbamates, health effects of, 300*t*
Carbon disulfide, health effects of, 296*t*
Carbon monoxide, health effects of, 299*t*
Carbon tetrachloride, health effects of, 296*t*
Cardiovascular disease (CVD)
    in men, 828–29
    prevention of, 799
    in women, 797
    world health issues, 392
Care, systems of, 16–17
Care management, 17
Care planning, 992
Caregivers
    assessment of, 864, 989
    burden of, 864
    burnout, 563, 862, 864
    in chronic illness, 560
    competence of, 864
    elderly persons as, 863–65
    for elders in the family, 862
    families as, 740

family, 988–89
Family Medical Leave Act of 1993, 810
    health care policy and, 811
    informal, 977
    non-nursing, 563
    paraprofessional, 562
    patient perceptions, 555
    for persons with chronic disease, 548–49
    respite services for, 562
    stress and, 549, 810–11, 989
    women as, 783
Caring
    definition, 230
    nursing value of, 771
    resource utilization and, 267
Carpal tunnel syndrome, 1043
Carter, Edith, 85
Carter, Jimmy, 591
Carter Center, Atlanta, Georgia, 49, 386, 390, 1082, 1083*b*–1084*b*
Cartilage products, 371
Case-control studies, 114*t*
Case finders, 729
Case management
    by advanced practice nurses, 1075–76
    community health nurses in, 730
    definition of, 722
    description of, 93, 146
    disability services and, 722–23
    in home health care, 986
    innovations, 1075–76
    nurses role in, 151
    in occupational health, 1050–52
    school nurse role in, 1004, 1014
    in shelters settings, 134–35
    for vulnerable populations, 628
Case-mix adjustment, 986
"Cassandra" (Nightingale), 74
Cat-scratch fever, 443
Categorical programs, insurance, 170–74
Categorically needy persons, 172
Caucasian populations
    caregiving responsibilities, 562
    elderly persons in, 860–61
    family structures, 783
Celiac disease, 554
Centers for Disease Control and Prevention (CDC)
    APHA partnership with, 309
    on barriers to immunization, 95
    Coordinated School Health Program (CSHP), 1004
    data from, 110
    description, 192–93, 194
    on emerging infectious disease threats, 438*t*
    funding for school health, *1011*
    Healthy Schools Initiative, 1010

    on Katrina cough, 591
    *Morbidity and Mortality Weekly Report,* 1020
    national public health performance standards, 946
    on premature mortality, 18
    preparation for disasters, 581–82
    REACH program, 547
    secondary data from, 45, 57
    study of chlorpyrifos levels, 276
    study of lead levels in children, 276
    on vaccines, 840
    Youth Risk Behavior Survey (YRBS), 679, 790
Centers for Medicare and Medicaid Services (CMS). *See also* conditions of participation (CoPs)
    access to health care and, 96
    conditions of participation, 979
    credentialing by, 147*b*
    home health care and, 981–82
    home health documentation, 979–80
    hospice regulation, 983
    regulation by, 983
    standards of participation, 159
    use by elderly populations, 861
Cerebral palsy
    etiology, 709*t*
    frequency, 709*t*
Cerebrovascular accidents, 786
Certification. *See also* accreditation; licensing
    of advanced practice nursing, 1065*b*, 1066–68
    of nurse practitioners, 1067
    of occupational health nurses, 1056
    of school nurses, 1012
Certified Managed Care Nurses (CMCNs), 152
Certified nurse midwives, 1064, 1066, 1068
Certified registered nurse anesthetists, 1066, 1068
Certified registered nurses, 1064
Cerumen, 871
Chadwick Report, 71
Chain of infection, 426–27
CHAMPUS (Civilian Health and Medical Program of the Uniformed Services), 173–74
Change
    agents of, 411–13, 559
    force field analysis, *412, 413*
Charity care, 169
Chemical addictions, in the elderly, 887
Chemotherapy, 557, 797
Chernobyl Nuclear Disaster, 603*b*
Child abuse, 515–16

Child Abuse Prevention and Treatment Act(CAPTA), 713*t*
Child fatality review, 838*b*
Child Nutrition Amendments, 212
Childbirth
    death risk, 25
    preventing maternal mortality, 839–40
    risks of, 785–86
Childcare, child health and, 852
Childfind, 729, 730
Childhood victimization, 684
Children
    abuse of, 516*b*
    alcohol use by, 481*b*
    allergies in, 846
    behavioral problems, 1020
    benefits of home visits, 961
    camp experiences for, 722
    chronic illness and, 554–55
    with disabilities, 712, 723
    as disaster survivors, 604
    disasters and, 600
    discharge planning, 1018
    environmental exposures, 285
    health impact of poverty on, 848–51
    health issues of, 838–55
    HIV-infected, 469–70
    home-based programs for, 843–44
    homeless, 637
    hospice care for, 995
    immunization of, 840
    incidence of disabilities in, 708
    indicators of abuse, 517*t*
    interventions with parents, 517*t*
    maltreatment of, 515–16
    mental health of, 840–41
    meth orphans, 665
    obesity in, 25
    prevention of injury to, 840
    resistance to stress, *763*
    respite care for, 469
    risk of HIV infection, 468
    in rural counties, 660–61
    school-based programs for, 842–43
    school nursing and, 1004
    substance abuse interventions, 493–94
    vulnerability of, 622–23
Children's Health Insurance Program (CHIP), 173, 620
Chillin' out, 44
Chiropractic medicine, 371
Chlamydia, 455
*Chlamydia trachomatis,* 455
Chlordane, health effects of, 300*t*
Chlordecone, health effects of, 300*t*
Chlorinated hydrocarbons, 300*t*
Chlorine gas, health effects of, 298*t*
Chlorpyrifos levels, 276

Cholesterol objectives, 551*t*
Chromium, health effects of, 293*t*
Chronic care model, 558–59
Chronic illnesses
    at-risk families and, 765
    caregivers for individuals with, 548–49
    challenges of, 544
    in children, 841, 1005–6
    clinical practice guidelines, 980
    community-based supports, 560
    community health nursing in, 559–60, 566
    coping mechanisms, 555
    costs of, 549*t*
    definition of, 551–52
    disability *versus,* 552
    economic burden of, 546*t*
    in the elderly, 867
    elderly persons with, 861
    experiences of, 552–55
    families in care during, 740
    financing for, 560–61
    gender-specific issues, 561–62
    health burden of, 546*t*
    health promotion in, 565–66
    in homeless people, 644*t*
    hospice care, 563
    immunization advice, 886
    institutionalization in, 564–65
    mainstreaming students with, 1011–12
    neglect of self and, 563
    nursing supervision, 562
    palliative care, 563
    prevention of, 548, 549
    quality of life and, 556–58
    self-help strategies and, 558–59
    support groups, 562–63
    surveillance of, 566
    in the United States, 545–48
    vulnerable populations, 549–55
    in women, 786–87
    world health issues, 392–93
Chronic kidney disease, 553
Chronic obstructive pulmonary disease (COPD), 393, 551*t*, 1038–39
Chronic renal failure
    disability and, 552
    *Healthy People 2010* objectives, 551*t*
    hypertension and, 555
    management of, 548
    trends in, 553
Chronic sorrow, chronic illness and, 554
Civil defense systems, 589
Civil Rights Act of 1964, 191
Civil Works Administration (CWA), 88
Classical era, history, 64–65
Client information management, 240, 331
Client rights, 263

Client-server technology, 334
Climate change, 936
Clinical Information Systems (CIS), 962
Clinical nurse leaders (CNLs), 1064
Clinical nurse specialists, 137, 1064, 1066–70
Clinical practice guidelines, 980
Clinical practice patterns, 168
Clinical studies, characteristics, 114*t*
Clinics, APNs in, 1073
Clinton, Hillary Rodham, 125–26
Clinton health care plan, 221–22
Clock Drawing test, 868
Coalition of Psychiatric Nursing Organizations (CPONO), 923–24
Coalitions, function of, 414
Cocaine, 481, 498
*Code of Ethics for Nurses with Interpretive Statements* (ANA), 22
Coenzyme 10 (CoQ10), 377
Coercive power, 189
Cognitive dissonance, 342*t*
Cognitive functioning, 878–81
Cognitive objectives, health education, 350–51
Cognitive skills, poverty and, 849–51
Cohesion, 407
Cohort studies, 114*t*
Cohorts, definition of, 859
Collaboration
    in community-focused interventions, 48, 49
    counterforces to, 178
    with families, 752
    in home health care, 987–88
    by missionary nurses, 1097
    by nurses, 628–29
    opportunities for, 177–78
    in policy development, 219
    by school health nurses, 1004, 1017, 1018–19, 1025
Commission on Accreditation of Allied Health Education Programs (CAAHEP), 127
Commission on Chronic Illness, 550–51
Commission on the Status of Women, 802–3
Commitment, to the homeless, 648
Committee on Medicine and Public Health, 177
Committees, congressional, 198–99
Common human experiences, 913*b*
Common law, 197
Commonwealth Fund, 936
Communicable diseases
    adult immunizations, 436*t*
    chain of infection, 426–27
    challenges of, 946

control of, 431–36
emerging and re-emerging, 436–47
global health issues, 391–92
immunity to, 428–29
occupational transmission of, 1040–41
prevention of, 429–31
public health interest in, 93
reportable, 110b, 431t
role of community health nursing,
    424–26
routes of infection, 426–28
in schools, 1020
screening in schools, 1017
susceptibility to, 428–29
transmission of, 426–29, 427t
vaccine-preventable, 428b
Communication
about complementary therapies, 368
about persons with disabilities, 715–17
among case managers, 722
cultural patterns of, 800b
definition, 747
devices for hearing impairment, 870–71
disaster planning and, 589
disaster warnings, 583
during disasters, 596
distractions in home visiting, 967–68
e-mail, 330, 338, 1028
in elderly populations, 876–78
of environmental risks, 282,
    284–85, 284b
during evacuations, 594
gaining entry into communities, 42–44
within groups, 406
during home visits, 959b
with legislators, 200b
nursing skills in, 767
open, 406
patterns of, 58–59
patterns within families, 747–49
for persons with disabilities, 726
QUAD Council Public Health Nursing
    competencies, 951t
skills of missionary nurses, 1097
skills of school nurses, 1013–14
technology-assisted, 992
transcultural nursing and, 231
trust and, 650
Communication technology, 335–36
Communitarian ethics, 256–57
Communities. *See also* community
    assessments
4+ model of wellness and, 320–21
accessibility issues, 720
collective trauma to, 604–5
competence of, 35t
cultural gatekeepers, 231
definition, 14

effect of disasters on, 582
elders in, 860–62
empowerment of women, 783–85
examples of, 33
forums in assessment of, 44, 45
gaining entry into, 42–44
geographic boundaries, 58
health care delivery innovations,
    1075–76
health education in, 353–59
health insurance ratings, 169
health learning by, 355–58
health measures for, 25
health promotion within, 306–7
impact of public health policies, 223–24
influences on health of, 20–23
nutritional assessment of, 57–58
occupational health nursing and,
    1051–52
partnerships with, 404
population-focused care and, 26t
profiles of, 56–57
response to disasters, 586
schools as, 1017
self-concept of, 57
service initiatives, 1087
with shared cultures, 940
structure of, 41t
substance abuse interventions, 497b
Community-as-partner model, 38–39, 39t
Community-as-patient, 32
Community assessments
community-as-partner model,
    38–39, 39t
community empowerment, 37
conducting, 41–46
description, 36–37
final reports on, 52
framework for, 37–41
general systems model, 39–41
identification of target systems, 40
interviews, 40b
Lundy—Barton model, 56–59
planning phase, 47
problem list, 59
of process, 40, 41t
review of systems, 58–59
team composition, 43
Community-based care settings,
    133–35, 561
Community-based cultural nursing,
    230–34
Community-based nursing, 6
Community-based patients, 16
Community competency, 35
Community dimensions of practice, 952t
Community education, 257, 356t
Community empowerment, 37

Community-focused interventions
boundary assessments in, 33
collaborative arrangements, 48
evaluation phase, 52
implementation phase, 47–51
nursing process and, 42b
prioritization, 47, 47b
Community health
history, 64–99
managed care and, 151–52
Community Health Accreditation Program
    (CHAP), 147b
Community Health Advisors (CHAs),
    783–85
Community health diagnosis, 46, 47
Community health nurses (CHNs)
attitude self-assessment, 488
ethical problems facing, 262–63, 262b
in hate crime prevention, 523–24
identifying environmental risks, 281–82
nursing informatics and, 328–29
roles of, 48–51
in STD prevention, 472–75
working with persons with disabilities,
    728–30
Community health nursing
acute care *versus,* 15–16
communication technology and, 335–36
complementary health and, 372–73
computer applications in, 330–31
definition of, 944
description, 6, 12
economics of, 180–81
faith communities and, 1090–92
Community living
for people with disabilities, 717–19
Community mental health centers
    (CMHCs), 903, 904, 906b, 908
Community Need Index (CNI), 47
Community nursing organizations
    (CNOs), 145–46
Community/population assessments, 32
Community/population-focused care, 33
Compassion, 252
Competence
of caregivers, 864
of communities, 35t
Competition, issues of, 159–60
Complementary and alternative medicine
    (CAM), 129–30
barriers to use of, 373–74
integration into community nursing,
    374–78
modalities of, 369–72
usage statistics, 368–69
Complementary health, attitudes toward,
    366–67
Compliance, paternalism and, 342

Comprehensive community initiatives (CCIs), 768

*Comprehensive Introduction to Managed Care Nursing* (AAMCN), 152

Comprehensive school health movement, 495

Computerization. *See* informatics

Conceptual models, 941

Conditions of participation (CoPs), 979, 981–82, 994

Condoms, 467, 682

Confidentiality, 44, 661, 669–71, 1021, 1022. *See also* privacy

Conflict management, 408, 410–11, 773

Confusion, description, 879

Congenital syphilis, 95

Congregate housing, 563

Congregational health partnerships, 1087

Congress, U. S.
    authorization of policies, 222
    policy implementation, 222
    responsibilities of, 196b
    types of committees, 198–99

Congressional Act of 1803, 591

Connection power, 189, 1086

Connections, interagency, 768

Consciousness of families, 745

Consent by parents, 1021

Consequentialism, theory of, 252–53, 253b

Constipation, 876, 877b

Constitution, U. S., 188, 190

Constitutional law, 197

Construct for Public Health Nursing (White), 941–43, *942*

Constructed knowledge, 808

Constructed surveys, 44

*Consumer Bill of Rights and Responsibilities,* 142–43, 143b

Consumerism, 130, 310–11

Consumers, 161, 260

Contact urticaria, work-related, 1038

Continuing education, 90, 95, 337, 378, 598, 1012, 1056

Continuity of care
    disease state management and, 980b
    documentation of the care process and, 93
    home health nurses and, 972, 973

Contraception
    adolescent pregnancy and, 696–97
    emergency forms of, 804
    history of, 810
    information about, 91, 176, 693t
    teen use of, 682, 684b, 791
    in young adulthood, 793

Contracting process, 752

Cooperation, policy development, 219

Coordinated School Health Program (CSHP), 1004, 1012

Coordination of care, 987, 992, 1014

Coping mechanisms
    adaptive, 559, 562
    assessment of, 354
    deficient, 134, 556
    powerlessness and, 555

Corporate cultures, 1051

Correctional nursing, 205

Cost analysis, cost containment and, 174–76

Cost-benefits analysis (CBA), 19–20, 175

Cost containment, 17, 160, 162
    strategies for, 174–76, 174b

Cost-effectiveness analysis (CEA), 175–76

Cost-of-illness analyses, 175

Cost sharing, 169

Council on Linkages between Academia and Public Health Practice (COL), 945, 949

Counseling, 628–29, 724, 1051

Courage, nursing value of, 771

Creativity, of the elderly, 881–82

Credentialing, 146–48, 147b

Crimean fever, 81

Criminal justice, violence and, 508–9

Crippled Children's Services, 89, 92

Crisis intervention model, 921

Cross-sectional studies, 114t

Crude rates, 109–10

Cryptosporidiosis, 445

*Cryptosporidium parvum,* 445

Cuba, 86, 400, 592, 960

Cults, violent behavior and, 525–26

Cultural backlash, 238

Cultural barriers, 237

Cultural biases, 236

Cultural blindness, 230

Cultural brokers, 43

Cultural care diversity and universality, Leininger's theory of, 238–42

Cultural clashes, 230

Cultural competency, 952t

Cultural factors
    alcohol consumption, 481–82, 492
    in community assessment, 41
    community health and, 21
    in domestic violence, 922
    of elderly populations, 860–61
    in home health nursing, 972
    information technology and, 329
    managed care and, 147
    mental health, 903
    Muslim faith, 1089
    nurse—family partnerships and, 963
    patient autonomy and, 708
    patterns of communication, 800b

prayers from world religions, 1093
    in rural communities, 661
    status of age in, 860
    substance abuse and, 486
    violence and, 511–12, 525–26
    women's health and, 799–800

Cultural imposition, 230, 236

Cultural lifeways, 230

Cultural pain, 237

Cultural shock, 236–37

Cultural values, 230, 236

Cultural variations, 230, 237

Culturally competent care, 230, 235–36

Culturally congruent care, 233

Culture, definition of, 230

Culture bound, 237–38

Cyanide, health effects of, 299t

Cycle of violence, 513

Cyclic rates, 113

**D**

Da Vinci, Leonardo, 68–69

Data, nursing-related, 326

*DATA 2010,* 309

Data analysis, 44, 59

Data collection
    about home health care, 983–85
    in community assessment, 44–46
    Lundy—Barton model, 56
    objective data, 59
    by occupational health nurses, 1055
    by school nurses, 1014–15
    sources of data, 110–11
    subjective data, 59

Data management, 138

Databases, 329, 330–31, 338

Date rape, 533, 541, 791, 793, 819

Dating violence, 527, 663

Daycare centers, 129

DDT, health effects of, 300t

Deaconesses, 67

Decision-making
    ethical, 263–64
    family processes, 746–47
    Home Care Bill of Rights, 991
    patient autonomy and, 372
    shared, 407–8

Declaration of Alma Ata, 395–96

Defensive medicine, 131

Dehydration, signs of, 873–74

Deinstitutionalization, mental health care, 908

Delano, Jane A., 82

Delegation, issues of, 1021, 1023

Delinquency, self-esteem and, 924

Delirium, 879

Delivery of care, technology and, 992

Demand, for products, 159

Dementias, 796, 879, 880*b*

Democracy, definition of, 189

Democratic leadership. *See* participatory leadership

Demographic data

community profiles, 56–57

comparisons of, 57

global, 384

health care costs and, 167–68

infectious disease spread and, 437

Denominators, definition, 107

Denver Developmental Screening Test (DDST), 92

Deontological theories, 253–56, 254*b*, 266–67

Department of Education (DOE), 194

Department of Health and Human Services (DHHS), 192, 192*b*

Department of Homeland Security (DHS), 592

Department of Labor (DOL), 194

Dependence, definition, 480

Depletion, sources of, 316*b*

Depression

after disasters, 602

in children, 1020

chronic illness and, 552

coping with, 909

in the elderly, 868–69, 880–81, 881*b*

geriatric, 555

in mature women, 796

in men, 817

post-partum, 918

Deregulation, of health care delivery, 130

Dermatitis, work-related, 1038

DETERMINE checklist, 871

Developmental Disabilities Assistance and Bill of Rights Act, 713*t*

Developmental disorders, 708, 712, 1017, 1039–40

Diabetes

age-specific prevalence, *109*

amputations, 980

costs of, 546*t*

erectile dysfunction and, 826

*Healthy People 2010* objectives, 551*t*

morbidity, 546*t*

mortality from, 546*t*

prevention of, 313

race/ethnicity and, 547

world health issues, 392–93

Diagnosis-related groups (DRGs), 92, 123, 978, 986

Diarrhea, in the elderly, 875–76, 876*b*

Dieldrin, health effects of, 300*t*

Diet. *See* nutrition

Diet sodas, 793

Diffusion theory, 345*t*

Digital media, impact of, 333

Dioxane, health effects of, 297*t*

Diquat, health effects of, 300*t*

Directly observed therapy (DOT), 94

Disabilities

caused by mental illnesses, 916–17

children with, 712

chronic illness *versus,* 552

current situation for, 711–12

definition of, 550, 708

effects, 709*t*

ethical issues related to, 727–28

etiologies, 709*t*

etiquette and common courtesies, 716–17

health promotion in, 565–66

incidence of, 708–10

mandated education for children, 1009–10

people with

community living needs of, 717–19

in homes of their own, 719–20

legislative milestones, 713*t*

recreation, 721–22

rehabilitation services, 724

relationships, 721

rights of persons with, 712

role of community health nursing, 566

stigma of, 1017

students with, 1014

support groups, 562–63

Disability rights movement, 713–15, 714*t*

Disability services, 710–11, 722–23, 729

Disadvantaged status, 618

Disaster declarations, 592

Disaster management, 589–90, 594–95

Disaster preparedness, 1025

Disaster Relief Act, 591

Disaster shelters, 134–35, 595–96, 598–99

Disaster syndrome, 602

Disasters. *See also* natural disasters

characteristics of, 577–80

controllability of, 579

definitions, 576

duration of impact, 579

emergency stage, 584–85

forewarning, 579

global issues, 580

health effects of, 582*b*

impact stage of, 583–84

interdisaster stage of, 583

isolation of populations, 584–85

major, definition of, 576

nature of, 576–83

nurses' reactions to, 605–8

outcomes of, 586

phases of, 573–74

planning for, 572, 586–89, 597–98, 727

predictability of, 578–79

predisaster stage of, 583

prevention of, 608

reconstruction stage, 585

recovery phase, 590, 599–608

resources in industrialized countries, 582*b*

response levels, 590

roles of community health nurses, 596–99

scope of impact, 579

search-and-rescue missions, 595

speed of onset, 579

stages of, 583–86

steps in disaster declarations, 586–87

stressors related to, 606

survivors of, 596, 601–4

team responses, 590

training for, 575

triage, 595

types of, 576

victim responses, 600

Discernment, definition of, 252

Discharge planning, 17

Discharge teaching, 353–54

Discrimination

against African-American nurses, 83

Americans with Disabilities Act and, 191, 485, 550, 1055–56

homelessness and, 641–43

against male nurses, 83

Disease state management (DSM), 980, 980*b*

Diseases, stages of, 24

Disenfranchised groups, 621, 625

Distractions, 967, 968

Distributed data processing (DDP), 334, *335*

Distributive justice, 262*b*

Division of Industrial Hygiene, U. S., 89

Dix, Dorothea Linde, 85–86

Do not resuscitate (DNR) orders, 728, 1021, 1022

Dock, Lavinia Lloyd, 81

Doctorate of Nursing Practice (DNP), 137, 1064, 1066*b*, 1076

Documentation

of the care process, 93

disaster planning and, 589

home health care and, 979–81

of home visits, 958*b*

for Medicare, 981–82

by occupational health nurses, 1055

by school nurses, 1014, 1022–23

vocabulary choices, 981*b*

Domains of learning, 350–51, 351*t*

Domestic violence, 513

animal abuse and, 766

community-based programs, 767

cultural-community context, 922

"red flags," 804–5

situational context, 922
structural context of, 922
Dossey, Barbara, 80
Down syndrome, 709*t*
Drinking water safety, 22, 23
Dropout rates, 1014–15
Drug abuse, 465, 819
Drug Abuse Resistance Education
    (DARE), 493
Drug Abuse Warning Network
    (DAWN), 493
Drug abusers, workforce, 481*b*
Drug histories, 488
Drug interactions, 499–500, 499*t*
Drug rehabilitation, 1052
Drugs, costs of, 167
Drugs of abuse, classes of, 480*b*
Duchenne's muscular dystrophy, 709*t*
Dysphagia, 871

**E**
E-mail, 330, 338, 1028
Early intervention, 723
Early Periodic Screening Diagnosis and
    Treatment (EPSDT), 92
Earthquakes, 578, 580, 608
Ebers Papyrus, 64
Ecology, health and, 272–73
*Ecomaps*, 315
Economic abuse, 520*b*
Economic Opportunity Act, 212
Economics, of chronic disease, 546*t*
Education
    for children with disabilities, 712
    in community-focused interventions,
        51–52
    of the elderly, 869
    groups, 413
    levels in elderly populations, 861
    role of nurses, 832
    transition planning, 724
    vulnerability and, 623–24
    of women in the U.S., 781
Education for All Handicapped Children
    Act, 713*t*, 1009
Educational systems, 59, 1010–12
Edward VI, 70
Egyptian culture, history, 64
Elder abuse, 865
Elderly populations
    assessment of, 867–69
    calculating the nutritional status of, 872*b*
    causes of mortality and morbidity, 867*t*
    chronic illness in, 867
    communication issues, 876–78
    definitions of abuse, 518–19
    dementia management in, 880*b*
    demographics of, 860–61
    as disaster survivors, 604

dreams of, 866
education levels in, 869
elimination problems, 874–76
employment for, 881–82
exercise in, 878*b*
family developmental tasks, 864*b*
fluid requirements, 873
government programs for, 863
home environments, 967
indicators of abuse, 519*b*
life cycle of aging family members, 864*b*
maltreatment of, 516–19, 865, 865*b*, 865*t*
mature women, 796–97
medication education for, 500*b*
mobility in, 876–78, 878*b*
nutrition requirements, 871*t*
nutritional status, 873*b*
preventive studies for, 868*t*
proprioception, 885
by race and ethnicity, 660*t*
retirement for, 881–82
risk of HIV infection, 468–69
in rural counties, 409, 666
safety precautions for, 883
sensory integrity, 869–71
sexuality in, 882–83
sleep requirements, 874
socioenvironmental assessments, 869
speech impairment, 879*b*
substance abuse interventions,
    499–500, 499*t*
toughness of, 587
vulnerability of, 623
website usability and, 337
women and aging, 800–802
Elders
    in the community, 860–62
    definition, 859
    as individuals, 865–69
    nursing of, 860–85
Elders, Jocelyn, 622
Electronic funds transfer (EFT), 332
Electronic health records (EHRs), 327,
    980*b*, 992
Electronic mail. *See* e-mail
Electronic spreadsheets, 331
Elementary and Secondary Education Act
    (EASA), 1010
Elimination problems, 874–76
Emergencies, disasters and, 576
Emergency care centers, 135
Emergency contraception, 804
Emergency Maternity and Infant Care
    (EMIC) program, 89–90
Emergency plans, family, 574
Emergency stage, disasters, 584–85
*Emerging Infections* (NAS), 436
Emic views, 230, 236
Emotional abuse, 514, 515, 517*t*, 519*b*, 520*b*

Emotional health screening, 1017
Emotional support, 738–39
Empedodes of Acragas, 65
Employee education, 1055
Employee Retirement Income Security
    Act, 169
Employers, health insurance and, 169–70
Employment. *See also* occupational health
    nursing; occupational therapy
    in the elderly, 881–83
    for people with disabilities, 711, 720–21
    preplacement examinations, 1048
    in schools, 1006
    supported, 720–21
    transition planning, 724
    of women in the U. S., 781–82
Empowerment
    of communities, 37
    definition, 342*t*
    disease state management and, 980*b*
    evaluation of, 769
    in groups, 412
    of patients, 37
    self-help strategies and, 558–59
    of women, 783–85, 809–10
Encouragers, for groups, 410
End-of-life issues, 887
Energy, of families, 744
Energy therapies, 371–72
Enterobiasis, 444
Entitlement programs, 171–72
Entrepreneurs, nurses as, 137–38
Environment
    assessing exposures, 283*b*, 973
    assessing risks in, 966
    communication of risks, 284*b*
    community health and, 21–22
    concept of, 273
    disease prevention and, 429
    of families, 737
    family boundaries and, 750–52
    hazards in the workplace, 1034*b*
    health hazards and, 272–300
    health impacts of, 11
    home assessments, 283*b*
    impact on health, 1020
    impact on men, 818
    infectious disease spread and, 437
    nursing's role, 279–81
    poverty and hazards in, 851
    religious, 1094
Environmental distractions, 967
Environmental health
    definition, 273
    information resources, 289*t*
    occupational health nursing and, 1058
    policies, 276–78
    upstream thinking in, 286
Environmental health nursing, 286–88

Environmental justice, 287–88
Environmental justice movement, 275–76
Environmental policies, 280–81
Environmental Protection Agency (EPA), 22, 191, 274, 289*t*
Environmental tobacco smoke (ETS), 115, 565
EnvRN, 289*t*
Epidemic, definition, 102
Epidemic curves, 113
Epidemiological process, 104*t*, *105,* 106–11
Epidemiological triad, *103*
Epidemiology
    analytic, 114–15, 114*t*
    definition of, 24–25, 102–3
    descriptive, 105–11
    environmental health and, 276
    history of, 72
    scope of, 103–4
Equality, freedom and, 189
Erectile dysfunction (ED), 825–28
Ergonomics, 1046, 1054*b*
*Escherichia coli* 0157:H7, 440
Essential public health services, 944, 945*t*
*Essentials of Baccalaureate Nursing*
    *Education for Entry Level*
    *Community/Public Health Nursing*
    *Practice,* 12, 36
Ethical issues. *See also* bioethics
    approach to drug abuse, 491
    community health and, 22–23
    cost containment and, 169
    dilemmas, 250
    disability-related, 727–28
    in group leadership, 416
    in health education, 359–60
    HIV risk behaviors and, 466
    in home health care, 989–91
    in hospice care, 996
    informed consent, 728
    insurance coverage, 126
    for Israeli community health
        nurses, 262*b*
    for Louisiana public health nurses, 262*b*
    managed care-related, 148–49
    obesity-related, 105
    in occupational health nursing, 1052
    patient autonomy and, 372
    for school nurses, 1021–25
    vulnerable populations and, 626–27
Ethics
    agreement on norms of, 261*t*
    of caring, 261–62, 262*b*
    communitarian, 256–57
    decision-making and, 263–64
    definition, 250
    in environmental health nursing,
        286–88

    personal risk and, 263
    principle-based, 252–56
Ethnicity. *See* race/ethnicity
Ethnocentrism, 230, 236
Ethnographic interviews, 40*b*
Ethylene glycol ethers, 296*t*
Ethylene oxide, 297*t*
Etic views, definition, 230*b*, 234, 235, 236, 240
Etiquette, 716–17
Evacuations, 589, 593–97
Evaluation phase
    community assessments, 59
    for community education, 358
    formative measures, 52
    in group assessment, 416
    in health education, 352–53
    process-recording diagrams, *416–17*
    summative measures, 52
Evaluations, 42*b*, 768–69. *See also specific*
    assessments
Evidence-based practice
    chronic care model and, 559
    health care systems and, 12
    managed care and, 16
    nurse–family partnerships, 961–62
Executive branches, 191–92, 196
Executive function, elderly persons, 879
Exercise, 311, 878*b*, 888–89
Experience ratings, 169
Experimental studies, 114*t*
Expert power, 189
Exploitation, 519*b*, 520*b*, 712, 865
Exposure assessments, 282, 283*b*, 285–86

**F**
Facilitator roles, 833
Factor VIII, 463
Faith communities, 1085–87, 1090–98
Falls, in the elderly, 787–88
Families
    4+ model of wellness and, 320
    adolescent pregnancy and, 681
    of adolescents, 681
    assessment of, 743–52, 757
    at-risk groups, 763–66
    benefits of home visits, 961
    boundaries set by, 750–52
    caregiver issues, 549, 988–89
    communication patterns, 747–49
    community-based services, 763–66
    consciousness of, 745
    continuum of services for, *773*
    in crisis, 766
    decision-making processes, 746–47
    definition of, 736–37
    demographic changes in, 737
    elders in, 862–65

    emergency plans for, 574
    energy of, 744
    evaluation process, 753–54
    farmers, 672
    goal setting, 752–53
    health care for, 760–63
    health education for, 353–54
    health potential of, *744*
    health responsibilities of, 737–40, 743*b*
    with HIV, 469–70
    homeless, 645, 668
    identification of health needs, 752
    impact of teen pregnancy, 686
    interventions in, 494–95, 494*b*, 495*t*, 766–69
    population-focused care and, 26*t*
    promotion of child health, 838–41
    providers working with, 771*b*
    refugee, 765
    role structure of, 745–46
    roles of women in, 783–85
    in rural settings, 663
    structures of, 771, 783
    substance abuse and, 486, 487
    theoretical approaches to, 740–42
    value checkpoints, 771*b*
    values of, 749–50
    violence in, 513, 520, 520*b*, 803–5
    vulnerable, 617
Family development tasks, 742
Family development theory, 742
Family Education Rights and Privacy Act (FERPA), 1022
Family Medical Leave Act of 1993, 810, 1056
Family nurse practitioners (FNPs), 1012, 1069
Family planning services, 93. *See also* contraception
Family systems theory, 741–42
Farr, William, 102
Fatigue, responses to, 553
Fecal elimination, 875–76
Federal budget deficits, 94
Federal Communications Commission (FCC), 337
Federal Disaster Assistance Administration, 591
Federal Emergency Management Agency (FEMA), 586–87, 591, 599
Federal Emergency Relief Administration (FERA), 640
Federal government branches, 191–96
Federal poverty level (FPL), 172
*Federal Register,* 203
Fee-for-service, 123, 143, 986. *See also* indemnity plans
Female condom, 467

Feminism, 809
Feminization of poverty, 783
Ferraro, Geraldine, 195
Fertility, 825, 1039–40
Fetal alcohol syndrome, 709*t*
Fetal growth retardation, 849
Financial planning, 953*t*
Fiscal policies, 210
Five Gap Model, 1083*b*
Floods, 577, *577*
Focus groups, 44, 50, 57, 414
Folstein Mini-Mental State
    Examination, 894*t*
Food and Agriculture Organization
    (FAO), 386*b*
Food and Drug Administration (FDA), 192
Food-borne diseases, 438–40
Food poisoning, 947
Footwear, 878
Force field analysis, 412–13
Forensic nursing, 205, 511
Formaldehyde, 295*t*
Formative measures, 52
Fomites, definition, 426–27
*Forward Plan for Health 1977-1981*
    (DHHS), 311
4+ model of wellness, 312, 314–21,
    *315, 315b*
Fragile X syndrome, 709*t*
Free market system, 159–60
Freedom, definition of, 189
Frontier Nursing Service, 87
Function, of families, 741

**G**

Gait retraining, 878
Galen of Pergamum, 66
Gallup Polls on nursing, 67
Gangs, 525–26, 926, 927
Gastroenteritis, 849
Gatekeepers, 410, 494
Gay-related immune deficiency syndrome
    (GRID). *See* HIV/AIDS
Gender differences, 561–62, 786, 816, 840
Gender roles, 799–800
General systems model, 39–41, 56–59
*General Systems Model for Community
    and Population Assessment and
    Intervention* (Lundy and Barton),
    39–40
Generic care, 236
Genetic engineering, 333
Genetics screening programs, 93
Genital herpes, 456
Genital warts, 456–57
Genograms, 862, 909, 925
Geriatric care competencies, 896–97
Geriatric depression, 555

Geriatric Depression scale, 868, 895*t*
Geriatrics, definition, 859
Gerontological nursing, 859, 859*b*
Gerontology, 859
Ghetto countercultures, 634
*Giardia lamblia,* 444–45
Giardiasis, 444–45
Gingivitis, in the elderly, 871
"Glass ceilings," 782
Global health
    contagious diseases and, 544
    initiatives, 395–96
    issues-related to, 391–95
    nursing role in, 384, 396–97
    population-focused care and, 26*t*
    three Ps of, 24*t*
Globalization, global health and, 384
Goal attainment tasks, 410, 411
Goal setting theory, 344*t*
Goldmark Report, 80–81
Gonorrhea, 455–56
Goodrich, Annie, 82
Goth culture, 839
Government
    agencies for the homeless, 642*t*, 643*t*
    authority of, 188–91
    environmental policies, 278–81
    federal, 191–96
    health care delivery and, 136
    in health promotion, 309
    influence on occupational health
        nursing, 1054–56
    local, 197
    poverty and, 620
    programs for the elderly, 863
    roles in public health, 940
    state, 196
Government, state branches of, 196–97
Great Depression, The, 88, 936
Greek American families, 241–42
Greek era, history, 65–66
Gross domestic profit (GDP), 163–64, *164*
Group B streptococcal disease, *108*
Group initiation phase, 408
Groups
    definition, 353
    dissolution of, 410
    effective, 406–8
    functions of, 410–13
    health education for, 353–54
    maintenance of, 409–10
    member roles, 410–11
    membership decisions, 408
    stages of development, 408–13, 408*t*, 410
    stakeholder analysis, 409, 410*b*
    team building, 414–15
    types of, 413–15
    working with, 404, 405, 415–17

Guardianship process, 712
Guide dogs, 726
*Guide to Clinical Preventive Services,* 312
Gujarat earthquake, 578
Gun control, 527, 528
Gynecological age, 694

**H**

*Haemophilus influenzae B* (HIB)
    vaccine, 840
Hallucinogens, 481
Handicaps, definition of, 550, 716. *See also*
    disabilities
Hantavirus, 274*b*, 442
Hardiness, 627
Harm reduction model, 344*t*
Hate crimes, 523–24
Head injuries, 115–16
Head lice, 1022
Head Start programs, 620, 852, 1004
Healing, holistic frameworks, 367
Healing touch (HT), 378, 1075
Health
    determinants of, 942
    ecological world view, 272–73
    responsibility for, 310
    WHO definition, 10
Health adjusted life expectancy
    (HALE), *164*
Health belief model, 312, 344*t*
Health care
    costs
        gross domestic profit and, *164*
        influences on, 166*b*, 167–68
        reimbursement of, 123–26
        sources of payment, *168*, 168–69
        trends, 158, 162–68
        in the U. S., 11
    economic approach to, 159–62
    economic indicators, 163–64
    market failure in, 160–62
    payment for, 168–74
    private payment for, 983
    proxies, 990
    sources of payment for, *163*
    women's issue policies, 810–11
Health care–associated infections (HAIs),
    437–38
Health care calendar, 792*t*
Health care delivery systems
    Canadian, 399–400
    chronic care model in, 558–59
    community-based settings, 133–35
    Cuban, 400
    current U.S. system for, 126–30
    defensive medicine in, 131
    development of, 123*b*
    education for families, 739

evolution of, 122–26, 946
health care providers within, 127–28
health care settings, 128–31
health promotion and, 308
improving child health, 844–48
innovations in, 1075–76
issues affecting, 130–31, 131b
Jordanian, 401
levels of care, 126
managed care, 131–36
management software, 332–35
private, 123–24
reinvention of, 16–17
satisfaction by country, 175
telecommunications technology
        and, 204
U. S. providers, 127–28
utilization by men, 821–23
Health care reform
    cost of chronic illness and, 560–61
    history of, 125–26, 936–37
    impact of the media on, 221–22
    initiatives, 16–17
    legislative processes and, 198–203
    nursing's agenda for, 16
    school nursing services in, 1019
Health education
    assessment tasks, 348–50, 349t
    in the church community, 1087
    in communities, 353–59
    concepts, 342–43
    disease prevention and, 431
    domains of learning and, 350–51, 351t
    ethical issues in, 359–60
    learning goals, 350
    learning theories and, 343–44
    objectives, 350
    planning, 350–51
    pointers for, 352b
    process of, 346–53, 347t–348t
    purposes of, 342
    in schools, 1016
    theoretical bases, 342–46
    for women, 808
Health Education Act of 1978, 1009
Health fairs, 1090, 1096
Health-hazard risk evaluation, 312
Health indicators, 921b
Health information, policies, 220–21
Health Insurance Portability and
        Accountability Act, 169, 713t, 1022
Health insurance purchasing cooperatives
        (HIPCs), 169
Health law, U.S., 191b
Health maintenance organizations
        (HMOs), 97, 132, 144
Health management information systems
        (HMIS), 327, 328b

Health ministries, 1080–1102
    in action, 1086–90
    development of, 1082–84
    health education and, 1090
    models of, 1087
    organization of, 1091
    structures of, 1087–90
    wellness committees, 1088
Health policies
    child health and, 852
    choices of, 211–12
    description of, 210
    ethical issues, 165
    history in the U.S., 212–13
    politics and, 136–37
    stakeholders in, 212b
    values and, 259–61
Health promotion
    behaviors, 304
    in chronic illness, 565–66
    community-level, 306–7
    concepts of, 304–7
    definitions of, 305–6, 306b
    in disability, 565–66
    employee health and, 311
    factors influencing, 307–8
    government initiatives, 309
    models of, 311–21
    occupational health nurses and, 1052
    public—private partnerships, 309–10
    in the workplace, 1059
Health questionnaires, 1100–1102
Health Resources and Services
        Administration, 193
Health systems, community-level
        review, 58
Health visiting, history of, 78–79
Healthy Cities initiative, 35–36, 309, 635
Healthy communities, characteristics, 34–36
Healthy Communities 2000, 404b
Healthy for Life circle, 313, 313–14
Healthy People 2000, 210, 404b, 912
Healthy People 2010 objectives
    access-related, 167
    child-related, 839
    chronic illness-related, 551t
    clinical nurse specialist use of, 1070
    communicable disease-related, 425
    cultural diversity-related, 231
    for the elderly, 861–62
    on environmental health, 279
    family-related, 761
    goals of, 20, 20t, 136, 635
    health education-related, 360
    HIV-related, 470
    injury-related, 532
    law-related, 203
    leading health indicators, 907

men's health-related, 820–21
mental health-related, 912, 915
for the nation, 103, 210
nurse practitioners use of, 1070
occupational safety and health-related,
        1043–44
related to disabilities, 728, 729
on responsibility for change, 404b
rural life-related, 672
school-related, 1015–17
secondary data from, 44
STD-related, 459
substance abuse-related, 489–90
teen pregnancy prevention-related,
        868, 869
tobacco-related, 490
violence prevention-related, 532
women's health-related, 790
Healthy People in Healthy Communities
        (DHHS), 309
Healthy Schools Initiative (CDC), 1010
Hearing dogs, 726
Hearing impairments
    assessment, 870–71
    in elders, 870b
    etiology, 709t
    etiquette with people with, 717
    frequency, 709t
    hearing dogs, 726
    mobility issues, 878
    screening in schools, 1017
    work-related, 1037, 1040
Heart attacks, warning signs, 796. See also
        myocardial infarction
Heart disease
    costs of, 546t, 549t
    death in women and, 786, 796
    morbidity, 546t
    mortality from, 546t
Heart failure, 553, 982, 985
Heat-related deaths, 111
Hebrew culture, classical era, 64
Helmet laws, 115–16
Helminths, 444–45
Henry Street Settlement, 84, 979, 1007
Henry VIII, 70
Hepatitis viruses, 95, 432–34, 554, 1040–41
Heptachlor, health effects of, 300t
Herbal therapies, 377
Herd immunity, 429
Heroin, 481
Herpes simplex virus, 456
Heterosexism, 800
Hexamethylene diisocyanate, 298t
High-risk behaviors, 1006
Highly active antiretroviral therapy
        (HAART), 459, 460, 467, 468–69
Hill–Burton Act, 123, 190

Hip hop culture, 829

Hippocrates of Cos, 65

Hispanic populations
  college enrollment statistics, 781
  elderly persons in, 860–61
  family structures, 783
  in rural areas, 660–61
  STDs among adolescents, 806

History
  after the War years, 89–91
  bibliography, 82
  challenges of the 1930s, 89
  classical era, 64–65
  of communities, 57
  of community health, 64–99
  dark period of nursing, 70–71
  decades of change 1945-1960, 95–96
  early colonists, 188
  of environmental health policy,
      274–75, 276
  era of managed care, 96–97
  The Great Depression, 88
  Greek era, 65–66
  healing traditions, 367–69
  of health care delivery, 123–24
  of health care reform, 125–26
  health policy in the U.S., 212–13
  Industrial Revolution, 71–72
  influence of the 1960s, 91–93
  influence of the 1970s, 91–93
  Middle ages, 65–69
  milestones, 90b
  milestones for the 21st century, 97b
  of nursing, 10–11
  nursing in the Americas, 71
  of public health nursing, 64–99, 93–95
  The Reformation, 69–70
  The Renaissance, 68–69
  revolution, protest and order,
      1961–2000, 96
  Roman era, 66
  World War II, 88

HIV/AIDS, 445–46
  adolescent pregnancy and, 917
  challenges of, 544
  confidentiality issues, 669–71
  connection with tuberculosis, 447
  definitions, 458
  early detection, 19
  in elderly populations, 883
  empowerment evaluation in, 769
  first cases, 94
  in homeless populations, 643–44
  men with, 829–30
  mortality rates, 391
  natural history of, 104–5
  populations at risk for, 463–69
  prevention of, 926

race/ethnicity and, 464–65, 464t,
    465t, 547
  risk factors, 94
  scope of the problem, 459–62, 460,
      461, 462
  substance abuse and, 483
  survival trends, 548
  transmission of, 463, 645–46

HMOs. *See* health maintenance
    organizations

Holistic frameworks
  in advanced practice nursing, 1076
  for health ministries, 1082–84
  of home health nursing, 972
  home visits and, 957
  for hospice care, 995–96
  for nursing, 367, 368b
  in psychiatric-mental health
      nursing, 901

Holistic wellness, 312–14

Home-based programs, 843–44
  for people with disabilities, 711

Home Care Bill of Rights, 990, 991

Home health agencies
  accreditation of, 985–86
  classification of, 978–81, 978b
  government, 978
  institution-based, 978, 978b
  Medicare filings, 981
  nonprofit, 978, 978b
  proprietary, 978, 978b

Home health agency (HHA) care, 171

Home health aides, 977, 988b

Home health care
  definition, 972
  diagnoses referred to, 977b
  discharge to, 997
  documentation, 979–81, 982b
  economics of, 976–77
  ethical issues, 989–91
  evolution of, 956
  family caregivers, 988–89
  future of, 996–97
  growth of, 18, 977
  hospice, 993–96
  information technology in, 992–93
  insurance coverage, 166, 982–83
  legal issues, 989–91
  licensure, 983
  managed care and, 986–87
  Medicare criteria for patients, 983b
  monitoring systems, 984
  multidisciplinary approach to,
      987–88, 988b
  nursing interventions, 15t
  paraprofessionals in, 562
  quality assurance, 983–86
  regulation, 983

reimbursement programs, 983t
  technology in, 992–93
  therapies available, 977

Home Health Care Classification
    (HHCC), 329t

Home Health Compare, 984

Home health nursing, 956, 972
  coordination of care, 987
  experience of, 997b
  federal grants for, 91–92
  Medicare-certified agencies, 976
  public health nurses and, 91
  role description, 978b
  sample schedule, 973b, 974b–975b
  services, 972–76
  standards of, 975–76, 976b
  support groups for, 990

Home Health Quality Initiative, 984

Home safety checklist, 896t

Home visits, 955–69
  advantages of, 957–61
  assessing environmental risks, 966
  challenges of, 963–67
  challenges of the home setting, 958b
  distractions in the environment, 967–68
  economics of, 962–63
  effectiveness of, 961–63
  environmental assessments, 283b
  global connections, 960
  history of, 69
  for newborns, 179
  for persons with disabilities, 724
  process of, 956–57, 958b
  professional conversation and, 959b
  by public health nurses, 937
  purposes of, 957b
  teaching during, 354
  transcultural nursing and, 232

Homeless shelters, 133–34, 638, 914

Homelessness
  assessment of problems, 650–51
  causes of, 643b
  characteristics of, 637t
  chronic, 639
  definition, 639
  definition of, 639
  discrimination and, 641–43
  episodic, 639
  government influences, 640–41
  governmental agencies for, 642t, 643t
  health problems of, 643–46, 644t
  historical perspectives, 639–43
  ill health and, 641
  mental health and, 904
  nursing care for, 647–48
  reflecting on experience with, 925
  rights of, 649–50
  in rural areas, 667–69

serious mental illnesses in, 918
societal influences, 640–41
street ethnography, 910
temporary, 639
trends, 639*b*
urban, 636–46
of women, 806
Homeopathy, 370
Homer, 65
Homicides, 803–5, 918
Homophobia, 800, 816
Homosexual populations, 463–64, 829–32,
    882–83
Honesty, nonmalficence and, 262*b*
Hookworm infections, 444
Hormone-replacement therapy
    (HRT), 795
Hospice care
    for children, 995
    in chronic illnesses, 563
    concerns of recipients, 977
    goals of, 995
    in the home, 993–96
    mean survival times, 997
    under Medicare, 171
    Medicare coverage, 976
    Medicare mandates, 994–95
    multidisciplinary teams, 983*b*
    patient certification, 994
    philosophy of, 995*b*
    quality assurance, 993–95
    roles of, 129
    stresses involved in, 976
Hospital and Reconstruction Act of
    1946, 937
Hospital care
    discharge timing, 978
    health ministries and, 1082
    home health care and, 977
    infant transition to home, 841
    nursing turnover and, 937
    utilization by men, 822–23
Housing, 661, 667–69. *See also*
        environment; home visits;
        homelessness
    for persons with disabilities, 717–20
Human ecology theory, 740–41, 760, *762,*
    762–63
Human-generated disasters, 576, 576*b*
Human immunodeficiency virus.
        *See* HIV/AIDS
Human papillomavirus (HPV), 456–57
Human resources, disaster planning
    and, 589
Human rights, nursing and, 396–97
Hume, David, 258
Hurricane Andrew, 600
Hurricane Camille, 596

Hurricane Celia, 607
Hurricane Hugo, 608
Hurricane Katrina
    environmental effects of, 587
    health ministries after, 1082
    home health care and, 995
    Katrina cough, 591
    lessons learned from, 6, 579, 601
    personal experience of, 578
    population health after, 32
    roles of nurses during, 595
    scope of damage, 572
    shelter management, 598–99
    vulnerability to, 584
Hurricane Rita, 995
Hydration, in the elderly, 869, 873–74
Hydrochloric acid gas, 297*t*
Hydrofluoric acid gas, 297*t*
Hydrogen sulfide, 299*t*
Hypertension, 359, 551*t*, 826
Hyperthermia, 884, 884*b*
Hypothermia, 884, 884*b*

**I**

Identity, of groups, 406
*Iliad* (Homer), 65–66
Imagery, 376–77
Immigrants, 238, 1006
Immune system, humor and, 367
Immunity, 428–29
Immunization Action Coalition, 840
Immunizations. *See also* vaccinations
    for adults, 436*t*
    barriers to, 95
    of children, 840
    in the elderly, 886
    against hepatitis B, 95
    by public health nurses, 91
    screening in schools, 1017
    vaccine-preventable diseases, 431–35
Impact evaluations, 416
Impact of Events Scale-Revised
    (IES-R), 606
Impact stage, of disasters, 583–84
Impairments, definition of, 550
Imperfect markets, 163
Implementation phase, 42*b*, 47–51, 352,
    357–58
Impressing, community assessment, 43
*In loco parentis,* 1021
Incidence rates, 108–9
Inclusion
    community living and, 717
    federal mandates, 1009
    nursing value of, 771–72
    value of, 770–71
Incompetent to proceed (ITP), 917
Incubation periods, 426

Indemnity plans, 143. *See also* fee-for-
        service
Indian Health Service (IHS), 125, 193
Indicators, of community/population
        health, 34
Individualized educational plans (IEPs),
        723, 1018
Individualized family service plans (IFSPs),
        723, 1013, 1018
Individualized health plans (IHPs), 1018
Individuals
    4+ model of wellness and, 317, 320
    competence of, 35
    description of, 111
    health education for, 353–54
    obese, 317, 320
    population-focused care and, 26*t*
    respect for the autonomy of, 255
Individuals with Disabilities Education Act
        (IDEA), 712, 713*t*, 844–45, 1010
Industrial health services, 1035
Industrial hygiene, 1054*b*
Industrial Revolution, history, 71–72, 619
Industrialized countries, disaster resources
    in, 582*b*
Infant mortality
    community profiles, 56–57
    congenital syphilis and, 95
    by country, *165*
    prevention of, 839–40
    quality of life and, 93
    risks of STDs in, 458
    in the U. S., 11
    work-related, 1039–40
Infants. *See also* children; newborns
    environmental exposures, 285
    HIV transmission to, 467, 468
    transition from hospital to home, 841
Infectious diseases. *See* communicable
        diseases
Inflation, 167
Influenza viruses
    avian (H5N1), 442
    death in women and, 786
    pandemic, 430
    symptoms, 434–35
    types of, 435
    vaccination, 435
Informal caregivers, 977
Informant interviews, 44
Informatics, 326–28, 336–38, 992–93
Information
    nursing-related, 326
    power of, 189
Information technology, 992–93
Informed consent, 728
Injection drug users (IDUs), 465
Insomnia, 874

Institute of Medicine (IOM), 939–40
Institutionalization, 710
Instrumental activities of daily living (IADLs), 864
Insurance coverage. *See also* reimbursement
   ABCs of, 144*t*–145*t*
   access to care and, 166
   for advanced practice nurses, 1071–72
   cost of chronic illness and, 560–61
   employment-based insurance, 169–70
   for home health care, 979–83
   lack of, 122
   Medicare, 938
   for mental illnesses, 906–7
   private, 166, 169, 982–83
   in the U. S., 11, 126
   for women, 788
Integrated health care systems, 133
Integrity, definition of, 252
Intensive services, family-focused, 763
Intentional injuries, 662–63
Interdependence, of families, 737
Interdisaster stage, of disasters, 583
Internal maintenance tasks, 410
International Association of Forensic Nurses (IAFN), 205
International Atomic Energy Agency (IAEA), 386*b*
International Civil Aviation Organization (ICAO), 386*b*
International Council of Nurses, 396
International Decade for Natural Disaster Reduction (IDNDR), 581
International Fund for Agricultural Development (IFAD), 386*b*
International Healthy Cities Foundation (IHCF), 635–36
International Labor Organization (ILO), 386*b*
International Maritime Organization (IMO), 386*b*
International Monetary Fund (IMF), 386*b*
International Red Cross, 86, 592–93
International Society of Psychiatric— Mental Health Nurses (ISPN), 924
International Telecommunications Union (ITU), 386*b*
Internet
   access to, 964
   advocacy tools and, 224
   on children in disasters, 600
   community-based nursing and, 332
   connectedness and, 563
   drug sales over, 790
   impact of, 333
   in schools, 338
   technology in home care, 992

teens and, 789
   website usability, 337
Internet Protocol (IP) video systems, 964
Intervention studies
   characteristics, 114*t*
   intensity of, 766–67
   timing of, 766–67
Interviews, 40*b*
Intimate partner violence (IPV), 514, 515*b*, 805, 915
*Investing in Health* (World Bank), 389
Iowa Intervention Project, 329, 329*t*
Iowa Outcomes Project, 329, 329*t*
Irritant dermatitis, 1038
Isocyanates, 298*t*
Isolation
   in disasters, 584–85
   of infected persons, 429–30
   in rural communities, 661, 666
*Ixodes scapularis*, 440

**J**
Jenner, Edward, 69
Joint Commission, 147*b*, 327
Joint Statement on School Health, *1008*
Jordan, health care system in, 401
*Journal of Managed Care Medicine* (AAMCN), 152
*Journal of Nursing Research*, 95
Journaling, 910, 925
Judicial branch, federal, 194, 196
Judicial branch, state, 196–97
Judicial law, 197
Justice
   definition, 255
   distributive, 262*b*
   environmental justice movement, 275–76
   principles of, 257–59, 258*b*
Juvenile offenders, 927

**K**
Kahun Papyrus, 64
Kaiserwerth Institute, 74
Kant, Immanuel, 253–54
Kennedy, Edward, 16
Kepone, 300*t*
Ketones, 295*t*
Key informants, 41, 44
Kidney disease, 826. *See also* chronic renal failure
King, Coretta Scott, 794
Klebs, Edwin, 69
Knowledge, types of, 808
Knowledge deficits, 684
Koch, Robert, 69
Kübler-Ross, Elisabeth, 994, 1089

**L**
Labor Day holiday, 1059
Land mines, 392
Language
   diversity in, 940–41
   people-first, 715
   vocabulary choices, 981*b*
Latex allergies, 1038
Lawsuits, 204–5
Lay advisors, 50
Lead levels, 276, 293*t*
Leadership
   within groups, 415–16
   QUAD Council Public Health Nursing competencies, 953*t*
   styles of, 407, 415–16, 415*t*
   working with the homeless, 648–49
Learned helplessness, 514
Learned hopefulness, 514
Learning goals, 350, 881–82
Learning groups, 413
Learning theories, 343–44
Least possible contribution theory, 769–70
Legal issues
   in home health care, 989–91
   in occupational health nursing, 1052
   in school nursing, 1021–25
   vulnerable populations and, 626–27
Legislation
   adult protective services laws, 865
   in community-focused interventions, 50
   concerned with older adults, 863*b*
   creation of, 198–203
   of disability services, 710–11
   enforcement strategies, 943
   for environmental health, 274
   *Healthy People 2010 objectives*, 203
   influence on occupational health nursing, 1054–56
   Megan's law, 516
   mental health-related, 904*b*
   nursing practice and, 204–5
   for people with disabilities, 713*t*
   protecting people with disabilities, 712–14
   related to school health, 1007*b*, 1009–10, 1019
   types of, 197
Legislative branches, 194, 196
Legitimate power, 189
Leininger's theory of cultural care diversity and universality, 238–42, *241*
Lesbians, 800
Letters to the editor, 50
Level of consciousness, families, 745
Levels of prevention, 304–7
Lewin, Kurt, 411–13
Liability insurance, 1021

Libertarianism, 258
Liberty, freedom and, 189
Lice, 1022
Licensing. *See also* accreditation;
    certification
    of advanced practice nursing, 1065b
    examinations, 204
    of home health care, 983
    for nurses, 78
    of nursing practice, 203
    provisions of, 204
    of school nurses, 1012
Life cycle, aging family members, 864b
Life-cycle transitions, 738–39
Life expectancies
    community/population health and, 34
    by country, *170*
    definition, 858–59
    of men, 832t
    race and, 861
    in the U. S., 11
Life option approaches, 690
Life review process, 882
Life span, definition, 858
Life support, 728
Lifestyles, healthy, 11, 131
Lip reading etiquette, 717
Listening skills, 349–50, 768, 869
Lister, Joseph, 69
*Listeria monocytogenes*, 439
Listeriosis, 439
Literacy, assessment of, 350
Living wills, 990
Lobbying, 200, 203
Local government, 197
Locations, for assessments, 349
Loma Prieta earthquake, California, 608
Long-term care, 972
    advanced practice nurses in, 1073–74
    chronic illness and, 564–65
    *Healthy People 2010* objectives, 551t
    roles of, 128–29
    safety issues, 564–65
    selection of, 565
    women in, 802
Longevity
    of Americans, 131
    definition, 859
    public health efforts and, 939
Longitudinal studies, 114t
Low back disorders, work-related,
    1041–42
Low-birth-weight infants, 687, 849,
    1039–40
Lundy-Barton Model, 40–41, 41t, 56–59,
    60–61
Lung cancer, 783, 797
Lyme disease, 440–41, 440b

**M**
Macronutrients, 871t
Mainstreaming, 1009, 1011–12
Malaria, 441–42, 441b
Male nurses, 83
Malnutrition, 871. *See also* nutrition
Malpractice lawsuits, 204–5
Maltreatment of elders, 865, 865b, 865t
Mammography, 780, 787
Managed care
    barriers to care in, 149b
    community health and, 151–52
    competition among providers, 19
    concept of, 132
    consumer driven, 180–81
    credentialing, 146–48, 147b
    definition, 132, 142
    era of, 96–97
    financing of, 142
    health care delivery through, 131–36
    health promotion and, 308
    home health care and, 986–87
    managed competition and, 96
    management mechanisms, 146
    market-driven, 152
    models of, 143–45
    nurses' role in, 149–51
    nursing's future and, 16–17
    opportunities for nurses, 150t
    principles of, 142–43
    public health efforts and, 176–77,
        947–48
    stakeholders in, 142
    substance abuse denials and, 485
Managed care organizations (MCOs), 132
Managed competition, 136
Management skills, 953t
Manipulative therapies, 371
*Manual for Midwives* (Osborne), 87
Maps, data presentation using, 112
Marijuana use, 481, 482
Marine Hospital Service, 190
Market failures, 160–62, 161b
Market health care mode, 260t
Market justice approach, 180–81
Market shares, 144t, 159
Marriage, roles of women in, 783–85
Marxism, 258
Mass media. *See also* public opinion
    in community-focused interventions,
        50–51, 51b
    effect on policy making, 220
    health care reform and, 221–22
    impact on school health, 1027–28
    influence on adolescents, 789
    influence on substance abuse, 484
    information through, 220
    portrayal of disabilities, 710t

role in disaster management, 594–95
role in policy development, 215, *216*
violence and, 528–29
Massage therapy, 371
Mature women, 796–97, 810b
MCOs. *See* managed care organizations
    (MCOs)
Meaning, roles of the family, 738
Measles, 93
Mechanical vector-borne transmission, 426
Media advocacy, 51
Medicaid (Title XIX). *See also* Centers for
    Medicare and Medicaid Services
    (CMS)
    creation of, 16
    description, 172–73
    enrollment in, 176
    establishment of, 92, 162
    expansion in the 1980s, 93
    for home health care, 983t
    poverty and, 620
    for pregnant adolescents, 791
    reimbursement under, 173, 982, 1071
    Web site, 984
    for women, 807
Medical assistive devices, 724–25
*Medical Education in the United States and
    Canada* (Flexner), 368
Medical insurance, private, 92. *See also*
    insurance coverage; reimbursement
Medical management, 145t
Medical product safety, 551t
Medical professionalism model, 260
Medical social workers, 988b
Medical technologies, 724–25
Medically fragile children, 1009
Medically indigent persons, 626
Medically needy persons, 173
Medicare (Title XVIII)
    creation of, 16, 91
    criteria for home care patients, 983b
    criteria for hospice care, 983b
    description, 170–72
    establishment of, 162
    home health bill of rights, 990
    for home health care, 981–82, 983t
    home health nursing and, 976–78
    hospice care, 994–95
    Hospital Insurance (Part A), 171
    inpatient hospital care, 171
    Medicare+Choice program (Part C),
        171–72
    payment for an episode of care, 981–82
    Social Security Act of 1935 and, 938
    Supplementary Medical Insurance
        (SMI, Part B), 171
Medicare+Choice program (Part C),
    171–72

Medications. *See also* over-the-counter
drugs; prescription drugs
chemical addictions, 887
costs of, 167
drug interactions, 499–500
in the elderly, 886, 886b
Medicine wheel, 313, *313*
Medigap insurance, 172
Mediterranean fever, 81
Megan's law, 417
*Megatrends* (Naisbitt), 311
Melanoma in children, 841
Men
aging by, 816
at-risk populations, 829–32
behavioral factors, 818–20
diets of, 818–19
health issues, 816–35
health research issues, 833
homeless, 910
homicide rates, 918
impact of environmental factors, 818
impact of ethnic factors, 816–18
impact of sociocultural factors,
816–18
life expectancy, 832t
osteoporosis in, 821
risk from STDs, 458
socialization processes, 816–18
stay-at-home fathers, 831
Mental health care
assessment of the elderly, 868
of children, 840–41, 1006
classification of disorders, 915
college response to issues, 1011
in the community, 903–7
definitions of, 902–3
economics of, 905
leading indicators of, 921b
National Health Objectives for, 927t
public health model, 922
public status assessments, 915–19
public—private split, 908–9
school-based programs for, 843
in women, 788
Mental health reform, 904–7
Mental illnesses
definitions, 903
in farmers, 671–72
in homeless people, 644t
inpatient services, 906–7
prevention of, 927
stigma of, 928
vulnerable populations, 905b
Mental impairment, 708
Mental institutions, discharge from, 905
Mental retardation, 712, 728, 850
Mercury, 294t

Mesopotamia, history, 64
Methamphetamine use, 482, 484, 665
Methicillin-resistant *S. aureus* (MRSA),
429, 437–38, 438, 444, 990
Methylene diphenyldisocyanate
(MDI), 298t
Metropolitan Life Insurance Company, 85
Metropolitan statistical areas
(MSAs), 658
Micronutrients, 871t
Middle ages, 65–69
Midlife, research areas, 810b
Midwives, history in the U.S., 87
Migraine headaches, 545, 557
Migrant farm workers, 667, 1058–59
Migrant health, 1058–59
Mild cognitive impairment (CMI), 879
Military health care, 88, 125
Mill, John Stuart, 72, 252
Millbank Report, 941
Millennium Developmental Goals,
396, 397b
Mind–body interventions, 370
Mini-Mental State Examination (MMSE),
868, 894t
Minoan culture, history, 64
Miosis, 870
Missionary nursing, 1095, 1097–98
Mobile computing, 327
Mobile phones, 333
Mobility impairments, 716, 876–78
Monitoring devices, 725
Monitoring the Future study, 482
Monopolies, free markets and, 161
Moral imagination, 264–65
Moral rules, development of, 252–56
Morbidity, prevalence and, 109
*Morbidity and Mortality Weekly Report*
(MMWR), 110
Mortality rates, 56–57, 108, 111,
527–28
Mothers, deaths of, 839–40
Motivation, definition, 342t
Motorcycles, 872
MRSA. *See* methicillin-resistant *S. aureus*
(MRSA)
Multidrug resistance, 444
Multidrug-resistant tuberculosis
(MDR-TB), 447
Multiple intelligence practices, 723
Musculoskeletal disorders, 1042
Music therapy, 375–76, 377, 724
Muslim faith, 1089
Mutual Recognition Model, 204
*Mycobacterium tuberculosis*, 446–47
Myelomeningocele, 709t
Myocardial infarction, 553. *See also* heart
attacks, warning signs

**N**
NA-TECH disasters, 577
NANDA (North American Nursing
Diagnosis Association), 329t
Natinal Environmental Policy Act, 191
National Alliance for Caregiving, 988
National Alliance for the Mentally Ill
(NAMI), 912–13
National Association for Home Care and
Hospice, 994
National Association of Colored Graduate
Nurses, 96
National Association of Home Care and
Hospice, 990
National Association of Insurance
Commissioners (NIAC), 147b
National Association of School Nurses
(NASN), 1012, 1023
National Center for Child Fatality
Review, 838b
National Center for Complementary and
Alternative Medicine (NCCAM),
130, 369
National Center for Environmental Health
(NCEH), 289t
National Center for Health Statistics, 44
National Center on Educational Outcomes
(NCEO), 1010
National Center on Elder Abuse, 518
National Committee for Quality Assurance
(NCQA), 146–47, 147b
National Disaster Medical System
(NDMS), 590
National Environmental Education and
Training Foundation, 289t
National Food Safety Initiative (NFSI),
438–39
National Health and Education
Consortium (NHEC), 1015
National Health Interview Survey, 368–69
National Health Objectives for Mental
Health, 927t
National Health Service Corps
(NHSC), 1073
National Health Survey, 110
National Institute for Occupational Safety
and Health (NIOSH), 1036,
1054, 1057t
National Institute of Environmental Health
Sciences (NIEHS), 289t
National Institute of Mental Health, 90
National Institutes of Health (NIH),
192, 369
National Law Center on Homeless and
Poverty, 649–50
National League for Nursing (NLN), 81
National Longitudinal Study of Healthy
Adolescents (NLSHA), 1006, 1017

National Nursing Coalition for School Health, 1015
National Occupational Research Agenda (NORA), 1036b
National Organization of Nurse Practitioner Faculties (NONPF), 1069
National Partnership for Immunization (NPI), 48
National Public Health Performance Standards (NPHPS), 946
National Quality Forum (NQF), 984
National Research Council (NRC), 518–19
National Rural Health Association (NRHA), 668
National School Lunch Amendment, 212
National Survey on Drug Use and Health (NSDUH), 481
Native American nations
    access to care, 1073
    community health interventions, 125
    elderly persons in, 861
    medicine wheel, 313
    rural populations, 661
    understanding of existence, 313
Natural disasters. See also disasters
    categories of, 576b
    definition, 576
    distribution by type, 575
    people killed by, 575
    recovery of communities, 57
    reduction efforts, 581
Natural history of disease, 104–5, 106t
Natural therapies, 377
Naturopathy, 370
Nazi medical experimentation, 254
Near poor, 620, 626
Needle exchange programs, 465
Negative feedback, 742
Neglect
    of children, 515
    of elders, 519b, 865
    protection from, 712
    of self, 563
Negligence, lawsuits, 204–5
Neighborhoods, 497, 851–52
Nepal, home visiting in, 960
Networked client care, 333–35
Neural tube defects, 1039–40
Neurons to Neighborhoods (IOM), 841
New Deal, 936
Newborns. See also infants
    care of, 697
    early discharge of, 179
    health status of, 697
    outcomes of teen pregnancy, 687
    screening of, 727
    status of, 693t

Newton, Isaac, 68
NIC (Nursing Intervention Classification), 329t
Nickel, 294t
Nicotine addiction, 561
Nightingale, Florence, 10, 72–77
    British Nurses Association and, 78
    "Cassandra," 74
    on community assessments, 32
    on community health, 78–79
    in the Crimea, 74, 102
    definition of health, 10
    on environmental health, 1058
    as epidemiologist, 102–3
    legacy of, 79–80, 1084–85
    military reform efforts, 77
    Notes on Hospitals, 76
    Notes on Nursing, 77
    polar-area diagram, 103
    political reform efforts, 77
    public health initiatives and, 181–82
    on public health nursing, 941
    on sanitation, 75–77
    work of, 10
Nightingale School of Nursing at St. Thomas, 77–78
Nitrogen oxides, 298t
No Child Left Behind (NCLB) legislation, 1010, 1020
NOC (Nursing Outcomes Classification), 329t
Non-governmental organizations (NGOs), 386
Noncompliance, 989
Nonhealth systems, 58
Nonmalficence, 255, 256, 262b
Nonsummativity, concept of, 741
Norms, definition, 406
Noroviruses (NoV), 426
North American Nursing Diagnosis Association (NANDA), 329t
Nosocomial infections, 437
Not guilty by reason of insanity (NGI), 917
Notes on Hospitals (Nightingale), 76
Notes on Nursing (Nightingale), 21, 77
Nuclear power, 332–33
Nuclear Regulation Commission, 274
Numerators, definition, 107
Nurse anesthetists, 1066
Nurse-Family Partnerships (NFPs), 961–62, 963
Nurse–initiated distractions, 968
Nurse Licensure Compact (NLC), 204
Nurse midwives, 1066
Nurse Multistate Licensure Mutual Recognition Model, 204
Nurse practice acts, 204, 1021

Nurse practitioners (NPs), 1064
    authority of, 1069–70
    early roles of, 96
    education of, 1069–70
    Healthy People 2010 objectives, 1070
    history of, 1067
    in occupational health, 1053
    prescriptive authority of, 1074
    roles of, 1065
    school nurses and, 1027
    scope of practice, 1069–70
    specialization by, 1074
    workloads, 1074
Nurse–family interventions, 752–55
Nurse–Family Partnerships (NFPs), 843–842
Nurse–patient relationships, 15
Nurses
    in the disaster response, 590
    as entrepreneurs, 137–38
    health care delivery by, 127
    in the political process, 200, 203
    public health policies proposed by, 223–24
    reactions to disaster, 605–8
    shortages of, 396
    specialization by, 96
    substance abuse interventions, 500–502
    substance-abusing, 501b
    who smoke, 501t
Nursing
    conceptual models for, 921t
    core values of, 771
    definition, 230
    of elders, 860–85
    family-focused, 742–43
    family-oriented, 742–43
    global connection, 923
    health policy and, 137
    history of, 67, 907
    human rights and, 396–97
    new opportunities in, 137–38
    public opinion of, 67
    in the twenty-first century, 11–12
    use of reflection in, 924–26
Nursing Center for School Health, 1015
Nursing centers, 1075
Nursing classification systems, 328–29, 329t
Nursing data, 326
Nursing diagnoses, 42b, 46, 59
Nursing for the Future (Brown), 81
Nursing home workers, 1037
Nursing homes, selection of, 565
Nursing informatics, 326–28, 328–29
Nursing information systems, 326, 327
Nursing Intervention Classification (NIC), 329t

Nursing knowledge, 326
Nursing Outcomes Classification
(NOC), 329*t*
Nursing process
for the community, 41–52
community health, 59
data collection, 44–46
diagnosis, 59
evaluation, 59
gaining entry into communities,
42–44
Lundy–Barton model, 56
planning, 59
steps in, 104*t*
Nursing shortages, 944–45, 1056
*Nursing's Agenda for Health Care Reform,*
16, 96
Nurture, sources of, 316*b*
Nutrition. *See also* diet; malnutrition
in adolescent pregnancy, 694*b*
assessments, **57–58**, 371, 483
barriers to, 872
chronic illnesses and, 371
in chronic renal disease, 553
deficits in the elderly, 872*t*
*Healthy People 2010* objectives, 551*t*
of men, 818–19
requirements of the elderly,
871–73, 871*t*
Nutting, Mary Adelaide, 82

**O**

Obesity
among children, 25
chronic illness and, 565
costs of, 546*t*, 549*t*
in the elderly, 873
*Healthy People 2010* objectives, 551*t*
morbidity, 546*t*
mortality from, 546*t*
school-based programs for, 842
in schools, 1014
urban environments and, 38
in the U.S., 105
world health issues, 392
Observation, of communities, 44, 58
Obsessive–compulsive disorders
(OCD), 912
Occupational and environmental health
history form, 1047*b*–1048*b*
Occupational hazard exposures, 1050
Occupational health
categories of illnesses, 1037*t*
fatal traumatic injuries, 1043
latency period of illnesses, 1037
nonfatal traumatic injuries, 1043
nurse-managed models of, 1056–58
risks for women, 807–8

Occupational health nurse case
manager, 1052
Occupational health nurse clinician, 1052
Occupational health nurse consultants,
1053, 1057–58
Occupational health nurse corporate
directors, 1053
Occupational health nurse educators, 1053
Occupational health nurse health
promotion specialists, 1052
Occupational health nurse managers,
1052–53
Occupational health nurse
practitioners, 1053
Occupational health nurse researchers, 1053
Occupational health nursing
certification of, 1056
code of ethics, 1046*b*
education for, 1056
employee education, 1055
future of, 1058–60
history of, 1034–36
interdisciplinary fields of practice, 1054*b*
practice of, 1044–54
professionalism in, 1056–58
research priorities, 1035*b*, 1036*b*
roles of, 1032–61, *1053*
scope of practice, 1046–57
standards of practice, 1044
Occupational medicine, 1054*b*
Occupational Safety and Health Act of
1970, 1035, 1054
Occupational Safety and Health
Administration (OSHA), 665–66,
1035, 1054
Occupational therapists, 988*b*
Occupational therapy, 724
Office of Alternative Medicine (OAM), 369
Office of National Preparedness, 592
Office of Personal Management
(OPM), 147*b*
Oklahoma City bombings, 600, 603*b*,
605, 1025
Older Americans Act Amendments, 713*t*
Omnibus Reconciliation Act (OBRA),
145, 1071
Oral assessments, 872
Organ transplants, 332, 728
Organization policies, 211
Organophosphates, 299*t*
Orthomolecular medicine, 371
Osborne, Mary D., 87, 936
Osteopathic manipulation, 371
Osteoporosis
caregivers for individuals with, 548–49
in the elderly, 878
*Healthy People 2010* objectives, 551*t*
impact of, 556

management of, 986
in men, 821
nursing interventions by setting, 15*t*
prevention of, 879*b*
risk profile for women, 798*t*
signs and symptoms, 798
in women, 797–99
Outcome evaluations, 416
Outcomes. *See also* patient care
outcomes
care management and, 17
evaluation of policies, 223
lack of insurance and, 166
measures of community health, 25
Outcomes and Assessment Information
Sets (OASIS), 981, 982, 984, 986
Outputs, evaluation of policies, 223
Over-the-counter drugs. *See also*
medications; prescription drugs
documentation of, 982
drug interactions, 499
use by adolescents, 790
Overweight, 551*t*, 873
Oxycontin, 481
Ozone, 298*t*

**P**

Pain management, 555
Palliative care, 563, 972, 976, 995
Pan American Health Organization
(PAHO), 457, 461*t*
Pap smears, 787
Paraquat, 300*t*
Parasitic diseases, 444–45
Parental rights, 712
Parent–child interactions, 533–34
Parenting education, 693*t*, 695
Parents, 517*t*, 529, 691*b*
Parish nursing, 1090–92, 1092*b*,
1100–1102
Participation, 406–7
Participatory leadership, 415–16, *416*
Partnerships, by nurses, 404, 628–29
Passive immunity, 429
Pasteur, Louis, 69
*Pasteurella pestis,* 67
Paternalism, theory of, 258, 342
Pathogenicity, 426
Patient advocates, 148–49, 712. *See also*
advocacy
Patient care outcomes, 133–36. *See also*
outcomes
Patient education
disease state management and, 980*b*
nurses' role in, 149
role of school nurses, 1014
technology in home care, 992
for vulnerable populations, 628–29

Patients
  empowerment of, 37
  resources of, 627
  responsibilities of, 989
  rights of, 263, 989
  strengths of, 627
Paxil, side effects, 1021
Peer education, 690
Peer pressures, 1017
Peer review organizations (PROs), 147b
Penicillin, 87, 454
Pentagon attacks, 579
People-first language, 715
Perimenopausal period, 780, 793–96, 810b
Period of infectivity, 426
Period prevalence, 109
Periodic rates, 113
Person, description of, 111
Person-centered planning, 717
Personal care attendants, 719
Personal computers, 333. See also
    informatics
Personal-digital assistants (PDAs), 327,
    331, 1067. See also informatics
Personal health promotion, 305
Personal identity, 737–38
Personal surveillance, 430
Persons with special needs, 616
Pesticides, 299t
Pets, 726, 846
Phenomena of concern, 919, 920b
Phenomenological perspective, 926–27
Phenylketonuria (PKU) screening, 727
Philippine American families, 242
Phosgene, 298t
Photovoice, 784
Physical abuse
  of adolescents, 684
  of children, 515, 516b, 517t
  of elders, 519b
  in families, 520b
  intimate partner violence, 514
  of women, 803–5
Physical assessments, 58, 868
Physical fitness, community-level, 58
Physical impairment, 708. See also
    disabilities
Physical therapists, 988b
Physical therapy
  for persons with disabilities, 724
Physician assistants, 127
Physician hospital organizations
    (PHOs), 146
Physicians
  advanced practice nurses and, 1073
  health care delivery by, 127
  as part of a team, 988b
  reimbursement for, 172
Phytotherapy, 371

Pilot studies, 48
Pinworm infections, 444
Places, rates related to, 111–112
Planned Parenthood of America, 81
Planning phase
  community assessments, 46–47, 59
  for community education, 357
  community-focused interventions,
      42b, 59
  for health education, 350–51
  prioritization steps, 47
Plans of care (POCs)
  in hospice, 995
  for individuals, 982
  multidisciplinary teams and,
      987–88, 988b
Plasmodium spp., 441–42
Plato, 65
PLISSIT model, 883
Pneumococcal diseases, 435
Pneumonia, death in women and, 786
Point-of-service providers (POSs), 133,
    143–44
Point prevalence, 109
Poison Prevention Packaging Act, 274
Polar-area diagram, 103
Policies
  in community-focused interventions, 50
  corporate cultures and, 1051
  development strategies, 219–22
  environmental, 280–81
  on environmental health, 276–78
  evaluation of, 222–23
  Home Care Bill of Rights, 991
  for the homeless, 649–50
  implementation of, 222–23
  information needed for, 219
  QUAD Council Public Health Nursing
      competencies, 951t
  on substance abuse, 485
Policy environments, 215
Policy instruments, 217
Policy research, 175–76
Polio, 709t
Polio epidemics, 937
Polio vaccine, 91
Political action committees (PACs), 203
Political power, definition of, 189
Political systems, 58, 188–89
Politics, 136–37, 260t, 358–59. See also
    government; legislation
Pollution Prevention Act, 274
Polychlorinated biphenyls (PCBs), 297t
Polypharmacy, 886, 890
Population-focused care, 6, 19, 26t
Population-level interventions, 36
Populations
  4+ model of wellness and, 320–21
  assessment of, 36, 37, 41, 56–59

  definition, 14
  demographics, 167
  descriptive epidemiology, 105–11
  examples of, 33
  growth, 275, 384, 385b
  of interest, 20
  isolation in disasters, 584–85
  self-awareness of, 33
  worldwide, 275
Positive feedback, 742
POSs. See point-of-service providers
    (POSs)
Post-traumatic stress disorder (PTSD), 585,
    602, 606, 917, 1025
Postpartum care, 693t, 918
POTS video, 964
Poverty
  at-risk families and, 765
  child health impacts, 848–51
  cultural perspectives, 619–20
  definition, 394
  elderly persons in, 861
  environmental hazards and, 851
  feminization of, 783
  health-related perspectives, 620–21
  homelessness and, 641
  nutritional requirements and, 872
  in rural areas, 660
  vulnerability and, 618–19
  women and, 624–25, 807
  women in the U. S., 782–83
  world health and, 394
Poverty index, 620
Power
  concepts of, 189
  politics and, 188
  resources and, 555
  role of the family, 738
  sources of, 189
Powerlessness, 555
PPOs. See preferred provider organizations
Prayer, 375
Predisaster stage, of disasters, 583
Preferred provider organizations (PPOs),
    97, 132, 145
Pregnancy, 458, 458t, 498. See also
    adolescent pregnancies
Prenatal care, 166, 685, 693t, 694–95, 791
Prenatal diagonses, 727
Presbycusis, 870
Prescription drugs, 790, 1020. See also
    medications
Prescriptive authority, 1074, 1076
Presence, concept of, 901
Press releases, 50–51, 51b. See also mass
    media
Pressure sores, 884–85, 885b
Preterm infants, 849, 1039–40
Prevalence rates, calculation of, 109

Prevention. *See also* primary prevention; secondary prevention; tertiary prevention
  collaboration in, 177
  of communicable diseases, 429–31
  of food-borne illnesses, 439
  of hate crimes, 523–24
  of HIV/AIDS, 511
  of homelessness, 649
  levels of, 304
  of mental disorders, 912
  of NIDDM, 313
  of sexually-transmitted diseases, 472
  of substance abuse, 489
  of violence, 532–37
Preventive care
  access by men, 823
  acute care *versus*, 19
  community-based care and, 17–23
  components of, 126
  in correctional facilities, 205b
  disease state management and, 980b
  economics of, 176–79
  for the elderly, 869–85
  family-based programs, 763–64
  by home health nurses, 972
  home visits and, 961–62
  occupational health nursing and, 1051
  school-based programs, 1007
  strategies for, 211t
Prices, of products, 159
Primary aging, 858
Primary care
  advanced practice nurses in, 1076
  centers for, 135
  components of, 126
  concept of, 395
  *Healthy People 2010* objectives, 551t
  nurse practitioners in, 1069
  nurses as providers of, 151
  nursing model, 923
  school-based clinics and, 1027
Primary mental health care model, 923–24
Primary prevention, 105. *See also* prevention
  of communicable diseases, 429–30
  description of, 24
  of elder abuse, 865b
  health promotion and, 304
  in the history of disease, 106t
  of mental illness, 922
  of MRSA, 438
  of pregnancy, 687–89
  of substance abuse, 490–91
  of violence, 533–34
*Principles and Consumer Bill of Rights*, 142
Principles of the Ethical Practice of Public Health, 255
Prisons, 205, 540–41, 806–7

Privacy, 991, 1022. *See also* confidentiality
Problem-Oriented Medical Recording (POMR), 59
Problem solving, 408, 767
Procedural knowledge, 808
Process, as measure of health, 34
Process evaluation, 416
Professional care, 236
Professional health promotion, 305
Professional stranger concept, 43
Program planning, 951t
Proportions, use of, 107
Proprioception, 885
Prospective payment systems (PPSs), 123–24
Prospective studies, 114t
Prostate cancer, 823–24, 823t
Prostate-specific antigen, 823
Protozoans, 444–45
Provider liaisons, 151
Psychiatric disorders, 487. *See also* mental health
Psychiatric–mental health nursing, 900
  ethical issues, 919
  frameworks for, 920–21
  future of, 927–28
  history of, 907–13, 908b
  individuals and groups needing, 913–15
  levels of practice, 911–13
  models for, 921–27
  perspective of, 901–2
  phenomena of concern, 919, 920b
  phenomenological perspective, 926–27
  primary care model of, 923
  primary mental health care model of, 923–24
  state of, 909–11
Psychiatric–mental health services, 919
Psychomotor objectives, 350–51
Psychotropic medications, 1020
Public direct care programs, 173–74
Public health
  definition of, 124–25
  education about AIDS, 94
  essential services, 944
  goals of, 124b
  violence and, 508–9
Public Health Association, 124
Public health infrastructure, epidemics and, 588
Public health model, 922
Public health nursing. *See also* community health nursing
  challenges for, 944–49
  community activism and, 83–85
  competencies, 949–50, 951t–953t
  conceptual basis of, 940–43
  description, 6, 12, 1044
  early education, 88–89

  early health outcomes, 937–38
  ethical conflicts faced in, 262b
  geographic areas covered by, 940
  health outcomes, 937–38
  history, 64–99, 936–39
  nurse shortages, 944
  philosophy of, 939–44
  research studies, 93
  standardization of practice, 88–89
  USPHS Division of, 90
  values of, 942
Public Health Nursing Practice Model (ASTDN), *943*, 944, 945t
Public health policies, 213–15, 223–24
Public health professionals, defined, 97
Public health sciences, 952t
Public opinion. *See also* mass media
  environment movement, 277–78
  health policy and, 136–37
  mass media and, 220
  on substance abuse, 484–85
Public policies
  description of, 210
  development of, 215–22, *216*
  goals of, 217–18
  public health and, 214–15
  purpose of, 211
  shaping of, 217
Public Services International (PSI), 389
Public–private partnerships, 309–10
Puerto Rican populations, 562
Pulmonary emboli, 785
Pure Food and Drug Act (1906), 212
Pyle, Ernie, 88

**Q**

Quad Council of Public Health Nursing Organizations, 12, 944, 945–46, 949–50, 951t–953t
Quality assurance
  in home health care, 983–85
  hospice-related, 993–95
Quality Compass (NCQA), 147
Quality of care, 991
Quality of life
  aging and, 557–58
  biases related to, 728
  chronic illness and, 556–58
  cognitive functioning and, 878–79
  indicators of, 93
Quarantine, use of, 430
Quasi-markets, health care, 163
Questions, assessment use of, 349, 349t

**R**

Rabies, 443–44
Race/ethnicity. *See also specific* groups
  adolescent pregnancy and, 681
  birth mothers' age and, 789t

caregiving burdens and, 562
child mortality rates and, 840
chronic disease burden and, 547, 550
community health and, 20–23
elderly populations, 860–61
HIV/AIDS and, 464–65, 464*t*, 465*t*
homelessness and, 641
of migrant farm workers, 667
in rural counties, 660–61, 660*t*
rural—urban poverty and, *661*
socialization of men, 816–18
vulnerability and, 623–24
Racial and Ethnic Approaches to
    Community Health (REACH), 547
Railroad Retirement disability
    benefits, 171
Rap music, 786
Rape, forensic nursing, 511. *See also* date
    rape
Rates
    adjusted, 109–10
    age-specific, 111
    calculation of, 108
    crude, 109–10
    definition, 107
    presentation of, 111, 112*t*
    specific, 109–10
    use of, 106–11
Rathbone, William, 78
Ratios, use of, 107
Readiness, definition, 342*t*
Reading levels, 350
Reasoned action, theory of, 345*t*
Reconstruction stage of disasters, 585
Recreation therapy
    for persons with disabilities, 724, 729
Referent power, 189
Referrals, 989
Reflective thinking, 771, 772, 924–26
The Reformation, 69–70
Refugees, 238, 765
Registered nurses, 7
Regulation
    competition *versus,* 159–60
    health plan coverage and, 144*t*
    legislative process and, 203
    of managed care organizations, 146–48
    of nursing practice, 203
Rehabilitation, 721, 724
Rehabilitation Act, 713*t*
Reiki, 1092
Reimbursement programs
    for advanced practice nurses, 1071–72
    computerization of, 334
    for home health care, 981–83, 983*t*,
        986–87
    telehealth care and, 337
Relationship-focused care, 766, 767, 902

Relationships
    abusive, 514, 533, 803–5
    with adolescents, 789
    ethical dilemmas and, 263
    of people with disabilities, 721
Relative value scales, 172
Relaxation exercises, 377
Religion. *See also* spirituality
    church access, 722
    historical view of illness, 64–65
    Muslim faith, 1089
    prayers, 1093
    review of systems, 59
    spirituality and, 1085
    spirituality in the elderly, 885
Religiosity, 1085
Religious attendance, 1086
Religious communities, 1082
The Renaissance, history, 68–69
Renal diet, 553
Renal insufficiency, 548
Reno, Janet, *547*
Repetitive trauma injuries, 1037–38
*Report of the Sanitary Commission of
    Massachusetts* (Shattuck),
    71, 124
*Report on an Inquiry into the Sanitary
    Conditions of the Laboring
    Population of Great Britain*
    (Chadwick), 71
Reproductive health
    education in, 91
    risks and, 785–86
    STDs and, 457–58
    work-related hazards, 1039–40
    world health issues, 392
Reproductive rights, 728
*The Republic* (Plato), 65
"Rescue fantasies," 767
Research
    by missionary nurses, 1097–98
    NIOSH centers for, 1057*t*
    by occupational health nurses,
        1052, 1053
    opportunities for nurses in, 138
    process of, 104*t*
Reservoirs, infectious disease, 426
Resource management
    ethical issues, 266
    for homeless populations, 649
    managed care barriers, 149*b*
    nurses' role in, 150
Resource utilization groups, version 3
    (rIG-III), 172
Respiratory infections, 842, 849
Respite care, 562, 720, 864–65
Restorative care, 126
Restraints, use of, 564–65

Retired Senior Volunteer Program
    (RSVP), 881
Retirement, in the elderly, 881–83
Retirement communities, 129
Retrospective studies, 114*t*
Return-to-work contracts, 501–2
Review of systems, community-level, 58–59
Reward power, definition of, 189
Risk
    assessment of, 281–82
    factors in, 106
    management of, 150–51, 282
    vulnerability and, 616–17
Risky lifestyle behaviors, 618
RN No Harm, 289*t*
Robb, Isabel Hampton, 81
Robots, 332
Rockefeller Foundation, 89
Role modeling, 257
Roman era, history, 66
Roundworm infections, 444
Roy's Adaptation Model, 984
Rule making, 222
Rural communities
    adolescents in, 662–66
    agricultural hazards, 665–66
    definition of, 658–59, 659
    demographics, 560–661
    elderly populations, 666, 861
    growth of, 660
    HIV/AIDS in, 670
    personal biases about, 661
    risks and lifestyle in, 662
    schematic of, *658*
    school children in, 1004
    substance abuse interventions, 496, 496*b*
Rural health centers, 129, 409
Rural Nursing Incentive Act of 1991, 1071
Rural populations, 659–61
Rural—urban continuum, 658
Ryan White AIDS Drug Assistance
    Program (ADAP), 201
Ryan White CARE Act, 462, 463*b*

**S**
Safety, occupational health nurses and,
    1054*b*
Sago mining disaster, 1042
Salivation, in the elderly, 871
Salk, Jonas, 429
Salk vaccine, 937
*Salmonella,* 427, 439, 443
Salmonellosis, 439
Salvation Army disaster services, 593
"Sandwich generation," 863
SANE nurses, forensics and, 511
Sanger, Margaret, 81–82
Sanitation, history of, 65

Saunders, Cicely, 994
Scales, Jessie Sleet, 85
School-based clinics, 1009, 1028–27
School-based services, 842–43, 1025–27
School health care
    accountability for, 1023
    advanced practice nurses and, 1074–75
    business involvement in, 1024
    CDC funding for programs, *1011*
    components of, 1007
    funding of, 1019, 1020, 1023–24
    mental health, 1011
    practical issues in, 1019–20
    role of the media in, 1027–28
    supervision of, 1023
    types of service, 1013*t*
School Health Resource Services
        (SHRS), 1028
School Nurse Practitioners (SNPs), 1009
School nurses, 1002–31
    advocacy by, 1026
    case finding by, 1018–19
    collaborative roles, 1017
    continuing education, 1012
    credentials of, 1012
    description, 1004
    education of, 1012
    as first responders, 1025
    history of, 93, 1007–10
    legal issues, 1021–25
    role definition of, 1012–15, *1013*
    shortages of, 1020
    technology innovations, 1028
    typical day of, 1005
School–health linkages, 1025–27
Schools
    absenteeism, 844, 1011
    at-risk populations, 1017
    attendance data, 1014
    clinics in, 847
    health curriculum, 1007
    *Healthy People 2010* objectives, 360
    numbers of children in, 1020
    peer pressure in, 1017
    as research sites, 1015
    substance abuse interventions, 495
    teen pregnancy prevention programs,
        691–92
    violence in, 521, 1024–25
Scoliosis, screening, 1017
Screening
    Denver Developmental Screening Test
        (DDST), 92
    Early Periodic Screening Diagnosis and
        Treatment (EPSDT), 92
    genetics programs, 93
    for phenylketonuria, 727
    potential for abuse, 533

in schools, 1017, 1019
    secondary prevention and, 24
    for sexually-transmitted diseases, 472
    for syphilis, 454
Seacole, Mary, 75, 77, 83
Search-and-rescue missions, 595
Secondary aging, 858
Secondary analysis of existing data, 44
Secondary care, 126, 130
Secondary data, 44, 56–57
Secondary prevention, 105
    of communicable diseases, 430–31
    description of, 24
    of elder abuse, 865*b*
    health promotion and, 304
    in the history of disease, 106*t*
    of homelessness, 652
    of mental illness, 922
    of substance abuse, 492, 492*b*
    of teen pregnancy, 692
    of violence, 534–35
Segregation, disease prevention and, 430
Self-as-patient reflection, 925
Self-assessment quizzes, 771*b*
Self-care
    consumerism and, 310–11
    cost effectiveness of, 1075
    deficits, 902
    by nurses, 901, 1049
    promotion of, 708
    reflection on, 925
    in young adulthood, 792–93
Self clinical reflection, 925–26
Self-concept, in the elderly, 880
Self-determination, 561, 965–66
    for persons with disabilities, 712, 718
Self-disclosure, 965
Self-efficacy, 342*t*, 752–55
Self-employment, 881
Self-esteem
    chronic illness and, 555
    substance abuse and, 483
    violence prevention and, 533, 924
Self-examination
    breast, 797
    testicular, 824, 825*b*
Self-help groups, 414
Self-help strategies, 558
Self-identity, *770*, 816
Self-insurance, 169
Self-reflection, 901, 925
Self-regulation, 742
Self-worth, 737–38
Senescence, 859
September 11 attacks, 1025. *See also* World
        Trade Center attacks
Serious mental illnesses (SMIs), 900,
        916–17

Service learning, 264–65
Seventh Day Adventist Church, 1082
Sex education, 20
Sex offenders, 516
Sexual abuse
    of adolescents, 684
    of children, 515, 516*b*, 517*t*
    of elders, 519*b*
    in families, 520*b*
    of women, 803–5
Sexual activity
    adolescent pregnancy and, 696–97
    age of onset, 791
    among adolescents, 678–79
    of people with disabilities, 721
    by rural adolescents, 664
    in schools, 1020
    by teens, 791
Sexual aggression, 833
Sexual orientation, 800, 804
Sexual rights
    of persons with disabilities, 728
Sexual violence, 514
Sexuality, in the elderly, 882–83
Sexually transmitted diseases (STDs)
    access to care and, 470
    in adolescents, 791, 806, 1021
    basic facts, 454*b*
    clinical presentation of, 454*b*
    common diseases, 454–57
    in elderly populations, 882–83
    health consequences of, 457–58
    health services for, 470, 472
    increased incidence, 94–95
    in pregnancy, 458, 458*t*
    risk assessments, 473
    risk factors, 455*t*
    scope of the problem, 454
    screening, 472
Shattuck Report, 71
Shelter nurses, 133–35
Short-term specialized care facilities, 128
Sick roles, 554, 786
Sildenafil citrate (Viagra), 827–28
*Silent Spring* (Carson), 274
Silica exposure, 1039
Silicosis, 1039
Skilled nursing facilities (SNFs), 171, 172
Skilled nursing visits (SNVs), 976
Skin disorders, 644*t*
Skin integrity, 884–85
Sleep deprivation, 874
Sleep requirements, 874
Sleet, Jessie, 85
Smoking, 482
    absenteeism and, 1040
    costs of, 546*t*
    by men, 818, 819

morbidity, 546*t*

mortality from, 546*t*

nicotine addiction, 561

by nurses, 501*t*

Smoking cessation programs, 19–20, 175

Snow, John, 72, 102

Snowmobile injuries, 662

SOAP format, 59

Social change, 49–50

Social cognitive theory, 786

Social control, 494

Social justice approaches, 181, 286–87

Social learning theory, 345*t*

Social marketing theory, 345*t*–346*t*

Social modeling theory, 494

Social responsibility, 771, 772

Social Security Act of 1935, 88, 89, 92, 124, 162, 212, 938

Social Security Disability Income (SSDI), 711

Social systems, review of, 58

Social workers, 128

Socialization

    chronic illness and, 554–55

    of men, 816–18, 828

    role of the family in, 739

    substance abuse and, 486

Societal expectations, 307–8

Socioeconomic status, 623–24, 849–51

Space flight, 333

Spanish-American War, 86

Special-interest groups, 136–37

Specialization, nursing, 96

Specific rates, 109–10

Speech impairments, 717

Speech therapists, 988*b*

Speech therapy, 724

Spina bifida, 709*t*

Spinal cord injuries, 709*t*

Spiritual domains

    in the 4+ model of wellness, 316

    health ministries, 1082–84

    of hospice care, 995–96

    medicine and, 366

Spirituality

    in the elderly, 885

    nursing assessment of, 375

    nursing interventions and, 841–42

    religion and, 1085

Spontaneous abortions, 1039–40

Spreadsheets, 331, 338

Stakeholders

    analysis of, 409, 410*b*

    in managed care, 142

    in policy development, 218–19

    in U.S. health policies, 212*b*

Standard metropolitan statistical areas (SMSAs), 110

Standard setters/testers, 411

Standards of care, 975–76, 976*b*

Standards of participation, 159

Standards of practice, 1044

*Staphylococcus aureus*

    methicillin-resistant (MRSA), 429, 437–38

    nosocomial infections, 437

    penicillin-resistant, 424

State Children's Health Insurance Program (SCHIP), 1019

Status, as measure of health, 34

Statutory laws, 197

Stay-at-home fathers, 831

Stereotyping, 230, 237

Stewart B. McKinney Homeless Assistance Act of 1987, 641–42

Stoddard solvent, 296*t*

Strategic information, policies and, 219

Street ethnography, 910

Strength-based approaches, 763–64

Stress

    anticipatory counseling, 608

    caregiving and, 810–11

    children with resistance to, *763*

    coping by men, 817

    coping with, 909

    disaster-related, 606

    erectile dysfunction and, 826

Stroke, 546*t*, 786, 878

Structural violence, 510, *510*

Structure

    of families, 741, 771

    as measure of health, 34

Struthers, Lina Rogers, 1009

Student health records, 1022–23

Substance Abuse and Mental Health Services Administration (SAMHSA), 193

Substance use. *See also* alcohol consumption

    among adolescents, 683

    among nurses, 500–502, 501*b*

    among rural adolescents, 663–64

    as a community problem, 480–83

    definition, 480–83

    depression and, 1020

    drug histories in, 488

    impacts of, 483

    interventions, 489–502

    intimate partner violence and, 915

    personal factors in, 487

    risk factors for, 484–87, 487*b*

    in schools, 1014

    scope of, 481–83

    serious mental illness and, 916

    signs of, 488–89, 488*b*, 489*b*

    treatment options, 493*b*

    vulnerable populations, 487*b*

    workplace signs of, 495*b*

Subsystems, community structure and, 41*t*

Suffering, chronic illness and, 554–55

Suicide, 527–28

    adolescent, 917

    among the elderly, 881, 881*b*

    living with suicidality, 916

    by men, 819–20

    by rural adolescents, 663

    in young adulthood, 917

Sulfur dioxide, 298*t*

Summative evaluations, 353

Summative measures, 52

Summerians, history, 64

"Superbugs," 444

Supplemental Security Income (SSI), 172, 666

Supplementary Medical Insurance (SMI, Part B), 171

Supplier-influenced demand, 161

Supply, of products, 159

Support groups, 413–14

    attendance at, 911

    for cancer patients, 799*b*

    growth of, 562–63

    for home health professionals, 990

    for mental health issues, 906*b*

    networks for patients, 627

    for professional caregivers, 990

    reflecting on experience with, 925

Support services, 763–64

Suprasystems, 41*t*

Surveillance, 430, 566

Surveys, community assessment, 44, 45

Swapping, community assessment, 43–44

Syphilis

    epidemiology, 89, 107

    increased incidence, 94–95

    public health approaches, 937

    screening for, 454

    symptoms, 454

    Tuskegee experiments, 254

Systems issues, ethical issues and, 263

Systems of care, 844

Systems thinking skills, 953*t*


T

Tanning, 788–89

Target populations, 319

Target systems, 41*t*

Targeted programs, 764–66

Task groups, 414

Taste changes, 871

Tattoos, wearing of, 243–44

Tax credits, 213–14

Tax Equity and Fiscal Responsibility Act of 1982 (TEFRA), 123

Teachers, medical procedures and, 1024

Teaching, 354. *See also* health education; learning

Team building, 414–15
Team work, disaster planning and, 589
Technicians, care delivery by, 127–28
Technology
    assessment in policy research, 175–76
    health care costs and, 167
    in home health care, 992–93
    home visit facilitation, 956, 963–65
    impact on health care delivery, 130
    life-changing advances in, 332–33
    for persons with disabilities, 724–25
    school health nursing and, 1028
    telecommunications, 204
    use by advanced practice nurses, 1067
Technology-Related Assistance Act for
        Individuals with Disabilities, 713t
Teen health clinics, 405
Telecommunications technology, 204
Telehealth, 335–36, 336–38
Telemedicine, 335, 993, 1028
Telephones, connectedness and, 563
Television, school health and, 1027
Temporary Assistance for Needy Families
        (TANF), 173, 194, 848
Terminal illnesses, 977. *See also* hospice
        care
Terrorism, 946, 1004, 1024–25
Tertiary care, 126, 130, 922
Tertiary prevention, 105
    description of, 24–25
    in the history of disease, 106t
    of homelessness, 652
    of infectious diseases, 431
    of substance abuse, 493
    of teen pregnancy, 692, 697
Testicular cancer, 824–25
Testosterone, violence and, 816
Therapeutic touch (TT), 378, 1075
Therapists, care delivery by, 127–28
Therapy groups, 414
Thermal regulation, 883–84
Third-party payers, 124, 158, 161. *See also*
        insurance coverage; reimbursement
        programs
Ticket to Work Incentives Improvement
        Act, 713t
Ticks, 440–41
Time, rates related to, 112–14, 113t
Timing, assessments, 349
Titanic disaster, 573–74
Title V grants, 91
Title XIX. *See* Medicaid
Title XVIII. *See* Medicare (Title XVIII)
Tobacco, 217, 482, 490, 496b, 546t. *See also*
        smoking
Toluene, 295t
Toluene diisocyanate (TDI), 298t, 1038
Tornados, impact of, 586
Tort law, 204–5

Torture, war and, 531
Touch therapy, 378
Toxic Release Inventory, 274
Toxicology, 279, 1045
Toxins, exposures to, 272
Traditional Chinese medicine, 370
Transcultural nursing, 234–35, 235b, 246
Transcultural Nursing Society, 246
Transition planning, 17, 724
Transportation, disaster planning and, 589
Transtheoretical model, 346, 473–75
Trauma centers, 135
Traumatic brain injuries, 115–16, 709t
Traumatic disorders, 644t
Traumatic injuries, work-related, 1043
Travel, disease transmission and, 426
Trends, reporting rates, 113, 114t
Triage, during disasters, 595
Triage nurses, 149–50
Trichoroethylene (TCE), 295t–296t
Truck driving, 1044
Truman, Harry, 16
Trust, 349, 789
Trustworthiness, 252
Tsunami, Indian Ocean, 572, 574,
        579–81
Tuberculosis (TB)
    age-specific rates, 112t
    death from, 83
    directly observed therapy, 94
    historical impact, 424, 446
    morbidity threat of, 938
    mortality rates, 391
    multidrug-resistant, 446, 447
    occupational transmission of, 1041
    transmission, 446
Tunnel vision, 870
Tuskegee experiments, 254
TWEACK test, 887
Tyler, Elizabeth, 84, 85

**U**
Ultraviolet light exposure, 788–89
Underinsured groups, 621, 625–26
Underweight in the elderly, 873
Unemployment, 765
Unified Nursing Language System
        (UNLS), 329
Uninsured groups, 621, 625–26
Unintentional injuries, 662
United Nations (UN)
    agencies linked to, 386b
    Children's Emergency Fund (UNICEF),
        386–87
    Commission on the Status of Women,
        802–3
    Educational, Scientific, and Cultural
        Organization (UNESCO), 386b
    global health initiatives, 384–86

    International Decade for Natural
        Disaster Reduction, 581
    Millennium Developmental Goals, 396
    Platforms for Action for women,
        809–10
United States
    abortion statistics, *107*, 694t
    access to care in, 941
    adults with chronic conditions, 552
    birth rates, 785–86
    causes of death 1900 *vs.* 2000, 104t
    chronic illness in, 545–48
    current health care delivery system,
        126–30
    healing traditions in, 367–69
    health care costs, 122
    health care statistics, 11
    labor force by industry, 1034t
    labor force by job, 1034t
    longevity, 131
    obesity in, 105
    population trends, 660t
    problem of homelessness, 653
    reportable infectious diseases, 431t
    rural populations, 660t
    school violence in, 521
    teen birth rates, 678
    types of violence at, 513–32
    urban populations, 634, 660t
    women in poverty in, 782–83
    women's health in, 780–89
United States Census data, 44, 110
United States Public Health Service
        (USPHS), 44, 89, 175, 193–94, 430,
        937, 1010
Unity, nursing theme of, 923
Universal human experiences, 910–11
Universal moral conceptualization, theory
        of, 232
Universal Postal Union (UPO), 386b
Unlicensed assistive personnel, 1023
Upper extremities, musculoskeletal
        disorders of, 1042
Upstream thinking, 286, 760–61
Urban environments
    development projects, 636
    elderly persons in, 861
    homeless populations, 636–46
    improvement of, 652
    largest cities, 645
    obesity and, 38
    urban sprawl, 636
    water supplies for, 635
Urban populations, 634
Uridine, 300t
Urinary incontinence, 796, 874–75, 875b
Utilitarianism, 252–53, 253b, 266
Utilization, managed care barriers, 149b
Utilization review, 150

**V**

Vaccinate Alaska Coalition (VAC), 48
Vaccinations, 424, 431–32. *See also*
    immunizations
Vaccines, 428*b*, 435–36, 436*t*, 457
Value checkpoints, 771*b*
Values, of families, 749–50
Vancomycin, 444
Vector-borne diseases, 440–42
Vehicle-borne transmission, 426
Veterans, 625, 808
Veteran's Administration, 92, 125, 174–75,
    190, 563
Viagra (sildenafil citrate), 827–28
Vicodin, 481
Vincent de Paul, Saint, 69
Violence. *See also* behavioral violence;
    domestic violence; intimate partner
    violence (IPV)
    community concerns, 541
    in community settings, 525–26
    definitions, 509–12
    in families, 520, 520*b*
    HIV risk and, 466–67
    injuries due to, 662–63
    levels of, 393
    by men, 819–20
    mental illness and, 917
    microlevel interventions, 533–35
    nursing in prisons, 540–41
    prevention of, 532–37
    public health issues, 508–9
    in schools, 1024–25
    serious mental illnesses and, 918
    testosterone and, 816
    threatened egotism and, 924
    in the United States, 513–32
    victims of, 395
    war and, 393–94, 530–32
    against women, 803–5
    in the workplace, 529–30
    youth-based, 521–29
Virtue ethics, 251–52
Virulence, infectious disease, 426
Visial impairments, 716–17
Vision, assessment, 869–70
Vision impairment, 709*t*
Visiting nurses, 956
Visiting Nurses Association of Omaha
    Community Health Problem and
    Intervention system, 329*t*
Visual impairment, 726, 1017, 1037
Visually-impaired elders, 870*b*, 878
Vital statistics, 56–57, 110
Vitamin D, 788
Vitamin E, 13
Vocational rehabilitation, 721
Vocational Rehabilitation Act, 710

Vulnerability, 616–17, 965
Vulnerable families, 617
Vulnerable populations
    community perspectives, 621
    cultural perspectives, 619–20
    health-related perspectives, 620–21
    historical perspectives, 619
    home visits to, 962
    mental health care for, 927
    mental illnesses, 905*b*
    persons with special needs, 616, 621–26
    poverty and, 618–19
    risks shared by, 616–17
    in schools, 1017, 1018–19
    support services for, 763–64

**W**

Wald, Florence, 994
Wald, Lillian, 82, 83–85, 936, 979, 1007
War
    epidemiology of, 531
    health problems, 531*b*
    impact on children, 532, 1004, 1025
    mass violence and, 530–32
    refugees, 531–32
    roles of nurses, 531–32
    on terror, 909
    victims of, 510
    violence and, 393–94
    women speak about, 522
Water Pollution Control Act of 1948, 212
Weapons, 663, 1016, 1024–25
Web of causation model, *617*, 617–18
Websites, usability of, 337
Weight loss, 873
Welfare programs, 172–73
Welfare-to-Work programs, 620
Wellness
    community-level, 306–7
    definitions of, 305–6, 306*b*
    high-level, 305
    holistic, 312
    importance of, 304
    models of, 311–21
Wellness committees, 1088
West Nile virus, 442
Wheelchairs, 716
*Who Will Keep the Public Healthy*
    (IOM), 97
Whole Communities Collaborative, 1084*b*
Wide area networks (WANs), 333–34
Windshield surveys, 44, 45–46
Witch craze, Middle Ages, 68
*Witches, Midwives, and Nurses* (Ehrenrich
    and English), 69
Women
    about wars, 522
    adolescent years, 789–92

    aging and, 800–802
    births by age and race, 789*t*
    cancer in, 797
    cardiovascular disease in, 797
    as caregivers, 783, 863–65
    causes of death in, 786–87
    delay in seeking care by, 787
    education in the U.S., 781
    elderly, 860
    employment in the U. S., 781–82
    empowerment of, 783–85, 809–10
    expectancy in the U. S., 780–81
    feminism and, 809
    health care policy and, 810–11
    health profiles of, 780–89
    health-promotion activities, 792*b*
    homeless, 646, 806, 910
    incarcerated, 806–7
    issues affecting health of, 803–8
    mature, 796–97
    mental health, 788
    in multiproblem families, 765
    osteoporosis in, 797–99, 798*t*
    patterns of health, 786–89
    patterns of illness, 786–89
    in poverty, 782–83, 807
    reproductive risks to, 785–86
    research areas, 810*b*
    risk of HIV infection, 466–69
    roles in marriage, 783–85
    sexual orientation, 800
    substance abuse interventions, 497–99
    veterans, 808
    violence against, 514–15
    vulnerability and, 624–25
    ways of knowing, 808–11
    workplace health, 807–8
Women, Infants and Children's
    Supplemental Food Program
    (WIC), 23, 212, 222, 620, 769, 791
Women's Health Equity Act of 1990, 810
Women's Health Study, 13
Women's rights, world health and, 394–95
Work-related hazards, 1034*b*, 1036–43
Work-related injuries, 1037, 1037*t*
Worker/workplace assessment and
    surveillance, 1046–57
Workers' Compensation, 1038, 1056
Workforce, demographic trends, 1043–44
Working poor, vulnerability of, 626
Workplace changes, 1043–44
Workplaces
    assessments, 1048*b*
    drug abusers in, 481*b*
    health hazards, 1034*b*
    health promotion in, 311
    signs of drug abuse, 495*b*
    substance abuse and, 486–87

substance abuse interventions, 495–96
substance-abusing nurses, 501*b*
violence in, 529–30
women's health issues, 807–8
Works Progress Administration
(WPA), 640
World Bank Group (WBG), 386*b*, 388–90,
389*t*
World Conference on Women, 810*b*
World Development Report (WDR), 389
World Health Organization (WHO)
achievements of, 387*b*
on community empowerment, 37
on community health, 47
definition of health, 10
definition of violence, 509
on elder abuse, 518
function of, 387–88
goals of, 386*b*

Healthy Cities initiative, 35–36, 635
International Classification of
Functioning, Disability and
Health, 550
regional offices, 388*b*
on skin cancers, 788–89
World Intellectual Property Organization
(WIPO), 386*b*
World Meteorological Organization
(WMO), 386*b*
*World Report on Violence and Health*
(WHO), 393
World Tourism Organization (WTO), 386*b*
World Trade Center attacks, 579, 585, 604,
851, 1051. *See also* September 11
attacks; terrorism
World War II, 88, 641

**X**
Xerophthalmia, 870
Xylene, 295*t*

**Y**
Young adulthood
causes of death during, 793
research areas related to, 810*b*
suicide in, 917
women's health needs, 792–93
Youth Risk Behavior Survey (YRBS), 679,
790, 1015*t*, 1016
Youth violence, 521–29, 521*b*, 524*b*,
528–29, 532

**Z**
Zinc oxide, 294*t*
Zoonoses, 426, 442–44

# Photo Credits